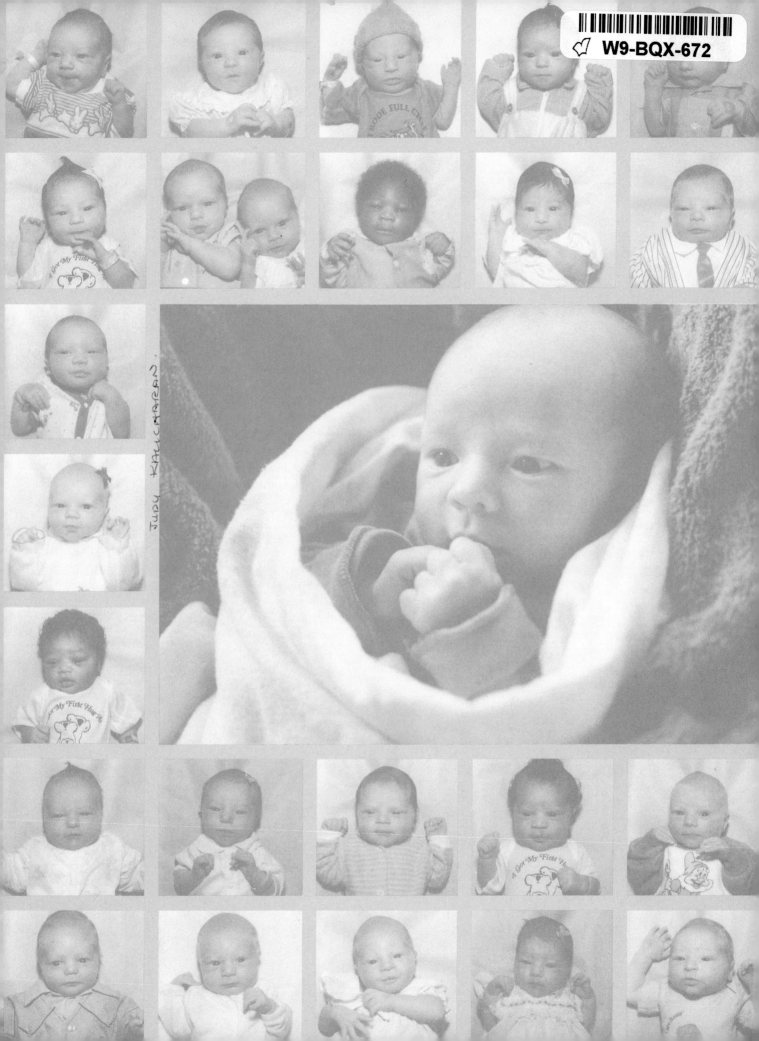

JUDY KALLENBACH

About Our Cover...

Featured on our cover is the dramatic quilt, *The Tide,* by Miwako Kimura, which appears in the book *Japanese Quilt* by Jill Widell and Yuko Watanabe. To us, the quilt seems to epitomize the childbearing family experience and the connectedness that one family has with another, generation to generation, Miwako Kimura as an artist/quilter has made the quilt her canvas, and using color, shape, and texture has given it life. Brilliant hues and subtle shading are all connected together by hundreds of stitches, each created one by one. The quilt captures a feeling of great movement and change yet remains peaceful, calm, and comforting. The blue tones suggest water and sky. For many people, the crane is a cultural symbol of life and happiness.

It is not only the exquisite beauty of this quilt that has touched us. That this beauty is found in an object that has been a part of families and of women's lives is particularly special. For more than 700 years women have been creating quilts to provide warmth and comfort for their families. In every possible type of setting and circumstance, women have pieced together the material, connecting each one with tiny stitches. To us, the stitches symbolize the strength, work, and love that holds the family together. Just as each family touches the future as each child is born, the quilt reaches the future as it is passed from one generation to another.

Maternal-Newborn Nursing

A Family-Centered Approach

Fourth Edition

Sally B. Olds, RNC, MS
Marcia L. London, RNC, MSN, NNP
Patricia W. Ladewig, PhD, RNC, NP

ADDISON-WESLEY NURSING
A Division of The Benjamin/Cummings Publishing Company, Inc.

Redwood City, California • Menlo Park, California
Reading, Massachusetts • New York • Don Mills, Ontario
Wokingham, U.K. • Amsterdam • Bonn • Sydney
Singapore • Tokyo • Madrid • San Juan

Sponsoring Editor: Patti Cleary; *Developmental Editor:* Jamie Northway; *Production Coordinator:* Cathy Lewis; *Book Designer:* Detta Penna; *Cover Designer:* Yvo Riezebos; *Designer, color chart:* Rudy Zehntner; *Illustrator, color chart:* Charles W. Hoffman III: *Photography Research:* Wendy Earl; *Photographers:* Suzanne Arms Wimberley, Elizabeth Elkin, and Amy Snyder (photos from earlier editions by William Thompson and George B. Fry III); *Endpaper photos:* Joe Tysl; *Illustrators:* Elizabeth Morales-Denney (medical), Merry Finley (technical), Jack P. Tandy (line), Charles W. Hoffman III (tonal); *Copy Editor:* Tärna Rosendahl; *Proofreader:* Holly McLean Aldis; *Indexer:* William Richardson Associates; *Manufacturing Supervisor:* Casimira Kostecki; *Composition:* G & S Typesetters, Inc.

Cover quilt: *The Tide* by Miwako Kimura

Library of Congress Cataloging-in-Publication Data
Olds, Sally B., 1940–
   Maternal-newborn nursing: a family-centered approach / Sally B. Olds, Marcia L. London, Patricia A. Ladewig.—4th ed.
      p. cm
   Includes bibliographical references and index.
   ISBN 0-8053-5580-4
      1. Obstetrical nursing. 2. Neonatology. I. London, Marcia L. II. Ladewig, Patricia A. III. Title
      [DNLM: 1. Neonatology—nurses' instruction. 2. Obstetrical Nursing. WY 157.3 044m]
   RG951.043   1992
   610.73'678—dc20
   DNLM/DLC
   for Library of Congress   91-22036
                                                        CIP

Care has been taken to confirm the accuracy of information presented in this book. The authors, editors, and publisher, however, cannot accept any responsibility for errors or omissions or for consequences from application of the information in this book and make no warranty, express or implied, with respect to its contents.

The authors and publisher have exerted every effort to ensure that drug selections and dosages set forth in this text are in accord with current recommendations and practice at the time of publication. However, in view of ongoing research, changes in government regulations, and the constant flow of information relating to drug therapy and drug reactions, the reader is urged to check the package inserts of all drugs for any change in indications of dosage and for added warnings and precautions. This is particularly important when the recommended agent is a new and/or infrequently employed drug. Mention of a particular generic or brand name drug is not an endorsement, nor an implication that it is preferable to other named or unnamed agents.

ISBN 0-8053-5580-4
12345678910-RN-9594939291

Addison-Wesley Nursing
A Division of the Benjamin/Cummings Publishing Company, Inc.
390 Bridge Parkway
Redwood City, California 94065

First, Second and Third Edition Contributors

Martha Cox Baily, RN
Elizabeth M. Bear, CNM, MS
Irene Bobak, RN, CNP, MN, MSN
Joyce Boles, RN, MN, CPNP
Rena Brescia, RNC, MS
Sallye P. Brown, RN, MN
Penelope Childress, RN
Pamela Crispin, RN
Marilyn Doenges, RN, MA
Nancy Donaldson, RN, MSN
Joan Edelstein, RN, PNP, MSN, MPH
Mildred R. (Holly) Emrick, RN, MSN
Jack Ford, MD, FACOG
Laurel Freed, RN, PNP, MN
Sandra L. Gardner, RN, PNP, MS
Sharon Glass, RN, BS, NNP
Pauline Goolkasian, RN, MSN
Effie A. Graham, RN, PhD
Janet Griffith-Kenney, RN, PhD
Ann Kelley Havenhill, RN, MN
Louise Westberg Hedstrom, RN, CNM, MSN
Patricia Hemak, RN, MS
Linda Andrist Hereford, RN, MSN, NP
Loretta C. Cermely Ivory, RN, CNM, MS
L. Jean Johns, RN, MS
E. JoAnne Jones, RN, MEd, MSN
Emma K. Kamm, RN
Lynette Karls, BS, MS
Janet Kennedy, DN, DNSc
Joy M. Khader, RN, MSN
JoAnn Kilb, RN, MSN, NNP
Stephan Kilb, RN, NNP
Jean Theirl King, RD, BS
Virginia Gramzow Kinnick, RN, CNM, MSN
Kathleen Knafl, RN, PhD
Nancy Ellen Krauss, RN, MS
Joan Kub, RN, MS
Eleanor Latterell, RD, MS
Eileen Leaphart, RNC, MN
Mary Ann Leppink, RN, MS
Dietra Lowdermilk, RN, MEd
Anne L. Matthews, RN, MS
Mary Ann McClees, RN, MS
Nancy McCluggage, RN, CNM, MA
Cynthia A. McMahon, RN, MSN
Anne Garrard McMath, RN, MSN, PNP
Caryl E. Mobley, RN, MSN
Donna Rae Meirath Moriarty, RN, MSN
Karen Rooks, Nauer, RN, BS
Mary Ann Neihaus, RN, MSN, CEN, EMT-A
Shannon Perry, RN, PhD
Sally J. Phillips, RN, MSN
Lovena L. Porter, RN, MS
Carol Freeman Rosenkrantz, RN, MN
Carol Hawthorne Rumpler, RN, MS
Joanne F. Ruth, RN, MS
Madrean Schober, RNC, BGS
M. Carole Schoffstall, RN, MS
Paula Shearer, RN, MSN
Constance Lawrenz Slaughter, RN, BSN
Mari Lou Steffen, RN, EdD
Deborah Sweeney, RN, CNM, MS
Marie Swigert, RN, MSN
Elvira Szigeti, RN, MN
Janel N. Timmins, RN, MA
Linda Ungerleider, RN, MSN
Marcia Vavich, RN, MA
Janet Veatch, RN, MN
Betty Blome Winyall, RN, MSN

To *women of the world*
for the life they give, nurture, and sustain—sometimes at the cost of their own life,
sometimes when they are too young or too old or too sick or too poor
for the exquisite joy or despair their life brings them
and to a special woman, my daughter Allison Olds

To *men*
for their willingness to take an active part in the childbearing experience and to father
and to some special young men, our sons: Scott Olds, Craig and Matthew London, and Ryan and Erik Ladewig

To *love*
and the sense of wonder it gives to the world and to those who love us,
Joe Olds, David London, and Tim Ladewig

To *students*
who have the courage and energy to learn and who touch our lives

To *us*
three rugged individualists who are bound together in our love for childbearing families
and who have been given this wonderful opportunity to grow together

We raise our cup to life.

SBO, MLL, PWL

*P*reparing nurses to assume their increasingly important role in family-oriented maternity care continues to be the primary goal of this fourth edition. More than ever before, today's nurses play a central role in the planning for and experience of birth, and in how families feel about the experience afterward. Nurses today are client advocates and educators. Women now have choices about how and where they give birth and, in some cases, about whether their caregiver will be a physician or a nurse-midwife.

Designed for use in undergraduate nursing programs, this text encompasses the entire childbearing process, from preconception planning through pregnancy, birth, and the postpartum period. Content progresses from normal to at-risk information within each phase: pregnancy, labor and birth, care of the newborn, and the postpartum period. Cultural aspects of childbearing and material on the childbearing adolescent are integrated appropriately throughout.

Every page of this new edition has been updated to reflect the most current research and technology. The underlying philosophy of the text, however, remains unchanged: that pregnancy and birth are normal life processes and that members of the family are co-participants in care. Each of the learning aids reflected in this new edition has been grounded in that philosophy and in our commitment to a family-centered approach.

New Features

Emphasis on Critical Thinking Skills

Maternal-newborn nurses use critical thinking in all aspects of their nursing practice, from the initial building of a knowledge base as a beginning student, to the expert nurse's application of nursing standards of care and research findings. Because of its importance in providing excellent nursing care, we have emphasized critical thinking skill-building throughout this new edition.

● Chapter 2, "Tools for Critical Thinking in Maternal-Newborn Nursing," presents many of the components of critical thinking that nurses use in their everyday practice, including a comprehensive knowledge base, the nursing process, nursing standards, statistics, and nursing research.

● Critical Thinking exercises appear throughout the text, set off by a colored barhead to encourage students to stop and think about the information they have already learned and to make decisions based on that information.

● Research Notes summarize current research studies and incorporate critical thinking questions to heighten students' awareness of the application of research to nursing practice.

Increased Emphasis on Client/Family Teaching

A central responsibility of the maternal-newborn nurse is the teaching that nurses do at all stages of pregnancy and the childbearing process—including the important postpartum teaching that is done before and immediately after families are discharged from the hospital. To highlight and emphasize this important role, we have incorporated several new features:

● New apple logos 🍎 highlight discussion of client/family teaching throughout the text.

● Teaching Guides include more detailed discussions of client/family teaching. Examples include *What to Expect During Labor* on page 000 and *What to Tell Parents about Daily Infant Care* on page 000.

● Client/Family Teaching Cards, found opposite page 176, are handy tools for the student to use while studying or in the clinical setting for quick reference.

Increased Application of the Nursing Process

The nurse's role in all aspects of the childbearing process is clearly delineated throughout this text and is presented within the framework of the nursing process. Chapters are organized around the five steps of the nursing process: assessment, diagnosis, planning, implementation, and evaluation. In addition, numerous special features reinforce the nursing process as a framework for learning and for nursing care:

● Assessment Guides summarize assessment findings, alterations and possible causes, and nursing responses to assessment data.

● New Key Nursing Diagnoses to Consider boxes highlight the most important nursing diagnoses for specific conditions, using the most current NANDA diagnoses.

● Nursing Care Plans have been modified to increase the emphasis on client goals, rationale for nursing interventions, and evaluation of outcome criteria.

● Procedures describe interventions specific to maternal-newborn nursing care in illustrated, step-by-step fashion.

Content New to This Edition
● Chapter 2, Tools for Critical Thinking in Maternal-Newborn Nursing

● Chapter 3, The Contemporary Family: Structure, Function, and Dysfunction

● Chapter 15, The Expectant Family: Age-Related Considerations

● Chapter 18, Pregnancy at Risk: Pregestational Problems

● Chapter 19, Pregnancy at Risk: Gestational Onset

● Condensed and reorganized unit on Women's Health

- Expanded and updated content on pregnancy-induced hypertension, diabetes mellitus, AIDS and substance abuse

Very Special Learning Aids

- The blood and body fluid alert logo 🩸 reinforces awareness of CDC body fluid precautions.

- A full-color, fold-out chart depicts maternal-fetal development month-by-month. Client teaching and anticipatory guidance are noted below each developmental phase, giving the student an excellent learning tool and a ready reference.

- Full-color photographs included on the reverse side of the development chart vividly show particular visual aspects of pregenancy, childbirth, and the newborn.

Enhanced Visual Appeal

For today's visually oriented students, we have developed an attractive new two-color design that highlights the key information they need to learn at the same time that it commands their interest. Students are brought closer to the childbearing experience through the use of dramatic photographs and the poignant personal reflections of childbearing women and families from many cultures.

Pedagogical Features

Since the first edition of this text, instructors and students alike have praised the wealth of in-text learning aids provided. In this edition, we have once again created a book that is both easy to learn from and easy to use as a reference. Each chapter begins with clear, measurable **Objectives** and ends with a summary of **Key Concepts,** as well as lists of **References** and **Additional Readings.** Throughout the text **Key Terms** are highlighted in boldfaced type, with definitions included in a **Glossary** at the back of the text.

Throughout the text, **Contemporary Issues** boxes highlight legal and ethical dilemmas in maternal-newborn nursing. In addition, where appropriate, we have included **Drug Guides** for those medications commonly used in maternity nursing, to guide students in correctly administering medications. All new nursing **Research Notes** highlight current nursing research issues and now emphasize application of critical thinking skills.

Complete Teaching/Learning Package

To help instructors make the best use of this new edition, we have developed a comprehensive new supplements package with the following components:

- **Student Workbook** This popular workbook has been revised and updated in keeping with the changes made in this revision. It incorporates strategies for students to increase synthesis of their knowledge.
- **1000-item Test Bank** Available in booklet form or as computer software for IBM or Apple, this updated and revised test bank helps faculty quickly and easily create numerous unique examinations. Test items are classified by cognitive level and nursing process step.
- **Clinical Handbook (New)** Written by the authors, this new clinical handbook serves as a portable, succinct quick-reference to guide students in the clinical area.
- **Instructor's Manual** Written by Virginia Kinnick, RN, MSN, this timesaving aid has been thoroughly revised and includes transparency masters.
- **Transparency Acetates** Forty 2-color transparencies present enlarged versions of important text figures.

Acknowledgments

The clinicians, teachers and scholars who reviewed this text helped us immeasurably with their eye for detail, their suggestions for content to be included, and their dedication to helping us develop a text that is relevant and current. And so we extend our sincere thanks to the following reviewers:

- Bernadine Adams, RN, BSN, MN
  Associate Professor
  Northeast Louisiana University
  School of Nursing
  Monroe, LA

- Kathleen H. Allen, RN, MA
  Contra Costa College
  San Pablo, CA

- Janet L. Andrews, RNC, MSN
  Emory University
  Atlanta, GA

- Donna Burleson, RN, BSN, MS
  Director of Health Occupations
  Cisco Junior College
  Abilene, Texas

- Karen Cobb, RN, BSN, MA, MSN, Doctoral Candidate
  Assistant Professor
  Indiana University School of Nursing
  Indianapolis, IN

- Patricia Diehl, RN, BSN, MA
  West Virginia School of Nursing
  Health Sciences Center
  Morgantown, West Virginia

- Marguerite Jackson, RN, MS, CIC
  Director, Medical Center Epidemiology Unit
  Assistant Clinical Professor of Community Medicine
  University of California
  San Diego, CA

- Alice Pappas, RN, BSN, MSN, PhD, RNC
  Baylor University School of Nursing
  Dallas, TX

- Cheryl Pope Long, RN, BSN, MSN, EdD
  School of Nursing
  Georgia College
  Milledgeville, GA

- Faith M. Reierson, RN, MN
  Former Coordinator, Nursing Program
  Olympic College
  Bremerton, WA

- Mary Van Allen, RN, BSN, MSN
  Indiana University
  Indianapolis, IN

- Aubrey Wade, RN
  Berkeley Non-Interventive Birth Advocates
  Association
  Berkeley, CA

Each time we undertake a revision of our text we are committed to offering students the best that we can of nursing theory and practice so that our book captures the essence and warmth of the childbearing experience. We draw from our own experiences and practice, we speak with other educators and practitioners, we meet with students, we talk with childbearing families—all to gain greater insight into the current state of the art in our field. As we revise and update the content we also seek to organize the material in a way that is both logical for the reader and visually appealing. In this effort we were blessed to have the support and assistance of a marvelous developmental editor, Jamie Northway. Jamie challenged us to look at familiar content in a new way; she helped us develop learning aids that enhance a students' understanding of content; and she brought a wonderful attention to detail that helped us maintain the highest level of internal consistency. She did this with humor, grace, talent and zest. We consider her a special friend.

Taking a final manuscript through all the stages necessary to produce a text requires someone with an eye for detail and the ability to coordinate and bring together a variety of pieces into a meaningful whole. This is the job of the production coordinator. Only occasionally do you find someone who can handle all these pieces in a seemingly effortless way. Cathy Lewis, our production coordinator, is such a person. She remained consistently unflappable, gracious, and calm throughout the lengthy, often hectic process. She is quite a lady!

Once again Detta Penna brought her unique talent and creativity to this project in designing a look that is warm, approachable, and alive. She has a magical touch.

Over the years we have sought to incorporate photos that show the essence of the childbearing experience and of women's health. The photographs of Suzanne Arms Wimberley are justly renowned for their sensitive portrayal of human life and we are honored to include many of her pieces in this text. We are also delighted to include photographs from three other talented photographers, Elizabeth Elkin, Amy Snyder and Joe Tysl. Wendy Earl, who coordinated photography research, brought to the book an understanding of composition and an awareness of the importance of a photo in conveying a message. She was committed to helping us achieve excellence.

Elizabeth Morales-Denney and Merry Finley, both skilled illustrators joined us for the first time in this edition. Their creativity and understanding of the field enabled them to render important ideas in a clear, simple way that promotes student learning.

We wish to extend a sincere word of thanks to Tärna Rosendahl for her skillful copyediting of the text and to Holly McLean-Aldis for proofreading the material so carefully.

William Richardson Associates developed the high quality index found in this edition.

Bradley Burch, editorial assistant, and Alyssa Weiner, production assistant, worked closely with us throughout the process. They both are talented, energetic, supportive, and unfailingly cheerful.

And finally we wish to thank our sponsoring editor, Patti Cleary. It is difficult to convey the sense of trust, respect, and deep affection that we feel for this special woman. She has worked closely with us as mentor, cheerleader, and friend. Her vision has inspired us, her humor has sustained us. We love her enthusiasm and her unrestrained joy in life. She is an incredible woman.

Many thanks to all of you who have taken the time to share your thoughts and ideas about previous editions of the text. Your input is invaluable and reflects the commitment you feel to the childbearing family and to women's health. Our primary goal, our deepest commitment, is to bring you a text that is usable, readable and relevant. We are honored by your support.

Sally B. Olds
Marcia L. London
Patricia W. Ladewig

Dear Students:

We believe that working with childbearing families gives you the opportunity to experience the essence of nursing at its best. You can play a vital role in helping families learn what they need to know in order to be as independent as possible; you can have countless opportunities to improve and refine your assessment skills as you work with essentially healthy women and infants, and those with complications; and you can use the other nursing skills you have learned in a variety of acute care settings.

We love this field and we know that many of you will as well. Some of you, on the other hand, may find that this area of nursing is not your first interest, and that's OK, too. We would have a real problem if every nurse loved the same area!

We do hope that you will use this opportunity to grow in professional ability and to appreciate the importance of all you do as nurses—not just the technical and organizational tasks, although they are undoubtedly crucial, but also the caring you bring to the role of nurse. When you hold the hand of a laboring woman or help an adolescent plan a way to tell her parents of her pregnancy; when you provide accepting care to a woman with AIDS or gently stroke the skin of a pre-

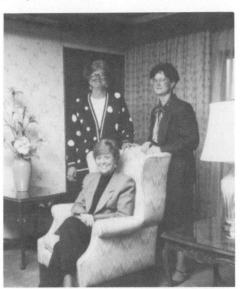

Standing at left, Sally Olds; at right, Marcia London; sitting, Pat Ladewig

term infant; when you rejoice with a delighted father or console a grieving one; you are practicing the heart of nursing.

Caring in an optimal environment is not difficult but caring in today's practice setting is more of a challenge. Finding a way to maintain a caring environment when you are overworked and stretched by fiscal constraints and a lack of adequate staffing requires great dedication, creativity, and personal resolve. We have attempted to help you translate caring into practice throughout this text through the tone of the book, the photos and art work, the personal quotes, and the content itself with its emphasis on holistic care.

As you work to translate what you learn into practice, please take care of yourselves as well. Providing excellent nursing care is infinitely rewarding and can be energizing, but it is also draining both physically and emotionally. Make time to play, rest, exercise, be with loved ones, and participate in things that rejuvenate you.

We think that nurses are very special people and we are proud to be counted among them. Good luck with your studies! We wish you well.

Sally Olds
Marcia London
Patricia Ladewig

Contributors to the Fourth Edition

Authors

Sally B. Olds, RNC, MS
Associate Professor
Beth-El College of Nursing
Colorado Springs, Colorado

Marcia L. London, RNC, MSN, NNP
Associate Professor and
Director of Neonatal Nurse Practitioner Program
Beth-El College of Nursing
Colorado Springs, Colorado

Patricia W. Ladewig, PhD, RNC, NP
Professor and Dean
School for Health Care Professions, Regis University
Denver, Colorado

Contributors

Emily Coogan Bennett, BSN, MSN, RNC
Medical College of Virginia
Virginia Commonwealth University
Richmond, VA   *Contributed to Chapter 7*

Ellen E. Biebesheimer, RN, MSN, PHP
Beth-El College of Nursing
Colorado Springs, CO   *Contributed to Chapters 29 and 30*

Rena Brescia, RN, MS, CRNP
OB/GYN Nursing Consultant
Adult Nurse Practitioner
Baltimore, MD   *Contributed to Chapter 26*

Patricia Budd, RN, BSN, PhD Candidate
Associate Professor
Beth-El College of Nursing
Colorado Springs, CO   *Contributed the Research Boxes*

Jane Congleton, RN, MS
Memorial Hospital
Colorado Springs, CO   *Contributed to the genetics section*

Louise Westberg Hedstrom, RN, MSN, CNM
Associate Professor, Division of Nursing
North Park College
Chicago, IL   *Contributed to Chapters 18 and 19*

Virginia Gramzow Kinnick, BSN, MSN, EdD, CNM
Associate Professor
School of Nursing
University of Northern Colorado
Greeley, CO   *Contributed to Chapter 15*

Vicki A. Lucas, RNC, PhD, OGNP
Division Head, Nursing Care of Women and Childbearing
   Families
Director, Women's Health Care Graduate Program
School of Nursing
University of Texas Health Science Center-Houston
Houston, TX   *Contributed to Chapter 10*

Nancy A. McCluggage, RN, BSN, MA, CNM
Staff Nurse-Midwife
Clinical Instructor
University of California/Naval Nurse-Midwifery Program
Department of Reproductive Medicine
Naval Hospital
San Diego, CA   *Contributed to Chapters 20 and 21*

Kathy Miller, RNC, MNP, BSN, MS
The Penrose Saint Francis Healthcare System
Colorado Springs, CO   *Contributed to Chapter 31*

Janet Pepper, RN, BSN, MS
University of Colorado
Health Sciences Center
Denver, CO   *Contributed to Chapter 5*

Deborah Wooley Perlis, RN, CNM, PhD, FACCE
Assistant Professor
School of Nursing
University of Colorado
Graduate Nurse-Midwifery Program
                                Contributed to Chapter 23

Mary Ann Rhode, RN, CNM, MS
Presbyterian/St. Lukes Medical Center
Denver, CO   *Contributed to Chapter 36*

Timothy R. Sauvage, CRNA, MS
Director, Anesthesia Nursing
Clinical Specialization
University of North Dakota
Grand Forks, ND   *Contributed to Chapter 24*

Constance Lawrenze Slaughter, RN, BSN, MSN
Medical Office Administrator
Kaiser Permanente Health Center East
Portland, OR   *Contributed to Chapter 25*

Elvira Szigeti, RN, BSN, MN, PhD
University of North Dakota
Grand Forks, ND   *Contributed to Chapter 9*

Candice J. Tolve, RN, MSN, Doctoral Candidate
Instructor, Program in Nursing,
Regis University
Denver, CO   *Contributed to Chapter 22*

Linda Salsman Ungerleider, RN, MSN, ACCE
North Park College
Chicago, IL   *Pregnancy at Risk Chapter*

Contents in Brief

Assessment Guides

 Contemporary Issues

 Drug Guides

 Teaching Guides

Nursing Care Plans

Procedures

Research Notes

Contents in Detail

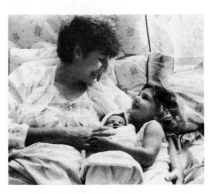

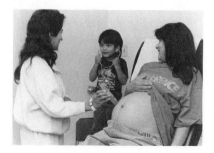

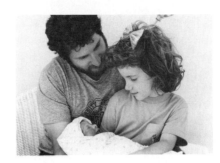

PART ONE

Contemporary Maternity Nursing

CHAPTER 1
Current Issues In Maternal-Newborn Nursing

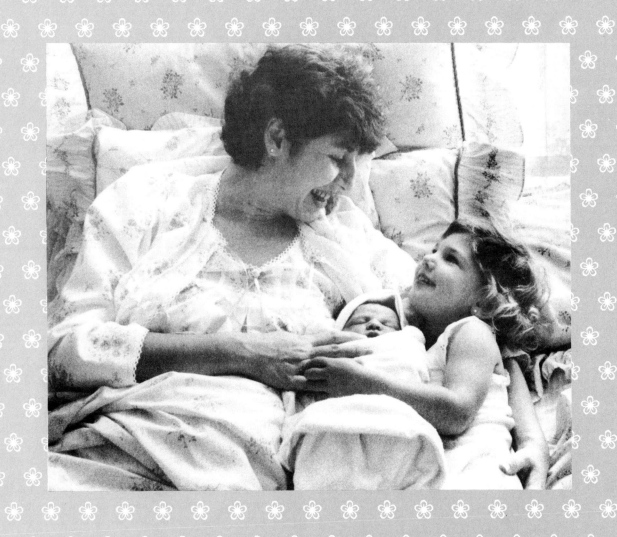

OBJECTIVES

Relate the concept of the expert nurse to nurses caring for childbearing families.

Discuss the impact of the self-care movement on contemporary childbirth.

Compare the nursing roles available to the maternal-newborn nurse.

Summarize the similarities and differences between certified nurse-midwives (CNMs) and lay midwives.

Discuss the concept of childbirth as a business.

Describe significant legal and ethical issues for nurses caring for childbearing families.

Evaluate the potential impact of some of the special situations in contemporary maternity care.

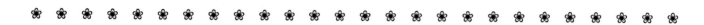

When I started out in practice by myself, I didn't fully appreciate that when I went single-handedly to deliver babies at home—one midwife in the midst of at least three generations of a family—that I would be, in many respects, at their mercy. The qualities of their lives and relationships crowded in on the relatively simple act of birth, making it rich with possibilities, some beneficial, some not. (A Midwife's Story)

I've worked labor and delivery, helping families have their children, for 18 years now. My friends ask me how it is that I seem to know as soon as I see a woman get off the elevator whether I have time for a slow, low-key admission with lots of teaching and support, or whether I had better take care of the essentials first. It's not just how a woman's acting, although behavior is certainly a useful cue. I seem to have a sense of what is to come and the actions I need to take.

I like what I do. I like working with couples, involving them in the decision making and working with them for the kind of experience they planned for. I recall one birth experience vividly. I was working nights. The elevator door opened, and two ambulance attendants rushed out pushing a stretcher and calling for help. The woman on the cart was wearing a blue parka and pushing. The ambulance attendants were so scared they had trouble getting the stretcher into the room and kept bumping into things. Then they were all concerned about getting her into bed and doing paperwork. I could see there was no time for moving her to the bed or anything. I had to take over. I told them to wait outside for a little bit and told her I would take care of things. She had looked frightened, but when everyone left she calmed down.

I think she knew it was safe with me. I pulled back the cover and found her naked from the waist down. The parka on top and nothing else. I wanted to laugh but there was no time. The head was coming. She did really well—pushed when I asked and then panted—and that baby just eased into the world. We were both thrilled. We'd shared something special. We didn't get that parka messy either!

A minute or so later her husband rushed in. He had followed the ambulance to the hospital. She looked up at him, smiled, and said, "Look, Dad, at what we've got!"

The nurse in the preceding anecdote will probably always remember the woman in the blue parka. Why? Because this nurse made a difference in the woman's life. Many nurses can recall special moments, shared experiences, in which they felt that they practiced the essence of nursing and, in so doing, touched a life.

What is the essence of nursing? It can be stated simply: Nurses care for people, care about people, and use their expertise to help people help themselves.

All nurses who provide care and support to childbearing women, their infants, and their families can make a difference. But how does this happen? How do nurses develop expertise in nursing and become skilled, caring practitioners?

Benner (1984) suggests that as nurses develop their skills in making clinical judgments and intervening appropriately, they progress through five levels of competence. Beginning as a novice, the new nurse progresses to advanced beginner and then to competent, proficient, and, finally, expert nurse.

The novice, lacking in experience, relies on rules to guide actions. As a nurse gains experience, he or she begins to draw on that experience to view situations more holistically, becoming increasingly aware of subtle cues that indicate physiologic and psychologic changes. The expert nurse has a clear vision of what is possible in a given situation. This holistic perspective is based on a wealth of knowledge bred of experience and enables the nurse to act "intuitively" to provide effective care.

In nursing practice, intuition is "the ability to experience the elements of a clinical situation as a whole, to solve a problem or reach a decision with limited concrete information. It is not the guessing of the beginning practitioner" (Schraeder & Fischer 1986, p 161). The use of intuitive perception is an important part of the "art of nursing," especially in areas such as maternal-newborn nursing, where change occurs quickly and families look to the nurse for help and guidance. Labor nurses become attuned to a woman's progress or lack of progress; nursery nurses detect subtle changes in their small charges; antepartal and postpartal nurses become adept at assessing and teaching. Thus, skilled nursing practice depends on a solid base of knowledge and clinical expertise delivered in a caring, holistic manner. Benner and Wrubel (1989) emphasize the primacy of caring in nursing practice. The following situation provides an example of an expert nurse demonstrating this important caring dimension:

My first pregnancy ended in spontaneous abortion at eight weeks, so this time I decided not to tell anyone I was pregnant until I was three months along. We had just told both families the news the preceding day when it happened again. I began bleeding heavily and we rushed to the ER. Here I was, a maternal-newborn nursing instructor, and I couldn't seem to handle a pregnancy. I was in the bathroom when I passed the fetus into the johnny cap. My poor baby—so small, maybe 3 or 4 inches long. I began to sob uncontrollably as I rang for the nurse. I told her what happened and she helped me to bed. My husband sat with his arm around me as I cried while the nurse took our baby out. A few minutes later she came back and said, "I saw on your record that you are Catholic. Would you like me to baptize your baby?" I said "Oh, yes, please," and she left. I've never forgotten how that made me feel. She saw me as a total person. I'm still teaching and now I have two children. Whenever I teach high-risk pregnancy I tell that story to the students. I want them to know what a difference a nurse can make.

We believe that many nurses who work with childbearing families are experts: They are sensitive, intuitive, and technically skilled. Such nurses do make a difference in the quality of care childbearing families receive.

Contemporary Childbirth

As anyone who has practiced in maternal or newborn nursing for several years will tell you, the field has changed dramatically. Today's maternal-newborn nurse has far broader responsibilities than the nurse of 25 years ago. Today nurses focus more on the specific goals of the individual childbearing woman and her family. The use of the nursing process has helped bring this about.

Not only has maternal-newborn nursing changed, so has the whole experience of childbirth. No longer do laboring women leave their partners and family at the labor room door while they work to give birth without the family's loving presence; no longer are newborns routinely whisked away for a prescribed period, to reappear magically for feedings every four hours and then return to the safe atmosphere of a central nursery; no longer are young siblings treated like walking sources of infection that threaten every infant. Today fathers are active participants in the birth experience. Families and friends are also often included. Siblings are encouraged to visit and meet their newest family member and may even attend the birth, although this practice is controversial. Today the concept of "family-centered childbirth" is accepted and encouraged.

Childbearing women now have many choices. They can choose to give birth in hospital labor rooms, birthing rooms or birthing centers (attached to the hospital or freestanding), or even at home. The primary caregiver may be a physician, a nurse-midwife, or even a lay midwife. More choices are available with regard to use of analgesia, position for labor, and position for birth. Women may elect to give birth sitting, squatting, on hands and knees, sidelying, standing, or in the more traditional position.

Unfortunately, some of the new choices open to educated consumers may also have a negative side. This is especially true with regard to the concept of early discharge. Until a few years ago, even women with uncomplicated births were required to stay in the hospital for several days. However, many women who had supportive families were eager to return home as soon as possible following birth. They had the time and resources to return to the hospital or clinic for any necessary follow-up care and were well-prepared to care for themselves and their newborns. In a somewhat unanticipated development, as hospitals have attempted to control costs, early discharge has become the norm, and women with little knowledge, experience, or support now find themselves discharged 24 or 48 hours after giving birth. To compensate, nurses need to work hard to do necessary teaching and discharge preparation while the woman is in the birthing facility. In this early postpartal period, however, women are often less ready emotionally to learn.

In some areas, follow-up care is provided to women who are discharged early. Nurses visit the women at home to assess their health and that of their infants and to do any necessary teaching. This trend toward home care is a positive one, and we hope that this method of meeting the needs of families becomes standard practice.

The Self-Care Movement

At the end of the 19th century most individuals were self-reliant consumers. No standardization of medical education existed, and M.D. following the name gave no guarantee of the nature of the education, if any, or experience and background of the practitioner. Numerous syrups and nostrums were available for self-treatment, including many products that contained opium or morphine. Home doctor books were available, and even the Sears Roebuck catalog of 1897 included a "Consumers Guide" containing 16 pages of medical instruments and drugs for both humans and animals (Mumford 1983). By the 1920s this situation had changed significantly. Medical education reform resulted in well-trained physicians with far more scientific knowledge than the average layperson. The more powerful medications were obtainable only through a physician. Thus, the age of the physician-reliant consumer began. Increasing medical specialization and evolving technology also contributed to the trend toward consumer reliance on physicians. Phrases such as "whatever the doctor says" or "I just need to see the doctor and get a shot to fix it" characterized the prevailing attitude. The health care provider assumed the major portion of responsibility for health maintenance (Hill & Smith 1985).

The self-care movement began to emerge in the late 1960s as new consumers sought to understand technology and take an interest in their own health and basic self-care skills. Toffler (1980) refers to these new consumers as "prosumers of medicine" because they are "people who are at the same time producers and consumers of health benefits." These prosumers exercise, control their diet, monitor their psychologic and physiologic status, and, in some cases, even do their own diagnostic tests. They thus assume many primary care functions. Furthermore, today's health care consumers are requiring greater information and accountability from their health care providers (Inlander 1990). These consumers recognize that information, indeed, is power.

In evaluating this trend toward self-care, Naisbitt (1982) refers to it as a move toward self-help and away from institutional help (medicine). He stresses the return to self-reliance, with a focus on holistic care, wellness, and preventive medicine.

Practicing self-care—assuming responsibility for one's own health—often requires assertiveness and taking an active role in seeking necessary information. This assertiveness is sometimes difficult for women. Abrums (1986) points out that health care providers develop their role expectations of women from previous experiences. If most of a health care provider's experience is with women who approach their health care passively, the provider may be disconcerted by an assertive woman who seeks to assume

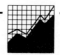

Research Note

Clinical Application of Research

Because little research has been done on Cambodian childbearing beliefs and practices, Judith Klug (1990) designed an ethnographic study to explore this perspective. She wanted to identify the cultural knowledge of Cambodian refugees about conception and fetal development as well as to determine how this knowledge related to birth control and prenatal care.

The women learned about conception by "'overhearing' elder women's conversations" (Klug 1990, p 111). Several of the women believed that a woman needed to be "cool" to conceive. Only one of the twelve women interviewed knew that a woman could become pregnant on a monthly basis, and most did not know when ovulation occurred or what was involved in the process. Information about herbal medicines included use of *wuchi paifeng* to alleviate "stuck blood" from a menstrual period, use of *cho plag* to abort the fetus by increasing the heat of the woman's body, and use of other herbal medicines to cool the body and facilitate pregnancy.

Information about fetal development included the fact that babies born in odd months, that is, the seventh or ninth month of gestation, will be viable, while babies born in even months, including the eighth month of gestation, will die. Physical deformities such as a missing limb occurred because the woman behaved improperly during pregnancy, the baby had acted improperly during a prior life, or the woman had fallen during her pregnancy.

Beliefs about birth control included the use of tubal ligation even though the women did not know what the procedure involved. Although most of the women knew about birth control pills, only one of them knew that the pills needed to be taken daily to prevent pregnancy. Prenatal care incorporated the use of Western medical personnel as well as midwives and herbal medicines.

Critical Thinking Applied to Research

Strengths: Prolonged engagement with the population group and a detailed, rich description of findings.

Concerns: Categories appear to have been identified by researcher rather than emerging from the data.

Klug J: Childbearing beliefs among Cambodian refugee women. *West J Nurs Res* 1990; 12(1):108.

responsibility for her own health. Abrums suggests that nurses can play an important role in bringing about change in this area. As nurses grow to value self-care, they will also begin to reward assertive behavior in women. This will, in turn, encourage women to continue such behavior. Thus physicians and other health care providers will become more familiar with assertive women who seek to be active participants in their own care and will eventually consider such behavior the norm.

Maternal-newborn care offers a special opportunity to promote active participation in health care because it is essentially health focused; in most cases clients are well when they enter the system; and the consumer movement that has already influenced childbirth encourages people to speak up for preferences in dealing with health care providers.

Self-care has gained an even broader appeal in recent years because literature suggests that it can significantly reduce health care costs. We believe that self-care will be a vital part of health care for years to come. Obviously, self-care is not always realistic or appropriate, especially in acute emergencies, but in many situations self-care is appropriate. With this in mind, we have attempted throughout this book to suggest ways in which nurses might offer health education that would enable the childbearing woman or the parents of a newborn to meet their own health care needs. We see this as one of nursing's most important functions and one that nurses are especially well qualified to perform.

Because of our support of self-care we have used the term **client** rather than patient when referring to the childbearing woman. The term client implies an active, rather than a passive, role. The client seeks assistance from individuals who have special skills and knowledge that the client does not. Information and suggestions for a plan of action regarding the client's particular problem are offered to the client by the health care professional. The client can choose not to accept the professional's advice. Furthermore, the health care professional cannot proceed with the plan of action without the client's consent. In this relationship the client assumes responsibility for his or her decisions.

The nursing profession has been at the forefront in recognizing that people who are able should take an active role in their own health care, and the term client best fits this concept. Nurses involved in a maternity client–health care professional relationship must understand that it is their professional expertise and skill that is being sought. Any attempt to make decisions for the client is therefore inappropriate.

Nursing Roles

The contemporary maternal-newborn nurse has a variety of roles. In our opinion the most important roles are care giver, advocate, educator, researcher, change agent, and political activist.

Care Giver

The nurse uses professional expertise to help maintain and, when possible, maximize the health of the childbearing woman and her family. The nurse accomplishes this by making assessments, formulating nursing diagnoses, planning and providing care, and providing comfort and support when necessary. This may involve direct physical and emotional care of the childbearing woman or aid to the family caring for the mother.

Advocate

As a client advocate, the nurse supports the client's rights and assists him or her in making informed judgments. The maternity nurse advocate informs clients by clearly identifying all the options available, as well as the risks of each one; by explaining simply but completely the nursing actions; and by answering all questions with facts and not personal opinions. The maternity nurse advocate then supports the client's decision by adhering to it and ensuring that others do the same.

The nurse advocate can enhance the consumer–health care provider relationship by giving individuals complete information about desired services so that the consumer's expectations are realistic. The client–health care professional relationship can also be enhanced by helping individuals understand that their participation in their health care is desired and indeed necessary.

Educator

As discussed in the preceding section on self-care, the nurse has an important role as **educator.** The nurse assesses the need for education and information based on personal observation and input from the woman or her family. The nurse provides information at the client's level of understanding and confirms with the client that the information is understood. The nurse then provides any additional information necessary based on the individual's goals for learning. Nurses in maternity settings are especially active in client education. Nurses on many postpartum units, mother-baby units, and newborn nurseries have developed teaching checklists, a variety of handouts and literature, and teaching programs. However, individualized teaching between nurse and client is still the cornerstone of education for the maternal-newborn nurse (Figure 1–1).

Researcher

More and more often nurses in clinical settings are becoming involved in nursing research. Some agencies hire doctorally prepared nurses to work with staff nurses and assist them in developing research proposals and implementing the planned research. Barnard (1985) states that the challenge for nursing lies in developing research to evaluate

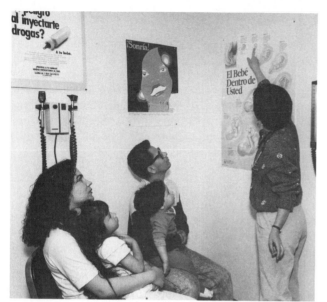

Figure 1–1   Individualized education for child-bearing women and their families is one of the prime responsibilities of the maternal-newborn nurse.

the effectiveness of nursing interventions that are sometimes taken for granted. A recent study found, for example, that research-based nursing interventions produced 28% better outcomes for 72% of the patients studied. These improved outcomes resulted in shorter hospital stays and a concurrent financial savings (Heater et al 1990). Because of our belief in the value of nursing research, we have incorporated research boxes into most of the chapters throughout this text.

CRITICAL THINKING

Can you think of ways in which nurses might function as change agents? Do you know of any specific examples?

Change Agent

Today's nurse is a change agent who works within the health care setting to effect change that will ensure safe, satisfying childbirth experiences for families and guarantee competent care for women and their babies. Nurses accomplish this change in a variety of ways: by working on utilization, quality assurance, peer review, and protocols and procedures committees; by becoming active in a professional organization; and, informally, by sharing pertinent articles and workshop information with colleagues to help them become more aware and concerned.

Political Activist

Nurses must become more involved in the political arena. This involvement may begin simply with becoming active in one's professional organization and keeping abreast of political issues that affect nursing. Some nurses find a broader base for expressing concerns when they become members of their political party caucuses and are elected as delegates to their party conventions. Some nurses find that they can be most effective by writing logical, factual, and concerned letters to legislators about important health care issues. Nurses can also take action by contributing to the campaigns of representatives who are attuned to health care issues. The contributions should be accompanied by a letter specifying why the support was given. Political representatives are always eager to know which of their actions gained them constituent support. Some nurses can best serve nursing by helping to develop public policy (by working in regulatory agencies or by running for political office). This level of involvement provides visibility and, more importantly, opportunities to make a difference through the laws of the country.

Barry (1990) explored the characteristics of nurses involved in public policy (in state legislatures, congressional offices, or regulatory agencies) and found that in comparison to other employed nurses they tended generally to be older, had more formal education, were more likely to be unmarried, and were less likely to have children. These characteristics could certainly change if more nurses become active in the public policy arena.

Nurse-Physician Relationships

Today's professional nurse is being taught to function with physicians and other members of the health care team as a peer, not as the passive handmaiden of the past. Nursing students are learning to view their relationships as collegial rather than dependent. Relationships between nurses and physicians vary widely. In situations in which there is a high level of mutual confidence and respect, nurses find their work especially satisfying, and clients benefit from the high quality of the rapport (Figure 1–2)

A birthing area nurse recalls a situation in which she worked closely with a caring physician for the good of a childbearing woman and her family.

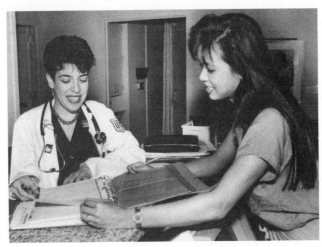

Figure 1–2 A collaborative nurse-physician relationship contributes to excellent client care.

This happened several years ago before it was common to have families attend cesarean deliveries. I was working evenings and was caring for a woman—I'll call her Mrs V. She was 39 weeks along and her membranes had been ruptured for 26 hours. We tried to induce labor but it wasn't working. In those days the rule was that membranes should never be ruptured for more than 24 hours, so we were stretching it already. Finally her doctor decided that due to her failure to progress a cesarean was necessary. He went in to discuss it with Mrs V and her husband and to get the permit signed. Dr Waters was a really caring doctor and he spent a long time explaining, but she became terribly upset and just sobbed. He came out to the desk and said, "Mrs King, I can't seem to reach Mrs V. You have a good relationship with her. Will you please try?" I went in, let her cry for awhile, and then talked to her about her feelings. She said that she had taken childbirth classes with her husband and they had planned how they would share the birth of their baby. She couldn't stand the thought of facing surgery alone. I remembered reading that several hospitals throughout the country had started letting fathers attend nonemergency cesareans, but we had never done it at our hospital. I went out and told Dr Waters about her feelings and about the literature I had read on the subject. He had done some reading on it too and said, "I'm willing to try it if you are and if you feel you can support Mr V." The evening supervisor agreed to circulate so I could stay near Mr V. Dr Waters and I talked to the family together, explaining what would happen and giving them the choice. They were so excited; Mrs V was like a

new woman. She had an epidural so she would be awake, and her husband sat at the head of the table near her. When their daughter was born, he held her for a while as he sat near his wife, and then carried the baby to the nursery while Dr Waters finished the surgery. I'm not a big trend setter or nursing leader, but that night Dr Waters and I took a risk together and we made a difference. Afterward we sat in the nurses' station, had a cup of coffee, and just grinned at each other. I'll never forget it.

As the vignette shows, nurses and physicians working together as peers can have a tremendous positive impact on the quality of care provided. Moreover, one of the unexpected benefits of the current nursing shortage is the realization it has brought to many health care providers and consumers of the vitally important role nurses play in providing excellent care to clients and families. As medicine becomes demystified, as consumers become active participants in their care, and as financial constraints demand cooperation, it is evident that a truly collegial relationship between nurses and physicians will benefit everyone.

Professional Options in Maternal-Newborn Nursing Practice

Nursing is unique in its adaptability and flexibility in providing maternity care in various settings. Nurses are found

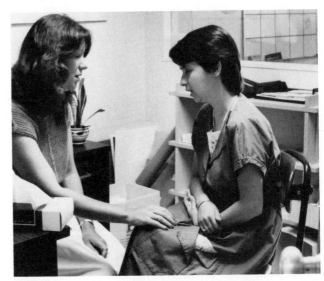

Figure 1–3 Among other choices, a nurse may choose to work in volunteer community services or in public health departments.

in the maternity departments of acute care facilities, in physicians' offices, in public health department clinics, in college health services, in family planning clinics, in school nursing programs dealing with sex education or adolescent pregnancies, in volunteer community health services, in abortion clinics, and in any other setting where a client has a need for maternity care. The depth of nursing involvement in various settings is determined by the qualifications and the role or function of the nurse employed. Many different titles have evolved to describe the professional requirements of the nurse in various maternity care roles. These titles include the following:

- **Professional nurses** are graduates of an accredited basic program in nursing who have successfully completed the nursing examination (NCLEX) and are currently licensed as registered nurses. Professional nurses use the nursing process and employ their clinical skills in a variety of settings to provide basic nursing care. Today's nurse assumes a collaborative role with the physician and other members of the health care team and is competent, assertive, and willing to take risks in the role of client advocate.

- **Nurse practitioners** are professional nurses who have received specialized education in either a master's degree program or a continuing education program. They function in a newer, expanded role, most often as providers of ambulatory care services. They focus on physical and psychosocial assessment, including health history, physical examination, and certain diagnostic tests and procedures. The nurse practitioner makes clinical judgments and begins appropriate treatments, seeking physician consultation when necessary. Within the scope of his or her clinical practice and expertise, the nurse practitioner is well qualified to clinically manage a client whose illness has stabilized.

- **Clinical nurse specialists** are professional nurses with master's degrees who have additional specialized knowledge and competence in a specific clinical area. They assume a leadership role within their specialty and work to improve client care both directly and indirectly.

- **Certified nurse-midwives (CNMs)** are educated in the two disciplines of nursing and midwifery and possess evidence of certification according to the requirements of the American College of Nurse-Midwives (ACNM). Nurse-midwifery practice is the independent management of care of essentially normal women and newborns, antepartally, intrapartally, postpartally, and/or gynecologically. The nurse-midwife works within a health care system that provides for medical consultation, collaborative management, or referral in accord with the *Standards for the Practice of Nurse-Midwifery* as defined by the American College of Nurse-Midwives (1987).

The nurse-midwife practices within the framework of a medically directed health service. The CNM functions in private practice or as a member of the obstetric team in medical centers, institutions, universities, birth centers, and community health projects with active programs of nurse-midwifery.

CNMs and Lay Midwives

When nurse-midwifery began in the United States it provided quality maternity care to those unable to afford physicians. Time and again CNMs demonstrated that the care they provided significantly lowered perinatal mortality. Today, as consumers of health care seek more involvement in decisions about their birth experience, an exciting trend is evolving: Women who can afford a choice of health care providers are choosing nurse-midwives. These women feel that CNMs recognize that the childbearing family wants to share an experience, to feel close and supported, and to control the birth experience.

The importance of nurse-midwives has been increasingly acknowledged. Nurse-midwives have prescription writing privileges in the District of Columbia and about one-half of the states and are receiving hospital privileges in many areas (Rooks 1990). This is due, in part, to a 1988 recommendation of the Institute of Medicine that physicians and state laws encourage hospital privileges for CNMs. Moreover, the National Commission to Prevent Infant Mortality urged state universities to expand their

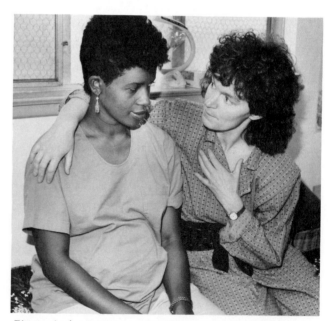

Figure 1–4   A nurse–midwife comforts her client.

nurse-midwifery programs (The Commission, 1988). Unfortunately, training slots are not being filled in all programs. In 1989, 9% of slots were unfilled and only 172 new nurse-midwives were certified (Rooks 1990).

Lay midwives, or direct-entry midwives, usually are non-nurses who enter midwifery because of a desire to assist families to participate in home births. Lay midwives and nurse-midwives share many values: Both have a philosophy of nonintervention; both value a family-centered birth experience. However, nurse-midwives are concerned about the level of education of the lay midwife. Originally most lay midwives were experientially trained and unlicensed. Some states, such as Arizona, require that they must now be licensed. Lay midwives have begun efforts to improve their own standards and education, and a direct-entry midwifery school is now in existence in Seattle (Rooks 1990).

Many nurse-midwives believe that the education they received as nurses enhances their ability to function as midwives. Their nursing background helps CNMs function effectively in an emergency situation; it helps them deal with some of the broader health problems of the families they serve; it helps them understand how and when to collaborate with health professionals from other specialties; and it enables them to negotiate the health care system on behalf of their clients (Rooks 1983). Certification by the ACNM provides the public with some reassurance about the qualifications of a nurse-midwife.

Currently, the ACNM is working to develop more cordial relationships with the Midwives Alliance of North America (MANA), which is the association of lay midwives. Many CNMs support the idea of sharing continuing education course offerings with lay midwives because it is the childbearing woman who ultimately will benefit. Is there a place for a limited-focus care giver such as the lay midwife in this country? There has been in the past, and many states seem to be saying that a place exists today. Regardless of the outcome, there is a place for the CNM in today's process of childbirth. Midwifery helps provide balance, a recognition of the magic of a process that has become increasingly technical. Flanagan (1986) sums it up well: "It is the humanity tempering the science of obstetrics" (p 198).

The Business of Childbirth

As the consumer movement has gained momentum, hospitals have become aware that the revenue generated from maternity units is a significant factor in a hospital's success and stability. In fact, childbirth has become big business. Hospitals proudly proclaim their commitment to women's health and boast of their women's "center," "hospital," "pavilion," or "core." Mention is made of the availability of birthing rooms, Jacuzzis to labor in, tape decks to provide soothing music, double beds or birthing chairs for the birth, and celebration steak dinners for the woman and her partner.

This advertising has both positive and negative effects. On the positive side it is exciting to see the changes in care for the childbearing family. Women are now recognized as consumers of a service and, as such, have clout. It is far less common for childbearing couples to feel they have to "fight the system" to have the birth experience for which they planned. The system wants childbirth to be satisfying, and health care agencies are more willing to work with couples within the boundaries of good health care.

However, Nathan Boring (1986) raises an important question about the trend toward hospital advertising: Who pays for health care ads? Initially the costs of advertising are borne by the hospital but the costs eventually filter down to consumers of that care. The inescapable question is whether all the advertising is really necessary. Are the differences between accredited hospitals as great as their advertising suggests?

Physicians are also facing the rising specter of competition. Physicians are enrolling in marketing and practice management classes, hiring consultants, and taking major steps to restructure their practices. These changes are related to a more than adequate supply of physicians (currently there are 237 physicians for every 100,000 people as compared to 148 physicians per 100,000 in 1965) and a reported decline in physician income (although physicians' income did rise faster than inflation throughout the 1980s) (Priester 1990). They are also related to a decreased demand for health care services as employers and insurance companies limit medical services; and a decline in client satisfaction. This development may represent an advantage to the financially solvent consumer who can enjoy the additional service engendered by competition but may interfere with adequate access to health care for the uninsured and those unable to bear the expense.

Health maintenance organizations (HMOs) are proclaimed by some as the way to provide high-quality care while containing rising health care costs. Others suggest that the structure of HMOs may lead to economizing at the client's expense. Since a member of an HMO pays an annual fee and sees group doctors, choice of care giver may be limited, especially in a smaller organization. Because of the wide range of quality possible among different HMOs and the doctors within the group, it certainly behooves the consumer to investigate an organization carefully before joining. An alternative, related approach is the preferred provider organization (PPO). In a PPO the health care provider has an agreement or contract with a purchaser (often an insurance company) to provide services at an agreed, generally discounted, charge. This guarantees a portion of the health care market for the provider and helps contain costs (Priester 1990).

Nurses are playing a role in both kinds of organizations because their services are less expensive than a physician's and nursing services often decrease the need for other, more costly services, including hospitalization (Griffith 1985).

Thus, nurses often provide prenatal care, staff well-baby clinics, and do counseling in family planning.

Malpractice and the Cost of Insurance

One of the most significant influences on maternity care today involves the ever-increasing specter of litigation and the rising cost of malpractice insurance, especially in specialties such as obstetrics. In the United States, malpractice insurance costs approximately 5% of a physician's gross income; however, obstetricians in major metropolitan areas such as New York may pay annual fees of $100,000, approximately 28% of their gross income (Forum 1990). Physicians are organizing to protest such high rates and are urging states to pass legislation limiting the size of awards in malpractice cases. Indiana, for example, has enacted legislation limiting to $500,000 the amount a plaintiff can recover (Vevaina & Burns 1990). Vocal consumers, especially those who have been victims of malpractice, are fighting such limiting legislation as unfair.

Meanwhile, the increases in insurance rates have caused more and more physicians to drop the obstetrics portion of their practices or to almost double the fees they charge (Vevaina & Burns 1990). In many areas, family practitioners have given up obstetrics completely. Thus, communities find themselves with no physician willing to assist with childbirth. In some cases, women must drive 100 miles or more to receive qualified obstetric care. The implications of this trend for the high-risk woman are frightening.

What factors have contributed to the malpractice insurance problem? Lander (1978) stated that three conditions are necessary for a malpractice action to occur: (1) an angry client, (2) an error by the physician or the hospital, and (3) injury to the client as the result of the medical intervention. Today's physicians suggest that a fourth factor must also be considered: the desire for money on the part of an attorney or patient. Physicians suggest that careful doctors must bear the financial burden for the mistakes of careless or negligent colleagues. However, physicians do relatively little to police their ranks and remove the incompetent or impaired. Attorneys suggest that physicians should pay for their mistakes because these mistakes have such a lasting impact. The phrase "doctors bury their mistakes" has become their battle cry. Although lawsuits can force physicians to pay for serious errors, one can also argue that many frivolous lawsuits are filed that waste the courts' time and cost the physician and insurance company time and money in preparation.

It is easy to focus on the physicians and attorneys and lose sight of the insurance companies. These companies claim their rate increases are financially necessary because of the large financial awards made to victims by the courts. However, outspoken critics of the insurance industry suggest the increases are necessary because of poor financial management. Thomas G. Goddard, a former official with the Association of Trial Lawyers, suggests that the cause is even more devious: Insurance companies claim financial necessity while spiriting profits away in tax writeoffs and reserve funds (Newsweek Feb 17, 1986).

The malpractice crisis has become so visible that many state legislatures have now passed legislation to attempt to control the problem. It seems obvious that something must be done to keep the many people who need skilled medical care from being penalized because of the crisis in the malpractice insurance industry that has developed.

In the mid-1980s nurse-midwives faced a similar insurance crisis when, despite the fact that fewer than 6% of the members of the American College of Certified Nurse-Midwives had ever had a claim filed against them (compared to 60% of obstetricians and gynecologists), and less than 1% had lost suits, they were notified that their insurance would not be renewed (*Am J Nurs* 1986). Fortunately, the Risk Retention Act passed by Congress in 1986 enabled groups to band together to self-insure, and nurse-midwifery was saved. The cost of premiums did increase significantly, however. Rate schedules are now determined by claims lost data. Consequently, CNMs as a group must "give a high priority to the development of and adherence to standards for midwifery practice" (Sinquefield 1986, p 67).

Nurse-midwifery has received some benefit from the crisis. Nurse-midwives recognize the impact that each has on other CNMs. They have recognized anew the importance of maintaining positive, open relations with clients; of involving clients in decision making; of obtaining informed consent; and of carefully documenting their actions. In addition the ACNM has learned that the group can be influential; the members can mobilize, present a positive image to the public and to legislators, and make a difference politically (Sinquefield 1986).

Legal and Ethical Aspects of Maternal-Newborn Nursing

The maternal-newborn nurse must be aware of the many legal and ethical issues that affect nursing practice today. These issues are important and cannot be ignored, because ignorance is not considered adequate justification for failure to comply with current standards of care.

Scope of Practice

The scope of practice is the limits of nursing practice as defined by state statutes. Nurse practice acts broadly describe the practice of professional nursing. The practice of nursing includes such activities as observing, recording, and administering medications and therapeutic agents. Many nurse practice acts identify functions and actions that are appropriate for nurses functioning in expanded roles such as nurse-midwife and OB/GYN or neonatal nurse practitioner. Such actions may include diagnosis and prenatal management of uncomplicated pregnancies (nurse-midwives may also manage births), and prescribing and dispensing medications under protocols in specified circumstances. A nurse must function within the scope of practice or run the risk of being accused of practicing medicine without a license.

Standard of Care

A minimum standard of care is required of all professional nurses. The standard against which practice is compared is the care that a reasonably prudent nurse would provide under the same or similar circumstances.

There are a number of examples of written standards of practice. The American Nurses' Association (ANA) has published standards of professional practice written by the ANA Congress for Nursing Practice. In addition, Divisions of Practice of the ANA have published standards including the standards of practice for maternal-child health. The Council of Perinatal Nurses has published standards for perinatal nursing. Specialty organizations, such as the Nurses' Association of the American College of Obstetricians and Gynecologists (NAACOG) and the Association of Operating Room Nurses (AORN), have developed standards for specialty practice. Agencies have policy and procedure books. Other guidelines for care include standardized procedures, that is, policies and protocols—developed through collaboration among administrators, physicians, and nurses within health care facilities—that cover overlapping functions of nurses and physicians. Nurses on units may develop standard care plans. Books and articles are another source of standards, as are common practice and those functions that have common acceptance. The identified standards range from those having the force of law to those that are suggestions or guidelines for care. Some standards may be goals to strive for, others may define minimums, violations of which may provide grounds for accusations of nursing negligence. Nurse managers have a responsibility to keep the policy and procedure books on their units up to date so that the written standards are consistent with current practice in their agency. By the same token, practicing nurses must follow the established policies and procedures. When a nurse acts outside the guidelines, he or she invites litigation and faces the difficult task of convincing a jury he or she was practicing competently.

Right to Privacy

The right to privacy is the right of a person to keep her or his person and property free from public scrutiny. Maternity nurses must remember that this includes avoiding unnecessary exposure of the childbearing woman's body. To protect the woman, only those responsible for her care should examine her or discuss her case.

The right to privacy is protected by state constitutions, statutes, and common law (Baer 1985). Professional standards protecting the privacy of clients have been adopted by the American Nurses' Association (ANA), the National League for Nursing (NLN), and the Joint Commission on Accreditation of Hospitals (JCAHO). Each health care agency should also have a written policy dealing with the privacy of its clients.

These laws, standards, and policies specify that information about the treatment, condition, and prognosis of a client can be shared only by health professionals responsible for his or her care. Information that is considered "vital statistics" (name, age, occupation, and so on) may be revealed legally but often is withheld because of ethical considerations. For example, revealing information about the admission of a single or divorced woman to the maternity unit may be legal but not in the best interests of the woman. Problems can be prevented by talking with the client to learn what information may be released and to whom. When the client is a celebrity or one who is considered newsworthy, inquiries by the media are best handled by the public relations department of the agency.

There are some instances when the public good takes precedence over the right to privacy. For example, state laws require the reporting of gunshot wounds, child abuse, animal bites, and communicable diseases.

Confidentiality

Confidential communications exist between persons in a trusting relationship, and such persons cannot be forced to divulge the information even in a court of law. Privileged communications exist between attorney and client, husband and wife, and clergy and those who seek their counsel. In many states physician-client privilege is also protected by law. Privilege is predicated on the idea that it is necessary for the client to disclose personal information for the physician to provide adequate care. Nurses are protected by laws of privilege in only a few states.

A client may waive his or her right to confidentiality of the medical record by action or by words. For example, if a childbearing woman sues a physician or hospital for negligence, she waives the right to confidentiality of the medical record because the medical record is an important source of evidence of the quality of care. In addition, clients commonly consent to disclose information to insurance companies or employers.

Informed Consent

Informed consent is consent given by a competent person who is of age and has had an explanation of the treatment or procedure. A person must give informed consent prior to receiving any medications or treatments. An individual should not even be touched unless permission to do so has been given.

The explanation of the treatment or procedure must include a description of the procedure, a statement of the benefits and risks associated with the procedure, and a discussion of the alternatives (including no treatment). Sufficient time must be provided for client questions. Some balance is necessary between too little information and an excessively detailed description of a treatment including all possible risks no matter how remote. Omitting necessary information may induce a person to give consent that might not be given if the risks were known. On the other hand, graphic details may so frighten the person that consent cannot be given. How much information is enough to enable a person to make an informed decision is not clear. In some jurisdictions medical custom dictates the amount of information; in other jurisdictions the person is entitled to the information needed by a reasonable person to make the decision.

The physician is responsible for obtaining informed consent; the nurse may witness the signature on the consent form. If the nurse determines that the client does not understand the procedure or the risks, she or he must notify the physician, who must then provide additional information in order that the consent be informed. Anxiety, fear, pain, and medications that alter consciousness may influence a client's ability to give informed consent. An oral consent is legal, but a written consent is easier to defend in court.

Parents have the authority and responsibility to give consent for their minor children. Since the age of majority varies from state to state, nurses must be aware of the law in the state where they practice. Special problems can occur in maternity nursing when a minor gives birth. The minor may be able to consent to treatment for her infant but not for herself. In many states a pregnant teenager is considered an "emancipated minor." Emancipated minors and married minors are usually able to give consent for themselves.

A married woman may give consent for her own treatment; however, when the procedure involves sterilization or threatens the life of a fetus, it is customary in some areas also to secure the consent of her spouse.

The childbearing woman usually signs a general consent form on admission to an agency. This consent covers ordinary obstetric and nursing care, treatments, laboratory tests, and medications. Separate informed consent must be obtained for surgery, for unusual or experimental treatments, or for participation as a subject in research.

Common situations in maternity nursing in which separate consent is necessary include administration of anesthesia, cesarean birth, and tubal ligation.

When a medication or procedure is indicated and the client makes an informed choice to refuse the medication or treatment, the client is usually required to sign a form to release the doctor and hospital from liability resulting from the effects of such refusal. For example, Jehovah's Witnesses commonly refuse blood transfusions or Rho (D) immune globulin.

Reporting and Recording

The medical record (1) provides a basis for client care planning and for continuity in evaluation of the condition and treatment of the client; (2) provides written evidence of the client's course of evaluation, treatment, and changes in condition; (3) documents communications among the care givers; (4) protects the legal interest of the client, care giver, and hospital; and (5) furnishes data for research and continuing education (Joint Commission 1985).

Documentation should be viewed as an integral part of quality care. It is a clinical responsibility, not just a clerical one. Nurses' notes are important because, unlike other parts of the client's record, they are in chronological order and document the medications and treatments given and how the woman or infant responded. Chagnon and Easterwood (1986) point out that five types of nursing error frequently appear in maternity charts that come to litigation. These errors are (p 303):

- Incomplete initial history and physical
- Failure to observe and take appropriate action
- Failure to communicate changes in a client's condition
- Incomplete and/or inadequate documentation
- Failure to use or interpret fetal monitoring appropriately

The chart offers the only evidence that a nurse made appropriate assessments, provided quality care, took necessary action, notified physicians as quickly and clearly as necessary, and met the standards of care.

Good nurses' notes are clear, concise, and legible. They document what the nurse did, saw, heard, felt, and smelled. They contain objective descriptions rather than subjective labels. For example, it is far more effective to chart "Fundus firm, in the midline, 1 fingerbreadth below the umbilicus. No clots expressed." than to chart "Fundus normal." In addition to describing what the nurse observed, nurses' notes should describe interventions provided, responses to the interventions, safety measures, and when the physician was notified about the woman's condition or change in condition. When a treatment or medication is omitted, the reason should be charted.

Only accepted abbreviations should be used. Errors should be corrected appropriately (by drawing a line through the error and writing *error* and the initials of the person who made and recorded the error). Correct grammar and spelling are important.

When a nurse forgets to record some information, the information can be recorded later as a late entry and identified as such. For example,

3/12/92 3:20 PM. Late entry. On 3/11/92 at 4:05 PM cesarean incision dressing removed per Dr's order. Scant amount serosanguinous drainage present. Incision clean, dry. Edges well approximated. No redness or edema noted. S. Perry, RN.

Nursing Negligence

Negligence is defined as negligent conduct, that is, omitting or committing an act that a reasonably prudent person would not omit or commit under the same or similar circumstances. *Malpractice* is negligent action of a professional person. The elements of negligence are (1) there was a duty to provide care, (2) the duty was breached, (3) injury occurred, and (4) the breach of duty caused the injury (proximate cause).

The duty to provide care arises when the client arrives at the agency. By virtue of their employment at the agency nurses have a duty to provide care. Duty may be breached by omission—failing to give a medication, failing to assess properly, failing to notify a physician of a change in a laboring woman's condition, and so on—or by commission—giving the wrong medication, giving a medication incorrectly, placing the wrong infant in a crib, and so on. The injury that results may be physical—for example, an eclamptic woman who is left unattended and with the siderails down falls and breaks a leg during a convulsion—or mental—the injury causes pain and suffering. Finally, the breach of duty must cause the injury: If a client falls, for example, it must be *proved* that negligence, such as failure to take seizure precautions, was directly responsible for the fall.

There are some exceptions to this definition of negligence. Such incidents are covered by the doctrine of *res ipsa loquitur:* The thing speaks for itself. For example, leaving a sponge in a cesarean birth client or cutting the ureters instead of the fallopian tubes would be covered under this doctrine.

In determining whether nursing negligence occurred, the care that was given is compared to the standard of care. If the standard was not met, negligence occurred. Birth injuries are common situations in which accusations of medical malpractice or nursing negligence are made. Because anoxia in the fetus can have such serious and long-lasting effects (such as death, cerebral palsy, or mental retardation), judgments against defendants have run into the millions of dollars, contributing to the high cost of malpractice insurance, the practice of defensive medicine, and the rise in the rate of cesarean births.

There have been many suits involving childbearing families. For example, a nurse in Utah did not do a vaginal examination on a woman admitted for induction of labor (*Nelson v Peterson,* 542 P2d 1075 [Utah 1975]). The nurse did an external examination and listened to fetal heart tones. She left to assist with another birth. When she returned, she proceeded with the induction procedure. When the doctor examined the woman, he noted the umbilical cord was protruding from the vagina and the fetus was dead. If the nurse had examined the woman vaginally, the tragedy might have been avoided.

Another instance involved a woman who was admitted to a hospital for the birth of her second child (*Hiatt v Groce,* 215 Kans 14, 523 P2d 320 [1974]). The cervix was dilated to 7 cm. Her first child was born shortly after reaching 8 cm dilatation. The husband urged the nurse to call the physician. The nurse said she would decide when to call the physician. The infant was born a few minutes later and the mother had several lacerations. To compound the problems for the defense, the nurse inaccurately recorded that a physician delivered the baby since she had been instructed never to chart that she had delivered a baby. The jury determined that the nurse acted negligently and awarded damages to the woman.

Failure to call a physician in time can be considered negligence. A woman was in strong labor for seven hours with no documented progress (*Samii v Baystate Medical Center, Inc.,* 395 NE2d 455 [1979]). The woman started vomiting and had other signs of distress. At this point the nurse had difficulty hearing the fetal heartbeat. She did not call the physician until she was unable to hear the heartbeat. An emergency cesarean was performed at that time, but the baby died. The parents won the lawsuit.

In other cases, nurses and/or hospitals have been found liable when equipment failed (oxygen did not work during a resuscitation effort), was missing (no bulb syringe on delivery tray), or was used improperly (steam from a vaporizer too close to the infant caused burns). Many problems can be prevented if the nurse makes proper assessments, anticipates problems, calls for help when necessary, and ensures that equipment is available, in working order, and used properly.

Risk Management

Effective management of risks of liability includes recognizing the occurrence of incidents and promptly taking action to prevent recurrence. Many hospitals employ a risk manager, often an attorney, who examines incident reports and records of problems for trends and recommends changes in policy or procedure to reduce such occurrences. The risk manager may work with managers in high-risk areas, such as the emergency department, operating rooms, and critical care units, to plan programs of prevention. In the obstetrics area effectively reducing risks includes being aware of the woman's history, taking time to record findings on the physical examination, keeping good records, giving medications accurately and noting the woman's response, accurately interpreting fetal monitor tracings, recording descent of the presenting part as well as dilatation, noting the date and time the physician was notified, recording teaching provided, and recording telephone calls and the advice given (Cohn 1984). The essence of risk management is anticipating problems and taking steps to prevent the problem from occurring.

Basic Ethical Principles

In caring for childbearing families, nurses need to be aware of the numerous ethical dilemmas they may face. These dilemmas may involve questions about maternal rights, fetal rights, paternal rights, and even the rights of society. In attempting to resolve these dilemmas it is crucial to have a clear understanding of basic ethical principles.

Among the schools of ethical thought, two theories are commonly cited—utilitarianism and deontology. *Utilitarianism* (also called teleological or consequentialist theory), simply put, states that an action should provide the greatest good for the greatest number. If the end product of an action is positive, the action is viewed as good and the means to that end are justifiable. Conversely, *deontology* states that certain acts are inherently right and others are inherently wrong regardless of their consequences (Beauchamp & Childress 1983). Deontologists also believe that human beings should never be used by others as a means to an end.

Several important ethical principles often apply to nursing practice: autonomy, nonmaleficence, beneficence, and justice. *Autonomy* refers to self-governance or the right of a person to make her or his own choices. The doctrine of informed consent arises out of this right. How can an individual function autonomously in decision making unless he or she possesses all the necessary information?

The principle of *nonmaleficence* states that "above all, do no harm." It is the duty to avoid intending or causing harm to another. The principle of *double effect* arises out of the concept of nonmaleficence. It states that some actions have both good and evil outcomes. However, if the intended outcome of the action is good and the evil outcome is unintended or indirect, the action is morally permissible. The classic example of double effect is the case of a pregnant woman with cancer of the uterus. If hysterectomy is performed with the intent of removing the cancer and saving the woman's life, the loss of the fetus becomes the unintended consequence (Beauchamp & Childress 1983).

Beneficence is closely related to nonmaleficence and refers to the responsibility to do good. This belief in an ethical responsibility to benefit others when possible is one of the hallmarks of health care ethics. The practice of medical paternalism stems from the principle of beneficence: It suggests a benevolent father who wishes the best for his children and therefore makes decisions for them rather than letting them make their own decisions. Commonly, a physician acts paternalistically when he or she withholds information—such as the diagnosis of a fetal anomaly—from a client. Paternalism raises a moral question as to whether beneficence should take precedence over autonomy (Beauchamp & Childress 1983).

The principle of *justice* states that each should receive what is his or her right or due—that is, that "equals should be treated equally and those who are unequal should be treated differently according to their differences" (Bushy et al, 1989).

Ethical decision making is based on the application of ethical principles and a consideration of rights. One of the greatest dilemmas, however, arises from the question of whose rights should prevail. In making ethical decisions, the rights of the individual and the rights of society are considered and the risks and benefits are weighed. It is evident from the hot debate sparked by so many of the ethical dilemmas found in caring for childbearing families that, in many cases, there are no clear-cut solutions to be found.

Special Situations in Maternity Care

Maternal-Fetal Conflict

Until fairly recently, the fetus was viewed legally as a nonperson. However, advances in technology have increasingly enabled physicians to treat the fetus and monitor fetal development. This, in turn, has "fostered the emergence of the fetus as a patient apart from the mother, with separate medical needs which the physician may feel obligated to meet (Sise 1988, p 263). Religious values also influence this discussion. The Catholic Church and certain Protestant groups view the fetus as human from the moment of fertilization. Other Protestant denominations consider the fetus in terms of potential human life and assign the fetus greater value as the pregnancy progresses. Orthodox Judaism, on the other hand, considers that full human status is not reached until 30 days after birth (Sise 1988).

Thus, the question of rights is far from clear. Therapeutic interventions on behalf of the fetus may take several forms: forced cesarean birth for the good of the fetus, coercion of mothers who practice high-risk behaviors such as substance abuse to enter treatment, and, perhaps most dramatically, mandating that women undergo experimental in utero therapy or surgery in an attempt to correct a specific birth defect (Evans et al 1990). Each of these interventions infringes on the right of autonomy of the mother if she is an unwilling participant.

Is it appropriate to violate a mother's right to autonomy for the good of her fetus? Legally the courts had been moving in that direction by mandating cesarean births for women who have not consented using the rationale that it is necessary for fetal well-being (Allen 1990). Perhaps the most famous case involved a terminally ill woman who was required by the court to undergo a cesarean birth against her will to save the life of her 26.5-week fetus. The newborn died a few hours after birth and the mother died two days later. In April 1990, the District of Columbia Court of Appeals issued its opinion on the case. In *In Re A.C.* (1990), the court stated that "in virtually all cases the question of what is to be done is to be decided by the patient—the pregnant woman—on behalf of herself and the fetus." This position provided unprecedented legal acknowledgement of the pregnant woman's right to autonomous decision making (Allen 1990).

Authorities agree that most women are strongly motivated to take action to protect the health and well-being of their fetus. However, attempts have been made to criminalize the behavior of pregnant women who fail to follow a physician's advice or who engage in activity (such as substance abuse) considered detrimental to the fetus. Experts suggest that such punitive and repressive measures will only serve to drive from the health care system those women who could benefit most from receiving care (Ryan 1990).

The American College of Obstetricians and Gynecologists (ACOG) Committee on Ethics 1987 Position Statement *Patient Choice: Maternal-Fetal Conflict* supports the position that "Every reasonable effort should be made to protect the fetus, but the pregnant woman's autonomy should be respected." The statement points out that acts of coercion threaten the physician-patient relationship, limit maternal freedom of choice, and violate the basic principles of informed consent. It states, "Resort to the courts is almost never justified." Care givers should rely on education, counseling, and exhortation to encourage a woman to modify high-risk behaviors (Ryan 1990).

Fetal Research

Research with fetuses has been responsible for remarkable advances in the care and treatment of fetuses with health problems. For example, the treatment of Rh-sensitized infants and the evaluation of lung maturity by determining the lecithin/sphingomyelin ratio has been developed through such research (Committee on Research 1984). Federal regulations currently specify that experimentation is limited to meeting the health needs of an individual fetus. In nontherapeutic research there must be minimal risk to the fetus, and the knowledge must be important and not obtainable by other means (Elias & Annas 1983). Consent must be obtained from both parents, and an institutional review board must review the protocol.

The federal regulations also require that proposals involving fetal research and in vitro fertilization be reviewed by the National Ethics Advisory Board. Funding for the board expired in 1980 and, since no national review can be done, research has been severely restricted (Fletcher & Schilman 1985).

State laws may be more restrictive than the federal regulations. Some states have outlawed fetal research altogether while in other states therapeutic research may be permissible.

Intrauterine Fetal Surgery

Intrauterine fetal surgery, an example of therapeutic research, is a therapy for anatomic lesions that can be corrected surgically but are incompatible with life if not treated (Inturrisi et al 1985). Examples of such lesions are bilateral hydronephrosis due to obstruction, congenital diaphrag-matic hernia, and obstructive hydrocephalus. The surgery involves opening the uterus during the second trimester (before viability), treating the fetus, and replacing it in the uterus. The risks to the fetus are substantial, and the mother is committed to cesarean births for this and subsequent pregnancies (because the upper, active segment of the uterus is entered). The parents must be informed of the experimental nature of the treatment, the risks of the surgery, the commitment to cesarean birth, and alternatives to the treatment. The parents must have the opportunity to ask questions and time to make a considered choice.

An established ethical principle states that a client does not need to consent to any experimental procedure. This principle, coupled with the woman's right to autonomy, should protect her from efforts to coerce her into agreeing to unwanted experimental surgery. Health care providers must be careful that their zeal for new technology does not lead them to focus unilaterally on the fetus at the expense of the mother (Evans et al 1990).

Abortion

Since the 1973 Supreme Court decision in *Roe v Wade,* abortion has been legal in the United States. Abortion can be performed until the period of viability. After that time abortion is permissible only when the life or health of the mother is threatened. Before viability the rights of the mother are paramount; after viability the rights of the fetus take precedence. There are continuing efforts by individuals and states to limit or abolish abortion by prohibiting Medicaid funding of abortions and putting other restrictions on the procedure. These include restricting abortions to hospitals (which significantly increases the cost of the procedure) and requiring agencies to provide graphic details of the procedure, ostensibly to provide informed consent. At present the decision for abortion is to be made by the woman and her physician. Care givers have the right to refuse to perform an abortion or to assist with the procedure if abortion is contrary to their moral and ethical beliefs.

Artificial Insemination

Artificial insemination (AI) is accomplished by depositing into a woman sperm obtained from the husband or other donor. The sperm can be deposited into the vagina, the cervical canal, or the uterus. Homologous insemination (AIH) involves the husband's (or partner's) sperm; donor insemination (AID) involves a donor other than the husband (or partner). No states prohibit AIH. There is no question of adultery by the wife, and the child is legitimate. Legal problems may occur with AID, however. Since the child is a biologic child of the mother, legal concerns center around the donor. A donor must sign a form waiving all parental rights. The donor must also furnish accurate health information, particularly about genetic traits or diseases. The husband often also signs a form agreeing to the insemination. The husband must agree to assume parental responsibility for the child. Some men may legally adopt the child so there is no question of parental rights and responsibilities. Several states have legislation regarding paternity of the child conceived by AID.

Surrogate Childbearing

Surrogate childbearing is one example of "collaborative reproduction" (Robertson 1983). In this instance a woman agrees to bear a child for a couple who are unable to have a child of their own. The child is conceived by artificial insemination with sperm from the husband in the couple desiring the child, and the child is therefore the husband's biologic offspring. The biologic mother agrees to relinquish the child at birth, the wife of the father of the child agrees to adopt the child, and the biologic mother receives payment for the expenses associated with the pregnancy and birth and, usually, a lump sum payment for her participation.

There are many arguments for and against surrogate childbearing. Those in favor of it recount the biologic mother's altruism in providing a couple who desperately want a child with the opportunity to be parents, the benefits and joys to the couple who receive the child, and the birth of a child who would otherwise not be born. They suggest that the problems and risks are no different from other instances of artificial insemination by donor (AID) and the emotional trauma of separating an infant from a birth mother for adoption.

Those who are against surrogate childbearing cite the possibility of the birth of a defective newborn that no one wants, a biologic mother who refuses to relinquish the newborn, the risks of a pregnancy to the biologic mother with no benefits, the appearance of buying a child (which is illegal in all states), and the identity problems when the child discovers she or he is adopted and wonders why he or she was relinquished by the birth mother. Others oppose surrogate childbearing on moral, ethical, or legal grounds and assert that questions of heritage and the legality of AID have not been resolved. The case of Baby M (1987) caused several states to establish laws limiting surrogacy.

In Vitro Fertilization and Embryo Transfer

In vitro fertilization (IVF) and embryo transfer (ET) is a therapy offered to selected infertile couples. In this process ovulation is induced, one or more oocytes are retrieved by transvaginal ultrasound scanning in conjunction with transvaginal aspiration and fertilized with sperm from the husband or a donor. Three to four embryos are transferred to the wife when they reach the four- to six-cell stage. The success rate of the procedure is low; clinical pregnancies result in 20% to 25% of oocyte retrievals (Rosenwaks & Davis 1990). Legal issues associated with this procedure include questions of paternity if donor sperm is used, what to do with embryos that are not implanted, and what to do when a multiple pregnancy occurs.

Oocyte Donation

Oocyte donation provides an alternative approach for women who lack oocytes, usually because of premature ovarian failure. The oocyte donor may be known to the recipient or may be a stranger. Her oocytes are fertilized with sperm from the recipient's partner in a way similar to that for IVF-ET. The endometrium of the recipient is stimulated with hormones to prepare it to receive the fertilized oocytes, which are transferred as described previously. The success rate exceeds 25% per transfer in some centers (Rosenwaks & Davis 1990). The procedure is subject to all the legal and ethical issues associated with surrogate childbearing, except that the development of a maternal-child relationship is not an issue.

Gamete Intrafallopian Transfer

Gamete intrafallopian transfer (GIFT) is used in women with at least one functioning tube whose infertility is due to unknown causes or male factors such as low sperm count. In GIFT, multiple oocytes are retrieved at laparoscopy from the woman or a donor and transferred with sperm directly into the fallopian tubes. The resulting pregnancy is considered in vivo fertilization.

A variety of ethical questions emerge: What are the rights and responsibilities of the donors? What should be done with surplus fertilized oocytes? To whom do the frozen embryos belong—the parents together or separately? The hospital? Who is liable if a woman contracts AIDS from donated sperm? Should children be told the method of their conception?

❀ ❀

KEY CONCEPTS

Many nurses working with childbearing families are expert practitioners who are able to serve as role models for nurses who have not yet attained the same level of competence.

Contemporary childbirth is family centered, offers choices about birth, and recognizes the needs of siblings and other family members.

The self-care movement, which emerged in the late 1960s, emphasizes personal health goals, a holistic approach, and an emphasis on preventive care.

Nurses function in a variety of roles, including care giver, advocate, educator, researcher, change agent, and political activist.

A nurse must practice within the scope of practice or be open to the accusation of practicing medicine without a license.

The standard of care is that of a reasonably prudent nurse.

The right to privacy is protected by state constitutions, statutes, and common law.

Informed consent—based on knowledge of a procedure and its benefits, risks, and alternatives—must be secured prior to providing treatment.

Documentation is an integral part of providing quality nursing care.

Nursing negligence is omitting or committing some action that a reasonable, prudent nurse would not omit or commit.

Risk management involves anticipating problems and taking steps to prevent them from occurring.

Intrauterine fetal surgery is a therapy for anatomic lesions that can be corrected surgically and are incompatible with life if left untreated.

Abortion can be performed until the age of viability. There are continuing efforts to restrict or abolish abortion. Care givers have the right to refuse to perform an abortion or assist with the procedure.

❀ ❀

References

Abrums M: Health care for women. *JOGNN* May/June 1986;15:250.

Allen AE: *In Re A.C.*—An affirmation of ACOG committee opinion number 55: Maternal-fetal conflict. *Women's Health Issues* Fall 1990; 1:37.

American College of Nurse-Midwives: *What is a Nurse-Midwife?* Washington DC: The College, 1979.

Annas GJ: Redefining parenthood and protecting embryos: Why we need new laws. *Hastings Cent Rep* 1984; 14:25.

Baer OJ: Protecting your patient's privacy. *Nurs Life* 1985; 5(3):50.

Barnard KE: MCN keys to research: Blending the art and science of nursing. *MCN* January/February 1985; 10:63.

Barry CT: Profiles of nurses involved in public policy. *Nurs Economics* May/June 1990; 8(3):174.

Beauchamp TL, Childress JF: *Principles of Biomedical Ethics,* 2nd ed. New York: Oxford University Press, 1983.

Benner P: *From Novice to Expert.* Menlo Park, CA: Addison-Wesley, 1984.

Benner P, Wrubel J: *The Primacy of Caring.* Menlo Park, CA: Addison-Wesley, 1989.

Boring NL: Health care ads—Who pays? *US News & World Report* February 17, 1986, p 73.

Bushy A et al: Ethical principles: Application to an obstetric case. *J Obstet Gynecol Neonatal Nurs* May/June 1989; 18(3):207.

Chagnon L, Easterwood B: Managing the risks of obstetrical nursing. *MCN* September/October 1986; 11:303.

Cohn SD: The nurse-midwife: Malpractice and risk management. *J Nurse-Midwifery* 1984; 24:316.

Committee on Research: Fetal research. *Pediatrics* 1984; 74:440.

Curry MA, Howe CL: Nurses made a difference. *MCN* July/August 1985; 10:225.

Department of Health and Human Services, Secretary's Commission on Nursing: *Final Report* (1988). Vol. I. Washington, DC.

Elias S, Annas GJ: Perspectives on fetal surgery. *Am J Obstet Gynecol* 1983; 145:807.

Evans MI et al: Fetal therapy: The next generation. *Women's Health Issues* Fall 1990; 1:31.

Flanagan JA: Childbirth in the eighties: What next? *J Nurse-Midwifery* July/August 1986; 31:194.

Fletcher JC, Schilman JD: Fetal research: The state of the question. *Hastings Cent Rep* 1985; 15:6.

Forum: The malpractice crisis in ob/gyn: Is there a solution? *Female Patient* February 1990; 15:63

Griffith H: Who will become the preferred providers? *Am J Nurs* May 1985; 85:538.

Heater BS et al: Helping patients recover faster. *Am J Nurs* October 1990; 90:19.

Hill L, Smith N: *Self Care Nursing.* Norwalk, CT: Appleton-Century-Crofts, 1985.

Inlander CB: Medicine and the consumer revolution. *The World and I* August 1990; p 515.

Inturrisi M et al: Fetal surgery for congenital hydronephrosis. *J Obstet Gynecol Neonatal Nurs* 1985; 14:271.

Joint Commission on Accreditation of Hospitals: Medical Record Services. *Accreditation Manual for Hospitals.* Chicago: Joint Commission, 1985.

Lander L: *Defective Medicine: Risks, Anger, and the Malpractice Crisis.* New York: Farrar, Straus, and Giroux, 1978.

The malpractice mess. *Newsweek* February 17, 1986; p 74.

Mumford E: *Medical Sociology.* New York: Random House, 1983.

Naisbitt J: *Megatrends.* New York: Warner Books, 1982.

New insurers' consortium will cover nurse-midwives practice. *Am J Nurs* September 1986; 86:1051.

Pace-Owens S: In vitro fertilization and embryo transfer. *J Obstet Gynecol Neonatal Nurs* 1985; 14 (Suppl):44s.

Priester R: From cottage industry to big business: Impact on medical practice. *The World and I* August 1990; p 467.

Robertson JA: Surrogate mothers: Not so novel after all. *Hastings Cent Rep* 1983; 13:28.

Rooks JP: Nurse-Midwifery: The window is wide open. *Am J Nurs* December 1990; 90:31.

Rooks JP: The context of nurse-midwifery in the 1980s: Our relationship with medicine, nursing, lay-midwives, consumers, and health care economists. *J Nurse-Midwifery* September/October 1983; 28:3.

Rosenwaks Z, Davis OK: *In vitro* fertilization and related techniques. In: *Danforth's Obstetrics and Gynecology,* 6th ed. Scott JR et al (editors). Philadelphia: Lippincott, 1990.

Ryan KJ: Erosion of the rights of pregnant women: In the interest of fetal well-being. *Women's Health Issues* Fall 1990; 1:21.

Schraeder BD, Fischer DK: Using intuitive knowledge to make clinical decisions. *MCN* May/June 1986; 11:161.

Sinquefeld G: The medical malpractice insurance crisis: Implications for future practice. *J Nurse-Midwifery* March/April 1986; 31:65.

Sise CB: Maternal rights versus fetal interests: An ethical issue with nursing implications. *J Prof Nurs* July/August 1988; 4(4):262.

Stickney J: Two cheers for HMOs. *Money* May 1985; p 155.

The National Commission to Prevent Infant Mortality: *Death Before Life: The Tragedy of Infant Mortality.* Washington, DC: The Commission, August 1988.

Toffler A: *The Third Wave.* New York: Morrow, 1980.

Vevaina JR, Burns SA: The malpractice dilemma. *The World and I* August 1990; p 529.

Weitz R, Sullivan DA: Licensed lay midwifery in Arizona. *J Nurse-Midwifery* January/February 1984; 29:21.

Additional Readings

Atrash HK et al: Legal abortion trends in the US. *Contemp OB/GYN* February 1990; 35:58

Heland KV: Failure to diagnose breast cancer malpractice claims: A new threat to obstetrics and gynecology? *Women's Health Issues* Winter 1991; 1:96.

Holzemer WL: Quality and cost of nursing care: Is anybody out there listening? *Nurs Health Care* October 1990; 11:412.

Mahoney D: Under oath: Testifying against a physician. *Am J Nurs* February 1990; 90:23.

Popkess-Vawter S: Wellness nursing diagnoses: To be or not to be? *Nurs Diagnosis* January/March 1991; 2(1):19.

Rooks JP: Let's admit we ration health care—then set priorities. *Am J Nurs* June 1990; 90:38.

Schorr T: Winds of autonomy. *MCN* January/February 1991; 16(1):38.

Stimpson M, Hanley B: Nursing policy analyst: Advanced practice role. *Nursing and Health Care* January 1991; 12(1):10.

Styles M: Challenges for nursing in this new decade. *MCN* November/December 1990; 15:347.

CHAPTER 2

Tools for Critical Thinking in Maternal-Child Nursing

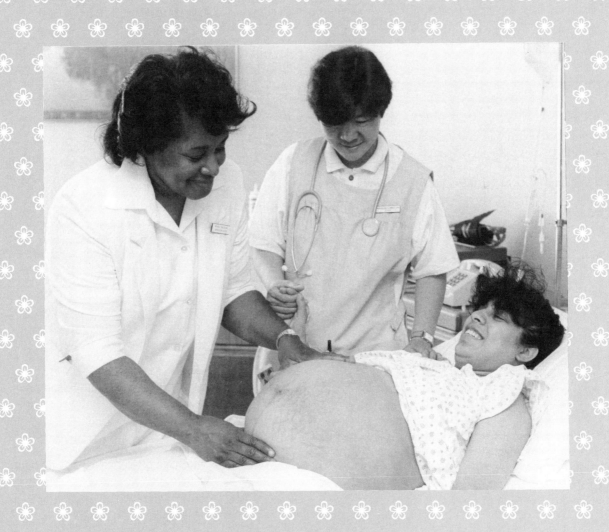

OBJECTIVES

Discuss critical thinking as it applies to the maternal-newborn nurse.

Describe the application of the nursing process in the maternal-newborn setting.

Compare descriptive and inferential statistics.

Relate the availability of statistical data to the formulation of further research questions.

Discuss the application of nursing research in the maternal-newborn setting.

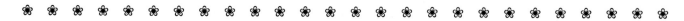

Statistics have never been so real for me as when I used them to prepare my speech to prospective legislators on "Meet the Candidates" night. I wanted them to acknowledge prevention of preterm birth as an important area that deserved funding. When I told them how many preterm babies were born in our state—and how much it cost taxpayers—the candidates listened and asked how they could help.

Most people are able to learn new information and consider factual data, but a more complex mental process is needed in order to use the facts learned and arrive at new insights and conclusions. This more complex process is critical thinking. **Critical thinking** involves separating fact from opinion, identifying prejudice and stereotypes that may influence information, exploring differing ideas and views, and coming to new conclusions or insights because of the thinking process.

Maternal-newborn nurses use critical thinking in all aspects of their nursing practice. From the initial building of a knowledge base as a beginning student to the expert nurse's application of research findings and nursing standards of care, maternal-newborn nurses continually use critical thinking skills to analyze data and make decisions.

This chapter presents many of the tools (or components) for critical thinking that nurses use in their everyday practice. One of the most important tools is a comprehensive knowledge base. This knowledge base incorporates information from a variety of disciplines:

1. The nursing process provides a systematic way of processing and analyzing data.
2. Communication skills are important in obtaining necessary data and in maintaining communication during the provision of care.
3. Standards of care developed by professional groups ensure that nurses provide quality care.
4. Knowledge of statistical data assists the nurse in identifying trends and problems.

5. Interpretation and application of nursing research findings provide the nurse with a scientific basis for nursing practice.

Critical Thinking

Nurses have used a problem-solving process in approaching the organization and implementation of nursing care for a long time. In the past, the nurse observed particular aspects of a client; then, working from a sound knowledge base, the nurse arrived at conclusions. Today the process of decision making has become more complex. Nurses have a myriad of data at their disposal, and it is important to be able to sort out the pertinent information. In today's health care setting, the nurse uses critical thinking to analyze the client's situation and to devise a plan or approach to care. The nurse analyzes available data by asking questions: What is important? What data clusters together? What pieces of information are missing? Does the picture I see make sense intellectually? Does it "feel right"? What do I expect? What other experience do I have that I can draw on?

Each beginning professional nursing student gains experience in critical thinking as basic decisions are made regarding client care. To make these basic decisions, the student asks: Are the client's vital signs within normal limits? Should I expect them to be? If the vital signs are not "normal," what factors may be influencing them? As the student gains experience and faces additional challenges from more complex client care situations, the process of critical thinking becomes expanded and yet refined. Consider the following: A 22-year-old woman named Isabella Johnson is in her third pregnancy and has been hospitalized for preterm labor. Her care involves remaining in bed at all times and lying on either her left or right side. Four times a day, a monitor is used to assess whether she is having uterine contractions and to assess characteristics of the fetal heartbeat. Although the woman has smoked for the last five years and states that she smokes to relieve her stress, she has been forbidden to smoke in the hospital. She has been hospitalized for four weeks and has been told that she will need to remain in the hospital on bedrest for the remaining seven weeks of her pregnancy. She has a two-year-old and a one-year-old at home. Her mother and a friend are sharing the responsibility of caring for her two children, although both women work full time. Isabella misses her children desperately and says that she has not been separated from them until this pregnancy.

In considering the nursing care for Isabella, a simplistic view would dictate that the nurse carry out the physician's orders and ensure that Isabella is compliant with the medical plan of care. However, the experienced nurse recognizes that the complex process of devising a plan of care involves considering the unique factors that Isabella brings to the situation. As the plan of care is devised the nurse will consider: What does the hospitalization mean for Isabella? Are the child-care provisions working? Are other resources available? Are back-up systems available for periodic relief or in the case of illness? How does the stress of worrying about her children and their care affect Isabella's course of treatment? What signs of stress are present now? What cultural and/or sociological values and beliefs does Isabella bring to the situation? How can her beliefs and values be incorporated into her plan of care? If smoking has been a part of the pregnancy to date, is there scientific evidence to support cessation now? If Isabella stops smoking now, will additional stress be added? Could other arrangements be made for Isabella to be monitored in the home if child care and help with cleaning and cooking could be arranged? Are there research studies that would support alternative arrangements for her care?

Once these questions are considered, the nurse pulls together the common threads of information; that which does not apply is discarded, and the relevant aspects are kept. For example, the nurse may be concerned about the child care arrangements; however, Isabella knows both care givers and is comfortable with the arrangements. Throughout the process, the nurse has used critical thinking to explore different ideas and values, to differentiate opinions and facts, and to consider the factors that are involved in Isabella Johnson's care.

Knowledge Base

The maternal-newborn nurse founds her practice on a comprehensive knowledge base that includes information regarding pregnancy, labor and birth, the postpartal period, and the newborn period. Information includes normal anatomic, physiologic, and psychologic processes; factors that place the woman at risk; and complications that may occur in the childbearing period.

Nursing theories related to adaptation, stress, locus of control, human caring, and care of individuals may also be a part of the maternal-newborns nurse's knowledge base. In addition to the content/nursing theory knowledge base, the maternity nurse synthesizes knowledge from other disciplines. Knowledge of family development is obtained from sociology and psychology. Anthropology provides insights into other cultural patterns, which increases understanding of the various women and their families who come into the childbearing health care setting.

Acquisition of knowledge is a life-long process for today's professional nurse. New technology is being discovered and implemented at a rapid rate; change and progress are inevitable. Maternal-newborn nurses, and nurses in other fields, find it a challenge to keep their knowledge base current with this information explosion; therefore, specialization has become prevalent. Specialization provides a narrower focus and helps direct the learning process.

Nursing Process

The *nursing process* is the foundation for nursing practice. This approach to problem identification and resolution has been in use for more than two decades (Grant et al 1990). The nursing process consists of five steps—assessment, analysis/nursing diagnosis, planning, implementation and evaluation—and is analogous to the problem-solving process used by nurses since Florence Nightingale.

Assessment

In the assessment phase, the maternal-newborn nurse gathers both subjective and objective data about the health status of the childbearing woman. Subjective information may be obtained from the woman and family members and includes their perception of the health impairment or problem and its management. Objective data are measurable and include physical assessment findings and laboratory test results.

Analysis and Nursing Diagnosis

The second step in the process is the analysis, assimilation, and clustering of assessment data into relevant categories from which nursing diagnoses are derived. Each nursing diagnosis describes a specific health problem, either actual or potential; its etiology; and the associated signs and symptoms. The formulation of a nursing diagnosis is the crucial step in the process, for the resulting plan of care is based on the problems as the nurse perceives them. In contrast to the medical diagnosis, which generally remains the same throughout the woman's health problem, the nursing diagnosis will reflect the changing response of the woman as her condition improves or worsens and as she and her family adjust to those changes (NAACOG 1989).

Consider the following nursing diagnosis: Knowledge deficit related to inadequate knowledge of normal anatomic, physiologic, and psychologic changes in pregnancy. The general health problem, knowledge deficit, is presented with the specific areas of knowledge deficit. Knowledge deficit is a client health problem that is clearly in the realm of nursing care, not in that of medical diagnosis.

Once established, nursing diagnoses serve to direct the nursing plan of care. The nurse identifies expected outcomes (goals) and priorities of care as well as nursing interventions necessary to achieve the specified goals. Nursing interventions are directed at altering or eliminating the etiologic and/or contributing factors of the health problem, and the related signs and symptoms serve as a baseline for evaluation of the effectiveness of care.

Nursing diagnoses are incorporated in this text in several ways. In most chapters nursing diagnosis appears clearly as a part of the nursing process. The chapters devoted to high-risk situations present examples of nursing diagnoses that may apply to specific problems being discussed. In addition, nursing diagnoses are emphasized in the nursing care plans, which focus on selected conditions or situations. These nursing diagnoses are used as the basis for organizing and directing nursing care.

Planning

Once the analysis is completed and nursing diagnoses are formulated, the nurse establishes outcome goals. The nurse identifies interventions that will help the client meet the established goals and develops outcome criteria that will signify that the goals have been met. Lastly the nurse prioritizes the care needed. The beginning nurse usually works through this process step by step, while the more experienced nurse is frequently able to develop an intricate plan of care covering all the steps simultaneously.

Implementation

In the fourth step of the nursing process, the maternal-newborn nurse implements the identified plan of care and specific nursing interventions. The nurse uses many skills that are common to other areas of nursing, as well as many skills specific to the maternal-newborn setting. Common interventions include auscultation of fetal heart rate, Leopold maneuvers to determine fetal position in the uterus, measurement of the uterus to determine growth, sterile vaginal examinations to determine the woman's labor progress, and use of electronic monitors that provide continuous data regarding the fetal heart rate and uterine contractions.

Evaluation

The woman's progress or lack of progress toward the identified expected outcomes (goals) is evaluated by the woman and the nurse. The evaluation process includes asking questions: Have expected outcomes been met? Is reassessment needed? Are new problems present? Are changes in any part of the process necessary? Do new priorities need to be identified? Is revision of the plan of care required?

Evaluation is a logical end step, but it is also used continuously throughout the nursing process. The nurse continually evaluates the assessments that have been made, the priorities of care, and the effectiveness of the nursing interventions as nursing care is delivered. See Table 2–1 for an example illustrating application of the nursing process.

Table 2–1 Application of the Nursing Process

The following brief example illustrates the application of the nursing process.

Sarah, a 16-year-old adolescent, comes to the school nurse's office and asks why she seems to be having trouble with her pregnancy. She states she doesn't have any energy and can't keep her weight down. She is in her sixth month of pregnancy and has gained 3 pounds. She exercises every day for one hour, smokes one pack of cigarettes a day, and has trouble sleeping because of the pressure of homework and a part-time job each evening.

The nurse applies the nursing process as follows:

Assessment: Subjective data—Sarah states "I have trouble with my pregnancy; I have no energy, have trouble keeping my weight down, and lots of trouble sleeping." Objective data—3-pound weight gain in six months of pregnancy (below recommended rate). Sarah appears underweight for her height, pale with dark circles under her eyes.

Analysis/nursing diagnosis: The objective and subjective data support problems with adequate nutrition and the statements regarding her weight suggest the need for information regarding nutritional needs during pregnancy. Sarah also needs to understand the need to obtain adequate rest and to clarify her perception of the role of exercise in pregnancy. The nurse ascertains that Sarah is going to the prenatal clinic on a fairly regular basis. The nurse decides the highest priority nursing diagnosis is knowledge deficit related to adequate nutritional needs during pregnancy. The nurse could have selected a nursing diagnosis directed toward the sleep disturbance or the potential for alterations in nutrition related to inadequate intake for pregnancy needs. But overall she decided that giving Sarah complete information about her pregnancy would address a number of problems.

Planning: The goals of care include: Client will be able to verbalize the nutritional requirements in pregnancy, will not lose any further weight, and will begin gaining at least 3 pounds per month.

Implementation: The nurse and Sarah plan sessions for the next few weeks during which there will be time for discussion and information to be shared. She gives Sarah some booklets designed for pregnant adolescents regarding nutritional and general care needs. The nurse obtains a current weight, and together they create a graph to record her weight each week. Sarah's interest in cartooning makes this a fun and creative project. The nurse asks her to keep a food intake record for three days and to drop it off at the end of the week.

Evaluation: As the relationship builds and they work together, the success of the interventions will be measured by Sarah's ability to verbalize nutritional needs and the objective data provided by her weight each week. The food intake record provides specific data to work with to encourage a diet to meet pregnancy needs.

❀ ❀ ❀ ❀ ❀ ❀ ❀ ❀ ❀ ❀ ❀ ❀

Nursing Care Plan

The outcome of the nursing process is the creation of a nursing care plan. In this text, nursing care plans on selected conditions or problems will be presented within various chapters. The nursing care plan begins with a section entitled "Client Assessment" that includes nursing history, physical examination, and diagnostic studies. The remainder of the nursing care plan is divided into columns in which nursing diagnoses, interventions, rationale for the interventions, and evaluation appear. (See Table 2–2 for sample nursing care plans.)

Table 2–2   Sample Nursing Care Plan Outline

NURSING CARE PLAN
Example: **Hemorrhage** (the condition or problem to be discussed)

CLIENT ASSESSMENT

Nursing History	**Physical Examination**	**Diagnostic Studies**
Presents key aspects that the nurse focuses on for the identified condition or problem.	Includes physical evidence that the nurse may find.	Includes pertinent diagnostic studies.

Nursing Diagnosis	Nursing Intervention	Rationale	Evaluation
NANDA approved nursing diagnoses are listed in this column. Example: Knowledge deficit related to adequate nutritional needs during pregnancy	Includes specific nursing interventions to address the nursing diagnosis and achieve the client outcome.	Contains rationale for each nursing intervention.	Identifies evidence that demonstrates achievement of client goals.

Communication

The maternal-newborn nurse uses communication skills in all interactions with the childbearing woman and her family. The nurse begins by establishing rapport and a sense of trust with the client. Rapport and trust are enhanced when the client's individuality and beliefs are respected, when privacy is provided, and when the nurse is nonjudgmental.

The nurse uses therapeutic communication techniques (Table 2–3) during assessment, interventions, and all teaching activities. In order to ensure successful communication, the nurse may need to use a variety of techniques.

Networking

Networking is a term that is used to describe the interaction of individuals. Networking may refer to the mechanism used by members of groups to exchange information or to establish new contacts. Although nurses have a long history of talking with each other, the process of creating a network of associates, acquaintances, and other professionals around a common goal is somewhat new. Currently, nurses are using networks to exchange information and ideas, to implement interventions suggested through research, and to collaborate on personal, professional, and client-care issues (Harter et al 1989).

Networking for professional nurses in the maternal-newborn setting include the following (Harter et al 1989):

1. Taking part in discussion groups through informal meetings or through a journal club

2. Telephoning or writing to colleagues to share information

Table 2–3   Examples of Therapeutic Communication Techniques in Maternal-Newborn Nursing

Technique	Example
Listening attentively	The nurse faces the woman, maintains eye contact, and positions herself so that she is leaning slightly toward the client. The nurse concentrates her attention on the interaction with the client.
Using open-ended questions	The nurse asks questions such as: "How do you feel about exercise during pregnancy?"
Clarifying	The nurse confirms the meaning of a comment.
	Client: "One person said to do exercises this way, and another person said I was not doing them right."
	Nurse: "So you feel you are getting conflicting instructions from us?"
	Client: "Yes, it's hard not knowing what to do."
Paraphrasing	The nurse restates the client's message in the nurse's own words.
	Client: "I can't exercise in the morning, and the evening seems so full, and. . . ."
	Nurse: "You are having difficulty exercising."
Focusing	The nurse helps the woman focus on a particular aspect of the conversation.
	Client: "I am having strange feelings in my body, mostly in my abdomen."
	Nurse: "Describe the feeling."

3. Participating in opportunities to meet other nurses at professional meetings and conferences
4. Getting involved with others in the community around a common cause

Standards of Care

In the midst of a rapidly changing health care system and widely divergent approaches to basic nursing education, nursing standards provide direction and information for the practicing nurse. Standards of care identify the basic expectations and functions of a particular nursing role and therefore provide a framework for accountability in nursing practice. The standards of care also provide guidelines for ethical practice, as discussed in Chapter 1. In addition they provide a basis for identifying quality in specific health care settings. The Organization for Obstetric, Gynecologic, and Neonatal Nurses (NAACOG) has These standards have played an integral part in providing direction for the development of high-quality maternity services in the United States. Because the health care setting may vary from one region to another, the standards are used as a basis for developing individualized policies and protocols.

Standards of Nursing Care: The NAACOG Nursing Standard

Standard Comprehensive obstetric, gynecologic, and neonatal (OGN) nursing care shall be provided to the client and her family and shall utilize all components of the nursing process, including assessment, nursing diagnosis, planning, implementation, and evaluation; it shall reflect informed consent and respect for the rights of the client and her family.

Interpretation The nurse has the responsibility for collecting pertinent data and assessing the client's needs in order to determine the nursing intervention necessary to assist the client and her family. The care plan should take into consideration psychosocial as well as physical aspects of the client's history and should include active involvement of the client and her family.

The OGN nurse should support the client and family members' desires to participate in the nursing process as appropriate. In addition, the client and her family should be supported throughout the nursing process by assessing the potential for individual or family crisis and evaluating their resources for coping, by use of supportive services, and by family interaction.

The OGN nurse should be familiar with the type of client records required and should share the responsibility for accurate and complete record keeping, maintaining appropriate confidentiality, to provide for continuity and co-ordination of nursing care, medical treatment, and client progress. The documentation of nursing care given should reflect the achievement or nonachievement of predetermined goals. Records should be retained for the appropriate interval of time as governed by law and local regulations (NAACOG 1991).

Application Ms Gayle works in the mother-baby unit in a local hospital and has been participating on a committee to revise the chart forms. In reviewing the standards, the committee found the forms reflected the standards in using and documenting the nursing process and client care goals. The one area not clearly reflected involved documentation of informed consent and client/family wishes for the birth experience. A place was added to the Kardex, and each nurse was instructed to ask and record specific client/family wishes.

In addition to standards of care, the NAACOG Committee on Practice develops OGN Nursing Practice Resources as an aid to maternal-newborn nursing practice. The Nursing Practice Resources do not define a standard of care, rather, they present techniques of practice that are currently accepted and recommended by leading authorities. For example, in March 1990 an OGN Nursing Practice Resource entitled *Fetal Heart Rate Auscultation* became available. The resource guide provides information regarding the techniques for monitoring fetal heart rate, guidelines for the frequency of fetal heart rate assessment, and information on documentation. (See Chapter 22 for information regarding the incorporation of these guidelines into intrapartal nursing assessment.

Statistics

Evaluation of the health care system relies on *statistics,* the collection and analysis of pertinent numerical data. Health-related statistics provide an objective basis for projecting client needs, allocating resources, and analyzing new data for evaluation of effectiveness of treatment.

There are two major types of statistics—descriptive and inferential. Descriptive statistics describe or summarize a set of data: they report the facts—what *is*—in a concise and easily retrievable way. An example of a descriptive statistic is the birth rate in the United States. How the data are compiled and presented is determined by the question being asked. Although no conclusion about *why* some phenomenon has occurred may be drawn from these "vital" statistics, certain trends can be identified, high-risk "target groups" delineated, and research questions generated that will provoke further investigation using more sophisticated statistical testing.

Inferential statistics allow the investigator to draw conclusions or inferences about what is happening between two or more variables in a population and to establish or refute causal relationships between them. For example, descriptive statistics show that the infant mortality rate in the United States has declined over the past decade. Exactly *why* that trend has occurred cannot be answered by simply looking at these data, however. More data and inferential statistics, using smaller samples of the population of pregnant women, are needed to determine whether this finding is due to earlier prenatal care, improved maternal nutrition, use of electronic fetal monitoring during labor, and/or any number of factors potentially associated with maternal-fetal survival.

Descriptive statistics are the starting point that allows the formulation of research questions. Inferential statistics answer specific questions and generate theories to explain relationships between variables. Theory applied in nursing practice can help make changes in the specific variables that may be causing or contributing to certain health problems. The following section deals primarily with descriptive statistics, although inferential considerations are addressed through the use of possible research questions that may assist in identifying relevant variables.

Descriptive Statistics

Birth Rate   Birth rate refers to the number of live births per 1000 population. After a peak in rate for all races of 25.0 in 1955, there has been a decline until the rate remained constant in 1975 and 1976—14.6 live births per 1000 population. This is the lowest recorded birth rate in the history of the United States. Beginning in 1975–1976, there was a small yearly increase through 1982 and then another decrease was recorded in 1983–1984. Since 1985 there has been a small increase in the birth rate each year, with 16.2 live births per 1000 reported in 1989 and 17.5 in June 1990 (US Dept of Health and Human Services 1990).

Live births and birth rate for Canada are presented in Table 2–4. The birth rate in Canada remains lower than in the United States.

Table 2–4   Live Births and Birth Rates, Canada, 1980–1990

Year	Live births[†]	Birth rate[‡]
**1990 (preliminary)	384,430	14.5
1985	375,727	14.8
1980	370,709	15.5

[†]*Live births = per 1000 population*
[‡]*Live birth rate = per 1000 population*

Modified from Vital Statistics. *Vol. I. Births and deaths. 1985. Canada Health Division Vital Statistics and Disease Registry. Cat. 84–204. Minister of Supply and Services. November 1986. Table 1, p 2.*
**Preliminary data. Personal contact. Statistics Canada. Publications Sales and Service. Ottawa, Canada. November 1, 1990.*

Inferential considerations regarding birth rate may be identified by posing some of the following research questions:

- Is there an association with changing societal values?
- Is the difference in birth rate between various age groups reflective of education? Does it represent availability of contraceptive information?
- Since women are averaging 1.8 children apiece and the replacement rate is 2.1 per couple, what are the future implications of the declining rate?

Age of Mother   In the United States in 1988 the highest birth rate (113.4) for the first child was in women 25–29 years of age, followed by a birth rate of 111.5 for women 20–24 years of age. The next highest rate was for 18- to 19-year-olds (81.7) and then for 30- to 34-year-olds (73.7) (see Table 2–5). There has been an increase in the birth rate for all age categories above 20 years of age since 1986 (see Figure 2–1). However, the largest increase has occurred in women 25–44 years of age who were born during the baby boom after World War II (US Dept of Health and Human Services 1990).

The number of women in the 15–19 years of age category has declined, as has the number of births to this group. As the 15- to 19-year-old reaches age 20–29, the peak years of childbearing, the total number of births could stabilize or even decline.

Inferential considerations regarding birth rate may be identified by posing some of the following research questions:

- Is there an association with changing societal values? With changing roles of women? With changing national economic conditions and financial status?
- Is there a correlation between years of education? Availability of contraceptive information for different age groups and races?

Weight at Birth   In 1988 the median birth weight of infants was 3420 grams (7 pounds, 9 ounces) for white babies and 3180 grams (7 pounds) for black babies. Both of these weights have remained unchanged since 1984. The median weight for all babies was 3370 grams (7 pounds, 7 ounces). The newborn posing the most concern to health professionals is the low-birth-weight (less than 2500 grams) infant. In the United States in 1988, low-birth-weight infants comprised 6.9% of all births. This rate is unchanged from 1987 and is the same as it was in 1976. As in previous years, a substantial racial difference in low-birth-weight infants persists, with 5.6% for white births, 13.0% for black births, and 11.5% for all other races. Teenagers and women between 40 and 49 years of age are most likely to bear low-

Table 2–5   Birth rates by age of mother, live-birth order, and race of child: United States, 1988*
[Rates are live births per 1,000 women in specified age and racial group. Live-birth order refers to number of children born alive to mother]

Live-birth order and race of child	15–44 years†	10–14 years	Age of mother								
				15–19 years							
			Total	15–17 years	18–19 years	20–24 years	25–29 years	30–34 years	35–39 years	40–44 years	45–49 years
All races											
Total	67.2	1.3	53.6	33.8	81.7	111.5	113.4	73.7	27.9	4.8	0.2
First child	27.6	1.3	41.0	29.1	57.9	53.1	41.2	19.1	5.7	0.8	0.0
Second child	22.0	0.0	10.3	4.2	18.9	38.0	40.8	26.4	8.4	1.1	0.0
White											
Total	63.0	0.6	43.7	25.5	69.2	102.5	111.6	72.9	26.9	4.4	0.2
First child	26.2	0.6	34.8	22.7	51.7	51.4	41.9	19.3	5.7	0.8	0.0
Second child	21.1	0.0	7.6	2.5	14.7	35.2	41.1	26.7	8.3	1.0	0.0
All other											
Total	87.5	4.0	95.3	67.6	137.4	152.3	122.3	77.8	33.4	7.0	0.4
First child	34.3	3.9	67.1	55.0	85.6	60.7	37.5	17.9	5.8	1.1	0.0
Second child	26.3	0.1	21.6	10.9	38.0	50.5	39.7	24.7	9.1	1.4	0.1
Black‡											
Total	86.6	4.8	105.9	76.6	150.5	157.5	112.8	66.0	27.5	5.6	0.3
First child	33.5	4.7	74.1	62.1	92.4	60.4	29.8	12.4	4.0	0.8	0.0
Second child	25.8	0.1	24.3	12.5	42.3	52.9	37.3	19.8	6.8	1.0	0.0

†*Rates computed by relating total births, regardless of age of mother, to women aged 15–44 years.*
‡*Included in All other.*

National Center for Health Statistics: Advance report of final natality statistics, 1988. Monthly Vital Statistics Report. Vol. 39, No. 4, Supp. Hyattsville, MD: Public Health Service, 1990. Modified from Table 3, p 17.

birth-weight infants (US Dept of Health and Human Services 1990) (Table 2–6).

Inferential considerations regarding weight at birth may be explored by posing the following questions:

- Are there factors that affect different age and racial groups?
- Nutritional status before and during pregnancy?
- Educational level?
- Length of time between pregnancies?
- Availability of prenatal care?
- Desire and ability to seek prenatal care?
- Physical health of the mother?
- Presence of environmental factors such as high population levels or high altitude?

Infant Mortality   The *infant death rate* is the number of deaths of infants under one year of age per 1000 live births in a given population. *Neonatal mortality* is the number of deaths of infants less than 28 days of age per 1000 live births. *Perinatal mortality* encompasses both

neonatal deaths and fetal deaths per 1000 live births. (Fetal death is death in utero at 20 weeks or more gestation.) For statistical purposes the period from 28 days to 11 months of age is designated the *postneonatal period*. Table 2–7 delineates infant mortality by age.

The 1989 rate of 9.7 per 1000 live births was the lowest rate ever recorded in the United States. The infant mortality rate in blacks has been approximately twice the rate in whites since the early 1900s (US Dept of Health and Human Services 1990).

Infant mortality for 1979 and 1980 in Canada is presented in Table 2–7. Comparison of Canadian and U.S. infant mortality reveals a lower rate for Canada.

The U.S. infant mortality rate has continued to be an area of concern, yet the United States has fallen to 19th place among industrialized nations in infant mortality rankings. In 1985, Japan ranked first with an infant mortality rate of 6.0 while the United States had an infant mortality rate of 10.6. Health care professionals, policy makers, and the public have continued to stress the need in the United States for better prenatal care, coordination of health services, and the provision of comprehensive maternal-child services. However, as many as one-third of pregnant women

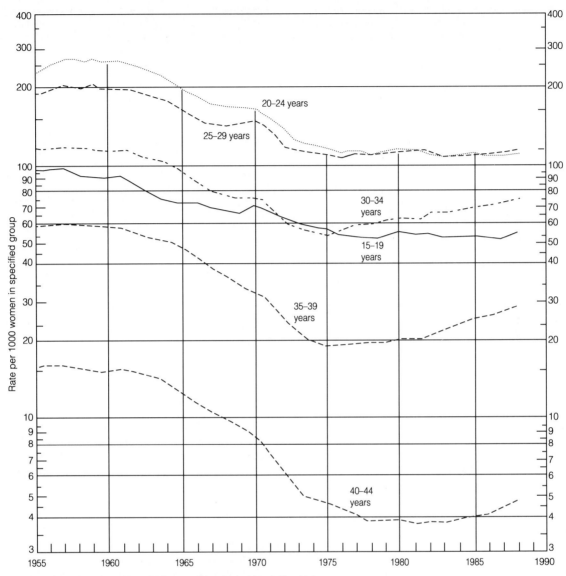

Note: Beginning with 1959, trend lines are based on registered live births;
trend lines for 1955–59 are based on live births adjusted for underregistration.

Figure 2–1   1 Birth rates by age of mother: United States 1955–1988. (Source: National Center for Health Statistics: Advance report of final natality statistics, 1988. Monthly Vital Statistics Report. *Vol. 39, No. 4, Supp. Hyattsville, MD: Public Health Service, 1990. Figure 2, p 3.)*

in some United States communities do not receive prenatal care, and our global ranking continues to fall (Arnold et al 1989). The National Commission to Prevent Infant Mortality (1988) has made several recommendations to ensure universal access to prenatal care including the following:

1. Broaden private and public health insurance for women of childbearing age.
2. Extend Medicaid coverage.
3. Provide better coordination between public agencies.

4. Establish a national council on children's health and well-being (US National Commission 1988).

Additional factors affecting the infant mortality rate may be identified by considering the following research questions:

● Does infant mortality correlate with a specific maternal age?
● Is it associated with the time in pregnancy that the woman seeks prenatal care? Number of prenatal visits?

Table 2–6 Infant Mortality Rates by Age: United States, 1950,[†] 1960,[†] 1970,[†], 1980,[†] and 1989

Year	Under 1 year	Under 28 days	28 days– 11 months
1990 (June)	9.5*	5.9*	3.5*
1989	9.7**	6.2**	3.4**
1980	12.6	8.4	4.1
1970	20.0	15.1	4.9
1960	26.0	18.7	7.3
1950	29.2	20.5	8.7

[†]*National Center for Health Statistics: Annual summary of births, marriages, divorces, and deaths, United States, 1985. Monthly Vital Statistics Report. Vol. 34, No. 13, DHHS Pub. No. (PHS) 86–1120. Public Health Service, Hyattsville, MD. September 19, 1986.*

National Center for Health Statistics: Births, marriages, divorces, and deaths for June 1990. Monthly Vital Statistics Report. Vol. 39, No. 6. Hyattsville, MD: Public Health Service, 1990
**National Center for Health Statistics: Annual summary of births, marriages, divorces, and deaths: United States, 1989. Monthly Vital Statistics Report. Vol. 38, No. 13. Hyattsville, MD: Public Health Service, 1990.*

Table 2–7 Infant Mortality (Total Infant Death Rate per 1000 Live Births): Canada, 1980, 1985, and 1988*

Year	Under 1 year
1988[†]	7.2
1985	8.0
1980	10.4

[†]*Personal contact. Statistics Canada Publications, Sales and Services. Ottawa, Ontario. Nov. 1, 1990.*

Modified from Vital Statistics. Vol. I. Births and deaths. 1985. Canada Health Division Vital Statistics and Disease Registry. Cat. 84–204. Minister of Supply and Services. November 1986. Table 22, p 54.

- Is there a difference between racial groups? If so, is it associated with an educational level? Availability of prenatal care?

Maternal Mortality The maternal death rate in the United States has decreased steadily in the last 25 years (Table 2–8). The 1987 maternal mortality rate of 6.6 is only one-third the 1970 rate of 21.5. As with other statistics, such as infant mortality rate, there continues to be a discrepancy between whites and blacks with regard to maternal mortality rate. In 1987, 2.8 times more black women than white women died in childbirth (US Dept of Health and Human Services 1990). In the past, the leading causes of death were hemorrhage, sepsis, and hypertensive disorders of pregnancy. Currently the leading causes are em-

Table 2–8 Maternal Mortality Rate per 100,000 Live Births: United States, 1950–1987*

Year	Rate
1987[†]	6.6
1980	9.2
1970	21.5
1960	37.1
1950	83.3

[†]*Latest maternal mortality rate. Personal Conversation. National Center for Health Statistics. November 1, 1990.*

National Center for Health Statistics: Advance report of final mortality statistics, 1984. Monthly Vital Statistics Report. Vol. 35, No. 6, Supp. (2). DHHS Pub. No. (PHS) 86–1120. Public Health Service, Hyattsville, MD. September 26, 1986.

bolism, hypertensive disorders of pregnancy, hemorrhage, ectopic pregnancy, and infection (Scott et al 1990).

Factors influencing the decrease in maternal mortality include development of obstetrics as a recognized medical specialty; increased numbers of certified nurse-midwives; the establishment of high-risk centers for mother and newborn care; the prevention and control of infection with antibiotics and improved techniques; the availability of blood and blood products for transfusions; lowered rates of anesthesia-related deaths; and the application of research for the prevention of maternal deaths.

Additional data affecting maternal mortality may be identified by asking the following:

- Is there a correlation with age? Availability of health care? Economic status? Access to health care?

- Is there adequate federal funding to reach women in need?

The maternal mortality rate in Canada was 5 in 1988. (Statistics Canada. Personal contact 11/1/1990).

Implications of Statistics for Nursing
The successful implementation of the nursing process depends on the appropriate application of statistics. Nurses can make use of statistics in a number of ways. For example, statistical data may be used to:

- Determine populations at risk
- Assess the relationship between specific factors
- Help establish a data base for different client populations
- Determine the levels of care needed by particular client populations
- Evaluate the success of specific nursing interventions
- Determine priorities in case loads

- Estimate staffing and equipment needs of hospital units and clinics

Descriptive statistics may also be used to help decide whether a problem actually exists. For example, a nurse working in a large maternity center that has 6,000 births per year (500 births per month) notes that 2 babies with diaphragmatic hernia have been born in the last year. She wonders whether this number reflects the projected incidence and whether the rate is higher than normal.

The rate of the defect can be determined by dividing the number of cases by the number of births.

$$\frac{2 \text{ (number of cases)}}{6,000 \text{ (number of births)}} = 0.0003 \text{ (rate)}$$

By calculating the hospital's rate, the nurse can demonstrate that although the number of cases has seemed excessive, it is within the "normal" rate of incidence, which is 1:3000 live births (rate 0.0003).

If the rate had been higher than normal, then additional questions would need to be asked. Is there a correlation with a particular maternal age? Diet? Illness during pregnancy? Place of residence? Treatment during pregnancy? Exposure to toxic materials?

Statistical information is available through many sources, including professional literature; state and city health departments; vital statistics sections of private, county, state, and federal agencies; special programs or agencies (family-planning agencies); and demographic profiles of specific geographic areas. Nurses who make use of this information will find themselves well prepared to protect the health needs of maternity clients and their families.

Nursing Research

Research is a vital step in expanding the science of nursing. It is also a means of improving client care and continuing to advance the profession of nursing.

Once research is accomplished it must be translated into the clinical practice setting, that is, it must be made useful to nurses taking care of clients. Success in this effort ultimately depends on the willingness and ability of nurses to transfer research-generated knowledge into practical nursing interventions. This practical application can consist in reading completed research studies of relevance to the specific health problem or client need and trying out the methods that worked for the investigator. Of course this example is an oversimplification, but we would like to emphasize that the process of applying research findings to improve client care can and should be made a relatively simple exercise in problem solving; otherwise, the gap between research and action will remain wide.

Application of Research

The best way to begin the application of research to daily practice is to read research studies relevant to the prac-

---

Research Note

Comparing and Contrasting Types of Qualitative Research

Ethnography examines a culture or subculture (Germain 1986). Ethnography focuses on context and uses interviews, historical documents, and participant observation to develop description. Data are coded and analyzed to determine categories and themes.

"Grounded theorists search for social processes present in human interaction" (Hutchinson 1986, p 113). Grounded theory, as ethnography, uses interviews, participant observation, and examines documents to collect data. However, the data are analyzed by a constant comparative technique in which every piece of data is compared to every other piece of data. Data collection continues until all of the categories are saturated or no new categories emerge and data becomes redundant.

Phenomenology primarily uses interviews because the focus is on the meaning of the experience, not the context. The data are analyzed in a manner consistent with the branch of phenomenology to which the researcher adheres.

Although each of these qualitative methods utilize similar methods of data collection, the underlying question and the purpose of the research is different in each method. "The aim of phenomenology is to describe experience as it is lived by people" (Oiler 1986, p 70). The outcome may be a theory or description of the meaning of lived experience. Ethnography as product generates detailed, rich description that may be developed into theory. The purpose of grounded theory research is to identify core variables or basic social processes and to develop theory.

Germain C: Ethnography: The method. In Munhall P, Oiler C (editors): *Nursing Research: A Qualitative Perspective*. Norwalk, CT: Appleton-Century-Crofts, 1986.
Hutchinson S: Grounded theory: The method. In Munhall P, Oiler C (editors): *Nursing Research: A Qualitative Perspective*. Norwalk, CT: Appleton-Century-Crofts, 1986.
Oiler C: Phenomenology: The method. In Munhall P, Oiler, C (editors): *Nursing Research: A Qualitative Perspective*. Norwalk, CT: Appleton-Century-Crofts, 1986.

---

tice setting. The following two brief examples specific to maternal-newborn nursing help to illustrate how the findings of a research study might be applied to improve client care and how clinical nurses and nursing faculty may collaborate on research studies.

Example 1: Clinical Implications Assessment of fetal movement has been recognized as a method to provide some reassurance of fetal well-being and also to alert the expectant mother to possible fetal compromise. Some maternal-newborn health providers believe that assessment of fetal movement is appropriate for high-risk pregnancies but that it should not be recommended in low-risk pregnancies because it will increase maternal anxiety.

Gibby (1988) investigated whether the use of a fetal assessment method increased maternal anxiety. The study subjects were low-risk pregnant women who completed the State-Trait Anxiety Inventory at specified times during the pregnancy. The experimental group also completed daily fetal movement assessment. Gibby found that there was no significant difference between the two groups and that the group who completed daily fetal movement assessment did not indicate increased anxiety.

Although the study sample was small, the findings imply that fetal movement records may be used to provide information about the fetus without increasing maternal anxiety. The study results may be used to support the teaching of daily fetal movement assessment to low-risk women in many settings.

The clinical and/or research nurse may also identify future study questions such as: does the time in pregnancy affect the findings? Is there a difference between various fetal movement assessment methods? What methods of teaching provide the most effective use of assessment tools? What other maternal factors might enhance the daily use of a fetal assessment method?

Example 2: Collaborative Research Lyons et al (1990) report the results of a collaborative descriptive/correlational study designed to identify nursing diagnoses selected by postpartum mothers and their nurses. The investigators consisted of two hospital-based clinical nurse specialists, two nurse managers, and a university-based nursing professor. Working together, they submitted a proposal to Sigma Theta Tau, and each nurse pursued institutional approval. The study spanned approximately one year and provided a variety of benefits. The nursing staff identified an increased appreciation of nursing research, increased morale, and improvement of nursing care. Benefits for the institution included more effective uses of resources, visibility in research conferences and at conferences where data were reported, and enhanced recruitment opportunities. The researchers identified personal satisfaction and achievement and opportunities to work together as some of the benefits of the collaborative process.

The Lyons et al study may be used as an impetus to nurses in searching out other professionals who are interested in research. The collaborative process allows many investigators to share ideas, resources, talents, and the task of completing the study.

The examples just given are meant to illustrate how a practitioner might begin to think about using nursing research to improve maternal care. Of course, much time passes and much work will be required before an idea becomes an implemented practice. Change must be regarded in terms of costs and benefits before old ways are discarded for new ones.

Critical Thinking: An Example

Each of the tools of critical thinking—knowledge base, nursing process, nursing standards, statistics, and nursing research—can exist separately, but in practice they overlap and build upon each other. An example of just one possible situation is presented in the following case study.

Two birthing unit nurses express concerns to each other about the seemingly high numbers of adolescents who have been giving birth in their unit.

At the next staff meeting they voice their concerns and raise questions about whether the number of teenage mothers seen in their unit is higher than normal. After discussion the nurses decide that they need to formulate a plan to gather more information. Each nurse volunteers to pursue a particular aspect of a plan of action. Their plan includes contacting the local public health department for local and national statistics on this age group; looking at the availability of health care for adolescents in their community; investigating the particular health problems of the pregnant teenager and risks to their infants; checking the availability of prenatal education groups for adolescents; finding out whether their community has school health programs and what the program content is; looking at national statistics regarding when adolescents seek prenatal care; talking with community nurse-midwives, physicians, and prenatal clinic personnel to see if the national statistics apply to their community; collecting information about current legislative issues affecting adolescent health care; seeking further information about the needs of adolescents during pregnancy and delivery by doing a library search; and looking for continuing education programs dealing with the pregnant adolescent client.

At subsequent staff meetings each nurse shares information, and other areas are investigated as the need is identified. How they evaluate the data and apply them will depend on the requirements of their maternity unit and the unique needs of their community.

Possible outcomes may include developing a research study; volunteering in local adolescent clinics; developing and teaching prenatal classes for adolescents; volunteering to teach in community school health programs; organizing a continuing education program on the adolescent mother for community hospitals; and forming a network within their professional nursing organizations to stay informed about legislative issues pertaining to adolescents.

As the example illustrates, the application of the tools of critical thinking assists the nurse in analyzing data and planning a course of action.

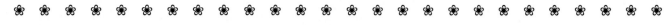

KEY CONCEPTS

Today's nurse uses a variety of nursing skills in applying the critical thinking process in the setting of maternal-newborn nursing.

A comprehensive nursing knowledge base forms the basis for nursing activities.

The nursing process, composed of assessment, analysis and nursing diagnosis, plan of care, implementation, and evaluation, provides a systematic method of approaching nursing practice.

Communication skills are important in obtaining client data and in providing nursing care.

Nursing standards provide information and guidelines for nurses in their own practice, in developing policies and protocols in health care settings, and in directing the development of quality nursing care.

Descriptive statistics describe or summarize a set of data. Inferential statistics allow the investigator to draw conclusions about what is happening between two or more variables in a population.

Nursing research is vital to add to the nursing knowledge base, expand clinical practice, and expand nursing theory.

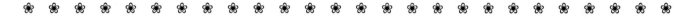

References

Arnold LS, Brecht MC, Hockett A et al: Lessons from the past. *MCN* March/April 1989; 14(2):75.

Gibby NW: Relationship between fetal movement charting and anxiety in low-risk pregnant women. *J Nurse-Midwifery* July/Aug 1988; 33(4):185.

Gordon M: *Nursing Diagnosis: Process and Application.* New York: McGraw-Hill, 1987.

Grant J, Kinney M, Guzzetta C: A methodology for validating nursing diagnoses. *Adv Nurs Sci* 1990;12(3):65.

Lyons NB, Stein M, Blackburn S et al: Too Busy for Research? Collaboration: An Answer. *MCN* March/April 1990; 15(2):67.

NAACOG: *OGN Nursing Practice Resource: Nursing Diagnoses.* Washington, DC: NAACOG, 1989.

NAACOG: *Standards for the Nursing Care of Women and Newborns.* 4th ed. Washington, DC: NAACOG, 1991.

North American Nursing Diagnosis Association: *Classification of Nursing Diagnoses: Proceedings of the Seventh Conference.* St. Louis: Mosby, 1987.

Scott JR, DiSaia PJ, Hammond CB et al: *Danforth's Obstetrics and Gynecology.* 6th ed. Philadelphia: Lippincott, 1990.

U.S. National Commission To Prevent Infant Mortality: *Death Before Life: The Tragedy of Infant Mortality.* Washington, DC: The Commission, 1988.

Additional Readings

Boyd CO: Critical appraisal of developing nursing research methods. *Nurs Science Quarterly.* Spring 1990; 3(1):42.

Gleeson RM, McIlvain-Simpson G, Boos ML et al: Advanced practice nursing: A model of collaborative care. *MCN* January/February 1990; 15(1):9.

Harter C, Grossman LK: Networking to implement effective health care. *MCN* November/December 1989; 14(6):387.

Lee PP, Estes CL: The Nation's Health. 3rd ed. Boston: Jones and Bartlett Pub. 1991.

NAACOG: *OGN Nursing Practice Resource. Fetal Heart Rate Auscultation.* Washington, DC: NAACOG, March 1990.

Rip MR, Hunter JM: The community perinatal health care system of urban Cape Town, South Africa—I. Characteristics of mothers and birth outcomes. *Soc Sci Med* 1990; 30(1):111.

Schwartz RM: What price prematurity? *Fam Plann Perspect* July/August 1989; 21(4):170.

Torres A, Kenney AM: Expanding Medicaid coverage for pregnant women: Estimates of the impact and cost. *Fam Plann Perspect* January/February 1989; 21(1):19.

PART TWO

The Contemporary Family and Reproductive Issues

CHAPTER 3

The Contemporary Family:

Structure, Function, and Dysfunction

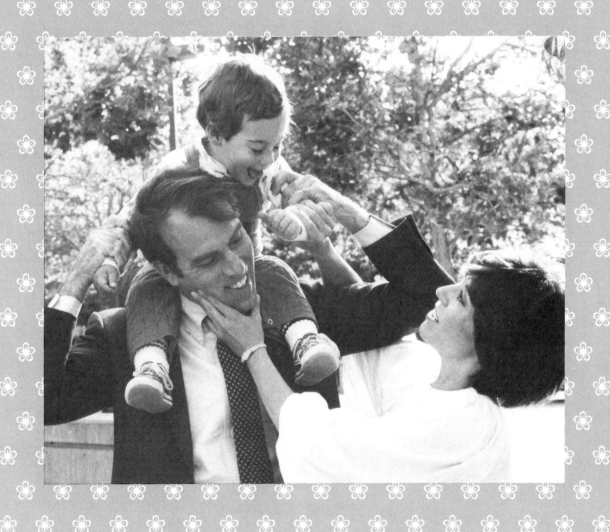

OBJECTIVES

Summarize the status of the family in today's society.

Identify major variations in family structure and function.

Compare different approaches of conceptualizing family life as it relates to the childbearing family.

Develop an overview of instruments for assessing family functioning.

Discuss the implications for nursing practice of treating the family as a unit of care.

Describe the types and extent of family violence.

List the social, psychologic, political, and cultural factors that contribute to the occurrence of spouse abuse.

Describe the myths and facts about spouse abuse.

Discuss the role of the nurse who cares for battered women.

Identify the factors that place parents at risk for child abuse.

Delineate the short- and long-term effects of child abuse on the child and other members of the family.

Identify the responsibilities of the nurse who suspects child abuse.

Describe the community resources available to violence-prone families.

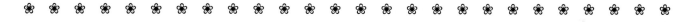

He didn't know what kind of father he'd make. He was so afraid our closeness and incredible happiness together would be cut into by a child—but of course he wanted us to have a baby more than anything in the world, he just would have to get used to the idea. (Lauren Bacall, By Myself)

Family health, long the domain of public health professionals, is now becoming a primary concern of all health care providers. Consumer pressures, professional initiatives, and research on the family-illness relationship have increased the emphasis on family-centered health care. As people become better educated about their own health, they want to know more about the purpose and consequences of health care services for themselves and their families. Changing consumer needs and escalating health care costs have created consumer demand for alternative services and health care personnel. Growing awareness of the interdependence of stress and illness, as well as of physical fitness and health, has heightened interest in both individual and family self-care.

Family-centered care is also widely endorsed by health care professionals, who recognize the family as the primary source of physical and emotional support for individual members and as the primary influence on its children's development. Research on childbearing families has shown that family involvement during pregnancy and birth can enhance the birth experience, attachment between parents and infants, and parenting skills.

The recognition that effective health care of individuals requires the involvement of their support network has necessitated an expanded role for the nurse. The nurse now includes the family in health teaching, explanations of medical and surgical interventions, and coordination of health care activities. In addition, as the focus shifts from the parental unit to the entire family, nurses are incorporating siblings, grandparents, and other family members into the plan of care. The nurse can assist the entire family's adjustment to the arrival of a new infant by helping them to improve their communication patterns. For example, the family members may be encouraged to discuss their feelings and perceptions and identify potential role changes that may occur. When a family experiences a loss, such as the birth of a stillborn, disabled, or preterm infant, the maternal-newborn nurse can work with the entire family to assist them in coping with the event (Ross & Cobb 1990).

The ability to work effectively with a variety of families requires both understanding of how families function and willingness to consider the difficult issues inherent in achieving family-centered care. This chapter provides an introduction to varying family forms and functions, acquaints the reader with major conceptualizations of family life, and describes the instruments used to assess family functioning. It also focuses on understanding families and the major issues the nurse is likely to encounter in working with them.

The Contemporary Family

What is "the typical family?" In the 1950s and early 1960s (in the United States), that phrase evoked an image of a happily married, white, middle-class couple with two or three children, with the man as breadwinner and the woman as housewife. The children were fairly well behaved and well adjusted. Divorce was infrequent because it was socially unacceptable. An aura of stability, contentment, and complacency surrounded the family.

Families responded to the political and social movements of the 1960s and 1970s in different ways. Some families remained virtually untouched by all that was going on around them; others responded by rethinking the values and assumptions underlying their views of family life. They questioned long-standing beliefs about what it meant to be a parent, a spouse, or a child and explored new forms of family grouping and ways of being a family.

People have learned valuable lessons from this chaotic time. A great difference clearly exists between the "typical" family created from statistical information (or wishful thinking) and real families. Real families are dynamic and unique. Many do indeed consist of two adults and two or three children. However, the couple may not necessarily be married, or white, or middle class, or even of opposite sexes. A woman may be the breadwinner; a man, the "househusband." It is not unlikely that one or both adults have been or will be divorced. The children may be siblings by marriage (that is, stepsiblings), not by blood ties. The children may also be far less childlike than their counterparts of 20 years ago owing to their early and continued exposure (via television) to world events, technology, and varied life-styles. This phenomenon is sometimes referred to as "accelerated" childhood.

Contemporary family life is complex, with little room for complacency. What is typical about the typical family is that its members are faced with the difficult but usually gratifying task of coexisting with one another and their environment. In order to do this, each family must maintain itself as a functioning unit in the face of an everchanging situation. Hill (1974) captured the essence of the demands most families confront when he noted:

> The family is perhaps more subject to disturbance than any other organization because of its rapidly changing age composition and frequently changing plurality patterns. Its curious age and sex composition make it an inefficient work group, a poor planning committee, an unwieldy play group, and a group of uncertain congeniality. Its leadership is shared by two relatively inexperienced amateurs for most of their incumbency, new to the role of spouse and parent. They must work with a succession of disciples having few skills and lacking in judgment under conditions which never seem to remain stable long enough to bring about a settled organization (p 374).

A logical place to begin an exploration of this complex, changing entity called the family is with a definition. Not surprisingly, there is no single, generally accepted definition of **family**. Some authors focus on family structure or the configuration of actors and roles comprising the family. Others emphasize the activities or functions in which family members are engaged. The increase in nontraditional family forms has fostered a trend toward defining families in terms of the members' emotional ties to one another. Friedman (1986), for example, defined the family as two or more individuals who are emotionally involved and live in geographic proximity. This is a fairly broad definition, but it still does not include the single adult who lives alone (see below) or the "bicoastal" couple in which each partner lives in a different part of the country. Bicoastal couples consider themselves a family even though they may be geographically separated.

Stanhope and Lancaster (1988) define the family as "two or more individuals coming from the same or different kinship groups, who are involved in a continuous living arrangement, usually residing in the same household, experiencing common emotional bonds, and sharing certain obligations toward others" (p 353).

Regardless of the definition one chooses, a family has certain common characteristics. The members are joined emotionally and/or legally. Cultural values and beliefs are a part of every family, and these values and beliefs are transmitted by family members from generation to generation. The family unit is an interdependent group of individuals with definite role relationship and communication patterns that form a small social system. In addition, the family serves as a buffer between the individual members and the larger society (Friedman 1986; Clark 1984). The concepts of family structure and function are discussed in more detail in the following section.

Family Structure

Many trends and changes in attitudes have contributed to the increase in the kinds of family configurations we see today. These configurations represent an array of family structures (Figure 3–1). One of the primary reasons for the growing number of different family forms is that our society is becoming increasingly pluralistic and highly differentiated. The "typical" family structure of the past no longer fulfills the needs of this varied and dynamic society.

The term *family structure* refers to the organization of the family unit. In the past, the dominant form of family structure, the **nuclear family**, was composed of husband, wife, and children. Although this remains the most prevalent family form in the United States today (U.S. Bureau of the Census 1987), alternative family forms are increasing, and many families do not fit this pattern. The sexual revolution, the women's movement, "no fault" divorce laws and high divorce rates, increases in single-parent families (U.S. Bureau of the Census 1987), and economic changes have all influenced how families are structured in our society.

According to Hymovich (1980) and Friedman (1986) most families belong to one of the following types of family configurations:

> *Single adult.* According to Friedman's definition, the unmarried adult living alone is not considered to be a family configuration because the proximity, interaction, and support that are part

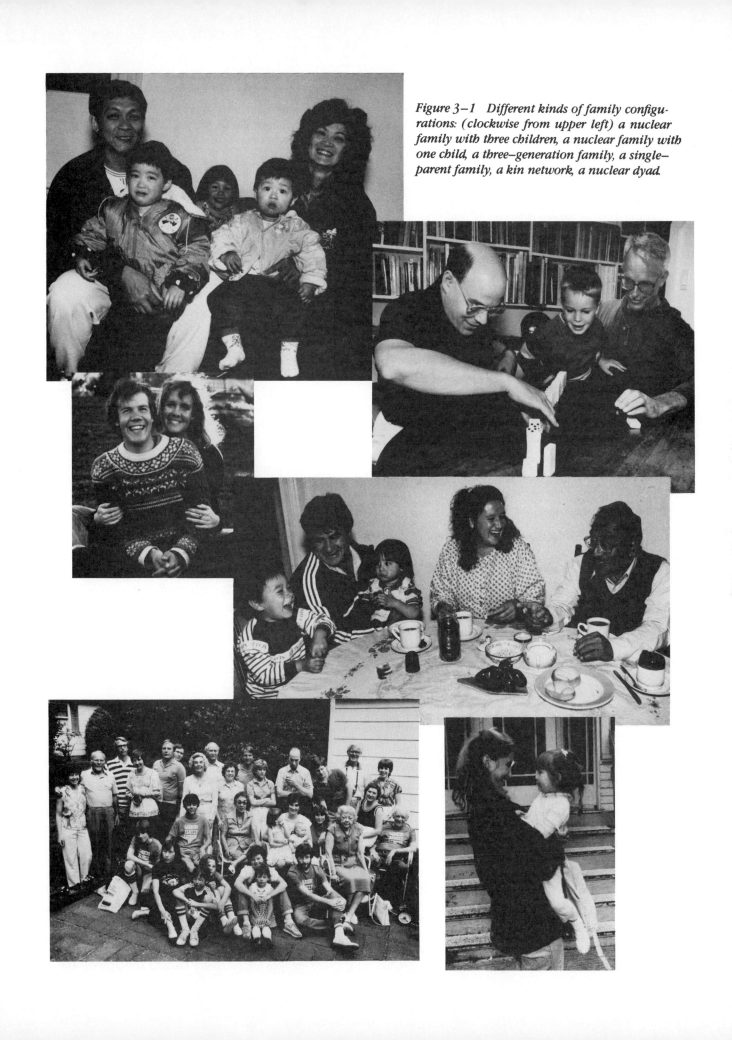

Figure 3–1   Different kinds of family configurations: (clockwise from upper left) a nuclear family with three children, a nuclear family with one child, a three-generation family, a single-parent family, a kin network, a nuclear dyad.

of family life are not present. The person living alone must perform functions typically ascribed to the family, however, such as finding suitable housing and income and organizing relationships with the extended family and community.

A variation of the single-adult family configuration that the maternal-newborn nurse may encounter is the *unmarried-parent* family, usually consisting of a mother and a child. These parents either do not desire marriage at all or do not desire it in the near future. With society's increasingly liberal attitudes toward sexuality, a large number of unmarried women are choosing to keep a child rather than giving it up for adoption. In addition, an increasing number of single adults are adopting children. This family configuration is the same as that of the single-parent family, discussed later, with the important exception that the latter involves a disrupted family, in which one of the parents is no longer living in the immediate household.

Nuclear dyad. Frequently referred to as the *beginning family,* the nuclear dyad consists of a husband and wife living in a single-family residence. One or both partners are employed outside the home, and there are either no children or, in the case of an older couple, no children at home.

Single parent. One-parent families are becoming far more prevalent, as the rate of divorce and separation is beginning to stabilize at a relatively high rate. One adult is left alone either (by separation, divorce, or death of a spouse) to raise minor children in a separate household with no other adults. Also in this category are single parents who adopt or who have never been married. If no other source of family income exists, or if the adult prefers, he or she may seek outside employment, adding even more responsibilities to family life. Many single parents eventually remarry, creating a need for additional role changes for both the former and the new family units.

A majority of single-parent families are headed by women (U.S. Bureau of the Census 1987). Lack of adequate earning power, plus a lack of financial support from the fathers, continue to plague single-parent families headed by women. See Chapter 6 for further discussion of related issues. A small percentage (2.5%) of single-parent families are headed by men (U.S. Bureau of the Census 1987), but the number headed by men is increasing (Moynihan 1987). Divorced fathers are often separated from their children, causing hardship and conflicts. Depending on the nature of the parents' relationship after divorce, collaborative parenting may or may not

be possible. If the father's contact with the children is infrequent, the father-child relationship may suffer.

Nuclear family. The traditional family structure in our society is the nuclear family. It includes husband, wife, and all minor children living together in a single household. Dual employment may or may not be a component of this family. In this chapter the nuclear family is generally the structure referred to, although many of the concepts discussed can be applied to other family types. Lamb (1980) found that nuclear families were more effective and reliable socializing situations than single-parent families but only when the nuclear families' marital relationships and overall emotional environments were harmonious.

Three-generation family. In the three-generation structure, one or more dependent grandparents live in a household with either a single-parent family or a nuclear family. Such a family can benefit from the grandparents' wisdom and experience; the grandmother's role may also include assisting with child care, freeing the mother to seek employment. This arrangement is a feature of many Asian families.

Kin network (or extended family). The *extended* family includes two or more nuclear or unmarried households or any of the previously described configurations living in proximity, exchanging goods, and looking to each other for interaction and support. Although the parents have authority within their single households, the other adults are often consulted for advice, support, and authority in intrafamily affairs. A newly formed nuclear family may in fact be part of a *kin network* if relatives by blood or marriage are nearby and are part of the family's social group. For some families, the trend for mothers to return to work has revived the need to depend on relatives living in separate households to care for children while parents are working (Ross & Cobb 1990). Many families are rediscovering the advantages of a well-maintained kinship system.

Blended (reconstituted, stepparent) *families.* Recently, the nuclear family has been rocked by an increasing number of marital separations and divorces, often resulting in a variation of the nuclear family known as the blended family (Gelliss et al 1989). This trend has been accompanied by a high rate of remarriage. *Reconstituted,* or *blended,* families are established through remarriage, raise children from previous marriages and/or from the current marriage, and in many instances create larger kinship systems for the child. According to McCubbin and Dahl (1985), the most common issues facing reconstituted families include winning acceptance, integrating the stepparent into an established family, and resolving the mixed allegiance that the biologic parent has toward the new mate and existing children.

In addition to the more common forms outlined above, the nurse may encounter clients who are members of other types of family structures. Ross and Cobb (1990) described communal, cohabitation, and homosexual (gay) forms, all characterized by comparatively atypical configurations of positions and patterned relationships. While it is impossible to identify and describe all the new sizes and shapes in which families now come, it is important to recognize the extent to which such variation exists and to be open to family structures that differ radically from one's own.

Family Function

The concept of family function focuses on the family as a task performance group. By accomplishing certain goals, the family contributes to the survival of the wider social system of which it is a part, the family unit as a whole, and the individual members of that unit. In a broader sense, *function* refers to the consequences or outcomes that a family's interrelated motives and subsequent behavior have for the family as a unit (Ritzer 1983), that is, what the family does. While there is some variation among authors regarding specific family functions, the following are often cited as important goals that families must achieve to continue functioning.

Friedman (1986) has identified five major functions, plus an underlying mechanism by which these functions are achieved. These include (1) the *affective function*, which forms the primary basis for continuation of the family as a unit by meeting the family members' emotional needs; (2) the *reproductive function*, which provides for continuity within the family system and society; (3) the *socialization function*, which socializes children to their roles in society; (4) the *health care function* and provision of food, shelter, clothing and warmth; and (5) the *economic function*, which provides the family with economic resources for survival (Table 3–1).

Family coping strategies provide the mechanism for carrying out these functions. Internal family coping strategies include (1) family group reliance, (2) humor, (3) greater family sharing, (4) reframing or controlling the meaning of a problem, (5) joint problem solving, and (6) flexible roles. External family coping strategies include (1) seeking out information or knowledge about the stressor, (2) increasing linkages with community groups such as clubs and organizations, (3) using social support systems, (4) using self-help groups, and (5) seeking spiri-

tual support. Without effective family coping strategies, the family's functions cannot be accomplished (Friedman 1986).

Given a particular configuration of members and a set of general tasks or goals that must be accomplished if the family is to survive, families develop rules and roles that characterize their day-to-day functioning. This means that much of family life has a taken-for-granted quality about it. A *role* is a cluster of interpersonal behaviors, attitudes, and activities associated with an individual in a certain situation or position. The behaviors tend to be learned through interactions with parents and siblings. *Attitudes* are the expectations of the society in which the child is raised; they affect and can be modified by the individuals' behaviors. Role activities are governed by expectations and behavior patterns of friends, relatives, and others outside the individual. Role behaviors, attitudes, and activities are learned to a large extent through the process of socialization.

Each family must define its role in the community and the roles of its individual members within the family unit. These roles are learned through interaction and imitation. Children learn the roles of their parents while learning their own roles and form their self-concepts on the basis of how well they execute their own roles. The roles that children assume affect their psychosocial development into adulthood.

Once the roles of family members are developed, family processes usually continue in a predictable pattern. When interruptions occur in the expected personal roles, family processes will also be interrupted. In most cases, one person will assume the other's role. For example, when the wage earner is disabled for a period, the spouse may need to find a job to replace the lost income, and the children may have to add more household duties and responsibilities to their roles.

Theoretical Frameworks for Understanding the Family

By defining and interrelating concepts, theoretical frameworks provide a tool for understanding and analyzing families. Numerous different frameworks are available for viewing family life, including the structural-functional, interactional, psychoanalytic, anthropologic, and developmental frameworks. The purpose of these various frameworks is to provide a nurse with a lens for viewing the family. Depending on which lens is selected, the nurse sees a somewhat different entity. Just as certain definitions of family focus attention on composition of the family, and others focus on function, theoretical frameworks provide a foundation for understanding family life, family assessment, and nursing care.

Table 3–1 Guidelines for Functional Family Assessment *

Affective Function

1. Do the family members display signs of affection for one another?

2. Do the family members appear to trust and respect one another?

3. Is the family supportive of its members?

4. What events or situations within the family could influence the parents' ability to provide nurturance of the children?

5. Do any of the children appear to be assuming adult or parenting roles that can influence how well their own emotional needs are being met?

Reproductive Function

1. Is the number of children within the family acceptable to both partners?

2. Are the family members comfortable with their own sexuality?

3. How is sexuality and reproductive information conveyed to the children?

4. Do members of the family use birth control? Are these methods satisfactory?

5. Do any of the family members have concerns related to sexuality and reproduction?

Socialization Function

1. Who in the family is primarily responsible for child care?

2. Who in the family is primarily responsible for discipline, rewards, or punishment?

3. What cultural influences affect the family's childrearing practices?

4. How does the family's socioeconomic class influence the family's childrearing practices?

5. What other variables influence the family's childrearing practices?

6. Does the family identify problem areas related to childrearing and discipline?

Health Care Function

1. Who in the family makes decisions related to the members' health care needs? Illness needs?

2. What health care facilities are available to the family?

3. What health care facilities are used by the family?

4. What is done when a family member becomes ill?

5. Does the family have adequate resources for health care needs? Does the family have health insurance?

6. Does the family have a private physician? Or do they visit a health clinic?

7. Are there specific health/illness practices related to the family's culture (ie, folk medicine practices)?

8. Is the "health practitioner" identified within the family's culture (ie, "granny," herbalist)?

9. What preventive health care practices are incorporated into the family's life-style?

10. What barriers to health care are perceived by the family?

Economic Function

1. What are the sources of the family income? Who in the family provides the economic resources?

2. Does the family have adequate income and/or resources to provide food, shelter, and clothing for the family members?

3. Does the family have health insurance or resources to pay for health care services?

4. What agencies need to be contacted to assist the family in the provision of adequate health care, food, clothing, or shelter?

Coping Function

1. What events or situations is the family experiencing that are potentially stressful? How does the family perceive these events or situations?

2. What resources or assets exist within the family to deal with the stressful events or situations?

3. Does the family have adequate support systems?

4. Does the family use humor? Is there joint problem solving?

5. Are the family roles flexible?

6. Is there family group reliance?

7. Is the family denying that a problem exists?

8. Does anyone in the family try to exploit the family members?

9. What is the family's level of adaptation?

Adapted from Friedman MM: Family Nursing: Theory and Assessment 2nd Ed., *Norwalk, CT: Appleton-Century-Crofts, 1986.*

Overview of Frameworks

Three frameworks have been especially popular in nursing's study of the family: the *interactional framework*, the *systems framework*, and the *developmental framework*. The last has been especially influential in family nursing. The interactional framework looks at family members' subjective views of their situation, emphasizing internal family dynamics. In contrast, the systems view of family is directed toward the relationship between the family and the larger social system. It is also concerned with how families maintain stability within an everchanging environment. The developmental framework emphasizes changing family structures and functions across the various stages of the family life cycle. Following a brief introduction to the interactionist and systems frameworks, the remainder of this section focuses on a more detailed presentation of the developmental framework.

Interactional Framework

The interactional framework centers on understanding within the family by discovering how individual members define their situation (internal dynamics). Interactions focus on subjective meaning as indicated by the three basic premises on which the framework is grounded:

1. Human beings act toward things on the basis of the meaning these things have for them.
2. The meaning of such things is derived from or arises out of the social interaction one has with others.
3. Meanings are modified through an interpretive process used by the person in dealing with the things he/she encounters.

The concepts of self, interaction, and role are central to the framework. The self is viewed as a constantly changing process that arises from interaction with others. Roles are seen as emergent rather than static entities. Interactionists focus on understanding how individuals define their roles and the implications of these definitions for how they enact them.

Knafl (1985) used an interactional perspective to study how families responded to a child's routine hospitalization. Consistent with the interactional orientation, one aspect of the study was to discover how families defined the child's hospitalization and their parenting role within the hospital setting. The data revealed wide variations in parents' views of the hospitalization; some described it as a "normal," expectable part of childhood, and others depicted it as a full-scale family crisis. Moreover, parents held quite differing views of what their parenting role should be in the hospital. Some preferred to delegate all caretaking and decision making to the professional staff, while others actively negotiated with staff to remain involved in caretaking and decision making.

The interactional framework is an appropriate lens for viewing families from the family's point of view. One can use data on these subjective views to identify common processes that family members use to define and manage various family situations. The framework is helpful in isolating specific potential sources of difficulties as family members relate to one another and to their community.

Systems Framework

The systems framework emphasizes the concepts of structure, function, boundary maintenance, and change. Aldous (1978, p 26) identified four fundamental characteristics of the family as a social system:

1. The positions occupied by family members are interdependent.
2. The family maintains boundaries and therein constitutes an identifiable unit.
3. The family performs certain tasks both for the larger social system and for family members.
4. The family as a unit is capable of change.

Family structure is defined by the patterned interactions that develop over time among individuals occupying the various positions in the family. The positions (such as wife-mother and husband-father) that comprise the family are viewed as interdependent, although the degree of interdependence may vary both across families and within a single family over time. For example, children typically become less dependent on their parents as they grow older, while parents may become increasingly dependent on their children.

Regarding the concept of boundaries, Hill (1974) conceptualized the family as a semiclosed system, maintaining links to other social systems and exercising control over the nature and frequency of those links. The family's ability to maintain control over its boundaries is linked to the previously described family functions. For example, if a family is unable to control a certain member's behavior, it may have to open its boundaries to law enforcement officials whether it wants to or not.

The family both reacts to and initiates change. In systems terminology, these two processes are referred to as *positive* and *negative* feedback, respectively. Following a systems perspective, change is conceptualized in terms of goal attainment and information exchange. Families exchange information and receive feedback from their environment. Such feedback is processed by family members who interpret it in terms of the family's goals and tasks. Depending on the "fit" between the feedback and the intended goal, the family may respond by altering either its behaviors or its goals. In a negative feedback situation, the family takes a reactive stance and alters its behavior in response to outside input. For example, a couple changes their usual division of labor after their first child is born when they realize their former way of dividing household chores is no longer suitable. The change occurs only after a series of disruptive arguments in which each partner vehemently argues a different point of view. Such a change is reactive since it follows the birth of the baby and is made in the context of threatened family stability due to increased conflict between husband and wife. In a positive feedback situation, the family takes a proactive stance and initiates change in response to an anticipated situation. In a proactive situation, a couple anticipates that the birth of a baby will require a change in their established division of labor, and therefore they negotiate and try out several different arrangements before the baby is born.

The systems perspective is ideally suited to exploring family goal orientations, boundary maintenance, patterns of communication, and exchanges between the family and other social systems. It provides the nurse with a framework for understanding these aspects of family life.

Developmental Framework

The developmental framework looks at the family over time as it progresses through predictable stages of the life cycle. Duvall (1977) views the family as having universal tasks as well as specific developmental tasks that must be accomplished at eight different stages. Each stage is determined by the age and school placement of the oldest child. Each family member is involved in meeting his or her own individual tasks as well as contributing to the developmental tasks of the family as a unit. The first two stages, married couples/beginning families and childbearing families, are discussed in more detail.

The developmental approach has been criticized because of its lack of attention to diverse family forms, such as the childless family, and for what is described as its middle-class bias (Friedman, 1986). Carter and McGoldrick (1989) for example, have developed a framework for studying families of varying forms. Dislocations of the family life cycle, such as divorce, require systematic changes in order for the family to proceed developmentally. However, the developmental framework can be useful for nurses and other health professionals because it allows the nurse to assess whether or not the developmental tasks are being accomplished and to anticipate change as the nuclear family progresses through the life cycle (Bradshaw 1988).

Married Couple Stage

The first stage of Duvall's developmental family life cycle is the married couple/beginning family stage, which starts when the couple enters marriage and ends with the birth or adoption of the first child.

The primary family tasks of the married couple/beginning family are establishing a mutually satisfying marriage relationship, forming a new household, and deciding whether to become parents. For the remarried, an additional critical task is acceptance of the termination of the previous marriage in order to establish a healthy conjugal relationship with a new mate. In meeting the developmental tasks, the newly formed couple must learn to live with and compromise with each other and to relate to each other's kin. Methods for resolving conflicts, as well as communication patterns and support of one another, must be developed. If the methods for resolving conflict and communication patterns are healthy, the couple is more likely to achieve a satisfactory marital relationship.

A couple may experience difficulty in sexual adjustment because of inaccurate or incomplete information resulting in unrealistic expectations of each other. The degree of sexual experience, particularly the amount of factual knowledge the partners bring to the marriage, affects their adaptation to the relationship. If a couple brings their own unresolved needs and desires into the relationship, it can have an adverse effect on the sexual relationship (Goldenberg & Goldenberg 1985). Marriage partners who recognize each other's varying needs and expectations are able to cooperate to achieve a mutually fulfilling sexual relationship.

One of the primary roles of the nurse working with families in this stage is that of health educator. The nurse can provide accurate information about family planning, pregnancy, sexuality concerns, role changes, and functional communication methods.

Couples who remain childless because of infertility will need support and education regarding their options. Infertility is often viewed as a crisis, and the nurse needs to be aware that the couple's relationship may be affected. The nurse can assist the couple by allowing them to verbalize their frustrations and concerns. The nurse can also provide the couple with information about various options, such as surgical or pharmacologic therapies. If these interventions are not successful, the nurse can discuss other options, such as in vitro fertilization, artificial insemination, and adoption, with the couple. Couples who choose to remain childless need to be supported in their decision. These couples must still work through the developmental tasks of establishing themselves as a unit.

Beginning Family Stage

In the latter part of the first stage in the family life cycle, a couple's expectations of having their own child may be fulfilled. This marks the beginning family stage. Although this stage may cover the shortest time span in the cycle, this period is filled with many intense and diverse feelings. When the couple is told that conception has occurred, they may either accept or reject the pregnancy. Some pregnancies are unplanned, although either partner may subconsciously desire pregnancy. Others are planned and may even have been anticipated for months or years before conception actually takes place.

After their initial reactions to the fact that the wife is pregnant, the couple must accomplish certain tasks that are an offshoot of those from the earlier part of the married couple phase. For example, arrangements must be made for the physical care of the baby. These arrangements may mean drastic changes for the family if they have to move into larger quarters or to a place where children are accepted.

In the beginning family period, the couple must make adjustments in *patterns of earning and spending*. Generally, the man is in the early phase of his career, and his salary may be low. The woman's salary, which may be a necessary part of the family income, may come to an end during the pregnancy. Many mothers choose to return to work after the baby is born, requiring that child care costs be added to the budget. Health care during the pregnancy and birth also requires large amounts of money, especially with rising medical costs.

Work loads and designation of authority in the household also change out of necessity during pregnancy. The man may assume more of the heavy household chores, as it is difficult for the woman to bend and move about. At the same time, pregnant women do not find that their physical state prohibits them from pursuing many of the activities they enjoy, such as working, entertaining, or even participating in sports.

Sexual activities must also be altered to accommodate the physical and emotional changes of pregnancy. The pregnancy may have positive, negative, or no effects on the couple's sexual relationship. Husbands are as likely to feel changes in their sexual responses as their wives are. Because of changes in breast and abdominal size, the couple will need to alter their normal sexual activities.

As soon as the couple knows they are expecting a child, a new focus of interaction becomes evident, enlarging their need for and use of communication. Most couples feel a sense of fulfillment as they feel pride in their ability to conceive a child, as the wife begins to show signs of pregnancy, and as they make plans for the child's arrival. Husband and wife undergo changes in self-concepts in terms of masculinity, femininity, and parenthood. All of these tasks are accomplished with greater ease if the husband and wife develop communication patterns that help them cope with new responsibilities.

Communication with significant others also takes on a new perspective. Relatives and close friends may have a prominent role in helping the young couple with their baby after birth; they can give physical and emotional support to the wife as she undertakes the new tasks of child care. On the other hand, significant others can interfere with the couple's adjustment to pregnancy and childbirth by telling "old wives' tales" and frightening myths. Reorienting relatives and friends to the kind of relationship that is most desirable for new parents and their child is a major task of the beginning expectant family.

Reorientation must also occur in *relationships with friends and in community activities*. Recreational and social activities can continue to be a major part of the couple's life, curtailed only to the extent that the pregnancy decreases the woman's ability to participate. The mother-to-be may be more sensitive about her partner's ability to continue his activities because his mobility is not affected. She may believe that he is seeking outside inter-

Research Note

Clinical Application of Research

Janice Rustia and Douglas Abbott (1990) examined the expected behaviors of first-time fathers through role theory concepts. This 2-year longitudinal study explored four aspects of perceived paternal behaviors. The four aspects encompassed what the father considered to be appropriate behavior, personally expected behaviors, prior knowledge about parenting, and what behaviors the mother expected. A standardized interview, used for data collection, addressed the perceptions of appropriate paternal behaviors, behaviors the father would do, and the actual behaviors performed by the father. Paternal behaviors included physical or socioemotional activities of caretaking such as bathing, dressing, and playing with the infant. Fathers answered questions about paternal modeling from their childhood as well as interest or participation in parent education.

The fathers' scores for expected behavior and performed behavior were similar but changed over time, increasing in areas such as playing with or cuddling the infant. Fathers did less than what they had expected they would do, but both scores, actual and expected, increased over time. What the father actually did and what the mother expected of the father changed over time but not exactly in the same way.

Critical Thinking Applied to Research

Strengths: Longitudinal study over two years, well-constructed conceptual framework, clear operational definitions of predictors of paternal role behavior, discussion section which placed this study within the context of other associated research.

Concerns: Lack of clarity about the number of couples used for data analysis, minimal reporting of validity and reliability for the instruments used, and when ANOVA results have both significant interaction effects as well as significant main effects, the results are difficult to interpret.

Rustia J, Abbott D: Predicting paternal role enactment. *West J Nurs Res* 1990; 12(2): 145.

ests as she becomes more introspective about the birth of the child. The man may feel left out of many of the woman's activities as she visits the physician and attends groups to discuss the care and rearing of children. Planning joint activities while continuing to respect each other's needs for autonomy can help the couple make a comfortable transition to the complementary relationship that will be needed in future years.

An expectant couple is open to and eager for knowledge about pregnancy, labor and delivery, and child care. Their background knowledge may be based more on hearsay than fact. They may have had little or no experience with infants and small children.

The couple must also resolve their questions about whether they are prepared to bring a child into their lives, how the baby will fit into their lives, and how they will alter their pattern of living for their child. As mentioned earlier, both partners feel emotions that are new to them and seek understanding from each other. The more one partner is able to meet the other's emotional needs, the more love each will be able to give to their child.

Childbearing Family Stage

The arrival of the first child marks a time of both crisis and great joy for the young family. Again the family faces a period of reorganization. Duvall explains that during the *childbearing family stage* (from the birth of the first child until that child is 30 months old), the baby and family become stabilized in their schedules and relationships with each other. The parents feel great joy about the birth of their first child and share their joy with their family and friends; the new mother feels a sense of accomplishment and is ready to relax and let others care for her and her baby for a few days. At the same time, the young couple has a feeling of great responsibility for their child's growth and development.

The first task of the childbearing family is *to arrange the home to meet the needs of the newborn infant.* The primary responsibility of the parents is to provide a safe, comfortable environment for the infant. A primary need of the newborn is a quiet, clean place to sleep. As children grow and become more mobile, their immediate environment enlarges even though they are still unable to protect themselves from many of its dangers.

Costs of raising a child are drastically increasing, creating additional problems for a couple already dealing with the increased costs of daily living. Even in the United States, where prosperity is relatively common, many families are below poverty level and children are raised with a minimum of economic expenditure.

The birth of the first child requires a *reworking of responsibility and accountability patterns.* A baby requires round-the-clock care, much of which is assumed by the mother, particularly if she is breast-feeding the child. The father may assume more of the household tasks, such as shopping and running errands outside the home. The partners share in seeking solutions to problems that arise during the day. The child also has accountability to parents as he or she grows older. The approval or disapproval of parents teaches him or her what parents consider good and bad, and he or she recognizes good acts as pleasing ones.

Reestablishing a satisfying sexual relationship with one's partner is another task of the childbearing family stage. Sexual activity usually decreases or ceases during the postnatal period. The new mother becomes absorbed in her child, and her close physical relationship with the baby may decrease her sexual needs. The responsibilities of caring for a newborn may leave her physically exhausted. Her partner may feel rejected as the new mother focuses on the baby's needs instead of his. Much mutual patience and understanding is necessary as the couple strives to reunite to meet each other's needs.

Two stresses occur in the childbearing family period that can hinder or further the *development of effective communication:* the newborn's crying and the decreased sharing between the parents. Crying, the newborn's only means of communication, can be extremely disconcerting until the new parents are able to interpret what the various types of cries mean and until they learn to anticipate their infant's needs. When the parents believe they have met the needs of their child and the crying continues for no apparent reason, their frustration increases. However, as the parents attempt to meet the baby's needs lovingly, the baby's trust in them increases, and other methods of communication emerge such as smiling, cooing, and eventually talking.

The other strain on effective communication is decreased sharing between the parents. Their tasks may be more separately defined as the father works outside the home while the mother remains busy caring for their new baby and the house. They participate in different activities and have less time to be alone together. Instead of the one relationship of the couple, three relationships have developed to include the infant in the family circle. If the new mother returns to work soon after the baby is born, both parents may experience additional strain. However, even though the parents may have distinct tasks, they can share more as they watch their baby grow.

Relationships with relatives are also a facet of the development of the childbearing family. The new parents will receive much advice on how to care for the child. If they are mature and have successfully completed their previous developmental tasks, they are able to sift through this information and use what is most meaningful to them. The greater the difference between the two parental families, the greater the likelihood of conflicting advice, because each set of grandparents will want the child to be raised according to the traditions of their family. And, of course, the parental families can also supply a great deal of support and comfort to the new parents, who are trying to establish their own traditions.

The young family must participate in *community activities to establish relationships outside the home.* They are more involved in their home life than they were before their baby's birth and must find suitable babysitting arrangements if they desire to go out together. Their interests may change as they seek out congenial couples with young children who can share similar experiences.

A further responsibility of the childbearing family is to *decide whether or when to have more children* and to take appropriate measures. Having children in quick succession may prove to be a tremendous strain for both parents, although some couples prefer to have their children close together. If the first child has a defect or dies shortly after birth, the decision about whether or when to have another child becomes paramount.

Maintenance of motivation and morale in the childbearing family may become difficult. The repetitive tasks of everyday child care may overshadow the basic satisfactions of parenthood. Values placed on material objects may need to be changed, becoming dependent on what is good for the young child. The parents need to continue their independence as a couple while recognizing the child's dependence on them. The developmental needs of the child and those of the parents may be in conflict, so priorities must be set. The young family may need to accept assistance from relatives and friends at a time when they are still striving to be a separate unit.

The early childbearing and childrearing years have a significant influence on the ultimate strength of the family unit. Many crises occur that can either divide or unite the family. A division or conflict may not be evident while the children are still dependent but may manifest itself after the children have left home and there is little else to hold the parents together. Yet these same stresses can unite the family more solidly if they are faced as mutual problems and if individual needs and priorities are taken into account in family interrelationships.

The nurse can assist the family during this phase of family development by providing health teaching related to family planning, infant care, child development, and safety. The nurse can also give the couple support as they adjust to the physical and emotional demands of being parents. If other children are born during this phase, the nurse can assist the couple with problems related to sibling rivalry and time management. Drastic role changes accompany parenthood, and often the couple has little preparation. The nurse assists the family to communicate in an open manner about the various role changes that are occurring. Since wellness behaviors are learned at an early age, the nurse should provide the family with information related to stress management, nutrition, dental care, immunizations, exercise, and healthy life-style practices.

Factors Affecting Family Structures and Functions

Regardless of its structure, the family does not function in isolation. The well-being of a family can be promoted or hindered by the acts or policies of other persons or institutions. Characteristics such as race and ethnicity or a less common family configuration may affect the family's social status, income level, and community acceptance. Religion often has a strong influence on the values, beliefs, and moral concepts of the family. Many religions also dictate behavioral codes, rituals, traditions of family life, and childrearing practices.

The implications of these and other factors differ for each family. Members within each family can also be af-

fected to varying degrees. The following sections explore the concepts of and factors affecting family life-style.

Family Life-Style

Families are characterized by diversity. As mentioned earlier, families come in widely varying sizes and behave in widely varying ways. While every family is unique, certain factors, such as socioeconomic status, race, and ethnicity, can have an important impact on the family's life-style. Levin and Idler (1981) describe life-style as "this webbing material of values, beliefs, expectations, criteria of choice, problem solving, communication, and commitment that is unique to the family" (p 68).

Traditionally, a family's socioeconomic status was determined by certain characteristics of the husband-father, including his occupation, education, and income. A more recent trend has been to include information from both parents in determining the family's socioeconomic status. (See Chapter 6 for discussion of the socioeconomic problems faced by single-parent families headed by women.) Social scientists consider education and occupational position to be the two main components of social class. Income is also a factor but is of less importance.

Family life across social classes has been shown to vary with regard to both structural and functional characteristics. There is an inverse relationship between social class and family size: The more affluent the family, the smaller it is. Differences have been noted as well in communication style and childrearing practices in families of differing social classes.

Kohn's (1979) conclusion speaks to the importance of discerning the values on which parents' interactions with their children are based. It is important for health care professionals to learn how families and their individual members subjectively define their situations in order to understand the dynamics of family life.

Ethnic identity also influences family life. Ross and Cobb (1990) define ethnic identity as the way that an individual or family perceives themselves in relation to the larger society. Ethnic groups subdivided into early ethnic minorities (such as Irish and German), recent and continuing ethnic minorities (such as Vietnamese and Cuban), historically subjugated ethnic minorities (such as black and native American), and socioreligious ethnic minorities (such as Mormon and Greek Orthodox). Structural and functional differences have often been associated with families of varying ethnic backgrounds. Members of a specific ethnic group share a distinct linguistic, social, and cultural background.

Nurse anthropologists and ethnographers such as Tripp-Reimer (1983), and Leininger (1985) have provided valuable insights into the family life and health care beliefs and practices of various ethnic groups. Speaking to the importance of understanding ethnomedical practices, Tripp-Reimer (1983) said: "While it is crucial to be sensitive to cultural beliefs and practices, it is just as essential not to overgeneralize and assume that all members of the sub-culture hold to a particular belief or practice" (p 101). In a similar vein, Levin and Idler (1981) stressed the need for health care professionals to recognize the health care functions of the family in general.

> Many indigenous practices have emerged from historical test and may depend for their effectiveness on an integrated, interacting set of values and beliefs. It may well be that their effective power lies in the family's commitment to them and their symbolic contribution to family identity (p 66).

It is virtually impossible to describe in a meaningful way the socioeconomic and ethnic variations that exist in American families. However, such differences do exist. It is reasonable to expect that the young, professional couple will have a different way of being a family than their working- or lower-class counterparts. Likewise, it is reasonable to expect a recent Cuban immigrant to differ in her ideas about parenting from a third-generation Mormon from Salt Lake City. However, there is an important difference between "reasonable expectations" and stereotyping. On the one hand, professionals want to be sensitive to clients' diverse needs and expectations; on the other hand, they don't want to attribute needs or expectations based on preconceived notions of what families in a given socioeconomic or ethnic group membership are like. In keeping with those words of caution, the reader is directed to the Additional Readings section at the end of this chapter for sources of information on different family types.

Societal Trends

Status of Women
The traditional role for a woman in our society gave her dominance in the home. Her role had value for the family but did not have prestige in the greater society. The lack of prestige made it a safe role for women, one in which their men would not intervene. Thus the home became the stronghold for women.

Similarly, the man has traditionally been considered the head of the household, and the status and life-style of those within the home have depended to a large extent on him. But now more women are becoming part of the work force to supplement family income, to satisfy chosen career goals, or to work voluntarily in charitable organizations. As women move out into the working world, in addition to contributing income so that their families can enjoy a higher standard of living, they are gaining more status for themselves within their families and in the community.

In recent years, women have moved into the labor force in increasing numbers. It is estimated that by 1990 only 14% of American families now fit into the traditionally prescribed roles of father-breadwinner and mother-housewife ("On the Home Front" 1986). As women move into the work force, three areas of family life are likely to be

influenced: division of labor within the home, marital adjustment, and parenting. For a more detailed discussion of women and societal issues, see Chapter 6.

It is difficult to determine how the wife's employment affects marital satisfaction. Of the many variables likely to influence the relationship, two of the most important are the family's financial situation and each partner's values or beliefs regarding the woman's participation in the labor force. Dissatisfaction is most likely when partners hold conflicting beliefs in this area.

Value of Children
The value of children varies greatly, depending on the meaning each society attaches to children. In addition, the reaction of individual family members to a child is personalized and subjective (Figure 3–2). Historically, the motivations for having children have been religious, political, and cultural. Some individuals want children for their own gratification—to have someone to guide and control, to reap economic gains, to improve one's status, to ensure one is cared for in old age, to satisfy cultural requirements, or to provide a means of personal immortality.

Many historical changes have influenced the importance of children in society. In agrarian societies, children are valued for the economic gain they bring to their family and society. Industrialization and urbanization in North America have reduced the economic necessity of having

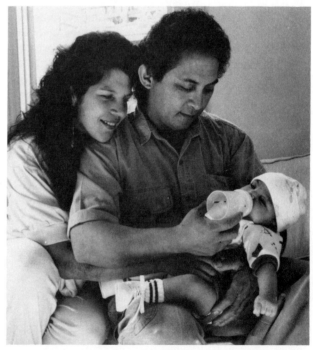

Figure 3–2 The value of a child to a family is personalized and depends on socioeconomic, religious, and cultural factors (From Mott SR, James SR, Sperhac AM: Nursing Care of Children and Families, *2nd ed. Menlo Park, CA: Addison-Wesley, 1990, p 475.)*

children. As a result, children have become less "valuable" and more valued.

Environmental Factors

Environmental factors influencing the family are closely interrelated with the cultural and socioeconomic factors discussed previously. The environment includes outside forces that may alter the behaviors and activities of family members and the family group. Forces such as relatives, friends, and significant others; home, neighborhood, and community settings; and social, religious, and governmental institutions within the community all influence the family.

In childbearing families, environmental factors are most significant in terms of their effects on parents. Parents, based on their experience and background, interpret the meaning of the interaction between environmental forces and the family for their children. If their explanations are positive, they transmit to their children feelings of security, stability, and well-being. However, if the parents feel negative toward or threatened by their surroundings, they may transmit feelings of danger, hostility, and anger. The way that the family interacts with its environment is likely to have a direct effect on the family's ability to meet members' needs, individually and collectively.

The physical setting in which the family lives also affects family functioning. Poor housing may adversely influence family and member attitudes, behaviors, motivational levels, and self-esteem, which in turn increases stress and the risk of illness and accidents. The overcrowding of a home may interfere with privacy and result in inadequate childrearing and housekeeping practices. Chaotic, disorganized homes may produce children with developmental delays or deviancies, which may be permanent. If family functioning continues to be impaired as the child's environment expands to settings outside the home, problems may become evident in the child's ability to communicate, solve problems, and form relationships.

Within the neighborhood and community, families tend to associate freely with community groups and other institutions to identify resources and receive services as needed. The family's ability to seek help through contact with others appears related in part to the family's perception of itself as a part of a whole and to its successful dealings with the larger community in meeting physical, psychologic, and social requirements.

Nursing Implications

There are no simple "recipes" for working with families. Theories and research provide a basis for understanding families and suggest important areas of concern, typical patterns of behavior, and the range of variation surrounding the typical. Theories and research, however, do not prescribe what the nurse should do in a given situation. These decisions emanate from thoughtful interactions with family members in which the nurse interprets the family's definition of the situation in light of his or her own knowledge.

A major goal of family-centered maternity care is to help each member of an expectant family achieve optimal health by preventive, maintenance, and restorative measures. Nurses have the additional role of assisting families to accomplish appropriate developmental tasks at each family stage.

The success of the family depends on the achievement of these tasks. At times the family may find that success comes easily; at other times, they must overcome delay or failure. Since failure tends to follow failure just as success follows success, the nurse may need to intervene to break a family's cycle of failures in performing tasks and to guide them toward success.

When giving care to a client, the nurse should keep in mind the long-term, intimate relationships among family members. The person receiving care has performed a unique role within the family group that must be acknowledged if the family is to function optimally. Thus families have the right to examine the kind of care and service a family member is receiving, to complain when the service is unsatisfactory, and to seek other sources of services when they are dissatisfied.

To ensure the provision of appropriate individualized care, the maternity nurse uses the nursing process as the framework for planning and implementing responsible health care.

The Family as Client

Because the individual develops as a member of a family unit, the nurse must understand the family to understand the individual. This is especially important in the maternity setting because the nurse is directly responsible for the well-being of two members of the same family—mother and child.

The concept of the family as a client is one of the most important components of family-centered maternity nursing. Ideally, the family gives each member love and trust and responds consistently so that he or she may mature into an individual who is able to give these qualities to others.

Friedman (1986) identifies the family unit as being the critical resource for the delivery and success of health care services for the following reasons:

1. In a family unit a dysfunction of one or more family members generally affects each individual as well as the family unit. If the nurse considers only the individual, the nursing assessment is fragmented rather than complete and holistic.

2. Assessing the family helps the nurse understand the individual functioning within his or her primary social context. With the expectant and childbear-

ing family, the nurse is able to assist the prospective parents to prepare for the new family member.

3. A strong interrelationship exists between the health status of a family as a unit and that of the individuals who constitute the family. By emphasizing health promotion and maintenance in the family, the nurse should have a positive effect not only on the individuals in the family but also on the family unit.

4. In considering the family as a whole, the nurse identifies potential risk factors, thereby facilitating the nurse's role in illness prevention.

5. When illness occurs, the family is instrumental in seeking health care and in determining members' sick-role behaviors.

In family-centered maternity nursing, the nurse generally focuses on health promotion and maintenance and prevention of illness, primarily with the beginning or childbearing family. To interact effectively with the wide variety of families she or he is likely to encounter, the nurse needs to do the following:

● Reevaluate personal cultural beliefs and values.

● Recognize personal biases and beliefs about a particular culture (stereotyping).

● Assess the individual/family carefully and openly, without judgment.

● Avoid generalizations and assumptions based on personal ideas and knowledge about a particular culture. There is diversity *within* every culture.

In view of these suggestions, it is a good idea for the nurse to confirm any assumptions regarding the particular culture or group by speaking tactfully with the individual or family. The nurse's goal is to provide excellent care based on a complete biopsychological assessment that includes a cultural component.

Through the assessment process discussed in the next section, the nurse identifies risk factors that may lead to health problems. Planning with the family determines health goals that may require the involvement of other health team members. Assessment, intervention, and evaluation should be viewed as negotiative, interactive processes. Nurses and family members each bring unique knowledge and skills to a given health care situation. Ideally, they work together to achieve goals that are mutually acceptable.

❀ *APPLYING THE NURSING PROCESS* ❀

Family Assessment

Assessment of the beginning or childbearing family's status is the first step in determining the family's level of functioning. Data may be gathered in a variety of settings, including the home, clinic, and hospital. When assessing the family of a maternity client, the nurse should be comprehensive but focused on areas of particular relevance to the family. In-

depth data collection is necessary in those areas that pose a problem for the family or are of concern to the nurse.

To collect valid, pertinent data, the nurse must establish a positive relationship with the client, a family member, and/or the family group. The use of empathy, positive regard, and active listening enables the nurse to gather complete, yet selective, information about the family. The nurse should obtain the following:

● Basic identifying information, including the names, ages, gender, and relationships of all family members

● Religious and cultural associations

● Type of family configuration

● Data about the members of the extended family who are closest to the nuclear family, especially if they reside nearby and form a strong support group for each other

● Individual and family perception of family functioning: communication patterns, division of labor

Health History

The nurse records a health history of the entire family since family health problems have potential effects on children. The nurse gathers information about the extended and nuclear family regarding past acute and chronic illnesses, congenital defects, mental health, obesity, or the occurrence of accidents. A family pedigree may be helpful in summarizing this information visually (see Chapter 5 on genetic counseling). With the beginning expectant family or the childbearing family, data about all pregnancies become significant. Knowledge of experiences of family members with health care delivery systems or hospitalization helps in deciding which approach to the family will be most helpful.

The nurse also needs to obtain data about the current health status of each family member. With the beginning and childbearing family, the nurse assesses the family's strengths and limitations in promoting and maintaining health by learning about the family's definitions of health and illness, their nutritional status, attitudes toward medicine use (prescription and nonprescription), recreational and exercise activities, exposure to environmental hazards, and sleep and rest practices. When a client is pregnant, prenatal assessment is essential (see Chapter 13). Other important information includes data on each family member's allergies, health problems requiring prescription medications, environmentally and genetically related illnesses, the family's knowledge about these disorders, and treatments that have been recommended and implemented.

Health Practices

Assessing the competency of the family to promote and maintain health, care for ill members, and carry out health care instructions is vital in determining the nurse's interaction with the family. Many families use preventive health measures such as obtaining routine medical, dental, hearing, and ophthalmic examinations and immunizations and participating in other screening programs. If the family does not use such preventive measures, the nurse needs to assess the family's knowledge about or access to such measures. The nurse may find it necessary to identify health care facilities that are accessible to the family and to discuss how they are used.

Home Environment

A valid assessment of the family may require several home visits. Some families feel that a home visit by a nurse is an invasion of privacy but most become more amenable as rapport is established. When assessing the characteristics of a home, the nurse must make objective observations; personal standards and values should not be allowed to distort evaluation of the living conditions. Living space that provides all family members with privacy and comfortable sleeping arrangements and permits each person to pursue interests and needs is important. If a new baby is expected, preparation for arrival should be evident. Adequate heat, light, cooking facilities, water, storage facilities, and hygienic equipment are necessary for maintaining the well-being of all family members. Toys, books, and other recreational and educational equipment should be available for any children in the home. Play areas should be away from safety hazards and should be adequately supervised. The distance of the home from health care facilities and the availability of transportation to them should also be investigated.

Appraisal of the home environment gives only some indication of the economic status of the family. Knowledge about the sources and amounts of family income and about the work skills of individual members aids in assessing health behavior and needs. Information about the allocation of income to shelter, clothing, food, savings, insurance, education, recreation, and health care reveals the family's economic priorities and its ability to meet the needs of all family members.

The home assessment may also include observations of the population characteristics and resources of the neighborhood and the larger community in which the family lives, taking into account the family's associations and transactions within the community. How parents view their interaction with their neighborhood and community is significant because their children tend to relate in a similar fashion. Certain health problems can also have broad effects within a community. For example, diseases can be transmitted by children to other children in schools and from them to the rest of the family. After identifying such situations, a nurse can make recommendations to help families cope with such problems.

Assessment Tools

In addition to the sources of information just described, several tools for objective data collection can be used to measure various aspects of family functioning. Some assessment tools concentrate on mother-infant interactions and needs for teaching and support. The Maternal Attachment Assessment Strategy provides a system of observing maternal-child behavior and establishing a profile of the mother's attachment behaviors (Avant 1982). The Mother-Infant Play Interaction Scale (MIPIS) is another tool that measures response reciprocity between mother and infant during unstructured play (Walker 1982).

The Feetman Family Functioning Scale (Roberts & Feetman 1982) assesses parents' views of relationships among family members and between the family and other social systems. It is a systematic method of assessing family functioning under stress. By identifying specific stressors, the maternal-newborn nurse can proceed to identify sources of support that will help diminish the stress. The Family APGAR test (Smilkstein 1984) assesses family functioning in the areas of adaptability, partnership, growth, affection, and resolve. The Family Environment Scale (Moos & Moos 1976) measures three components of family life: relationships, personal growth, and family system maintenance. The tool provides data that help the nurse compare parent and child perceptions and actual and preferred family environment and to assess and facilitate change. The Family Assessment Device (FAD) is a self-reporting measure that identifies family strengths and limitations so that the nurse can reinforce family strengths or correct limitations (Epstein et al 1983).

Speer and Sachs (1985) provide an excellent overview and evaluation of nine family assessment tools. Their evaluation is based on the following criteria: understandable, easily administered and scored, reliable and valid, appropriate for all types of families, and clinically relevant. Such tools can facilitate the nurse's assessment of the family.

Analysis and Nursing Diagnosis

After completing the assessment of the family, the nurse analyzes the data to formulate nursing diagnoses. Goals based on each nursing diagnosis are then established for the family. These are divided into short- and long-range goals and should be a joint enterprise between the family and the nurse. Without this cooperative interaction, the goals may not meet the needs that the family believes are important, may not be realistic for the family, or may not be accepted by the family as its responsibility.

The priority of these goals must then be determined. This is a highly individualized process; input from the family continues to have great importance. A severe illness, an unplanned child, and lack of funds for a needed purchase can all be crucial matters. The family may consider obtaining funds to be the most pressing goal, whereas the nurse may believe that accepting the child should receive immediate attention, and the physician may think that the treatment of the illness should be given top priority. Factors that affect priorities include the family's perceptions of its needs, the number of problems that require attention, the feasibility of goals set, the readiness of the family to meet the goals, and the amount of preparation or education necessary before the goals can be met. Working with the family, the nurse must validate the goals and their importance to gain the family's support in achieving them.

Planning

Planning interventions is the next step in the nursing process. The nursing care plan must be based on the goals set in consultation with the family. There are generally many approaches to every problem, and the nurse needs to identify the one that seems most likely to work in the family's particular framework of attitudes, beliefs, and values. Family participation in planning can be valuable, because the family knows about its ability to deal with the situation. Therefore, the nursing plan must be accepted by the family prior to putting it into action.

During the planning stage, decisions must be made about those health care workers, other professionals, and community agencies that will be of greatest value to the family. The nurse can explain the services available from these agencies. The family's needs may be best satisfied by several agencies, which will require interagency cooperation and coordination of efforts. The nurse may serve as the coordinator of these activities, assuring continuity of services to the family. One long-range goal for the family should be to strengthen its knowledge of community resources to meet its own health needs.

Implementation

In implementing a care plan, the nurse must constantly keep in mind the short- and long-range goals that have been set for the family. Therapeutic interaction continues to be of primary importance. Changes in family needs often produce stress on some or all members. The recommendations and teaching of the nurse or other professionals may cause more stress, as any change always causes some tension and anxiety. Family members may feel guilty about having certain needs and may be concerned about how these needs will be accepted by others. Any serious difficulties have probably already disrupted the family, and its members may have had to take on roles and responsibilities with which they are unfamiliar.

The nurse needs to be aware not only of the family's changing situation but also of its members' changing views regarding their situation. In this sense, assessment is ongoing and cuts across the intervention and assessment stages of the nursing process. Further resources may be needed to help the family cope in dealing with any problems.

When working with beginning and childbearing families, the nurse assumes many roles, including teacher, counselor, coordinator, researcher, and advocate. In these roles, the nurse is careful to communicate in a manner that is understandable and meaningful to the family. Knowledge of the family's developmental level, internal processes, socio-

economic status, and cultural background helps in determining the most effective approach to use. A collaborative effort is necessary for learning to occur: The nurse assists the family to define change strategies, and the family decides how to apply the learning primarily through their own resources. In some circumstances the nurse supports the family's position or initiates plans to foster further development, thus ensuring continued learning.

The nurse acts primarily as a teacher, counselor, and advocate in helping a couple determine their family-planning needs. The nurse offers information in a manner that the family can understand and use, demonstrating understanding and respect for needs and belief systems. Some families hesitate to use family-planning techniques because of fears or dislike of, or misunderstanding about, contraception; because of worries that they cannot afford family planning; or because of beliefs that others are trying to limit the size of their ethnic group.

The nurse's responsibilities to the beginning expectant family include preparing the couple for the woman's physical and emotional condition and needs, and planning for the man's desires for involvement. Teaching expectant couples about pregnancy, labor, and birth and counseling them about child care and the parental role are important nursing responsibilities.

After the child is born, a primary concern of the nurse is to make sure that the family can meet the needs of the newborn infant. The nurse assumes the roles of teacher and counselor when discussing the needs of the infant and demonstrating infant care to the parents. In addition, the nurse acts as the family advocate by giving emotional support to new parents and by providing guidance on effective use of health care professionals.

Evaluation

To interpret the success or failure of the nursing care plan, the nurse takes into account the goals set for the family and the effects produced. Again, the family should play an important part in this evaluation, as it has in other steps of the nursing process. Members need to be encouraged to respond freely and openly.

If a goal has been fully achieved, the nursing interventions have been successful. If a goal has not been attained, the nurse should explore the reasons for the failure and devise a new plan that might meet with greater success. If a goal has been partially achieved, the nurse and family determine whether the plan is realistic and simply needs more time or whether modifications are necessary. The nurse may find that changes in the family necessitate adjustments and adaptations in the nursing care plan at any point during its implementation. Even when all goals appear to have been attained, periodic reevaluation and encouragement are necessary for the family to continue to function at the best level.

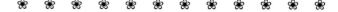

Application of the Nursing Process: A Case Example

The following example illustrates the integration of theory and research in an application of the nursing process.

Situation

Mr and Mrs Hunter, both in their early thirties, have been married for seven years. They have a three-year-old son, Brian, and Mrs Hunter is in her second trimester of pregnancy. In the 12 months preceding the pregnancy, she experienced two spontaneous abortions, both during the first eight weeks of pregnancy. Mr Hunter is a mechanic for a local car dealer, and Mrs Hunter works three mornings a week as a receptionist in a real estate office. Her work schedule coincides with Brian's nursery school schedule. Since becoming pregnant, Mrs Hunter has been seen by a nurse-midwife at the HMO to which the family belongs. She and Mr Hunter plan to attend the HMO's childbirth and parenting classes during her last trimester. Mrs Hunter is in excellent physical health and has had a problem-free pregnancy. Nonetheless, during her last checkup with the nurse-midwife, she indicated two major areas of concern: (1) pressure from her husband and close relatives to quit her job and (2) negative comments from Brian about having a new family member. Mrs Hunter reported that she and her husband had had several "blowups" over her desire to continue working. In addition, both Mr and Mrs Hunter felt Brian should share their excitement about the new baby and were concerned about his "bad" behavior whenever they encouraged him to show enthusiasm about the baby.

❧ *APPLYING THE NURSING PROCESS* ❧

Nursing Assessment

Working from an interactionist perspective, the nurse-midwife decided to elicit more detailed information from family members regarding their "definition of the situation." She suggested that Mrs Hunter schedule an appointment in the next two weeks for her and Mr Hunter to talk to the nurse-midwife about "plans for the new baby." During this family session, the nurse-midwife learned that Mr and Mrs Hunter viewed Mrs Hunter's working quite differently. For Mrs Hunter, work was a social outlet and source of income. She said she had always worked and felt proud to contribute to the family income even though it wasn't absolutely necessary. She hoped to move back into full-time employment as her children got older. Moreover Mrs Hunter identified physical benefits because she walked the half mile to and from work every day. Mrs Hunter resented her husband's efforts to "control her life" and noted that this was an aspect of his personality she had not experienced before.

In contrast Mr Hunter cited his wife's two previous spontaneous abortions as evidence that she should "take care of herself." He felt he had a responsibility to both his wife and the unborn child to make sure his wife took care of herself. He was confused by his wife's anger about what he saw as "good intentions."

With regard to Brian's behavior, Mr and Mrs Hunter feared that his negative outbursts probably were a prelude to even worse behavior after the baby was born. They described how they had intensified their efforts to convince Brian that having a new baby in their home would be wonderful. They mentioned that Brian's grandfather liked to tease him about having to cook his own meals after the baby was born since his mother would be too busy to prepare meals.

Analysis and Nursing Diagnosis

The nurse-midwife concluded that the Hunters did not have a shared definition of Mrs Hunter's work and that their views were the source of escalating conflict as the pregnancy progressed. While the couple had a shared view of their son's behavior, the nurse-midwife concluded that their definition of that situation and subsequent actions probably were contributing to Brian's negative feelings about the pregnancy.

Based on her interactions with the Hunters, the nurse-midwife identified two tentative nursing diagnoses:

- Ineffective family coping; related to increased family conflict over Mrs Hunter's desire to continue working outside the home
- Potential altered parenting of siblings related to inexperience with sibling responses to birth of a baby

Implementation

The nurse-midwife pointed out to Mr and Mrs Hunter that they viewed Mrs Hunter's job in quite different ways although both believed that they were doing what was best for both Mrs Hunter and the baby. The HMO had several family therapists on staff and the Hunters agreed with the nurse-midwife that it would be a good idea to get some help to resolve any conflicts between them prior to the baby's birth.

The nurse-midwife was knowledgeable in the area of child development and sibling behavior. Through teaching and discussion, she was able to begin to alter the Hunters' definition of Brian's behavior. She provided them with several articles on sibling relationships from popular magazines and assured them that Brian's behavior was quite normal even if it seemed "bad" to them. She suggested that they deemphasize talk about the baby around Brian and that they gently encourage Brian's grandfather to stop teasing him.

Evaluation

At a subsequent prenatal checkup, Mrs Hunter reported that she and her husband still disagreed about her working, but the therapist had helped them to appreciate each other's viewpoint. She indicated that they no longer had "big battles," only "minor skirmishes" over the issue. She also indicated that the therapist had been helpful in getting them to anticipate possible issues regarding Mrs Hunter's return to work.

Mrs Hunter said she and her husband had been skeptical about the advice regarding Brian but had been desperate enough to try anything. While still not overjoyed at the thought of a new brother or sister, Brian was described as considerably less negative than he had been. Mrs Hunter laughingly reported that he had volunteered to "lend" the baby some of his old stuffed toys.

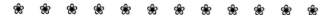

Family Life Cycle and Developmental Task: Potential for Dysfunction

In the ideal family, every family member is kind and considerate toward the others in the family. Everyone acts in loving ways toward each other. The parents respect, nurture, and support each other and each of their children. In times of crisis, the family members work together to resolve the difficulty. Everyone in the ideal family flourishes because his or her physical and emotional needs are met.

Although many families try, it is very difficult to be an ideal family. This is not an ideal world, and the stresses and worries of daily living can provoke even the best-intentioned person to behave toward others in less-than-loving ways. Moreover, families are made up of all kinds of people. Some of these individuals have physical and emotional problems that can impair their ability to interact with others in positive and adaptive ways.

A family, like a child, is born, develops, and matures. At each stage, families are faced with new developmental tasks requiring a reorganization of roles, communication patterns, and goals. Families are also affected by situational crises (such as illness, change or loss of income, or change in family composition), maturational crises of individual members, or changes in social and environmental conditions (such as economic inflation or a move to a new locale).

Understanding the goals, structure, roles, functions, and tasks of families and the changes inherent in periods of transition from one life stage to another can be useful to the nurse providing care to families in times of crisis. During times of stability, the nurse uses this knowledge base to anticipate the needs of families and their members. The nurse can help them identify ways to satisfactorily perform their roles and to adapt to role changes with minimal stress.

Nurses can also help families recognize their strengths and can support their developmental efforts as a growing healthy family unit. During times of family crisis, the nurse applies this knowledge base to help the family identify the strengths it can use to deal with the problem. Interventions include supporting family members and providing positive reinforcement for attempts to develop these strengths.

Beavers and Voeller (1983) developed a framework to study healthy families. In their studies, they identify a number of significant variables for an optimally functioning family. Healthy families were found to have the following characteristics:

- The ability to express feelings openly
- A strong parental coalition with a flexible structure within the family
- Members who perceived themselves as others did
- High levels of initiative
- An attitude of affiliation toward human encounters
- The ability to respect the views of others
- A high degree of personal autonomy within the family
- The ability to be humorous and hopeful

When the health or development of a family member—whether it be a parent or child—is threatened, the entire family system is at risk for abnormal development or dysfunction. Based upon this knowledge, the nurse needs to be alert to cues that signal a troubled or potentially troubled family so that dysfunction or disintegration of the family can be averted through prompt intervention (Figure 3–3).

Dysfunctional families are unable to carry out society's accepted family tasks, and they are unable to pro-

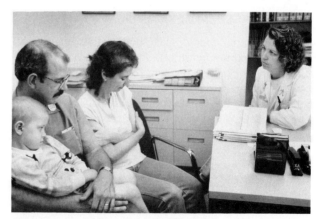

Figure 3–3   The nurse assesses parent-child interactions, including verbal and nonverbal cues, during discussion of family roles, expectations, and relationships (From Mott SR, James SR, Sperbac AM: Nursing Care of Children and Families, 2nd ed. Menlo Park, CA: Addison-Wesley, 1990, p 565.)

Table 3–2 Indicators of Families at Risk for Dysfunction

Family Structure

Single-parent family with inadequate supports
Blended family with inadequate supports
Adoptive family with inadequate supports
Teenage family
Young family with several children close in age
Single parent with changing live-in partner
Family with peripheral spouse—viewed by spouse as unreliable, incompetent, tyrannical
Parental separation

Family Environment

Impoverished family
Multiproblem family
Immature parents
Member(s) with handicapping, chronic, or fatal disease
Migrant or highly mobile family
Employment instability of key family members
Violence-prone family
Chemically dependent family member(s)
Chronic marital discord

vide for the physical or emotional needs of their members. Such families display behaviors that place all family members at risk, physically, emotionally, socially, and intellectually. Certain structural and environmental stressors have a high correlation with placing a family at risk to become dysfunctional. These stressors are listed in Table 3–2. Adult members of dysfunctional families are unable or unwilling to assume responsibility for their own actions.

Possibly the most serious result of unhealthy interpersonal interactions within a family is family violence—the threatened or actual use of physical force by one family member against another. In a violence-prone family, anyone can be the target: a spouse, a child, a grandparent. But in the end the entire family is the victim.

Family violence has serious immediate and long-term effects on all members of the family. The individual who is abused suffers mental and physical injury, possibly death. Children who witness violence often come to accept its use and often perpetuate it in their adult relationships. If the abuse comes to the attention of the legal system, the abuser may face charges of criminal assault and a jail sentence. In cases of child abuse, the children may be removed from their parents' care and placed in foster homes.

Family violence occurs in some form in more than half of the households in the United States (Mott et al 1990). It occurs in families of all races, religions, and socioeconomic and educational levels. The family may be loosely structured with unclear role differentiation, or it may be highly structured, with rigid, traditional, patriarchal roles. The adults in these families seldom share power or make decisions jointly or equally. Communication is poor, and partners often send hidden or double messages. Children may be overprotected and treated with extreme attention and love by one partner or neglected by both parents. Children

may become the parents' scapegoats and may be subjected to harsh discipline and abuse.

Types of Family Violence

The most common types of family violence are spouse abuse and child abuse. **Spouse abuse** is the physical and/or emotional battering of one partner, typically the woman, by the other. The exact incidence of wife abuse and battering in North America is unknown. Official statistics indicate that one out of ten women is abused by the man with whom she lives, but experts believe this figure underestimates the problem. The actual ratio may be closer to one in five. One study estimated that violence occurs in over one third of the marriages in the United States (O'Leary et al 1989).

Child abuse refers to physical, emotional, or sexual harm done to a child either by the child's parents or caretakers or by older siblings. As with spouse abuse, the exact incidence of child abuse is unknown. From 1980 to 1988, reporting of child abuse cases quadrupled, and the number is expected to increase (Mott et al 1990).

Historical Factors Contributing to Family Violence

Family violence is not new. Wife battering is as old as the institution of marriage. Child abuse, ranging from neglect to infanticide, has occurred in almost every society.

Throughout history, both wives and children were considered "property." A woman was the property of her husband; he had the "right"—even the duty—to "keep her in line," even to kill her. Outsiders "kept out of it"; battering was a family matter. Children were the property of their parents. Parents had the right to send their children to work in unsafe conditions, to transfer ownership to others as in child slavery or arranged marriages, even to dispose of them if they wished (Mott et al 1990). Severe disciplinary measures used by parents were acceptable and considered family business.

The legal status of women and children has improved over the years. Even so, in some states it is still legal to administer corporal punishment to children in school. And many people still hold on to the traditional views of male dominance in marriage, which can contribute to the occurrence of spouse abuse (Bohn 1990).

Spouse Abuse

Spouse abuse, particularly wife battering, is the most common form of violence in the United States but the least reported serious crime (Bullock et al 1989). The women's movement and heightened public sensitivity to violence against women have stimulated recognition of the extent of this problem.

Spouse abuse may take many forms including the following:

- Verbal attacks and insults
- Emotional deprivation and aggravation
- Social isolation and economic deprivation
- Intellectual derision and ridicule
- Sexual demands or deprivation
- Physical pain and injury

According to Walker (1979) and Helton and Snodgrass (1987), a battered woman is one who has suffered one or more episodes of battery from her male partner or ex-partners. Battery includes slapping, kicking, shoving, punching, forms of torture, and sexual assault. Women who are physically abused can also suffer psychologic and emotional abuse.

Wife abuse and battering occur in all ages, races, lifestyles, socioeconomic groups, educational levels, and occupations (Bullock et al 1989).

Studies found that battering is more prevalent among lower-income groups, urban families, blue-collar workers, minority racial groups, people who have not completed high school, families in which the husband is unemployed, families with more than three children, and individuals with no religious affiliation. It is likely that the problem of battering is simply better hidden among the middle- and higher-income groups, where women have access to private health care providers, psychiatrists, and attorneys.

Contributing Factors

Spouse abuse is a result of the complex and dynamic interaction of social, cultural, political, and psychologic factors. King and Ryan (1989) and Mahon (1981) identified these factors as follows:

- *Childhood experiences.* Children who witness or experience abuse and battering are more likely to become batterers (males) or to be abused (females) in their own marriages.
- *Sex role conditioning.* Traditionally females have been socialized to believe they are inferior, inadequate, and dependent on males for approval. Women are often expected to seek male approval by being nurturing and submissive. Males have traditionally been socialized to expect these behaviors of females and to expect to be financially successful, aggressive, and independent.
- *Economic insecurity of women.* Women typically receive less education and fewer job skills than men. Those with children are often financially dependent on their husbands because their own earning power is limited. When they leave the relationship, they frequently fall into poverty.

- *Fear of humiliation.* Family members, friends, and neighbors may think the woman brought abuse on herself or may not understand why she does not leave the batterer. These personal supports may desert the battered woman in fear of their own safety.
- *Ages of children.* Families with young children are subject to more stress and demands; mothers may be more dependent on their husbands for economic and emotional support for themselves and their children.
- *Institutional indifference.* Law enforcement personnel, social service agencies, and the judicial system often do not understand. They feel frustrated and impotent when battered women repeatedly return to their husbands.
- *Belief that violence among family members is a private matter.* Belief in the sacredness and privacy of the family has contributed to lack of intervention by legal, social, and medical agencies (King & Ryan 1989).
- *Malperception of inequity of power.* Men who perceive they lack power or resources in their homes or jobs may feel the need to prove themselves and resort to violence against those they perceive as less powerful to assert their superiority (King & Ryan 1989).
- *Religious traditions.* Most religions support the inferiority of women and believe that women should be dependent on their husbands. Laws and statutes based on these doctrines protect battering husbands from prosecution. Religion supports patriarchy, which is written into the laws and economic system to enforce the order of society.

Common Myths About Battering and Battered Women

Numerous myths about battering and battered women are believed by both professionals and the public. These myths often reinforce misunderstanding of battering and perpetuate the problem by keeping battered women silent. Myths range from the belief that the battered woman is a passive, innocent victim to the belief that she asked for and desires the beating. Professionals who provide services for battered women need to recognize and counteract these myths. Some commonly accepted myths are discussed here.

Battering occurs in a small percentage of the population. The statistics on reported cases underrepresent the true incidence. Battering is a seriously underreported crime: It generally occurs at night, in the home, and without witnesses. It is estimated that only one in ten women report battering assaults.

Battering is a lower-class problem. It is true that lower-class families have a higher incidence of reported battering and are more likely to have contact with community agencies concerning this problem, but wife abuse also occurs in middle- and upper-income families. Lower-class families have more unemployment and less education and may have a tradition of expressing anger physically rather than verbally. Middle- and upper-class women may hide their battering, and nurses may ignore or minimize abuse in these women (King & Ryan 1989).

Battered women provoke males to beat them; women push men beyond the breaking point and incite physical violence. Women are often socialized to feel responsible for the state of their relationship. Mahon (1981) observed that battered women blamed their husbands for their beatings and tried to distance themselves from them and others. These women had difficulty understanding that their silence and distancing maneuvers were part of the interplay that may have led to violent behavior; they tended to blame outside sources such as alcohol or their husband's unemployment. These blaming but aloof patterns of battered women can also contribute to violent scenes and continued battering.

It is important to recognize that people are individually responsible for their behavior: Batterers lose self-control because of their own internal inadequacies and not because of what the women did or did not do. To accept responsibility for another's actions or to place the blame entirely on another person negates each individual's responsibility in an interaction.

Alcohol and drug abuse cause battering. Studies do show a relationship between battering incidents and alcohol use by batterers. In many cases alcohol is viewed as the primary trigger precipitating the battering. However, alcohol use may be an underlying problem in the relationship. King & Ryan (1989) proposed that batterers use alcohol as an excuse to carry out a violent act and shift the blame from themselves to the alcohol. Others suggest that alcohol reduces the batterers' inhibitions, increasing the likelihood of violent acts. Battered women often blame the violence on the batterer's drunkenness and think that the abuse will stop if their husbands stop drinking. Unfortunately, this usually does not happen.

Battered women were battered children. This myth holds true in only a few cases; the majority did not grow up in violent homes (Bohn 1990). Most women report that their husbands were the first person to beat them. Many battered women, however, were exposed to sex-role stereotyping that reinforced their own belief in their inability to take care of themselves. Consequently, they assumed a dependent role with men.

Battered women can easily leave the situation. Leaving is easier said than done. Women assume they are responsible for their marriages and children; they may still love their husbands, rely on them for financial support, and feel their children need a father. Usually battered women have been psychologically abused and have come to believe that family problems are their fault. They usually have isolated themselves from family, friends, and agencies that could assist them. They may fear retaliation and more severe beatings from their husbands if they leave. Many women with children have no place to go, and shelters have long waiting lists.

Batterers and battered women cannot change. If psychosocial learning theory is accurate, both batterers and battered women can be resocialized and can learn more effective ways of relating and interacting. Batterers can learn to verbalize their feelings, rechannel their aggressions, and accept the fact that women are not their property to punish or beat. Battered women can be resocialized to recognize their self-worth and develop assertive skills. They can learn to relate with men in more productive ways.

Characteristics of Battered Women

Battered women hold similar traditional views of sex roles. Many were raised to be submissive, passive, and dependent and to seek approval from male figures. Whereas some battered women were exposed to domestic violence between their parents, others first experience it from their husbands. Battered women are likely to accept the traditional female role in their marriage and believe their husbands will love and protect them. As traditionalists, they believe in family unity and accept prescribed female sex-role stereotypes, believing it is a woman's responsibility to keep her man happy. They believe that they are responsible for the marriage; they have an investment in it and want to make it work. If the marriage fails, they think they have failed as women, that it is their fault, and that their "punishment" is justified.

Battered women typically attribute their beatings to some personal shortcoming or inadequacy. Battered women report that they believed their partners' insults and accusations of being bad wives and negligent mothers. As these women become more isolated, it becomes harder for them to judge who is right. Convinced that they are to blame, they find it easier to admit their guilt than to confront their husbands. For years the men they love and trust have been telling them how bad or incompetent they are. Eventually they fully believe in their inadequacy; they are psychologically destroyed. They feel worthless. Their low self-esteem reinforces their belief that they deserve to be beaten.

Many battered women do not work outside the home. They are isolated from their families, friends, and neighbors and totally dependent on their husbands for financial and emotional needs. Their extreme dependency makes them their husbands' victims. They do not believe they can be independent or self-sufficient.

After repeated beatings, a woman's self-esteem is virtually nonexistent. She feels depressed and guilty about a situation over which she has no control. Her sense of hopelessness and helplessness reduces her problem-solving ability. Women who have depended on others most of their lives often feel incapable of handling their abusive situation. Ignorance of available resources and personal despondency further contribute to their sense of powerlessness.

Battered women often feel a pervasive, undefined guilt. They may internalize their anger at their husbands and the situation into depression or may express it indirectly with severe stress reactions and psychophysiologic symptoms. Some women live in constant fear that their husbands will strike again more severely than the last time or that they will strike the children. Fear permeates the woman's every action; she feels she cannot trust anyone because she no longer can trust the man who supposedly loves and protects her. Fear becomes part of her daily life because she knows that the slightest provocation, suspicion, or jealousy may incite another attack. Caught between their terror of remaining in the home and fear of the unknown if they leave, trapped by psychologic paralysis and complete dependency on their husbands, some women attempt suicide. Bohn (1990) reported that 20% to 50% of battered women attempt suicide.

Characteristics of Batterers

Batterers come from all racial, ethnic, and religious groups and all professions, occupations, and socioeconomic groups. Physical abuse may be seen in the batterer's history and is only one of the many power tactics abusers may use to control their partner (Bohn 1990). Battering is also more common in families where the husband is experiencing difficulty at work or is unemployed.

Many of the frustrations that abusive men cannot handle are related to their jobs, their perceptions of themselves and their wives, and their inability to achieve their goals. Their feelings of socioeconomic inferiority, powerlessness, and helplessness conflict with their assumptions of male supremacy. Emotionally immature or aggressive men may express these overwhelming feelings of inadequacy through violence.

Many batterers feel undeserving of their wives, yet they blame and punish the very person they value. Extreme jealousy and possessiveness are the hallmarks of the abuser. They characteristically express their ambivalence by alternating episodes of unmerciful beatings with periods of remorse and loving attention. Extremes in behavior and overreacting are typical patterns.

Battered women often describe their husbands as lacking respect toward women in general, having come from homes where they have witnessed abuse of their mothers or were themselves abused as children, and having a hidden rage that erupts occasionally. Batterers accept conventional "macho" values, yet when they are not angry or aggressive, they appear childlike, dependent, seductive, manipulative, and in need of nurturing. This dual personality of batterers reflects the conflict between their belief that they must live up to their macho image and their feelings of inadequacy and insecurity in the role of husband or provider. Combined with low frustration tolerance, and poor impulse control, their pervasive sense of powerlessness leads them to strike out at life's inequities by abusing women.

The Battered Woman and the Role of the Nurse

Increased publicity and public sensitivity and heightened awareness of women's rights are encouraging battered women to leave their homes and seek shelter and community assistance. In the past decade, almost every community has developed domestic violence programs, shelters, and resources for battered women (The Battered Woman 1989). State and federal funds have assisted these efforts with the development of the National Domestic Violence Hotline (1-800-333-SAFE), but the needs of battered women and their children are still insufficiently met.

Battered women enter the health care system in many different settings. Nurses may see these women in the physician's office with minor trauma or in the emergency room with multiple severe injuries. Battered women are frequently seen in obstetric services since battering often begins and occurs more frequently during a woman's pregnancy. Nurses in psychiatric–mental health services frequently counsel women who have been battered, and community health nurses may find battered women during home visits (Tilden & Shepherd 1987). Unfortunately, emergency rooms, hospitals, and social service agencies do not routinely recognize and report battering cases to the legal authorities for action and followup, although some states are initiating this policy.

Wife abuse is a major social problem that ignorance and lack of resources allow to continue. Former Surgeon General C. Everett Koop (1989) stated that domestic violence is "an overwhelming moral, economic, and public health burden that our society can no longer bear." Society and health professionals now need to move beyond mere

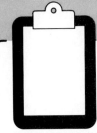

Nursing Care Plan:
The Battered Woman

Nursing History

History of delay between time of injury and time when treatment sought

Vague or evasive accounts of the cause of injuries

Inappropriate affect for situation

History of drug or child abuse

Type and sites of injuries

History of emotional complaints

Increased anxiety in presence of possible batterer

Physical Examination

Complete physical examination

Injuries at multiple sites, especially in area of head, face, neck, chest, abdomen, and upper extremities.

Nursing Diagnosis	Nursing Interventions	Rationale	Evaluation
Ineffective individual coping related to low self-esteem secondary to ongoing abusive relationship. *Client Goal:* Woman can identify her areas of strength and need for self-determination.	Provide supportive counseling and reassurance. Accept and acknowledge woman's state of confusion. Encourage woman to express her feelings and concerns. Assist woman in identifying her strengths and re-establish her feelings of control.	Women may have come to believe that they are to blame for abuse or are dependent on abuser. Battered women can be assisted in recognizing their self-worth and developing assertive skills.	Woman is able to verbalize her feelings.
Knowledge deficit related to available community resources and support services.	Identify the woman's support systems. Discuss the woman's options with her. Identify available community resources such as shelters, financial aid, child care, job training, or employment counseling.	Women's support system may include her family, friends, or neighbors. Woman may feel she is trapped in the relationship and has no options. Women are often unaware of available resources for support or assistance.	The woman discusses resources and support services that are available within the community.

recognition of the problem to develop a better understanding of the dynamics of battering. Nurses can intervene in the cycle of violence by helping battered women recognize their options and take appropriate action.

The Nurse's Attitudes and Characteristics

Nurses in many different health care settings often come in contact with battered and abused women but fail to recognize them, especially if their bruises are not visible. Nurses who wish to help battered women need advanced knowledge of the dynamics of battered women, assessment skills for recognizing subtle cues of battering, and appropriate intervention skills in counseling and referral. Nurses need to be sensitive to battered women's problems and able to tolerate their own empathic feelings of fear and terror as battered women describe their violent experiences and abusive situations. Other skills required by the nurse include compassion, a sense of reality, and a sense of humor, along with the ability to set limits in decision making. Lichtenstein (1981, p 243) suggested that nurses assess their feelings about helping battered women cope by asking themselves:

1. To what extent am I meeting my own personal needs rather than those of the client?

2. Do my feelings include inappropriate ones such as pity and a sense of helplessness?

3. Am I inadvertently attempting to cope with my feelings about a person's level of progress by withdrawing, blaming her, prematurely confronting her, or prematurely pressuring her to make a decision?

4. Do I believe that she has the resources, strength, interests, and abilities to mobilize herself sufficiently to cope constructively with her difficulties?

Working with battered women is often frustrating, and many health care providers feel impotent when these women repeatedly return to their abusive situations without developing sufficient ego strength or coping abilities. Many health care workers are reluctant to become involved, knowing that battered women require long-term assistance and counseling, often for many years, before they are able to change or leave the situation. They become frustrated by spending their time and energy assisting women who remain in a violent situation and then return to the agency in a few months in worse condition than before. It is important for nurses to realize that they cannot rescue battered women; these women must decide on their own how to handle the situation. The effective nurse provides battered women with information that empowers them in decision making and supports their decision, knowing that incremental assistance over the years may be the only alternative until they are ready to explore other options.

❀ *APPLYING THE NURSING PROCESS* ❀

Nursing Assessment

Victims of family violence may be clients in any setting, yet they are difficult to identify because they rarely admit their problems. Women who are at high risk of battering often have a history of alcohol or drug abuse, child abuse, or abuse in the previous or present marriage. Other signs of possible abuse include the following:

- Expressions of helplessness and powerlessness: an attitude that the woman lacks control over her life
- Low self-esteem, as seen in the woman's dress, her appearance, and the way she relates to health care providers
- Signs of depression in remarks about fatigue, hopelessness, and somatic problems such as headache, insomnia, choking sensations, or chest, back, or pelvic pain.

During the assessment of female clients, the nurse should be alert to the following cues of abuse:

- *Hesitancy in providing detailed information about the injury and how it occurred.* The woman may appear timid and evasive and may avoid eye contact; she may seem embarrassed about having been injured.
- *Inappropriate affect for the situation.* The woman may appear overly frightened, disoriented, or depressed over minor injuries. She may display extremes in behavior by minimizing the importance of significant injuries or appearing fragile with minor injuries.
- *Delayed reporting of symptoms.* Considerable time may elapse between the injury and the woman's seeking treatment. She may have waited until the batterer left home to come in for treatment, or she may have hoped that her symptoms would disappear.
- *Types and sites of injuries.* The usual injuries are bruises, abrasions, or contusions to the head (eyes and back of neck), throat, chest, breast, abdomen, or genitals. Usually there are multiple injury sites. Nonbattered women's injuries are usually located at one or two sites and on the extremities such as sprains and strains.
- *Inappropriate explanation.* The woman's account of the cause does not fit the type and location of the injuries. She may state she fell down the stairs or walked into a door, although she has abrasions and contusions around her eyes and throat.
- *Increased anxiety in the presence of the possible batterer.* The woman may look to him for approval before answering questions about her injury and its cause. He may hang around her, appear reluctant to

leave her alone for fear she will talk, or demand to be present during the examination.

Since battering is now so prevalent, it is important to include questions about domestic violence in all primary care encounters.

The nurse who suspects a woman has been abused or beaten should try to interview and counsel her in a quiet, safe place, away from the man or anyone else who brought her in. Different approaches to verify battering can be used by the nurse. Lichtenstein (1981) suggested obtaining an extensive history of family communication patterns, arguments, and conflict resolution; the article provides an excellent list of history questions. Other nurses prefer to share their observations concerning the inconsistency of the injuries with the nature of the cause, hoping the woman will change her story and admit to being beaten. Some nurses wait until the woman is willing to say she has been beaten, whereas others prefer direct confrontation and may ask, "Have you ever been physically hurt by anyone?" Nurses can analyze the woman's behavior and their own feelings to determine the most appropriate and effective approach.

The assessment of the woman should include information about her strengths and support system. Strengths may include education, employment history, activities in the home, community involvement, and her ability to cope or handle past problems. The woman's support system may include her family, friends, neighbors, and community agencies or organizations.

During the assessment phase, the nurse begins building a relationship with the woman based on trust, understanding, and advocacy. A woman may feel ashamed and embarrassed about her injuries and situation. It is important to assure her that all information she provides will be kept confidential. Trust begins as the nurse conveys an attitude of unconditional acceptance, empathy, and positive regard for the woman's worth and dignity. The woman may need to be asked or given permission to discuss her problems before she shares them. Asking questions with sensitivity is better than avoiding the issues. A gentle, firm approach is useful. Nurses should show that they recognize the woman's feelings and that they accept her right to feel as she does. If and when a woman reveals that she has been beaten, she may begin crying and pouring out details of her years of abuse. Empathic listening, support, and possibly some light nourishment, such as coffee, tea, or a soft drink with crackers, may be helpful.

Nursing Diagnosis

Analysis of the woman's history and physical examination reveals patterns that may lead the nurse to suspect abuse and battering. If the woman's story of how she received her injuries is inconsistent with her symptoms, the nurse should record the woman's statements and the evidence, noting that the inconsistency suggests possible abuse and that further follow-up is recommended. The nurse can write in the chart, "injuries are inconsistent with her account of the accident" or "injuries are consistent with assault" if that is the case or "She denies being beaten" if the woman was asked directly and so responded.

In cases where the woman states she has been beaten, kicked, punched, or attacked but does not identify the assailant, the nurse should record the extent of injuries, note the woman's exact words, and describe the incident with a diagnosis of probable battering. Those cases in which the woman states she was beaten by a husband or mate may be diagnosed as battering with all evidence recorded, including the woman's statements.

When abuse or battering is suspected or determined, the nurse should formulate nursing diagnoses based on the assessment findings. Nursing diagnoses related to nonphysical components of abuse or battering may include the following:

- Disturbance in self-concept related to feelings of worthlessness and powerlessness
- Knowledge deficit related to available community resources secondary to social isolation

Nursing Plan and Implementation

Provide Psychologic and Emotional Support

When a battered woman comes in for treatment, she needs to feel safe physically and safe in talking about her injuries and problems. If a man is with her, ask or tell him to wait in the waiting room while you examine the woman. This may reduce her fear, help in establishing trust, and facilitate her expressions of guilt, shame, and embarrassment, along with pent-up anger, rage, and terror about her battering situation. Anger may be directed toward herself, the batterer, or health professionals.

A battered woman also needs to reestablish a feeling of control over her world. She needs to regain a sense of predictability by knowing what to expect and how she can interact. The nurse should provide sufficient information about what to expect in terms the woman can understand. Simple explanations about how long she will stay, whom she will see, and what will be done are important. Some women ask no questions, whereas others produce a barrage of questions. Giving the woman control can be accomplished by asking her permission to do simple tasks and providing her with choices whenever possible. Inform her that her record will be kept confidential and not released or seen by anyone outside the hospital or agency without her permission.

The nurse encourages the woman to talk about her injuries and home situation by asking, "How did this happen to you?" or saying, "We often see injuries like yours when a woman has been beaten. Has this happened to you?" Directly confronting the injuries and possible battering may provide the opening for the woman who is trying to cope in private; she may feel less ashamed and frightened when offered this lead in a relaxed, supportive, and nonjudgmental manner. A woman may continue to deny her battering if she has resigned herself to living with the situation.

Supportive counseling and reassurance are professional skills nurses use throughout each phase of the nursing process with a battered woman. The nurse should:

- Let the woman work through her story, problems, and situation at her own pace.

- Anticipate her ambivalence in the love-hate relationship with the batterer; after all, she knows he may be loving and contrite after the incident if she has been through the cycle of violence before.

- Respect the woman's capacity to change and grow when she is ready.

- Assist her in identifying specific problems and support realistic ideas for reducing or eliminating those problems.

- Help clarify her beliefs and myths and provide information to change her false beliefs.

For example, if the woman feels that she is responsible for or deserves the beating, the nurse assures her that her husband or male friend is totally responsible for his own actions and that she cannot be held responsible for another person's behavior. If the woman thinks that all men beat their women and that there is no way to avoid this problem, the nurse explains that this is not so and that both people in a relationship can change. If the woman thinks that she is the only one who is beaten, the nurse tells her that many women are battered and that until recently their problems were ignored, but that now various community agencies are available to assist battered women. If, having been through the cycle of violence, a woman thinks her husband will change, the nurse tells her that the abuse and beatings usually continue to get worse over time until the woman takes the initiative and changes the situation with the help of community resources. If a woman continues to see the positive side of the family situation, such as that the marriage is still intact; the children have a father, home, and food; and she loves the man, she needs to examine the benefits and consequences of remaining in the situation. The appropriate intervention is not to tell her what to do but to help her recognize her options and resources and exercise her own decisions. Advising or encouraging a woman to leave an abusive situation is not always in the woman's best interest; leaving the home is a major decision with long-lasting consequences. The woman may be economically unable to leave the situation, especially if she has young children. If the woman leaves and then later returns home, both husband and wife may become more frustrated, increasing the possibility of further beatings and even homicide. The most acceptable course of action is one that the woman freely chooses.

Provide Information About Community Resources

Besides offering emotional support, medical treatment, and counseling, the nurse should inform any woman she suspects may be in an abusive situation of the services available in the hospital, agency, and community. Battered women have many needs that require the assistance and coordination of different community agencies. Unfortunately, many battered women are unaware of community agencies that can assist them.

Battered women may need the following:

- Medical treatment for injuries

- Temporary shelter to provide a safe environment for themselves and their children

- Counseling to raise their self-esteem and assist them in understanding the dynamics of family violence

- Legal assistance for protection and/or prosecution

- Financial assistance to provide shelter, food, and clothing

- Job training or employment counseling

- An ongoing support group with counseling on relationships with males and children

A network of community agencies can meet these numerous, varied needs of women, children, and batterers. It is important that employees in these agencies understand the complex dynamics of family violence and wife battering as well as how their services and those of other agencies can assist these families. Services that are available to the battered woman are discussed in the following sections.

Emergency Room Services Many battered women are first seen and diagnosed in the emergency rooms of their neighborhood hospitals. Approximately 20% to 50% of all female emergency room clients are battered women (Campbell & Sheridan 1989).

Emergency room nurses and personnel need to be alert to symptoms of battering, recognize these cues, and encourage women to seek assistance from community agencies. Some states require that suspected cases of abuse and battering be reported to the legal authorities or social service agencies.

Shelter and Housing Since family violence has been recognized as a major social problem, many community agencies have sought federal and state funds to provide needed services and shelters.

Shelters differ in the services they provide, depending on the governing body, financial resources and funding agencies, organizational structure, staff qualifications, and range of available community services. Typical shelters provide battered women and their children with a room, beds, food, clothing, and other basic necessities. If professional staff are available, the shelter may offer crisis counseling, individual and group counseling or therapy, and information about and networking with community agencies such as legal aid, welfare, job training, financial and employment agencies, and women's counseling or support groups.

For safety reasons, the location of most shelters is undisclosed, but they can be contacted through a community crisis line. Unfortunately, admission requirements usually state that the woman must have been beaten in the past; this eliminates those women in potentially violent situations until they have been beaten.

Legal Services and Options   During incidents of domestic violence, the police are frequently called by the victim or neighbors. Family violence typically occurs on the weekend or in late evening when most social service agencies are closed; therefore, the police department is often the first major agency involved. A few police officers are trained to intervene in domestic violence disputes, and many dislike responding to these calls, which are extremely dangerous and often result in death or injury to police officers (Sherman 1983). Many police officers do not understand the complex dynamics of family violence. They may fear for their own safety or believe that they should only try to defuse the situation. Some may feel that these calls are not important because they seldom arrest anyone and most women do not press charges. Because an officer must see the crime committed before arresting anyone on misdemeanor charges, and wife beating usually occurs in the privacy of the home before the police arrive, the police usually just warn the batterer to cool down. This leaves the woman in a more vulnerable position for having sought outside assistance.

Legal options for battered women vary according to state laws and services. In some states a woman may seek a restraining order from the family court or a domestic relations court to protect herself from the batterer. This restraining order specifies that the man may not physically abuse his wife or other family members but does not give the man a criminal record. If the battered woman decides to prosecute, the case is usually heard in criminal court, which handles crimes of assault, harassment, and battery. Criminal court hearings may result in a fine, probation, and/or a jail sentence if the batterer is convicted; then the man would have a criminal record. The prosecution process is often lengthy and may last more than a year. Some state judicial systems are introducing more lenient options such as mandatory counseling for batterers in lieu of prosecution. Divorce is another legal recourse a woman may choose, but divorce may take several months to a year.

Most battered women are unaware of their legal options. They fear further beatings if they prosecute the batterer. Limited financial resources may also keep them from seeking legal assistance. Some women do not understand the complex judicial process and their options within it. Therefore, few battered women press charges against the batterer, so their fear and vulnerability to repeated beatings continue, with minimal assistance from the police and legal system. Some communities provide legal advocacy services to help battered women understand the judicial process and its consequences to the woman, children, and batterer.

Financial Services   Once battered women leave their homes or seek legal assistance, they usually receive no financial support from the batterer. Without funds, battered women and their children are at the mercy of community social service agencies, and it usually takes weeks for papers to be processed before any money is forthcoming. Agencies that may provide financial assistance to battered women include their county welfare department, Aid to Families with Dependent Children, The United Way, women's support groups, religious organizations, and possibly the Salvation Army. There may be other local groups to assist these women in various ways such as providing food or clothing.

Employment Training or Placement   Many battered women are full-time mothers who lack advanced education, training, and job experience. High unemployment rates, minimal skills, and inadequate transportation make it difficult for these women to obtain employment with an adequate salary. Women who have children must consider where to place them during working hours as well as the added cost of child care. Often the woman's choice is restricted to accepting welfare or taking a low-paying job. Either choice usually means lowering the standard of living to subsistence. Avoiding beatings at such a cost may not seem like a viable option.

Some women do seek job training if the opportunities are available, but training provides no guarantee of future job placement. A woman may still have to arrange for financial support and child care while obtaining advanced employment skills or an education.

Counseling   Battered women may need a variety of counseling services, such as crisis intervention, short-term individual therapy, group therapy, or peer support groups, over an extended period. Counseling and therapy may be provided by nurses, social workers, psychologists, mental health specialists, or clergy with special training.

Evaluation

After interacting with a battered woman, the nurse may wonder how to judge the effectiveness of her actions. It is helpful to remember that the average battered woman endures the situation for years before seeking meaningful assistance. The nurse may see the woman at the beginning of this long process when she is not yet ready to change her situation. Most women return home in resignation after each battering. Some seek temporary shelter several times before taking final steps to change their situation.

It takes a long time for a woman to concede that life may be better outside the battering situation and that there are effective ways to change the situation. Each woman needs to plan her own life when she has sufficient strength and knowledge of her options and consequences. The nurse should remember that if the woman decides to return home, it is the woman's decision and not the nurse's problem. Having recognized the battered woman, provided counsel, and properly referred her, the nurse has planted the seed for release from the cycle of violence. The seed may lie dormant for years; at a critical moment in the woman's life, it may sprout and change her life.

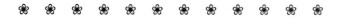

Child Abuse

One of the most disastrous results of dysfunctional parenting is child abuse. Child abuse arises in part from the cultural sanctioning of physical discipline of children by their parents. Among the many serious effects of child abuse are physical handicaps, poor self-image, inability to love others, antisocial or violent behavior in later life, and death.

A small number of abusing parents are mentally ill, but most abusing parents have less serious problems that respond to intervention. Parents at risk for abusive behavior may manifest one or more of the risk factors identified in Table 3–3.

Patterns of Abuse

Child abusers are found among all socioeconomic, religious, and ethnic groups. Some child abusers are irrational or even psychotic, but most are ordinary people who feel trapped in stressful life situations with which they cannot cope satisfactorily. Many abusive parents are simply confused and overwhelmed by parenthood or by life in general and vent their frustrations on their children. Because all parents have negative feelings about their children at one time or another, the difference between parents who abuse and those who do not is often only a matter of degree. All parents are at risk occasionally, but most parents are able to channel their frustration and anger appropriately.

The parent with a potential for abuse is one who feels isolated, is unable to trust others, is too passive to be able to give, or has very unrealistic expectations for children. Parents at risk for abuse tend to expect their children to perform for their gratification, and they tend to use severe physical punishment to ensure a child's proper behavior (Kempe & Kempe 1984). As mentioned earlier, parents who abuse their children are likely to have been abused as children. This multigenerational pattern of child abuse, although disturbing, does help in identifying families in need of prevention.

Table 3–3	Parental Risk Factors for Child Maltreatment*	
Risk factor	**Assessment finding**	
Lack of nurturing experience	Inadequate experience with parenting (eg, multiple foster homes)	
	Parent neglected or abused as a child	
	Parent expected to meet high demands of own parents as a child	
Lack of knowledge or normal growth and development	Inability to read "cues" of child	
	Impatience when child does not respond as expected; unreasonable discipline	
	Unrealistically high expectations for the child	
Isolation	Inadequate use of supports	
	Inability to identify resources	
	Unknown to others in community	
Low self-esteem	Lack of trust, particularly of authority figures	
	Expect rejection	
High vulnerability to criticism	History of family violence in family of origin or in current family system (eg, spouse abuse)	
	Impulsive	
Many unmet needs	Feelings of being unloved or having unresponsive spouse, unstable marriage, or no marriage at all	
	Youthful marriage, forced marriage, unwanted pregnancy	
Multiple stressors	Poverty, unemployment, substandard housing, lack of job opportunities	
	Inadequate clothing and insufficient food	
Substance abuse	Abuse of alcohol or drugs	
Role reversal	Emotional immaturity, lack of patience, inability to make judgments	
	Preoccupied with self	
	Depression	
	Dependent on others	

Adapted from Mott SR, James SR, Sperhac AM: Nursing Care of Children and Families, 2nd ed. Menlo Park, CA: Addison-Wesley, 1990, p 589.

Many abusive parents also have unrealistic expectations for themselves and unknowingly contribute to their problems. For example, one parent waxed the kitchen floor during a snowstorm and then abused the child who tracked mud into the house. The parent's behavior and expectations for the child clearly contributed to the problem.

Parents with a potential for abuse often expect their children to meet their needs and therefore are most likely to abuse a child who is viewed as "different."

Children at risk for abuse may be the result of difficult pregnancies or births or those born at inconvenient times, born out of wedlock, the "wrong" sex, or too active or too passive. Some children are abused because they are the result of a forced pregnancy with an unloved partner or the result of rape or incest. Others have characteristics, such as looks and mannerisms, that evoke negative associations in the abusing parent. Children who have been separated from their families because of prematurity or neonatal disease are more likely to be at risk for abuse. Children with congenital anomalies, mental retardation, hyperactivity, or chronic illness are also at risk. Children with abnormal sleep-wake patterns or feeding difficulties and those who are unresponsive to caregiving might also be at risk if they are living in a family with other risk factors (Mott et al 1990). Only a small percentage of premature or difficult children, however, are abused, and for all abused children, it is the combination of parental deficiencies and characteristics of the child that create the problems leading to abuse.

Child abuse is most likely to occur during times of crisis. The parent's loss of a job, for example, might be just enough to make the crying of a fretful infant unbearable. Some families hover on the brink of perpetual crisis, living with constant changes that contribute to feelings of inadequacy. The magnitude of the crisis is not always in proportion to the abuse. A relatively minor crisis might be viewed as the "last straw" in an unhappy situation.

Solving a crisis for troubled families is not enough if new crises and stressors merely reestablish dysfunctional patterns. Instead, the nurse teaches parents to develop their own coping strategies and to identify when and how to seek help. Parents who learn the problems inherent in isolation, for example, will then seek assistance when under stress and will avoid the patterns of behavior that cause them to abuse their children.

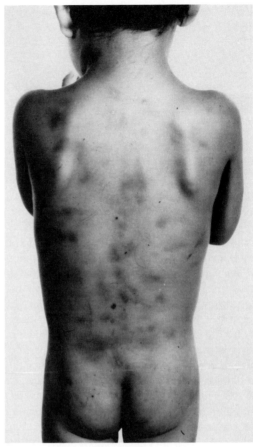

Figure 3–4   Abused child

Types of Abuse

There are several prevalent types of child abuse or maltreatment; some are more visible than others. The nurse needs to assess for all forms of abuse (Figure 3–4). The consequences of emotional and sexual abuse are not as obvious as those of physical abuse, but the effects of these types of abuse may last longer and be more damaging to the personal development of the child. Table 3–4 describes the types and characteristics of abuse.

Munchausen syndrome by proxy is an unusual type of child abuse in which the parent invents or directly induces the child's illness or injury symptoms. The factitious

Table 3–4 Types of Child Abuse*		
	Definition	**Characteristics**
Physical abuse	Nonaccidental injury of a child	Physical injury at variance with history or explanation given; repeated pattern of physical punishment with short- or long-term effects
Emotional abuse	Nonphysical, often verbal, assault on a child—usually critical, demeaning, and emotionally devastating	Attack inflicted by parent or other adult, often as part of a continuing pattern
Sexual abuse	Use of a child for sexual purposes, including incest, rape, molestation, prostitution, or pornography	Nonabusing parent or other family members often aware of the abuse (and might be criminally liable if they do nothing to stop it)
Adolescent abuse	Physical, emotional, or sexual abuse inflicted on an adolescent	Adolescent who runs away from home; abusing parent often considers abuse justified

*Adapted from Mott SR, James SR, Sperhac AM: Nursing Care of Children and Families, 2nd ed. Menlo Park, CA: Addison-Wesley, 1990, p 592.

symptoms usually result in the child undergoing unnecessary and extensive medical tests and procedures (Kahan & Yorker 1990; Mott et al 1990). The parent appears to need the child to be ill. Care of these families requires a multidisciplinary approach and long-term therapy.

Documentation

Child *neglect* can be defined as failure by parents or other custodian to meet the medical, emotional, physical, or supervisory needs of a child, whereas child *abuse* is nonaccidental physical or threatened harm and includes mental and emotional injury, sexual abuse, and sexual exploitation (Allen & Hollowell 1990). In situations of child abuse and neglect, documentation of evidence is vital.

Records provide the legal basis for intervening on behalf of the child. Nursing history and daily notes need to be accurate, timely, and objective. The goal of documentation is to provide a written account of each visit or contact. If the nursing records become part of a court proceeding, they need to portray a family by specifying behaviors that indicate progress or failure in providing a safe, nurturing environment for the child. In some neglect cases, much of the evidence is intangible and difficult to prove; therefore, input from many professionals is necessary to convince the court that a child is actually at risk for abuse or neglect. Evidence of risk might include the doctor's and nurse's notes on the child, the school nurse's report, and the social worker's impressions during a home visit regarding the child's physical appearance; interactions with parents, peers, and other adults; ability to respond to questions; and general development (Figure 3–5). Evidence of neglect might include developmental delays, substance abuse, poor medical care, poor school attendance, or lack of supervision. Careful documentation and recorded evidence are essential when presenting a case to the judicial system. See Table 3–5.

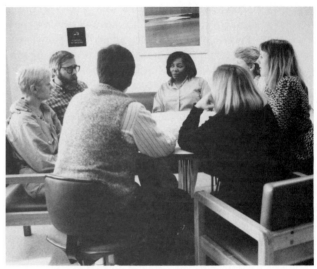

Figure 3–5   Parents explore ideas and ways to cope with stress in parenting classes and group therapy sessions (From Mott SR, James SR, Sperbac AM: Nursing Care of Children and Families, *2nd ed. Menlo Park, CA: Addison-Wesley, 1990, p 603.)*

Child Abuse and the Role of the Nurse

By the nature of their work, nurses in a variety of settings are involved in the identification, treatment, and prevention of child abuse and neglect. Nurses who see medical problems that suggest abuse or neglect or who see children and parents whose behavior indicates the potential for abuse or neglect are called on to collaborate with members of other disciplines in protecting children at risk and advocating care for both children and families. Because

Table 3–5   Components of Report of Child Maltreatment*

Aspect of report	Example
Reason for suspicion or assessment of incident	Child's comments; nature or extent of injury
Behaviors observed and by whom	Teacher's report; circumstances of discovery (eg, "child found alone by police in car")
Quality of parent-child relationship (if observed)	Any comforting measure noted or lacking (eg, "father speaks in loud tones and uses threatening language")
What family has been told (to assist in follow-up for all team members)	Purpose of Child Protective Services (if family is unaware of report, explain rationale)
What protection team should do first	Possible interventions (eg, assess home and risks to siblings; investigate and enlist possible community supports)

*Adapted from Mott SR, James SR, Sperbac AM: Nursing Care of Children and Families, 2nd ed. Menlo Park, CA: Addison-Wesley, 1990, p 592.

each family is part of a community system, nurses also need to be aware of community resources. The nurse's early detection of child abuse and neglect may lead to the first attempts to intervene and provide services to the child and family.

❀   *APPLYING THE NURSING PROCESS*   ❀

Nursing Assessment

Childhood accidents are a common source of injuries; thus every parent who brings a child in for treatment of an injury should not automatically be suspected of abuse. Certain physical and behavioral findings are indicative of abuse, however, and it is important for the nurse to be aware of these clues. Tables 3–6 and 3–7 list the findings indicative of physical and sexual abuse.

In all cases of suspected abuse or neglect, the nurse needs to ask the child and family members present the following questions:

1. How did the accident (or incident) happen?
2. When did the accident happen?

Table 3–6   Signs and Symptoms of Physical Abuse*

Indication of abuse	Assessment findings
Bruises or welts on ears, eyes, mouth, lips, torso, buttocks, genital areas, calves	Injuries may be in shape of object used to produce them (eg, sticks, belts, hairbrushes, buckles)
	Injuries located on parts of body not usually injured, such as bruising behind the ear, bleeding into the conjunctiva or retina, pinch marks on genitals (normal bruises commonly appear on forehead, shins, knees, elbows)
	Injuries often in various stages of healing
Burns	Shape suggests type of burn
Immersion burns	Immersion burns on feet have "socklike," on hands "glovelike," on buttocks or genitalia "donutlike" appearance
Pattern burns	Pattern suggests object used (eg, iron, stove grate, electric burner, heater); small, circular burns on feet, face, hands, chest, or buttocks suggest cigar or cigarette
Friction burns	Friction burns on legs, arms, neck, or torso may be caused by child having been tied up with rope
Scald burns	Caused by hot liquid poured over trunk or extremities; multiple splash marks may appear on body; depth of burn varies with temperature of liquid, length of contact, and presence of clothing
Fractures of skull, face, nose, orbit, long bones, ribs	Multiple or spiral fractures caused by twisting motion
	Evidence of epiphyseal separations and periosteal shearing
	Shaft fractures from direct blows
	Fractures may be in various stages of healing if earlier fractures went untreated
Lacerations or abrasions on mouth, lips, gums, eyes, genitals	Human bite marks, especially those of adult size, may be evident
	Torn frenulum in infant from forcing object into mouth
	Puncture wounds or deep scratch marks from fingernails around face or genital area
Head trauma	Evidence of increased intracranial pressure in infant (eg, bulging fontanelle)
	Subdural hematomas from being dropped on the head or from receiving blows to the head; if abuse is repetitive, separation of cranial sutures may be evident due to chronic subdural hematoma
	Areas of baldness and swelling from hair being pulled out when dragging the child by the hair
Neck trauma	Limited range of motion from whiplash injury due to being shaken
	Dislocation or subluxation of neck
Somatic	Persistent vomiting or abdominal pain
	Rigid abdomen due to internal bleeding
	Shock
Child's behaviors	Extreme aggressiveness or withdrawal; wariness of adults; fear of going home; apprehension when other children cry
	Appears disinterested or frightened of parents, shows no emotion when parents leave or return
	Indiscriminate friendliness and immediate affection shown toward anyone providing attention
	Vacant stare; no eye contact
	Surveys environment but remains motionless
	Stiffens when approached as if expecting punishment of a physical nature
	Inappropriate response to painful procedures

*Adapted from Mott SR, James SR, Sperhac AM: Nursing Care of Children and Families, *2nd ed.* Menlo Park, CA: Addison-Wesley, 1990, p 593.*

Table 3–7 Signs of Sexual Abuse *	
Physical Signs	**Behavioral Signs**
Laceration of labia, vagina, or perineum	Advanced knowledge of adult sexual behavior
Irritation, pain, or injury to genital area	Discussion of or implied involvement in sexual activity
Hematomas in genital area	Expression of severe emotional conflict at home with fear of intervention
Vaginal or penile discharge	Reluctance to participate in sports, showers, changing of clothes
Dysuria or urinary frequency	
Sexually transmitted disease in young child (on eyes, mouth, anus, or genitals)	Excessive bathing
Pregnancy	Sitting carefully because of injuries
Itching, bruises, or bleeding in genital area	Unusual interest in genital area (eg, "French kissing" or fondling of genitals, excessive masturbation)
Unexplained vaginal or rectal bleeding	
Enlarged vaginal or rectal orifice	Sexual acting out with peers
Foreign objects in vagina or rectum	Sleep disturbances (eg, nightmares, fear of sleeping alone)
Increased rectal pigmentation	
Gait disturbance	Reluctance to participate in activities with a particular person or at a particular place
	Increased number of new fears
	Fear of being alone
	Poor peer relations
	Depression
	Change in performance at school
	Eating disorders
	Vague somatic complaints
	Extreme shyness
	Increased aggressive or hostile behavior
	Encopresis
	Enuresis
	Self-destructive or suicidal behaviors
	Substance abuse
	Runaway behaviors

*Adapted from Mott SR, James SR, Sperhac AM: Nursing Care of Children and Families, *2nd ed. Menlo Park, CA: Addison-Wesley, 1990, p 597.*

3. Where were the child and other family members at the time?
4. Who was caring for the child at the time?
5. Who saw the accident?
6. What did the child do after the accident?
7. What measures were taken by the parent?

After recording answers to these questions, the nurse proceeds with the physical assessment, noting the location, color, and characteristics of all cutaneous lesions. Photographs might be needed as legal evidence. Orthopedic, surgical, ophthalmologic, and gynecologic examinations also might be needed depending on the type of injuries. Gynecologic examination includes cultures for gonorrhea and other sexually transmitted diseases, microscopic ex-amination for blood and sperm, pregnancy testing, and clothing examination for semen, blood, or pubic hairs. Strict procedures must be followed in collecting evidence and specimens to provide data the courts will accept.

The most important determination to make during the assessment is the risk of reinjury to the victim or injury to other children in the household. Assessment of family functioning, coping strategies, and current state of crisis provides valuable data for such determination. Sometimes, even when the injuries are not severe, hospitalization or foster home placement is necessary. Protection of the child (or children) is always the priority.

An interview with parents or extended family members is essential. Interviewing adult family members separately allows the interviewer to compare the facts and check the validity of the data.

In assessing neglected or abused children and their families, the nurse considers the long-term consequences of neglect and their possible effects on family cooperation in meeting goals. Assessment of neglected or abused children and their families include the following:

- The parents' emotional ability to accept services
- Communication patterns within the family
- The range and availability of services
- The family's use of services
- Supportive counseling for all family members
- The children's growth and developmental patterns
- The parents' attempts to diminish isolation
- The parents' responses to expectations to change behaviors
- The quality of nurturance within the family
- Family dynamics and other risk factors such as substance abuse or violence
- Environmental stressors such as inadequate housing, hygiene, or nutrition

Analysis and Nursing Diagnosis

Once it has been determined that a child has been abused by a parent, the nurse should formulate nursing diagnoses based on the assessment findings. Examples of nursing diagnoses related to dysfunctional parenting are:

- Ineffective parental coping related to stress
- Knowledge deficit regarding the normal process of growth and development of children
- Disturbance in self-concept related to parent's low self-esteem

Examples of nursing diagnoses related to the abused child are:

- Developmental vulnerability related to dysfunctional parent-child interaction
- Potential for disturbance in self-concept related to parental abuse

Nursing Plan and Implementation

Provide Support to Dysfunctional Parents

Providing parental supports to marginally functioning parents is preferable to removing the child from the home. Removing children is traumatic, and most communities lack adequate foster care homes. Foster care is more expensive than maintaining the family system. Dysfunctional parents also tend to continue the cycle of dysfunctional parenting with other children in the family.

Although both professionals and nonprofessionals acknowledge intense feelings concerning child abuse and neglect, they have little concern for the abusive parents. Jolly

K, a former abusive parent (and the founder of Parents Anonymous), identified that abusive parents are afraid. They are afraid of what they are doing and of what will happen if they do not go for help.

Working with neglectful and abusive parents is emotionally draining and disturbing for all people involved. Seeing a child victimized calls forth strong emotions, particularly among nurses, who might be required to provide nursing care during the time of the acute injury. The tendency is to protect the victim, the innocent child, and to punish the parent, who after all is the offender, but the nurse who perceives the family as a system understands that both child and parent are victims (Wissow 1990). The etiology of abuse is complex and multifaceted.

> [Parents] bring to the family and to their roles as parents developmental histories that may predispose them to treat their offspring in an abusive/neglectful manner. Stress-promoting social forces both within the family (eg, handicapped child, marital conflict) and beyond (eg, social isolation, unemployment) increase the likelihood that parent-child conflict will occur (Wissow 1990).

Nurses need to avoid "rescuer fantasies," which can stem from caring for a child and wanting to save that child from harm. Unless recognized, these fantasies can blind the nurse to the real needs of the child and family. If the focus is the child's injuries, negative feelings toward the parent can multiply and ultimately affect interventions. Some nurses employ both overt (deliberately ignoring the parent or making accusatory remarks) and covert (supplying information in an offhand manner) behaviors toward abusive parents, thereby inhibiting rapport and parent teaching. One approach to this problem might be to have two nursing teams, one to care for the child and one to interact with the parent, to help channel some negative feelings and maintain communication. Periodic discussions can help nurses focus on the identified needs of both the parent and child and allow for the appropriate release of tension. Nurses need to recognize and affirm that child abuse is not simply the problem of a disturbed parent but is a social problem of vast dimensions.

Nurses can avoid judgmental attitudes by first examining their own thoughts, feelings, and beliefs about poverty, neglect, alternative life-styles, and different ethnic and cultural groups. Nurses need to understand the complex relationships among poverty, alienation, and neglect, not only to identify risk factors but also to recognize the social forces that keep some families locked in a cycle of dysfunction.

Assist Parents in Coping with Stress

A major task for the nurse is helping dysfunctional parents understand the impact of stress and crises in their lives and the appropriate responses to these crises. In a family that is providing only marginal child care, any stress, however small, might create a crisis. Illness; separation of a family member; or problems with housing, heating, cooking, or laundry might trigger further neglect or apathy in an already fragile parent. The nurse who identifies stress in dysfunctional families therefore needs to assess coping strategies. Successful coping patterns suggest growth and motivation. The nurse might be able to praise parents for positive coping behaviors or may need to teach appropriate ways to cope with stress. A family's reaction to stress is often a measure of the family's strength as a system.

Most parents need support services as they learn to develop new coping techniques. Group therapy, which provides peer support, might assist abusive parents because finding others with similar problems minimizes isolation (Figure 3–5). Nurse therapists can address and help parents verbalize common fears and misconceptions about parenting. The first signs of dysfunctional parenting, however, must be discussed with the family. The nurse needs to guard against becoming so involved with the family that early indicators of serious parenting problems go unrecognized. Progress might be slight at times but must always be identified, especially to the parent with low self-esteem.

Nurses and other professionals often need to make contracts and establish realistic deadlines in working with families. This in turn is good role modeling. Dysfunctional families need to be informed that the pattern of child care is inadequate and not acceptable to the community or school system. Facts of legal consequence, including removal of the children, need to be both verbalized and written out. These measures might seem drastic, but if they are handled in too gentle a manner and the family misinterprets the message, valuable time may be lost in mixed messages and conflicts.

Some parents appear to be docile, cooperative, and open but have merely learned responses that please. The nurse therefore is careful to identify concrete changes that indicate progress. Otherwise the therapeutic contact might end too early for a family that appears to have changed. Periodic evaluation of family dynamics and interagency accomplishments and conflicts should ensure that the family does not manipulate workers or agencies and decrease the effectiveness of the plan. In some instances a child protective worker is needed to function as coordinator.

Provide Information About Community Resources

Intervention at all levels is more effective when multiple resources are available and the family can help choose which resources to use. Most families need to draw on a variety of resources to break the cycle of a dysfunctional life-style (Broome & Daniels 1987). Nurses and other health professionals therefore need to be aware of the services available within their communities (Table 3–8). They need to help families find those programs most geared to their needs and then coordinate the program goals and the family's progress.

Formerly abusive parents often report increased self-

Table 3–8 Community Services Commonly Needed by Families Demonstrating Health-Threatening Parenting*
Public housing
Welfare
Mental health centers
Emergency shelters
Subsidized child care
Homemaker services
WIC program
Food stamps
Free medical or dental care
Family and/or marital counseling
Vocational rehabilitation, employment services
Foster care
Parents Anonymous
Fuel assistance agencies
Child guidance centers
Child development clinics
Housing authorities
Alcoholics Anonymous, Al-Anon, Ala-Teen, Ala-Tot
Visiting Nurse Association
Juvenile authorities
DCYS (Division of Child and Youth Services)
Ambulatory care settings
Occupational health settings
Religious-affiliated groups

*Adapted from Mott SR, James SR, Sperhac AM: Nursing Care of Children and Families, *2nd ed. Menlo Park, CA: Addison-Wesley, 1990, p 607.*

esteem as they assist other parents in distress. Some continue to attend Parents Anonymous meetings long after their initial needs are met, and many parents report pleasurable relationships with their children for the first time in their lives.

Provide Support to the Child

If significant changes in the family are unavoidable, the child needs assistance in working through feelings of having caused the changes. Siblings also need to be included in the treatment plan of an abused or neglected child. If the child is hospitalized, fears of pain or violence are intensified by the unfamiliar surroundings and people. If a parent does visit, the parent is often unsupportive and may be angry with the child. The child is often confused, hurt, and frightened. Nurses and other hospital staff can identify pain, fear, and confusion and help the child discuss those feelings. The child needs to be told what will happen in developmentally appropriate terms and be reassured, as much as possible, that the parent will be back. The fewer the number of care givers, the more likely it is that the child will establish trusting relationships.

Some children have never heard their names spoken in a gentle voice, and a slow, gentle approach is essential to build any degree of trust. Children who withdraw from human contact must be allowed a reasonable period of time in which to grieve and appraise new people. If the child regresses, the regressive behavior needs to be accepted un-til the child can ease into a more appropriate developmental stage.

Younger children are likely to need nurturing in the form of rocking, cuddling, and soothing. The child initially might appear to reject any comforting, however, or become aggressive in response to overwhelming anxiety. The aggressive behaviors are learned responses to chaotic living and can become a problem if the child manages to manipulate many people. Team members need to set consis-

Table 3–9 Evaluation of Interventions to Alter At-Risk Parenting *	
Goal for parental behavior	**Evaluation**
Identifies problems in the family system	Parent develops insight into the emotional climate of the family
Identifies factors that contribute to potential or actual abusive behaviors	
Demonstrates ability to meet own needs	
Finds alternatives to present coping strategies by first identifying external stressors	
Describes feelings toward self and children	
Demonstrates alternative coping strategies in stressful situations	
Demonstrates realistic expectations of children by identifying age-appropriate behaviors	Parent improves parenting skills
Identifies methods of discipline	
Demonstrates some consistency and appropriate use of discipline	
Identifies a person or agency to contact in a crisis	
Provides a safe environment for children by identifying an adequate caregiver during parental absence, identifying and correcting environmental hazards, providing ongoing health care for children	
Identifies family members and friends available for support	Parent establishes and uses a positive support system
Indicates frequency of visits to family and friends	
Identifies ways in which family, friends, community supports (eg, church, school) can be helpful	
Identifies ways in which health care system can be helpful	
Demonstrates appropriate use of health care system and other agencies by keeping appointments	
Earns income above the poverty level or receives and manages public assistance optimally (eg, food stamps used to buy food that is then allocated appropriately among family members)	Parent has adequate income to maintain family
Manages budget to purchase appropriate low-cost clothing for family members	
Provides adequate housing that meets minimal requirements (heat, electricity, cooking and refrigeration facilities, some furnishings)	
Remains at same residence without frequent moves	

*Adapted from Christensen ML, Schommer BL, Velasquez J: An interdisciplinary approach to preventing child abuse. Matern/Child Nurs J March/April 84 (2). Copyright © 1984, American Journal of Nursing Co.

tent limits in a firm but kindly manner and help the child learn more acceptable behaviors. Aggressive children usually have feelings of deprivation, sadness, and loneliness and may believe themselves to be unworthy and bad. Such children have little faith in their ability to inspire approval and affection.

Individual therapy may help aggressive children to discuss the expectations their parents have for them and family dynamics. The therapeutic approach is to face reality honestly and not to arouse expectations in the child that the parent cannot or will not fulfill (Kempe & Kempe 1984). Children who have been severely abused or have witnessed severe abuse of a sibling also need support in developing future relationships that are free of fears, guilt, and anxieties. Children facing loss or separation from their parents need therapeutic assistance to handle the loss and time to mourn the loss.

Long-term follow-up of dysfunctional families has no set time frame for completion. In some instances services are required until the children reach adulthood. Periodic evaluation of parental progress and family growth includes monitoring the behaviors of the children, who might exhibit anger, anxiety, intense loneliness, or apathy. The children's progress in school must also be assessed, together with their response to authority figures. Dysfunctional behaviors suggest that the child needs individual attention. Communication and caring, although time-consuming for the team members, does assist both parents and children in coping with the normal stress of development.

Evaluation

The nurse who is caring for dysfunctional families must evaluate care on an ongoing basis. The nurse needs to see the family at regular intervals to identify specific evidence of progress or failure. Informing the parents of the consequences of failure to meet expectations and deadlines is a delicate and crucial issue for the nurse because most nurses find it difficult to discuss removing children from the family. Parents must know, however, that children's safety and security are of primary importance. The parents' failure to meet goals indicates a need for more intervention.

With a parent who has a history of inflicting trauma in response to personal stress, the expected behaviors need to be defined immediately. Table 3–9 lists specific goals for parental behavior. These can be used to determine the success of nursing interventions.

❀ ❀

KEY CONCEPTS

The evolution of today's family is a result of social, political, economic, and philosophical changes.

Family structure describes the number of family members and the relation of each family member to the others; family function describes the effects of the family behaviors on the family unit.

The development of the family is defined by a set of developmental tasks that the family undertakes at various times during its life cycle.

Common types of families include nuclear, single-parent, reconstituted (blended), and extended families.

Family assessment is the process of gathering and analyzing data about a family and its members. During the process the nurse collects data about the family structure, function, roles, and knowledge about infant-child care.

The overall goal of family assessment is to promote family growth by identifying teaching and referral needs.

Family violence occurs, with women and children being the most frequent targets, in families of all socioeconomic levels, races, and structure.

Family violence may result in physical and psychologic trauma to family members, removal of children from the parents' care, and legal proceedings against the perpetrators of the violence.

Wife battering is a common occurrence, but it is the least reported serious crime in the United States.

Nurses are in an excellent position to intervene and assist battered women by recognizing their cues, diagnosing their problems appropriately, and understanding the complex dynamics of the battering family. The nurse provides information about available community resources, medical attention, and emotional support.

All members of a violence-prone family are affected by the violent behavior; interventions should be directed at both victims and abusers.

Child abuse is physical violence or verbal assaults directed against a child.

Parents who abuse their children often feel isolated, are unable to trust others, have few supports for coping with stress, or have unrealistic expectations for their children's behavior.

Indicators of physical abuse include a series of injuries in various stages of healing (especially a series of similar injuries), the family's delay in seeking treatment, use of multiple treatment facilities, and attempts to hide or minimize the abuse, sometimes with special clothing.

The nurse documents evidence of child abuse by noting and specifically describing parent and child behaviors.

Nursing actions in cases of child abuse include providing support to the parents and child and providing information about the referrals to community resources.

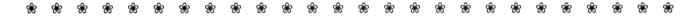

References

Aldous J: *Family Careers.* New York: Wiley, 1978.

Allen JM, Hollowell EE: Nurses & child abuse/neglect reporting: Duties, responsibilities, and issues. *J Pract Nurs* June 1990; 56.

Avant P: A maternal attachment assessment strategy, in Humenick S (editor): *Analysis of Current Assessment Strategies in the Health Care of Young Children and Childbearing Families.* New York: Appleton-Century-Crofts, 1982.

Beavers W, Voeller M: Family models: Comparing and contrasting the Olsen Circumplex model with the Beavers system model. *Fam Process* 1983; 22(3):85.

Bohn DK: Domestic violence and pregnancy: Implications for practice. *J. Nurse-Midwifery* 1990; 35(2):86.

Bradshaw MJ (editor): *Nursing of the Family in Health and Illness: A Developmental Approach.* Norwalk, CT: Appleton & Lange, 1988.

Broome ME, Daniels D: Child abuse: A multidimensional phenomenon. *Holistic Nurs Pract* 1987; 1(2):13.

Bullock LFC, Sandella JA, McFarlane J: Breaking the cycle of abuse: How nurses can intervene. *J Psychosoc Nurs* 1989; 27(8):1113.

Campbell JC, Sheridan DJ: Emergency nursing interventions with battered women. *J Emerg Nurs* 1989; 15(1):12.

Carter B, McGoldrick M (editors): *The Changing Family Life Cycle: A Framework for Family Therapy.* New York: Allyn & Bacon, 1989.

Clark MJD: *Community Nursing: Health Care for Today and Tomorrow.* Reston, VA: Prentice-Hall, 1984.

Duvall EM: *Marriage and Family Development,* 5th ed. Philadelphia: Lippincott, 1977.

Epstein NB et al: The McMaster Family Assessment Device. *J Marital Fam Ther* 1983; 9:171.

Friedman MM: *Family Nursing Theory and Assessment,* 2nd ed. New York: Appleton-Century-Crofts, 1986.

Gelliss CL et al: *Toward a Science of Family Nursing.* New York: Addison-Wesley, 1989.

Goldenberg I, Goldenberg H: *Family Therapy, an Overview,* 2nd ed. Monterey, CA: Brooks/Cole, 1985.

Helton AS, Snodgrass FG: Battering during pregnancy: Intervention strategies. *Birth* 1987; 14(3):142.

Hill RL: Modern systems theory and the family: A confrontation, in Sussman MB (editor): *Sourcebook of Marriage and the Family,* 2nd ed. Boston: Houghton Mifflin, 1974.

Hymovich DP: *Child and Family Development: Implications for Primary Health Care.* New York: McGraw-Hill, 1980.

Kahan BB, Yorker BC: Munchausen syndrome by proxy. *J School Health* 1990; 60(3):108.

Kempe RS, Kempe CH: *Child Abuse.* Cambridge, MA: Harvard Univ Press, 1984.

King MC, Ryan J: Abused women: Dispelling myths and encouraging intervention. *Nurse Pract* 1989; 14(5):47.

Knafl KA: How families manage a pediatric hospitalization. *West J Nurs Res* 1985; 7:151.

Kohn ML: The effects of social class on parental values and practices, in Reiss D, Hoffman H (editors): *The American Family: Dying or Developing.* New York: Plenum, 1979.

Koop CE: Doctors announce campaign to combat domestic violence. *ACOG News Release.* January 3, 1989.

Lamb M: What can research experts tell parents about effective socialization? In Fantini MD, Cardenas A (editors): *Parenting in a Multicultural Society.* White Plains, NY: Longman, 1980.

Leininger M: Transcultural care diversity and universality: A theory of nursing. *Nurs Health Care* 1985; 209.

Levin S, Idler E: *The Hidden Health Care System.* Cambridge: Ballinger, 1981.

Lichtenstein VR: The battered woman: Guidelines for effective nursing intervention. *Issues Ment Health Nurs* July-September 1981; 3:237.

Mahon L: Common characteristics of abused women. *Issues Ment Health Nurs* January-June 1981; 3:137.

McCubbin H, Dahl B: *Marriage and Family: Individuals and Life Cycles.* New York: Wiley, 1985.

Moos RW, Moos BS: A typology of family social environments. *Fam Process* 1976; 15:357.

Mott SR, James SR, Sperhac AM: *Nursing Care of Children and Families,* 2nd ed. Menlo Park, CA: Addison-Wesley, 1990.

Moynihan DP: *Family and Nation.* San Diego: Harcourt, Brace, Jovanovich, 1987.

O'Leary KD et al: Prevalence and stability of spousal aggression. *J Consult Clin Psychol* 1989; 57:263.

On the home front. San Francisco *Chronicle,* August 28, 1986.

Ritzer G: *Contemporary Sociological Theory.* New York: Knopf, 1983.

Roberts C, Feetman S: Assessing family functioning across three areas of relationships. *Nurs Res* April 1982; 231.

Ross B, Cobb KL: *Family Nursing: A Nursing Process Approach.* Redwood City, CA: Addison-Wesley, 1990.

Sherman KO: The battered woman. *Dimens Crit Care Nurs* 1983; 2(January/February):30.

Smilkstein G: The physician and family function assessment. *Fam Systems Med* Fall 1984; 263.

Speer J, Sachs B: Selecting the appropriate family assessment tool. *Pediatr Nurs* 1985; 11:349.

Stanhope M, Lancaster J: *Community Health Nursing: Process and Practice for Promoting Health.* St. Louis: Mosby, 1988.

The battered woman: Breaking the cycle of abuse. *Emerg Med* June 15, 1989, p 104.

Tilden UR, Shepherd P: Battered women: The shadow side of families. *Holistic Nurs Pract* 1987; 1(2):25.

Tripp-Reimer T: Retention of a folk health practice among four generations of urban Greek immigrants. *Nurs Res* 1983; 32:97.

U.S. Bureau of the Census: *Statistical Abstract of the United States.* Washington DC: Government Printing Office, 1987.

Walker LE: *The Battered Woman.* New York: Harper & Row, 1979.

Walker T: Mother-infant play. in Humenick S (editor): *Analysis of Current Assessment Strategies in the Health Care of Young Children and Childbearing Families.* New York: Appleton-Century-Crofts, 1982.

Wissow L: *Child Advocacy for the Clinician.* Baltimore, MD: Williams & Wilkins, 1990.

Additional Readings

Campbell DW: Family paradigm theory and family rituals: Implications for child and family health. *Nurse-Pract.* February 1991; 16:22.

Duvall EM, Miller BC: *Marriage and Family Development,* (6th ed). New York: Harper & Row, 1985.

Fox PG: Stress related to family change among Vietnamese refugees. *J Community Health Nurse.* 1991; 8(1):45.

Hammond J, Perez-Stable A, Ward CG: Predictive value of historical and physical characteristics for the diagnosis of child abuse. *South Med J* February 1991; 84:166.

Herrick CA: Neuman's Systems Model for nursing practice as a conceptual framework for a family assessment. *J Child Adolesc Psychiatr Ment Health Nurs* April/June 1989; 2:61.

Torres S: A comparison of wife abuse between two cultures: perceptions, attitudes, nature, and extent. *Issues Ment Health Nurs* January/March 1991; 12:113.

Wright LM, Leahey M: *Nurses and Families: A Guide to Family Assessment and Intervention.* Philadelphia: Davis, 1989.

CHAPTER 4

The Reproductive System

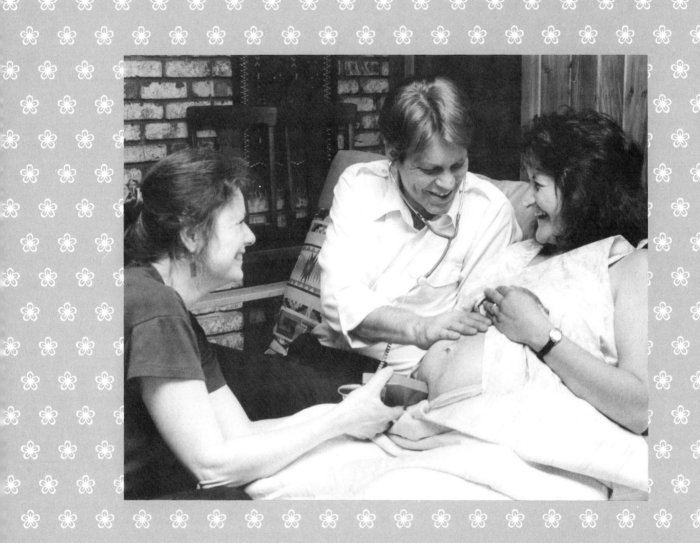

OBJECTIVES

Delineate the major changes in the reproductive system that occur during puberty.

Identify the structures and functions of the female and male reproductive systems.

Summarize the action of the hormones that affect reproductive functioning.

Describe the menstrual cycle, correlating the phases of the cycle with their dominant hormones and the changes that occur in each phase.

Explain the physiologic aspects of the female reproductive cycle.

Discuss the significance of specific female reproductive structures during childbirth.

ℐ always thought it was so boring to study anatomy and physiology. Who cares how many bones there are in the pelvis, or the muscles involved. But now I'm with mothers having babies and now it all makes sense. (A nursing student)

Understanding childbearing requires more than understanding sexual intercourse or the process by which the female and male sex cells unite. One must also become familiar with the structures and functions that make childbearing possible and the phenomena that initiate it. This chapter considers the anatomic, physiologic, and sexual aspects of the female and male reproductive systems. Information regarding basic embryologic development is also presented in order to increase understanding of anatomy, physiology, and function.

The female and male reproductive organs are *homologous*; that is, they are fundamentally similar in function and structure. The primary functions of both the female and male reproductive systems are to produce sex cells and to transport the sex cells to locations where their union can occur. The sex cells, called **gametes**, are produced by specialized organs called **gonads**. A series of ducts and glands within both the male and female reproductive systems contribute to the production and transport of the gametes.

Early Development of Reproductive Structures and Processes

Although the genetic sex of an embryo is determined at fertilization, for about the first eight weeks of gestation, the male and female reproductive systems are undifferentiated. This undifferentiated period is followed by a period of rapid, dramatic changes as the reproductive organs differentiate and develop into recognizable structures.

Ovaries and Testes

During the fifth week of gestation, a primitive gonad arises from the urogenital ridge. The gonad develops a medulla and cortex as primary sex cords appear in the underlying mesenchyme. In genetic males, during the seventh and eighth week the medulla develops into a testis, and the cortex regresses. In genetic females, by about the tenth week the cortex develops into an ovary and the medulla regresses.

The testis produces the male gametes, called **spermatozoa** or *sperm*, by a process called **spermatogenesis**. This process will be described in Chapter 11. Spermatogenesis of mature sperm does not occur until the onset of puberty.

Every egg available for maturation in a woman's reproductive life is present at her birth. During fetal life, the ovary produces *oogonia*, cells that become primitive eggs called *oocytes*, by the process of **oogenesis** (see Chapter 11). No oocytes are formed after fetal development. About 150,000 oocytes are contained in the ovaries at birth (Scott et al 1990). Each oocyte is contained in a small ovarian cavity called a *primitive follicle*.

During a female's reproductive years, every month one of the oocytes undergoes a process of cellular division and maturation that transforms it into a fertilizable egg, or **ovum**. At **ovulation**, the ovum is released from its follicle. The remaining follicles and oocytes degenerate over time.

Figure 4–1 illustrates the embryologic development of the gonads and other internal reproductive organs.

Other Internal Structures

During the undifferentiated, or indifferent period—the first seven weeks—two pairs of genital ducts develop: the *mesonephric* and *paramesonephric* ducts.

In genetic females, the fallopian tubes are formed from the unfused portions of the paramesonephric ducts, and the fused portions give rise to the epithelium and uterine glands. The endometrial stroma and the myometrium develop from the adjacent mesenchyme.

The vagina is derived from more than one embryologic structure. The vaginal epithelium develops from the

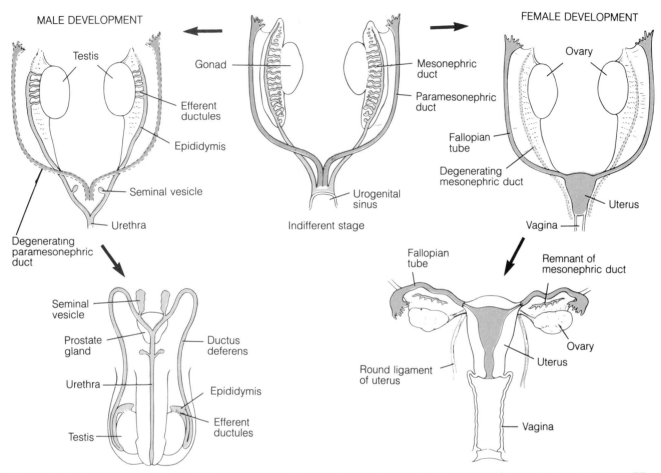

Figure 4–1 Embryonic differentiation of male and female internal reproductive organs (From Spence AP, Mason EB: Human Anatomy and Physiology, 3rd ed. Menlo Park, CA: Benjamin/Cummings, 1987.)

endoderm of the urogenital sinus, and the musculature develops from the uterovaginal primordium.

The urethral and paraurethral glands develop from outgrowths of the urethra into the surrounding mesenchyme. Bartholin's glands arise from similar structures.

In genetic males, the fetal testes secrete two hormones: Testosterone stimulates the mesonephric ducts to develop into the male genital tract, and the other hormone (müllerian regression factor) suppresses the development of the paramesonephric ducts, which would otherwise develop into the female genital tract.

From the mesonephric ducts comes development of the efferent ductule, vas deferens, epididymis, seminal vesicle, and ejaculatory duct. Both the prostate and the bulbourethral glands develop from endodermal outgrowths of the urethra.

External Structures

Genetic males and females possess the same external genitals until the end of the ninth week. By the twelfth week, differentiation of the external genitals is complete.

If fetal testosterone is not present, the indifferent external genitals are feminized. The phallus becomes the clitoris, and the urogenital folds remain open, forming the labia minora. The labioscrotal folds form the labia majora.

If fetal dihydrotestosterone is present, the indifferent external genitals become masculine. The phallus elongates, forming the penis. The fusion of the urogenital folds on the ventral surface of the penis forms the penile urethra, with the urethral meatus moving forward toward the glans penis.

Puberty

The term **puberty** refers to the developmental period between childhood and attainment of adult sexual characteristics and functioning. Its onset is never sudden, although it may appear so to parents or to the young person who is not prepared for the physical and emotional changes of puberty. Boys generally mature physically about two years later than girls. In boys the age of onset of puberty ranges from 10 to 19 years; 14 years is the average age of onset. In girls the age of onset ranges from 9 to 17 years; 12 years is the average age of onset.

Puberty occurs over a period lasting 1½ to 5 years and involves profound physical, psychologic, and emotional changes. These changes result from the interaction of the central nervous system and the endocrine organs.

Major Physical Changes

In both boys and girls, puberty is preceded by an accelerated growth rate called *adolescent spurt.* Widespread body system changes occur at this time, including maturation of the reproductive organs.

The pattern of physical changes varies among individuals. Girls experience a broadening of the hips, then budding of the breasts, the appearance of pubic and axillary hair, and the onset of menstruation, called **menarche.**

The average time between breast development and menarche is 2 years (Speroff et al 1989). The physical changes of puberty manifest themselves differently in every person. The age at onset and progress of puberty vary widely, physical changes overlap, and the sequence of events can also vary from person to person. This diversity results from people's different degrees of response to hormonal stimulation.

Boys usually first note such changes as an increase in the size of the external genitals; the appearance of pubic, axillary, and facial hair; the deepening of the voice; and nocturnal seminal emissions without sexual stimulation (mature sperm are not usually contained in these earliest emissions).

Physiology of Onset

Puberty is initiated by input from the central nervous system. The process, which begins during fetal life, is sequential and complex.

The central nervous system releases a neurotransmitter that stimulates the hypothalamus to synthesize and release **gonadotropin-releasing factor (GnRF)** (Tanner 1990). GnRF is transmitted to the anterior pituitary, where it causes the synthesis and secretion of the gonadotropins, **follicle-stimulating hormone (FSH)** and **luteinizing hormone (LH).**

Although the gonads do produce small amounts of estrogens (female sex hormones) and androgens (male sex hormones) before the onset of puberty, FSH and LH stimulate increased secretion of these hormones. Androgens and estrogens influence the development of secondary sex characteristics. FSH and LH stimulate the processes of spermatogenesis and maturation of ova.

Other hormones are involved in the onset of puberty. Although less direct, their action is essential. Abnormally high or low levels of adrenocorticotropic hormone (ACTH), thyroid hormone, or growth hormone (GH) can disrupt the onset of normal puberty (Tanner 1990).

Female Reproductive System

The female reproductive system consists of the external and internal genitals and the accessory organs of the breasts. The structure of the bony pelvis is also discussed in this section because of its importance in childbearing.

External Genitals

All the external reproductive organs, except the glandular structures, can be directly inspected. The size, color, and shape of these structures vary extensively among races and individuals.

The female external genitals, referred to as the **vulva** or pudendum, include the following structures (Figure 4–2):
- Mons pubis
- Labia majora
- Labia minora
- Clitoris
- Urethral meatus and opening of the paraurethral (Skene's) glands
- Vaginal vestibule (vaginal orifice, vulvovaginal glands, hymen, and fossa navicularis)
- Perineal body

Although not true parts of the female reproductive system, the urethral meatus and perineal body are considered here because of their proximity and relationship to the vulva.

The vulva has a generous supply of blood and nerves and is influenced by estrogenic hormones. As a woman ages, hormonal activity decreases, causing the vulvar organs to atrophy and become subject to a variety of lesions.

Mons Pubis
The *mons pubis* is a softly rounded mound of subcutaneous fatty tissue beginning at the lowest portion of the anterior abdominal wall. Also known as the mons veneris, this structure covers the anterior portion of the symphysis pubis. The mons pubis is covered with pubic hair, typically with the hairline forming a transverse line across the lower abdomen (Figure 4–2). The hair is short and varies from sparse and fine in the Asian woman to heavy, coarse, and curly in the black woman.

The mons pubis protects the pelvic bones, especially during coitus.

Labia Majora
The *labia majora* are longitudinal, raised folds of pigmented skin, one on either side of the vulvar cleft (Figure 4–2). As the pair descend, they narrow, enclosing the vulvar cleft, and merge to form the posterior junction of the perineal skin.

With each pregnancy, the labia majora become less prominent. The labia majora are covered by stratified squamous epithelium containing hair follicles and sebaceous glands with underlying adipose and muscle tissue. Immediately under the skin is a sheet of dartos muscle, which is responsible for the wrinkled appearance of the labia majora as well as for their sensitivity to heat and cold.

The inner surface of the labia majora in women who have not had children is moist and looks like a mucous membrane, but after many births it is more skinlike (Cunningham et al 1989).

Arterial blood is supplied by the internal and external pudendal arteries. Because of the extensive venous network in the labia majora, varicosities may occur during pregnancy and obstetric or sexual trauma may cause hematomas.

The labia majora share an extensive and diffuse lymphatic supply with the other structures of the vulva. Understanding this supply is important in understanding malignancies of the female reproductive organs. Because of the nerves supplying the labia majora (from the first lumbar and third sacral segment of the spinal cord) certain regional anesthesia blocks will affect them.

The chief function of the labia majora is protection of the structures lying between them.

Labia Minora

The *labia minora* are soft folds of skin within the labia majora that converge near the anus, forming the *fourchette* (Figure 4–2).

Each labium minus has the appearance of shiny mucous membrane, moist and devoid of hair follicles. The labia minora are rich in sebaceous glands. Because sebaceous glands do not open into hair follicles but directly onto the surface of the skin, sebaceous cysts are common in this area. The labia minora are composed of erectile tissue containing loose connective tissue, blood vessels, numerous large venous spaces, and involuntary muscle tissue. Vulvovaginitis in this area is very irritating because of the many tactile nerve endings.

The functions of the labia minora are to lubricate and waterproof the vulvar skin and to provide bactericidal secretions. The labia minora increase in size at puberty and decrease after menopause due to changes in estrogen levels.

Clitoris

The clitoris is the most erotically sensitive part of the female genital tract and is a common site of masturbation. The clitoris, located between the labia minora, is about 5 to 6 mm long and 6 to 8 mm across. Its tissue is essentially erectile.

The clitoris consists of the glans, the corpus or body, and two crura (Figure 4–2). The glans is partially covered by a fold of skin called the *prepuce*. This area often appears as an opening to an orifice, and may be confused with the urethral meatus. Attempts to insert a catheter here produce extreme discomfort.

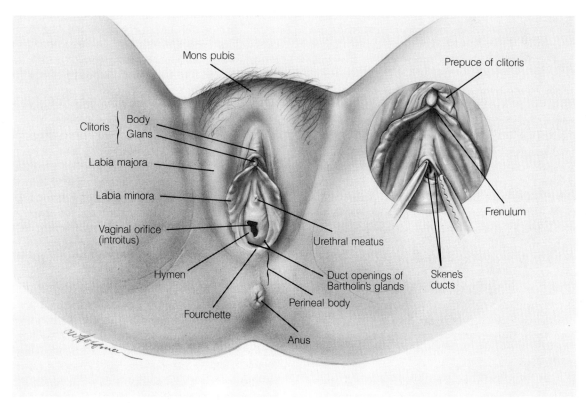

Figure 4–2 Female external genitals, longitudinal view

The clitoris has very rich blood and nerve supplies. Overall, the clitoris has a richer nerve supply than the penis.

The clitoris exists primarily for female sexual enjoyment. In addition, it produces *smegma.* Along with other vulval secretions, smegma has a unique odor that may be sexually stimulating to the male.

Urethral Meatus and Paraurethral Glands

The *urethral meatus* is located 1 to 2.5 cm beneath the clitoris in the midline of the vestibule (Figure 4–2). At times the meatus is difficult to see because of the presence of blind dimples, small mucosal folds, or wide variance in location. Its appearance is often puckered and slitlike.

The *paraurethral glands*, or *Skene's glands*, open into the posterior wall of the urethra close to its orifice (Figure 4–2). Their secretions help lubricate the vaginal vestibule, facilitating sexual intercourse.

Vaginal Vestibule

The vaginal vestibule is a boat-shaped depression enclosed by the labia majora and visible when they are separated. The vestibule contains the vaginal opening, or *introitus*, which is the border between the external and internal genitals.

The **hymen** is a thin, elastic membrane that partially closes the vaginal opening. Its strength, shape, and size vary greatly among women. The hymen is essentially avascular. The belief that the intact hymen is a sign of virginity and that it is broken at first sexual intercourse with resultant bleeding is not valid. The hymen can be broken through strenuous physical activity, masturbation, menstruation, or the use of tampons. Once it is broken, the irregular tags of tissue that remain are called the myrtiform or hymenal carbuncles.

External to the hymenal ring at the base of the vestibule are two small papular elevations containing the orifices of the ducts of the *vulvovaginal (Bartholin's) glands.* They lie under the constrictor muscle of the vagina. The vulvovaginal glands are not generally palpable upon examination, being placed deep in the perineal structures. These glands secrete a clear and viscous mucus with an alkaline pH that enhances the viability and motility of sperm deposited in the vaginal vestibule.

These ducts of the vulvovaginal glands can harbor *Neisseria gonorrhoeae* and other bacteria, which can cause suppuration and Bartholin's gland abscesses (Cunningham et al 1989).

Innervation of the vestibular area is mainly by the perineal nerve from the sacral plexus. The area is not sensitive to touch generally; however, the hymen contains numerous free nerve endings as receptors to pain.

Perineal Body

The **perineal body** is a wedge-shaped mass of fibromuscular tissue, measuring about $4 \times 4 \times 4$ cm, found between the lower part of the vagina and the anal canal (Figure 4–2). This area between the anus and the vagina is referred to as the **perineum**.

The muscles that meet at the perineal body are the external sphincter ani, both levator ani (the superficial and deep transverse perineal) and the bulbocavernosus. These muscles mingle with elastic fibers and connective tissue in an arrangement that allows a remarkable amount of stretching.

The perineal body is much larger in the female than in the male. It is subject to laceration and is the site of episiotomy during childbirth (see Chapter 26).

Internal Genitals

The female internal reproductive organs—the vagina, uterus, fallopian tubes, and ovaries—are target organs for estrogenic hormones. These organs play a unique part in the reproductive cycle (Figure 4–3). The internal reproductive organs can be palpated during vaginal examination and assessed through use of a speculum, laparoscope, or culdoscope.

Vagina

The **vagina** is a muscular and membranous tube that connects the external genitals with the center of the pelvis (Figure 4–3). It extends from the vulva to the uterus in a position nearly parallel to the plane of the pelvic brim. The vagina is often referred to as the *birth canal* because it forms the lower part of the axis through which the presenting part of the fetus must pass during birth.

Because the cervix of the uterus projects into the upper part of the anterior wall of the vagina, the anterior wall is approximately 2.5 cm shorter than the posterior wall. Measurements range from 6 to 8 cm for the anterior wall and 7 to 10 cm for the posterior wall.

In the upper part of the vagina, which is called the vaginal vault, there is a recess or hollow around the cervix. The area is referred to as the vaginal *fornix.*

The walls of the vaginal vault are very thin. This thinness facilitates pelvic examination. Various structures can be palpated through the walls and fornix of the vaginal vault, including the uterus, a distended bladder, the ovaries, the appendix, the cecum, the colon, and the ureters.

When a woman lies on her back, the space in the fornix permits the pooling of semen after intercourse. The collection of a large number of sperm near the cervix in a favorable environment increases the chances of impregnation.

The walls of the vagina are covered with ridges, or **rugae**, crisscrossing each other. These rugae allow the vagina to stretch during the descent of the fetal head.

A rich blood supply is needed to maintain a high glycogen content in the epithelial cells as well as to nourish the underlying musculofascial layer, through which the vaginal vault has strong attachments to the cervix. These muscle layers are continuous with the superficial muscle fibers of the uterus. A thin band of striated muscle, the sphincter vaginae, is found at the lowest extremity of the vagina. However, the levator ani is the principal muscle that closes the vagina.

During a woman's reproductive life, an acidic vaginal environment is normal (pH 4.0 to 5.0). Secretion from the vaginal epithelium provides a moist environment. The acidic environment is maintained by a symbiotic relationship between lactic acid-producing bacilli (Döderlein bacillus or lactobacillus) and the vaginal epithelial cells. These cells contain glycogen, which is broken down by the bacilli into lactic acid. The amount of glycogen is regulated by the ovarian hormones. Any interruption of this process can destroy the normal self-cleansing action of the vagina. Such interruption may be caused by antibiotic therapy, douching, or use of vaginal sprays or deodorants. For further discussion, see Chapter 7.

The acidic vaginal environment is normal only during the mature reproductive years and in the first days of life when maternal hormones are operating in the infant. A relatively neutral pH of 7.5 is normal from infancy until puberty and after menopause.

Each third of the vagina is supplied by a distinct vascular and lymphatic pattern. Venous drainage is accomplished by the venous plexus, which is also anastomosed to the vertebral venous plexus. This anastomosis makes it possible for a pelvic embolism or carcinoma to bypass the heart and lungs and lodge in the brain, spine, or other remote part of the body.

Lymphatic drainage in the upper third of the vagina drains into the external and internal iliac nodes; the middle third, into the hypogastric nodes; and the lower third, into the inguinal glands. The posterior wall drains into nodes lying in the rectovaginal septum. Any vaginal infection follows these routes.

The vagina is a relatively insensitive organ, with meager somatic innervation to its lower third by the pudendal nerve and virtually no special nerve endings. Sensation during sexual excitement and coitus is minimal and pain during the second stage of labor is less than if somatic innervation were greater. Nervous supply to the vagina is predominantly autonomic.

The vagina functions to:

- Serve as the passage for sperm and for the fetus during birth.
- Provide passage for the menstrual products from the uterine endometrium to the outside of the body
- Protect against trauma from sexual intercourse and infection from pathogenic organisms

Uterus

As the core of reproduction and hence continuation of the human race, the uterus, or womb, has been endowed with a mystical aura. Numerous customs, taboos, mores, and values have evolved about women and their reproductive function. Although scientific knowledge has replaced much of this folklore, remnants of old ideas and superstitions persist. The nurse must be able to recognize and deal with such attitudes and beliefs so that nursing care can be effective.

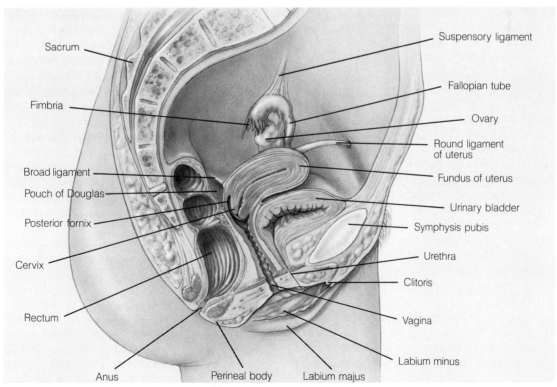

Figure 4–3 Female internal reproductive organs

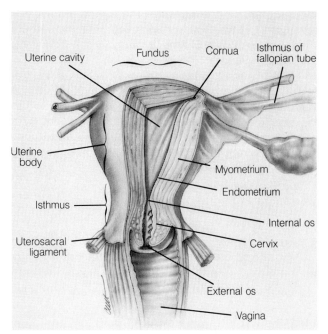

Figure 4–4   Structures of the uterus

The **uterus** is a hollow, muscular, thick-walled, pear-shaped organ lying centrally in the pelvic cavity between the base of the bladder and the rectum and above the vagina (Figure 4–4). It is level with or slightly below the brim of the pelvis, with the external opening of the cervix (the external os) about the level of the ischial spines. The mature organ weighs about 60 g and is approximately 7.5 cm long, 5 cm wide, and 1 to 2.5 cm thick.

Many uterine anomalies are thought to be congenital. Between the sixth and ninth week of embryonic development, the paramesonephric ducts, which are adjacent to the mesonephric ducts, grow caudally (toward the head). Their ultimate fusion gives rise to the fallopian tubes, uterine fundus, cervix, and upper vagina. A normal uterus therefore requires two symmetric, parallel, equal-sized paramesonephric ducts to meet in the midline. Anomalies represent the absence of either one or both of the ducts, degrees of failure to fuse, or canalization defects. Uterine malformations such as the bicornuate ("two-horned") and didelphys ("double uterus") uterus are associated with habitual abortion. Because both the urinary and reproductive systems develop from the common urogenital fold in the embryo, anomalies in one system are frequently accompanied by anomalies in the other. Problems of infertility and premature labor and birth are common.

The uterus is kept in place by three sets of supports. The upper supports are the broad and round ligaments. The middle supports are the cardinal, pubocervical, and uterosacral ligaments. The lower supports are those structures considered to be the pelvic muscular floor.

The position of the uterus can vary, depending on a woman's posture, number of children borne, bladder and rectal fullness, and even normal respiratory patterns. Only

the cervix is anchored laterally. The body of the uterus can move freely forward or backward. The axis also varies. The uterus generally bends forward, forming a sharp angle with the vagina. There is a bend in the area of the isthmus of the uterus; from there the cervix points downward. The uterus is said to be anteverted when it is in this position. The anteverted position is considered normal.

The isthmus, referred to earlier in this section, is a slight constriction in the uterus that divides it into two unequal parts. The upper two-thirds of the uterus is the **corpus**, or body, composed mainly of a smooth muscle layer (myometrium). The lower third is the **cervix**, or neck. The rounded uppermost portion of the corpus that extends above the points of attachment of the fallopian tubes is called the **fundus**. The elongated portion of the uterus where the fallopian tubes open is called the **cornua**.

The isthmus is about 6 mm above the internal os, and it is in this area that the uterine endometrium changes into the mucous membrane of the cervix. The isthmus takes on importance in pregnancy because it becomes the lower uterine segment. With the cervix, it is a passive segment and not part of the contractile uterus. At birth, this thin lower segment, situated behind the bladder, is the site for lower-segment cesarean births (see Chapter 26).

The blood and lymphatic supplies to the uterus are extensive (Figure 4–5). Innervation of the uterus is entirely by the autonomic nervous system and seems to be more regulatory than primary in nature. Even without an intact nerve supply, the uterus can contract adequately for birth, as illustrated by the fact that hemiplegic women have adequate uterine contractions.

Pain of uterine contractions is carried to the central nervous system by the eleventh and twelfth thoracic nerve roots. Pain from the cervix and upper vagina passes through the ilioinguinal and pudendal nerves. The motor fibers to the uterus arise from the seventh and eighth thoracic vertebrae. Because the sensory and motor levels are separate, caudal and spinal anesthesia can be used during labor and birth.

The function of the uterus is to provide a safe environment for fetal development. The uterine lining is cyclically prepared by steroid hormones for implantation of the embryo (nidation). Once the embryo is implanted, the developing fetus is protected until it is expelled.

Both the body of the uterus and the cervix are changed permanently by pregnancy. The body never returns to its prepregnant size, and the external os changes from a circular opening of about 3 mm to a transverse slit with irregular edges.

The Corpus   The corpus of the uterus is made up of three layers. The outermost layer is the *serosal layer* or **perimetrium**, which is composed of peritoneum. The middle layer is the *muscular uterine layer* or myometrium. This muscular uterine layer is continuous with the muscle layer of the fallopian tubes and with that of the vagina. This helps these organs present a unified reaction to various stimuli—ovulation, orgasm, or the deposit of sperm in the vagina. These muscle fibers also extend into the ovarian, round, and cardinal ligaments and minimally into the uterosacral ligaments, which helps explain the vague but disturbing pelvic "aches and pains" reported by many pregnant women.

The myometrium has three distinct layers of uterine (smooth) involuntary muscles (Figure 4–6). The outer layer, found mainly over the fundus, is made up of longitudinal muscles especially suited to expel the fetus during birth. The middle layer is thick and made up of interlacing muscle fibers in figure eight patterns. These muscle fibers surround large blood vessels, and their contraction pro-

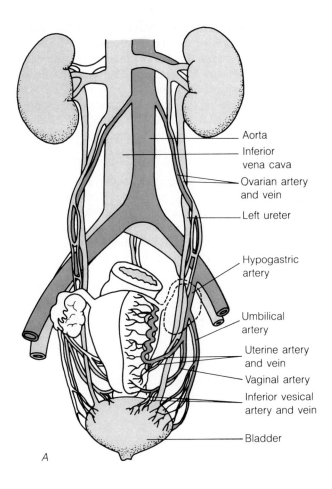

A

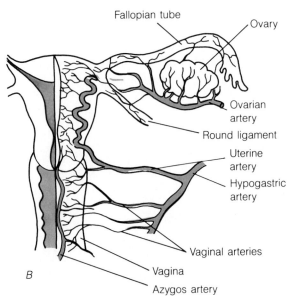

B

Figure 4–5   Blood supply to internal reproductive organs: A Pelvic blood supply. B Blood supply to vagina, ovary, uterus, and fallopian tubes

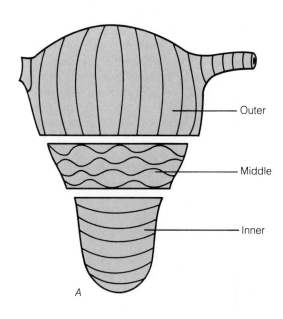

A

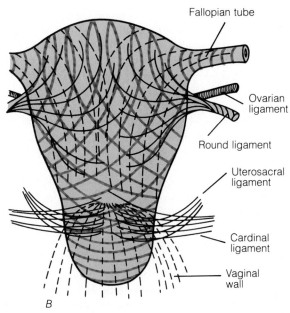

B

Figure 4–6   Uterine muscle layers: A Muscle fiber placement B Interlacing of uterine muscle layers

duces a hemostatic action. The inner muscle layer is made up of circular fibers, which form sphincters at the fallopian tube attachment sites and at the internal os. The internal os sphincter inhibits the expulsion of the uterine contents during pregnancy but stretches in labor as cervical dilatation occurs. An incompetent cervical os can be caused by a torn, weak, or absent sphincter at the internal os. The sphincters at the fallopian tubes prevent menstrual blood from flowing backward into the fallopian tubes from the uterus.

Although each layer of muscle has been discussed as having a unique function, it must be remembered that the uterine musculature works as a whole. The uterine contractions of labor are responsible for the dilatation of the cervix and provide the major force for the passage of the fetus through the pelvic axis and vaginal canal at birth. The mucosal layer, or **endometrium,** of the uterine corpus is the innermost layer. This layer is composed of a single layer of columnar epithelium, glands, and stroma. From menarche to menopause, the endometrium undergoes monthly degeneration and renewal in the absence of pregnancy. As it responds to a governing hormonal cycle and prostaglandin influence as well, the endometrium varies in thickness from 0.5 to 5 mm.

The glands of the endometrium produce a thin, watery, alkaline secretion that keeps the uterine cavity moist. This "*endometrial milk*" not only assists the sperm on their journey to the fallopian tubes but also provides nourishment to the blastocyst prior to implantation in the endometrium (Chapter 11).

The unique blood supply to the endometrium is important. In the myometrium, the radial arteries branch off from the arcuate arteries at right angles. Once inside the endometrium, they become the basal arteries supplying the zona basalis (a layer of the endometrium) and ultimately become the coiled arteries supplying the zona functionalis (also part of the endometrium). The straighter basal arteries are smaller than the coiled arteries; they are not sensitive to cyclic hormonal control. Hence the zona basalis portion remains intact and is the site of new endometrial tissue generation. The coiled arteries are extremely sensitive to cyclic hormonal control. Their response is alternate relaxation and constriction during the ischemic or terminal phase of the menstrual cycle. This response allows for other endometrial tissue to be shed during menstruation.

When pregnancy occurs and the endometrium is not shed, the reticular stromal cells surrounding the endometrial glands become the decidual cells of pregnancy. The stromal cells are highly vascular, channeling a rich blood supply to the endometrial surface.

The Cervix The cervix is about 2.5 cm in both length and diameter. It is canal-like; its exit into the vagina is called the **external os**, and its entrance into the corpus is called the **internal os** (Figure 4–4).

The cervix is a protective portal for the body of the uterus as well as the connection between the vagina and the uterus. The cervix is divided by its line of attachment into the vaginal and supravaginal areas. The *vaginal cervix* projects into the vagina at an angle of from 45° to 90° and ends at the external os. The *supravaginal cervix* is surrounded by the attachments that give the uterus its main support: the uterosacral ligaments, the transverse ligaments of the cervix (Mackenrodt's ligaments), and the pubocervical ligaments.

The vaginal cervix appears pink. The cervical canal appears rosy red and is lined with columnar ciliated epithelium, which contain mucus-secreting glands. Most cervical cancer begins at this squamocolumnar junction. Its exact location varies with age and number of pregnancies. Figure 4–7 shows this junction at various stages of a woman's life.

The cervix is highly elastic as a result of the high fibrous and collagenous content of the supportive tissues and the vast number of folds in the cervical lining.

The cervical mucosa has three functions: (1) to provide lubrication for the vaginal canal, (2) to act as a bacteriostatic agent, and (3) to provide an alkaline environment to shelter deposited sperm from the acidic vagina. At ovulation, cervical mucus is clearer, thinner, and more alkaline than at other times.

Uterine Ligaments The uterine ligaments support and stabilize the various reproductive organs. The ligaments shown in Figures 4–6 and 4–8 are described in this section.

1. The **broad ligament** keeps the uterus centrally placed and provides stability within the pelvic cavity. It is a double mesenteric layer that is continuous with the abdominal peritoneum. The broad ligament covers the uterus anteriorly and posteriorly and extends outward from the uterus to enfold and stabilize the fallopian tubes. The round

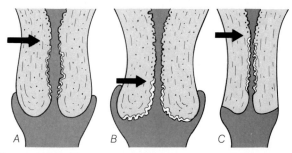

Figure 4–7 Changes in squamocolumnar function (arrows) at various stages of life. A Childhood. B Reproductive years. C Post-menopausal years (Modified from Beller FK et al: Gynecology: A Textbook for Students, 3rd ed. New York: Springer-Verlag, 1980, p 34.)

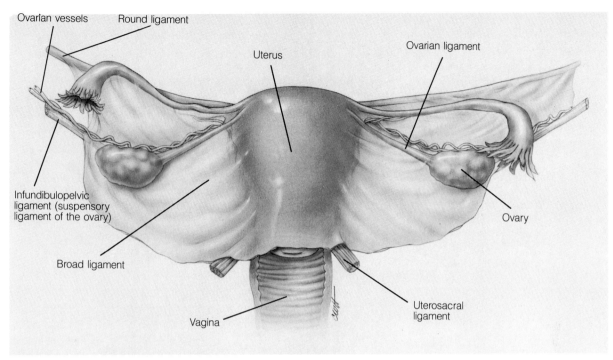

Figure 4–8   Uterine ligaments (cardinal ligaments not shown)

and ovarian ligaments are at the upper border of the broad ligament. At its lower border, it forms the cardinal ligaments. Between the folds of the broad ligament are connective tissue, involuntary muscle, blood and lymph vessels, and nerves.

2. The **round ligaments** help the broad ligament keep the uterus in place. Each of the round ligaments arises from the sides of the uterus near the fallopian tube insertion. They extend outward between the folds of the broad ligament, passing through the inguinal ring and canals and eventually fusing with the connective tissue of the labia majora. The round ligaments are made up of longitudinal muscle and enlarge during pregnancy. During labor the round ligaments steady the uterus, pulling downward and forward, so that the presenting part of the fetus is forced into the cervix.

3. The **ovarian ligaments** anchor the lower pole of the ovary to the cornua of the uterus. They are composed of muscle fibers that allow the ligaments to contract. This contractile ability influences the position of the ovary to some extent, thus helping the fimbriae of the fallopian tubes to "catch" the ovum as it is released each month.

4. The **cardinal ligaments** are the chief uterine supports, suspending the uterus from the side walls of the true pelvis. These ligaments, also known as *Mackenrodt's*, or *transverse cervical ligaments*, arise from the sides of the pelvic walls and attach

to the cervix in the upper vagina. These ligaments prevent uterine prolapse and also support the upper vagina.

5. The **infundibulopelvic ligament** suspends and supports the ovaries. Arising from the outer third of the broad ligament, the infundibulopelvic ligament contains the ovarian vessels and nerves.

6. The **uterosacral ligaments** provide support for the uterus and cervix at the level of the ischial spines. Arising on each side of the pelvis from the posterior wall of the uterus, the uterosacral ligaments sweep back around the rectum and insert on the sides of the first and second sacral vertebrae. The uterosacral ligaments contain smooth muscle fibers, connective tissue, blood and lymph vessels, and nerves. Providing support for the uterus and cervix at the level of the ischial spines, they also contain sensory nerve fibers that contribute to dysmenorrhea.

Fallopian Tubes

The **fallopian tubes**, also known as *oviducts*, arise from each side of the uterus and reach almost to the side of the pelvis, where they turn toward the ovaries (Figure 4–9). Each tube is 8 to 13.5 cm long, lying in the superior border of the broad ligament (mesosalpinx). A short section of each fallopian tube is inside the uterus; its opening into the uterus is 1 mm in diameter. The fallopian tubes link the peritoneal cavity with the external environment through

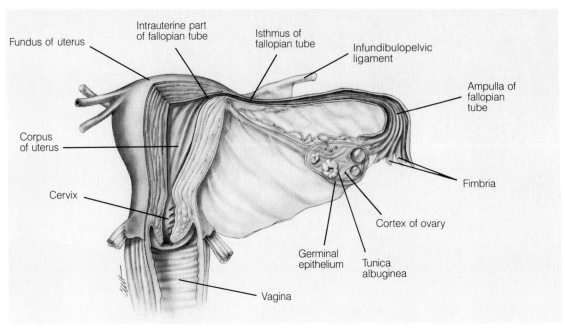

Figure 4–9   Fallopian tube and ovary

the uterus and vagina. This linkage increases a woman's biologic vulnerability to disease processes.

Each tube may be divided into three parts: the isthmus, the ampulla, and the infundibulum or fimbria. The **isthmus** is straight and narrow, with a thick muscular wall and an opening (lumen) 2 to 3 mm in diameter. It is the site of tubal ligation (a surgical procedure to prevent pregnancy; see Chapter 7).

Next to the isthmus is the curved **ampulla**, which comprises the outer two-thirds of the tube. Fertilization of the secondary oocyte by a spermatozoon usually occurs here. The ampulla ends at the fimbria, which is a funnel-like enlargement with many moving fingerlike projections (fimbriae) reaching out to the ovary. The longest of these, the *fimbria ovarica,* is attached to the ovary to increase the chances of intercepting the ovum as it is released.

The wall of the fallopian tube is made up of four layers: peritoneal (serous), subserous (adventitial), muscular, and mucous tissues. The peritoneum covers the tubes. The subserous layer contains the blood and nerve supply, and the muscular layer is responsible for the peristaltic movement of the tube. The mucosal layer, immediately next to the muscular layer, is composed of ciliated and nonciliated cells with the number of ciliated cells more abundant at the fimbria. Nonciliated cells are goblet cells that secrete a protein-rich, serous fluid that nourishes the ovum. The constantly moving tubal cilia propel the ovum toward the uterus. Because the ovum is a large cell, this ciliary action is needed to assist the tube's muscular layer peristalsis. Any malformation or malfunction of the tubes could result in infertility or even sterility.

A well-functioning tubal transport system involves active fimbriae close to the ovary; peristalsis of the tube

created by the muscular layer; ciliated currents beating toward the uterus; and the proximal contraction and distal relaxation of the tube caused by different types of prostaglandins (Scott et al 1990).

Each fallopian tube is richly supplied with blood by the uterine and ovarian arteries. Thus the fallopian tubes have an unusual ability to recover from any inflammatory process. Lymphatic drainage occurs through the vessels close to the ureter into the lumbar nodes along the aorta. The functions of the fallopian tubes are as follows: to provide transport for the ovum from the ovary to the uterus (transport through the fallopian tubes varies from 3 to 4 days); to act as a site for fertilization; and to serve as a warm, moist, nourishing environment for the ovum or *zygote* (a fertilized egg; see Chapter 11).

Ovaries

The *ovaries* are two almond-shaped glandular structures just below the pelvic brim. One ovary is located on each side of the pelvic cavity. Their size varies among women and according to the stage of the menstrual cycle. Each ovary weighs 6 to 10 g and is 1.5 to 3 cm wide, 2 to 5 cm long, and 1 to 1.5 cm thick. The ovaries of girls are small but become larger after puberty. They also change in appearance from a smooth-surfaced, dull white organ to a pitted gray organ because of scarring due to ovulation. It is rare for both ovaries to be at the same level in the pelvic cavity. The ovary is held in place by the ovarian, broad, and infundibulopelvic ligaments (Figure 4–8) which were discussed earlier in the chapter.

There is no peritoneal covering for the ovaries. Although this lack of covering assists the mature ovum to erupt, it also allows easier spread of malignant cells from

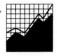

Research Note

Clinical Application of Research

Premenstrual syndrome (PMS) consists of a set of cyclically recurring symptoms which may be grouped in one of four categories: anxiety, edema, appetite, and depression. Ruth Seideman (1990) theorized that a health education program, based at least in part on Orem's theory of self-care, would reduce the symptoms of PMS.

Forty-seven women with moderate to severe PMS kept health diaries about their PMS symptoms for 3 months prior to being randomly assigned to either a control group or an experimental group. The experimental group then participated in a PMS educational program that primarily included information about nutritional treatment of the syndrome.

The author used analysis of covariance (ANCOVA) to determine if the change that occurred in the experimental group was due to the nutritional treatment or to a preexisting difference in the two groups. Findings included a significant difference between the experimental group and the control group. The experimental group had a reduction in occurrence of PMS symptoms associated with anxiety and appetite, as well as a reduction in severity of symptoms related to edema and a decrease in the number of days with premenstrual symptoms.

Critical Thinking Applied to Research

Strengths: Related findings back to conceptual framework and recommended a larger sample size for future study.

Concerns: With both groups coming from the same workplace, there could have been some sharing of information which might have diluted the effect of the treatment. When interpreting ANCOVA, the degree of freedom for the groups are the number of groups minus one, or in this case, two minus one (Munro et al, 1986). The author used $F_2(44)$ instead of $F_1(44)$.

Munro B, Visintainer M, Page E: *Statistical methods for health care research.* Philadelphia: Lippincott, 1986.

Seideman R: Effects of a premenstrual syndrome education program on premenstrual symptomatology. *Health Care Women Internat* 1990; 11:491.

cancer of the ovaries. A single layer of cuboidal epithelial cells, called the germinal epithelium, covers the ovaries. The ovaries are composed of three layers: the tunica albuginea, the cortex, and the medulla. The *tunica albuginea* is dense and dull white and serves as a protective layer. The *cortex* is the main functional part because it contains ova, graafian follicles, corpora lutea, degenerated corpora lutea (corpora albicantia), and degenerated follicles. The *me-*

dulla is completely surrounded by the cortex and contains the nerves and the blood and lymphatic vessels. The ovaries are relatively insensitive unless they are squeezed or distended.

The ovary is a crucial component of reproduction. Even a small part of a functioning ovary will ovulate, providing an ovum for fertilization monthly. Close to a million oocytes are locked in the first meiotic division at birth. See Chapter 11 for a more detailed discussion of meiotic division.

The ovaries are the primary source of two important hormones: the estrogens and progesterone. *Estrogens* are associated with those characteristics contributing to femaleness including breast alveolar lobule growth and duct development. The ovaries secrete large amounts of estrogen, while the adrenal cortex (extraglandular sites) produces minute amounts of estrogen in nonpregnant women.

Progesterone is often called the *hormone of pregnancy* because its effects on the uterus allow pregnancy to be maintained. This hormone also inhibits the action of prolactin in α-lactalbumin synthesis, thereby preventing lactation during pregnancy (Cunningham et al 1989).

The interplay between the ovarian hormones and other hormones such as FSH and LH is responsible for the cyclic changes that allow pregnancy to occur. The hormonal and physical changes that occur during the female reproductive cycle will be discussed later in this chapter. When a woman reaches the age of 45 to 55 years, the ovaries no longer secrete estrogen. Ovulatory activity ceases and menopause occurs.

Bony Pelvis

The female *bony pelvis* has two unique functions:

- To support and protect the pelvic contents
- To form the relatively fixed axis of the birth passage

Because the structural aspects of the pelvis are so important to childbearing, its structures must be understood clearly.

Bony Structure

The pelvis is made up of four bones: two innominate bones, the sacrum, and the coccyx. The pelvis resembles a bowl or basin; its sides are the innominate bones, and its back is composed of the sacrum and coccyx. Lined with fibrocartilage and held tightly together by ligaments, the four bones join at the symphysis pubis, the two sacroiliac joints, and the sacrococcygeal joints (Figure 4–10).

The **innominate bones,** also known as the *hip bones* or *os coxae*, are made up of three separate bones: the ilium, the ischium, and the pubis. These bones fuse to form a circular cavity, the *acetabulum,* which articulates with the femur.

The *ilium* is the broad, upper prominence of the hip. The *iliac crest* is the margin of the ilium. The *iliac spine,*

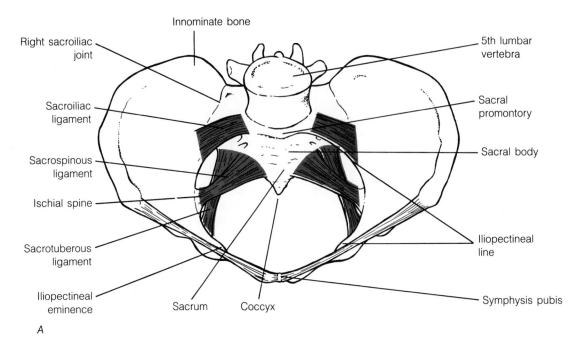

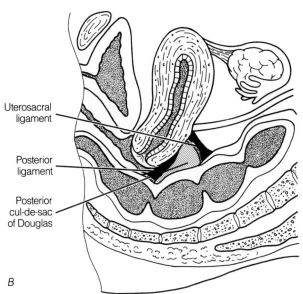

Figure 4–10 Pelvic bones A With supporting ligaments B Midsagittal view in supine position

the foremost projection nearest the groin, is the site of attachment for ligaments and muscles.

The *ischium*, the strongest bone, is under the ilium and below the acetabulum. the L-shaped ischium ends in a marked protuberance, the *ischial tuberosity*, on which the weight of a seated body rests. The **ischial spines** arise near the junction of the ilium and ischium and jut into the pelvic cavity. The shortest diameter of the pelvic cavity is between the ischial spines. The ischial spines can serve as a reference point during labor to evaluate the descent of the fetal head into the birth canal.

The **pubis** forms the slightly bowed front portion of the innominate bone. Extending medially from the acetabulum to the midpoint of the bony pelvis, the two pubic bones meet to form a joint, the **symphysis pubis**. The triangular space below this junction is known as the *pubic arch*. The fetal head passes under this arch during birth. The symphysis pubis is formed by heavy fibrocartilage and the superior and inferior pubic ligaments. The mobility of the inferior ligament, also known as the *arcuate pubic ligament*, increases during pregnancy and to a greater extent in subsequent pregnancies than in first pregnancies.

The sacroiliac joints also have a degree of mobility that increases near the end of pregnancy as the result of an upward gliding movement. The pelvic outlet may be increased by 1.5 to 2 cm in the squatting, sitting, and dorsal lithotomy positions. These relaxations of the joints are induced by the hormones of pregnancy.

The *sacrum* is a wedge-shaped bone formed by the fusion of five vertebrae. On the anterior upper portion of the sacrum is a projection into the pelvic cavity known as the **sacral promontory**. This projection is another obstetric guide in determining pelvic measurements. (For further discussion of pelvic measurements, see Chapter 13.)

The small triangular bone last on the vertebral column is the *coccyx*. It articulates with the sacrum at the sacrococcygeal joint. The coccyx usually moves backward during labor to provide more room for the fetus.

Pelvic Floor

The muscular **pelvic floor** is designed to overcome the force of gravity exerted on the pelvic organs. It acts as a buttress to the irregularly shaped pelvic outlet, thereby providing stability and support for surrounding structures.

Deep fascia and the levator ani and coccygeal muscles form the part of the pelvic floor known as the **pelvic dia-**

phragm. Above it is the pelvic cavity; below and behind it is the perineum. Laterally, the walls of the pelvis are composed of the obturator internus muscles and fascia, which form a band called the arcus tendineus. The sacrum is located posteriorly.

The *levator ani muscle* makes up the major portion of the pelvic diaphragm and consists of four muscles: ileococcygeus, pubococcygeus, puborectalis, and pubovaginalis. Forming a sling for the pelvic structures, the levator ani is interrupted by the urethra, vagina, and rectum. The ileococcygeal muscle, a thin muscular sheet underlying the sacrospinous ligament, assists the levator ani to support the abdominal and pelvic organs. Muscles of the pelvic floor are shown in Figure 4–11 and discussed in Table 4–1. Endopelvic fascia covers the pelvic diaphragm. The component parts function as a whole, yet they are able to move over one another. This feature provides an exceptional capacity for dilatation during birth and return to pre-pregnant condition following birth.

The *urogenital triangle* (diaphragm) is external to the pelvic diaphragm, in the triangular area between the ischial tuberosities and the hollow of the pubic arch. It is made up of superficial and deep perineal membranes. Most tending from the rami of the ischial and pubic bones. Most important in this region are the deep transverse perineal muscles, which are flat bands of muscle arising from the ischiopubic rami and intertwining in the midline to form a seam, or raphe. These muscles are modified to encircle both the urinary meatus and the vaginal orifice, forming the urethral and vaginal sphincters.

Pelvic Division

The pelvic cavity is divided into the false pelvis and the true pelvis (Figure 4–12).

The **false pelvis** is the portion above the pelvic brim, or linea terminalis, bounded by the lumbar vertebrae posteriorly, the iliac fossae laterally, and the lower abdominal wall anteriorly. Its primary function is to support the weight of the enlarged pregnant uterus and direct the presenting fetal part into the true pelvis below.

The **true pelvis** lies below the pelvic brim and is bounded above by the promontory and alae of the sacrum and the upper margins of the pubic bones and below by the pelvic outlet. The true pelvis represents the bony limits of the birth canal. It measures about 5 cm at its anterior wall at the symphysis pubis and about 10 cm at its posterior wall. When a woman is standing upright, the upper portion of the pelvic cavity or canal is directed downward and

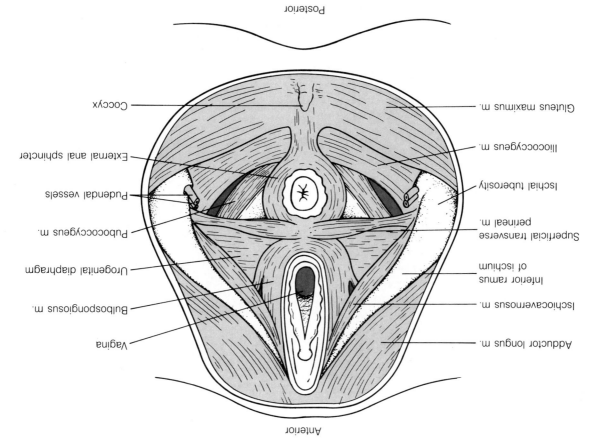

Posterior

Coccyx

External anal sphincter

Pudendal vessels

Pubococcygeus m.

Urogenital diaphragm

Bulbospongiosus m.

Vagina

Gluteus maximus m.

Iliococcygeus m.

Ischial tuberosity

Superficial transverse perineal m.

Inferior ramus of ischium

Ischiocavernosus m.

Adductor longus m.

Anterior

Figure 4–11 Muscles of the pelvic floor. The puborectalis, pubovaginalis, and coccygeal muscles cannot be seen from this view.

Table 4–1　Muscles of the Pelvic Floor

Muscle	Origin	Insertion	Innervation	Action
Levator ani	Pubis, lateral pelvic wall, and ischial spine	Blends with organs in pelvic cavity	Inferior rectal, second and third sacral nerves, plus anterior rami of third and fourth sacral nerves	Supports pelvic viscera; helps form pelvic diaphragm
Iliococcygeus	Pelvic surface of ischial spine and pelvic fascia	Central point of perineum, coccygeal raphe, and coccyx		Assists in supporting abdominal and pelvic viscera
Pubococcygeus	Pubis and pelvic fascia	Coccyx		
Puborectalis	Pubis	Blends with rectum; meets similar fibers from opposite side		Forms sling for rectum, just posterior to it; raises anus
Pubovaginalis	Pubis	Blends into vagina		Supports vagina
Coccygeus	Ischial spine and sacro- spinous ligament	Lateral border of lower sacrum and upper coccyx	Third and fourth sacral nerves	Supports pelvic viscera, helps form pelvic dia- phragm; flexes and ab- ducts coccyx

backward and its lower portion, downward and forward. This forms an axis or curved canal through which the presenting part of the baby must pass during birth (Figure 4–12). The inclination of the pelvis is the angle formed by two planes, a horizontal one through the tip of the coccyx and the superior border of the symphysis pubis and an inclined one through the sacral promontory and the superior border of the symphysis pubis. This pelvic angle of inclination usually measures 50° to 60° (Figure 4–13).

The bony circumference of the true pelvis is made up of the sacrum, coccyx, and innominate bones below the linea terminalis. This area is extremely important in obstetrics because its size and shape must be adequate for normal fetal passage during labor and at birth. The relationship of the fetal head to this cavity is of critical importance. The true pelvis is considered to have three parts: the inlet, the pelvic cavity, and the outlet. The pelvic planes are imaginary flat surfaces drawn across the three parts of the true pelvis at strategic levels (Figure 4–14). Associated with each part are distinct obstetric measurements that aid in evaluating the adequacy of the pelvis for childbirth.

The dimensions of the true pelvis and their obstetric implications are described here. Measurement techniques are discussed in Chapter 13. The effects of inadequate or abnormal pelvic diameters on labor and birth are further considered in Chapter 22.

The **pelvic inlet** is the upper border of the true pelvis and typically is round in the female. The size and shape of the pelvic inlet are determined by assessing three antero-posterior diameters: the diagonal conjugate, obstetric conjugate, and conjugate vera (see Chapter 13). The **diagonal conjugate** extends from the subpubic angle to the middle of the sacral promontory and is 12.5 cm. The diagonal con-

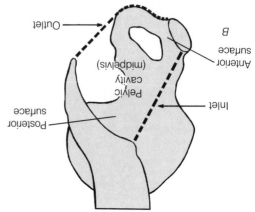

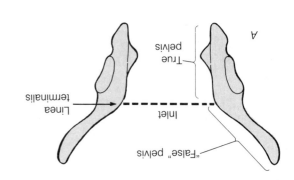

Figure 4–12　Female pelvis: A False pelvis is shallow cavity above inlet; true pelvis is deeper portion of the cavity below inlet. B True pelvis consists of inlet, cavity (midpelvis), and outlet.

jugate can be measured manually during a pelvic examination. The **obstetric conjugate** extends from the middle of the sacral promontory to an area approximately 1 cm below the pubic crest. Its length is estimated by subtracting 1.5 cm from the diagonal conjugate. The fetus passes through the obstetric conjugate, and the size of this diameter determines whether the fetus can move down into the birth canal in order for engagement to occur. The true (anatomic) conjugate, or **conjugate vera**, extends from the middle of the sacral promontory to the middle of the pubic crest (superior surface of the symphysis). One additional measurement, the **transverse diameter**, helps determine the shape of the inlet. The transverse diameter is the largest diameter of the inlet and is measured using the linea terminales as the points of reference. This diameter assists in determining the shape of the inlet.

The **pelvic cavity** (canal) has varying diameters. The largest part of the pelvis is called the **plane of the greatest dimensions** (Figure 4–14). It is a curved canal with a longer posterior than anterior wall. A change in the lumbar curve can increase or decrease the pelvic inclination and can influence the progress of labor since the fetus has to adjust itself to a curved path as well as to the different diameters of the true pelvis (Figure 4–12).

The smallest part of the pelvis is called the **plane of the least dimensions**, or the midpelvic plane (Figure 4–14). Arrest of labor occurs most frequently because of contracture (narrowing) in this plane, so its diameters are of great importance. The plane extends from the lower margin of the symphysis pubis, through the ischial spines, to the junction of the fourth and fifth sacral vertebraes. The anteroposterior diameter extends from the lower margin of the symphysis pubis to the junction of the fourth and fifth sacral vertebrae. The transverse (interspinous) diameter ex-

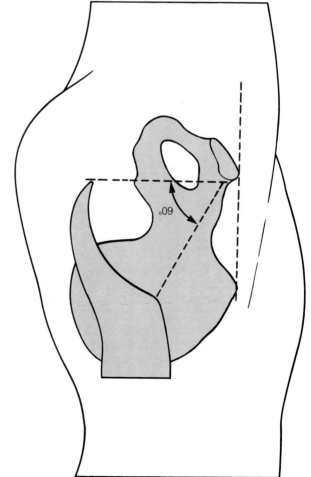

Figure 4–13 *Pelvic angle of inclination while woman is standing*

60°

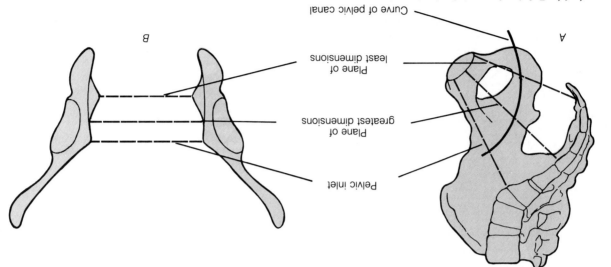

Pelvic inlet

Plane of greatest dimensions

Plane of least dimensions

Curve of pelvic canal

A

B

Figure 4–14 *Pelvic planes: A Sagittal section B Coronal section*

tends between the ischial spines and measures about 10.5 cm; it is the shortest pelvic diameter. The posterior sagittal diameter extends from the bispinous diameter to the junction of the fourth and fifth sacral vertebrae. At the midpelvic plane, the curve of the pelvic canal begins, and the axis of the birth canal changes. Until it reaches the ischial spines, the fetal head descends in a straight line. Then it curves forward toward the pelvic outlet (Figure 4–14).

The pelvic outlet is at the lower border of the true pelvis. The anteroposterior diameter of the pelvic outlet increases during birth as the presenting part pushes the coccyx posteriorly at the mobile sacrococcygeal joint. Decreased mobility, a large fetal head, and/or a forceful birth can cause the coccyx to snap. As the infant's head emerges, the long diameter of the head (occipital frontal) parallels the long diameter of the outlet (anteroposterior).

The transverse diameter (*bi-ischial* or *intertuberous*) extends from the inner surface of one ischial tuberosity to the other. It is the shortest diameter of the pelvic outlet and becomes shorter as the pubic arch narrows. The anterior sagittal diameter extends from the middle of the transverse diameter to the suprapubic angle. The posterior sagittal diameter extends from the middle of the transverse diameter to the sacrococcygeal junction. This is the most significant diameter of the outlet because it is the smallest diameter through which the infant must pass as it descends through the pelvic canal. The pubic arch has great importance, because the baby must pass under it. If it is narrow, the baby's head may be pushed backward toward the coccyx, making the extension of the head difficult. This situation is known as *outlet dystocia*, and forceps (outlet) assisted birth is required. The clinical assessment of each of these obstetric diameters is discussed further in Chapter 13.

Pelvic Types

The Caldwell-Moloy classification of pelves (Figure 4–15) is widely used to differentiate types of bony pelves (Caldwell & Moloy 1933). *Gynecoid, android, anthropoid*, and *platypelloid* are the four basic types. However, variations in the female pelvis from plane to plane are so great that classic types are not usual.

An imaginary line drawn through the greatest transverse diameter of the inlet divides it into anterior and posterior segments. The pelvis type is determined by assessing the posterior segment of the inlet; the anterior segment of the inlet names variations. For example, an android pelvis with an anthropoid variation means that the posterior segment of the inlet is android and the anterior segment is anthropoid. Consideration is given to the size of the sacrosciatic notch, flaring of the pelvic brim, the shape of the inlet, and the relationship of the greatest anteroposterior diameter to the greatest transverse diameter.

Each type of pelvis has a characteristic shape, and each shape has implications for labor and birth. The types are described briefly here and the implications for labor and birth in detail in Chapter 13.

Gynecoid Pelvis   The most common female pelvis is the gynecoid type. The inlet is rounded, with the anteroposterior diameter a little shorter than the transverse diameter. All the inlet diameters are at least adequate. The posterior segment is broad, deep, and roomy, and the anterior segment is well rounded. The gynecoid midpelvis has nonprominent ischial spines, straight and parallel side walls, and a wide, deep sacral curve. The sacrum is short and slopes backward. All of the midpelvic diameters are at least adequate. The gynecoid pelvic outlet has a wide and round pubic arch, the inferior pubic rami are short and concave. The anteroposterior diameter is long and the transverse diameter adequate. The capacity of the outlet is adequate. The bones are of medium structure and weight. Approximately 50% of female pelves are classified as gynecoid.

Android Pelvis   The normal male pelvis is the android type. The inlet is heart-shaped. The anteroposterior and transverse diameters are adequate for birth, but the posterior sagittal diameter is too short and the anterior sagittal diameter is long. The posterior segment is shallow because the sacral promontory is indented, resulting in a reduced capacity. The anterior segment is narrow, and the forepelvis is sharply angled. The android midpelvis has prominent ischial spines, convergent side walls, and a long, heavy sacrum inclining forward. All the midpelvic diameters are reduced. The distance from the linea terminalis to the ischial tuberosities is long, yet the overall capacity of the midpelvis is reduced. The android outlet has a narrow, sharp, and deep pubic arch, the inferior pubic rami are straight and long. The anteroposterior diameter is short and the transverse diameter is narrow. The capacity of the outlet is reduced. The bones are of medium to heavy structure and weight.

Approximately 20% of female pelves are classified as android. The influence of an android pelvis on labor is not favorable. Descent into the pelvis is slow. The fetal head usually engages in the transverse or occipital posterior diameter in asynclitism (oblique presentation) with extreme molding. Arrest of labor is frequent, requiring difficult forceps manipulation (rotation and extraction), and the deep, narrow pubic arch may lead to extensive perineal lacerations. Cesarean birth may be required.

Anthropoid Pelvis   The anthropoid pelvis inlet is oval, with a long anteroposterior diameter and an adequate but rather short transverse diameter. Both the posterior and anterior segments are deep; the posterior sagittal diameter is extremely long, as is the anterior sagittal diameter. The anthropoid midpelvis has variable ischial spines, straight side walls, and a narrow and long sacrum that inclines backward. The midpelvic diameters are at least adequate. The anthropoid outlet has a normal or moderately narrow pubic arch, the inferior pubic rami are long and narrow. The outlet capacity is adequate, and the bones are of medium weight and structure.

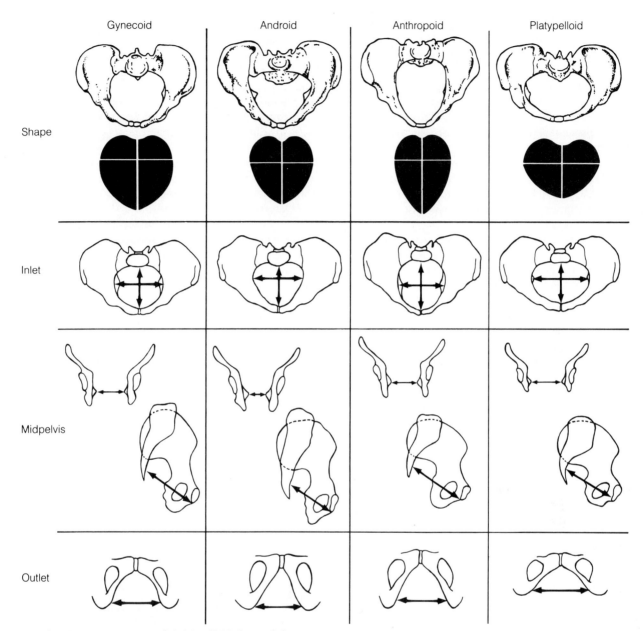

	Gynecoid	Android	Anthropoid	Platypelloid

Figure 4–15   Comparison of Caldwell-Moloy pelvic types

Approximately 25% of female pelves are classified as anthropoid.

Platypelloid Pelvis   The platypelloid type refers to the flat female pelvis. The inlet is distinctly transverse oval, with a short anteroposterior and extremely short transverse diameter. The posterior sagittal and anterior sagittal diameters are short. Both the anterior and posterior segments are shallow. The platypelloid midpelvis has variable ischial spines, parallel side walls, and a wide sacrum with a deep curve inward. Only the transverse diameter is adequate; thus, the midpelvic capacity is reduced. The platypelloid outlet has an extremely wide pubic arch; the inferior

pubic rami are straight and short. The transverse diameter is wide but the anteroposterior diameter is short. The outlet capacity may be inadequate. The platypelloid bones are similar to the gynecoid type. Only 5% of female pelves are classified as platypelloid.

Breasts

The **breasts**, or *mammary glands*, considered accessories of the reproductive system, are specialized sebaceous glands. They are conical and symmetrically placed on the sides of the chest. The greater pectoral and anterior serratus muscles underlie each breast. Suspending the breasts are fibrous tissues, called *Cooper's ligaments*, that extend from the deep fascia in the chest outward to just under the skin covering the breast. The left breast is frequently larger than the right.

In the center of each mature breast is the **nipple**, a protrusion about 0.5 to 1.3 cm in diameter. The nipple is composed mainly of erectile tissue, which becomes more rigid and prominent during the menstrual cycle, sexual excitement, pregnancy, and lactation. The nipple is surrounded by the heavily pigmented **areola**, 2.5 to 10 cm in diameter. Both the nipple and areola are roughened by small papillae called *Montgomery's tubercles*. As an infant suckles, these tubercles secrete a fatty substance that helps lubricate and protect the breasts.

The breasts are composed of glandular, fibrous, and adipose tissue. The glandular tissue consists of acini or alveoli (Figure 4–16), which are arranged in a series of 15 to 24 lobes separated from each other by adipose and fibrous tissue.

Each lobe is made up of several lobules, which are comprised of many grapelike clusters of alveoli around minute ducts. They are lined with a single layer of cuboidal epithelium, which secretes the various components of milk. The ducts from several lobules combine to form larger lactiferous ducts, or sinuses, which open on the surface of the nipple. The smooth muscle of the nipple causes erection of the nipple on contraction.

Cyclic hormonal control of the mature breast is complex. Essentially, estrogenic hormones stimulate the growth and development of the ductal epithelium. Progesterone, in association with estrogen, is responsible for the acinar and lobular development during the luteal phase of menstruation. In addition, adrenal corticosteroids, prolactin, somatotropin (growth hormone), and thyroxine are necessary for estrogen and progesterone to act.

The arterial, venous, and lymphatic systems communicate medially with the internal mammary vessels and laterally with the axillary vessels. Therefore, in cancer of the breast, metastasis follows the vascular supply both medially and laterally (Figure 4–17).

The biologic function of the breasts is to provide nourishment and protective maternal antibodies to infants through the lactation process. They are also a source of pleasurable sexual sensation.

Female Reproductive Cycle

Menstruation is a physiologic event shared by all women, yet each woman's experience is unique. How a woman experiences menstruation depends on sociocultural factors and her attitudes about her body, sexuality, and reproductive function.

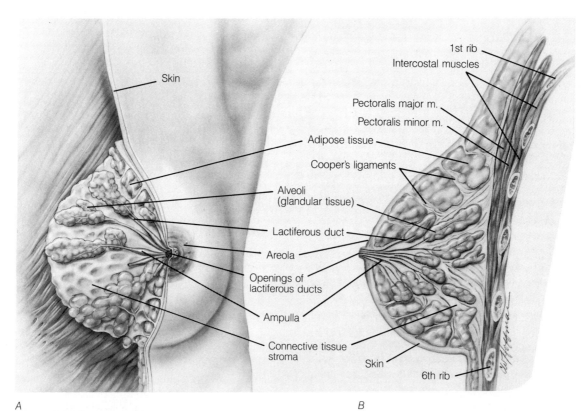

Figure 4–16 *Anatomy of the breast: A Anterior view of partially dissected left breast. B Sagittal view.*

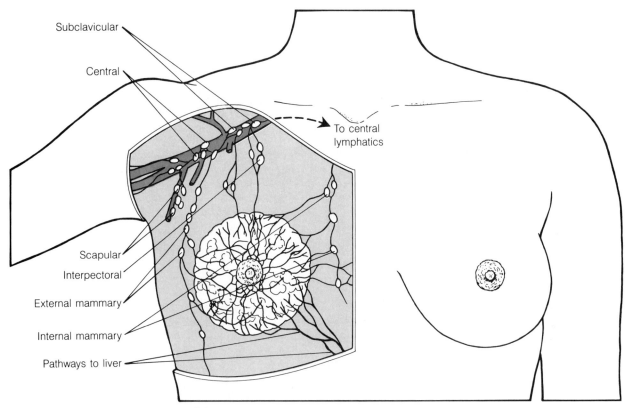

Subclavicular

Central

To central
lymphatics

Scapular
Interpectoral
External mammary
Internal mammary
Pathways to liver

Figure 4–17   Lymphatic drainage of the breast

The monthly rhythmic changes in sexually mature females is usually called the menstrual cycle. A more accurate term is the **female reproductive cycle (FRC)**. The FRC is composed of the *ovarian cycle*, during which ovulation occurs, and the *menstrual cycle*, during which menstruation occurs. These two cycles take place simultaneously (Figure 4–18).

Menstruation is cyclic uterine bleeding in response to cyclic hormonal changes. (Secondary sex characteristics associated with the hormonal changes are discussed earlier in this chapter.) Menstruation occurs when the ovum is not fertilized and begins about 14 days after ovulation in a 28-day cycle. The menstrual discharge, also referred to as the *menses* or *menstrual flow*, is composed of blood mixed with fluid, cervical and vaginal secretions, bacteria, mucus, leukocytes, and other cellular debris. The menstrual discharge is dark red and has a distinctive odor.

A review of the endometrium and its arterial blood supply will provide further understanding of the menstrual process. Blood flow from the spiral arterioles in the superficial endometrium is reduced, leading to a lack of blood and oxygen, which in turn produces tissue death (necrosis) and discharge of the superficial endometrium (menses). At the same time, the straight arterioles provide the basal endometrium with sufficient blood flow to maintain this layer of the endometrium and the endometrial glands (or seeds) that are responsible for the generation of the endometrium in the next female reproductive or menstrual cycle (Figure 4–19). Bleeding is controlled by vasospasm of the straight basal arterioles, resulting in coagulative necrosis at the vessel tips.

Menarche—the onset of menstruation—usually occurs when a girl is about 12 to 13 years of age. Frequently, ovulation does not occur in early cycles; these are called anovulatory cycles. Early cycles also are often irregular in frequency, amount of flow, and duration. Within several months to two to three years, a regular cycle becomes established.

Menstrual parameters vary greatly among individuals. Generally, menstruation occurs every 28 days, plus or minus five to ten days. Emotional and physical factors such as illness, excessive fatigue, stress or anxiety, and rigorous exercise programs can alter the cycle interval. In addition, certain environmental factors such as temperature and altitude may affect the cycle.

The duration of menses is from two to eight days, with the blood loss averaging 30 to 100 mL and the loss of iron averaging 0.5 to 1 mg daily.

Physiologic Aspects of the Female Reproductive Cycle

Effects of Female Hormones

After menarche, a female undergoes a cyclic pattern of ovulation and menstruation (if pregnancy does not occur)

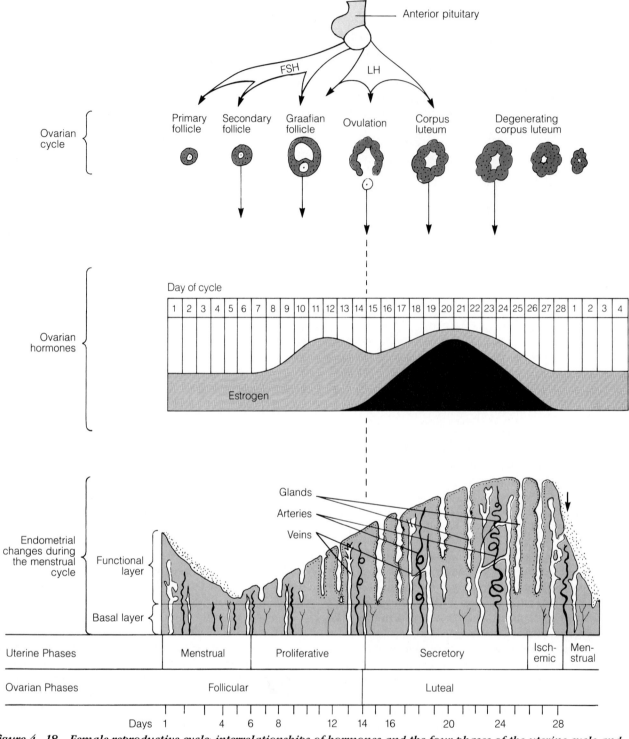

Figure 4–18 Female reproductive cycle: interrelationships of hormones and the four phases of the uterine cycle and the two phases of the ovarian cycle

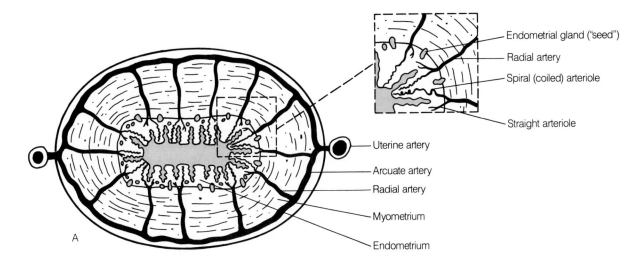

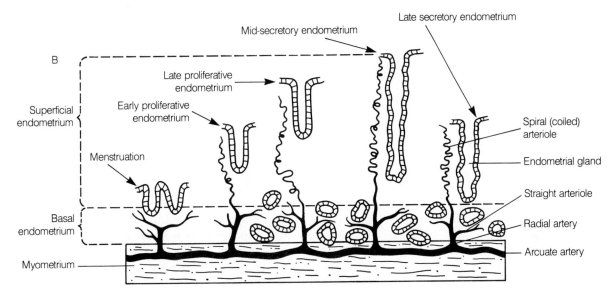

Figure 4–19   A blood supply to the endometrium (cross-section view of the uterus). B Schematic representation of blood supply during complete menstrual cycle (Modified from Bloom ML, Van Doungen L: Clinical Gynaecology: Integration of Structure and Function. *London: William Heinemann, 1972, p 144.)*

for a period of 30 to 40 years. This cycle is an orderly process under neurohormonal control: Each month one oocyte matures, ruptures from the ovary, and enters the fallopian tube. The ovary, vagina, uterus, and fallopian tubes are major target organs for female hormones. Each organ undergoes changes indicative of the exact point in time of any menstrual cycle.

The ovaries produce mature gametes and secrete hormones. Ovarian hormones include the estrogens, progesterone, and testosterone. The ovary is sensitive to FSH and LH. The uterus is sensitive to estrogen and progesterone. The relative proportion of these hormones to each other controls the events of both ovarian and menstrual cycles.

Estrogens   *Estrogens* are associated with those characteristics contributing to "femaleness." The major estrogenic effects are due primarily to three classical estrogens: estrone, β-estradiol, and estriol. β-Estradiol is the major estrogen. Estrogens are secreted in large amounts by the ovaries in nonpregnant women.

Estrogens control the development of the female secondary sex characteristics: breast development, widening of the hips, and adipose deposits in the buttocks and mons pubis. The growth of body hair in females is also influenced by estrogen. Estrogens assist in the maturation of the ovarian follicles and cause the endometrial mucosa to proliferate following menstruation. The amount of estrogens is greatest during the proliferative (follicular or estrogenic) phase of the menstrual cycle. Estrogen also causes the uterus to increase in size and weight because of increased glycogen, amino acids, electrolytes, and water. Blood supply is expanded as well. Under the influence of estrogens, myometrial contractility increases in both the uterus and the fallopian tubes, and there is increased uterine sensitivity to oxytocin. Estrogens inhibit FSH production and stimulate LH production.

Estrogens have effects on many hormones and other carrier proteins. This explains, for example, the increased amount of protein-bound iodine in pregnant women and in women who use oral contraceptives containing estrogen.

Estrogens may increase libidinal feelings in humans. They decrease the excitability of the hypothalamus, which may cause an increase in sexual desire.

For many years estrogens have been considered a preventive factor for coronary artery disease in women up to menopause, in the absence of diabetes or hypertension. Both lipoprotein and triglyceride metabolism are altered by estrogens. Although low estrogen levels do decrease serum cholesterol and β-lipoprotein levels and increase phospholipids and α-lipoprotein levels, numerous other factors must be considered in the development of coronary artery disease. Recent studies indicate that persistent high stress, coupled with specific types of personality patterns, diet (excessive calories, sodium, and saturated fats), smoking (especially in women taking oral contraceptives), obesity, and lack of exercise are influencing today's rise in incidence of coronary artery disease in women.

Progesterone   *Progesterone* is secreted by the corpus luteum and is found in greatest amounts during the secretory (luteal or progestational) phase of the menstrual cycle. It decreases the motility and contractility of the uterus caused by estrogens, thereby preparing the uterus for implantation after fertilization of the ovum. The endometrial mucosa is in a ready state as a result of estrogenic influence. Progesterone causes the uterine endometrium to further increase its supply of glycogen, arterial blood, secretory glands, amino acids, and water. This hormone is often called the *hormone of pregnancy* because its effects on the uterus allow pregnancy to be maintained.

Under the influence of progesterone, the vaginal epithelium proliferates and the cervix secretes thick, viscous mucus. Breast glandular tissue increases in size and complexity. Progesterone also prepares the breasts for lactation.

The temperature rise of about $0.35°C$ ($0.5°F$) that accompanies ovulation and persists throughout the secretory phase of the menstrual cycle is probably due to progesterone.

Prostaglandins   Prostaglandins (PGs) (oxygenated fatty acids), which are also classified as hormones, have a varied action in the body. The different types of prostaglandins (PGs) are indicated by Roman letters and either numbers (PGE_1) or Greek alphabet letters ($PGF_{2\alpha}$). Generally PGEs relax smooth muscles and are potent vaso-

dilators; PGFs are potent vasoconstrictors and increase the contractility of muscles and arteries. While their primary actions seem antagonistic, their basic regulatory functions in cells are achieved through an intricate pattern of reciprocal events. The discussion here will summarize their role in ovulation and menstruation.

Certain PGs are known to have a major role in the regulation of reproductive processes. For example, PGE_1 and PGE_2 appear to affect gonadotropin secretion by acting on the hypothalamus (Scott et al 1990).

Prostaglandin formation increases during follicular maturation, is dependent on gonadotropins, and is essential to ovulation. Extrusion of the ovum, resulting from the increased contractility of the smooth muscle in the theca layer of the mature follicle, is thought to be caused by $PGF_{2\alpha}$ (Wallach 1988). Significant amounts of PGs are found in and around the follicle at the time of ovulation.

While the exact mechanism by which the corpus luteum degenerates in the absence of pregnancy remains obscure, $PGF_{2\alpha}$ is thought to induce progesterone withdrawal, the lowest point of which coincides with the onset of early menses.

Endometrium and menstrual fluid are known to be rich sources of PGs. Studies (Franz 1988) suggests that the ratio of $PGF_{2\alpha}$ to PGE is a critical factor in the endometrial cycle.

During the late secretory phase the level of $PGF_{2\alpha}$ is higher than that of PGE. This event increases vasoconstriction and contractility of the myometrium, which contributes to the ischemia preceding menstruation. High concentration of PGs may also account for the vasoconstriction of the endometrium venous lacunae allowing for platelet aggregation at vascular rupture points, thereby preventing a rapid blood loss during menstruation. The menstrual flow's high concentration of PGs may also facilitate the process of tissue digestion, which allows for an orderly shedding of the endometrium during menstruation.

Neurohumoral Basis of the Female Reproductive Cycle

The FRC is controlled by complex interactions between the nervous and endocrine systems and their target tissues. These interactions involve the hypothalamus, anterior pituitary, and ovaries; their functions are reciprocal.

The hypothalamus secretes gonadotropin-releasing hormone (GnRH) to the pituitary gland in response to signals received from the central nervous system. This releasing hormone is often called both luteinizing hormone–releasing hormone (LHRH) and follicle-stimulating hormone–releasing hormone (FSHRH). The hypothalmus responds to positive and negative feedback from the ovarian hormones.

In response to GnRH, the anterior pituitary secretes the gonadotropic hormones FSH and LH. The ovaries contain specialized FSH and LH receptor cells. These receptor cells activate the production of adenylcyclase, causing increased cell growth and hormone secretion through the cyclic adenosine monophosphate (cAMP) mechanism. FSH is primarily responsible for the maturation of the ovarian follicle. As the follicle matures, it secretes increasing amounts of estrogen, which enhance the development of the follicle. (This estrogen also is responsible for the rebuilding/proliferation phase of the endometrium after it is shed during menstruation.)

Final maturation of the follicle will not come about without the action of LH. The anterior pituitary's production of LH increases sixfold to tenfold as the follicle matures. About 18 to 24 hours after the peak production of LH, ovulation occurs (Franz 1988).

The LH is also responsible for the "luteinizing" of the theca and granulosa cells of the ruptured follicle. As a result, estrogen production is reduced and progesterone secretion continues. Thus estrogen levels fall a day before ovulation; tiny amounts of progesterone are in evidence. Ovulation takes place following the very rapid growth of the follicle, as the sustained high level of estrogen diminishes, and progesterone secretion begins.

The ruptured follicle undergoes rapid change; luteinization is accomplished and the mass of cells becomes the corpus luteum (Hatcher et al 1990). The lutein cells secrete large amounts of progesterone with smaller amounts of estrogen. (Concurrently, the excessive amounts of progesterone are responsible for the secretory phase of the uterine cycle.) Seven or eight days following ovulation, the corpus luteum begins to involute, losing its secretory function. The production of both progesterone and estrogen is severely diminished. The anterior pituitary responds with increasingly large amounts of FSH; a few days later LH production begins. As a result, new follicles become responsive to another ovarian cycle and begin maturing.

Ovarian Cycle

The ovarian cycle has two phases: the follicular phase (days 1–14) and the luteal phase (days 15–28) in a 28-day cycle. Usually only the length of the follicular phase varies in menstrual cycles of varying duration because the luteal phase is of fixed length. During the *follicular phase,* the immature follicle matures as a result of FSH. Within the follicle, the oocyte grows. A mature **graafian follicle** appears about the 14th day under dual control of FSH and LH.

In the mature graafian follicle, the cells surrounding the antral cavity are granulosa cells. The oocyte and follicular fluid are enclosed in the cumulus oophorus. The stromal elements of the ovary are condensed around the follicle in two layers: the *theca interna,* a vascular, hypertrophied layer; and the *theca externa,* an avascular layer of connective tissue. The theca interna cells resemble the luteal cells of the corpus luteum. The *zona pellucida* (oolemma), a thick elastic capsule, develops around the oocyte. The fully mature graafian follicle is a large structure, measuring 5 to 10 mm. The mature follicle produces increasing amounts of estrogen.

Just before ovulation, the mature oocyte completes its first meiotic division (see Chapter 11 for a description of meiosis). As a result of this division, two cells are formed: a small cell called a **polar body** and a larger cell called the **secondary oocyte.** The secondary oocyte matures into the ovum.

As the graafian follicle matures and enlarges, it comes close to the surface of the ovary. The ovary surface has a blisterlike protrusion 10 to 15 mm in diameter, and the follicle's walls become thin. Extrusion of the ovum is aided by proteolytic enzyme formation by the theca externa and prostaglandin secretion into the follicular tissues. The secondary oocyte, polar body, and follicular fluid are pushed out. The ovum is discharged near the fimbria of the fallopian tube and is pulled into the tube to begin its journey.

Occasionally, ovulation is accompanied by midcycle pain, known as *mittelschmerz.* This pain may be caused by a thick tunica albuginea or by a local peritoneal reaction to the expelling of the follicular contents. Vaginal discharge may increase during ovulation, and a small amount of blood (midcycle spotting) may be discharged as well.

The body temperature increases about 0.3–0.6°C (0.5–1.0°F) 24 to 48 hours after the time of ovulation. It remains elevated until the day before menstruation begins. There may be an accompanying sharp basal body temperature drop just before the increase. These temperature changes are useful clinically to determine the approximate time ovulation occurs.

Generally, the ovum takes several minutes to travel through the ruptured follicle to the fallopian tube opening. The contractions of the tube's smooth muscle and its ciliary action propel the ovum through the tube. The ovum remains in the ampulla, where it may be fertilized and cleavage can begin. The ovum is thought to be fertile for only 6 to 24 hours. It reaches the uterus 72 to 96 hours after its release from the ovary.

The *luteal phase* begins when the ovum leaves its follicle. Under the influence of LH, the **corpus luteum** develops from the ruptured follicle. Within two or three days, the corpus luteum becomes yellowish and spherical and increases in vascularity. If the ovum is fertilized and implants in the endometrium, the fertilized egg begins to secrete **human chorionic gonadotropin (hCG),** which is needed to maintain the corpus luteum. If fertilization does not occur, within about a week after ovulation the corpus luteum begins to degenerate, eventually becoming a connective tissue scar called the *corpus albicans.* With degeneration comes a decrease in estrogen and progesterone. This allows for an increase in LH and FSH, which trigger the hypothalamus. Approximately 14 days after ovulation (in a 28-day cycle), in the absence of pregnancy, menstruation

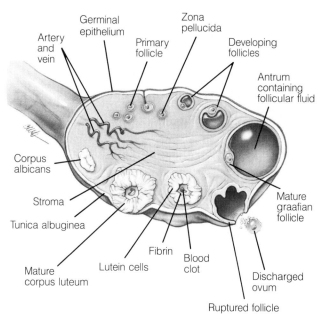

Figure 4–20 Various stages of development of the ovarian follicles

begins. Figure 4–20 depicts the changes that the follicle undergoes during the ovarian cycle.

Menstrual Cycle

The menstrual cycle has four phases: the menstrual phase, proliferative phase, secretory phase, and ischemic phase (see Table 4–2). Menstruation occurs during the *menstrual phase*. Some endometrial areas are shed, while others remain. Some of the remaining tips of the endometrial glands begin to regenerate. The endometrium is in a resting state following menstruation. Estrogen levels are low, and the endometrium is 1 to 2 mm deep. During this part of the cycle, the cervical mucosa is scanty, viscous, and opaque.

The *proliferative phase* begins when the endometrial glands enlarge, becoming tortuous and longer, in response to increasing amounts of estrogen. The blood vessels become prominent and dilated, and the endometrium increases in thickness sixfold to eightfold. This gradual process reaches its peak just before ovulation. The cervical mucosa becomes thin, clear, watery, and more alkaline, making the mucosa more favorable to spermatozoa. As ovulation nears, the cervical mucosa shows increased elasticity, called *spinnbarkheit*. At ovulation, the mucus will stretch more than 5 cm. The cervical mucosa pH increases from below 7.0 to 7.5 at the time of ovulation. On microscopic examination, the mucosa shows a characteristic ferning pattern (see Figure 5–4B). This ferning pattern is a useful aid in assessment of ovulation time (Table 4–3). For in-depth discussion, see Chapter 5.

The *secretory phase* follows ovulation. The endometrium, under estrogenic influence, undergoes slight cellular growth. Progesterone, however, causes such marked swelling and growth that the epithelium is warped into folds

Table 4–2 Characteristics of Menstrual Cycle and Ovulation

Menstrual phase (days 1–5)	Estrogen levels are low Cervical mucus is scanty, viscous and opaque Endometrium is shed
Proliferative phase (days 6–14)	Endometrium and myometrium thickness increases
	Estrogen peaks just before ovulation
	Cervical mucosa at ovulation: Is clear, thin, watery, and alkaline Is more favorable to sperm Has *spinnbarkheit* greater than 5 cm Shows ferning pattern on microscopic exam
	Just prior to ovulation body temperature drops, and then at ovulation BBT increases 0.3 to 0.6°C, and *mittelschmerz* and/or midcycle spotting may occur
Secretory phase (days 15–26)	Estrogen drops sharply, and progesterone dominates
	Vascularity of entire uterus increases
	Tissue glycogen increases, and the uterus is made ready for implantation
Ischemic phase (days 27–28)	Both estrogen and progesterone levels fall
	Spiral arteries undergo vasoconstriction
	Endometrium becomes pale
	Blood vessels rupture
	Blood escapes into uterine stromal cells

Table 4–3 Signs of Ovulation

The cervical mucosa changes in the following ways:
- The amount of mucus increases
- It appears thin, watery, and clear
- *Spinnbarkheit* greater than 5 cm is present
- A ferning pattern appears on microscopic examination

Basal body temperature increases 0.3 to 0.6°C 24 to 48 hr after ovulation

Mittelschmerz may be present

Midcycle spotting may occur

(Figure 4–21). The amount of tissue glycogen increases. The glandular epithelial cells begin to fill with cellular debris, become tortuous, and dilate. The glands secrete small quantities of endometrial fluid in preparation for a fertilized ovum. The vascularity of the entire uterus increases greatly, providing a nourishing bed for implantation. If implantation occurs, the endometrium, under the influence of progesterone, continues to develop and become even thicker (Figure 4–22, see Chapter 11 for an in-depth discussion of implantation).

If fertilization does not occur, the *ischemic phase* begins. The corpus luteum begins to degenerate, and as a result both estrogen and progesterone levels fall. Areas of ne-

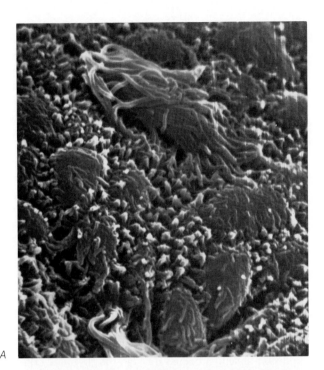

A

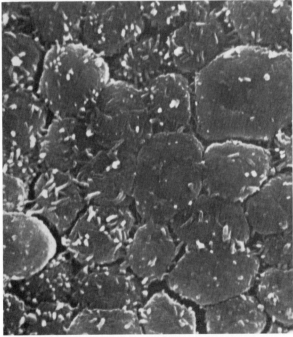

B

Figure 4–21   Scanning electron micrographs of the uterine lining during different phases of the uterine cycle. During the luteal phase (A) some of the cells have cilia and some are secreting droplets. The secreting cells are covered with microvilli. In the secretory phase (B), microvilli are still present on the surface of the secreting cells, but the general surface of the lining has a lumpier appearance than during the proliferative phase, and the cilia appear shorter and less numerous. The named phases refer to the uterine condition at the time the photographs were taken. (Courtesy Dr E S E Hafez, Wayne State University, Detroit, Michigan)

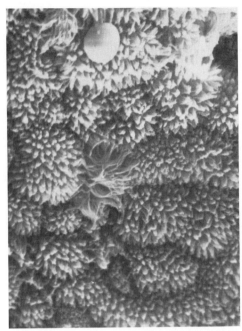

Figure 4–22   Scanning micrograph of the inner lining of the uterus at the time of implantation of the blastocyst. The blastocyst is an embryo at an early stage of development. (Courtesy Dr. E S E Hafez, Wayne State University, Detroit, Michigan)

crosis appear under the epithelial lining. Extensive vascular changes also occur. Small blood vessels rupture, and the spiral arteries constrict and retract, causing a deficiency of blood in the endometrium, which becomes pale. This ischemic phase is characterized by the escape of blood into the stromal cells of the uterus. The menstrual flow begins, thus beginning the menstrual cycle again. After menstruation the basal layer remains, so that the tips of the glands can regenerate the new functional endometrial layer. See Table 4–4 for a summary of the FRC.

Table 4–4   Summary of Female Reproductive Cycle

Ovarian Cycle

- *Follicular phase* (days 1–14): Primordial follicle matures under influence of FSH and LH up to the time of ovulation

- *Luteal phase* (days 15–28): Ovum leaves follicle; corpus luteum develops under LH influence and produces high levels of progesterone and low levels of estrogen

Menstrual Cycle

- *Menstrual phase* (days 1–5)

- *Proliferative phase* (days 6–14): Estrogen peaks just prior to ovulation. Cervical mucus at ovulation is clear, thin, watery, alkaline, and more favorable to sperm; shows ferning pattern; and has *spinnbarkheit* greater than 5 cm. At ovulation body temperature drops, then rises sharply and remains elevated

- *Secretory phase* (days 15–26): Estrogen drops sharply and progesterone dominates

- *Ischemic phase* (days 27–28): Both estrogen and progesterone levels drop

---

Male Reproductive System

To date, the male organs have not been studied in the same depth as their female counterparts. New techniques are being applied to the study of male factors in such areas as infertility, contraception, congenital anomalies, and reproduction in general.

The primary reproductive functions of the male genitals are to produce and transport the male sex cells (sperm) through and eventually out of the genital tract into the female genital tract. The male reproductive system consists of the external and internal genitals (Figure 4–23).

External Genitals

The two external reproductive organs are the penis and the scrotum.

Penis

The *penis* is an elongated, cylindrical structure consisting of a body, termed the shaft, and a cone-shaped end called the glans. The penis lies in front of the scrotum.

The shaft of the penis is made up of three longitudinal columns of erectile tissue: the paired corpora cavernosa and a third, the corpus spongiosum. These columns are covered by a dense fibrous connective tissue and then enclosed by an elastic tissue. The penis is covered by a thin outer layer of skin.

The corpus spongiosum contains the urethra and extends beyond the corpora cavernosa to become the glans at the distal end of the penis. The urethra widens within the glans and ends in a slitlike orifice, located in the tip of the glans, called the *urethral meatus.* A circular fold of skin arises just behind the glans and covers it. Known as the *prepuce*, or *foreskin*, it is frequently removed by the surgical procedure of circumcision (Chapter 29). If the corpus spongiosum does not surround the urethra completely, the urethral meatus may occur on the ventral aspect of the penile shaft (hypospadias) or on the dorsal aspect (epispadias).

The penis is innervated by the pudendal nerve. Sympathetic fibers come from the hypogastric and pelvic plexuses, while parasympathetic fibers from the third and fourth sacral nerves form the splanchnic nerves. When the parasympathetic fibers are stimulated, the ischiocavernous muscle contracts, preventing the return of venous blood from the cavernous sinuses. The blood vessels of the penis engorge, causing the penis to become erect. During *erection*, the penis elongates, thickens, and stiffens.

Sexual stimulation causes the penis to become erect. If stimulation is intense enough, the forceful and sudden expulsion of semen occurs through the rhythmic contractions of the penile muscles. This phenomenon is called *ejaculation*.

The penis serves both the urinary and reproductive systems. Urine is expelled through the urethral meatus. The primary function of the penis is to deposit sperm in the female vagina during sexual intercourse so that fertilization of the ovum can occur.

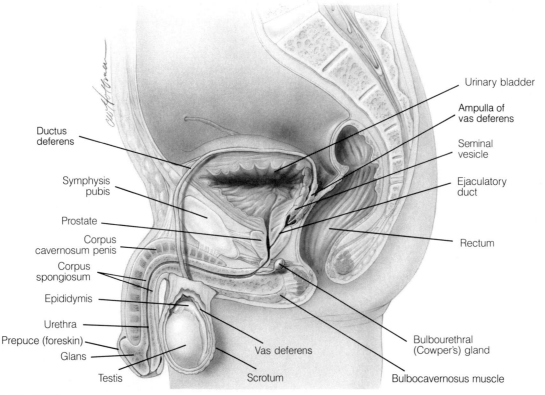

Figure 4–23   Male reproductive system

Scrotum

The *scrotum* is a pouchlike structure that hangs in front of the anus and behind the penis and may extend below it. Composed of skin and the *dartos* muscle, the scrotum shows increased pigmentation and scattered hairs. The sebaceous glands open directly onto the scrotal surface; their secretion has a distinctive odor. Contraction of the dartos and cremasteric muscles shortens the scrotum and draws it closer to the body, thus wrinkling its outer surface. The degree of wrinkling is greatest in young men and at cold temperatures and is least in older men and at warm temperatures.

Inside the scrotum are two lateral compartments separated by a medial septum derived from the dartos muscle. Each compartment contains a testis with its related structures. Because the left spermatic cord grows longer during embryologic development, the left testis and its scrotal sac hang lower than the right. A ridge (raphe) on the external scrotal surface marks the position of the medial septum and continues anteriorly on the urethral surface of the penis but disappears in the perineal area.

The function of the scrotum is to protect the testes and the sperm by maintaining a temperature lower than that of the body. Spermatogenesis will not occur if the testes fail to descend and thus remain at body temperature. Because it is sensitive to touch, pressure, temperature, and pain, the scrotum defends against potential harm to the testes.

Internal Genitals

The male internal reproductive organs include the gonads (testes or testicles), a system of ducts (epididymis, vas deferens, ejaculatory duct, and urethra), and accessory glands (seminal vesicles, prostate gland, bulbourethral glands, and urethral glands). See Table 4–5 for a summary of male reproductive organ functions.

Testes

The *testes* are a pair of oval, compound glandular organs contained in the scrotum (Figure 4–24). In the sexually mature male, they are the site of spermatozoa production and the secretion of several male sex hormones.

Each testis is 4 to 6 cm long, 2 to 3 cm wide, and 3 to 4 cm deep. Each weighs 10 to 15 g. It is covered by a serous membrane and an inner capsule that is tough, white, and fibrous. The connective tissue sends projections inward to form septa, dividing the testis into 250 to 400 lobules. Each lobule contains one to three tightly packed, convoluted *seminiferous tubules* containing sperm cells arranged in layers in all stages of development.

The seminiferous tubules are surrounded by loose connective tissue, which houses abundant blood and lymph vessels and the *Leydig's (interstitial) cells*. The cells produce testosterone, the primary male sex hormone. The seminiferous tubules come together to form the 20 or 30

Table 4–5 Summary of Male Reproductive Organ Functions

- The testes house seminiferous tubules and gonads
- Seminiferous tubules contain sperm cells in various stages of development and undergoing meiosis
- Sertoli's cells nourish and protect spermatocytes (phase between spermatids and spermatozoa)
- Leydig's cells are the main source of testosterone
- Epididymides provide an area for maturation of sperm and a reservoir for mature spermatozoa
- The vas deferens connects the epididymis with the prostate gland, then connects with ducts from the seminal vesicle to become an ejaculatory duct
- Ejaculatory ducts provide a passageway for semen and seminal fluid into the urethra
- Seminal vesicles secrete yellowish fluid rich in fructose, prostaglandins, and fibrinogen. This provides nutrition that increases motility and fertilizing ability of sperm. Prostaglandins also aid fertilization by making the cervical mucus more receptive to sperm
- The prostate gland secretes thin, alkaline fluid containing calcium, citric acid, and other substances. Alkalinity counteracts acidity of ductus and seminal vesicle secretions
- Bulbourethral (Cowper's) glands secrete alkaline, viscous fluid into semen, aiding in neutralization of acidic vaginal secretions

---

straight tubules, which in turn form an anastomosing network of thin-walled spaces, the *rete testis*. The rete testis forms 10 to 15 efferent ducts that empty into the duct of the epididymis. Prior to this, the efferent ducts enlarge and become convoluted.

Most of the cells lining the seminiferous tubules undergo a process of maturation called *spermatogenesis*. (See Chapter 11 for further discussion of spermatogenesis.) Sperm production varies among and within the tubules, with cells in different areas of the same tubule undergoing different stages of spermatogenesis. The seminiferous tubules also contain *Sertoli's cells*, which nourish and protect the spermatocytes. The sperm are eventually released from the tubules into the epididymis, where they mature further.

Like the female reproductive cycle, the process of spermatogenesis and other functions of the testes are the result of complex neural and hormonal controls. The hypothalamus secretes releasing factors, which stimulate the anterior pituitary to release the gonadotropins FSH and LH. These hormones cause the testes to produce **testosterone**, which maintains spermatogenesis, increases sperm production by the seminiferous tubules, and stimulates production of seminal fluid (Guyton 1991).

Along with testosterone and the other androgens, FSH maintains the spermatogenic function of the testes. LH is called *interstitial cell-stimulating hormone* (ICSH) in males because it stimulates the interstitial cells of the testes (Leydig's cells) to synthesize testosterone from cholesterol. Testosterone in turn inhibits the secretion of ICSH by the anterior pituitary. Most of the circulating testosterone is converted in the liver to 17-ketosteroids, which are secreted in the urine. About one-third of these ketosteroids are metabolized from testicular testosterone; the rest are adrenal in origin.

Testosterone is the most prevalent and potent of the testicular hormones. Its target organs are the testes, prostate, and seminal vesicles. In addition to being essential for spermatogenesis, it increases sperm production by the seminiferous tubules, stimulates production of seminal fluid, and is responsible for the development of secondary male characteristics and certain behavioral patterns. The effects of testosterone include structural and functional development of the male genital tract, emission and ejaculation of seminal fluid, distribution of body hair, promotion of growth and strength of long bones, increased muscle mass, and enlargement of the vocal cords. The action of testosterone on the central nervous system is thought to produce aggressiveness and sexual drive. The action of testosterone is constant, not cyclic like that of the female hormones. Its production is not limited to a certain number of years, but is thought to decrease in quantity with age.

In summary, the primary functions of the testes are to serve as the site of spermatogenesis and to produce testosterone.

Epididymis

The epididymis (plural, *epididymides*) is a duct about 6 m (20 feet) long, although it is convoluted into a compact structure about 3.75 cm long. An epididymis lies behind each testis. It arises from the top of the testis, extends downward, and then passes upward, where it becomes the vas deferens.

The epididymis provides a reservoir where spermatozoa can survive for a long period. When discharged from the seminiferous tubules into the epididymis, the sperm are immotile and incapable of fertilizing an ovum. The spermatozoa remain in the epididymis for 2 to 10 days. As the sperm are transported along the tortuous course of the epididymis, they become both motile and fertile (Marieb 1989).

Vas Deferens and Ejaculatory Duct

The *vas deferens*, also known as the *ductus deferens*, is about 40 cm long and connects the epididymis with the prostate. One vas deferens arises from the posterior border of each testis. It joins the spermatic cord and weaves over and between several pelvic structures until it meets the vas deferens from the opposite side. Each vas deferens terminus expands to form the *ampulla* and joins with the seminal vesicle (a gland) duct to form the *ejaculatory duct*, which passes through the prostate gland and merges with the urethra. The ejaculatory ducts serve as a passageway for semen and fluid secreted by the seminal vesicles. The main function of the ductus deferens (vas deferens) is to rapidly squeeze the sperm from their storage sites (the epididymis and distal part of the ductus deferens) into the urethra.

Men who choose to take total responsibility for birth control may elect to have a vasectomy. In this procedure the scrotal portion of the ductus deferens is surgically incised or cauterized. Although sperm continues to be produced for the next several years, they can no longer reach the outside of the body. Eventually, they deteriorate and are reabsorbed (Marieb 1989).

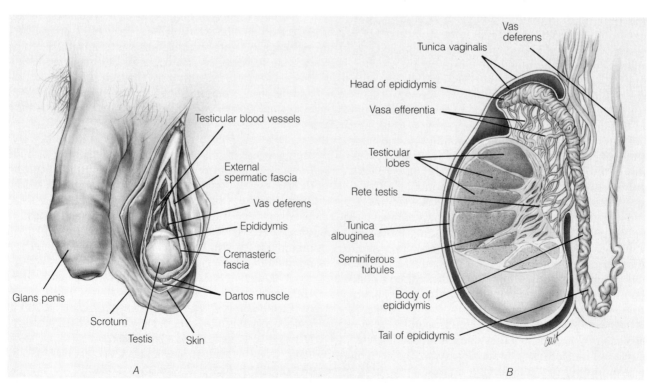

Figure 4–24   The testes: A External view. B Sagittal view showing interior anatomy

Urethra

The male urethra is a passageway for urine and semen. The urethra begins in the bladder and passes through the prostate gland, where it is called the *prostatic urethra*.

The urethra emerges from the prostate gland to become the *membranous urethra*. It terminates in the penis, where it is called the *penile urethra*. In the penile urethra, goblet secretory cells are present, and smooth muscle is replaced by erectile tissue.

Accessory Glands

The male accessory glands are specialized structures under endocrine and neural control. Each secretes a unique and essential component of the total seminal fluid in an ordered sequence.

The *seminal vesicles* are two glands composed of many lobes. Each vesicle is about 7.5 cm long. They are situated between the bladder and rectum and immediately above the base of the prostate. The epithelium lining the seminal vesicles secretes a yellow, viscous fluid rich in high-energy fructose, prostaglandins, fibrinogen, and amino acids. During ejaculation, this fluid mixes with sperm in the ejaculatory ducts. An activating principle is present in the secretions that acts on the sperm to increase their motility. This fluid (about 60% of the semen fluid volume) helps provide an environment favorable to sperm motility and metabolism.

The *prostate gland* encircles the upper part of the urethra and lies below the neck of the bladder. Made up of several lobes, it measures about 4 cm in diameter and weighs 20 to 30 g. The prostate is made up of both glandular and muscular tissue. It secretes a thin, milky, alkaline fluid containing high levels of zinc, calcium, citric acid, and acid phosphatase (Marieb 1989). This fluid protects the sperm from the acidic environment of the vagina and the male urethra, which could be spermicidal.

The *bulbourethral* or *Cowper's glands* are a pair of small round structures on either side of the membranous urethra. The glands secrete a clear, thick mucus that becomes part of the semen. This secretion also lubricates the penile urethra during sexual excitement and neutralizes the acid in the male urethra and the vagina, thereby enhancing sperm mobility.

The *urethral* or *Littre's glands* are tiny mucous-secreting glands found throughout the membranous lining of the penile urethra. Their secretions add to those of the bulbourethral glands.

Semen

The male ejaculate, *semen* or *seminal fluid*, is made up of spermatozoa and the secretions of the accessory glands. The seminal fluid transports viable and motile sperm to the female reproductive tract. Effective transportation of sperm requires adequate nutrients, an adequate pH (about 7.5), a specific concentration of sperm to fluid, and an optimal osmolarity.

A spermatozoon is made up of a *head* and a *tail* (Figure 4–25). The tail is divided into the middle piece and end piece. The head's main components are the *acrosome, nucleus,* and *nuclear vacuoles*. The head carries the male's 23 chromosomes, and it is the part that enters the ovum at fertilization (Chapter 11). The tail, or *flagellum,* is specialized for motility.

Sperm may be stored in the male genital system up to 42 days, depending primarily on the frequency of ejaculations. The average volume of ejaculate following abstinence for several days is 2 to 5 mL but may vary from 1 to 10 mL. Repeated ejaculation results in decreased volume. Once ejaculated, sperm can live only two or three days in the female genital tract.

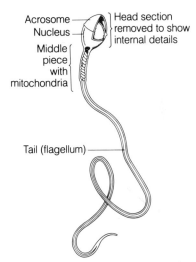

Figure 4–25 Schematic representation of a mature spermatozoon

KEY CONCEPTS

Reproductive system activities include developmental changes that lead to puberty, gametogenesis (spermatogenesis and oogenesis), sexual intercourse, development of sense of sexuality, pregnancy, embryo development, parturition, and lactation.

Reproductive activities require a complex interaction between the reproductive structures, the central nervous system, and such endocrine glands as the pituitary, hypothalamus, testes, and ovaries.

At puberty, an alteration in brain sensitivity leads to an increased release of GnRH, which stimulates LH and FSH. In the male, this stimulation leads to an increase in testosterone; in the female, it leads to an increase in estrogen and progesterone.

Estrogen is the principal cause of the events of puberty (maturation of ova, enlargement of the uterus and fallopian tubes, deposition of fat in the breasts and hips, and characteristic hair growth) in females.

Puberty changes for the male (onset of spermatogenesis; enlargement of the penis, scrotum, and testes; voice changes; and characteristic hair growth) occur as a result of increased testosterone production by the testes.

The female reproductive system consists of: the ovaries, where female germ cells and female sex hormones are formed; the fallopian tubes, which capture the ovum and allow transport to the uterus; the uterus, whose lining is shed during menstruation or is the implantation site for the fertilized ovum (blastocyst); the cervix, which is a protective portal for the body of the uterus and the connection between the vagina and the uterus (it must thin and dilate to allow passage of a baby); and the vagina, which is the passageway from the external genitals to the uterus and provides for discharge of menstrual products to the outside of the body.

The female reproductive cycle is composed of the ovarian cycle, during which ovulation occurs, and the menstrual cycle, during which menstruation occurs.

These two cycles take place simultaneously and are under neurohumoral control.

The ovarian cycle has two phases: the follicular phase and the luteal phase. During the follicular phase the primordial follicle matures under the influence of FSH and LH until ovulation occurs. The luteal phase begins when the ovum leaves the follicle and the corpus luteum develops under the influence of LH. The corpus luteum produces high levels of progesterone and low levels of estrogen.

The menstrual cycle has four phases: menstrual, proliferative, secretory, and ischemic. Menstruation is the actual shedding of the endometrial lining, when estrogen levels are low. The proliferative phase begins when the endometrial glands begin to enlarge under the influence of estrogen and cervical mucosa changes occur; the changes peak at ovulation. The secretory phase follows ovulation and under the influence primarily of progesterone the uterus increases its vascularity to make it ready for possible implantation. The ischemic phase is characterized by degeneration of the corpus luteum, fall in both estrogen and progesterone levels, constriction of the spiral arteries, and escape of blood into the stromal cells of the endometrium.

The male reproductive system consists of: the testes, where male germ cells and male sex hormones are formed; a series of continuous ducts through which spermatozoa are transported outside the body; accessory glands that produce secretions important to sperm nutrition, survival, and transport; and the penis, which serves as the organ of copulation.

✿ ✿

References

Caldwell WE, Moloy HC: Anatomical variations in the female pelvis and their effect on labor with a suggested classification. *Am J Obstet Gynecol* 1933; 26:479.

Cunningham FG, MacDonald PC, Gant NF (editors): *Williams Obstetrics,* 18th ed. Norwalk, CT: Appleton & Lange, 1989.

Franz WB: Basic Review: Endocrinology of the normal menstrual cycle. *Primary Care* 1988; 15(3):607.

Guyton AC: *Textbook of Medical Physiology,* 8th ed. Philadelphia: Saunders, 1991.

Hatcher RA et al: *Contraceptive Technology: 1990–1991,* 15th ed. New York: Irvington, 1990.

Marieb EN: *Human Anatomy and Physiology.* Redwood City, CA: Benjamin/Cummings, 1989.

Scott JR et al: *Danforth's Obstetrics and Gynecology,* 6th ed. Philadelphia: Lippincott, 1990.

Speroff L et al: *Clinical Gynecologic Endrocrinology and Infertility,* 4th ed. Baltimore: Williams & Wilkins, 1989.

Tanner JM: *Fetus into Man: Physical Growth from Conception to Maturity,* 2nd ed. Boston: Harvard University Press, 1990.

Wallach EE: The mechanism of ovulation. In Sciarra JL et al

Additional Readings

Cumming DC, Cumming CE, Kieren DK: Menstrual mythology and sources of information about menstruation. *Am J Obstet Gynecol* February 1991; 164:472.

Drife JO: Breast modifications during the menstrual cycle. *Int J Gynecol Obstet* 1989; 1 (Suppl.):19.

Hodgen GD: Neuroendocrinology of the Normal Menstrual Cycle. *J Reprod Med* 1989; 34(1) (Suppl.):68S.

MacLennan AH: The role of the hormone relaxin in human reproduction and pelvic girdle relaxation. *Scand J Rheumatol Suppl* 1991; 88:7.

Odell WD, Griffin J.: Pulsatile secretion of chorionic gonadotropin during the normal menstrual cycle. *J Clin Endocrinol Metab* 1989; 69(3):528.

Shukovski L, Healy DL, Findlay JK: Circulating immunoreactive oxytocin during the human menstrual cycle comes from the pituitary and is estradiol dependent. *J Clin Endocrinol Metab* 1989; 68(2):455.

Zhou JP et al: Reproductive hormones in menstrual blood. *J Clin Endocrinol Metab* 1989; 69(2):338.

CHAPTER 5
Special Reproductive Concerns

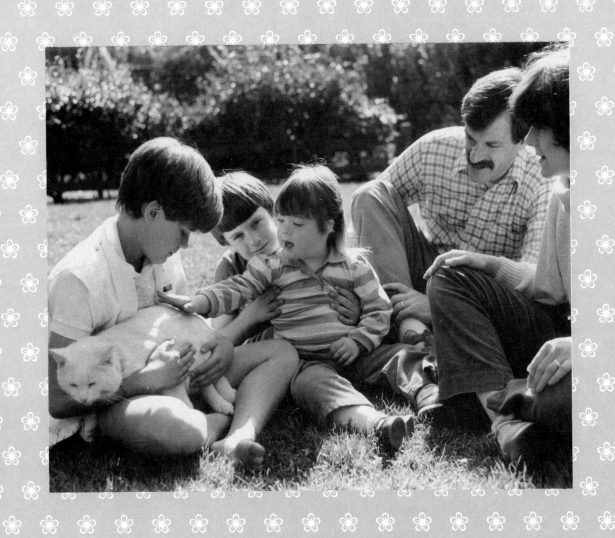

OBJECTIVES

Describe how variations in the male and female reproductive systems contribute to a couple's inability to conceive.

Summarize the physiologic and psychologic effects of infertility on a couple.

Identify the various tests done in an infertility workup.

Discuss the indications for chromosomal analysis and genetic amniocentesis.

Relate the significance of the Barr chromatin body to identifying sex chromosome abnormalities.

Identify the general characteristics of an autosomal dominant disorder.

Compare autosomal recessive disorders with X-linked (sex-linked) recessive disorders.

Compare prenatal and postnatal diagnostic procedures that may be used to determine the presence of genetic disease.

Explore the emotional impact on a couple undergoing genetic testing and/or the birth of a baby with a genetic disorder.

Explain the nurse's responsibility in genetic counseling.

✿ ✿

As my husband and I were sitting in the waiting room at the in vitro clinic, I felt great apprehension. For four years, we had been unable to conceive a child. I'd been through 2 surgeries, dozens of blood tests, hormone drugs that made me irrational and emotional, and many difficult times of blaming myself, feeling out of control and having surprisingly painful reactions to seeing mothers and newborns together. After many long discussions, we had decided that, if in vitro didn't work for us, we would adopt a child. But still, somehow, we both felt that we wanted to experience childbirth together, to bring our own child into the world.

We were on the brink of the most expensive treatment in the infertility process, the treatment that is the last resort for most infertile couples. Each month's treatment would involve nearly $10,000 of uninsured costs; 50 injections, many of which I would have to administer to myself; two procedures under anesthesia; 4 or 5 ultrasounds; a dozen blood tests; and only a 30% chance of conceiving a child. Was I doing the right thing? Was this the right clinic for us? After so many months of disappointments, did I dare to get my hopes up once again?

A young nurse burst into the office, tremendously excited and out of breath. She'd just come from the lab, having done a blood test, and had discovered that a patient, Judy, was pregnant. Watching the thrill and caring of these nurses' faces helped me to decide. Yes, I was in the right place. Yes, it was

worth hoping again. Even if in vitro didn't work for us, we had to try.

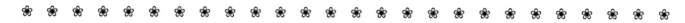

Most couples who want children are able to have them with little trouble. Pregnancy and childbirth usually take their normal course, and a healthy baby is born. But some couples are not so fortunate and are unable to fulfill their dream of having a healthy baby because of special reproductive problems.

This chapter explores two particularly troubling reproductive problems facing some couples; the inability to conceive and the risk of bearing babies with genetic abnormalities.

Infertility

Infertility is defined as lack of conception after one year of unprotected sexual intercourse (Speroff et al 1989). Infertility has had a profound emotional, psychologic, and economic impact both on the affected couples and on society. Approximately 10% to 15% of couples in their reproductive years are infertile.

Primary infertility identifies those women who have never conceived, whereas *secondary infertility* indicates those who have formerly been pregnant but have not conceived during one or more years of unprotected intercourse (Hammond 1987; Speroff et al 1989). *Sterility* is a term applied when there is an absolute factor preventing reproduction.

The incidence of infertility appears to be increasing and may be related to the following factors:

1. More couples are delaying marriage and postponing childbearing until they have passed the suggested age of optimal fertility in women (20–25 years of age).

2. Anovulation may be prolonged after using birth control pills, although this is rare with the low-dose pills now in common use.

3. Infections associated with intrauterine devices or following abortions can affect fertility.

4. Sexually transmitted diseases may cause obstructive disease of the male and female reproductive systems (Hammond 1987).

Essential Components of Fertility

Understanding the elements essential for normal fertility can help the nurse identify the many factors that may cause infertility. The following essential components must be presented for normal fertility:

Female partner:

1. The vaginal, cervical, uterine, and tubal mucus must be favorable to the survival of spermatozoa.

2. There must be clear passage between the cervix and the fallopian tubes.

3. Fallopian tubes must be patent and have normal peristaltic movement to allow ascent of spermatozoa and descent of ova (ovum). The fimbriated ends of the fallopian tubes must be able to "pick up" and transport ova.

4. Ovaries must produce and release normal ova in a timely manner.

5. There must be no obstruction between the ovaries and the uterus.

6. The endometrium must be in a normal physiologic state to allow implantation of the blastocyst and to sustain normal growth.

Male partner:

1. The testes must produce adequate numbers of motile sperm.

2. The male genital tract must not be obstructed.

3. The male genital tract secretions must be normal.

4. Ejaculated spermatozoa must be deposited in the female genital tract in such a manner that they reach the cervix.

These normal findings are correlated with possible causes of deviation in Table 5–1. In addition to these nec-essary elements, certain general physiologic and psychologic conditions must be present to support conception.

With intricacies of timing and environment playing such a crucial role, it is an impressive natural phenomenon that approximately 85% of couples in the United States are able to conceive (Diamond 1988). Of the remaining 15% of couples who are unable to conceive, their cause is either a problem in the male partner, or a hormonal, tubal, or cervical problem in the female partner. In 10% to 20% of these couples the cause of infertility cannot be identified (Speroff et al 1989). In 35% there are multiple etiologies. Professional intervention can help 30% to 50% of infertile couples achieve pregnancy.

Couples should be referred for infertility evaluation if they have been unable to conceive after at least one year of attempting to achieve pregnancy. If the woman is over 35 years old, it may be appropriate to refer the couple after only 6 to 9 months of unprotected intercourse without conception. At 25 years of age, the age at which couples are the most fertile, the average length of time needed to achieve conception is 5.3 months. The average 20- to 30-year-old American couple has intercourse one to three times a week, a frequency that should be sufficient to achieve pregnancy if all other factors are satisfactory. In about 20% of cases, conception occurs within the first month of unprotected intercourse. There continues to be an increase in the number of women who gave birth to their first child after the age of 30. Delaying parenthood appears to increase the possibility that one or more of the physiologic processes necessary for conception will be adversely affected (Collins & Rowe 1989; Speroff et al 1989).

Care of the Couple with Inability to Conceive

The easiest and least intrusive infertility testing approach is used first. Extensive testing is avoided until data confirm that the timing of intercourse and the length of coital exposure have been adequate. The couple should be informed of the most fertile times to have intercourse during the menstrual cycle. Teaching the couple the signs of and timing of ovulation within the cycle and effective sexual techniques may solve the problem before extensive testing needs to be initiated (see Table 5–2). Primary assessment, including a comprehensive history and physical examination for any obvious causes of infertility, is done before a costly, time-consuming, and emotionally trying investigation is initiated. During the first visit for the preliminary investigation, the basic infertility workup is explained. The basic investigation for the couple depends on the individuals' history and usually includes assessment of ovarian function, cervical mucosal adequacy and receptivity to sperm, sperm adequacy, tubal patency, and the general condition of the pelvic organs. Since approximately 40% of infertility

Table 5–1 Possible Causes of Infertility

Necessary norms	Deviations from normal
Female	
Favorable cervical mucus	Cervicitis, immunologic response (inhospitable mucus), use of coital lubricants, antisperm antibodies
Clear passage between cervix and tubes	Myomas, adhesions, adenomyosis, polyps, endometritis, cervical stenosis, endometriosis, congenital anomalies (for example, septate uterus, Asherman syndrome)
Patent tubes with normal motility	Pelvic inflammatory disease, peritubal adhesions, endometriosis, IUD, salpingitis (for example, tuberculosis), neoplasm, ectopic pregnancy, tubal ligation
Ovulation and release of ova	Primary ovarian failure, polycystic ovarian disease, hypothyroidism, pituitary tumor, lactation, periovarian adhesions, endometriosis, medications (for example, oral contraceptives), premature ovarian failure, hyperprolactinemia, Turner syndrome
No obstruction between ovary and uterus	Adhesions, endometriosis, pelvic inflammatory disease
Endometrial preparation	Anovulation, luteal phase defect, IUD, malformation, uterine infection
Male	
Normal semen analysis	Abnormalities of sperm or semen, polyspermia, congenital defect in testicular development, mumps after adolescence, cryptorchidism, infections, gonadal exposure to x rays, chemotherapy, smoking, alcohol abuse, malnutrition, chronic or acute metabolic disease, medications (for example, morphine, ASA, ibuprofen, and cocaine), marijuana use, constrictive underclothing, heat
Unobstructed genital tract	Infections, tumors, congenital anomalies, vasectomy, strictures, trauma, varicocele
Normal genital tract secretions	Infections, autoimmunity to semen, tumors
Ejaculate deposited at the cervix	Premature ejaculation, hypospadias, retrograde ejaculation (for example, diabetic), neurologic cord lesions, obesity (inhibiting adequate penetration)

Table 5–2 Self-Care: Fertility Awareness

Avoid douching and artificial lubricants. Prevent alteration of pH of vagina and introduction of spermicidal agents.

Promote retention of sperm. The male superior position with female remaining recumbent for at least one hour after intercourse maximizes the number of sperm reaching the cervix.

Avoid leakage of sperm. Elevate the woman's hips with a pillow after intercourse. Avoid getting up to urinate for one hour after intercourse.

Maximize the potential for fertilization. Have intercourse one to three times per week around the time of ovulation and at intervals of no less than 48 hours.

Avoid emphasizing conception during sexual encounters to decrease anxiety and potential sexual dysfunction.

Maintain adequate nutrition and reduce stress. Using stress reduction techniques and good nutrition habits increases sperm production.

Explore other methods to increase fertility awareness, such as home assessment of cervical mucus and basal body temperature recordings.

is related to a male factor, the noninvasive examination of semen should be one of the first diagnostic tests prior to moving on to the more invasive diagnostic procedures involving the woman.

It is never easy to discuss one's sexual activity, especially when potentially irreversible problems with fertility may exist. The mutual desire to have children is central to many marriages. A fertility problem is a deeply personal, emotion-laden area in a couple's life (Blenner 1990). The self-esteem of one or both partners may be threatened if the inability to conceive is seen as a lack of virility or femininity. The nurse can provide comfort to couples by offering a sympathetic ear, a nonjudgmental atmosphere, and appropriate information and instructions. The nurse should encourage the presence of both partners. Since counseling includes discussion of very personal matters, nurses who are comfortable with their own sexuality are more capable of establishing rapport and eliciting relevant information.

Health care interventions in cases of infertility are illustrated in Figure 5–1. Following the initial interview with the couple, a comprehensive history is taken and a physical examination is performed. The historical data base for the couple should include the following information.

A. Female
1. Medical/surgical history
   a. Current/past illness
   b. Radiation exposure
   c. Past surgical history including abdominal surgeries (such as appendectomy)
   d. Medications

e. Adult weight history
f. Rubella immunity

2. Gynecologic history
   a. Menstrual/ovulation history, including age of menarche; interval, duration and quantity of menses; dysmenorrhea (medications used); impact on daily activities; date of last menstrual period; premenstrual changes such as mood swings, breast tenderness, acne; mittelschmertz (midcycle ovulation pain); intermenstrual spotting; amenorrhea (primary or secondary)

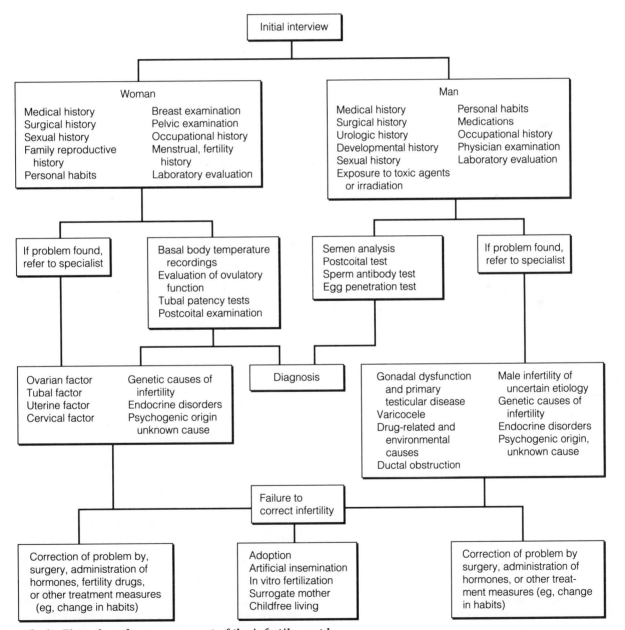

Figure 5–1   Flow chart for management of the infertile couple

   b. Current or recent lactation, galactorrhea (milky breast discharge), hirsutism
   c. Last Pap smear, history of abnormal Pap smears and treatment (cone biopsy, cryosurgery)
   d. History of endometriosis
   e. History of in utero exposure to di-ethylstilbestrol (DES)
   f. History of sexually transmitted disease and treatment, history of pelvic inflammatory disease

3. Family history
   a. Genetic history
   b. History of birth defects
   c. History of reproductive problems
   d. Ethnic background and religion (screen for Tay-Sachs disease, sickle-cell disease, or thalassemia)

4. Social History
   a. Religion
   b. Occupation (exposure to toxic substances, work hours may conflict with adequate intercourse)
   c. Exercise (strenuous exercise such as long-distance running or professional dancing may contribute to amenorrhea)
   d. Educational background
   e. Cigarette smoking, alcohol or non-prescribed drug use
   f. Dietary habits (current or past history of eating disorders)

5. Pregnancy/fertility history
   a. Number of pregnancies, age at conception, outcome, number of partners, number of spontaneous abortions or therapeutic abortions.
   b. Complications, history of ectopic pregnancy and treatment (ruptured, tube removed), history of preterm labor/birth, cesarean births, infant birth weights
   c. Duration of infertility (length of time without conception)
   d. Past contraceptive measures used and when (type, duration, complications)

6. Sexual history: practices and knowledge
   a. Frequency and timing of intercourse, satisfaction
   b. Use of lubricants, positions used, douching practices.

B. Male
1. Medical/surgical history
   a. Current medications and past long-term medications
   b. History of groin injury, mumps after adolescence, tuberculosis, sexually transmitted diseases, acute viral illness in the last three months
   c. Surgical history, including hernia repair, vasectomy or vasectomy reversal, varicocele repair

2. Developmental history
   a. History of endocrine disease
   b. Age of growth spurt, appearance of facial hair and other secondary sexual characteristics

3. Family history
   a. Genetic history
   b. History of birth defects
   c. History of reproductive problems
   d. Ethnic background and religion (screen for Tay-Sachs disease, sickle-cell disease, or thalassemia

4. Social history
   a. Religion
   b. Occupation (exposure to toxic substances, work hours, sitting for extended hours (eg, truck drivers)
   c. Exercise (strenuous? marathon runner? use of hot baths after exercise?)
   d. Educational background
   e. Cigarette smoking, alcohol or non-prescribed drug use

5. Sexual/fertility history
   a. Previous fertility history
   b. History of infertility
   c. Sexual practices
   d. Knowledge, satisfaction

Following completion of the couple's histories, a complete physical examination of each partner is performed. See Table 5–3.

Tests for Infertility

After a thorough history and physical examination of both partners, tests may be initiated to identify other causes of infertility. Infertility may be related to a female problem, to a male problem, or to multifactorial problems.

A thorough history and physical evaluation of the female includes assessment of the structure and function of the cervix, uterus, fallopian tubes, and ovaries. Evaluation of the male includes at least two careful semen analyses and possible evaluation of immunologic causes of infertility and sperm penetration. The female fertility assessments will be discussed first. For review of female reproductive cycle characteristics, see Table 5–4 and Figure 5–2.

Table 5–3 Infertility Physical Workup and Laboratory Evaluation

Female	Male
1. Physical examination a. Assessment of height, weight, blood pressure, temperature, and general health status b. Endocrine evaluation of thyroid for exophthalmos, lid lag, tremor, or palpable gland c. Fundus evaluation for presence of increased intracranial pressure especially in oligomenorrheal or amenorrheal women (possible pituitary tumor) d. Reproductive features (including breast and external genital area) e. Physical ability to tolerate pregnancy	1. Physical examination a. General health (assessment of height, weight, blood pressure) b. Endocrine evaluation (for example, presence of gynecomastia) c. Visual fields evaluation for bitemporal hemianopia d. Abnormal hair patterns
2. Pelvic examination a. Papanicolaou smear b. Culture for gonorrhea, if indicated, also possible chlamydia or mycoplasma culture (opinions vary) (Risi & Sanders 1989; Speroff 1989) c. Signs of vaginal infections (see Chapter 10) d. Shape of escutcheon (for example, does pubic hair distribution resemble that of a male?) e. Size of clitoris (enlargement caused by endocrine disorders) f. Evaluation of cervix: old lacerations, tears, erosion, polyps, condition and shape of os, signs of infections, cervical mucus (evaluate for estrogen effect of spinnbarkheit and cervical ferning)	2. Urologic examination (includes presence or absence of phimosis; location of urethral meatus; size and consistency of each testis, vas deferens, and epididymis; presence of varicocele) 3. Rectal examination a. Size and consistency of the prostate, with microscopic evaluation of prostate fluid for signs of infection b. Size and consistency of the seminal vesicles
3. Bimanual examination a. Size, shape, position, and mobility of uterus b. Presence of congenital anomalies c. Presence of endometriosis d. Evaluation of adnexa: ovarian size, cysts, fixations, or tumors	4. Laboratory examination a. Complete blood count b. Sedimentation rate if indicated c. Serology d. Urinalysis e. Rh factor and blood grouping f. Semen analysis (two to three separate analyses) g. If indicated, testicular biopsy, buccal smear
4. Rectovaginal examination a. Presence of retroflexed or retroverted uterus b. Presence of rectouterine pouch masses c. Presence of possible endometriosis	
5. Laboratory examination a. Complete blood count b. Sedimentation rate if indicated c. Serology (hepatitis antibody and HIV if indicated) d. Urinalysis e. Rh factor and blood grouping, rubella titer f. If indicated, thyroid function tests, prolactin glucose tolerance test, 17-ketosteroid assay, 17-hydrocorticoid assay, testosterone or dihydroepiandrestenedrone levels	

Table 5–4 Female Reproductive Cycle

FRC includes the ovarian cycle and the menstrual cycle

Ovarian Cycle

Follicular phase (days 1–14): Primordial follicle matures under influence of FSH and LH up to the time of ovulation.

Luteal phase (days 15–28): Ovum leaves follicle, corpus luteum develops under LH influence and produces high levels of progesterone and low levels of estrogen.

Menstrual Cycle

Menstrual phase (days 1–5)

Proliferative phase (days 6–14): Estrogen peaks just prior to ovulation. Cervical mucus at ovulation is clear, thin, watery, alkaline, and more favorable to sperm; shows ferning pattern; and has spinnbarkheit greater than 5 cm. At ovulation body temperature drops, then rises sharply and remains elevated.

Secretory phase (days 15–26): Estrogen drops sharply and progesterone dominates.

Ischemic phase (days 27–28): Both estrogen and progesterone levels drop.

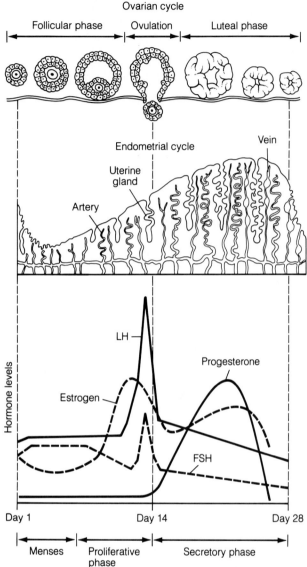

Figure 5–2 Sequence of events in a normal reproductive cycle showing the relationship of hormone levels to events in the ovarian and endometrial cycles. From Ovulation Induction: Clinical Aspects/Practical Applications, A Nursing Perspective, 1988:11, with permission of Serono Laboratories, Inc., Norwell, Massachusetts.

Evaluation of Ovulatory Factors

Ovulation problems account for approximately 25% of infertility (Seibel 1990). One basic test of ovulatory function is the **basal body temperature recording (BBT)**, which aids in identifying follicular and luteal phase abnormalities. At the initial visit, the woman is instructed in the technique of recording basal body temperature, which may be taken with a BBT thermometer. This special kind of thermometer measures temperature between 96F and 100F and is calibrated by tenths of a degree, thereby facilitating identifica-

tion of slight temperature changes. The woman may choose the site to obtain the temperature. Possible sites include oral, axillary, rectal, or vaginal, and the same site should be used each time. For best results the thermometer should be kept beside the bed, and the woman should take her temperature upon awakening, before any activity. After obtaining her temperature, she shakes the thermometer down to prepare it for use the next day. This step is important, as even the activity of shaking the thermometer immediately before use can cause a small increase in the basal temperature. Other factors that may produce temperature variation are sleeplessness, digestive disturbances, illness, fever, and emotional upset. Daily variations should be recorded on a temperature graph. The temperature graph typically shows a biphasic pattern during ovulatory cycles, whereas in anovulatory cycles it remains monophasic. The temperature graph and the readings are used for detecting timing of ovulation and the best time for intercourse (Figure 5–3).

Basal temperature for females in the preovulatory phase is usually below 98F (36.7C). As ovulation approaches, production of estrogen increases and at its peak may cause a slight drop, then rise, in the basal temperature. When ovulation occurs, there is a surge of luteinizing hormone (LH), and progesterone is produced by the corpus luteum, causing a 0.5F to 1.0F (0.3C to 0.6C) rise in basal temperature. These changes in the basal temperatures create the typical biphasic pattern. Figure 5–3B shows a biphasic ovulatory BBT chart. Progesterone is thermogenic (it produces heat) thereby maintaining the temperature increase during the second half of the menstrual cycle. Temperature elevation does not predict the day of ovulation but provides supportive evidence of ovulation about a day after it has occurred. Actual release of the ovum probably occurs 24 to 36 hours prior to the first temperature elevation (Speroff et al 1989).

With the additional documentation of coitus, serial BBT charts can be used to indicate if, and approximately when, the woman is ovulating and if intercourse is occurring at the proper time to achieve conception. A proposed schedule for intercourse based on serial BBT charts might be to recommend sexual intercourse *every other day* in the period of time beginning 3 to 4 days prior to and continuing for 2 to 3 days following the expected time of ovulation.

Hormonal assessments of ovulatory function fall into two categories:

1. *LH assays.* A more sensitive assay of ovulatory function is measurement of serum or urine LH. Daily sampling of LH at midcycle can detect the LH surge. The day of the LH surge is believed to be the day of maximum fertility. Urine testing can be done at home. Serum LH levels can be tested by radioimmune assay (RIA). Normal serum values vary depending on the phase of the menstrual cycle.

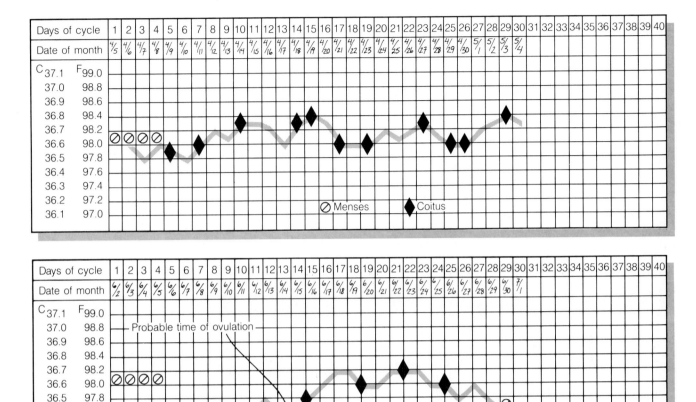

Figure 5–3 *A A monophasic, anovulatory basal body temperature chart. B A biphasic basal body temperature chart illustrating ovulation, the different types of testing, and the time in the cycle that each would be performed*

2. *Progesterone assays.* Progesterone levels furnish the best evidence of ovulation and corpus luteum functioning. Plasma progesterone levels begin to rise with the LH surge and peak about eight days after the LH surge. Two blood samples, on days 8 and 21, showing an increase of from less than 1 ng/mL to greater than 5 ng/mL indicates ovulation. A normal serum progesterone level is 10 ng/mL or higher on day 21 (Seibel 1990). Urinary pregnanediol reaches levels of 4 to 6 mg at 24 hours after ovulation; a level of 2 mg at 24 hours or greater indicates ovulation. Serum progesterone levels may be assayed in conjunction with an endometrial biopsy.

Biopsy of the endometrium provides information regarding the effects of progesterone produced by the corpus luteum after ovulation.

The biopsy is usually performed in a physician's office 2 to 6 days before menstruation since this is the time of the greatest luteal function. A sample of endometrium from the fundal area of the uterus is obtained with a special small tubular curet, which is attached to either electric, water, or syringe suction. The woman should be informed that she will experience cramping similar to menstrual cramps at the time the actual specimen is taken.

A dysfunction may exist if the endometrial lining does not show the expected amount of secretory tissue for that day of the woman's menstrual cycle. Endometrial biopsies and serum progesterone assay may both be necessary to confirm luteal phase dysfunction.

Ultrasound is now being used as an important adjunct in determining changes in follicular development and detecting timing of ovulation (Hecht & Hoffman 1989). This is extremely useful in defining timing of intercourse or artificial insemination. Ultrasound in conjunction with labo-

TEACHING GUIDE
Self-Care Methods of Determining Ovulation

Assessment The nurse focuses on the woman's knowledge of her own body functions, mucus secretions, and menstrual cycle.

Nursing Diagnosis The key nursing diagnosis will probably be: Knowledge deficit related to normal body changes occurring with menstruation and ovulation.

Nursing Plan and Implementation The teaching plan will include information on expected changes in cervical mucus and body temperature related to menstrual cycle, how to recognize that ovulation has occurred, and self-care methods for determining fertility days.

Client Goals At the completion of the teaching session, the woman will be able to:

1. Accurately identify cervical mucus changes.
2. Accurately take and record BBT temperature.
3. Discuss the changes in BBT and cervical mucus that indicate ovulation has occurred.
4. Summarize physical symptoms that may indicate ovulation has occurred.

Teaching Plan

Content

Basal Body Temperature (BBT) Expected findings: The BBT can sometimes drop 12 to 24 hours before ovulation but a sustained rise *almost always* follows for several days, or a biphasic pattern with temperature elevation for 12 to 14 days prior to menstruation can be seen. At ovulation, temperature will rise 0.4−0.8F above baseline pre-ovulatory level. Some women notice a drop in temperature 24 hours prior to ovulation. Once a 0.4−0.8F rise has occurred for three consecutive days a woman can safely have intercourse since her fertile days have passed. All three days should have higher temperature readings than any of the previous days in the cycle. A woman needs to take her BBT for three to four months to develop a consistent pattern.

Procedure: The woman should take her temperature for five minutes every morning before she gets out of bed (needs at least three hours of sleep) and before starting any activity (including smoking). She should choose one site (oral, vaginal, rectal) and use same site each time. A BBT thermometer is preferable. After five minutes she should record her temperature on special BBT chart (with 0.1 markings). The temperature dots for each day are connected to see baseline temperature readings. (See Figure 5−3.)

Special considerations: Situations that can disturb body temperature: large alcohol intake, sleeplessness, gastrointestinal or other illness, immunization, warm or hot climate, jet lag, or use of electric blanket.

Teaching Method Discuss BBT changes.

Demonstrate BBT thermometer and chart.

Provide pictures of anovulation cycle and biphasic cycle.

(continued)

TEACHING GUIDE (continued)

Teaching Plan

Cervical Mucus Method Expected findings: Pre- and postovulatory mucus is yellow, thick, and dry; or absent; or white and cloudy. Close to or during ovulation, mucus is clear, slippery (like egg whites), and elastic (can be stretched between two fingers—spinnbarkheit). Ovulation most likely occurs about 24 hours after the last day of abundant, slippery discharge (Hatcher et al 1990). Four days after peak mucus or when it is again dry, thick, and cloudy, the woman has passed her fertile days and may resume intercourse.

Mucus changes: During menstruation blood covers up sensation of wetness or mucus. For a few days after menstruation the vagina feels moist but is not distinctly wet (called "dry" days). The next mucus stage is thick, cloudy, whitish or yellowish, and sticky mucus. Vagina still doesn't feel wet and this lasts for several days. As ovulation nears, mucus usually becomes more abundant, accompanied by an increasingly wet sensation. Next the clear slippery mucus decreases until it is no longer detectable and either the thick, cloudy, sticky mucus returns or there is no mucus at all until the next menstrual period.

Procedure: The woman should check her vagina each day when she uses the bathroom, either by dabbing the vaginal opening with toilet paper or by putting a finger inside the opening. She should note the wetness (presence of mucus), collect mucus, and look at its color and consistency. Findings are recorded on chart each day. Several cycles of mucus changes are recorded to become familiar with the pattern before relying on this method.

Special considerations: Presence and consistency of mucus is altered by vaginal infection, vaginal medications such as creams or suppositories, spermicides, lubricants, douching, sexual arousal, or semen.

Some advise complete abstinence throughout the *first* cycle a woman charts her mucus changes to help her avoid confusing mucus with semen and normal sexual lubrication.

Other Additional physical findings that may indicate ovulation has occurred include slight vaginal spotting, mittelschmertz, increased libido.

Evaluation Teaching has been effective if the nurse discussed BBT and cervical mucus changes associated with ovulation, demonstrated BBT procedure and charting of BBT and cervical mucus changes. The woman feels comfortable with BBT and cervical mucus procedure and completion of charting. The woman is able to describe her body functions, how they change, and how they can be used to identify fertile periods and the time at which ovulation may occur.

Show woman posters of mucus changes, spinnbarkheit of different elasticity.

Discuss feelings about actual procedure.

Discuss rationale for physical changes. Answer questions?

ratory hormone assays is critical for clients preparing for in vitro fertilization (IVF) or gamete intrafallopian transfer (GIFT). These procedures are discussed later in this chapter.

Evaluation of Cervical Factors

The cervical mucus cells of the endocervix consist predominantly of water. As ovulation approaches, the ovary increases its secretion of estrogen and produces changes in the cervical mucus. The amount of mucus increases tenfold and the water content rises significantly.

Mucus elasticity or **spinnbarkheit** increases and the viscosity decreases at ovulation. Excellent spinnbarkheit exists when the mucus can be stretched 8 to 10 cm or longer (Speroff et al 1989). This is accomplished by using two glass slides (Figure 5–4A) or by grasping some mucus at the external os and stretching it in the vagina toward the introitus. Studies are exploring the possibility of cervical mucus strand size and spacing as causes of infertility (Poon & McCoshen 1985).

The **ferning capacity** (Figure 5–4B) of the cervical mucus also increases as ovulation approaches. Ferning, or crystallization, is caused by decreased levels of salt and water interacting with the glycoproteins in the mucus during the ovulatory period and is thus an indirect indication of estrogen production. To test for ferning, mucus is obtained from the cervical os, spread on a glass slide, allowed to air dry, and examined under the microscope.

To be receptive to sperm, cervical mucus must be thin, clear, watery, profuse, alkaline, and acellular. As shown in Figure 5–5, the mazelike microscopic mucoid strands align in a parallel manner to allow for easy sperm passage. The mucus is termed inhospitable if these changes do not occur.

Cervical mucus inhospitable to sperm survival can have several causes, some of which are treatable. For example, estrogen secretion may be inadequate for the development of receptive mucus. Therapy with supplemental estrogen for approximately six days before expected ovulation encourages the formation of suitable spinnbarkheit (Speroff et al 1989). In addition, use of oral guaifenesin during the follicular phase may help decrease the viscosity of cervical mucus. Cervical infection, another cause of mucosal hostility to sperm, can be treated, depending on the type of infection. Cone biopsy, electrocautery, or cryosurgery of the cervix may remove large numbers of mucus-producing glands, creating a "dry cervix" that decreases sperm survival (Hammond & Talbert 1985).

The cervix can also be the site of secretory immunologic reactions in which antisperm antibodies are produced, causing agglutination or immobilization of sperm. A mucus-sperm contact or sperm penetration test has been developed in which initial interaction is observed microscopically. The most widely used serum-sperm bioassays are the gelatin agglutination tests, the sperm immobilization test, and radioimmunoassays, which have been developed to detect specific classes of antibodies in serum and seminal fluid. The treatment for antisperm antibodies

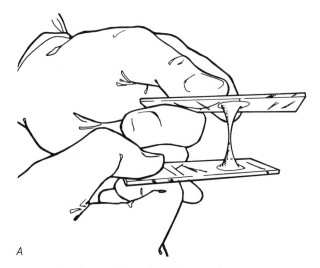

A

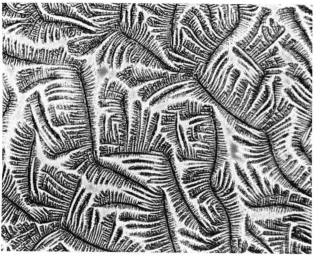

B

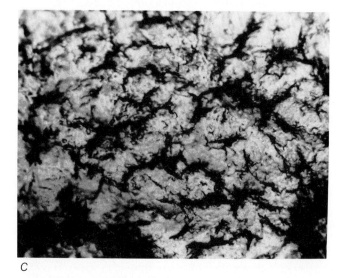

C

Figure 5–4 A Spinnbarkheit (elasticity). B Ferning pattern. C Lack of ferning pattern (From Speroff L et al: Clinical Gynecologic Endocrinology and Infertility, *4th ed. Baltimore: Williams & Wilkins, 1989, p 520.)*

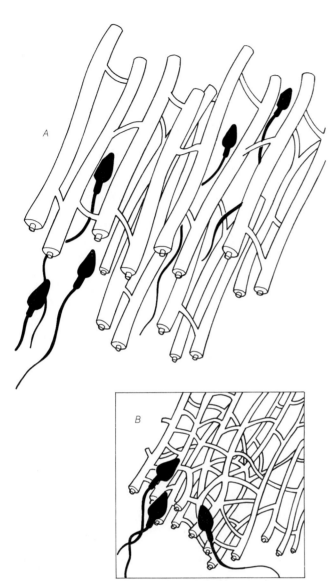

Figure 5–5 Sperm passage through cervical mucus. A Receptive mucus under estrogen influence coincides with ovulation. B Nonreceptive mucus under influence of progesterone, endogenous or exogenous (From Fogel CL, Woods NP: Health Care of Women. *St. Louis: Mosby, 1981)*

remains an area of controversy. Treatments include the following:

- Intrauterine insemination of the male's washed sperm (Smarr et al 1988)
- Corticosteroid therapy for immunosuppression to reduce antibody concentrations (Smarr et al 1988)
- When only the woman has a positive antibody titer, condom use for six months to reduce the titer by decreasing the exposure to the antigen (Speroff 1989)

The **postcoital examination (Huhner test)** is performed one or two days prior to the expected date of ovu-

lation. This examination evaluates the cervical mucus and the number and motility of the sperm at the endocervix. The procedure assesses the sperm's ability to negotiate the cervical barrier and the interaction of sperm and mucus.

The couple is asked to have intercourse four to six hours before examination. A small plastic catheter, attached to a 10-mL syringe, is placed in the cervix. Mucus is aspirated from the internal and external os, measured, and examined microscopically for signs of infection, spinnbarkheit, ferning, number of active spermatozoa per highpowered field, and number of spermatozoa with poor or no motility.

Evaluation of Male Factors

A semen analysis is the most important initial diagnostic study of the male. It is one of the first steps in infertility testing because it is relatively simple and precludes unnecessary exposure of the female partner to high-risk painful procedures.

To obtain adequate results the specimen is collected after two to three days of abstinence. If the male has difficulty producing sperm other than during intercourse, special condoms are available to collect the sperm. Regular condoms should not be used because they contain spermicidal agents and sperm can be lost on the condom. The specimen should be placed in a glass container and brought to the laboratory within an hour of collection if possible (2 to 3 hours maximum). It should be marked with the time of collection and date of previous ejaculation and maintained at body temperature. Repeated semen analysis may be required to identify the male's fertility potential adequately, a minimum of two separate analyses is recommended. Semen collections should be repeated at least 74 days apart to allow for new germ cell maturation. (Speroff et al 1989).

Sperm analysis provides information about sperm motility and morphology as well as a determination of the absolute number of spermatozoa present (Table 5–5). Debate exists over the absolute number of sperm required for fertility. An infertile specimen is one that reveals fewer than 10 million sperm per milliliter, less than 50% to 60% active sperm, motility at 6 hours or less than 35%, or less than 60% normal sperm forms (Seibel 1990).

Table 5–5 Normal Semen Analysis

Factor	Value
Volume	2 to 6 cc
pH	7.0 to 8.0
Total sperm count	20 million
Liquefaction	Complete in one hour
Motility	50% or greater
Normal forms	60% or greater

(Source: Speroff L, Glass RH, Kase NG: Clinical Gynecologic Endocrinology and Infertility, *4th ed. Williams & Wilkins, 1989.*

Spermatozoa have been shown to possess intrinsic antigens that can provoke male immunologic infertility. This is especially apparent following vasectomy reversals or genital trauma such as testicular torsion in which autoimmunity to sperm develops (the male produces antibodies to his own sperm) (Igbal et al 1989). Research now indicates that it is the actual presence of antibodies on the spermatozoal surface (not just the presence of antibodies in the serum) that affects sperm function and thus leads to subfertility). Treatment for the presence of sperm antibodies in the male may include immunosuppression, and sperm washing-dilution insemination techniques. Other tests of sperm function, including sperm penetration assay (SPA) or hamster egg penetration tests, are available (Grunfeld 1989). The efficacy of these tests in predicting penetration by the sperm of the human egg is still unclear (Chan et al 1989; Daya et al 1989).

Evaluation of Uterine Structures and Tubal Patency

Tubal patency tests are usually done after BBT evaluation, semen analysis, and the other less invasive tests have been done and results evaluated. Tubal patency and uterine structure are evaluated usually by hysterosalpingography. Other invasive tests of tubular function are laparoscopy and hysteroscopy. Hysteroscopy may be performed earlier in the evaluation if the woman's history suggests possible tubal damage or uterine abnormalities.

Hysterosalpingography, or **hysterogram**, involves an instillation of a radiopaque substance into the uterine cavity. As the substance fills the uterus and fallopian tubes and spills into the peritoneal cavity, it is viewed with x-ray techniques. This procedure can reveal tubal patency and any distortions of the endometrial cavity. Hysterosalpingography has also been known to have a therapeutic effect. This effect may be caused by the flushing of debris, breaking of adhesions, or induction of peristalsis by the instillation.

The hysterosalpingogram should be performed in the proliferative phase of the cycle to avoid interrupting an early pregnancy. This timing also avoids the lush secretory changes in the endometrium that occur after ovulation, which may prevent the passage of the dye and present a false picture of cornual obstruction. Hysterosalpingography causes moderate discomfort. The pain is referred from the peritoneum, which is irritated by the subdiaphragmatic collection of gas, to the shoulder.

Hysteroscopy allows the physician to further evaluate any areas of suspicion within the uterine cavity that have been revealed by the hysterosalpingogram. It is often done in conjunction with a laparoscopy but can be done independently and does not require general anesthesia. A fiberoptic instrument is placed into the uterus for further evaluation of polyps, myomata, or structural variations (Speroff et al 1989).

Laparoscopy enables direct visualization of the pelvic organs and is usually done six to eight months after the hysterosalpingogram unless symptoms suggest the need for earlier evaluation. The woman usually is given a general anesthetic for this procedure. Entry is generally made through an incision in the umbilical area, although it is occasionally done suprapubically. The peritoneal cavity is distended with carbon dioxide gas, and the pelvic organs can be directly visualized with a fiberoptic instrument. Tubular function can be assessed by instillation of dye into the uterine cavity through the cervix. The pelvis is evaluated for endometriosis, adhesions, organ fixations, pelvic inflammatory disease, tumors, and cysts. Visualization is best when the procedure is performed in the early follicular stage of the cycle (Siebel 1990). The intraperitoneal gas is usually manually expressed at the end of the procedure. Routine preanesthesia instructions should be given. The woman is told she may have some discomfort from organ displacement and shoulder and chest pain caused by gas in the abdomen lasting 24 to 48 hours after the procedure. She should be informed that she can resume normal activities after resting for about two days. Using postoperative pain medication and assuming a "knee-chest" position may help relieve discomfort.

Culdoscopy is sometimes used to assess tubular function. Culdoscopic examination of pelvic structures is accompanied by injecting indigo, carmine, or similar dyes through a cannula inserted into the cervix after local anesthetic infiltration.

Methods of Infertility Management

Pharmacologic Methods

If an ovulatory defect has been detected during the fertility testing, the treatment depends on the specific cause of the problem. In the presence of normal ovaries and an intact pituitary gland, *clomiphene citrate (Clomid)* is often used (see Drug Guide: Clomid). This medication induces ovulation in 80% of women by actions at both the hypothalamic and ovarian levels, and 40% of these women will become pregnant. Approximately 5% of women develop multiple gestation pregnancies, almost exclusively twins. Clomiphene works by increasing the secretion of LH, which stimulates follicle growth (Archer et al 1989).

The woman is instructed to take the medication daily for five days, usually beginning on day 5 of the menstrual cycle. She is informed that if ovulation occurs, it will be on cycle day 14 to 16. The presence of ovulation and evaluation of the response to therapy is assessed by BBT or LH monitoring, ultrasound evaluation, and possibly progesterone assays in conjunction with an endometrial biopsy.

A pelvic exam should be done to rule out ovarian enlargement, hyperstimulation syndrome, or the presence of pregnancy before another cycle is begun. Ovarian enlargement and abdominal discomfort may result from follicular growth and development of multiple corpus luteum formation. Persistence of ovarian cysts is a contraindication for further clomiphene administration. Other side effects in-

DRUG GUIDE
Clomid (Clomiphene Citrate)

Overview of Action

Clomid stimulates follicular growth by increasing secretion of FSH and LH. Ovulation is expected to occur five to ten days after last dose. Used when anovulation is caused by hypothalamic suppression, luteal phase dysfunction, oligo-ovulation and in vitro fertilization.

Route, Dosage, Frequency

Administered orally. Fifty mg/day to 250 mg/day from day 5 to day 9 (total of five days) of the menstrual cycle. Usually start with 50 mg/day and increase dose 50 mg each time (Kennedy & Adashi 1987). May need to give estrogen simultaneously if decrease in cervical mucus occurs.

Contraindications

Presence of ovarian enlargement, ovarian cysts, hyperstimulation syndrome, liver disease, visual problems, pregnancy.

Side Effects

Antiestrogenic effects may cause decrease in cervical mucus production.

Other side effects include: vasomotor flushes; abdominal distention and ovarian enlargement secondary to follicular growth and development and multiple corpus luteum formation; bloating, pain, soreness, breast discomfort; nausea and vomiting; visual symptoms (spots, flashes); headaches; dryness or loss of hair; multiple pregnancies.

Nursing Considerations

Determine if couple has been advised to have sexual intercourse every other day for one week beginning five days after the last day of medications.

Instruct couple on use of BBT chart to assess if ovulation has occurred. Also inform couple that plasma progesterone, cervical mucus, and vaginal cytology may be done.

Remind couples that if the woman doesn't have a period she must be checked for the possibility of pregnancy before another trial of Clomid is started.

clude vasomotor flushes, abdominal distention, bloating, breast discomfort, nausea and vomiting, vision problems (such as visual spots), headache, and dryness or loss of hair. Supplemental low-dose estrogen may be given to ensure appropriate quality and quantity of cervical mucus, since clomiphene has been shown to inhibit mucus production (Chong et al 1987).

 Self-Care Measures Women can assess the presence of ovulation and possible response to clomiphene therapy by doing BBT and evaluating cervical mucus. The woman should be knowledgeable about side effects and call her health care provider if they occur. When visual disturbances (flashes, blurring, spots) occur, the woman should avoid brightly lit rooms. This side effect disappears within a few days or weeks after discontinuation of therapy (Kennedy & Adashi 1987). The occurrence of hot flashes may be due to the antiestrogenic properties of Clomid. Some relief can be obtained through increased intake of fluids and use of fans.

Human menopausal gonadotropin (hMG) also referred to as menotropin, is a combination of FSH and LH obtained from postmenopausal women's urine and administered intramuscularly every day for varying periods of time during the first half of the cycle to stimulate follicular development (Speroff et al 1989). The most common commercial preparation is Pergonal. Ovarian overstimulation syndrome may develop with this form of therapy. Follicle size and number must be monitored by real-time ultrasound and serum estradiol assays, and hMG is administered to match the LH surge and follicle development. When follicle maturation has occurred, human chorionic gonadotropin (hCG) may be administered by intramuscular injection to stimulate ovulation. The couple is advised to have intercourse on the day of the hCG administration and for the next two days. The multiple birth rate is reported to be about 20% with 15% twins. Women who elect to have hMG medication usually have passed through all other forms of management without conceiving. Strong emotional support and thorough education are needed because of the numerous office visits and injections resulting in potentially significant stress in the couple's relationship.

When hyperprolactinemia accompanies anovulation, the infertility may be treated with *bromocriptine.* This medication acts directly on the prolactin-secreting cells in the anterior pituitary. It inhibits the pituitary's secretion of prolactin—thus preventing suppression of the pulsatile secretion of FSH and LH. This restores normal menstrual cycles—and induces ovulation by allowing FSH and LH production. High prolactin levels may impair the glandular production of FSH and LH and/or block their action on the ovaries. If treatment is successful, the tests of ovulatory function will indicate that ovulation is occurring and a normal biphasic pattern will result. Bromocriptine should be discontinued if pregnancy is suspected or at the anticipated time of ovulation because of its possible teratogenic effects. Other side effects include nausea, diarrhea, dizziness, headache, and fatigue.

When endometriosis is determined to be the cause of the infertility, *danazol* (Danocrine) may be given to suppress ovulation and menstruation and to effect atrophy of the ectopic endometrial tissue. Other pharmologic treatments involve use of oral contraceptives or oral medoxyprogesterone acetate, and GnRH agonists (Friedman et al 1989). For in-depth discussion of the management and care needed for endometriosis see Chapter 8.

Gonadotropin-releasing hormone is a new therapeutic tool for ovulation stimulation. It is used for women who have insufficient endogenous release of GnRH. Administration is usually by continuous intravenous infusion accomplished by a portable infusion pump with a pulsatile mechanism worn on a belt around the waist. The length of treatment varies from two to four weeks and hCG is also given to stimulate ovulation. The risk of multiple gestation and hyperstimulation is less than with hMG therapy, and the treatment is also less expensive (Speroff et al 1989). Significant client education and support are necessary for effective use of the pump. Some women find the pump cumbersome.

Progesterone therapy for luteal phase defects may also be effective. This may be given alone or in conjunction with clomiphene (Murray et al 1989).

Artificial Insemination

Artificial insemination, with either the husband's semen (AIH) or that of a donor (AID), is the depositing of semen at the cervical os or in the uterus by mechanical means. The conception rates are approximately 30% for AID and 15% for AIH. AIH is used in cases of too small or too large a volume of sperm, too few or too many sperm, low levels of spermatozoal motility, anatomic defects accompanied by inadequate deposition or penetration of semen, or retrograde ejaculation (Jacobs & Ory 1989; American Fertility Society 1990).

AID is considered in cases of total lack of sperm motility or combination of inadequate motility and viability of sperm or inherited disorders affecting only males. AID is not appropriate therapy in cases of women with antibodies, since they have antibodies against antigens common to all human sperm cells, not just to their partner's sperm.

Numerous factors need to be evaluated before AID is performed. Has every possible effort been made to diagnose and treat the cause of the male infertility? Do tests indicate normal fertility and sperm/ovum transport in the woman? Is each member psychologically stable? Is this a voluntary decision on the part of the male partner? Are there any religious constraints? Does the donor have any disease or genetic problems? If insemination by donor is being considered, screening for HIV infection needs to be considered as well (Quagliarello 1988).

Artificial insemination is accomplished by collecting semen from the male in a glass container. The semen then is drawn into a syringe and placed in a small plastic cervical cup. The cup is put in place at the cervical os, and the woman remains in the supine position with the hips elevated for about 30 minutes. An alternative method is to instill the semen directly into the uterus using a small plastic catheter on a syringe. The semen must first be chemically cleansed and centrifuged. This method enables the semen to bypass possible cervical or immunologic factors.

In Vitro Fertilization

The first birth conceived by *in vitro fertilization (IVF)* was achieved in Great Britain in 1978. This procedure is selectively used in cases in which infertility has resulted from tubal factors, mucus abnormalities, male factors, and immunity to spermatozoa in either partner and when infertility is long-term and unexplained.

Ovulation is induced using fertility drugs, and ovarian function is monitored daily with blood tests, cervical mucus tests, and ultrasound. Just before ovulation, the ripened ova are aspirated from the ovaries during laparoscopy or through a transvaginal or transurethral approach (Speroff et al 1989). The ova are fertilized with the prospective father's sperm and transferred to the mother's uterus when they reach the four- to eight-cell stage of development. A series of progesterone injections are given to assist the process of implantation.

In vitro fertilization is an invasive method of treating infertility. The risk to offspring can only be assessed with more experience. Controversy concerning IVF has elicited concern, criticism, opinions, and condemnation from a variety of church leaders and scientists. In spite of the ethical and legal issues, it has found fairly wide acceptance with childless couples. It should be noted that IVF costs several thousand dollars and the chances of success are about 10%.

Other Assisted Reproductive Techniques

Other assisted reproductive technologies are being developed, including gamete intrafallopian transfer (GIFT) and zygote intrafallopian transfer (ZIFT) (Medical Research International 1990; Devroey et al 1990). In GIFT, ovulation is induced similarly to IVF. However, after eggs are retrieved they are placed directly into the fallopian tube alone with the male's sperm, usually via laparoscopy. In ZIFT, eggs are retrieved and incubated with the male's sperm similarly to IVF. However, eggs are transferred back to the woman's body at a much earlier stage of cell division and, as in GIFT, are placed in the fallopian tube or tubes and not the uterus.

Contemporary Issue
How Many Is Too Many?

In vitro fertilization has been an answer for many couples who are unable to conceive. The procedure involves retrieval of the woman's ovum at the time of ovulation. After conception occurs, using the husband's sperm, the fertilized ovum is replaced in the woman's uterus. The chance of success is increased when more than one ovum is removed and fertilized.

Although in vitro fertilization has been viewed as a tremendous new development by many childless couples, some groups have raised questions about the procedure. Some of the issues include the following:

- If more than one fertilized ovum is returned to the uterus, it may be possible for the woman to have a multiple pregnancy of two to eight fetuses. This multiple pregnancy creates problems when birth occurs long before the estimated date of birth. The financial and emotional costs are great when the parents have more than one baby in an intensive care setting.

- If more than one ovum is fertilized and they are not returned to the uterus, what should be done with them? If they are kept, are the embryos entitled to inheritance from their family? If the embryos are destroyed, is it murder?

- Should "extra" embryos be made available for implantation into another woman's uterus?

- Should research be allowed on the extra embryos? If so under what conditions and for what purposes? Who should approve the research that is done? Is approval needed?

- If extra embryos are frozen and kept, how long should the facility be required to keep them? Does prolonged freezing harm the embryo?

- If sperm other than the husband's is used to fertilize the ovum, does it create special problems? Who does the child belong to? Does the husband need to adopt the child?

- With a success rate of approximately 10 to 20 percent, does in vitro fertilization take advantage of childless couples rather than helping them?

- Does the procedure move conception out of the human range entirely?

Success rates for these procedures are generally high, and GIFT may be more acceptable by adherents of some religions, since fertilization does not occur outside the woman's body (Medical Research International 1990).

Adoption

The adoption of an infant can be a difficult and/or frustrating experience for all persons involved (Arms 1990). A waiting period as long as seven years even to begin the adoption process is not uncommon. The decrease in number of available infants has occurred because many infants are reared by their single mothers instead of being relinquished for adoption as was customary in the past. In addition, many unwanted pregnancies are being terminated by elective abortion. Some couples seek international adoptions or consider adopting older children, children with handicaps, or children of mixed parentage because the adoption process in such cases is quicker and more children are available. The nurse can assist couples considering adoption by providing information on community resources for adoption as well as by providing support through the adoption process. Couples also need support if they choose to remain childless (Menning 1988).

The Nurse's Role

Approximately 15% of the childbearing population in the United States (one out of six couples) is unable to conceive or carry a pregnancy to term. The couple may incur tremendous emotional and physical stress as well as financial expense for infertility testing. Treatment can cost over $20,000 a year and insurance coverage may be limited. Years of effort and numerous evaluations and examinations may take place before a conception occurs, if one occurs at all. In a society that values children and considers them to be the natural result of marriage, infertile couples may face a myriad of tensions and discrimination.

The nurse needs to be constantly aware of the emotional needs and sometimes irrational thoughts and fears of the couple with a fertility problem. The emotional aspect of infertility is often more difficult for the couple than the testing and treatment. Constant attention to temperature charts and instructions about their sex life from a person outside the relationship naturally affects the spontaneity of a couple's interactions. Their relationship will be stressed by these and other intrusive but necessary measures. The tests may heighten feelings of frustration or anger between the partners. Correction of infertility may require surgery, administration of hormones, and other treatment measures. The need to share this intimate area of a relationship may cause feelings of guilt and shame. Throughout the evaluations and emotional-financial strains one or both partners may undergo at this time, the nurse plays a major role in teaching and offering emotional support. An assessment tool such as the infertility questionnaire (Table 5–6)

Table 5–6　Infertility Questionnaire*

Self-image

1. I feel bad about my body because of our inability to have a child.
2. Since our infertility, I feel I can do anything as well as I used to.
3. I feel as attractive as before our infertility.
4. I feel less masculine/feminine because of our inability to have a child.
5. Compared with others, I feel I am a worthwhile person.
6. Lately, I feel I am sexually attractive to my wife/husband.
7. I feel I will be incomplete as a man/woman if we cannot have a child.
8. Having an infertility problem makes me feel physically incompetent.

Guilt/Blame

1. I feel guilty about somehow causing our infertility.
2. I wonder if our infertility problem is due to something I did in the past.
3. My spouse makes me feel guilty about our problem.
4. There are times when I blame my spouse for our infertility.
5. I feel I am being punished because of our infertility.

Sexuality

1. Lately I feel I am able to respond to my spouse sexually.
2. I feel sex is a duty, not a pleasure.
3. Since our infertility problem, I enjoy sexual relations with my spouse.
4. We have sexual relations for the purpose of trying to conceive.
5. Sometimes I feel like a "sex machine," programmed to have sex during the fertile period.
6. Impaired fertility has helped our sexual relationship.
7. Our inability to have a child has increased my desire for sexual relations.
8. Our inability to have a child has decreased my desire for sexual relations.

The questionnaire is scored on a Likert scale with responses ranging from "strongly agree" to "strongly disagree." Each question is scored separately, and the mean score is determined for each section (Self-Image, Guilt/Blame, Sexuality). The total mean score is then divided by 3. A final mean score of greater than 3 indicates distress. From Bernstein, J., Assessment of psychological dysfunction associated with infertility. JOGNN (14) supplement. 1985.

Research Note

Clinical Application of Research

Janet Blenner (1990) used grounded theory to explore the perceptions of 25 couples undergoing infertility assessment and treatment. The emergent theory of self-care was substantive in nature. "Substantive theories are generated for a specific, circumscribed and empirical area of inquiry" (Hutchinson 1986, p 111).

According to the self-care theory which emerged from the data, all but one set of couples started in a passive, traditional patient role. Some patients remained in this role even when they recognized that their physicians lacked a complete picture of their (the couple's) problem. However, other patients, upon perception of fragmentation of their care created by the physician's inability to give complete attention to the problem, moved into an assertive role of actively acquiring knowledge.

The acquisition of knowledge moved the patient into a more equal role with the health professional and led to a third phase of active participation or "taking control" of their own treatment. The participants, in this phase, perceived the plan of care to be mutually derived and assumed more responsibility for the outcome of the care.

The fourth phase consisted of more satisfaction with the treatment and perception of better relationships with the health care providers. Passive couples who did not progress through these phases reported feelings of vulnerability and two of the couples actually stopped treatment.

Critical Thinking Applied to Research

Strengths: Description of grounded theory process, theoretical basis, sample and original interview questions. Identification of aspects of qualitative rigor including member checking.

Blenner J: Attaining self-care in infertility treatment. *Appl Nurs Res* 1990; 3(3): 98.

Hutchinson S: Grounded theory: The method. In: Munhall P, Oiler C: *Nursing Research: A Qualitative Perspective.* Norwalk, CT: Appleton-Century-Crofts, 1986.

---

can assist the nurse in determining the support needs of the couple. Extensive and repeated explanations may be necessary to help relieve anxiety.

Infertility may be perceived as a loss by one or both partners, and as in the loss of a loved one who dies, this situation is attended by feelings of grief and mourning. Each couple passes through several stages of feelings, not unlike those identified by Kübler-Ross: surprise, denial, anger, isolation, guilt, grief, and resolution (Menning 1988). It is important to remember that each partner may progress through the stages at different rates. Nonjudgmen-

tal acceptance and a professional caring attitude on the nurse's part can go far to dissipate the negative emotions the couple may experience while going through this process. This is also a time when the nurse may assess the quality of the couple's relationship: Are they able and willing to communicate verbally and share feelings? Are they mutually supportive? The answers to such questions may help the nurse identify areas of strength and weakness and construct an appropriate plan of care. At times, individual or group counseling with other infertile couples may facilitate the couple's resolution of feelings brought about by

Table 5–7 Tasks of the Infertile Couple

Tasks	Nursing interventions
1. Recognition of how infertility affects their lives and expression of feelings (may be negative toward self or mate)	1. Supportive: help to understand and facilitate free expression of feelings
2. Grieving the loss of potential offspring	2. Help to recognize feelings
3. Evaluation of reasons for wanting a child	3. Help to understand motives
4. Decision making about management	4. Identify alternatives; facilitate partner communication

(Source: Sawatzky M: Tasks of the infertile couple. JOGNN *1981; 10:132.)*

their own difficult situation. Sawatzky (1981) has identified the essential tasks of the infertile couple (Table 5–7).

Genetic Disorders

Even when conception has been achieved, families can have special reproductive concerns. The desired and expected outcome of any pregnancy is the birth of a healthy "perfect" baby. Unfortunately, a small but significant number of parents experience grief, fear, and anger when they discover that their baby has been born with a defect or a genetic disease. Such an abnormality may be evident at birth or may not appear for some time. The baby may have inherited a disease from one parent, creating guilt and strife within the family.

Regardless of the type or scope of the problem, parents will have many questions: "What did I do?" "What caused it?" "Will it happen again?" The nurse must anticipate the parents' questions and concerns and guide, direct, and support the family. To do so, the nurse must have a basic knowledge of genetics and genetic counseling. Many congenital anomalies and diseases are genetic or have a strong genetic component. Others are not genetic at all. The genetic counselor attempts to categorize the problem and answer the family's questions. Professional nurses can help expedite this process if they already have an understanding of the principles involved and are able to direct the family to the appropriate resources.

Chromosomes and Chromosomal Abnormalities

All hereditary material is carried on tightly coiled strands of DNA known as **chromosomes**. The chromosomes carry the genes, the smallest unit of inheritance, as discussed in greater detail in Chapter 11.

All **somatic** (body) cells contain 46 chromosomes, which is the **diploid** number, while the sperm and egg contain half as many (23) chromosomes, or the **haploid** number (see Chapter 11). There are 23 pairs of *homologous* chromosomes (a matched pair of chromosomes, one inherited from each parent). Twenty-two of the pairs are known as **autosomes** (nonsex chromosomes), and one pair are the **sex chromosomes**, X and Y. A normal female has a 46,XX chromosomes constitution; the normal male, 46,XY (Figures 5–6 and 5–7).

The **karyotype**, or pictorial analysis of an individual's chromosomes, is usually obtained from specially treated and strained peripheral blood lymphocytes. Once obtained, the cells are stimulated to undergo mitosis. The mitotic process is stopped during a phase called metaphase, the preparation is then stained and the chromosomes become visible

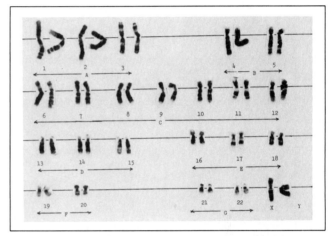

Figure 5–6 Normal female karyotype (Courtesy Dr Arthur Robinson, National Jewish Hospital and Research Center, Denver, CO)

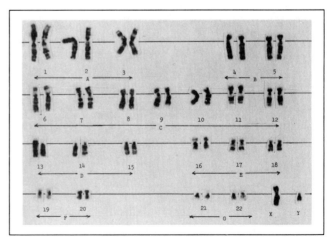

Figure 5–7 Normal male karyotype (Courtesy Dr Arthur Robinson, National Jewish Hospital and Research Center, Denver, CO)

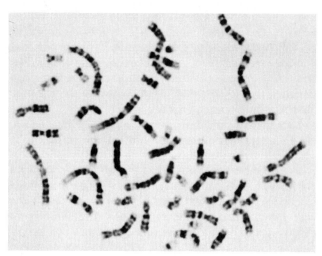

Figure 5–8   Chromosomes in metaphase spread (Courtesy Dr Arthur Robinson, National Jewish Hospital and Research Center, Denver, CO)

(Figure 5–8). Although the use of peripheral blood is an easy, convenient method of obtaining chromosomes, almost any tissue can be examined to get this information. In the case of a stillbirth or perinatal death in which there are multiple congenital abnormalities and there is a question of diagnosis or cause, karyotypes of cells in the child's internal organs (such as kidney, gonad, or thymus), rib, or skin can be examined if the tissues have not been fixed in formalin. In addition, a piece (1 mm x 1 mm) of placenta taken from near the insertion of the cord and deep enough to include chorion may be sent for karyotyping. In the case of fetal death, obtaining placental tissue may yield results when fetal tissue does not.

Chromosome abnormalities can occur in either the autosomes or the sex chromosomes and can be divided into two categories: abnormalities of number and abnormalities of structure. With the advent of quinacrine mustard staining of chromosomes, begun by Caspersson in 1970, it is possible to identify not only those cases in which an entire chromosome has been added or deleted but also those in which the addition or deletion of chromosomal material has been very small.

Even small alterations in chromosomes can cause problems, especially those associated with slow growth and development or with mental retardation. The child does not need to have obvious major malformations to be affected. Some of these abnormalities can also be passed on to other offspring. In some cases, chromosomal analysis is appropriate even if clinical manifestations are mild. Whatever the case, too much or too little genetic material usually produces adverse effects on normal growth and development.

Indications for chromosomal analysis include the following:

- Chromosome syndrome suspected (or clients with a clinical diagnosis of Down syndrome)

- Mental retardation and congenital malformations
- Abnormal sexual development (primary amenorrhea, lack of secondary sex characteristics)
- Ambiguous genitalia
- Multiple miscarriages
- Possible balanced translocation carrier (see discussion of abnormalities of chromosome structure in this chapter).

Autosome Abnormalities

Abnormalities of Chromosome Number   Abnormalities of chromosome number are most commonly seen as trisomies, monosomies, and as mosaicism. In all three cases, the abnormality is most often caused by *nondisjunction.* Nondisjunction occurs when paired chromosomes fail to separate during cell division. If nondisjunction occurs in either the sperm or the egg before fertilization, the resulting zygote (fertilized egg) will have an abnormal chromosome makeup in all of the cells (trisomy or monosomy). If nondisjunction occurs after fertilization, the developing zygote will have cells with two or more different chromosome makeups, evolving into two or more different cell lines (mosaicism).

Trisomies are the product of the union of a normal gamete (egg or sperm) with a gamete that contains an extra chromosome. The individual will have 47 chromosomes and is trisomic (has three chromosomes the same) for whichever chromosome is extra. Down syndrome (formerly called mongolism) is the most common trisomy abnormality seen in children (Figure 5–9). The presence of the extra chromosome 21 produces distinctive clinical features (see Table 5–8 and Figure 5–10). With the advent of modern surgical techniques and antibiotics, children with

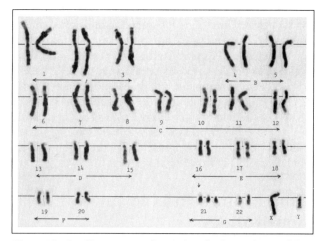

Figure 5–9   Karyotype of a male who has trisomy 21, Down syndrome: Note the extra 21 chromosome. (Courtesy Dr Arthur Robinson, National Jewish Hospital and Research Center, Denver, CO)

Table 5–8 Chromosomal Syndromes

Altered chromosome	Genetic defect and incidence	Characteristics
21	Trisomy 21 (Down syndrome) (secondary to nondisjunction or 14/21 unbalanced translocation) 1 in 700 live births (Figure 5–10)	CNS: Mental retardation 　　　Hypotonia at birth Head: Flattened occiput 　　　Depressed nasal bridge 　　　Mongoloid slant of eyes 　　　Epicanthal folds 　　　White speckling of the iris (Brushfield's spots) 　　　Protrusion of the tongue 　　　High, arched palate 　　　Low-set ears Hands: Short fingers 　　　Abnormalities of finger and foot 　　　Dermal ridge patterns (dermatoglyphics) 　　　Transverse palmar crease (simian line) Other: Congenital heart disease
21	2° mosaicism (Down syndrome) Incidence 1%	Classic symptoms as described in trisomy 21 except that the child has normal intelligence
18	Trisomy 18 1 in 3000 live births (Figure 5–11)	CNS: Mental retardation 　　　Severe hypertonia Head: Prominent occiput 　　　Low-set ears 　　　Corneal opacities 　　　Ptosis (drooping of eyelids) Hands: Third and fourth fingers overlapped by second and fifth fingers 　　　Abnormal dermatoglyphics 　　　Syndactyly (webbing of fingers) Other: Congenital heart defects 　　　Renal abnormalities 　　　Single umbilical artery 　　　Gastrointestinal tract abnormalities 　　　Rocker-bottom feet 　　　Cryptorchidism 　　　Various malformations of other organs
18	Deletion of long arm of chromosome 18	CNS: Severe psychomotor retardation Head: Microcephaly 　　　Stenotic ear canals with conductive hearing loss Other: Various other organ malformations
13	Trisomy 13 1 in 5000 live births (Figure 5–12)	CNS: Mental retardation 　　　Severe hypertonia 　　　Seizures Head: Microcephaly 　　　Microphthalmia and/or coloboma 　　　Malformed ears 　　　Aplasia of external auditory canal 　　　Micrognathia 　　　Cleft lip and palate Hands: Polydactyly (extra digits) 　　　Abnormal posturing of fingers 　　　Abnormal dermatoglyphics Other: Congenital heart defects 　　　Hemangiomas 　　　Gastrointestinal tract defects 　　　Various malformations of other organs
5	Deletion of short arm of chromosome 5 (cri du chat—cat cry syndrome) 1 in 20,000 live births (Figure 5–15)	CNS: Severe mental retardation 　　　A catlike cry in infancy Head: Microcephaly 　　　Hypertelorism 　　　Epicanthal folds 　　　Low-set ears Other: Failure to thrive 　　　Various organ malformations

(continued)

Table 5–8 (continued)

Altered chromosome	Genetic defect and incidence	Characteristics	
X (sex chromosome)	Only one X chromosome in female (Turner syndrome) 1 in 300 to 7000 live female births (Figure 5–13)	CNS:	No intellectual impairment Some perceptual difficulties
		Head:	Low hairline Webbed neck
		Trunk:	Short stature Cubitus valgus (increased carrying angle of arm) Excessive nevi Broad shieldlike chest with widely spaced nipples Puffy feet No toe nails
		Other:	Fibrous streaks in ovaries Underdeveloped secondary sex characteristics Primary amenorrhea Usually infertile Renal anomalies Coarctation of the aorta
X	Extra X in male (Klinefelter syndrome) 1 in 1000 live male births, approx. 1%–2% of institutionalized males	CNS:	Normal intelligence to mild mental retardation
		Trunk:	Occasional gynecomastia Eunochoid body proportions
		Other:	Small, soft testes Underdeveloped secondary sex characteristics Usually sterile

Down syndrome are now living into their fifth or sixth decade of life.

Trisomies can occur among other autosomes, the two most common being trisomy 18 and trisomy 13 (see Table 5–8 and Figures 5–11 and 5–12). The prognosis for children with trisomy 13 and 18 is extremely poor. Most children (70 percent) die within the first three months of life.

Monosomies occur when a normal gamete unites with a gamete that is missing a chromosome. In this case, the individual will have only 45 chromosomes and is said to be monosomic. Individuals with monosomy of an entire autosomal chromosome cannot survive. The only exception is in the sex chromosomes. A female can survive with only one X chromosome; this condition is known as *Turner syndrome* (Table 5–8 and Figure 5–13).

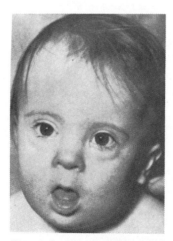

Figure 5–10   A child with Down syndrome (From Smith, DW: Recognizable Patterns of Human Malformations. Philadelphia: Saunders, 1982.)

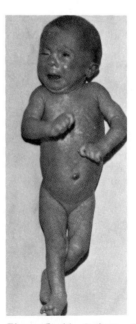

Figure 5–11   Infant with trisomy 18. (From Smith, DW: Recognizable Patterns of Human Malformations. Philadelphia: Saunders, 1982.)

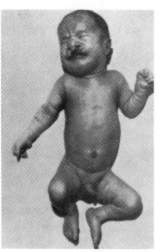

Figure 5–12   Infant with trisomy 13. (From Smith, DW: Recognizable Patterns of Human Malformations. *Philadelphia: Saunders, 1982.)*

Mosaicism occurs after fertilization and results in an individual with two different cell lines, each with a different chromosomal number. Mosaicism tends to be more common in the sex chromosomes, but when it does occur in the autosomes, it is most common in Down syndrome.

Different body tissues may have different chromosome makeups, depending on when the nondisjunction occurs. Or the tissue may have a mixture of cells, and the ratio of normal to abnormal cells may vary from one tissue to the next. For instance, in Down syndrome, one cell line contains the normal 46 chromosomes while the other cell line contains 47 chromosomes, that is, an extra number 21. Or within a single tissue, some of the cells may be normal while others contain the extra chromosome 21.

Clinical signs and symptoms may vary if mosaicism is present. In Down syndrome the clinical signs may be classic, minimal, or not apparent, depending on the number and location of the abnormal cells. An individual with many of the classic signs of Down syndrome but with normal intelligence should be investigated for the possibility of mosaicism. In such cases, more than one tissue may have to be examined to make the diagnosis. The peripheral blood may contain 46 chromosomes while the skin fibroblasts contain 47, +21.

Abnormalities of Chromosome Structure Abnormalities of chromosome structure involving only parts of the chromosome generally occur in two forms: translocation and deletions and/or additions. As the technology improves, more of these chromosomal structural abnormalities can be detected. Again, Down syndrome is one of the most common syndromes described (see Table 5–8).

Not all children born with Down syndrome have trisomy 21. Instead, they may have an abnormal rearrangement of chromosomal material known as a *translocation.*

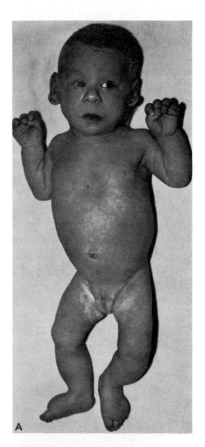
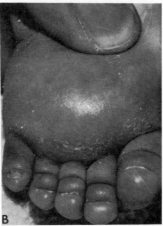

Figure 5–13   Infant with Turner syndrome at one month of age. Note: A Prominent ears. B Lymphedema (From Lemli L, Smith DW: The XO syndrome: A study of the differentiated phenotype in 25 patients. J Pediatr *1963; 63:577.)*

Clinically, the two types of Down syndrome are indistinguishable. What is of major importance to the family is that the two different types have significantly different risks of recurrence. The only way to distinguish between the two is to do a chromosome analysis.

The translocation occurs when the carrier parent has 45 chromosomes, usually with one chromosome fused to another. A common translocation is one in which one number 21 chromosome is fused to a number 14 chromosome. The parent has one normal 14, one normal 21, and one 14/21 chromosome. Since all the chromosomal material is present and functioning normally, the parent is clinically normal. This individual is known as a *balanced translocation carrier.*

When a person who is a balanced translocation carrier has a child with a person who has a structurally normal chromosome constitution, there are several possible outcomes (Figure 5–14). The offspring can receive the carrier parent's normal number 21 and normal number 14 chromosomes in combination with the noncarrier parent's normal chromosomes 21 and 14. In this case the offspring is chromosomally normal. Or the child may receive one of the balanced translocations, thus becoming a carrier like the carrier parent—chromosomally abnormal but clinically normal. If, however, the offspring receives the carrier parent's normal number 21 chromosome and the 14/21 chromosome and the noncarrier parent's normal chromosomes, the offspring receives two functioning number 14 chromosomes and three functioning number 21 chro-

mosomes. At first glance, the child seems to have 46 chromosomes but actually has an extra chromosome 21. Thus the child has an *unbalanced translocation* and has Down syndrome. Other types of translocations can occur. But regardless of the chromosome involved, any person having a balanced chromosome rearrangement (translocation) has the potential of having a child with an unbalanced chromosome constitution. This usually means a substantial negative effect on normal growth and development.

The other type of structure abnormality seen is caused by *additions and/or deletions* of chromosomal material. Any portion of a chromosome may be lost or added, generally leading to some adverse effect. Depending on how much chromosomal material is involved, the clinical effects may be mild or severe. Many types of additions and deletions have been described, such as a deletion of the short arm of chromosome 5 (cri du chat syndrome) or the deletion of the long arm of chromosome 18 (see Table 5–8 and Figure 5–15).

Sex Chromosome Abnormalities   To better understand normal X chromosome function and thus abnor-

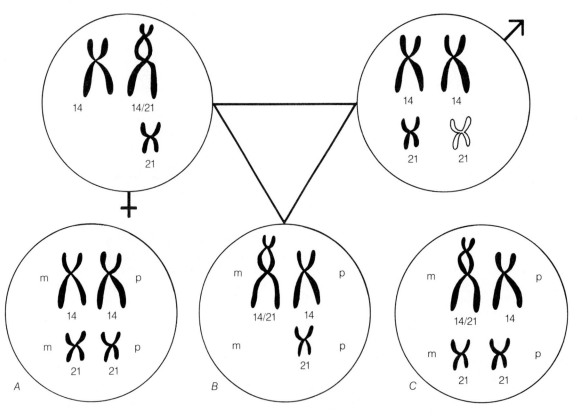

m = maternal origin
p = paternal origin

Figure 5–14   Diagram of various types of offspring when mother has a balanced translocation between 14 and 21 and father has a normal arrangement of chromosomal material. A Normal offspring. B Balanced translocation carrier. C Unbalanced translocation: Child has Down syndrome.

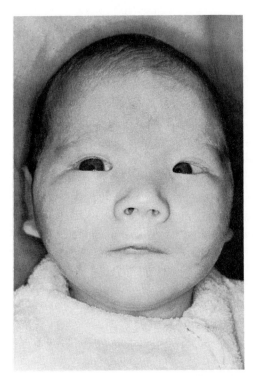

Figure 5–15 Infant with cri du chat syndrome resulting from deletion of part of the short arm of chromosome 5. Note characteristic facies with hypertelorism, epicanthus, and retrognathia. (From Thompson JS, Thompson MW: Genetics in Medicine, 4th ed. Philadelphia: Saunders, 1986.

malities of the sex chromosomes, the nurse should know that in females, at an early embryonic stage, one of the two normal X chromosomes becomes inactive. The inactive X chromosome forms a dark staining area known as the **Barr body**, or sex *chromatin body* (Figure 5–16).

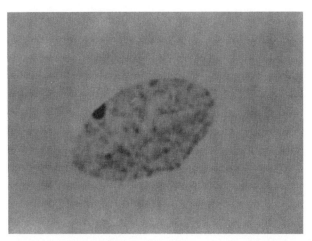

Figure 5–16 Nucleus with one Barr body; the patient is sex chromatin positive. (Courtesy Dr Arthur Robinson, National Jewish Hospital and Research Center, Denver, CO)

The Barr body may be seen by examining the cells scraped from the inside of a woman's mouth. This procedure, the *buccal smear*, will show the number of inactive X chromosomes or Barr bodies present. The normal female has one Barr body, since one of her two X chromosomes has been inactivated. The normal male has no Barr bodies, since he has only one X chromosome to begin with. The number of Barr bodies seen on the buccal smear is *always* one less than the number of X chromosomes present in the woman's cells.

When Y cells are stained and viewed, the Y chromosome appears as a bright body within the nucleus. The number of Y bodies present is equal to the number of Y chromosomes present. Males should have one Y body, and females should have none.

The most common sex chromosome abnormalities are **Turner syndrome** in females (45, X with no Barr bodies present) and **Klinefelter syndrome** in males (47, XXY with one Barr body present). See Table 5–8 for clinical description of these abnormalities. During the newborn period, clinical signs and symptoms of Turner syndrome are lymphedema of the back of the hands and top of the feet and excessive skin on the neck.

Other sex chromosome abnormalities may occur. Whether it is an increased number of X chromosomes or Y chromosomes or both, the affected individual generally has an increased number of abnormalities and increased severity of mental retardation.

Patterns of Inheritance

Many inherited diseases are produced by an abnormality in a single gene or pair of genes. In such instances, the chromosomes are grossly normal. The defect is at the gene level. Some of these gene defects can be detected by new technologies, including DNA and biochemical assays. The pattern of inheritance for a particular disease or defect is often determined by two methods: (1) close examination of the family in which the disease appears and (2) knowledge of how disease has been previously inherited, when no laboratory methods of detection are available.

There are two major categories of inheritance: **Mendelian** or **single-gene inheritance**, and **non-Mendelian**, or **multifactorial inheritance**. Each single-gene trait is determined by a pair of genes working together. These genes are responsible for the observable expression of the traits (eg, blue eyes, fair skin), referred to as the **phenotype**. The total genetic makeup of an individual is referred to as the **genotype** (pattern of the genes on the chromosomes). One of the genes for a trait is inherited from the mother; the other, from the father. An individual who has two identical genes at a given locus is considered to be **homozygous** for that trait. An individual is considered to be **heterozygous** for a particular trait when he or she has two different **alleles** (alternate forms of the same gene) at a given locus on a pair of homologous chromosomes.

The well-known modes of single-gene inheritance are autosomal dominant, autosomal recessive, and X-linked (sex-linked) recessive. There is also a less-common, X-linked dominant mode of inheritance and a newly identified mode of inheritance, the fragile-X syndrome.

Autosomal Dominant Inheritance

An individual is said to have an autosomal dominantly inherited disorder if the disease trait is heterozygous. That is, the abnormal gene overshadows the normal gene of the pair to produce the trait. It is essential to remember that in autosomal dominant inheritance:

1. An affected individual generally has an affected parent. The family pedigree (graphic representation of a family tree) usually shows multiple generations having the disorder (Figure 5–17).

2. The affected individual has a 50% chance of passing on the abnormal gene to each of his or her children (Figure 5–17).

3. Both males and females are equally affected, and a father can pass the abnormal gene on to his son. This is an important principle when distinguishing autosomal dominant disorders from X-linked disorders.

4. An unaffected individual in most cases cannot transmit the disorder to his or her children.

5. A mutation or a change of a normal gene into a dominant abnormal gene is possible. In this case, this is the first time the disorder is seen in the family; an affected child is born to parents who are

unaffected. In such instances, there is not an increased risk of future children of the same parents to be affected. The child, however, now has a 50% chance of passing the abnormal gene on to each of his or her offspring.

6. Autosomal dominant inherited disorders have varying degrees of presentation. This is an important factor when counseling families concerning autosomal dominant disorders. Although a parent may have a mild form of the disease, the child may have a more severe form. Unfortunately there is no method for predicting whether a child will be only mildly affected or more severely affected. The geneticist or health care provider must be thorough in the examination of family members to discern whether any of those individuals are indeed affected. They may express the disease in such a mild form that a cursory examination may miss clinical signs of the disease.

Some common autosomal dominantly inherited disorders are Huntington chorea, polycystic kidney disease, neurofibromatosis (von Recklinghausen disease), and achondroplastic dwarfism.

Autosomal Recessive Inheritance

An individual has an autosomal recessively inherited disorder if the disease manifests itself only as a homozygous trait. That is, because the normal gene overshadows the abnormal one, the individual must have two abnormal genes to be affected. The notion of a *carrier state* is appropriate

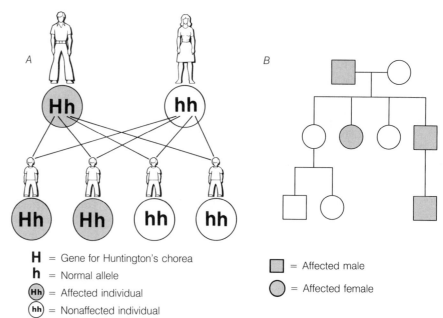

Figure 5–17 A Autosomal dominant inheritance. One parent is affected. Statistically, 50% of offspring will be affected, regardless of sex. B Autosomal dominant pedigree

H = Gene for Huntington's chorea
h = Normal allele
(Hh) = Affected individual
(hh) = Nonaffected individual

■ = Affected male
● = Affected female

here. An individual who is heterozygous for the abnormal gene is clinically normal. It is not until two individuals mate and pass on the same abnormal gene that affected offspring may appear. It is essential to remember that in autosomal recessive inheritance:

1. An affected individual has clinically normal parents, but they are both carriers of the abnormal gene (Figure 5–18).

2. Parents who are both carriers of the same abnormal gene have a 25% chance of both passing the abnormal gene on to *any* of their children (Figure 5–18).

3. If the child of two carrier parents is clinically normal, there is a 50% chance that he or she is a carrier of the gene (Figure 5–18).

4. Both males and females are equally affected.

5. The family pedigree usually shows siblings affected in a horizontal fashion (Figure 5–18). Future generations are not affected unless both parents carry the same abnormal gene.

6. There is an increased history of consanguineous matings. Parents who are closely related are more likely to have the same genes in common than two parents who are unrelated.

7. Recessively inherited disorders tend to be more severe in their clinical manifestations. Clinically normal carrier parents pass on the disorder, and the affected offspring will often not reproduce. If an affected individual does reproduce, all the children will be carriers for the disorder.

8. The presence of the abnormal gene for some autosomal recessively inherited disorders can be detected in a normal carrier parent. For instance, Tay-Sachs disease is caused by an inborn error of metabolism—that is, a deficiency of the enzyme hexosaminidase A. An affected individual has little or no enzyme activity present, whereas a carrier parent usually has 50% normal enzyme activity present. The carrier is biochemically abnormal but phenotypically normal. The heterozygous state can be detected, even though it is asymptomatic.

Some other common autosomal recessive inherited disorders are cystic fibrosis, phenylketonuria (PKU), galactosemia, sickle-cell anemia, and most metabolic disorders.

X-Linked Recessive Inheritance

X-linked or sex-linked disorders are those for which the abnormal gene is carried on the X chromosome. A female may be heterozygous or homozygous for a trait carried on the X chromosome, since she has two X chromosomes. A male, however, has only one X chromosome. The male in this case is considered to be *hemizygous,* having only one alternate form of the gene instead of a pair for a given trait or disorder. Thus an X-linked disorder is manifested in a male who carries the abnormal gene on his X chromosome. His mother is considered to be a carrier when the normal gene on one X chromosome overshadows the abnormal gene on the other X chromosome. It is essential to remember that in X-linked recessive inheritance:

1. There is no male-to-male transmission. Fathers pass only their Y chromosomes to their sons and their

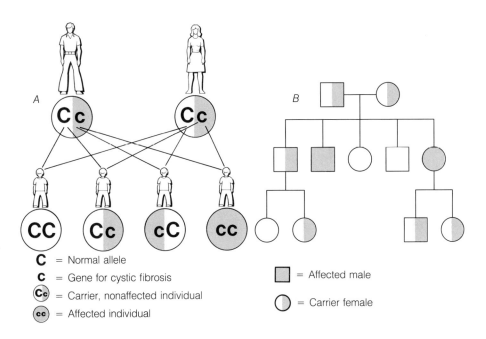

Figure 5–18 A Autosomal recessive inheritance. Both parents are carriers. Statistically, 25% of offspring are affected, regardless of sex. B Autosomal recessive pedigree

C = Normal allele

c = Gene for cystic fibrosis

Cc = Carrier, nonaffected individual

cc = Affected individual

☐ = Affected male

◯ = Carrier female

X chromosomes to their daughters. Daughters receive one X chromosome from the mother and one from the father.

2. Affected males are related through the female line (Figure 5–19B).

3. There is a 50% chance that a carrier mother will pass the abnormal gene to each of her sons, who will thus be affected. There is a 50% chance that a carrier mother will pass the normal gene to each of her sons, who will thus be unaffected. There is a 50% chance that a carrier mother will pass the abnormal gene to each of her daughters, who become carriers like their mother (Figure 5–19). There is also a 50% chance that a carrier mother will pass on her normal gene to her daughter, who will thus not be a carrier.

4. Fathers affected with an X-linked disorder cannot pass the disorder to their sons, but *all* their daughters become carriers of the disorder.

5. Occasionally, a female carrier may show some symptoms of an X-linked disorder. This situation is probably due to random inactivation of the X chromosome carrying the normal allele. Thus a heterozygous female may show some manifestation of an X-linked disorder.

Common X-linked recessive disorders are hemophilia, Duchenne muscular dystrophy, and color blindness.

X-Linked Dominant Inheritance

X-linked dominant disorders are extremely rare, the most common being vitamin D-resistant rickets. When X-linked dominance does occur, the pattern is similar to X-linked recessive inheritance except that heterozygous females are affected. It is essential to remember that in X-linked dominant inheritance:

1. The abnormal gene is dominant and overshadows the normal gene on the female's other X chromosome.

2. There is no male-to-male transmission. An affected father will have affected daughters but no affected sons.

Fragile-X Syndrome

A newly identified chromosomal disorder is the *fragile-X syndrome*. It is a central nervous system disorder linked to a "fragile site" on the X chromosome. This fragile site is seen when cells are grown in a folic acid–deficient media and detectable in both affected males and heterozygote carrier females (Shapiro 1988). Fragile-X syndrome is characterized by moderate mental retardation, large protuberant ears, and large testes after puberty (Thompson & Thompson 1986).

Multifactorial Inheritance

Many common congenital malformations, such as cleft palate, heart defects, spina bifida, dislocated hips, clubfoot, and pyloric stenosis are caused by an interaction of many genes and environmental factors. They are, therefore, multifactorial in origin. It is essential to remember that in multifactorial inheritance:

1. The malformations may vary from mild to severe. For example, spina bifida may range in severity

Figure 5–19 A X-linked recessive inheritance. The mother is the carrier. Statistically, 50% of male offspring are affected, and 50% of female offspring are carriers. B X-linked pedigree

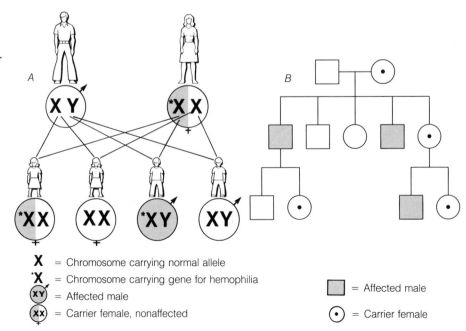

X = Chromosome carrying normal allele
˙X = Chromosome carrying gene for hemophilia
(XY) = Affected male
(XX) = Carrier female, nonaffected

☐ = Affected male
⊙ = Carrier female

from mild, as spina bifida occulta, to more severe, as a myelomeningocele. It is believed that the more severe the defect, the greater the number of genes present for that defect.

2. There is often a sex bias. Pyloric stenosis is more common in males, whereas cleft palate is more common among females. When a member of the less commonly affected sex shows the condition, a greater number of genes must usually be present to cause the defect.

3. In the presence of environmental influence (such as seasonal changes, altitude, irradiation, chemicals in the environment, or exposure to toxic substances), it may take fewer genes to manifest the disease in the offspring.

4. In contrast to single-gene disorders, there is an additive effect in multifactorial inheritance. The more family members who have the defect, the greater the risk that the next pregnancy will also be affected.

5. Risk factors are determined by the distribution of cases found in the general population. The risk of recurrence is usually 2% to 5% for all first-degree relatives (ie, parents, siblings, and children) if one family member is affected. The recurrence figure decreases with second-degree relatives (ie, grandparents, grandchildren, aunts, and uncles) and so forth. Generally the recurrence risks increase the more family members who are affected.

Although most congenital malformations are multifactorial traits, a careful family history should always be taken, since occasionally cleft lip and palate, certain congenital heart defects, and other malformations can be inherited as autosomal dominant or recessive traits. Other disorders thought to be within the multifactorial inheritance group are diabetes, hypertension, some heart diseases, and mental illness.

Nongenetic Conditions

Not all disorders or congenital malformations are inherited or have an inherited component. Malformations present at birth may be caused by an environmental insult during pregnancy, such as exposure to a drug or an infectious agent (see Chapter 14). Some malformations, however, cannot be explained by genetic mechanisms or teratogens. These disorders are considered to have a developmental cause. A couple who has a child with phocomelia (abnormality of the limbs), in the absence of any other problems or family history, may be reassured that the problem is developmental in etiology and the risk for future pregnancies is low. Such reassurance is also appropriate for families concerned about a child's seizures or developmental delays, if they can be attributed to an acquired problem.

Prenatal Diagnosis

Parent-child and family planning counseling have become a major responsibility of professional nurses. To be effective counselors, nurses need to have the *most* current knowledge available concerning prenatal diagnosis.

It is essential that the couple be completely informed as to the known and potential risks of each of the genetic diagnostic procedures. The nurse needs to recognize the emotional impact on the family of a decision to have or not to have a genetic diagnostic procedure.

The ability to diagnose certain genetic diseases by various diagnostic tools has enormous implications for the practice of preventive health care. Several methods are available for prenatal diagnosis, although some are still being used on an experimental basis.

Genetic Ultrasound

Ultrasound may be used to assess the fetus for genetic and/or congenital problems. With ultrasound, one can visualize the fetal head for abnormalities in size, shape, and structure. Craniospinal defects (anencephaly, microcephaly, hydrocephalus), gastrointestinal malformations (omphalocele, gastroschisis), renal malformations (dysplasia or obstruction), and skeletal malformations are only some of the disorders that have been diagnosed in utero by ultrasound. Screening for congenital anomalies is best done at 18 to 20 weeks, when fetal structures have completed development (DeVore & Hobbins 1989). There is no information documenting harm to the fetus or long-term effects with exposure to ultrasound. However, there is no guarantee of complete safety; therefore, the practitioner and the parents must evaluate the risks against the benefits on an individual basis (Lewin & Goldberg 1989; Lizzi 1988).

Genetic Amniocentesis

The major method of prenatal diagnosis is genetic amniocentesis (Figure 5–20). The procedure is described in Chapter 20. The indications for genetic amniocentesis include:

1. Advanced maternal age. Any woman 35 or older is at greater risk for having children with chromosome abnormalities. Approximately 85% of all amniocentesis is done because of advanced maternal age (Verp 1989). See Chapter 20 for further discussion. Half of the chromosomal abnormalities due to maternal age are trisomy 21, and half are other abnormalities of chromosome number, such as trisomy 13, 18, XXX, XXY, etc. The risk of having a liveborn infant with a chromosome problem is 1 in 200 for a 35-year-old woman; the risk for trisomy 21 is 1 in 400. At age 45, the risks are 1 in 20 and 1 in 40, respectively (Hook et al 1988). Table 5–9 presents maternal age-related risks at different gestational ages.

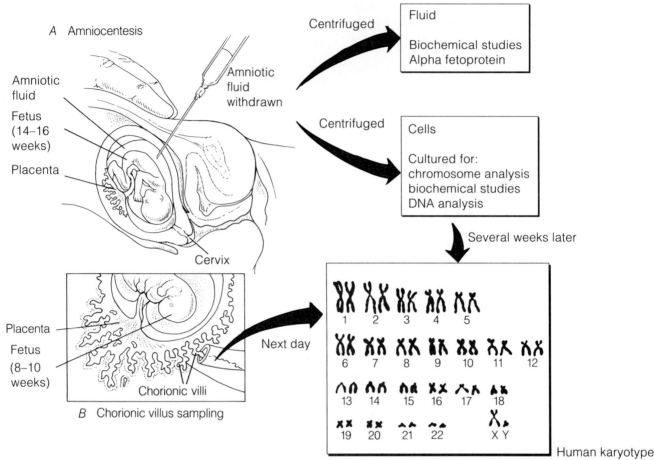

Figure 5–20   A genetic amniocentesis for prenatal diagnosis is done at 14 to 16 weeks' gestation. B Chorionic villus sampling is done at 8–10 weeks and the cells are karyotyped immediately. (Adapted from Marieb EN: Human Anatomy and Physiology, Redwood City CA: Benjamin/Cummings, 1989, p. 992.

2. Previous child born with a chromosomal abnormality. Young couples who have had a child with trisomy 21, 18, or 13 have approximately a 1% to 2% risk of a future child having a chromosome abnormality. Genetic amniocentesis is made available to any couple who has already had a child with a chromosome abnormality.

3. Parent carrying a chromosomal abnormality (balanced translocation). Any couple in which one of the partners is a carrier of a balanced translocation should be considered for prenatal diagnosis. Although the person with the chromosome rearrangement is clinically normal, he or she has the potential for conceiving a child with an unbalanced chromosome constitution, which usually has substantial adverse effects on normal development. For example, a woman who carries a balanced 14/21 translocation has a risk of approximately 10% to 15% that her children will be affected with the

unbalanced translocation of Down syndrome; if the father is the carrier, there is a 2% to 5% risk.

4. Mother carrying an X-linked disease. In families in which the woman is a known or possible carrier of an X-linked disorder, such as hemophilia or Duchenne muscular dystrophy, genetic amniocentesis, chorionic villus sampling (CVS), or percutaneous umbilical blood sampling (PUBS) may be appropriate options for the family. Increasingly, these disorders can be diagnosed in utero. For a known female carrier, the risk of an affected male fetus is 50%. With new technologies such as DNA testing, it may be possible to identify affected males from the nonaffected males in some disorders. In disorders where female carriers can be distinguished from noncarriers, only the carrier females would be offered prenatal diagnosis.

5. Parents carrying an inborn error of metabolism that can be diagnosed in utero. The number of in-

Table 5–9 Risk for Chromosomal Abnormalities Due to Maternal Age at Different Stages of Pregnancy *

Maternal age (years)	10 weeks rates noted with CVS	17 weeks rates noted with amniocentesis	Birth	
			Chromosomal anomalies	Down syndrome**
33		1/200	1/300	1/600
34		1/170	1/250	1/500
35	1/110	1/130	1/200	1/400
36	1/80	1/100	1/170	1/340
37	1/65	1/80	1/130	1/260
38	1/50	1/65	1/100	1/200
39	1/35	1/50	1/80	1/160
40	1/30	1/40	1/65	1/130
41	1/20	1/30	1/50	1/100
42	1/15	1/25	1/40	1/80
43	1/13	1/20	1/30	1/60
44	1/10	1/15	1/25	1/50
45	1/7	1/12	1/20	1/40
46	1/6	1/10	1/16	1/32
47	1/4	1/8	1/12	1/24
48	1/3	1/6	1/10	1/20

Approximate (rounded) estimates from Hook EB, Cross PK, Jackson L, et al: Maternal age-specific rates of 47, +21 and other cytogenetic abnormalities diagnosed in the first trimester of pregnancy in chorionic villus biopsy specimens: Comparison with rates expected from observations at amniocentesis. Am J Hum Genet 1988; 42:797 and Hook EB, Cross PK, Schreimachers DM: Chromosomal abnormality rates at amniocentesis and in live-born infants. JAMA 1983; 249:2034. Rates for maternal ages >45 years are based on very small numbers
** Risk for Down Syndrome is approximately half of each number listed above, eg, age 33 risk for liveborn Down syndrome is 1 in 600.*

herited metabolic disorders that can be diagnosed in utero is increasing at a rapid rate (Crawford 1988).

Metabolic disorders detectable in utero include (partial list): argininosuccinicaciduria, cystinosis, fabry disease, Galactosemia, Gaucher disease, Homocystinuria, Hunter syndrome, Hurler disease, Krabbe disease, Lesch-Nyhan syndrome, maple syrup urine disease, Metachromatic leukodystrophy, Methylmalonic aciduria, Niemann-Pick disease, Pompe disease, Sanfilippo syndrome, Tay-Sachs disease.

6. Both parents carrying an autosomal recessive disease. When both parents are carriers of an autosomal recessive disease, there is a 25% risk for each pregnancy that the fetus will be affected. Diagnosis is made by testing the cultured amniotic fluid cells (enzyme level, substrate level, product level, or DNA) or the fluid itself. Autosomal recessive diseases identified by amniocentesis are hemoglobinopathies such as sickle-cell anemia and thalassemia. Most research to date has been in the prenatal diagnosis of hemoglobinopathies. Both sickle-cell anemia and β-thalassemia once were diagnosed using fetal blood samples obtained by amnioscopy, which has a 3% to 5% risk of fetal

demise and spontaneous abortion. Now prenatal diagnosis of these conditions can be accomplished on uncultured amniotic fluid from an amniocentesis using a restriction endonuclease analysis of DNA and, in some cases, by direct detection of the DNA mutation (Ostrer & Hejtmancik 1988). With the detection of the deletion that causes 70% of the cases of cystic fibrosis, carrier testing and prenatal diagnosis are available for some families. It is theorized that the other 30% of the cases of cystic fibrosis are caused by numerous different deletions (Kerem et al 1989; Lemna et al 1990). For those families without a known deletion but with a living affected relative, carrier detection and prenatal diagnosis may be possible with DNA testing by restriction endonuclease and/or biochemical analysis of amniotic fluid with the microvillar enzyme activity (Brock 1988).

7. Family history of neural tube defects. Genetic amniocentesis is available to those couples who have had a child with neural tube defects or who have a family history of these conditions, which include anencephaly, spina bifida, and myelomeningocele. Neural tube defects are usually multifactorial traits.

Regardless of the statistical risk for a given family, whether for an isolated neural tube defect or a

---

Table 5–10   Couples to Be Offered Prenatal Diagnosis

Nurses should consider prenatal diagnosis for:

Women 35 or over at time of conception and birth

Couples having a balanced translocation (chromosomal abnormality)

Mother carrying X-linked disease, eg, hemophilia

Couples having a previous child with chromosomal abnormality

Couples in which either partner or a previous child is affected with a diagnosable metabolic disorder

Couples in which both partners are carriers for a diagnosable metabolic or autosomal recessive disorder

Family or personal history of neural tube defects

Ethnic groups at increased risk for specific disorders

Couples with history of two or more first trimester spontaneous abortions

---

disorder in which a neural tube defect is a constant feature, the risk of recurrence can be reduced (possibly by as much as 90%) through α-fetoprotein (AFP) determination of the amniotic fluid (Cohen 1987). α-Fetoprotein is a substance produced in fetal liver, kidney, and gastrointestinal tract. In pregnancies in which the fetus has an open neural tube defect, α-fetoprotein leaks into the amniotic fluid and levels are elevated (Lemire 1989). Thus, genetic amniocentesis allows those families for whom the risk of a neural tube defect is increased the opportunity to choose whether to have a child affected with such a disorder (see Table 5–10).

Chorionic Villus Sampling (CVS)

Chorionic villus sampling is a new technique that is used in selected regional centers. Its diagnostic capability is similar to amniocentesis. Its advantage is that diagnostic information is available before the completion of the first trimester of pregnancy. (For further discussion, see Chapter 20).

Percutaneous Umbilical Blood Sampling

Percutaneous umbilical blood sampling (PUBS) is a technique used for obtaining blood which allows for more rapid chromosome diagnosis, for genetic studies, or for transfusion for Rh isoimmunization or hydrops (Dunn et al 1988). For more in-depth discussion see Chapter 20.

Implications of Prenatal Diagnostic Testing

It is imperative that counseling precede any procedure for prenatal diagnosis. Many questions and points must be considered if the family is to reach a satisfactory decision.

With the advent of diagnostic techniques such as amniocentesis, couples at risk, who would not otherwise have additional children, can decide to conceive. The percentage of therapeutic abortions after amniocentesis is small; most couples find peace of mind throughout the remainder of the pregnancy after prenatal diagnosis.

After prenatal diagnosis, a couple can decide not to have a child with a genetic disease. For many couples, however, prenatal diagnosis is not a solution, since the only method of preventing a genetic disease is preventing the birth by aborting the affected fetus. This decision can only be made by the family.

Genetic counselors do, however, discuss with the family all available options if an abnormal fetus is discovered or suspected. Every pregnancy has a 3% to 4% risk for an infant to be born with a birth defect, some of which can be diagnosed before birth. When an abnormality is detected or suspected, an attempt is made to determine the diagnosis by assessing the family health history (via the pedigree) and the pregnancy history and by evaluating the fetal anomaly or anomalies. The parents are then presented with options.

Prenatal diagnosis cannot guarantee the birth of a normal child. It can only determine the presence or absence of specific disorders (within the limits of laboratory error). Many disorders can be prenatally diagnosed; the list has grown and continues to grow almost daily. Experts on a specific disorder should be consulted before information is given to couples and before options regarding prenatal diagnosis are discussed.

Treatment of prenatally diagnosed disorders may begin during the pregnancy, thus possibly preventing irreversible damage. For example, a galactose-free diet may be given to a mother carrying a fetus with galactosemia. In light of the philosophy of preventive health care, information that can be obtained prenatally should be made available to all couples who are expecting a baby or who are contemplating pregnancy.

Postnatal Diagnosis

Questions concerning genetic disorders, cause, treatment, and prognosis are most often first discussed in the newborn nursery or during the infant's first few months of life. When a child is born with anomalies, has a stormy neonatal period, or does not progress as expected, a genetic evaluation may well be warranted.

Accurate diagnosis and optimal treatment plan incorporate the following:

- Complete and detailed histories to determine if the problem is prenatal (congenital), postnatal, or familial in origin.

- Thorough physical examination, including dermatoglyphic analysis (Figure 5–21).

- Laboratory analysis, which includes chromosome analysis; enzyme assay for inborn errors of metabolism (see Chapter 29 for further discussion on these specific tests); and antibody titers for infectious teratogens, such as toxoplasmosis, rubella, cytomegalovirus, and herpes virus (TORCH) (see Chapter 19).

To make an accurate diagnosis the geneticist consults with other specialists and reviews the current literature. This permits the geneticist to evaluate all the available information before arriving at a diagnosis and plan of action.

Physical Examination

The physical examination is essential in helping to establish the diagnosis. The geneticist must attend to minute details and look for specific patterns of abnormalities. Two major questions should be kept in mind: Is just one organ system involved or are multiple systems involved? Does the abnormality have a prenatal or postnatal onset? If only a single malformation is present, such as cleft palate, or only one organ system is involved (the skin), the geneticist tends to think in terms of multifactorial, single-gene disorders, or developmental causes. If multiple malformations are present, chromosomal and teratogenic causes are often the first possibilities to consider. Many chromosomal abnormalities and single-gene disorders are associated with a specific pattern of malformations. Thus, one must have expertise in syndrome recognition to be able to arrive at an accurate diagnosis.

Dermatoglyphic Analysis

Dermatoglyphics (Figure 5–21) are the patterns of the ridged skin found on the fingers, palms, toes and soles (Thompson & Thompson 1986). Although each individual has a unique ridge pattern, specific types of patterns exist that can be systematically classified. Since differentiation of dermal ridges is complete by the end of the fourth month of gestation, many genetic disorders that affect multiple systems also affect the dermatoglyphics. Thus, a child with a chromosomal abnormality often exhibits certain characteristic dermatoglyphics.

Pattern combinations and frequencies considered together are more significant than pattern types alone. In Down syndrome or any other abnormality, any one of the particular specified patterns seen can also be found in normal individuals. It is when these patterns are in *combination* that they are associated with a specific disorder, such as Down syndrome.

Children with Down syndrome often have a single flexion crease (single transverse palmar crease) on the palms, an increased number of ulnar loops on the fingertips (often on all ten fingers), and a characteristic pattern on the soles of the feet (the hallucal pattern), known as an arch tibial (Figure 5-21). Children with trisomy 13 are found to have an increase in the number of arch patterns on the fingertips and single flexion creases of the palms (Thompson & Thompson 1986). Chromosome abnormalities are only one area in which unusual dermatoglyphics have been described and can be associated with other single-gene or multifactorial disorders.

Laboratory Analysis

Laboratory studies include chromosome analysis (discussed on p 130), enzyme assays, and serologic and microscopic studies. Enzyme assays are performed to diagnose inherited metabolic diseases. These usually are done if the result on newborn screening is abnormal or if the child has any combination of the following: nausea and vomiting, enlarged viscera, poor feeding, lethargy, and seizures. Metabolic abnormalities should also be considered in any child who does well during the neonatal period with normal developmental milestones but then deteriorates, particularly in CNS functioning. The major assays done are of amino and organic acids. Other specific enzyme assays are performed only if the clinical picture warrants doing them.

As mentioned, some genetic disorders are identified on newborn screening. The major purpose of screening programs is to identify affected newborns as soon as possible after birth so that corrective treatment can be insti-

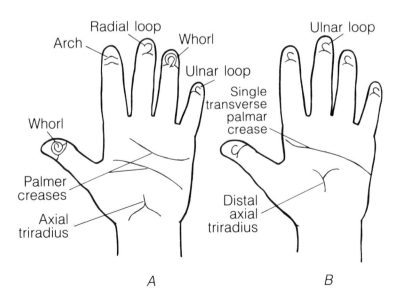

A   *B*

Figure 5–21 Dermatoglyphic patterns of the hands in A, a normal individual and B, in a child with Down syndrome. Note the single transverse palmar crease, distally placed axial triradius, and increased number of ulnar loops.

tuted before irreversible damage is done. Many institutions now screen for six inborn errors of metabolism: PKU, galactosemia, hypothyroidism, sickle-cell anemia, maple syrup urine disease, and homocystinuria. (See Chapter 32 for further discussion of these conditions.)

The Family, The Nurse, and The Genetic Counseling Process

Genetic counseling is a communication process in which the genetic counselor tries to provide a family with the most complete and accurate information on the occurrence or the risk of recurrence of a genetic disease in that family. The goals inherent in this definition are threefold. First, genetic counseling allows families to make informed decisions about reproduction. Second, it assists families in assessing the available treatments, examining appropriate alternatives to decrease the risk, learning about the usual course and outcome of the genetic disease or abnormality, and dealing with the psychologic and social implications that often accompany such problems. Finally, it is hoped that genetic counseling will help decrease the incidence and impact of genetic disease. The use of a team approach and appropriate timing are important considerations in genetic counseling.

Team Approach

Because genetic counseling is a complex and multidimensional process, it cannot be done efficiently or effectively in isolation. The genetics team usually includes a medical geneticist, a genetic associate, and/or a nurse-geneticist. Often a social worker is directly involved. This group works closely with cytogeneticists, biochemists, and other specialty groups to clarify the situation for families. Many genetics groups also work closely with clergy and family support groups to provide the family with additional resources.

The genetics team continually tries to inform and assist the primary health care provider before, during, and after counseling. Ideally, the primary physician or nurse clinician will feel free to consult the genetics team as a resource group for information, assistance, and support in the care of their clients.

Timing

Timing is an important aspect of the counseling process. Preferably, counseling should be *prospective*—before the birth of an affected child. Increasing numbers of young couples who are contemplating childbearing are seeking genetic counseling to discover their risk of having children with an abnormality or genetic disease. However, many genetic diseases do not present themselves until after an affected child is born. Genetic counseling in this case is *retrospective*.

In retrospective genetic counseling, time is a crucial factor. One cannot expect a family who has just learned that their child has a birth defect or has Down syndrome to

assimilate any information concerning future risks. However, the couple should never be "put off" from counseling for too long a period, only to find that they have borne another affected child. Here the nurse can be instrumental in directing the parents into counseling at the appropriate time. At the birth of an affected child, the nurse can inform the parents that genetic counseling is available before they attempt having another child. Asking one or two members of a genetics team to introduce themselves to the family is often enough to bring up the subject of genetic counseling. When the parents have begun to recover from the initial shock of bearing a child with an abnormality, or when they begin to contemplate having more children, the nurse can encourage the couple to seek counseling.

The Nurse's Role

Nurses who are aware of families at an increased risk for having a child with a genetic disorder are in an ideal position to make referrals. Genetic counseling is an appropriate course of action for any family wondering, "Will it happen again?" The nursery nurse frequently has the first contact with the family and newborn with a congenital problem. The family nurse practitioner or family-planning nurse is in an excellent position to reach at-risk families before the birth of another baby with a congenital problem. Genetic counseling referral is advised for any of the following categories:

1. *Congenital abnormalities, including mental retardation.* Any couple who has a child or a relative with a congenital malformation may be at an increased risk and should be so informed. If mental retardation of unidentified cause has occurred in a family, there may be an increased risk or recurrence.

   In many cases, the genetic counselor will identify the cause of a malformation as a teratogen (see Chapter 14). The family should be aware of teratogenic substances so they can avoid exposure during any subsequent pregnancy.

2. *Familial disorders.* Families should be told that certain diseases may have a genetic component and that the risk of their occurrence in a particular family may be higher than that for the general population. Such disorders as diabetes, heart disease, cancer, and mental illness fall into this category.

3. *Known inherited diseases.* Families may know that a disease is inherited but not know the mechanism or the specific risk for them. An important point to remember is that family members who are not at risk for passing on a disorder should be as well informed as family members who are at increased risk.

4. *Metabolic disorders.* Any families at risk for having a child with a metabolic disorder or biochemical

defect should be referred. Because most inborn errors of metabolism are autosomal recessively inherited ones, a family may not be identified as at risk until the birth of an affected child.

Carriers of the sickle-cell trait can be identified before pregnancy is begun, and the risk of having an affected child can be determined. Prenatal diagnosis of an affected fetus is available on an experimental basis only.

5. *Chromosomal abnormalities.* As discussed previously, any couple who has had a child with a chromosomal abnormality may be at an increased risk of having another child similarly affected. This group would include families in which there is concern for a possible translocation.

The process of genetic counseling usually begins after the birth of a child diagnosed as having a congenital problem or genetic disease. After the parents have been referred to the genetic clinic, they are sent a form requesting information on the health status of various family members. At this time, the nurse can help by discussing the form with the family or clarifying the information needed to complete it. A pedigree and family health history facilitate identification of other family members who might also be at risk for the same disorder. The family being counseled may wish to notify those relatives at risk so that they, too, can be given genetic counseling. When done correctly, the family history and pedigree become one of the most powerful and useful tools for determining a family risk.

A screening pedigree generally includes the affected individual, siblings, parents, aunts, uncles, and grandparents (Figure 5–22). If the family does not have all the necessary information at hand, the nurse can urge them to obtain the information in time for their first genetic counseling session, when a more complete pedigree will be taken.

The pedigree is a fairly easy and productive method for screening families. The nurse can obtain the necessary information and draw a screening pedigree in approximately 15 minutes. Information that should be obtained when drawing the family pedigree includes names (maiden names if appropriate) and birth dates of members of the immediate family; names and ages of the remainder of the family (including deceased members), with a description of their health status; causes of death of family members; and any other information the family feels is significant. In discussing the affected individual, the nurse should obtain information on the pregnancy history of the mother (including miscarriages), medications and drugs taken during pregnancy, x-ray exposure, infections or illness during pregnancy, the type of birth control used prior to pregnancy, and the method used to diagnose the pregnancy. A

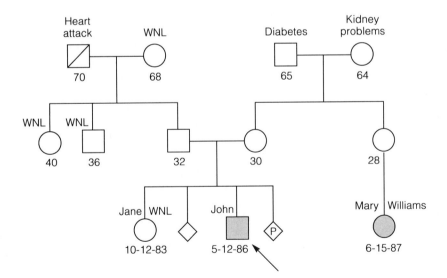

Figure 5–22 Screening pedigree. Arrow indicates the nearest family member affected with the disorder being investigated. Basic data have been recorded. Numbers refer to the ages of the family members.

Key:

☐ = Male

▨ = Affected male

○ = Female

◉ = Affected female

⬦ = Pregnant

WNL = Within normal limits

◹ = Deceased male

◇ = Spontaneous abortion

☐—○ = Mating line

⊔ = Sibship line

complete childbirth history should be taken, including a description of any complications. It is also appropriate for the nurse to ask the family when the problem was evident to them or was diagnosed.

The nurse should inquire about the affected child's growth and development. The information obtained should include developmental milestones, growth in comparison to siblings or other children the same age, symptoms of a problem, school records, and any previous testing.

Finally, information concerning ethnic background, family origin, and/or religion should be elicited. Many genetic disorders are more common among certain ethnic groups or more commonly found in particular geographic areas. For example, families from the British Isles are at higher risk of having children with neural tube defects; the Ashkenazi Jews are at higher risk of sickle-cell anemia; and people of Mediterranean heritage have a higher risk of thalassemias.

Follow-up Counseling   When all the data have been carefully examined and analyzed, the family returns for a follow-up visit. At this time, the parents are given all the information available, including the medical facts, diagnosis, probable course of the disorder, and any available management; the inheritance pattern for this particular family and their risk of recurrence; and the options or alternatives for dealing with the risk of recurrence. The remainder of the counseling session is spent discussing the course of action that seems appropriate to the family in view of their risk and family goals.

Among those options or alternatives are prenatal diagnosis and early detection and treatment, and in some cases, adoption, artificial insemination, or delayed childbearing.

The family may consider *artificial insemination by donor (AID),* discussed earlier in this chapter. This alternative is appropriate in several instances; for example, if the male partner is affected with an autosomal dominant disease, AID would decrease the risk of having an affected child to zero, since the child would not inherit any genes from the affected parent. If the man is affected with an X-linked disorder and does not wish to continue the gene in the family (all his daughters will be carriers), AID would be an alternative to terminating all pregnancies with a female fetus. If the man is a carrier for a balanced translocation and if termination of pregnancy is against family ethics, AID is the most appropriate alternative. AID is also appropriate if both parents are carriers of an autosomal recessive disease. AID lowers the risk to a very low level or to zero if a carrier test is available. Finally, AID may be appropriate if the family is at high risk for a multifactorial disorder.

Couples who are young and at risk may decide to delay childbearing for a few years. Medical science and medical genetics are continually making breakthroughs in early detection and treatment. These couples may find in a few years that prenatal diagnosis will be available or that a disease can be detected and treated early to prevent irreversible damage.

Table 5–11   Nursing Responsibilities in Genetic Counseling

Identify families at risk for genetic problems.

Assist families in acquiring accurate information about the specific problem.

Act as liaison between family and genetic counselor.

Assist the family in understanding/dealing wtih information received.

Aid families in coping with this crisis.

Provide information about known genetic factors.

Ensure continuity of nursing care to the family.

The family may return to the genetic counselor a number of times to air their questions and concerns. It is desirable for the nurse working with the family to attend many or all of these counseling sessions. Since the nurse has already established a rapport with the family, the nurse can act as a liaison between the family and the genetic counselor. Hearing directly what the genetic counselor says helps the nurse clarify issues for the family, which in turn helps them formulate questions.

When the parents have completed the counseling sessions, the counselor sends them and their physician a letter detailing the contents of the sessions. The family keeps this document for reference. See Table 5–11.

Perhaps one of the most important and crucial aspects of genetic counseling in which the nurse is involved is follow-up counseling. The nurse with the appropriate knowledge of genetics is in an ideal position to help families review what has been discussed during the counseling sessions and to answer any additional questions they might have. As the family returns to the daily aspects of living, the nurse can provide helpful information on the day-to-day aspects of caring for the child, answer questions as they arise, support parents in their decisions, and refer the family to other health and community agencies.

If the couple is considering having more children or if siblings want information concerning their affected brother or sister, the nurse should recommend that the family return for another follow-up visit with the genetic counselor. Appropriate options can again be defined and discussed, and any new information available can be given to the family. Many genetic centers have found the public health nurse to be the ideal health professional to provide such follow-up care.

Care must be taken not to assume a diagnosis, determine carrier status or recurrence risks, or provide genetic counseling without adequate information and training. Inadequate, inappropriate, or inaccurate information may be misleading or harmful. Health care professionals need to learn the appropriate referral systems and options for care in their region.

❦ ❦

KEY CONCEPTS

A couple is considered infertile after one year of unprotected coitus.

At least 15% of couples in the United States have undesired infertility.

A thorough history and physical examination of both partners is essential as a basis for infertility investigation.

General areas of fertility investigation are evaluation of ovarian function, cervical mucus adequacy and receptivity to sperm, sperm number and function, tubal patency, general condition of the pelvic organs, and certain laboratory tests.

Among cases of infertility, 40% involve male factors, 40% involve female hormonal defects, 30% to 50% involve female tubal disorders, 10% involve cervical factors, 10% to 20% have no identifiable cause, and 35% have multifactorial etiologies.

Medications may be prescribed to induce ovulation, facilitate cervical mucus formation, reduce antibody concentration, increase sperm count and motility, and suppress endometriosis.

The emotional aspect of infertility may be more difficult for the couple than the testing and therapy.

The nurse should be prepared to provide accurate information about infertility and dispel myths.

The nurse assesses coping responses and initiates counseling referrals as indicated.

Based on a sound knowledge base regarding common genetic problems, the nurse should prepare the family for counseling and act as a resource person during and after the counseling sessions.

Some genetic conditions that can currently be diagnosed prenatally are craniospinal defects; renal malformations; hemophilia; fragile-X syndrome; thalassemia; cystic fibrosis; many inborn errors of metabolism, such as Tay-Sachs disease or maple syrup urine disease; and neural tube defects. This list expands daily as new technology allows more conditions to be detected.

Autosomal dominant disorders are characterized by an affected parent who has a 50% chance of having an affected child and affects males and females equally. The characteristic presentation will vary in each individual with the gene. Some of the common autosomal dominant inherited disorders are Huntington chorea, polycystic kidney, and neurofibromatosis (von Reckinghausen disease).

Autosomal recessive disorders are characterized by both parents being carriers; each offspring having a 25% chance of having the disease, a 25% chance of not being affected, and a 50% chance of being a carrier; and males and females being equally affected. Some common autosomal recessive inheritance disorders are cystic fibrosis, PKU, galactosemia, sickle-cell anemia, Tay-Sachs disease, and most metabolic disorders.

X-linked recessive disorders are characterized by no male-to-male transmission, effects limited to males, a 50% chance that a carrier mother will pass the abnormal gene to her son, a 50% chance that a carrier mother will not transmit the abnormal gene to her son, a 50% chance that a daughter will be a carrier, and a 100% chance that daughters of affected fathers will be carriers. Common X-linked recessive disorders are hemophilia, color blindness, and Duchenne muscular dystrophy.

Multifactorial inheritance disorders include cleft lip and palate, spina bifida, dislocated hips, clubfoot, and pyloric stenosis.

The chief tools of prenatal diagnosis are ultrasound, amniocentesis, chorionic villus sampling, and percutaneous umbilical blood sampling.

❦ ❦

References

American Fertility Society: New guidelines for the use of semen donor insemination. *Fertil Steril* 1990; 53(3)(Suppl):1s.

Archer DF et al: Effects of clomiphene citrate on episodic luteinizing hormone secretion throughout the menstrual cycle. *Am J Obstet Gynecol* September 1989; 161(3):581.

Arms S: *Adoption: A Handful of Hope.* Berkeley, CA: Celestial Arts, 1990.

Blenner JL: Attaining self-care in infertility treatment. *Applied Nursing Research* 1990; 3(3):98.

Brock DJH: Prenatal diagnosis of cystic fibrosis. *Arch Dis Child* 1988; 63:701.

Chan SYW et al: Predictive value of sperm morphology and movement characteristics in the outcome of in vitro fertilization of human oocytes. *J In Vitro Fertil Embryo Transfer* 1989; 6(3):142.

Chong AP et al: Identification and management of clomiphene citrate response. *Fertil Steril* 1987; 48(6):941.

Cohen FL: Neural tube defects: Epidemiology detection and prevention *JOGNN* March/April 1987; 16(2):105

Collins JA, Rowe TC: Age of the female partner is a prognostic factor in prolonged unexplained infertility: A multicenter study. *Fertil Steril* 1989; 52(1):15.

Crawford MA: Prenatal diagnosis of common diseases. *Br Med J* 1988; 297:502.

Daya S, Gunby J, Kohut J: Semen predictors of in vitro fertilization and embryo cleavage. *Am J Obstet Gynecol* November 1989; 161:1284.

DeVore GR, Hobbins JC: Ultrasound diagnosis of congenital birth defects. In: *Gynecology and Obstetrics*. Vol. 3. Sciarra JJ et al (editors). Hagerstown, MD: Harper & Row, 1989.

Devroey P et al: Zygote intrafallopian transfer as a successful treatment for unexplained infertility. *Fertil Steril* 1989; 52(2):246.

Diamond MP: Surgical aspects of infertility. In: *Gynecology and Obstetrics*. Vol. 5. Sciarra JJ et al (editors). Hagerstown, MD: Harper & Row, 1988.

Dunn PA, Weiner S, Ludomirski A: Percutaneous umbilical blood sampling. *JOGNN* 1988; 5:308.

Friedman AJ et al: A randomized placebo-controlled, double-blind study evaluating the efficacy of leuprolide acetate depot in the treatment of uterine leiomyomata. *Fertil Steril* 1989; 51(2):251.

Grunfeld A: Workup for male infertility. *J Reprod Med* 1989; 34(2):143.

Hammond ME: Evaluation of the infertile couple. *Obstet Gynecol Clin North Am* 1987; 14(4):821.

Hammond M, Talbert L: *Infertility*. Oradell, NJ: Medical Economics Books, 1985.

Hatcher RA et al: *Contraceptive Technology: 1990–1992*, 15th ed. New York: Irvington, 1990.

Hecht BR, Hoffman DI: The use of ultrasound in infertility. *Clin Obstet Gynecol* 1989; 32(3):541.

Hook EB et al: Maternal age-specific rates of 47, +21 and other cytogenetic abnormalities diagnosed in the first trimester of pregnancy in chorionic villus biopsy specimens: Comparison with rates expected from observations at amniocentesis. *Am J Hum Genet* 1988; 42:797.

Igbal PK et al: Clinical characteristics of subfertile men with antisperm antibodies. *Br Obstet Gynecol* 1989; 96:107.

Jacobs LA, Ory SJ: Changes in artificial insemination regimens for male factor infertility. *Clin Obstet Gynecol* 1989; 32(3):586.

Kennedy JL, Adashi EY: Ovulation induction. *Obstet Gynecol Clin North Am* December 1987; 14(4):831.

Lemire RJ: Neural tube defects. *JAMA* 1988; 259(4):558.

Lemna WK et al: Mutation analysis for heterozygote detection and the prenatal diagnosis of cystic fibrosis. *N Engl J Med* 1990; 322(5):291.

Lewin PA, Goldberg BB: Ultrasound bioeffects for the perinatologist. In *Gynecology and Obstetrics* Vol. 3. Sciarra JJ et al (editors). Hagerstown MD: Harper and Row, 1989.

Medical Research International: In vitro fertilization-embryo transfer in the United States: 1988 results from the IVF-ET registry. *Fertil Steril* 1990; 53(1):13.

Menning E: *Infertility: A guide for the childless couple* 2nd ed. New York: Prentice Hall, 1988.

Murray DL et al: Oral clomiphene citrate and vaginal progesterone suppositories in the treatment of luteal phase dysfunction: A comparative study. *Fertil Steril* 1989; 51(1):35.

Oster H, Hejtmancik JF: Prenatal diagnosis and carrier detection of genetic diseases by analysis of deoxyribonucleic acid. *J Pediatri* 1988; 112(5):679.

Quagliarello J: Artificial insemination. In: *Gynecology and Obstetrics* Vol 5. Sciarra JL et al (editors). Hagerstown, MD: Harper & Row, 1988.

Sawatzky M: Tasks of the infertile couple. *JOGNN* 1981; 10(2):132.

Seibel MM: *Infertility-A Comprehensive Text.* Norwalk, Conn: Appleton & Lange, 1990.

Shapiro LR et al: Experience with multiple approaches to the prenatal diagnosis of the fragile X syndrome: Amniotic fluid, chorionic villi, fetal blood and molecular methods. *Am J Med Genet* 1988; 30:347.

Sherrod RA: Coping with infertility: A personal perspective turned professional. *MCN* 1988; 13:191.

Smarr SC et al: Effect of therapy on infertile couples with antisperm antibodies. *Am J Obstet Gynecol* 1988; 158:969.

Speroff L, Glass R, Kase N: *Clinical Gynecologic Endocrinology and Infertility,* 4th ed. Baltimore: Williams & Wilkins, 1989.

Thompson JS, Thompson MW: *Genetics in Medicine,* 4th ed. Philadelphia: Saunders, 1986.

Verp MS: Antenatal diagnosis of chromosome abnormalities. In: *Gynecology and Obstetrics,* Vol. 3. Sciarra JJ et al (editors). Hagerstown MD: Harper & Row, 1989.

Additional Readings

Annas GJ, Elias S: The treatment of infertility: Legal and ethical concerns. *Clin Obstet Gynecol* 1989; 32(3):614.

Bernstein J: Parenting after infertility. *J Perinat Neonat Nurs*. September 1990; 4:11.

Bernstein J: Parenting after infertility. *J Perinat Neonat Nurs*. September 1990; 4:11.

Kardon NB: Genetic abnormalities: Their role in amenorrhea and infertility. *Female Patient* 1989; 14:17.

Keleher KC: Occupational health: How work environments can affect reproductive capacity and outcome. *Nurse Pract* 1991; 16(1):23.

Medical Research International: In vitro fertilization-embryo transfer (IVF-ET) in the United States: 1989 results from the IVF-ET registry. *Fertil Steril* 1991; 56(1):14.

Rojas FJ, Djannati E, Rojas IM: The effect of bromocriptine on the motility of human spermatozoa and its capacity to penetrate the cervical mucus. *Fertil Steril* 1991; 55(1):48.

Wright J, Duchesne C, Sabourin S: Psychological distress and infertility: Men and women respond differently. *Fertil Steril* 1991; 55(1):100.

PART THREE

Women's Health Throughout the Lifespan

CHAPTER 6

Women's Care:

Social Issues

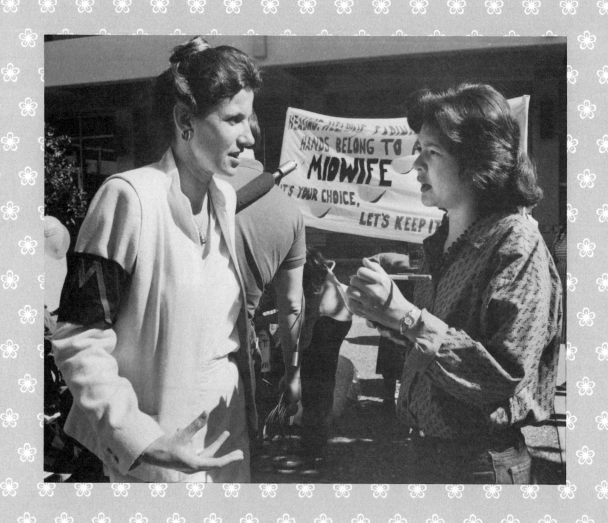

OBJECTIVES

Describe the concept of feminization of poverty.

Discuss the current work environment and the factors that affect women's wages.

Discuss work benefits that affect the childbearing woman.

Describe environmental hazards present in the childbearing woman's work setting.

Discuss briefly the philosophical differences in the question of abortion.

❀ ❀

I don't think there has ever been a more exciting time for women. There are many challenges that face us; work, wage and role issues, safety in pregnancy and childbearing, and conflict over women's rights. On the other hand, women have never been more active and involved in the issues that affect them. The 1990's hold much promise for our future.

Women of today have the opportunity to be dynamic, challenging, and challenged individuals. They have opportunities for personal and professional growth that did not exist 20 years ago. Because of political and social changes that have occurred in this country since the early 1970s women's options have expanded dramatically. Although many women still choose the traditional "women's" careers and become nurses, teachers, and mothers, others are entering occupations that until recently were filled almost exclusively by men. More women than ever have joined the ranks of lawyers and judges, managers and corporate heads, scientists, journalists, legislators, construction workers, plumbers, and other laborers. Women can be found in almost all occupations and thus are sharing in many of the benefits that come with these positions.

Progress has its costs, however. For example, the woman with a career and a family may have difficulty maintaining both. The woman who would like nothing more than to be a wife and mother may be forced by the high cost of living to work outside the home and entrust the care of her children to others. The woman who has devoted her prime childbearing years to establishing a career rather than a family may find herself feeling pressure to find a partner and have children before it is too late.

Nurses must deal with many of the issues facing women, if not personally, then in their dealings with women as they come into the health care setting for maternal-newborn care. To help nurses better understand their clients' concerns and problems, this chapter addresses a few of the more serious issues facing women today.

Women and Poverty

The economic plight of many women is reflected in the phenomenon referred to as the *feminization of poverty,* a term suggested by Diana Pearce (1983). Simply stated, a growing number of women live on incomes below the poverty level, which in 1990 was $12,092 for a family of four and $8,020 for a family of two (Denver Post 1990). The extent of this problem is enormous and increasing at a rapid rate. Compared to men, women are 51% more likely to be living in poverty, and children are 121% more likely to be poor than men (Bassi 1988). Two-thirds of all poor people in this country are women and children, and it is projected that by the year 2000, nearly all people living in poverty will be women and children (Figure 6–1).

The feminization of poverty extends beyond the United States. Females make up over half of the approximately 23.4% of people living in absolute poverty (Brown et al 1990), and women are expected to continue to be the

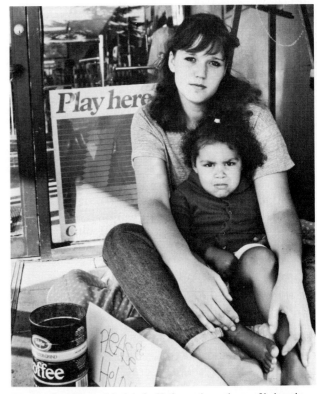

Figure 6–1 Two-thirds of all those Americans living in poverty are women and children.

Table 6–1 Some Facts About Poverty in the United States

The rate of poverty in the general population is 15.2%.

78% of all the poor are women.

5% of male-headed couple households live at or below the level of poverty.

36% of female-headed households live at or below the level of poverty.

30% of white families are headed by a woman. (Kilman & Poteet 1989), and 27% of those families live at or below the level of poverty (Ellis 1990).

51% of black children live in female-headed households, and 52% of these families live at or below the level of poverty (Ellis 1990).

53.4% of Hispanic female-headed households live at or below the level of poverty.

Source: Leslie & Swider 1986, Sidel 1986, Ellis 1990, Kilman & Poteet 1989.

---

majority of the over 50% worldwide poverty rate in 2050–2075 (Brown et al 1990). Women must cope with some special problems: they live with the burden of working more than men but are paid less for the same work; they are expected to bear, raise, and feed many (preferably male) children; they are frequently abused and beaten in their own home; often they have few legal rights. The literacy rate for females is lower than that for males, and education—when available—is more frequently provided for men (Brown et al 1990).

The statistics on the poverty of children are even more shocking. It is estimated that one in four preschoolers in our country lives in poverty (Sidel 1986). More than 25% of our children are now being raised in single-parent families, and that number is expected to double in the 1990s (Tager 1990). More than 53.9% of children living in families headed by a woman are below the poverty level (Sidel 1986). Some sources suggest that the children of female-headed families may be destined for persistent poverty in adulthood. Children of poverty face a future of continued system dependence and homelessness (Bowdler 1989). See Table 6–1.

Although the statistics on poverty may be shocking, they reveal little about what living with poverty is like. It is a day-by-day experience fraught with struggle and hardship:

I thought this would never happen to me. Things were so good for us and our daughter that I thought we would not be another one of those divorced families. Two months after I became pregnant with our second child, it was over. My husband left us. Suddenly, I am the sole support of myself and my children. It's like I'm dreaming, like a nightmare. I'm a teacher, and I've always had a good job, but I have taken time off to stay with our first child and haven't worked for the last two years. I thought it

was important to stay at home and take care of our baby, and Jim felt that way too. Since he left I haven't been able to get a teaching position or any job. So now I don't have medical insurance or any benefits to help with this pregnancy. Applying for Medicaid has to be one of the most humiliating experiences I have ever had. I'm an intelligent woman with a college degree and I couldn't figure out the forms. I'm smart really, surely I am, but I felt so dumb. The lines and the impersonal treatment that I had heard about but never believed in was there. I was a number and felt shuttled from one place to the next. You know, they don't do it on purpose. I know they have heard so many awful stories, but you know it hurt. It will take six weeks to qualify, and that means I will be more than halfway through the pregnancy. I've called and no one will accept me now, without paying money I don't have. I feel really caught. I know I should be getting prenatal care, I had problems with the last pregnancy and I know care is important. I'm caught, I can't get care without money, and I'm afraid when I start care they will be angry with me because I waited so long. It seems there is no way to win. There are only two doctors in our town that will accept Medicaid and they are clear across town. It's all right. I'm thankful that I can get some help now when I need it, but it is so hard. I never dreamed I'd be in this position. I just never dreamed.

Contributing Factors

The feminization of poverty has occurred as a result of three major factors:

- The increase of families headed by females (Leslie & Swider 1986) and the fact that women bear almost all the economic burden of raising the children (Pearce 1983)
- A labor market in which the largest percentage of women work in low-paying, low-status occupations with few benefits and little chance of advancement (Leslie & Swider 1986) and the sex discrimination and occupational segregation that occur in these positions (Pearce 1983)
- The welfare system

Abowitz (1986) has identified similar reasons for the feminization of poverty in Canada.

Increase in Female-Headed Households

The increase in the number of female-headed families is closely associated with divorce. Almost one out of every two marriages end in divorce (Sidel 1986). As a result of divorce the woman's standard of living generally decreases approximately 73% and the male's increases by 41% (Leslie & Swider 1986). This dramatic change in the standard of living is usually associated with the lower earning capacity of women and the fact that the children remain with the

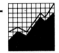

Research Note

Clinical Application of Research

Ferne Franks and Sandra Faux (1990) determined the levels of depression among Chinese, Vietnamese, Portuguese, and Latin American immigrant women. Additionally, they investigated the relationship among demographic variables, stress, mastery (the extent to which the individual perceives control over life's course), and symptoms of depression.

Results showed that depression scores for all four groups were high, with the Portuguese scores reaching diagnostic levels. Regression analysis for the total group demonstrated that the variables of perceived stress, level of education, financial status, and mastery explained 38% of the variance of the depression scale. Each of the four groups differed from each other in terms of predictor variables. Perceived stress and number of friends within reach determined 47% of the depression variable variance for Chinese women; life events and age explained 75% for Vietnamese; perceived English skills and perceived social support decided 50% for the Portuguese women; and employment and financial status accounted to 87% of the variance in Latin American immigrant women.

Researchers raised questions about the reliability and validity of their instruments when attempting to determine significant predictors of depression across cultural groups. Implications for nursing included the identification of different predictors of depression for each cultural group.

Critical Thinking Applied to Research

Strengths: Extensive literature review of current status of research on depression in immigrants. Performed power analysis to determine needed number of subjects to obtain desired level of statistical significance and effect size. Gave internal consistency or Cronbach's alpha scores for several of the tools used to measure variables. Also identified validity for multicultural use with some tools.

Concerns: Although each group of subjects was randomly selected from an ethnic master list, the origin of the master lists is not described.

Franks F, Faux S: Depression, stress, mastery, and social resources in four ethnocultural women's groups. *Res Nurs Health* 1990; 13:283.

woman. Women receive custody of the children in 90% of the cases (Enrenreich & Piven 1984), and the economic assistance provided by the father is minimal. Approximately 4% of women receive alimony; approximately 60% of non-custodial fathers are legally obligated to pay child support, and only half of those pay the full amount mandated. One in four fathers who are ordered to pay child support pay nothing (Klitsch 1989). There are differences for black mothers and for mothers who were never married. Only one-third of black mothers were awarded child support, and on the average the amount was about 20% less than for non-blacks (Beller & Graham 1988). Approximately 11% of never-married mothers were awarded child support (Beller & Graham 1988).

Labor Market

The dual labor market is also associated with the prevalence of poverty in women. There are two sectors in the labor market. The primary sector is characterized by good pay and fringe benefits, job security, and a large number of union groups. The secondary sector has lower-paying jobs, less unionization, and fewer benefits. Women are concentrated in the secondary sector, and the characteristics of this sector tend to keep women in poverty even with full-time employment (Leslie & Swider 1986).

Welfare System

The welfare system provides much-needed assistance to many women. The amount of assistance, however, does not even raise the family to the poverty level. In an effort to assist families and women receiving benefits from the welfare system, including Aid for Families of Dependent Children (AFDC), some states have devised programs to provide job training. Wisconsin offers female heads of families a program that includes job training, child care, and health care during one year of job training. After the woman enters the job market, the health care benefits continue for one year. The program lasts two years, after which time all public monies are withdrawn. Benefits of the program include its focus on increasing job market skills and providing support through monthly funding, child care, and health care to achieve this goal. Disadvantages center on the fact that most of the women will only qualify for a minimum-wage job when it is very difficult if not impossible to maintain a family's home, transportation, child care, and health care on a full-time, minimum-wage job. (See Nursing Care Plan 6–1.)

Homelessness

For many individuals, the thought of a homeless person conjures up a vision of an older man curled in a doorway or making a home under a bridge. However, this vision is less accurate nowadays than in the past; today's homeless have very different characteristics. Of the approximately three million homeless (Bowdler 1990), most are white, female, and young (Bader 1990); approximately 20% are families (Bowdler 1989; Weitzman 1989); and as many as 15% may be under the age of five (King 1989). It has been noted that of the total homeless population, families with children are the fastest growing group (Whitman & Friedman 1990).

Health risks and problems of the homeless are greater than in the general population. Malnutrition predisposes the homeless to a variety of respiratory and nutritional diseases. Bowdler (1989) reports that in a study of homeless people in Boston, tuberculosis—which has an incidence of 13 per 100,000 in the general population—occurred at a rate of 1700 per 100,000. Substance abuse had an incidence of 30%, while alcoholism affected more than 50% of the individuals. Of the children under five years of age, almost half had developmental delays in language, motor, and social skills. Clinical depression and anxiety affected over half of the children over five years of age (Bowdler 1989).

Effects on Health Care

The effects of poverty on health care are extensive. Since 1981, many funding cuts have directly affected programs that benefited those living in poverty. Funding cuts to Aid to Families with Dependent Children and Medicaid have resulted in more than 500,000 people losing their eligibility. The food stamp program has lost 1,000,000 due to decreased funding. The Women, Infants and Children nutrition program (WIC) is currently providing assistance to only one-third of the people who are eligible. These cuts come at a time when the benefits of adequate nutrition and prenatal care have been documented to save $2 to $11 for each $1 spent (Mundinger 1986).

Women living in poverty are also frequently without any kind of health insurance. Overall, over 25% of the population is without any type of health insurance, which is a 25% to 35% increase since 1977. Since health insurance is used to obtain care and for preventive health measures, the implication is that the health of the general population will decline.

Statistical data already is beginning to reflect the change in health insurance coverage and funding cuts. Women who do not receive prenatal care are three times more likely to have low-birth-weight babies, and the incidence of low-birth-weight babies is increasing. Overall, infant mortality has decreased fairly rapidly throughout this century until 1980. At that time the infant mortality rate continued to decline but at a much slower rate. In the late 1980s there was no further decline and the overall rate even showed some trend toward a slight increase. In poor areas the increase in infant mortality has been marked.

The effects of poverty on women's health care will require continued investigation. Currently the status of the mothers and babies is being studied by the Public Health Service Task Force on women's health issues, which is considering not only childbearing but also other factors that affect women's health. They have identified general recommendations such as promoting safe and healthful physical and social environments; providing services for the prevention and treatment of illness; coordinating research and evaluation; educating and informing the public; disseminating research information; and designing guidance for legislative and regulatory measures.

Suggestions for Nursing Action

The issue of women and poverty is critical, and the implications for childbearing care are very real. A pregnant woman who is suffering economically may also suffer physically. The physical and psychologic states of the woman depend on her access to health care and her financial ability to act on her health care providers' recommendations. In the end, it is often the children who suffer the most, bearing the physical and psychological scars of their mothers' struggles.

Nurses should be concerned about the issue of women and poverty for two primary reasons. One reason is related to the nurse's professional role. The health care system and thus nursing is intricately woven into the political and social structures of society. Nurses often work with women on welfare; they *see* the effects of poverty on childbearing families and the pain and struggles of these families. Because of the limited resources of these women, nurses' efforts to provide quality care may be stymied.

The other reason for concern is largely personal. The majority of nurses are women, and like the teacher on p. 153, some nurses may find themselves in financial difficulty, frequently due to circumstances beyond their control.

What can nurses do about the growing problem of female poverty? The following sections include suggestions for action that nurses can take to ease this crisis.

Personal Action

Be aware of your own beliefs about poverty and the women who need public assistance.

Explore your feelings regarding the myths of poverty (see Table 6–2)

Remain knowledgeable about the impact of poverty on the childbearing woman and her family.

Speak out to inform others of the facts; correct misconceptions.

Client Action

Be sensitive in assessing a woman's economic status during intake interviews. Use the knowledge of the current extent of this problem to predict other women who may be at risk.

Provide supportive counseling and determine the woman's ability to follow a treatment plan, especially when extra expenditure of funds is required.

Be alert for women who are not able to follow a treatment plan or accomplish self-care measures due to economic problems.

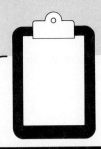

Nursing Care Plan for
Care of Expectant Woman with Limited Resources

Nursing History

Elicit which of the following are present in her life:

Limited financial resources

Lack of secure housing

Limited accessibility of transportation

Limited money for food

Limited emotional support

Limited recreational opportunities

Social Assessment

Educational level

Work setting

Primary language

Nursing Diagnosis	Nursing Interventions	Rationale	Evaluation
Powerlessness related to limited resources *Client Goal:* The client will experience increased sense of control over her own life.	Provide opportunities for client to talk with health care providers to establish rapport and feeling of support. Provide opportunities for decision making to enhance self-esteem. Assist the woman in establishing priorities in terms of her own needs, and assist her in locating resources to get needs met. Provide information regarding community resources for available financial support; housing resources; food supplements such as WIC, food stamps; transportation resources such as city, bus, ride sharing; neighborhood community activities; church groups. Provide information regarding health care settings such as: community health clinic, prenatal classes through the clinic, and future well-baby/nurturing classes. Discuss resources for spiritual support such as church groups. Explore child-care potential in neighborhood such as baby-sitting cooperatives, day care. Investigate community loan programs for maternity clothes, child-care equipment. Loan programs may be available in the Salvation Army or at thrift stores.	A sense of rapport enhances the health care relationship and provides a basis for communication, support, and counseling. A sense of control over one's life may increase self-esteem. Knowledge of available resources will enhance the woman's ability to select those that will best meet her needs. Prenatal care is available at low cost through community health clinics. Depending on the support available, a church group may be a useful resource. Some communities have a loan program for maternity needs.	The woman verbalizes increased sense of power and control over her life.

Table 6–2 Myths About Poverty

Myth	Reality
People living in poverty are black urban females who have been on welfare for many years.	Approximately two-thirds of the people on welfare are white (Sidel 1986).
Poverty is perpetuated from parents to children to grandchildren in a never-ending cycle.	Slightly over half of the individuals living in poverty do so from one year to the next. Only 2% of the poor are classified as permanently poor. Recurrent poverty is rare and is generally not passed from one generation to the next (Hill 1985).
People in poverty are a different breed from the rest of us.	People who are temporarily poor are not different from the population as a whole (Sidel 1986).
People on welfare programs do not try to get off the programs and get a job.	Over 60% of poor adults work (Whitman et al 1988). The majority of women living in poverty sought employment even when the employment meant they lost benefits and were at an even lower economic level (Zinn & Sarri 1984).

Stay knowledgeable about community resources to assist the woman with financial need and be prepared to offer suggestions and counseling regarding possible resources. It is much more helpful to give a group name and a phone number than to send the woman out to search on her own.

Community Action

Identify resources in your community that are pertinent to the needs of the childbearing woman.

When possible, work with community organizations and planners to identify financial needs of childbearing women in the community.

Offer your nursing knowledge expertise to community groups to help them meet the financial and health needs of childbearing women and their families.

Political Action

Know your legislators and their views. Be available to discuss issues and act as a resource for them as they become more knowledgeable about issues that affect childbearing women.

Make your opinions and ideas known to your legislator.

Support programs that benefit childbearing women and help identify areas that need to be addressed.

Educate the legislators about the alarming increase of poverty among women.

Research Action

Investigate the impact of poverty on the health and welfare of childbearing women and their families. When women are unable to obtain adequate care, document it so it will be available for future use.

Conduct research projects to dispel myths associated with poverty.

Women in the Workplace

Women have been entering the work force in increasing numbers since the mid-1940s. In 1990, 70% of all women with children between the ages of six and seventeen worked outside the home, and by 2000, 70% of women between the ages of 45 and 54 will be working (Tager 1990). Women will take two-thirds of the new jobs created in the 1990s (Naisbitt & Aburdene 1990).

The number of women in high-ranking professions is changing. Women represented 4% of the total number of lawyers in 1971 and 40% in 1987. The percentage of female physicians rose from 7% in 1966 to 32.3% in 1987. Women engineers increased from 1% of the total number of engineers in 1971 to 13% in 1987 (Naisbitt & Aburdene 1990). Women comprise almost 50% of accountants and 50% of office managers, and they hold nearly 40% of executive, administrative, and management jobs.

Although more women are choosing high-ranking careers, a large number are still employed in low-level occupations and are not highly paid. In addition, there is wage discrimination in some jobs. There has been a discrepancy between men's and women's wages since women first entered the work force in the mid-1800s. For more than 100 years, women's wages have been approximately 50% to 60% of men's wages. This situation has improved in the past few years. In the 1970s, with the rapid influx of women into the work force, women's wages were about 57% of men's. In the 1980s, women's wages rose to about 70% of men's; however, this rise occurred because men's wages fell by about 22% (Phillips 1990).

The discrepancy between men's and women's wages is caused by many factors. From the beginning, women's wages were purposely set lower than men's, simply because it was a woman doing the job (Sidel 1986). The work of men and women was not valued equally. Unfortunately, this belief still affects women in the workplace.

Another factor is that women's education and experience have not generally been equal to men's, and this has affected women's ability to draw comparable salaries (Pennar & Merrosh 1985). This discrepancy in education and experience has its origins in the socialization process of girls and boys.

Young women traditionally have been socialized in ways that affect their opportunities and expectations. Girls are not expected to do as well as boys in technologic fields such as the sciences (Eccles & Jacobs 1986), so they may not be encouraged to enter these fields. Boys are encouraged to develop a competitive spirit first in sports and then in other areas of their lives. They learn that "being a winner" and "knowing how to play the game" are valued qualities. Girls, on the other hand, are usually not encouraged to develop a competitive spirit; many cultures do not view competitiveness as an important or desirable trait for a girl to have. Girls learn from parents, the media, their peers, and others that physical attractiveness is the key to success since it is more likely to earn popularity than being smart (Pogrebin 1980; Muff 1982). Fearing loss of femininity, girls pull back from intellectual endeavors beginning at the secondary level and continuing into the college years (Pogrebin 1980). By the time these girls are women and ready to enter the work force, most do not have the educational training or the competitive skills to "play the game" that men of equal age and intelligence have.

Certainly all these factors have contributed to the wage discrepancy between men and women. Currently, there are several factors exerting a positive force on the issue of wage discrimination.

- The number of women obtaining a college education continues to increase, and these women influence the work environment as they enter the work force.

- Many working women are holding their jobs for extended periods and are not as likely to work for short periods. They are gaining more experience in performing their jobs, and this has a positive effect on their productivity. As productivity rises, wages generally rise.

- Women have become more involved in the political arena and are raising the issue of comparable worth.

The basic premise of comparable worth is that the same wages should be paid for work that requires comparable skills, responsibility, education, and experience. This issue has created much controversy. The National Committee on Pay Equity believes that work can be equated based on evaluative studies. They agree that the Equal Pay Act has ended blatant discrimination but indirect discrimination continues (Arnold 1985). The National Association of Manufacturers, on the other hand, believes that instituting comparable worth standards would raise costs excessively. The projections of the resulting cost to manufacturers and business and individuals vary. Some believe that the increased financial burden would close business (Arnold 1985), and others believe that all women would lose because there would be fewer jobs available for women (Chavez 1985).

In some companies, comparable worth is a reality. Major companies such as IBM, AT&T, and Bank of America have instituted some forms of comparable worth. At least 30 states have comparable worth legislation pending or have commissions studying the issue.

Nurses' Pay

Nurses as a group experience many of the same problems that confront women in the general work force. The average starting salary of a staff nurse in 1990 was $24,768 and the average maximum salary was $37,168 (despite gains, the shortage hangs on in 1991). Nurses' salaries are still below what other professionals with similar education and responsibilities are paid. There are a variety of reasons for the continuing low wages for nurses (Wright 1986):

- 97% of nurses are women, and as with other professions or job categories that are held mainly by women, wages stay in the low range.

- The majority of nurses are employed in hospitals, and in many communities there is only one hospital. Because of this lack of competition, the hospitals are in a position to keep wages low.

- There are only a few organized collective-bargaining groups for nurses.

- The recent federal, state, and local efforts to cut and contain health care costs have created a climate in which jobs are eliminated and pay increases are delayed.

Suggestions for Nursing Action

What can nurses do about wage discrimination in the health care system? What can nurses do to help clients who are suffering financially because of wage discrimination? The following sections include suggestions for actions nurses can take.

Personal Action

Seek information regarding the wages for nurses in your community.

Share wage information with other nurses so more people will be informed. When wages are kept secret, disparities are more likely to exist.

Validate what it is that you do as a nurse and why you are cost-efficient so you will know your own worth and will be better able to discuss wages.

Help other nurses maintain their self-esteem and feelings of worth.

Client Action

Encourage women to push for wage equity.

Encourage women to talk together about wages so inequities can be identified.

Community Action

Work with community leaders and groups to identify the lack of adequate jobs and wage inequity in your community.

Political Action

Educate legislators about the status of womens' wages and the impact low wages have on health care for the childbearing woman and her family.

Support programs that enhance employment opportunities for fair wages for women.

Maternity Leaves and Child-Care Benefits

Maternity Leaves

Combining a career with childbearing can be a challenging task. However, leaving a job to have a child results at the very least in lost experience, most commonly in lost benefits, perhaps a lost opportunity for promotion, and sometimes loss of the job completely.

Parental leave for childbearing has been a national issue for a number of years. At this time, "only 40% of working women are allowed as much as six weeks of paid disability leave after childbirth . . . " (Brophy 1986 p 57). Business, child development, and labor experts have recommended that some form of uniform parental leave be established in our country. Some type of child care is guaranteed by many other countries and at least 75 other industrialized countries provide some kind of parental leave (Lamm 1986). The United States is the only industrialized country that does not provide some statutory maternity leave or parental benefit (Sidel 1986). European countries offer six months leave as a standard (Brophy 1986). In most countries the woman's wage continues during the leave. For instance, Sweden grants a 52-week leave for either parent with 100% of wages for 38 weeks; Canada grants a maternal leave for 37 weeks with 60% of wages for 15 weeks; and Chile allows either parent an 18-week leave at 100% of wages (Brophy 1986)

Congressional Representative Patricia Schroeder of Colorado introduced a national bill in 1986 to provide a minimum of 18 weeks of unpaid leave for parents. This leave could be used with the birth or adoption of a newborn or in the event of a child's serious illness (Kantrowitz

et al 1986). In Spring 1991 parental leave legislation was still being discussed.

Although there is no standard national leave policy, women need to be aware of their rights, which were established by The Pregnancy Discrimination Act of 1978. This act provides guidelines regarding pregnancy, including the following (Brophy 1986):

- A pregnant woman cannot be denied a job if she is able to perform major job functions.
- The same procedure for using sick-leave pay or disability benefits must be used for the pregnant woman as for other employees.
- Employee medical coverage must include pregnancy benefits.
- The mother can use all her maternity benefits without penalty.

When a woman is planning a pregnancy, it would be wise for her to acquire information regarding pregnancy benefits in her work setting. The state in which she lives will also have guidelines or regulations regarding pregnancy. Questions that the woman may need to address include (California Department of Justice 1983):

Can I be forced to go on leave because I am pregnant?

What are my rights to sick leave or disability leave with my pregnancy?

Can I lose my job for taking disability leave associated with pregnancy?

Do I have any rights concerning infant care?

Is my employer required to provide maternity benefits and insurance coverage?

Recently the Supreme Court upheld the Pregnancy Discrimination Act by determining that a woman is guaranteed her job after returning from maternity leave (Court guarantees job . . . 1987).

Child-Care Benefits

Child care has been a working woman's problem for years. In our country, less than 10% of infants and about 24% of children under 3 are in licensed day-care centers (Belsky 1986). Almost half (45%) of the care of children under 3 is by a relative (Belsky 1986). In France, however, 95% of 3- to 6-year-olds are taken care of in free public schools (Kantrowitz et al 1986). The number of companies in the United States that provide day care is approximately 3500, which is an increase of 40% since 1984 (Naisbitt and Aburdene 1990).

Some women work out arrangements for combining their careers with childbearing by taking a creative approach to hours and tasks. A full-time job may be shared by two women, with each one working 2½ days, or one working mornings and other afternoons. At times, a work schedule can be temporarily reduced to two or three days a week for a few months.

Given increased attention from citizens, legislators, and business, a uniform policy may not be far away. Until that occurs, women need to know their rights in the workplace. As women continue to remain in the work force, continued attention will be focused on the needs of parents for child care.

CRITICAL THINKING

What benefits will be important for you as you enter your professional career?

Suggestions for Nursing Action

Personal Action

Examine the benefits in your own work environment. When questions arise or unmet needs are identified, follow the guidelines in your facility to suggest changes or additions in benefit policies.

Be knowledgeable about the current status of wage inequity and the effect this has on the childbearing woman's ability to afford adequate child care.

Once prepared with accurate knowledge, speak out when needed to provide information and correct inaccurate information about women's wages.

Client Action

Talk with women to identify whether their benefit packages are useful.

Encourage women to investigate the benefits in their own work setting.

Provide resources that can be used to learn about regulations regarding benefits on the community, state, and national levels.

Encourage women to pursue their questions regarding benefits until they are answered satisfactorily.

Community Action

Provide community leaders with information about the need for comprehensive maternal and child-care benefits for childbearing women and their families.

Work within the community to identify benefits for the nursing profession.

Work with community and professional nursing groups to enhance the status of nursing.

Work with your professional nursing organizations to improve benefits for nursing.

Political Action

Write your legislator and support legislation that addresses and corrects wage inequities. Let your legislator know if you do not support legislation and why. Educate legislators about the importance of a national policy on parental leaves and child care.

Environmental Hazards in the Workplace

As more women enter the work force they are exposed to an ever-increasing number of chemicals and environmental pollutants. Of the approximately 50,000 chemicals used today in industry, about 500 have been implicated as having potentially hazardous effects on reproduction (Bernhardt 1990).

1. *Hazards of the microelectronic industry.* Study of the microelectronic industry has indicated that there is a link between various substances used in this field and birth defects, spontaneous abortions, and other reproductive problems. Among the "high-tech" hazards are glycol ethers, arsenic, lead, and radiation (Hembree 1986).

2. *Lead.* Lead was one of the first agents found to have adverse effects on reproduction. Lead contamination causes an increased rate of spontaneous abortions, stillbirths, and prematurity; surviving children are more likely to have impaired growth and neurologic damage (Bang et al 1983). A study of 35,000 female factory workers in Finland (Hembree 1986) demonstrated an increased spontaneous abortion rate in women who worked in electronics and with lead soldering.

Changes related to the reproductive system have also been reported in male workers who are exposed to lead. Several studies have indicated decreased libido, decreased sperm count, and abnormal sperm morphology. There is also an increased number of spontaneous abortions or stillbirths in pregnancies fathered by male workers exposed to lead (Winder 1989). The effects on the male reproductive system have been observed with high-level exposure and also with exposure that is within current recommendations of regulatory authorities for the workplace (Winder 1989).

Although research suggests that lead has adverse effects on the reproductive function of both female and male workers, only women are now excluded from exposure to lead in the workplace. This exclusion is based on the idea that a woman's exposure to lead can directly intoxicate the fetus. This view also underlies the formation of fetal protection policies that have been developed in industrial settings. Under a fetal protection policy, a woman in her reproductive years may be excluded from working with lead (Scialli 1989).

3. *Vinyl chloride.* Vinyl chloride is used in the manufacture of plastics and resin (Bernhardt 1990). There is an increased incidence of spontaneous abortion and stillbirth in wives of workers exposed to vinyl chloride. Studies indicate that the fetal death may be caused by chromosomal changes in the male germ cell (Schnorr 1988).

4. *Halogenated hydrocarbons.* Polychlorinated biphenyls (PCBs) are the most widely known halogenated hydrocarbons. They are used in the manufacture of plastics and as heat-exchange fluids in the electrical industry (Lione 1988). High-level exposure to PCBs has been associated with an increased spontaneous abortion rate, low birth weight, hyperpigmentation at birth (cola-colored skin), gingival hyperplasia, and tooth eruption at birth (Lione 1988). Low-level exposure, which may occur from eating fish caught from PCB-contaminated waterways, may also cause low birth weight and reduced infant head size. PCBs may also be transferred to newborns through breast milk (Lione 1988).

5. *Antineoplastic drugs.* Nurses who administer antineoplastic drugs may be at increased risk for adverse effects if exposed during the childbearing years. A study of Finnish nurses exposed to antineoplastic drugs revealed an increase in spontaneous abortions and fetal anomalies (Selevan et al 1985). Menstrual irregularities and amenorrhea have also been reported (Shortridge 1988).

6. *Video display terminals.* Questions regarding the use of video display terminals (VDTs) have arisen in recent years. Several studies have suggested that VDT operators have increased spontaneous abortion rates and cardiovascular malformations (Kurppa et al 1985; Ericson & Kallen 1986; Schnorr 1990), while other researchers have not been able to document the same findings (Brix & Butler 1986; McDonald et al 1986). Marcus (1990) suggests that further studies should include measurement of electromagnetic radiation and job stress and that criteria to establish the presence of pregnancy should be more uniformly applied in order to more clearly investigate the effects of VDTs.

7. *Anesthetics.* Exposure to anesthetic agents such as nitrous oxide has been associated with increased spontaneous abortion rates and increased numbers of congenital anomalies (Schumann 1990).

8. Nurses have an occupational hazard in the exposure inherent in providing care for sick people. Exposure to toxoplasmosis, rubella, cytomegalovirus, herpes simplex and hepatitis B may affect pregnancy and fetal outcome (Bernhardt 1990). Exposure to HIV infection has also been a concern to health care professionals.

Environmental hazards are increasing with the discovery and development of new products, and they exert their effect on everyone in that environment. Women are at particular risk while they are in the childbearing years. While no work environment is without risks, it is becoming more important for each woman to become knowledgeable about her own workplace. Information can be obtained from libraries, the Public Health Department, and special agencies that collect data regarding environmental hazards.

Suggestions for Nursing Action

Environmental hazards are an area of particular interest and importance to maternal-newborn nurses. Not only does the health care environment carry some risk to each nurse, but also the nurse needs to be knowledgeable about the possible risks to which childbearing women are exposed. Nurses can be influential in encouraging more investigation of chemical substances and environmental hazards so that work environments will be safer for all.

Personal Action

Be knowledgeable about hazards in your own work environment.

Collect information regarding the effects of various environmental hazards on the childbearing woman and her family.

Follow guidelines and procedures in the work setting to decrease your risk.

Client Action

Obtain information about environmental hazards in the woman's work environment.

Suggest resources to the woman to enhance her knowledge.

Recommend resource groups to obtain more information.

Community Action

Work with community leaders and groups to identify environmental hazards in your community.

Provide education regarding the hazards to childbearing women.

Political Action

Provide information about environmental hazards in your community to your legislator.

Educate your legislator regarding the special effects of environmental hazards on the childbearing woman and her family.

Support legislation that addresses and solves problems involving environmental hazards.

Research Action

Document problems that are observed during your care of clients.

Abortion

Abortion is a highly charged issue, and people both for and against legalized abortion are known for their heated confrontations. Even the terms used to refer to those with differing philosophic opinions about abortion are cause for argument. The antiabortion philosophy is dubbed "prolife" and the proabortion philosophy is called "prochoice." This seems to suggest that the prochoice philosophy would not be in favor of life. It is partly this politicizing terminology that works to polarize opposing viewpoints.

The abortion issue is one that different factions have dealt with in one way or another for centuries. For the past 200 years the policies and philosophies in the United States have been directed primarily by the medical community. Through the first half of this century, abortion was a topic not to be discussed; it was a private matter. An important result of this privacy was that even though people held many divergent opinions about abortion, each philosophic position believed that its opinions were those of the majority. In the 1960s an effort to clarify laws and philosophies made the issue of abortion an open one; it was no longer a private issue that one could quietly hope that others would solve in the "right way." More importantly, people discovered that their opinion was not necessarily that of the majority.

There are many different opinions and many issues associated with abortion. One study on abortion (Luker 1984) identified four major arguments that are the basis of differing feelings about the rightness or wrongness of abortion:

1. The moral status of the embryo. Historically, the status of the embryo has been ambiguous from philosophic, religious, and moral viewpoints. Questions of the legal status of the fetus, the use of medical technology, and the value of children are central to this argument.

2. The moment that life begins. The fact that the heartbeat of a developing embryo can be observed by the end of the first month of gestation is accepted by both sides. However, there is no agreement on what this fact means. A heartbeat is necessary for life but the ability to breathe is also critical to maintain life. Does the fact that there is a heartbeat prove that life exists, or does life require a heartbeat and the ability to breathe?

3. The personhood of the embryo. Personhood carries with it inalienable rights to due process in our society. The question, then, is whether the embryo is a person. An additional issue is the allocation of scarce resources, which also involves the worth and value of an individual person but in a different way. If an embryo can be destroyed and denied care, what is to stop our society from deciding that another should not receive care?

4. The woman's role in our society. The ability to have an abortion gives the woman control over her reproductive life. But in establishing this control, the role of motherhood becomes just one role that women might choose. Some opponents fear that legal abortion devalues the role of motherhood and remaining in the home to raise children.

The abortion issue is clearly a complex one involving many philosophic points, values, and opinions. Table 6–3 presents some of the basic differences between those who support abortion and those who are against it. The belief systems are the result of extensive research (Luker 1984) and are characteristics identified by the majority of people on both sides of this issue. The differences are presented in general and may not be pertinent for individuals. A person who feels he or she is prolife may think the items listed are too narrow and may find items in both columns appropriate to their personal beliefs; a prochoice person may also identify with items from both lists.

The moral, legal, and ethical questions regarding abortion continue into the 1990s. The public debate continues as groups with both philosophic views speak out and protest publicly against those with perceived opposing views. The Supreme Court continues to consider cases that challenge the 1973 *Roe v Wade* decision, such as *Webster v Reproductive Health Services* (1989). Individual states are also striving to enact abortion policies that address at what point an abortion may be done and under what circumstances, where it may be done, and if spousal or parental permission is required. Some states are adding a required informational session that precedes the abortion decision and a waiting period between the informational session and the abortion procedure. The debate extends into the development of new contraceptive techniques and has focused on the introduction of RU 486 (a French drug that has been used to cause abortion) into the United States.

One of the questions that concerns both prochoice and prolife groups is the possible psychologic impact of having an abortion or of carrying an unwanted pregnancy to term (Rogers & Stoms 1989). Clearly, on the public

Table 6–3 Belief Systems Associated with Abortion	
For Abortion as a Choice	**Against Abortion**
Role:	*Role:*
Men and women are essentially equal. Women's reproductive and family roles are not "natural" or required. The reproductive function can be a barrier to full equality.	Men and women are intrinsically different and have distinctly different roles in life. Abortion devalues the traditional roles of men and women.
Abortion:	*Abortion:*
Control over reproduction is essential to full equality.	Abortion is intrinsically wrong because it takes a human life. If a woman has control over her fertility it upsets basic social relationships between men and women.
Contraceptives:	*Contraceptives:*
Contraceptives should be very safe, effective, and readily available and preferably should not interfere with the spontaneity of sexual relations.	Contraceptives interfere with the potential to become pregnant, which disturbs the true meaning of sexual relations. The use of natural family-planning methods is preferred in that the potential for procreation exists.
Sex:	*Sex:*
Sex is natural and positive.	Sex is serious and filled with responsibility.
Parenting:	*Parenting:*
People should plan for beginning a family and fit children into family and life goals. They should attend parenting seminars and classes and seek information about effective parenting styles. The parent's duty is to prepare the child for the future. Optional parenting enhances the quality of parents. It is important for a child to be wanted.	Parenting is a natural role and does not need to be studied. The goal of marriage is to have children, not material things. Setting goals disturbs the reason for marriage. When a couple have financial and educational preparation, their values regarding family and childbirth may change. There is an antichild sentiment in the world today.

Note: The views delineated in this table are general and not meant to categorize individuals in either group. Each individual will probably find that his or her personal beliefs and philosophies are a blend of those held by both groups.

Source: From Luker K. Abortion and the Politics of Motherhood, Berkeley, University of California Press, 1984.

scene, in the legislative arena, and in people's private beliefs, the abortion issue is one that continues to raise many questions (Annas 1989; Mahowald 1989).

The implications of abortion for maternal-newborn nurses are also complex. Each nurse will have many opportunities over the course of a professional nursing career to examine her or his personal feelings and opinions, and there is a good chance that these opinions will change over time as the nurse has new experiences and insights.

The philosophies of nurses mirror those of the society at large, and it may be difficult to provide care for an individual who is participating in a procedure with which the nurse disagrees. If a client is having an abortion, the nurse who does not support abortion may be faced with a decision about whether to provide care. In some settings, nurses do not have to provide care for women having an abortion if it is against their own personal philosophy and if another nurse is available to provide care. The nurse with a prochoice philosophy may have difficulty understanding how a professional colleague could possibly choose not to care for a client based on the client's personal beliefs. If a nurse can choose not to care for a woman having an abortion, can the nurse also choose not to provide care for an alcoholic? A drug addict? A person of another race or religion? The questions facing nurses about the abortion issue have implications for other areas of nursing.

Suggestions for Nursing Action

Personal Action

Explore your own feelings and beliefs regarding abortion.

Talk with others and gather information about abortion.

Be knowledgeable about the issues involved.

Client Action

If your beliefs allow you to care for women considering abortion, provide counseling and support to women as they seek information. If your beliefs do not allow you to care for women who choose abortion, avoid imposing your opinions on them. Provide factual information.

Be nonjudgmental when working with women who have abortions.

Community Action

Work with community groups that support your views.

Support adequate health care for women regardless of the option that the woman chooses (to seek an abortion or to continue with the pregnancy).

Political Action

Provide education, support, and assistance to legislators in order to attain legislation that promotes your philosophy and ensures safe care for women.

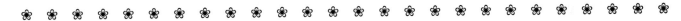

KEY CONCEPTS

The number of women living in poverty is increasing at a rapid rate. Childbearing women seem to be at particular risk due to current trends in the divorce rate, the frequency with which the mother gains custody of children, and factors in the work environment that make it difficult for women to earn a good wage.

Women's wages have always been lower than men's because of demand, education, skills, discrimination, and underlying philosophies that deem women's work as less valuable. Women are working to change the wage system by pushing for comparable worth legislation.

Work benefits that affect women pertain especially to maternity leave and child care. The United States does not have a standard policy regarding maternity benefits and leave.

The chemical compounds present in the workplace are numerous and are increasing by 1000 each year. The implications of exposure during the childbearing years are known in some instances, and others are currently being investigated.

The belief systems and philosophies regarding abortion are complex. Some general characteristics can be identified in people for and against abortion.

Nurses need to be aware of some of the current issues affecting the childbearing woman so they can better understand the client as she comes to the maternal-newborn health care setting.

References

Abowitz DA: Data indicate the feminization of poverty in Canada, too. *Sociol Social Res* April 1986; 70:209.

Annas GJ: Webster and the politics of abortion. *Hastings Center Report* March/April 1989; p 36.

Arnold B: Why can't a woman's pay be more like a man's? *Business Week,* January 28, 1985, p 83.

Bader EJ: The "Housing Now" march on Washington. *The Humanist* January/February 1990; 50:5.

Bang KM, Lockey JM, Keye W: Reproductive hazards in the work place. *Fam Commun Health* May 1983; 6:44.

Bassi LJ: Poverty among women and children: What accounts for the change? *Am Econ Rev* May 1988; 78:91.

Beller AH, Graham JW: The feminization of poverty: Child support payment—evidence from repeated cross sections. *Am Econ Rev* May 1988; 78:81.

Bernhardt JH: Potential workplace hazards to reproductive health: Information for primary prevention. *JOGNN* January/February 1990; 19:53.

Bowdler JE: Health problems of the homeless in America. *Nurs Pract* July 1989; 14:44.

Brophy B: Expectant moms, office dilemma. *U.S. News & World Report,* March 10, 1986, p 57.

Brown LR, Flavin C, Postel S et al: *State of the World 1990: A Worldwatch Institute Report on Progress Toward a Sustainable Society.* New York: Norton, 1990.

California Department of Justice: *Women's Rights.* Sacramento, CA: 1983.

Chavez L: Pay equity is unfair to women. *Fortune* March 1985; 111:161.

Court guarantees job in maternity leave. *Denver Post,* January 14, 1987, p 1.

Despite gains, shortage hangs on. *The American Nurse.* Official Newspaper of The American Nurses Association. March 1991; p 18.

Eccles JS, Jacobs FE: Social forces shape math attitudes and performances. *Signs* 1986; 11:367.

Ellis JE: What black families need to make the dream come true. *Business Week* January 22, 1990; p 29.

Enrenrich B, Piven FF: The feminization of poverty. *Dissent* Spring 1984; 31:162.

Hembree D: High-tech hazards. *Ms* March 1986; 14:79.

Kantrowitz B et al: Changes in the workplace. *Newsweek,* March 31, 1986, p 57.

Kilman C, Poteet, GW: Child care needs of nursing personnel: the challenge for the future. *J Ped Nurs* December 1988; 3:369.

Klitsch M: Noncustodial fathers can probably afford to pay far more child support than they now provide. *Fam Plann Perspect* November/December 1989; 21:278.

King CE: Homelessness in America. *The Humanist* May/June 1989; 49:8.

Lamm D: Best and brightest: They should be encouraged to have children. *Denver Post,* Contemporary, June 29, 1986.

Leslie LA, Swider SM: Changing factors and changing needs in women's health care. *Nurs Clin North Am* March 1986; 21:111.

Lione A: Polychlorinated biphenyls and reproduction. *Repro Toxicology.* 1988; 2(2):83.

Luker K: *Abortion and the Politics of Motherhood.* Berkeley: University of California Press, 1984.

Mahowald MB: Abortion: Searching for common ground. *Hastings Center Report* July/August 1989; p 22.

Muff J: *Socialization, Sexism and Stereotyping.* St. Louis: Mosby, 1982.

Mundinger MO: Health service funding cuts and declining health of the poor. *N Engl J Med* July 1986; 313:44.

Naisbitt J, Aburdene P: *Megatrends 2000: Ten New Directions for the 1990s.* New York: Morrow, 1990.

Pearce DM: The feminization of ghetto poverty. *Society* November/December 1983; 21:70.

Pennar K, Merrosh E: Women at work. *Business Week,* January 28, 1985, p 80.

Phillips K: *The Politics of Rich and Poor.* New York: RanJom House, 1990.

Pogrebin LC: *Growing Up Free.* New York: McGraw-Hill, 1980.

Rogers JL, Stoms GB, Phifer JL: Psychological impact of abortion: Methodological and outcomes summary of empirical research between 1966 and 1988. *Health Care for Women International* 1989; 10:347.

Schnorr TM: NIOSH epidemiologic studies of pregnancy outcomes. *Repro Toxicol* 1988; 2:247.

Schnorr TM The NIOSH study of reproductive outcomes among video display terminal operators. *Repro Toxicol.* 1990; 4:61.

Schrader A: Medicaid opened up to thousands. *Denver Post* April 1, 1990, 1C.

Schumann D: Nitrous oxide anaesthetic: Risks to health personnel. *Int Nurs Rev* January/February 1990; 37:214.

Scialli AR: Who should paint the nursery? *Reprod Toxicol* 1989; 3(3):159.

Shortridge LA: Assessment of menstrual variability in working populations. *Reprod Toxicol.* 1988; 2:171.

Sidel R: Women and Children Last. New York: Viking 1986.

Tager MJ: Work and family issues: A new frontier for health promotion. *Am J Health Promotion* January/February 1990; 4:237.

Weitzman BC: Pregnancy and childbirth: Risk factors for homelessness? *Fam Plann Perspect* July/August 1989; 21:175.

Whitman D, Friedman D, Thomas L: The return of skid row. *U.S. News & World Report,* January 15, 1990, p 27.

Whitman D, Thornton J, Shapiro JP et al: America's hidden poor. *U.S. News & World Report* January 11, 1988, p 18.

Winder C: Reproductive and chromosomal effects of occupational exposure to lead in the male. *Reprod Toxicol.* 1989; 3:221.

Wright BW: Nurses' pay: Why so low? *U.S. News & World Report,* March 17, 1986, p 72.

Zinn DK, Sarri RC: Turning back the clock on public welfare. *Signs* Winter 1984; 10:355.

Additional Readings

Cairns JA: The demand for abortion in England and Wales. *Soc Sci Med* 1989; 29(5):653.

Harvey FB: A new enterprise. *The Humanist* May/June 1989; 49(3):14.

Here are the women to watch in corporate America. *Business Month* April 1989; 133:38.

Novak M: The truth about poverty. *Forbes,* December 11, 1989, p 82.

Prows CA: Ribavirin's risks in reproduction: How great are they? *MCN* November/December 1989; 14:400.

Samuelson RJ: Racism and poverty. *Newsweek,* August 7, 1989, p 46.

Shapiro JP: A conservative war on poverty. *U.S. News & World Report.* February 27, 1989; p 20.

Tribe LH. *Abortion: The Clash of Absolutes* New York: WW Norton & Company 1990.

CHAPTER 7

Women's Care:

Health Promotion Through the Lifespan

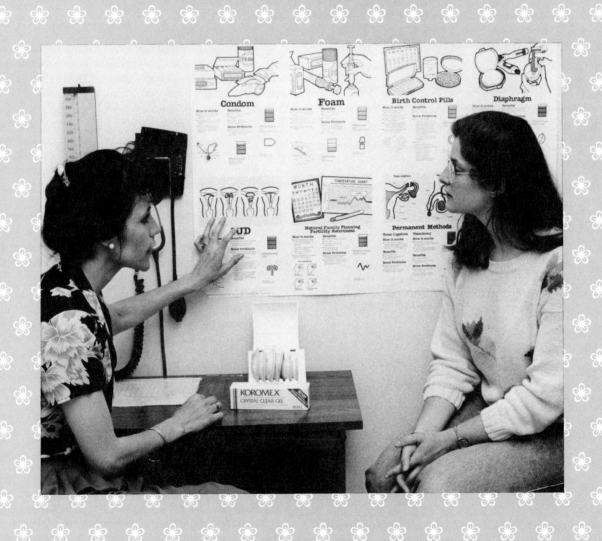

OBJECTIVES

Summarize the factors that influence the development of attitudes about sexuality.

Compare the sexual responses of males and females as identified by Masters and Johnson.

Describe techniques a nurse can use to be more effective when taking a sexual history.

Relate the basic content of preconception counseling to its rationale.

Compare the various methods of fertility control with regard to advantages, disadvantages, and effectiveness.

Develop a teaching plan that could be used to instruct a woman about a specific method of contraception.

Delineate the physical and psychologic aspects of menopause.

Discuss hormone replacement therapy in menopausal women with regard to purpose, procedures, benefits, and risks.

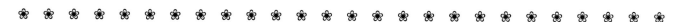

Our daughter and her family were visiting us from out of town for the holidays and we had our four children and their families for a festive family dinner. I found myself sitting back and enjoying their good-natured ribbing and camaraderie and could sense the love and closeness among them. It was interesting noting the similarities and also differences in each offspring's personality. I remembered each of their births and my feelings 45 years ago of incredible awe at the sight of my first baby girl. I could hardly believe the beautiful, perfect little person came from my husband and me. This same emotion persisted at the birth of another daughter and son. When our fourth child was born we learned to our great sorrow she had many health problems and would not survive very long. After 10 days on this earth she was called to heaven. We were blessed four years later when our second son was born well and healthy. Oh yes, there is a great emotional risk having a family and I learned I must cope with the sorrows as well as the great joy. In rearing my family I ran the gamut of emotions. There were times of intense pride; times of impatience and aggravation when my perfect little angels weren't so perfect; times of guilt when Mother wasn't so perfect either; times I felt fiercely protective but had to let them go so they could become self-sufficient, independent people. As I watched and studied my family I suddenly realized I not only love them all completely but I LIKE THEM as people in their own right, because they are good and caring as well as wonderful parents to our grandchildren. I experienced such a feeling of thankfulness because my husband and I were truly blessed. Would I be willing to do it again? Yes! Yes! Yes!

People are sexual beings. Men and women develop sexual identities, make sexual choices, and establish personal standards of appropriate sexual behavior. Human sexuality begins developing at conception and evolves throughout an individual's life. The sexual experimentation and exploration of children gives way to the more urgent activities of the adolescent. With maturity, sexual contact becomes part of a broader and usually more meaningful relationship.

People make many choices related to their sexual activity. They can choose to be sexually active or celibate. They can choose a monogamous relationship or relationships with many partners. They can choose heterosexual or homosexual activity. They can choose to be parents or to remain childless. They can choose unprotected intercourse, or they can use contraceptives. They can continue in a sexual relationship, or they can end it.

This chapter focuses on the concept of sexuality particularly as it relates to people of childbearing age and provides information on preconception planning for women or couples who choose to become parents. The chapter also focuses on available methods of contraception and on the needs of the menopausal woman.

Development of Sexuality

Sexual development begins at conception, when biologic sex is determined: XX, a female, XY, a male. As the embryo becomes a fetus and development continues, sexual differentiation takes place (see Figure 4-1), and the sex organs begin functioning. Even as the sex organs are developing, other senses and systems are developing that enable the infant to react to sexual stimuli at birth. The sense of touch, for example, which is fundamental in the development of sexuality, is highly developed by eight weeks' gestation.

The stimuli, experiences, and relationships that are essential to the development of sexuality come into play at birth. The infant learns to find satisfaction through oral stimuli, through contact with another, and through cuddling and holding. Young infants learn to touch their genitals and seem to be capable of sexual arousal.

Toddlers facing toilet training become even more aware of their bodies and may more consciously practice masturbation although their parents often discourage it. By age 3 most children are aware of their sexual identity as a result of consistent parental and social reinforcement. During the childhood years, from 5 through 12, sexual activity and interest may be less apparent but it has not disappeared. Games such as "playing house" or "playing doctor" help children learn sex roles and more about the differences between the sexes. Children show a preference for playmates of the same sex, although they may also show some romantic interest in members of the opposite sex.

Puberty and adolescence are a time of transition from childhood to adulthood. Adolescence finds physically and sexually mature young people trying to cope with new situations and sensations while they are still psychologically immature. Sexual experimentation begins, and masturbation accompanied by fantasy is common. Homosexual experiences may occur, and mutual masturbation for boys is not uncommon. Heterosexual contacts progress over four or five years from initial kissing and fondling, to mutual body exploration and masturbation, to sexual intercourse.

With adulthood comes responsibility and choice. Because sexual expression in marriage has the most legitimacy in our society, many adults choose to marry. However, new life-styles, changing morality, and contraceptive choices have made available other situations in which sexuality can be expressed.

Sexual Attitudes

Attitudes about sex are influenced by a variety of factors. The home environment is one of the greatest influences. Children raised by parents who are comfortable with and open about sexuality will probably be more comfortable with their sexuality than children raised in more restrictive environments. The following anecdote from a young mother provides an example.

When I was growing up, my parents always showed affection for each other and for us. Hugs, kisses, and pats on the shoulder were common. In discussing sexual issues with me, my mother was very direct and always used correct terminology. She never seemed embarrassed to answer questions. My closest girlfriend couldn't talk to her mother about anything. She told me once that she had never seen her parents show any physical affection for each other. They never kissed or hugged her either. She had an older sister, but they weren't close, so I ended up telling her what my mother told me. When we started high school and had so

many questions, it was harder. One day a neat thing happened. My mom made some cocoa, and the three of us sat and talked all afternoon. Mom answered our questions about sex and got us thinking about more abstract aspects of sexuality like ethics and choices. It was one of the most special times I ever shared with my mother. I hope I can do the same for my children.

Even if parents are not openly demonstrative, they can convey to children that sexuality is a natural, acceptable, and satisfying part of life by creating a positive home atmosphere.

Cultural background can profoundly influence the home and environment and thereby have a major impact on the child's socialization. Individuals raised in a male-dominated or strongly moralistic culture will usually have very different attitudes from those of individuals raised in a culture that views sexual expression as a shared experience between equals. People can reject cultural norms as adults, but doing so is often difficult and may cause stress.

Attitudes about sex are influenced by education and socioeconomic level. People with more income and education tend to be more comfortable with a wider variety of sexual activities. Sexual attitudes can be profoundly affected by previous sexual experiences, especially very intense experiences such as incest, rape, or severe punishment for sexual experimentation.

The personal characteristics of the individual are influential in the development of sexual attitudes. Although it is difficult to negate the influence of environment, people are born with different personality characteristics: Some are shy, others more adventuresome, and so forth. There are also variations in sex drive or libido that significantly influence an individual's view of sexuality.

Ethics and Sexuality

Sexuality must be considered within the context of a person's life and life choices. Sex is a major focus to some and a minor consideration to others. Some feel sex is only appropriate in a close and loving relationship; others feel that love and sex are separate and do not necessarily have to occur together.

Opinions also vary about the purpose of sexual intercourse. More traditional views hold that the sole purpose of sex is procreation. Pleasure may be experienced, but it is not essential. While it is obviously necessary for the man to experience an orgasm, a woman may or may not achieve one. Some believe that any sexual activities engaged in for pleasure only are selfish and immoral. Others believe that the purpose of sex is pleasure: If an action brings pleasure it is good. Nothing is unacceptable as long as it provides pleasure and release. Sex is only "bad" if it does not bring satisfaction to either or both parties. Sexual expression can also be viewed as a means of expression, a sharing of feelings, a union of two individuals seeking to communicate. This communication may involve demonstration of a variety of messages: tenderness, domination, passion, or even anger.

Although the basic patterns of psychosexual development are established by the end of adolescence, a person continues to develop and modify beliefs and attitudes throughout life. Many adults broaden their attitudes about sexual activities and experiment with different sexual lifestyles. During adulthood an individual usually resolves any psychosexual conflicts and develops a set of sexual values.

Sexual Response Cycle

People obtain sexual satisfaction in a variety of ways. A person alone may find sexual pleasure in a book, a film, or a stirring musical piece; he or she may also derive pleasure from fantasy or masturbation. Couples may experience sexual pleasure through a shared experience, through physical closeness such as holding each other or cuddling together; through touching, kissing, and stroking each other; through mutual masturbation; or through sexual intercourse.

Many terms are used to describe the sexual mating of a sexually mature male and female. These include coitus, sexual intercourse, copulation, making love, and the sex act. **Coitus** is defined as the insertion of the erect penis into the vagina. After repeated thrusting movements of the penis, the man experiences ejaculation of semen concurrent with orgasm. **Orgasm** is the involuntary climax of the sexual experience, involving a series of muscular contractions, profound physiologic bodily response, and intense sensual pleasure. Orgasm may be achieved by other methods of sexual stimulation besides sexual intercourse, such as masturbation and oral stimulation. Although the basic events of coitus are the same for all couples, wide variation exists in sexual positions, technique, duration, intent, meaning, and reactions among individuals.

Coitus is a personal act between two consenting adults. It can signify a variety of feelings, beliefs, and attitudes. It may reflect their mutual commitment and caring, or it may be a more immediate interaction for the purpose of personal pleasure or merely temporary companionship. In our society, sexual intercourse ideally is the sharing by two persons of their emotions and bodies in the context of the larger sharing of their lives. Such sexual interactions are the result of mutual caring and love.

Physiology of Sexual Response

Masters and Johnson (1966) have identified and described the physiology of the sexual response in both males and females. All the responses can be classified as either vasocongestive or myotonic. *Vasocongestion* involves the congestion or engorgement of blood vessels and is the most common physiologic response to sexual arousal.

Myotonia, a secondary physiologic response, is increased muscular tonus, which produces tension.

Human sexual response occurs in four separate phases: excitement, plateau, orgasm, and resolution. Female (Table 7–1) and male (Table 7–2) anatomic and physiologic reactions are similar. Wide variations occur, however, in duration and intensity of response.

Female sexual response varies considerably. Not all women experience orgasm consistently; they are influenced by their psychologic state, health, current sexual motivation, and environmental distractions. A woman may not experience orgasm during a particular act of coitus, or she may experience one or multiple orgasms of varying intensity (Figure 7–1A). Such variation is usual in a woman of "normal" sexual activity, interest, and response.

The male physical response is relatively constant, resulting in orgasm if erection and sexual stimulation are maintained (Figure 7–1B).

Women and men exhibit several identical responses. The *sex flush* is a maculopapular rash that usually begins in the epigastric area and spreads quickly to the breasts. More than half of women experience sex flush, whereas less than half of men do. Heart rate and blood pressure increase in

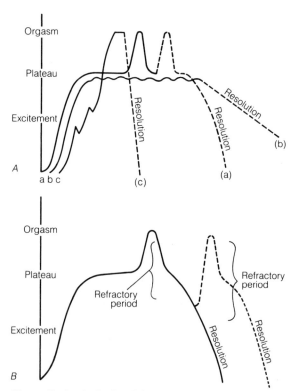

Figure 7–1 A Cycle of female sexual response: (a) reaction pattern with single or multiple orgasms; (b) reaction pattern without orgasm; (c) reaction pattern without distinct plateau. B Cycle of male sexual response. (From Masters WH, Johnson VE: Human Sexual Response. Boston: Little, Brown, 1966, p 5.)

Table 7–1 Anatomic and Physiologic Summary of Female Sexual Response

Organ	Excitement (foreplay)	Plateau (entry and coital movements)	Orgasm (climax)	Resolution (relaxation)
Clitoris	Size of glans increases; engorgement of dorsal vein occurs; shaft elongates	Glans retracts under hood after erection	Rhythmic muscular contractions occur, ranging from mild to intense	Returns to normal; no refractory period; multiple orgasms possible
Labia majora	Vasocongestion and swelling occurs; nulliparous: flatten and widen; multiparous: widen by movement from vaginal introitus	Increases		Return to normal size and color
Labia minora	Vasocongestion of erectile tissue occurs; color darkens; extension of tissue	Increases		Return to normal size and color
Vagina	Vaginal lubrication appears; in 10–30 seconds, widens and lengthens 1 cm; walls become purplish; progressive distention occurs; upper portion "tents"; rugae become smooth	Engorgement occurs; outer third of vagina swells; "orgasmic platform" develops; interior lumen decreases to "grasp" penis	Outer third has spasm, then rhythmic contractions; perivaginal muscles contract	Outer third relaxes after clitoris returns to normal; remaining portion returns to normal
Cervix	Moves upward and backward posteriorly	Cervical os opens slightly		Returns to normal position; os closes in 20–30 minutes
Uterus	Moves upward and backward	Increases in size	Rhythmic contractions from fundus to cervix occur	Returns to precoital size slowly
Breasts	Areolae increase in size; nipples become erect and size increases; sex flush may appear		Sex flush most pronounced	Slow return to normal; sex flush disappears

Table 7–2 Anatomic and Physiologic Summary of Male Sexual Response

Organ	Excitement (foreplay)	Plateau (entry and coital movements)	Orgasm (climax)	Resolution (relaxation)
Scrotum	Skin thickens; scrotal sac elevates and flattens against body (spermatic cord contracts)	Remains tense and close to body		
Testes	Elevate with scrotum	May increase in size by 50%; remain elevated		
Penis	Engorgement and erection is rapid; size increases; position changes; angle of protrusion created	Coronal ridge size increases; glans becomes purplish	Contracts	Becomes flaccid; refractory period: erection may not be experienced
Urethra	Moistened with mucus	Mucus increases; becomes distended with semen just before orgasm	Semen ejected with force as bulb contracts	Minor contractions persist even after semen is ejected
Seminal vesicles			Semen is discharged into urethral bulb	
Prostate			Contracts, expelling fluid into urethral bulb	
Bulbourethral glands		Few drops of fluid may be discharged (contain sperm)		
Breasts	Nipples may become erect; sex flush may appear		Sex flush most pronounced	Slow return to normal; sex flush fades slowly

proportion to the degree of sexual excitement. Muscles tense beginning in the excitement phase. This tension increases during the plateau phase. Hyperventilation occurs just before and during orgasm. At orgasm, muscle tension is extreme. The face may contort, while muscles of the neck, extremities, abdomen, and buttocks contract tightly. Individuals may moan, murmur, or cry out and will experience a total surrender to bodily responses, accompanied by acute pleasure and relief.

During resolution the body returns to the unaroused state. Muscular tension is dramatically reduced, and blood is released from the engorged tissues. If orgasm did not occur, the lingering vasocongestion may cause feelings of pelvic fullness and pressure that take a longer time to resolve.

Although women are capable of achieving multiple orgasms, men are more limited in that respect. Practically all men experience a refractory period as part of their resolution phase. During this period, which may last from a few minutes in young men to several hours in older men, a man is physiologically unable to achieve another erection. Some men, however, can achieve two or more ejaculations with such a short refractory time between that it may be compared to multiple orgasm.

The Nurse as Counselor on Sexuality and Reproduction

On occasion most people experience concern and even anxiety about some aspect of sexuality. Societal standards and pressures can cause people to evaluate and compare with others their sexual attractiveness, technical abilities, the frequency of sexual interaction, and so on. The reproductive implications of sexual intercourse are also a source of concern. Some people desire conception; others wish to avoid it at all costs. Health factors are another consideration. The increase in the incidence of sexually transmitted diseases, especially AIDS, human papilloma virus (HPV), and herpes, have caused many people to modify their sexual practices and activities.

Because sexuality and its reproductive implications are such an intrinsic and emotion-laden part of life, people have many concerns, problems, and questions about sex roles, sexual behaviors, sex education, family planning, sexual inhibitions, sexual morality, and related areas.

To be effective in providing sexual health care, nurses must develop an awareness of their own feelings, values, and attitudes about sexuality. Often people believe that their own sexual values and patterns of sexual behavior are the best ones, the "right" ones. This of course implies that all other attitudes and practices are not as good or are "wrong." Nurses must recognize their own beliefs and attitudes so that they can be more sensitive and objective when confronted with the beliefs of others. The nurse who recognizes that he or she is not comfortable dealing

with issues related to sexuality should avoid situations that require sexual counseling or should refer the client to a nurse who is more at ease in this area.

Many nurses who care for childbearing families will be faced with questions about sexuality, sexual practices, and so forth. These nurses need to have accurate, up-to-date knowledge about these topics. They should also know about the structure and functions of the male and female reproductive systems.

Continuing education for the practicing nurse and appropriate courses in undergraduate and graduate nursing education programs can teach nurses about sexual values, attitudes, alternative life-styles, cultural factors, and misconceptions and myths about sex and reproduction. The nurse can then maintain this knowledge by regular reading so that he or she is familiar with current literature on the subject.

Self-awareness and a sound knowledge base are not, by themselves, sufficient to make the nurse an effective counselor. The nurse also needs to develop skills in listening, communicating, interviewing, assessing, and intervening. Nurses today are often responsible for taking a woman's initial history. Opening the discussion with a brief explanation of the purpose of such questions is often helpful. For example the nurse might say,

> As your nurse I'm interested in all aspects of your well-being. Often women have concerns or questions about sexual matters, especially when they are pregnant (starting to be sexually active). I will be asking you some questions about your sexual history as part of your general health history.

The nurse may find the following additional suggestions useful when taking a sexual history:

- Provide a quiet, private place, free of distractions.
- Approach the situation in a relaxed unhurried way and with an attitude of honesty and acceptance.
- Use direct eye contact as much as possible unless you know that this is culturally unacceptable to the woman.
- Fit the taking of the sexual history into the gynecologic and obstetric history rather than isolating it.
- Do little if any writing during the discussion, especially if the woman seems ill at ease or is discussing very personal issues.
- Avoid sitting across a desk. Sit as close to the woman as seems comfortable to you both.
- Pay attention to nonverbal cues and body language.
- Ask open-ended questions. Often nurses develop the habit of asking questions that require a "yes" or "no" response. Open-ended questions often elicit far more information. For example, "What, if any-

thing, would you change about your current sex life?" will produce more information than "Are you happy with your sex life now?"

- If the woman has no questions or concerns, it is not necessary to press for a lengthy discussion. It may be that she is satisfied, or that your relationship has not reached the point where she is comfortable with such a discussion.

- Clarify terminology. If the woman uses a slang term find out what she means by it. If the word she uses is not comfortable for you, use one that is comfortable without being too clinical.

- Proceed from easier topics to those that are more difficult to discuss. Often it is easier to discuss the menstrual history, for example, before considering sexually transmitted diseases or unusual sexual practices.

- Before asking direct questions it is often useful to make a generality or normalcy statement such as "Many women worry about . . ." or "Often women have questions about . . ."

- Try to determine whether the woman has already identified specific concerns or if she attributes problems to something specific. For example, you might ask, "Do you feel that anything is affecting your sexual health or happiness in any way?"

- The phrase "How do you feel about that?" is used so often that it has become trite. Instead try "What would you like to change about that situation?" or "You seem uncomfortable. What are you thinking about now?"

- Self-disclosure can occasionally help the woman be more at ease. Before making any self-disclosure statement, however, the nurse should internally question whose needs will be met by the disclosure and whether there is any sense of being in competition with the client.

A complete sexual history may not be necessary in every situation and the depth of the information obtained will vary with the client's situation. It may take several encounters to complete a sexual history. Clients may not share such personal information until they have developed a trusting relationship with the care giver.

Applying the Nursing Process

After completing the sexual history, the nurse assesses the information obtained. If the nurse identifies a problem that requires further assessment, referral to a nurse practitioner, nurse-midwife, physician, or counselor may be necessary. In many instances the nurse alone will be able to develop a nursing diagnosis and then plan and implement therapy. For example, if the nurse determines that a woman who is interested in conceiving a child does not have a clear understanding of when she ovulates, the nurse may formulate the nursing diagnosis: Knowledge deficit related to the timing of ovulation. The nurse could then evaluate the woman's knowledge through discussion and review and work with the woman to provide necessary knowledge. The nurse might also suggest that the woman keep a menstrual calendar and monitor basal body temperatures and cervical mucus to identify the time of ovulation.

It is important for the nurse to be realistic in making assessments and planning interventions. It requires insight and skill to recognize when a woman's problem requires interventions that are beyond a nurse's preparation and ability. In such situations, appropriate referrals should be made.

Sociocultural Aspects of Menstruation

The consistent and somewhat mysterious recurrence of menstruation over the millennia has engendered menstrual belief systems that remain with us and become the social reality. Cultural, religious, and personal attitudes about menstruation are part of the menstrual experience and, unfortunately, often reflect negative attitudes toward women.

CRITICAL THINKING

How have you been influenced by attitudes and customs about menstruation? How is menstruation a part of your life now?

Some cultures have isolated women entirely (in menstrual huts, for example), or restricted them to the company of other women during menstruation because they believed that menstrual blood was "unclean" and dangerous. Some beliefs emanating from this myth are that menstruating women have the ability to harm growing crops, wither flowers, and cause bread not to rise. A common belief is that menstruating women are able to contaminate their husbands, so sexual intercourse is contraindicated (see Leviticus 15 and the Talmud). Menstruating women have been accused of having supernatural powers (because of the association of bleeding with death)—sometimes good but more often destructive.

Although many of these myths have disappeared, there is a tendency to regard the menstruating woman as vulnerable or less capable. Current customs include refraining from exercise, showers, and sexual intercourse and hiding the fact of menstruation entirely.

Some people have used these myths to deny jobs to women and treat them as inferior. The belief that women lose a lot of time from work is largely unsupported.

Women still work where they are needed at home, in factories, or in offices with no concessions in schedules or routines to take account of individual differences in cycles. It is interesting to note that men, who are more prone to incapacitating and unpredictable diseases such as heart problems, are encouraged to continue in highly responsible positions. The theme that women are less capable and vulnerable is constantly evolving into new applications. For example, lawyers in Britain and the United States used the premenstrual syndrome for a mental incompetence alibi (Tybor 1982). In post–World War II Japan, the legislative body passed laws allowing for a "menstrual leave" for the supposed incapacity of women at this time (Dan 1983). Orthodox Judaism still prescribes the ritual bath (mikvah) following menstruation (Siegel 1983), and fear of contamination occurs in other societies as well.

Fortunately the 1990s have afforded a more enlightened view of menstruating women in the United States. As they have appeared in increasing numbers in the work force, women have shown their competence in a male-dominated world. Women have worked hard to gain equal treatment and should make every effort to avoid using their menstrual cycle as a reason to avoid work or responsibility.

Male Attitudes and Sexual Activity

Most women have been socialized to refrain from discussing menstruation with men. In a survey of midwestern preteen girls, 85% expressed the belief that menstruation should not be discussed with boys, although 59% felt it was all right to discuss it with their fathers (Williams 1983). This cultural taboo is usually supported by the tendency to separate into gender groups for school discussions of growth and development.

Cultural taboos against coitus during menses are of long duration, but the health reasons for such taboos have been found to be invalid. Nurses discussing this area with clients may want to confirm that sexual activity during menses is common practice and is not contraindicated; however, not all couples desire it.

Many men, even male physicians, lack information about menstruation. It is important to be open and tell both daughters and sons about the many changes of the life cycle so that they can be comfortable and open about these changes and maturational processes.

The Role of the Nurse in Menstrual Counseling

Girls today begin to learn about puberty and menstruation at a surprisingly young age. Unfortunately the source of their "information" is sometimes their peers, and thus the information may be incomplete, inaccurate, and sensationalized. Nurses who work with young girls and adoles-

cents recognize this and are working hard to provide accurate health teaching and to correct misinformation about **menarche** (the onset of menses) and the menstrual cycle.

Assisting the Woman to Understand Her Menstrual Experience

The nurse provides information about what is normal and expected. Some of the objective data needed to assess individual women and determine normalcy include:

- *Length of the average cycle.* Early in a female's menstrual life, the median cycle length is 29 days; this will decrease slightly to a median of 25+ days prior to menopause. Cycle length that varies from 21 to 35 days is considered normal. Cycle length is calculated by counting the number of days from the onset of one menses to the onset of the next menses. There is a wide variation among women.

- *Individual variability.* The typical month-to-month variation in an individual's cycle is plus or minus two days, although greater normal variations are frequently noted. No woman's cycle is exactly the same length every month.

- *Amount of flow.* The average flow is approximately 30 mL in a period; users of IUDs will usually have double this amount. The average woman can characterize the amount of flow by the number of pads or tampons used. Increase or decrease in the number of pads or tampons used is a good subjective indicator of changes in menstrual flow.

- *Length of menses.* The length of the menses is usually from two to eight days. Here again, there is wide variability. The number of days is another indicator of amount of flow.

Information of a subjective nature may be elicited by general questions such as, "How do you feel?" "Has there been any change?" "Do you have any problems with your menstrual period?" Skilled interviewing will yield information about the social, environmental, and biophysical impacts of the individual's menstrual cycle.

Promotion of Successful Adaptation to Menarche

Many young women find it embarrassing or stressful to discuss the menstrual experience, both because of the many taboos associated with the subject and because of their immaturity. The young woman who matures earlier than her peers is especially likely to be at a disadvantage; because the event has not been expected to occur so soon, she is less likely to have an adequate knowledge base for coping with her experience. A girl 10 or 11 years of age is also limited by her cognitive immaturity; the "magical thinking" typical of her developmental stage may lead to such thoughts as "everyone will know I have my period."

The most critical factor in successful adaptation to menarche is the adolescent's level of preparedness. Rierdan (1983) reported a direct relationship between adequacy of preparation and the degree to which the menarcheal experience is positive. The nurse should make it clear that, within limits, variations in age at menarche, length of cycle, and duration of menses are normal because girls are likely to become concerned if they are not "on time" as compared with their peers. Rierdan (1983) also reported that it is helpful to acknowledge the negative aspects of menstruation (messiness, embarrassment), as well as its positive role as a symbol of maturity and womanhood.

The menarcheal client encountered by a nurse may be his or her own daughter, a hospitalized adolescent, a camper or student, or the client of a community health program. School nurses, especially, relate both to young women and their parents as part of planning for health and family life education curricula. Nursing assessment should address the stage of physical development, the client's need for information, and the needs of parents.

Education About Comfort Measures and Issues During Menstruation

 Menstrual fluid contains blood; cervical mucus; vaginal secretions, mucus, and cells; and degenerated endometrial particles. It is important to remember that this fluid usually does not smell until it makes contact with bacteria on the skin or in the air.

Tampons and Pads
Women in different cultures have handled their menstrual flow in many ways. Since early times, women have made tampons and pads from cloths or rags, which required washing but were reusable. Some women made them from gauze or cotton balls. Commercial tampons were introduced in the 1930s.

Today's adhesive stripped mini- and maxipads and flushable tampons have made life easier. Unfortunately, in their zeal to perfect a comfortable, convenient, leak- and odorproof product, manufacturers have added deodorants to both sanitary napkins and tampons and have increased their absorbency. (Consider why women need to deodorize internally if odor occurs only when the flow comes in contact with the air.)

Both these "improvements" may prove harmful. The chemical used to deodorize can create a rash on the vulva and can do worse damage to the tender mucous lining of the vagina itself. Excessive or inappropriate use of superabsorbent tampons can produce dryness and even small sores or ulcers in the vagina.

Superabsorbent tampons are to be used only for exceptionally heavy menstrual flow, not during the whole period. In the absence of a heavy menstrual flow, these tampons will absorb all moisture, leaving the vaginal walls dry and subject to injury. The absorbency of even regular tampons can vary. If the tampon is hard to pull out or shreds when removed or if the vagina becomes dry, the tampon is probably too absorbent. If a woman is worried about accidental spotting, she should check the diagrams on the packages of regular tampons. Those that expand in width are better able to prevent leakage without being too absorbent.

A woman may want to use tampons only during the day and switch to pads at night to avoid vaginal irritation. Tampons should be avoided on the last spotty days of the period. If a woman experiences vaginal irritation, itching, soreness, unusual odor, or bleeding while using tampons, she should stop using them or change brands or absorbencies to see if that helps.

There has been a question about the link between toxic shock syndrome (TSS) and tampon use. It is postulated that small vaginal ulcers or sores may allow or be the route by which harmful bacteria enter the bloodstream, causing TSS. Warning signs of TSS include the following:

- Fever (temperature of 101F or more)
- Diarrhea
- Vomiting
- Muscle aches
- Sunburn–like rash

A woman should be advised to seek *immediate* medical attention if these symptoms occur during a menstrual cycle, while wearing a diaphragm, or when using a contraceptive sponge.

The choice of sanitary protection must meet the individual's needs, and she should feel comfortable using it whether it be pads or tampons.

Vaginal Sprays and Douches
Another comfort issue is the use of douches and vaginal sprays. Many women have been led to believe that regular douching is as fundamental as a morning shower and that use of hygiene spray deodorant is as essential as use of underarm deodorant. In fact these douches and deodorants are not only unnecessary, but they also can be harmful. Vaginal sprays can cause infections, itching, burning, irritation, vaginal discharge, rashes, and other problems.

Women should carefully follow the directions for proper use of feminine deodorant sprays. It is recommended that these sprays be used externally only and not be used with sanitary napkins or applied to broken, irritated, or itching skin. The two circumstances in which women may be most concerned with vaginal odor are during menstruation and during intercourse, and these are times when use of feminine deodorant sprays is clearly contraindicated.

Douching is unnecessary since the vagina cleanses itself; simply wiping the vaginal lips is sufficient for cleanliness. Douching washes away the natural mucus and upsets the vaginal ecology, which can make the vagina more susceptible to infection. Douching with one of the perfumed or flavored douches can cause allergic reactions, and too frequent use of an undiluted or strong douche solution can induce severe irritation and even tissue damage. Propelling water up the vagina may also erode the antibacterial cervical plug and force bacteria and germs from the vagina into the uterus. Women should not douche during menstruation because the cervix is slightly dilated to permit the downward flow of menstrual flow from the uterine lining. It may be easier to introduce infection at this time, resulting in endometritis.

Women need to remember that there is nothing offensive about a healthy vagina. The mucous secretions that continually bathe the vagina are completely odor-free while they are in the vagina; only when they mingle with perspiration and hit the air does odor develop. Keeping one's skin clean and free of bacteria with plain soap and water is the most effective method of controlling odor. A soapy finger should be used to wash gently betwen the vulvar folds. Bathing is as important (if not more so) during the menstrual period as at any other time. There is no evidence that bathing will bring on cramps or interrupt blood flow. On the contrary, a long leisurely soak in a warm tub will promote menstrual blood flow and relieve cramps by relaxing the muscles.

Keeping the vaginal area fresh throughout the day means keeping it dry and clean. After bathing or showering and patting herself dry a woman should wear cotton panties. She should make sure that her clothes are loose enough to permit the vaginal area to breathe. After using the toilet, a woman should always wipe herself from front to back and if necessary, follow up with a moistened paper towel or toilet paper.

The most important thing to remember is that if an unusual odor persists despite these efforts, it may be a sign that something is awry. Certain conditions such as vaginitis produce a foul-smelling discharge.

Relief of Discomfort

Cramping and general discomfort may be alleviated by instituting certain nutritional practices, exercise, and use of heat and massage.

Nutritional self-care The B-complex vitamins, especially vitamin B_6, play a role in neutralizing the excessive amounts of estrogen produced by the ovaries during the course of a normal menstrual cycle and therefore may prevent against the bloating and irritability that sometimes occurs premenstrually. Vitamin E, a mild prostaglandin inhibitor, may help decrease menstrual discomfort. Vitamin E is also able to improve circulation, which reduces muscular spasms and pain by reducing the uterus's need for oxygen. Supplements may be taken, but these vitamins are also available in a well-balanced diet. Women should avoid salt because it can contribute to fluid retention.

Exercise Exercise, if performed daily, can relieve existing discomfort and help prevent menstrual cramps and associated complaints. It relieves constipation by increasing intestinal activity and curbs bloating by increasing perspiration. The deep breathing required during exercise brings more oxygen to the blood, which relaxes the uterus and helps ease discomfort. Exercise helps alleviate anxiety and tension. Helpful exercises include jogging, swimming, fast-paced walking, or bicycling. Menstrual relaxation exercises may also be beneficial.

Heat and Massage Heat is soothing and promotes increased blood flow. Any type of warmth, from sipping herbal tea to soaking in a hot tub or using a heating pad may be helpful during painful periods. Massage can also soothe aching back muscles and promote relaxation and blood flow.

Associated Menstrual Conditions

Premenstrual Syndrome

Premenstrual syndrome (PMS) refers to a symptom complex associated with menses. The symptoms must, by definition, occur between the time of ovulation and the onset of menses. They are repetitive in each menstrual cycle during the same time frame.

The exact cause of PMS is unknown, but a multitude of theories have been postulated to explain it. These range from hormone imbalance to nutritional deficiency and include prostaglandin deficiency, prostaglandin excess, vitamin B_6 deficiency, and endorphin deficiency. A great deal of research is currently being done on PMS, and it is likely that our understanding of the condition will increase in the future.

Women over age 30 are more likely to develop PMS than those under 30. It has been estimated that 30% to 50% of ovulating women have some of the following symptoms (Parisier et al 1985):

- *Psychologic*—irritability, lethargy, depression, low morale, anxiety, sleep disorders, crying spells, and hostility
- *Neurologic*—classic migraine, vertigo, syncope
- *Respiratory*—nasal congestion, hoarseness, asthma
- *Gastrointestinal*—nausea, vomiting, constipation, abdominal bloating, diarrhea, craving for sweets
- *Urinary*—retention and oliguria
- *Dermatologic*—acne
- *Mammary*—swelling and tenderness

Most women experience only some of these symptoms. The most disconcerting symptoms, and the ones that most women seek treatment for, are the psychologic ones. The symptoms usually are most pronounced two or three days before the onset of menstruation (although they may be present for up to two weeks before the onset of menstruation) and subside as menstrual flow begins, with or without treatment.

Nursing Care

The nurse can help the woman to identify specific symptoms and to develop healthy behavior. After assessment, counseling for PMS may include restriction of foods containing methylxanthines (eg, chocolate and coffee), fat, salt, and sugar; increased intake of complex carbohydrates and protein; and increased frequency of meals. Supplementation with B complex vitamins, especially B_6, may reduce anxiety and depression. A dose of 25 to 50 mg twice daily is recommended. Megadoses should be avoided because of B_6 toxicity (Stewart 1987). Vitamin E supplementation may reduce breast tenderness, and a program of aerobic exercises such as fast walking, jogging, and aerobic dancing is suggested.

Pharmacologic treatments for PMS have varied greatly. The more widely known remedies include progesterone suppositories, diuretics, prostaglandin inhibitors, and vitamin supplements. All have been effective in some women and not in others. Alprazolam (Xanax), a potent tranquilizer, is somewhat effective in reducing symptoms of PMS. However, the risk of using an addictive drug must be carefully weighed against the benefits (Smith et al 1987).

An empathetic relationship with a health care professional to whom the woman feels free to voice her concerns is highly beneficial. Encouragement to keep a diary may help the woman identify life events associated with PMS. Self-care groups and self-help literature may help women gain control over their bodies. Group members share helpful therapies including nutrition information and exercise and relaxation techniques. Biofeedback techniques can be learned and used to treat specific symptoms such as headache. Nurses can assist women who feel the negative aspects of the PMS publicity that focuses on labeling menstruating women as ill and not having control over their bodies. Support groups also assist in reducing the stress women may feel.

Dysmenorrhea

Dysmenorrhea, or painful menses, usually occurs a day or two prior to the onset of menstruation and subsides by the end of menses. Sloane (1985) reported that 90% of women experience some pain with menses, and 50% to 60% require analgesia some of the time. Cramps may be accompanied by headache, dizziness, backache, leg pain, nausea, vomiting, or diarrhea. Typically, a young girl's menstrual cycle is irregular and painless until regular ovulation is established. At that time, dysmenorrhea may occur in a cyclic fashion until a woman reaches her late 20s or until after a full-term pregnancy, when menstrual cramps often subside.

Primary dysmenorrhea is defined as cramps without underlying disease. Prostaglandin hormones (F_2 and $F_{2\alpha}$), which are produced by the uterus in higher concentrations during menstruation, are the cause of primary dysmenorrhea. Prostaglandins increase uterine contractions and decrease uterine artery blood flow, causing ischemia. The end result is the painful sensation of cramps.

Secondary dysmenorrhea is associated with an underlying pathologic condition of the reproductive tract and usually appears after menstruation has been established. Conditions that most frequently cause secondary dysmenorrhea include endometriosis, pelvic inflammatory disease, anatomic anomalies such as cervical stenosis, imperforate hymen, uterine displacement, ovarian cysts, and the presence of an IUD. Because primary and secondary dysmenorrhea may coexist, accurate differential diagnosis is essential for appropriate treatment.

Effective treatment for primary dysmenorrhea includes prostaglandin inhibitors and oral contraceptives. Prostaglandin inhibitors work by reducing the amount of local uterine release of prostaglandins, thereby reducing cramping. Oral contraceptives work primarily by blocking ovulation. A variety of prostaglandin inhibitors are available. These include aspirin, ibuprofen, mefenamic acid, and naproxen. Some are over-the-counter medications and others require a prescription. Oral contraceptives, too, are numerous, and a physical examination of the client is required before they can be prescribed. Women should consult their health care provider for advice about the best therapy for them.

Nursing Care

The nurse can assist women by becoming informed about self-care measures for dysmenorrhea. Self-care measures include starting an exercise program; using the pelvic rock exercise, which can decrease the pain; using heat in the form of baths, showers, or heating pads to relieve discomfort by increasing blood flow and decreasing muscle spasm; and getting more rest during menstruation. Hot drinks such as soups or spiced or herbal teas are soothing and relaxing and can help break the pain-tension cycle. Good nutrition can also promote a sense of well-being.

Biofeedback has been used against dysmenorrhea with some success (Heczy 1980; Balick et al 1982). Clients using biofeedback techniques perceived some control over their bodies and also appeared more relaxed.

Menstrual Cycle Variations

Amenorrhea, the absence of menses, is classified as primary or secondary. *Primary amenorrhea* is said to occur if menstruation has not been established by age 18 years. *Secondary amenorrhea* is said to occur when an established menses (of longer than three months) ceases. Any of the functional causes of delayed menarche may also cause secondary amenorrhea.

Primary amenorrhea necessitates a thorough assessment of the young woman to determine its cause. Identified causes include congenital obstructions, congenital absence of the uterus, testicular feminization, or absence or imbalance of hormones. Successful treatment is determined by causative factors. Many causes are not correctable, and infertility will result.

Secondary amenorrhea is caused most frequently by pregnancy. Aditional causes include lactation, hormonal imbalances, poor nutrition (anorexia nervosa, obesity, fad dieting), ovarian lesions, strenuous exercise (associated with long-distance runners with low body fat ratios), debilitating systemic diseases, stress of high intensity and/or long duration, stressful life events, a change in season or climate, use of oral contraceptives, the phenothiazine and chlorpromazine group of tranquilizers, and syndromes such as Cushing and Sheehan. Treatment is dictated by causative factors (Griffith-Kenney 1986). If the cause is related to such conditions the nurse can explain that once the underlying condition has been corrected—for example, when sufficient body weight is gained—menses will resume. Female athletes and women who participate in strenuous exercise routines may be advised to increase their caloric intake or reduce their exercise levels for a month or two to see whether a normal cycle ensues. If it does not, medical referral is indicated.

An abnormally short menstrual cycle is termed *hypomenorrhea*; an abnormally long one is called *hypermenorrhea*. Excessive, profuse flow is called *menorrhagia*, and bleeding between periods is known as *metrorrhagia*. Infrequent and too frequent menses are termed *oligomenorrhea* and *polymenorrhea*, respectively. Such irregularities should be investigated to rule out any disease process.

Anovulatory Cycle

An anovulatory cycle is a cycle in which ovulation does not occur, even though the woman is not taking oral contraceptives. These cycles are noted for their irregularity, the absence of any symptoms of menstrual distress, and (often) heavy bleeding (Charpentier 1983). In cases of this kind, estrogen excess results in the proliferation of endometrial growth because the secretory changes stimulated by progesterone fail to occur.

In women taking oral contraceptives, however, an ovulation-suppressed cycle occurs. Although administration of the birth control pill is interrupted each month so that cyclic withdrawal bleeding can occur, these episodes of bleeding are unlike normal menses in some respects.

Preconception Counseling

Pregnancy is often unplanned and unexpected. It may be the result of a contraceptive failure or a decision by the woman and her partner not to use any method of fertility control. For many women this decision is made for religious or philosophic reasons; some women get caught up in a romantic sexual encounter that they failed to anticipate and have no method of contraception available; and some women have unprotected intercourse because they are the victims of sexual assault.

Not all people wish to become parents. Society still puts pressure on couples to have children. Couples who choose to remain childless are often labeled "selfish" and "short-sighted." Despite the pressure, more couples are beginning to speak up for the right of choice.

Thus one of the first questions a couple should ask prior to conception is whether they wish to have children. This involves consideration of each person's personal goals, expectations of their relationship, and desire to be a parent. Often one individual wishes to have a child while the other does not. In such situations open discussion is essential to reach a mutually acceptable decision. In some cases this may require marital counseling.

Couples who wish to have children face a decision about the timing of pregnancy. At what point in their lives do they believe it would be best to become parents? Pregnancy comes as a surprise even when the decision about timing is made, but at least the couple has some control over it.

For couples who have religious beliefs that do not support contraception or who feel that fertility planning is unnatural and wrong, issues of timing of pregnancy are unacceptable and irrelevant. These couples can still take steps to ensure that they are in the best possible physical and mental health when pregnancy occurs.

Preconception Health Measures

If a couple has decided to have a child or if the couple does not find planning acceptable, they may make an effort to maximize the quality of their health. This effort should include making life-style changes to avoid known or potential health risks such as alcohol.

Because there is no definite safe level for alcohol consumption during pregnancy, and because the woman is often pregnant before she realizes it, a woman planning to become pregnant should be advised to stop drinking totally if possible. Because the effects on the embryo of heavy drinking by the father are not as well understood, less emphasis has been placed on male drinking. However, studies suggest that heavy alcohol consumption may decrease a man's fertility. Furthermore, his partner may find it more difficult to avoid alcohol if the man continues to drink. Thus it is helpful if the man, too, restricts his alcohol intake.

Smoking has been linked to increased miscarriage risk, placental abruption, preterm labor, and intrauterine growth retardation in the fetus. The woman is advised to cease smoking if possible or at least limit her intake to less than half a pack a day. Because exposure to cigarette smoke from another smoker also poses a risk and because of the

Contemporary Issue
Sex Selection: Possible? Yes. But Ethical?

For couples who strongly desire a child of a certain sex, the possibility of sex selection holds tremendous appeal. Earlier theories, such as Dr Landrum B Shettles belief that sex could be determined by controlling the time within a woman's cycle when conception occurred, were controversial and not always successful.

Recently Ronald Ericsson developed a procedure for sperm separation, which is marketed by Gametrics. The technique uses a filtering process based on the superior swimming ability of sperm bearing the Y chromosome. The filtration process eliminates the slower-swimming X sperm, leaving a solution that is composed of about 80% Y sperm. If a couple strongly desires a boy, the man obtains a specimen of his semen near the time when the woman ovulates. The specimen undergoes the filtration process and is artificially inseminated into the woman at the time of ovulation. Another process is being developed for isolating X sperm.

For couples unable to afford the Gametrics procedure, a home fertility lab kit is now available for determining sex. The kit is based on the Billings method of timing ovulation and the work of Dr Shettles; its success rate is not yet clear.

Proponents suggest that the process offers choice for couples and will improve family relationships because a child of the desired sex will be especially cherished.

Opponents believe that the process is unnatural and demeaning to babies. They suggest that in a male-dominated world with its recognized preference for boy children, the process is another indication of a deep-seated, if unconscious, prejudice against women.

The availability of this technique raises several difficult questions:

- If the process becomes widespread, will the balance of world population shift to males?

- Will the availability of the process strengthen and foster negative attitudes about women?

- Will religious groups view the technique as another form of unnatural technology and speak out against it? (The Catholic Church has already spoken out against the process of artificial insemination, which forms part of this procedure.)

- What will be the impact on a child born following the procedure if he or she is not the desired sex?

- Is the next step amniocentesis or chorionic villus sampling (CVS) to confirm the sex, followed by abortion if the fetus is not the desired sex? (Currently most medical facilities refuse to do amniocentesis or CVS solely for sex selection, except in cases of serious sex-linked disorders such as hemophilia.)

---

difficulty most people have in stopping smoking, it is especially helpful if the man doesn't smoke either.

The effects of caffeine are less clearly understood. Because it poses a potential risk, women are advised to stop drinking beverages containing caffeine completely if possible, or at least limit them to two drinks per day. In addition to coffee, tea, colas, and chocolate, caffeine is found in medications such as Excedrin, Anacin, fiorinal and many appetite suppressants.

Many of the social (cocaine, marijuana, LSD) and street (heroin, crack, etc) drugs pose a real threat to a fetus. Prescription drugs can also be hazardous. A woman who uses any drugs or medications should discuss the implications of their use with her health care provider. In most cases it is best to avoid the use of medication whenever possible.

Certain jobs result in exposure to agents that can reduce a man's or woman's fertility or that might cause harm to the fetus if the woman becomes pregnant. This is especially true of exposure to radiation, photographic chemi-

cals, and anesthetic agents. When a couple is contemplating pregnancy, they should carefully consider whether they are exposed to any environmental hazards at work or in their community.

Physical Examination

It is advisable for both partners to have a physical examination to identify any health problems so that they can be corrected if possible. These might include medical conditions such as high blood pressure or obesity; problems that pose a threat to fertility, such as certain sexually transmitted diseases; or conditions that keep the individual from achieving optimal health, such as anemia or colitis. If the family history indicates previous genetic disorders or if the couple is planning pregnancy when the woman is over age 35, the health care provider may suggest that the couple consider genetic counseling (see Chapter 5 for further discussion). In addition to the history and physical exam, the woman should have the following laboratory tests: urinalysis, complete blood count, Rh factor, VDRL, Pap smear, gonorrhea culture, rubella and hepatitis screens (Rosen 1990).

Prior to conception the woman is also advised to have a dental examination and any necessary dental work to avoid exposure to x-rays and the risk of infection.

Nutrition

Prior to conception it is advisable for the woman to be at a suitable weight for her body build and height. She should follow a nutritious diet that contains ample quantities of all the essential nutrients. Some nutritionists advocate emphasizing the following nutrients: calcium, protein, iron, B complex vitamins, vitamin C, folic acid, and magnesium. Excessive vitamin intake can cause severe fetal problems and should be avoided.

Exercise

A woman is advised to establish a regular exercise plan beginning at least three months before she plans to attempt to become pregnant. The exercise chosen should be one she enjoys and will continue. It should provide some aerobic conditioning and some general toning. Exercise improves the woman's circulation and general health and tones her muscles. Once an exercise program is well-established, the woman is generally encouraged to continue it during pregnancy. For a discussion of exercise during pregnancy see p 363.

Contraception

Women who wish to conceive and who take birth control pills are advised to stop the pill and have two or three normal menses before attempting pregnancy. This allows the natural hormonal cycle to return and facilitates dating the subsequent pregnancy. Women using an intrauterine device are advised to have it removed and wait one month before attempting to conceive. This allows the endometrium to be resterilized. During the waiting period, barrier methods of contraception (condoms, diaphragm, cervical cap, sponge, and spermicides) are recommended.

Conception

Most preconception recommendations focus on helping the couple attain their best possible health state so that they do not enter pregnancy with unnecessary risks. Conception is a personal and emotional experience, and even if a couple is prepared they may feel some ambivalence. This is a normal response, but they may require reassurance that the ambivalence will pass. A couple may get so caught up in preparation and in their efforts to "do things right" that they lose sight of the pleasure they derive from each other

and their lives together and cease to value the joy of spontaneity in their relationship. It is often helpful for the health care provider to remind an overly zealous couple that moderation is always appropriate and that there is value in taking "time to smell the roses."

Contraceptive Methods

A couple's decision to use a method of contraception is often motivated by a desire to gain control over the number of children they will conceive and/or to determine the spacing of future children. In choosing a specific method, consistency of use outweighs the absolute reliability of a given method. Other factors to be considered are the side effects and contraindications for use of a particular contraceptive method.

The nurse often assists the couple in selecting a contraceptive method. To be able to suggest a method that has practical application and is compatible with the couple's health and physical needs, the nurse must assess the couple to gather relevant data. The woman's past medical, surgical, menstrual, and obstetric history, including former contraceptive use, should be reviewed. The history should include immediate family incidences of diabetes, bleeding or clotting problems, heart problems or high blood pressure, migraine headaches or seizure disorders, kidney or liver disease, anemia, tuberculosis, stroke, cancer, or mental problems. This information provides a baseline of risk factors that could influence or contraindicate the prescription of oral contraceptives.

A precontraception physical examination should include, at a minimum, thyroid, breast, and pelvic examinations. Weight, age, and blood pressure can indicate risk factors that may preclude prescribing certain forms of birth control. Minimal laboratory testing includes a hemoglobin/ hematocrit analysis; dipstick urine for sugar and protein; Pap smear; endocervical culture for *Neisseria gonorrhoeae* and chlamydia; serologic test for syphilis; and any other test identified during the history or physical exam as being appropriate.

The couple's decisions about contraception should be made voluntarily, with full knowledge of options, advantages, disadvantages, effectiveness, side effects, and long-range effects; with access to alternatives; without pressure by health professionals; and with the strictest confidentiality. Many outside factors influence a couple's choice, including cultural influences, religious beliefs, personality, cost, effectiveness, misinformation, practicability of method, and self-esteem. Different methods of contraception may be appropriate at different times in a couple's life.

Following is a review of the major contraceptive methods available, with an examination of their advantages and disadvantages. Table 7–3 identifies first-year failure rates for the various birth control methods.

Table 7–3   Lowest expected, typical, and lowest reported failure rates during the first year of use of a method and first-year continuation rates. United States.*

Method	Percentage of women experiencing an accidental pregnancy in the first year of use			Percentage of women continuing use at one year[4]	
	Lowest expected[1]	Typical[2]	Lowest reported[3]	Exc. preg.	Inc. preg.
Chance[5]	85	85	43.1		
Spermicides[6] (foams, vaginal suppositories)	3	21	0.0	55	43
Periodic abstinence		20		84	67
Calendar	9		14.4[6]		
Ovulation method	3		10.5[6]		
Symptothermal[7]	2		12.6		
Postovulation	1		2.0[6]		
Withdrawal	4	18	6.7[6]		
Cap (with spermicidal cream or jelly)	6	18	8.0	77	63
Sponge					
Parous women	9	28	27.7	73	53
Nulliparous women	6	18	13.9	73	60
Diaphragm (with spermicidal cream or jelly)	6	18	2.1	69	57
Condom (without spermicides)	2	12	4.2	73	64
IUD		3		75	73
Progestasert®	2.0		1.9		
Copper T 380A	0.8		0.5		
Pill		3		75	73
Combination	0.1		0.0		
Progestogen only	0.5		1.1		
Injectable progestogen				70	70
DMPA	0.3	0.3	0.0		
NET	0.4	0.4	0.0		
Implants				90	90
NORPLANT® (6 capsules)	0.04	0.04	0.0		
NORPLANT®-2 (2 rods)	0.03	0.03	0.0		
Female sterilization	0.2	0.4	0.0		
Male sterilization	0.1	0.15	0.0		

*Adapted from Trussell J, et al: Contraceptive failure in the United States: An update. Stud Fam Plann *January/February* 1990; 21:207.

[1]Among couples who initiate use of a method (not necessarily for the first time) and who use it perfectly (both consistently and correctly), an estimate of the percentage expected to experience an accidental pregnancy during the first year if they do not stop use for any other reason.

[2]Among typical couples who initiate use of a method (not necessarily for the first time), the percentage who experience an accidental pregnancy during the first year if they do not stop use for any other reason.

[3]In the literature on contraceptive failure, the lowest reported percentage who experienced an accidental pregnancy during the first year following initiation of use (not necessarily for the first time) if they did not stop use for any other reason. However, see Note 7.

[4]Among couples attempting to avoid pregnancy, the percentage who continue to use a method for one year, under the alternative assumptions that no one becomes pregnant (Exc. Preg.) and that the proportion becoming pregnant is shown under Inc. Preg.

[5]The lowest expected and typical percents are based on data from populations where contraception is not used and from women who cease using contraception in order to become pregnant. These represent an estimate of the percent who would conceive among women now relying on reversible methods of contraception if they abandoned contraception altogether. The lowest reported percent is based on U.S. women who use no contraception even though they do not wish to become pregnant. This group is selected for low fecundity or low coital frequency, and some fraction may use an unreported variant of periodic abstinence.

[6]Too low, because rate is based on more than one year of exposure.

[7]Cervical mucus (ovulation) method supplemented by calendar in the preovulatory and basal body temperature in the postovulatory phases.

Fertility Awareness Methods

Fertility awareness methods, also referred to as natural family planning, are based on an understanding of the changes that occur throughout a woman's ovulatory cycle. All these methods require periods of abstinence and recording of certain events throughout the cycle; hence, cooperation of the partner is important.

Advantages of fertility awareness methods include the following: the methods are free, safe, acceptable to many whose religious beliefs prohibit other methods, provide an increased awareness of the body, involve no artificial substances or devices, encourage a couple to communicate about sexual activity and family planning, and are also useful in helping a couple plan a pregnancy.

Disadvantages include the following: they require extensive initial counseling to use effectively; they may interfere with sexual spontaneity; they require extensive maintenance of records for several cycles prior to beginning to use them; they may be difficult or impossible for women with irregular cycles to use; and, although theoretically they should be very reliable, in actual practice they may not be as reliable in preventing pregnancy as other methods.

The *basal body temperature (BBT) method* to detect ovulation requires that a woman take her BBT every morning upon awakening (before any activity such as drinking, smoking, or going to the bathroom) and record the readings on a temperature graph. After three to four months of recording temperatures, the woman with regular cycles should be able to predict when ovulation will occur. The method is based on the fact that the temperature sometimes drops just prior to ovulation and almost always rises and remains elevated for several days after. The temperature rise occurs in response to the increased progesterone levels that occur in the second half of the cycle. Figure 7–2 shows a sample BBT chart. To avoid conception, intercourse is avoided on the day of the temperature rise and for three days after. Because the temperature rise does not occur until after ovulation, a woman who had intercourse just prior to the rise is at risk of pregnancy. To decrease this risk, some couples abstain from intercourse for several days before the *anticipated* time of ovulation and then for three days after.

The *calendar method*, also referred to as the rhythm method, is based on the assumptions that ovulation tends to occur 14 days (plus or minus two days) before the start of the next menstrual period, sperm are viable for 48 to 72 hours, and the ovum is viable for 24 hours (Hatcher et al 1988). To use this method the woman must record her menstrual cycles for six to eight months, so that the shortest and longest cycles can be identified. The first day of menstruation is the first day of the cycle. The fertile phase is calculated from 18 days before the end of the shortest recorded cycle through 11 days from the end of the longest recorded cycle (Hatcher et al 1988). For example, if a woman's cycle lasts from 24 to 28 days, the fertile phase would be calculated as day 6 through day 17. Once this information is obtained, the woman can identify the fertile and infertile phases of her cycle. For effective use of this method, she must abstain from intercourse during the fertile phase.

The calendar method is the least reliable of the fertility awareness methods and has largely been replaced by the other, more scientific approaches.

The *cervical mucus method*, sometimes called the *ovulation method* or the *Billings method*, involves the assessment of cervical mucus changes that occur during the menstrual cycle. The amount and character of cervical mucus change as a result of the influence of estrogen and progesterone on the mucous secretory glands present in the cervix.

At ovulation, estrogen-dominant mucus is greatest in amount and stretchability. The woman notices a feeling of wetness around the vagina. This mucus shows a ferning pattern that becomes apparent when the mucus is placed on a glass slide and allowed to dry (see Figure 5-4). The stretchability (spinnbarkheit) of the cervical mucus is greatest at the time of ovulation and may vary from 5 to 20

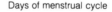

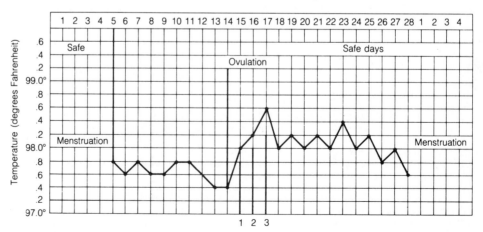

Figure 7–2   Sample basal body temperature chart. (Reprinted with permission from Crooks R, Baur K: Our Sexuality, 4th ed. Redwood City, CA: Benjamin/Cummings, 1990, p 387.)

cm. This type of mucus allows increased permeability to sperm.

During the luteal phase, the characteristics of the cervical mucus change. Progesterone-dominant mucus becomes thick and sticky and forms a network in the cervical canal that traps the sperm and makes their passage more difficult.

To use the ovulation method, the woman should abstain from intercourse for the first menstrual cycle. Cervical mucus should be assessed on a daily basis for the woman to become more familiar with varying characteristics. After a pattern has been established, abstinence from intercourse is necessary when estrogen-dominant mucus predominates and for four days following ovulation.

The *symptothermal method* consists of various assessments that are made and recorded by the couple. They use a chart to record information regarding cycle days, coitus, cervical mucus changes, and secondary signs such as increased libido, abdominal bloating, mittelschmerz, and basal body temperature. Through the various assessments, the couple learns to recognize signs that indicate ovulation. This combined approach tends to improve the effectiveness of fertility awareness contraception methods.

Coitus interruptus, or the withdrawal method of birth control, allows couples to have sexual intercourse until ejaculation is imminent. At that time the man withdraws his penis and ejaculates completely away from the external genitalia of his female partner. The method is available in any situation and requires no medication or devices. However, because of its high failure rate, it is not recommended. The failure rate among typical couples is 18% (Hatcher et al 1989).

Failure tends to occur for two reasons: First, this method demands great self-control on the part of the man, who must withdraw just as he feels the urge for deeper penetration with impending orgasm. Second, some preejaculatory fluid, which can contain sperm, may escape from the penis during the excitement phase prior to ejaculation. Because the quantity of sperm in this preejaculatory fluid is increased after a recent ejaculation, this is especially significant for couples who engage in repeated episodes of orgasm within a short period of time.

Abstinence can also be considered a situational contraceptive and, because of changing values and the increased risk of infection with intercourse, is gaining increased acceptance as a viable alternative to intercourse.

Douching after intercourse is an ineffective method of contraception and is not recommended. It may actually facilitate conception by pushing the sperm farther up the birth canal. Furthermore, sperm have been identified in the fallopian tubes as soon as 90 seconds after ejaculation.

Mechanical Contraceptives

Mechanical contraceptive methods act either as barriers preventing the transport of sperm to the ovum or by preventing implantation of the ovum/zygote.

Condom

Condoms are an effective means of contraception when used consistently and properly (Figure 7–3). Acceptance has been increasing, as a growing number of men are assuming responsibility for regulation of fertility. Another reason for the increased use of condoms is the protection they afford against some sexually transmitted infections, especially AIDS. Condoms are applied to the erect penis,

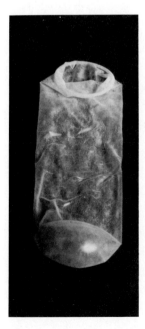

A

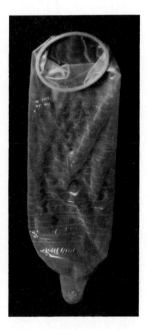

B

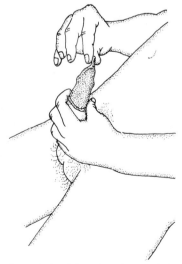

The end of a plain-end condom needs to be twisted as it is rolled onto the penis in order to leave space at the tip.

C

Figure 7–3 Condoms: A Unrolled condom with plain end. B Unrolled condom with reservoir tip. C Correct use of a plain-end condom. (© William Thompson; condoms courtesy of Planned Parenthood Association, San Mateo County, CA)

rolled from the tip to the end of the shaft, before vulvar or vaginal contact is made. A small space must be left at the end of the condom to allow for collection of the ejaculate so that the condom will not break at the time of ejaculation. Water-soluble lubricants, such as K-Y Jelly, should be used if the condom and/or vagina are dry to prevent irritation and possible condom breakage. For optimum effectiveness, the penis should be withdrawn from the vagina while still erect and the condom rim held to prevent spillage. If after ejaculation the penis becomes flaccid while still in the vagina, the male should hold onto the edge of the condom while withdrawing from the vagina to avoid spilling the semen and to prevent the condom from slipping off. The effectiveness of condoms is largely determined by their use. The condom is small, lightweight, disposable, and inexpensive; has no side effects; requires no medical examination or supervision; offers visual evidence of effectiveness; and protects against some sexually transmitted infections. For women, infection with a sexually transmitted infection increases the risk of pelvic inflammatory disease and resultant infertility. Many women now insist that their sexual partners use condoms, and many women carry condoms with them. In fact, some manufacturers report that women are now buying 40% of all condoms (Connell 1988).

With their increasing popularity comes increased choice. Condoms are now available with ribbed sides or smooth sides, tapered or straight-sided, lubricated or unlubricated, with spermicide and without. Condoms called "skin condoms" made from lamb's intestines are also available and are preferred by some men, especially those who have difficulty tolerating latex. They are not considered effective in preventing the spread of infection. Latex condoms are superior in that regard. Spermicidal condoms or concurrent use of a vaginal spermicide increases overall effectiveness.

Breakage, displacement, possible perineal or vaginal irritation, and dulled sensation are cited as disadvantages of the condom.

Currently a condom for women, the WPC-333, is being tested. This condom sheath fits in the vagina and has two rings: one stabilizes it in the vagina; the other remains outside the vagina. The manufacturer suggests that because the outer ring protects the labia and the base of the penis, it offers more protection from sexually transmitted infections than the male condom (Connell 1988).

Diaphragm

The **diaphragm** (Figure 7–4) is used with spermicidal cream or jelly and offers a good level of protection from conception. The woman must be fitted with a diaphragm

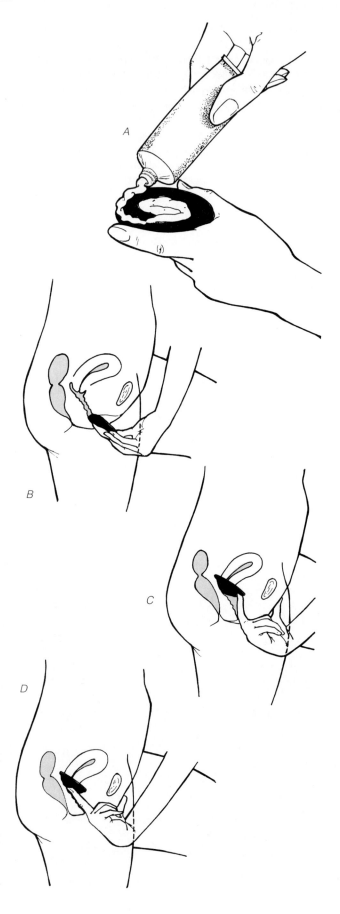

Figure 7–4 A Applying jelly to the rim and center of the diaphragm. B Inserting the diaphragm. C Pushing the rim of the diaphragm under the symphysis pubis. D Checking placement of the diaphragm. Cervix should be felt through the diaphragm.

and instructions given by trained personnel. The diaphragm should be rechecked for correct size after each childbirth and if a woman has gained or lost 15 pounds or more.

The diaphragm must be inserted prior to intercourse, with approximately one teaspoonful (or 1 1/2 inches from the tube) of spermicidal jelly placed around its rim and in the cup. This serves as a chemical barrier to supplement the mechanical barrier of the diaphragm. The diaphragm is inserted through the vagina and covers the cervix. The last step is to push the edge of the diaphragm under the symphysis pubis, which may result in a "popping" sensation. When fitted properly and correctly in place, the diaphragm should not cause discomfort to the woman or her partner. Correct placement of the diaphragm can be checked by touching the cervix with a fingertip through the cup. The cervix feels like a small rounded structure and has a consistency similar to that of the tip of the nose. The center of the diaphragm should be over the cervix. If more than four hours elapse between insertion of the diaphragm and intercourse, additional spermicidal cream should be used. It is necessary to leave the diaphragm in place for at least six to eight hours after coitus. If intercourse is desired again within the six hours, another type of contraception must be used or additional spermicidal jelly placed in the vagina with an applicator, taking care not to disturb the placement of the diaphragm. The diaphragm should be carefully held up to the light periodically and inspected for tears or holes.

Some couples feel that the use of a diaphragm interferes with the spontaneity of intercourse. The nurse can suggest that the partner insert the diaphragm as part of foreplay.

Diaphragms are an excellent contraceptive method for women who are lactating, who cannot or do not wish to use the pill (oral contraceptives), or who wish to avoid the increased risk of pelvic inflammatory disease associated with intrauterine devices. They are also a good choice for older women who smoke but don't wish to be sterilized.

Women who object to manipulating their genitals to insert the diaphragm, check its placement, and remove it may find this method unsatisfactory. It is not recommended for women with a history of urinary tract infection because pressure from the diaphragm on the urethra may interfere with complete bladder emptying and lead to recurrent urinary tract infections (UTIs). Women with a history of toxic shock syndrome should not use diaphragms or any of the barrier methods because they are left in place for prolonged periods. For the same reason the diaphragm should not be used during a menstrual period or if a woman has abnormal vaginal discharge.

Cervical Cap

The **cervical cap** (Figure 7–5) is a cup-shaped device, used with spermicidal cream or jelly, that fits snugly over the cervix and is held in place by suction. Effectiveness rates are similar to those for the diaphragm. Widely used in Europe, it is beginning to gain popularity in the United States. Use of the cervical cap is similar to that of the diaphragm. Unlike the diaphragm, however, the cap may be left in place for up to 48 hours. The cervical cap may be more difficult to fit because of limited size options. It also tends to be more difficult for women to insert and remove (Connell 1988).

Contraceptive Sponge

The **contraceptive sponge**, available without a prescription, is a small pillow-shaped polyurethane sponge with a concave cupped area on one side designed to fit over the

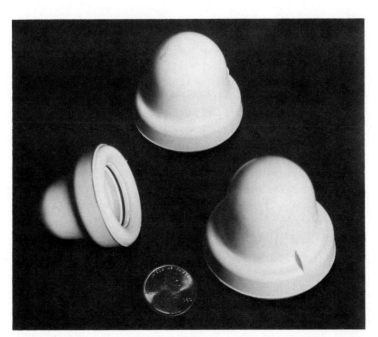

Figure 7–5 Cervical caps (© William Thompson; cervical caps courtesy of Planned Parenthood Association, San Mateo County, CA)

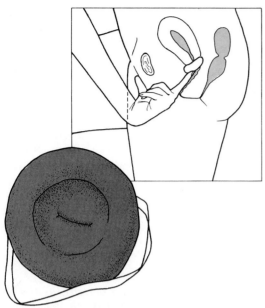

Figure 7–6 *Contraceptive sponge is moistened well with water and inserted into the vagina with concave portion over the cervix.*

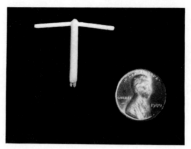

Figure 7–7 *The Progestasert T IUD (© William Thompson; IUD courtesy of Planned Parenthood Association, San Mateo County, CA)*

cervix. The sponge currently available, the Today® Vaginal Contraceptive Sponge, contains spermicide. The sponge is moistened thoroughly with water prior to use and inserted into the vagina so that the cupped area fits snugly over the cervical os (Figure 7–6). This decreases the chances of the sponge being dislodged during intercourse. The sponge may be worn for up to 24 hours. It should be left in place for six hours after intercourse. It is then discarded.

Advantages of the sponge include the following: professional fitting is not required; it may be used for multiple acts of coitus up to 24 hours; one size fits all; and it acts as both barrier and spermicide. Although data are limited, the sponge may provide some protection against chlamydia and gonorrhea. Problems associated with the sponge include difficulty removing the sponge, cost (approximately one dollar and fifty cents per sponge), and irritation or allergic reactions. Some women also report that vaginal dryness is sometimes a problem because the sponge absorbs vaginal secretions. Women with a history of toxic shock syndrome should not use vaginal sponges (Hatcher et al 1988).

Intrauterine Device

An **intrauterine device (IUD)** is designed to be inserted into the uterus and left in place for prolonged periods of time, providing continuous contraceptive protection. IUDs are thought to work by producing an inflammatory reaction in the endometrium and tubes. This, in turn, reduces the chances of fertilization and implantation. Because of numerous lawsuits, major manufacturers have withdrawn their IUDs from the market. Currently two IUDs are available. Both are medicated, containing either copper (Cu38OT—

ParaGard) or progesterone (Progestasert) (Figure 7–7). The Progestasert must be changed every year. The Para-Gard was originally approved by the FDA to be changed every four years; recently, however, it was approved for six years' use (Connell et al 1990).

Advantages of IUDs include high rate of effectiveness, continuous contraceptive protection, no need for coitus-related activity, and relative inexpensiveness over time. The possible adverse effects of IUDs limit their use somewhat. These include pelvic inflammatory disease, severe dysmenorrhea, irregular menses, increased bleeding during menses, uterine perforation, and expulsion. In addition, if the IUD fails and a pregnancy results, there is an increased incidence of ectopic pregnancy (Connell 1990).

IUDs are best suited to women who are multiparous and in a stable monogamous relationship. It is not recommended for women who have multiple sexual partners and are thus at risk for STDs (Tatum 1988).

The IUD is inserted into the uterus with its string or tail protruding through the cervix into the vagina. It may be inserted during a menstrual period or during the four- to six-week postpartum check. After insertion, the woman should be instructed to check for the presence of the string once a week for the first month and then after each menses. She is told that she may have some cramping and/or bleeding intermittently for two to six weeks and that her first few menses may be irregular. Follow-up examination is suggested four to eight weeks after insertion.

Recent advances may make it possible to insert an IUD postpartally immediately after expulsion of the placenta. The IUD is inserted into the uterus and held in place with absorbable chromic catgut suture placed into the myometrium. By the time the suture is absorbed, uterine involution has occurred and good retention of the IUD is possible (Connell 1990).

Oral Contraceptives

The use of hormones, specifically the combination of estrogen and progesterone, is a very successful birth control method. **Oral contraceptives** work by inhibiting the release of an ovum and by maintaining cervical mucus which is inhibitory to the passage of sperm. Numerous oral contraceptives are available. The "pill" is taken daily for 21 days beginning on the Sunday after the first day of the menstrual cycle. In most cases menses will occur one to four days after the last pill is taken. Seven days after completing her last pill, the woman restarts the pill. Thus the woman always begins the pill on the same day. Some companies offer a 28-day pack with seven "blank" pills so that the woman never stops taking a pill. The pill should be taken at approximately the same time each day for optimum effectiveness—usually upon arising or before retiring in the evening.

Although they are highly effective, oral contraceptives may produce side effects ranging from breakthrough bleeding to thrombus formation. Side effects from oral contraceptives may be either progesterone- or estrogen-related (Table 7–4). The use of low-dose (35 μg or less estrogen) preparation has reduced many of the side effects, but the threat of potential risk is sufficient to deter some women from using oral contraceptives.

Another oral contraceptive is the seldom-used progesterone-only pill, also called the *minipill*. It is used primarily by women who have a contraindication to the estrogen component of the combination preparation, such as history of thrombophlebitis, but are strongly motivated toward this form of contraception. The major problems with this preparation are amenorrhea or irregular spotting and bleeding patterns.

Contraindications to the use of oral contraceptives include pregnancy, previous history of thrombophlebitis or thrombolic disease, acute or chronic liver disease of cholestatic type with abnormal function, presence of estrogen-dependent carcinomas, undiagnosed uterine bleeding, heavy smoking, hypertension, diabetes, and hyperlipidemia. In addition, women with the following conditions who use oral contraceptives should be examined every three months: migraine headaches, epilepsy, depression, oligomenorrhea, and amenorrhea. Women who choose this method of contraception should be fully advised of potential side effects.

It is now recognized that oral contraceptives have some important noncontraceptive benefits. Many women experience relief of uncomfortable menstrual symptoms. Cramps are lessened, flow is decreased, and cycle regularity increased. Mittelschmerz is eliminated and the incidence of functional ovarian cysts is decreased. More importantly, there is a substantial reduction in the incidence of ectopic pregnancy, ovarian cancer, endometrial cancer, iron-deficiency anemia, and benign breast disease (Connell et al 1989). In addition, the FDA recently revised the oral contraceptive labeling material to state that for healthy, nonsmoking women over age 40, the benefits of oral contraceptives may outweigh possible risks. The FDA also urged that all women use the lowest-dose pill possible (The Contraception Report 1990).

Spermicides

Spermicides, available as creams, jellies, foam, vaginal film, and suppositories, are inserted into the vagina prior to intercourse. They destroy sperm or neutralize vaginal secretions and thereby immobilize sperm. Spermicides that effervesce in a moist environment offer more rapid protection, and coitus may take place immediately after they are inserted. Suppositories may require up to 30 minutes to dissolve and will *not* offer protection until they do so. The woman should be instructed to insert these spermicide preparations high in the vagina and maintain a supine position.

Spermicides are minimally effective when used alone, but their effectiveness increases in conjunction with a condom. They provide a high degree of protection from exposure to gonorrhea and are also useful against chlamydia, trichomonas, and herpes (Hatcher et al 1988).

The major advantages of spermicides are their wide availability and low toxicity. While some studies have suggested that the use of spermicides at the time of conception or early in pregnancy may be associated with an increased risk of congenital anomalies, recent studies show

---

Table 7–4 Side Effects of Oral Contraceptives

Estrogen component	Progestin component
Altered carbohydrate metabolism	Acne
Altered clotting factors—thrombophlebitis	Amenorrhea
Altered convulsive threshold	Anabolic weight gain
Altered lipid metabolism	Depression and altered libido
Breast tenderness or engorgement	Fatigue
Chloasma	Hirsutism
Edema and cyclic weight gain	Increased appetite
Excessive menstrual flow	Loss of hair
Headache	Oligomenorrhea
Hypertension	Increased low-density lipoprotein (LDL) cholesterol
Irritability, nervousness	Decreased high-density lipoprotein (HDL) cholesterol
Leukorrhea, cervical erosion, or polyposis	
Nausea, bloating	
Venous or capillary engorgement (spider nevi)	

no increased incidence. Researchers suggest that the early studies contained several design flaws, including the problem of recall bias (Brenner & Mishell 1990).

Long-acting Progestin Contraceptives

In 1990, levonorgestrel **subdermal implants** (Norplant) were approved for contraceptive use in the United States. Six silastic capsules containing levonorgestrel, a progestin, are implanted in the woman's arm. They are effective for up to five years (Figure 7–8).

Norplant acts by preventing ovulation in most women. It also stimulates the production of thick cervical mucus, which inhibits sperm penetration (Kaunitz 1990). Norplant provides effective continuous contraception that is removed from the act of coitus. Possible side effects include spotting, irregular bleeding or amenorrhea, an increased incidence of ovarian cysts, weight gain, headaches, acne, hirsutism, and depression (Kaunitz 1990). Women should be advised that the implant may be visible, espe-

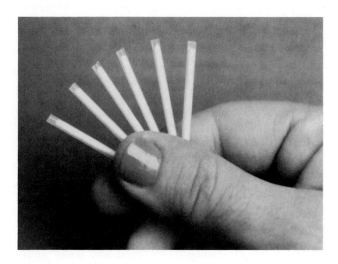

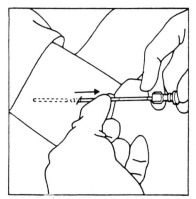

Figure 7–8   Norplant, a long-acting progestin contraceptive, is implanted in a woman's upper arm. (Photo courtesy of Wyeth-Ayerst Laboratories, Philadelphia, PA)

cially in very slender users, and that it requires a minor surgical procedure to insert and remove the implants.

Medroxyprogesterone acetate (Depo-Provera), another long-acting progestin, has not been approved for contraceptive use in the United States. For contraception, a single injection is given every 3 months. Depo-Provera has not been approved because of concerns about an association with breast cancer and possible teratogenicity.

Male Contraception

The vasectomy and the condom are currently the only forms of male contraception available in the United States. Hormonal contraception for men remains a problem although studies are under way.

Future Trends

A wide variety of contraceptive methods are currently being investigated for use in the United States. Many are already available in other countries, but the FDA requires extensive study to determine efficacy and safety prior to marketing in this country.

Potential future methods of contraception for women include progesterone-containing vaginal rings, LH-releasing hormone agonists, RU-486 (a once-a-month oral contraceptive that is a progesterone antagonist), and an antifertility vaccine. For men, research is focusing on glossypol, which interrupts spermatogenesis, and LH-releasing hormone analogues, which disrupt spermatogenesis.

Operative Sterilization

Before sterilization is performed on either partner, a thorough explanation of the procedure should be given to both. Each should understand that sterilization is not a decision to be taken lightly or entered into when psychologic stresses, such as separation or divorce, exist. Even though male and female procedures are theoretically reversible, the permanency of the procedure should be stressed and understood. All forms of reversible contraception should be explained and discussed in detail to assist the client in making an informed decision.

Male sterilization is achieved by a relatively minor procedure called a **vasectomy**. Under local anesthesia, a 2- to 3-cm incision is made over the vas deferens on each side of the scrotum. The ducts are isolated; severed; and occluded by ligation of the ends, by coagulation of the lumen, by burial of the cut ends, or by use of clips or polyethylene tubing with a stopcock for potentially reversible procedures. Absorbable sutures are used to close the skin. The man is instructed to apply ice when pain or swelling occurs and to use a scrotal support for a week. It takes about 4 to 6 weeks and 6 to 36 ejaculations to clear remaining sperm from the vas deferens. During that period, the couple is advised to use another method of birth control and to bring in two or three semen samples for a sperm count. The man is rechecked at 6 and 12 months to ensure that fertility has not been restored by recanalization. Side effects of a vasectomy include hematoma, sperm granulomas, and spontaneous reanastomosis.

Vasectomies can be reversed with the use of microsurgery techniques. Restored fertility, as measured by subsequent pregnancy, ranges from 30% to 85% (Hatcher et al 1989).

Female sterilization (**tubal ligation**) can be accomplished by several abdominal and vaginal procedures. The fallopian tubes are transected or occluded by electrocautery. Postpartal laparotomy is done 1 to 3 days after childbirth, under general anesthesia and usually with a small subumbilical incision. The tubes are isolated and may then be crushed, ligated, electrocoagulated, banded, or plugged (in the newer reversible procedures). The interval minilaparotomy uses a suprapubic incision with similar techniques for interrupting tubal patency.

Laparoscopic sterilization may be done at any time. One or two incisions are made in the subumbilical area. The abdomen is distended with carbon dioxide gas, the laparoscope is introduced through a trocar, and the fallopian tube is visualized. The isthmic portion of the tube is grasped and coagulated, transected, clipped, or banded. The procedure is repeated on the other tube.

Complications of female sterilization procedures include coagulation burns on the bowels, bowel perforation, infection, hemorrhage, and adverse anesthesia effects. Reversal of a tubal ligation depends on many factors, including the portion of the tube excised, the presence or absence of the fimbriae, and the length of the tube remaining. Microsurgical techniques are now the standard reversal approach, with successful pregnancy rates of 40% to 75%.

No reversible form of sterilization holds promise of widespread use at the present time. However, a reversible form of sterilization is currently being investigated. It incorporates the use of a hysteroscope for direct visualization of the tubal openings into the uterus. The openings are injected with a silicone substance that hardens and occludes the cornual section of the fallopian tube. Hysterosalpingography confirms the success of the procedure and a thread is left in the uterine cavity for future removal.

I think I'm like a lot of women. During my life I've used a variety of contraceptive methods. I took the pill back when the doses were higher, I used foam alone and had a baby, then used spermicidal cream and condoms more successfully. I never wanted a tubal and my husband refuses to consider vasectomy, so the IUD was a perfect alternative. I'm 41 and I like something I don't have to think about every time we want to make love. Women my age need choices, too.

Nursing Care

In most cases the nurse who provides information and guidance about contraceptive methods works with a woman because most contraceptive methods are female oriented. Since a man can purchase condoms without seeing a health care provider, only in the case of vasectomy does a man require counseling and interaction with a nurse. The nurse can play an important role in helping a woman choose a method of contraception that is acceptable to her and to her partner (Table 7–5).

In addition to the assessments described on page (176), the nurse can spend time with the woman learning about her life-style, personal attitudes about particular contraceptive methods, and plans for future childbearing. If a woman has multiple sexual partners and a high rate of sexual activity, for example, a spermicide alone offers only limited protection against pregnancy, while an IUD greatly increases her chances of developing pelvic inflammatory disease. Birth control pills may provide the greatest protection for this woman if future childbearing ability is important to her.

Religious beliefs are often important in selecting a method of fertility control, and the nurse counseling women about contraception should be sensitive to its importance. Some women accept only fertility awareness methods of contraception. The nurse working with these women can help by providing them with the information and support they need to follow this method effectively.

Personal bias also plays a role in selection of method. Some women are reluctant to take birth control pills because they fear the associated risk factors. If the woman remains fearful even after careful explanation and reassurance that the risks of the pill are limited in women who are good candidates for the pill, the nurse should recommend

Table 7–5   Factors to Consider in Choosing a Method of Contraception

Effectiveness of method in preventing pregnancy

Safety of the method:
Are there inherent risks?
Does it offer protection against STDs or other conditions?

Client's age and future childbearing plans

Any contraindications in client's health history

Religious or moral factors influencing choice

Personal preferences, biases, etc

Life-style:
How frequently does client have intercourse?
Does she have multiple partners?
Does she have ready access to medical care in the event of complications?
Is cost a factor?

Partner's support and willingness to cooperate

Personal motivation to use method

TEACHING GUIDE
Using a Method of Contraception

Assessment The nurse determines the woman's general knowledge about contraceptive methods, identifies the methods the woman has used previously (if any), identifies contraindications or risk factors for any methods, discusses the woman's personal preferences and biases about various methods, and discusses her commitment (and her partner's commitment if appropriate) to a chosen method.

Nursing Diagnosis Knowledge deficit related to correct use of chosen method of contraception.

Nursing Plan and Implementation The teaching plan will focus on confirming that a chosen method of contraception is a good choice for the woman. The nurse will then help the woman learn the method so that she can use it effectively.

Client Goals At the completion of teaching the woman will be able to:

1. Confirm for herself that the chosen method of contraception is appropriate for her.
2. List the advantages, disadvantages, and risks of the chosen method.
3. Describe (or demonstrate) the correct procedure for using the chosen method.
4. Cite warning signs that should be reported to the care giver.

Teaching Plan

Content Discuss the factors that a woman should consider in choosing a method of contraception (Table 7–5). Stress that the different methods may be appropriate at different times in the woman's life. Review the woman's reasons for selecting a particular method and confirm any contraindications to specific methods.

Discuss the advantages, disadvantages, and risks of the chosen method.

Describe the correct procedure for using a method. Go through step-by-step. Periodically stop and have the woman review the information for you. If a technique is to be learned (as with inserting a diaphragm or charting BBT), demonstrate and then have the woman do a return demonstration as appropriate. (Note: If certain aspects are beyond the nurse's level of expertise, the nurse can review the content and confirm that a woman has the opportunity to do a return demonstration. For example, an office nurse who does not do cervical cap fittings may cover information on its use, have the woman try inserting the cap herself, and then have the placement checked by the nurse practitioner or physician.)

Teaching Method Contraception is a personal decision, so the discussion should take place in a private area free of interruptions.

The nurse should create a supportive, warm, and comfortable atmosphere by her or his attitude and communication style—both verbal and nonverbal.

The nurse needs to consciously recognize that her or his personal preferences about contraception may be very different from those of the woman she or he is counseling. The nurse has the responsibility to provide accurate information in an open, nonjudgmental way.

Focus on open discussion. It may help to have written information about the method chosen. If a signed permit is required (as with sterilization or IUD insertion), the physician should also discuss the advantages, disadvantages, and risks.

Learning is best accomplished when material is broken down into smaller steps.

People learn best when multiple approaches are used, so it is helpful to have a model or chart to enable the woman to visualize what is being described. The nurse can also have a sample of the chosen method available: a package of oral contraceptives, an open IUD, or a symptothermal chart.

(continued)

TEACHING GUIDE (continued)

Teaching Plan

Provide information on what the woman should do if unusual circumstances arise: she forgets a pill, she misses a morning temperature, etc.

Stress warning signs that require immediate action on the part of the woman and explain why these signs indicate a risk. Carefully delineate the actions the woman should take: Should she contact her care giver? Stop the method? and so forth.

Arrange to talk with the woman again soon, either on the phone or at a return visit to determine if she has any questions about the method and to ensure that no problems have arisen.

Provide a written handout identifying the warning signs and listing the actions a woman should take. The handout should also cover actions the woman should take if an unusual situation develops. For example, what should she do if she vomits or has diarrhea while taking oral contraceptives? What action should she take if she and her partner are using a condom and it breaks? and so forth.

The woman should know that she is free to call if she has questions or concerns once she starts using the method. This increases her comfort level and enables you to detect potential problems early.

---

another method. By the same token, if a woman is uncomfortable with touching her genitals and thus finds the diaphragm distasteful, she should choose another method.

Personal bias can also influence the nurse unless care is taken. Nurses tend to recommend the methods they prefer and have confidence in. While this is understandable, it could also interfere with the effectiveness of the counseling the nurse provides. It is important for nurses to examine their own feelings, attitudes, and biases about contraceptive choices.

Once a method is chosen, the nurse can help the woman learn to use it effectively (see Teaching Guide—Using a method of contraception). Often it is the nurse who is available to answer questions about a particular method.

If a woman is considering a tubal ligation or her partner is considering a vasectomy, careful preoperative preparation and explanation is essential. The couple should clearly understand the risks and the surgical techniques used and should accept the idea that the method is essentially irreversible. Although the physician does much of the counseling for these procedures, nurses are often responsible for reinforcing the information and for answering questions.

The nurse also reviews any possible side effects and warning signs of the method chosen and counsels the woman about what action to take if she suspects she is pregnant. In many cases the nurse may become involved in telephone counseling for women who call with questions and concerns. Thus, it is vital that the nurse be knowledgeable about this topic and have resources available to find answers to less common questions.

Menopause

Menopause, the cessation of menses, marks a developmental transition in a woman's life. It signals the end of reproductive potential and implies aging, if not old age. The current median age of menopause in the United States is 50 years. Approximately one third of the entire female population of the Western world is postmenopausal (Mishell 1987). **Climacteric**, or change of life, a word often used synonymously with menopause, refers to the host of psychologic and physical alterations that occur around the time of menopause.

Psychologic Aspects

The impact of menopause on a woman's emotional state is undergoing an enlightened reconceptualization (Breen 1988). The traditional view held that menopause was a time of crisis, emotional struggle, depression, anxiety, and loss of self-esteem. In certain cultures, women no longer able to bear children were considered "used up" and "useless" (Griffith-Kenney 1986). Thankfully, as the number of women reaching menopause increases, researchers are taking a new look. Attitudes toward menopause relate to social expectations. In cultures where attitudes toward aging and the elderly are positive, menopause is less stressful. Research suggests, for example, that menopausal women who are productive and employed experience less emotional distress than women who are unemployed (Severne 1982).

Clearly, a woman's psychologic adaptation to menopause and the climacteric is multifactorial. She is influenced by her own expectations and knowledge, her physical well-being, family views, marital stability, and sociocultural expectations.

Physical Aspects

The physical characteristics of menopause are linked to the shift from a cyclic to a noncyclic hormone pattern. The age of onset may be influenced by nutritional, cultural, or genetic factors. The physiologic mechanisms initiating its onset are not exactly known. The onset of menopause occurs when ovarian function ceases. This results in diminished estrogen levels to the point that menstruation stops.

Generally, ovulation ceases prior to menopause. Individual variations exist and as much as 6 to 8 years of transition prior to menopause has been noted. The change is usually gradual, and normal menstrual irregularities do not include menorrhagia or metrorrhagia. Atrophy of the ovaries occurs gradually; FSH levels rise and less estrogen is produced. Menopausal symptoms include atrophic changes in the vagina, vulva, and urethra and in the trigonal area of the bladder.

Menopausal women often experience certain vasomotor disturbances that are clearly related to hormonal changes and the cessation of menstruation. Fifty percent of women report symptoms of heat arising on the chest and spreading to the neck and face (caused by vasodilation), sweating (mild to drenching), sleep disturbances, and occasional chills. This cluster of symptoms is often called hot flashes. There may be 20 to 30 of these a day, lasting 3 to 5 minutes. Dizzy spells, palpitations, and weakness are also reported by some women. Increased perspiration may occur at night as well as during the hot flash. Vasomotor symptoms in menopausal women vary widely. Some women have severe hot flashes as described, while others experience few, if any, at all.

Vulvar atrophy occurs late, and the pubic hair thins, turns gray or white, and may ultimately disappear. The labia lose substance and their heightened pigmentation. Pelvic fascia and muscles atrophy, resulting in decreased pelvic support. The breasts become pendulous and decrease in size and firmness.

The uterine endometrium and myometrium atrophy, as do the cervical glands. The uterine cavity becomes stenosed. The fallopian tubes atrophy extensively. The vaginal mucosa becomes smooth and thin and the rugae disappear, leading to loss of elasticity. As a result, intercourse may be painful. Dryness of the mucous membrane can lead to burning and itching. The vaginal pH level increases as the number of Döderlein's bacilli decreases.

Menopausal women remain orgasmic, although the excitement phase of the female sexual response cycle may be prolonged. Sexual interest and activity may even improve as the need for contraception disappears and personal growth and awareness increase.

The estrogen deprivation that occurs in menopausal women may significantly increase their risk of coronary heart disease. Estrogens improve the lipid profile by increasing high-density lipoprotein (HDL) and triglycerides and decreasing low-density lipoprotein (LDL) and total cholesterol. Furthermore, researchers speculate that estrogens may act directly on coronary arteries in a way not understood (Bowman 1990).

Hormone Replacement Therapy (HRT)

Hormone replacement therapy (HRT), also called estrogen replacement therapy (ERT), for menopausal women has been controversial for many years, but currently the American College of Obstetricians and Gynecologists recommends HRT in menopause. Estrogen replacement is helpful in stopping hot flashes and night sweats and in reversing atrophic vaginal changes. Perhaps most significantly, HRT may reduce the incidence of cardiovascular heart disease by 50% to 66% (Bowman 1990) and is effective in retarding bone loss and decreasing the fractures associated with osteoporosis.

Osteoporosis is a condition characterized by loss of bone mass, which puts an individual at risk for nontraumatic fractures. Osteoporosis is more common in women who are middle-aged or older. The following risk factors are also associated with osteoporosis:

- White or Asian
- Small-boned and thin
- Family history of osteoporosis
- Lack of regular exercise
- Nulliparous
- Early onset of menopause
- Consistently low intake of calcium
- Cigarette smoking
- Moderate to heavy alcohol intake

Pre- or postmenopausal women with four or more risk factors for osteoporosis should have bone mass measurements done. The woman's height should be measured at each visit because a loss of height is often an early sign that vertebrae are being compressed because of reduced bone mass (Miller 1988). A variety of conditions, including malabsorption syndrome, cancer, cirrhosis of the liver, chronic use of cortisone, and rheumatoid arthritis, can cause secondary arthritis, which resembles osteoporosis. If these secondary causes have been eliminated treatment for osteoporosis is instituted.

Prevention of osteoporosis is a primary goal of care. Women are advised to maintain an adequate calcium intake. Approximately 1200 mg of elemental calcium is recommended for premenopausal women and 1500 mg for postmenopausal women (Miller 1990). To achieve this level most women require supplements. Vitamin D supplements are also recommended. Women are also advised to participate regularly in exercise, to consume only modest quantities of alcohol and caffeine, and to stop smoking. This is especially important because alcohol and smoking have a negative effect on the rate of bone resorption (Mezrow & Rebar 1988). Women with no contraindications to estrogen who are showing evidence of bone loss are good candidates for ERT.

When estrogen is given alone it can produce endometrial hyperplasia and increase the risk of endometrial cancer. Thus, in women who still have a uterus, estrogen is opposed by giving a progestin for a portion of the cycle. Currently opinion varies as to the number of days that progesterone (Provera) should be included. Typically estrogen is given the first 25 days of the month with 10 mg Provera added for days 13 to 25 (Mezrow & Rebar 1988). (Some care givers still prefer to add the Provera for days 16 to 25.) An alternative approach involves the daily administration of 0.625 mg estrogen with 2.5 mg Provera. This regimen is associated with less vaginal bleeding, is sufficient to prevent endometrial hyperplasia and osteoporosis, and also retains most of the cardiovascular protective effects of the estrogen (Bowman 1990).

While most women take estrogen orally in tablet form, some women prefer the transdermal estrogen skin patch, which is applied twice a week to an area of skin free of hair.

A thorough history, physical examination including Pap smear, and baseline mammogram are indicated before starting HRT. An initial endometrial biopsy is no longer recommended for all women beginning HRT but is indicated for women with an increased risk of endometrial cancer and in those with irregular vaginal bleeding. The frequency of endometrial biopsies for women on HRT is controversial at this time. Some recommend them every two years or after any episodes of abnormal bleeding (Mezrow & Rebar 1988).

Women taking estrogen should be advised to stop immediately if they develop headaches, visual changes, signs of thrombophlebitis, or chest pain.

Some postmenopausal women with osteoporosis have shown increases in bone mass when they received a daily dose of thyrocalcitonin. Thyrocalcitonin, a hormone, inhibits osteoclastic bone resorption and is FDA-approved for this therapy. It is expensive, however, and requires daily subcutaneous injections. Sodium fluoride, taken daily, has also increased bone mass in some women by stimulating osteoblast activity (Miller 1990).

Etidonate diphosphate is a promising new treatment that is administered in an intermittent, cyclic fashion. It acts by inhibiting bone resorption and increasing bone mass. The drug, currently approved in the United States for the treatment of Paget's disease, may become a major agent in postmenopausal osteoporosis therapy (Miller 1990).

Nursing Care

Menopausal women may need assistance, in the form of counseling, to adjust successfully to this developmental phase of life. Reaction to menopause is determined to a large extent by the kind of life the woman has lived, by the

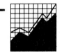

Research Note

Clinical Application of Research

To expand the knowledge base about women's healthy functioning, Janet Rose (1990) designed a phenomenologic study to examine women's experience of inner strength. Each of the nine participants discussed the manifestations of inner strength within her life.

Inner strength was found to be dynamic and complex with a "paradoxical coalescence of vulnerability with safety, tenacity with flexibility, resolution with ambiguity, movement with stillness and emotion with logic" (Rose 1990, p 61). Nine themes arose from the data.

One emergent theme was that of quintessencing, or the process of recognizing, becoming, accepting, and being one's real self. Centering, another theme, included the process of focusing and balancing outside events with the inner self. Quiescencing alluded to the renewal of energy and understanding through the processes of becoming, seeking, and developing an inner calm. Apprehending intrication encompassed the understanding and acceptance of complications and multiple viewpoints. Introspecting comprised an awareness of one's psychologic processes, of being curious and taking risks in spite of possible fear. Using humor released tension, increased ability to focus, and allowed for the visualization of both sides of a process. Interrelating incorporated open, meaningful, reciprocal interactions with others. Having capacity encompassed the ability to solve problems, call upon inner reserves, to persevere in spite of adversity. Embracing vulnerability involved acknowledgement of one's humanness and imperfections while still growing and developing.

Critical Thinking Applied to Research

Strengths: Identification of bracketing process or the setting aside of researcher's own biases and assumptions prior to starting research. Specific and explicit description of data analysis process.

Concerns: Due to the format of the article, explication of the nine essential themes from identified subcomponents is somewhat difficult.

Rose J: Psychologic health of women: A phenomenologic study of women's inner strength. *Adv Nurs Sci* 1990; 12(2): 56.

security she has in her feminine identity, and by her feelings of self-worth and self-esteem.

Nurses or other health professionals can help the menopausal woman achieve high-level functioning at this time in her life. Of paramount importance is the nurse's ability to understand and provide support for the woman's views and feelings. Whether the woman expresses "relief and delight" or "tearfulness and fear," the nurse needs to use an empathetic approach in counseling, health teaching, or providing physical care. Touch and caring as nursing measures may enhance the self-actualization of both nurse and client.

Nurses should explore the question of comfort during sexual intercourse. In counseling the woman the nurse may say, for example, "After menopause many women notice that their vagina seems dryer and intercourse can be uncomfortable. Have you noticed any changes?" This gives the woman information and may open discussion. The nurse can then go on to stress that dryness and shrinking of the vagina can cause discomfort and difficulty during intercourse. Lubrication with a water-soluble jelly will help provide relief. Use of estrogen, orally or in vaginal creams, may also be indicated. Increased frequency of intercourse will maintain some elasticity in the vagina.

When assessing the menopausal woman, the nurse should address the question of sexual activity openly but tactfully because many woman in this age group may have been socialized to be reticent in discussing sex.

The crucial need of women in the perimenopausal period of life is adequate information about the changes taking place in their bodies and their lives. Supplying that information provides both a challenge and an opportunity for nurses. A woman at menopause looks forward to about 30 more years of life. As she accomplishes the developmental tasks of the climacteric period and adjusts to changes that her life brings, she can affirm her worth and go on to an exciting and challenging future.

KEY CONCEPTS

Sexual development begins at conception. The development of sexuality continues throughout an individual's lifetime.

Attitudes about sex are influenced by a variety of factors including family and home environment, culture, education, socioeconomic level, previous sexual experiences, and individual personality characteristics.

Masters and Johnson (1966) have identified four phases in the human sexual response cycle: excitement, plateau, orgasm, and resolution.

To be effective as a counselor on sexual matters nurses must be aware of and comfortable with their feelings and attitudes; have accurate up-to-date knowledge; and be skilled in communicating, and be insightful enough to recognize those occasions when a woman's problem requires more specialized intervention so that appropriate referral can be made.

Girls and women should be provided with clear information about comfort issues, such as tampons (deodorant and absorbency); vaginal spray and douching practices; and self-care comfort measures, such as nutrition, exercise, and use of heat and massage during menstruation.

Premenstrual syndrome occurs most often in women over 30. Symptoms occur 2 to 3 days before onset of menstruation and subside as menstruation starts with or without treatment. Medical management includes progesterone agonists and prostaglandin inhibitors. Self-care measures include improved nutrition (vitamin B complex and E supplementation and avoidance of methylxanthines, such as in chocolate and caffeine), a program of aerobic exercise, and participation in self-care support groups.

Dysmenorrhea usually begins at, or a day before, onset of menses and disappears by the end of menstruation. Therapy with hormones, such as oral contraceptives, or with nonsteroidal anti-inflammatory drugs or prostaglandin inhibitors is useful. Self-care measures include improved nutrition, exercise, applications of heat, and extra rest.

Preconception counseling focuses on the decision to have children (if this decision is morally acceptable to the couple). It also includes counseling about health measures, physical examination, nutrition, exercise, and contraception.

Fertility awareness methods are "natural," noninvasive methods often used by people whose religious beliefs keep them from using other methods of contraception.

Mechanical contraceptives such as the diaphragm, cervical cap, contraceptive sponge, and condom act as barriers to prevent the transport of sperm. These methods are used in conjunction with a spermicide.

The IUD is another mechanical contraceptive that works primarily by preventing fertilization and implantation.

Oral contraceptives (the "pill") are combinations of estrogen and progesterone. When taken correctly they are the most effective of the reversible methods of fertility control.

Spermicides are less effective in preventing pregnancy when they are not used with a barrier method.

Permanent sterilization is accomplished by tubal ligation for women and vasectomy for men. Clients are advised that the method should be considered irreversible.

Menopause is a physiologic maturational change in a woman's life that may be associated with emotional attributes. It is a time of reflection on a woman's life up to this point and gives impetus to evaluate desired future directions. Physiologic changes include the cessation of menses and decrease in circulating hormones. The more common physiologic symptoms are "hot flashes," palpitations, dyspareunia, dizziness, and increased perspiration at night. The woman's anatomy also undergoes changes such as atrophy of the vagina, reduction in size and pigmentation of the labia, and myometrial atrophy. The risk of developing osteoporosis or coronary heart disease increases.

Current management of menopause still centers around estrogen replacement and calcium supplementation therapy.

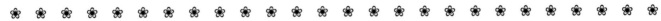

References

American Pharmaceutical Association: *Handbook of Non-Prescription Drugs*, 9th ed. Washington, DC, 1990.

Andersch B, Milson I: An epidemiologic study of young women with dysmenorrhea. *Am J Obstet Gynecol* 1982; 144:655.

Balick L et al: Biofeedback treatment and dysmenorrhea. *Biofeedback Self-Regul* 1982; 7:499.

Bowman M: Hormone replacement therapy: A new look at the combination regimen. *Female Patient* September 1990; 15:63.

Breen JL: *The Gynecologist and the Older Patient.* Rockville, MD: Aspen Publishers, 1988.

Brenner PF, Mishell DR: Control of human reproduction: Contraception, sterilization, and pregnancy termination. In: *Danforth's Obstetrics and Gynecology,* 6th ed. Scott JR et al (editors). Philadelphia: Lippincott, 1990.

Calderone MS: Fetal erection and its message to us. *SIECUS Rep,* May/June, 1983.

Connell EB et al: Contraceptive advances. Part I. Hormonal methods. *Female Patient* December 1989; 14:29.

Connell EB et al: Contraceptive advances. Part II. IUDs and barrier methods. *Female Patient* January 1990; 15:21.

Contraceptive use in older women—The rationale underlying new labeling. *The Contraceptive Report* 1990; 1(2):4.

Dan A: The law and women's bodies: Menstruation leave in Japan. Presented at Socio-Cultural Issues in Menstrual Cycle Research, an Inter-Disciplinary Conference/Workshop, University of California, San Francisco, May 20–21, 1983.

Delaney J, et al: *The Curse: A Cultural History of Menstruation.* New York: New American Library, 1976.

Faich G et al: Toxic shock syndrome and the vaginal contraceptive sponge. *JAMA* 1986; 225:216.

Fioretti P et al: *Postmenopausal Hormone Therapy: Benefits and Risks.* New York: Raven Press, 1987.

Fromer MJ: *Ethical Issues in Sexuality and Reproduction.* St. Louis: Mosby, 1983.

Glatt AE, et al: The prevalence of dyspareunia. *Obstet Gynecol* March 1990; 75:433.

Golub S: Sex differences in attitudes and beliefs regarding menstruation. In: *The Menstrual Cycle.* Vol. 2. Komnenich P et al (editors). New York: Springer, 1981.

Griffith-Kenney J: *Contemporary Women's Health.* Menlo Park, CA: Addison-Wesley, 1986.

Hatcher R et al: *Contraceptive Technology 1988–1989,* 14th ed. New York: Irvington Publishers, 1988.

Hatcher R et al: *Family Planning at Your Fingertips.* Dallas: Essential Medical Information Systems, Inc., 1990.

Hawkins JW et al: *Protocols for Nurse Practitioners in Gynecologic Settings.* New York: The Tiresian Press, 1987.

Heczy MD: Effects of biofeedback and autogenic training on dysmenorrhea. In: *The Menstrual Cycle.* Vol. 1. Dan A, Graham E, Beecher C (editors). New York: Springer, 1980.

Hogan RM: *Human Sexuality.* New York: Appleton-Century-Crofts, 1980.

Jones EF, Forrest JD: Contraceptive failure in the United States: Revised estimates from the 1982 National Survey of Family Growth. *Fam Plann Perspect* May/June 1989; 21:103.

Kaunitz AM: Long-acting progestin contraceptives. *Contemp OB/GYN* October 15, 1990; 35(special issue):59.

Masters WH, Johnson VE: *Human Sexual Response.* Boston: Little, Brown, 1966.

Miller PD: New hope for osteoporosis. *Female Patient* January 1990; 15:49.

Mishell DR: *Menopause: Physiology and Pharmacology.* Yearbook: Chicago, 1987.

Morris NM: Menstruation and marital sex. *J Biosoc Sci* 1983; 15:173.

Murata JM: Abnormal genital bleeding and secondary amenorrhea. *JOGNN* January/February 1990; 19:26.

Rierdan J: Variations in the experience of menarche as a junction of preparedness. In: *Menarche.* Golub S (editor). Lexington, MA: Lexington Books, 1983.

Riis B et al: Does calcium supplementation prevent postmenopausal bone loss? *N Engl J Med* January 1987; 316:173.

Rosen MG: Preconception care: Why it is necessary. *Female Patient* May 1990; 15:73.

Severne L: Psychologic aspects of menopause. In: *Changing Perspectives on Menopause.* Voda A et al (editors). Austin: University of Texas Press, 1982.

Siegel SJ: The effect of culture on the way women experience menstruation: Jewish women and mikvah. Presented at Socio-Cultural Issues in Menstrual Cycle Research, an Inter-Disciplinary Conference/Workshop, University of California, San Francisco, May 20–21, 1983.

Smith S et al: Treatment of premenstrual syndrome with alprazolam: Results of a double-blind placebo-controlled randomized crossover clinical trial. *Obstet Gynecol* 1987; 37:43.

Stewart F et al: *Understanding Your Body.* New York: Bantam Books, 1987.

Thiederman SB: Ethnocentrism: A barrier to effective health care. *Nurse Pract* August 1986; 11:52.

Trussel J et al: Contraceptive failure in the United States: An update. *Stud Fam Planning* January/February 1990; 21:207.

Tybor JR: Premenstrual tension tested as legal defense. *Chicago Tribune* May 23, 1982.

Williams LR: Beliefs and attitudes of young girls regarding menstruation. In: *Menarche.* Golub S (editor). Lexington, MA: Lexington Books, 1983.

Additional Readings

Adlersberg M, Thorne S: Emerging from chrysalis: Older widows in transition. *J Gerontol Nurs* 1990; 16(1):4.

Cohn SD: The evolving law of adolescent health care. *NAACOG'S Clin Issues Perinatal Women's Health Nurs* 1991; 2(2):201.

Fehring RV: New technology in natural family planning. *JOGNN* May/June 1991; 20:199.

Glatt AE et al: The prevalence of dyspareunia. *Obstet Gynecol* 1990; 75(3, part 1):433.

Hatasaka HH, Wentz AC: Hirsutism—Facts and folklore Part II: Management. *Female Patient* February 1991; 16(2):11.

Jarrett ME, Lethbridge DJ: The contraceptive needs of midlife women. *Nurse Pract* December 1990; 15:34.

Youngkin EQ: Estrogen replacement therapy and the estraderm transdermal system. *Nurse Pract* May 1990; 15:19.

Yuzpe AA: Current status of OCs. *Contemp OB/GYN* March1991; 36 (3):77.

CHAPTER 8

Women's Care:
Common Health Problems

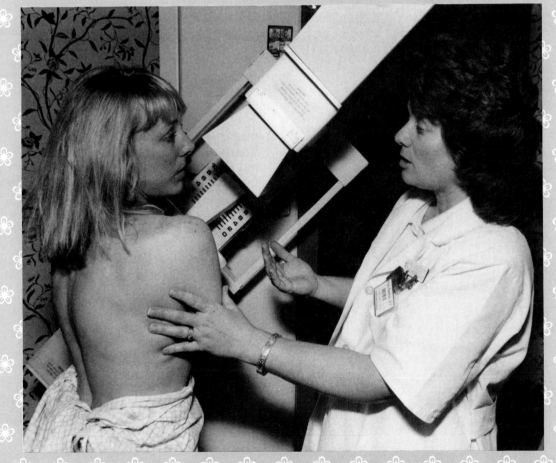

OBJECTIVES

Differentiate the common benign breast disorders.

Describe the tests available to diagnose carcinoma of the breast.

Identify the nursing needs of a woman with cancer of the breast.

Discuss the signs, symptoms, and treatment of endometriosis.

Describe toxic shock syndrome with regard to diagnosis, treatment, and health teaching.

Compare the common sexually transmitted infections with regard to causative organism, signs and symptoms, treatment, and long-term implications.

Summarize health teaching the nurse should provide to a woman with a sexually transmitted infection.

Relate the development and progression of pelvic inflammatory disease to the possible development of infertility.

Identify diagnostic measures that should be employed to establish a diagnosis when a woman has an abnormal finding during a pelvic examination.

Compare lower urinary tract infections with upper urinary tract infections.

❀ ❀

I was 35 when my husband divorced me for another woman. During the following year I had sex with only two men, but one of them gave me herpes. I was devastated when my nurse practitioner diagnosed it. I felt embarrassed, ashamed, dirty. My self-esteem had never been lower. My nurse practitioner was wonderful. She explained the disease and how it was spread and helped me find ways to relieve the symptoms. More than that, though, I always knew she cared about me personally. She helped me realize I was still a worthwhile person. Knowing she still liked and respected me helped me start feeling good about myself again. When I met a man I really cared about, she helped me figure a way to tell him about my herpes. He was able to accept it and still love me. We are married now and I've never been happier. We've followed my practitioner's advice about ways to avoid infecting my husband and he hasn't had any sign of infection. When I think about all the changes and stress in my life I can't imagine how I would have coped without my practitioner. She gave me support when I needed it and encouraged me to stand alone when I was ready. She's a special woman.

Women's health refers to a holistic view of women and their health-related needs within the context of their everyday lives. It is based on the awareness that a woman's physical, mental, and social status are interdependent and determine her state of health or illness. The woman's view of her situation, her assessment of her needs, her values, and her beliefs are valid and important factors to be incorporated into any health care intervention.

The contemporary woman is likely to encounter various gynecologic or urinary problems during her lifetime. Nurses can assist women by providing them with accurate, sensitive, and supportive health education and counseling. This information will empower women to become knowledgeable consumers of health care. The nurse's role is to assess the woman's needs, determine nursing diagnoses, plan interventions and follow-up, and evaluate the effectiveness of care provided. As part of this process the nurse can clarify misconceptions and address psychosocial aspects of specific health problems that concern the woman.

To meet the woman's needs, nurses need up-to-date information about health care practices and about available diagnostic and treatment options. This chapter provides basic information about a variety of gynecologic disorders. To simplify learning, information is presented according to specific disease processes and female body parts. It is essential to remember, however, that women are multidimensional, complex beings who are entitled to holistic health care.

The Female Breast

The female breast has for centuries assumed an importance far out of proportion to its natural purpose—the nourishment of an infant. Sexual interest in breasts is peculiar to humans and is a long-standing cultural phenomenon, as can be seen in the paintings and sculpture displayed in museums throughout the world (Sloane 1985) and in the idealized images of "perfect" breasts that are frequently used by the media to sell a variety of products and services. These cultural attitudes have perpetuated the belief among women that breasts are their "badge of femininity."

A complex interaction of cultural and psychosocial factors determine the significance of the breasts for each woman. Because people develop their body images in part via external feedback, the disproportionate glorification of the breasts may have profound effects on a woman's body image. Some women are willing to subject themselves to potentially disfiguring surgeries in order to improve the appearance of their breasts. Some women even choose the loss of life over the loss of a breast in their delay or refusal to seek medical care for a breast lump.

Breasts develop as a secondary sex characteristic during puberty. For the developing adolescent, her breasts are a visible symbol of her feminine identity and an important part of her body image and self-esteem. Because a woman's primary sexual organs cannot be observed, breast development provides visual confirmation that the adolescent is becoming a woman. Breasts are a source of erotic stimulation for many women, and they play a role in the expression of women's sexuality. Their size, shape, and appearance are unique to each woman.

Normal Cyclic Changes in the Nonlactating Breast

Like the uterus, the breast functions dynamically in a cyclic process that is regulated by the nervous and hormonal systems. Each month, in rhythm with the cycle of ovulation, the breasts become engorged with fluid in anticipation of pregnancy. The contours of the breasts' lobular structure become apparent, producing the sensations of lumpiness, tenderness, and perhaps pain. *Mastodynia* (premenstrual swelling and tenderness of the breasts) is common. It usually lasts for 3 to 4 days prior to the onset of menses, but the symptoms may persist throughout the month. Such symptoms may be diagnosed erroneously as fibrocystic breast disease but are more properly identified as increased physiologic nodularity, an exaggerated response to normal cyclic changes. If conception does not occur, the accumulated fluid drains away via the lymphatic network.

After menopause, adipose breast tissue atrophies and is replaced by connective tissue. Elasticity is diminished, and breasts tend to hang more loosely from the chest wall because of these tissue changes and relaxation of the suspensory ligaments. The nipples become smaller, flatter, and lose some erectile ability. The skin over the breasts may take on a relatively dry, thin texture. Cyclic engorgement of the breast tissue is absent after menopause but may resume with estrogen replacement therapy.

Care of the Woman with Fibrocystic Breast Disease

Fibrocystic breast disease (FBD) is the most common of the benign breast disorders. *Mammary dysplasia* or *chronic cystic mastitis* are also terms used to describe this benign condition. It is estimated that 50% of women of childbearing age will have palpable evidence of cystic disease sometime during their reproductive years (Norwood 1990). There is an increased risk for subsequent breast cancer in women with dysplastic fibrocystic changes. *Dysplasia* is determined by histologic examination and is seen as irregular cell growth. Multiple or solitary cysts occurring in fibrocystic disease that are not found to be dysplastic are not a risk factor for breast cancer.

FBD appears to be a problem for some women during the childbearing years, improving during pregnancy and lactation and resolving with menopause. Early cystic changes have been found in teenagers and women in their twenties; however, the occurrence of breast cysts is most prevalent in women 30 to 50 years of age (Norwood 1990).

Fibrosis is a thickening of normal breast tissue. The breast may become multinodular with a periodic mass. Cyst formation that may accompany fibrosis is considered a later change in fibrocystic disease. Cyst formation may result when normal secretions within the ductal network are unable to drain away. Their accumulation can then create a fluid-filled sac or cyst.

FBD is probably caused by an imbalance in estrogen and progesterone, which distorts the normal breast changes of the menstrual cycle. Current theories suggest that unopposed estrogen in the luteal phase related to progesterone deficiency may be the cause of fibrocystic breast disease. Because the condition responds to the changes of the menstrual cycle, a woman may actually observe a lessening in the size of a lump with the onset of her menstrual cycle. The symptoms often increase as the woman approaches menopause, while the condition generally improves following menopause. However, if a postmenopausal woman is treated with hormone replacement therapy, the cyclic breast changes may resume (Norwood 1990).

Medical Therapy

The woman often complains of pain, tenderness, and swelling that occurs cyclically and is most pronounced just before her menses begins. Physical examination may reveal only mild signs of irregularity, or the breasts may feel dense, with areas of irregularity and nodularity. Women often refer to this as "lumpiness." Some women may also have clear, milky, straw-colored, or greenish nipple discharge. Unilateral discharge and serosanguinous discharge should be evaluated further (Marchant 1990).

If the woman has a large, fluid-filled cyst she may experience a localized painful area as the capsule containing the accumulated fluid distends coincident with her cycle. However, if small cyst formation occurs, the woman may experience not a solitary tender lump but a diffuse tenderness.

Mammography, palpation, and fine-needle aspiration are used to confirm fibrocystic breast disease. Often, fine-needle aspiration is the treatment as well, affording relief from the tenderness or pain.

Diagnostic criteria for fibrocystic breast disease are as follows:

- A palpable, fluid-filled mass is felt.
- The mass can be aspirated.
- Histologic examination confirms cystic disease.
- Mammography indicates cystic formation.

Physical examination reveals that cysts are round, movable, and well delineated in appearance. Specific characteristics that differentiate a cyst from a malignant neoplasm are mobility, tenderness, and the absence of skin retraction (or pulling) in surrounding tissue.

Fine-needle aspiration, an office procedure, is used in conjunction with physical examination for diagnosis. Fluid withdrawal confirms the presence of a cyst. The fluid aspirated is sent for cytologic examination. If aspiration is incomplete, yielding no fluid, or yields bloody fluid, a biopsy is necessary. If the physical findings remain unclear, a mammogram is ordered to clarify the diagnosis. A mammogram revealing an unexplained or suspicious area warrants surgical exploration or biopsy (Norwood 1990).

Treatment of palpable cysts is conservative; invasive procedures such as biopsy are used only if the diagnosis is questionable. If a question persists, surgical exploration of the tissue and removal of the affected area are scheduled as an outpatient procedure. The mass or affected area is reexamined after four weeks to determine if the cyst has refilled.

Women with mild symptoms may benefit from restricting sodium intake and taking a mild diuretic during the week before the onset of menses. This counteracts fluid retention, relieves pressure in the breast, and helps decrease the pain. In other cases a mild analgesic is necessary.

Controversy surrounds the practice of limiting caffeine to relieve symptoms. Some recent studies have found a positive correlation between intake of methylxanthines (found in caffeine products such as coffee, tea, cola, chocolate, and some medications) and breast pain in women with FBD (Bullough et al 1990). Other studies reported no change when methylxanthines were limited, and one study reported that symptoms worsened when caffeine was eliminated (Norwood 1990).

Other approaches that are occasionally advocated include daily intake of 50 to 100 mg of thiamine daily. Thiamine plays a role in the detoxification of estrogen and might decrease levels of available estrogen. This method is not yet supported by good clinical trials (Havens et al 1986). Treatment with 600 IU of vitamin E daily has been beneficial to some women. This dose is safe and is not associated with the side effects found with higher doses. Vitamin A is also advocated by some clinicians but its value is questionable (Ellerhorst-Ryan 1988).

In severe cases of FBD, the hormone inhibitor danazol (Danocrine) is the drug of choice. It produces marked relief within four to six months. In most cases the medication is discontinued after six months and the improvement lasts for nine to twelve months. Symptoms, when they recur, do not tend to reach the level of pretreatment severity (Tobiassen 1984). Danazol does have some troubling side effects, especially weight gain, amenorrhea, and masculinization.

Additional medical therapies that have been found beneficial in varying degrees include oral contraceptives, progestins, and bromocriptine (Norwood 1990). These all work on the principle of estrogen suppression and progesterone stimulation or augmentation.

❈ *APPLYING THE NURSING PROCESS* ❈

Nursing Assessment

The nurse assesses the woman's understanding of fibrocystic breast disease and the importance of regular breast self-examination. Some specially trained nurses perform breast examinations of healthy women. The nurse reviews the woman's history for close relatives with fibrocystic breast disease or cancer of the breast. The nurse also obtains information on relief measures that have been effective for the woman.

Nursing Diagnosis

Nursing diagnoses that may apply to a woman with fibrocystic breast disease include the following:

Knowledge deficit related to lack of understanding of self-care measures

Pain related to the cyclic breast changes that occur premenstrually

---

CRITICAL THINKING

Why do you suppose so many women are unwilling to do monthly breast self-examination despite its value in detecting cancer early?

Nursing Plan and Implementation

Breast Self-Examination

Monthly **breast self-examination** (BSE) is the best method for detecting breast masses early. A woman who knows the texture and feel of her own breasts is far more likely to detect changes that develop. All health professionals need to include breast examination and the teaching of routine BSE in regular checkups. Often, the nurse, particularly in a clinic, office, or community health setting, assumes responsibility for teaching BSE to women. Nurses also have the opportunity to teach BSE in hospital settings.

Women often are reluctant to perform BSE and it is sometimes difficult to convince them to do it. Factors associated with effective teaching include individualized teaching by a nurse or physician, explanation of the technique of BSE, demonstration of correct technique, sensory information such as directing the woman's hand to touch and identify the "normal lumps" in her own breasts, and return demonstration. Other factors that contribute to success (but are somewhat less effective than those mentioned previously) include printed materials, reminder postcards, films and monthly logs (Champion 1989; Lauver 1989; Nettles-Carlson 1988; Olson et al 1989). The incorporation of these successful teaching techniques is essential in a nursing teaching plan for BSE. See Teaching Guide—Teaching Breast Self-Examination.

All premenopausal women should perform BSE monthly approximately one week after their menses. Pregnant women, women who have had a hysterectomy, and postmenopausal women should pick a certain day of the month—perhaps the first day or the date of their birth—as their regular day to do BSE. Postmenopausal women who are on cyclic hormone replacement therapy should perform BSE at the end of the week they do not take hormones.

The American Cancer Society has a pamphlet, "How to Examine Your Breasts," that can be obtained free of charge for distribution to clients.

 Education for Self-Care In addition to teaching BSE, the nurse suggests measures the woman can employ to help alleviate her discomfort. These include the following:

- Wearing a well-fitting, supportive bra, at night as well as during the day when symptoms are severe
- Applying ice packs to tender areas of the breasts
- Using nonprescription salicylates or anti-inflammatory medication
- Limiting caffeine and salt intake

Provision of Psychologic Support

By carefully explaining FBD and its relationship to the monthly cycle, the nurse can alleviate the woman's anxiety while reinforcing the importance of having any suspected abnormality investigated promptly. The major concern is that, because of the lumpiness of the breasts, small malignant neoplasms will be missed. In reality, women with FBD make up a minority of breast cancer cases, and the breast cancer risk is not uniform in all women with FBD. Breast cancer tends to be concentrated in those women with proliferative lesions, especially with atypia, and a contributory family history (Dupont & Page 1985).

The nurse can also point out that frequent professional breast examination and regular mammograms are tools that help detect any abnormalities, and that the woman who practices monthly BSE, follows her care giver's advice, and is examined regularly has taken positive action to protect her health.

Evaluation

Anticipated outcomes of nursing care include the following:

- The woman incorporates monthly BSE into her personal routine.

- The woman implements measures to help alleviate her discomfort.

- The woman understands fibrocystic breast disease, deals with her anxiety over the potential complications, and takes positive action to protect her health.

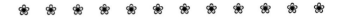

Care of the Woman with a Benign Disorder of the Breast

Table 8–1 summarizes common breast disorders. Mastitis is discussed in Chapter 36.

Fibroadenoma

The *fibroadenoma* is a common benign tumor seen in women in their teens and early twenties. It is the third most common tumor of the breast; its incidence is exceeded only by carcinoma and fibrocystic disease. The cause of fibroadenomas found in adolescent breasts appears closely linked to that of breast hypertrophy, which may occur during the pubertal growth spurt. Fibroadenomas will respond to hormonal influence and are known to increase in size and secrete milk during pregnancy. Unlike cystic disease, fibroadenoma has not been significantly associated with malignant neoplasms.

Fibroadenomas are solid tumors that are well defined, sharply delineated, and rounded, with a rubbery firmness. These tumors can be moved freely within the breast tissue and are not associated with any fibroblastic response in surrounding tissue. A solitary nodule is common, but multiple tumors have been observed in about 15 percent of cases (Ellerhorst-Ryan et al 1988). The size of a fibroadenoma ranges from 1 to 5 cm, with the nodule commonly occurring around the nipple or in the upper quadrant of the breast along the lateral side. Fibroadenomas are asymptomatic and nontender. They are usually discovered by accident.

Medical Therapy

Fibroadenomas are characterized by their appearance on physical examination. They are well-outlined, rounded, lobulated in appearance, rubbery, and relatively movable.

If there are any disquieting features to the appearance of the lump, fine-needle biopsy and/or excision of the mass may be indicated. Caution is exercised when deciding upon biopsy because excision of the mass in a young girl may interfere with normal breast development. Watchful observation and possible surgical excision are the only treatments for fibroadenomas. Surgery is often deferred, but if surgery is indicated, it is performed under local anesthesia on an outpatient basis. Surgical removal of a fibroadenoma concludes its treatment.

Teaching Breast Self-Examination

Assessment: The nurse determines the woman's general knowledge about BSE, identifies previous experience with BSE, identifies risk factors for breast cancer (See Table 8–2), determines the woman's general knowledge about breast cancer, discusses the woman's feelings about her breasts and BSE, identifies barriers to BSE and discusses her commitment to practice BSE.

Nursing Diagnosis: Knowledge deficit related to breast self-examination.

Nursing Plan and Implementation: The teaching plan will focus on assisting the woman to learn BSE so that she can use it effectively.

Client Goals: At the completion of teaching, the woman will be able to:

1. Discuss her risk of breast cancer.
2. Describe the use of BSE in breast cancer detection.
3. Demonstrate the correct procedure for BSE.
4. List warning signs of breast cancer to be reported to the care giver.
5. Incorporate monthly BSE into her personal routine.

Teaching Plan

Content: Discuss the risk factors associated with breast cancer (see Table 8–2).

Stress the unique risk factors associated with the woman's personal history and life-style.

Discuss the use of BSE in breast cancer detection.

Describe and demonstrate the correct procedure for BSE. A. Instruct the woman to inspect her breasts by standing or sitting in front of a mirror. She needs to inspect her breasts in three positions: with both arms relaxed down at her side, both arms stretched straight over her head, and both hands placed on her hips while leaning forward (Figure 8–1)

Teaching Method: This should be discussed in a private area free of interruptions. The room needs to have a mirror, bed, couch, or examining table; pillows, a patient gown and a private area for the woman to disrobe.

The nurse should create a supportive, warm, and comfortable atmosphere by attitude and communication style—both verbal and nonverbal. A discussion of breast cancer may bring forth many emotions in the woman, including grief for previous breast cancer–related losses.

Focus on open discussion. A brochure with statistics and illustrations may be useful. Stress the positive outcomes of early detection to counterbalance fears.

Learning is best accomplished when material is broken down into smaller steps and presented with multiple approaches. Prior to asking the woman to perform BSE, the nurse should use a model or a chart to demonstrate the procedure. Then the nurse should have the woman perform BSE. The nurse should be very supportive and give a lot of positive feedback, as some women may be embarrassed. The nurse needs to demonstrate a nonjudgmental, accepting attitude.

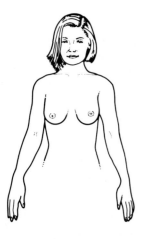
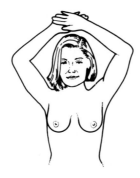
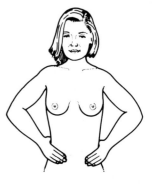

Figure 8–1   Positions for inspection

Teaching Plan

Advise the woman to look at the breasts individually and in comparison with one another. Note and record the following characteristics for each position:

Size and Symmetry of the Breasts

1. Breasts may vary, but the variations should remain constant during rest or movement—note abnormal contours.
2. Some size difference between the breasts is normal.

Shape and Direction of the Breasts

1. The shape of the breasts can be rounded or pendulous with some variation between breasts.
2. The breasts should be pointing slightly laterally.

Color, Thickening, Edema, and Venous Patterns

1. Check for redness or inflammation.
2. A blue hue with a marked venous pattern that is focal or unilateral may indicate an area of increased blood supply due to tumor. Symmetric venous patterns are normal.
3. Skin edema observed as thickened skin with enlarged pores ("orange peel") may indicate blocked lymphatic drainage due to tumor.

Surface of the Breasts

1. Skin dimpling, puckering, or retraction (pulling) when the woman presses her hands together or against her hips suggests malignancy.
2. Striae (stretch marks) red at onset and whitish with age are normal.

Nipple Size and Shape, Direction, Rashes, Ulcerations, and Discharge

1. Long-standing nipple inversion is normal, but an inverted nipple previously capable of erection is suspicious. Note any deviation, flattening, or broadening of the nipples.
2. Check for rashes, ulcerations, or discharge.

B. Instruct the woman to palpate (feel) her breasts.

Instruct woman as follows:

1. Lie down. Put one hand behind your head. With the other hand, fingers flattened, gently feel your breast. Press lightly (Figure 8–2A) Now examine the breast.

2. Figure 8–2B shows you how to check each breast. Begin as you see in C and follow the arrows, feeling gently for a lump or thickening. Remember to feel all parts of each breast.

3. Now repeat the same procedure sitting up, with the hand still behind your head (Figure 8–2C).

4. Squeeze the nipple between your thumb and forefinger. Look for any discharge—clear or bloody (Figure 8–2D).

(continued)

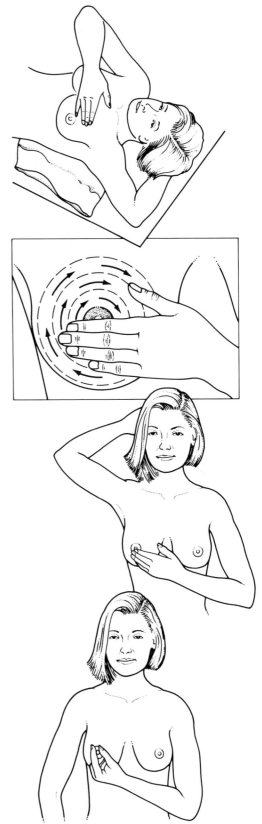

Figure 8–2   Breast self-examination

TEACHING GUIDE (continued)

Teaching Plan

C. Take the woman's hand and help her to identify her "normal lumps." For example: mammary ridge, ribs and nodularity in the upper outer quadrants.

Demonstrate "normal lumps" on the woman herself while guiding her hand and identifying the area.

D. After she examines her breasts and identifies her normal lumps, instruct her to palpate her breasts once more to identify any areas that she may have questions about. If questions arise, the nurse should palpate the area and attempt to identify if it is normal.

Allowing the woman to differentiate normal from abnormal lumps on herself and a model will increase confidence that she will recognize an abnormal finding. Having the nurse check her immediately afterwards will positively reinforce her and diminish the fear associated with BSE.

E. If a breast model is available, instruct the woman to palpate it and identify the lumps.

Provide information on the warning signs of breast cancer and what she should do if she identifies any of these signs during BSE.

Provide a written handout on the warning signs of breast cancer. The handout should also cover actions that she should take if a warning sign is discovered. Stress the positive effects of early detection.

Timing: Instruct the woman to perform BSE on a monthly basis. Be specific if she is premenopausal, pregnant, postmenopausal, or postmenopausal receiving hormone replacement therapy.

Teaching Method: Provide the woman with a reminder symbol for monthly BSE. The American Cancer Society provides such items to hang in the shower, place on a refrigerator, etc. Ask her when she plans to do BSE each month. This will serve as a method of evaluation and reinforcement. Praise her commitment to do monthly BSE. Give the woman a follow-up telephone number, eg, American Cancer Society, to use if she needs additional information or has questions. This will increase her comfort level with BSE and enable her to detect potential problems early.

Source: American Cancer Society: Breast Self-Examination and the Nurse, No. 3408 PE. New York, 1973.

Intraductal Papilloma

Although *intraductal papillomas* are relatively uncommon, they constitute the primary cause of nipple discharge in women who are not pregnant or lactating. Intraductal papillomas are primarily a disease of the menopausal years, although they may be found in women of any age.

Papillomas are fragile, fingerlike projections into the duct lumen that result from proliferation of the duct epithelium. Minimal trauma will cause blood or serum to collect in the involved duct and will result in spontaneous serous or bloody nipple discharge. No evidence currently exists linking a solitary intraductal papilloma with breast cancer. Multiple intraductal papillomas, however, have been associated with malignant transformation (Ohuchi 1984).

Medical Therapy

The majority of papillomas present as solitary nodules. These small, ball-like lesions may be detected on mammography but are most often nonpalpable, although palpation may elicit some tenderness. The presence of a papilloma is often frightening to the woman because her primary symptom is a discharge from the nipple that may be serosanguinous or brownish-green due to the presence of old blood.

If the woman reports a nipple discharge, the breast should be milked to obtain fluid. The fluid obtained is sent for a Papanicolaou (Pap) smear. The diagnosis is confirmed if papilloma cells are present (Havens et al 1986). The diagnosis may also be confirmed by a ductogram, which involves injecting radiopaque dye into the duct followed by a mammogram. The lesion may be excised and histologically examined to differentiate between a benign papilloma and a papillary carcinoma.

Treatment for benign papilloma is excision. Medical follow-up visits may be more frequent because of the possibility of recurrence and the similarity of papillary carcinoma to the benign condition.

Duct Ectasis (Comedomastitis or Plasma Cell Mastitis)

Mammary *duct ectasia* is a benign condition that involves inflammation of the ducts behind the nipple, duct enlarge-

Table 8–1 Summary of Common Breast Disorders

Condition	Age	Pain	Nipple discharge	Location	Consistency and mobility	Diagnosis and treatment
Duct ectasia	35–55 years; median age 40	Burning around nipple	Sticky, multi-colored; usually bilateral	No specific location	Retroareolar mass with advanced disease	Open biopsy; local excision of diseased portion of breast
Fibroadenoma	15–39 years; median age 20	No	No	No specific location	Mobile, firm, smooth, well delineated	Mammography, surgical or needle biopsy; excision of the tumor
Fibrocystic breast disease	20–49 years; median age 30 (may subside with menopause)	Yes	No	Upper outer quadrant	Bilateral multiple lumps influenced by the menstrual cycle	Needle aspiration; observation; biopsy if there is an unresolved mass or mammographic changes
Intraductal papilloma	35–55 years; median age 40	Yes	Serous or sero-sanguineous; usually unilateral from one duct	No specific location	Usually soft, poorly delineated	Pap smear of nipple discharge; biopsy; wedge resection
Mastitis	Childbearing years	Tenderness, pain	No	No specific location	Generalized redness of overlying skin	Antibiotic therapy; incision and drainage if mastitis progresses to an abscess

Source: Modified from Fogel CI, Woods NF (editors): Health Care of Women: A Nursing Perspective. *St. Louis: Mosby, 1981, p 337.*

ment, and collection of cellular debris and fluid in the involved ducts. The disease is most commonly seen in women ages 45 to 55, although it can be found in younger women. It was previously thought that breast-feeding and multiparity place women at increased risk for the disease, but studies do not substantiate this (Dixon 1983).

Breast pain and a palpable mass are common symptoms in premenopausal women; nipple discharge predominates in perimenopausal women; and nipple retraction is more often noted in postmenopausal women. This disease is not associated with cancer.

Medical Therapy

The woman will report a thick, sticky nipple discharge with burning pain, pruritus, and inflammation. The drainage may be green, greenish-brown, or blood-stained. Masses associated with duct ectasia may be poorly circumscribed. Nipple retraction, bloody nipple discharge, and axillary lymphadenopathy accompanying inflammation further complicate accurate differentiation of the disease from breast cancer. Treatment is conservative, with drug therapy aimed at symptomatic relief. The major central ducts of the breast occasionally have to be excised. Local excision of the in-

volved ducts has been effective in controlling symptoms. Treatment plans are dependent upon the severity of the problem. The vast majority of women will require nothing more than routine follow-up with physical examination. In the early stages of inflammation, women should be advised to keep their nipples clean to minimize the risk of infection. The symptoms may be frightening, and the woman may need emotional support in addition to reassurance that this disorder is not associated with cancer.

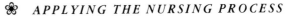 ❀ *APPLYING THE NURSING PROCESS* ❀

Nursing Assessment

During the period of diagnosis, the woman may be anxious about a possible change in body image or a diagnosis of cancer. The nurse can use therapeutic communication to assess the significance the woman places on her breasts; her current emotional status, coping mechanisms used during periods of stress, and knowledge and beliefs about cancer; and other variables that may influence her coping and adjustment.

Nursing Diagnosis

Nursing diagnoses that may apply to a woman with a benign disorder of the breast include the following:

- Knowledge deficit related to a lack of understanding of diagnostic procedures
- Anxiety related to threat to body image

Nursing Plan and Implementation

Provision of Emotional Support During the Period of Diagnosis

During the prediagnosis period the woman should be encouraged to express her anxiety. Misconceptions need to be clarified, and the woman should be allowed to express her fears. The woman may find herself considering the implications for her personal life, her family, and the future if the diagnosis is cancer. This "what if" concern helps the woman consider the implications of cancer and enables her to begin planning. It is tempting to disregard these concerns by simply responding, "Oh, don't think like that. Everything will be fine." Such an approach, however, invalidates the woman's concerns and denies her the opportunity to begin considering the future. The sensitive nurse will avoid unnecessary pessimism while recognizing that the woman's concerns are valid.

Evaluation

Anticipated outcomes of nursing care include the following:

- The woman feels comfortable discussing her fears, concerns, and questions during the period of diagnosis.
- The diagnosis is made accurately and quickly.

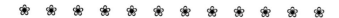

Care of the Woman with Carcinoma of the Breast

An estimated 43,000 deaths from breast cancer occur every year in the United States, compared to 23,000 deaths from cancer in all other female reproductive organs. Breast cancer is second only to lung cancer as a cause of cancer deaths in women. Furthermore, despite advances in treatment technology, no overall change in the rate of breast cancer deaths has occurred in the United States in the past 30 years (Nettles-Carlson 1989). Breast cancer accounts for nearly 26% of all years of potential life lost among women (Centers for Disease Control 1987). Early detection seems to influence the outcome of breast cancer more than does the particular type or combination of treatment

used; a woman's chances of survival are directly linked to the stage of the disease at diagnosis (Nettles-Carlson 1989).

Risk Factors for Breast Cancer

Factors placing women at risk for breast cancer have been studied extensively by epidemiologists and other clinical researchers. The risk factors associated with carcinoma of the breast in women are summarized in Table 8–2. The most significant risk factors have been identified as female gender, older age, and positive family history in a first-degree relative. Unfortunately, these risk factors cannot be modified with life-style changes. A woman's age is the most important risk factor in determining when to begin screening. Ninety percent of breast cancers occur in women aged 40 and older. Mammography screening should begin 5 years before a first-degree female relative was diagnosed with breast cancer in women with a family history (Nettles-Carlson 1989). Some studies, however, suggest that modifiable risk factors, including consumption of alcohol and high intakes of dietary fats, contribute to the risk of breast cancer. Additional risk factors associated with breast cancer are previous cancer in one breast, postmenopausal obesity (premenopausal obesity is not related), and certain specific cases of fibrocystic breast disease that have an atypical biopsy report (Hulka 1987). Studies have not shown that breast cancer risk is increased with the use of oral contraceptives and estrogen replacement therapy (ACOG 1989). Oral contraceptives are clearly contraindicated in women with a personal history of breast cancer.

A woman who has never been pregnant has an increased risk of breast cancer, but a recent study on delayed childbearing did not reveal an association between the trend toward delayed childbearing and an increased risk of breast cancer (White 1987).

Nurses need to assist women in assessing their risk for breast cancer. They also need to teach women about risk reduction through life-style modifications and through screening techniques. Although 95% of breast lumps are discovered by women themselves, they may delay seeking health care. The most significant indicator of breast cancer survival is stage of disease at diagnosis. The earlier the detection, the greater the chances of cure. Women delay seeking health care when a lump is detected for a variety of reasons: threats to body image, favorable attitude toward delay, perceived social pressure to delay, maintaining control over one's life, avoiding disruptions of one's life and others' lives and fear of negative health outcomes (Timko 1987). Nurses must break through these barriers to early detection and intervention if the incidence of breast cancer is to be reduced.

Pathophysiology of Breast Cancer

Theories about the causes of breast cancer include hormonal mechanisms, viral agents, and immunologic pro-

Table 8–2 Summary of Risk Factors for Breast Cancer

Factor	Higher risk	Lower risk
Age	≥40	<40
History of cancer in one breast	yes	no
Family history of premenopausal bilateral breast cancer	yes	no
Country of residence	North America Northern Europe	Asia Africa
Any first-degree relative with breast cancer	yes	no
History of fibrocystic condition with atypical hyperplasia	yes	no
Alcohol consumption	>9 drinks/wk	<9 drinks/wk
History of primary cancer in ovary or endometrium	yes	no
Radiation to chest	large doses	minimal exposure
Socioeconomic class	upper	lower
Age at first full-term pregnancy	>30	<20
Oophorectomy	yes	no
Postmenopausal body build	obese	thin
Race	white	black
Marital status	never married	never married
Age at menarche	early	late
Age at menopause	late	early
U.S. place of residence	urban Northern	rural Southern

cesses. Because breast cancer does not occur in the prepubertal female, it is thought that prior conditioning of the breast tissue by endogenous steroids may be essential for development of cancer.

A malignant breast neoplasm may originate either in a duct or in the epithelium of the breast lobes. It may be infiltrating (penetrating the limiting basement membranes) or noninfiltrating (nonpenetrating). All forms of breast cancer can spread locally by invasion. A breast tumor tends to adhere to the pectoral muscles or deep fascia of the chest wall beneath the breast and the skin overlying the breast. This adherence of the tumor can cause an appearance of skin dimpling and retraction in the later stages of the disease ("orange peel sign"). About 50% of all breast cancers originate in the upper outside quadrant and spread or metastasize to the axillary lymph nodes. Approximately 25% of all breast cancers arise in the central portion of the breast and metastasize to the mammary lymph node chain.

In more than half of all women with breast cancer,

systemic metastasis either has occurred by the time the woman seeks professional assistance or develops later. Malignant breast neoplasms spread from the breast to the axillary nodes, to the internal mammary nodes, and to the supraclavicular nodes. Of the women seeking medical care for a breast mass, 50% with a palpable lump of one month's duration have positive axillary nodes and 68% with a palpable lump of six months' duration have positive axillary nodes. Wider dissemination of the breast neoplasm is primarily through the bloodstream, with the common sites of distant metastasis being the lymph nodes, lungs, bone marrow, liver, brain, and bone (Nettles-Carlson 1989).

Cancer of the breast is often discovered accidentally by the woman or her sexual partner. During the early stages of development, the lump is usually isolated, movable, and painless. A hard, distinct mass that is not freely movable also suggests malignancy. More advanced signs, such as fixation to the skin, skin edema, nipple retraction, or deep fixation, are further evidence of cancer.

Screening, Detection, and Diagnosis

The purpose of breast screening programs is to identify women who have no clinical signs of breast cancer but have covert signs suggestive of the disease. The chances of cure are greatest when breast cancer is detected when the tumor is small and located in only one breast.

The primary screening tools currently available include regular breast self-examination, examination by a health professional, and mammography. Mammography is also used as a diagnostic tool in women with a palpable lump, as is ultrasonography. Thermography and diaphanography are used occasionally. Fine-needle aspiration or open biopsy are necessary for definitive diagnosis. However, prior to the collection of objective data, a thorough history on BSE findings, risk factors, and relevant historical data should be completed.

Monthly Breast Self-Examination

Monthly BSE has been shown to be the most effective method for early detection of breast cancer (American Cancer Society, 1988). Approximately 95% of breast lumps are found by women themselves.

Mammogram

A **mammogram** is a soft-tissue x-ray image taken of the breast without the injection of a contrast medium. It can detect lesions in the breast before they can be felt. A mammogram also serves as a diagnostic tool in making a differential diagnosis.

Currently the American Cancer Society, the AMA Council on Scientific Affairs (1989), and the American College of Radiology suggest the following mammogram screening guidelines:

- Baseline mammogram between ages 35 and 40

- Mammogram every 1 to 2 years between ages 40 and 49

- Mammogram annually for all women over age 50

Mammography is less effective for the diagnosis of abnormalities in younger, denser breast tissue. In light of the low incidence of breast cancer in women under age 30, it is suggested that sonography and aspiration are of greater benefit in evaluating breast masses in these women. A screening mammogram should only be used in this age group on women with a strong clinical suggestion of cancer (Ellerhorst-Ryan et al 1988). Controversy exists about the benefit of a screening mammogram in young women who have undergone augmentation mammoplasty. Concern exists that, because 22% to 83% of breast tissue is obscured by the implants, a lump may not be felt, even during professional examination (Hayes et al 1988). Thus, mammography may be recommended for this group.

Mammography is a useful tool, but it cannot replace BSE or physical examination. Up to 15% of early-stage breast cancers are detected by physical examination and

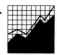

Research Note

Clinical Application of Research

Breast self-examination (BSE) can lead to early detection and treatment of breast cancer, yet only 30% of women regularly practice this technique. Mary Wyper (1990) used variables from the Health Belief Model in an effort to determine what factors contribute to the performance of BSE.

The model hypothesized two constructs that impacted the practice of BSE. The first construct, perceived threat of breast cancer, developed from combining the modifying factors of perceived susceptibility to breast cancer and perceived seriousness of breast cancer. The second construct incorporated the modifying factors of perceived benefits of BSE weighed against perceived barriers to BSE. The performance of BSE was examined through the variables of frequency, thoroughness, and a variable called BSE practice which was created by multiplying frequency by thoroughness.

Correlations between the health belief variables and the breast self-exam variables showed some correlation between susceptibility and both thoroughness and practice as well as correlation between benefits and the variables of frequency, thoroughness, and practice. However, the strongest correlations were between barriers and all three BSE variables and between the net perceived efficacy variable and the three variables of BSE. Multiple regression showed that barriers contributed 19% of the total explained variance of 22% for BSE. Some barriers to the performance of BSE included forgetting to perform the task, feeling unmotivated, creating worry about outcome, and not being certain of how to perform the procedure.

Critical Thinking Applied to Research

Strengths: Thorough review of research literature regarding breast self-examination. Development of theoretical model from literature. Reporting of tests for reliability and validity for this study.

Wyper M: Breast self-examination and the health belief model: Variations on a theme. *Res Nurs Health* 1990; 13: 421.

are not detected by mammogram (Ellerhorst-Ryan et al 1988).

Breast Examination by a Health Care Provider

The American Cancer Society and the American College of Obstetricians recommend that all women have their breasts examined annually by a trained health care provider. A woman at increased risk of breast cancer should have her breasts examined more frequently. If a woman finds a suspicious lump during BSE, she should be examined as soon as possible. If the health care provider finds a suspicious lump during breast examination, the care giver may order additional testing, or referral may be made to a surgeon, oncologist, or breast specialist. Figure 8–3 shows a decision tree for evaluating a palpable breast mass.

The physician also felt the lump and thickening, and now I'm waiting for my mammogram. In these few days my thoughts and feelings have been a roller coaster. I'm 46, and I'm wondering if this is it. Am I dying? Now? I'm afraid as I have not been afraid since one of our children was very ill. Try as I may to fill my head with other thoughts, it keeps slipping back to this.

Ultrasonography

Ultrasound of the breast is a painless, noninvasive method of detecting breast abnormalities. It can distinguish cysts from solid masses but cannot differentiate between malignant and nonmalignant cells. Ultrasound is used primarily to determine the location of cysts for needle aspiration. It is useful in women under 30 for whom mammography is not indicated and can be used to evaluate breast masses in women who are pregnant. It is especially useful in women with multiple cysts who need repeated examinations and in whom multiple aspirations would be prohibitive.

Thermography

Thermography is a pictorial representation of heat patterns on the surface of the breast. Breast cancer tends to have a higher metabolic rate and may appear as a "hot spot" on the film. Because of the high incidence of false results, thermography has not gained wide acceptance.

Diaphanography

Diaphanography, also known as transillumination, is a painless, noninvasive imaging technique that involves shining a light source through the breast tissue to visualize its interior. It is a valuable tool in diagnosing benign and malignant lesions when used in combination with mammography and physical examination. It appears to be more sensitive than mammography in evaluating younger, dense breast tissue, but its reliability is not sufficiently established to justify its use independent of mammography (Ellerhorst-Ryan 1988).

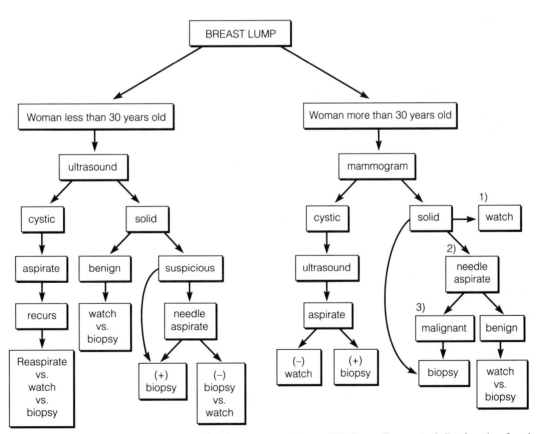

Figure 8–3   Decision tree for evaluating palpable breast mass. From Ellerhorst-Ryan et al: Evaluating benign breast disease. Nurse Pract *1988; 13(9):24.*

Needle Biopsy

Definitive diagnosis of a suspicious mass beyond the non-invasive preliminary screening and diagnostic techniques already mentioned always involves biopsy of some kind, by either aspiration or incision.

A fine-needle aspiration (biopsy) is accomplished by inserting a needle into the mass to withdraw cells or cystic fluid for microscopic examination. A fine needle on a hypodermic syringe is typically used by physicians to aspirate cystic fluid. Aspiration biopsy may be done in the physician's office or as an outpatient procedure. A wider needle may be used when removing a biopsy sample of cells from a solid mass. Needle biopsy is not always a definitive diagnostic procedure, and surgical (incisional) biopsy may still be necessary. Needle biopsies cannot conclusively rule out the presence of cancerous cells. Hence aspiration biopsy has been viewed by practitioners as only a supplemental diagnostic technique.

Surgical (Incisional) Biopsy

Incisional biopsy is the primary diagnostic technique for confirming the presence of cancer in a solid breast mass. Incisional biopsy involves direct examination of a portion of the tumor for microscopic evaluation by either frozen section or permanent section. Staging the cancer to determine its extent may follow the biopsy.

Surgical biopsy is performed on an outpatient basis with the woman under local anesthesia, the use of which has eliminated the postoperative complications common with general anesthesia. The tissue sample obtained during biopsy is sent out as a permanent section, and a pathologist's report is sent to the surgeon within a few days. During a follow-up office visit to the surgeon, the woman is given the results and the opportunity to discuss the best breast cancer treatment alternative for her. This two-step approach to breast cancer diagnosis has gained support from women and health care professionals alike. Participation in decision-making incorporates women, and possibly their families, as active partners. A decision made in this fashion is less likely to be regretted later.

Treatment of Breast Cancer

Within the medical profession, controversy persists regarding the treatment alternatives for breast cancer. What the physician decides is the best treatment for a woman with a newly diagnosed breast cancer may not be what the woman wishes. The physician's major concern may be the attainment of cure, necessitating a more radical surgical treatment, whereas the woman may feel that the threatened loss of a valued body part is equally important.

The treatment of breast cancer is based upon the following combination of treatment modalities: surgery, chemotherapy, radiation therapy, and hormone therapy (Knorr et al 1987). As stated previously, the treatment protocol is based upon the staging of the cancer at the time of di-

agnosis as well as regional cancer center protocols and philosophies.

If a woman is diagnosed with breast cancer during pregnancy, much more conservative treatment modalities are used. Treatment depends on the stage of the disease at the time of diagnosis. If possible, treatment is delayed until after childbirth. If waiting until then is not possible, the surgical treatment modality is initiated with special attention to the anesthesia utilized during the surgery. Radiation therapy, chemotherapy, and hormone therapy should be avoided during pregnancy, if at all possible, due to potential damage to the fetus.

Surgical Treatment Alternatives

As early as 1650, treatment of breast cancer involved removal of the affected breast (Weber 1983). The standard American surgical treatment was established in the 1890s when Halsted described the procedure now known as the Halsted radical mastectomy. This procedure entailed the removal of the entire breast, skin, pectoralis major and minor muscles, lymph nodes of the axilla, and surrounding fat tissue.

The unfortunate aspect of radical breast surgery is its mutilation. Breast cancer treatment has a significant emotional impact on the woman's integrity, body image, self-concept, and sexual identity. Because of the possibility of residual cancer cells after surgical intervention, many surgeons believe it is logical to remove the greatest amount of tissue in the hope of curative treatment. However, recent studies (Mann et al 1988) have offered proof that conservative breast surgery in early disease, combined with radiotherapy, gives five–year survival results that are as satisfactory as the modified radical mastectomy. It is important for the nurse to realize that the aim of surgical breast cancer treatment is threefold:

1. To preserve the woman's life
2. To minimize recurrence
3. To provide the best cosmetic results possible

Currently available surgical approaches include various types of mastectomy, local wide excision, and breast reconstruction.

Radical mastectomy is the procedure previously described. It is less commonly used today.

Extended radical mastectomy uses the Halsted radical mastectomy procedure plus the removal of the internal mammary lymph nodes.

Modified radical mastectomy involves removing the entire breast and the axillary contents; however, the pectoralis major muscle is preserved. Currently it is the surgical treatment of choice in many cases.

Total (simple) mastectomy refers to the surgical removal of the breast but not the pectoral muscle. This procedure is used for early-stage breast cancer and is usually followed by postoperative irradiation of regional lymph nodes. Breast reconstruction can be combined with the mastectomy or done at a later time.

Subcutaneous mastectomy evolved as a procedure to complement breast reconstruction. The internal breast tissue is removed and the skin of the breast remains. An implant is then inserted to restore breast shape. It is best used in breast cancers that are noninvasive and located away from the nipple.

Partial (segmental) mastectomy removes the tumor and 2 to 3 cm of surrounding tissue. Some of the breast remains. Axillary node dissection and the removal of at least a portion of the nodes are recommended. Current trends support the use of both radiation and chemotherapy in women who have positive lymph nodes when segmental mastectomy is done (Margolese 1986).

Wide local excision (tylectomy or lumpectomy) removes only the tumor mass and a narrow margin of normal tissue surrounding the mass. In early-stage breast cancer, simple excision followed by definitive radiation yields local tumor control and survival rates that compare favorably with those of other treatments (Knorr et al 1987). The procedure is done for cosmetic effect in women who are highly motivated to preserve the breast. However, many women are not suitable candidates for excision and irradiation because of the stage or type of cancer they have. Another advantage of the lumpectomy is that, depending on the size of the area excised and the duct involvement, women may be able to breast-feed following future pregnancies.

Breast reconstruction may be done using a variety of implants and surgical approaches. Candidates for breast reconstruction are women with a mass less than 2 cm and fewer than three positive nodes. Women who have received a radical mastectomy or the extended mastectomy are not good candidates because they lack sufficient amounts of skin and muscle. Table 8–3 lists the advantages and disadvantages of reconstructive surgery; Table 8–4 summarizes breast reconstruction procedures.

Additional Therapy

Radiation therapy to the breast is recommended for women who have had wide local excision (conservative treatment) and is started as soon as the incision has healed (Marchant 1990).

An assay of the breast cancer can be done to determine whether the malignant cells are estrogen-receptor–positive or negative. In premenopausal women with estrogen-receptor–positive tumors, oophorectomy can provide about a 65% chance of tumor remission (Duanne 1988).

Additive hormonal therapy involves administering large doses of estrogen, androgen, or progestin in postmenopausal women. High doses of these hormones have been observed to cause tumor regression, although the exact mechanism of interaction is unknown. Antiestrogen therapy has produced responses in about 70% of women who had estrogen-receptor–positive tumors or had previously responded to hormone therapy (Duanne 1988). Tamoxifen, an antiestrogen, is now commonly used in adjuvant therapy of postmenopausal women with receptor-positive neoplasms (Duanne 1988).

Adjuvant chemotherapy is recommended to cure microscopic metastatic disease in women with positive lymph nodes. Opinion varies as to the value of using chemotherapy or tamoxifen in women with negative lymph nodes, and at present there is no consensus as to the best approach (Marchant 1990).

Metastatic Disease

Metastatic breast cancer is characterized by the presence of cancer cells in distant parts of the body. Four sites of me-

---

Table 8–3 Advantages and Disadvantages of Reconstructive Breast Surgery

Advantages	Disadvantages
Improved physical appearance	The reality that the reconstructed breast is never identical to the unaffected breast
An invaluable psychologic lift and improvement of body image	The expense and risk of further surgical procedures
The ability to wear normal clothing without worrying about exposing a prosthesis	The possibility of an unsatisfactory result or surgical complications
The opportunity to resume more strenuous activities (eg, sports) without being concerned about exposing a prosthesis	The fact that the reconstructed breast will never replace the lost one

Table 8–4 Breast Reconstruction Procedures

Type	Procedure	Surgical Treatment amenable to reconstruction	Treatment considerations
Implant methods Silicone get implants	Internal prosthesis is inserted through a small incision at the base of the fold area of the affected breast. The implant is positioned underneath the breast skin.	Used with modified radical mastectomy, simple mastectomy, partial mastectomy, subcutaneous mastectomy, or lumpectomy	1. General side effects of surgery, including hemorrhage, infection, and edema. 2. Necrosis of the covering skin or discoloration of the skin over the implant. 3. The breast may harden into a baseball shape as a result of a fibrous capsule of scar tissue. 4. Improper placement may lead to an undesirable shape. 5. Inflatable implants can leak and deflate, necessitating their removal. 6. The size and shape of the remaining breast may need alteration, requiring a subsequent procedure to reduce/increase the unaffected breast. 7. Several basic surgical procedures allow the implant to be inserted at the time of the cancer surgery. 8. This is the least expensive and complicated of breast reconstruction surgeries.
Inflatable implants	After the implant is inserted in the above fashion, a saline solution is injected into the saucer-shaped form, and the wound is closed.		
Flaps	Series of procedures: 1. A flap is created from upper/lower abdomen, thigh, buttocks, or back into a tube of skin (pedicle). 2. Pedicle is attached to the chest. 3. Lower end of the pedicle is severed, and the tube of tissue is twisted and sutured over the missing breast area. 4. After the skin covering is sufficiently thick, an incision is made at the base of the skin mound, and an implant is inserted.	Used with Halsted radical mastectomy or extended radical mastectomy	1. General side effects of surgery, including hemorrhage, infection, and edema. 2. Flap methods can result in infection and tissue rejection. 3. More scarring occurs due to the numerous surgeries. 4. Symmetry between the breasts is difficult to achieve, and augmentation or reduction of the unaffected breast is usually necessary. 5. Flap method involves four to five hospitalizations and is very expensive.
Areola-nipple reconstruction	Nipple may be removed at the time of cancer surgery and checked for malignant cells. If it is free of carcinoma, it may then be sewn on the thigh or abdomen for transplantation later. Nipples also have been removed and put in a nipple bank until reconstruction is done The nipple is grafted onto the reconstructed breast as a separate procedure.	Used with any of the breast cancer surgeries following other reconstruction	1. General side effects of surgery, including hemorrhage, infection, and edema. 2. Nipple may become discolored. 3. Nipple graft may not take. 4. A new nipple may need to be created using skin from the labia or earlobe, and tatooing can be necessary to achieve pigmentation. 5. Many women are content with a created breast form and don't choose to have the additional procedure of nipple grafting. 6. Because of the potential problems and the risk that the woman's nipple may contain malignant cells, there is a trend toward constructing a new nipple rather than using the woman's nipple.

tastasis are the lungs, the viscera (liver), the brain, and bone. The woman with breast cancer metastasis has a shortened life expectancy, and her survival is frequently contingent on the organ systems involved in the metastasis and her response to therapy. In metastatic disease endocrine manipulation and chemotherapy are used to interrupt the cellular growth and spread of the cancer cells. Radiation therapy directed at a specific area and surgery are used palliatively to relieve the pain or obstruction associated with metastatic tumor spread. Metastatic disease is considered to be advanced or terminal when the cancer spread cannot be controlled by any of the therapeutic interventions previously discussed.

Metastatic breast cancer can cause various symptoms, depending in part on the organ affected. Metastasis to bone can cause a great deal of pain that is exacerbated by movement. Analgesics must be taken on a regular schedule to maintain a constant serum level of analgesia. Radiation therapy of affected areas may alleviate skeletal pain. Visceral metastasis can involve ascites, which require diuretic therapy and possibly paracentesis. Lung metastasis often results in pleural effusions and difficulty in breathing. Brain metastasis can produce an alteration in sensorium, particularly memory loss, headaches, visual disturbances, seizures, and ataxic gait.

Psychosocial issues related to metastatic breast cancer change from those related to cure and restoration of body image to those related to the achievement of quality survival and symptom control. In the presence of a disease that is not yet curable, hope takes on new meaning. Hope for cure is replaced by hope for continuing availability of therapeutic options, treatment responsiveness, long-term survival, freedom from symptoms, and hope that life-style patterns and interpersonal relationships will remain intact.

Psychosocial Concerns of the Woman with Breast Cancer

Sometimes a woman does not seek medical attention following the discovery of a breast lump. Factors that appear to be significant in delay include attempts to deny the presence of a lump, lack of knowledge about breast disorders, fear of mutilating surgery, fear of body image change, fear of relationship changes, and reluctance to submit to diagnostic and therapeutic procedures. Compared with women who seek treatment promptly, women who delay tend to believe more strongly that the condition is not serious, experience a greater sense of powerlessness, and use more avoidance defenses in coping. They are also more likely to be depressed. Related psychosocial problems of delaying women have included marital problems, rejection by family members, and a general sense of isolation related to living alone.

When a woman is confronted with a breast mass she initiates a decision-making process about her diagnostic and treatment options and her approach to her condition. The optimal solution for her is more likely to be achieved if she uses reason, acts systematically, and makes a decision consistent with her preferences and beliefs. The most consistent influence on a woman's decision making is her physician. Nevertheless, the woman is the only person who can decide what benefits of surgery are worth what personal risks. Despite the seriousness of the diagnosis, the time constraints, and the expense involved, the woman should be encouraged to seek a second opinion, which is now paid for by many third-party payment plans.

In the early phases of treatment an emotional dichotomy often prevails: The woman experiencing a mastectomy deals with both the potential loss of life due to cancer and the loss of a breast or a portion of it. Yet in the period immediately preceding and following mastectomy, health professionals tend to emphasize treatment of the cancer so that the woman will comply with her therapeutic regimen. The issue of breast loss is postponed. In the early postoperative phase, the woman may experience strong pressure from her partner, family, friends, and health care team to "do well" by adjusting quickly and easily to the surgery. Most American women have been socialized to be "good" by pleasing others. To please her mate or her physician, a woman may begin to deny some of her feelings, particularly about the loss of the breast. She may hold back her questions and refrain from talking about her feelings to make a good impression. Nurses need to encourage women to discuss breast loss and body disfigurement. Otherwise the natural grieving associated with this loss may be delayed.

The course of adjustment confronting the woman with breast cancer has been described as four phases: shock, reaction, recovery, and reorientation (Gyllenskold 1982). In the shock phase women make statements like "Everything is unreal" or "I can't understand what is happening to me." Shock extends from the discovery of the lump through the process of diagnosis.

Reaction occurs in conjunction with the initiation of treatment. As treatment begins, the woman is compelled to face what has occurred and begins to take in what has happened. Coping mechanisms become evident during this phase. Reaction coincides with the length of treatment, and for many women radiation treatment ·or chemotherapy prolongs this period to months. During the phases of shock and reaction the woman is completely absorbed with what has caused the problem. Treatment reinforces the diagnosis of cancer and the immediate consequences of the disease. Denial of breast loss and the reality of the illness is common during the periods of diagnosis and treatment. Denial protects the woman, making therapy tolerable.

Recovery begins during convalescence following the completion of medical treatment. Anxiety about her illness diminishes and the woman looks to the future once more. She turns outward and gradually resumes her former activities. Conversely, depression and social isolation occur if the woman is unable to negotiate the recovery phase successfully.

A woman's family and friends significantly influence her recovery. Women often perceive their partners as their primary source of support. However, both members of a couple must adjust to her condition and its implications, as well as to the effect of therapy on their sexual intimacy. Difficulties with psychosocial adjustment to breast cancer tend to be similar for women and their partners except in the area of role adjustments, where women have more difficulty. Research suggests that both the women and their partners show improvements in mood and adjustment over time, although symptoms of distress remained elevated for up to 30 days after surgery (Northouse & Swain 1987).

Friends and relatives may be reluctant to initiate social interaction during the recovery period. The woman's own uncertainty about resuming previous activities coupled with friends' reticence about "pushing her" may result in a more withdrawn lifestyle.

Reorientation follows recovery and is unending. It is accomplished when the woman can acknowledge that breast cancer is a part of her life, yet living, for her, has returned to or perhaps exceeded its former fullness and meaning.

Nursing Care of the Woman with Breast Cancer

Nursing care of the woman with breast cancer is multidimensional. It involves meeting the educational, psychosocial, psychosexual, and physical needs of the woman, and to a certain extent, those of her family. In meeting these needs the nurse functions as care giver, counselor, educator, liaison, and advocate. The nursing care changes as the woman progresses from the period of diagnosis to the recovery period.

Nursing Care During the Diagnostic Period

Nursing care begins before a woman faces a diagnosis of breast cancer. Indeed, the nurse can significantly affect the woman's prognosis by encouraging early detection of malignant tumors. Health teaching can assist the woman in understanding breast cancer treatment alternatives before disease occurs. If breast cancer is diagnosed, awareness of possible choices enables a woman to select the treatment regimen she perceives is best for her individual needs.

Nursing Assessment

The woman seeking health care following discovery of a lump is likely to be apprehensive. She may hold unfounded beliefs about breast cancer. Holistic health assessment should be conducted in an understanding, unhurried, emotionally supportive atmosphere. Such an assessment has therapeutic value in itself. It should include:

- A systems review emphasizing the reproductive system, particularly the breast
- The significance the woman attributes to her breasts
- The woman's knowledge and beliefs about breast cancer
- Identification of social support (family, friends, clergy, etc)
- The woman's emotional status and coping mechanisms she has used during periods of stress
- Environmental factors that may influence coping and adjustment

Assessment of the woman facing a diagnosis of breast cancer must be an ongoing process. Sufficient data must be obtained to provide the nurse and other health team members with increasing insight into the client's biophysical, mental, emotional, and social situation.

Nursing Diagnosis

Nursing diagnoses that may apply during the diagnostic period include the following:

- Knowledge deficit related to the diagnostic procedures
- Fear related to the possibility of a diagnosis of cancer

Nursing Plan and Implementation

The nurse should assure the woman that she will be able to participate in decision making about her treatment once the biopsy results are known. Nursing advocacy involves supporting the woman's right to make the best decision for her. With the assistance of the nurse the woman can explore her fears, clarify her values, and identify the treatment options that would be personally acceptable. Once the woman has made an informed decision, the nurse's role becomes one of support. The woman and her partner should be told the treatment alternatives together once the results of the biopsy are known.

Nursing Care During the Preoperative Period

If a diagnosis of cancer is made and the woman elects to have a surgical intervention, nursing care is directed to the assessments and care typically indicated prior to any surgery, as well as the assessments indicated by the woman's condition.

Nursing Assessment

The nurse assesses the woman's health status with regard to any evidence of infection, especially respiratory infection, which would increase her risk of complications. The nurse inquires about medication allergies, previous experience with surgery, and any factors in the woman's history (for example, previous episodes of thrombophlebitis or routine use of steroid medication) that increase her risk.

The nurse also assesses the woman's knowledge of her condition, what to expect from surgery, and what postoperative care involves. Finally the nurse assesses the woman's and her family's emotional state and attitude toward the surgery.

Nursing Diagnosis

Nursing diagnoses that might apply preoperatively include the following:

- Knowledge deficit related to the surgical procedure
- Anxiety related to possible change in body image following surgery
- Ineffective individual coping related to inability to accept the reality of the cancer diagnosis

Nursing Plan and Implementation

The nurse explains the routines, equipment, and procedures that are pertinent to the woman's hospital stay, including preoperative preparation and the care and assessments that are done postoperatively. The nurse may also have the woman practice deep breathing and coughing and leg exercises. The nurse provides the woman and her family with opportunities to ask questions and express their feelings. It is important for the woman to feel that she is receiving care from individuals who are not only skilled technically but also concerned about her as a person.

Nursing Care During the Postoperative Period

Nursing care during the postoperative period changes as the woman progresses and adapts following surgery. The woman's needs in the immediate postoperative period, for example, are somewhat different from those on the third postoperative day.

Nursing Assessment

The nurse assesses the woman's condition postoperatively to detect any potential complications. Vital signs are assessed regularly for evidence of change, and the nurse is alert to other signs that might indicate shock. The dressing is inspected and reinforced as necessary, and the quantity of drainage in the wound suction device (Hemovac) is monitored.

In addition, other routine postoperative assessments are made. The nurse auscultates the woman's lungs, assesses the abdomen for distention, evaluates urinary output, monitors the intensity of the woman's discomfort, and regulates the intravenous fluids.

After the immediate postoperative period, the nurse continues to assess the woman for evidence of infection, discomfort, and emotional problems. Throughout the postoperative period the nurse evaluates the woman's teaching needs and plans appropriate interventions.

Nursing Diagnosis

Nursing diagnoses that may apply during the postoperative period include the following:

- Potential alteration in respiratory function related to the effects of anesthesia and immobility
- Potential for infection related to surgical intervention
- Pain related to surgery

Nursing Plan and Implementation

Following surgery the woman receives appropriate postoperative care. This includes nursing actions to prevent respiratory and circulatory complications and to prevent infection. The nurse is alert to the woman's level of pain and uses medication and nursing techniques to help the woman be comfortable and obtain rest. The woman who has had lymph nodes removed as part of her surgical treatment is at risk of swelling and pain in the arm on her affected side. This is especially true if a radical or modified radical mastectomy was done. The nurse keeps the arm elevated, measures the circumference of the limb, and encourages the woman to use the affected arm for feeding, washing, and hair combing. The nurse also teaches arm exercises such as wall climbing, forward and lateral arm lifts, pendulum swinging, exaggerated deep breathing, and pulley exercises.

The nurse who assumes primary responsibility for helping the woman deal with the psychosocial aspects of her breast loss should provide the woman with opportunities to express her feelings about her breast and its loss. The nurse must be sensitive to the woman's cues as to when it is acceptable to involve the sexual partner in the observation of the woman's incision and in counseling about the woman's altered appearance. The nurse can also discuss the types of prostheses available if reconstruction is not possible or if the woman has decided against it. Even if the woman will be having reconstruction at a later time, she will probably be interested in using a prosthesis temporarily.

Nursing Care During Discharge Planning

Nursing care for discharge planning begins the day that the woman is first encountered in the health care system. It is a long-term planning process the involves the health care team and family. The focus is on follow-up care and resumption of a normal life-style.

Nursing Assessment

The nurse assesses the woman's and family's readiness for discharge planning and teaching. In addition to physical readiness for discharge, the nurse assesses emotional readiness for learning and for discharge. The nurse ascertains if the woman's condition is stable and if she is free of physical and psychosocial complications. Family resources are assessed in order to determine the need for follow-up nursing care and support services in the home.

Nursing Diagnosis

Nursing diagnoses that may apply during discharge planning include the following:

- Potential sexual dysfunction related to loss of body part
- Knowledge deficit related to lack of understanding of the importance of follow-up care
- Knowledge deficit related to community resources

Nursing Plan and Implementation

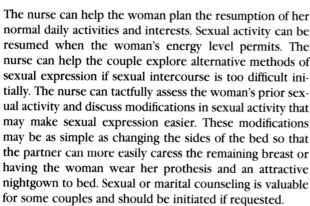

The nurse can help the woman plan the resumption of her normal daily activities and interests. Sexual activity can be resumed when the woman's energy level permits. The nurse can help the couple explore alternative methods of sexual expression if sexual intercourse is too difficult initially. The nurse can tactfully assess the woman's prior sexual activity and discuss modifications in sexual activity that may make sexual expression easier. These modifications may be as simple as changing the sides of the bed so that the partner can more easily caress the remaining breast or having the woman wear her prothesis and an attractive nightgown to bed. Sexual or marital counseling is valuable for some couples and should be initiated if requested.

Prior to discharge the woman should clearly understand her follow-up treatment and care. The nurse can collaborate with the physician regarding planned postoperative therapy so that the woman understands what is involved in any scheduled therapies such as chemotherapy. The woman should thoroughly understand the importance of preventive health care such as BSE and the need to comply with follow-up examinations.

Referrals to either a community health nurse or a "Reach to Recovery" volunteer should be initiated and the date of the visit confirmed with the woman. A "Reach to Recovery" volunteer from the American Cancer Society is invaluable in helping the woman adjust to her mastectomy. Each volunteer has had a mastectomy herself and often serves as a role model for the woman with a new mastectomy. The American Cancer Society volunteer can provide the woman with information about breast prostheses and guidelines for arm exercises and self-care.

Evaluation

Anticipated outcomes of nursing care include the following:

- The woman copes successfully with the diagnosis of breast cancer and the therapy she chooses.
- The woman clearly understands her diagnosis and treatment, her therapy, and her long-term prognosis.
- If she receives surgery, the woman has a successful recovery period. If complications do occur they are quickly recognized and treatment is begun.
- The woman participates in planning her recovery program.
- The woman completes planned exercises, activities, follow-up, and additional therapy.

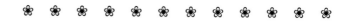

Care of the Woman with Endometriosis

Endometriosis is a condition characterized by the presence of endometrial tissue outside the endometrial cavity. This tissue responds to the hormonal changes of the menstrual cycle and bleeds in a cyclic fashion. This bleeding results in inflammation, fibrosis, and formation of adhesions. The most common symptoms include progressive dysmenorrhea, dyspareunia (painful intercourse), and infertility.

Endometriosis may occur at any age after puberty, although it is most common in women between 30 and 40 and is rare in postmenopausal women. A familial tendency does seem to exist.

The exact cause of endometriosis is unknown. Proposed theories of etiology include retrograde menstrual flow and inflammation of endometrium, hereditary tendency, and most recently, an immunologic defect (Talbert & Kauma 1990).

The pelvic pain associated with endometriosis is cyclic in nature, due to the normal monthly fluctuations in hormones. It is postulated that estrogen and progesterone stimulate endometrial-like tissue growth, like that which occurs in the uterus during the menstrual cycle. The tissue even becomes secretory in nature and bleeds just like a menstrual period. The bleeding causes pressure and inflammation in the adjacent tissues, causing pain (Treybig 1989).

The most common sites of endometriosis are the ovaries, the uterosacral ligaments, and the cul-de-sac. However, endometriosis can involve many body organs remote from the pelvis and thus produce a host of complications. For example, intrathoracic endometriosis can result in pneumothorax (Chagares 1987).

Women with certain menstrual characteristics are more at risk for developing endometriosis. A woman with a menstrual cycle length of 27 days or less and a menstrual flow lasting a week or more has twice the risk compared to a woman with longer cycle length and shorter flow duration (Treybig 1989).

The long-term sequelae of endometriosis are many and range from minor to the most serious complication, infertility. This is caused by interference with ovum release and tubal movement secondary to tubal adhesions.

Medical Therapy

Somewhat paradoxically, the extent of a woman's symptoms does not necessarily indicate the extent of her endometriosis. A woman may have extensive involvement with few symptoms or only a few lesions with severe incapacitation. The most common symptom is pelvic pain, which is often a dull ache or cramping sensation. It is often related to menstruation and generally ceases following the completion of the woman's menses. Dyspareunia, another common symptom, occurs most frequently if the uterus is retroverted and lesions are present in the area of the posterior vaginal fornix or the uterosacral ligaments.

Another frequently cited symptom is abnormal uterine bleeding. No specific pattern exists, although it may be frequent, prolonged, and excessive.

Endometriosis is often diagnosed when a woman seeks treatment or evaluation for infertility. Bimanual examination may reveal a fixed, tender, retroverted uterus and palpable nodules in the cul-de-sac. The diagnosis can be confirmed by laparoscopy or laparotomy.

Treatment may be medical, surgical, or a combination of the two. During the laparoscopic examination, the physician may surgically resect any visible implants of endometrial tissue, taking care to avoid damaging any organs. Laser vaporization can be used for all but the deepest implants (Batt & Severino 1990). This allows for more exact removal of tissue, less adjacent tissue damage, and decreased bleeding. If the woman does not desire pregnancy at the present time, she may be started on oral contraceptives. In women with minimal disease and symptoms, treatment includes observation, analgesics, and nonsteroidal anti-inflammatory medication (NSAID). The woman who desires pregnancy and has been unsuccessful in her attempts to conceive is treated with a six-month course of danazol. (See Drug Guide on danazol.) Nasal Nafarelin (400 μg/d) is also useful in reducing the size of implants and in relieving pain. The drug is a gonadotropin–releasing hormone agonist (GnRH) (Batt & Severino 1990). Nafarelin has an action and side effects similar to those of danazol.

In more advanced cases surgery may be done to remove implants and break up adhesions. If severe dyspareunia or dysmenorrhea are symptoms, the surgeon may perform a presacral neurectomy. In advanced cases in which childbearing is not an issue, a hysterectomy with bilateral salpingo-oophorectomy may be done.

❀ *APPLYING THE NURSING PROCESS* ❀

Nursing Assessment

The nurse should be aware of the common symptoms of endometriosis and elicit an accurate history if a woman mentions these symptoms. If a woman is being treated for endometriosis, the nurse should assess the woman's understanding of the condition, its implications, and the treatment alternatives.

Nursing Diagnosis

Nursing diagnoses that may apply to a woman with endometriosis are listed in the Nursing Care Plan.

Nursing Plan and Implementation

The nurse can be available to explain the condition, its symptoms, treatment alternatives, and prognosis. The nurse can help the woman evaluate treatment options and make choices that are appropriate for her. If medication is begun, the nurse can review the dosage, schedule, possible side effects, and any warning signs. Women are often advised to avoid delaying pregnancy because of the risk of infertility. The woman may wish to discuss the implications of this decision on her life choices, relationship with her partner, and personal preferences. The nurse can be a nonjudgmental listener and help the woman consider her options. (See Nursing Care Plan—Endometriosis.)

Evaluation

Anticipated outcomes of nursing care include the following:

- The woman clearly understands her condition, its implications for fertility, and her treatment options.

- The woman successfully copes with the discomfort and long-term implications of her diagnosis.

- After considering her options, the woman chooses appropriate treatment options and therapy.

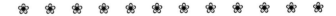

Care of the Woman with Toxic Shock Syndrome

Toxic shock syndrome (TSS) was first described in children (Todd et al 1978). Two years later the association between TSS and menstruation was identified (Johnson 1985). Although TSS has been reported in children, postmenopausal women, and men, it is primarily a disease of women

DRUG GUIDE
Danazol (Danocrine)

Overview of Action

Danazol is a testosterone derivative with a mild androgenic effect. The drug has an antigonadotropic effect that results in the suppression of both follicle-stimulating hormone (FSH) and luteinizing hormone (LH). As a consequence, ovulation is suppressed and amenorrhea develops. Danazol also reduces levels of sex steroids by inhibiting the enzymes responsible for their production, and binds steroid hormone receptors on endometrial tissue implants (Hill & Herbert 1988). This results in atrophy of endometrial tissue implants and endometrium within the uterus. Dose-related menstrual changes have been associated with this drug. At lower dosages (50–100 mg), menstrual bleeding may be regular or irregular. With dosages of 200–400 mg, 40% to 90% of women experience amenorrhea. Progress of endometriosis is stopped and the woman's pain is relieved. The drug may also be used to treat fibrocystic breast disease.

Route, Dosage, Frequency

Endometriosis: 400 mg, orally, two times per day for three to six months. Therapy is begun if pregnancy test is negative or during woman's menstrual period. Treatment may be extended for nine months or restarted if symptoms recur.

Breast disease: 400 mg/day orally. Long-term effects of treatment not known.

Contraindications

Pregnancy

Breast-feeding women

Impaired kidney, heart, or liver function

Undiagnosed abnormal vaginal bleeding

Side Effects

Vaginal bleeding	Acne
Vasomotor instability	Oily skin and hair
Hirsutism	Weight gain

Reduced libido	Decreased breast size
Voice changes, hoarseness	Irritability, depression
Edema	Sleep disorders, fatigue
Muscle cramps	Gastroenteritis
Headaches	Signs of atrophic vaginitis
Nausea	Alopecia
Clitoral enlargement	Amenorrhea

Changed lab values including: reduced high-density lipoprotein (HDL); increased low-density lipoprotein (LDL); increased liver enzyme levels (serum glutamic-oxaloacetic transaminase [SGOT], serum glutamic-pyruvic transaminase [SGPT], creatinine phosphokinase [CPK], lactic dehydrogenase [LDH])

Nursing Considerations

1. Inform woman about potential side effects; stress that menses and ovulation usually resume within two to three months after discontinuing therapy.

2. Continue routine breast examinations and report any enlarged or hardened breast nodules.

3. Obtain baseline and other liver function tests as ordered.

4. Voice changes should be reported immediately and the medication stopped to avoid permanent damage.

5. Observe woman for signs of virilization.

6. Since ovulation may not be suppressed, a back-up, nonhormonal form of birth control should be used if the woman wishes to avoid conception (Govoni & Hayes 1988).

of reproductive age, especially at or near menses or during the postpartum period. The causative organism is a strain of *Staphylococcus aureus* that produces a specific toxin called TSST-1. Although the vast majority of women have antibodies to *S. aureus,* only a few ever develop signs of the disease. Research indicates a possible link between high levels of estradiol and inhibition of toxin production. If this is the case, it would explain the higher incidence of

TSS during menstruation and the postpartal period when estradiol levels are low.

The use of high-absorbency tampons has been widely related to an increased incidence of TSS. However, occluding the cervical os with a contraceptive device such as a diaphragm or contraceptive sponge, especially if they are left in place for more than 24 hours, may also increase the risk of TSS.

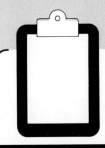

Nursing Care Plan
Endometriosis

Nursing History:

1. Predisposing risk factors include:
   a. Single
   b. Delayed childbearing
   c. Positive familial history
   d. Higher socioeconomic class
   e. Retroflexed uterus
   f. Underweight

2. Symptoms:
   a. Onset typically 30 to 40 years of age (may appear at younger age)
   b. Suprapubic pain may start a few days to a few weeks before onset of menses—associated with a late decline of symptoms, which may last until day 6; pain may eventually last the entire month.
   c. Dyspareunia
   d. Painful defecation
   e. Rectal pressure
   f. Abnormal uterine bleeding
   g. ≤27-days of menstrual cycle and seven days of menses

3. Menstrual history:
   a. Menarche—normal age
   b. Frequency—every 27 days or less
   c. Duration—7 days or more
   d. Associated symptoms such as pain, rectal bleeding, intermenstrual bleeding
   e. Amount—normal or excessive

4. History of Symptoms
   a. Cyclic, associated with menstrual cycle
   b. Increased severity over time
   c. Infertility after 6 months to one year unprotected intercourse
   d. Long-term oral contraceptive use—symptoms begin after discontinued

5. Physical Examination
   a. External genitalia may have small bluish lesions on the labia or perineal area.
   b. Speculum examination may reveal lesions on the cervix and vaginal wall.
   c. Bimanual examination may reveal the following:
      i. Tender nodes palpable along the uterosacral ligaments, cul-de-sac of Douglas, and above the posterior fornix of the vagina
      ii. Ovaries may be enlarged, tender, fixed
      iii. May have adnexal thickening and nodularity
      iv. Uterus retroverted and fixed; pain elicited with movement

Diagnostic Studies:

a. Negative pregnancy test, chlamydia culture, gonorrhea culture; nonreactive serology
b. Normal Pap smear, CBC, and u/a
c. Positive radioimmunoassay for cell surface antigens and endometrial antibodies

Nursing Diagnosis	Nursing Interventions	Rationale	Evaluation
Pain related to dysmenorrhea *Client Goal:* Woman will obtain relief of pain as evidenced by her verbal expressions of comfort, ability to sleep, ability to participate in activities of daily living.	Promote comfort through: 1. Judicious use of analgesics and nonsteroidal anti-inflammatory medications (NSAIDs) 2. Adequate rest periods 3. Provision of emotional support 4. Use of supportive nursing measures such as backrubs, relaxation techniques, diversional activities.	Comfort is essential to enable the woman to function optimally in her daily activities.	Woman states she is free of pain. She is able to rest well and participate in daily activities.

(continued)

Nursing Care Plan (continued)

Nursing Diagnosis	Nursing Interventions	Rationale	Evaluation
	5. Application of heat to affected areas.		
	6. Promotion of physical exercise—aerobics and pelvic tilt.		
	7. Diet modification including: a. Decreased salt b. Increased intake of foods that are natural diuretics: peaches, watermelon, cranberry juice, asparagus		
Knowledge deficit related to lack of understanding of disease process. *Client Goal:* Woman will be able to discuss her condition, its treatment, and her care needs.	Provide effective client education by: 1. Explaining anatomy and physiology of the reproductive tract, the diagnosis, associated symptomatology, treatment alternatives, and progress. 2. Discussing daily living alternatives. 3. Instructing woman regarding NSAIDs: start medication at the onset of symptoms or at least one day before scheduled menses; maintain consistent pattern for taking medication. 4. Discussing potential side effects and contraindications of NSAIDs. 5. Explaining the use of the symptom diary and basal body temperature chart. 6. Instructing woman to contact her care-giver if symptoms worsen. 7. Giving woman specific information on the medication prescribed for her: a. Danazol (see Drug Guide) b. Ibuprofen 400 mg po q4h.	Women have the right and the responsibility to be actively involved in their own health care to the extent that they are able to actively participate. The woman needs appropriate information to make decisions.	The woman clearly understands her condition, its implications and the treatment options as evidenced by her discussion of these topics and her cooperation with care (demonstrated in her use of the symptom diary).

(continued)

Nursing Care Plan (continued)

Nursing Diagnosis	Nursing Interventions	Rationale	Evaluation
	c. Naproxen sodium 500 mg po initially followed by 250 mg q6–8h d. Mefenamic acid 500 mg po initially followed by 250 mg q4–6h. e. 6-month course of nafarelin acetate nasal spray (400 g/d) f. 3–6 month course of leuprolide acetate 0.5 mg subcutaneously daily g. Suppression therapy with oral contraceptives.		
Ineffective individual coping related to depression secondary to infertility. *Client Goal:* The woman successfully copes with the discomfort and long-term implications of the diagnosis.	Promote effective coping by: 1. Discussing life choices and relationship with partner. 2. Discussing personal preferences, values, etc. 3. Discussing treatment options for infertility (See Chapter 9) 4. Identifying positive coping skills 5. Demonstrating a non-judgmental attitude by supportive listening. 6. Identifying positive coping skills. 7. Referring the woman to a counselor and/or support group (if needed). 8. Encouraging the woman to express and deal with grief related to infertility. 9. Referring the woman to community resources as needed.	Woman with endometriosis may become depressed not only because of the disease itself but also because of the secondary infertility. Positive coping skills will allow her to feel fulfilled and satisfied with her life.	The woman successfully copes with the diagnosis as evidenced by verbal expression of satisfaction, a positive affect, and active participation in her life.

Medical Therapy

Early diagnosis and treatment are important in preventing a fatal outcome. The case-to-fatality ratio has decreased from 15% to 3% (Eschenbach 1990).

The most common signs of TSS include fever (often greater than 38.9C [102F]); desquamation of the skin, especially the palms and soles, which usually occurs one to two weeks after the onset of symptoms; a sunburn-like rash; hypotension; and dizziness. Systemic symptoms often include vomiting, diarrhea, severe myalgia, and inflamed mucous membranes (oropharyngeal, conjunctival, or vaginal). In addition, disorders of the central nervous system, including alterations in consciousness, disorientation, and coma, may occur.

Laboratory findings reveal elevated BUN, creatinine, SGOT, SGPT, and total bilirubin, while platelets are often less than 100,000/mm³. Blood, throat, and CSF cultures are negative, as are tests for Rocky Mountain spotted fever (Colls 1986).

Women with TSS are generally hospitalized and given supportive therapy, including intravenous fluids to maintain blood pressure. Severe cases may require dialysis, administration of vasopressors, and intubation. Penicillinase-resistant antibiotics, while of limited value during the acute phase, do help reduce the risk of recurrence (Eschenbach 1990).

❀   *APPLYING THE NURSING PROCESS*   ❀

Nursing Assessment

Nurses caring for women should ask about their clients' tampon use practices. The nurse should pay special attention to women who customarily wear their tampons for extended periods of time or who leave a diaphragm or contraceptive sponge in place longer than six hours after intercourse. The nurse should also be alert for early signs of TSS and refer women with them to a physician for further evaluation.

Nursing Diagnosis

Nursing diagnoses that may apply to a woman with TSS include the following:

- Knowledge deficit related to ways of preventing the development of TSS
- Pain related to severe myalgia secondary to TSS

Nursing Plan and Implementation

Nurses play a major role in helping educate women about ways of preventing the development of TSS. Women should understand the importance of avoiding prolonged use of tampons. Tampons should be changed every 3 to 6 hours,

and super-absorbency tampons should be avoided. Some women may choose to use other products, such as sanitary napkins or minipads. The woman who chooses to continue using tampons may reduce her risk by alternating them with napkins and by avoiding overnight use of tampons.

Postpartal women are advised to avoid the use of tampons for six to eight weeks after childbirth. Women with a history of TSS should totally refrain from using tampons (Eschenbach 1990).

Women who use barrier contraceptives such as diaphragms or contraceptive sponges should avoid leaving them in place for prolonged periods. These devices should not be used during the postpartum period or when the woman is menstruating.

Nurses can also help make women aware of the signs and symptoms of TSS so that women will seek treatment promptly if signs occur.

Evaluation

Anticipated outcomes of nursing care include the following:

- The woman understands the cause of toxic shock syndrome and modifies any personal practices that might increase her risk of developing TSS.
- If a woman develops TSS, treatment is effective and any potential problems are quickly identified and corrected.
- A woman with a history of TSS does not have a recurrence.

❀   ❀   ❀   ❀   ❀   ❀   ❀   ❀   ❀   ❀   ❀   ❀

Care of the Woman During a Pelvic Examination

Women have a pelvic examination performed for a variety of reasons ranging from health maintenance to disease diagnosis. The pelvic exam is often perceived by women as an uncomfortable and embarrassing procedure. The negative feelings may cause women to delay having yearly gynecologic examinations, and this avoidance may pose a threat to life and health.

To make the pelvic examination less threatening, and thus improve health-seeking behavior, more health care providers are performing what is called an educational pelvic examination. During this type of exam the woman becomes an active participant and has an opportunity to learn about her body, voice her concerns, and share decisions regarding her care.

The educational exam includes offering the woman a mirror to watch the procedure, pointing out anatomic parts to her, and positioning and draping her to allow eye-to-eye contact with the practitioner. The woman is encouraged to participate by asking questions and giving feedback.

Nurse practitioners, nurse-midwives, and physicians all perform pelvic examinations. Nurses assist the practitioner and the woman during the examination. Procedure 8–1 provides information on assisting with a pelvic examination.

Vulvar Self-Examination

During the pelvic examination many care givers also provide education about self-examination of the vulva. This procedure, like the self-examination of the breast, permits early detection of abnormalities, thereby maximizing the possibility of cure and the use of conservative treatment approaches (Lawhead 1990).

Self-examination of the vulva is simple to perform. The woman is advised to assume a sitting position on a bed or chair. In good light she holds a mirror in one hand and uses her other hand to expose the tissue of her perineum while she carefully inspects and palpates the area. Pregnant or obese women may find it easier to inspect the area while standing with one foot placed on a low stool (Lawhead 1990). Any abnormalities or changes should be reported to the woman's health care provider.

The examination should be performed monthly at the same time as the BSE in all sexually active asymptomatic women or women over age 18. Women with a history of vulvar lesions or women with symptoms should inspect their vulva more frequently.

Care of the Woman with a Vaginal Infection

Candida albicans (Moniliasis)

Moniliasis (often called "yeast infection") is the most common form of vaginitis affecting the vagina and vulva. Recurrences are frequent for some women. Factors that contribute to occurrence of this infection are use of oral contraceptives, use of antibiotics, pregnancy, diabetes mellitus, presence of human immunodeficiency virus (HIV), use of feminine hygiene products, and other premenstrual factors that are unclear. A gram-positive fungus (*Candida albicans*) is the causative organism. *Candida* is a resident of the mouth, intestines, and vagina in 25% to 50% of healthy women (Horowitz et al 1987). Infection seems to occur when there is overgrowth of this organism.

Medical Therapy

The goal of medical therapy is to diagnose the infection and treat it effectively. The woman will often complain of thick, white, curdy vaginal discharge; severe itching; dys-

uria; and dyspareunia. A male sexual partner may experience a rash or excoriation of the skin of the penis, and possibly pruritus. The male may be symptomatic and the female asymptomatic.

On physical examination the woman's labia may be swollen and excoriated if the pruritus has been severe. A speculum examination reveals thick, white, tenacious cheeselike patches adhering to the vaginal mucosa. Diagnosis is confirmed by microscopic examination of the vaginal discharge; hyphae and spores will usually be seen on a wet mount preparation (Figure 8–4).

Medical treatment of monilial vaginitis includes intravaginal insertion of miconazole, butaconazole, teraconazole, or clotrimazole suppositories or cream at bedtime for 3 days to one week. Recently clotrimazole vaginal inserts and cream have become available over-the-counter. It is indicated for women with a history of yeast infection who clearly recognize the symptoms. If the vulva is also infected, the cream is prescribed and may be applied topically. Nystatin and single-dose therapy are less effective than recommended therapies. Pregnant women are treated the same as nonpregnant women (Centers for Disease Control 1989). Infection at the time of childbirth may cause thrush in the neonate.

Because *Candida* may be harbored in the folds of the skin of the penis, it may be necessary to treat the sexual partner to prevent recurrence of the vaginitis in the woman. Topical miconazole usually eliminates the yeast infection

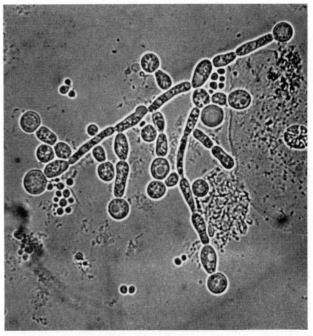

Figure 8–4 *The hyphae and spores of* Candida albicans *(Courtesy Centers for Disease Control)*

Nursing Responsibilities During Pelvic Examination

Nursing action	Rationale
Objective: Assemble and prepare equipment.	
Prepare and arrange following equipment so that they are easily accessible:	Examination is facilitated.
	Warmed speculum assists in lubrication and facilitates initial insertion when culture and smears are to be taken. Do not use lubricant on speculum prior to insertion. This may alter findings or cultures.
1. Various-sized vaginal specula, warmed with water or on a heating pad prior to insertion.	
2. Gloves.	
3. Water soluble lubricant.	
4. Materials for Pap smear and cultures.	
5. Good light source.	
Objective: Prepare woman.	Explanation of procedure decreases anxiety.
Explain procedure.	Comfort is promoted during internal examination. She may feel more comfortable with shoes on rather than supporting her weight with bare heels against cold stirrups.
Instruct woman to empty her bladder and to remove clothing below waist. She may be encouraged to keep her shoes on and will be given a disposable drape or sheet to place on her lap. Encourage her to sit on the end of the examining table with the drape across her lap prior to examination. Provide a warm environment either through overhead heat lights or through central heat. If a woman has never had a pelvic examination before, show her the equipment and explain the procedure prior to examination.	
Position woman in lithotomy position with thighs flexed and adducted. Place her feet in stirrups. Buttocks should extend slightly beyond end of examining table (Figure 15–3).	
Drape woman with a sheet, leaving flap so perineum can be exposed.	
Objective: Provide support to woman as physician or nurse practitioner carries out examination.	
Explain each part of examination as it is performed: inspection of external genitals, vagina, and cervix: bimanual examination of internal organs. Instruct woman to relax and breathe slowly.	Relaxation is promoted.
Advise woman when speculum is to be inserted and ask her to bear down.	When speculum is inserted, woman may feel intravaginal pressure. Bearing down helps open vaginal orifice and relax perineal muscles.
Lubricate examiner's finger well prior to bimanual examination.	Lubrication decreases friction and eases insertion.
Objective: Provide for woman's comfort at end of examination.	
Move to the end of the examining table and face woman's perineum. Cover the woman with the drape. Apply gentle pressure to the woman's knees and encourage her to move toward the head of the table. Offer your hand to the woman, remove her heels from the stirrups, and assist the woman to a sitting position. Be sure that she is not dizzy and that she is sitting or standing safely before you leave the room.	Supine position may create postural hypotension.
Provide tissues to wipe lubricant from perineum.	Upon assuming sitting position, vaginal secretions along with lubricant may be discharged.
Provide privacy for woman to dress.	Comfort and sense of privacy is promoted.

from the male. However, the CDC states that treatment of the sex partner is not necessary unless candidal balanitis is present or chronicity is a problem. Women with frequent unexplained infections should be evaluated for predisposing conditions and the diagnosis confirmed with a culture (Centers for Disease Control 1989). Colposcopic examination of the region will rule out condylomatous lesions as a contributing factor (Deitch & Smith 1990).

If miconazole cream is being used by both partners, sexual intercourse is permitted and may assure the spread of the cream throughout the vagina. With other methods of treatment, abstinence is recommended until both partners are cured.

Nursing Assessment

The nurse caring for the woman should suspect monilial vaginitis if the woman complains of intense vulvar itching and a curdy, white discharge. Because the woman with diabetes mellitus during pregnancy is especially susceptible to this infection, the nurse should be alert for symptoms in these women. In some areas, nurses are trained to do speculum examinations and wet mount preparations and can, therefore, confirm the diagnosis themselves. In most cases, however, the nurse who suspects a vaginal infection reports this to the woman's physician, nurse practitioner, or certified nurse-midwife.

Nursing Diagnosis

Nursing diagnoses that might apply to the woman with monilial vaginitis include the following:

- Potential impaired skin integrity related to scratching secondary to the effects of the monilial infection
- Knowledge deficit related to ways of preventing the development of monilial vaginitis

Nursing Plan and Implementation

If the woman is experiencing discomfort due to the pruritus, the nurse can recommend gentle bathing of the vulva with a weak sodium bicarbonate solution. If a topical treatment is being used, the woman should bathe the area before applying the medication.

The nurse also discusses with the woman the factors that contribute to the development of monilial vaginitis and can suggest ways to prevent recurrences, such as wearing cotton underwear, careful wiping front to back following elimination, and avoiding the use of panty hose, tight jeans, and feminine hygiene products such as vaginal powders, vaginal sprays, deodorant tampons, deodorant pads, douches, bubble bath, deodorant soap, and perfumed lubricants. Some women report that the addition of yogurt to the diet or the use of activated culture of plain yogurt as a

vaginal douche helps prevent recurrence by maintaining high levels of lactobacillus.

Evaluation

Anticipated outcomes of nursing care include the following:

- The woman's symptoms are relieved and the infection is cured.
- The woman is able to identify self-care measures to prevent further episodes of monilial vaginitis.

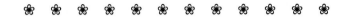

Bacterial Vaginosis (*Gardnerella vaginalis* Vaginitis)

Many flora normally inhabit the vagina of the healthy woman. Some of these organisms are potentially pathogenic. In some women these bacteria begin to "overgrow," causing a vaginitis. The cause of this overgrowth is not clear, although tissue trauma and sexual intercourse are sometimes identified as contributing factors. The *Gardnerella vaginalis* organism (formerly referred to as *Hemophilus vaginalis*) has been found in the vast majority of cases, along with an increased concentration of anaerobic bacteria. The infected woman often notices an excessive amount of thin, watery, yellow-gray vaginal discharge with a foul odor described as "fishy." The characteristic "clue" cell is seen on a wet mount preparation (Figure 8–5). Also, there is a positive amine "whiff" test. When the discharge is mixed with the potassium hydroxide on a wet mount, a "fishy odor" is emitted.

The nonpregnant woman is generally treated with metronidazole (Flagyl). Because of its potential teratogenic effects, metronidazole is avoided during pregnancy. 300

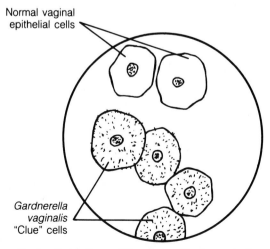

Figure 8–5 Depiction of the clue cells characteristically seen in bacterial vaginosis (Gardnerella vaginalis)

mg clindamycin twice a day for 7 days is used instead (Centers for Disease Control 1989). Clindamycin has been shown to be as effective as metronidazole in the treatment of bacterial vaginosis but without the concerns of teratogenesis or the side effects (Greaves et al 1988). Recent studies suggest that bacterial vaginosis in pregnancy may be a factor in premature rupture of membranes and preterm birth. These studies require confirmation, however (Centers for Disease Control 1989).

Asymptomatic infections are common in nonpregnant women and generally are not treated. No clinical counterpart of bacterial vaginosis exists in males, and treatment of male sex partners has not shown to be beneficial for the woman or the male partner (Centers for Disease Control 1989).

Care of the Woman with a Sexually Transmitted Infection

The occurrence of **sexually transmitted infection (also called a sexually transmitted disease [STD])** has increased over the past few decades. The terms *venereal disease* and *VD* are being used less frequently; they appear outdated and carry value-laden, negative connotations. No matter how these infections are classified, women often feel anxious, guilty, embarrassed, or fearful when they have or suspect they have vaginitis or a sexually transmitted infection. Vaginitis and sexually transmitted infections are the most common reasons for outpatient treatment of women.

Table 8–5 provides a summary of sexually transmitted infections and their treatment. Precautions specific to a particular sexually transmitted infection are noted with discussion of that infection.

Trichomoniasis

Between 15% and 20% of all women are infected with trichomoniasis at some time. This infection is most frequently seen in females 16 to 35 years of age. Women are usually symptomatic, although some women who are carriers have no noticeable discomfort. Between 60% and 90% of the male partners may be asymptomatic. Worldwide, trichomoniasis infects an estimated 180 million people annually (Thomason & Gelbart 1989).

Trichomonas is a microscopic motile protozoan that thrives in an alkaline environment. Most infections are acquired through sexual intimacy. Transmission by shared

Table 8–5 Summary of Sexually Transmitted Diseases

Disease	Organism	Diagnosis	Treatment Nonpregnant	Pregnant
Vulvovaginal candidiasis	*Candida albicans*	Wet-mount hyphae	Miconazole	Miconazole
Bacterial vaginosis	Anaerobic normal flora	Wet-mount clue cells	Metronidazole	Clindamycin
Trichomoniasis	Trichomonads	Wet-mount trichomonads	Metronidazole	None
Syphilis	*Treponema pallidum*	Dark-field examination VDRL or RPR	Benzathine Penicillin G	Benzathine Penicillin G
Herpes genitalis	Herpes simplex virus	Herpes culture	Acyclovir	None
Chlamydia	*Chlamydia trachomatis*	Chlamydia culture	Doxycycline	Erythromycin base
Gonorrhea	*Neisseria gonorrhoeae*	Gonorrhea culture	Ceftriaxone and Doxycycline	Ceftriaxone and Erythromycin base
Acquired immunodeficiency syndrome	Human immunodeficiency virus	ELISA test	Varies	Varies
Condyloma acuminata	Human papilloma virus	Virapap Biopsy Pap smear	Cryotherapy Podophyllin	Cryotherapy Trichloracectic acid
Pediculosis pubis	*Phthirus*	Microscopic identification of lice or nits	Permethrin 1% Creme Rinse or Lindane 1% shampoo	Permethrin 1% Creme Rinse
Scabies	*Sarcoptes scabiei*	Confirmation of symptoms or scraping of furrows	Lindane 1% lotion	Crotamiton 10% lotion

bath facilities, wet towels, or wet swimsuits may be possible (Centers for Disease Control 1989). In women, this parasite lives only in the genitourinary tract—on squamous epithelial cells lining the vagina, Skene's glands, and urethra. In men, it lives in the urethra, prostate gland, and—in uncircumcised males—under the foreskin. *Trichomonas* can change the normal vaginal environment, promoting growth of anaerobic bacteria and resulting in the development of bacterial vaginosis. It may also serve as a carrier (or vector) for transmission of human viral diseases because it ingests cells containing virus particles (Thomason & Gelbart 1989).

Medical Therapy

Symptoms of trichomoniasis include a yellow-green, frothy, odorous discharge frequently accompanied by inflammation of the vagina and cervix, dysuria, and dyspareunia. Visualization of *Trichomonas* under the microscope on a wet-mount preparation of vaginal discharge will confirm the diagnosis (Figure 8–6).

Prescriptive treatment for trichomoniasis is metronidazole administered over 7 days or in a single 2-g dose for both male and female sexual partners. Intercourse should be avoided until both partners are cured.

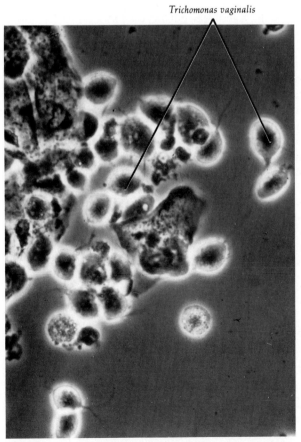

Trichomonas vaginalis

Figure 8–6 Microscopic appearance of Trichomonas vaginalis *(Courtesy of Centers for Disease Control)*

The woman should be informed that metronidazole is contraindicated in the first trimester of pregnancy because of possible teratogenic effects on the fetus. However, no other adequate therapy exists. For women with severe symptoms *after the first trimester*, treatment with 2 g of metronidazole in a single dose may be considered (Centers for Disease Control 1989). The woman and her partner should be cautioned to avoid alcohol while taking metronidazole; the combination has an effect similar to that of alcohol and Antabuse—abdominal pain, flushing, or tremors (Centers for Disease Control 1989).

Various vaginal creams, suppositories, or douches may decrease symptoms without clearing up the infection. The only treatment proven to be effective is metronidazole. Therefore, other methods are not recommended.

Chlamydial Infection

Chlamydial infection, caused by *Chlamydia trachomatis*, is the most common STD in the United States. The organism is an intracellular bacterium with several different immunotypes. Immunotypes of *Chlamydia* are responsible for lymphogranuloma venereum and trachoma, which is the world's leading cause of preventable blindness.

Chlamydia is a major cause of nongonococcal urethritis (NGU) in men. In women it can cause infections similar to those that occur with gonorrhea. It can infect the fallopian tubes, cervix, urethra, and Bartholin's glands. Pelvic inflammatory disease, infertility, and ectopic pregnancy are also associated with chlamydia (Bourcier & Seidler 1987).

The infant of a woman with untreated chlamydia is at risk of developing ophthalmia neonatorum, which, although responsive to erythromycin ophthalmic ointment, does not respond to silver nitrate eye prophylaxis. The newborn may also develop chlamydial pneumonia. In fact, approximately 30,000 cases of pneumonia in infants 6 months old or less are traceable to chlamydial infections. Pregnant women with asymptomatic cases of chlamydia have a 40% to 70% incidence of neonatal chlamydial infection. Chlamydia may also be responsible for premature labor and fetal death.

Symptoms of chlamydia include a thin or purulent discharge, burning and frequency of urination, and lower abdominal pain. Women, however, are often asymptomatic. Diagnosis is frequently made after treatment of a male partner for NGU or in a symptomatic woman with a negative gonorrhea culture. Moreover, 25% to 60% of heterosexual women with gonorrheal infections also have chlamydia (Centers for Disease Control 1989). Laboratory detection is now simpler due to the availability of a test to detect monoclonal antibodies specific for *Chlamydia.* However, as is the case with syphilis and gonorrhea, women are not routinely screened for chlamydia due to the added expense of the test. The Centers for Disease Control (1989) has identified priority groups for chlamydia screening, including high-risk pregnant women, adolescents, and women with multiple sexual partners.

The usual prescribed treatment for chlamydia is tetracycline or doxycycline. Any woman diagnosed with gonorrhea should also be treated with one of these medications because of the high risk of co-infection with *Chlamydia*. The male sexual partner should also be tested and treated (Centers for Disease Control 1989). Pregnant women should be treated with erythromycin ethyl succinate (Centers for Disease Control 1989). Many authorities are recommending routine treatment of newborns with tetracycline or erythromycin eye ointment to avoid the possibility of conjunctivitis. Barrier contraceptives, especially contraceptive sponges and spermicidally treated condoms, offer some protection against chlamydia (Queenan 1987).

Herpes Genitalis (Herpes Simplex Virus)

Herpes infections are seen in private offices more often than gonorrhea. It is estimated that between 5 and 20 million people in the United States have genital herpes and that 500,000 new cases occur each year (Breslin 1988). The herpes simplex virus is the causative organism. There are two types of herpes:

- Type 1—usually noted to be present above the waist and not usually sexually transmitted (the "cold sore" is the most common herpes type 1 lesion). This type may occur in the genital area, usually as a result of oral-genital sexual contact.

- Type 2—usually associated with genital infections. This type can occur as oral lesions after oral-genital sexual contact if genital lesions are present.

The clinical symptoms and treatment of type 1 and type 2 herpes are the same when they occur in the genital area.

Primary Episode

Multiple blisterlike vesicles appear, usually in the genital area and sometimes affecting the vaginal walls, cervix, urethra, and anus. The vesicles may appear within a few hours to 20 days after exposure and rupture spontaneously to form extremely painful, open, ulcerated lesions. Inflammation and pain secondary to the presence of herpes lesions can cause difficult urination and urinary retention. Inguinal lymph node enlargement may be present. Flulike symptoms and genital pruritus or tingling also may be noticed. A severe primary episode does not necessarily indicate that a woman will be predisposed to frequent or severe recurrences. Primary episodes usually last the longest and are the most severe. Lesions heal spontaneously in 2 to 4 weeks (Netting & Kauffman 1990).

Recurrent Episodes

After the lesions heal, the virus enters a dormant phase, residing in the nerve ganglia of the affected area. Some individuals never have a recurrence, whereas others have regular recurrences. Recurrent lesions usually occur at the site of the primary episode. Recurrences are usually less severe than the initial episode and seem to be triggered by emotional stress, menstruation, ovulation, pregnancy, frequent or vigorous intercourse, poor health status or a generally rundown physical condition, tight clothing, or overheating. Some genital herpes infections may be asymptomatic. It has been reported that 14% to 43% of women with cytologically detected herpes simplex virus may have asymptomatic viral shedding. It is assumed that asymptomatic viral shedding may transmit the herpes infection; this could explain the acquisition of the disease from individuals with no history of genital lesions (Breslin 1988). Diagnosis is made on the basis of the appearance of the lesions, Pap smear or culture of the lesions, and sometimes blood testing for antibodies.

Medical Therapy

There is no known cure for herpes. Prescriptive treatment is available to provide relief from pain and prevent complications from secondary infection. Women may apply acyclovir (Zovirax) ointment to reduce viral shedding and healing time of the lesions. Oral acyclovir can be considered for women with primary episodes and for recurrences. Acyclovir should not be used for pregnant women because its safety has not be established for that group (Centers for Disease Control 1989).

Self-help suggestions include cleansing with povidone-iodine (Betadine) solution to prevent secondary infection and Burow's solution to relieve discomfort. Use of vitamin C or lysine is frequently suggested to prevent recurrence, although studies have not documented the effectiveness of these supplements. Keeping the genital area clean and dry, wearing loose clothing, and wearing cotton underwear or none at all will promote healing. Primary or recurrent lesions will heal without prescriptive therapies.

Women should be advised to abstain from sexual activity while lesions are present. Genital herpes and other diseases causing genital ulcers have been associated with an increased risk of acquiring HIV infection; therefore, condoms should be used during all sexual contact (Centers for Disease Control 1989).

Syphilis

Syphilis is a chronic infection caused by a spirochete, *Treponema pallidum*. Syphilis can be acquired congenitally, through transplacental inoculation, and can result from maternal exposure to infected exudate during sexual contact or from contact with open wounds or infected blood. The incubation period varies from 10 to 90 days, and even though no symptoms or lesions are noted during this time, the woman's blood contains spirochetes and is infectious.

Syphilis is divided into early and late stages. During the early stages (primary), a painless chancre appears at the site where the *Treponema pallidum* organism entered the body. Symptoms include slight fever, loss of weight, and malaise. The chancre persists for about four weeks and then disappears. In six weeks to six months, secondary symptoms appear. Skin eruptions called condylomata lata, which resemble wartlike plaques, may appear on the vulva. Other secondary symptoms are acute arthritis, enlargement of the liver and spleen, iritis, and a chronic sore throat with hoarseness. When infected in utero, the newborn will exhibit secondary stage symptoms of syphilis (Netting & Kauffman 1990). Transplacentally transmitted syphilis, if not treated, can result in stillbirth, preterm birth, and neonatal death (Benoit 1988).

The incidence of syphilis declined after the discovery of penicillin, but since 1958 the incidence has been increasing. More than 40,000 cases were reported in the United States in 1988 (Centers for Disease Control 1989). As a result of the increased incidence and the disease's impact on the fetus in utero, serologic testing of every pregnant woman is recommended; testing is required by some state laws. Testing is done at the initial prenatal screening and repeated in the third trimester.

With adequate early treatment congenital syphilis is preventable. However, one of the following outcomes can occur in the presence of untreated maternal syphilis: (a) second trimester abortion, (b) a stillborn infant at term, (c) a congenitally infected infant born prematurely or at term, or (d) an uninfected live infant. The clinical manifestations and treatment of the syphilitic newborn are discussed in Chapter 32.

Medical Therapy

The goal of medical therapy is to identify women with syphilis and begin antibiotic treatment.

Diagnosis is made by dark-field examination for spirochetes. Blood tests such as VDRL (Venereal Disease Research Laboratories), RPR (Rapid Plasma Reagin), or the more specific FTA-ABS (fluorescent treponemal antibody absorption test) are commonly done. Blood studies may be negative if blood is drawn too early.

For women with syphilis of less than a year's duration, the Centers for Disease Control (CDC) recommend 2.4 million units of benzathine penicillin G intramuscularly. If syphilis is of long (more than a year) duration, 2.4 million units of benzathine penicillin G is given intramuscularly once a week for three weeks. If a woman is allergic to penicillin, doxycycline can be given. Maternal serologic testing may remain positive for eight months, and the newborn may have a positive test for three months.

In the pregnant woman, treatment with penicillin should begin after the first positive test rather than waiting for further testing. Pregnant women who are allergic to penicillin should not be treated with doxycycline or tetracycline. Erythromycin has not been found to be effective in treating pregnant women. Therefore, it is recommended that allergic women be skin-tested to validate their allergy to penicillin and be desensitized in order to be treated with penicillin (Centers for Disease Control 1989). All sexual partners need to be screened and treated.

Gonorrhea

Gonorrhea (popularly called "clap," "GC," "drip," or "dose") is an infection caused by the bacteria *Neisseria gonorrhoeae.* Over 900,000 cases of gonorrhea were reported in the United States in 1988 (Centers for Disease Control 1989). If a nonpregnant woman contracts the disease, she is at risk of developing pelvic inflammatory disease. If a woman becomes infected after the third month of pregnancy, the mucus plug in the cervix will prevent the infection from ascending, and it will remain localized in the urethra, cervix, and Bartholin's glands until the membranes rupture. Then the disease can spread upward.

Medical Therapy

The majority of women with gonorrhea are asymptomatic. Thus it is accepted practice to screen for this infection by doing a cervical culture during the initial prenatal examination. Cultures of the urethra, throat, and rectum may also be required for diagnosis, depending on the body orifices used for intercourse.

The most common symptoms of gonorrheal infection include a purulent, greenish-yellow vaginal discharge; dysuria; and urinary frequency. Some women also develop inflammation and swelling of the vulva. The cervix may appear swollen and eroded and may secrete a foul-smelling discharge in which gonococci are present.

Treatment consists of antibiotic therapy with 250 mg ceftriaxone intramuscularly once plus 100 mg doxycycline by mouth twice a day for 7 days. If the woman is allergic to ceftriaxone, spectinomycin is given followed by the doxycycline. Additional treatment may be required if the cultures remain positive 7 to 14 days after completion of treatment. All sexual partners must also be treated or the woman may become reinfected. Pregnant women should be treated with 250 mg ceftriaxone intramuscularly once plus 500 mg erythromycin by mouth twice a day for 7 days (Centers for Disease Control 1989).

Women should be informed of the need for reculture to verify cure and the need for abstinence or condom use until cure is confirmed. Both sexual partners should be treated if either has a positive test for gonorrhea. It is important to explain why treatment is necessary even if the client has a negative culture or is asymptomatic. For example, false-negative reports are possible. Gonorrhea may be asymptomatic. Untreated infections are associated with the following risks:

- The possibility of pelvic inflammatory disease and secondary infertility.

- Disseminated gonorrhea can involve joints or cause septicemia.

- Infection present at the time of birth causes ophthalmia neonatorum in the infant.

Acquired Immunodeficiency Syndrome (AIDS)

Acquired immunodeficiency syndrome (AIDS) is a fatal disorder caused by a virus. The care of a person with AIDS is primarily supportive, although some medications are being developed that seem to prolong life. The reader is referred to a medical-surgical text for description of this care.

However, because the diagnosis of AIDS or the presence of the AIDS antibody has profound implications for a fetus if the woman is pregnant, AIDS is discussed in greater detail in Chapter 18.

Condyloma Acuminata (Venereal Warts)

Venereal warts occur in all age groups and develop in more than 50% to 70% of sexual partners of infected individuals. They are relatively common, with an incidence of 50 per 100,000 population (Netting & Kauffman 1990). The causative organism is human papilloma virus (HPV). A woman often seeks medical care after noting "bumps" in the genital area. Single or multiple soft, grayish-pink, cauliflowerlike lesions may be observed (Figure 8–7).

The moist warmth of the genital area is conducive to the growth of condyloma, which may be present on the vulva, vagina, cervix, and anus. The virus is transmitted through sexual contact. The incubation period following exposure is 3 weeks to 3 years.

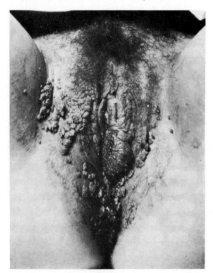

Figure 8–7 *Condylomata acuminata on the vulva (From Danforth's Obstetrics and Gynecology, Scott, JR, Disaia PJ, Hammond, CB, Spellacy, WN, (eds.) 6th ed., 1990, Fig. 47–1, p. 935.*

Approximately 50 HPV types have been identified so far, and a number of these types are associated with malignant transformation resulting in cancer of the anogenital tract (Lucas 1988). In women with abnormal Pap smears, the prevalence of HPV is 80% to 96% (Lucas 1990). HPV proliferates during pregnancy due to immunosuppression, increased hormonal activity and increased vascularity. HPV in pregnancy has been associated with laryngeal papilloma in the newborn (Lucas 1990).

Medical Therapy

Because condyloma sometimes resembles other lesions and malignant transformation is possible, all atypical, pigmented, and persistent warts should be biopsied and treatment should be instituted promptly. The treatment of choice for pregnant and nonpregnant women is cryotherapy with liquid nitrogen to destroy the lesions (Centers for Disease Control 1989). An alternative therapy is topically applied podophyllin, which the woman is instructed to wash off four hours after application. The drug is not used during pregnancy because it is thought to be teratogenic and in large doses has been associated with fetal death. If the woman is pregnant or if the lesions do not respond to podophyllin, trichloroacetic acid (TCA) may be used. Carbon dioxide laser therapy, performed under colposcopy, has a good success rate. This is probably because use of the colposcope aids in detecting tiny "satellite" lesions (Centers for Disease Control 1989).

Generally HPV is asymptomatic, although recently it has been associated with monilialike symptoms (Enterline & Leonardo 1989). Women with chronic yeast infections with a negative monilia culture should be screened for HPV with colposcopy. HPV is most commonly detected by Pap smear and the visualization of external lesions. The type of HPV virus may be identified using the recently developed Virapap test (Irwin 1990).

Medical literature has indicated a link between the occurrence of condyloma and abnormal cell changes of the cervix or possibly cervical cancer. Women with abnormal Pap smears, especially if condyloma is identified, should be screened for HPV with a colposcopic examination. During the colposcopy, biopsies are taken to confirm the diagnosis. If the cellular atypia is due to HPV, treatment is initiated promptly with cryotherapy or laser therapy (McQuistan 1989). All male sex partners need to be screened and treated because of the high rate of transmission and recurrence (Lucas 1988). Pregnant women are treated with cryotherapy, laser therapy, or TCA. A cesarean birth is not necessary because the perinatal rate of transmission is low (Lucas 1990).

Pediculosis Pubis (Pubic or Crab Louse)

Pubic lice occur more commonly in adults than in children. Pediculosis pubis is caused by *Phthirus,* a grayish parasitic "crab" louse that lays eggs that attach to the hair shaft. Transmission is primarily by sexual contact, but transmission through shared towels and bed linens is possible.

Medical Therapy

Symptoms include intense pruritus in areas covered by pubic hair. Occasionally lice are present in chest hair, armpits, eyelashes, and eyebrows. "Crabs" or brown-red spots may be noted in the underwear. Diagnosis is made by clinical and microscopic identification of adult lice or nits (eggs). Pediculosis is treated with 1% Permethrin creme rinse applied to the affected area for 10 minutes, plus combing of the pubic hair with a fine-tooth comb. Over-the-counter medications are safe but less effective. Women should be instructed to launder or dry clean all contaminated linens or clothing. All sexual partners or members of the household should be treated. The woman should be warned of possible toxicity with overuse of the medication. Women should be cautioned not to use medication in or around their eyes. Pediculosis of the eyelashes should be treated by the application of occlusive ophthalmic ointment to the eyelid margins, 2 times a day for 10 days, to smother lice (Centers for Disease Control 1989).

Clients should be reevaluated in 1 week if symptoms persist. Retreatment may be necessary if lice are found or eggs are observed at the hair-stem junction. Alternative treatment is with pyrethrins and piperonyl butoxide applied to the affected area and washed off after 10 minutes or lindane 1% (Kwell) shampoo applied for 4 minutes and thoroughly washed off. Lindane is not recommended in pregnant or lactating women (Centers for Disease Control 1989).

Scabies

Sarcoptes scabiei is an ectoparasitic itch mite. The female mite burrows under the skin to deposit her eggs. Transmission is by intimate sexual contact and contact with household members.

Medical Therapy

Symptoms include pruritus that worsens at night or when the individual is warm. Noticeable erythematous, papular lesions or furrows may be present. Diagnosis is made by confirmation of the symptoms or scraping of the furrows to obtain mites. Prescriptive therapy is 1% lindane (Kwell) lotion applied from the neck down after taking a bath and thoroughly washed off after eight hours. This treatment is not recommended in pregnant or lactating women. In the pregnant woman, crotamiton 10% should be applied to the entire body from the neck down for 2 nights and thoroughly washed after 24 hours after the second application. Clothing and bed linen should be washed and dried in a hot dryer or dry cleaned (Centers for Disease Control 1989). The woman should be advised that sexual partners and other household members should also be treated.

Clothing and household linens should be laundered and air dried or dry cleaned. Persistent pruritus often occurs after treatment; the woman should be aware that pruritus does not signify that the treatment is ineffective. She should be cautioned that overuse of lotion can cause toxicity.

General Principles of Nursing Intervention

❀ *APPLYING THE NURSING PROCESS* ❀

Nursing Assessment

The nurse working with women must become adept at taking a thorough history and identifying women at risk for sexually transmitted infections. Factors that place a woman at risk for STDs are multiple sexual partners, partners with high-risk behaviors, a partner's involvement with other sexual partners, use of feminine hygiene products, high-risk sexual activities such as intercourse without barrier contraception or anal intercourse, treatment with antibiotics while taking oral contraceptives, and young age at onset of sexual activity. The nurse should be alert for signs and symptoms of sexually transmitted infections and familiar with diagnostic procedures if infection is suspected.

While each STD has certain distinctive characteristics, the following complaints suggest the possibility of infection and warrant further investigation:

- Presence of a "sore" or lesion on the vulva
- Increased vaginal discharge or malodorous vaginal discharge
- Burning with urination
- Dyspareunia
- Bleeding after intercourse
- Pelvic pain

In many instances the woman is asymptomatic but may report symptoms in her partner, especially painful urination or urethral discharge. It is often helpful to ask the woman whether her partner is experiencing any symptoms.

Nursing Diagnosis

Nursing diagnoses that may apply when a woman has a sexually transmitted disease include the following:

- Altered family processes related to the effects of a diagnosis of STD on the couple's relationship
- Knowledge deficit related to the long-term effects of the diagnosis on childbearing status

- Personal identity disturbance related to difficulty in accepting the knowledge that the condition is sexually transmitted

Nursing Plan and Implementation

Education for Self-Care

In a supportive and nonjudgmental way the nurse provides the woman who has a sexually transmitted infection with information about the disease, methods of transmission, implications for pregnancy or future fertility, and importance of thorough treatment. If treatment of her partner is indicated, the woman must understand that it is important to prevent a continuous cycle of reinfection. She should also understand the need to abstain from sexual activity, if necessary, during treatment.

The woman should be instructed about the correct procedure for taking her medication and should clearly understand the importance of any follow-up assessments. Prevention of STDs should be stressed with all women. Women in a monogamous relationship with a low-risk partner are at least risk for STD. Multiple sexual partners, previous history of STD, and IV drug use are associated with higher risk, as are high-risk activities such as anal intercourse and exchange of body fluids. Women should be encouraged to require partners, especially new partners, to use a condom.

If a woman suspects she has an infection she should abstain from intercourse and seek testing. Disappearance of symptoms does not mean the infection is cured. If medication is prescribed it is important to complete the full prescription. Treatment of sexual partners is an important part of therapy to prevent recurrence or spread.

Provision of Psychologic Support

Some sexually transmitted infections such as trichomoniasis or chlamydia may cause a woman concern but once diagnosed are rather simply treated. Other STDs may also be fairly simple to treat medically but may carry a stigma and be emotionally devastating for the woman. Diseases such as pediculosis pubis may cause a woman to feel "unclean," while syphilis, since it is reportable, may leave the woman feeling exposed and vulnerable. Herpes can be especially difficult to deal with emotionally because it causes discomfort and is not presently curable.

The sensitive nurse can be especially helpful in encouraging the woman to explore her feelings about the diagnosis. She may experience anger or feel "betrayed" by a partner; she may feel guilt or see her diagnosis as a form of "punishment"; or she may feel concern about the long-term implications for future childbearing or ongoing intimate relationships. She may experience a myriad of differing emotions that she never expected. Opportunities to discuss her feelings in a nonjudgmental environment can be especially helpful. The nurse can offer suggestions about

support groups if indicated and assist the woman in planning for her future with regard to sexual activity.

More subtly, the nurse's attitude of acceptance and matter-of-factness conveys to the woman that she is still an acceptable person who happens to have an infection.

Evaluation

Anticipated outcomes of nursing care include the following:

- The infection is identified and cured if possible. If not, supportive therapy is provided.
- The woman and her partner understand the infection, its method of transmission, its implications, and the therapy.
- The woman copes successfully with the impact of the diagnosis on her self-concept.

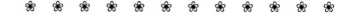

Care of the Woman with Pelvic Inflammatory Disease

Pelvic inflammatory disease (PID) occurs in approximately 1% of women between 15 and 39, although sexually active young women between 15 and 24 have the highest infection rate (Eschenbach 1990). Fifteen percent to 40% of all infertility is attributed to PID (Shattuck 1988). The disease is more common in women who have had multiple sexual partners, a history of PID, early onset of sexual activity, recent gynecologic procedure, or an intrauterine device. It usually produces a tubal infection (salpingitis) that may or may not be accompanied by a pelvic abscess. However, perhaps the greatest problem of PID is that postinfection tubal damage is associated with a high incidence of infertility.

The organisms most frequently identified with PID include *Chlamydia trachomatis*, *Neisseria gonorrhoeae*, and *Mycoplasma hominis*, although other aerobic and anaerobic organisms that are often part of the normal vaginal flora have also been found in women with PID (Centers for Disease Control 1989).

Medical Therapy

Symptoms of PID include bilateral sharp, cramping pain in the lower quadrants, fever, chills, purulent vaginal discharge, irregular bleeding, malaise, dysuria, nausea, and vomiting. However, it is possible to be asymptomatic and have normal laboratory findings.

Women with chlamydia–associated PID are young (75% are younger than 25 years of age), asymptomatic, experience only low-grade pelvic pain, rarely have an elevated temperature, and frequently have irregular bleeding.

Women with gonorrhea–associated PID have a more pronounced clinical picture (fever, initial pain at menstrual bleeding, and palpable adnexal swelling) (Bourcier & Seidler 1987). Cervical motion tenderness (Chandelier sign) and adnexal swelling are also common with PID, but these signs also occur in appendicitis and ectopic pregnancy, which must be ruled out (Centers for Disease Control 1989).

Diagnosis consists of a clinical examination to define symptoms plus blood tests and a gonorrhea culture and test for chlamydia. Other diagnostic procedures that may be helpful in confirming the diagnosis include the following:

- Elevated white blood count and sedimentation rate
- Wet prep of vaginal secretions that reveals the presence of numerous inflammatory cells and coccoid bacteria
- Culdocentesis that provides fluid containing an elevated white blood count
- Ultrasound to detect the presence of a pelvic abscess
- Laparoscopy to confirm the diagnosis and enable the examiner to obtain cultures from the fimbriated ends of the fallopian tubes

In stressing the accuracy of confirming a diagnosis of PID by the use of laparoscopy, Eschenbach (1986) states:

> It is estimated that for every 100 times a clinical diagnosis of pelvic inflammatory disease is made without visual confirmation, four patients with ectopic pregnancy and three patients with appendicitis are treated for pelvic inflammatory disease, resulting in a critical delay in the correct diagnosis (p 992).

Except in very mild cases, the woman is hospitalized and treated with intravenous antibiotics. Antibiotics such as doxycycline and cefoxitin are used if the causative organism is either *Chlamydia trachomatis* or *Neisseria gonorrhoeae*, while an abscess or the presence of anaerobes or gram-negative rods indicates treatment with clindamycin and an aminoglycoside such as gentamicin. In addition, supportive therapy is often indicated for severe symptoms. The sexual partner should also be treated. If the woman has an IUD, it is generally removed 24 to 48 hours after antibiotic therapy is started (Eschenbach 1990).

After the infection is treated, microsurgical techniques are sometimes used to release any adhesions and repair tubal damage if the woman desires to bear children.

✺ *APPLYING THE NURSING PROCESS* ✺

Nursing Assessment

The nurse is alert to factors in a woman's history that put her at risk for PID. Even though fewer IUDs are available, many women still have them, and the nurse should question the woman about possible symptoms, such as aching pain in the lower abdomen, foul-smelling discharge, malaise, and the like. The woman who is acutely ill will have obvious symptoms, but a low-grade infection is more difficult to detect.

Nursing Diagnosis

Nursing diagnoses that may apply to a woman with PID include the following:

- Pain related to peritoneal irritation
- Knowledge deficit related to a lack of understanding of the possible effects of PID on fertility

Nursing Plan and Implementation

The nurse plays a vital role in helping to prevent or detect PID. The nurse should discuss risk factors related to this infection with clients. The woman who uses an IUD for contraception and has multiple sexual partners should clearly understand the risk she faces. The nurse should discuss signs and symptoms of PID and stress the importance of early detection should the woman develop symptoms.

The woman who develops PID should understand the importance of completing her antibiotic treatment and of returning for follow-up evaluation. She should also understand the possibility of decreased fertility following the infection. If appropriate, the nurse can answer the woman's questions about microsurgical techniques.

The care of the woman who is acutely ill with pelvic abscess is discussed in Chapter 36.

Evaluation

Anticipated outcomes of nursing care include the following:

- The woman clearly understands her condition, her therapy, and the possible long-term implications of PID on her fertility.
- The woman completes her course of therapy, and the PID is cured.

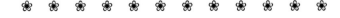

Care of the Woman with Vulvitis

Genital pruritus and soreness may be secondary to a nonpathogenic process. Common causes are:

- Frequent douching or use of over-the-counter douches
- Feminine deodorant spray
- Detergents or harsh soaps

- Colored or perfumed toilet paper
- Contraceptive creams, foams, or suppositories
- Dye as in new clothing
- Synthetic clothing that traps moisture, such as nylon underwear, polyester slacks
- Intercourse without proper lubrication
- Deodorant menstrual pads or tampons
- Estrogen deprivation after menopause

Education for Self-Care

Although women are often told that the practices listed above contribute to vaginitis, this is not necessarily so. In many cases the woman may be experiencing vulvitis without vaginitis.

The nurse can inform women of the possible factors contributing to local irritation and encourage them to avoid practices that contribute to symptoms. Suggestions for good genital hygiene are advisable. The nurse should encourage medical evaluation if symptoms persist. Specifically, a medical evaluation is warranted in postmenopausal women with symptoms because they are at increased risk for vulvar cancer. The nurse should discourage women from treating themselves with over-the-counter anti-inflammatory creams and douches.

Care of the Woman with Cervicitis

Cervicitis is an inflammation of the cervix. It may be caused by an infective process such as gonorrhea, herpes, *Trichomonas*, *Candida*, or *Gardnerella*. Chemical or hygienic products used in the vagina or the presence of foreign bodies may cause cervicitis.

Medical Therapy

Symptoms of cervicitis include yellow discharge with odor, dyspareunia, postcoital bleeding, and irregular bleeding. A woman may be asymptomatic. Diagnosis consists of a clinical examination and appropriate wet mount smear, cultures, or Pap smear. Appropriate treatment is antibiotic therapy, cryotherapy, or removal of any foreign object (IUD or tampon).

Education for Self-Care

The woman should be advised to avoid possible vaginal irritants such as douches or tampons. Medical care should be sought if the woman is symptomatic. If an abnormal reading occurs on a Pap smear report, the nurse should clarify the report for the woman. If the inflammatory finding or Pap smear indicates HPV or condylomata, a colposcopy is performed for further evaluation. It is reassuring to inform

women that an infectious process and cervical irritants can result in an abnormal Pap smear reading. The Pap smear should be repeated after these problems are eliminated.

Care of the Woman with an Abnormal Finding During Pelvic Examination

Abnormal Pap Smear Results

Women tend to expect a report of negative or normal when having a Pap smear done, but various abnormal finding are common. The original purpose of the Pap smear was to detect the presence of cellular abnormalities by obtaining a smear containing cells from the cervix and the endocervical canal. Precancerous or potentially cancerous conditions, as well as cervical cancer, can be identified by microscopic identification.

Cervical dysplasia and cervical carcinoma are known sexually transmitted diseases probably caused by HPV. The increase in sexual activity among teenagers has resulted in increased HPV and abnormal Pap smears in that age group. Thus, annual Pap smears and the use of barrier contraception should be stressed in sexually active women (Spitzer & Krumholz 1988).

Early detection of abnormalities allows early changes to be treated before cells reach a precancerous or cancerous stage. Noncancerous changes in cervical cells may be found, or a false-negative report may occur. Some findings that are classified as abnormal, such as inflammatory or "atypical" cells, are not indicative of cancer. Table 8–6 describes Pap smear classifications and the appropriate response.

Medical Therapy

Diagnostic or therapeutic procedures employed in cases of cellular abnormalities include repetition of Pap smears at shorter intervals, colposcopy and endocervical biopsy, cryotherapy, or laser conization. Decisions for management are based on the specific report.

Colposcopy has evolved as an appropriate "second step" in many cases when a Pap smear is abnormal. The examination, typically done in an office or clinic, permits more detailed visualization of the cervix in bright light using a microscope with magnification six to 40 times (Stafl 1990). The cervix can be visualized directly and again following application of 3% acetic acid. The acetic acid causes abnormal epithelium (dysplasia or carcinoma) to assume a characteristic white appearance. Using the colposcope, a lesion can be localized to obtain a "directed biopsy" (DiSaia 1990).

Women who have multiple sexual partners or a history of herpes, condyloma acuminata, or other STDs have an increased risk of abnormal cell changes and cervical cancer. Some researchers believe that precancerous cer-

Table 8-6 Classification of Pap Smears

Class	Description	Response
1	Negative for malignant cells	Repeat smear annually.
	with *Candida albicans*	Treat with antifungal cream; repeat in three months.
	with *Trichomonas vaginalis*	Treat client and partner with metronidazole; repeat in three months.
	with inflammation	Culture for *Chlamydia trachomatis, Neisseria gonorrhoeae*; treat appropriately.
2	Inflammatory squamous or endocervical atypia	Controversial—if possible refer for colposcopy and biopsy. Otherwise, treat the apparent source of inflammation and repeat in three months. If still atypical, refer for colposcopy.
	Koilocytotic or condylomatous atypia	Refer for colposcopy and biopsy.
3	Dysplasia—mild, moderate, or severe	Refer for colposcopy and biopsy.
4	Positive for in situ carcinoma	Refer for colposcopy and biopsy.
5	Positive for invasive carcinoma	Refer for colposcopy and biopsy.

Source: Spitzer M, Krumholz BA: Pap screening for teenagers: A lifesaving precaution. Contemp OB/GYN *January 1988; 31:33.*

vical cell changes are more common in women who have been exposed to diethylstilbestrol (DES), but other researchers disagree.

If a pregnant woman has an abnormal Pap smear (dysplasia), a colposcopy and biopsies are done to evaluate the disease further. If the biopsy shows anything less than invasive cancer, treatment is postponed until after birth. However, continued evaluation during pregnancy is recommended with Pap smears and colposcopic exams every 3 to 6 months (McGee 1987).

Ovarian Masses

Between 70% and 80% of ovarian masses are benign. More than 50% are functional cysts occurring most commonly in women 20 to 40 years of age. Functional cysts are rare in women who take oral contraceptives.

Ovarian cysts usually represent physiologic variations in the menstrual cycle. Dermoid cysts (cystic teratomas) comprise 10% of all benign ovarian masses. Cartilage, bone, teeth, skin, or hair can be observed in these cysts. Endometriomas, or "chocolate cysts," are another common type of ovarian mass.

Medical Therapy

A woman with an ovarian mass may be asymptomatic; the mass may be noted on a routine pelvic examination. She may experience a sensation of fullness or cramping in the lower abdomen (often unilateral), dyspareunia, irregular bleeding, or delayed menstruation.

Diagnosis is made on the basis of a palpable mass with or without tenderness and other related symptoms.

Radiography or ultrasonography may be used to assist or confirm the diagnosis. Transvaginal ultrasonography has been found to provide a sharper image of the ovaries than abdominal ultrasonography (Modica & Timor-Tritsch 1988). The diagnosis may be confirmed using laparoscopy or laparotomy.

The woman is frequently kept under observation for a month or two because most cysts will resolve on their own and are harmless. Alternatively, oral contraceptives may be prescribed for one or two months to suppress ovarian function. If this regimen has been effective, a repeat pelvic examination should be normal. If the mass is still present after 60 days of observation and oral contraceptive therapy, a diagnostic laparoscopy or laparotomy may be considered. Tubal or ovarian lesions, ectopic pregnancy, cancer, infection, or appendicitis also must be ruled out before a diagnosis can be confirmed.

Surgery is not always necessary but will be considered if the mass is larger than 6 to 7 cm in circumference; if the woman is over 40 years of age with an adnexal mass, a persistent mass, or continuous pain; and if the woman is taking oral contraceptives. Surgical exploration is also indicated when a palpable mass is found in an infant or young girl or in a postmenopausal woman.

Women who are taking oral contraceptives should be informed of their preventive effect against ovarian masses. Women may need clear explanations about why the initial therapy is observation. A discussion of the origin and resolution of ovarian cysts may clarify this treatment plan. If surgery should involve removal or impaired function of one ovary, the woman should be assured that the remaining ovary should take over ovarian functioning and that pregnancy is still possible.

Uterine Masses

Fibroid tumors, also called leiomyomas, are among the most common benign disease entities in women and are the most common reason for gynecologic surgery. Between 20% and 50% of women develop leiomyomas by 40 years of age. The potential for cancer is minimal. Leiomyomas are more common in black women.

Medical Therapy

Smooth muscle cells are present in whorls and arise from uterine muscles and connective tissue. The size varies from 1 to 2 cm to the size of a 10-week fetus. Frequently the woman is asymptomatic. Lower abdominal pain, fullness or pressure, menorrhagia, metrorrhagia, or increased dysmenorrhea may occur, particularly with large leiomyomas. Ultrasonography, especially transvaginal ultrasonography, revealing masses or nodules can assist in and confirm the diagnosis. Leiomyoma is also considered as possible diagnosis when masses or nodules involving the uterus are palpated on a pelvic examination.

The majority of these masses require no treatment and will shrink after menopause. Close observation for symptoms or an increase in size of the uterus or the masses may be the only management most women will require. Routine repeat pelvic examinations every three to six months are commonly recommended unless there are other symptoms. Of particular concern is a mass that does not shrink postmenopausally or that develops postmenopausally and is associated with postmenopausal bleeding. This concern does not apply to postmenopausal women on hormone replacement therapy.

If a woman notices symptoms, or pelvic examination reveals that the mass is increasing in size, surgery (myomectomy, dilation and curettage, or hysterectomy) will be recommended. The choice of surgery depends on the age and reproductive status of the woman and/or the significance of the noted changes. There are no medications or therapies to prevent fibroids. However, fibroids are estrogen-dependent tumors; estrogen supplementation (premarin) can stimulate their growth and antiestrogen medications (danazol) can prevent their growth.

General Principles of Nursing Intervention

❀ *APPLYING THE NURSING PROCESS* ❀

Nursing Assessment

Except for those nurses specially trained to do pelvic examinations and Pap smears, these procedures are not routinely done by nurses. In most cases, nursing assessment is directed toward an evaluation of the woman's understanding of the findings, their implications, and her psychosocial response.

Nursing Diagnosis

Nursing diagnoses that might apply to a woman with an abnormal finding from pelvic examination include the following:

- Anxiety related to the significance of the finding
- Fear related to the possibility of cancer
- Knowledge deficit related to the meaning of the diagnosis

Nursing Plan and Implementation

Research indicates that women undergoing colposcopy have questions about the procedure (such as timing of events), the sensations they will experience, the meaning of the results, and treatment options (Barsevick & Lauver 1990). Nurses are able to provide information about colposcopy and other diagnostic procedures the woman will undergo. In addition, the woman needs accurate information on etiology, symptomatology, and treatment options. She should be encouraged to report symptoms and keep appointments for follow-up examination and evaluation. The woman needs realistic reassurance if her condition is benign; she may require counseling and effective emotional support if a malignancy is likely. If the management plan includes surgery, she may need the nurse's support in obtaining a second opinion and making her decision.

Evaluation

Anticipated outcomes of nursing care include the following:

- The woman understands the abnormal finding, the diagnostic procedures that are indicated, and the possible causes of the abnormal finding.
- The woman copes successfully with the stress associated with waiting for a definite diagnosis.
- If surgery is warranted, the woman and her family cope successfully with the surgical procedure.

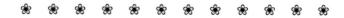

Care of the Woman with a Urinary Tract Infection

A urinary tract infection (UTI) may be a mere inconvenience or may reach life-threatening severity. Bacteria usually enter the urinary tract at its distal end; that is, by way of the urethra. The organisms are capable of migrating against the downward flow of urine. The shortness of the female urethra facilitates the passage of bacteria into the bladder. Other conditions that facilitate bacterial entry are relative incompetence of the urinary sphincter, frequent enuresis (bedwetting) prior to adolescence, and urinary catheterization. A habit of wiping from the back to front after urination may transfer bacteria from the anorectal area to the urethra.

About 5% of women have at least one UTI before becoming sexually active. The prevalence increases 1% per decade of life (Millette-Petit 1988). Voluntarily suppressing the desire to urinate is a predisposing factor. Elderly women who have more difficulty in the awareness of the urge to void and the ability to hold urine have a significantly higher incidence of UTI than younger women (Whippo & Creason 1989). Retention overdistends the bladder and can lead to an infection. For reasons that are unclear, there seems to be a relationship between recurring UTI and sexual intercourse. General poor health or lowered resistance to infection can also increase a woman's susceptibility to UTI. Stasis of urine, compression of ureters (especially the right ureter), decreased bactericidal capabilities of leukocytes in the urine, and vesicoureteral reflux (backward urine flow) make the pregnant woman even more susceptible to UTI.

The highest prevalence of UTI is among women of high parity in the low socioeconomic level, women with a history of UTI, and women with sickle cell disease or sickle cell trait.

Asymptomatic bacteriuria (ASB) (bacteria in the urine actively multiplying without accompanying clinical symptoms) constitutes about 6% to 8% of cases of UTI. This becomes especially significant if the woman is pregnant. Between 25% and 30% of pregnant women with untreated ASB will go on to develop pyelonephritis (Cruikshank 1990). Asymptomatic bacteriuria is almost always caused by a single organism. If more than one type of bacteria is cultured, the possibility of urine culture contamination must be considered.

The most common cause of ASB is *Escherichia coli.* Other commonly found causative organisms include *Klebsiella* and *Proteus.*

A woman who has had a UTI is more susceptible to a recurrent infection. If a pregnant woman develops an acute UTI, especially with high temperature, amniotic fluid infection may develop and retard the growth of the placenta.

Lower Urinary Tract Infection (Cystitis)

Because urinary tract infections are ascending, it is important to recognize and diagnose a lower UTI early to avoid the sequelae associated with upper UTI.

Interstitial cystitis is a relatively uncommon type of cystitis that is frequently misdiagnosed as either bacterial, urologic, or gynecologic in origin. It is a chronic inflammatory condition of unknown etiology involving the bladder wall. Women between the ages of 20 and 70 are most often affected. Clients complain of bladder pain, urgency, frequency, genital pain, dyspareunia, and sleep disturbances. The urine culture is negative and the only physical finding may be some urethral or vaginal tenderness. Interstitial cystitis does not respond to antibiotic therapy and no effective treatment regimen has been found (McCormick & Vinson 1988; Fletcher 1988).

Medical Therapy

Symptoms of frequency, pyuria, and dysuria without bacteriuria may indicate urethritis caused by *Chlamydia trachomatis.* It has become a common pathogen in the genitourinary system.

When cystitis develops, the initial symptom is often dysuria, specifically at the end of urination. Urgency and frequency also occur. Cystitis is usually accompanied by a low-grade fever (101F or lower), and hematuria is seen occasionally. Urine specimens usually contain an abnormal number of leukocytes and bacteria.

Oral sulfonamides, particularly sulfisoxazole, are generally effective against lower UTI. If the woman is pregnant these should only be used in early pregnancy since they interfere with protein binding of bilirubin in the fetus. Use of sulfonamides in the last few weeks of pregnancy can lead to neonatal hyperbilirubinemia and kernicterus. Other drugs that are usually effective (and apparently safe for a fetus) are ampicillin and nitrofurantoin (Furadantin). Nitrofurantoin crosses the placenta, but no harm to the fetus has been demonstrated.

❀   *APPLYING THE NURSING PROCESS*   ❀

Nursing Assessment

During each visit the nurse notes any complaints from the woman of pain on urination or other urinary difficulties. If any concerns arise, the nurse obtains a clean catch urine specimen from the woman.

Nursing Diagnosis

Nursing diagnosis that may apply to a woman with a lower UTI include the following:

- Pain related to dysuria secondary to the urinary tract infection
- Knowledge deficit related to a lack of understanding of self-care measures to help prevent recurrence of UTI

Nursing Plan and Implementation

Education for Self-Care   The nurse should make sure the woman is aware of good hygiene practices, since most

Table 8–7 Measures for Preventing Cystitis
If you use a diaphragm for contraception try changing methods or using another size of diaphragm.
Avoid bladder irritants such as alcohol, caffeine products, and carbonated beverages.
Increase fluid intake, especially water, to a minimum of six to eight glasses per day.
Make regular urination a habit; avoid long waits.
Practice good genital hygiene including wiping from front to back after urination and bowel movements.
Be aware that vigorous or frequent sexual activity may contribute to urinary tract infection.
Urinate before and after intercourse to empty the bladder and cleanse the urethra.
Complete medication regimens even if symptoms decrease.
Do not use medication left over from previous infections.
Drink cranberry juice to acidify the urine. This has been found to relieve symptoms in some cases.

bacteria enter through the urethra after having spread from the anal area. Table 8–7 identifies measures for preventing cystitis. The nurse should also reinforce instructions or answer questions regarding the prescribed antibiotic, the amount of liquids to take, and the reasons for these treatments. Cystitis usually responds rapidly to treatment, but follow-up urinary cultures are important.

Evaluation

Anticipated outcomes of nursing care include the following:

- The woman implements self-care measures to help prevent cystitis as part of her personal routine.
- The woman can identify the signs, symptoms, therapy, and possible complications of cystitis.
- The woman's infection is cured.

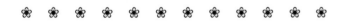

Upper Urinary Tract Infection (Pyelonephritis)

Pyelonephritis (inflammatory disease of the kidneys) is less common but more serious than cystitis and is often preceded by lower UTI. It is more common during the latter part of pregnancy or early postpartum and poses a serious threat to maternal and fetal well-being. Women with symptomatic pyelonephritis during pregnancy have an increased risk of premature births as well as intrauterine growth retardation.

Medical Therapy

The goal of medical intervention is to diagnose acute pyelonephritis and begin treatment as soon as possible. Acute pyelonephritis has a sudden onset with chills, high fever of 39.6–40.6C (103–105F), and flank pain (either unilateral or bilateral). The right side is almost always involved if the woman is pregnant because the large bulk of intestines to the left pushes the uterus to the right, putting pressure on the right ureter and kidney. Nausea, vomiting, and general malaise may ensue. With accompanying cystitis, frequency, urgency, and burning with urination may be experienced.

Edema of the renal parenchyma or ureteritis with blockage and swelling of the ureter may lead to temporary suppression of urinary output. This is accompanied by severe colicky pain, vomiting, dehydration, and ileus of the large bowel. The woman with acute pyelonephritis will generally have increased diastolic blood pressure, positive fluorescent antibody titer (FA-test), low creatinine clearance, significant bacteremia in urine culture, pyuria, and presence of white blood cell casts.

During pregnancy, acute pyelonephritis can lead to maternal sepsis, and is life threatening to both the woman and her unborn child. Consequently the woman is hospitalized and started on intravenous antibiotic therapy as soon as an acute upper UTI is diagnosed by symptoms and urine culture. In the case of obstructed pyelonephritis, a blood culture is necessary. The woman is kept in bed. After a sensitivity report, the antibiotic may be changed to one more specific for the infecting organism. Ampicillin, or nitrofurantoin, or one of these in combination with a sulfonamide, is commonly prescribed. Other antibiotics considered safe during pregnancy include cephalexin, sulfisoxazole, and methenamine.

If signs of urinary obstruction occur or continue, the ureter may be catheterized to establish adequate drainage.

With appropriate drug therapy, the woman's temperature should return to normal. The pain subsides and the urine shows no bacteria within two to three days. Follow-up urinary cultures are needed to ensure that the infection has been eliminated completely.

Nursing Assessment

During the woman's visit the nurse obtains a sexual and medical history to identify the woman at risk for UTI. A clean-catch urine specimen is evaluated for evidence of ASB.

Education for Self-Care The nurse provides the woman with information to help her recognize the signs of UTI, so she can contact her care giver as soon as possible. The nurse also discusses hygiene practices, the advantages of wearing cotton underwear, and the need to void frequently to prevent urinary stasis.

The nurse stresses the importance of maintaining a good fluid intake. Drinking cranberry juice daily and taking 500 mg Vitamin C both help acidify the urine and may help prevent recurrence of infection. Women with a history of

UTI find it helpful to drink a glass of fluid prior to sexual intercourse and void before and afterward.

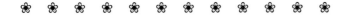

Cystocele and Pelvic Relaxation

A cystocele is the downward displacement of the bladder, which appears as a bulge in the anterior vaginal wall. Arbitrary classifications of mild to severe are frequently given. Genetic predisposition, vaginal childbearing, obesity, and increased age are factors that may contribute to cystocele (Samples et al 1988).

Medical Therapy

Symptoms of stress incontinence are most common, including loss of urine with coughing, sneezing, laughing, or sudden exertion. Vaginal fullness, a bulging out of the vaginal wall, or a dragging sensation may also be noticeable.

If pelvic relaxation is mild, Kegel exercises are helpful in restoring tone. The exercises involve contraction and relaxation of the pubococcygeal muscle. Women have found these exercises helpful before and after childbirth in maintaining vaginal muscle tone. Estrogen may improve the condition of vaginal mucous membranes—especially in menopausal women (see Chapter 7). Vaginal pessaries or rings may be used if surgery is undesirable or impossible or until surgery can be scheduled. Surgery may be considered for cystoceles considered moderate to severe.

Education for Self-Care

The nurse may instruct the woman in the use of Kegel exercises. Information on the causes and contributing factors and discussion of possible alternative therapies will greatly assist the woman.

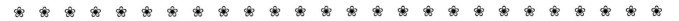

KEY CONCEPTS

The breasts function in a cyclic process that is regulated by nervous and hormonal systems. Thus many women experience breast tenderness and swelling premenstrually.

In fibrocystic breast disease the cysts tend to be round, mobile, and well delineated. The woman generally experiences increased discomfort premenstrually. Because of the increased risk of developing breast cancer, women with FBD should understand the importance of monthly BSE.

Factors that increase a woman's risk of developing breast cancer include advancing age (most occur after age 40), family history (especially mother or sister) of breast cancer, early menarche, late menopause, personal history of cancer in one breast, high levels of dietary fat, and high-protein and low-selenium diet.

Recommendations for frequency of screening mammograms are:

• Baseline mammogram between ages 35 and 40

• Mammogram every one to two years between ages 40 and 50

• Mammogram annually for all women after age 50

Diagnosis of suspicious breast mass is made by fine-needle biopsy.

A variety of surgical treatment alternatives now exist for women with breast cancer, including radical mastectomy, modified radical mastectomy, simple mastectomy, subcutaneous mastectomy, partial mastectomy, and lumpectomy. Breast reconstruction following surgery is becoming a more common alternative. Other treatment modalities for breast cancer include radiation therapy, chemotherapy, and endocrine therapy.

A woman with breast cancer faces many psychologic concerns including fear of the diagnosis, altered body image, and the response of family and friends. She must also deal with the long-term prognosis and her physical response to the treatment she receives. Nurses play a vital role in providing information and psychologic support.

Endometriosis is a condition in which endometrial tissue occurs outside the endometrial cavity. This tissue bleeds in a cyclic fashion in response to the menstrual cycle. The bleeding leads to inflammation, scarring, and adhesions. The prime symptoms include dysmenorrhea, dyspareunia, and infertility.

Treatment of endometriosis may be medical, surgical, or a combination. For the woman not desiring pregnancy at present, oral contraceptives are used. Women desiring pregnancy are treated with a course of danazol.

Toxic shock syndrome, caused by a toxin of *Streptococcus aureus,* is most common in women of childbearing age. There is an increased incidence in women who use tampons or barrier methods of contraception such as the diaphragm and sponge.

Moniliasis, a vaginal infection caused by *Candida albicans,* is most common in women who use oral contraceptives, are on antibiotics, are currently pregnant, or have diabetes mellitus. It is generally treated with intravaginal miconazole or clotrimazole suppositories.

Chlamydial infection is difficult to detect in a woman, but may result in PID and infertility. It is treated with doxycycline.

Herpes genitalis, caused by the herpes simplex virus, is a recurrent infection with no known cure. Acyclovir (Zovirax) may provide a reduction in symptoms.

Syphilis, caused by *Treponema pallidum,* is a sexually transmitted infection that is treatable if diagnosed. The characteristic lesion is the chancre. Syphilis can also be transmitted in utero to the fetus of an infected woman. The treatment of choice is penicillin.

Gonorrhea, a common sexually transmitted infection, may be asymptomatic in women initially but may cause PID if not diagnosed early. The treatment of choice is ceftriaxone and doxycycline.

Condyloma accuminata (venereal warts) is transmitted by a virus. Treatment is indicated because research suggests a possible link with cervical cancer. The treatment chosen depends on the size and location of the warts.

Nurses caring for women with an STD should discuss methods of prevention, signs and symptoms, and treatment alternatives in a supportive, nonjudgmental way.

Women with an abnormal finding on a pelvic examination will need careful explanation of the finding and techniques of diagnosis and emotional support during the diagnostic period.

The classic symptoms of a lower UTI are dysuria, urgency, frequency, and sometimes hematuria. Oral sulfonamides are the treatment of choice.

An upper UTI is a serious infection that can permanently damage the kidneys if untreated. Generally the woman is acutely ill and may require supportive therapy as well as antibiotics.

A cystocele is a downward displacement of the bladder into the vagina. Often it is accompanied by stress incontinence. Kegel exercises may help restore tone in mild cases.

❧ ❧

References

Abrums M: Health care for women. *JOGNN* 1986; 15(3):250.

American Cancer Society: *Cancer Facts and Figures 1988.* American Cancer Society, New York 1988.

Barsevick AM, Lauver D: Women's informational needs about colposcopy. *Image* Spring 1990; 22(1):23.

Batt RE, Severino MF: Endometriosis: A comprehensive approach. *Female Patient* March 1990; 15:77.

Benoit JA: Sexually transmitted diseases in pregnancy. *Nurs Clin North Am* 1988; 23(4):937.

Berkley SF et al: The relationship of tampon characteristics to menstrual toxic shock syndrome. *JAMA* 1987; 258(7):917.

Bourcier KM, Seidler AJ: Chlamydia and condylomata acuminata: An update for the nurse practitioner. *JOGNN* 1987; 16(1):71.

Breslin E: Genital herpes simplex. *Nurs Clin North Am* 1988; 23(4):907.

Buechner J et al: Use of mammography for breast cancer screening: Rhode Island 1987. *Morbid Mortal Weekly Rep* 1988; 37(23):357.

Bullough B et al: Methylxanthines and fibrocystic breast disease: A study of correlations. *Nurse Pract* 1990; 15(3):36.

Centers for Disease Control: 1989 Sexually transmitted disease treatment guidelines. *Morbid Mortal Weekly Rep* 1989; 38(5–8):1.

Centers for Disease Control: Sexually Transmitted Disease Statistics. Atlanta, GA: US Dept. of Health and Human Services, 1989.

Centers for Disease Control: Screening for cervical and breast cancer—Southeastern Kentucky. *Morbid Mortal Weekly Rep* 1988; 36(52):845.

Chagares R: Intrathoracic endometriosis: A woman's health issue. *Heart Lung* 1987; 16(2):183.

Colls JP: Toxic shock syndrome: In perspective. *NAACOG Update Series* 1986; 3(17):2.

Council on Scientific Affairs: Mammographic screening in asymptomatic women aged 40 years and older. *JAMA* 1989; 26(17):2535.

Cruikshank DP: Cardiovascular, pulmonary, renal, and hematologic diseases in pregnancy. In: *Danforth's Obstetrics and Gynecology,* 6th ed. Scott JR et al (editors). Philadelphia: Lippincott, 1990.

Deitch KV, Smith JE: Symptoms of chronic vaginal infection and microscopic condyloma in women. *JOGNN* 1990; 19(2):133.

Denny MS et al: Gynecologic health needs of elderly women. *J Gerontol Nurs* 1989; 15(1):33.

Desmond M et al: When to suspect chlamydia. *Patient Care* 1987; 21(18):64.

Diokno A et al: Urinary incontinence in elderly women: Urodynamic evaluation. *J Am Geriatr Soc* 1987; 35(10):940.

DiSaia PJ: Disorders of the uterine cervix: Benign lesions. In: *Danforth's Obstetrics and Gynecology,* 6th ed. Scott JR et al (editors). Philadelphia: Lippincott, 1990.

Dixon JM et al: Mammary duct ectasia. *Br J Surg* 1983; 70(10):601.

Dodd MJ: Patterns of self-care in patients with breast cancer. *West J Nurs Res* 1988; 10(1):7.

Duanne C: Hormonal therapy for breast cancer. *Cancer Nurs* 1988; 11(5):288.

Dupart W, Page D: Risk factors for breast cancer in women with proliferative breast disease. *N Engl J Med* 1985; 312:146.

Eddy D et al: The value of mammography screening in women under age 50 years. *JAMA* 1988; 259(10):1512.

Eddy DM: Screening for breast cancer. *Ann Intern Med* 1989; 111(5):389.

Ellerhorst-Ryan JM et al: Evaluating benign breast disease. *Nurse Pract* 1988; 13(a):13.

Engelking C: Breast cancer recurrence: Demystifying risk and outcome projections. *Innovations Oncology Nurs* 1989; 5(3):1.

Engelking C: Recurrent breast cancer: Physical and psychosocial sequelae. *Innovations Oncology Nurs* 1989; 5(3):1.

Enterline JA, Leonardo JP: Condylomata acuminata. *Nurse Pract* 1989; 14(4):8.

Eschenbach DA: Pelvic infections and sexually transmitted diseases. In: *Danforth's Obstetrics and Gynecology,* 6th ed. Scott JR et al (editors). Philadelphia: Lippincott, 1990.

Fletcher S: Interstitial cystitis: Painful bladder syndrome. *Nurse Pract* 1988; 13(10):7.

Fogel CI: Gonorrhea: Not a new problem but a serious one. *Nurs Clin North Am* 1988; 27(4):885.

Goldwyn R: Breast reconstruction after mastectomy. *N Engl J Med* 1987; 317(27):1711.

Govoni LE, Hayes JE: *Drugs and Nursing Implications,* 6th ed. Norwalk, CT: Appleton-Century-Crofts, 1988.

Grady KE: Older women and the practice of breast self-examination. *Psychol Women Q* 1988; 12(4):473.

Greaves W et al: Clindamycin versus metronidazole in treatment of bacterial vaginosis. *Obstet Gynecol* 1988; 72(5):799.

Hayes H et al: Mammography and breast implants. *Plast Reconstr Surgery* 1988; 82(1):1.

Henderson J, Taylor K: Age as a variable in an exercise program for the treatment of simple urinary stress incontinence. *JOGNN* 1987; 16(4):266.

Henzi MP et al: Administration of nasal nafarelin as compared to oral danazol for endometriosis: A multicenter, double-blind comparative trial. *N Engl J Med* 1988; 318(8):485.

Hill GA, Herbert CM: Endometriosis—Drug therapy or surgery? *Female Patient* October 1988; 13:69.

Himmelstein LR: Evaluation of inflammatory atypia: A literature review. *J Reprod Med* 1989; 34(9):634.

Horowitz BJ et al: Sexual transmission of candida. *Obstet Gynecol* 1987; 69(6):883.

Hulka B: What influences breast cancer risk: *Contemp OB/GYN* 1987; 29(4):91.

Irwin M: Life technologies' virapap test approved for distribution. *ONF* 1990; 17(1):137.

Jacob T et al: Breast self-examination knowledge, attitudes and performance among black women. *J Nat Med Assoc* 1989; 81(7):769.

Knorr C et al: Treatment options in breast cancer. *Patient Care* 1987; 21(14):108.

Krieger J et al: Diagnosis of trichomoniasis. *JAMA* 1988; 259(8):1223.

Kuhns-Hastings J: Management of female incontinence with Kegel exercises. *Am Assoc Occup Health Nurs* 1988; 36(2):78.

Lauver D: Theoretical perspectives relevant to breast self-examination. *Adv Nurs Sci* 1987; 9(4):16.

Lauver D: Instructional information and breast self-examination practice. *Res Nurs Health* 1989; 12(1):11.

Lawhead RA: Vulvar self-examination: What your patient should know. *Female Patient* January 1990; 15:33.

Levine MN et al: The thrombogenic effect of anticancer drug therapy in women with stage II breast cancer. *N Engl J Med* 1988; 318(7):404.

Lucas VA: Medicalization of women's health care. Unpublished manuscript, 1988.

Lucas VA: Human papillomavirus infections: A potentially carcinogenic sexually transmitted disease. *Nurs Clin North Am* 1988; 23(4):917.

Lucas VA: Clinical implications of perinatal and childhood human papillomavirus infections. *Nurse Pract Forum* 1990; 1(1):7.

The Ludwig Breast Cancer Study Group: Combination adjuvant chemotherapy for node positive breast cancer: Inadequacy of a single perioperative cycle. *N Engl J Med* 1988; 319(11):677.

McCormick N, Vinson R: Sexual difficulties experienced by women with interstitial cystitis. *Women Therapy* 1988; 792(3):109.

McGee J: Management of cervical dysplasia in pregnancy. *Nurse Pract* 1987; 12(3):34.

McQuistan CM: The relationship of risk factors for cervical cancer and HPV in college women. *Nurse Pract* 1989; 14(4):18.

McWhorter WP, Mayer WJ: Black/white differences in type of initial breast cancer treatment and implications for survival. *Am J Public Health* 1987; 77(12):1515.

Mann BK et al: Changing treatment of breast cancer in New Mexico from 1969 through 1985. *JAMA* 1988; 259(23):3413.

Markowitz L et al: Toxic shock syndrome. *JAMA* 1987; 278(1):75.

Millette-Petit JM: Urinary tract infections in older adults. *Nurse Pract* 1988; 13(12):21.

Minkoff HL, Landesman SH: The case of routinely offering prenatal testing for human immunodeficiency virus. *Am J Obstet Gynecol* 1988; 159(4):793.

Modica MM, Timor-Tritsch IE: Transvaginal sonography provides a sharper view into the pelvis. *JOGNN* 1988; 17(2):89.

Murray P et al: Oral contraceptive use in women with a family history of breast cancer. *Obstet Gynecol* 1989; 73(6):977.

Netting SL, Kauffman FH: Diagnosis and management of sexually transmitted genital lesions. *Nurse Pract* 1990; 15(1):20.

Nettles-Carlson B et al: Effectiveness of teaching breast self-examination during office visits. *Res Nurs Health* 1988; 11(1):41.

Nettles-Carlson B: Early detection of breast cancer. *JOGNN* 1989; 5(18):373.

Northouse LL, Swain MA: Adjustment of patients and husbands to the initial impact of breast cancer. *Nurs Res* 1987; 36(4):221.

Norwood SL: Fibrocystic breast disease: An update and review. *JOGNN* 1990; 19(2):116.

Office of Surveillance and Analysis, Centers for Disease Control: Trends in screening mammograms for women 50 years of age and older. *Morbid Mortal Weekly Rep* 1989A; 38(9):137.

Office of Surveillance and Analysis, Center for Disease Control: State-by-state variation in screening mammograms for women 50 years of age and older. *Morbid Mortal Weekly Rep* 1989B; 38(10):157.

Ohuchi N et al: Possible cancerous change of intraductal papilloma of the breast. *Cancer* 1984; 54(4):605.

Olson RL et al: Self-confidence as a critical factor in breast self-examination. *JOGNN* 1989; 18(6):476.

Queenan JT et al: Contraceptive sponge offers protection against chlamydia, gonorrhea but increases risk of candida. *Natl Women Health Rep* 1987; 8(1):1.

Redeker N: Health beliefs, health locus of control and the frequency of practice of breast self-examination in women. *JOGNN* 1989; 18(1):45.

Report from Centers for Disease Control: Premature mortality due to breast cancer, United States, 1984. *Morbid Mortal Weekly Rep* 1987; 36(44):736.

Rice MA, Szopa JJ: Group interventions for reinforcing self-worth following mastectomy. *Oncology Nurs Forum* 1988; 15(1):33.

Rubin LN, Borucki R: The intrauterine device and pelvic inflammatory disease revisited: New results from the Women's Health Study. *Obstet Gynecol* 1988; 72(1):1.

Russell L: Caffeine restriction as initial treatment for breast pain. *Nurse Pract* 1989; 14(2):36.

Rutledge DN: Factors related to women's practice of breast self-examination. *Nurse Res* 1987; 36(2):117.

Samples JT et al: The dynamic characteristics of the circumvaginal muscles. *JOGNN* 1988; 17(3):194.

Seidel HM: *Mosby's guide to physical examination.* St. Louis: Mosby, 1987, p 343.

Selvaggi SM: Spatula/cytobrush vs. spatula/cotton swab detection of cervical condylomatous lesions. *J Reprod Med* 1989; 34(9):629.

Shattuck JC: Pelvic inflammatory disease: Education for maintaining fertility. *Nurs Clin North Am* 1988; 23(4):899.

Shuttleworths: Female circulation: Medical discourse and popular advertising in the mid-victorian era. In *Body/Politics: Women and the Discourses of Science.* Jacobus M et al (editors). New York: Routhledge, 1990, pp 47–68.

Sloane E: *Biology of Women.* New York: Wiley, 1985, pp 181–182.

Spitzer M, Krumholz B: Pap screening for teenagers: A lifesaving precaution. *Contemp OB/GYN* 1988; 31(1):33.

Stafl A: Disorders of the uterine cervix: Colposcopy. In: *Danforth's Obstetrics and Gynecology,* 6th ed. Scott JR et al (editors). Philadelphia: Lippincott, 1990.

Szechtman PA et al: Recurrent and metastatic breast cancer treatment. *Innovations Oncology Nurs* 1989; 5(3):6.

Taylor P et al: The screening Papaniocolau smear: Contributions of the endocervical brush. *Obstet Gynecol* 1987; 70(5):734.

Timko C: Seeking medical care for breast cancer symptoms: Determinants of intentions to engage in prompt or delay behavior. *Health Psychol* 1987; 6(4):305.

Tobiassen T et al: Danazol treatment of severely symptomatic fibrocystic disease of the breast and long-term follow-up: The Hjorring Project. *Acta Obstet Gynecol Scand* (Suppl) 1984; 123:159S.

Treybig M: Primary dysmenorrhea or endometriosis. *Nurse Pract* 1989; 14(5):8.

The American College of Obstetricians and Gynecologists: *Statement by the ACOG on Estrogen, Estrogen-Progestin, and Breast Cancer.* Washington, DC: ACOG, 1989.

Vorherr H: Fibrocystic breast disease: Pathophysiology, pathomorphology, clinical picture and management. *Am J Obstet Gynecol* 1986; 154(1):161.

Webster D, Lipetz M: Women's health: changing definitions; changing times. *Nurs Clin North Am* 1986; 21(1):89.

Wells T et al: Urinary incontinence in elderly women: Clinical findings. *J Am Geriatr Soc* 1987; 35(10):933.

Whippo CC, Creason NS: Bacteriuria and urinary incontinence in aged female nursing home residents. *J Adv Nurs* 1989; 14(3):217.

White E: Projected changes in breast cancer incidence due to the trend toward delayed childbearing. *Am J Public Health* 1987; 77(4):495.

Additional Readings

Amankwaa LC; Frank DI: Vulvovaginal candidiasis: A study of immediate vs. delayed treatment on patient comfort. *Nurse Pract* June 1991; 16(6):23.

Barber HRK et al: Geriatric gynecology. *Female Patient* March 1990; 15:35.

Hamwi DA: Screening mammogram: Increasing the effort toward breast cancer detection. *Nurse Pract* December 1990; 15:27.

Hindle WH: Clinical dialogue: Fine needle aspiration of breast masses. *Contemp OB/GYN* October 15, 1990; 35(s):25.

Martens MG: Cystitis: Improving patient compliance. *Contemp OB/GYN* June 1991; 36(6):65.

Payton CE: Improving utilization of mammography screening in the physician's office practice. *Women's Health Issues* Winter 1991; 1(2):90.

Swehla M: Identifying and validating nursing diagnoses in a gynecologic ambulatory-care setting. *JOGNN* 1990; 19(5):439.

Tabor A, Berget A: Cold-knife and laser conization for cervical intraepithelial neoplasia. *Obstet Gynecol* 1990; 76(4):633.

Tinkle MB: Genital humanpapillomavirus infection: A growing health risk. *JOGNN* 1990; 19(6):501.

CHAPTER 9

Women's Care:
Reproductive Surgery

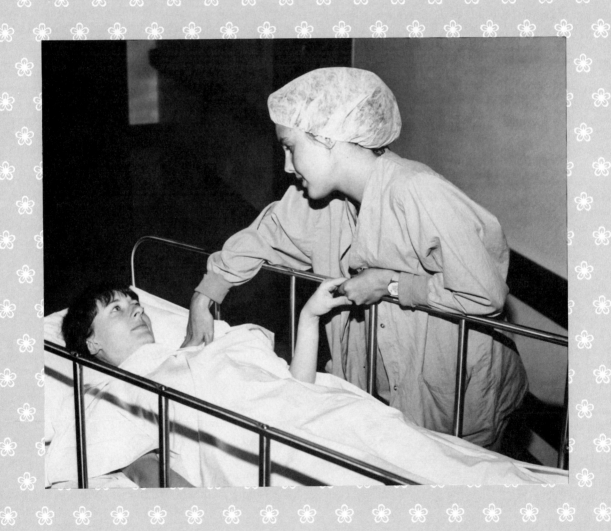

OBJECTIVES

Discuss the issues and concerns surrounding gynecologic surgery.

Describe the most common gynecologic surgical procedures.

Discuss the nursing care of women during gynecologic surgery.

❀ ❀

Before I was faced with cancer, I thought that doctors were the people with all the information. But it was the nurse who explained the test results and the diagnosis the doctor had given me. Because of my nurse, I know just what to expect and how to take care of myself. I think nurses should speak up more, so people know all the wonderful things they do.

The women's health movement has increased public and professional awareness of issues related to gynecologic problems and treatments. Information on new, improved diagnostic and surgical techniques that may be used as alternatives to major surgery is being disseminated to consumers and nurses by various groups. The field of reproductive surgery has changed considerably since the late nineteenth century when an oophorectomy was performed to treat "female unruliness" and hysterectomies were used to treat backaches and "prevent" cancer (Ammer 1989).

Continuing increases in the number of reproductive surgical procedures being performed, particularly hysterectomies, are still cause for concern, however. This chapter identifies gynecologic surgery issues of interest to nurses and women facing the prospect of surgery. It provides an overview of the most common reproductive surgical procedures, including dilation and curettage, hysterectomy, tubal surgery, and termination of pregnancy. It describes indications for surgery, techniques, risks and complications, pre- and postoperative nursing interventions, and psychosexual responses to surgery. It also explains evaluation and treatment of women having surgery because of abnormal cytologic findings and presents an overview of surgical management for gynecologic cancer.

Issues and Concerns for Women Facing Surgery

There are many components to an informed decision to undergo reproductive surgery. The first question that should be addressed is: What are the indications for having the surgery? An explanation of the surgical procedure and the reasons it was selected over other available alternative procedures should be given to the woman. Effects on childbearing ability and/or sexual performance should be explained, as well as effects on the general functioning of the body. An explanation of the risks of the surgery should include the common risks, the nonserious risks, the rare or unusual complications, and the risk of not surviving (Brunner & Suddarth 1988).

The question whether a second opinion on the necessity for surgery should be sought is somewhat controversial. In the case of elective surgery, different physicians may have different opinions. A woman should be encouraged to consult other physicians when there is controversy about a treatment (such as, for example, treatment of early cervical cancers) or when the surgeon is unknown to the woman. A specialist in gynecology is the preferred source for a second opinion (Ammer 1989). Some third-party payment plans encourage second opinions. The woman can analyze the information and discuss her concerns with the nurse or physician before she signs a written consent that acknowledges the information given and the authorization for the surgery.

Other concerns that may influence the decision to have reproductive surgery may be categorized as general concerns about surgery and specific concerns related to gynecologic surgery. General concerns include the following:

- Anesthesia: fear of general anesthesia because of loss of control; fear of regional anesthesia because of possible postoperative problems and concern about being awake during surgery
- Anticipation of postoperative pain
- Fear of death or disability
- Concerns about limitation of normal functioning and dependency during recovery
- Financial coverage for hospitalization
- Family members: welfare of family members while the woman is undergoing surgery (eg, child care, loss of wages, help for household chores) (Brunner & Suddarth 1988)

Specific concerns related to gynecologic surgery are related to the significance of the reproductive organs for the woman. Surgery to alter or remove a reproductive organ may be perceived as a threat to self-concept.

Body image is affected whenever a body part is lost. The degree of mourning for that loss is related to the significance attached to it. Even though there is no outwardly apparent change with a hysterectomy, the loss may be felt strongly. Many women fear postoperative changes such as masculinization, weight gain, and loss of sexuality. Reproductive surgery may also be seen as a threat to femininity in our society, which emphasizes childbearing and motherhood. A woman whose self-esteem comes from sources other than attractiveness and the ability to bear children will usually adjust better to reproductive surgery.

Issues and Concerns for Nurses

Two major areas of concern to the nurse advocate are:

What information does the woman need to make an informed decision about surgery?

What assessment data about the woman are needed to implement a plan of care?

The nurse needs a broad knowledge of gynecology to assist women in making informed decisions. The practitioner must be able to explain a planned surgical intervention at the woman's level of understanding. Before providing explanations, the nurse may have to assess what the woman has already been told by the physician and whether she has any misconceptions about the procedure or its effects.

The nurse needs physical and psychosexual assessment data to plan comprehensive care of the woman. The nurse considers the woman as a total person from the woman's point of view. Her self-concept is assessed in terms of body image and feelings of self-worth as influenced by family, society, and culture. For example, religion may be an important factor in a woman's decision making. A woman who is a Jehovah's Witness may decline surgery because according to her beliefs she must refuse to accept blood transfusions. However, major gynecologic surgery can be performed with minimum morbidity and mortality, and the woman should have this information (Ammer 1989). The nurse needs to assess the woman's feelings about the surgery or its effects and encourage her to express her concerns.

Care of the Woman During Gynecologic Surgery

Hysterectomy

A hysterectomy involves the removal of the uterus through an abdominal incision or through the vagina. When the fallopian tubes and both ovaries are also removed, the procedure is called a total abdominal hysterectomy with bilateral salpingo-oophorectomy (TAH-BSO) or panhysterectomy. At this time, approximately 650,000 patients undergo total abdominal hysterectomies annually (Stovall et al 1990).

The necessity for such a large number of hysterectomies has recently been questioned. When a hysterectomy is recommended, the woman needs to be aware of her right to a second opinion before making her final decision. The nurse has an important role in providing information to women about issues such as hysterectomy and other reproductive surgery.

Indications
Hysterectomy is the usual treatment for several conditions, although there is no medical consensus about absolute indications. Abdominal hysterectomies are generally performed for cancer of the cervix, endometrium, and ovary; fibroids; endometriosis; chronic pelvic inflammatory disease (PID); and adenomyosis.

Surgical Procedure
The types of hysterectomy include those already described and total vaginal hysterectomy (TVH), the removal of the uterus through the vagina. An anterior and/or posterior repair of the vaginal walls may also be performed with vaginal hysterectomy. This surgical repair is done when weakened pelvic supports have displaced one or more of the pelvic organs (urethra, bladder, rectum), causing urinary incontinence, constipation, or defecation problems.

Abdominal procedures are usually performed in women who have had previous pelvic surgery with resulting adhesions, scarring, or endometriosis, and in nulliparous women whose fallopian tubes and ovaries are also to be removed. Abdominal hysterectomy is also preferred when malignancy is suspected or confirmed because the procedure allows exploration of the abdomen and pelvis to locate tumor extension. Disadvantages of the abdominal procedure over the vaginal procedure include scarring, more postoperative pain, slower recovery, and more problems with bowel functions.

Vaginal hysterectomy is usually the preferred treatment for uterine prolapse and pelvic relaxation. The advantages of vaginal hysterectomy include earlier ambulation, less postoperative pain, less anesthesia and operative time, less blood loss, no visible scar, and a shorter hospital stay. The vaginal route is preferred for the elderly, obese, or debilitated woman who is a poor risk for abdominal surgery. The major disadvantage of a vaginal hysterectomy is the increased risk of deep vein thrombosis (DiSaia & Walker 1990).

Removal of the ovaries with the uterus remains controversial. Some surgeons recommend that the ovaries never be removed in premenopausal women because bilateral oophorectomy results in surgical castration and menopause. Other physicians recommend removal of the ovaries in all hysterectomy patients over 40 years of age because of the risk of ovarian cancer. Still others recommend removal of ovaries at the time of a hysterectomy if the woman has a family history of ovarian cancer (Ravnikar 1990). In any case, oophorectomy should not be considered routine with hysterectomy. The woman should be informed about the alternatives so that she can decide which alternative she prefers. If the ovaries are removed in a premenopausal woman, estrogen replacement therapy needs to be considered. Further discussion of this treatment appears in the following section on oophorectomy.

Preoperative preparation for the hysterectomy generally includes the following:

- Laboratory work (complete blood count, hemoglobin, hematocrit, type and cross-match of blood, urinalysis, chest radiographs, electrocardiogram)
- Vaginal examination and/or complete physical examination
- Surgical preparation (enema, douche, abdominal-pubic or perineal shave)
- Maintaining NPO status for 8 hours prior to surgery
- Emptying of bladder just prior to surgery
- Preoperative medication and intravenous fluids

❀ *APPLYING THE NURSING PROCESS* ❀

Nursing Assessment

Nursing assessment of the woman undergoing a hysterectomy will include psychosocial aspects and determination of the learning needs of the woman.

The initial reaction to the need for hysterectomy has been related to the grief responses identified by Kübler-Ross and described by Gitlin et al 1989. The first response may be shock, disbelief, or denial, especially if the surgery is an emergency procedure. The woman may not realize the impact of the surgery. Anger may result when there is a waiting period between diagnosis and surgery. This anger often results from the loss of reproductive function or conceptual loss of femininity. A bargaining stage may be noted in childless women who express the desire to have a child before having surgery. Depression can occur preoperatively if the woman is very sensitive about her impending loss and is upset by the sight of a pregnant woman or comments about attractiveness.

It is important for the nurse to thoroughly assess the physiologic, psychosocial, and sexual needs of the woman. Factors known to affect psychologic adjustment after surgery include the age of the woman, her cultural background and educational level, the attitude of her husband or sexual partner, her family situation, her preoperative preparation, and whether or not cancer is involved. The significance of the uterus in the woman's self-image will be reflected in her attitudes about menstruation, childbearing, body image, and sexuality. If the woman equates her uterus with femininity, she may feel an acute loss. She may feel that she will become an "empty shell." If she sees childbearing as a major role in life, loss of reproductive ability

can cause distress. The loss of menses is viewed with relief if there has been dysmenorrhea or other menstrual problems but with sadness if menses is seen as a cleansing process or a sign of youth. The woman may feel that sexual ability and desire depend on the presence of the uterus and that hysterectomy will affect satisfaction and ability (Gitlin et al 1989).

Misconceptions and fears about the effects of hysterectomy need to be identified preoperatively so that correct information is provided to the woman and reassurances are given that assist her in making a positive emotional adjustment to surgery.

Nursing Diagnosis

Examples of nursing diagnoses that may apply include the following:

- Knowledge deficit related to need for hysterectomy
- Knowledge deficit related to preoperative routines, postoperative exercises/activity, and/or postoperative alterations/sensations
- Fear related to unknown outcome of surgery

Nursing Plan and Implementation

Provision of Preoperative Teaching

During teaching sessions, the nurse can be a counselor, support person, listener, and teacher. Involvement of the woman's partner or significant others in the discussions can help them accept the surgery and support the woman. Techniques that will encourage the woman to express her feelings and concerns include sitting down with the woman and using active listening, eye contact, open-ended questions, nonverbal communication, and touch.

Preoperative information and teaching can be done individually or in groups. Being informed about hysterectomy prior to surgery can decrease anxiety and prepare the woman for the procedure and the postoperative period. The preoperative information given should include the consequences of the surgery (what is removed, effect on reproductive ability, and so on), the type of anesthesia used, possible risks and complications, postoperative care routines, convalescence, and when activities can be resumed.

Promotion of Physical Well-Being in the Postoperative Period

Routine postoperative care includes monitoring vital signs, temperature, and fluid intake and output; checking the amount of bleeding by assessing the abdominal dressing and/or perineal pads; assessing the need for pain relief; and encouraging early ambulation, leg exercises, turning, coughing, and deep breathing. In addition to these routine interventions, the diet will be advanced from clear liquids to a regular diet when bowel sounds are present. Sitz baths, heat lamps, and ice packs may be used to relieve perineal discomfort, decrease swelling, and promote healing (for vaginal hysterectomy). Foley catheters are usually discontinued 8 to 10 hours after surgery unless anterior repairs were done with vaginal hysterectomy, in which case the Foley or suprapubic catheter may remain in place for up to seven days even though the woman returns home 24 to 48 hours after surgery.

Postoperative complications can occur with both abdominal and vaginal hysterectomies. Hemorrhage, urinary tract complications, and wound infections occur more frequently with the vaginal procedure. Complications associated more frequently with abdominal procedures include intestinal obstruction (paralytic ileus), thromboembolism, pulmonary embolism, atelectasis, pneumonia, and wound dehiscence. Emotional complications can occur with both procedures (see the following section on psychosexual reactions).

Discharge planning begins prior to admission. The nurse and other members of the health care team should discuss and reinforce information concerning physical and emotional recovery. Topics to be covered include physical changes the woman can expect, physical limitations or restrictions during convalescence, anticipatory guidance, and emotional reactions that can occur.

Anticipated physical changes include weakness and fatigue, cessation of menses, inability to become pregnant, possibility of painful intercourse after vaginal hysterectomy with repair (until vaginal walls are stretched); possible bowel irregularity, possible lack of appetite, possible phantom pain (uterine cramps), and possible temporary loss of vaginal sensation after vaginal hysterectomy. Restrictions after surgery may include avoidance of heavy lifting, strenuous housework, or active sports for at least one month; avoidance of tub baths, douches, and sexual intercourse for three to six weeks; and avoidance of sitting for long periods of time to prevent pelvic congestion. Anticipatory guidance is given to stress the need for the postoperative checkup in four to six weeks. The woman also should be taught the signs of infection, hemorrhage, and bladder problems because these complications can occur after she leaves the hospital. Discussions about possible emotional responses should clear up any misconceptions about hysterectomy causing masculinization, detrimental effects on sexual responses, or mental illness (Cohen 1989).

Addressing Psychosexual Concerns

A variety of feelings may be associated with a hysterectomy. Fear, anxiety, lowered self-esteem, and depression may be felt by the woman. Depression is more frequently seen in women who have had a hysterectomy for treatment of cancer—because these clients must also face the possibility of death from the disease—and in women who have an abdominal hysterectomy rather than a vaginal procedure (Cohen 1989).

There are wide variations in sexual adjustment after a hysterectomy. Cohen (1989) reported that preoperative levels of sexual activity and satisfaction together were the best predictors of postoperative sexual function. Greater involvement by nurses in convalescent counseling is important. Such involvement includes preoperative assessment of the woman's sexual behavior and identifying postoperative needs. Specific information that may assist with sexual adjustment after surgery includes the following:

- The vagina shrinks temporarily postoperatively and coitus will help stretch it.
- Using water-soluble lubricants may make coitus more comfortable.
- Clitoral orgasm may be encouraged.
- The goal is overall sensual enjoyment.

Nurses who are not comfortable with or knowledgeable about sexual counseling should either seek more education in human sexuality or refer the client to someone who is more comfortable discussing it.

Evaluation

Anticipated outcomes of nursing care include the following:

- The woman understands the reason for the hysterectomy, the alternatives, the expected outcome of surgery, the risks, and aspects of self-care after surgery.
- The woman has an uneventful recovery without complications.
- The woman feels she is able to ask questions and obtain support.
- The woman is able to participate in decision making as she desires.

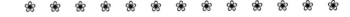

Dilation and Curettage

Dilation and curettage (D & C) is the most frequently performed minor gynecologic surgical procedure. Indications for D & C can be diagnostic or therapeutic. Diagnostic indications include checking for uterine malignancy, evaluating infertility causes, and investigating dysfunctional uterine bleeding. Therapeutic indications include treatment of heavy bleeding, incomplete abortion, therapeutic abortion, dysmenorrhea, and removal of polyps.

Salpingectomy

Salpingectomy is the unilateral or bilateral removal of the fallopian tubes. Indications include diseases of the tubes, sepsis, malignancy, and tubal pregnancy. Salpingectomy for tubal pregnancy is generally an emergency procedure because the placenta erodes the fallopian tube and can cause hemorrhage once the fallopian tube is completely eroded.

Tubal Reconstruction

Microsurgery has significantly affected gynecologic surgery primarily in the treatment of infertility and reversal of sterilization. The procedure involves "unblocking" the tubes and reconnecting the remaining portions (tubal reanastomosis), using magnification and microsurgical techniques to obtain proper alignment and accurate approximation of the tubes. The success rate in reversal of sterilization surgery is 60% (Rosenwaks & Davis 1990).

Oophorectomy

Oophorectomy is unilateral or bilateral removal of the entire ovary. Indications may include severe pelvic inflammatory disease, malignancy, ectopic pregnancy, and ovarian cysts. Ovaries may be removed when a hysterectomy is performed if the woman is menopausal but may not be removed in premenopausal women, depending on the indication for the hysterectomy. An oophorectomy may be performed at the time of hysterectomy to reduce the risk of ovarian cancer. The reasons for not performing oophorectomy are related to the superiority of hormones produced by the body over hormone replacement therapy in younger women.

When both ovaries are removed in premenopausal women, abrupt surgical menopause occurs. This may cause decreased libido, decreased vaginal lubrication, and decreased sensations in the lower vaginal tract. Symptoms of menopause—such as hot flashes and atrophy of the vaginal epithelium—may be treated with hormone replacement therapy. Women at risk for developing osteoporosis or who have a strong family history of cardiovascular disease are prime candidates for hormone replacement therapy (London & Hammond 1990). Estrogen is usually given orally on a cyclic basis, in the lowest doses compatible with effective treatment of symptoms (0.3 to 0.625 mg) to reduce severe menopausal symptoms and the risk of osteoporosis. Women on hormone replacement therapy with estrogen are at risk for hypertension, gallbladder disease, angina pectoris, breast cancer, and endometrial cancer (if they have not had a hysterectomy). Topical application of estrogen may relieve vaginal atrophy and difficult or painful coitus (dyspareunia), although water-soluble lubricants may work as well (Stumpf 1990). There is no consensus on the risk factors, benefits, or side effects of the use of estrogen replacement in women who have had hysterectomies. Some clinicians advocate administration of progesterone for a portion of each cycle to oppose the estrogen effects. Whether or not a woman who does not have a uterus should receive progestin is

controversial (Stumpf 1990). There is a need for further research on this issue.

Nursing Care

The nurse assesses the woman's knowledge of the surgery, the indications for it, the risks, and self-care information. The nurse also assesses the woman's knowledge of the need for estrogen replacement and the associated problems of this therapy.

The nurse gives the woman information regarding the expected surgery, the expected benefit, the risks, and associated complications. The woman will need to know the expected activities during hospitalization and how to perform self-care after discharge. The woman will also need information about hormone replacement therapy in order to make an informed decision about whether she wants to receive it.

Surgical Interruption of Pregnancy

Although for centuries abortion was banned by both church and public law, many women still sought to terminate their pregnancies. Because of the illegal status of abortion, however, the procedure was always dangerous. Illegal abortions became the single highest cause of maternal death in this country. Since 1973, when induced abortion became a legal option, the maternal mortality rate has declined steadily.

Although legalized abortion has been in effect for several years, the controversy over the moral and legal issues continues. This controversy is as readily apparent in the medical and nursing professions as among other groups. See Chapter 6 for further discussion of the belief system and social issues surrounding abortion.

Factors Influencing the Decision to Seek Abortion

A number of physical and psychosocial factors influence a woman's decision to seek an abortion. The presence of a disease or health state that jeopardizes the mother's life and serious, life-threatening fetal problems are frequently suggested as indications for abortion. In other instances, the timing or circumstance of the pregnancy creates an inordinate stress on the woman and she chooses an abortion. Some of these situations may involve contraceptive failure, rape, or incest. In all cases, the decision is best made by the woman or couple involved. A mother whose life is threatened by the pregnancy may choose to continue the pregnancy while one with no obvious threat may choose abortion. Many feel this is as it should be because the decision must rest with the individuals who bear the impact of the continuance or termination of the pregnancy.

Methods

The method of abortion differs depending on the length of gestation. See Table 9–1 for various techniques.

 APPLYING THE NURSING PROCESS ❁

Nursing Assessment

The nurse must assess the woman's knowledge base regarding the abortion and her emotional status in order to devise a teaching plan and provide emotional support.

Nursing Diagnosis

Examples of possible nursing diagnoses include the following:

- Knowledge deficit related to the abortion procedure, alternatives, risks, and associated self-care
- Pain related to the procedure and uterine cramping

Nursing Plan and Implementation

As the woman makes her decision about having an abortion she will need information about the types of abortion and

Table 9–1 Methods Used in Termination of Pregnancy

First-trimester abortion	Complications
Dilation and Curettage	
Dilation and curettage is the oldest method. It involves the use of a metal curette to scrape out the inside of the uterus. It is not done frequently now because other methods are deemed safer and less traumatic.	Perforation of the uterus, laceration of the cervix, systemic reaction to the anesthetic agent, hemorrhage
Minisuction	
A minisuction is accomplished with a small-bore cannula and a 50-mL syringe as a vacuum source. This technique is also called menstrual regulation or menstrual extraction.	Perforation of the uterus, laceration of the cervix, systemic reaction to the anesthetic agent, hemorrhage
Vacuum Curettage	
After a paracervical block, the cervix is dilated and a vacuum suction cannula is inserted to remove the contents of the uterus. Laminaria may be inserted into the cervix the day before to dilate the cervix.	Perforation of the uterus, laceration of the cervix, systemic reaction to the anesthetic agent, hemorrhage (Brenner & Mishell 1990)
Second trimester (mid-trimester)	**Complications**
Hypertonic Saline	
Hypertonic saline is still a common method after 20 weeks. A laminaria is inserted the day before. Hypertonic saline is injected or infused into the amniotic cavity. The procedure takes an average of 33 to 35 hours to completion. Some clinicians begin intravenous oxytocin a few hours after the instillation of hypertonic saline. In this case the procedure takes an average of 25 hours (Brenner & Mishell 1990). The addition of oxytocin increases the risk to the woman.	Cervical laceration, uterine rupture, cardiovascular collapse, pulmonary and/or cerebral edema, renal failure, failed abortion, hemorrhage, infection, embolism
Dilation and Extraction (D&E)	
Laminaria are inserted one or two days before the procedure. During the D&E an IV is started, local anesthesia is administered, and the contents are removed with a combination of suction and forceps. The procedure usually takes 10 to 20 minutes.	Perforation of the uterus with bladder or intestinal injury, amniotic fluid embolism, disseminated intravascular coagulation (Brenner & Mishell 1990)
Systemic Prostaglandins	
Prostaglandin E_2 vaginal suppositories or 15-methyl $PGF_{2\alpha}$ (Prostin 15M) may be used. The average time for either of these procedures is 13 to 15 hours.	Nausea, vomiting, fever (Brenner & Mishell 1990)
Intrauterine Prostaglandins	
Insertion of laminaria is done the night before. Prostaglandin $F_{2\alpha}$ is injected into the amniotic sac. The abortion procedure usually averages about 14 hours after the $PGF_{2\alpha}$ is instilled. In some instances, urea is also instilled.	Vomiting, diarrhea, fever, cervical rupture, hemorrhage, infection (Brenner & Mishell 1990)

the associated risks. The woman needs to understand the available alternatives and the possible problems. The debate about abortion is frequently impassioned, which makes it very difficult to obtain accurate, unbiased facts on which to base a decision. The nurse helps provide valuable information so that the woman can make an informed choice.

The need for teaching continues during the procedure and for self-care measures afterward.

Provision of Support

Important aspects of care include allowance for verbalization by the woman; support before, during, and after the procedure; monitoring of vital signs, intake, and output; providing for physical comfort and privacy throughout the procedure; and health teaching regarding self-care, the importance of the postabortion checkup, and contraception review.

Evaluation

Anticipated outcomes of nursing care include the following:

- The woman understands the procedure, the alternatives, and the associated risks.

- The woman has been able to participate in informed decision making.

- The woman has not suffered any complications of the procedure.

- The woman has a support base and is aware of resources in her community that she may use if needed.

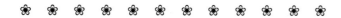

Surgical Interventions for Abnormal Cytology

Whenever there are abnormal findings on a woman's Pap smear report, the cytologic study should be repeated. If an abnormal smear is reported again, a colposcopy can be performed to examine the cervix more closely. If the initial Pap report reveals mild dysplasia or a more serious finding, colposcopy should be done immediately. If abnormal tissue is detected, punch biopsies and endocervical curettage (ECC) are carried out. If cervical intraepithelial neoplasia (CIN) is detected, five possible treatments are suggested based on whether the ECC was negative or positive and whether invasive cancer was found. Treatment alternatives are colposcopy, biopsy, laser therapy, conization, cryosurgery, and surgical management.

Colposcopy

Colposcopy is a medical examination used to diagnose precancerous changes of the cervix or cervical intraepithelial neoplasia (CIN) (Barsevick & Lauver 1990). In addition, it

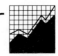

Research Note

Clinical Application of Research

In order to examine the relationship between information-seeking behavior and either preference for information or preference for involvement, Andrea Barsevick and Jean Johnson (1990) asked women who were undergoing colposcopy to participate in a research project. The study also investigated the association between information seeking and emotional responses of the women to a stressful situation, that of undergoing colposcopy.

Measurement of information seeking included recording the number of questions asked during the colposcopy as well as whether or not the woman requested an information sheet. When the procedure was scheduled, the woman was told that the sheet was available upon request. The request was an indication of information seeking about the procedure.

Results showed positive correlations between the number of questions asked and one of the scales for preference for information and between the preference for behavioral involvement and requesting an information sheet. Additionally, semipartial correlations showed that women who asked more questions had a higher degree of confidence about the examination.

Critical Thinking Applied to Research

Strengths: Excellent description of validity for the two scales used to identify preference for information. Other psychometric properties described for all tools, including the tool to determine emotional responses developed for this study. Identification of limitations of the study.

Concerns: Having one of the researchers with the participant during the examination to record the number of questions asked might impact internal validity through the communication of experimenter expectations.

Barsevick A, Johnson J: Preference for information and involvement, information seeking and emotional response of women undergoing colposcopy. *Res Nursing Health* 1990; 13:1.

is a diagnostic tool for women exposed to diethylstilbestrol (DES).

The woman first empties her bladder. With the woman in a lithotomy position, a speculum is inserted into the vagina and the cervix is cleaned with a solution of 3% acetic acid, which softens the cervical mucosa and causes the tissues to swell. The examiner looks through a stereoscopic viewing instrument (which is not inserted into the vagina). The examiner looks for areas of irregular punctuation or mosaic white epithelium in the transformation zone, the area of the cervix where columnar epithelium has been changed by the process of metaplasia to squamous epithelium. Dysplasia, CIN, and carcinoma in situ (CIS) usually originate in this area. If abnormal tissue is detected, a punch biopsy of the tissue is performed, and the woman may experience a pinching or stinging sensation.

Colposcopy is performed as an outpatient procedure. Specific nursing care includes the following (Barsevick & Lauver 1990):

- Providing concrete, objective information about the examination and self-care instruction
- Anticipating the need for information about the cause and meaning of abnormalities
- Answering general questions about treatment options and procedures
- Assisting and encouraging slow breathing or other relaxation techniques during the procedure

Biopsy

A cervical biopsy is performed to investigate suspicious cervical tissue to diagnose or rule out cancer of the cervix at its earliest stages. An endometrial biopsy is used to diagnose functional menstruation disorders, infertility problems related to ovulation, and benign or malignant lesions.

The woman may experience moderate to severe cramplike pains during the procedure and afterward. A small amount of bleeding also may occur after the biopsy and may continue for up to two weeks. Bleeding as heavy as a menstrual period should be reported to the physician or clinic.

An endocervical curettage is performed prior to biopsies to confirm the presence or absence of disease in the endocervix. The endocervical canal is scraped from the internal to external os. The woman needs to be prepared for some cramping and pain during the procedure.

Laser Therapy

The laser is used to treat both CIN and vaginal and vulvar intraepithelial neoplasia. It is reported to be safer, less mutilating, and less costly than conization and hysterectomy. The laser is used when all boundaries of the lesion are visible on colposcopy and the endocervical curettage is negative. The invisible, highly concentrated beam is absorbed by water in the tissues, and the energy is converted to heat, causing evaporation of the cellular water and cellular death. Normal tissue remains intact (DiSaia & Stafl 1990).

The laser can be used in outpatient settings. No anesthesia is necessary for cervical lesions, and there is minimal bleeding. The woman may experience minor cramping and a slight discharge for 5 to 7 days. She should avoid the use of tampons, douching, and sexual intercourse for two weeks. Healing may take 6 to 12 weeks. Laser is specific to the lesion and should not affect fertility. (DiSaia & Stafl 1990).

Conization

A conization is generally performed when the entire lesion cannot be visualized by colposcopic examination. In this procedure a cone of tissue, the size and length of which are determined by the extent of the lesion, is surgically removed. A large amount of normal tissue is removed along with the abnormal tissue. Conization can be performed as an inpatient or outpatient procedure and under local or general anesthesia (DiSaia & Stafl 1990). There is a risk of postoperative infection and hemorrhage, and premature labor and abortion may be experienced in future pregnancies. A prolonged or profuse menstrual period can occur with the next two or three cycles.

Cryosurgery

Cervical dysplasia, endocervicitis, and nabothian cysts may be treated by cryosurgery. The procedure uses freezing to cause tissue necrosis. A double freeze method is advocated, with nitrous oxide or carbon dioxide as the refrigerant. The freezing also can destroy normal tissue. The failure rate for treatment of stage II and III CIN is as high as 30%.

The procedure is usually performed a week after the menstrual period to avoid disturbing a pregnancy and to allow new tissue to generate before the next period. Cryosurgery can be performed in the physician's office or clinic without anesthesia. It is not a painful procedure, although the woman may experience some cramping.

The woman should be told to expect a heavy, persistent watery discharge for several weeks. She should not use tampons and should avoid sexual intercourse while the discharge is present, because the cervix is easily damaged.

Surgical Management of Gynecologic Cancer

Reproductive malignancies can be treated with surgery, radiation, chemotherapy, or a combination of the three methods depending on the type of cancer and the extent of disease. A discussion of reproductive oncology and all the treatment modalities is beyond the scope of this chapter; this discussion focuses on surgical management, emphasizing radical surgery and its physiologic, psychosocial, and sexual implications.

Types of Cancer

Cervical Cancer Microinvasive cancer of the cervix (depth of penetration of the tumor into submucosal tissues up to 3 mm) is treated with hysterectomy. Invasive cancer of the cervix is treated according to the extent of the cancer, the woman's health, and her age. Staging of the cancer is an evaluation process that identifies the extent of spread of the tumor based on routine studies such as intravenous pyelography (IVP), complete blood count, barium enema, cystoscopy, lymphangiography, bone scan, and proctoscopy (Table 9–2). TAH and bilateral lymphadenectomy

Table 9–2	Staging of Cervical Cancer

Stage 0:	Carcinoma in situ, intraepithelial carcinoma
Stage I:	Carcinoma strictly confined to the cervix (extension to the corpus should be disregarded)
Stage II:	Carcinoma extends beyond the cervix but has not extended to the pelvic wall; vagina involved, but not as far as the lower third.
Stage III:	Carcinoma extends to pelvic wall. On rectal examination there is no cancer-free space between the tumor and the pelvic wall. The tumor involves the lower third of the vagina. All cases with hydronephrosis or nonfunctioning kidney are included.
IIIa:	No extension to the pelvic wall
IIIb:	Extension to the pelvic wall and/or hydronephrosis or non-functioning kidney
Stage IV:	Carcinoma extends beyond the true pelvis or clinically involves the mucosa of the bladder or rectum. Bullous edema as such does not permit a case to be allotted to stage IV.
IVa:	Spread of the growth to adjacent organs
IVb:	Spread to distant organs

From: DiSaia PJ, Stafl A: Disorders of the uterine cervix. In: Danforth's Obstetrics and Gynecology, 6th ed. Scott JR et al (editors). Philadelphia: Lippincott, 1990, p 1006.

Table 9–3	Staging of Endometrial Cancer

Stage Ia	G123:	Tumor limited to endometrium
Ib	G123:	Invasion to less than one-half the myometrium
Ic	G123:	Invasion to more than one-half the myometrium
Stage IIa	G123:	Endocervical glandular involvement only
IIb	G123:	Cervical stromal invasion
Stage IIIa	G123:	Tumor invades serosa and/or adnexa, and/or positive peritoneal cytology
IIIb	G123:	Vaginal metastases
IIc	G123:	Metastases to pelvic and/or para-aortic lymph nodes
Stage IVa	G123:	Tumor invasion of bladder and/or bowel mucosa
IVb:		Distant metastases including intra-abdominal and/or inguinal lymph nodes

Graded according to the degree of histologic differentiation:

G1: 5% or less of a nonsquamous or nonmorular solid growth pattern
G2: 6% to 50% of a nonsquamous or nonmorular solid growth pattern
G3: More than 50% of a nonsquamous or nonmorular solid growth pattern

From: Creasman WT: New gynecologic cancer staging. Obstet Gynecol February 1990; 75:287. Reprinted with permission from the American College of Obstetricians and Gynecologists.

are recommended for stage Ib and Ic. Stage Ia cancer of the cervix is treated with hysterectomy or radiotherapy. In this stage the cancer is confined to the cervix. Stages IIa through IV involve tumor growth beyond the cervix (ie, vagina, pelvis, ureters, and outside the reproductive organs), and the treatment of choice is radiotherapy. (DiSaia & Stafl 1990).

Ovarian Cancer   Ovarian cancer is very difficult to diagnose and frequently it has spread before it has been detected. All stages of ovarian cancer are treated with a total abdominal hysterectomy and bilateral salpingo-oophorectomy. Radiation and chemotherapy are often used following surgery.

Endometrial Cancer   Stage I tumors, which involve only the corpus, are treated with TAH-BSO (Table 9–3). Stage II tumors, which involve the corpus and cervix, require TAH-BSO with lymph node dissection and radiation therapy. Stages III and IV are usually treated with external and/or intracavitary irradiation (Kneisl & Ames 1986).

Vulvar Cancer   Cancer of the vulva is more common in women between 70 and 80 years of age who have had chronic vulvitis. Treatment usually includes vulvectomy and removal of superficial inguinal lymph nodes.

Vulvectomy

A simple vulvectomy is performed for leukoplakia and intractible pruritus, whereas a radical procedure is done for malignant disease. A simple vulvectomy is the removal of the labia majora and minora and the clitoris. Radical vulvectomy is the removal of the whole vulva, the skin and fat of the femoral triangle, and the pelvic lymph nodes. Skin grafts may be necessary.

This disfiguring procedure is associated with marked psychosexual disturbances. Most women report greatly decreased sexual arousal levels and low self-image (Hacker et al 1984). The woman may express grief over her loss by crying, withdrawing, or becoming depressed or angry.

Sexual activity can be resumed within three months but adjustments are necessary owing to the loss of sensory perception for foreplay. Stimulation of the breast, thighs, buttocks, or anterior abdominal wall can be suggested.

Pelvic Exenteration

A pelvic exenteration is performed for recurrence of cervical cancer. Only about 5% of women with recurrence are candidates for the procedure, which is not performed if there is any evidence of tumor outside the pelvis, if the cancer has metastasized to the lymph nodes, or if all of the tumor cannot be removed.

Exenteration can be of the anterior or posterior pelvis or of the total pelvis. *Anterior exenteration* is the removal of the uterus, ovaries, fallopian tubes, vagina, bladder, urethra, and pelvic lymph nodes. Urine is diverted through an ileal conduit. *Posterior exenteration* is the removal of the uterus, fallopian tubes, ovaries, descending colon, rectum, and anal canal. A colostomy is created. A *total exenteration* is a combination of the anterior and posterior procedures. A vagina can be reconstructed from split-thickness skin grafts or a segment of small bowel.

Complications associated with exenteration include intestinal and urinary obstruction, thrombophlebitis, pulmonary embolism, pyelonephritis, hypovolemia, peritonitis, pneumonia, and wound infection.

Nursing Care

The nurse frequently has contact with the woman shortly after she has been told of the possible diagnosis. The woman may be confused and stunned by the diagnosis or unclear about what is happening. The nurse can provide support as she begins to establish a relationship with the client. Initial assessments may focus on the information the woman has and desires, on clarifying information, and on assessing her coping style and strengths. It may be helpful to ask the woman to explain her diagnosis and anticipated treatment in order to determine her understanding and the need for further information. After these beginning assessments the nurse extensively assesses preoperative physical and emotional states and potential problems with adjustment related to the woman's body image. A woman's self-concept and feelings of self-worth are associated with her appearance or ability to have normal body functions. The sociocultural (religious, racial) influences on the woman also need to be assessed. Another major assessment area is the impact of the surgery on sexual functioning, particularly when alteration of excretory function and obliteration of the vagina have occurred with pelvic exenteration. The feelings and reactions of the sexual partner are crucial to the woman's adjustment. The nurse or counselor should explore with the woman and her partner new ways of physical contact. Often the woman is so anxious about the recurrence of her cancer that she is willing to accept the body changes preoperatively because she is hopeful for a cure. The best predictor for how a woman will respond after surgery is how she reacted prior to surgery (Gitlin 1989).

Postoperative care for vulvectomy includes urinary drainage via an indwelling catheter to prevent wound contamination and meticulous wound care to debride and provide healing. Wound care usually consists of debriding with a solution of half-strength peroxide followed by normal saline. The wound is then dried with either a heat lamp or a hair dryer (cold air) (Brunner & Suddarth 1988).

Postoperative care for the woman with pelvic exenteration usually begins with three or four days in the intensive care unit because of the risk of shock, cardiac changes, and kidney failure. Once the woman returns to the regular postoperative unit, care includes the usual postoperative interventions, as well as care for the ileal conduit and/or colostomy. The nurse needs to continue to assess the woman for a grief reaction to the drastic changes in her body and should expect emotional fluctuations.

❀ ❀

KEY CONCEPTS

Components of an informed decision regarding reproductive surgery include an explanation of the indications for the surgery, the surgical procedure, the treatment and alternatives, the risks and the effects on the woman.

The nurse focuses on the information the woman needs to make an informed decision and on the assessment of data and implementation of nursing care.

A hysterectomy involves the removal of the uterus. It may be done abdominally or vaginally.

Dilation and curettage is the most frequently performed minor gynecologic surgical procedure. It is done for heavy bleeding, incomplete abortion, therapeutic abortion, dysmenorrhea, or removal of a polyp.

A number of physical and psychological factors influence a woman's decision to seek an abortion.

When abnormal Pap smear results are discovered, associated procedures may include colposcopy, biopsy, laser surgery, conization, or cryosurgery.

Gynecologic cancer involves carcinoma of the cervix, ovaries, uterus, endometrium, and/or vulva.

❀ ❀

References

Ammer C: *The New A to Z of Women's Health: A Concise Encyclopedia.* New York: Facts on File, 1989.

Barsevick AM, Lauver D: Women's informational needs about colposcopy. *Image* Spring 1990; 22(1):23.

Brunner LS, Suddarth DS: Management of patients with gyneco-logic disorders. In: Brunner LS, Suddarth DS: *Textbook of Medical-Surgical Nursing,* 6th ed. Philadelphia: Lippincott, 1988.

Cohen SM et al: Another look at psychologic complications of hysterectomy. *Image* Spring 1989; 21(1):51.

DiSaia PJ, Stafl A: Disorders of the uterine cervix. In: *Danforth's Obstetrics and Gynecology,* 6th ed. Scott JR et al (editors). Philadelphia: Lippincott, 1990.

Gitlin MJ et al: Psychiatric syndromes linked to reproductive function in women: A review of current knowledge. *Am J Psychiatry* November 1989; 146(11):14.

Kneisel CR, Ames SA: *Adult Health Nursing.* Menlo Park, CA: Addison-Wesley, 1986.

London SN, Hammond CB: The climacteric. In: *Danforth's Obstetrics and Gynecology,* 6th ed. Scott JR et al (editors). Philadelphia: Lippincott, 1990.

Ravnikar V: Physiology and treatment of hot flushes. *Obstet Gynecol* 1990; 75(4):3S.

Reiner IJ: Early discharge after vaginal hysterectomy. *Obstet Gynecol* March 1988; 71:416.

Rosenwaks Z, Davis OK: In vitro fertilization and related techniques. In: *Danforth's Obstetrics and Gynecology,* 6th ed. Scott JR et al (editors). Philadelphia: Lippincott, 1990.

Stovall TG et al: Hysterectomy for chronic pelvic pain of presumed uterine etiology. *Obstet Gynecol* 1990; 75(4):676.

Stumpf PG: Pharmacokinetics of estrogen. *Obstet Gynecol* 1990; 75(4):95.

Utian WH: Current perspectives in the management of the menopausal and postmenopausal patient: Introduction. *Obstet Gynecol* 1990; 75(4):15.

Webb C: Professional and lay social support for hysterectomy patients. *J Adv Nurs* 1986; 11:167.

Additional Readings

Bachmann GA: Psychosexual aspects of hysterectomy. *Women's Health Issues* Fall 1990; 1(1):41.

Brenner PF, Mishell DR: Control of human reproduction: Contraception, sterilization, and pregnancy termination. In: *Danforth's Obstetrics and Gynecology,* 6th ed. Scott JR et al (editors). Philadelphia: Lippincott, 1990.

Crestman WT: New gynecologic cancer staging. *Obstet Gynecol* February 1990; 75:287.

Langer R et al: The effect of total abdominal hysterectomy on bladder function in asymptomatic women. *Obstet Gynecol* 1989; 74(2):205.

Moore J: Vaginal hysterectomy: Its success as an outpatient procedure. *AORNJ* 1988; 48(6):1114.

Pearse WH: Maternal-Fetal conflict. *Women's Health Issues* Fall 1990; 1(1):12.

Reiner IJ: Early discharge after vaginal hysterectomy. *Obstet Gynecol* 1988; 131(4):446.

Stotland NL: Social change and women's reproductive health care. *Women's Health Issues* Fall 1990; 1(1):4.

CHAPTER 10

Women's Care:

The Crisis of Rape

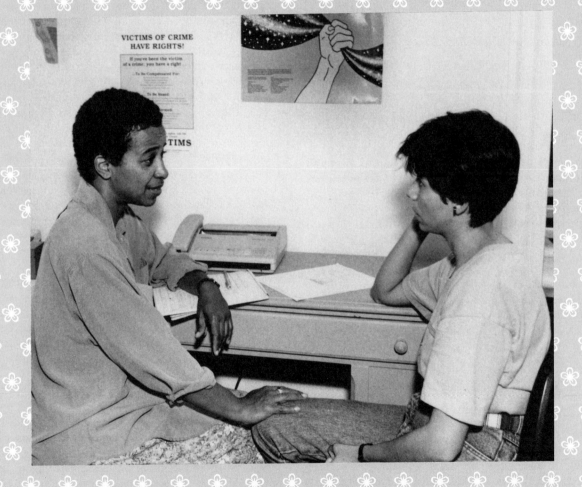

OBJECTIVES

Contrast the nonsexual and sexual aspects of rape.

Compare the types of rape.

Identify the phases of the rape trauma syndrome.

Discuss the importance of values clarification for nurses caring for rape survivors.

Discuss the nurse's role as client advocate and counselor with rape survivors.

Summarize the procedures for collecting and preserving physical evidence of sexual assault.

Discuss the preventive and legal responsibilities of the community.

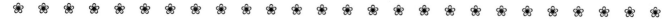

If you really want to help her, the first thing you must do is believe her—even if no weapons were used, she knew the single assailant, she didn't make a police report, and/or there is no evidence of harm. It is not necessary for you to decide if she was "really raped." She says she was raped and that's enough. She feels raped, and she needs your support.

(Linda E. Ledray, Recovering from Rape*)*

Rape can happen to women of all ages, ethnic backgrounds, and walks of life. No woman is immune. As rape is being recognized as one of today's most serious violent crimes, rape crisis counseling centers are emerging to meet the needs of rape survivors. Nevertheless, society continues to harbor many myths and misconceptions about rape and rape survivors. Fear related to these myths may discourage the rape survivor from reporting the assault and may deprive her of the care she needs.

To assist the rape survivor in overcoming this horrifying trauma, the nurse must be able to refute societal myths and must understand the legal definitions of rape, the personality patterns of rapists, and the ways in which survivors are likely to respond. With this information, the nurse can apply specific nursing strategies to benefit the rape survivor and her loved ones.

Definitions and Perspectives

In its broadest sense, **rape** is involuntary sexual contact with another person. However, the legal definition varies according to state. In some states rape involves vaginal penetration by a penis. In other states, all types of forced sex, including oral or anal sex or vaginal penetration by a hand or object, are included in the definition (Parrot 1988). The term *sexual assault* is also used to label such acts. Legally, three elements are necessary for a charge of rape: nonconsent of the victim; the use of force, threat, or deception; and vaginal penetration, however slight.

The person who rapes may be a stranger, acquaintance, husband, or employer. Rape is an act of violence expressed sexually. The act is not motivated by sexual desire but by issues of power, anger, or control. It is a man's aggression and rage acted out against a female.

Rape has been reported against females from age 6 months to 93 years. It is the fastest growing reported crime of violence in the United States (Dennis 1988), occurring once every six minutes (Newsweek, 1990). In 1986 the FBI reported that there were 90,434 rapes, which is a rate of 73 rapes per 100,000 women. However, rape is considered one of the most underreported crimes in this country, and estimates of the actual incidence vary from 4 to 20 times greater than reported (Burge 1989). Rape by an assailant known to the woman occurs approximately 75% of the time (Newsweek, 1990) although it is especially likely to be unreported. The National Center for the Prevention and Control of Rape estimates that one out of every three women will be raped at some time in her life. The incidence of rape in the United States is four times the rate in Germany, 13 times that of England, and 20 times that of Japan (Newsweek, 1990).

Rape is more common in the summer (especially during August) and in large metropolitan areas, although the rate of rape is increasing more rapidly in midsize cities than in large metropolitan areas. Younger women are more likely to be victims, as are black women, but no group is immune (Gordon & Riger 1989).

Myths About Rape

Many people believe the myths that rape commonly occurs at night, to provocatively clothed, promiscuous women. They believe that rapists are sex-starved lunatics who were provoked by the clothing or appearance of the woman. Furthermore, it is a common misconception that no truly virtuous woman can be raped against her will, so that if rape occurs, the woman must have "asked for it." Conversely, the myth continues, since there is nothing a woman can do about rape, she should just relax and enjoy it.

The belief in some or all of these myths has shaped people's response to the rape survivor. Research indicates that blacks, males, and people with traditional views of women's roles tend to believe more that women are responsible for causing rape and are less desirable after the rape; they consider rapists as madmen driven by passion, and favor harsh punishment for rapists (Gordon & Rigor 1989). Culture plays an important role in people's response to rape. "In cultures in which virginity is viewed as a "prized possession" of single women, rape victims are blamed and punished for losing their family honor" (Mollica & Son 1989, p 375). Fortunately, education does seem to be changing societal views about these myths to some extent.

Societal Views of Rape

Rape As Conquest

The act of rape is ages old. Traditionally, it was viewed, not as an act of a man against a woman, but as an act of aggression against another man—the woman's husband or father; that is, her "owner." To rape a man's daughter or wife was the ultimate insult, an act of power. On conclusion of a battle, rape of the wives and daughters of the losers symbolized the triumph of the conquerors and the humiliation of the vanquished.

The Victim As Temptress

Recently, rape survivors have been accused of provoking the assault by their appearance or behavior or merely by being present in a secluded area. This neomedieval concept of rape portrays woman as a temptress preying on men's susceptibility to passion, destroying their always tenuous control, until she "gets what she is asking for."

Various studies have refuted the myth that rape is passion out of control. Groth and Burgess (1977), for example, interviewed 170 convicted rapists. Virtually none of these men reported sexual dysfunction in consenting sexual relations, but 59% reported sexual dysfunction during the rape. Moreover, 9% of these men admitted that coitus was not their intent.

Rape has also been portrayed as a universal female fantasy—the secret dream of every American girl. Sudden attack, physical abuse, and the threat to her life were believed to "turn her on." Actually, rape appears to be the fantasy of some men. Malamuth (1981) asked male students at the University of California whether they would rape a woman if they knew they would not be caught and punished. Approximately 35% said they might.

Rape As a Means of Control

Violence against women is also viewed as a means of control by society. Men are generally physically stronger than women and, in a patriarchal society, have greater power and influence. Many women grow up knowing a vague sense of fear that limits their choices and activities as they feel the need always to be on guard. Thus they look to males to serve in the role of "protector," keeping women safe from harm. Unfortunately, these protectors are the very ones who may perpetrate the acts of violence, but, because society often fails to hold men accountable, the violence continues. Sanday studied reports of primitive tribal societies and concluded that rape is not integral to male nature; rather, it is "the means by which men programmed for violence express their sexual selves" (Garrison 1983, p 6).

Who Commits Rape—and Why

Characteristics of Rapists

Like their victims, rapists come from all ethnic backgrounds and walks of life. More than half are under 25 years of age, and three out of five are married and leading "normal" sex lives. Why do these men rape? Of the many theories proposed in answer to this question, none provides a concrete explanation.

Groth and Burgess (1977) found that 33% of the rapists they interviewed had been sexually abused as children. Their assaults appeared to replicate their childhood experiences. Groth and Burgess's study has been criticized as being biased because all their subjects were incarcerated and therefore not representative of male sexual offenders, the vast majority of whom are not imprisoned.

Rapists also have been examined for biologic abnormalities; for example, the extra Y chromosome (XYY) phenomenon. The extra Y chromosome is thought to cause elevated levels of testosterone, leading to increased aggression. The finding that few incarcerated rapists had extremely high levels of testosterone appears to invalidate this theory (Rada et al 1976).

CRITICAL THINKING

Why do you think the incidence of date rape is increasing? What can women do to protect themselves from acquaintance rape?

Types of Rape

Rape has been categorized in different ways. One method considers whether the rapist was known to the survivor. In **blitz rape**, the assailant and victim are strangers, and the rape is sudden and unexpected. In blitz rape the rapist is more likely to use a weapon and threaten violence or murder.

Confidence rape (also called **acquaintance rape**) involves an assailant with whom the victim had previous nonviolent interaction. The attacker uses deception and trust to gain access to the victim and then betrays that trust. **Date rape** is a type of confidence rape. This type of rape is commonly found on college campuses and occurs between a dating couple. In date rape situations the male has usually planned to have sex and will do what he feels necessary if denied. Thus, in this case, the primary motivation of the rapist is sexual gratification (Crooks & Baur 1990). Research suggests that men tend to justify rape more when the woman initiated the date, when the man paid the expenses, and when they went to the man's residence (Muehlenhard 1988). In confidence rape, the victim is more likely to have consumed drugs or alcohol prior to the attack and tends to delay in reporting the attack (Silverman et al 1988).

Rape has also been categorized as **power rape**, **anger rape**, or **sadistic rape**. The purpose of power rape is control or mastery. The male uses sexual intercourse to place a woman in a powerless position so that he can feel dominant, potent, and strong. He often believes his victim enjoys the assault, and he exerts only the amount of force necessary to subdue his victim. Often power rape is a planned blitz attack, but most acquaintance rapes are also power rapes (Parrot 1988).

Anger rape is the use of a sexual act to express feelings of rage. Typically, the assailant feels abused and mistreated by significant women in his life, and the rape becomes a symbolic act of revenge. Often the act is characterized by considerable brutality and degradation. Attacks on older women often are a form of anger rape.

The sadistic rapist has an antisocial personality and sadism usually characterizes all his relationships. He delights in torture and mutilation and is aroused by his victim's struggles and pain. In this type of rape, the victim and assailant are generally strangers, and the assault is planned. This type of rape, while fortunately rare, usually receives media attention.

Gang rape is more common in younger men who are responding to peer pressure. Typically only one or two of the men may have a rapist mentality but they are able to incite the others to commit acts they would not do individually. Often gang rape can escalate to severe violence and sadistic behavior as the young men seek to outdo each other (Newsweek 1990). The 1989 rape of the Central Park jogger is a well-known example.

The foregoing classifications are not mutually exclusive; they categorize the dominant motive in a given rape. Regardless of the style of attack, anger, power, and sadism are components of any rape, which is essentially the use of sexual behavior to meet nonsexual needs.

Rape Trauma Syndrome

Rape is viewed as a situational crisis; that is, an unanticipated traumatic event that the victim generally is unprepared to handle because it is unforeseen. Following rape,

Table 10–1 Phases of the Rape Trauma Syndrome

Phase	Response
Acute phase	Fear, shock, disbelief, desire for revenge, anger, denial, anxiety, guilt, embarrassment, humiliation, helplessness, dependency; survivor may seek help or may remain silent.
Outward adjustment phase	Survivor appears outwardly composed, denying and repressing feelings; for example, she returns to work, buys a weapon, adds security measures to her residence, and denies need for counseling.
Reorganizational phase	Survivor experiences sexual dysfunction, phobias, sleep disorders, anxiety, and a strong urge to talk about or resolve feelings; victim may seek counseling or may remain silent.

the survivor may experience a cluster of symptoms described by Burgess and Holmstrom (1979) as "**rape trauma syndrome**." Burgess and Holmstrom originally described this syndrome as having two phases: the acute phase and the adjustment or reorganization phase. Sutherland and Scherl proposed an intermediate "outward adjustment" phase (Golan 1978). These phases are summarized in Table 10–1. Other authors have described an alternative "silent reaction." Survivors also suffer long-term effects.

Although the phases of response are discussed individually in the following sections, they often overlap. Individual responses and their duration vary greatly.

Acute Phase

The acute phase of rape trauma syndrome begins during the rape and may last for a few days or up to three weeks (Gordon & Riger 1989). The woman may experience fear, shock, and disbelief and sometimes denial. The woman may feel embarrassed, humiliated, guilty, and unclean; her wish to cleanse herself by bathing or douching may be overpowering, even if she knows that by doing so she is destroying evidence. She may feel angry or anxious, powerless or helpless. Some women blame themselves and feel guilty or feel compelled to "play the scene over and over in their minds."

The rape survivor may suppress her emotions or may reveal them by crying, sobbing, or acting tense and restless. Survivors who control or mask their emotions may appear calm, composed, or subdued. Physical manifestations of rape trauma syndrome include (Burgess & Holmstrom 1979, p 234):

- *Circulatory*—flushing, perspiration, feeling hot or cold.
- *Respiratory*—sighing respirations, hyperventilation, dizziness.

- *Gastrointestinal*—abdominal pain, nausea, anorexia, diarrhea, constipation.
- *Genitourinary*—urinary frequency; interference with sexual function.
- *Mental*—impaired attention, poor concentration, poor memory, changes in outlook and planning.

Many rape survivors also experience alterations in sleep patterns such as insomnia, nightmares, or crying out at night.

Outward Adjustment Phase

Once the acute stage has passed, the survivor may appear adjusted. She returns to work or school and resumes her usual roles. But although she appears composed she is actually coping by denial and suppression (Fogel & Woods 1981). Sutherland and Scherl suggested that the survivor needs the outward adjustment phase to cope with the experience of rape; it is a means of regaining control of her life (Golan 1978). During this time, she may move to a different residence or may institute security measures such as installing extra locks or requesting an unlisted telephone number. She may buy a weapon or take a course in self-defense. These activities do not resolve her emotional trauma; they simply push it further into her subconscious. In addition, she may get less support from others who perceive her as being "over it."

Reorganizational Phase

Because the rape experience had not been resolved, denial and suppression cannot sustain the survivor for long. These coping mechanisms deteriorate; she becomes depressed and anxious and feels a strong urge to talk about the rape. At this point, the woman enters the reorganizational phase of the rape trauma syndrome. She must alter her self-concept and resolve her feelings about the rape.

During this phase, the rape survivor experiences numerous difficulties. Survivors frequently report prolonged menstrual and/or gynecologic disorders. The woman may develop phobias. Fears of being indoors or outdoors or of being attacked from behind—depending on how the attack took place—are common. Because of these fears, the woman may alter her life-style. If she is afraid of crowds, of being out after dark, or of returning to an empty house, she may become a virtual recluse.

Rape survivors frequently report sexual dysfunction. Some women become totally averse to sexual activity. Those who do try to engage in sex often report a decrease in vaginal lubrication, inability to be aroused, unusual sensations in the genital area, and inability to achieve orgasm (Foley & Davies 1983).

Sleep disorders persist. Survivors report repeated nightmares in which they either relive the rape or thwart the rapist's attempt. In either case the dream contains disturbing violence. The woman repeatedly replays the role of victim until she comes to terms with the experience.

The Silent Reaction

Women who do not report the rape go through the phases of the rape trauma syndrome without using available support systems. Their reasons for keeping silent vary; a woman may be embarrassed, she may accept society's "temptress view" and blame herself, or she may fear retaliation. Her experience may be discovered much later, perhaps when she seeks professional help in resolving a different crisis.

Research Note

Clinical Application of Research

Barbara Brown and Carole Garrison (1990) used the information obtained from nonreporting incest survivors who had been admitted to a sexual assault crisis center to investigate patterns of physical and psychosocial symptoms and correlations among several variables. Nonreporting incest survivors were women who had been sexually abused before the age of 18 and had never received treatment. A second group of nonabused women also completed a similar self-reporting questionnaire. At least 30% of the abused women reported sexual dysfunction, alcohol abuse, and drug abuse while only slightly over 1% of the nonabused women described these findings. Psychosocial symptoms such as suicidal thoughts, depression, relationship problems, and guilt were identified by the abused group, while the nonabused group reported 11% or less in each of these categories. The researchers found positive correlations between age and additional episodes of abuse, age and physical symptoms, onset age and duration of incest and duration and number of offenders.

Critical Thinking Applied to Research

Strengths: Description of characteristics of a group of women, nonreporting incest survivors, who are not often studied.

Concerns: One of the purposes of the study was to design an assessment instrument which would assist in the identification of nonreporting survivors of incest. A questionnaire was developed but psychometric properties were not identified and this purpose was not specifically addressed in either the results or the implications. The text stated that results from nonabused women were used in the correlation statistics but the N of the correlation table corresponds only to the number of abused women. The study might have been stronger as two separate studies with two well-defined groups.

Brown B, Garrison C: Patterns of symptomatology of adult women incest survivors. *West J Nurs Res* 1990; 12(5):587.

Some women seek medical help for their physical injuries without disclosing that a rape was the cause. The nurse who suspects that a woman has been raped should seek validation through sympathetic questioning. Public health nurses are often able to identify silent victims by their observations of violent family interactions.

Long-Term Effects

Although not enough research has been devoted to determining the long-term effects of rape, the most prevalent sequelae appear to be sexual problems, fear, and anxiety. In summing up the few studies conducted to date, Ferris (1983) compared the long-term reactions of survivors with those related to war, hurricanes, floods, or similar major disasters.

The Rape Survivor and the Role of the Nurse

Rape survivors often enter the health care system by way of the emergency room; nurses are often the first to counsel them. It is essential to remember that the rape survivor is not sick; she is in a crisis state. Counseling should follow the crisis intervention pattern outlined in Table 10–2.

Clarifying the Nurse's Reaction

The values, attitudes, and beliefs of a care giver will necessarily affect the competency and focus of the care that that person gives. Interaction with a rape survivor may provoke

Table 10–3	Nursing Actions Appropriate to Phases of the Rape Trauma Syndrome
Phase	**Nursing action**
Acute phase	Creating a safe milieu
	Explaining the sequence of events in the health care facility
	Allowing the woman to grieve and express her feelings
	Providing care for significant others
Outward adjustment phase	Providing advocacy and support at the level requested by the woman
	Providing assistance to significant others
Reorganizational phase	Establishing a trusting relationship
	Assisting the woman to understand her role in the assault
	Clarifying and enhancing the woman's feelings
	Assisting the woman in planning for her future

anxiety, ambivalence, or feelings of personal vulnerability to rape. The nurse may feel overwhelmed by sympathetic feelings or by a sense of inadequacy. Conversely, the nurse may consciously or subconsciously accept the view that a woman was "asking for it." Such feelings interfere with the nurse's ability to give empathic, advocative assistance. Moreover, the nurse may silently convey these feelings to the woman, thus increasing her distress.

Nurses who work with rape survivors must understand their own attitudes and beliefs about rape. With the aid of a skilled facilitator, nurses can discuss their feelings about rape and rape survivors and resolve any conflicts.

Acute Phase

Policies for admitting and examining rape survivors vary among institutions. A woman who has been raped is under great stress and needs the sensitive care of professionals who are aware of her special needs. The manner in which she is treated at this crucial time will strongly affect her ability to function in the future. Table 10–3 outlines the general principles of nursing actions during the various phases of the rape trauma syndrome.

The first priority is creating a safe, secure milieu. Admission information should be gathered in a quiet, private room. The woman should be reassured that she is not alone and will not be abandoned and that she is safe from a second attack. During this time, the nurse can develop a relationship so that the rape survivor has a person to whom she can relate consistently throughout her hospital experience.

The survivor's level of emotional distress must be assessed, both for the purpose of planning care and as possible courtroom evidence. Scrupulous documentation is

Table 10–2	Nursing Strategies to Assist the Client in Crisis

The nurse:

Listens actively and with concern

Encourages the open expression of feelings

Assists the woman in gaining an understanding of the crisis

Assists the woman to accept reality gradually

Assists the woman to explore new ways of coping with her problems

Links the woman to a social network

Assists the woman to make decisions about:
  What problem needs to be solved
  How it is to be solved
  When and where it should be solved
  Who should be solving it

Reinforces newly learned coping strategies

Encourages follow-up contact

Source: Adapted from Kozier B, Erb G: Fundamentals of Nursing, 3rd ed. Menlo Park, CA: Addison-Wesley, 1987.

essential because the survivor's medial record is often used in the courtroom to verify her testimony if the rapist is prosecuted. The mental status examination includes the following:

- *General appearance and behavior.* What is the woman's attitude? Her posture? What mannerisms does she display?
- *Consciousness/awareness.* Is the woman oriented to time, place, and identity? Is she able to focus on a subject, theme, or event?
- *Affectivity and mood.* Is the woman depressed? Anxious? Displaying elation anxiety? Is she fearful or apathetic? Is she expressing her feelings or controlling them?
- *Motor behavior.* Is the woman inactive, hyperactive, or underactive?
- *Thought control.* How logical is the woman's flow of ideas and associations?
- *Intellectual functioning.* How intelligent does the woman appear? What is her level of general knowledge? How well does she remember events? How sound is her judgment?

It is imperative that control be returned to the woman as quickly as possible. She has suffered trauma in which all control was taken from her. The nurse can return control by encouraging the woman to make contact. When feasible, the woman should decide on the sequence of hospital events. In this way the nurse helps her deal with her crisis in small, manageable increments.

The woman should be encouraged to express her feelings and reassured that anger and fear are normal, appropriate responses. The nurse can also address expressed or unexpressed guilt by assuring the woman that the rape was not her fault.

By explaining the medical examination and the sequence of events in the emergency department, the nurse alleviates anxiety related to fear of the unknown. The woman should know what is going to happen and why, and how she can assist in each phase of the examination. (Examination of the rape survivor and collection of evidence are discussed later in this chapter.)

Throughout the experience, the nurse acts as the survivor's advocate, providing support without usurping decision making. The nurse need not agree with all the survivor's decisions but should respect and defend the survivor's right to make them.

The family members or friends on whom the survivor calls also need nursing care. Like the survivor, the reactions of the family will depend on the values to which they ascribe. Sonstegard et al (1982) reported that the most common reaction is to regard rape as a sexual act rather than an act of violence. Many families or mates blame the survivor for the rape and feel angry with her for not being more careful. They may feel personally wronged or attacked and

see the survivor as being devalued or unclean. These reactions compound the survivor's crisis.

By spending some time with family members before their first interaction with the survivor, the nurse can reduce their anxiety and absorb their frustrations, sparing the woman further trauma.

Outward Adjustment Phase

A survivor who is in the outward adjustment phase may deny any need for counseling. The nurse, respecting the woman's wishes, does not force counseling on her. The family, however, may still be in need of assistance in coping with anger or guilt. The survivor's behavior may confuse them. By providing information and support, the nurse can assist them in examining and reconciling their feelings.

Reorganizational Phase

As the woman enters the reorganizational phase, she usually feels a strong urge to discuss and resolve her feelings about herself and her assailant. "This means that she must come to terms intellectually and viscerally (her head and heart) by acknowledging the impact of the rape on her life and incorporating it as a stressful memory in her total life experience" (Burgess & Holmstrom 1979, p 330). During this phase, the survivor may benefit from counseling.

Rape Counseling

Foley and Davies (1983) identified three phases of rape counseling: self-exploration, self-understanding, and action.

Self-Exploration
Counselor and survivor explore the survivor's feelings and establish rapport. Feelings that have been denied and suppressed are brought into the woman's awareness. She should be encouraged to express those feelings openly, identify their source, and understand that they belong to her. The nurse employs a nondirective therapeutic use of self, responding empathically to the survivor's feelings and demonstrating perception of and sensitivity to the woman's feelings, thoughts, and experiences. Acceptance of the woman and respect for her are essential. The woman must feel that she can come to the nurse in a safe, stable, nonjudgmental environment to express her feelings fully and get in touch with them.

Self-Understanding
Having identified the woman's feelings, she and the nurse go on to clarify them and understand their source. Understanding the reasons for her feelings enables the woman to decide on actions that will resolve her problems. The nurse can assist her in understanding the larger context of the rape. It is important for the nurse to avoid reinforcing the prevalent myth that rape is the survivor's "fault." Rather,

the nurse can use questions and discussion to encourage the woman to conclude that the blame lies with the rapist. Similarly, the nurse assists the individual in formulating strategies for returning to her prerape level of functioning.

Action

In this phase the survivor makes specific plans for overcoming her problems and tests them with the nurse's support. With the nurse, the woman explores her thoughts and feelings about self-care, celebrates her victories, and evaluates her defeats. It is important to emphasize that the loss of control that occurred during the rape was temporary and that the woman does have control over other aspects of her life. "The counselor can conclude that the victim has come to terms with the rape when the victim can honestly say that the memory is not as frequent, the physical distress is not as great, and the intensity of the memory has decreased" (Burgess & Holmstrom 1979, p 331).

Physical Care of the Rape Survivor

Traditionally, the health care system has met the physical needs of the rape survivor (often to the detriment of emotional needs). Repair of tissue damage and prevention of complications are primary concerns. Because rape is a crime as well as a traumatic emergency, however, some aspects of medical care are governed by the need to collect and preserve legal evidence for use in prosecuting the assailant. In so doing, health care providers must respect the rights of the rape survivor, which are summarized in Table 10–4. To better meet women's needs, many emergency departments use multidisciplinary teams to provide effective care to rape survivors and their families.

Detailed History

Obtaining a detailed history is an essential first step in acquiring necessary medical and forensic data, but it can also be a therapeutic tool if done in a sensitive, caring way. Because rape survivors may appear relaxed and normal when first seen, care givers may underestimate the woman's needs, but it is essential that rape survivors receive immediate attention (Robinson 1990). An explicit sexual history is usually taken immediately after the woman has received any necessary emergency care. Because care givers often lack experience in obtaining the necessary information in enough depth and detail, many agencies use a standardized history flow sheet to record information.

The care giver should use a nonjudgmental approach and avoid leading or coaching the woman. Once the sheet

---

Table 10–4   The Rights of the Rape Survivor

The rape victim has the right:

1. To transportation to a hospital when incapacitated.
2. To emergency room care with privacy and confidentiality.
3. To be listened to carefully and treated as a human being, with respect, courtesy, and dignity.
4. To have an advocate of choice accompany her through the treatment process.
5. To be given as much credibility as a victim of any other crime.
6. To have her name kept from the news media.
7. To be considered a victim of rape regardless of the assailant's relationship to her.
8. Not to be exposed to prejudice against race, age, class, life-style, or occupation.
9. Not to be asked questions about prior sexual experience.
10. To be treated in a manner that does not usurp her control but enables her to determine her own needs and how to meet them.
11. To be asked only those questions that are relevant to a court case or to medical treatment.
12. To receive prompt medical and mental health services, regardless of whether the rape is reported to the police.
13. To be protected from future assault.
14. To accurate collection and preservation of evidence for court in an objective record that includes the signs and symptoms of physical and emotional trauma.
15. To receive clear explanations of procedures and medication in language she can understand.
16. To know what treatment is recommended, for what reasons, and who will administer the treatment.
17. To know any possible risks, side effects, or alternatives to proposed treatments, including all drugs prescribed.
18. To ask for another physician, nurse practitioner, or nurse.
19. To consent to or refuse any treatment, even when her life is in serious danger.
20. To refuse to be part of any research or experiment.
21. To make reasonable complaints and to leave a care facility against the physician's advice.
22. To receive an explanation of and understand any papers she agrees to sign.
23. To be informed of continuing health care needs after discharge from the emergency room, hospital, physician's office, or care facility.
24. To receive a clear explanation of the bill and review of charges and to be informed of available compensation.
25. To have legal representation and be advised of her legal rights, including the possibility of filing a civil suit.

Reprinted with permission of author from Foley TS, Davies MA: Rape: Nursing Care of Victims. St. Louis, Mosby, 1983.

is completed, the woman can be given her own copy to take home (Renshaw 1989).

Collection of Evidence

The collection of evidence may, in itself, be traumatic for the woman. It is valuable to have someone available to provide support and act as an advocate during these procedures. This person may be a family member or close friend, but often it is a nurse.

The woman should receive a thorough explanation of the procedures to be carried out and should sign a consent form. An important legal concept when dealing with rape survivors is the need to preserve the *chain of evidence*, meaning that all physical evidence and specimens should remain in the hands of a professional until they are turned over to a police officer. Preserving the chain of evidence is done to prevent confusion and the possibility of tampering with evidence (Beckmann & Groetzinger 1989). Most agencies have special sexual assault kits that contain all necessary supplies for collection and labeling of evidence.

Vaginal and rectal examinations are performed, along with a complete physical examination for trauma. Any lacerations of the vaginal wall are repaired and noted.

Clothing

Clothing is inspected for the presence of semen, because often the rapist ejaculates outside the vagina. Clothing should be placed in a paper bag, sealed, and labeled appropriately.

Swabs of Stains and Secretions

Swabs of body stains are analyzed for semen or sperm. Because victims are often forced to commit fellatio, oral swabs are examined for semen. Gonorrhea cultures also are taken from oral swabs. Specimens of the woman's saliva are examined to determine whether she is a secretor or nonsecretor of certain blood-group antigens. If she is a nonsecretor—that is, if these antigens are not present in her saliva—the presence of antigens in her mouth and/or vagina may be evidence of semen from the assailant (Foley & Davies 1983).

Vaginal and rectal swabs are necessary to document the presence of sperm. Because sperm are sensitive to air and do not survive for long periods, a screen for vaginal sperm is performed as soon as possible. A vaginal smear is placed on a wet mount and stained; any sperm that are present will appear light blue. The absence of sperm, however, does not signify that no rape has occurred. As discussed earlier, many rapists suffer from sexual dysfunction during the rape and do not ejaculate.

Hair and Scrapings

Clippings or scrapings of the woman's fingernails are examined for blood or tissue from the assailant. Approximately 15 hairs are pulled from her head to analyze the root structure and identify foreign hairs. Her pubic hair is combed to check for loose pubic hair that may have been transferred from the rapist.

Blood samples

Blood is drawn to be tested for gonorrhea and syphilis and to determine whether the woman is pregnant.

Photographs

The procedure for taking photographs, if any, is determined by institutional policy.

Prevention of Sexually Transmitted Disease

The survivor is offered prophylactic treatment for sexually transmitted diseases (STDs). Usually 250 mg ceftriaxone is given intramuscularly, followed by 100 mg doxycycline orally, twice daily for seven days (Beckmann & Groetzinger 1989). In addition, any identified STDs are treated. The woman should be offered human immunodeficiency virus (HIV) testing at the time she seeks care and again in three to six months. If she tests positive, she should be referred to a center specializing in the treatment of AIDS. Some agencies advocate treating the woman with a vaginal application of nonoxynol-9 as a possible anti-HIV (anti-AIDS) treatment (Foster & Bartlett 1989). If the survivor chooses not to receive prophylactic treatment, the nurse should instruct her to return in two weeks to be tested for gonorrhea and again in four to six weeks to be tested for syphilis.

Prevention of Pregnancy

The woman is questioned about her menstrual cycle and contraceptive practices. If she could become pregnant as a result of the rape, postcoital therapy is offered. Treatment involves 5 mg ethinyl estradiol orally, twice daily for five days with 10 mg prochlorperazine (Compazine) orally or by suppository every eight hours to control nausea (Beckmann & Groetzinger 1989). Other side effects include vomiting, headache, breast tenderness, and menstrual irregularities. Estrogen therapy should begin within 72 hours of intercourse to be effective. Because the estrogen may be teratogenic, a pregnancy test should be performed first. The woman should be advised that if she becomes pregnant despite the therapy, one of her options is a therapeutic abortion.

Rape As a Community Responsibility

Preventive education, funding of rape crisis counseling centers, and prosecution of the rapist are community responsibilities.

Preventive Education

Community colleges or local rape awareness groups may offer courses in preventive strategies. Some classes focus on increasing women's awareness of situations in which they are at risk. Others are concerned with changing societal attitudes about rape and rape survivors. Because rape is a considerable risk for any woman, courses in what to do during and after a rape may also be helpful. Nurses are well qualified to initiate or participate in preventive instruction.

Rape Crisis Counseling

Most rape crisis counseling centers operate 24 hours a day, seven days a week. Their services are invaluable. Properly trained telephone counselors can help the woman regain control early in the crisis. Early crisis intervention often encourages the woman to seek professional treatment and assistance. Many rape crisis centers offer free counseling to rape survivors or can refer them to qualified counselors. Information on sexually transmitted disease and pregnancy alternatives may also be obtained from these centers.

Prosecution of the Rapist

Legally, rape, like any criminal action, is considered a crime against the state rather than against the victim. Therefore, prosecution of the assailant is a community responsibility in which the district attorney will act on the victim's behalf. The victim, however, must initiate the process by reporting the crime and pressing charges against her assailant. Once authorities have apprehended the alleged rapist, the judicial system is set into motion.

Procedures vary from state to state. A judge or magistrate generally conducts a hearing to determine whether there is sufficient evidence that a crime has in fact been committed and that the accused has committed it. If so, the alleged assailant will be bound over for the grand jury. The grand jury will hear the state's evidence (not the defense), again to determine whether the evidence is sufficient for trial. If so, the defendant is indicted; if not, he is acquitted. Once indicted, a defendant must stand trial unless he waives this right. He may elect to have his case heard by a judge rather than a jury. Either a judge or a jury will find the defendant guilty or not guilty, and he will be retained or set free accordingly.

Many rape survivors who have gone through the judicial process refer to it as a second rape—and sometimes a more damaging one. The survivor will be repeatedly asked to identify the assailant and describe the rape in intimate detail. Throughout the pretrial period, the defense attorney may use delaying tactics, obtaining continuances or postponements, further frustrating the survivor and her support system. Publicity may intensify her feelings of humiliation, and if the assailant is released on bail, she may fear retaliation.

During the trial itself, cross-examination by the defense attorney can be a severely degrading experience in which the "victim as temptress" myth is continually evoked. Although some states have altered their laws so that the survivor's sexual history may not be made public, others have not. The defense attorney will try to discredit her testimony, causing her to feel victimized a second time. Consider, for example, the case of a New York investment banker who was attacked, beaten and gang-raped in New York City's Central Park by a gang of youths engaged in a "wilding." During their trial, the woman was accused of lying, faking amnesia, and inviting the attack because she was out at night (Newsweek, 1990).

The nurse acting as a counselor needs to be aware of the judicial sequence to anticipate rising tension and frustration in the survivor and her support system. They will need consistent, effective support at this crucial time.

✿ ✿

KEY CONCEPTS

A rape occurs every six minutes in the United States, yet a majority of rapes are unreported. The assailant is known to the woman 75% of the time. Estimates suggest that one out of every three women will be raped at some time in her life.

Why men rape remains a mystery, although it has been established that rape is an act of eroticized aggression.

Following rape, the survivor will usually experience an assortment of symptoms known as the rape trauma syndrome.

The nursing actions to assist rape survivors are encompassed in the roles of advocate, educator, and counselor.

Nurses inform the woman of the sequence of events and her options and support the survivor's decisions.

The counseling process used by the nurse follows the crisis intervention model because the survivor is in a situational crisis rather than being ill.

Nursing research is needed on the long-term effects of rape on survivors and their families, positive coping mechanisms used by past survivors, and effective counseling strategies.

Widespread education is also needed to abolish societal myths surrounding rape.

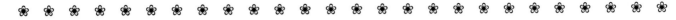

References

Beckmann CRB, Groetzinger LL: Treating sexual assault victims: A protocol for health professionals. *Female Patient* May 1989; 14:78.

Burge SK: Violence against women as a health care issue. *Fam Med* September/October 1989; 21:368.

Burgess AW, Holmstrom LL: *Rape: Crisis and Recovery.* Englewood Cliffs, NJ: Prentice-Hall, 1979.

Crooks R, Baur K: *Our Sexuality,* 4th ed. Redwood City, CA: Benjamin/Cummings, 1990.

Dennis LI: Adolescent rape: The role of nursing. *Issues Comprehensive Pediat Nurs* 1988; 11:59.

Fogel CI, Woods NF: *Health Care of Women: A Nursing Perspective.* St. Louis: Mosby, 1981.

Foley TS, Davies MA: *Rape: Nursing Care of Victims.* St. Louis: Mosby, 1983.

Foster IM, Bartlett J: Anti-HIV substances for rape victims (letter). *JAMA* 1989; 261(23):3407.

Garrison J: *Research on Rapists: Response to Violence in the Family and Sexual Assault.* Vol. 6, No. 2, Rockville, MD: National Center for the Prevention and Control of Rape, March/April, 1983.

Golan N: *Treatment in Crisis Situations.* New York: Free Press, 1978.

Gordon MT, Riger S: *The Female Fear.* New York: Free Press, 1989.

Groth AN, Burgess AW: Sexual dysfunction during rape. *N Engl J Med* 1977; 297(14):764.

Malamuth N: Rape proclivity among males. *J Soc Issues* 1981; 37:138.

Mollica RF, Son L: Cultural dimensions in the evaluation and treatment of sexual trauma. *Psych Clin North Am* June 1989; 12:363.

Muehlenhard CL: Misinterpreted dating behaviors and the risk of date rape. *J Soc Clin Psychol* 1988; 6(1):20.

Parrot A: *Coping with Date Rape and Acquaintance Rape.* New York: Rosen Publishing Group, 1988.

Rada RT et al: Plasma testosterone levels in the rapist. *Psychosom Med* 1976; 38(4):257.

Renshaw DC: Treatment of sexual exploitation: Rape and incest. *Psych Clin North Am* June 1989; 12:257.

Robinson JC: Rape—A crime with health consequences. *Female Patient* March 1990; 15:25.

Silverman DC et al: Blitz rape and confidence rape: A typology applied to 1,000 consecutive cases. *Am J Psychiatry* November 1988; 145:1438.

Sonstegard LJ et al: *Women's Health: Ambulatory Care.* Vol. I. New York: Grune & Stratton, 1982.

The mind of the rapist. *Newsweek,* July 23, 1990, p 46.

Additional Readings

Candib IM: Violence against women: No more excuses. *Fam Med* September/October 1989; 21:339.

Campbell JC: Using nursing research to change the law . . . marital rape exemption. *Am J Nurs* July 1989; 89:948.

Cartwright PS, Moore RA: The elderly victim of rape. *South Med J* August 1989; 82:988.

Koss M: The women's mental health research agenda: Violence against women. *Am Psychol* 1990; 45(3):374.

Minden P: The victim care service: A program for victims of sexual assault. *Arch Psych Nurs* February 1989; 3:41.

Moore KA et al: Nonvoluntary sexual activity among adolescents. *Fam Plann Persp* May/June 1989; 21:110.

Myers MF: Men sexually assaulted as adults and sexually abused as boys. *Arch Sex Behav* June 1989; 18:203.

Nathanson DL: Understanding what is hidden: Shame in sexual abuse. *Psych Clin North Am* June 1989; 12:381.

Osborn M, Bryan S: Evidentiary examination in sexual assault. *J Emerg Nurs* May/June 1989; 15:284.

Schetky DH, Benedek E: The sexual abuse victim in the courts. *Psych Clin North Am* June 1989; 12:471.

Pregnancy

Conception and Fetal Development

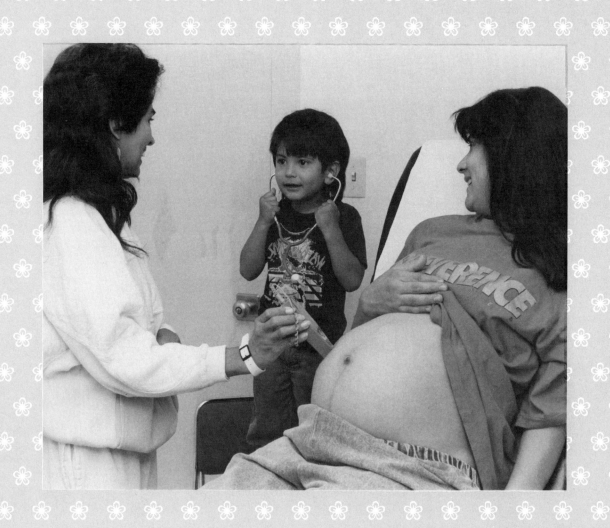

OBJECTIVES

Explain the difference between mitotic cellular division and meiotic cellular division.

Describe the components of the process of fertilization.

Describe the development, structure, and functions of the placenta and umbilical cord during intrauterine life.

Summarize the significant changes in growth and development of the fetus in utero at 4, 6, 12, 16, 20, 24, 28, 36, and 40 weeks' gestation.

Identify the vulnerable periods during which teratogenesis of the various organ systems may occur, and describe the resulting congenital malformations.

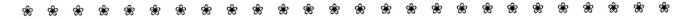

Every person is unique. What is interesting about this uniqueness is that all of us have most if not all the same "parts," and these parts usually function similarly. Even our chromosomes, those determinants of the structure and function of our organ systems and traits, are made of the same biochemical substances. How do we become unique, then? The answer lies in the physiologic mechanisms of heredity, the processes of cellular division, and the environmental factors that influence our development from the moment we are conceived. This chapter explores the processes involved in conception and fetal development—the basis of our uniqueness.

Chromosomes

The body (somatic) cells of each individual contain within their nuclei threadlike bodies known as **chromosomes**, which are composed of strands of **deoxyribonucleic acid (DNA)** and protein. *Genes* are regions in the DNA strands that contain coded information used to determine the unique characteristics of the individual; they are arranged in linear order on the chromosomes.

As the storage place for genetic information, DNA does not leave the cell nucleus. The DNA strand splits and forms the basis for a ribonucleic acid (RNA) molecule. The RNA passes out of the nucleus and carries coded information to the cytoplasm of the cell. An error in the "reading" of the code can cause a change that may have serious effects on the functioning of the organism.

Each chromosome contains two longitudinal halves called *chromatids*, which are joined together at a point called the centromere. Each animal species has a constant number of chromosomes in each of its body cells. Humans have 46 chromosomes divided into 23 pairs: 22 pairs of chromosomes are called autosomes and one pair (23rd pair) of sex chromosomes (designated either XX or XY). Each member of a pair carries either similar genes referred to as *homologous* (homozygous) or dissimilar, allelic, genes referred to as *heterozygous* (Figure 11–1A).

The chromosomes are classified according to their length and to the position of their centromere. When the centromere is centrally located, the longitudinal halves are divided into arms of approximately equal length, and the chromosome resembles an X (Figure 11–1B).

Cellular Division

All humans begin life as a single cell (fertilized ovum). This single cell reproduces itself, and in turn each new cell also reproduces itself in a continuing process. The new cells are similar to the cells from which they came.

Cells are reproduced by either mitosis or meiosis, two different but related processes. **Mitosis** results in the production of additional diploid body (somatic) cells. Mitosis makes growth and development possible, and in mature individuals it is the process by which our body cells continue to divide and replace themselves. **Meiosis**, by contrast, is the cell division process by which sexual reproduction occurs, leading to the development of a new organism.

Mitosis

During mitosis the cell undergoes several changes, ending in cell division. Although mitosis is a continuous process, it is generally divided into five stages: interphase, prophase, metaphase, anaphase, and telophase (Figure 11–2).

During interphase, before cell division takes place, the DNA within the chromosomes replicates so that the genes will be doubled. Mitosis begins when the cell enters prophase. The chromosomes condense and form the shape we usually recognize as a chromosome. Next comes the appearance of a mitotic apparatus known as a spindle, in which fine threads extend from the top and bottom poles of the nucleus. At each pole of the spindle, a body known as the centriole is formed, so that the threads of the spindle extend from one centriole to the other. Next the nuclear membrane, which separates the nucleus from the cytoplasm, disappears; the nucleus as a separate entity disappears, and the cell enters metaphase.

During metaphase, the chromosomes line up at the equator (midway between the poles) of the spindle. Meta-

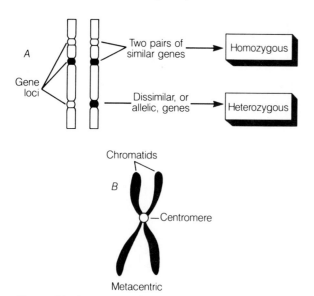

Figure 11–1 A Pair of chromosomes with similar (homozygous) and dissimilar (heterozygous) genes. B Classification of chromosomal joining (From Whaley LE: Understanding Inherited Disorders. St. Louis: Mosby, 1974, p 6)

phase is followed by anaphase, in which the two chromatids of each chromosome separate and move to opposite ends of the spindle, where they cluster in masses near the two poles of the cell.

Telophase is essentially the reverse of prophase. A new nuclear membrane forms, separating each newly formed nucleus from the cytoplasm. The spindle disappears and the centrioles relocate outside of each new nucleus. Within the nucleus the nucleolus again becomes visible, and the chromosomes lengthen and become thread-like. As telophase nears completion, a furrow develops in the cytoplasm at the midline of the cell and divides it into two daughter cells, each with its own nucleus. Daughter cells have the same **diploid number of chromosomes** (46) and the same genetic makeup as the cell from which they came.

In other words, after a cell with 46 chromosomes goes through mitosis, the result is two identical cells, each of them having 46 chromosomes.

Meiosis occurs during **gametogenesis**, the process by which germ cells, or **gametes**, are produced. The gametes must have a haploid number (23) of chromosomes so that when the female gamete (the egg or ovum) and the male gamete (sperm or spermatozoon) unite to form the **zygote**, the normal human diploid number of chromosomes (46) is reestablished.

Meiosis

Meiosis consists of two successive cell divisions (see Figure 11–2). In the first division, the chromosomes replicate.

Next, a pairing takes place between homologous chromosomes (Sadler 1985). Instead of separating immediately as in mitosis, the similar chromosomes become closely intertwined. An exchange of parts between chromatids (the arms of the chromosomes) often takes place. At each point of contact, there is also a physical exchange of genetic material between the chromatids. New combinations are provided by the newly formed chromosomes; these combinations account for the wide variation of traits, such as hair or eye color, in people. The chromosome pairs then separate, each member of a pair moving to opposite sides of the cell. (In contrast, during mitosis the chromatids of each chromosome separate and move to opposite poles.) The cell divides, forming two daughter cells, each with 23 replicated chromosomes—the same amount of DNA as a normal somatic cell. In the second division, the chromatids of each chromosome separate and move to opposite poles of each of the daughter cells. Cell division occurs, resulting in the formation of four cells, each containing 23 single chromosomes (the **haploid number of chromosomes**). These daughter cells contain only half the DNA of a normal somatic cell (Moore 1988).

Occasionally during the second meiotic division, two of the chromatids may not move apart rapidly enough when the cell divides. The still-paired chromatids are carried into one of the daughter cells and eventually form an extra chromosome. This condition is referred to as an *autosomal nondisjunction* (chromosomal mutation) and is harmful to the offspring that may result should fertilization occur. The implications of nondisjunction are discussed in Chapter 5.

Another type of chromosomal mutation can occur if chromosomes break during meiosis. If the broken segment is lost, the result is a shorter chromosome; this situation is known as deletion. If the broken segment becomes attached to another chromosome, it is called translocation, which often results in harmful structural mutations (Thompson & Thompson 1986). The effects of translocation are described in Chapter 5.

Gametogenesis

Oogenesis

Oogenesis is the process by which female gametes are produced. As discussed in Chapter 4 the ovaries begin to develop early in the fetal life of the female. All the ova that the female will produce in her lifetime are formed by the sixth month of fetal life. The ovary gives rise to oogonial cells, which develop into *oocytes*. Meiosis begins in all oocytes before the female infant is born but stops before the first division is complete and remains in this arrested phase until puberty. During puberty the mature primary oocyte continues through the first meiotic division in the graafian follicle of the ovary.

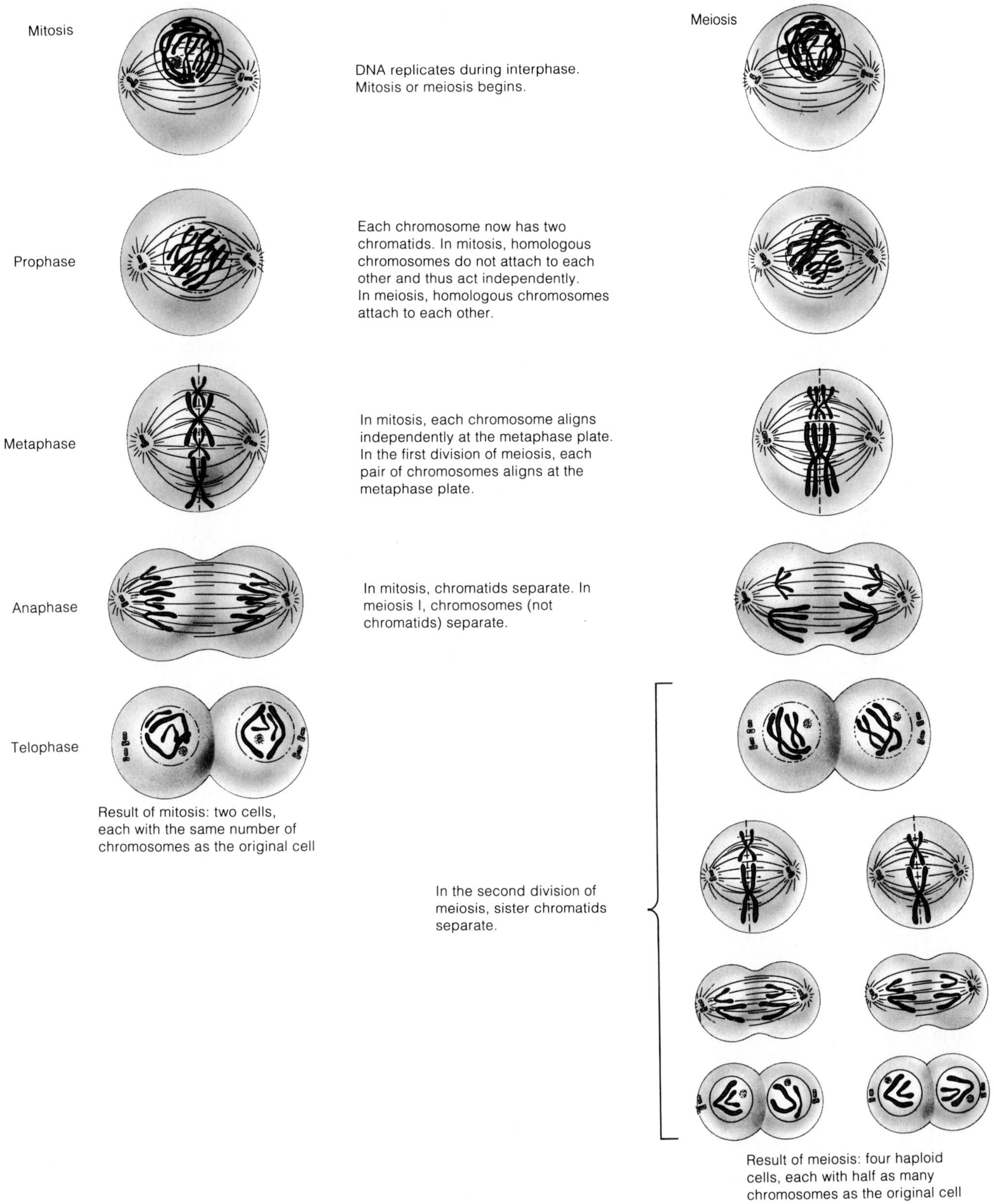

Mitosis

Meiosis

DNA replicates during interphase.
Mitosis or meiosis begins.

Prophase

Each chromosome now has two
chromatids. In mitosis, homologous
chromosomes do not attach to each
other and thus act independently.
In meiosis, homologous chromosomes
attach to each other.

Metaphase

In mitosis, each chromosome aligns
independently at the metaphase plate.
In the first division of meiosis, each
pair of chromosomes aligns at the
metaphase plate.

Anaphase

In mitosis, chromatids separate. In
meiosis I, chromosomes (not
chromatids) separate.

Telophase

Result of mitosis: two cells,
each with the same number of
chromosomes as the original cell

In the second division of
meiosis, sister chromatids
separate.

Result of meiosis: four haploid
cells, each with half as many
chromosomes as the original cell

Figure 11–2   Comparison of mitosis and meiosis. (Adapted From Becker WM, Deamer DW:
The World of the Cell, *2nd ed. Redwood City, CA: Benjamin/Cummings, 1991, p 435, 490)*

The first meiotic division produces two cells of unequal sizes with unequal amounts of cytoplasm but the same number of chromosomes. These two cells are the *secondary oocyte* and a minute *polar body*. Both the secondary oocyte and the first polar body contain 22 replicated autosomal chromosomes and one replicated sex chromosome (X). At the time of ovulation, second meiotic division begins immediately and proceeds as the oocyte moves down the fallopian tube. Division is again not equal. The secondary oocyte proceeds to metaphase where its meiotic division is arrested.

Only when fertilized by the sperm does the secondary oocyte complete the second meiotic division, becoming a mature ovum with the haploid number of chromosomes and having virtually all the cytoplasm. The second polar body is also formed at this time (Figure 11–3). The first polar body has now also divided, producing two additional polar bodies. Thus, when meiosis is completed, four haploid cells have been produced: three small polar bodies, which eventually disintegrate, and one ovum (Sadler 1985) (Figure 11–4).

Spermatogenesis

During puberty the germinal epithelium in the seminiferous tubules of the testes begins the process of spermatogenesis, which produces the male gamete (sperm) and continues into senescence. As the diploid spermatogonium enters the first meiotic division, it is called the *primary spermatocyte*. During this first meiotic division, the spermatogonium replicate and form two haploid cells termed *secondary spermatocytes*, each of which contains 22 autosomal chromosomes and either an X sex chromosome or a Y sex chromosome. During the second meiotic division they divide to form four spermatids, each with the haploid number of chromosomes (Figure 11–4). The spermatids undergo a series of changes during which they lose most of their cytoplasm and become sperm (spermatozoa). The nucleus becomes compacted into the head of the sperm, which is covered by a cap called an acrosome. A long tail is produced from one of the centrioles (see Figure 4–25).

Sex Determination

The two sex chromosomes of the twenty-third pair determine the sex of an organism. The larger of the sex chromosomes is designated X, and the smaller sex chromosome is called Y. Females have two X chromosomes, and males have an X and Y chromosome. Because male cells contain both an X and a Y chromosome, meiosis in the male produces two gametes with an X chromosome and two gametes with a Y chromosome from each primary spermatocyte. The sex chromosomes in oocytes are both X, and thus the mature ovum can have only one type of sex chromosome. To produce a female child each parent must contribute an X chromosome. To produce a male, the mother must contribute an X chromosome and the father a Y chromosome.

The Y chromosomes contain mainly genes for maleness. The X chromosomes carry several genes other than those for sexual traits. As discussed in Chapter 5, these other traits are termed *sex linked* because they are controlled by the genes of the X chromosome. Two examples of sex-linked traits are color blindness and hemophilia, seen primarily in males.

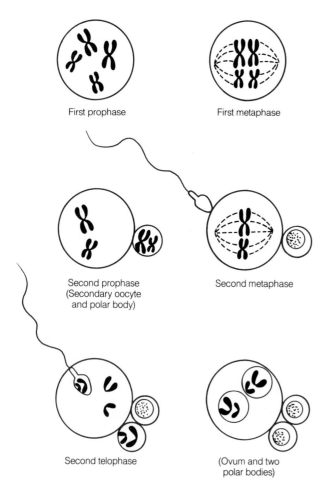

First prophase

First metaphase

Second prophase
(Secondary oocyte
and polar body)

Second metaphase

Second telophase

(Ovum and two
polar bodies)

Figure 11–3   Human oogenesis and fertilization (From Thompson JS, Thompson MW: Genetics in Medicine, *4th ed. Philadelphia: Saunders, 1986, p 23)*

It seems that I knew the moment you began. We had been planning and wanting the pregnancy for months. We carefully kept track of my menstrual periods and calculated the time of ovulation, and yet pregnancy kept eluding us. Then suddenly one night, I knew that you were there. This had been the moment, and even as I lay quietly I somehow could sense your presence.

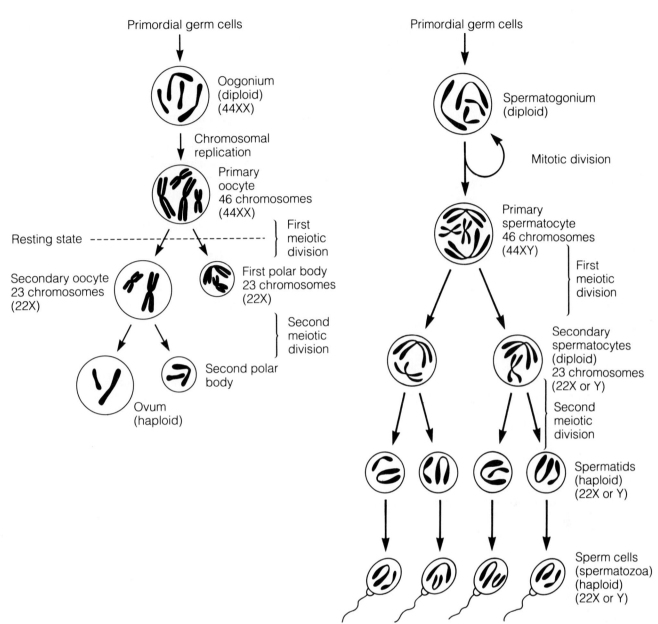

Figure 11–4 Gametogenesis involves meiosis within the ovary and testis. Note that during meiosis, each oogonium produces a single haploid ovum, whereas each spermatogonium produces four haploid spermatozoa. (Adapted from Becker WM, The World of the Cell, *1st ed. Menlo Park CA: Benjamin/Cummings, 1986, pp 620, 622)*

That feeling never changed, it just grew stronger as you grew inside me.

I haven't told many people about this. People look at me like I'm crazy. But I think if we would ask mothers, we would be surprised to find out just how many know exactly the moment that conception occurs.

Fertilization

The process of **fertilization**, or the joining of ovum and sperm, takes place in the ampulla (or outer third) of the fallopian tube. High estrogen levels during ovulation increase the contractility of the fallopian tubes, which helps move the ovum down the tube. The high estrogen levels also cause a thinning of the cervical mucus, facilitating penetration by the sperm.

The ovum's cell membrane is surrounded by two layers of tissue. The layer closest to the cell membrane is called the *zona pellucida*. It is a clear, noncellular layer whose function is not known. Surrounding the zona pellucida is a ring of elongated cells, called the *corona radiata* because they radiate from the ovum like the gaseous corona around the sun. These cells are held together by hyaluronic acid.

The mature ovum and spermatozoa have only a brief time to unite. Ova are considered fertile for about a 24-hour period after ovulation (Glass 1987). Sperm can survive in the female reproductive tract for up to 72 hours but are believed to be healthy and highly fertile for only about 24 hours (Moore 1988).

In a single ejaculation the male deposits approximately 200 to 400 million spermatozoa in the female's vagina, of which fewer than 200 actually reach the ampula (Moore 1988). The spermatozoa move up the female tract by the flagellar movements of their tails. Transit time from the cervix into the fallopian tube can be as short as five minutes but usually takes an average of four to six hours after ejaculation (Cunningham et al 1989). Prostaglandins in the semen may increase uterine smooth muscle contractions, which help transport the sperm (Spence & Mason 1987). The fallopian tubes have a dual ciliary action that facilitates movement of the ovum toward the uterus and movement of the sperm from the uterus toward the ovary. The ovum has no inherent power of movement.

The sperm must undergo two processes before fertilization can happen: capacitation and the acrosomal reaction (Overstreet et al 1988). *Capacitation* is the removal of the plasma membrane overlying the spermatozoa's acrosomal area and loss of seminal plasma proteins and glycoprotein coat. If the glycoprotein coat is not removed the sperm will not be able to fertilize the ovum. Capacitation occurs in the female reproductive tract (aided by uterine tube enzymes) and is thought to last up to seven hours.

The acrosomal reaction follows capacitation. The acrosomal covering of the head of the sperm contains the enzyme hyaluronidase. As millions of sperm surround the ovum, they deposit minute amounts of hyaluronidase in the corona radiata, the outer layer of the ovum. This activity is the *acrosomal reaction*. The hyaluronidase breaks down hyaluronic acid in the corona radiata layer of the ovum, resulting in perforations that allow one spermatozoon to penetrate the zona pellucida of the ovum (Figure 11–5). At the moment of penetration, a cellular change occurs in the ovum that renders it impenetrable by other spermatozoa (called the block to polyspermy); thus only one spermatozoon enters a single ovum (Wassarman 1988). The cellular change that blocks other sperm from entering the ovum is mediated by release of materials from the cortical granules, organelles found just below the ovum's surface.

At the moment of penetration the second meiotic division is completed in the nucleus of the oocyte, and the second polar body is produced. At the union of the gametes, each containing a haploid number of chromosomes (23), the diploid number (46) is restored. Also at this time, the sex of the new individual is established. Within the cell the nuclei of the spermatozoon and oocyte unite, and their individual nuclear membranes disappear. Their chromosomes pair up, and a new cell, the zygote, is created. The

---

Research Note

Clinical Application of Research

Margarete Sandelowski and her associates (1990) used a grounded theory methodology to explore the process of conception for infertile couples. This process was prolonged and progressed from having a pregnancy to being pregnant.

The components of the process of conception for infertile couples included the forcing of conception, resolution of conceptual ambiguity, and reconciliation of conception as both an idea and an event. For the fertile couples, conception was usually the result of a romantic interlude. Also a dichotomous view of pregnancy incorporated the concept of either/or not "a little pregnant." The result of conception for the fertile couple was, after a short wait for confirmation, an in-body, with-baby pregnancy.

For the infertile couples, conception usually was a labor with lovemaking becoming a "chore" that could include intrusive tasks such as temperature taking or self-administering hormones. The conception could even occur outside the natural process, through artificial insemination or in vitro fertilization.

Unlike the fertile couples and their either/or pregnancy, the infertile couples had to resolve several areas of conceptual ambiguity, such as the idea of serial positive pregnancy tests but no baby or a nongrowing pregnancy. To the infertile couple, pregnancy became a continuum, not a dichotomous event.

The reconciliation of conception as both idea and event occurred because many of the usual cues (in the fertile couples) that pregnancy has occurred are used to monitor successful continuation of the conception. Or, the symptoms are created prior to conception as a chemically induced state of pregnancy in order for the woman's body to maintain the fertile egg.

Critical Thinking Applied to Research

Strengths: Excellent description of sample, data analysis process, and research protocol. Discussion of criteria used to ensure qualitative rigor.

Sandelowski M, Harris B, Holditch-Davis D: Pregnant moments: The process of conception in infertile couples. *Res Nurs Health* 1990; 13:273.

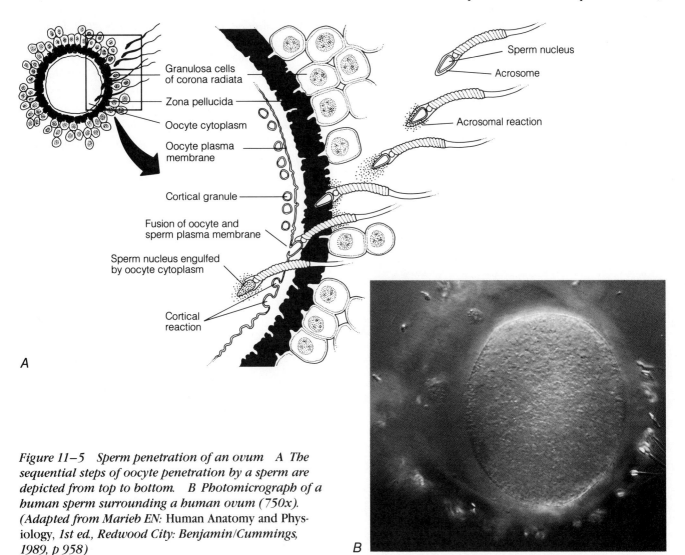

Figure 11–5 Sperm penetration of an ovum A The sequential steps of oocyte penetration by a sperm are depicted from top to bottom. B Photomicrograph of a human sperm surrounding a human ovum (750x). (Adapted from Marieb EN: Human Anatomy and Physiology, 1st ed., Redwood City: Benjamin/Cummings, 1989, p 958)

zygote contains a new combination of genetic material, which creates an individual different from either parent and from anyone else.

Twins

Twins have been reported to occur more often among black than among white women and more often among white individuals than among women of Asian origin. Among all groups, as parity (having given birth to a viable infant) increases so does the chance for multiple births.

Twins may be either fraternal or identical. If they are fraternal, they are *dizygotic*, which means they arise from two separate ova fertilized by two separate spermatozoa (Figure 11–6). There are two placentas, two chorions, and two amnions; however, the placentas sometimes fuse together and look as if they are one. Despite their birth relationship, fraternal twins are no more similar to each other

than they would be to siblings born singly. They may be the same or different sex.

Dizygotic twinning increases with maternal age up to about 35 years of age and then decreases abruptly. The chance of dizygotic twins increases with parity, in conceptions that occur in the first three months of marriage, and with coital frequency; the chance of dizygotic twinning decreases during periods of malnutrition. Studies indicate dizygotic twins occur in certain families, perhaps because of genetic factors leading to double ovulation (Creasy & Resnik 1988).

Identical, or *monozygotic*, twins develop from a single fertilized ovum. They are of the same sex and have the same genotype (appearance). Identical twins usually have a common placenta (Figure 11–6).

Monozygotic twins originate from division of the fertilized ovum at different stages of early development (Cunningham et al 1989). Division of the single fertilized ovum occurs only after the embryo consists of thousands of cells.

Complete separation of the cellular mass into two parts is necessary for twin formation. The number of amnions and chorions present depends on the timing of the division:

1. If division occurs within the first 72 hours after fertilization (before the inner cell mass and chorion are formed), two embryos, two amnions, and two chorions will develop. This occurs about 20% to 30% of the time, and there may be distinct placentas or a single fused placenta.

2. If division occurs between four and eight days after fertilization (when the inner cell mass is formed and the chorion cells have differentiated but those of the amnion have not), two embryos develop with separate amnionic sacs. These sacs will eventually be covered by a common chorion.

3. If the amnion has already developed approximately eight days after fertilization, division results in two embryos with a common amnionic sac and a com-

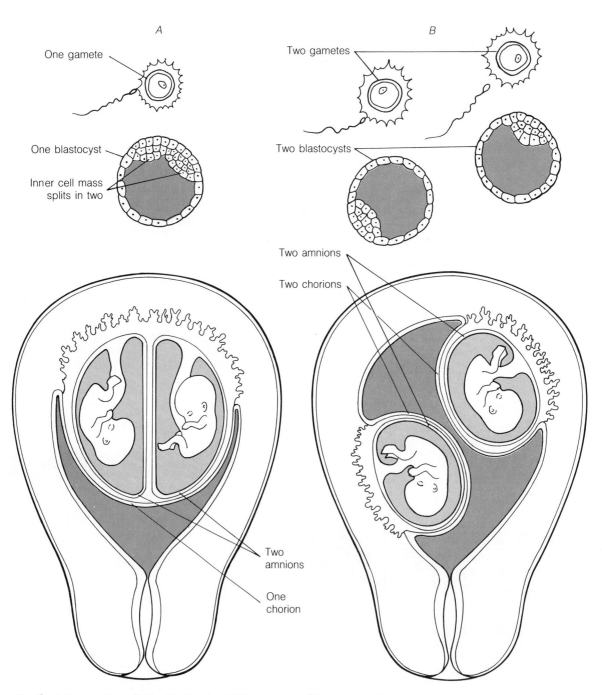

Figure 11–6 A Formation of identical twins. B Formation of fraternal twins

mon chorion. This type occurs about 1% of the time (Creasy & Resnik 1988).

Monozygotic twinning is considered a random event and occurs in approximately 1 of 250 births. The survival rate of monozygotic twins is 10% lower than that of dizygotic twins, and congenital anomalies are more prevalent. Both twins may have the same malformation (Oxorn 1986).

Intrauterine Development

Development after fertilization can be divided into three phases: cellular multiplication, cellular (embryonic membrane) differentiation, and development of organ systems. These phases and the process of implantation will be discussed next.

Cellular Multiplication

Cellular multiplication begins as the zygote moves through the fallopian tube into the cavity of the uterus. This transportation takes three days or more (Cunningham et al 1989) and is accomplished mainly by a very weak fluid current in the fallopian tube resulting from the beating action of the ciliated epithelium that lines the tube.

The zygote now enters a period of rapid mitotic divisions called **cleavage**, during which it divides into two cells, four cells, eight cells, and so on. These cells, called *blastomeres*, are so small that the developing cell mass is only slightly larger than the original zygote. The blastomeres are held together by the zona pellucida. The blastomeres will eventually form a solid ball of cells called the **morula**. Upon reaching the uterus, the morula floats freely for a few days, and then a cavity forms within the cell mass.

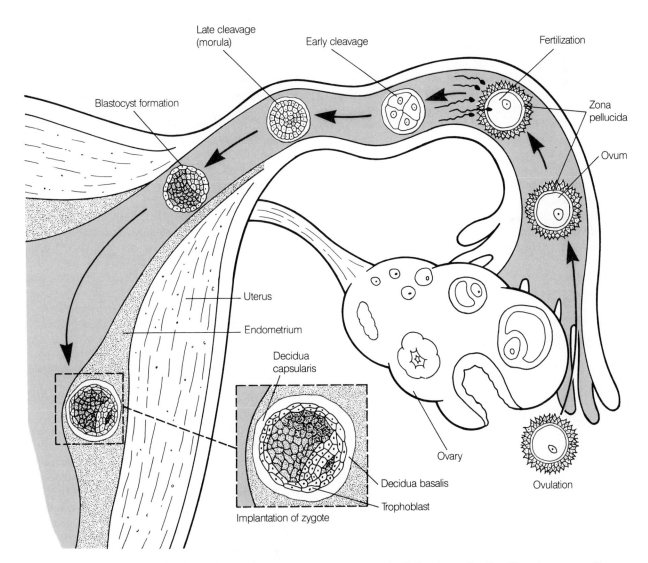

Figure 11–7   During ovulation the ovum leaves the ovary and enters the fallopian tube. Fertilization generally occurs in the outer third of the fallopian tube. Subsequent changes in the fertilized ovum from conception to implantation are depicted.

The inner solid mass of cells is called the **blastocyst**. The outer layer of cells that surround the cavity and have replaced the zona pellucida is the **trophoblast**. Eventually, the trophoblast develops into one of the embryonic membranes, called the chorion. The blastocyst develops into the embryo and the other embryonic membrane called the amnion. The journey of the fertilized ovum to its destination in the uterus is illustrated in Figure 11–7.

Implantation

While floating in the uterine cavity, the blastocyst is nourished by the uterine glands, which secrete a mixture of lipids, mucopolysaccharides, and glycogen. The trophoblast attaches itself to the surface of the endometrium for further nourishment. The most frequent site of attachment is the upper part of the posterior uterine wall (Figure 11–7). Between days 7 and 9 after fertilization the blastocyst implants itself by burrowing into the uterine lining and penetrating down toward the maternal capillaries until it is completely covered. In order for implantation to occur, the zona pellucida must disappear (Moore 1988). The lining of the uterus thickens below the implanted blastocyst, and the cells of the trophoblast grow down into the thickened lining, forming processes called *villi*.

Under the influence of progesterone, the endometrium increases in thickness and vascularity in preparation for implantation and nutrition of the ovum. After implantation the endometrium is called the *decidua*. The portion of the decidua that covers the blastocyst is called the **decidua capsularis**; the portion directly under the implanted blastocyst is the **decidua basalis**; and the portion that lines the rest of the uterine cavity is the **decidua vera (parietalis)** (see Figure 11–7 inset). The decidua basalis is the area where the chorionic villi (the chorion frondosum) will develop to form the fetal component of the placenta. The maternal part of the *placenta* develops from the decidua basalis, which contains large numbers of blood vessels.

Cellular Differentiation

Embryonic Membranes

The **embryonic membranes** begin to form at the time of implantation (Figure 11–8). These membranes protect and support the embryo as it grows and develops inside the uterus. The first membrane to form is the **chorion**, the outermost embryonic membrane that encloses the amnion, embryo, and yolk sac. The chorion is a thick membrane that develops from the trophoblast and has many fingerlike projections, called *chorionic villi*, on its surface. The villi begin to degenerate, except for those just under the embryo, which grow and branch into depressions in the uterine wall, forming the fetal portion of the placenta. By the fourth month of pregnancy, the surface of the chorion is smooth except at the place of attachment to the uterine wall.

The second membrane, the **amnion**, originates from the ectoderm, a primary germ layer, during the early stages of embryonic development. The amnion is a thin protective membrane that contains amniotic fluid. The space between the amniotic membrane and the embryo is the *amniotic cavity*. This cavity surrounds the embryo and yolk sac, except where the developing embryo (germ layer disk) attaches to the trophoblast via the umbilical cord. As the embryo grows, the amnion expands until it comes in contact with the chorion. These two slightly adherent membranes form the fluid-filled amniotic sac (or **bag of waters**) that protects the floating embryo.

Amniotic Fluid

Amniotic fluid functions as a cushion to protect against injury. It also helps control the embryo's temperature, permits symmetric external growth of the embryo, prevents adherence to the amnion, and allows freedom of movement so that the embryo-fetus can change position freely, thus aiding in musculoskeletal development.

The amount of amniotic fluid is about 30 mL at 10 weeks and increases to 350 mL at 20 weeks. After 20 weeks, the volume ranges from 500 to 1000 mL (Moore 1988). The amniotic fluid volume is constantly changing as the fluid moves back and forth across the placental membrane. As the pregnancy continues, the fetus contributes to the volume of amniotic fluid by excreting urine. The fetus also swallows up to 400 mL of the fluid every 24 hours. Between 600 and 800 mL of amniotic fluid flows in and out of the fetal lung each day (Creasy & Resnik 1988). Amniotic fluid is slightly alkaline and contains albumin, urea, uric acid, creatinine, lecithin, sphingomyelin, bilirubin, fat, fructose, leukocytes, proteins, epithelial cells, enzymes, and fine hair called lanugo. Abnormal variations in amniotic fluid volume are oligohydramnios (less than normal amount of amniotic fluid) and hydramnios (over 2000 mL of amniotic fluid). Hydramnios is also called polyhydramnios. See Chapter 25 for in-depth discussion of alterations in amniotic fluid volume.

Moore (1988) postulates that some amniotic fluid is formed by the amniotic membrane cells. Other sources suggest that amniotic fluid may be a transudate of maternal plasma. More probably, it is a transudate of fetal plasma, since a close relationship exists between fetal size and amount of amniotic fluid up to 20 weeks' gestation.

Water and solutes must pass between the amniotic fluid and fetus; Figure 11–9 summarizes the major pathways of exchange. During the first half of pregnancy water is transported across the highly permeable skin of the fetus, because the amniotic fluid composition resembles fetal extracellular fluid. After 24 weeks, thickening of the fetal skin inhibits the diffusion. A major pathway for intrauterine water accumulation in pregnancy appears to be across the chorionic villi between the maternal and fetal compartments (Marieb 1989).

Yolk Sac

In humans the yolk sac is small and functions only in early embryonic life. It develops as a second cavity in the blastocyst, about day 8 or 9 after conception, and forms primitive red blood cells during the first six weeks of development until the embryo's liver takes over the process. As the embryo develops, the yolk sac is incorporated in the umbilical cord, where it can be identified as a degenerate structure.

Primary Germ Layers

About day 10 to 14 after conception the homogenous mass of blastocyst cells differentiate into the primary germ layers. These layers, the **ectoderm**, **mesoderm**, and **endoderm**

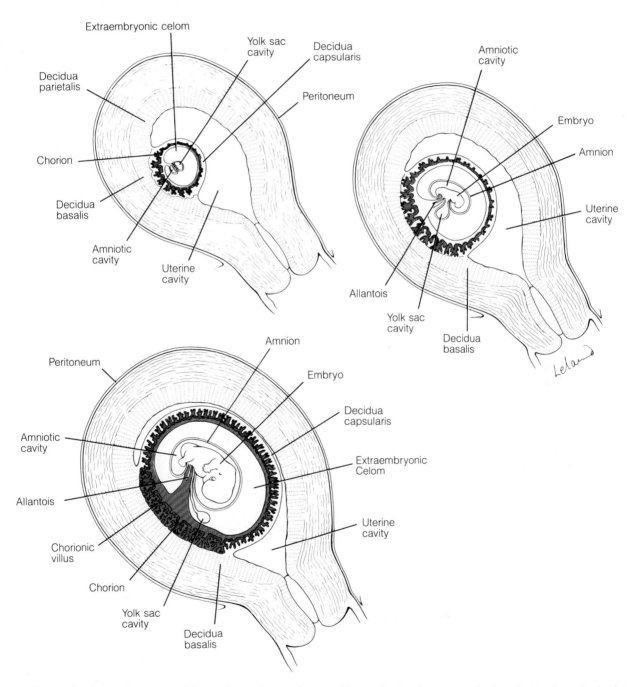

Figure 11–8 Early development of the embryonic membranes. The early development of selected structures is depicted starting at the top left and moving clockwise. The time sequence is from day 10 to day 14 after conception to approximately eight weeks. (From Spence AP, Mason EB: Human Anatomy and Physiology, 3rd ed. Menlo Park, CA: Benjamin/ Cummings, 1987, p 851)

(Figure 11–10), are formed at the same time as the embryonic membranes. From these primary germ cell layers, all tissues, organs, and organ systems will develop (Table 11–1).

How and why differentiation occurs is not clearly understood. Differentiation is believed to be a gene-directed phenomenon that originates in the DNA of the zygote and is carried out in the cytoplasm by an elaborate set of chemical reactions caused by the RNA-controlled synthesis of specific enzymes.

Intrauterine Organ Systems

Placenta

The **placenta** is the means of metabolic and nutrient exchange between the embryonic and maternal circulations. Placental development and circulation does not begin until the third week of embryonic development. The placenta develops at the site where the developing embryo attaches to the uterine wall. Expansion of the placenta continues until about 20 weeks, when it covers about one-half the inside of the uterus. After 20 weeks' gestation, the placenta becomes thicker but not wider. At 40 weeks' gestation, the placenta is about 15 to 20 cm (5.9 to 7.9 in.) in diameter and 2.5 to 3.0 cm (1.0 to 1.2 in.) in thickness. At that time, it weighs about 400 to 600 g (14 to 21 oz).

The placenta has two parts: the maternal portion and the fetal portion. The maternal portion consists of the decidua basalis and its circulation. Its surface is red and fleshlike. The fetal portion consists of the chorionic villi and their circulation. The fetal surface of the placenta is covered by the amnion, which gives it a shiny, gray appearance. (See Color Plates III and IV)

Development of the placenta begins with the chorionic villi. The trophoblast cells of the chorionic villi form spaces in the tissue of the decidua basalis. These spaces fill with maternal blood, and the chorionic villi grow into these spaces. As the chorionic villi differentiate, two tro-

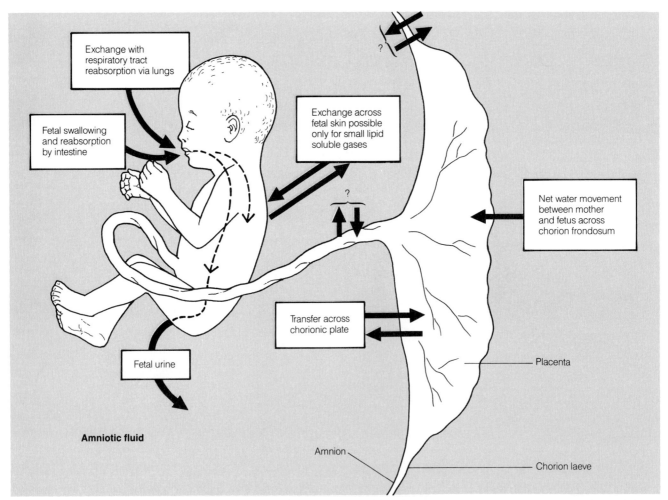

Figure 11–9   Summary of the significant pathways of water and solute exchange between the amniotic fluid and fetus (From Seeds AE: Current concepts of amniotic fluid dynamics. Am J Obstet Gynecol November 1980; 138:575)

phoblastic layers appear: an outer layer called the *syncytium* (consisting of syncytiotrophoblasts) and an inner layer known as the *cytotrophoblast* (Chavez 1987) (Figure 11–11). The cytotrophoblast thins out and disappears about the fifth month, leaving only a single layer of syncytium covering the chorionic villi. The syncytium is in direct contact with the maternal blood in the intervillous spaces. It is the functional layer of the placenta and secretes the placental hormones of pregnancy.

A third, inner layer of connective mesoderm develops in the chorionic villi, forming *anchoring villi*. These anchoring villi eventually form the *septa* (partitions) of the placenta. These septa divide the mature placenta into 15 to 20 segments called **cotyledons**. In each cotyledon, the

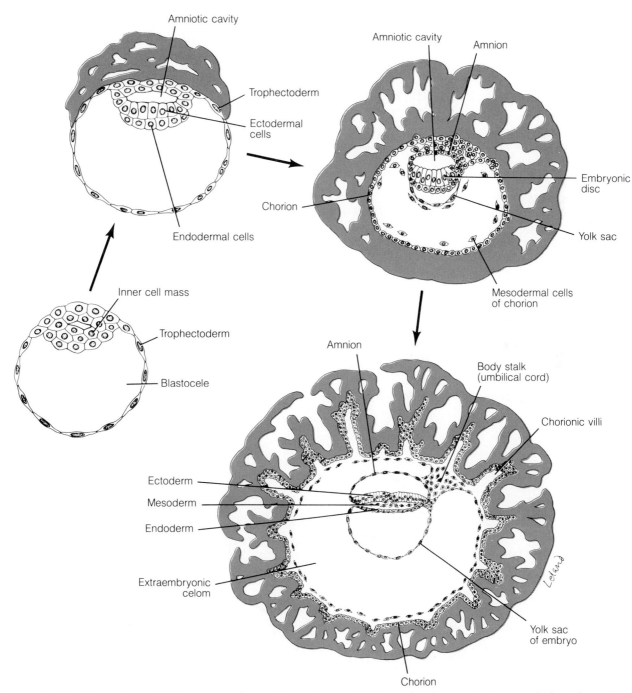

Figure 11–10   Formation of primary germ layers (From Spence AP, Mason EB: Human Anatomy and Physiology, 3rd ed. Menlo Park, CA: Benjamin/Cummings, 1987, p 849)

Table 11–1 Derivation of Body Structures from Primary Cell Layers

Ectoderm	Mesoderm	Endoderm
Epidermis	Dermis	Respiratory tract epithelium
Sweat glands	Wall of digestive tract	Epithelium (except nasal), including pharynx, tongue, tonsils, thyroid, parathyroid, thymus, tympanic cavity
Sebaceous glands	Kidneys and ureter (suprarenal cortex)	
Nails	Reproductive organs (gonads, genital ducts)	Lining of digestive tract
Hair follicles	Connective tissue (cartilage, bone, joint cavities)	Primary tissue of liver and pancreas
Lens of eye		Urethra and associated glands
Sensory epithelium of internal and external ear, nasal cavity, sinuses, mouth, anal canal	Skeleton	Urinary bladder (except trigone)
	Muscles (all types)	Vagina (parts)
Central and peripheral nervous sytems	Cardiovascular system (heart, arteries, veins, blood, bone marrow)	
Nasal cavity		
Oral glands and tooth enamel	Pleura	
Pituitary glands	Lymphatic tissue and cells	
Mammary glands	Spleen	

branching villi form a highly complex vascular system that allows compartmentalization of the uteroplacental circulation. The exchange of gases and nutrients takes place across these vascular systems.

Exchange of substances across the placenta is minimal during the first three to five months of development because of limited permeability. The villous membrane is initially too thick. As the villous membrane thins, the placental permeability increases until about the last month of pregnancy, when permeability begins to decrease as the placenta ages.

Placental Circulation After implantation of the blastocyst, the cells distinguish themselves into fetal cells and trophoblastic cells. The proliferating trophoblast successfully invades the decidua basalis of the endometrium, first opening the uterine capillaries and later opening the larger uterine vessels. The chorionic villi are an outgrowth of the blastocystic tissue. As these villi continue to grow and divide, the fetal vessels begin to form. The intervillous spaces in the decidua basalis develop as the endometrial spiral arteries are opened.

By the fourth week the placenta has begun to function as a means of metabolic exchange between embryo and mother. The completion of the maternal–placental–fetal circulation occurs about 17 days after conception when the embryonic heart begins functioning (Cunningham et al 1989).

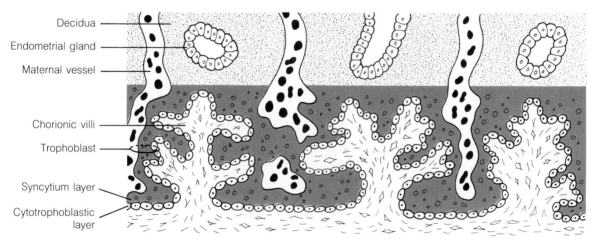

Decidua
Endometrial gland
Maternal vessel

Chorionic villi
Trophoblast

Syncytium layer
Cytotrophoblastic layer

Figure 11–11 Longitudinal section of placental villus. Spaces formed in the maternal decidua are filled with maternal blood; chorionic villi proliferate into these maternal-blood-filled spaces and differentiate into a syncytium layer and a cytotrophoblast layer.

By 14 weeks, the placenta is a discrete organ. The placenta has grown in thickness as a result of growth in the length and size of the chorionic villi and accompanying expansion of the intervillous space.

The *cotyledons* of the maternal surface contain branches of a single placental mainstem villus, allowing for some compartmentalization of the uteroplacental circulation. Each cotyledon is a vascular unit containing branching vessels which are distributed throughout a particular lobule and partially separated from other lobules by the cotyledon's thin septal partitions.

In the fully developed placenta, fetal blood in the villi and maternal blood in the intervillous spaces are separated by three or four thin layers of tissue. The capillaries of the villi are lined with an extremely thin endothelium and are surrounded by a layer of mesenchymal (connective) tissue. This connective tissue is covered by chorionic epithelium consisting of cytotrophoblast and syncytiotrophoblast (see Figure 11–11). As previously discussed, the cytotrophoblast thins out and disappears after the fifth month.

Fetal blood flows through the two umbilical arteries to the capillaries of the villi, and oxygen-enriched blood flows back through the umbilical vein to the fetus (Figure 11–12). Late in pregnancy a soft blowing sound (*funic souffle*) can be heard over the area of the umbilical cord of the fetus. The rate of the sound is synchronous with the fetal heartbeat and the flow of fetal blood through the umbilical arteries.

Maternal blood, rich in oxygen and nutrients, spurts from the spiral uterine arteries into the intervillous spaces. These spurts are produced by the maternal blood pressure. The spurt of blood is directed toward the chorionic plate, and as the blood flow loses pressure, it becomes lateral (spreads out). Fresh blood continually enters and exerts pressure on the contents of the intervillous spaces, pushing blood toward the exits in the basal plate. Blood is then drained through the uterine and other pelvic veins. A *uterine souffle* is also heard in the later months of pregnancy. This uterine souffle, which is timed precisely with the mother's pulse and heard just above the mother's symphy-

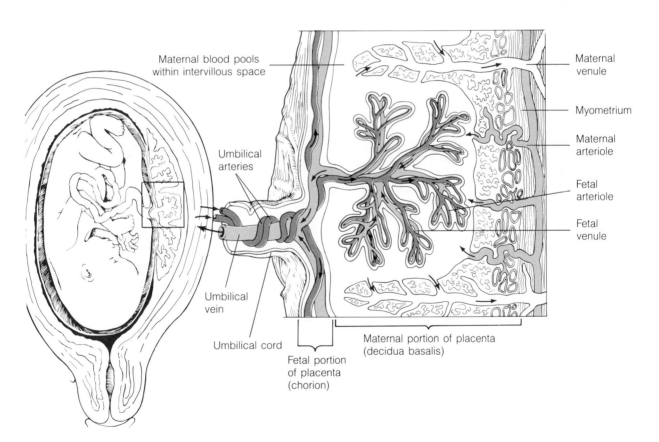

Figure 11–12 Vascular arrangement of the placenta. Arrows indicate the direction of blood flow. Maternal blood flows through the uterine arteries to the intervillous spaces of the placenta and returns through the uterine veins to maternal circulation. Fetal blood flows through the umbilical arteries into the villous capillaries of the placenta and returns through the umbilical vein to the fetal circulation. (From Spence AP, Mason EB: Human Anatomy and Physiology, *3rd ed. Menlo Park, CA: Benjamin/Cummings, 1987, p 850)*

sis pubis, is caused by the augmented blood flow entering the dilated uterine arteries.

Circulation within the intervillous spaces depends on maternal blood pressure producing a gradient between arterial and venous channels. The lumen of the spiral uterine artery is narrow when it pierces the chorionic plate and enters the intervillous space, resulting in an increased blood pressure. The pressure in the arteries forces the blood into the intervillous spaces and bathes the numerous small villi in oxygenated blood. As the pressure decreases, the blood flows back from the chorionic plate toward the decidua where it enters the endometrial veins.

Ahokas (1985) postulated that prostaglandins are implicated in the regulation of uterine and placental blood flow because of their vasoconstrictive and vasodilative effects.

Braxton Hicks contractions (Chapter 12) are believed to facilitate placental circulation by enhancing the movement of blood from the center of the cotyledon through the intervillous space.

Placental Functions Placental exchange functions occur only in those fetal vessels in intimate contact with the covering syncytial membrane. The syncytium villi have brush borders containing many microvilli, which greatly increase the exchange rate between maternal and fetal circulation (Sadler 1985).

The placental functions, many of which begin soon after implantation, include fetal respiration, nutrition, and excretion. To carry out these functions, the placenta is involved in metabolic and transfer activities. It also has endocrine functions and special immunologic properties.

Metabolic Activities The placenta produces glycogen, cholesterol, and fatty acids continuously for fetal use and hormone production. The placenta also produces numerous enzymes required for fetoplacental transfer, and it breaks down certain substances, such as epinephrine and histamine. In addition, it stores glycogen and iron.

Transport Function The placental membranes actively control the transfer of a wide range of substances by five major mechanisms:

1. *Simple diffusion* moves substances from an area of higher concentration to an area of lower concentration. Substances that move across the placenta by simple diffusion include: water, oxygen, carbon dioxide, electrolytes (sodium and chloride), anesthetic gases, and drugs. Insulin and steroid hormones originating from the adrenals and thyroid hormones also cross the placenta but at a very slow rate. The rate of oxygen transfer across the placental membrane is greater than that allowed by simple diffusion, indicating that oxygen is also transferred by facilitated diffusion of some type (see below).

2. *Facilitated transport* involves a carrier system to move molecules from an area of greater concentration to an area of lower concentration. Molecules such as glucose, galactose, and some oxygen are transported by this method. The glucose level in the fetal blood ordinarily is approximately 20% to 30% lower than the glucose level in the maternal blood because glucose is being metabolized rapidly by the fetus. This in turn causes rapid transport of additional glucose from the maternal blood into the fetal blood.

3. *Active transport* can work against a concentration gradient and allows molecules to move from areas of lower concentration to areas of higher concentration. Amino acids, calcium, iron, iodine, water-soluble vitamins, and glucose are transferred across the placenta this way. The measured amino acid content of fetal blood is greater than that of maternal blood, and calcium and inorganic phosphate occur in greater concentration in fetal blood than in maternal blood (Eden & Boehm 1990)

4. *Pinocytosis* is important for transferring large molecules, such as albumin and gamma-globulin. Materials are engulfed by amoeba−like cells forming plasma droplets.

5. *Hydrostatic* and *osmotic pressures* allow the bulk flow of water and some solutes.

Other modes of transfer exist as well. For example, fetal red blood cells pass into the maternal circulation through breaks in the placental membrane, particularly during labor and birth. Certain cells, such as maternal leukocytes, and microorganisms, such as viruses (for example, the human immunodeficiency virus [HIV], which causes acquired immunodeficiency syndrome [AIDS]) and the bacterium *Treponema pallidum* (which causes syphilis), can also cross the placental membrane, but the exact mechanism is not known. Some bacteria and protozoa infect the placenta by causing lesions and then entering the fetal blood system.

Several factors affect transfer rate:

- Molecular size
- Electrical charge
- Lipid solubility
- Placental area
- Diffusion distance
- Maternal-fetal-placental blood flow
- Blood saturation with gases and nutrients
- pka of the substance
- Maternal-placental-fetal metabolism of the substance

Substances that have a molecular weight of 1000 daltons or more have difficulty crossing the placenta by simple diffusion. Therefore heparin, with a molecular weight above 6000, does not cross the placenta, while warfarin sodium (Coumadin), which has a molecular weight in the 300 to 400 range, crosses easily.

Electrically charged molecules pass across the placenta more slowly. An example is the muscle relaxant, succinylcholine. A lipid-soluble substance moves quickly across the placenta into the fetal circulation. Reduction of the placental surface area, as with abruptio placentae (partial or complete premature separation of a normally implanted placenta) will lessen the area that is functional for exchange. Placental diffusion distance also affects exchange. In conditions such as diabetes and placental infection, edema of the villi increases the diffusion distance, thus increasing the distance the substance has to be transferred.

Changes in blood flow between the fetus and maternal intervillous space blood is dependent upon the transfer rate of substances, the ratio of blood on each side of the placenta and by the binding and dissociation abilities of carrier molecules in the blood. Decreased intervillous space blood flow is seen during labor and with certain maternal disease conditions such as hypertension. Mild fetal hypoxia increases the umbilical blood flow, but severe hypoxia results in decreased blood flow.

As the maternal blood picks up fetal waste products and carbon dioxide, it drains back into the maternal circulation through the veins in the basal plate. Fetal blood is hypoxic by comparison; it therefore attracts oxygen from the mother's blood. In addition, affinity for oxygen increases as the fetal blood gives up its carbon dioxide, which also decreases its acidity.

Endocrine Functions The placenta produces hormones that are vital to the survival of the fetus. These include human chorionic gonadotropin (hCG); human placental lactogen (hPL); and two steroid hormones, estrogen and progesterone.

The hormone *hCG* is similar to LH and prevents the normal involution of the corpus luteum at the end of the menstrual cycle (see Chapter 4). If the corpus luteum stops functioning before the 11th week of pregnancy, spontaneous abortion occurs. The hCG also causes the corpus luteum to secrete increased amounts of estrogen and progesterone.

After the 11th week the placenta produces enough progesterone and estrogen to maintain pregnancy. In the male fetus hCG also exerts an interstitial cell-stimulating effect on the testes, resulting in the production of testosterone. This small secretion of testosterone during embryonic development is the factor that causes male sex organs to grow. Human chorionic gonadotropin may play a role in the trophoblast's immunologic capabilities (ability to exempt the placenta and embryo from rejection by the mother's system). Human chorionic gonadotropin is used as a basis for pregnancy tests (for discussion of pregnancy tests, see Chapter 12).

Human chorionic gonadotropin is present in maternal blood serum eight to ten days after fertilization, just as soon as implantation has occurred, and is detectable in maternal urine a few days after the missed menses. Chorionic gonadotropin reaches its maximum level at 50 to 70 days' gestation and then begins to decrease as placental hormone production increases.

Progesterone is a hormone essential for pregnancy. It increases the secretions of the fallopian tubes and uterus to provide appropriate nutritive matter for the developing morula and blastocyst. It also appears to aid in ovum transport through the fallopian tube (Ahokas 1985). Progesterone causes decidual cells to develop in the uterine endometrium, and it must be present in high levels for implantation to occur. Progesterone also decreases the contractility of the uterus, thus preventing uterine contractions from causing spontaneous abortion.

Prior to stimulation by hCG, the production of progesterone by the corpus luteum reaches a peak about seven to ten days after ovulation. Implantation occurs at about the same time as this peak. At 16 days after ovulation, progesterone reaches a level between 25 and 50 mg per day and continues to rise slowly in subsequent weeks (Cunningham et al 1989). After ten weeks the placenta (specifically, the syncytiotrophoblast) takes over the production of progesterone and secretes it in tremendous quantities, reaching levels late in pregnancy of more than 250 mg per day.

By seven weeks the placenta produces more than 50 percent of the *estrogens* in the maternal circulation. Estrogens serve mainly a proliferative function, causing enlargement of the uterus, breasts, and breast glandular tissue. Estrogens also have a significant role in increasing vascularity and vasodilation, particularly in the villous capillaries near the end of pregnancy. Placental estrogens increase markedly toward the end of pregnancy, to as much as 30 times the daily production in the middle of a normal monthly menstrual cycle. The primary estrogen secreted by the placenta is different from that secreted by the ovaries: The placenta secretes mainly *estriol,* whereas the ovaries secrete primarily *estradiol.* The placenta by itself cannot synthesize estriol. Essential precursors are provided by the adrenal glands of the fetus and are transported to the placenta for the final conversion to estriol.

The hormone *hPL* (human placental lactogen; sometimes referred to as human chorionic somatomammotropin or hCS) is similar to human pituitary growth hormone; hPL stimulates certain changes in the mother's metabolic processes, which ensure that more protein, glucose, and minerals are available for the fetus. Secretion of hPL can be detected by about four weeks. Human placental lactogen is a useful indicator of fetal growth retardation (Eden & Boehm 1990). Recently new placental proteins have been identified which may have clinical uses. These include SP 1, PP 5 (placental protein 5) and others (Eden & Boehm 1990; Cunningham et al 1989).

Immunologic Properties The placenta and embryo are transplants of living tissue within the same species and are therefore considered *homografts.* Unlike other homografts, the placenta and embryo appear exempt from immunologic reaction by the host. Most recent data suggests that there is a suppression of cellular immunity by the placental hormones (progesterone and hCG) during pregnancy. One theory used to explain this phenomenon suggests that trophoblastic tissue is immunologically inert. It may contain a cell coating that masks transplantation antigens and that repels sensitized lymphocytes.

Umbilical Cord

As the placenta is developing, the **umbilical cord** is also being formed from the amnion. The **body stalk**, which attaches the embryo to the yolk sac, contains blood vessels that extend into the chorionic villi. The body stalk fuses with the embryonic portion of the placenta to provide a circulatory pathway from the chorionic villi to the embryo. (See Figure 11–12.) As the body stalk elongates to become the umbilical cord, the vessels in the cord decrease to one large vein and two smaller arteries. About 1% of umbilical cords have only two vessels, an artery and a vein; this condition may be associated with congenital malformations. A specialized connective tissue known as **Wharton's jelly** surrounds the blood vessels. This tissue, plus the high blood volume pulsating through the vessels, prevents compression of the umbilical cord in utero. At term, the average cord is 2 cm (0.8 in.) across and about 55 cm (22 in.) long. The cord can attach itself to the placenta in various sites. Central insertion into the placenta is considered normal. (See Chapter 19 for a discussion of the various attachment sites.)

Umbilical cords appear twisted or spiraled. This is most likely caused by fetal movement. A true knot in the umbilical cord rarely occurs and, if it does, the cord is usually long. More common are so-called false knots. False knots are caused by the folding of cord vessels. A *nuchal cord* is said to exist when the umbilical cord encircles the fetal neck.

Fetal Circulatory System

The circulatory system of the fetus has several unique features which, by maintaining the blood flow to the placenta, provide the fetus with oxygen and nutrients while removing carbon dioxide and other waste products.

Most of the blood supply bypasses the fetal lungs, since they do not carry out respiratory gas exchange. The placenta assumes the function of the fetal lungs by supplying oxygen and allowing the fetus to excrete carbon dioxide into the maternal bloodstream. Figure 11–13 shows the fetal circulatory system. The blood from the placenta flows through the umbilical vein, which penetrates the abdominal wall of the fetus. It divides into two branches, one of which circulates a small amount of blood through the fetal liver and empties into the inferior vena cava through the hepatic vein. The second and larger branch, called the

ductus venosus, empties directly into the fetal vena cava. This blood then enters the right atrium, passes through the **foramen ovale** into the left atrium, and pours into the left ventricle, which pumps it into the aorta. Some blood returning from the head and upper extremities by way of the superior vena cava is emptied into the right atrium and passes through the tricuspid valve into the right ventricle. This blood is pumped into the pulmonary artery, and a small amount passes to the lungs and provides nourishment only. The larger portion of blood passes from the pulmonary artery through the **ductus arteriosus** into the descending aorta, bypassing the lungs. Finally, blood returns to the placenta through the two umbilical arteries, and the process is repeated.

The fetus receives oxygen via diffusion from the maternal circulation because of the gradient difference of PO_2 of 50mm Hg in maternal blood in the placenta to a 30 mm Hg PO_2 in the fetus. At term the fetus receives oxygen from the mother's circulation at a rate of 20 to 30 mL/min (Sadler 1985). Fetal hemoglobin facilitates obtaining oxygen from the maternal circulation, since it carries as much as 20% to 30% more oxygen than adult hemoglobin. For further discussion see Chapter 27.

Fetal circulation delivers the highest available oxygen concentration to the head, neck, brain, and heart (coronary circulation) and a lesser amount of oxygenated blood to the abdominal organs and the lower body. This circulatory pattern leads to *cephalocaudal* (head-to-tail) development in the fetus.

Fetal Heart

The heart of the fetus, as in the adult, is under the control of its own pacemaker. The sinoatrial (S-A) node sets the rate and is supplied by the vagus nerve. Bridging the atrium and the ventricle is the atrioventricular (A-V) node. It is also supplied by the vagus nerve. Baseline changes in the fetal heartbeat have been shown to be under the influence of this nerve. Atropine will block this effect.

Under the influence of the sympathetic nervous system, norepinephrine is released when the fetus is stressed, causing an increase in the fetal heart rate. To counteract the increase in blood pressure, baroreceptors, which respond to stretch, are present in the vessel walls at the junction of the internal and external carotid arteries. When stimulated, these receptors, under the influence of the vagus and glossopharyngeal nerves, cause the fetal heart rate to slow.

Chemoreceptors in the fetal peripheral and central nervous systems respond to decreased oxygen tensions and to increased carbon dioxide tensions, leading to fetal tachycardia and an increase in blood pressure. The central nervous system (CNS) also has control over heart rate. Increased activity of the fetus in a wakeful period is exhibited in an *increase in the beat-to-beat variability* of the fetal heart baseline. Sleep patterns demonstrate a *decrease in*

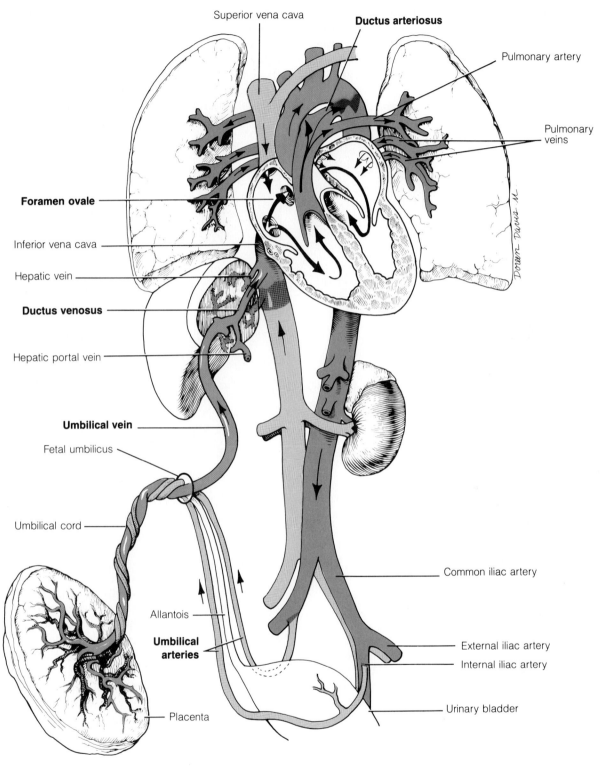

Figure 11–13   Fetal circulation. Blood leaves the placenta and enters the fetus through the umbilical vein. After circulating through the fetus the blood returns to the placenta through the umbilical arteries. The ductus venosus, the foramen ovale, and the ductus arteriosus allow the blood to bypass the fetal liver and lungs. (From Spence AP, Mason EB: Human Anatomy and Physiology, *3rd ed. Menlo Park, CA: Benjamin/Cummings, 1987, p 862)*

the beat-to-beat baseline variability. In cases of severe hypoxia, increased levels of epinephrine and norepinephrine act on the fetal heart to produce a faster and stronger rate.

Embryonic and Fetal Development and Organ Formation

Pregnancy is calculated to last an average of ten lunar months: 40 weeks, or 280 days. This period of 280 days is calculated from the beginning of the last menstrual period to the time of birth. EDB (estimated date of birth) is usually calculated by this method. The fertilization age or post-conception age of the fetus is calculated to be about two weeks less, or 266 days (38 weeks). The latter measurement is more accurate because it measures time from the fertilization of the ovum, or conception. The basic events of organ development in the embryo and fetus will be discussed in the following sections. The time periods used are **postconception age periods**.

Human development follows three stages. The preembryonic stage consists of the first 14 days of development after the ovum is fertilized; the embryonic stage covers the period from day 15 until approximately the eighth week; and the fetal stage extends from the end of the eighth week until delivery.

Preembryonic Stage

The first 14 days of human development, starting on the day the ovum is fertilized (conception), are referred to as the *preembryonic stage* or the *stage of the ovum.* This period is characterized by rapid cellular multiplication and differentiation and the establishment of the embryonic membranes and primary germ layers, discussed earlier.

Embryonic Stage

The stage of the **embryo** starts on day 15 (begins the third week after conception or fertilization) and continues until approximately eight weeks or until the embryo reaches a crown-to-rump length of 3 cm or 1.2 in. This length is usually attained about 49 days after fertilization. The embryonic stage is a period of differentiation of tissues into essential organs and development of the main external features. It is during this period that the embryo is most vulnerable to teratogens.

Three Weeks

In the third week the embryonic disk becomes elongated and pear-shaped, with a broad cephalic end and a narrow caudal end (Figure 11–14). The ectoderm has formed a long cylindrical tube for brain and spinal cord develop-

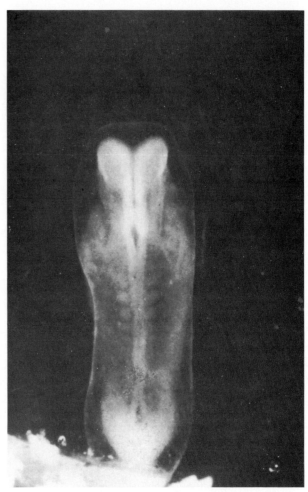

Figure 11–14   The embryo at three weeks (Courtesy Drs Roberts Rugh and Landrum B Shettles)

ment. The gastrointestinal tract, created from the endoderm, appears as another tubelike structure communicating with the yolk sac. The most advanced organ is the heart. At three weeks a single tubular heart forms just outside the body cavity of the embryo.

Four to Five Weeks

During days 21 to 32, *somites,* a series of mesodermal blocks, form on either side of the embryo's midline. The vertebrae that form the spinal column will develop from these somites. Prior to 28 days, arm and leg buds are not visible, but the tail bud is present. The pharyngeal arches—which will form the lower jaw (mandibular arch), hyoid bone, and cartilage of the larynx—develop at this time. The pharyngeal pouches appear now; these pouches will form the eustachian tube and cavity of the middle ear, the tonsils, and the parathyroid and thymus glands. The primordia of the ear and eye are also present. By the end of 28 days, the tubular heart is beating at a regular rhythm and

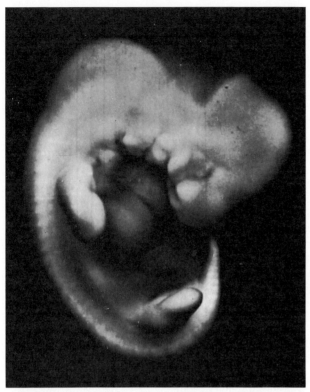

Figure 11–15 The embryo at five weeks (Courtesy Drs Roberts Rugh and Landrum B Shettles)

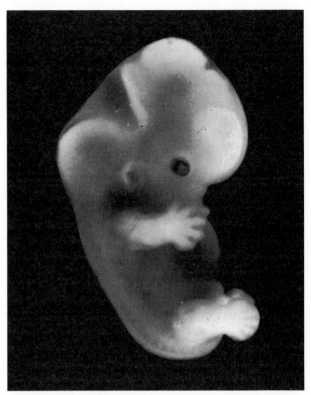

Figure 11–16 The embryo at six weeks (Courtesy Drs Roberts Rugh and Landrum B Shettles)

pushing its own primitive blood cells through the main blood vessels.

During the fifth week, the optic cups and lens vesicles of the eye form and the nasal pits develop. Partitioning in the heart occurs with the dividing of the atrium. The embryo has a marked C-shaped body, accentuated by the rudimentary tail and the large head folded over a protuberant trunk (Figure 11–15). By day 35, the arm and leg buds are well developed, with paddle-shaped hand and foot plates. The heart, circulatory system, and brain show the most advanced development. The brain has differentiated into five areas, and ten pairs of cranial nerves are recognizable.

Six Weeks

At six weeks the head structures are more highly developed and the trunk is straighter than in earlier stages (Figure 11–16). The upper and lower jaws are recognizable, and the external nares are well formed. The trachea has developed, and its caudal end is bifurcated for beginning lung formation. The upper lip has formed, and the palate is developing. The ears are developing rapidly, as are the other postbrachial body parts. The arms have begun to extend ventrally across the chest, and both arms and legs have digits, although they may still be webbed. There is a slight elbow bend in the arm, and the arm is more advanced in development than the leg. Beginning at this stage the prominent tail will recede. The heart now has most of its definitive characteristics, and fetal circulation begins to be established. The liver begins to produce blood cells.

Seven Weeks

At seven weeks the head of the embryo is rounded and nearly erect (Figure 11–17). The eyes have shifted from their original lateral position to a forward location, where they are closer together, and the eyelids are beginning to form. The palate is nearing completion, and the tongue is developing in the formed mouth. The gastrointestinal and genitourinary tracts undergo significant changes during the seventh week. Prior to this time the rectal and urogenital passages formed one tube that ended in a blind pouch; they now separate into two tubular structures. The intestines enter the extraembryonic coelom in the area of the umbilical cord (called umbilical herniation) (Moore 1988). At this point the beginnings of all essential external and internal structures are present.

Eight Weeks

At eight weeks the embryo is approximately 3 cm (1.2 in.) long crown to rump (C–R) and clearly resembles a human being (Figure 11–18). Facial features continue to develop. The eyelids begin to fuse. Auricles of the external ears begin to assume their final shape, but they are still set low (Moore 1988). External genitals appear but are not discernible, and the rectal passage opens with the perforation

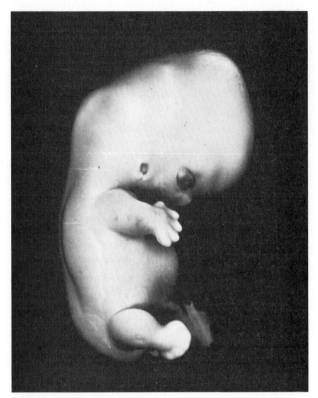

Figure 11–17   The embryo at seven weeks (Courtesy Drs Roberts Rugh and Landrum B Shettles)

of the anal membrane. The circulatory system through the umbilical cord is well established. Long bones are beginning to form, and the large muscles are now capable of contracting.

Fetal Stage

By the end of the eighth week the embryo is sufficiently developed to be called a **fetus**. Every organ system and external structure that will be found in the full-term newborn is present. The remainder of gestation is devoted to refining structures and perfecting function.

Nine to Twelve Weeks

By ten weeks the fetus reaches a C–R length of 5 cm (2 in.) and weighs about 14 g. The head is large and comprises almost half of the fetus's entire size (Figure 11–19). The neck is distinct from the head and body, and both the head and neck are straighter than in previous stages of development.

By 12 weeks, the fetus reaches an 8-cm (3.2-in.) C–R

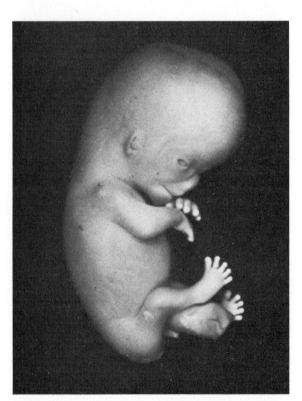

Figure 11–18   The fetus at eight weeks (Courtesy Drs Roberts Rugh and Landrum B Shettles)

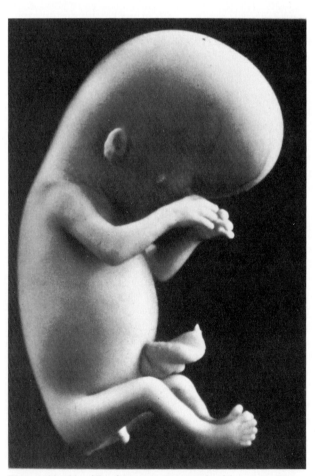

Figure 11–19   The fetus at nine weeks (Courtesy Drs Roberts Rugh and Landrum B Shettles)

length and weighs about 45 g (1.6 oz). The face is well formed, with the nose protruding, the chin small and receding, and the ear acquiring a more adult shape. The eyelids close at about the tenth week and will not reopen until about 28 weeks. Some reflex movements of the lips suggestive of the sucking reflex have been observed at three months. Tooth buds now appear for all 20 of the child's first teeth (baby teeth). The limbs are long and slender, with well-formed digits. The fetus can curl the fingers toward the palm and make a tiny fist. The legs are still shorter and less developed than the arms. The urogenital tract completes its development, well-differentiated genitals appear, and the kidneys begin to produce urine. Red blood cells are produced primarily by the liver. Spontaneous movements of the fetus now occur. Fetal heart tones can be ascertained by electronic devices between 8 and 12 weeks.

Thirteen to Sixteen Weeks

This is a period of rapid growth. At 13 weeks the fetus weights 55 to 60 g and is about 9 cm (3.6 in.) in C–R length. **Lanugo**, a fine, downy hair, begins to develop, especially on the head. The fetal skin is so transparent that blood vessels are clearly visible beneath it. More muscle tissue and body skeleton have developed, which tend to hold the fetus more erect. Active movements are present—the fetus stretches and exercises its arms and legs. It makes sucking motions, swallows amniotic fluid, and produces meconium in the intestinal tract. Bronchial tubes are branching out in the primitive lungs, and sweat glands are developing. The liver and pancreas now begin production of their appropriate secretions. By the beginning of week 16, skeletal ossification is clearly identifiable.

Twenty Weeks

The fetus doubles C–R length and now measures about 19 cm (8 in.). Fetal weight is between 435 and 465 g. Lanugo hair covers the entire body and is especially prominent on the shoulders. Subcutaneous deposits of brown fat, which has a rich blood supply, makes the skin a little less transparent. Nipples now appear over the mammary glands. The head sports fine, "wooly" hair, and the eyebrows and eyelashes are beginning to form. The fetus has nails on both fingers and toes. Muscles are well developed, and the fetus is active. Fetal movement, known as *quickening*, is felt by the mother. The heartbeat is audible with the use of a stethoscope. Quickening and fetal heartbeat can help in reaffirming maternal estimated date of birth.

Twenty-four Weeks

The fetus at 24 weeks reaches a crown-to-heel (C–H) length of 28 cm (11.2 in.). It weighs about 780 g (1 lb, 10 oz). The hair on the head is growing long, and eyebrows and eyelashes have formed. The eye is structurally complete and will soon open. The fetus has a reflex hand grip (grasp reflex) and, by the end of six months, a startle reflex. Skin covering the body is reddish and wrinkled, with little

subcutaneous fat. Skin on the hands and feet has thickened, with skin ridges on palms and soles forming distinct footprints and fingerprints. The skin over the entire body is covered with a protective cheeselike fatty substance secreted by the sebaceous glands called **vernix caseosa.** The alveoli in the lungs are just beginning to form.

Twenty-five to Twenty-eight Weeks

At six calendar months the fetal skin is still red, wrinkled, and covered with vernix caseosa. During this time the brain is developing rapidly, and the nervous system is complete enough to provide some degree of regulation of body functions. The eyelids open and close under neural control. If the fetus is a male, the testes begin to descend into the scrotal sac. Respiratory and circulatory systems have developed sufficiently. Even though the lungs are still physiologically immature, they are sufficiently developed to provide gas exchange. A fetus born at this time will require immediate and prolonged intensive care in order to survive and to decrease the risk of major handicap. The fetus at 28 weeks (Figure 11–20) is about 35 to 38 cm (14

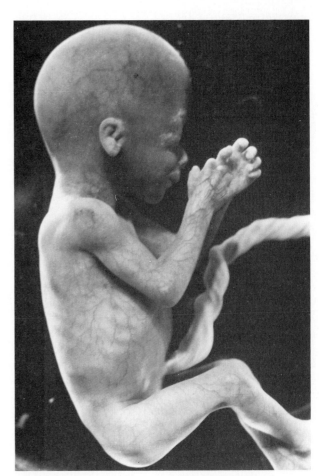

Figure 11–20   The fetus at 28 weeks (Courtesy Drs Roberts Rugh and Landrum B Shettles)

to 15 in.) long C-H and weighs about 1200 to 1250 g (2 lbs, 10.5 oz to 2 lbs, 12 oz).

Twenty-nine to Thirty-two Weeks

At 30 weeks the pupillary light reflex is present (Moore 1988). The fetus is gaining weight from an increase in body muscle and fat and weights about 2000 g (4 lbs, 6.5 oz) with a length of about 38 to 43 cm (15 to 17 in.) by 32 weeks of age. The CNS has matured enough to direct rhythmic breathing movements and partially control body temperature. However, the lungs are not yet fully mature. Bones are now fully developed but are soft and flexible. The fetus begins storing iron, calcium, and phosphorus. In males the testicles may be located in the scrotal sac but are often still high in the inguinal canal.

Thirty-six Weeks

The fetus is beginning to get plump with less-wrinkled skin covering the deposits of subcutaneous fat. Lanugo hair is beginning to disappear, and the nails reach the edge of the fingertips. By 35 weeks the fetus has a firm grasp and exhibits spontaneous orientation to light. By 36 weeks of age the weight is usually 2500 to 2750 g (5 lb, 12 oz to 6 lb, 11.5 oz), and the C–H length of the fetus is about 42 to 48 cm (16 to 19 in.). An infant born at this time has a good chance of surviving but may require some special care, especially if there is intrauterine growth retardation.

Thirty-eight to Forty Weeks

The fetus is considered full term at 38 weeks after conception. The C–H length varies from 48 to 52 cm (19 to 21 in.) with males usually longer than females. Males also usually weigh more than females. The weight at term is about 3000 to 3600 g (6 lb, 10 oz to 7 lb, 15 oz). The skin is pink and has a smooth polished look. The only lanugo hair left is on the upper arms and shoulders. The hair on the head is no longer woolly but coarse and about an inch long. Vernix caseosa is present, with heavier deposits remaining in creases and folds of the skin. The body and extremities are plump, with good skin turgor, and the fingernails extend beyond the fingertips. The chest is prominent but still a little smaller than the head, and mammary glands protrude in both sexes. The testes are in the scrotum or are palpable in the inguinal canals. As the fetus enlarges, amniotic fluid diminishes to about 500 mL or less, and the fetal body mass fills the uterine cavity. The fetus assumes what is referred to as its *position of comfort*, or lie. The head is generally pointed downward following the shape of the uterus and also possibly because the head is heavier than the feet. The extremities and often the head are well flexed. After five months, feeding patterns, sleeping patterns, and activity patterns become established, so that at term the fetus has its own body rhythms and individual style of response.

Table 11–2	Fetal Development: What Parents Want to Know
4 weeks:	The fetal heart begins to beat.
8 weeks:	All body organs are formed.
8–12 weeks:	Fetal heart tones can be heard by Doppler device.
16 weeks:	Baby's sex can be seen. Although thin, looks like a baby.
20 weeks:	Heartbeat can be heard with fetoscope. Mother feels movement (quickening). Baby develops a regular schedule of sleeping, sucking, and kicking. Hands can grasp. Assumes a favorite position in utero. Vernix (lanolinlike covering) protects the body and lanugo (fine hair) keeps oil on skin. Head hair, eyebrows, and eyelashes present.
24 weeks:	Weighs 1 lb 10 oz. Increasing activity. Fetal respiratory movements begin.
28 weeks:	Eyes begin to open and close. Baby can breathe at this time. Surfactant needed for breathing at birth is formed. Baby is two-thirds its final size.
32 weeks:	Has fingernails and toenails. Subcutaneous fat being laid down. Baby appears less red and wrinkled.
38–40 weeks:	Fills total uterus. Gets antibodies from mother.

Table 11–2 lists some important developmental milestones.

Factors Influencing Embryonic and Fetal Development

Among factors that may affect embryonic development are the quality of the sperm or ovum from which the zygote was formed and the genetic code established at fertilization. In addition, the adequacy of the intrauterine environment is important for optimal growth. If the environment is unsuitable before cellular differentiation occurs, all the cells of the zygote are affected. The cells may die, which causes spontaneous abortion, or growth may be slowed, depending on the severity of the situation. When differentiation is complete and the fetal membranes have formed, an injurious agent has the greatest effect on those cells undergoing the most rapid growth. Thus the time of injury is critical in the development of anomalies.

Because organs are formed primarily during embryonic development, the growing organism is considered most vulnerable to hazardous agents during the first months of pregnancy (Paul & Himmelstein 1988). Table 11–3 lists

Table 11–3 Developmental Vulnerability Timetable

Weeks since conception	Potential teratogen-induced malformation
3	Ectromelia (congenital absence of one or more limbs) Ectopedia cordis (heart lies outside thoracic cavity)
4	Omphalocele Tracheoesophageal fistula (4–5* weeks) Hemivertebra (4–5* weeks)
5	Nuclear cataract Microphthalmia (abnormally small eyeballs; 5–6* weeks) Facial clefts Carpal or pedal ablation (5–6* weeks)
6	Gross septal or aortic abnormalities Cleft lip, agnathia (absence of the lower jaw)
7	Interventricular septal defects Pulmonary stenosis Cleft palate, micrognathia (smallness of the jaw) Epicanthus Brachycephalism (shortness of the head; 7–8* weeks) Mixed sexual characteristics
8	Persistent ostium primum (persistent opening in atrial septum) Digital stunting (shortening of fingers and toes)

May occur in several different time periods after conception.

Source: Modified from Danforth DN, Scott JR: Obstetrics and Gynecology, 5th ed. Philadelphia: Lippincott, 1986, p. 319.

potential malformations related to the time of insult. Any agent, such as a drug, virus or radiation, that can cause development of abnormal structures in an embryo is referred to as a **teratogen**. Chapter 12 discusses the effects of specific teratogenic agents on the developing fetus.

Adequacy of the maternal environment is also important during the periods of rapid embryonic and fetal development. Maternal nutrition can affect brain development. The period of maximum brain growth and myelination begins with the fifth lunar month before birth and continues during the first six months after birth. During the first six months after birth there is a twofold increase in myelination; in the second six months to two years of age there is a 50% further increase (Volpe 1987). Amino acids, glucose, and fatty acids are considered to be the primary dietary factors in brain growth. A subtle type of damage that affects the associative capacity of the brain, possibly leading to learning disabilities, may be caused by nutritional deficiency at this stage. (Maternal nutrition is discussed in depth in Chapter 16.)

Another prenatal influence on the intrauterine environment is maternal hyperthermia associated with sauna baths or hot tub use (Jones & Chernoff 1984). Studies of the effects of maternal hyperthermia during the first trimester have raised concern about possible central nervous system defects and failure of neural tube closure. The effects of substance abuse on fetal development are discussed in Chapters 18 and 31.

❀ ❀

KEY CONCEPTS

Humans have 46 chromosomes, which are divided into 23 pairs—22 pairs of autosomes and one pair of sex chromosomes.

Meiosis is the process by which new organisms are formed. It occurs during gametogenesis and consists of two successive cell divisions (reduction division), which produce a gamete with 23 chromosomes (22 chromosomes and 1 sex chromosome)—the haploid number of chromosomes.

Gametes must have a haploid number (23) of chromosomes so that when the female gamete (ovum) and the male gamete (spermatozoon) unite (fertilization) to form the zygote, the normal human diploid number of chromosomes (46) is reestablished.

Sex chromosomes are referred to as X and Y. Females have two X chromosomes and males have an X and a Y chromosome. Y chromosomes are carried only by the sperm. To produce a male child the mother contributes an X chromosome and the father contributes a Y chromosome.

An ovum is considered fertile for about a 24-hour period after ovulation, and the sperm is capable of fertilizing the ovum for only about 24 hours after it is deposited in the female reproductive system.

Both capacitation and acrosomal reaction must occur for the sperm to fertilize the ovum.

Intrauterine development first proceeds via cellular multiplication in which the zygote undergoes rapid mitotic division called cleavage. As a result of cleavage the zygote divides and multiplies into cell groupings called blastomeres, which are held together by the zona pellucida. The blastomeres will eventually become a solid ball of cells called the morula. When a cavity forms in the morula cell mass, the inner solid cell mass is called the blastocyst.

After implantation the endometrium is called the decidua. Decidua capsularis is the portion that covers the blastocyst. Decidua basalis is the portion that is directly under the blastocyst. Decidua vera is the portion that lines the rest of the uterine cavity.

Embryonic membranes are called the amnion and the chorion. The amnion is formed from the ectoderm and is a thin protective membrane that contains the amniotic fluid and the embryo. The chorion is a thick membrane that develops from the trophoblast and encloses the amnion, embryo, and yolk sac.

Amniotic fluid cushions the fetus against injury, controls the embryo's temperature, allows symmetrical external growth, prevents adherence to the amnion, and permits freedom of movement.

Amniotic fluid is made up of albumin, creatinine, lecithin, sphingomyelin, fat, bilirubin, proteins, epithelial cells, and lanugo. Normal volume is 500 to 1000 mL/day after about 20 weeks. The fetus contributes to the amniotic fluid via urination.

Primary germ layers give rise to all tissues, organs, and organ systems. The three primary germ cell layers are ectoderm, endoderm, and mesoderm.

The placenta develops from the chorionic villi and has two parts: The maternal portion, consisting of the decidua basalis, is red and fresh-looking. The fetal portion, consisting of chorionic villi, is covered by the amnion and appears shiny and gray. The placenta is made up of 15 to 20 segments called cotyledons.

The placenta serves endocrine (production of hPL, hCG, estrogen, and progesterone), metabolic, and immunologic functions; it acts as the fetus' respiratory organ, is an organ of excretion, and aids in the exchange of nutrients.

The umbilical cord contains two umbilical arteries, which carry deoxygenated blood from the fetus to the placenta, and one umbilical vein, which carries oxygenated blood from the placenta to the fetus. The umbilical cord usually has a central insertion into the placenta. Wharton's jelly, a specialized connective tissue, prevents compression of the umbilical cord in utero.

Twins are either monozygotic (identical) or dizygotic (fraternal). Dizygotic twins arise from two separate ova fertilized by two separate spermatozoa. Monozygotic twins develop from a single fertilized ovum.

Fetal circulation is a unique circulatory system that provides for oxygenation of the fetus while bypassing the fetal lungs.

Stages of fetal development include the preembryonic stage (the first 14 days of human development starting at the time of fertilization), the embryonic stage (from day 15 after fertilization, or the beginning of the third week, until approximately eight weeks after conception), and the fetal stage (from 8 weeks until delivery at approximately 40 weeks postconception).

Some significant events that occur during the embryonic stage are: at four weeks, the fetal heart begins to beat and at six weeks, fetal circulation is established.

The fetal stage is devoted to refining structures and perfecting function. Some significant developments during the fetal stage are:
At 8–12 weeks all organ systems are formed and now require maturation.
At 16 weeks sex can be determined visually.
At 20 weeks fetal heartbeat can be auscultated by a fetoscope, and the mother can feel movement (quickening).
At 24 weeks vernix caseosa covers the entire body.
At 26 to 28 weeks the eyes reopen.
At 32 weeks skin appears less wrinkled and red since subcutaneous fat has been laid down.
At 36 weeks fingernails reach the ends of fingers.
At 40 weeks vernix caseosa is apparent only in creases and folds of skin, and lanugo hair remains on upper arms and shoulders only.

The embryo is particularly vulnerable to teratogenesis during the first 8 weeks of cell differentiation and organ system development.

❀ ❀

References

Ahokas RA: Development and physiology of the placenta and membranes. In: *Gynecology and Obstetrics*. Vol. 2. Sciarra JL et al (editors). Hagerstown, MD: Harper & Row, 1985.

Chavez DJ: Implantation. In: *Gynecology and Obstetrics*. Vol. 5. Sciarra JL et al (editors). Hagerstown, MD: Harper & Row, 1987.

Creasy RK, Resnik JR: *Maternal–Fetal Medicine Principles and Practice*. Philadelphia: Saunders, 1988.

Cunningham FG, MacDonald PC, Gant NG: *Williams Obstetrics*. Norwalk, CT: Appleton & Lange, 1989.

Eden RD, Boehm FH (editors): *Assessment and Care of the Fetus: Physiological, Clinical, and Medicolegal Principles*. Norwalk CT: Appleton & Lange, 1990.

Glass RH: Egg transport and fertilization. In: *Gynecology and Obstetrics*. Vol. 2. Sciarra JL et al (editors). Hagerstown, MD: Harper & Row, 1987.

Jones KL, Chernoff GF: Effects of chemical and environmental agents. In: *Maternal-Fetal Medicine Principles and Practice*. Creasy RK, Resnik JR (editors). Philadelphia: Saunders, 1984, p 190.

Marieb EN: *Human Anatomy and Physiology*. Redwood City, CA: Benjamin/Cummings, 1989.

Moore KL: *The Developing Human: Clinically Oriented Embryology,* 4th ed. Philadelphia: Saunders, 1988.

Overstreet JW, Katz DF, Cross NL: Sperm transport and capacitation. In: *Gynecology and Obstetrics*. Vol 5. Sciarra JL et al (editors). Hagerstown, MD: Harper & Row, 1988.

Oxorn H: *Human Labor and Birth,* 5th ed. Norwalk, CT: Appleton-Century-Crofts, 1986.

Paul M, Himmelstein J: Reproductive hazards in the workplace: What the practitioner needs to know about chemical exposures. *Obstet Gynecol* June 1988; 71(6):921.

Sadler TW: *Langman's Medical Embryology,* 5th ed. Baltimore: Williams & Wilkins, 1985.

Spence AP, Mason EB: *Human Anatomy and Physiology*. 3rd ed. Menlo Park, CA: Benjamin/Cummings, 1987.

Thompson JS, Thompson MW: *Genetics in Medicine,* 4th ed. Philadelphia: Saunders, 1986.

Volpe JJ: *Neurology of the Newborn,* 2nd ed. Philadelphia: Saunders, 1987.

Wassarman PM: Fertilization in mammals. *Sci Am* December 1988; 259(6):78.

Additional Readings

Cranz-Svalenius E, Jorgensen C, Mariscal U-B: Intrauterine growth of the fetus at term: A prospectus and longitudinal study with real-time ultrasound. *J Ultrasound Med* 1990; 9:35.

Epel D: The initiation of development at fertilization. *Cell Differentiation and Development* 1990; 29:1–12.

Feinberg RF, Kliman HJ, Lockwood CJ: Is oncofetal fibronectin a trophoblast glue for human implantation? *Am J Pathol* March 1991; 138:537.

Jack BW, Culpepper L: Preconception care. *J Fam Pract* March 1991; 32(3): 306.

Navot D, Bergh PA, Williams M et al: An insight into early reproductive processes through the in vivo model of ovum donation. *J Clin Endocrinol Metab* February 1991; 72:408.

Pellicer A, Calatayud C, Mirio F et al: Comparison of implantation and early development of human embryos fertilized in vitro verus in vivo using transvaginal ultrasound. *J Ultrasound Med* January 1991; 10:31.

Riduan Joesoef M, Beral V, Rolfs RT, Aral SO, Cramer DW: Are caffeinated beverages risk factors for delayed conception? *Lancet* January 20, 1990; 335:136.

CHAPTER 12

Physical and Psychologic Changes of Pregnancy

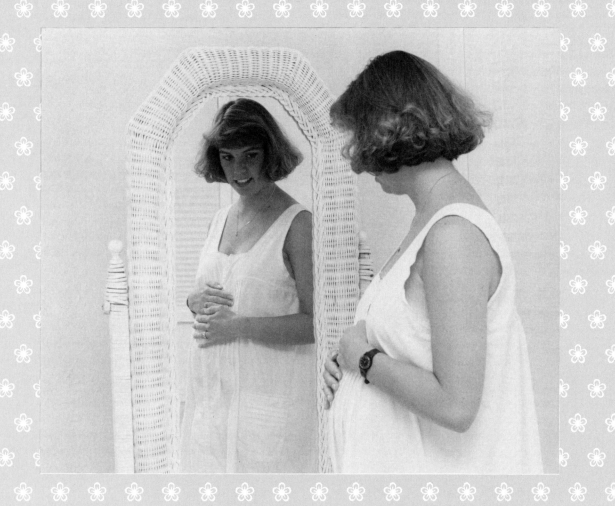

OBJECTIVES

Identify the anatomic and physiologic changes that occur during pregnancy.

Relate the physiologic and anatomic changes that occur in the body systems during pregnancy to the signs and symptoms that develop in the woman.

Compare subjective (presumptive), objective (probable), and diagnostic (positive) changes of pregnancy.

Contrast the various types of pregnancy tests.

Discuss the emotional and psychologic changes that commonly occur in a woman, her partner, and her family during pregnancy.

Summarize cultural factors that may influence a family's response to pregnancy.

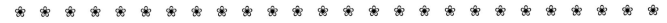

The atmosphere of approval in which I was bathed—even by strangers on the street, it seemed—was like an aura I carried with me. . . . This is what women have always done.
(Adrienne Rich, Of Woman Born)

Through modern technology and highly evolved research methods, we know a great deal about how pregnancy occurs and what happens to the fetus and the woman's body during gestation. Yet no matter how much we learn about this event, it never ceases to amaze us. First, it is nothing short of a miracle that the union of two microscopic entities—an ovum and a sperm—can produce a living being. Second, the woman's body must undergo extraordinary physical changes to sustain a pregnancy. A pregnant woman's body changes in size and shape, and all her organ systems modify their functions to create an environment that protects and nurtures the growing fetus.

Pregnancy is divided into three trimesters, each a three-month period. Each trimester has its own predictable developments in both the fetus and the mother. This chapter describes both obvious and subtle physical and psychologic changes caused by pregnancy. It also discusses the various cultural factors that can affect a woman's well-being during pregnancy.

Anatomy and Physiology of Pregnancy

The changes that occur in the pregnant woman's body are caused by several factors. Many changes are the results of hormonal influences, some are caused by the growth of the fetus inside the uterus, and some are a result of the mother's physical adaptation to the changes that are occurring.

Reproductive System

The changes in the body during pregnancy are most obvious in the organs of the reproductive system.

Uterus

The changes in the uterus during pregnancy are phenomenal. Before pregnancy the uterus is a small, semisolid, pear-shaped organ measuring approximately 7.5 × 5 × 2.5 cm and weighing about 60 g (2 oz). At the end of pregnancy the dimensions are approximately 28 × 24 × 21 cm, with an organ weight of approximately 1000 g (2.2 lb). Its capacity increases from 10 mL to 5 L or more.

The enlargement of the uterus is primarily a result of an increase in size (*hypertrophy*) of the preexisting myometrial cells. There is only a limited increase in cell number (*hyperplasia*). Individual cells have been shown to increase 17 to 40 times their prepregnancy size as a result of the stimulating influence of estrogen and the distention caused by the growing fetus. The amount of fibrous tissue between the muscle bands increases markedly, which adds to the strength and elasticity of the muscle wall.

The uterine walls are considerably thicker during the first few months of pregnancy than during the nonpregnant state. The initial changes are stimulated by increased estrogen and progesterone levels and not by mechanical distention by the products of conception. After approximately the third month, intrauterine pressure begins to be exerted by the uterine contents. The myometrial hypertrophy continues during the first few months of pregnancy. Then the musculature begins to distend, resulting in a thinning of the muscle wall to a thickness of about 5 mm or less at term. The ease of palpating the fetus through the abdominal wall attests to this thinning.

The circulatory requirements of the uterus increase as the uterus enlarges and the fetus and placenta develop. The size and number of the blood vessels and lymphatics increase greatly. By the end of pregnancy, one-sixth the total maternal blood volume is contained within the vascular system of the uterus.

Braxton Hicks contractions—irregular, generally painless contractions of the uterus—occur intermittently throughout pregnancy. They begin near the end of the first trimester (Kochenour 1990) and may be palpated bimanually beginning about the fourth month of pregnancy. During a contraction, the previously relaxed uterus becomes firm or hard and then returns to the relaxed state. These contractions help stimulate the movement of blood through the intervillous spaces of the placenta (Cunningham et al 1989). In late pregnancy these contractions become uncomfortable and may be confused with true labor contractions.

Cervix

Estrogen stimulates the glandular tissue of the cervix, which increases in cell number and becomes hyperactive. The endocervical glands occupy about half the mass of the cervix at term, as compared to a small fraction in the nonpregnant state. They secrete a thick, tenacious mucus, which accumulates and thickens to form the mucus plug that seals the endocervical canal and prevents the ascent of bacteria or other substances into the uterus. This plug is expelled when cervical dilatation begins. The hyperactive glandular tissue also causes an increase in the normal physiologic mucorrhea, at times resulting in a profuse discharge. Increased vascularization causes both softening and a blue-purple discoloration of the cervix (Chadwick's sign). Increased vascularization is a result of hypertrophy and engorgement of the vessels below the growing uterus.

Ovaries

The ovaries cease ovum production during pregnancy. Many follicles develop temporarily but never to the point of maturity. The cells lining these follicles, the thecal cells, become active in hormone production and have been called the *interstitial glands of pregnancy.*

The corpus luteum persists and produces hormones until about week 10 to 12 of pregnancy. It engulfs approximately a third of the ovary at its peak of hypertrophy. By the middle of pregnancy, it has regressed to almost complete obliteration. The progesterone it secretes maintains the endometrium until adequate progesterone is produced by the placenta to maintain the pregnancy.

Vagina

The vaginal epithelium undergoes hypertrophy, increased vascularization, and hyperplasia during pregnancy. As with the cervical changes, these changes are estrogen-induced and result in a thickening of mucosa, a loosening of connective tissue, and an increase in vaginal secretions. The secretions are thick, white, and acidic (pH 3.5–6.0). The acid pH plays a significant role in preventing infections. However, it also favors the growth of yeast organisms, resulting in moniliasis, a common vaginal infection during pregnancy.

As in the uterus, the smooth muscle cells of the vagina become hypertrophied, with an accompanying loosening of the supportive connective tissue. By the end of pregnancy, the vaginal wall and perineal body have become sufficiently relaxed to permit distention of the tissues and passage of the infant.

Because the blood flow to the vagina is increased, it may show the same blue-purple color (Chadwick's sign) seen in the cervix.

Breasts

Soon after the first menstrual period is missed, estrogen- and progesterone-induced changes are noted in the mammary glands. Increases in breast size and nodularity are the result of glandular hyperplasia and hypertrophy in preparation for lactation. By the end of the second month superficial veins are prominent, nipples are more erectile, and pigmentation of the areola is obvious. Hypertrophy of Montgomery's follicles is noted within the primary areola. Striae may develop as the pregnancy progresses. Breast changes are often most noticeable in the woman who is pregnant for the first time.

Colostrum, an antibody-rich, yellow secretion, may be expressed manually by the 12th week and may leak from the breasts during the last trimester of pregnancy. Colostrum gradually converts to mature milk during the first few days following childbirth.

Respiratory System

Pulmonary function is modified throughout pregnancy. Pregnancy induces a small degree of hyperventilation as the tidal volume (amount of air breathed with ordinary respiration) increases steadily throughout pregnancy. There is a 30% to 40% rise from nonpregnant values in the volume of air breathed each minute. Between weeks 16 and 40, oxygen consumption increases approximately 15% to 20% to meet the increased needs of the mother as well as those of the fetus and placenta. The vital capacity (maximum amount of air that can be moved in and out of the lungs with forced respiration) increases slightly, while lung compliance and pulmonary diffusion remain constant. Measurements of airway resistance show a marked decrease in pregnancy in response to elevated progesterone levels. This permits increases in oxygen consumption, in carbon dioxide production, and in the respiratory functional reserve.

The diaphragm is elevated and the substernal angle is increased as a result of pressure from the enlarging uterus. This change causes the rib cage to flare, with a decrease in the vertical diameter and increases in the anteroposterior and transverse diameters. The circumference of the chest may increase by as much as 6 cm. The increase compensates for the elevated diaphragm, and there is no significant loss of intrathoracic volume. Breathing changes from abdominal to thoracic as pregnancy progresses, and descent of the diaphragm on inspiration becomes less possible.

Nasal "stuffiness" and epistaxis are not uncommon. They occur because of estrogen-induced edema and vascular congestion of the nasal mucosa.

Cardiovascular System

The growing uterus exerts pressure on the diaphragm, pushing the heart upward and to the left and rotating it forward. This lateral displacement makes the heart appear somewhat enlarged on x-ray examination.

Blood volume progressively increases throughout pregnancy, beginning in the first trimester and peaking in the middle of the third trimester at about 45% above nonpregnant levels. This increase is due to increases in both plasma and erythrocytes. No increase occurs in pulmonary capillary wedge pressure or in central venous pressure despite the increase in blood volume. This is due to decreases in both systemic vascular resistance (21%) and pulmonary vascular resistance (34%), which enable the circulation to adapt to higher blood volume while maintaining normal vessel pressures (Clark et al 1989).

During pregnancy organ systems receive additional blood flow according to their increased workload. Thus blood flow to the uterus and kidneys increases, while hepatic and cerebral flow remains unchanged.

The pulse rate frequently increases during pregnancy, although the amount varies from almost no increase to an increase of 10 to 15 beats per minute. The blood pressure decreases slightly during pregnancy, reaching its lowest point during the second trimester. The blood pressure then gradually increases during the third trimester and is near prepregnant levels at term (when the baby is due).

The femoral venous pressure slowly rises as the uterus exerts increasing pressure on return blood flow. There is an increased tendency toward stagnation of blood in the lower extremities, with a resulting dependent edema and tendency toward varicose vein formation in the legs, vulva, and rectum late in pregnancy. The pregnant woman becomes more prone to develop postural hypotension because of the increased blood volume in the lower extremities.

The enlarging uterus may cause pressure on the vena cava when the woman lies supine, resulting in the **vena caval syndrome** or *supine hypotensive syndrome* (Figure 12–1). This pressure interferes with returning blood flow and produces a marked decrease in blood pressure with ac-

companying symptoms of dizziness, pallor, and clamminess, which can be corrected by having the woman lie on her left side.

The total red blood cell volume increases by 18% to 30% (Hume & Killam 1990). This increase is necessary to transport the additional oxygen required during pregnancy. Because the plasma volume increase is greater than the erythrocyte increase, however, the hematocrit, which measures the portion of whole blood that is composed of erythrocytes, decreases by an average of about 7%. This decrease is referred to as the **physiologic anemia of pregnancy** (pseudoanemia).

Iron is necessary for hemoglobin formation, and hemoglobin is the oxygen-carrying component of erythrocytes. Thus the increase in erythrocyte levels results in an increased need for iron by the pregnant woman. Even though the gastrointestinal absorption of iron is moderately increased during pregnancy, it is usually necessary to add supplemental iron to the diet to meet the expanded red blood cell and fetal needs.

Leukocyte production equals or is slightly greater than the increase in blood volume. The average cell count is 5000 to 12,000/mm³, with an occasional woman developing a physiologic leukocytosis of 15,000/mm³. During labor and the early postpartum period these levels may reach 25,000/mm³. Although an estrogen-related cause has been suggested, the reason for this dramatic increase remains unknown.

The fibrin level in the blood is increased by as much as 40% at term, and the plasma fibrinogen has been known to increase by as much as 50%. The increased fibrinogen accounts for the nonpathologic rise of the sedimentation rate. Although the clotting time of the pregnant woman does not differ significantly from that of the nonpregnant woman, blood factors VII, VIII, IX, and X are increased so that pregnancy becomes a somewhat hypercoagulable state.

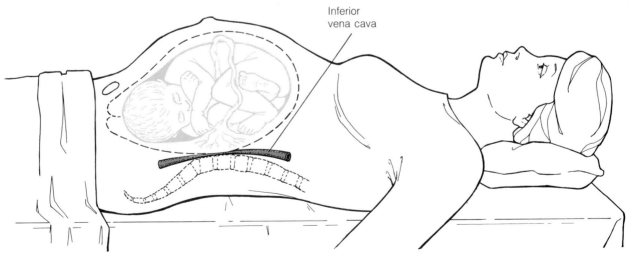

Inferior vena cava

Figure 12–1   Vena caval syndrome. The gravid uterus compresses the vena cava when the woman is supine. This reduces the blood flow returning to the heart and may cause maternal hypotension.

These changes, coupled with venous stasis in late pregnancy, place the pregnant woman at increased risk of developing venous thrombosis.

Gastrointestinal System

Many of the discomforts of pregnancy are attributed to changes in the gastrointestinal system. Nausea and vomiting during the first trimester are associated with the hCG secreted by the implanted ovum and with a change in carbohydrate metabolism that occurs in early pregnancy. Peculiarities of taste and smell are common and can further aggravate gastrointestinal discomfort. Gum tissue may become softened and may bleed when only mildly traumatized. The secretion of saliva may increase or even become excessive (*ptyalism*). The gastric contents become more acidic as a result of elevated gastrin levels (produced by the placenta) (Camann & Ostheimer 1990).

During the second half of pregnancy, numerous gastrointestinal symptoms are attributable to the pressure of the growing uterus and smooth muscle relaxation caused by elevated progesterone levels. The intestines are displaced laterally and posteriorly and the stomach superiorly. Heartburn (pyrosis) is caused by the reflux of acidic secretions from the stomach into the lower esophagus as a result of relaxation of the cardiac sphincter. Gastric emptying time and intestinal motility are delayed, leading to frequent complaints of bloating and constipation, which can be aggravated by the smooth muscle relaxation and increased electrolyte and water reabsorption in the large intestine. Hemorrhoids frequently develop if constipation is a problem or, in the second half of pregnancy, from pressure on vessels below the level of the uterus.

Only minor liver changes occur with pregnancy. Plasma albumin concentrations and serum cholinesterase activity decrease with normal pregnancy as with certain liver diseases.

The emptying time of the gallbladder is prolonged during pregnancy as a result of smooth muscle relaxation from progesterone. Hypercholesterolemia may follow, and it can predispose the woman to gallstone formation.

Urinary tract

The kidneys, ureters, and bladder undergo striking changes in both structure and function. The growing uterus puts pressure on the bladder and bladder irritation is present until the uterus rises out of the pelvis. Near term, when the presenting part engages in the pelvis, pressure is again exerted on the bladder. This pressure can impair the drainage of blood and lymph from the hyperemic bladder, rendering it more susceptible to infection and trauma. The bladder, normally a convex organ, becomes concave from the external pressure, and its retention capacity is greatly reduced.

Dilation of the kidneys and ureter may occur, most frequently on the right side above the pelvic brim, due to the lie of the uterus. This dilation is accompanied by elongation and curvature of the ureter. There appears to be no single factor accounting for this anatomic variation; instead, a combination of ureteral atonia and hypoperistalsis, possibly caused by the placental progesterone and by pressure from the enlarging fetus, seem to be involved. The same type of hydroureter and bladder relaxation can be produced in the nonpregnant female with massive doses of progesterone.

The glomerular filtration rate (GFR) and renal plasma flow (RPF) increase early in pregnancy. The GFR rises by as much as 50% by the beginning of the second trimester and remains elevated until birth. The increase in RPF is slightly less and decreases somewhat during the third trimester (Cunningham et al 1989). The mechanism for these rises remains unclear, but hPL may play a part as it possesses properties similar to the pituitary growth hormone and has been shown experimentally to produce rises in GFR. Changes in posture definitely affect excretion of sodium and water in late pregnancy. However, the influence of posture on GFR and RPF is more variable (Cunningham et al 1989).

An increased renal tubular reabsorption rate compensates for the increased glomerular activity. Amino acids and water-soluble vitamins are excreted in greater amounts than in the nonpregnant woman. Glycosuria is not uncommon or necessarily pathogenic during pregnancy but is merely a reflection of the kidneys' inability to reabsorb all of the glucose filtered by the glomeruli. However, pregnancy can be diabetogenic, so the possibility of diabetes mellitus cannot be disregarded.

The increased renal function during pregnancy results in an increased clearance of urea and creatinine and in a lowering of the blood urea and nonprotein nitrogen values. Because of this, measurement of creatinine clearance provides an accurate test of renal functioning during pregnancy.

Skin and Hair

Changes in skin pigmentation commonly occur during pregnancy. These changes are stimulated by elevated levels of melanocyte-stimulating hormone, which may be caused by increased estrogen and progesterone levels.

The pigmentation of the skin increases primarily in areas that are already hyperpigmented: the areola, the nipples, the vulva, the perianal area, and the linea alba. The **linea alba** refers to the midline of the abdomen from the pubic area to the umbilicus and above. During pregnancy increased pigmentation may cause this area to darken. It is then referred to as the **linea nigra** (See Color Plate II). Some women also develop facial **chloasma** or the "mask of pregnancy." This is an irregular pigmentation of the cheeks, forehead, and nose that occurs in many women during pregnancy and is accentuated by sun exposure. Similar changes may occur in women who are taking oral contraceptives. Facial chloasma is more prominent in dark-haired women and is occasionally disfiguring. Fortunately it fades, or at least regresses, soon after birth when the hormonal influence of pregnancy has stopped. In addition, the sweat and sebaceous glands are frequently hyperactive during pregnancy.

Striae, or stretch marks, are reddish, wavy, depressed streaks that may occur over the abdomen, breasts, and thighs as pregnancy progresses. They are caused by reduced connective tissue strength due to elevated adrenal steroid levels.

Vascular spider nevi may develop on the chest, neck, face, arms, and legs. They are small bright-red elevations of the skin radiating from a central body. They may be caused by increased subcutaneous blood flow in response to increased estrogen levels. This condition frequently occurs in conjunction with palmar erythema and is of no clinical significance. Both usually disappear shortly after the termination of pregnancy, when there is a decrease in estrogen levels in the tissues.

Hair growth may also be altered during pregnancy due to the effects of estrogen. The rate of hair growth may be decreased, and the number of hair follicles in the resting or dormant phase is also decreased. After birth the number of hair follicles in the resting phase increases sharply and the woman may notice increased shedding of hair for three to four months. Practically all hair is replaced within six to nine months, however (Key & Resnik 1986).

Musculoskeletal System

No demonstrable changes occur in the teeth of the pregnant woman. No demineralization takes place. The fairly common occurrence of dental caries during pregnancy has led to the myth, "A tooth for every pregnancy." The dental caries that may accompany pregnancy are likely to be caused by inadequate oral hygiene and dental care.

The sacroiliac, sacrococcygeal, and pubic joints of the pelvis relax in the later part of the pregnancy, presumably as a result of hormonal changes. This often causes a waddling gait. A slight separation of the symphysis pubis can often be demonstrated on radiologic examination.

As the pregnant woman's center of gravity gradually changes, the lumbodorsal spinal curve is accentuated and the woman's posture changes (Figure 12–2). This posture change compensates for the increased weight of the uterus anteriorly and frequently results in low backache. Late in pregnancy, neck, shoulder, and upper extremity aching may occur from shoulder slumping and anterior flexion of the neck accompanying the lumbodorsal lordosis.

Often pressure of the enlarging uterus on the abdominal muscles causes the rectus abdominis muscle to separate, producing **diastasis recti**. If the separation is severe and muscle tone is not regained postpartally, subsequent pregnancies will not have adequate support and the woman's abdomen may appear pendulous.

Metabolism

Most metabolic functions accelerate during pregnancy to support the additional demands of the growing fetus and its support system. The expectant mother must meet her own tissue replacement needs, those of the fetus, and those preparatory for labor and lactation. No other event in life induces such profound metabolic changes.

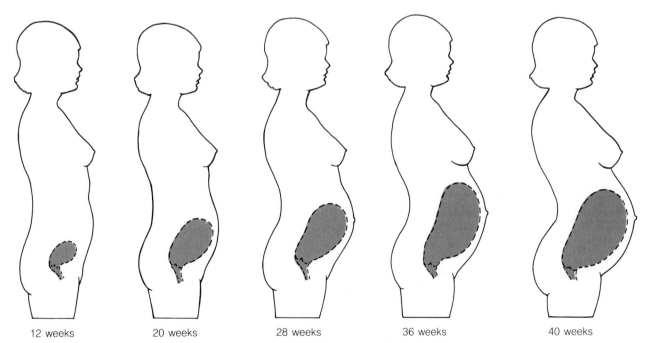

| 12 weeks | 20 weeks | 28 weeks | 36 weeks | 40 weeks |

Figure 12–2   Postural changes during pregnancy. Note the increasing lordosis of the lumbosacral spine and the increasing curvature of the thoracic area.

Weight Gain

The average weight gain during a normal pregnancy is 25 to 30 lb or 11.0 to 13.6 kg. Weight may decrease slightly during the first trimester due to the nausea, vomiting, and food intolerances of early pregnancy. The lost weight is soon regained, and an average increase of 3, 12, and 12 lb occurs in the first, second, and third trimesters, respectively. The average weight gain is distributed as follows: 11 lb, fetus, placenta, amniotic fluid; 2 lb, uterus; 4 lb, increased blood volume; 3 lb, breasts; 5 to 10 lb, maternal stores.

Adequate nutrition and weight gain are important during pregnancy. Maternal nutrition is discussed in detail in Chapter 16.

Water Metabolism

Increased water retention is a basic chemical alteration of pregnancy. Several interrelated factors cause this phenomenon. The increased level of steroid sex hormones affects sodium and fluid retention. The lowered serum protein also influences the fluid balance, as do the increased intracapillary pressure and permeability. The products of conception—fetus, placenta, and amniotic fluid—account for an average increase of 3.5 L of water. Another increase of 3.5 L is contained within the mother's hypertrophied organs and augmented blood volume and interstitial fluids. The extracellular fluid is distributed primarily below the uterus, the area of elevated venous pressure.

Nutrient Metabolism

The fetus makes its greatest protein and fat demands during the last half of gestation, doubling in weight in the last 6 to 8 weeks. The increased nitrogen (*protein*) retention that begins in early pregnancy is initially used for hyperplasia and hypertrophy of maternal tissues, such as the uterus and breasts. Nitrogen must be stored during pregnancy to maintain a constant level within the breast milk and to avoid depletion of maternal tissues.

Fats are more completely absorbed during pregnancy, resulting in a marked increase in the serum lipids, lipoproteins, and cholesterol and decreased elimination through the bowel. Fat deposits in the fetus increase from about 2% at midpregnancy to almost 12% at term. The excess nitrogen and lipidemia are considered to be a preparation for lactation.

The demand for *carbohydrate* increases, especially during the last two trimesters. Ketosis can be a problem, especially with the diabetic woman, due to glycosuria, reduced alkaline reserves, and lipidemia. Intermittent glycosuria is not uncommon during pregnancy. When it is not accompanied by a rise in blood sugar levels, glycosuria is a physiologic entity secondary to the increased glomerular filtration rate. Fasting blood sugar levels tend to fall slightly, returning to more normal levels by the sixth postpartal month. The oral glucose tolerance test shows no change with pregnancy.

The possibility of diabetes must not be overlooked during pregnancy. Plasma levels of insulin are increased during pregnancy (probably due to hormonal changes), and rapid destruction of insulin takes place within the placenta. Insulin production must be increased by the mother, and any marginal pancreatic function quickly becomes apparent. The diabetic woman often experiences increased exogenous insulin demands during pregnancy.

The demand for *iron* during pregnancy is accelerated, and the pregnant woman needs to guard against anemia. Iron is necessary for the increase in erythrocytes, hemoglobin, and blood volume, as well as for the increased tissue demands of both woman and fetus.

Iron transfer takes place at the placenta in only one direction—toward the fetus. It has been demonstrated that approximately five-sixths of the iron stored in the fetal liver has been assimilated during the last trimester of pregnancy. This stored iron in the fetal liver compensates in the first four months of neonatal life for the normal inadequate amounts of iron available in breast milk and non-iron-fortified formulas.

The progressive absorption and retention of *calcium* during pregnancy has been noted. The maternal plasma concentration of bound calcium decreases as the levels of bindable plasma proteins fall. Approximately 30 g of calcium is retained in maternal bone for fetal deposition late in pregnancy.

Pregnancy produces little change in the metabolism of most other minerals other than retention of amounts needed for fetal growth.

Vitamin metabolism does not change appreciably with pregnancy (see Chapter 16 for requirements of minerals and vitamins).

Endocrine System

Thyroid

Pregnancy influences the thyroid gland's size and activity. Often a palpable change is noted, which represents an increase in vascularity and hyperplasia of glandular tissue. Serum-free thyroxine (T_4) increases in early pregnancy and thyroid-stimulating hormone (TSH) decreases. These changes indicate that the thyroid is activated physiologically, and this activation may be due to hCG (Kimura et al 1990). The elevated T_4 levels continue until 6 to 12 weeks postpartum. Increased thyroxine-binding capacity is represented by the change in serum protein-bound iodine (PBI) from a nonpregnant level of 5 to 12 μg/dL to a pregnant level of 9 to 16 μg/dL. The cause is probably the increase in circulating estrogens; the same situation can be stimulated by the administration of estrogens, including oral contraceptives, to the nonpregnant woman.

The basal metabolic rate (BMR) increases by as much as 25% in late pregnancy. Most of the increase in oxygen consumption is a result of fetal metabolic activity. Blood studies and BMR indicate the existence of hyperthyroidism, but it is not present clinically. It should be noted that spontaneous abortion often occurs in the presence of hypothyroidism.

Parathyroid

The concentration of the hormone secreted by the parathyroids and the size of the glands increase, paralleling the fetal calcium requirements. Parathyroid hormone concentration reaches its highest level of approximately twofold between 15 and 35 weeks of gestation, returning to a normal or even subnormal level before childbirth.

Pituitary

During pregnancy, the pituitary gland enlarges somewhat, but it returns to normal size after birth. There is no significant change in the posterior lobe of the gland, although the anterior lobe increases in weight with each successive pregnancy.

Pregnancy is made possible by the hypothalamic stimulation of the anterior pituitary hormones: FSH, which stimulates ovum growth, and LH, which effects ovulation. Pituitary stimulation prolongs the corpus luteal phase of the ovary, which maintains the secretory endometrium for development of the pregnancy. Two additional pituitary hormones, thyrotropin and adrenotropin, alter maternal metabolism to support the pregnancy. Prolactin, also an anterior pituitary secretion, is responsible for initial lactation. (Continued lactation depends on the suckling of the infant.)

The posterior pituitary contains the mechanism for the release of oxytocin and vasopressin, which exert oxytocic, vasopressor, and antidiuretic effects. The main effects of oxytocin are the promotion of uterine contractility and the stimulation of milk ejection from the breasts. Vasopressin causes vasoconstriction, which results in increased blood pressure; it also has an antidiuretic effect and plays an important role in the regulation of water balance. Vasopressin secretion is controlled by changes in plasma osmolarity and blood volume.

Adrenals

Little structural change occurs in the adrenal glands during a normal pregnancy. Estrogen-induced increases in the levels of circulating cortisol result primarily from lowered renal excretion. The circulating cortisol levels regulate carbohydrate and protein metabolism. A normal level resumes one to six weeks postpartum.

The adrenals secrete increased levels of aldosterone by the early part of the second trimester. The levels of secretion are even more elevated in the woman on a sodium-restricted diet. This increase in aldosterone in a normal pregnancy may be the body's protective response to the increased sodium excretion associated with progesterone (Cunningham et al 1989).

Pancreas

The pregnant woman has increased insulin needs. The islets of Langerhans are stressed to meet this increased demand, and a latent deficiency may become apparent during pregnancy, producing symptoms of gestational diabetes (see Chapter 18).

Hormones in Pregnancy

Several hormones are required to maintain pregnancy. Most of these are produced initially by the corpus luteum; production is then assumed by the placenta. The hormones produced during pregnancy are human chorionic gonadotropin, human placental lactogen, estrogen, progesterone, and relaxin. (For an in-depth discussion of placental hormones, see Chapter 11.)

Human Chorionic Gonadotropin (hCG) The trophoblast secretes hCG in early pregnancy. This hormone stimulates progesterone and estrogen production by the corpus luteum to maintain the pregnancy until the placenta is developed sufficiently to assume that function.

Human Placental Lactogen (hPL) Also called human chorionic somatomammotropin (hCS), hPL is produced by the syncytiotrophoblast. This hormone is an antagonist of insulin; it increases the amount of circulating free fatty acids for maternal metabolic needs and decreases maternal metabolism of glucose.

Estrogen Secreted originally by the corpus luteum, estrogen is produced primarily by the placenta as early as the seventh week of pregnancy. Estrogen stimulates uterine development to provide a suitable environment for the fetus. It also helps to develop the ductal system of the breasts in preparation for lactation.

Progesterone Progesterone, also produced initially by the corpus luteum and then by the placenta, plays the greatest role in maintaining pregnancy. It maintains the endometrium and inhibits spontaneous uterine contractility, thus preventing early spontaneous abortion due to uterine activity. Progesterone also helps develop the acini and lobules of the breasts in preparation for lactation.

Relaxin Relaxin is detectable in the serum of a pregnant woman by the time of the first missed menstrual period. Relaxin inhibits uterine activity, diminishes the strength of uterine contractions, aids in the softening of the cervix, and has the long-term effect of remodeling collagen. Its primary source is the corpus luteum, but small amounts are believed to be produced by the placenta and decidua.

Prostaglandins in Pregnancy

Prostaglandins (PGs) are lipid substances that can arise from most body tissues but occur in high concentrations in the female reproductive tract and are present in the decidua during pregnancy. The exact functions of PGs during pregnancy are still unknown, although it has been proposed that they are responsible for maintaining reduced placental vascular resistance. Decreased prostaglandin levels may contribute to hypertension and pregnancy-induced hypertension (PIH). Prostaglandins are also believed to play a role in the complex biochemistry that initiates labor (Wallach & Zacur 1990).

Subjective (Presumptive) Changes

The subjective changes of pregnancy are the symptoms the woman experiences and reports. They can be caused by other conditions (Table 12–1) and therefore cannot be considered proof of pregnancy. The following can be diagnostic clues when other signs and symptoms of pregnancy are also present.

Amenorrhea is the earliest symptom of pregnancy. In a healthy woman whose menstrual cycles are regular, missing one or more menstrual periods leads to the consideration of pregnancy.

Nausea and vomiting are experienced by almost half of all pregnant women during the first three months of pregnancy and result from elevated hCG levels and changed carbohydrate metabolism. The woman may feel merely a distaste for food or may suffer extreme vomiting. These symptoms frequently occur in the early part of the day and

Table 12–1 Differential Diagnosis of Pregnancy—Subjective Changes

Subjective changes	Possible causes
Amenorrhea	Endocrine factors: early menopause; lactation; thyroid, pituitary, adrenal, ovarian dysfunction Metabolic factors: malnutrition, anemia, climatic changes, diabetes mellitus, degenerative disorders, long-distance running Psychologic factors: emotional shock, fear of pregnancy or sexually transmitted infection, intense desire for pregnancy (pseudocyesis), stress Obliteration of endometrial cavity by infection or curettage Systemic disease (acute or chronic), such as tuberculosis or malignancy
Nausea and vomiting	Gastrointestinal disorders Acute infections such as encephalitis Emotional disorders such as pseudocyesis or anorexia nervosa
Urinary frequency	Urinary tract infection Cystocele Pelvic tumors Urethral diverticula Emotional tension
Breast tenderness	Premenstrual tension Chronic cystic mastitis Pseudocyesis Hyperestrinism
Quickening	Increased peristalsis Flatus ("gas") Abdominal muscle contractions Shifting of abdominal contents

disappear within a few hours and hence are commonly called **morning sickness**. Some women may complain of nausea or vomiting in late afternoon and evening, especially in association with fatigue. This gastrointestinal disturbance usually appears about the end of the first month of pregnancy and disappears spontaneously six to eight weeks later, although it may be prolonged in some instances. Recent research suggests that women who vomit in early pregnancy have a decreased incidence of spontaneous abortion, stillbirth, or premature labor (Klebanoff et al 1985).

Excessive fatigue may be noted within a few weeks after the first missed menstrual period and may persist throughout the first trimester.

Urinary frequency is experienced during the first trimester. In the early weeks of pregnancy the enlarging uterus is still a pelvic organ and exerts pressure on the bladder. The increased vascularization and pelvic congestion that occurs in each pregnancy can also cause frequent voiding. This symptom decreases during the second trimester, when the uterus is an abdominal organ, but reappears during the third trimester when the presenting part descends into the pelvis.

Changes in the breasts are frequently noted in early pregnancy. Some women report significant breast changes prior to missing their first menses. Engorgement of the breasts due to the hormone-induced growth of the secretory ductal system results in the subjective symptoms of tenderness and tingling, especially of the nipple area.

Quickening, or the mother's perception of fetal movement, occurs about 18 to 20 weeks after the **last menstrual period (LMP)** in a primigravida but may occur as early as 16 weeks in a multigravida (woman who has been pregnant more than once). Quickening is a fluttering sensation in the abdomen that gradually increases in intensity and frequency.

Objective (Probable) Changes

An examiner can perceive the objective changes that occur in pregnancy. They are more diagnostic than the subjective symptoms. However, their presence does not offer a definite diagnosis of pregnancy (Table 12–2).

Changes in the pelvic organs caused by increased vascular congestion are the only physical signs detectable within the first three months of pregnancy. These changes are noted on pelvic examination. There is a softening of the cervix, called **Goodell's sign**. **Chadwick's sign** is the deep red to purple or bluish coloration of the mucous membranes of the cervix, vagina, and vulva due to increased vasocongestion of the pelvic vessels. (Cunningham et al [1989] consider Chadwick's sign a subjective sign, while Scott et al [1990] consider it an objective sign.) **Hegar's sign** is a softening of the isthmus of the uterus, the area between the cervix and the body of the uterus, which occurs at six to eight weeks of pregnancy. This area may become so soft that on a bimanual exam there seems to be

Table 12–2   Differential Diagnosis of Pregnancy—
Objective Changes

Objective changes	Possible causes
Changes in pelvic organs	Increased vascular congestion
Goodell's sign	Estrogen-progestin oral contraceptives
Chadwick's sign	Vulvar, vaginal, cervical hyperemia
Hegar's sign	Excessively soft walls of nonpregnant uterus
Uterine enlargement	Uterine tumors
Braun von Fernwald's sign	Uterine tumors
Piskacek's sign	Uterine tumors
Enlargement of abdomen	Obesity, ascites, pelvic tumors
Braxton Hicks contractions	Hematometra, pedunculated, submucous, and soft myomas
Uterine souffle	Large uterine myomas, large ovarian tumors, or any condition with greatly increased uterine blood flow
Pigmentation of skin	Estrogen-progestin oral contraceptives
Chloasma	Melanocyte hormonal stimulation
Linea nigra	
Nipples/areola	
Abdominal striae	Obesity, pelvic tumor
Ballottement	Uterine tumors/polyps, ascites
Pregnancy tests	Increased pituitary gonadotropins at menopause, choriocarcinoma, hydatidiform mole
Palpation for fetal outline	Uterine myomas

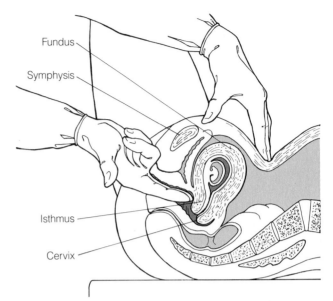

Figure 12–3   Hegar's sign, a softening of the isthmus of the uterus

nothing between the cervix and the body of the uterus (Figure 12–3). **Ladin's sign** is a soft spot anteriorly in the middle of the uterus near the junction of the body of the uterus and cervix (Figure 12–4*A*). **McDonald's sign** is an ease in flexing the body of the uterus against the cervix.

The uterus assumes an irregular globular shape during the early months of pregnancy. Irregular softening and

enlargement at the site of implantation, known as **Braun von Fernwald's sign,** occurs about the fifth week (Figure 12–4*B*). Occasionally an almost tumorlike asymmetrical enlargement occurs, called **Piskacek's sign** (Figure 12–4*C*). Generalized enlargement and softening of the body of the uterus are present after the eighth week of pregnancy. The fundus of the uterus is palpable just above the symphysis pubis at approximately 10 to 12 weeks' gestation and at the level of the umbilicus at 20 to 22 weeks' gestation (Figure 12–5).

Enlargement of the abdomen during the childbearing years is usually regarded as evidence of pregnancy, especially if the enlargement is progressive and is accompanied by a continuing amenorrhea. It is usually more pronounced in a woman whose abdominal musculature has lost some of its tone because of previous childbirth.

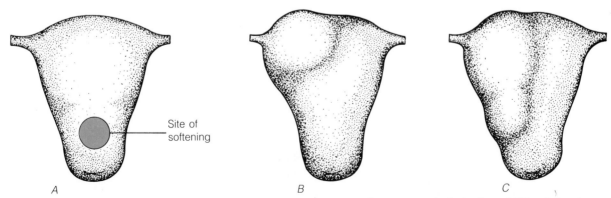

Figure 12–4   Early uterine changes in pregnancy. A Ladin's sign, a soft spot anteriorly in the middle of the uterus near the junction of the body of the uterus and the cervix. B Braun von Fernwald's sign, irregular softening and enlargement at the site of implantation. C Piskacek's sign, a tumorlike, asymmetrical enlargement

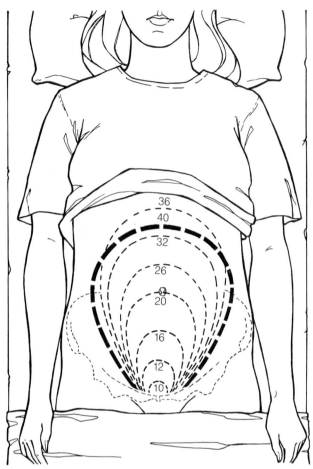

Figure 12–5 Approximate height of the fundus at various weeks of pregnancy.

As mentioned earlier, **Braxton Hicks contractions** are ordinarily painless contractions that occur at irregular intervals throughout pregnancy but are felt with abdominal palpation after week 28. As the woman approaches the end of the pregnancy, these contractions may become more uncomfortable and are then often called "false labor."

Uterine souffle may be heard when auscultating the abdomen over the uterus. It is a soft blowing sound at the same rate as the maternal pulse and is due to the increased uterine vascularization and the blood pulsating through the placenta. It is sometimes confused with the funic souffle, which is a soft blowing sound of blood pulsating through the umbilical cord. The *funic souffle* is at the same rate as the fetal heart rate.

Changes in pigmentation of the skin and the *appearance of abdominal striae* are common manifestations in pregnancy. Facial *chloasma* occurs in varying degrees in pregnant women after week 16. The pigmentation of the nipple and areola may darken, especially in primigravidas and dark-haired women. The Montgomery glands of the areola may become enlarged. The skin in the midline of the abdomen may develop a pigmented line, the *linea nigra* (Color Plate II), which may also include the umbilicus and

surrounding area. As the uterus enlarges, striae appear on the abdomen and buttocks as the underlying connective tissue breaks down. These changes occur in about one-half of all pregnant women.

The *fetal outline* may be identified by palpation in many pregnant women after 24 weeks of gestation, becoming easier to distinguish as term approaches. **Ballottement** is the passive fetal movement elicited by pushing up against the cervix with two fingers. This pushes the fetal body up and, as it falls back, the examiner feels a rebound.

Pregnancy tests are based on analysis of maternal blood or urine for the detection of human chorionic gonadotropin, the hormone secreted by the trophoblast. These tests are not considered positive signs of pregnancy because the similarity of hCG and the pituitary-secreted LH occasionally results in cross-reactions. In addition, certain conditions other than pregnancy can cause elevated levels of hCG.

Pregnancy Tests

Most pregnancy tests in the past were bioassays that used laboratory animals. These tests were time-consuming and subject to error. Consequently they have been replaced by immunoassays and radioreceptor assay tests.

Immunoassay

The immunologic pregnancy tests are based on the antigenic property of hCG. There are three types of tests:

1. *Agglutination-inhibition test (Pregnosticon R).* No clumping of cells occurs when the urine of a pregnant woman is added to the hCG-sensitized red blood cells of sheep.

2. *Latex agglutination tests (Gravindex and Pregnosticon slide test).* Latex particle agglutination is inhibited in the presence of urine containing hCG.

The agglutination-inhibition test and the latex agglutination tests are approximately 95% accurate in diagnosing pregnancy and 98% accurate in determining the absence of pregnancy. The tests become positive approximately 10 to 14 days after the first missed menstrual period. The specimen used for the tests is the first early morning midstream urine because it is adequately concentrated for accuracy. The presence of protein substances (such as blood) in the specimen should be avoided because false-positive results may occur.

3. β *subunit radioimmunoassay or RIA.* This test uses an antiserum with specificity for the β subunit of hCG in blood plasma. This is a very accurate pregnancy test. It requires about one hour to complete and becomes positive a few days after presumed implantation, thereby permitting earlier diagnosis of pregnancy. This test is also used in the diagnosis of ectopic pregnancy or trophoblastic disease.

4. *Enzyme-Linked Immunosorbent Assay (ELISA).*
This assay is useful for detecting and quantifying small amounts of material. A blue color develops, the intensity of which is related to the amount of hCG present (Cunningham et al 1989).

Radioreceptor Assay (RRA)

Radioreceptor assay (Biocept-G) uses the principle of high-affinity receptors to detect pregnancy. It is a sensitive test and can be performed in one hour, but because it fails to distinguish between hCG and LH, cross-reactions may occur.

Over-the-Counter Pregnancy Tests

CRITICAL THINKING

What factors might cause a woman to choose a home pregnancy test rather than have a pregnancy test done in a health care facility?

Over-the-counter pregnancy tests are available at a reasonable cost. These tests, performed on urine, employ the hemagglutination-inhibition or the β subunit antibody principle. The false-positive rate of these tests is low, however, the false-negative rate is much higher. One study of users found the false-negative rate to be almost 25%. Furthermore, only one-third of the users complied with the test kit instructions (Cunningham et al 1989).

Home pregnancy test instructions are quite explicit and should be followed carefully to get optimum results. Best results are obtained when the first morning-voided clear urine specimen is collected in a new container or in a clean container free of detergents or contaminants. Exact measurements must be made of urine and reagents. The test tube must remain undisturbed for the appropriate time, free of heat, vibration, or direct sunlight, although the newer kits do state that they are not sensitive to vibration. The reading must be made at the appropriate time. The tests vary in their ability to identify a pregnancy, ranging from three to nine days after the expected last menstrual period.

Opinion varies about the advisability of making these tests available to the general public. Proponents suggest that the results will encourage women to seek care earlier in the event of pregnancy. Opponents suggest that once a woman has her pregnancy confirmed she may delay seeking care. They also believe that false results may lead to unnecessary anxiety or, more importantly, a false sense of security or even relief.

Diagnostic (Positive) Changes

The positive signs of pregnancy are completely objective, cannot be confused with pathologic states, and offer conclusive proof of pregnancy, but they are usually not present until after the fourth month of pregnancy.

The *fetal heartbeat* can be detected with a fetoscope by approximately week 17 to 20 of pregnancy. With the electronic Doppler device, it is possible to detect the fetal heartbeat as early as week 10 to 12. The fetal heart rate is between 120 and 160 beats per minute and must be counted and compared with the maternal pulse for differentiation. Auscultation of the abdomen may reveal sounds other than that of the fetal heart. The maternal pulse, emanating from the abdominal aorta, may be unusually loud or a uterine souffle may be heard.

Fetal movements are actively palpable by a trained examiner after about 20 weeks' gestation. They vary from a faint flutter in the early months to more vigorous movements late in pregnancy.

Ultrasound is a technique that can be used for a positive diagnosis as early as the sixth week of pregnancy. The gestational sac can be observed by 5 to 6 weeks' gestation (3 to 4 weeks after conception); fetal parts and fetal heart movement can be seen as early as 10 weeks. Fetal movement can be detected with the real-time methods at approximately 12 weeks after the LMP (10 weeks after conception). (See Chapter 20 for further discussion.)

More recently ultrasound using a vaginal probe has been employed to detect a gestational sac as early as 10 days after implantation (Cunningham et al 1989).

Psychologic Response of the Expectant Family to Pregnancy

Pregnancy is a developmental challenge, a turning point, in a family's life and therefore is accompanied by stress and anxiety whether the pregnancy is desired or not. Pregnancy confirms one's biologic capabilities to reproduce. It is evidence of one's participation in sexual activity and as such is an affirmation of one's sexuality. For beginning families pregnancy is the transition period from childlessness to parenthood. If the pregnancy terminates in the birth of a child, the couple enters a new stage of their life together, one that is irreversible and characterized by awesome responsibilities.

The expectant couple may be unaware of the physical, emotional, and cognitive states peculiar to pregnancy. The couple may anticipate no problem from such a normal event as pregnancy and therefore may be confused and distressed by the feelings and behaviors commonly associated with childbearing.

If the expectant woman is married or has a stable partner, she no longer is only a mate but also must assume the role of mother. Her partner will soon be a father. Career goals and mobility may be altered or thwarted for one or both partners. Each partner begins to see the other in a different light. Their relationship takes on a different meaning to them and within the larger family and community. Their life-style changes. Role reorientation and re-identification are inevitable with each additional pregnancy and child. The set routines, family dynamics, and interactions are altered again with each pregnancy and require readjustment and realignment.

Even if a pregnant woman is without a stable partner, by design or circumstance, but plans to keep the baby or place it for adoption, she will still experience changes in role identity and psychobiologic maturation. The woman is no longer a separate individual. She must now consider the needs of another being who is totally dependent on her, at least during the pregnancy.

Decisions about financial matters need to be made at this time. Will the woman work during the pregnancy and return to work after the baby is born? If she chooses to return to work, how soon after the birth of the child will she return? Decisions may also need to be made about the division of tasks within the home. If the woman expects to share household and child-care tasks with the man, but he believes that women take care of home and children and men provide the income, conflicts will inevitably arise. Similarly, problems may also arise if a father wishes to assume an active parenting role but the mother feels she has the "final say" about parenting issues. When these differences are discussed openly, needs are identified, and solutions developed mutually, the newly forming family moves toward meeting the needs of its members.

Pregnancy can be a rewarding experience, especially if the couple has formed a trusting alliance and are sincere in their desire to share every aspect of the experience. However, a weak relationship is often in greater jeopardy during pregnancy, especially if the man is forced to become involved in childbirth education classes and to be the woman's coach during labor and her supporter during childbirth.

The couple must face the realities of labor and birth before parenthood can be realized. Many nonparents have little idea what labor entails. Their information is frequently based on experiences related to them by family members or friends, and these tales are often fraught with myths and exaggerations. Classes in prepared childbirth can help them overcome much of this lack of information or misinformation.

Labor is threatening in many respects. Pain, disfigurement, disruption of bodily function, and even death are potential threats for the woman. The man faces the potential disfigurement of his wife, impairment of her health, or her death. Both fear that the baby may be ill or disfigured. The expectant couple is subject to anxiety during this period, and no one can reassure them about the outcome.

For some couples pregnancy is more than a developmental stage; it is a crisis. *Crisis* can be defined as a disturbance or conflict in which the individual cannot maintain a state of equilibrium. Habitual problem-solving techniques are inadequate. Any natural turning point (courtship, pregnancy, parenthood, death, or loss of a loved one) that necessitates intrapersonal and interpersonal changes and reorganization can precipitate a crisis.

Pregnancy can be considered a *maturational crisis,* since it is a common event in the normal growth and development of the family. During such a crisis, the individual or family is in disequilibrium. Egos weaken, usual defense mechanisms lose their effectiveness, unresolved material from the past reappears, and relationships shift. The period of disequilibrium and disorganization is characterized by abortive attempts to solve the perceived problems. If the crisis is unresolved, it will result in maladaptive behaviors in one or more family members, and possible disintegration of the family. Families who are able to resolve a maturational crisis successfully will return to normal functioning and can even strengthen the bonds in the family relationship.

Crisis and its potential for successful resolution are affected by the individual or family's (a) present level of organization or disorganization; (b) past experiences of success or failure with crisis, stress, and anxiety; (c) established coping patterns, productive or unproductive; and (d) availability and effectiveness of resources and support persons. What one person considers a crisis may not be perceived as a crisis by another. Previous experience, for example, may alter an individual's perception of the event.

Pregnancy As a Developmental Stage

Pregnancy can be viewed as a developmental stage with its own distinct developmental tasks. Pregnancy can be a time of support or conflict for a couple, depending on the amount of adjustment each is willing to make to maintain the family's equilibrium. Family dynamics are an important factor in adjusting to pregnancy. Family strengths include the ability of the couple to talk about issues that are important to them, to resolve conflicts and make compromises, and to seek and receive assistance and support from loved ones (Tomlinson et al 1990).

During pregnancy the couple plans together for the first child's arrival, collecting information on how to be parents. At the same time each continues to participate in some separate activities with friends or family members. The availability of social support is an important factor in psychosocial well-being during pregnancy. For example, Cronenwett (1985) found that availability of emotional and material support (financial assistance, gifts, help with housework, etc) is positively associated with postpartum outcomes for couples. During this time relatives tend to dominate a couple's social network. While men derive most emotional support from relatives, however, women derive somewhat less support from relatives and somewhat more support from friends (Cronenwett 1985). The social network often is a major source of advice for the pregnant woman. Research suggests that both folk beliefs and sound information are given. The most commonly reported myth for women is that reaching above the head will cause the umbilical cord to wrap around the baby's neck (St. Clair & Anderson 1989).

Although individual activities are important, some conflict may arise if the couple's activities become too divergent. Thus they may find it necessary to limit their outside associations.

During pregnancy the expectant mother and father both face significant changes and must deal with major psychosocial adjustments (Table 12–3). Other family members, especially the couple's other children and the grandparents-to-be, must also adjust to the pregnancy.

The Mother

Pregnancy is a condition that alters body image and also necessitates a reordering of social relationships and changes in roles of family members. The way a particular woman meets the stresses of pregnancy is influenced by her emotional makeup, her sociologic and cultural background, and her acceptance or rejection of the pregnancy.

Many women manifest similar psychologic and emotional responses during pregnancy, including ambivalence, acceptance, introversion, mood swings, and changes in body image.

Ambivalence

Initially, even if the pregnancy is planned, there is an element of surprise that conception has occurred. This feeling is generally coupled with a feeling that the timing is wrong, that pregnancy is desirable "some day" but "not now." The reasons women cite may vary widely—long-term plans, job commitments, financial stress, the needs of an existing child—but the general feeling is that one is not ready to have a child at this time. This feeling accounts for much of the ambivalence commonly experienced by women during early pregnancy. Ambivalence may also be related to the

Table 12–3 Parental Reactions to Pregnancy

First trimester		Second trimester (continued)	
Mother's reactions	**Father's reactions**	**Mother's reactions**	**Father's reactions**
Informs father secretively or openly	Differ according to age, parity, desire for child, economic stability	Remains regressive and introspective; all problems with authority figures projected onto partner; may become angry as if lack of interest is sign of weakness in him	If he can cope, will give her extra attention she needs; if he cannot cope, will develop a new time-consuming interest outside of home
Feels ambivalent toward pregnancy; anxious about labor and responsibility of child	Acceptance of pregnant woman's attitude or complete rejection and lack of communication	Continues to deal with feelings as a mother and looks for furniture as something concrete	May develop a creative feeling and a "closeness to nature"
Is aware of physical changes; daydreams of possible miscarriage	Is aware of his own sexual feelings; may develop more or less sexual arousal	May have other extreme of anxiety and wait until ninth month to look for furniture and clothes for baby	May become involved in pregnancy and buy or make furniture
Develops special feelings for, renewed interest in mother, with formation of own mother identity	Accepts, rejects, or resents mother-in-law		
	May develop new hobby outside family as sign of stress		
Second trimester		**Third trimester**	
Mother's reactions	**Father's reactions**	**Mother's reactions**	**Father's reactions**
Feels movement and is aware of fetus and incorporates it into herself	Feels for movement of baby, listens to heartbeat, or remains aloof with no physical contact	Experiences more anxiety and tension, with physical awkwardness	Adapts to alternative methods of sexual contact
Dreams that partner will be killed, telephones him often for reassurance	May have fears and fantasies about himself being pregnant; may become uneasy with this feminine aspect in himself	Feels much discomfort and insomnia from physical condition	Becomes concerned over financial responsibility
Experiences more distinct physical changes; sexual desires may increase or decrease	May react negatively if partner is too demanding; may become jealous of physician and of his/her importance to partner and her pregnancy	Prepares for birth, assembles layette, picks out names	May show new sense of tenderness and concern; treats partner like doll
		Dreams often about misplacing baby or not being able to deliver it; fears birth of deformed baby	Daydreams about child as if older and not newborn; dreams of losing partner
		Feels ecstasy and excitement; has spurt of energy during last month	Renewed sexual attraction to partner
			Feels ultimately responsible for whatever happens

need to modify personal relationships or career plans, to fear coupled with excitement about assuming a new role, to unresolved emotional conflicts with one's own mother, and to fears about pregnancy, labor, and birth. Such feelings may be even more pronounced in the event of an unplanned or unwanted pregnancy. Women who feel comfortable addressing the issue of ambivalence tend to focus on two main areas: changed life-style, including the career-motherhood dilemma, and financial security. Indirect evidence of ambivalence includes complaints about depression, physical discomfort, and feeling "ugly" and unattractive (Lederman 1984).

During the early months the pregnant woman may seriously consider the possibility of an abortion if the pregnancy is unwanted. In the event of religious conflicts about induced abortion, the woman may experience guilt feelings about her thoughts or may tend to focus on the possibility of spontaneous abortion (miscarriage). Even when the pregnancy is consciously planned and desired, thoughts of abortion and miscarriage arise. The idea that the baby might be lost has a certain emotional appeal because it represents the possible relief of fears and ambivalence. Concurrently the pregnant woman may feel guilty for having such negative thoughts and may worry that, in some way, these thoughts will harm the baby (Robinson & Stewart 1990).

Acceptance

Acceptance of pregnancy is influenced by many factors. Lower acceptance tends to be related to an unplanned pregnancy and greater evidence of fear and conflict. The woman carrying an unplanned pregnancy tends to experience more physical discomfort and depression. When a pregnancy is well accepted, on the other hand, the woman demonstrates feelings of happiness and pleasure in the pregnancy. She experiences less physical discomfort and shows a high degree of tolerance for the discomforts associated with the third trimester (Lederman 1984).

During the *first trimester,* evidence of pregnancy is limited to amenorrhea and to the word of the care giver that the pregnancy test was positive. In an effort to verify her condition a woman may become minutely conscious of changes in her body that could validate the pregnancy. During the first trimester the woman's baby does not seem real to her and she focuses on herself and her pregnancy (Rubin 1984).

The *second trimester* is relatively tranquil. Morning sickness generally passes, the threat of spontaneous abortion diminishes, and the woman begins to accept the reality of her pregnancy (Figure 12–6). It is not unusual for an enthusiastic primagravida to don maternity clothes at the beginning of this trimester even when it is not truly necessary. The clothing serves as a verification of her pregnant state.

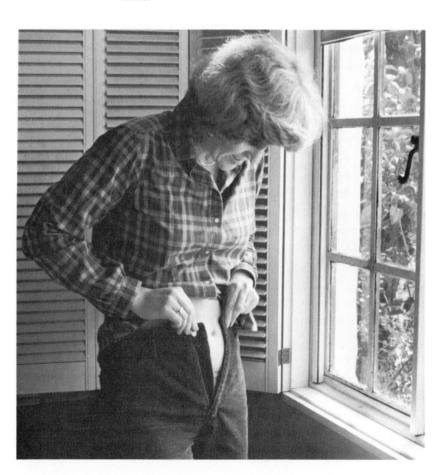

Figure 12–6 During the second trimester the most obvious evidence of pregnancy is the woman's expanding abdomen.

The highlight of the second trimester is quickening, which generally occurs about week 20—midway through the pregnancy. Actual perception of fetal movement frequently produces dramatic changes in the woman. She now perceives her baby as a real person and generally becomes excited about the pregnancy even if she hasn't been prior to this time.

As quickening and her altered physical appearance confirm her pregnant state, the woman adjusts to the idea of change and begins to prepare for her new role and her new set of relationships—with her partner and family, the child-to-be and other children, friends, and loved ones. When the pregnancy is well accepted, the woman takes pleasure in the sensations of pregnancy and attempts to picture her baby in order to know him or her better. The woman may avidly delve into folklore regarding the child's sex and may carefully study photos of herself and her partner to gain some clues about her child's appearance. She may ask her friends about childbirth and seek out other women who are pregnant or have recently given birth. She feels well, is excited, and may exhibit the "glow" so often attributed to pregnant women.

The *third trimester* combines a sense of pride with anxiety about what is to come in order for the child to be born. During this time the special prerogatives of pregnancy may be most marked. As her protruding abdomen proclaims her advanced pregnancy, the woman may find that others become more solicitous, that a chair may be offered in a crowded room, that others may carry her parcels. The woman may actually need this help, she may simply enjoy it as a privilege of pregnancy, or she may reject it if she fears that such gestures indicate she is helpless.

During the final trimester physical discomforts again increase, and adequate rest becomes a necessity. The woman, eager for the pregnancy to end, wonders if her baby's expected date of birth is accurate. She makes final preparation for the baby and may spend long periods considering names for the child. During this time the woman worries more about the health and safety of her unborn child and may have concerns that she will not behave well during childbirth (Robinson & Stewart 1990).

The woman may feel vulnerable to rejection, loss, or insult. She may worry about a variety of things and hesitate to go out unless accompanied by someone she is certain cares about her. She may withdraw into the security and quiet of her home. Toward the end of this period there is often a burst of energy as the woman prepares the "nest" for her expected infant. Many women report bursts of energy in which they vigorously clean and organize their homes.

Introversion

Introversion, or turning in on one's self, is a common occurrence in pregnancy. An active, outgoing woman may become less interested in previous activities and more concerned with needs for rest and time alone. This concentration of attention permits the woman to plan, adjust, adapt, build, and draw strength in preparation for her child's birth (Rubin 1975). As she becomes more aware of herself, her partner may feel she is being overly sensitive. He may perceive her introversion and passivity as exclusion of him and may in turn become unable to interact with her, either verbally or physically, or to provide the affection, support, and consideration she requires (Stickler et al 1978). This change in relationships may result in disequilibrium and stress for the entire family. It is essential that the couple work together to establish new, mutually acceptable patterns of response in order to overcome these blocks to communication.

I don't know if this is really considered a problem or not, but at times it seems like a problem. I'm really subject to drastic mood changes. That, or I'll be extremely emotional. For no reason at all I'll start crying or just laughing until I can hardly breathe. I don't know why; and if I can't understand it, it's twice as hard for John, especially if I'm bummed out or crying. It doesn't seem normal for a person to cry for no reason and I never did it before. (Quoted in Psychosocial Adaptation to Pregnancy)

Mood Swings

Throughout pregnancy the emotions of many women are characterized by mood swings, from great joy to deep despair. Frequently the woman will become tearful with little apparent cause. When asked why she is crying, she may find it difficult or impossible to give a reason. The situation is extremely unsettling for the partner, causing him to feel confused and inadequate. Because the man may feel unable to handle the woman's tears, he often reacts by withdrawing and ignoring the problem. Since the pregnant woman needs increased love and affection, she may perceive his reaction as unloving and nonsupportive. Once the couple understands that this behavior is characteristic of pregnancy, it becomes easier for them to deal with it more effectively—although it will be a source of stress to some extent throughout pregnancy.

Changes in Body Image

Body image refers to the mental image or picture one has of his or her body. It involves personal attitudes, feelings, and perceptions and may be influenced by environmental, cultural, temporal, physiologic, psychologic, and interpersonal factors. Thus it is dynamic and ever changing.

Pregnancy produces marked changes in a woman's body within a relatively short period of time. Women perceive that they require more body space as pregnancy progresses (Fawcett et al 1986). They also experience changes in body image. The degree of this change is related to a certain extent to personality factors, social network responses, and attitudes toward pregnancy. However, research suggests that women tend to feel somewhat negative about their bodies by the third trimester of pregnancy (Strang & Sullivan 1985).

Body boundary is another aspect of body image. It is the boundary that defines self, "containing and demarcating self as an entity separate from the surroundings" (Rubin 1984, p 17). When the body boundary is definite, the body is seen as firm, strong, and distinct from its environment. Body boundary vulnerability occurs when the body boundary is perceived as delicate, capable of being penetrated, and not readily distinguishable from its environment. The pregnant woman may feel both increased body boundary definitions and body boundary vulnerability during pregnancy, which suggests that the woman may perceive her body as vulnerable and yet as a protective container (Fawcett 1978).

Changes in body image are normal but can be very stressful for the pregnant woman. Explanation of the changes and discussion of the alterations in body image may help both the woman and her partner deal with the stress associated with this aspect of pregnancy.

Psychological Tasks of the Mother

Rubin (1984) has identified four major tasks that the pregnant woman undertakes to maintain her intactness and that of her family and at the same time incorporate her new child into the family system. These tasks form the foundation for a mutually gratifying relationship with her infant:

1. *Ensuring safe passage through pregnancy, labor, and birth.* The pregnant woman feels concern for both her unborn child and herself. She seeks competent maternity care to provide a sense of control and wishes to establish a relationship with her nurse-midwife or physician so that they "know" her and her needs. During this time the woman seeks knowledge from literature, observation of other pregnant women and new mothers, and discussion with others who have borne children. The pregnant woman also seeks to ensure safe passage by engaging in self-care activities related to diet, exercise, alcohol consumption, and so forth (Patterson et al 1990). In the third trimester, as her movements slow and her body mass increases, she becomes aware of external threats in the environment—a toy on a stair, the awkwardness of an escalator—that pose a threat to her intactness and represent hazards to be overcome. External threats become more significant, and the woman worries if her partner is late or she is home alone. Sleep becomes difficult and she begins to long for the baby's birth, even though it, too, is frightening.

2. *Seeking of acceptance of this child by others.* The birth of a child alters a woman's primary support group, her family, and her secondary affiliative groups. During the first trimester, the woman may feel sorrow at the anticipated changes, but in most cases the transition from existing social groupings to newer groupings occurs smoothly. The family generally makes the transition, and the woman slowly and subtly alters her secondary network to meet the needs of her pregnancy. In this adjustment the woman's partner is the most important figure. His support and acceptance influence her completion of her maternal tasks, the formation of her maternal identity, indeed the entire course of her pregnancy. If there are other children in the home the mother also works to ensure their acceptance of the coming child. Accepting the coming change in exclusive relationships—woman and partner or mother and first child—is sometimes stressful, and the woman will often work to maintain some special time with her partner or older child. Achieving social acceptance of the child and herself as mother may be more difficult for the adolescent mother or single woman. The child to come is not always wanted, and the woman often must direct her energies to changing this situation.

3. *Seeking of commitment and acceptance of self as mother to the infant (binding-in).* During the first trimester the child remains a rather abstract concept. With quickening, however, the child begins to become a real person, and the mother begins to develop bonds of attachment. The mother experiences the movement of the child within her in an intimate exclusive way, and out of this experience bonds of love form. The mother develops a fantasy image of her ideal child. This possessive love increases her maternal commitment to protect her fetus now and her child after he or she is born.

4. *Learning to give of oneself on behalf of one's child.* Childbirth involves many acts of giving. The man "gives" a child to a woman; she in turn "gives" a child to the man. Life is given to an infant, a sibling is given to older children of the family. The woman begins to develop a capacity for self-denial and learns to delay immediate personal gratification to meet the needs of another. Baby showers and baby gifts are acts of giving that help the mother's self-esteem while also helping her acknowledge the separateness and needs of the coming baby.

Accomplishment of these tasks helps the expectant woman develop her self-concept as mother. Often the expectant mother turns to her own mother during pregnancy because her mother is a source of information and can serve as a role model (Lederman 1984). A woman's self-concept as mother expands with actual experience and continues to grow through subsequent childbearing and childrearing. Occasionally a woman never accepts the mother role but plays the role of babysitter or older sister.

The Father

Until fairly recently, the expectant father was often viewed as a "bystander" or observer of his partner's pregnancy. He was necessary for conception, for bill-paying, and for providing male guidance as his child matured. Little attention was given to his needs, responses, and adjustments during pregnancy. Research suggests, however, that the father's stresses, adaptive behaviors, and developmental processes are as complex as those of his mate (Longobucco & Freston 1989).

In response to societal pressures, the influence of the woman's movement, and the economic pressures that result in more women employed outside the home, shared parenting and breadwinning have become more commonplace. Then, too, many men have actively sought to be more involved in the experience of childbirth and parenting. Jordan (1990) suggests that "the essence of the experience of expectant and new fatherhood is laboring for relevance. . . . He labors to incorporate the paternal role into his self-identity as a salient and integrated component of his personhood, and to be seen as relevant to childbearing and childrearing by others." (p 12).

Thus, the expectant father must first deal with the reality of the pregnancy, and then struggle to gain recognition as a parent from his partner, his family, friends, co-workers, society—and from his baby as well. The expectant mother can help her partner be a participant and not merely a helpmate to her if she has a definite sense of the experience as *their* pregnancy and *their* infant and not *her* pregnancy and *her* infant (Jordan 1990).

The expectant father faces psychologic stress as he makes the transition from nonparent to parent or from parent of one or more to parent of two or more. The stressor most frequently identified by expectant fathers has often been financial concern. Recent research suggests that major sources of stress include concern that the baby will not be healthy and normal and worry about the pain the partner will experience in childbirth, about unexpected events during pregnancy, and about the baby's condition at birth (Glazer 1989). Other sources of stress for expectant fathers include concern over the changing relationship with their partner, diminished sexual responsiveness in their partner or in themselves, change in relationships with their family or male friends, their role during labor and birth, and their ability to parent.

Expectant fathers experience many of the same feelings and conflicts experienced by expectant mothers when the pregnancy has been confirmed. Contradictory feelings may occur when men first become aware of the pregnancy. For example, with most men, there is an initial source of pride in their virility implicit with fertilization whether the pregnancy was planned or not. At the same time feelings of ambivalence are prevalent. The extent of ambivalence depends on many factors, such as whether the pregnancy was planned, his relationship with his partner, his previous experiences with pregnancy, his age, and his economic stability.

The expectant father must establish a fatherhood role just as the woman develops a concept of herself as mother. Fathers who are most successful at this generally like children, are excited about the prospect of fatherhood, are

Research Note

Clinical Application of Research

Pamela Jordan (1990) conducted a grounded theory study about expectant and new fatherhood. The primary process that emerged from the data was that of the father laboring for relevance in becoming a parent. Three developmental subprocesses unfolded from the primary process. One subprocess involved the father grappling with the reality of the pregnancy and child. The reality of the child became more substantial as the pregnancy progressed. Another subprocess was that of the father's struggle to be recognized as a parent. Fathers often felt that they became a supporting player, not a leading man. Mate, friends, health care providers, and even the baby were key recognition providers to the father. Key recognition providers could either reinforce the supporting role or assist the father to achieve a leading role. The third subprocess consisted of the father's role making in terms of becoming an involved parent. Data showed that men came to fatherhood with a lack of parenting behaviors or roles. Role making occurred when the man moved from being a provider and mate to being a sperm donor, and then to being a father of the product of childbirth. Some men moved beyond this phase to incorporate the child as a part of "me" and the role of parent as characteristic of self. However, key recognition providers could inhibit the actualization of involved parenthood.

Critical Thinking Applied to Research

Strengths: Adherence to the philosophic principles of qualitative research; description of sample, data collection, and analysis.

Concerns: Use of the terms validity and reliability for issues of qualitative rigor. Although the issues discussed under this heading were pertinent to and consistent with the principles of a qualitative study, these terms imply a concept of single reality and linearity rather than multiple realities and multidimensionality of time congruous with qualitative research.

Jordan P: Laboring for relevance: Expectant and new fatherhood. *Nurs Res* 1990; 39(1): 11.

eager to nurture a child, have confidence in their ability to be a parent, and share the experiences of pregnancy and childbirth with their partners (Lederman 1984).

First Trimester

After the initial excitement of the announcement of the pregnancy to friends and relatives and their congratulations, an expectant father may begin to feel left out of the pregnancy. He is also often confused by his partner's mood changes and perhaps bewildered by his responses to her changing body. He may resent the attention given to the woman and the need to change their relationship as she experiences fatigue and a decreased interest in sex.

During this time his child is a "potential baby." Fathers often picture interacting with a child of 5 or 6, rather than a newborn. Even the pregnancy itself may seem unreal until the woman shows more physical signs (Jordan 1990).

Second Trimester

The father's role in the pregnancy is still vague in the second trimester, but his involvement can be facilitated by his watching and feeling fetal movement. Many women report that their partner kisses them on the abdomen more in pregnancy than at any other time. Both may find this sexually arousing, and, during the second trimester especially, it can be a facilitator to increasing sexual activity.

It is helpful if the father, as well as the mother, has the opportunity to hear the fetal heartbeat. That involves a visit to the nurse-midwife's or physician's office. Involvement of fathers in antepartal care is increasing as fathers become more comfortable with this new role. For many men, seeing the infant on ultrasound is an important experience in accepting the reality of the pregnancy.

The expectant father needs to confront and resolve some of his own conflicts about the fathering he experienced. He will need to sort out those behaviors in his own fathering that he wants and does not want to imitate. This process usually occurs gradually as the pregnancy progresses. Since a more active involvement in childbirth and parenting by fathers is somewhat new, men may have few role models available to them. Fishbein (1984) suggests that the actual role a father assumes is less important than the process of negotiating between husband and wife to reach agreement on the father's role. Fishbein found that agreement was more important than actual degree of paternal involvement. Agreement between partners tended to increase with age and combined family income.

The woman's appearance begins to change at this time too, and men react differently to the physical change. For some it decreases sexual interest; for others it may have the opposite effect. A multitude of emotions are experienced by both partners, and it continues to be important for them to communicate and accept each other's feelings and concerns. In situations in which the expectant mother's demands dominate the relationship, the expectant father's resentment may increase to the point that he is spending more time at work, involved in a hobby, or with his friends. The behavior is even more likely if the expectant father did not want the pregnancy and/or if the relationship was not a good one prior to the pregnancy.

Third Trimester

If the couple have communicated their concerns and feelings to one another and grown in their relationship, the third trimester is a special and rewarding time. A more clearly defined role evolves at this time for the expectant father, and it becomes more obvious how the couple can prepare together for the coming event. They may become involved in childbirth education classes, and more concrete preparations for the arrival of the baby begin, such as shopping for a crib, car seat, and other equipment. If the expectant father has developed a detached attitude about the pregnancy prior to this time, however, it is unlikely that he will become a willing participant even though his role becomes more obvious.

Concerns and fears may recur. Many men are afraid of hurting the unborn baby during intercourse. Some feel uncomfortable with fetal activity during foreplay or after intercourse, which may make it seem that the unborn baby was an observer. The father may also begin to have anxiety and fantasies about what could happen to his partner and the unborn baby during labor and birth and feels a great sense of responsibility. The questions asked earlier in pregnancy emerge again. What kind of parents will he and his partner be? Will he really be able to help his partner in labor? Can they afford to have a baby?

Couvade

The term **couvade** traditionally has referred to the observance of certain rituals and taboos by the male to signify the transition to fatherhood. In non-Western society these taboos may have taken specific form—for example, the man may have been forbidden to eat certain foods or carry certain weapons. More recently, the term couvade has been used to describe the unintentional development of physical symptoms by the partner of a pregnant woman. The incidence of couvade has been cited as ranging from 11% to 65% (Longobucco & Freston 1989).

The most commonly occurring symptoms include fatigue, difficulty sleeping, increased appetite, anxiousness, and upset stomach (Brown 1988). Other symptoms include headache, backache, irritability, and depression (Clifton 1985). Research suggests that those men who demonstrate couvade syndrome tend to have a higher degree of paternal role preparation and are involved in more activities related to this preparation (Longobucco & Freston 1989).

Siblings

The introduction of a new baby into the family is often the beginning of sibling rivalry. Sibling rivalry results from children's fear of change in the security of their relationships with their parents. Some of the behaviors demonstrating feelings of sibling rivalry may even be directed toward the mother during the pregnancy as she experiences more fatigue and less patience with her toddler. Parents who recognize the problem early in pregnancy and begin constructive actions can help minimize the problems of sibling rivalry.

Preparation for the young child begins several weeks prior to the anticipated birth and is designed according to the age and experience of the child. Because they do not have a clear concept of time, young children should not be told too early about the pregnancy. From the toddler's point of view, "several weeks" is an extremely long time. The mother may let the child feel the baby moving in her uterus, explaining that this is "a special place where babies grow." The child can help the parents put the baby clothes in drawers or prepare the nursery. The child will probably be interested in trying on the clothes, lying in the crib, and trying out other baby items.

The concept of consistency is important in dealing with young children. They need reassurance that certain people, special things, and familiar places will continue to exist after the new baby arrives. The crib is an important though transient object in a child's life. If it is to be given to the new baby the parents should thoughtfully help the child adjust to this change (Honig 1986). Any move from crib to bed or from one room to another should precede the baby's birth.

If the child is ready for toilet training, it is most effectively done several months before or after the baby's arrival. Parents should know that the older toilet-trained child may regress to wetting or soiling because he or she sees the new baby getting attention for such behavior. The older weaned child may want to drink from a bottle again after the new baby comes. Lack of knowledge of these common occurrences can be frustrating to the new mother and can compound the stress that she feels during the early postpartum days.

During the pregnancy the older child should be introduced to a new baby for short periods to get an idea of what a new baby is like. This introduction dispels fantasies that the new arrival will be big enough to be a playmate.

Pregnant women may also find it helpful to bring their children to a prenatal visit after they have been told about the expected baby. The children are encouraged to become involved in prenatal care and to ask any questions they may have. They are also given the opportunity to hear the baby's heartbeat, either with a stethoscope or with the Doppler. This helps make the baby more real to them.

The school-age child should be involved in the pregnancy. If the pregnancy is viewed as a family affair, the child is not excluded from the experience. Teaching about the pregnancy should be based on the child's level of understanding and interest. Overeager parents may go into lengthier and more in-depth responses than the child is interested in. Some children are more curious than others. Books at their level of understanding can be made available in the home. Involvement in family discussions, attendance at sibling preparation classes, encouragement to feel fetal movement, and an opportunity to listen to the fetal heart supplement the learning process and help make the school-age child feel part of the pregnancy.

The older child may appear to have a sophisticated knowledge base, but it may be intermingled with many misconceptions. Thus, opportunities should be provided for discussion and participation.

Even after the birth siblings need to feel that they are part of a family affair. Changes in hospital regulations allowing siblings to be present at the birth or to visit their mother and the new baby facilitate this process. On arrival at home siblings can share in "showing off" the new baby.

Preparation of siblings for the arrival of a new baby is essential but other factors are equally important. These include the amount of parental attention focused on the new arrival, amount of parental attention given the older child after the birth of the new arrival, and parental reinforcement of regressive and/or aggressive behavior.

Grandparents

The first relatives told about a pregnancy are usually the grandparents. Although relationships with parents can be very complex, this period in a family's life most often promotes a closer relationship between the expectant couple and their parents. The expectant mother may find she is increasing contact with her mother, and anticipates finding the support she needs from the relationship. The expectant father may find he is doing the same with both of his parents. Usually the expectant grandparents become increasingly supportive of the expectant couple, even if disapproval of the couple's marriage and/or other conflicts were previously present.

Grandparents may be unsure about the amount of involvement they are "allowed" during the pregnancy and childbearing process. Most want to be helpful; some may bestow advice and/or gifts unsparingly. Since grandparenting can occur over a wide span of years, people's response to this role can vary considerably. For some this new role may occur at a relatively young age, and the connotation of aging that accompanies the role may affect their response to the pregnancy. The younger grandparent may also be active in work and other activities and may not demonstrate as much interest as the young couple would like.

It can be difficult for even sensitive grandparents to know how much involvement the couple want. Expectant couples want to feel in control of their new situation, which may be initially difficult in their changing roles. Grandparents find that this factor, as well as changing roles in their own life (for example, retirement, financial concerns, menopause of the expectant grandmother, death of a friend), may contribute to conflicts in the changing family structure. Some parents of expectant couples may already be grandparents and have already developed their own style of grandparenting, which will be an important factor in how they respond to the pregnancy.

Childbearing and childrearing practices are very different for today's childbearing couple. It helps family cohesiveness for young couples to share with interested grandparents what today's practices are and why they feel they are effective. Some couples may even choose to have grandparents attend the birth. At the same time, it is important for young couples to listen to any differences expectant grandparents want to explain. When grandparents give advice, it helps to remember that they care. When their recommendations seem effective, it is significant to grandparents that young couples do listen.

Occasionally young couples feel they are receiving more advice than they can tolerate. Too often they perceive parents' suggestions as criticizing their ability to prepare adequately for the childbearing process—and later as criticizing their care of the newborn. It is helpful for the young couple to discuss the problem and agree on a plan of action. The role of the helping grandparents when the new baby is brought home needs to be clarified before the event to ensure a comfortable situation for all.

In some areas classes are available to provide information for grandparents about changes in birth and parenting practices. These classes help familiarize grandparents with new parents' needs and may offer suggestions for ways in which the grandparents can support the childbearing couple.

Cultural Values and Reproductive Behavior

CRITICAL THINKING

How might nurses learn more about the cultural beliefs and practices of the ethnic groups that live in their area?

A universal tendency exists to create ceremonial rituals and rites around important life events. Thus pregnancy, childbirth, marriage, and death are often tied to ritual. Scott & Stern (1985) suggest that ritual is passed from one generation to another in three ways:

- *Formal teaching* such as childbirth preparation classes
- *Informal teaching* through role modeling and observation
- *Folktales or stories of advice or warning*, often passed on by the mother or grandmother of the family

The rituals, customs, and practices of a group are a reflection of the group's values. Thus the identification of cultural values is useful in predicting reactions. An understanding of male and female roles, family life-styles, or the meaning of children in a culture may explain reactions of joy or shame. Pregnancy is a joyful event in a culture that values children. In some cultures, however, pregnancy is a shameful event if it occurs outside of marriage.

Health values and beliefs are also important in understanding reactions and behavior. Certain behaviors can be expected if a culture views pregnancy as a sickness, whereas other behaviors can be expected if pregnancy is viewed as a natural occurrence. Prenatal care may not be a priority for women who view pregnancy as a natural occurrence.

Generalizations about cultural characteristics or cultural values are difficult since these characteristics may not be exhibited by every individual within a culture. Just as variations are seen *between* cultures, variations are also seen *within* cultures. These variations are often related to social and economic factors such as class, income, and education. For example, a third-generation Chinese-American family might have very different values and beliefs from a traditional Chinese family because of their exposure to the American culture. For this reason, the nurse needs to supplement a general knowledge of cultural values and practices with a complete assessment of the individual's values and practices.

Attitudes about pregnancy may vary somewhat among cultures. Black Americans, for example, usually consider pregnancy as a state of wellness. Mexican-Americans generally view pregnancy as a natural and desirable condition, while most Native American groups consider pregnancy a normal process. For the Asian family, pregnancy is a normal natural process, but it is also a time of anticipation and anxiety (Char 1981). In all these cultures, children are desired. Children ensure continuation of the family and cultural values. A woman who gives birth to a child, especially a son, often achieves higher status. This is true in traditional Chinese families, for example. In Mexican-American society and among many Hispanic groups, having children is evidence of the male's virility and is a sign of manliness or *machismo*, a desired trait.

Health Beliefs

Although pregnancy is perceived as a natural occurrence in many cultures, it may also be viewed as a time of increased vulnerability. In groups that adhere to beliefs in evil spirits, certain protective precautions are often followed. For example, pregnant Vietnamese women are warned to avoid funerals, places of worship, and streets at noon and five o'clock in the afternoon since spirits are present at these times (Stringfellow 1978). Many Vietnamese and Laotian women believe that overeating or inactivity during pregnancy leads to a difficult labor (Lee et al 1988). In the Mexican-American culture, the concept of *mal aire* or bad air is sometimes related to evil spirits. It is thought that air, especially night air, may enter the body and cause harm. Preventive measures, such as keeping the windows closed or covering the head, are used. For many Southeast Asians, "wind" represents a bad external influence that may enter a person when the body is vulnerable, such as during and after childbirth or during surgery (Lee et al 1988).

Most of the taboos stemming from the belief in evil spirits exist for fear of injuring the unborn child. Taboos also emanate from the fear that a pregnant woman has evil powers. For this reason pregnant women are sometimes prohibited from taking part in certain activities. For example, the pregnant Vietnamese woman cannot attend a wedding for fear of bringing bad luck to the newlyweds (Hollingsworth et al 1980).

The equilibrium model of health is based on the concept of balance between light and dark, heat and cold. Asian belief focuses on the notion of *yin* and *yang*. Yin represents the female, passive principle—darkness, cold, wetness—while yang is the masculine, active part—light, heat, and dryness. When the two are combined, they are all that can be. The hot-cold classification is seen in cultures in Latin America, the Near East, and Asia. The dimensions and meanings of this classification vary, however, and require further investigation.

Mexican-Americans often consider illness to be an excess of either hot or cold. To restore health, imbalances are often corrected by the proper use of foods, medications, or herbs. These substances are also classified as hot or cold. For example, an illness attributed to an excess of coldness will be treated only with hot foods or medications. The classification of foods is not always consistent, but it does conform to a general structure of traditional knowledge. Certain foods, spices, herbs, and medications are perceived to cool or heat the body. These perceptions do not necessarily correspond to the actual temperature; some hot dishes are said to have a cooling quality.

The Vietnamese also consider that pregnancy is a cold state because a great deal of body heat is lost. Therefore they avoid cold drinks and foods following birth (Calhoun 1985). Hindu women, on the other hand, consider pregnancy a "hot" period and eat "cool" foods to counterbalance the hot state (Wollett & Dosanjh-Matwala 1990).

The concepts of hot and cold are not as important in Native American or black American beliefs. There are some similarities, however, in all of these groups because of the emphasis on a balance in nature. Henderson and Primeaux (1981) state that black Americans believe that health is a harmony with nature and a balance between good and evil, whereas Native Americans have traditionally seen health as harmony with nature.

Health Practices

Health care practices during pregnancy are influenced by numerous factors, such as the prevalence of traditional home remedies and folk beliefs, the importance of indigenous healers, and the influence of professional health care workers. In an urban setting the age, length of time in the

---

Contemporary Issue
Do I Have a Right to Know?

For thousands of adults the decision to have a child is fraught with uncertainty because they have no knowledge of their family histories. Because they are adopted their decision is a form of medical Russian roulette. This lack of information becomes part of day-to-day existence for adopted people. They learn to live without the information so many of us take for granted—information about potential health problems that form part of a family's history. Would a man watch his diet and exercise program more carefully, for example, if he knew he had a strong family history of heart disease? How would a woman react if she knew her biologic mother, grandmother, and aunt all developed breast cancer? It is impossible to predict.

The problem changes subtly but significantly when the question of conceiving a child arises. People have no control over their genetic inheritance. They can, however, decide whether to pass their genetic inheritance on to a child, but only if they know what that inheritance entails.

Many adopted children are speaking up, urging that family histories be made available so that they can plan their lives more thoughtfully. In the future it is possible that a complete family history will be provided to parents who adopt a child to help them in raising the child and to help the child in adulthood. Unfortunately, unless a form of updating is available, health problems that develop for the

biologic parents or their families after the adoption would still be missed.

The problems and concerns that are being raised focus on several issues:

- Is it fair to ask the biologic mother, who made the difficult decision to relinquish her child, to step forward and become involved again? Aren't we "changing the rules" on her and violating her right to privacy and anonymity?

- Ethically, do people have a right to know their history? Does a moral obligation exist to inform family members of possible health problems?

- Should a system of family history reporting be developed? Who would maintain it? How would it be updated?

- Is there a way to meet the needs of adopted people to know their health histories? Should it be left up to the biologic parents to provide significant information for adoption agencies to pass along to the children? Do the children have a right to ask that adoption records be made public so that they can contact their biologic parents? What if the parents refuse to share information?

- What of the rights and needs of children conceived by parents who were adopted? How can they be helped?

city, marital status, and strength of the family may affect these patterns. Socioeconomic status is also important since modern medical services are more accessible to those who can afford it. The social network is an important source of information for a pregnant woman. Often the advice is sound, but sometimes the rationale is incorrect or the advice, if followed, could be harmful (St. Clair & Anderson 1989).

An awareness of alternative health sources is crucial for health professionals since these practices affect health outcomes. Many Mexican-American mothers are strongly influenced by familism and will seek and follow the advice of their mothers or older women in the childbearing period (Tamez 1981).

Indigenous healers are also important to specific cultures. In the Mexican-American culture the healer is called a *curandero*. In some Native American tribes the medicine man may fulfill the healing role. Herbalists are often found in Asian cultures, and faith healers, root doctors, and spiritualists are sometimes consulted in the black American culture.

Cultural Factors and Nursing Care

In recent years people from a variety of cultures have immigrated to North America. This influx of people has had a significant impact on the health care system. Numerous differences exist in beliefs, values, health care practices and expectations, language, world views, and etiquette between these newly arrived people and the majority of health care providers.

Health care providers are often unaware of the cultural characteristics they themselves demonstrate. Without cultural awareness care givers tend to project their own cultural responses onto foreign-born clients and assume that the clients are demonstrating a specific behavior for the same reason that they would. For example, health care providers sometimes label a pregnant or postpartum Filipino woman as "lazy" because of her rather sedentary lifestyle. In reality this style results from the cultural belief that inactivity is necessary to protect the mother and child (Stern et al 1985). Thiederman (1986) suggests that if health care providers fail to understand the reasons for a person's behavior, it is impossible for them to intervene appropriately and ensure cooperation.

To a certain extent most of us are guilty of ethnocentrism, at least some of the time. *Ethnocentrism* "involves the belief that the values and practices of one's own culture are the best ones, and, in some cases, the only ones of any worth" (Thiederman 1986, p 52). Thus the nurse who values stoicism during labor may be uncomfortable with the more vocal response of a Latin American woman. Another nurse may be disconcerted by the Vietnamese woman who is so intent on maintaining self-control that she smiles throughout labor (Calhoun 1985).

Health care providers sometimes believe that if members of other cultures do not share Western values, they should adopt them. This is especially difficult for some nurses caring for childbearing families if the nurse is a firm believer in the equality of the sexes and women's liberation. The nurse may find it difficult to remain silent if a woman from a Middle Eastern culture defers to her husband in decision making. It is important to remember that pressure to defy cultural values and beliefs can be stressful and anxiety provoking for these women (Thiederman 1986).

Members of minority culture groups are often found living in a certain area of a community. The nurse can begin developing cultural sensitivity by becoming knowledgeable about the cultural practices of local groups. For example, is it considered courteous to avoid eye contact? Should last names be used in conversation as a sign of respect? Is a female health care provider necessary?

Cultural assessment is an important aspect of prenatal care. The nurse should identify the main beliefs, values, and behaviors that relate to pregnancy and childbearing. This includes information about ethnic background, amount of affiliation with the ethnic group, patterns of decision making, religious preferences, language, communication style, and common etiquette practices (Tripp-Reimer et al 1984). The nurse can also explore the woman's (or family's) expectations of the health care system.

In planning care the nurse considers the extent to which the woman's personal values, beliefs, and customs are in accord with the values, beliefs, and customs of the woman's identified cultural group, the nurse providing care, and the health care agency. If discrepancies exist, the nurse then considers whether the woman's system is supportive, neutral, or harmful in relation to possible interven-

---

Table 12–4   Providing Effective Prenatal Care to Families of Different Cultures

Nurses who are interacting with expectant families from a different culture or ethnic group can provide more effective, culturally sensitive nursing care by:

- Identifying personal biases, attitudes, stereotypes, and prejudices
- Making a conscious commitment to respect the values and beliefs of others
- Learning the rituals, customs, and practices of the major cultural and ethnic groups with whom they have contact
- Including cultural assessment and assessment of the family's expectations of the health care system as a routine part of prenatal assessment
- Incorporating the family's cultural practices into prenatal care as much as possible
- Fostering an attitude of respect for and cooperation with alternative healers and care givers whenever possible
- Providing for the services of an interpreter if language barriers exist
- Learning the language (or at least several key phrases) of at least one of the cultural groups with whom they interact
- Recognizing that ultimately it is the woman's right to make her own health care choices

tions (Tripp-Reimer et al 1984). If the woman's system is supportive or neutral, it can be incorporated into the plan. For example, individual food practices or methods of pain expression may differ from those of the nurse or agency but would not necessarily interfere with the nursing plan. On the other hand, certain cultural practices might pose a threat to the health of the childbearing woman. For example, some Filipino women will not take any medication during pregnancy. The health care provider may consider a certain medication essential to the woman's well-being. In this case the woman's cultural belief may be detrimental to her own health. The nurse then faces two considerations:

1. identifying ways of persuading the woman to accept the proposed therapy; or
2. accepting the woman's rationale for refusing therapy if she is not willing to change her belief system (Tripp-Reimer et al 1984).

Table 12–4 summarizes the key actions a nurse can take to become more culturally aware.

❀ ❀

KEY CONCEPTS

Virtually all systems of a woman's body are altered in some way during pregnancy.

Blood pressure decreases slightly during pregnancy. It reaches its lowest point in the second trimester and gradually increases to near normal levels in the third trimester.

The enlarging uterus may cause pressure on the vena cava when the woman lies supine. This is called the vena caval syndrome.

A physiologic anemia may occur during pregnancy because the total plasma volume increases more than the total number of erythrocytes. This produces a drop in the hematocrit.

The glomerular filtration rate increases during pregnancy. Glycosuria may be caused by the body's inability to reabsorb all the glucose filtered by the glomeruli.

Changes in the skin include the development of chloasma; linea nigra; darkened nipples, areola, and vulva; striae; spider nevi; and palmar erythema.

Insulin needs are increased during pregnancy. A woman with a latent deficiency state may respond to the increased stress on the islets of Langerhans by developing gestational diabetes.

The subjective (presumptive) signs of pregnancy are those symptoms experienced and reported by the woman, such as amenorrhea, nausea and vomiting, fatigue, urinary frequency, breast changes, and quickening.

The objective (probable) signs of pregnancy can be perceived by the examiner but may be caused by conditions other than pregnancy.

The diagnostic (positive) signs of pregnancy can be perceived by the examiner and can only be caused by pregnancy.

During pregnancy the expectant woman may experience ambivalence, acceptance, introversion, emotional lability, and changes in body image.

Rubin (1984) has identified four developmental tasks for the pregnant woman: (1) ensuring safe passage through pregnancy, labor, and birth; (2) seeking acceptance of this child by others; (3) seeking commitment and acceptance of self as mother to the infant; and (4) learning to give of oneself on behalf of one's child.

Fathers also face a series of adjustments as they accept their new role.

Siblings of all ages require assistance in dealing with the birth of a new baby.

Cultural values, beliefs, and behaviors influence a couple's response to childbearing and the health care system.

Ethnocentrism is the belief that one's own cultural beliefs, values, and practices are the best ones, indeed the only ones worth considering.

A cultural assessment does not have to be exhaustive, but it should focus on factors that will influence the practices of the childbearing family with regard to their health needs.

❀ ❀

References

Brown MA: A comparison of health responses in expectant mothers and fathers. *West J Nurs Res* 1988; 10(5):527.

Calhoun MA: The Vietnamese woman: Health/illness attitudes and behavior. *Health Care Women Internat* 1985; 6:61.

Camann WR, Ostheimer GW: Physiological adaptations during pregnancy. *Internat Anesthesiol Clin* Winter 1990; 28(1):2.

Char EI: the Chinese American. In: *Culture and Childrearing*. Clark AL (editor). Philadelphia: Davis, 1981.

Clark SL et al: Central hemodynamic assessment of normal term pregnancy. *Am J Obstet Gynecol* December 1989; 161:1439.

Clifton F: Expectant fathers at risk for couvade. *Nurs Res* September/October 1985; 35:290.

Cronenwett LR: Network structure, social support, and psychological outcomes of pregnancy. *Nurs Res* March/April 1985; 34:93.

Cunningham FG, MacDonald PC, Gant NF: *Williams Obstetrics*, 18th ed. Norwalk, CT: Appleton & Lange, 1989.

Fawcett J: Body image and the expectant couple. *MCN* July/August 1978; 3:227.

Fawcett J et al: Spouses' body image changes during and after pregnancy: A replication and extension. *Nurs Res* July/August 1986; 35:220.

Fishbein EG: Expectant father's stress—Due to mother's expectations? *JOGNN* September/October 1984; 13:325.

Glazer G: Anxiety and stressors of expectant fathers. *West J Nurs Res* 1989; 11(1):47.

Hollingsworth AO et al: The refugees and childbearing: What to expect. *RN* November 1980; 43:45.

Honig JC: Preparing preschool-aged children to be siblings. *MCN* January/February 1986; 11:37.

Horn M, Manion J: Creative grandparenting: Bonding the generations. *JOGNN* May/June 1985; 14: 233.

Jordan PL: Laboring for relevance: Expectant and new fatherhood. *Nurs Res* January/February 1990; 39:11.

Kay MA: The Mexican American. In: *Culture, Childbearing, Health Professionals*. Clark AL (editor). Philadelphia: Davis, 1978.

Key TC, Resnik R: Maternal changes in pregnancy. In: *Obstetrics and Gynecology*, 5th ed. Danforth DN, Scott JR (editors). Philadelphia: Lippincott, 1986.

Kimura M et al: Physiologic thyroid activation in normal early pregnancy is induced by circulating hCG. *Obstet Gynecol* May 1990; 75:775.

Klebanoff R et al: Epidemiology of vomiting in early pregnancy. *Obstet Gynecol* November 1985; 66:612.

Lederman RP: *Psychosocial Adaptation in Pregnancy*. Englewood Cliffs, NJ: Prentice-Hall, 1984.

Lee RV et al: Southeast Asian folklore about pregnancy and parturition. *Obstet Gynecol* April 1988; 71:643.

Longobucco DC, Freston MS: Relation of somatic symptoms to degree of paternal-role preparation of first-time expectant fathers. *JOGNN* November/December 1989; 18:482.

Messer E: Hot-cold classification: Theoretical and practical applications of a Mexican study. *Soc Sci Med* 1981; 15B:133.

Patterson ET et al: Seeking safe passage: Utilizing health care during pregnancy. *Image* Spring 1990; 22(1):27.

Robinson GE, Stewart DE: Motivation for motherhood and the experience of pregnancy. *Can J Psychiatry* December 1990; 34:861.

Rubin R: *Maternal Identity and the Maternal Experience*. New York: Springer, 1984.

Rubin R: Maternal tasks in pregnancy. *Mat Child Nurs J* Fall, 1975; 4:143.

Scott MDS, Stern PN: The ethno market theory: Factors influencing childbearing health practices of Northern Louisiana black women. *Health Care Women Internat* 1985; 6:45.

St. Clair PA, Anderson NA: Social network advice during pregnancy: Myths, misinformation, and sound counsel. *Birth* September 1989; 16:103.

Stern PN et al: Culturally induced stress during childbearing: The Philippine-American experience. *Health Care Women Internat* 1985; 6:105.

Stickler J et al: Pregnancy: A shared emotional experience. *MCN* May/June 1978; 3:153.

Strang VR, Sullivan PL: Body image attitudes during pregnancy and the postpartum period. *JOGNN* July/August 1985; 14:332.

Strickland OL: The occurrence of symptoms in expectant fathers. *Nurs Res* May/June 1987; 36:184.

Stringfellow L: The Vietnamese. In: *Culture, Childbearing, Health Professionals*. Clark AL (editor). Philadelphia: Davis, 1978.

Tamez EG: Familism, machismo, and childbearing practices among Mexican Americans. *J Psychiatr Nurs* 1981; 19:21.

Thiederman SB: Ethnocentrism: A barrier to effective health care. *Nurse Pract* August 1986; 11:52.

Tomlinson B et al: Family dynamics during pregnancy. *J Adv Nurs* 1990; 15:683.

Tripp-Reimer T et al: Cultural assessment: Content and process. *Nurs Outlook* March/April 1984; 32:78.

Wallach EE, Zacur HA: The endocrine physiology of reproduction (adrenal, thyroid, prostaglandins, pineal). In: *Danforth's Obstetrics and Gynecology*, 6th ed. Scott JR et al (editors). Philadelphia: JB Lippincott, 1990.

Wollett A, Dosanjh-Matwala N: Pregnancy and antenatal care: The attitudes and experiences of Asian women. *Child Care Health Dev* 1990; 16:63.

Additional Readings

Ahmed F: Unmarried mothers as a high-risk group for adverse pregnancy outcomes. *J Community Health* February 1990; 15:35.

Coons SJ et al: The use of pregnancy test kits by college students. *J Am Coll Health* January 1990; 38:171.

Fawcett J: Spouses' experiences during pregnancy and the postpartum: A program of research and theory design. *Image* Fall 1989; 21:149.

Grace JT: Development of maternal-fetal attachment during pregnancy. *Nurs Res* July/August 1989; 38:228.

Joyce TJ et al: Pregnancy wantedness and the early initiation of prenatal care. *Demography* February 1990: 27:1.

Kisileuski BS et al: Maternal and ultrasound measurements of elicited fetal movements: a methodolic consideration. *Obstet Gyncol* June 1991; 77 (6):889.

Norbeck JS, Anderson NJ: Psychosocial predictors of pregnancy outcomes in low-income black, Hispanic, and white women. *Nurs Res* July/August 1989; 38:204.

Pratt D: The partner's role in pregnancy. *Nursing (London)* April 26, 1990; 4(9):23.

Yazigi RA et al: Hormonal therapy during early pregnancy. *Contemp Ob/Gyn* Jan 1991; 36:61.

CHAPTER 13

Antepartal Nursing Assessment

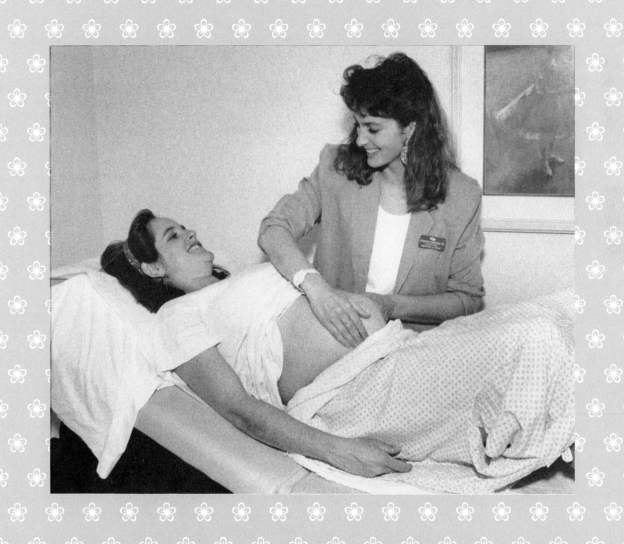

OBJECTIVES

Summarize the essential components of a prenatal history.

Explain the common obstetric terminology found in the history of a maternity client.

Identify factors related to the father's health that should be recorded on the prenatal record.

Describe the normal physiologic changes one would expect to find when performing a physical assessment on a pregnant woman.

Explain the use of Nägele's rule to determine estimated date of birth.

Develop an outline of the essential measurements that can be determined by clinical pelvimetry.

Describe areas that should be evaluated as part of the initial assessment of psychosocial factors related to a woman's pregnancy.

Relate the danger signs of pregnancy to their possible causes.

❀ ❀

Our daughter, one of the authors of this book, invited me to write a few paragraphs. What would I write about? How about comparing the father's role at childbirth, when she was born, to the role of today's father. The father of the 1940s. . . . Main objective, get your wife to the hospital on time. No delays. Don't wait too long. You're not schooled in delivering babies. Next, check her in and find the father's waiting lounge. You won't be needed until the baby is born. Fathers are really useless at this time. Try not to be nervous. Smoking is in fashion so you're well equipped with a fresh pack. Coffee is available. Lots and lots of coffee. This hospital is very considerate. The delivery may take a long time. It's always at night. It seems babies are never born in the daytime. You're tired. You try to nap but there is another expectant father who wants to gab. He's nervous. Calm him down. Act as though it's nothing. Maybe you can pace. It's hard to pace in a room ten foot square. Delivery may take anywhere from twenty minutes to twenty hours. Hope it's not twenty hours. More coffee, more cigarettes, no sleep. What a drain on the father. . . . The baby finally comes. Two hours later the doctor remembers the father is waiting. "It's a beautiful, healthy baby girl. Mother and baby are doing fine. You can see them now, but only for five minutes." What a relief. The pressure is finally off. Isn't nature wonderful? . . . Today's father, my son. Schooled in Lamaze. Drives his wife to the hospital. Dons his cap and gown while she is being prepped. When birth is about to begin they go to the birthing room together. His camera is ready. The baby is born. He cuts the cord. What a relief. The pressure is finally off. Isn't nature wonderful?

Today nurses are assuming a more important role in prenatal care, particularly in the area of assessment. The certified nurse-midwife has the education and skill to perform in-depth prenatal assessments. The nurse-practitioner may share the assessment responsibilities with a physician. An office nurse, whose primary role may be to counsel and meet the psychologic needs of the expectant family, performs assessments in those areas.

In the prenatal clinic or obstetrician's office, it is often the nurse who has the first contact with the pregnant woman, as the nurse performs initial assessments such as vital signs and weight. The nurse's attitude toward the woman during this early period can set the tone for the remainder of the visit.

An environment of comfort and open communication should be established with each antepartal visit. The nurse should convey concern for the woman as an individual and availability to listen and discuss the woman's concerns and desires. A supportive atmosphere coupled with the information found in the physical and psychosocial assessment guides in this chapter will enable the nurse to identify needed areas of education and counseling.

Client History

The course of a pregnancy depends on a number of factors, including the prepregnancy health of the woman, presence of disease states, emotional status, and past health care. Ideally, health care before the advent of pregnancy has been adequate, and antenatal care will be a continuation of that established care. One important method of determining the adequacy of a woman's prepregnancy care is a thorough history.

Definition of Terms

The following terms are used in the obstetric history of maternity clients:

Gestation: The number of weeks since the first day of the last menstrual period (LMP)

Abortion: Birth that occurs prior to the end of 20 weeks' gestation

Term: The normal duration of pregnancy

Preterm or premature labor: Labor that occurs after 20 weeks but before the completion of 37 weeks of gestation

Postterm labor: Labor that occurs after 42 weeks of gestation

Antepartum: Time between conception and onset of labor; usually used to describe the period during which a woman is pregnant. "Antepartum" is used interchangeably with "prenatal."

Intrapartum: Time from onset of labor until the birth of the infant and placenta.

Postpartum: Time from birth until the woman's body returns to an essentially prepregnant condition.

Gravida: Any pregnancy, regardless of duration, including present pregnancy

Primigravida: A woman who is pregnant for the first time

Multigravida: A woman who is in her second or any subsequent pregnancy

Nulligravida: A woman who has never been pregnant

Nullipara: A woman who has not given birth at more than 20 weeks' gestation

Primipara: A woman who has had one birth at more than 20 weeks' gestation, regardless of whether the infant is born alive or dead

Multipara: A woman who has had two or more births at more than 20 weeks' gestation

Stillbirth: A fetus born dead after 20 weeks of gestation

The terms *gravida* and *para* refer to pregnancies/births, not to the fetus.

The following examples illustrate how these terms are applied in clinical situations:

1. Jean Smith has one child born at 38 weeks and is pregnant for the second time. At her initial pre-
natal visit, the nurse indicates her obstetric history as "gravida 2 para 1 ab 0." Jean Smith's present pregnancy terminates at 16 weeks' gestation. She is now "gravida 2 para 1 ab 1."

2. Liz Alexander is pregnant for the fourth time. She has a child born at 35 weeks at home. She lost one pregnancy at 10 weeks' gestation and gave birth to another infant stillborn at term. At her prenatal assessment the nurse records Liz Alexander's obstetric history as "gravida 4 para 2 ab 1."

Because of the confusion that may result from this system when a multiple pregnancy occurs, a more detailed approach is used in some settings. Using the detailed system, gravida keeps the same meaning, while that of para is altered somewhat to focus on the number of infants born rather than the number of deliveries. A useful acronym for remembering the system is TPAL.

First digit, T—number of *term* infants; that is, the number of infants born at the completion of 37 weeks' gestation or beyond.

Second digit, P—number of *preterm* infants born; that is, the number of infants born before the completion of 37 weeks' gestation.

Third digit, A—number of pregnancies ending in either spontaneous or therapeutic *abortion*.

Fourth digit, L—number of currently *living* children to whom the woman has given birth.

Using this approach, Jean Smith (described in the first example) would initially have been classified as "gravida 2 para 1001." Following her spontaneous abortion she would be "gravida 2 para 1011." Liz Alexander would be described as "gravida 4 para 1111" (Figure 13–1).

Client Profile

The history is essentially a screening tool that identifies the factors that may detrimentally affect the course of a pregnancy. For optimal prenatal care the following information should be obtained for each maternity client at the first prenatal assessment:

1. Current pregnancy:
   a. First day of last normal menstrual period (LMP).

Name	Gravida	Term	Preterm	Abort	Living Child
Jean Smith	2	1	0	0	1
Liz Alexander	4	1	1	1	1

Figure 13–1 The TPAL approach provides more detailed information about the woman's pregnancy history.

b. Presence of cramping, bleeding, or spotting since LMP.

c. Woman's opinion about when conception occurred and when infant is due.

d. Woman's attitude toward pregnancy. (Is pregnancy planned? Wanted?)

e. Results of pregnancy test, if completed.

f. Any discomforts since LMP: nausea, vomiting, frequency, etc.

2. Past pregnancies:
   a. Number of pregnancies.
   b. Number of abortions, spontaneous or induced.
   c. Number of living children.
   d. History of preceding pregnancies: length of pregnancy, length of labor and birth, type of birth (vaginal, forceps or silastic cup, cesarean, etc.), woman's perception of the experience, complications (antepartal, intrapartal, postpartal).
   e. Perinatal status of previous children: Apgar scores, birth weights, general development, complications, feeding patterns (breast/bottle).
   f. Blood type and Rh factor (if negative—medication after birth to prevent sensitization).
   g. Prenatal education classes, resources (books).

3. Gynecologic history:
   a. Previous infections: vaginal, cervical, tubal, sexually transmitted.
   b. Previous surgery.
   c. Age of menarche.
   d. Regularity, frequency, and duration of menstrual flow.
   e. History of dysmenorrhea.
   f. Sexual history.
   g. Contraceptive history (If birth control pills were used, did pregnancy immediately follow cessation of pills? If not, how long after?)
   h. Date of last Pap smear; any history of abnormal Pap smear.

4. Current medical history:
   a. Weight.
   b. Blood type and Rh factor, if known.
   c. General health including nutrition, regular exercise program (type, frequency, duration).
   d. Any medications presently being taken (including nonprescription medications) or taken since the onset of pregnancy.
   e. Previous or present use of alcohol, tobacco, or caffeine. (Ask specifically about amount consumed each day.)
   f. Illicit drug use and/or abuse. (Ask about specific drugs such as cocaine, crack, marijuana.)
   g. Drug allergies and other allergies.

h. Potential teratogenic insults to this pregnancy, such as viral infections, medications, x-ray examinations, surgery, live cats in home (possible source of toxoplasmosis).

i. Presence of disease conditions, such as diabetes, hypertension, cardiovascular disease, renal problems.

j. Record of immunizations (especially rubella).

k. Presence of any abnormal symptoms.

5. Past medical history:
   a. Childhood diseases.
   b. Past treatment for any disease condition: Any hospitalizations? History of hepatitis? Rheumatic fever? Pyelonephritis?
   c. Surgical procedures.
   d. Presence of bleeding disorders or tendencies. (Has she received blood transfusions?)

6. Family medical history:
   a. Presence of diabetes, cardiovascular disease, hypertension, hematologic disorders, tuberculosis, preeclampsia-eclampsia (pregnancy-induced hypertension [PIH]).
   b. Occurrence of multiple births.
   c. History of congenital diseases or deformities.
   d. Occurrence of cesarean births.

7. Religious/cultural history:
   a. Does the woman wish to specify a religious preference on her chart? Does she have any religious beliefs or practices that might influence her health care or that of her child, such as prohibition against receiving blood products, dietary considerations, circumcision rites, etc.?
   b. Are there practices in her culture or that of her partner that might influence her care or that of her child?

8. Occupational history:
   a. Occupation.
   b. Does she stand all day, or are there opportunities to sit and elevate her legs? Any heavy lifting?
   c. Exposure to harmful substances.
   d. Opportunity for regular lunch, breaks for nutritious snacks.
   e. Provision for maternity leave.

9. Partner's history:
   a. Presence of genetic conditions or diseases.
   b. Age.
   c. Significant health problems.
   d. Previous or present alcohol intake, drug use, tobacco use.
   e. Blood type and Rh factor.
   f. Occupation.
   g. Educational level.
   h. Attitude toward the pregnancy.

10. Personal information:
  a. Age.
  b. Educational level.
  c. Race or ethnic group (to identify need for prenatal genetic screening or counseling).
  d. Stability of living conditions.
  e. Economic level.
  f. Housing.
  g. Any history of emotional or physical deprivation (herself or children).
  h. History of emotional problems.
  i. Support systems.
  j. Overuse or underuse of health care system.
  k. Acceptance of pregnancy.
  l. Personal preferences about the birth (expectations of both the woman and her partner, presence of others, and so on).
  m. Plans for care of child following birth.

Obtaining Data

A questionnaire like the one shown in Figure 13–2 is used in many instances to obtain information. The woman should complete the questionnaire in a quiet place with a minimum of distractions.

The nurse can obtain further information in a direct interview, which allows the pregnant woman to expand or clarify her responses to questions and gives the nurse and client the opportunity to begin developing a good relationship.

The expectant father should be encouraged to attend the initial and subsequent prenatal assessments. He is often able to contribute information to the history and may use the opportunity to ask questions and express concerns that may be of particular importance to him.

Prenatal High-Risk Screening

A highly significant part of the prenatal assessment is the screening for high-risk factors. **Risk factors** are any findings that have been shown to have a negative effect on pregnancy outcome, either for the woman or her unborn child. Many risk factors can be identified during the initial prenatal assessment; others may be detected during subsequent prenatal visits. It is important that high-risk pregnancies be identified early so that appropriate interventions can be instituted immediately.

All risk factors do not threaten the pregnancy to the same degree. Thus, many agencies use a risk scoring sheet to determine the degree of risk. The sheet is initiated at the first visit and becomes a permanent part of the woman's record. Information may be updated throughout the pregnancy as necessary. It is always possible that a pregnancy may begin as low risk and change to high risk because

of complications. Risk is also assessed intrapartally and postpartally.

Table 13–1 is an example of one risk-scoring protocol that evaluates the woman for factors that increase her risk of spontaneous preterm birth. Table 13–2 identifies the major risk factors currently recognized. The table describes maternal and fetal/neonatal implications should the risk be present in the pregnancy. In addition to the factors listed, the perinatal health team also needs to evaluate such psychosocial factors as ethnic background; occupation and education; financial status; environment, including living arrangements and location; and the woman's and her family's or significant other's concept of health, which might influence her attitude toward seeking health care.

Initial Physical Assessment

After a complete history is obtained, the woman is prepared for a thorough physical examination.

The Initial Prenatal Physical Assessment Guide beginning on p. 324 can be used by nurses involved in antepartal care. Nurses can use the information that is pertinent to them in their role, at their level of expertise, and based on the practices and policies of each agency.

The physical examination begins with assessment of vital signs and proceeds to a complete examination of the woman's body. The pelvic examination is performed last.

Before the examination, the woman should provide a clean voided urine specimen. After emptying her bladder, she is asked to disrobe and is given a gown and a sheet or some other protective covering. The woman who has emptied her bladder will be more comfortable during the pelvic examination, and the examiner will be able to palpate the abdominal organs more easily.

As a result of basic education programs or physical assessment or practitioner courses, increasing numbers of nurses are prepared to perform physical examinations. The nurse who has not yet fully developed specific assessment skills assesses the woman's vital signs, explains the procedures to allay apprehension, positions her for examination, and assists the examiner as necessary.

Each nurse is responsible for operating at the expected standard for someone with that individual nurse's skill and knowledge base. The following situation demonstrates this expectation.

Margo Cole is being seen in the clinic at 36 weeks' gestation. She began prenatal care at 12 weeks and her pregnancy to date has been uneventful. Pam Forbes graduated from her nursing program 9 months ago without having received any formal classes in physical assessment. Ms Forbes is doing the initial routine assessments for Ms Cole and observes that her weight gain has been exces-

Name _____ Age _____

Address _____ Home Telephone _____

What was the last year of schooling completed? _____

How old were you when your menstrual periods started? _____

How many days does a normal period last? _____

How many days are there between periods? _____

Do you have cramping with your periods? yes___no___

Is the pain: minimal _____

           moderate _____

           severe _____

What was the date of your last normal menstrual period? _____

Have you had bleeding or spotting

since your last menstrual period?   yes___no___

Have you been on birth control pills?   yes___no___

If yes, when did you stop taking them? _____

How many previous pregnancies have you had? _____

How many living children do you have? _____

Have you had any abortions or stillbirths?   yes___no___

If yes, how many? _____

Were any of your previous babies born prematurely? yes___no___

List the birth weight of all previous children.

1. _____   3. _____

2. _____   4. _____

Did any of your children have problems immediately after birth?

yes___no___

If yes, check the problems that occurred:

Respiratory _____   Feeding _____

Jaundice _____   Heart _____

Bleeding _____

Did you have any problems with:

previous pregnancies?   yes___no___

If yes, what was the problem? _____

previous labors?   yes___no___

If yes, what was the problem? _____

previous postpartal periods: yes___no___

If yes, what was the problem? _____

Are you Rh negative: yes___no___

Did you receive RhoGam after each pregnancy?   yes___no___

What is your present weight? _____

Are you presently taking any prescripton or nonprescription drugs?

yes___no___

If yes, please list medications:

1. _____   3. _____

2. _____   4. _____

Do you smoke?   yes___no___

If yes, how many cigarettes per day? _____

How much alcohol do you consume each day? _____

each week? _____

If you have had any of the following diseases,
place a check beside it.

_____ Chickenpox   _____ High blood pressure
_____ Mumps   _____ Heart disease
_____ Measles (3 day)   _____ Respiratory disease
_____ Measles (2 week)   _____ Kidney disease
_____ Asthma   _____ Frequent bladder
                                                        infections

If any of the following diseases is present in your family,
place a check beside the item.

_____ Diabetes   _____ Preeclampsia-eclampsia
_____ Cardiovascular disease   _____ Multiple pregnancies
_____ High blood pressure   _____ Congenital disorder
_____ Breast cancer

The following questions pertain to the father of this child.

What is the father's age? _____

Does he take prescription or nonprescription drugs?   yes___no___

If yes, please list the medications:

1. _____   3. _____

2. _____   4. _____

What is his alcohol intake each day? _____

each week? _____

Figure 13–2 Sample prenatal questionnaire

Table 13–1 System for Determining Risk of Spontaneous Preterm Birth*

Points assigned	Socioeconomic factors	Previous medical history	Daily habits	Aspects of current pregnancy
1	Two children at home Low socioeconomic status	Abortion × 1 Less than 1 year since last birth	Works outside home	Unusual fatigue
2	Maternal age < 20 years or > 40 years Single parent	Abortion × 2	Smokes more than 10 cigarettes per day	Gain of less than 5 kg by 32 weeks
3	Very low socioeconomic status Height < 150 cm Weight < 45 kg	Abortion × 3	Heavy or stressful work Long, tiring trip	Breech at 32 weeks Weight loss of 2 kg Head engaged at 32 weeks Febrile illness
4	Maternal age < 18 years	Pyelonephritis		Bleeding after 12 weeks Effacement Dilation Uterine irritability
5		Uterine anomaly Second trimester abortion DES exposure Cone biopsy		Placenta previa Hydramnios
10		Preterm birth Repeated second-trimester abortion		Twins Abdominal surgery

Score is computed by adding the number of points given any item. The score is computed at the first visit and again at 22 to 26 weeks' gestation. A total score of 10 or more places the woman at high risk of spontaneous preterm birth.

Adapted from Creasy RK, Gummer BA, Liggins GC: A system for predicting spontaneous preterm birth. Obstet Gynecol *1980;55:692.*

sive. When checking the vital signs Ms Forbes also notes a significant increase in Ms Cole's blood pressure. At this point Ms Forbes should be considering the possibility that Ms Cole may be developing PIH. Ms Forbes would continue her assessment by using a dipstick to check the urine for the presence of protein, query Margo Cole about any recent problems with swelling, and do at least an initial check for any edema. Ms Forbes is not expected to diagnose the condition, but her charting should reflect her findings in a logical manner so that the clinician will be alerted, an in-depth assessment will be made, and treatment initiated if necessary.

Thoroughness and a systematic procedure are the most important considerations when performing a physical exam. To promote completeness the assessment guide is organized into three columns: area to be assessed/normal findings, alterations and possible causes of the alterations, and nursing response to data. The nurse should be aware that certain organs and systems are assessed concurrently with other systems.

Nursing interventions based on assessment of the normal physiologic and psychologic changes associated with pregnancy and client teaching and counseling needs that have been mutually defined are discussed in more detail in Chapter 14.

Determination of Due Date

Childbearing families generally want to know the "due date," or the date around which childbirth will occur. Historically the due date has been called the estimated date of confinement (EDC). The concept of confinement is, however, rather negative, and there is a trend in the literature to avoid it by referring to the birth date as the EDD or *estimated date of delivery*. Childbirth educators often stress that babies are not "delivered" like a package, they are *born*. In keeping with a view that emphasizes the normality of the process, we have chosen to refer to the due date as the **EDB (Estimated Date of Birth)** throughout this text.

To calculate the EDB it is helpful to know the first day of the woman's last menstrual period (LMP). However, some women have episodes of irregular bleeding or fail to keep track of menstrual cycles. Thus other techniques also help to determine how far along a woman is in her pregnancy, that is, at how many weeks' gestation she is. Other techniques that can be used include evaluating uterine size, determining when quickening occurs, and auscultating fetal heart rate with a fetoscope.

(Text continues on page 331.)

Table 13–2 Prenatal High-Risk Factors

Factor	Maternal implication	Fetal/neonatal implication
Social-Personal		
Low income level and/or low educational level	Poor antenatal care Poor nutrition ↑ risk of preeclampsia	Low birth weight Intrauterine growth retardation (IUGR)
Poor diet	Inadequate nutrition ↑ risk anemia ↑ risk preeclampsia	Fetal malnutrition Prematurity
Living at high altitude	↑ hemoglobin	Prematurity IUGR
Multiparity > 3	↑ risk antepartum/postpartum hemorrhage	Anemia Fetal death
Weight < 100 lb	Poor nutrition Cephalopelvic disproportion Prolonged labor	IUGR Hypoxia associated with difficult labor and birth
Weight > 200 lb	↑ risk hypertension ↑ risk cephalopelvic disproportion	↓ fetal nutrition
Age < 16	Poor nutrition Poor antenatal care ↑ risk preeclampsia ↑ risk cephalopelvic disproportion	Low birth weight ↑ fetal demise
Age > 35	↑ risk preeclampsia ↑ risk cesarean birth	↑ risk congenital anomalies ↑ chromosomal aberrations
Smoking one pack/day or more	↑ risk hypertension ↑ risk cancer	↓ placental perfusion → ↓ O_2 and nutrients available Low birth weight IUGR Preterm birth
Use of addicting drugs	↑ risk poor nutrition ↑ risk of infection with IV drugs	↑ risk congenital anomalies ↑ risk low birth weight Neonatal withdrawal Lower serum bilirubin
Excessive alcohol consumption	↑ risk poor nutrition Possible hepatic effects with long-term consumption	↑ risk fetal alcohol syndrome
Preexisting Medical Disorders		
Diabetes mellitus	↑ risk preeclampsia, hypertension Episodes of hypoglycemia and hyperglycemia ↑ risk cesarean birth	Low birth weight Macrosomia Neonatal hypoglycemia ↑ risk congenital anomalies ↑ risk respiratory distress syndrome
Cardiac disease	Cardiac decompensation Further strain on mother's body ↑ maternal death rate	↑ risk fetal demise ↑ perinatal mortality
Anemia:* hemoglobin < 9 g/dL (white) < 29% hematocrit (white) < 8.2 g/dL hemoglobin (black) < 26% hematocrit (black)	Iron deficiency anemia Low energy level Decreased oxygen-carrying capacity	Fetal death Prematurity Low birth weight
Hypertension	↑ vasospasm ↑ risk CNS irritability → convulsions ↑ risk CVA ↑ risk renal damage	↓ placental perfusion → low birth weight Preterm birth

(continued)

Table 13–2 Prenatal High-Risk Factors (continued)

Factor	Maternal implication	Fetal/neonatal implication
Thyroid disorder Hypothyroidism	↑ infertility ↓ BMR, goiter, myxedema	↑ spontaneous abortion ↑ risk congenital goiter Mental retardation → cretinism ↑ incidence congenital anomalies
Hyperthyroidism	↑ risk postpartum hemorrhage ↑ risk preeclampsia Danger of thyroid storm	↑ incidence preterm birth ↑ tendency to thyrotoxicosis
Renal disease (moderate to severe)	↑ risk renal failure	↑ risk IUGR ↑ risk preterm birth
DES exposure	↑ infertility, spontaneous abortion ↑ cervical incompetence	↑ spontaneous abortion ↑ risk preterm birth
Obstetric Considerations *Previous Pregnancy*		
Stillborn	↑ emotional/psychologic distress	↑ risk IUGR ↑ risk preterm birth
Habitual abortion	↑ emotional/psychologic distress ↑ possibility diagnostic workup	↑ risk abortion
Cesarean birth	↑ probability repeat cesarean birth	↑ risk preterm birth ↑ risk respiratory distress
Rh or blood group sensitization	↑ financial expenditure for testing	Hydrops fetalis Icterus gravis Neonatal anemia Kernicterus Hypoglycemia
Large baby	↑ risk cesarean birth ↑ risk gestational diabetes	Birth injury Hypoglycemia
Current Pregnancy		
Rubella (first trimester)		Congenital heart disease Cataracts Nerve deafness Bone lesions Prolonged virus shedding
Rubella (second trimester)		Hepatitis Thrombocytopenia
Cytomegalovirus		IUGR Encephalopathy
Herpesvirus type 2	Severe discomfort Concern about possibility of cesarean birth, fetal infection	Neonatal herpesvirus type 2 2° hepatitis with jaundice Neurologic abnormalities
Syphilis	↑ incidence abortion	↑ fetal demise Congenital syphilis
Abruptio placenta and placenta previa	↑ risk hemorrhage Bed rest Extended hospitalization	Fetal/neonatal anemia Intrauterine hemorrhage ↑ fetal demise
Preeclampsia/eclampsia (PIH)	See hypertension	↓ placental perfusion → low birth weight
Multiple gestation	↑ risk postpartum hemorrhage	↑ risk preterm birth ↑ risk fetal demise
Elevated hematocrit* > 41% (white) > 38% (black)	Increased viscosity of blood	Fetal death rate 5 times normal rate
Spontaneous premature rupture of membranes	↑ uterine infection	↑ risk preterm birth ↑ fetal demise

Data from Garn SM, et al: Maternal hematologic levels and pregnancy outcomes. *Semin Perinatol* 1981; 5(April): 155.

Initial Prenatal Physical Assessment Guide

Assess/Normal Findings	Alterations and Possible Causes*	Nursing Responses to Data†
Vital Signs		
Blood pressure (BP): 90–140/60–90	High BP (essential hypertension; renal disease; pregestational hypertension; apprehension or anxiety associated with pregnancy diagnosis, exam, or other crises; PIH if initial assessment not done until after 20 weeks' gestation)	BP > 140/90 requires immediate consideration; establish woman's BP; refer to physican if necessary. Assess woman's knowledge about high BP; counsel on self-care and medical management.
Pulse: 60–90 beats/min. Rate may increase 10 beats/min during pregnancy	Increased pulse rate (excitement or anxiety, cardiac disorders)	Count for one full minute; note irregularities.
Respiration: 16–24 breaths/min (or pulse rate divided by four). Pregnancy may induce a degree of hyperventilation; thoracic breathing predominant	Marked tachypnea or abnormal patterns	Assess for respiratory disease.
Temperature: 36.2–37.6°C (98–99.6°F)	Elevated temperature (infection)	Assess for infection process or disease state if temperature is elevated; refer to physician/CNM.
Weight		
Depends on body build	Weight < 100 lb (45 kg) or > 200 lb (91 kg); rapid, sudden weight gain (PIH)	Evaluate need for nutritional counseling; obtain information on eating habits, cooking practices, foods regularly eaten, income limitations, need for food supplements, pica and other abnormal food habits. Note initial weight to establish baseline for weight gain throughout pregnancy.
Skin		
Color: Consistent with racial background; pink nail beds	Pallor (anemia); bronze, yellow (hepatic disease, other causes of jaundice)	The following tests should be performed: complete blood count (CBC), bilirubin level, urinalysis, and blood urea nitrogen (BUN).
	Bluish, reddish, mottled; dusky appearance or pallor of palms and nail beds in dark-skinned women (anemia)	If abnormal, refer to physician.
Condition: Absence of edema (slight edema of lower extremities is normal during pregnancy)	Edema (PIH); rashes, dermatitis (allergic response)	Counsel on relief measures for slight edema. Initiate PIH assessment; refer to physician.
Lesions: Absence of lesions	Ulceration (varicose veins, decreased circulation)	Further assess circulatory status; refer to physician if lesion severe.

*Possible causes of alterations are in parentheses.
†This column provides guidelines for further assessment and initial nursing intervention.

(continued)

Initial Prenatal Physical Assessment Guide (continued)

Assess/Normal Findings	Alterations and Possible Causes*	Nursing Responses to Data†
Spider nevi common in pregnancy	Petechiae, multiple bruises, ecchymosis (hemorrhagic disorders)	Evaluate for bleeding or clotting disorder.
Moles	Change in size or color (carcinoma)	Refer to physician.
Pigmentation: Pigmentation changes of pregnancy include linea nigra, striae gravidarum, chloasma		Assure woman that these are normal manifestations of pregnancy and explain the physiologic basis for the changes.
Café-au-lait spots	Six or more (Albright's syndrome or neurofibromatosis)	Consult with physician.
Nose		
Character of mucosa: Redder than oral mucosa; in pregnancy nasal mucosa is edematous in response to increased estrogen, resulting in nasal stuffiness and nosebleeds	Olfactory loss (first cranial nerve deficit)	Counsel woman about possible relief measures for nasal stuffiness and nose bleeds (epistaxis); refer to physician for olfactory loss.
Mouth		
May note hypertrophy of gingival tissue because of estrogen	Edema, inflammation (infection); pale in color (anemia)	Assess hematocrit for anemia; counsel regarding dental hygiene habits. Refer to physician or dentist if necessary.
Neck		
Nodes: Small, mobile, nontender nodes	Tender, hard, fixed or prominent nodes (infection, carcinoma)	Examine for local infection; refer to physician.
Thyroid: Small, smooth lateral lobes palpable on either side of trachea; slight hyperplasia by third month of pregnancy	Enlargement or nodule tenderness (hyperthyroidism)	Listen over thyroid for bruits, which may indicate hyperthyroidism. Question woman about dietary habits (iodine intake). Ascertain history of thyroid problems; refer to physician.
Chest and Lungs		
Chest: Symmetric, elliptical, smaller anteroposterior (A–P) than transverse diameter	Increased A–P diameter, funnel chest, pigeon chest (emphysema, asthma, chronic obstructive pulmonary disease [COPD])	Evaluate for emphysema, asthma, pulmonary disease (COPD).
Ribs: Slope downward from nipple line	More horizontal (COPD) Angular bumps Rachitic rosary (vitamin C deficiency)	Evaluate for COPD. Evaluate for fractures. Consult physician. Consult nutritionist.
Inspection and palpation: No retraction or bulging of intercostal spaces (ICS) during inspiration or expiration; symmetrical expansion	ICS retractions with inspiration, bulging with expiration; unequal expansion (respiratory disease)	Do thorough initial assessment. Refer to physician.

*Possible causes of alterations are in parentheses.
†This column provides guidelines for further assessment and initial nursing intervention.

(continued)

Initial Prenatal Physical Assessment Guide (continued)

Assess/Normal Findings	Alterations and Possible Causes*	Nursing Responses to Data†
Tactile fremitus	Tachypnea, hyperpnea, Cheyne-Stokes respirations (respiratory disease)	Refer to physician.
Percussion: Bilateral symmetry in tone	Flatness of percussion, which may be affected by chest wall thickness	Evaluate for pleural effusions, consolidations, or tumor.
Low-pitched resonance of moderate intensity	High diaphragm (atelectasis or paralysis), pleural effusion	Refer to physician.
Auscultation: Upper lobes: bronchovesicular sounds above sternum and scapulas; equal expiratory and inspiratory phases	Abnormal if heard over any other area of chest	Refer to physician.
Remainder of chest: vesicular breath sounds heard; inspiratory phase longer (3:1)	Rales, rhonchi, wheezes; pleural friction rub; absence of breath sounds; bronchophony, egophony, whispered pectoriloquy	Refer to physician.

Breasts

Assess/Normal Findings	Alterations and Possible Causes*	Nursing Responses to Data†
Supple; symmetric in size and contour; darker pigmentation of nipple and areola; may have supernumerary nipples, usually 5–6 cm below normal nipple line	"Pigskin" or orange-peel appearance, nipple retractions, swelling, hardness (carcinoma); redness, heat, tenderness, cracked or fissured nipple (infection)	Encourage monthly self-breast checks; instruct woman how to examine own breasts.
Axillary nodes unpalpable or pellet-sized	Tenderness, enlargement, hard node (carcinoma); may be visible bump (infection)	Refer to physician if evidence of inflammation.
Pregnancy changes:		Discuss normalcy of changes and their meaning with the woman.
1. Size increase noted primarily in first 20 weeks.		Teach and/or institute appropriate relief measures.
2. Become nodular.		Encourage use of supportive brassiere.
3. Tingling sensation may be felt during first and third trimester; woman may report feeling of heaviness.		
4. Pigmentation of nipples and areolas darkens.		
5. Superficial veins dilate and become more prominent.		
6. Striae seen in multiparas.		
7. Tubercles of Montgomery enlarge.		
8. Colostrum may be present after twelfth week.		
9. Secondary areola appears at 20 weeks, characterized by series of washed-out spots surrounding primary areola.		

*Possible causes of alterations are in parentheses.
†This column provides guidelines for further assessment and initial nursing intervention.

(continued)

Initial Prenatal Physical Assessment Guide (continued)

Assess/Normal Findings	Alterations and Possible Causes*	Nursing Responses to Data†
10. Breasts less firm, old striae may be present in multiparas.		
Heart Normal rate, rhythm, and heart sounds *Pregnancy changes:* 1. Palpitations may occur due to sympathetic nervous system disturbance. 2. Short systolic murmurs that ↑ in held expiration are normal due to increased volume.	Enlargement, thrills, thrusts, gross irregularity or skipped beats, gallop rhythm or extra sounds (cardiac disease)	Complete an initial assessment. Explain normalcy of pregnancy-induced changes. Refer to physician if indicated.
Abdomen Normal appearance, skin texture, and hair distribution; liver nonpalpable; abdomen nontender *Pregnancy changes:* 1. Purple striae may be present (or silver striae on a multipara). 2. Diastasis of the rectus muscles late in pregnancy.	Muscle guarding (anxiety, acute tenderness); tenderness, mass (ectopic pregnancy, inflammation, carcinoma)	Assure client of normalcy of diastasis. Provide initial information about appropriate postpartum exercises. Evaluate client anxiety level. Refer to physician if indicated.
3. Size: Flat or rotund abdomen; progressive enlargement of uterus due to pregnancy. 10–12 weeks: Fundus slightly above symphysis pubis. 16 weeks: Fundus halfway between symphysis and umbilicus. *20–22 weeks:* Fundus at umbilicus. *28 weeks:* Fundus three fingerbreadths above umbilicus. *36 weeks:* Fundus just below ensiform cartilage.	Size of uterus inconsistent with length of gestation (intrauterine growth retardation [IUGR] multiple pregnancy, fetal demise, hydatidiform mole)	Reassess menstrual history regarding pregnancy dating. Evaluate increase in size using McDonald's method. Use ultrasound to establish diagnosis.
4. Fetal heartbeats: 120–160 beats/min may be heard with Doppler at 10–12 weeks' gestation; may be heard with fetoscope at 17–20 weeks.	Failure to hear fetal heartbeat after 17–20 weeks (fetal demise, hydatidiform mole)	Refer to physician. Administer pregnancy tests. Use ultrasound to establish diagnosis.
5. Fetal movement not felt prior to 20 weeks' gestation by examiner.	Failure to feel fetal movements after 20 weeks' gestation (fetal demise, hydatidiform mole)	Refer to physician for evaluation of fetal status.

*Possible causes of alterations are in parentheses.
†This column provides guidelines for further assessment and initial nursing intervention.

(continued)

Initial Prenatal Physical Assessment Guide (continued)

Assess/Normal Findings	Alterations and Possible Causes*	Nursing Responses to Data†
6. Ballottement: During fourth to fifth month, fetus rises and then rebounds to original position when uterus is tapped sharply.	No ballottement (oligohydramnios)	Refer to physician for evaluation of fetal status.
Extremities		
Skin warm, pulses palpable, full range of motion; may be some edema of hands and ankles in late pregnancy; varicose veins may become more pronounced	Unpalpable or diminished pulses (arterial insufficiency); marked edema (PIH)	Evaluate for other symptoms of heart disease; initiate follow-up if woman mentions that her rings feel tight. Discuss prevention and self-treatment measures for varicose veins; refer to physician if indicated.
Spine		
Normal spinal curves: Concave cervical, convex thoracic, concave lumbar	Abnormal spinal curves: flatness, kyphosis, lordosis	Refer to physician for assessment of cephalopelvic disproportion (CPD).
In pregnancy, lumbar spinal curve may be accentuated	Backache	May have implications for administration of spinal anesthetics; see p 697 for relief measures.
Shoulders and iliac crests should be even	Uneven shoulders and iliac crests (scoliosis)	Refer very young women to a physician; discuss back-stretching exercises with older women.
Reflexes		
Normal and symmetrical	Hyperactivity, clonus (PIH)	Evaluate for other symptoms of PIH.
Pelvic Area		
External female genitals: Normally formed with female hair distribution; in multiparas, labia majora loose and pigmented; urinary and vaginal orifices visible and appropriately located	Lesions, hematomas, varicosities, inflammation of Bartholin's glands; clitoral hypertrophy (masculinization)	Explain pelvic examination procedure (Procedure 8–1). Encourage woman to minimize her discomfort by relaxing her hips. Provide privacy.
Vagina: Pink or dark pink; vaginal discharge odorless, nonirritating; in multiparas, vaginal folds smooth and flattened; may have episiotomy scar	Abnormal discharge associated with vaginal infections	Obtain vaginal smear. Provide understandable verbal and written instructions about treatment for woman and partner, if indicated.
Cervix: Pink color; os closed except in multiparas, in whom os admits fingertip	Eversion, reddish erosion, Nabothian or retention cysts, cervical polyp; granular area that bleeds (carcinoma of cervix); lesions (herpes, human papilloma virus [HPV])	Provide woman with a hand mirror and identify genital structures for her; encourage her to view her cervix if she wishes. Refer to physician if indicated.

*Possible causes of alterations are in parentheses.
†This column provides guidelines for further assessment and initial nursing intervention.

(continued)

Initial Prenatal Physical Assessment Guide (continued)

Assess/Normal Findings	Alterations and Possible Causes*	Nursing Responses to Data†
	Presence of string or plastic tip from cervix (intrauterine device [IUD] in uterus)	Advise woman of potential serious risks of leaving an IUD in place during pregnancy; refer to physician for removal.
Pregnancy changes: 1–4 weeks' gestation: Enlargement in anteroposterior diameter 4–6 weeks' gestation: Softening of cervix (Goodell's sign), softening of isthmus of uterus (Hegar's sign); cervix takes on bluish coloring (Chadwick's sign) 8–12 weeks' gestation: Vagina and cervix appear bluish-violet in color (Chadwick's sign)	Absence of Goodell's sign (inflammatory conditions, carcinoma)	Refer to physician.
Uterus: Pear-shaped, mobile, smooth surface	Fixed (pelvic inflammatory disease [PID]); nodular surface (fibromas)	Refer to physician.
Ovaries: Small, walnut-shaped, non-tender (ovaries and fallopian tubes are located in the adnexal areas)	Pain on movement of cervix (PID); enlarged or nodular ovaries (cyst, tumor, tubal pregnancy, corpus luteum of pregnancy)	Evaluate adnexal areas; refer to physician.
Pelvic Measurements		
Internal measurements: **1.** Diagonal conjugate at least 11.5 cm (Figure 13-7A)	Measurement below normal	Vaginal birth may not be possible if deviations are present. Consider possibility of cesarean birth. Determine CPD by radiological examination and ultrasound at term.
2. Obstetric conjugate estimated by subtracting 1.5–2 cm from diagonal conjugate	Disproportion of pubic arch	
3. Inclination of sacrum	Abnormal curvature of sacrum	
4. Motility of coccyx; external inter-tuberosity diameter > 8 cm	Fixed or malposition of coccyx	
Anus and Rectum		
No lumps, rashes, excoriation, tenderness; cervix may be felt through rectal wall	Hemorrhoids, rectal prolapse; nodular lesion (carcinoma)	Counsel about appropriate prevention and relief measures; refer to physician for further evaluation.

*Possible causes of alterations are in parentheses.
†This column provides guidelines for further assessment and initial nursing intervention.

(continued)

Initial Prenatal Physical Assessment Guide (continued)

Assess/Normal Findings	Alterations and Possible Causes*	Nursing Responses to Data†
Laboratory Evaluation		
Hemoglobin: 12–16 g/dL; women residing in high altitudes may have higher levels of hemoglobin	< 12 g/dL (anemia)	Hemoglobin < 12 g/dL requires iron supplementation and nutritional counseling.
ABO and Rh typing: Normal distribution of blood types	Rh negative	If Rh negative, check for presence of anti-Rh antibodies.
		Check partner's blood type; if partner is Rh positive, discuss with woman the need for antibody titers during pregnancy, management during the intrapartal period, and possible candidacy for RhIgG.
Complete blood count (CBC)		
Hematocrit: 38%–47%; physiologic anemia (pseudoanemia) may occur Red blood cells (RBC): 4.2–5.4 million/μL	Marked anemia or blood dyscrasias	Perform CBC and Schilling differential cell count.
White blood cells (WBC): 4500–11,000/μL Differential	Presence of infection; may be elevated in pregnancy and with labor	Evaluate for other signs of infection.
Neutrophils 40%–60%		
Bands up to 5%		
Eosinophils 1%–3%		
Basophils up to 1%		
Lymphocytes 20%–40%		
Monocytes 4%–8%		
Syphilis tests—serologic test for syphilis (STS), complement fixation test, Venereal Disease Research Laboratory (VDRL) test—nonreactive	Positive reaction STS—tests may have 25%–45% incidence of biologic false positive results; false results may occur in individuals who have acute viral or bacterial infections, hypersensitivity reactions, recent vaccination, collagen disease, malaria, or tuberculosis	Positive results may be confirmed with the fluorescent treponemal antibody absorption (FTA-ABS) tests; all tests for syphilis give positive results in the secondary stage of the disease; antibiotic tests may cause negative test results.
Gonorrhea culture: Negative	Positive	Refer for treatment.
Urinalysis (u/a): Normal color, specific gravity; pH 4.6–8.0	Abnormal color (porphyria, hemoglobinuria, bilirubinemia); alkaline urine (metabolic alkalemia, *Proteus* infection, old specimen)	Repeat u/a; refer to physician.
Negative for protein, red blood cells, white blood cells, casts	Positive findings (contaminated specimen, kidney disease)	Repeat u/a; refer to physician.
Glucose: Negative (small degree of glycosuria may occur in pregnancy)	Glycosuria (low renal threshold for glucose, diabetes mellitus)	Assess blood glucose; test urine for ketones.

*Possible causes of alterations are placed in parentheses.
†This column provides guidelines for further assessment and initial nursing interventions.

(continued)

Initial Prenatal Physical Assessment Guide (continued)

Assess/Normal Findings	Alterations and Possible Causes*	Nursing Responses to Data†
Rubella titer: hemagglutination-inhibition test (HAI) > 1:10 indicates woman is immune	HAI titer < 1:10	Immunization will be given on postpartum or within six weeks after childbirth. Instruct woman whose titers are < 1:10 to avoid children who have rubella.
Antibody screen: Negative	Positive	If results are positive, further testing should be done to identify specific antibodies; in addition, antibody titers may be done during pregnancy.
Sickle cell screen for black clients: Negative	Positive; test results would include a description of cells	Refer to physician.
Papanicolaou (Pap) test: Negative	Test results that show atypical cells	Refer to physician. Discuss the meaning of the various classes with the woman and importance of follow-up.‡

*Possible causes of alterations are placed in parentheses.
†This column provides guidelines for further assessment and initial nursing interventions.
‡The current trend is to report Pap test results as follows:
1. Negative
2. Atypical (this finding would describe the cells)
Some clinicians may still use Class I to Class V terminology, with Class I being negative and Class V cancer in situ. It is important to know the scoring system used by the laboratory doing the test.

Nägele's Rule

The most common method of determining the EDB is Nägele's rule. To use this method, one begins with the first day of the last menstrual period, subtracts three months, and adds seven days. For example:

First day of LMP	November 21
Subtract 3 months	− 3 months
	August 21
Add 7 days	+ 7 days
EDB	August 28

A simpler method is to change the months to numeric terms:

November 21 becomes	11−21
Subtract 3 months	− 3
	8−21
Add 7 days	+ 7
EDB	August 28

If a woman with a history of menses every 28 days remembers her LMP and was not taking oral contraceptives prior to becoming pregnant, Nägele's rule may be a fairly accurate determiner of her predicted birth date. However, if her cycle is irregular or 35 to 40 days in length, the time of ovulation may be delayed by several days. If she has been on oral contraceptives, ovulation may be delayed several weeks following her last menses. Ovulation usually occurs 14 days before the onset of the next menses, not 14 days after the previous menses. Thus, the accuracy of this method has been questioned. Mittendorf et al. (1990) found that the average length of gestation in uncomplicated pregnancies is longer than Nägele's rule suggests, especially for white primiparas (+7 days). They also reported that the Irish, for example, calculate the EDB from the last day of menses rather than the first day.

A gestation calculator or "wheel" permits the care giver to calculate the EDB even more quickly (Figure 13–3).

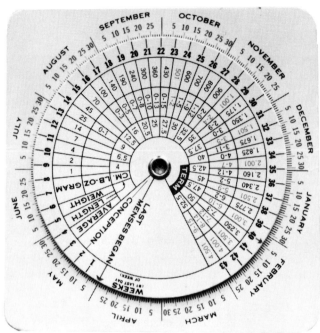

Figure 13–3 The EDB wheel can be used to calculate due date. The last menses began arrow is placed on the date of the woman's LMP. The EDB is then read at the arrow labeled 40. In this case, the LMP was April 30th and the EDB is February 4th.

Uterine Assessment

Physical Examination

When a woman is examined in the first 10 to 12 weeks of her pregnancy and the nurse practitioner, certified nurse-midwife, or physician thinks that her uterine size is compatible with her menstrual history, uterine size may be the single most important clinical method for dating her pregnancy. In many cases, however, women do not seek obstetric attention until well into their second trimester, when it becomes much more difficult to evaluate specific uterine size. In the case of the obese woman, it is most difficult to determine uterine size early in pregnancy.

Fundal Height

Fundal height may be used as an indicator of uterine size, although this cannot be used late in pregnancy. A centimeter tape measure is used to measure the distance from the top of the symphysis pubis over the curve of the abdomen to the top of the uterine fundus (McDonald's method) (Figure 13–4). Fundal height in centimeters correlates well with weeks of gestation between 20 and 31 weeks (Cunningham et al. 1989). At 26 weeks' gestation, for example, fundal height is probably about 26 cm. At 20 weeks' gestation the fundus is about 20 cm and at the level of the umbilicus in an average female. To be most accurate,

fundal height should be measured by the same examiner each time and the woman should have voided within 30 minutes of the exam (Engstrom 1988). If the woman is very tall or very short, fundal height will differ. In the third trimester, variations in fetal weight decrease the accuracy of fundal height measurements.

Measurements of fundal height from month to month and week to week may give indications of intrauterine growth retardation (IUGR), if there is a lag in progression, or indications of the presence of twins or hydramnios if there is a sudden increase in height. Unfortunately this method of dating a pregnancy can be quite inaccurate in obese women, in women with uterine fibroids, and in mothers who develop hydramnios.

Fetal Development

Quickening

Fetal movements felt by the mother may give some indications that the fetus is nearing 20 weeks' gestation. However, quickening may be experienced between 16 and 22 weeks' gestation, so this is not a completely accurate method. Because multiparous women have experienced quickening before, they often report it earlier than a primigravida does.

Fetal Heartbeat

The fetal heartbeat can be detected as early as week 16 and almost always by 19 or 20 weeks of gestation with an ordinary fetoscope. In the case of twins or the obese woman, it may be later than this before the fetal heartbeat can be detected. Fetal heartbeat may be detected with the ultrasonic Doppler device (Figure 13–5) at about 10 to 12 weeks' gestation.

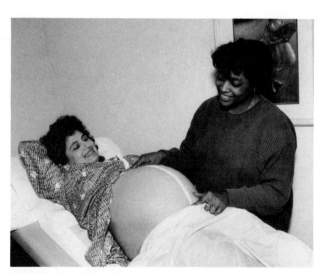

Figure 13–4 The nurse measures fundal height using McDonald's method.

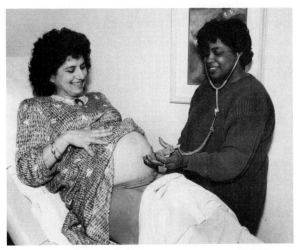

Figure 13–5 Listening to fetal heartbeat with Doppler device.

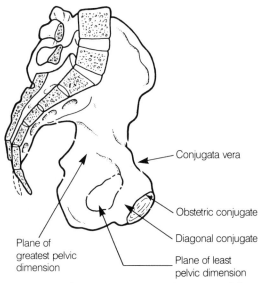

Figure 13–6 Anteroposterior diameters of the pelvic inlet and their relationship to the pelvic planes

Ultrasound

In the first trimester, ultrasound scanning can detect a gestational sac as early as 5 to 6 weeks after the LMP, fetal heart activity by 9 to 10 weeks and occasionally earlier, and fetal breathing movement by 11 weeks of pregnancy. Crown-to-rump measurements can be made for assessment of fetal age until the fetal head can be defined. Biparietal diameter measurements can be made by approximately 12 to 13 weeks, and are most accurate between 20 and 30 weeks, when rapid growth in biparietal diameter occurs. (See Chapter 20 for an in-depth discussion of ultrasound scanning of the fetus.)

Assessment of Pelvic Adequacy

The pelvis is assessed vaginally to determine whether its size is adequate for a vaginal birth. Nurses with special preparation may perform the vaginal assessment and interpret pelvimetry findings. This is sometimes referred to as clinical pelvimetry.

Pelvic Inlet

The important anteroposterior diameters of the inlet for childbearing are the diagonal conjugate, the obstetric conjugate, and the conjugata vera or true conjugate (Figure 13–6). Other diameters are the transverse (13.5 cm) and the oblique (12.75 cm).

The anteroposterior diameters of the pelvic inlet may be assessed by attempting to reach from the lower border of the symphysis pubis to the sacral promontory with the middle finger. The clinician should determine the length of the finger before attempting this. The diagonal conjugate can then be measured by marking the place where the proximal part of the hand makes contact with the pubis (Figure 13–7). Then the distance is measured (at least 11.5 cm or more). The obstetric conjugate can be estimated by subtracting 1.5 to 2.0 cm from the length of the diagonal conjugate. This is the smallest and thus the most important anteroposterior diameter through which the fetus must pass. It should measure 10.0 cm or more. It is measured by x-ray examination from the sacral promontory to the upper inner point on the symphysis that extends farthest back into the pelvis. The true conjugate extends from the upper border of the symphysis pubis to the middle of the sacral promontory. It can be determined by subtracting 1.0 cm from the diagonal conjugate.

Pelvic Cavity (Midpelvis)

Important midpelvic measurements include the plane of least dimension, or midplane (anteroposterior diameter, 11.5–12.0 cm; posterior sagittal diameter, 4.5–5.0 cm; and transverse diameter [interspinous], 10.0 cm). The planes of the midpelvis cannot be accurately measured by clinical examination. An evaluation of adequacy is made based on the prominence of the ischial spines and degree of convergence of the side walls.

Location of the sacrospinous ligament, a firm ridge of tissue, makes location of the ischial spines easier. When this ligament is located, the examiner should run the fingers along it laterally toward the anterior portion of the pelvis. The spines may range from a small firm bump like the knuckle of a finger (termed *not encroaching*) to a very prominent bone.

The sacrosciatic notch should admit two fingers. A wide notch means that the sacrum curves posteriorly, giving the anteroposterior diameter of the midpelvis a greater length. A narrow notch indicates a decreased diameter. The width of the sacrosciatic notch is more accurately evaluated through x-ray examination but can be estimated through vaginal examination.

The length of the sacrospinous ligament is measured by tracing the ligament from its origin on the ischial spines to its insertion on the sacrum. It is usually 4 cm or two to three finger breadths long.

The capacity of the cavity can be assessed by sweeping the fingers down the side walls bilaterally to evaluate the shape of the pelvic side walls—whether convergent, divergent, or straight. The curvature, inclination, and hollowness of the sacrum help indicate the capacity of the posterior pelvis. It is estimated digitally by palpating the sacrococcygeal junction and by inching up toward the promontory. The examiner then estimates the hollowness of the sacrum, which normally is hollow.

The plane of greatest pelvic dimensions represents the largest portion of the pelvic cavity and has no obstetric significance.

Pelvic Outlet

The anteroposterior diameter of the pelvic outlet (9.5–11.5 cm), which extends from the lower border of the symphysis pubis to the tip of the sacrum, can be measured digitally (Figure 13–7*B*). The transverse diameter of the outlet is measured by placing the fist between the ischial tuberosities. It usually measures 8 to 10 cm (Figure 13–8). The posterior sagittal diameter, the third important outlet diameter, normally measures at least 7.5 cm.

The mobility of the coccyx is determined by pressing down on it with the forefinger and middle finger during the initial vaginal examination. An immobile coccyx can decrease the diameter of the outlet.

The subpubic angle is estimated by palpating the bony structure externally. It should be 85° to 90°. The subpubic angle is estimated by placing two fingers side by side at the border of the symphysis (Figure 13–9). It is probably reduced if the examiner cannot separate his or her fingers.

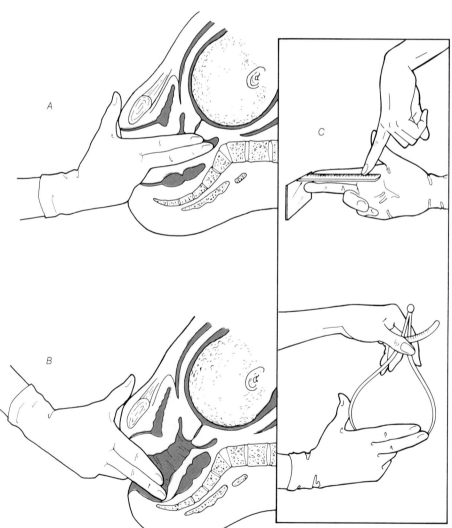

Figure 13–7 Manual measurement of inlet and outlet. A Estimation of diagonal conjugate, which extends from lower border of symphysis pubis to sacral promontory. B Estimation of anteroposterior diameter of the outlet, which extends from lower border of the symphysis pubis to tip of sacrum. C Methods that may be used to check manual estimation of anteroposterior measurements.

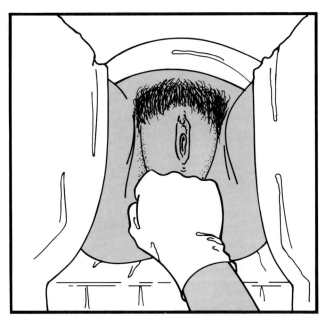

Figure 13–8 Use of closed fist to measure outlet. Examiner should know distance between first and last proximal knuckles.

The length and shape of the pubic rami affect the transverse diameter of the outlet. The pubic ramus is expected to be short and concave inward, as opposed to straight and long.

The height and inclination of the symphysis pubis are measured, and the contour of the pubic arch is estimated. Excessively long or angulated bone structure shortens the diameter of the obstetric conjugate. Height can be determined by placing the index finger of the gloved hand up to the superior border of the symphysis. The examiner should measure the length of the first phalanx of the index finger (normally about 2.5 cm). Inclination can be determined by externally placing one finger on the top of the symphysis while the internal finger palpates the internal margin. An imaginary line is drawn between the fingers and the angle is estimated.

A posterior inclination with the lower border of the pubis slanting inward decreases the anteroposterior diameter. The anteroposterior sagittal diameter is the most significant diameter of the outlet, as it is the shortest diameter through which the infant must pass. Estimating the contour of the pubic arch provides information on the width of the angle at which these bones come together. The pubic arch has obstetric importance; if it is narrow the infant's head may be pushed backward toward the coccyx, making extension of the head difficult.

Figure 13–9 (right) Evaluation of outlet. A Estimation of suprapubic angle. B Estimation of length of pubic ramus. C Estimation of depth and inclination of pubis. D Estimation of contour of suprapubic angle.

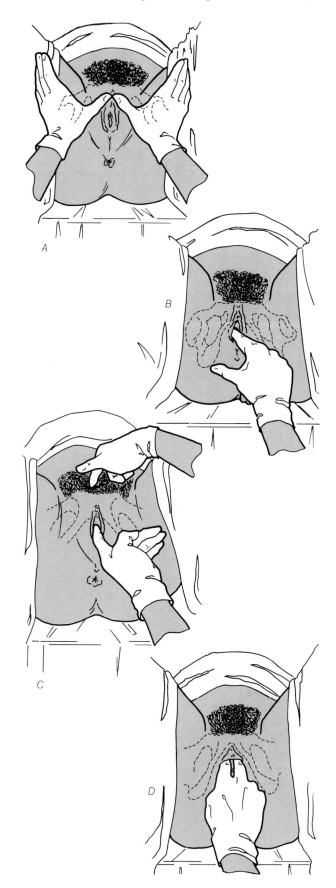

Initial Psychosocial Assessment

CRITICAL THINKING

What approaches might the nurse use to effectively assess the woman's psychosocial status at the initial visit? What behavioral cues in the woman might be helpful?

At the initial visit the woman may be most concerned with the diagnosis of pregnancy. However, during this visit she (and her partner, if he is present) is also evaluating the health team that she has chosen. The establishment of the nurse–client relationship will help the woman evaluate the health team and also provides the nurse with a basis for an atmosphere that is conducive to interviewing, support, and education. A psychosocial assessment is difficult to obtain if the woman does not feel free to talk.

Many women are excited and anxious on the initial visit. Because of this, the initial psychosocial assessment is general and the goal is to set the foundation for a trusting nurse–client relationship.

As part of the initial psychosocial assessment the nurse discusses with the woman any cultural factors that influence the woman's expectations about the childbearing experience. It is especially helpful if the nurse is familiar with common practices of various cultural groups that reside in the community. If the nurse gathers this data in a tactful, caring way it can help make the childbearing woman's experience a positive one.

Religious practices also require consideration. If the woman is a Jehovah's Witness, for example, she may be opposed to receiving blood products should the need arise. Other religious influences can also be discussed. Are there any religious ceremonies or practices that are generally performed during pregnancy or the postpartum period?

The Initial Psychosocial Assessment Guide on page 337 can be used as a basis for evaluating the woman's needs for education and support.

Subsequent Client History

At subsequent prenatal visits the nurse continues to gather data about the course of the pregnancy to date. The nurse asks specifically whether the woman has experienced any discomfort, especially the kinds of discomfort that are often seen at specific times during a pregnancy. Thus, in the first trimester, the nurse would consider discomforts such as nausea, vomiting, frequency, breast tenderness, and so forth. The nurse inquires about physical changes that relate directly to the pregnancy, such as fetal movement. Other pertinent information includes any exposure to contagious illnesses; medical treatment and therapy prescribed for nonpregnancy problems since the last visit; any prescription or over-the-counter medications that were not prescribed as part of the woman's prenatal care.

The danger signs that a woman should report immediately are generally discussed during the initial prenatal visit and reviewed when she comes for her second prenatal visit. Many care givers also provide printed information on the subject that is written in lay terms. Table 13–3 identifies the danger signs of pregnancy and possible causes for each.

Subsequent Physical Assessment

The recommended frequency of prenatal visits is as follows:

● Every 4 weeks for the first 28 weeks of gestation
● Every 2 weeks to week 36
● After week 36, every week until childbirth

The Subsequent Physical Assessment Guide on p. 339 provides a systematic approach to the regular physical examinations that the pregnant woman should undergo for optimal prenatal care.

Subsequent Psychosocial Assessment

Periodic prenatal examinations offer the nurse an opportunity to assess the childbearing woman's psychologic needs and emotional status. If the woman's partner attends the prenatal visits, his needs and concerns can also be identified.

The interchange between the nurse and woman will be facilitated if it takes place in a friendly, trusting environment. The woman should be given sufficient time to ask questions and to air concerns. If the nurse provides the time and demonstrates genuine interest, the woman will feel more at ease bringing up questions that she may believe are silly or concerns that she has been afraid to verbalize. The nurse who has an accurate understanding of all the changes of pregnancy is most able to answer questions and provide information. See the foldout color chart, "Maternal–Fetal Development," for vivid illustrations of some of this information.

During the prenatal period, it is essential to begin assessing the ability of the woman (and her partner, if possible) to successfully assume their responsibilities as parents. Table 13–4 identifies areas for assessment and provides some sample questions the nurse might use to obtain necessary information. If the woman's responses are primarily negative, interventions can be planned for the prenatal and postpartal periods.

Initial Psychosocial Assessment Guide

Assess/Normal Findings	Alterations and Possible Causes*	Nursing Responses to Data†
Psychologic Status		
Excitement and/or apprehension; ambivalence	Marked anxiety (fear of pregnancy diagnosis, fear of medical facility)	Establish lines of communication. Active listening is useful. Establish trusting relationship. Encourage woman to take active part in her care.
	Apathy Display of anger with pregnancy diagnosis	Establish communication and begin counseling. Use active listening techniques.
Educational Needs		
May have questions about pregnancy or may need time to adjust to reality of pregnancy		Establish educational, supporting environment that can be expanded throughout pregnancy.
Support Systems		
Can identify at least two or three individuals with whom woman is emotionally intimate (partner, parent, sibling, friend, etc.)	Isolated (no telephone, unlisted number); cannot name a neighbor or friend whom she can call upon in an emergency; does not perceive parents as part of her support system	Institute support system through community groups. Help woman to develop trusting relationship with health care professionals.
Cultural or Religious Considerations		
Any cultural or religious beliefs or practices that might influence pregnancy. Is able to express her personal preferences and beliefs about the childbearing experience. Identifies any people (mother, curandera, tribal healer, etc) that influence her.	Language barriers that prevent effective communication Cultural beliefs or practices that might endanger her health or that of fetus	Work with knowledgeable translator to provide information and answer questions. Have information printed in the language of different cultural groups that live in the area. Work with significant people to meet woman's health needs.
Family Functioning		
Emotionally supportive Communications adequate Mutually satisfying Cohesiveness in times of trouble	Long-term problems or specific problems related to this pregnancy, potential stressors within the family, pessimistic attitudes, unilateral decision making, unrealistic expectations of this pregnancy and/or child	Help identify the problems and stressors, encourage communication, discuss role changes and adaptations.
Economic Status		
Source of income is stable and sufficient to meet basic needs of daily living and medical needs	Limited prenatal care Poor physical health Limited use of health care system Unstable economic status	Discuss available resources for health maintenance and the birth. Institute appropriate referral for meeting expanding family's needs—food stamps, etc.
Stability of Living Conditions		
Adequate, stable housing for expanding family's needs	Crowded living conditions Questionable supportive environment for newborn	Refer to appropriate community agency. Work with family on self-help ways to improve situation.

*Possible causes of alterations are placed in parentheses.
†This column provides guidelines for further assessment and initial nursing intervention.

Table 13–3 Danger Signs in Pregnancy

The woman should report the following danger signs in pregnancy immediately:

Danger sign	Possible cause
1. Sudden gush of fluid from vagina	Premature rupture of membranes
2. Vaginal bleeding	Abruptio placentae, placenta previa Lesions of cervix or vagina, "Bloody show"
3. Abdominal pain	Preterm labor, abruptio placentae
4. Temperature above 38.3C (101F) and chills	Infection
5. Dizziness, blurring of vision, double vision, spots before eyes	Hypertension, preeclampsia
6. Persistent vomiting	Hyperemesis gravidarum
7. Severe headache	Hypertension, preeclampsia
8. Edema of hands, face, legs, and feet	Preeclampsia
9. Muscular irritability, convulsions	Preeclampsia, eclampsia
10. Epigastric pain	Preeclampsia—ischemia in major abdominal vessels
11. Oliguria	Renal impairment, decreased fluid intake
12. Dysuria	Urinary tract infection
13. Absence of fetal movement	Maternal medication, obesity, fetal death

During the subsequent psychologic assessments, a woman may exhibit psychologic problems such as the following:

- Increasing anxiety
- Inability to establish communication
- Inappropriate responses or actions
- Denial of pregnancy
- Inability to cope with stress
- Failure to acknowledge quickening
- Failure to plan and prepare for the baby (for example, living arrangements, clothing, feeding methods)
- Indications of substance abuse

If the woman appears to have these or other critical psychologic problems, the nurse should refer her to appropriate professionals.

The Subsequent Psychosocial Assessment Guide on p. 342 provides a model for the evaluation of both the pregnant woman and the expectant father.

Research Note

Clinical Application of Research

Ellen Lazarus and Elliot Philipson (1990) wanted to determine if race or ethnicity, as separate from social class, impacted prenatal care and pregnancy outcomes. Ethnicity meant "a particular cultural group or population distinguished by common customs, language, history, and self-identity" (Lazarus & Philipson 1990, p 6). In their descriptive study of cultural differences, use of perinatal clinics, and doctor-patient interactions of 27 Puerto Rican and 26 low-income white women, they found that ethnic considerations influenced foods eaten, circumcision, and breast-feeding patterns. Both groups were similar in social characteristics such as marriage, age, and education. The groups were also similar in percentage of unplanned pregnancies (over 75%) and birth outcomes, ie, birth weight, Apgar scores.

Three problems, common to both groups, emerged from the study of clinic use. There were long clinic waits of two to four hours, problems with continuity of care (staff rarely followed the same woman), and difficulties with communication between residents and patients.

The researchers found that advice from physicians and other health care providers was a much more important factor influencing both groups than advice from family and friends. Folk beliefs took priority only when information was not forthcoming from the health care providers. However, due either to clinic problems or intimidation by medical jargon, many times the patients were reluctant to ask questions of rushed doctors and thus were perceived as noncompliant or uninterested in their pregnancy. This research study resulted in a change in clinic function.

Critical Thinking Applied to Research

Strengths: Prolonged engagement of participants, over 18 months, with 500 interviews, and observation of at least 3 interactions between each woman and a health care provider.

Concerns: Although the conceptual framework developed a potential relationship between pregnancy risk factors and ethnicity, risk factors are not explicitly addressed in either the purpose or the results of the study.

Lazarus E, Philipson E: A longitudinal study comparing the prenatal care of Puerto Rican and white women. *Birth* 1990; 17 (1): 6.

Subsequent Physical Assessment Guide

Assess/Normal Findings	Alterations and Possible Causes*	Nursing Responses to Data†
Vital Signs		
Temperature: 36.2–37.6C (98–99.6F)	Elevated temperature (infection)	Evaluate for signs of infection. Refer to physician.
Pulse: 60–90/min Rate may increase 10 beats/min during pregnancy	Increased pulse rate (anxiety, cardiac disorders)	Note irregularities. Evaluate anxiety and stress.
Respiration: 16–24/min	Marked tachypnea or abnormal patterns (respiratory disease)	Refer to physician.
Blood pressure: 90–140/60–90 (falls in second trimester)	> 140/90 or increase of 30 mm systolic and 15 mm diastolic (PIH)	Assess for edema, proteinuria, hyperreflexia. Refer to physician. Schedule appointments more frequently.
Weight Gain		
First trimester: 2–4 lb *Second trimester:* 12 lb *Third trimester:* 12 lb	Inadequate weight gain (poor nutrition, nausea, IUGR) Excessive weight gain (excessive caloric intake, edema, PIH)	Discuss appropriate weight gain. Provide nutritional counseling. Assess for presence of edema or anemia.
Edema		
Small amount of dependent edema, especially in last weeks of pregnancy	Edema in hands, face, legs, feet (PIH)	Identify any correlation between edema and activities, blood pressure, or proteinuria. Refer to physician if indicated.
Uterine Size		
See Initial Physical Assessment Guide for normal changes during pregnancy	Unusually rapid growth (multiple gestation, hydatidiform mole, hydramnios, miscalculation of EDB)	Evaluate fetal status. Determine height of fundus (p 332). Use diagnostic ultrasound.
Fetal Heartbeat		
120–160/min Funic souffle	Absence of fetal heartbeat after 20 weeks' gestation (maternal obesity, fetal demise)	Evaluate fetal status.
Laboratory Evaluation		
Hemoglobin: 12–16 g/dL Pseudoanemia of pregnancy	< 12 g/dL (anemia)	Provide nutritional counseling. Hemoglobin is repeated at 7 months' gestation. Women of Mediterranean heritage need a close check on hemoglobin because of possibility of thalassemia.
Antibody screen.: Negative	Positive	Refer for further testing to identify specific antibodies. Titers may be indicated. If negative repeat at 7 months.

*Possible causes of alterations are in parentheses.
†This column provides guidelines for further assessment and initial nursing interventions.

(continued)

Subsequent Physical Assessment Guide (continued)

Assess/Normal Findings	Alterations and Possible Causes*	Nursing Responses to Data†
50 g, one-hour glucose screen (done between 24 and 28 weeks' gestation)	Plasma glucose level > 140 mg/dL (gestational diabetes mellitus [GDM])	Discuss implications of GDM. Refer for a diagnostic glucose tolerance test.
Urinalysis: See Initial Prenatal Physical Assessment Guide (p 330) for normal findings	See Initial Prenatal Physical Assessment Guide (p 330) for deviations	Repeat urinalysis at 7 months' gestation. Dipstick test at each visit.
Protein: Negative	Proteinuria, albuminuria (contamination by vaginal discharge, urinary tract infection, PIH)	Obtain dipstick urine sample. Refer to physician if deviations are present.
Glucose: Negative	Persistent glycosuria (diabetes mellitus)	Refer to physician.
Note: Glycosuria may be present due to physiologic alterations in glomerular filtration rate and renal threshold		

*Possible causes of alterations are in parentheses.
†This column provides guidelines for further assessment and initial nursing interventions.

Table 13–4 Prenatal Assessment of Parenting Guide*

Areas assessed	Sample questions

I. *Perception of Complexities of Mothering*
 	
A. Baby is desired for itself.
Positive:
  1. Feels positive about pregnancy.
Negative:
  1. Wants baby to meet own needs such as someone to love her, someone to get her out of unhappy home.
	1. Did you plan on getting pregnant?
	2. How do you feel about being pregnant?
	3. Why do you want this baby?

B. Expresses concern about impact of mothering role on other roles (wife, career, school).
Positive:
  1. Realistic expectations of how baby will affect job, career, school, and personal goals.
  2. Interested in learning about child care.
Negative:
  1. Feels pregnancy and baby will make no emotional, physical, or social demands on self.
  2. No insight that mothering role will affect other roles or lifestyle.
	1. What do you think it will be like to take care of a baby?
	2. How do you think your life will be different after you have your baby?
	3. How do you feel this baby will affect your job, career, school, and personal goals?
	4. How will the baby affect your relationship with boyfriend or husband?
	5. Have you done any reading, babysitting, or made any things for a baby?

C. Gives up routine habits because "not good for baby"; eg, quits smoking, adjusts time schedule, etc.† Positive: 1. Gives up routines not good for baby: quits smoking, adjusts eating habits, etc.	

II. *Attachment*
A. Strong feelings regarding sex of baby.
  Why?
Positive:
  1. Verbalizes positive thoughts about the baby.
Negative:
  1. Baby will be like negative aspects of self and partner.
	1. Why do you prefer a certain sex? (Is reason inappropriate for a baby?)
	2. Note comments client makes about baby not being normal and why client feels this way.

B. Interested in data regarding fetus, eg, growth and development, heart tones, etc. Positive: 1. As above.	

(continued)

Table 13–4 Prenatal Assessment of Parenting Guide* (continued)

Areas assessed	Sample questions

Negative:
1. Shows no interest in fetal growth and development, quickening, and fetal heart tones.
2. Negative feelings about fetus expressed by rejection of counseling regarding nutrition, rest, hygiene.

C. Fantasies about baby.
Positive:
1. Follows cultural norms regarding preparation.
2. Time of attachment behaviors appropriate to her history of pregnancy loss.
Negative:
1. Bonding is conditional depending on sex, age of baby, and/or labor and delivery experience.
2. Patient only considers own needs when making plans for baby.
3. Exhibits no attachment behaviors after critical period of previous pregnancy.
4. Failure to follow cultural norms regarding preparation.

Sample questions (for C. Fantasies about baby):
1. What did you think or feel when you first felt the baby move?
2. Have you started preparing for the baby?
3. What do you think your baby will look like—what age do you see your baby at?
4. How would you like your new baby to look?

III. Acceptance of Child by Significant Others

A. Acknowledges acceptance by significant other of the new responsibility inherent in child.
Positive:
1. Acknowledges unconditional acceptance of pregnancy and baby by significant others.
2. Partner accepts new responsibility inherent with child.
3. Timely sharing of experience of pregnancy with significant others.
Negative:
1. Significant others not supportively involved with pregnancy.
2. Conditional acceptance of pregnancy depending on sex, race, age of baby.
3. Decision making does not take in needs of fetus; eg, spends food money on new car.
4. Takes no/little responsibility for needs of pregnancy, woman/fetus.

Sample questions (for A):
1. How does your partner feel about pregnancy?
2. How do your parents feel?
3. What do your friends think?
4. Does your partner have a preference regarding the baby's sex? Why?
5. How does your partner feel about being a father?
6. What do you think he'll be like as a father?
7. What do you think he'll do to help you with child care?
8. Have you and your partner talked about how the baby might change your lives?
9. Who have you told about your pregnancy?

B. Concrete demonstration of acceptance of pregnancy/baby by significant others; eg, baby shower, significant other involved in prenatal education.†
Positive:
1. Baby shower.
2. Significant other attends prenatal class with client.

Sample questions (for B):
1. Note if partner attends clinic with client (degree of interest); eg, listens to heart tones, etc. Significant other plans to be with client in labor and delivery.
2. Is your partner contributing financially?

IV. Ensures Physical Well-being

A. Concerns about having normal pregnancy, labor and delivery, and baby.
Positive:
1. Client preparing for labor and delivery, attends prenatal classes, interested in labor and delivery.
2. Client aware of danger signs of pregnancy.
3. Seeks and uses appropriate health care: eg, time of initial visit, keeps appointments, follows through on recommendations.
Negative:
1. Denial of signs and symptoms that might suggest complications of pregnancy.
2. Verbalizes extreme fear of labor and delivery—refuses to talk about labor and delivery.
3. Fails appointments, failure to follow instructions, refuses to attend prenatal classes.

Sample questions (for A):
1. What have you heard about labor and delivery?
2. Note data about client's reaction to prenatal class.

B. Family/client decisions reflect concern for health of mother and baby; eg, use of finances, time.†
Positive:
1. As above.

† *When "Negative" is not listed in a section, the reader may assume that negative is the absence of positive responses.*

* *Modified and used with permission of the Minneapolis Health Dept., Minneapolis, MN.*

Subsequent Psychosocial Assessment Guide

Assess/Normal Findings	Alterations and Possible Causes*	Nursing Responses to Data†
Expectant Mother		
Psychologic status:		
First trimester: incorporates idea of pregnancy; may feel ambivalent, especially if she must give up desired role; usually looks for signs of verification of pregnancy, such as increase in abdominal size, fetal movement, etc.	Increasing stress and anxiety Inability to establish communication; inability to accept pregnancy; inappropriate response or actions; denial of pregnancy; inability to cope	Encourage woman to take an active part in her care. Establish lines of communication. Establish a trusting relationship. Counsel as necessary. Refer to appropriate professional as needed.
Second trimester: baby becomes more real to woman as abdominal size increases and she feels movement; she begins to turn inward, becoming more introspective		
Third trimester: begins to think of baby as separate being; may feel restless and may feel that time of labor will never come; remains self-centered and concentrates on preparing place for baby		
Educational needs:	Inadequate information	Teach and/or institute appropriate relief measures (see Chapter 14).
Self-care measures and knowledge about following:		
Breast care		
Hygiene		
Rest		
Exercise		
Nutrition		
Relief measures for common discomforts of pregnancy		
Danger signs of pregnancy (Table 13–3)		
Sexual activity: Woman knows how pregnancy affects sexual activity	Lack of information about effects of pregnancy and/or alternative positions during sexual intercourse	Provide counseling
Preparation for parenting: Appropriate preparation; See Table 13–4	Lack of preparation (denial, failure to adjust to baby, unwanted child) See Table 13–4	Counsel. If lack of preparation is due to inadequacy of information, provide information (see Chapter 14).
Preparation for childbirth: *Client aware of following:*		If couple chooses particular technique, refer to classes (see Chapter 17 for description of childbirth preparation techniques).
1. Prepared childbirth techniques		Encourage prenatal class attendance.
2. Normal processes and changes during childbirth		Educate woman during visits based on current physical status. Provide reading list for more specific information.

*Possible causes of alterations are placed in parentheses.
†This column provides guidelines for further assessment and initial nursing interventions.

(continued)

Subsequent Psychosocial Assessment Guide (continued)

Assess/Normal Findings	Alterations and Possible Causes*	Nursing Responses to Data†
3. Problems that may occur as a result of drug and alcohol use and of smoking	Continued abuse of drugs and alcohol; denial of possible effect on self and baby	Review danger signs that were presented on initial visit.
Woman has met other physician and/or nurse-midwife who may be attending her birth in the absence of primary care giver	Introduction of new individual at birth may increase stress and anxiety for woman and partner	Introduce woman to all members of group practice.
Impending labor: *Client knows signs of impending labor:*	Lack of information	Provide appropriate teaching, stressing importance of seeking appropriate medical assistance.
1. Uterine contractions that increase in frequency, duration, intensity		
2. Bloody show		
3. Expulsion of mucous plug		
4. Rupture of membranes		
Expectant Father		
Psychologic status:	Increasing stress and anxiety	Encourage expectant father to come to prenatal visits.
First trimester: may express excitement over confirmation of pregnancy and of his virility; concerns move toward providing for financial needs; energetic; may identify with some discomforts of pregnancy and may even exhibit symptoms	Inability to establish communication Inability to accept pregnancy diagnosis Withdrawal of support Abandonment of the mother	Establish lines of communication. Establish trusting relationship.
Second trimester: may feel more confident and be less concerned with financial matters; may have concerns about wife's changing size and shape, her increasing introspection		Counsel. Let expectant father know that it is normal for him to experience these feelings.
Third trimester: may have feelings of rivalry with fetus, especially during sexual activity; may make changes in his physical appearance and exhibit more interest in himself; may become more energetic; fantasizes about child but usually imagines older child; fears of mutilation and death of woman and child arise		Include expectant father in pregnancy activities as he desires. Provide education, information, and support. Increasing number of expectant fathers are demonstrating desire to be involved in many or all aspects of prenatal care, education, and preparation.

*Possible causes of alterations are placed in parentheses.
†This column provides guidelines for further assessment and initial nursing interventions.

KEY CONCEPTS

A complete history forms the basis of prenatal care and is reevaluated and updated as necessary throughout the pregnancy.

The initial prenatal physical assessment is a careful and thorough physical examination designed to identify physical variations and potential risk factors.

Laboratory tests completed at the initial visit, such as a complete blood count, ABO and Rh typing, urinalysis, Pap smear, gonorrhea culture, rubella titer, and various blood screens, provide information about the woman's health during early pregnancy and also help detect potential problems.

The estimated date of birth (EDB) can be calculated using Nägele's rule. Using this approach, one begins with the first day of the last menstrual period (LMP), subtracts three months, and adds seven days. A "wheel" may also be used to calculate the EDB.

Accuracy of the EDB may be evaluated by physical examination to assess uterine size, measurement of fundal height, and ultrasound. Perception of quickening and auscultation of fetal heartbeat are also useful tools in confirming the gestation of a pregnancy.

The diagonal conjugate is the distance from the lower posterior border of the symphysis pubis to the sacral promontory. The obstetric conjugate is estimated by subtracting 1.5 from the length of the diagonal conjugate.

As part of the assessment of the pelvic cavity (midpelvis) the prominence of the ischial spines is assessed, the sacrosciatic notch and the length of the sacrospinous ligament are measured, and the shape of the pelvic side walls is evaluated. Finally, the hollowness of the sacrum is determined.

The anteroposterior diameter of the pelvic outlet is determined, the mobility of the coccyx is assessed, the suprapubic angle is estimated, and the contour of the pubic arch is evaluated to assess the adequacy of the pelvic outlet.

The nurse begins evaluating the woman psychosocially during the initial prenatal assessment. This assessment continues and is modified throughout the pregnancy.

Cultural and ethnic beliefs may strongly influence the woman's attitudes and apparent compliance with care during pregnancy.

References

Cunningham FG et al: *Williams Obstetrics,* 18th ed. Norwalk, CT: Appleton & Lange, 1989.

Engstrom JL: Measurement of fundal height. *JOGNN* May/June 1988; 17:172.

Additional Readings

Diamond FB: Patients' prenatal medical record précis. *JOGNN* November/December 1990; 19:491.

Gardner MO et al: Effects of prenatal care on twin gestations. *J Reprod Med* May 1990; 35:519.

Harmon JS et al: Antenatal resting, mobile outpatient monitoring service. *JOGNN* January/February 1989; 18:21.

Heins HC JR et al: A randomized trial of nurse-midwifery prenatal care to reduce low birth weight. *Obstet Gynecol* 1990; 75 (3 Pt 1):341.

McGoldrick KE: Prenatal care: Investing in the future. *J Am Med Wom Assoc* March/April 1990; 45:35.

Mittendorf R et al: The length of uncomplicated human gestation. *Obstet Gynecol* June 1990; 75:929.

Poland ML et al: Quality of prenatal care: Selected social, behavioral, and biomedical factors, and birth weight. *Obstet Gynecol* April 1990; 75:607.

Schwethelm B et al: Risk status and pregnancy outcome among Medicaid recipients. *Am J Prev Med* May/June 1989; 5:157.

CHAPTER 14

The Expectant Family:
Needs and Care

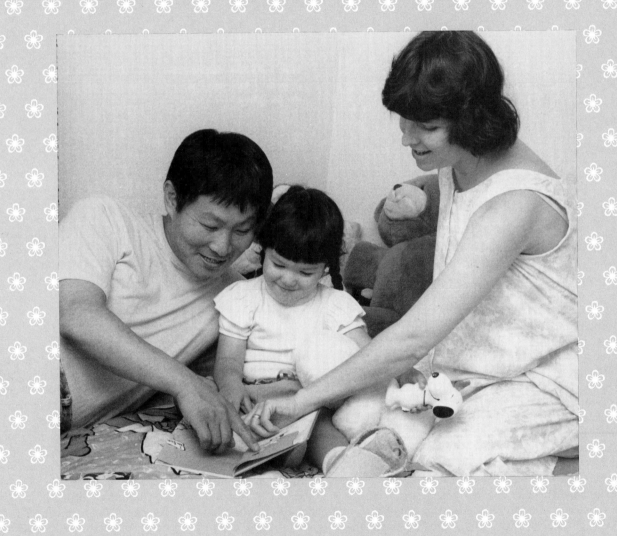

OBJECTIVES

Summarize the areas of assessment important in establishing a comprehensive data base for the expectant woman and her family.

Describe communication skills that nurses can use to enhance effectiveness in nursing assessments and implementation of care.

Explain the causes of the common discomforts of pregnancy and appropriate measures to alleviate these discomforts.

Develop a plan of care incorporating anticipatory guidance of the pregnant woman and her family to maintain and promote well-being for each trimester of pregnancy.

Discuss the significance of cultural considerations in managing nursing care during pregnancy and common practices of specific cultures.

Discuss the significance of using the nursing process to promote health in the woman and her family during pregnancy.

Compare similarities and differences in the needs of expectant women in various age groups.

❀ ❀

I don't know how I timed it, but my nursing program OB rotation finishes up right about on my due date. Watching all the births during my rotation has been really exciting. The labor and delivery nurses laugh and say my hormones should be hopping now, but I think this baby is subliminally telling me that we won't "hatch" until I take my last final exam!

From the moment a woman finds out that she is pregnant, she faces a future marked by dramatic changes. Her appearance will be altered. Her relationships will change. She will experience a variety of unique physical changes throughout the pregnancy. Even her psychologic state will be affected.

Her family must also adjust to the pregnancy. Roles and responsibilities of family members will be altered as the woman's ability to perform certain activities changes. They too must adapt psychologically to the situation.

The expectant woman and her family will probably have many questions about the pregnancy and its impact on her and the other members of the family. In addition, the daily activities and health care practices of the woman become of concern when she and her family realize that the well-being of the unborn child can be affected by what she does.

The nurse often assumes the dual roles of teacher and counselor for expectant families who desire information about pregnancy and the adjustments they must make. In particular, the nurse teaches the pregnant woman about the physical discomforts that may occur and the self-care measures that the woman can use to obtain relief.

This chapter provides the information necessary for nurses to teach and counsel pregnant women and their families. It describes the common discomforts of pregnancy, their causes, and self-care measures. The chapter also contains information and advice on general health practices and other activities that may affect, or be affected by, pregnancy.

❀   *USING THE NURSING PROCESS*   ❀

During the Antepartal Period

Pregnancy is a healthy process for most women. Thus, antepartal nursing care primarily involves anticipatory guidance and education. The nursing process provides a framework for the nurse to identify and meet the needs of the expectant woman and her family.

Nursing Assessment

Because most pregnant women are healthy, the purpose of assessment during pregnancy is to ensure that everything is progressing normally and to identify potential problems that may affect the well-being of the woman or her fetus.

The nurse must assess not only the woman's physical condition but also the psychosocial factors that affect her pregnancy experience. The population of pregnant women is diverse in age, life experiences, cultural beliefs, educational background, health practices, family structure, attitudes, and interests. Each of these factors needs to be assessed so that the nurse can develop a plan of care that considers the woman's specific needs and concerns.

The accuracy of the nurse's assessment often depends on the nurse's ability to develop rapport with the woman and use communication skills effectively. The nurse's comfort level in dealing with the concerns expressed by the pregnant woman and her family is also important. A nonjudgmental approach and knowledge about health promotion behaviors during pregnancy are essential. The nurse must remember that promotion of maternal well-being and optimum fetal outcome is the purpose of care. With this thought in mind, personal concerns should not be as difficult to assess.

Nursing Diagnosis

The nurse may see a specific woman only once every three to four weeks at the beginning of pregnancy. As a result, a written plan of care that incorporates the data base, nursing diagnoses, and goals is essential for continuity of care.

Several nursing diagnoses may apply to a woman with a healthy pregnancy. Examples of applicable nursing diagnoses include:

- Knowledge deficit related to the use of medication during pregnancy
- Constipation related to the physiologic effects of pregnancy
- Altered sexuality patterns related to changed sexual activity during pregnancy

Nursing Plan and Implementation

Once nursing diagnoses have been identified, the next step is to establish priorities of nursing care. Sometimes priorities of care are based on the most immediate needs or concerns perceived by the woman. For example, during the first trimester, when a woman is experiencing nausea or is concerned about sexual intimacy with her partner, she is not likely to be ready to hear about labor and birth.

The woman's priorities may not always be the same as the nurse's. If the safety of the woman or her fetus is at issue, however, that takes priority over other concerns of the woman or her family. It is the responsibility of medical and nursing care givers to help the woman and her family understand the significance of a problem and to plan appropriate interventions to deal with it. Suppose, for example, a woman with early signs of pregnancy-induced hypertension (PIH) is advised to enter the hospital immediately to begin bedrest. If she does not have hospital insurance, however, and there is no one to care for her young children, cooperation with the treatment advice may be impossible. As a result, the signs of PIH may become more severe. It is important for the nurse to assess the woman holistically and plan care accordingly.

The intervention methods most used by nurses in caring for the expectant woman and her family are communication techniques and teaching-learning strategies. These intervention methods are most obvious when used in groups, such as early pregnancy classes and childbirth education classes, but the nurse in the prenatal setting often applies these techniques on an individual basis.

The value of providing a primary care nurse to coordinate care for each childbearing family is beginning to be recognized. The nurse in a clinic or HMO may be the only source of continuity for the woman, who may see a different physician or nurse-midwife at each visit. The nurse can be extremely effective in working with the expectant family by providing them with necessary and complete information about pregnancy, self-care measures, and community resources or referral agencies that may be of help to them. Such education allows the family to assume equal responsibility with health care providers in working toward their common goal of a positive childbearing experience.

Evaluation

Evaluation is an ongoing process. At each prenatal visit the nurse evaluates the effectiveness of previous teaching by using information obtained from the woman and from various assessment tools. For instance, the woman's pattern of weight gain, her vital signs, her degree of comfort, and her success in implementing previously discussed strategies provide information about the success of previous nursing interventions. When the woman has been unable to follow an established treatment plan, it may be due to factors in the woman's environment that were not previously known. Thus, the cycle of the nursing process begins again with assessment as the nurse collects further data.

❋ ❋ ❋ ❋ ❋ ❋ ❋ ❋ ❋ ❋ ❋ ❋ ❋

Nursing Assessment of the Expectant Family

As described in Chapter 13, during the initial contact with the expectant mother or couple the nurse obtains a health history and client profile. The data base is completed with a description of body functioning, a complete physical examination, laboratory tests, and a psychologic evaluation (Chapter 13).

During subsequent visits, the nurse may ask the woman what *mother* means to her, what she thinks an average day with the baby will be like, and what she expects from the father. The nurse can ask the father similar questions about his expectations of himself and his partner as parents. The couple's answers will provide information about their progress in accomplishing the developmental tasks of pregnancy and will help the nurse determine whether their expectations are realistic.

From the health assessment, the nurse develops nursing diagnoses and an initial plan for interventions during the couple's preparation for childbearing and childrearing.

Nursing Diagnosis

The nurse can anticipate that for many women with a low-risk pregnancy, certain nursing diagnoses will be used more frequently than others. This will, of course, vary from woman to woman and according to the time in the pregnancy. Many of the more commonly used nursing diagnoses are identified in Key Nursing Diagnoses to Consider—Pregnancy. After formulating an appropriate diagnosis, the nurse then establishes goals to guide the nursing plan and interventions.

Nursing Plan and Implementation During Pregnancy

Relieving the expectant woman's discomforts and maintaining her physical health are important parts of the nursing plan. The plan also anticipates the need for information and guidance (Table 14–1). Interventions are timed to

Table 14–1	Topics for Client Teaching During Pregnancy

All three trimesters

Discomforts of pregnancy (see Table 14–4)

Nutrition and weight gain

Sexual activity

Sibling preparation

First trimester

Attitude toward pregnancy

Exercise and rest

Smoking; use of alcohol and other drugs

Traveling

Fetal growth and development

Danger signals associated with spontaneous abortion

Employment

Early pregnancy classes

Second trimester

Concerns related to changes in body

Fetal growth and development

Fetal movement

Clothing

Care of skin and breasts

Beginning preparation for care of the infant (equipment and room)

Decisions about infant feeding

Third trimester

Exercise and rest

Traveling

Danger signals

Preparation for labor and birth

Completion of preparation in home for new baby

Decisions about the infant (circumcision, method of feeding, etc.)

Decision making for the early postpartum period

Education about psychologic and physical expectations in the early postpartum period

Research Note

Clinical Application of Research

Because most studies of family functioning focus on the woman's point of view, Ramona Mercer and her associates (1990) planned a research inquiry which examined the effect of stress on family functioning from the standpoint of both the pregnant woman and her partner. The four groups studied included high-risk hospitalized women (HRW), partners of high-risk women (HRM), low-risk women (LRW), and partners of low-risk women (LRM).

The groups reported on perception of family functioning, and a causal model was examined to determine the direct and indirect effects on family functioning. While both the HRW and HRM reported less optimal family functioning than the low-risk couples, and the high-risk couples reported similar conditions of family functioning, the LRM related significantly less discrepant functioning than did the LRW.

Testing of causal models showed that for the HRW, a sense of mastery accounted for the most variance (17%) in the model. Trait anxiety and relationship with father as a child also had direct effects on family functioning, for a total explained variance of 33% in the model. The model for HRM explained 48% of the variance of family functioning, with direct effects from perceived social support (32%), positive relationship with mother as a teenager (12%), and negative life events (4%). The model for the LRW explained 23% of the variance and included depression (13%) and perceived support (10%) as direct effects. Several variables of this complex model had indirect effects upon the two direct variables. The model for the LRM included direct effects from perceived social support (16%), negative life events (8%), health perception (5%), and extent of current contact with father (3%).

Critical Thinking Applied to Research

Strengths: Extensive reporting, citing both current and prior studies, about the psychometric properties of research tools used. (Psychometric properties establish reliability and validity.) Description of data analysis procedure and identification of potential limitations of the study.

Mercer R, Ferketich S, DeJoseph J, et al: Effect of stress on family functioning during pregnancy. *Nurs Res* 1990; 37(5): 268.

coincide with the woman's (couple's) readiness and needs. In addition, because the woman's well-being is directly related to the well-being of those to whom she is closest, the nurse helps meet the needs of the woman's family to better maintain the harmony and integrity of the family unit. The nurse does this by providing support and prenatal education. If the nurse is effective, family members may gain greater problem-solving ability, self-esteem, self-confidence, and ability to participate in health care. Parents who feel good about themselves also have a solid foundation on which to build meaningful relationships with their children.

Promotion of Family Wellness

Father

Although the father of the baby is present in most cases, his presence cannot be assumed. If he is not a part of the family structure, it is important to assess the woman's support system to determine what significant persons in her life will play a major role during this childbearing experience.

When the father is part of the family or support system, providing anticipatory guidance to him is a necessary part of any plan of care. He may need information about the anatomic, physiologic, and emotional changes that occur during pregnancy and postpartum, the couple's sexuality and sexual response, and the reactions that he may experience. He may wish to express his feelings about breast- versus bottle-feeding, the sex of the child, and other topics. If it is culturally acceptable to the couple and personally acceptable to him, the nurse refers the couple to expectant parents' classes for further information and support from other couples.

The nurse assesses the father's intended degree of participation during labor and birth and his knowledge of what to expect. If the couple prefers that his participation be minimal or restricted, the nurse supports their decision. With this type of consideration and collaboration, the father is less apt to develop feelings of alienation, helplessness, and guilt during the intrapartal period. The relationship between the couple may be strengthened and his self-esteem raised. He is then better able to provide physical and emotional support to his partner during labor and birth.

Siblings

The nurse incorporates in the plan for prenatal care a discussion about the negative feelings that older children may have. Parents may be distressed to see an older child become aggressive toward the newborn. Parents who are unprepared for the older child's feeling of anger, jealousy, and rejection may respond inappropriately in their confusion and surprise. The nurse emphasizes that open communication between parents and children (or acting out feelings with a doll if the child is too young to verbalize) helps children master their feelings and may prevent them from hurting the baby when they are unsupervised. Children may feel less neglected and more secure if they know that their parents are willing to help with their anger and aggressiveness.

Parents may be encouraged to bring their children to antepartal visits. Seeing what is involved and listening to the fetal heartbeat may make the pregnancy more real to siblings. Many agencies also provide sibling classes geared to different ages and levels of understanding. "Hands on," experience-based classes seem to be especially effective for young siblings (Spadt et al 1990).

Prenatal Education

The nurse provides informal and formal education to the childbearing family throughout the prenatal period. This education is designed to help the family carry out self-care when appropriate and to report changes that may indicate a possible health problem. The nurse also provides anticipatory guidance to help the family plan for changes that will occur following childbirth. Issues that could be possible sources of postpartal stress should be discussed by the expectant couple. Some issues to be resolved beforehand may include the sharing of infant and household chores, help in the first few days, options for babysitting to allow the mother and couple some free time, the mother's return to work after the baby's birth, and sibling rivalry. Couples resolve these issues in different ways; however, postpartal adjustment is easier for a couple who agree on the issues beforehand than for a couple who do not confront and resolve these issues.

Cultural Considerations in Pregnancy

As discussed in Chapter 12, specific actions during pregnancy are often determined by cultural beliefs. Some beliefs that have been passed down from generation to generation may be called "old wives' tales." These beliefs certainly had some meaning at one time, but the meanings have often been lost with the passing of time. Other beliefs have definite meanings that are retained. Tables 14–2 and 14–3 present activities prescribed and proscribed by certain cultures. The tables are not meant to be all-inclusive; they offer a few examples of cultural activities encouraged or proscribed during the prenatal period.

In working with clients of another culture, the health care professional should be as open as possible to other beliefs. If certain activities are not harmful, there is no need to impose one's beliefs and practices upon a person of another culture. If the activities are harmful, the nurse can consult or work with someone within the culture or someone aware of cultural beliefs and values to help modify a client's behavior. (See Nursing Care Plan: Non-English-Speaking Woman at First Prenatal Visit.)

Relief of the Common Discomforts of Pregnancy

Common discomforts of pregnancy are often referred to as minor discomforts by health care professionals. These discomforts, however, are not minor to the pregnant woman.

Most of the discomforts of pregnancy are a result of physiologic and anatomic changes and are fairly specific to

Table 14–2 Activities or Rituals During Pregnancy

Culture	Activity	Cultural meaning or belief	Nursing intervention
Mexican American	Certain clothing worn (muneco-cord worn beneath the breasts and knotted over the umbilicus; Brown, 1976)	Ensures a safe birth	If practice does not cause any danger, do not interfere with it.
	Use of spearmint or sassafras tea or benedictine (Brown 1976)	Eases morning sickness	Assess use of herbs and determine safety of their use.
	Use of cathartics during the last month of pregnancy (Brown 1976)	Ensures a good birth of a healthy boy	Assess use of cathartics. Provide teaching about dangers of practice and explore culturally acceptable means of resolving constipation (high-fiber foods).
Black American	Use of self-medication for many discomforts of pregnancy (Epsom salts, castor oil for constipation; herbs for nausea and vomiting; vinegar and baking soda for heartburn) (Carrington 1978)	Improves health and builds resistance	Assess use of self-medication; discourage those practices that may present problems.
Native American (selected examples)	*Navajo* Meeting with medicine man 2 months prior to birth (Farris 1976)	Prayers ensure safe birth and healthy baby	Encourage the use of support systems.
	Exercise during pregnancy; concentrating on good thoughts, and being joyful (Farris 1976)	"Produce[s] efficiency and promote[s] joy" (Sevcovic 1979, p 39)	Encourage exercise as tolerated.
	Muckeshoot Keeping busy and walking a lot (Horn 1982)	Makes baby be born earlier, and labor and birth easier	Encourage walking as tolerated.
	Tonawanda Seneca Eating sparingly and exercising freely (Evaneshko 1982)	Makes birth easier	Assess nutritional patterns and provide teaching if needed.
Vietnamese	Consuming ginseng tea Conversing with and counseling fetus (Hollingsworth et al 1980)	Gives strength	Assess use and be certain it is not taken to the exclusion of necessary nutrients.
White American	Certain clothing worn	Promotes comfort	
	Self-medication for discomforts of pregnancy	Improves health	Counsel regarding effect of drugs on fetus.
	Seeks obstetric care	Ensures safe pregnancy and birth	
	Attends classes, reads books, attempts to gain more knowledge	Increases knowledge	Assist with pertinent books and topics.
	Concerned that maternity clothes make her look fat	Self-image	
	Oils & creams applied to avoid stretch marks	Self-image	Provide information regarding skin care.

each of the three trimesters. Some preexisting problems, such as hemorrhoids and varicose veins, are aggravated during pregnancy. These discomforts worsen with enlargement of the gravid uterus; they may appear in the second trimester and become intensified in the third trimester. For women who do not have these preexisting conditions, the second trimester of pregnancy may be a relatively comfortable time. The discomforts caused by the enlarging uterus do not affect them until the last trimester or even until the last month.

Table 14–4 identifies the common discomforts of pregnancy, their possible causes, and the self-care measures that might relieve the discomfort.

First Trimester

Nausea and Vomiting Nausea and vomiting are early symptoms in pregnancy. Some degree of nausea occurs in the majority of pregnant women. These symptoms appear sometime after the first missed menstrual period and usually cease by the fourth missed menstrual period. Approximately 50% to 80% of pregnant women experience some degree of nausea (DiIorio 1988). Some women develop an aversion only to specific foods, many experience nausea upon arising in the morning, and others experience nausea throughout the day or in the evening. Vomiting does not occur in the majority of these women.

Table 14–3   Proscribed Activities

Culture	Activity	Rationale
Mexican American	Pregnant woman should not look at the full moon (Brown 1976)	It will cripple or deform the unborn child
	She should not hang laundry or reach high	This will cause knots in the umbilical cord
	Baby showers should not be planned until time of birth (Kay 1978)	Earlier would invite bad luck or the "evil eye"
	The woman should not allow herself to quarrel or express anger (Kay 1978)	Consequences are spontaneous abortion, premature labor, or knots in the cord
Black American	Avoid any emotional fright (Carrington 1978)	Baby will have a birthmark
	Avoid reaching up	The umbilical cord may wrap around the baby's neck
Native American (selected examples)	*Navajo* Rug weaving is forbidden; carrying and lifting also avoided (Sevcovic 1979)	Puts unnatural strain on the body
	Avoid funerals or looking at dead animals (Sevcovic 1979)	Exposes the baby to the realm of the dead and may cause later illness to the baby
	Laguna Pueblo Do not sew with a bone or a needle (Farris 1976)	This will have an unkind effect on the baby
Vietnamese	Do not attend weddings or funerals (Hollingsworth et al 1980)	Bad luck for the newlyweds; the baby may cry
White American	Don't reach above head	Umbilical cord will wrap around baby's neck
	If frightened by snakes or other animals	May cause birthmark
	Don't lift heavy objects	May cause separation of the placenta

While the specific cause of nausea and vomiting in early pregnancy is not known, a common theory attributes the nausea to hormonal changes related to hCG levels in the body and changes in carbohydrate metabolism. HCG begins to be present in the body at about the time that symptoms of morning sickness usually begin, and hCG levels are subsiding when the discomfort of nausea and vomiting usually ends. Research has, as yet, failed to confirm this theory, however (Kochenour 1990). Fatigue and emotional factors may also play a role.

Education for Self-Care   Treatment of nausea and vomiting is not always successful, but the symptoms can be reduced. The nurse must assess when the nausea and/or vomiting occurs to be helpful in suggesting methods of relief. For some women, nausea may be relieved simply by avoiding the odor of certain foods or other conditions that precipitate the problem. If nausea occurs most frequently during early morning, the woman may find it helpful to eat dry crackers or toast before arising slowly. Arising slowly and avoiding sudden position changes throughout the day may also help prevent nausea due to hypotensive episodes.

It is generally helpful to eat small, frequent meals (sometimes as often as every two hours) throughout the day and to avoid greasy or highly seasoned foods. Eating dry meals and taking all liquids, including soups, between meals may help some women. Sudden changes in blood sugar levels can be avoided if the small meals are high in protein or complex carbohydrates. More recently, some women have obtained relief from acupressure wrist bands. While health care providers are reluctant to prescribe any medication during pregnancy, some women find 10–30 mg pyridoxine (vitamin B_6) daily helpful (Varner 1990).

Although some nausea is common, the woman who suffers from extreme nausea coupled with vomiting requires additional assessment. She should be advised to contact her health care provider if she vomits more than once per day or shows signs of dehydration such as dry mouth, decreased amounts of highly concentrated urine, and the like. In such cases the physician/certified nurse-midwife may order antiemetics. However, antiemetics should be avoided if at all possible during the first trimester because of the danger of teratogenic effects on embryo development.

Nausea and vomiting generally cease by the fourth month of pregnancy. If they do not, hyperemesis gravidarum (a complication of pregnancy discussed in Chapter 19) may develop.

Nasal Stuffiness and Epistaxis   Once pregnancy is well established, elevated estrogen levels may produce edema of the nasal mucosa resulting in nasal stuffiness, nasal discharge, and obstruction. Epistaxis may also result.

Education for Self-Care   Cool air vaporizers and normal saline nose drops may be helpful. However, the problem is often unresponsive to treatment. Women experiencing these problems find it difficult to sleep and may resort to nasal sprays and decongestants to relieve the problem.

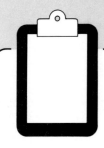

Nursing Care Plan
Non-English-Speaking Woman
at First Prenatal Visit

Nursing History:

1. Assess degree of communication possible. Determine if the woman understands some English, even if her verbal skills are limited.
2. Gather basic information as possible about course of pregnancy, estimated gestational age, sensitivity to medications, existing problems or concerns.

Physical Examination:

1. Vital signs, height and weight, general appearance.
2. Observe for signs of confusion, fear, anxiety.

Diagnostic Studies:

1. Urinalysis
2. CBC
3. Rubella titer, hepatitis screen if indicated.
4. Other lab work as appropriate.

Nursing Diagnosis/Goals	Nursing Interventions	Rationale	Evaluation
Nursing Diagnosis: Impaired verbal communication related to lack of understanding of care giver's language. *Client Goal:* The woman will have an opportunity to share information	Arrange for an interpreter—family member, friend, or staff person—to be present at this visit and subsequent visits as needed.	For effective ongoing communication, a shared language is essential.	The woman is comfortable communicating through the interpreter as evidenced by her willingness to answer questions and provide information and by her expressions of acceptance of the process.
Nursing Diagnosis: Impaired social interaction related to differing cultural practices and expectations between client and nurse. *Client Goal:* The woman will discuss her expectations.	Ask the woman to describe her expectations of the health care system. Ask her about customs and culturally specific practices that are important to her. Ask her to describe any practices that are specifically forbidden in her culture. Describe procedures usually performed during a prenatal visit and discuss her feelings about them. Postpone any nonessential procedures to a subsequent visit if she appears overloaded.	To provide effective, culturally sensitive care the nurse must gather information about acceptable and proscribed activities for the woman and her family.	The woman is able to discuss her expectations of the health care system and identify cultural practices that are important to her. She shows no evidence of fear or emotional distress about prenatal practices common to this country.

(continued)

Nursing Care Plan (continued)

Nursing Diagnosis/Goals	Nursing Interventions	Rationale	Evaluation
Nursing Diagnosis: Impaired social interaction related to culturally specific expectations of the role of the partner in the pregnancy and birth. *Client Goal:* The woman will have an opportunity to discuss her wishes regarding her partner's involvement.	Ask the woman about her partner's and her expectations of his degree of involvement. Is it preferable to them for him to be the primary support person, or do they prefer that a family member or close friend fill that role?	The role of the partner is often culturally specific and may vary greatly. The nurse should recognize this and respect the couple's wishes.	The woman is able to express her preferences about the partner's degree of involvement clearly and specifically.
Nursing Diagnosis: Knowledge deficit related to a lack of information about the changes associated with pregnancy and about prenatal care practices in this country. *Client Goal:* The woman will gain information regarding pregnancy changes and prenatal care.	Provide basic information about pregnancy and prenatal care. Plan additional sessions as needed so that the woman is not overwhelmed with information. Provide opportunities for questions and clarification. If possible provide printed information in the woman's language. Establish a mutually acceptable method for her to contact a care giver if she has questions or problems, or in an emergency.	All pregnant women have the right to clear, accurate information in order to be active participants in their health care.	The woman is able to ask questions and discuss areas of interest. She is willing to return for regular prenatal care.

Table 14–4 Self-Care Measures for Common Discomforts of Pregnancy

Discomfort	Influencing factors	Self-care measures
First Trimester		
Nausea and vomiting	Increased levels of hCG Changes in carbohydrate metabolism Emotional factors Fatigue	Avoid odors or causative factors. Eat dry crackers or toast before arising in morning. Have small but frequent meals. Avoid greasy or highly seasoned foods. Take dry meals with fluids between meals. Drink carbonated beverages.
Urinary frequency	Pressure of uterus on bladder in both first and third trimesters	Void when urge is felt. Increase fluid intake during the day. Decrease fluid intake *only* in the evening to decrease nocturia.
Breast tenderness	Increased levels of estrogen and progesterone	Wear well-fitting supportive bra.
Increased vaginal discharge	Hyperplasia of vaginal mucosa and increased production of mucus by the endocervical glands due to the increase in estrogen levels	Promote cleanliness by daily bathing. Avoid douching, nylon underpants, and pantyhose; cotton underpants are more absorbent; powder can be used to maintain dryness if not allowed to cake.
Nasal stuffiness and epistaxis	Elevated estrogen levels	May be unresponsive but cool air vaporizer may help; avoid use of nasal sprays and decongestants.
Ptyalism	Specific causative factors unknown	Use astringent mouthwashes, chew gum, or suck hard candy.
Second and Third Trimesters		
Heartburn (pyrosis)	Increased production of progesterone; decreasing gastrointestinal motility and increasing relaxation of cardiac sphincter; displacement of stomach by enlarging uterus; thus regurgitation of acidic gastric contents into esophagus	Eat small and more frequent meals. Use low-sodium antacids. Avoid overeating, fatty and fried foods, lying down after eating, and sodium bicarbonate.
Ankle edema	Prolonged standing or sitting Increased levels of sodium due to hormonal influences Circulatory congestion of lower extremities Increased capillary permeability Varicose veins	Practice frequent dorsiflexion of feet when prolonged sitting or standing is necessary. Elevate legs when sitting or resting. Avoid tight garters or restrictive bands around legs.
Varicose veins	Venous congestion in the lower veins that increases with pregnancy Hereditary factors (weakening of walls of veins, faulty valves) Increased age and weight gain	Elevate legs frequently. Wear supportive hose. Avoid crossing legs at the knees, standing for long periods, garters, and hosiery with constrictive bands.
Hemorrhoids	Constipation (see following discussion) Increased pressure from gravid uterus on hemorrhoidal veins	Avoid constipation. Apply ice packs, topical ointments, anesthetic agents, warm soaks, or sitz baths; gently reinsert into rectum as necessary.
Constipation	Increased levels of progesterone, which cause general bowel sluggishness Pressure of enlarging uterus on intestine Iron supplements Diet, lack of exercise, and decreased fluids	Increase fluid intake, fiber in the diet, exercise. Develop regular bowel habits. Use stool softeners as recommended by physician.
Backache	Increased curvature of the lumbosacral vertebras as the uterus enlarges Increased levels of hormones, which cause softening of cartilage in body joints Fatigue Poor body mechanics	Use proper body mechanics. Practice the pelvic tilt exercise. Avoid uncomfortable working heights, high-heeled shoes, lifting heavy loads, and fatigue.
Leg cramps	Imbalance of calcium/phosphorus ratio Increased pressure of uterus on nerves Fatigue Poor circulation to lower extremities Pointing the toes	Practice dorsiflexion of feet in order to stretch affected muscle. Evaluate diet. Apply heat to affected muscles.

(continued)

Table 14–4   Self-Care Measures for Common Discomforts of Pregnancy (continued)

Discomfort	Influencing factors	Self-care measures
Faintness	Postural hypotension Sudden change of position causing venous pooling in dependent veins Standing for long periods in warm area Anemia	Arise slowly from resting position. Avoid prolonged standing in warm or stuffy environments. Evaluate hematocrit/hemoglobin.
Dyspnea	Decreased vital capacity from pressure of enlarging uterus on the diaphragm	Use proper posture when sitting and standing. Sleep propped up with pillows for relief if problem occurs at night.
Flatulence	Decreased gastrointestinal motility leading to delayed emptying time Pressure of growing uterus on large intestine Air swallowing	Avoid gas-forming foods. Chew food thoroughly. Get regular daily exercise. Maintain normal bowel habits.
Carpal tunnel syndrome	Compression of median nerve in carpal tunnel of wrist Aggravated by repetitive hand movements	Avoid aggravating hand movements. Use splint as prescribed. Elevate affected arm.

Such interventions can exaggerate the nasal stuffiness, and create other discomforts. The use of any medication in pregnancy should be avoided if possible.

Urinary Frequency   Urinary frequency is a common discomfort of pregnancy. It occurs early in pregnancy because of the pressure of the enlarging uterus on the bladder. This condition subsides for a while when the uterus moves out of the pelvic area into the abdominal cavity around the twelfth week. Although the glomerular filtration rate increases in pregnancy, it does not cause a significant increase in urine output. Frequency recurs in the last trimester as the enlarging uterus begins to press on the bladder again. Coughing or sneezing in the last month may even cause leakage of urine.

As long as other symptoms of urinary tract infection do not appear, frequency of urination is considered normal during the first and third trimesters.

 Education for Self-Care   There are no methods of decreasing the frequency of urination in pregnancy. Fluid intake should never be decreased to prevent frequency. The woman should be encouraged to maintain an adequate fluid intake: at least 2000 mL/day. She should also be encouraged to empty her bladder frequently (approximately every two hours while awake).

Frequent bladder emptying helps decrease the incidence of leakage of urine. Since frequency often results in several trips to the bathroom each night, it is important to remind the woman to consider safety factors in the home such as a clear path to the bathroom, the use of a night light, and the like. The woman who leaks urine may choose to wear pantyliners during the day. If she does, she should change them as soon as they become damp to avoid peri-

neal excoriation and to avoid contamination of the perineum from the rectal area if the pads move back and forth as she walks. Tightening of the pubococcygeus muscle, which supports internal organs and controls voiding, can help maintain good perineal tone. This procedure, known as Kegel's exercise, is discussed on page 365.

While frequency is considered normal during the first and third trimesters, signs of bladder infection, such as pain, burning with voiding, or blood in the urine, should be reported to the woman's health care provider.

Breast Tenderness   Sensitivity of the breasts occurs early and continues throughout the pregnancy. Increased levels of estrogen and progesterone play large roles in the soreness and tingling sensation felt in the breasts and in the increased sensitivity of the nipples.

Education for Self-Care   A well-fitting, supportive brassiere gives the most relief for this discomfort. The qualities of a properly supportive brassiere are discussed in the section on breast care (p 360).

Ptyalism   Ptyalism is a rare discomfort of pregnancy in which excessive, often bitter saliva is produced. Causal theories are vague, and effective treatments are limited.

Education for Self-Care   Using astringent mouthwashes, chewing gum, or sucking on hard candy may minimize the problem of ptyalism.

Increased Vaginal Discharge   Increased vaginal discharge (**leukorrhea**) is common in pregnancy. The discharge is usually whitish and consists of mucus and exfoliated vaginal epithelial cells. It occurs as the result of

Key Nursing Diagnoses to Consider
Pregnancy

Early Pregnancy	Late Pregnancy
Impaired adjustment	Impaired adjustment
Anxiety	Anxiety
Ineffective family coping	Constipation
Ineffective individual coping	Ineffective family coping
Fear	Fear
Fluid volume deficit	Ineffective individual coping
Altered health maintenance	Altered family processes
Knowledge deficit	Knowledge deficit
Noncompliance	Noncompliance
Altered nutrition	Altered nutrition
Altered role performance	Altered role performance
Personal identity disturbance	Personal identity disturbance
Altered sexuality patterns	Altered sexuality patterns
Health-seeking behaviors	Sleep pattern disturbance
Decisional conflict	Situational low self-esteem
Fatigue	Fatigue
Sleep pattern disturbance	Health-seeking behaviors

hyperplasia of vaginal mucosa and increased production of mucus by the endocervical glands. In addition, the increased acidity of the secretions encourages the growth of *Candida albicans*, and the woman is thus more susceptible to monilial vaginitis.

 Education for Self-Care Cleanliness is important in preventing excoriation and vaginal infections. Daily bathing is adequate, and douching should be avoided during pregnancy if vaginal infections do not occur. Nylon underpants and pantyhose retain heat and moisture in the genital area; absorbent cotton underpants should be worn to help prevent problems. The pregnant woman should be encouraged to report any change in vaginal discharge and any irritation in the perineal area. These changes frequently indicate vaginal infections.

Second and Third Trimesters
It is difficult to classify discomforts as specifically occurring in the second or third trimester, since many problems are due to individual variations in women such as number of previously existing conditions. The symptoms discussed in this section usually do not appear until the third trimester in primigravidas but occur earlier with each succeeding pregnancy.

Heartburn (Pyrosis) Heartburn is the regurgitation of acidic gastric contents into the esophagus. It creates a burning or irritating sensation in the esophagus and radiates upward, sometimes leaving a bad taste in the mouth. Heartburn appears to be primarily a result of the displacement of the stomach by the enlarging uterus. The increased production of progesterone in pregnancy, decreases in gastrointestinal motility, and relaxation of the cardiac sphincter also contribute to heartburn.

Education for Self-Care Heartburn is aggravated by overeating, ingesting fatty and fried foods, and lying down soon after eating. These situations should therefore be avoided. The woman should be encouraged to drink an adequate amount of fluid (6 to 8 glasses) each day and to eat smaller and more frequent meals to accommodate the decreased size of her stomach. Good posture is important because it allows more room for the stomach to function. Antacids such as aluminum hydroxide (Amphojel) or a combination of aluminum hydroxide and magnesium hydroxide (Maalox) can be recommended. However, sodium bicarbonate (baking soda) and Alka-Seltzer should be avoided because of the potential for electrolyte imbalance.

Ankle Edema Most women experience ankle edema in the last part of pregnancy because of the increasing difficulty of venous return from the lower extremities. Prolonged standing or sitting and warm weather increase the edema. It is also associated with varicose veins. Ankle edema becomes a concern only when accompanied by hypertension or proteinuria or when the edema is not postural in origin.

Education for Self-Care The aggravating conditions just mentioned should be avoided. If the woman has to sit or stand for long periods, frequent dorsiflexion of her feet will help contract muscles, thereby squeezing the fluid back into circulation. The pregnant woman should not wear tight garters or other restrictive bands around her legs. During rest periods, the woman should elevate her legs and hips as described in the following section on varicose veins.

Varicose Veins Varicose veins are a result of weakening of the walls of veins or faulty functioning of the valves. Poor circulation in the lower extremities predisposes to varicose veins in the legs and thighs. With poor circulation stasis of the blood exerts pressure that gradually weakens the walls of the veins and causes varicosities. In other cases, faulty functioning of the valves causes pooling of blood in the lower extremities with concomitant pressure on the vein walls.

Pregnancy significantly increases the conditions that cause varicose veins. The weight of the gravid uterus in the pelvis aggravates the development of varicosities in the legs and pelvic area by preventing good venous return. Most women who do not have other predisposing factors can avoid the development of varicose veins in pregnancy with good preventive measures. Some women, however, experience obvious changes in the veins of their legs. Increased maternal age, excessive weight gain, a large fetus, heredity, and multiple pregnancy can all contribute to the problem.

Women with leg varicosities experience aching and tiredness in the lower extremities, with the discomfort increasing throughout the day. They frequently become discouraged by the discoloration in the veins of their legs and by obvious blemishes. Prevention or relief of the discomfort occurs when good venous return from the lower extremities is restored.

Vulvar varicosities may also be a problem in pregnancy, although they are less common. Varicosities in the vulva and perineum cause aching and a sense of heaviness. Support in these areas promotes relief.

Treatment of varicose veins by surgery or the injection method is not recommended during pregnancy. The woman should be aware that treatment may be needed after pregnancy because the problem will be aggravated by a succeeding pregnancy.

Phlebothrombosis and thrombophlebitis are possible complications of varicose veins, but they usually do not occur in a healthy pregnant woman. If these complications occur, the cause is often a local injury.

🍎 ***Education for Self-Care*** Regular exercise such as swimming, cycling, or walking promotes venous return, which helps prevent varicosities. Avoiding factors that contribute to venous stasis is also helpful. The pregnant woman should avoid standing or sitting for prolonged periods. She should also avoid crossing her legs at the knees because of the pressure on her veins. She should not wear garters or hosiery with constricting bands, such as knee-high hose. However, supportive hose or elastic stockings may be extremely helpful, depending on the amount of discomfort. Supportive hose should be put on in the morning and should be washed daily with soap and warm water to help retain its elasticity.

The pregnant woman should be encouraged to elevate her legs level with her hips when she sits. Comfort is enhanced if she supports the entire leg rather than simply propping her feet up on a stool, which may lead to hyperextension of the knees. The woman who sits or stands for long periods should walk around frequently to promote venous return to the heart. Venous return is most effec-

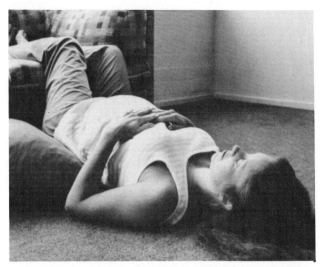

Figure 14–1 Swelling and discomfort from varicosities can be decreased by lying down with the legs and one hip elevated (to avoid compression of the vena cava).

tively promoted if the woman lies down with her feet elevated several times a day. To avoid difficulty related to pressure of the uterus on the vena cava, the woman can lie with her legs elevated on pillows and a pillow placed under one hip to displace the uterus to one side (Figure 14–1).

Support for vulvar varicosities can be provided by wearing two sanitary pads inside the underpants. Elevation of only the legs aggravates vulval varicosities by creating stasis of blood in the pelvic area. Therefore, it is important that the pelvic area also be elevated to promote venous drainage into the trunk of the body. More than one firm pillow under the hips may be needed to accomplish this elevation. Near the end of pregnancy, this position may be extremely awkward; the woman may best relieve uterine pressure on the pelvic veins by resting on her side. Blocks may also be placed under the foot of her bed to elevate it slightly.

Flatulence Flatulence results from decreased gastrointestinal motility, leading to delayed emptying, and from pressure upon the large intestine by the growing uterus. Air swallowing may also contribute to the problem.

Education for Self-Care The woman should be advised to avoid gas-forming foods and to chew her food thoroughly. Flatulence can be decreased by regular bowel habits and by exercise. 🍎

Hemorrhoids Hemorrhoids are varicosities of the veins around the lower end of the rectum and anus. In the nonpregnant state, hemorrhoids are usually caused by the straining that occurs with constipation. When a woman becomes pregnant, the gravid uterus creates pressure on the veins and thus interferes with venous circulation. As the pregnancy progresses and the fetus grows, greater pressure on the veins and displacement of intestines occur, increasing the problem of constipation and often resulting in hemorrhoids.

Some women may not be aware of hemorrhoids in pregnancy until the second stage of labor, when the hemorrhoids appear as they push just before birth. Hemorrhoids that occur in pregnancy or at birth usually subside, and they become asymptomatic after the early postpartal period.

Women who have hemorrhoids prior to pregnancy probably experience more difficulties with them during pregnancy because of the aggravating conditions just discussed.

Symptoms of hemorrhoids include itching, swelling, and pain, as well as hemorrhoidal bleeding. Internal hemorrhoids are located above the anal sphincter and are responsible for bleeding, usually with defecation. They are not usually painful unless they protrude from the anus. External hemorrhoids are located outside the anal sphincter. They are not usually the source of bleeding or pain; however, thrombosis of the hemorrhoids can occur, and in that case they become extremely painful. The thrombosis may resolve itself in 24 hours, or it can be treated in the physician's office by incising and evacuating the blood clot.

 Education for Self-Care Relief can be achieved by gently reinserting the hemorrhoid. Reinsertion is aided by gravity; it is more successful if the woman lies on her side or in the knee to chest position. She places some lubricant on her finger and presses against the hemorrhoids, pushing them inside. She holds them in place for 1 to 2 minutes and then gently withdraws her finger. The anal sphincter should then hold them inside the rectum. The woman will find it especially helpful if she can then maintain a side-lying position for a time, so this procedure is best done before bed or prior to a daily rest period.

Avoiding constipation is important in preventing and/or relieving the discomfort of hemorrhoids. Relief measures for existing hemorrhoid symptoms include ice packs, use of topical ointments and anesthetic agents, and warm soaks.

The woman should contact her health care provider if the hemorrhoids become hardened and noticeably tender to touch. Rectal bleeding that is more than spotting following defecation should also be reported.

Constipation Conditions in pregnancy that predispose the woman to constipation include general bowel sluggishness caused by increased progesterone and steroid metabolism; displacement of the intestines, which increases with the growth of the fetus; and oral iron supplements, which may be needed by the pregnant woman.

Education for Self-Care Increased fluid intake (at least 2000 mL/day), adequate roughage or bulk in the diet,

regular bowel habits, and adequate daily exercise can often maintain good bowel function in women who have not had previous problems. Some women find it helpful to drink a warm beverage or glass of prune juice in the morning. Women should leave sufficient time following breakfast so that the natural action of the body will produce defecation. Some women, rushing to leave for work or school, ignore or suppress the urge to defecate.

Women who try to develop good bowel habits during pregnancy will be prepared to maintain good bowel function after birth; meanwhile, they may need to use mild laxatives, stool softeners, and suppositories as recommended by their care giver. The nurse should help women with constipation to develop good daily bowel habits and to avoid becoming dependent on laxatives during pregnancy, a habit that may continue after birth.

Backache Many pregnant women experience backache. As the uterus enlarges, increased curvature of the lumbosacral vertebrae occurs. Circulating steroid hormones cause a softening and relaxation of pelvic joints, the growing uterus stretches the abdominal muscles, and the increasing weight creates a gradual tilt of the anterior portion of the pelvis. As the anterior portion of the pelvis tilts downward, the spinal curvature increases. If the woman does not learn how to correct this curvature, the strain on the muscles and ligaments will cause backache.

Education for Self-Care An exercise called the pelvic tilt can help restore proper body alignment. As the anterior pelvis is tilted upward, the curvature of the back is automatically decreased, relieving much of the discomfort. If proper body alignment is maintained throughout pregnancy, backaches can be relieved or even prevented. See discussion on exercises, page 364.

The use of proper posture and good body mechanics throughout pregnancy is important. The pregnant woman should not curve her back by bending over to lift or pick up items from the floor. The strain is felt in the muscles of the back. Leg muscles should be used to do the work instead. The woman can keep her back straight by bending her knees to lower her body into the squatting position (Figure 14–2). Her feet should be placed 12 to 18 inches apart to maintain body balance. When lifting a heavy object such as a child, she should place one foot flat on the floor, slightly in front of the other foot, and lower herself to the other knee. The object is held close to her body for lifting. This same principle of keeping the back straight and bending the knees applies when the woman sits down or gets out of a chair.

Work heights that require constant bending can contribute to backache and should be adjusted as necessary. Women who do not experience backache in pregnancy may become aware of it later as they bend to change a newborn's diaper.

A pendulous abdomen contributes to backache by in-

cramps, so the pregnant woman should be warned not to do so while doing exercises for childbirth preparation or when she is resting.

The exact cause of leg cramps is not known. Proposed contributing factors include an inadequate calcium intake, an imbalance in the calcium/phosphorus ratio, pressure of the enlarged uterus on the pelvic nerves leading to the legs, or pressure on the pelvic vessels causing impaired circulation.

Leg cramps are more common in the third trimester because of increased weight of the uterus on the nerves supplying the lower extremities. Fatigue and poor circulation in the lower extremities contribute to this problem.

Education for Self-Care Immediate relief of the muscle spasm is achieved by stretching the muscle. This is most effectively done with the woman lying on her back and another person pressing the woman's knee down to straighten her leg while pushing her foot toward her leg (Figure 14–3). Foot flexion techniques, massage, and warm packs can be used to alleviate discomfort from leg cramps.

The physician may recommend that the woman drink no more than a pint of milk daily and take calcium lactate, or the physician may suggest a quart of milk daily and prescribe aluminum hydroxide gel. Aluminum hydroxide gel stops the action of phosphorus on calcium by absorbing the phosphorus and eliminating it directly through the intestinal tract. The treatment recommendations depend on the frequency of the leg cramps.

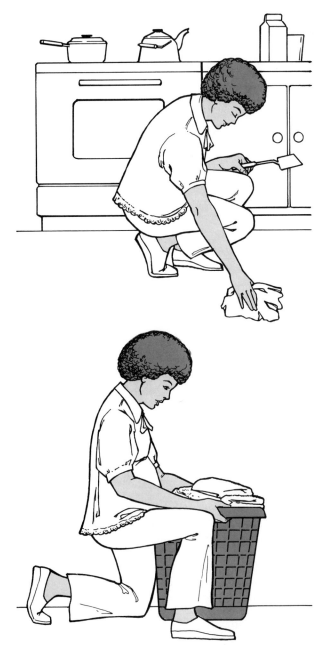

Figure 14–2 Proper body mechanics must be used by the pregnant woman when picking up objects from floor level or when lifting objects.

creasing the curvature of the spine. The use of a good supportive maternity girdle is discussed in the section on clothing, as is the role of high-heeled shoes in increasing the lumbosacral curvature (p 362).

Leg Cramps Leg cramps are painful muscle spasms in the gastrocnemius muscles. They occur most frequently at night after the woman has gone to bed but may occur at other times. Extension of the foot can often cause leg

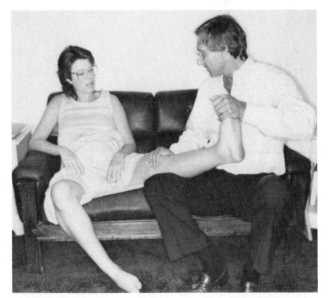

Figure 14–3 The expectant father can help relieve the woman's painful leg cramps by dorsiflexing the foot while holding her knee flat.

When planning a treatment regimen, one must be careful not to totally exclude milk from the woman's diet because it is an excellent source of other essential nutrients.

Faintness   Faintness is experienced by many pregnant women, especially in warm, crowded areas. The cause of faintness is a combination of changes in the blood volume and postural hypotension due to venous pooling of blood in the dependent veins. Sudden change of position or standing for prolonged periods can cause this sensation, and fainting can occur.

Education for Self-Care   The nurse should first be certain that the pregnant woman understands the symptoms of faintness. These include slight dizziness, a "swirling" or "floating" sensation, and a decreased ability to hear or focus attention. If faintness is experienced from prolonged standing or being in a warm, crowded room, the woman should sit down and lower her head between her legs. If this procedure does not help, the woman should be assisted to an area where she can lie down and get fresh air. When arising from a resting position, she should move slowly.

Shortness of Breath   Shortness of breath occurs as the uterus rises into the abdomen and causes pressure on the diaphragm. This problem worsens in the last trimester as the enlarged uterus presses directly on the diaphragm, decreasing vital capacity. The primigravida experiences considerable relief from shortness of breath in the last few weeks of pregnancy, when **lightening** occurs and the fetus and uterus move down in the pelvis. Because the multigravida does not usually experience lightening until labor, shortness of breath will continue throughout her pregnancy.

Education for Self-Care   During the day, relief can be found by sitting straight in a chair and using proper posture when standing. If distress is great at night, the woman can sleep propped up in bed with several pillows behind her head and shoulders.

Difficulty Sleeping   Although the pregnant woman may experience difficulty sleeping for many of the same psychologic reasons as the nonpregnant woman, many physical factors also contribute to this problem. The enlarged uterus may make it difficult to find a comfortable position for sleep, and an active fetus may aggravate the problem. The other discomforts of pregnancy such as urinary frequency, shortness of breath, and leg cramps may also be contributing factors.

Education for Self-Care   The pregnant woman may find it helpful to drink a warm (caffeine-free) beverage before bed and may benefit from a soothing backrub given by her partner or a family member. Pillows may be used to provide support for her back, between her legs, or for her upper arm when she lies on her side. Relaxation techniques may also help. The woman should avoid caffeine products, stimulating activity, and sleeping medication.

Round Ligament Pain   As the uterus enlarges during pregnancy, the round ligaments stretch, hypertrophy, and lengthen as the uterus rises up in the abdomen. Round ligament pain is attributed to this stretching.

Education for Self-Care   The woman may feel concern when she first experiences round ligament pain because it is often intense and causes a "grabbing" sensation in the lower abdomen and inguinal area. The nurse should warn women of this possible discomfort. Few treatment measures really alleviate this discomfort, but understanding the cause will help decrease anxiety. Once the care giver has ascertained that the cause of the discomfort is not related to a medical complication such as appendicitis or gall bladder disease, the woman may find that a heating pad applied to the abdomen brings some relief. She may also benefit from bringing her knees up on her abdomen.

Carpal Tunnel Syndrome   Carpal tunnel syndrome (CTS) results from compression of the median nerve in the carpal tunnel of the wrist. The syndrome is commonly bilateral but may be more pronounced in the dominant hand. Typically the woman with CTS awakens with numbness, tingling, or burning in the fleshy part of the palm near the thumb. She may also experience numbness in her fingers and mild hand weakness (Cunningham et al 1989). The syndrome is aggravated by repetitive hand movements such as typing. Symptoms often disappear following birth. Treatment involves splinting, avoidance of aggravating movements, and, in some cases, injection of steroids into the carpal tunnel. Surgery is indicated in severe cases (Varner 1990).

Education for Self-Care   Although the condition is not preventable, the woman should be advised to avoid aggravating activities and use her splint as directed.

Promotion of Maternal and Fetal Well-Being During Pregnancy

The pregnant woman is faced with the important responsibility of maintaining her health not only for her sake but also for the sake of her unborn child. Nurses can help promote maternal and fetal well-being by providing expectant couples with accurate and complete information about health behaviors that can affect pregnancy and childbirth.

Breast Care
Whether the pregnant woman plans to bottle or breast-feed her infant, proper support of the breasts is important

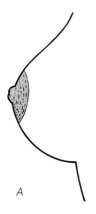

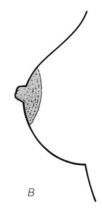

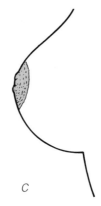

Figure 14–4 A When not stimulated, normal and inverted nipples often look alike. B When stimulated, the normal nipple protrudes. C When stimulated, the inverted nipple retracts. However, great variation exists. In some women, one or both nipples always appear inverted, even when not stimulated.

to promote comfort, retain breast shape, and prevent back strain, particularly if the breasts become large and pendulous. The sensitivity of the breasts in pregnancy is also relieved by good support.

A well-fitting, supportive brassiere has the following qualities:

- The straps are wide and do not stretch (elastic straps soon lose their tautness due to the weight of the breasts and frequent washing).

- The cup holds all breast tissue comfortably.

- The brassiere has tucks or other devices that allow it to expand, thus accommodating the enlarging chest circumference.

- The brassiere supports the nipple line approximately midway between the elbow and shoulder. At the same time, the brassiere is not pulled up in the back by the weight of the breasts.

Cleanliness of the breasts is important, especially as the woman begins producing colostrum. Colostrum that crusts on the nipples should be removed with warm water. The woman planning to breast-feed should not use soap on her nipples because of its drying effect.

Nipple preparation, begun during the third trimester, may help the breast-feeding mother by decreasing the amount of nipple soreness she experiences during the early days of breast-feeding. Nipple preparation promotes the distribution of the natural lubricants produced by Montgomery's tubercles, stimulates blood flow to the breast, and helps develop the protective layer of skin over the nipple. Women who are planning to nurse can begin by going braless when possible and by exposing their nipples to sunlight and air. Rubbing the nipples removes protective lubrication and should be avoided, but rolling the nipple may be beneficial. This is done by grasping the nipple between thumb and forefinger and gently rolling and pulling on it. A woman with a history of preterm labor is advised not to do this because nipple stimulation triggers the release of oxytocin. (See Chapter 19 for further discussion.)

Nipple-rolling is more difficult for women with flat or inverted nipples, but it is still a useful preparation for breast-feeding. Nipple inversion is usually diagnosed during the initial antepartal assessment. Occasionally a nipple appears inverted at all times. In other cases, the nipple appears normal initially but pressure on the alveoli with the examiner's thumb and finger causes the nipple to retract. The normal or flat nipple protrudes when this is done (Figure 14–4).

The woman with nipple inversion can increase nipple protractility by performing Hoffman's exercises (Figure 14–5) (Hoffman 1953). If the nipple is truly inverted,

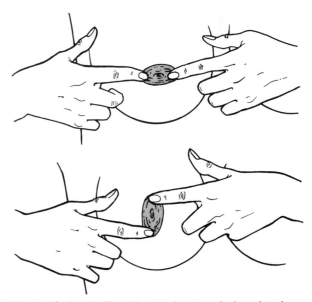

Figure 14–5 Hoffman's exercises are designed to increase nipple protractility. The woman is instructed to place her thumbs or index fingers opposite each other near the edge of the areola. She then presses into the breast and stretches outward to break any adhesions. This is done both horizontally and vertically.

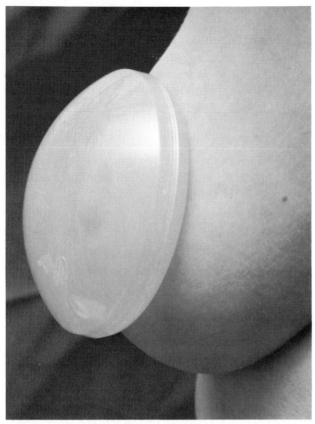

Figure 14–6 This breast shield is designed to increase the protractility of inverted nipples. These shields, worn the last three to four months of pregnancy, exert gentle pulling pressure at the edge of the areola, gradually forcing the nipple through the center of the shield. They may be used after birth if still necessary.

she can wear special breast shields (such as Woolrich or Eschmann shields) for the last three or four months of pregnancy (Figure 14–6). These shields tend to absorb moisture so they should not be worn more than a few hours at a time. Breast shields appear to be the only measure that really helps women with inverted nipples.

Oral stimulation of the nipple by the woman's partner during sex play is also an excellent technique for toughening the nipple in preparation for breast-feeding. The couple who enjoys this stimulation should be encouraged to continue it throughout the pregnancy.

Clothing

Maternity clothes are constructed with fuller lines to allow for the increase in abdominal size during pregnancy. Skirts and slacks have soft elastic waistbands and a stretchable panel over the abdominal area. Maternity clothes keep pace with fashion trends, enabling the woman to feel stylish. They are expensive and are worn for a relatively short time. Women can economize by sharing clothes with friends, sewing their own garments, or buying used maternity clothing.

Clothing should be loose and nonconstricting both for general comfort and to prevent some of the specific discomforts of pregnancy. For example, restricting bands such as garters can interfere with venous circulation and predispose to varicose veins or aggravate existing ones.

Maternity girdles are seldom worn today and are not necessary for most women. They are sometimes used by women athletes, such as runners, dancers, or gymnasts, who maintain a light workout schedule during pregnancy. Women with large pendulous abdomens may also benefit from a well-fitting supportive girdle. Without this support, the pendulous abdomen increases the curvature of the back and is a source of backache and general discomfort. Tight leg bands on girdles should be avoided.

High-heeled shoes aggravate back discomfort by increasing the curvature of the back and should not be worn if the woman experiences backache or problems with balance. Shoes should fit properly and feel comfortable.

Bathing

Daily bathing is important because of the increased perspiration and mucoid vaginal discharge that occurs in pregnancy. The woman may take either a shower or a tub bath according to her preference. Caution is needed during tub baths because balance becomes a problem as pregnancy advances. Rubber tub mats and hand grips are valuable safety devices. Moreover, vasodilation due to the warm water may cause the woman to experience some faintness when she attempts to get out of the tub. Thus, she may require assistance, especially in the third trimester. *To avoid introducing infection, tub baths are contraindicated in the presence of vaginal bleeding or when the membranes are ruptured.* Women are advised to avoid hot tubs or prolonged immersion in a very hot bath because of the possible harmful effects on the fetus when the maternal core temperature is elevated.

Employment

Studies of women who are employed during pregnancy show distinct differences. Women who work in office jobs tend to have slightly lower odds of having a small-for-gestational-age (SGA) baby than unemployed women. This may be because of better access to health care or because these women tend to be healthier as a group. However, women who work in strenuous manual jobs have a higher incidence of preterm or SGA infants than either office workers or unemployed women. This difference may be related to decreased uteroplacental perfusion as blood is shunted to muscle tissue or may reflect the fact that women who are better off tend to work in less strenuous jobs (Launer et al 1990). Similarly, women who work in occupations that require prolonged standing have a higher incidence of spontaneous abortion (McDonald et al 1988).

Major deterrents to employment during pregnancy include fetotoxic hazards in the environment, excessive physical strain, overfatigue and medical or pregnancy-related complications. In the last half of pregnancy occupations involving balance should be adjusted to protect the mother.

Fetotoxic hazards in the environment are always a concern to the expectant couple. If the pregnant woman or the woman contemplating pregnancy is working in industry, she should contact her company physician or nurse about possible hazards in her work environment and should do her own reading and research on environmental hazards. Some industrial products, such as turpentine and lead paint (which are also occasionally found in the home), are considered toxic substances during pregnancy. (See also Chapter 6 for a discussion of environmental hazards.)

Travel

The pregnant woman often has many questions about the effects of travel on her and on the fetus. If medical or pregnancy complications are not present, there are no restrictions on travel.

Travel by automobile can be especially fatiguing, aggravating many of the discomforts of pregnancy. The pregnant woman needs frequent opportunities to get out of the car and walk. A good pattern to follow is to stop every 2 hours and walk around for approximately 10 minutes.

Seat belts should be worn, including both lap and shoulder belts. The lap belt should fit snugly and be positioned under the abdomen. Seat belts play an important role in preventing maternal mortality with subsequent fetal loss. Fetal loss in car accidents is also caused by placental separation as a result of uterine distortion. Use of the shoulder belt decreases the risk of traumatic flexion of the woman's body, thus decreasing the risk of placental separation (Krozy & McColgan 1985).

As pregnancy progresses, travel by airplane or train is recommended for long distances. In the last weeks of pregnancy, sickle cell anemia, severe maternal anemia, or a history of thrombophlebitis may contraindicate flying (Barry & Bia 1989). To avoid the development of phlebitis, pregnant women should be advised to request an aisle seat and walk about the plane at regular intervals.

As pregnant women remain active and sometimes fly to more remote areas of the world, the availability of medical care at one's destination is another important consideration for the near-term woman. Travel should usually be avoided if there is a history of bleeding or pregnancy-induced hypertension or if multiple births are anticipated (Barry & Bia 1989).

Activity and Rest

What factors should be considered in advising a woman about exercise during pregnancy?

Exercise during pregnancy helps maintain maternal fitness and muscle tone, leads to improved self-image and sense of control, increases energy, improves sleep, relieves tension, helps control weight gain, promotes regular bowel function, and is associated with improved postpartum recovery. Normal participation in exercise can continue throughout an uncomplicated pregnancy.

Certain conditions do contraindicate exercise. These include ruptured membranes, maternal heart disease, history of/or existing preterm labor, multiple gestation, placenta previa, bleeding, incompetent cervix, or history of three or more spontaneous abortions (Leaf 1989).

Research related to the effects of maternal exercise on the fetus is varied and contradictory. In considering the effects of exercise on the fetus, however, two conditions are of possible concern: maternal hyperthermia and decreased uterine blood flow. Exercise can lead to increased maternal core temperature and hyperthermia. Studies have demonstrated an increased incidence of meningomyloceles among the infants of women who experienced heat stress due to vigorous exercise in the first trimester (Paisley & Mellion 1988). Uterine blood flow is reduced during exercise as blood is shunted from visceral organs to muscles. The fetus does seem able to withstand this stress, however, without developing hypoxia. Another area of concern is whether decreased uteroplacental blood flow during exercise compromises the ability of the fetus to dissipate heat via the placenta, especially since the fetus is not able to decrease temperature via perspiration or respiration (Fishbein & Phillips 1990).

In advising clients, many health care providers use the Guidelines for Exercise during Pregnancy and Postpartum formulated by the American College of Obstetricians and Gynecologists (1985). However, these guidelines have been criticized as not sufficiently taxing for physically fit, athletic women (Freyder 1989; Paisley & Mellion 1988). Current literature modifies the guidelines somewhat for aerobically conditioned women.

As our knowledge of the impact of exercise on pregnancy increases, the skilled sportswoman is no longer discouraged from participating in regular exercise. Pregnancy is not the time, however, to learn a new or strenuous sport.

The nurse may find the following guidelines useful in counseling women about exercise during pregnancy:

1. Before beginning an exercise program, a pregnant woman should be examined by her nurse-midwife/ physician. A woman already in an exercise program when pregnancy is confirmed should discuss her degree of participation with her care giver.

2. A moderate, rhythmic exercise routine involving large muscle groups such as found with swimming, cycling, walking, or cross-country skiing is best. As pregnancy progresses, non-weight-bearing exercises such as swimming and cycling are safe and provide fitness with comfort. Jogging or running is acceptable for women already conditioned to this activity. Certain sports, including all contact sports and horseback riding, are not recommended (Freyder 1989). High-speed falls while waterskiing have been associated with forceful entry of water into the uterus and miscarriage, while scuba diving may be associated with decompression sickness, fetal hypoxia, and hypercapnia (Sady 1989). Similarly, the woman should avoid high-risk activities such as skydiving, mountain climbing, racquetball, ice skating, and surfing. These activities require balance and coordination, but the woman's changed center of gravity and softened joints may decrease coordination.

   As pregnancy progresses, women should decrease the intensity of exercise. This helps compensate for the decreased cardiac reserve, increased respiratory effort, and increased weight of the pregnant woman (Paolone & Worthington 1985).

3. The woman is encouraged to exercise at least three times per week. Competitive sports are not recommended (ACOG, 1985).

4. To prevent hyperthermia, the woman should avoid prolonged overheating associated with vigorous exercise in hot, humid weather. By the same token, the woman should avoid hot tubs and saunas.

5. The woman should exercise for shorter intervals. ACOG guidelines recommend not longer than 15 minutes at a time with a maximum pulse rate of 140 beats per minute. Other authorities recommend that fit women can exercise for 30 minutes with maximum pulse rates of 150 beats per minute (Sady 1989).

6. The woman should warm up and stretch to help prepare the joints for activity and cool down with a period of mild activity to help restore circulation and avoid pooling of blood.

7. The woman should wear a supportive bra and appropriate shoes. She should take liquids liberally before and after exercising to avoid dehydration.

8. The woman should stop the activity and consult her care giver if unusual symptoms develop (ACOG, 1985). Symptoms such as dizziness, extreme shortness of breath, tingling, numbness, palpitations, abdominal pain, vaginal bleeding, or abrupt cessation of fetal movement should be reported.

9. Because of the risk of supine hypotensive syndrome, the woman should avoid lying flat on her back to exercise after the fourth month of pregnancy.

Adequate rest in pregnancy is important for both physical and emotional health. Women need more sleep throughout pregnancy, particularly in the first and last trimesters, when they tire easily. Without adequate rest, pregnant women have less resilience.

Finding time to rest during the day may be difficult for women who work or have small children. The nurse can help the expectant mother examine her daily schedule to develop a realistic plan for short periods of rest and relaxation.

Sleeping becomes more difficult during the last trimester because of the enlarged abdomen, increased frequency of urination, and greater activity of the fetus. Finding a comfortable position becomes difficult for the pregnant woman.

Figure 14–7 shows a position most pregnant women find comfortable. Progressive relaxation techniques similar to those taught in prepared childbirth classes can help prepare the woman for sleep (see Chapter 17).

Exercises to Prepare for Childbirth

Certain exercises help strengthen muscle tone in preparation for birth and promote more rapid restoration of muscle tone after birth. Some physical changes of pregnancy can be reduced considerably by faithfully practicing prescribed body-conditioning exercises. A great variety of body-conditioning exercises are taught, but only a few are discussed here.

The **pelvic tilt**, or pelvic rocking, helps prevent or reduce back strain and strengthens abdominal muscle tone. To do the pelvic tilt, the pregnant woman lies on her back and puts her feet flat on the floor. This bent position of the knees helps prevent strain and discomfort (Figure 14–8). She decreases the curvature in her back by pressing her spine toward the floor. With her back pressed to the floor, the woman tightens her buttocks and abdominal muscles as she tucks in her buttocks. The pelvic tilt can also be performed on hands and knees, while sitting in a chair, or while standing with the back against a wall. The body alignment achieved when the pelvic tilt is correctly done should be maintained as much as possible throughout the day.

Abdominal Exercises A basic exercise to increase abdominal muscle tone is tightening abdominal muscles in synchronization with respirations. It can be done in any position, but it is best learned while the woman lies supine. With knees flexed and feet flat on the floor, the woman expands her abdomen and slowly takes a deep breath. As she slowly exhales, she gradually pulls in her abdominal muscles until they are fully contracted. She relaxes for a few seconds and then repeats the exercise.

Partial sit-ups strengthen abdominal muscle tone and are done according to individual comfort levels. When doing a partial sit-up, the woman lies on the floor as described above (Figure 14–9). This exercise is done with the knees bent and the feet flat on the floor to avoid undue strain on the lower back. She stretches her arms toward her knees as she slowly pulls her head and shoulders off the floor to a comfortable level. (If she has poor abdominal muscle tone, she may not be able to pull up very far.) She then slowly returns to the starting position, takes a deep breath, and repeats the exercise. To strengthen the oblique abdominal muscles, she repeats the process, but stretches the left arm to the side of her right knee, returns to the floor, takes a deep breath, and then reaches with the right arm to the left knee.

These exercises can be done approximately five times in a sequence, and the sequence can be repeated at other times during the day as desired. It is important to do the exercises slowly to prevent muscle strain and overtiring.

Perineal Exercises Perineal muscle tightening, also referred to as **Kegel's exercises**, strengthens the pubococcygeus muscle and increases its elasticity (Figure 14–10). The woman can feel the specific muscle group to be exercised by stopping urination midstream. However, doing Kegel's exercises while urinating is discouraged because this practice has been associated with urinary stasis and urinary tract infection.

Childbirth educators sometimes use the following technique to teach Kegel's exercises. They tell the woman to think of her perineal muscles as an elevator. When she relaxes, the elevator is on the first floor. To do the exercises, she contracts, bringing the elevator to the second, third, and fourth floors. She keeps the elevator on the fourth floor for a few seconds, and then gradually relaxes the area (Fenlon et al 1986). If the exercise is properly done, the woman does not contract the muscles of the buttocks and thighs.

Kegel's exercises can be done at almost any time. Some women use ordinary events—for instance, stopping at a red light—as a cue to remember to do the exercise. Others do Kegel's exercises while waiting in a checkout line, talking on the telephone, or watching television.

Inner Thigh Exercises The pregnant woman should assume a cross-legged sitting position whenever possible. The *tailor sit* stretches the muscles of the inner thighs in preparation for labor and birth.

Sexual Activity

As a result of the physiologic, anatomic, and emotional changes of pregnancy, the couple usually has many questions and concerns about sexual activity during pregnancy. Often these questions are about possible injury to the baby or the woman during intercourse and about changes in the desire each partner feels for the other.

In the past, couples were frequently warned to avoid sexual intercourse during the last 6 to 8 weeks of preg-

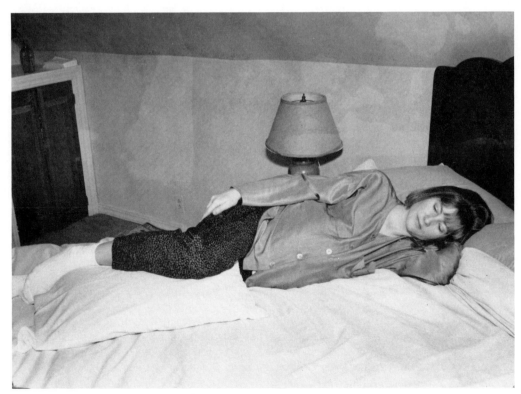

Figure 14–7 Position for relaxation and rest as pregnancy progresses.

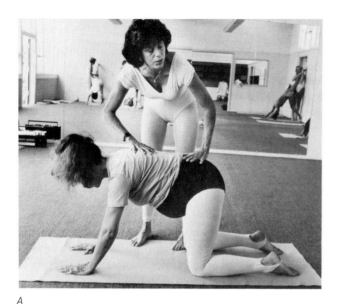

A

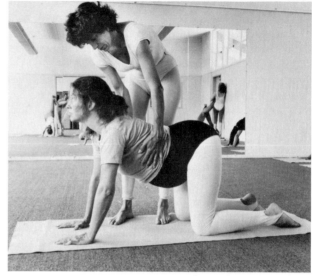

B

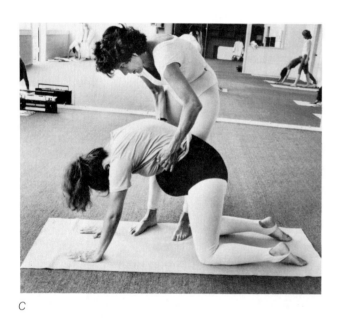

C

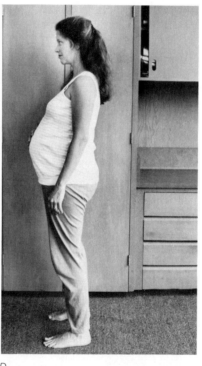

D

Figure 14–8 A Starting position when the pelvic tilt is done on the hands and knees. The back is flat and parallel to the floor, the hands are under the head, and the knees are directly under the buttocks. B A prenatal yoga instructor offers pointers for proper positioning for the first part of the tilt: head up, neck long and separated from the shoulders, buttocks up and pelvis thrust back, allowing the back to drop and release on an inhaled breath. C The instructor assists the woman in assuming the correct position for the next part of the tilt. It is done on a long exhalation, allowing the pregnant woman to arch her back, drop her head loosely, push away from her hands, and draw in the muscles of her abdomen to strengthen them. Note that in this position the pelvis and buttocks are tucked under and the buttock muscles are tightened. D Proper posture. The knees are not locked but slightly bent, the pelvis and buttocks are tucked under, thereby lengthening the spine and helping to support the weighty abdomen. With her chin tucked in, this woman's neck, shoulders, hips, knees, and feet are all in a straight line perpendicular to the floor. Her feet are parallel. This is also the starting position for doing the pelvic tilt while standing.

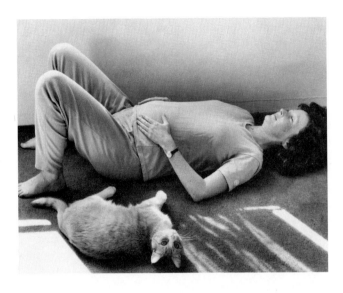

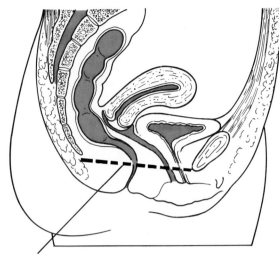
Pubococcygeus muscle with good tone

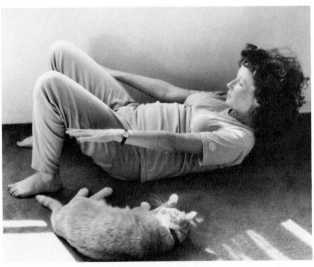

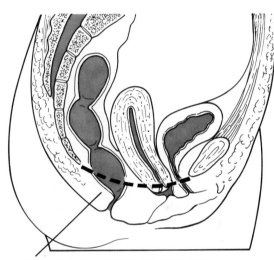
Pubococcygeus muscle with poor tone

Figure 14–9   The pregnant woman can strengthen her abdominal muscles by doing partial sit-ups.

Figure 14–10   Kegel's exercises. The woman learns to tighten the pubococcygeus muscle, which improves support to the pelvic organs.

nancy to prevent complications such as infection or premature rupture of the membranes. However, these fears seem to be unfounded. In a healthy pregnancy there is no valid reason to limit sexual activity (Reamy & White 1985). Intercourse is contraindicated when bleeding is present or the membranes are ruptured. Women with a history of preterm labor and those who experience strong uterine contractions following orgasm should be advised of the possible risks of coitus after 32 weeks' gestation (Kochenour 1990).

The expectant mother may experience changes in sexual desire and response. Often these are related to the various discomforts that occur throughout pregnancy. For instance, during the first trimester, fatigue or nausea and vomiting may decrease desire, while breast tenderness may make the woman less responsive to fondling of her breasts.

During the second trimester, many of the discomforts have lessened, and, with the vascular congestion of the pelvis, the woman may experience even greater sexual satisfaction than she experienced prior to pregnancy.

During the third trimester, interest in coitus may again decrease as the woman becomes more uncomfortable and fatigued. In addition, shortness of breath, painful pelvic ligaments, urinary frequency, and decreased mobility may lessen sexual desire and activity. If they are not already using them, the couple should consider coital positions other than male superior, such as side-by-side, female superior, and vaginal rear entry.

The pregnant woman may be alarmed by orgasmic changes in the last trimester. Instead of the rhythmic contractions of orgasm, she may experience longer contrac-

TEACHING GUIDE
Sexual Activity During Pregnancy

Assessment: Occasionally, a woman indicates her beliefs about sexual activity during pregnancy by asking a direct question. This is most likely to occur if the woman and the nurse have a good rapport. Often, however, the nurse must ask some general questions to determine the woman's level of understanding. A general statement may trigger a discussion and help the nurse in his or her determination. In many cases teaching about this topic is coupled with ongoing assessment of the woman's understanding of sexual activity during pregnancy.

Nursing Diagnosis: The key nursing diagnosis will probably be: knowledge deficit related to a lack of understanding about changes in sexuality and sexual activity during pregnancy.

Nursing Plan and Implementation: The teaching plan will generally focus on discussion or use a "question and answer" format. The presence of both partners may be beneficial in fostering communication between them and is acceptable unless personal or cultural factors indicate otherwise.

Client Goals: At the completion of the teaching the woman will:

1. Relate the changes in sexuality and sexual response that may occur during pregnancy to changes in technique, frequency, and response that may be indicated.

2. Explore personal attitudes, beliefs, and expectations about sexual activity during pregnancy.

3. Cite maternal factors that would contraindicate sexual intercourse.

Teaching Plan

Content: Begin by explaining that the pregnant woman may experience changes in desire during the course of pregnancy. During the first trimester, discomforts such as nausea, fatigue, and breast tenderness may make intercourse less desirable for many women.

Other women may have fewer discomforts and may find that their sexual desire is unchanged. In the second trimester, as symptoms decrease desire may increase. In the third trimester, discomfort and fatigue may lead to decreased desire in the woman.

Men may notice changes in their level of desire, too. Among other things, this may be related to feelings about their partner's changing appearance, their belief about the acceptability of sexual activity with a pregnant woman, or concern about hurting the woman or fetus. Some men find the changes of pregnancy erotic while others must adjust to the notion of their partner as a mother.

Explain that the woman may notice that orgasms are much more intense during the last weeks of pregnancy and may be followed by cramping. Because of the pressure of the enlarging uterus on the vena cava, the woman should not lie flat on her back for intercourse after about the fourth month. If the couple prefer that position, a pillow should be placed under her right hip to displace the uterus. Alternate positions such as side-lying, female-superior, or vaginal rear entry may become necessary as her uterus enlarges.

Teaching Method: Universal statements that give permission, such as "Many couples experience changes in sexual desire during pregnancy. What kind of changes have you experienced?" are often effective in starting discussion. Depending on the woman's (or couple's) level of knowledge and sophistication, part or all of this discussion may be necessary.

If the partner is present, approach him in the same nonjudgmental way used above. If not, ask the woman if she has noticed any changes in her partner or if he has expressed any concerns.

Deal with any specific questions about the physical and psychologic changes that the couple may have.

(continued)

TEACHING GUIDE (continued)

Teaching Plan

Stress that sexual activities that both partners enjoy are generally acceptable. It is not advisable for couples who favor anal sex to go from anal penetration to vaginal penetration because of the risk of introducing *E coli* into the vagina.

Alternative methods of expressing intimacy and affection such as cuddling, holding and stroking each other, and kissing may help maintain the couple's feelings of warmth and closeness.

If the man feels desire for further sexual release, his partner may help him masturbate to ejaculation or he may prefer to masturbate in private.

The woman who is interested in masturbation as a form of gratification should be advised that the orgasmic contractions may be especially intense in later pregnancy.

Stress that sexual intercourse is contraindicated once the membranes are ruptured or if bleeding is present. Women with a history of preterm labor may be advised to avoid intercourse because the oxytocin that is released with orgasm stimulates uterine contractions and may trigger preterm labor. Since oxytocin is also released with nipple stimulation, fondling the breasts may also be contraindicated in those cases.

A discussion of sexuality and sexual activity should stress the importance of open communication so that the couple feel comfortable expressing their feelings, preferences, and concerns.

Evaluation: The nurse determines the effectiveness of the teaching by evaluating the woman's (or couple's) response to information throughout the discussion. The nurse may also ask the woman to express information such as the contraindications to intercourse in her own words. Follow-up sessions and questions from the woman also provide information about teaching effectiveness.

Discussion about various sexual activities requires that the nurse be comfortable with his/her sexuality and be tactful. Often the nurse may find it advisable to volunteer such information to show that discussion of sexual variations is acceptable.

The couple may be content with these approaches to meeting their sexual needs or they may require assurance that such approaches are indeed "normal."

An explanation of the contraindications accompanied by their rationale provides specific guidelines that most couples find helpful.

Some couples are skilled at expressing their feelings about sexual activity while others find it difficult and can benefit from specific suggestions.

The nurse should provide opportunities for discussion throughout the talk.

Specific handouts on sexual activity are also helpful for couples and may address topics that were not discussed.

---

tions that may be followed by cramps and backache. Masturbation often creates a more intense contraction than occurs with intercourse (Masters & Johnson 1966). There is no evidence, however, that these contractions cause preterm labor in the large majority of pregnant women (Klebanoff et al 1984).

Sexual activity does not have to include intercourse. Many of the nurturing and sexual needs of the pregnant woman can be satisfied by cuddling, kissing, and being held. The warm, sensual feelings that accompany these activities can be an end in themselves. Her partner, however, may need to masturbate more frequently than before.

The sexual desires of men are also affected by many factors in pregnancy. These include the previous relationship with the partner, acceptance of the pregnancy, attitudes toward the partner's change of appearance, and concern about hurting the expectant mother or baby. Some men may withdraw from sexual contact because of a belief that sex with a pregnant woman is immoral. This may be especially true for the couple whose religious beliefs teach that sexual intercourse is only for procreation. Some men find it difficult to view their partners as sexually appealing while they are adjusting to the concept of her as a mother. On the other hand, some men find their partner's pregnancy arousing and experience feelings of increased happiness, intimacy, and closeness (Reamy & White 1985).

The expectant couple should be aware of their changing sexual desires, the normality of these changes, and the importance of communicating these changes to each other so that they can make nurturing adaptations. The nurse has an important role in helping the expecting couple adapt. The couple must feel free to express concerns about sexual activity, and the nurse must be able to respond and give anticipatory guidance in a comfortable manner (See Teaching Guide—Sexual Activity During Pregnancy).

Occasionally a woman initiates discussion about her sexual concerns, especially if she has good rapport with the nurse. More often, the nurse must broach the subject. A statement such as "Many couples experience changes in sexual desire during pregnancy" can initiate the discussion. This generalization can be followed by an exploration of the couple's personal experience. The question "What kind of changes have you experienced?" stimulates discussion more effectively than "Have you experienced any changes?"

The presence of both partners during sexual counseling is most effective in fostering communication between them.

Dental Care

Proper dental hygiene is important in pregnancy. In spite of such discomforts as nausea and vomiting, gum hypertrophy and tenderness, possible ptyalism, and heartburn, regular oral hygiene must not be neglected.

The pregnant woman is encouraged to have a dental checkup early in her pregnancy. Women who neglect to obtain dental care prior to pregnancy become aware of dental problems during this time and thus may associate these problems with pregnancy. General dental repair and extractions can be done during pregnancy, preferably under local anesthetic. The woman should inform her dentist of her pregnancy so that she is not exposed to teratogenic substances. Dental x-ray examinations and extensive dental work should be delayed when possible until after birth. Extensive dental care during pregnancy requires consultation between the dentist and the maternal health care professional.

Immunizations

All women of childbearing age need to be fully aware of the risks of receiving specific immunizations if pregnancy is possible. Expectant women, especially those who intend to travel throughout the world, should be aware of the immunizations that are contraindicated during pregnancy. In addition, it is important that expectant women clearly understand the recommendations that are made regarding other immunizations, such as those for influenza epidemics.

Immunizations with attenuated live viruses, such as rubella vaccine, should not be given in pregnancy because of the possible harmful effect of the live viruses on the developing embryo. Vaccinations using killed viruses can be used. Recommendations for immunizations during pregnancy are given in Table 14–5

Teratogenic Substances

Substances that adversely affect the normal growth and development of the fetus are called **teratogens**. Many of these effects are readily apparent at birth, but others may not be identified for years. A well-known example is the development of cervical cancer in adolescent females whose mothers took diethylstilbestrol (DES) during pregnancy.

Many suspected teratogenic substances exist. The harmful effects of others, such as some pesticides and expo-

---

Table 14–5 Summary of Recommendations for Immunization During Pregnancy

Live Virus Vaccines	**Inactivated Bacterial Vaccines**	**Hyperimmune Globulins**
Measles—contraindicated	Cholera—to meet international travel requirements	Hepatitis B—postexposure prophylaxis: give along with hepatitis B vaccine initially, then vaccine alone at 1 and 6 months
Mumps—contraindicated		
Poliomyelitis—not routine; increased risk exposure	Meningococcus—same as nonpregnant	Rabies—postexposure prophylaxis
	Plague—selective vaccination of exposed persons	Tetanus—postexposure prophylaxis
Rubella—contraindicated		
Yellow fever—travel to high-risk areas only	Typhoid—travel to endemic areas	Varicella—same as nonpregnant
Inactivated Virus Vaccines	**Toxoids**	**Pooled Immune Serum Globulins**
Influenza—serious underlying diseases	Tetanus-Diphtheria—same as nonpregnant	Hepatitis A—postexposure prophylaxis
Rabies—same as nonpregnant		Measles—postexposure prophylaxis

Modified from the American College of Obstetricians and Gynecologists. "Immunization During Pregnancy." ACOG Technical Bulletin No. 64, Washington D.C. May 1982.

sure to radiation (x rays, radioactive iodine, and atomic fallout) in the first trimester of pregnancy, have been documented.

Some environmental factors are also suspected to be teratogenic, but due to the complexities of the environment, causal relationships are difficult to demonstrate. For example, expectant women who live in high-altitude areas have been found to have an increased incidence of small-for-gestational-age babies.

Medications are perhaps the most likely documented teratogens, but other factors can also harm the fetus, including certain infections such as rubella, syphilis, herpesvirus type 2, toxoplasmosis, and cytomegalovirus (CMV). Hyperthermia (temperature greater than 39.4C [102.9F]) lasting 5 hours or more, especially if it occurs in the critical period of organ development, can cause CNS disorders such as anencephaly and meningomyelocele (Shepard 1984).

During pregnancy, women need to have adequate information available and a realistic perspective on potential environmental hazards. Factors that are suspected to be hazardous to the general population should obviously be avoided if possible. The expectant woman must remember that factors present in the environment for lengthy periods of time, such as pollution, have not resulted in epidemics of newborn defects.

Much research is being conducted on medications, alcohol, and cigarettes and their roles as teratogenic substances. This information is discussed in the following sections.

Medications

CRITICAL THINKING

What approaches might be effective in assessing medication use in a pregnant woman?

The prevalent use of medication in pregnancy is of great concern. Studies have demonstrated that the average pregnant woman takes many more medications than commonly believed, including over-the-counter (OTC) drugs as well as prescription drugs. Medications sold over the counter can be as dangerous as prescription drugs. For example, aspirin is known to inhibit prostaglandin synthesis. This may result in prolonged pregnancy or labor if the woman has used aspirin regularly. Aspirin also interferes with platelet functioning, which may increase the risk of bleeding antepartally or at birth (Niebyl 1990).

Over-the-counter cold and allergy preparations often contain a mixture of ingredients that may include an antipyretic, a cough suppressant, an expectorant, a decongestant, an antihistamine, an anticholinergic, and a topical anesthetic! When medication is needed, careful practitioners recommend preparations containing the fewest possible ingredients.

A major difficulty, even for women who attempt to eliminate all medication in pregnancy, involves ingestion of potential teratogenic medications for therapeutic purposes before pregnancy is diagnosed. It can be a problem for any woman, but especially for those with irregular menstrual cycles or for those who, because of great faith in their method of contraception, do not anticipate pregnancy. The classic period of teratogenesis extends from day 31 after the LMP (17 days after fertilization) to day 71 (54 days after fertilization) (Niebyl 1990). Table 14–6 identifies possible effects of selected drugs on the fetus or neonate.

To provide information for care givers and clients, the Food and Drug Administration has developed a classification system for medications administered during pregnancy:

Category A: Controlled studies in women have demonstrated no associated fetal risk. Few drugs fall into this category.

Category B: Animal studies show no risk but there are no controlled studies in women, or animal studies indicate a risk but controlled human studies fail to demonstrate a risk. Heparin and the penicillins fall into this category.

Category C: No adequate studies, either in animals or women, are available, or animal studies show teratogenic effects but no controlled studies in women are available. Many drugs fall into this category, which, because of the lack of information, is a problematic one for care givers. Epinephrine, beta–blockers, and acyclovir fall into this category.

Category D: Evidence of human fetal risk does exist, but the benefits of the drug in certain situations are thought to outweigh the risks. Examples of drugs in this category include tetracycline, vincristine, lithium, and hydrochlorothiazide.

Category X: The demonstrated fetal risks clearly outweigh any possible benefit. Examples of drugs in this category include isoretinoin (Accutane), estrogens, and clomiphene.

If a woman has taken a drug in category D or X, she should be informed of the risks associated with that drug and her alternatives. Similarly, a woman who has taken a drug in the safer categories can be reassured (Cunningham et al 1989).

As previously indicated, the first trimester is the time for greatest concern about gross structural defects in the fetus because it is the time of organ development. The effects of the medication on the fetus are influenced by medication dosage, timing of ingestion in relation to specific organ development, maternal absorption and metabolism, molecular size, lipid solubility, protein binding, and electrical charge. Some medications are harmful only if ingested in sufficient amounts for extended periods (Cunningham et al 1989).

Some medications are known to have teratogenic effects when ingested in the second and third trimesters.

Table 14–6 Possible Effects of Selected Drugs on the Fetus and Neonate *

Maternal drug	Effects on fetus and neonate
Risk outweighs benefits if the following drugs are given in the first trimester:	
Thalidomide	Limb, auricle, eye, and visceral malformations
Tolbutamide (Orinase)	Increase of anomalies
Streptomycin	Eighth nerve damage; multiple skeletal anomalies
Tetracycline	Inhibition of bone growth; syndactyly; discoloration of teeth
Iodide	Congenital goiter; hypothyroidism; mental retardation
Methotrexate	Multiple anomalies
Diethylstilbestrol	Clear-cell adenocarcinoma of the vagina and cervix; genital tract anomalies
Warfarin (Coumadin)	Skeletal and facial anomalies; mental retardation
Risk vs. benefits uncertain in the first trimester:	
Gentamicin	Eighth cranial nerve damage
Kanamycin	Eighth cranial nerve damage
Lithium	Goiter; eye anomalies; cleft palate
Barbiturates	Increase of anomalies
Quinine	Increase of anomalies
Septra or Bactrim	Cleft palate
Cytotoxic drugs	Increase of anomalies
Benefit outweighs risk in the first trimester:	
Clomiphene (Clomid)	Increase of anomalies; neural tube defects; Down syndrome
Glucocorticoids	Cleft palate; cardiac defects
General anesthesia	Increase of anomalies
Tricyclic antidepressants	CNS and limb malformations
Sulfonamides	Cleft palate; facial and skeletal defects
Antacids	Increase of anomalies
Salicylates	Central nervous system, visceral, and skeletal malformations
Acetaminophen	None
Heparin	None
Terbutaline	None
Phenothiazines	None
Insulin	Skeletal malformations
Penicillins	None
Chloramphenicol	None
Isoniazid (INH)	Increase of anomalies

Adapted from Howard FM, Hill JM: Obstet Gynecol Surv 1979;34:643.

For example, tetracycline taken in late pregnancy is associated with staining of teeth in children and has been shown to retard limb growth in premature infants; ingestion should be avoided during pregnancy. Sulfonamides taken in the last few weeks of pregnancy are known to compete with bilirubin attachment of protein-binding sites, resulting in jaundice in the newborn (Knoth & Dette 1985).

Other medications affect the fetus in much the same way that an adult is affected by an overdose. For example, the use of anticoagulants to treat thromboembolism in the mother can interfere with clotting factors in the fetus. However, this risk is lessened by frequent monitoring of prothrombin time in the mother, accompanied by appropriate changes in dosages of the anticoagulants. Because heparin does not cross the placenta, it is safer for the fetus than warfarin (Coumadin) and other anticoagulants. Moreover, warfarin is associated with multiple congenital anomalies when taken in early pregnancy (Niebyl 1990).

Many pregnant women need medication for definitive therapeutic purposes, such as the treatment of infections, allergies, or multiple other pathologic processes. In these situations, the problem of what to prescribe can be extremely complex. Known teratogenic agents are not prescribed and usually can be replaced by medications considered safe.

All medication should be avoided if possible. If no alternative exists, it is wisest to select a well-known medication rather than a newer drug whose potential teratogenic effects may not be known. When possible, the oral form of the drug should be used, and it should be prescribed in the lowest possible therapeutic dose for the shortest time possible. Finally, the care giver should carefully consider the multiple components of the medication (Whipkey et al 1984).

Consumers today are more aware of the potential risk of taking medications during pregnancy. They are asking for information and physicians are being held accountable to provide it.

A woman clearly has a right to the most comprehensive information available concerning medications. The nurse can assist her by suggesting appropriate references and helping her research information. Some fine reference books on drugs and pregnancy are currently available and should be part of the library of every office and clinic that provides prenatal care.

The nurse should also remind the woman of the importance of checking with her physician about medications she was taking when pregnancy occurred and about any nonprescription drugs she is contemplating using. A good rule to follow is that the advantage of using a particular medication must outweigh the risks. Any medication with possible teratogenic effects must be avoided.

Smoking

Infants of mothers who smoke tend to have a lower birth weight and a higher incidence of preterm birth than infants of mothers who do not smoke. These findings increase significantly as maternal age increases (Wen et al 1990). This may be related to the fact that older women have probably been smoking longer and may have some chronic vascular disease; they may consume more cigarettes daily, thus increasing their dose; or they may be more sensitive to the vasoconstrictive effects of cigarettes (Wen et al 1990). In addition, mothers who smoke have an increased risk of spontaneous abortion, placenta previa, abruptio placentae, and premature rupture of the membranes. This risk is related to the number of cigarettes smoked (Niebyl 1990).

The specific mechanism of smoking's effect on the fetus is not known. Smoking appears to decrease placental blood flow and plasma volume. In addition, changes found in the placentas of smokers suggest toxicity related to elements in tobacco smoke and ischemia due to the vasoconstrictive effects of nicotine on uterine vessels. Smoking may also interfere with maternal absorption or metabolism of calcium, vitamin C, vitamin B_{12}, and perhaps vitamins A, B_6, and B_1 (Aaronson & MacNee 1989).

Fewer women smoke today than did 20 years ago, and women who do smoke tend to stop smoking or at least reduce their intake once pregnancy is confirmed. When asked their reasons for changing their behavior, women most frequently cited concern for their child, concern for themselves, or social pressure (Waterson & Murray-Lyon 1989). Unfortunately, a majority of women who quit smoking during pregnancy do resume following birth, although this percentage is lower for women who quit early in pregnancy. This finding suggests that although women are aware of the potential impact of smoking on the fetus, they may be less knowledgeable about the effects of passive smoke on the baby (Fingerhut 1990).

As primary client educator, the prenatal nurse has a wonderful opportunity to provide individual or group teaching to help pregnant women reduce their smoking. Studies demonstrate that any decrease in smoking during pregnancy will result in a better fetal outcome. Pregnancy may be a difficult time for a woman to stop smoking, but she should be encouraged to reduce the number of cigarettes she smokes daily. The need to protect her unborn child may dramatically increase her motivation. The nurse can also provide information about the harmful effects of passive smoking so that the woman can encourage those close to her to limit their smoking.

Alcohol

Alcohol is now considered the primary teratogen in the Western world (Abel & Sokol 1988a). Fetuses of women who are heavy drinkers are at increased risk for developing **fetal alcohol syndrome (FAS)** (see Chapter 31). Worldwide, the incidence of FAS is between one and three per 1000 live births; however, certain populations such as Native Americans, Hispanics, and blacks, have a higher incidence (Stokes 1989).

The effects of moderate consumption of alcohol during pregnancy are not clearly known, but research suggests there is an increased incidence of lower birth weight and of some neurologic effects, such as attention-deficit disorder. Evidence suggests that the risk of teratogenic effects increases proportionately with increased average daily intake of alcohol. Pregnant women who have an occasional drink should not be unduly alarmed about the effect it will have on the fetus. However, binge drinking has been associated with fetal malformations (Cunningham et al 1989).

Alcohol passes the placental barrier within minutes after consumption, with fetal blood alcohol levels becoming equivalent to maternal blood alcohol levels. The effects of alcohol consumption vary according to the stage of fetal development. During the first trimester, alcohol probably alters embryonic development; throughout pregnancy, alcohol may disrupt the metabolism of protein, carbohydrates, and lipids, thereby interfering with cell division and growth; in the third trimester, the time of most rapid brain growth, alcohol may alter CNS development (Aaronson & MacNee 1989). The risk of neurologic damage is lessened if heavy drinking ceases in the third trimester, while decreased consumption of alcohol in midpregnancy is associated with a lower incidence of growth retardation. Malnutrition, common in heavy drinkers, and alcohol-induced maternal hypoglycemia may also contribute to fetal problems (Niebyl 1990).

Once women are aware of the pregnancy, most decrease their alcohol consumption because of concern for the fetus. In fact, women who consume alcohol reduce their drinking proportionately more than women who smoke reduce their smoking. This may be due to the habit-forming nature of smoking and to the fact that fetal alcohol syndrome has been so widely publicized (Rubin et al 1986).

Assessment of a woman's alcoholic intake should be a

chief part of each woman's medical history, with questions asked in a direct and nonjudgmental manner. All women should be counseled about the role of alcohol in pregnancy. When pregnant women become aware of the risk of alcohol to the fetus, most usually attempt to modify their alcoholic consumption. If heavy consumption is involved, these women should be referred early to an alcoholic treatment program. Since the drug disulfiram (Antabuse)—often used in the treatment of alcoholism—is suspected as a teratogenic agent, a woman in such a program should inform her counselor if she becomes pregnant.

Counseling about the effects of alcohol during pregnancy has been effective and should, of course, continue. Since the most profound impact of alcohol occurs in the first weeks after conception, nurses and other health care providers will see the most dramatic decrease in the effects of alcohol during pregnancy by increasing their teaching efforts in the period prior to conception. Teaching must take place in family-planning clinics, in preconception clinics, and during regular health care maintenance (Wright & Toplis 1986).

Caffeine

Current research reveals no evidence that caffeine increases reproductive or teratogenic risk in humans (Cunningham 1989). Previous studies that suggested a possible risk did not control well for the use of alcohol and tobacco (Niebyl 1990). During the third trimester, the half-life of caffeine triples. Thus, the same daily caffeine intake results in much higher blood levels. Until more definitive data is available, nurses should advise women of common sources of caffeine including coffee, tea, colas, and chocolate and suggest they use good judgment in moderating or limiting their caffeine intake.

Marijuana

Nearly 15% of pregnant women use marijuana (Abel & Sohol 1988b). The prevalence of marijuana use in our society raises many concerns about its effect on the fetus. Doing research on marijuana use in pregnancy is difficult, however, because it is an illegal drug. Unreliability of reporting, lack of a representative population, inability to determine strength or composition of the marijuana used, presence of herbicides, and use of other drugs at the same time are major factors complicating the research being done.

It is known that women who smoke or consume alcohol decrease their smoking or alcohol consumption once pregnancy is diagnosed. A recent study also included a comparison of heavy marijuana users with those who smoke and consume alcohol. Although the women who smoked cigarettes and consumed alcohol decreased their intake during pregnancy, the marijuana smokers did not alter their pattern of use during pregnancy (Fried et al 1985).

Perhaps the lack of conclusive results about the effects of marijuana in pregnancy lends a false sense of security.

Cocaine

A woman who uses cocaine during pregnancy is at increased risk for PIH, abruptio placentae, tachycardia, cardiovascular failure, intracerebral bleeding, paranoia, and death. Her fetus or neonate is at increased risk for IUGR, preterm birth, congenital malformations (CNS, cardiac, and genitourinary), behavioral abnormalities, fetal distress, and stillbirth (Dombrowski & Sokol 1990). These infants may show symptoms including poor feeding, increased respiratory and heart rates, irritability, irregular sleep patterns, and diarrhea (Newald 1986). (For further discussion see Chapter 18.)

As cocaine becomes more widely used by women of childbearing age, health care providers must become alert to early signs of cocaine use. It is often difficult for a nurse or physician to face the fact that a woman with whom they have a relationship may be using cocaine, but ongoing alertness and an open, nonjudgmental approach are important in early detection. Urine screening for cocaine is valuable, but because cocaine is metabolized rapidly, the drug screen is negative within 24 to 48 hours after cocaine use. Thus, it is probable that many abusers are missed. It is possible to use radioimmunoassays (RIA) of neonatal meconium to detect cocaine. This tool is valuable in detecting newborns of cocaine-abusing women (Dombrowski & Sokol 1990).

Maternal Assessment of Fetal Activity

Assessment of fetal movement patterns has been used as a screening procedure in the evaluation of fetal status since 1971 when the clinical significance of various types of fetal activity was first described. Clinicians now generally agree that vigorous fetal activity provides reassurance of fetal well-being and that marked decrease in activity or cessation of movement may indicate possible fetal compromise requiring immediate follow-up evaluation. The Cardiff-Count-to-Ten method is a noninvasive technique that permits the pregnant woman to monitor fetal well-being easily and without expense and then record her findings.

Sadovsky (1985a) noted that, although there is considerable variation among individuals, the average number of daily movements rises from about 200 at 20 weeks to a maximum of 575 at 32 weeks and gradually decreases to an average of 282 at term. In women with a multiple gestation, daily fetal movements are significantly higher. Connors et al (1988) found that the fetus has 90-minute rest and activity cycles during the last ten weeks of gestation.

Fetal activity is affected by many factors, including sound, drugs, cigarette smoking, sleep states of the fetus, blood glucose levels, and time of day. The expectant mother's perception of fetal movements and her commitment to completing a movement record may vary. When the woman understands the purpose of the assessment, how to complete the form, whom to call with questions, and what to report, and has the opportunity for follow-up during each visit, she will also see this as an important activity. (See Teaching Guide—What to Tell the Pregnant Woman About Assessing Fetal Activity.)

Case Study

Pamela Paulson is a 24-year-old gravida 2 para 0, whose first pregnancy ended in spontaneous abortion a year ago. Pam is a secretary for a construction firm and plans to continue working as long as possible. Her husband, Steve, is an electrician and has a fairly stable year-round income. Mrs Paulson was first seen in the clinic when she was nine weeks pregnant. Her first contact was Marie Carlson, an RN. Ms Carlson checked Mrs Paulson's vital signs, weight, and urine specimen; drew blood for laboratory tests; and completed the health history. She then asked Mrs Paulson if she had any questions or concerns. Mrs Paulson revealed that her pregnancy had been planned, and both she and her husband were eager to have a baby. However, she was constantly afraid that she would do something that might result in another miscarriage. Ms Carlson reassured her that it was not unusual for a woman to have one miscarriage. She then reviewed some of the big risk factors and asked Mrs Paulson if there was anything in her life-style or environment that might be a risk factor. Mrs Paulson stated she was an avid swimmer and generally stopped at the YWCA on her way home from work to swim. However, she had given that up once she suspected she was pregnant for fear of causing another miscarriage. Ms Carlson reassured her that as long as she was not having any bleeding or other problems that might interfere, swimming was a wonderful exercise that she certainly could continue. She was advised to monitor her level of fatigue to avoid overdoing it. They discussed Mrs Paulson's life-style further, and the nurse was able to reassure her that it was a healthy one. The remainder of the visit went well. Mrs Paulson's physician, Alice Warren, reported that the physical exam was normal and her pelvis appeared large enough for successful vaginal birth. Mrs Paulson was started on a vitamin and iron supplement; the warning signs of potential problems in pregnancy were reviewed; and she left with literature to read about all other aspects of pregnancy.

The early months of Mrs Paulson's pregnancy went smoothly. She did not suffer from nausea, and the urinary frequency she experienced eased in her fourth month. She continued prenatal visits every four weeks. As Mrs Paulson began wearing maternity clothes, her fear of miscarriage abated.

Mrs Paulson felt the first flutterings of fetal movement at 19 weeks, and the fetal heart tones (FHT) were auscultated a week later. She persuaded her husband to accompany her on a prenatal visit, and he obviously enjoyed hearing the baby's heartbeat with the Doppler.

In her seventh month, Mrs Paulson began to develop varicose veins in her legs and had problems with hemorrhoids. Ms Carlson and Mrs Paulson discussed her schedule and habits, identifying some changes she might make to ease her discomfort. Mrs Paulson began wearing maternity support hose to work and walking around her office every hour. During her breaks and at lunch, she lay on her side in the staff lounge with her feet elevated. She continued her evening swims. A review of Mrs Paulson's diet showed it had sufficient fiber, fresh fruit, and vegetables. She also drank several glasses of water every day. Nevertheless, constipation was still a problem. Ms Carlson reported these findings to Dr Warren and she prescribed a mild stool softener. Mrs Paulson continued to follow this regimen, and her symptoms eased.

At 37 weeks, Mrs Paulson began experiencing urinary frequency again, and physical assessment showed that lightening had occurred. Mrs Paulson reported to Ms Carlson that the nursery was ready and her suitcase was packed. She and her husband had taken the childbirth preparation classes offered at the clinic, and she felt well prepared.

Mrs Paulson and Ms Carlson spent some time talking about what being a parent meant, and Ms Carlson gave Mrs Paulson some interesting articles on adjusting to a new baby. They also spoke about some of the sexual changes Mrs Paulson might experience. At the end of the conversation, Mrs Paulson said, "I'm so glad you brought this up. I wondered what sex would be like afterward but felt a little embarrassed about asking."

One day before her EDB, Mrs Paulson went into labor and, following a 12-hour labor, gave birth to a 7 lb 2 oz son—Ryan Erik Paulson.

Evaluation

Throughout the antepartal period, evaluation is an essential part of effective nursing care. As nurses ask questions of the pregnant woman and her family or make observations of physical changes, they are evaluating the results of previous interventions. In evaluating the effectiveness of the interventions, the nurse should not be afraid to try creative solutions if they are logical and carefully thought out. This is especially important in dealing with families from other cultures. If a practice is important to a woman and not harmful, the culturally sensitive nurse will not discourage it.

In completing an evaluation, the nurse must also recognize situations that require referral for further evaluation. For example, a woman who has gained four pounds in one week does not require counseling about nutrition, she needs further assessment for pregnancy-induced hypertension (PIH). The nurse who has a sound knowledge of theory will recognize this and act immediately.

TEACHING GUIDE

What to Tell the Pregnant Woman About Assessing Fetal Activity

Assessment: The nurse focuses on the woman's prior knowledge and former use of fetal movement assessment methods, the week of gestation, and her communciation and ability to understand and process information.

Nursing Diagnosis: The key nursing diagnosis will probably be: Knowledge deficit related to fetal movement assessment methods.

Nursing Plan and Implementation:

Client Goals: At the completion of the teaching session the woman will be able to:

- Identify types of fetal assessment methods, reasons for assessment, how to accomplish the assessment, and methods of record keeping.

- Demonstrate the use of a movement record.

- List resources to call if questions arise.

- Discuss the importance of bringing the movement record to each prenatal visit.

Teaching Plan

General Content: The expectant woman needs to know that fetal movements are first felt around 18 weeks' gestation. From that time the fetal movements get stronger and easier to detect. A slowing or stopping of fetal movement may be an indication that the baby needs evaluation. The normal amount of movement varies considerably; however, most healthy babies move at least 10 times in 12 hours. The nurse teaches the woman a fetal assessment method and encourages her to complete the record each day. The record will be discussed at each prenatal visit and questions may be addressed at that time if desired.

Daily Fetal Movement Record (DFMR) (Figure 14–11): The low-risk woman begins at 27 weeks' gestation. The fetal movements are counted twice a day for 20–30 minutes each session. Five or six movements during each period of counting is looked on as reassuring.	**When to Contact the Care Provider:** If the woman has questions or concerns. If there are fewer than 10 fetal movements in a 12-hour period OR no movements in the morning OR less than three fetal movements in eight hours.	**What Happens Next:** The care provider will probably suggest a NST to further evaluate the baby. Additional testing may include a CST, tests for pulmonary maturity, and ultrasound (Gantes et al 1985, Chez & Sadovsky 1984).	**Teaching Method:** Verbal presentation Provide a sample DFMR.
The high-risk woman begins at 27 weeks of gestation. The fetal movements are counted three times a day for 30 minutes. Five or six movements during each period is desired. If there are less than three movements in a counting period the woman should continue counting for an hour or more.	Same as above		Verbal presentation Demonstrate how to palpate abdomen. Demonstrate how to record movements on DFMR scoring card.

(continued)

TEACHING GUIDE (continued)

Teaching Plan

Regardless of risk category, it will be advantageous for the woman to schedule the counting periods about one hour past eating and to combine the counting period with rest. A side-lying position provides optimal circulation to the uterus-placenta-fetus unit. In addition, the baby's movements are felt more readily while lying on the side. Later in the pregnancy, some women may be bothered by indigestion after eating. In this case they can prop up the upper body but still maintain a side-lying position.

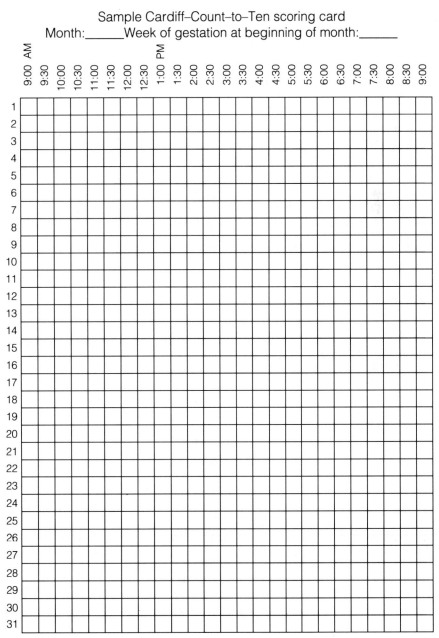

Figure 14–11   Fetal movement assessment method: The Cardiff-Count-to-Ten scoring card (adaptation).

(continued)

TEACHING GUIDE (continued)

Teaching Plan

**Cardiff-Count-to-Ten
(Figure 14–11):**

The woman begins these assessments in the 27th week of gestation. At 9:00 each morning, the woman begins counting the baby's movements. When there have been ten movements, an X is placed at the appropriate time on the card (Clark & Britton 1985; Eggertsen & Benedetti 1987).

When there are questions or concerns.

If there are fewer than ten movements by 9:00 PM (12 hours).

If overall the baby's movements are slowing and it takes much longer each day to note ten movements.

Same as above

Verbal presentation
Demonstrate how to record movements on Cardiff-Count-to-Ten scoring card.
Watch woman fill out record as examples are provided.

Evaluation: The nurse may evaluate learning by having the woman explain the method to the nurse and by asking the woman to fill the card in using a fictitious situation. At each prenatal visit, the expectant woman's record is reviewed and this provides another opportunity for evaluation of learning.

The ongoing and cyclic nature of the nursing process is especially evident in the prenatal setting. However, throughout the course of pregnancy certain criteria can be used to determine the quality of care provided. In essence, nursing care has been effective if:

- The common discomforts of pregnancy are quickly identified and are relieved or lessened effectively.

- The woman is able to discuss the physiologic and psychologic changes of pregnancy.

- The woman implements appropriate self-care measures if they are indicated during pregnancy.

- The woman avoids substances and situations that pose a risk to her well-being or that of her child.

- The woman seeks regular prenatal care.

❈ ❈

KEY CONCEPTS

The nursing process can be used effectively to plan and provide care to women during pregnancy.

Provision of anticipatory guidance about childbirth, the postpartum period, and childrearing is a primary responsibility of the nurse caring for women in an antepartal setting.

The nurse assesses the expectant father's knowledge level and intended degree of participation and then works with the couple to help ensure a satisfying experience.

Culturally based practices and proscribed activities may have a major impact on the childbearing family.

The common discomforts of pregnancy occur as a result of physiologic and anatomic changes. The nurse provides the woman with information about self-care activities aimed at reducing or relieving discomfort.

To make appropriate self-care choices and ensure healthful habits, a pregnant woman requires accurate information about a range of subjects from exercise to sexual activity, from bathing to immunizations.

Teratogenic substances are substances that adversely affect the normal growth and development of the fetus.

A pregnant woman should avoid taking medications or using over-the-counter preparations during pregnancy.

Evidence exists that smoking, consuming alcohol, or using social drugs during pregnancy may be harmful to the fetus.

Maternal assessment of fetal activity keeps the woman "in touch" with her fetus and provides ongoing assessment of fetal status.

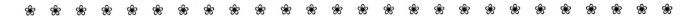

References

Aaronson LS, MacNee CL: Tobacco, alcohol, and caffeine use during pregnancy. *JOGNN* 1989; 18(4):279.

Abel EL, Sokol RJ: Alcohol use in pregnancy. In: *Drug Use in Pregnancy,* 2nd ed. Niebyl JR (editor): Philadelphia: Lea & Febiger, 1988a.

Abel EL, Sokol RJ: Marijuana and cocaine use during pregnancy. In: *Drug Use in Pregnancy,* 2nd ed. Niebyl JR (editor): Philadelphia: Lea & Febiger, 1988b.

American College of Obstetricians and Gynecologists (ACOG): *Exercise During Pregnancy and the Postnatal Period.* Washington DC: ACOG, 1985.

Barry M, Bia F: Pregnancy and travel. *JAMA* February 1989; 261:728.

Bernhardt JH: Potential workplace hazards to reproductive health: Information for primary prevention. *JOGNN* 1990; 19(1):53.

Brown MS: A cross-cultural look at pregnancy, labor, and delivery. *JOGNN* September/October 1976; 5:35.

Carrington BW: The Afro American. In: *Culture, Childbearing, Health Professionals.* Clark AL (editor). Philadelphia: Davis, 1978.

Connors G et al: Maternally perceived fetal activity from twenty-four weeks' gestation to term in normal and at-risk pregnancies. *Am J Obstet Gynecol* February 1988; 158:294.

Cunningham FG et al: *Williams Obstetrics,* 18th ed. Norwalk CT: Appleton & Lange, 1989.

DiIorio C: The management of nausea and vomiting in pregnancy. *Nurse Pract* May 1988; 13(5):23.

Dombrowski MP, Sokol RJ: Cocaine and abruption. *Contemp OB/GYN* April 1990; 35:13.

Evaneshko V: Tonawanda Seneca childbearing culture. In: *Anthropology of Human Birth.* Kay MA (editor): Philadelphia: Davis, 1982.

Farris LS: Approaches to caring for the American Indian maternity patient. *MCN* March/April 1976; 1:81.

Fenlon A et al: *Getting Ready for Childbirth,* 2nd ed. Boston; Little, Brown, 1986.

Fingerhut LA et al: Smoking before, during, and after pregnancy. *Am J Public Health* May 1990; 80(5):541.

Fishbein EG, Phillips M: How safe is exercise during pregnancy? *JOGNN* 1990; 19(1):45.

Freyder SC: Exercising while pregnant. *J Ortho Sports Phys Ther* March 1989; 10:358.

Fried PA et al: Marijuana use during pregnancy and decreased length of gestation. *Am J Obstet Gynecol* September 1984; 150:23.

Hoffman JB: A suggested treatment for inverted nipples. *Am J Obstet Gynecol* 1953; 66:346.

Hollingsworth AO, et al: The refugees and childbearing: What to expect. *RN* November 1980; 43:45.

Horn BM: Northwest coast Indians: The Muckleshoot. In: *Anthropology of Human Birth.* Kay MA (editor). Philadelphia: Davis, 1982.

Kay MA: The Mexican American. In: *Culture, Childbearing, Health Professionals.* Clark AL (editor): Philadelphia: Davis, 1978.

Klebanoff MA et al: Coitus during pregnancy: Is it safe? *Lancet* October 1984; 2:914.

Knothe H, Dette GA: Antibiotics in pregnancy: Toxicity and teratogenicity. *Infection* 1985; 13:49.

Kochenour NK: Normal pregnancy and prenatal care. In *Danforth's Obstetrics and Gynecology,* 6th ed. Scott JR et al (editors). Philadelphia: Lippincott, 1990.

Krozy RE, McColgan JJ: Auto safety . . . Pregnancy and the newborn. *JOGNN* January/February 1985; 14:11.

Launer LJ et al: The effect of maternal work on fetal growth and duration of pregnancy: A prospective study. *Br J Obstet Gynaecol* January 1990; 97:62.

Leaf DA: Exercise during pregnancy. *Postgrad Med* 1989; 85(1):233.

Masters WH, Johnson VE: *Human Sexual Response.* Boston: Little, Brown, 1966.

McDonald A et al: Fetal death and work in pregnancy. *Br J Ind Med* 1988; 45:148.

Niebyl JR: Teratology and drugs in pregnancy and lactation. In: *Danforth's Obstetrics and Gynecology,* 6th ed. Scott JR et al (editors). Philadelphia: Lippincott, 1990.

Paolone AM, Worthington S: Cautions and advice on exercise during pregnancy. *Contemp OB/GYN* May 1985; 25:150.

Paisley JP, Mellion MB: Exercise during pregnancy. *Am Fam Phys* November 1988; 38(5):143.

Rayburn WF: OTC drugs and pregnancy. *Perinatol Neonatol* September/October 1984; 8:21.

Reamy K, White SE: Sexuality in pregnancy and the puerperium: A review. *Obstet Gynecol* 1985; 40(1):1.

Sady SP et al: Aerobic exercise during pregnancy: Special considerations. *Sports Med* June 1989; 7(6):357.

Sevcovic L: Traditions of pregnancy which influence maternity care of the Navajo people. In: *Transcultural Nursing.* Leininger M (editor). New York: Masson, 1979.

Shepard TH: Teratogens: An update. *Hosp Pract* January 1984, p 191.

Spadt SK et al: Experiential classes for siblings-to-be. *MCN* May/June 1990; 15:184.

Stokes EJ: Alcohol abuse screening: What to ask your female patient. *Female Patient* December 1989; 14:17.

Stolte K: Nursing diagnosis and the childbearing woman. *MCN* January/February 1986; 13:13.

Varner M: General medical and surgical diseases in pregnancy. In: *Danforth's Obstetrics and Gynecology,* 6th ed. Scott JR et al (editors) Philadelphia: Lippincott, 1990.

Waterson SJ, Murray-Lyon IM: Drinking and smoking patterns among women attending an antenatal clinic: II. During pregnancy. *Alcohol Alcohol* 1989; 24(2):163.

Wen SW et al: Smoking, maternal age, fetal growth, and gestational age at delivery. *Am J Obstet Gynecol* 1990; 162:53.

Whipkey RR et al: Drug use in pregnancy. *Ann Emerg Med* 1984; 13:346.

Wright JT, Toplis PJ: Alcohol in pregnancy. *Br J Obstet Gynaecol* March 1986; 93:201.

Additional Readings

Amstey MS: Immunization in pregnancy. *Contemp OB/GYN* October 1989; 34:15.

Freidman JM et al: Potential human teratogenicity of frequently prescribed drugs. *Obstet Gynecol* April 1990; 75:594.

Hammond TL et al: The use of automobile safety restraint systems during pregnancy. *JOGNN* July/August 1990; 19:339.

Karboski, JA: Medication selection for pregnant women. *Female Patient* May 1991; 16:15.

Poland ML et al: Quality of prenatal care; selected social, behavioral, and biomedical factors; and birth weight. *Am J Obstet Gynecol* April 1990; 75:607.

Popkess S: Wellness nursing diagnosis: To be or not to be? *Nurs Diagnosis* January/March 1991; 2:19.

Rosen MG et al: Caring for our future: A report by the expert panel on the content of prenatal care. *Obstet Gynecol* May 1991; 77:82.

Starn J, Niederhauser V: An MCN model for nursing diagnosis to focus intervention. *MCN* May/June 1990; 15:180.

Van Denter MC: Ptyalism in pregnant women. *JOGNN* May/June 1991; 20:206.

CHAPTER 15

The Expectant Family:

Age-Related Considerations

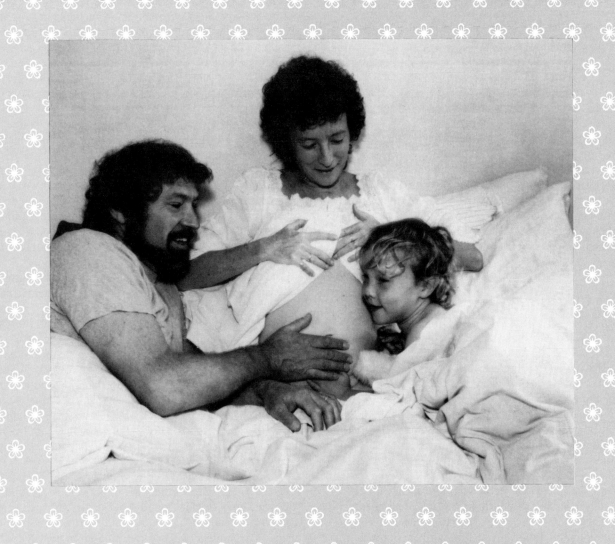

OBJECTIVES

Summarize the physical, psychologic, and sociologic risks faced by an adolescent who is pregnant.

Describe the reactions and needs of the adolescent father.

Discuss the reactions of the adolescent's family to her pregnancy.

Formulate a plan of care to meet the needs of a pregnant adolescent.

Identify the medical risks faced by an older expectant couple.

Relate the concerns of older expectant couples to their adaptation to pregnancy.

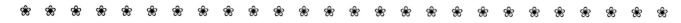

I am a freshman in college and so is my daughter. I had her when I was 15 and that forced me to grow up in a hurry. For years I've thought about being a nurse and now is my chance. Please understand, my daughter is very precious to me, but a part of me knows that if I had it to do over, I would change so much of my life—if only I had known!

Pregnancy is a challenging time for all women as they adjust to the changes they experience and prepare to assume a new role as mother of one child or of two or more children. Even if a woman chooses to terminate her pregnancy, the very fact of being pregnant has a lasting effect on her. Age at the time of pregnancy may be a factor in a woman's adjustment, both physically and psychologically. This chapter explores the special needs and concerns of pregnant adolescents and of women who become pregnant over age 35 years.

Care of the Pregnant Adolescent

Out of eleven million sexually active adolescent females in the United States, approximately one million become pregnant each year (Crooks & Baur 1990). For these young women pregnancy comes at a time when their physical development is incomplete, they have not yet completed the developmental tasks of adolescence, their available support systems may be limited, and their education is unfinished.

Adolescent pregnancy, long a concern of health care providers, is gaining increased attention from the general population as reflected in growing media coverage of the problem. This increased media attention began with the release of the results of a study done by Alan Guttmacher Institute (Wallis 1985). The study compared teenage birthrates in 37 countries and abortion rates in 13 other countries. The results demonstrated that the number of births per 1000 women under 20, as well as the incidence of abortion in the same age group, were significantly higher in the United States than in other developed countries in the study. However, the incidence of women having sexual intercourse during the teenage years is comparable to that in other countries (Jones et al 1985). A more recent study comparing teenage birth rates and abortion rates in England, Sweden, Finland, and the United States indicates that this trend continues (Wallace & Vienonon 1989). Researchers suggest that these countries may have lower adolescent pregnancy rates because of family influences, the greater availability of contraceptives, and the strong emphasis on sex education (Crooks & Baur 1990).

Authorities believe that many factors contribute to the increased incidence of adolescent pregnancy in the United States. Cohabitation and premarital sexual activity are becoming more commonplace and accepted in many parts of the country. Sexual innuendo permeates every aspect of the popular media, including music, music videos, television, and movies, while issues of sexual responsibility are commonly ignored. As a result of these trends, sexual activity is occurring at a younger age and is encouraged by peer pressure in the adolescent population.

Pregnancy risk taking (sexual activity without use of pregnancy prevention measures) is believed to stem from a variety of factors. Many teenage girls feel that they are not vulnerable to pregnancy, that because of their uniqueness, they are immune (Pete & DeSantis 1990; Kisker 1985). In the United States, it is reported that only one-third of sexually active teenagers between ages 15 and 19 always use contraception, and of those, only one-half rely on the most effective methods (Trussell 1988). Others, because of confusion or misinformation about conception, do not understand the risk ("I thought I was too young . . ." or "I don't make love that frequently . . ."). Still others fail to anticipate intercourse.

A woman's intrapsychic conflict about becoming pregnant is also cited as a factor in pregnancy risk taking (Flanigan et al 1990). The adolescent girl may use pregnancy for various subconscious or conscious reasons: to maintain dependence on her own mother; to punish her father and/or mother; to escape from an undesirable home situation; to gain attention; or to feel that she has someone to love and to love her. Some young women develop close relationships with their "mother-in-laws" and new extended family. For some, then, pregnancy provides the opportunity for a more stable family experience than is available with the girl's family of origin (Flanigan 1990).

Pregnancy may be a young woman's form of delinquency. Pregnant adolescents often have troubled family relationships, poor school achievement, and exposure to drug abuse (Palmore & Shannan 1988).

Pregnancy risk taking has also been linked to lack of knowledge about contraception. Because of this many health care providers advocate sex education in schools. Others feel that sex education is the responsibility of the parents. Recent research, however, suggests that neither knowledge nor sex education is related to changes in sexual behavior or in contraceptive use in adolescents under age 17 (Howard & McCabe 1990). Consequently, modified approaches, such as the use of slightly older, socially successful teens to provide information, teach assertiveness skills, and discuss pressures are being attempted (Howard & McCabe 1990).

Cultural values may cause a young woman to desire pregnancy. Many cultures, such as the Latino culture (including individuals from all Spanish-speaking countries), equate evidence of fertility with adult status. Duany and Pittman (1990) suggest that the formation of families and onset of employment occurs at an earlier age for Latinos than for either white or black youths and is a mark of adult success.

The incidence of teenage births is highest among low-income minority groups. However, in longitudinal studies that compare household income levels and basic skill deficits, the incidence of childbirth among white and minority teenagers is found to be essentially the same (Edelman 1988). Conversely, teens who are most likely to have abortions are from higher socioeconomic groups, are good students, have educational ambitions, and are less likely to have peers who are single parents. Their families also tend to have more favorable attitudes toward abortion and be less religious (Furstenburg et al 1989; Hofferth & Hayes 1987).

Teenage pregnancy can result from an incestuous relationship. The psychologic turmoil experienced by the incest victim may obliterate thought of the risk of pregnancy, especially for the young adolescent. Older adolescents may fear the possibility of pregnancy, but for a variety of psychologic reasons, may deny the reality. In the very young adolescent, incest or sexual abuse should be suspected as a possible cause of pregnancy (McAnarney & Hendee 1989).

Overview of the Adolescent Period

Physical Changes

Puberty, that period during which an individual becomes capable of reproduction, is a maturational process that can last from 1½ to 5 years. The major physical changes of puberty include a growth spurt, weight change, and the appearance of secondary sexual characteristics. Menarche, or the time of the first menstrual period, usually occurs in the

Research Note

Clinical Application of Research

Sharon Dormire and her associates (1989) examined adolescent parenthood to determine the impact of social support on the quality of parent-child interactions, the relationship of social support to parenting stress, and the impact of parenting stress on parent-infant reciprocity.

Comparison of the adolescents to normative samples for social support and adaptation to the parent role showed that the adolescents had lower scores on most of the scales; however, as noted by the authors, the normative samples were several years old. When adolescents were compared to a normative sample on stress, they consistently scored higher in terms of stress.

Spearman Rho correlations showed that several domains of the parent-child interaction, such as growth fostering and sensitivity to cues by the mother and responsivity by the infant, were positively correlated to several of the subcategories of both functional and network support. Also, a negative correlation was found between two factors from the stress scale: a sense of competence and acceptance of the infant and the areas of functional and network support. The most significant correlation between the parenting stress scale and the parent-infant interaction scale revealed that mothers who were less attached to their infants were less effective in responding to the distress cues given by their infant.

Critical Thinking Applied to Research

Strengths: Articulate statement of the research problem. Well developed conceptual framework.
Concerns: Spearman Rho might not have been the best statistical test to use with data that violated the underlying assumptions of normal distribution (Munro et al 1986). Comparison of adolescent mothers with adolescents who were not mothers on the stress scale might have determined if the higher stress levels were simply a function of adolescence and not motherhood.

Dormire S, Strauss S, Clarke B: Social support and adaptation to the parent role in first-time adolescent mothers. *JOGNN* July/August 1989; 327.

Munro B, Visintainer M, Page E: *Statistical Methods for Health Care Research.* Philadelphia: Lippincott, 1986.

last half of this maturational process, with the average age between 12 and 13. The range in age is between 9 and 17 years (Corbett & Meyer 1987).

The initial menstrual cycles are usually irregular and often anovulatory for the first 12 to 18 months; however, this is not true for all females. Some adolescents do not use contraception during this time with the false assumption that they cannot get pregnant. Even if their initial menstrual cycles are anovulatory, there is no certainty about when the first ovulatory cycle will occur; thus, contraception is important during this time for all adolescents who are sexually active.

Psychosocial Development

Although it is well documented that the onset of puberty now occurs at a younger age, there are no data to indicate that psychosocial development, particularly cognitive, occurs at an earlier age. In fact, authorities believe that there is a widening gap between psychologic and biologic maturation in adolescents (McAnarney & Hendee 1989; Orr et al 1988).

Developmental tasks of adolescence have been described by many writers and are based on a variety of classic theories. These tasks (Corbette & Meyer 1987, p 97) include:

1. Becoming comfortable with one's own body
2. Striving for independence
3. Building relationships with the same and opposite sexes
4. Seeking economic and social stability
5. Developing a value system
6. Learning to verbalize conceptually

This developmental process is reflected in the behaviors of youths during early, middle, and late adolescence. Although average ages for the completion of tasks have been identified, these ages are somewhat arbitrary and are affected by many factors such as. culture, religion, and socioeconomic status.

The early adolescent (age 14 and under) still sees authority in the parents. However, she begins the process of "leaving the family" by spending more time with friends, especially friends of the same sex. Conformity to peer group standards is reflected in her behavior and in the clothes she wears. During this phase the adolescent has a rich fantasy life. In addition, she is struggling to become comfortable with her changing body and body image and to fit this image with her fantasy life. Much time is spent in front of the mirror. The adolescent in this phase is very egocentric and is a concrete thinker. She has only minimal ability to see herself in the future or foresee the consequences of her behavior. She perceives her locus of control as external; that is, her destiny is controlled by others such as parents and school authorities.

Middle adolescence (15 to 17 years) is the time for challenging: Experimenting with drugs, alcohol, and sex is a common avenue for rebellion. The middle adolescent seeks independence and turns increasingly to her peer group. Peer group identification is obvious in her choice of dress, make-up, hair style, and music. During this phase the adolescent may believe that she is invincible and will not

suffer negative consequences from risk-taking behaviors. These years are often a time of great turmoil for the family as the adolescent struggles for independence and challenges the family's values and expectations.

The middle adolescent wants to be treated as an adult. However, fear of adult responsibility may cause fluctuation in behavior. At times she seems like a child, while at other times she is surprisingly mature. She is beginning to move from concrete thinking to formal operational thought but is not yet able to anticipate the long-term implications of all her actions.

In late adolescence (17 to 19 years) the young woman is more at ease with her individuality and decision-making ability. She can think abstractly and anticipate consequences. During this time she becomes more confident of her personal identity. The experiences of middle adolescence assist her in completing her developmental tasks. The late adolescent is capable of formal operational thought. She is learning to solve problems, to conceptualize, and to make decisions. These abilities help her see herself as having control, which leads to the ability to understand and accept the consequences of her behavior.

Table 15–1 suggests typical behaviors of the early, middle, and late adolescent when she becomes aware of her pregnancy. In reviewing these behaviors it is important to realize that other factors may influence the age at which these behaviors are seen.

The Adolescent Mother

Physiologic Risks

Adolescents over 15 years old who receive early, thorough prenatal care have no greater risk then women over 20 years old (Brucker & Mueller 1985; Piechnik & Corbett 1985). Unfortunately, many adolescents fail to seek early prenatal care. Those that do may fail to cooperate with recommendations especially those focusing on dietary practices either because of a lack of understanding of the importance of good nutrition or because of concerns related to body image. Thus risks for the pregnant adolescent include preterm births, low-birth-weight (LBW) infants, pregnancy-induced hypertension (PIH) and its sequelae, and iron-deficiency anemia.

In the adolescent population, prenatal care is the critical factor that most influences pregnancy outcome. Low-birth-weight babies are a common concern. Various studies indicate that early prenatal care, with emphasis on nutrition counseling, and coordination of agencies providing services significantly improves birth weights of babies of pregnant adolescents (Korenbrot et al 1989; McAnarney & Hendee 1989).

Pregnancy-induced hypertension represents the most prevalent medical complication in adolescents. Research suggests that this is related to parity, not age, since most pregnant adolescents are nulliparous and nulliparity is an important factor in the development of PIH (Cunningham

Table 15–1   Initial Reaction to Awareness of Pregnancy

	Adolescent behavior	Nursing implications
Early Adolescent (age 14 and under)	Fears rejection by family and peers. Enters health care system with an adult, most likely mother (parents still seen as locus of control). Value system still closely reflects that of parents, so still turns to parents for decision, or approval of decision. Pregnancy probably not result of intimate relationship. Self-conscious about normal adolescent changes in body. Self-consciousness and low self-esteem likely to increase with rapid breast enlargement and abdominal enlargement of pregnancy.	Nonjudgmental in approach to care. Focus on needs and concerns of adolescent teenager, but if parent accompanies daughter, parent needs to be included in plan of care. Encourage both to express concerns and feelings regarding pregnancy and options: abortion, maintaining pregnancy, adoption. Be realistic and concrete in discussing implications of each option. During physical exam of adolescent, respect increased sense of modesty. Explain in simple and concrete terms physical changes that are produced by pregnancy versus puberty. Explain each step of physical exam in simple and concrete terms.
Middle Adolescent (15–17 years)	Fears rejection by peers and parents. Unsure in whom to confide. May seek confirmation of pregnancy on own with increased awareness of options and services, such as over-the-counter pregnancy kits and Planned Parenthood. If in an ongoing, caring, relationship with partner (peer), may choose him as confidant. Economic dependence on parents may determine if and when parents are told. Future educational plans, perception of parental support or lack of support are significant factors in decision regarding termination or maintenance of the pregnancy. Possible conflict in parental and own developing value system.	Nonjudgmental in approach to care. Reassure regarding confidentiality. Help adolescent identify significant individuals in whom she can confide to help make a decision about the pregnancy. Need to be aware of state laws regarding requirement of parental notification if abortion intended. Also need to be aware of state laws regarding requirements for marriage: usually minimum age 18 for both parties; 16- and 17-year-olds only with consent of parents (Rhodes 1988). Encourage adolescent to be realistic about parental response to pregnancy.
Older Adolescent (17–19 years)	Most likely to confirm pregnancy on own and at an earlier date due to increased acceptance and awareness of consequences of behavior. Likely to use pregnancy kit for confirmation. Relationship with father of baby, future educational plans, own value system are among significant determinants of decision about pregnancy.	Nonjudgmental in approach to care. Reassure regarding confidentiality. Encourage adolescent to identify significant individuals in whom she can confide. Refer to counseling as appropriate. Encourage adolescent to be realistic about parental response to pregnancy.

et al 1989). Iron-deficiency anemia is a problem in all pregnant women. The adolescent who begins her pregnancy already anemic, however, is at increased risk and must be followed closely and counseled carefully regarding nutrition during pregnancy.

The increased risk of cephalopelvic disproportion (CPD) is a concern in adolescent pregnancy, especially with the younger adolescent because of a lack of pelvic maturity.

Teenagers 15 to 19 years old have the second highest incidence of sexually transmitted infections in the United States. The presence of herpes virus or gonorrhea during a pregnancy greatly increases the dangers. The incidence of chlamydial infection also increases (Osofsky 1985). Other problems seen in adolescents are cigarette smoking and drug use. The damage may be already done to the fetus by smoking or drug use by the time pregnancy is confirmed in young women.

Psychologic Risks

The most profound psychologic risk to the adolescent who maintains her pregnancy is the interruption of progress on her developmental tasks. Although adolescents have become sexually active at an earlier age and the incidence of adolescent pregnancy has increased, the developmental tasks of this age group remain the same. Add to this the tasks of pregnancy, and the young woman has an over-

whelming amount of psychologic work to do, the success of which will affect her own and her newborn's future.

Sociologic Risks

A substantial body of research indicates that the adolescent mother is at higher risk for social and economic disadvantages than her teenage counterpart who is not pregnant and lives in the same social environment. Being forced into adult roles before completing adolescent developmental tasks causes a series of events that affects the adolescent's entire life. These events may result in a prolonged dependence on parents, lack of stable relationships with the opposite sex, and lack of economic and social stability. In addition, the closer that pregnancy occurs to the changes of puberty and menarche, the more difficulty the teenager will have in becoming comfortable with her body image, given the continuing physical changes that do not fit her image of a "normal" teenager.

Many teenage mothers drop out of school during their pregnancy. Some researchers speculate that in some of these teenagers this tendency may have as much to do with low academic achievement and low academic commitment as it does with the pregnancy (Furstenberg et al 1989). Many never complete their education. Lack of education reduces the quality of jobs available to these individuals. Childbearing at an early age is a strong predictor for welfare dependency, especially in lower socioeconomic groups and when the pregnant adolescent's family will not support her (Furstenberg et al 1989).

There is evidence that, in the United States, the younger the adolescent at her first pregnancy, the more likely she is to become pregnant again while still an adolescent (Trussell 1988). These young women frequently fail to establish a stable family. Their family structure tends to be a single-parent, matriarchal family structure, often the same type in which the adolescent herself was raised.

Some pregnant adolescents choose to marry the father of the baby, who is often also a teenager. Unfortunately, the majority of adolescent marriages end in divorce (Hays 1987). This fact should not be surprising since pregnancy and marriage interrupt their "childhood" and basic education. Failure to be self-supporting logically follows lack of education and lost career goals. Lack of maturity in dealing with an intimate relationship also contributes to marital breakdown in this age group.

There is growing concern about children of teenage mothers. In general, these children are found to be at a developmental disadvantage compared to children whose mothers were older at the time of their birth. Many factors contribute to these differences, but the strongest evidence indicates that the adverse social and economic conditions facing teenage mothers are significant factors. These factors result in high rates of family instability, disadvantaged neighborhoods, and poor educational experiences for these children (Furstenberg et al 1989; Hays 1987).

The increased incidence of maternal complications, premature birth, and low-birth-weight babies among adolescent mothers also has an impact on society because many of these mothers are on welfare. The need for increased financial support for good prenatal care and nutritional programs remains critical.

Table 15–2 identifies the early adolescent's response to the developmental tasks of pregnancy. The early adolescent's response reflects her level of development, with

Table 15–2   The Early Adolescent's Response to the Developmental Tasks of Pregnancy

	Developmental tasks of pregnancy	Early adolescent's response to pregnancy	Nursing implications
1st Trimester	Pregnancy confirmation. Seeking early prenatal care as a confirmation tool. Begins to evaluate her diet and general health habits. Initial ambivalence common. Usually supportive partner.	May delay confirmation of pregnancy until late part of 1st trimester—unaware of pregnancy, fear of confiding in anyone, or denial. Rapid enlargement and sensitivity of breasts embarrassing and frightening to early adolescent—may be perceived as changes of puberty. If confiding in mother, may be experiencing family turmoil in response to pregnancy.	Explain physiologic changes of pregnancy versus those associated with puberty. Explain that ambivalence is normal with any pregnancy but recognize it as a much greater concern with adolescent pregnancy. Emphasize need for good nutrition as important for her well-being as much as infant's (prevention of PIH and anemia). Use simple explanations and lots of audio-visuals. Have adolescent listen to FHR with Doppler.
2nd Trimester	Quickening: Incorporates fetus as part of body image. Anxiety reduced. Buys maternity clothes. Looks at quality of own mothering and conflicts with mother as she begins to develop in her maternal role.	Some teenagers may delay validation of pregnancy until second trimester with family turmoil occurring at this time. Abdominal enlargement and quickening may be perceived as loss of control over body image. May try to maintain prepregnant weight and wear restrictive clothing to control and conceal changing body. Becomes dependent on her own mother for support. Egocentric. Still primarily a care receiver and identifies as such instead of developing in role of caregiver (Corbett 1987).	Continue to discuss importance of good nutrition and adequate weight gain as noted above. Discuss ways of utilizing common teenage clothing (large sweatshirts, blouses, etc) to promote comfort but preserve adolescent image to some degree. Discuss plans being made for baby, continued educational plans, and role of teen's parents.
3rd Trimester	At end of 2nd trimester, begins to view fetus as separate from self. Buys baby clothes and supplies. Prepares a place for the baby. Realistic about what baby is like. Prepares to give birth to infant. Anxiety increases as labor and birth approach and has concerns about well-being of fetus.	May focus on "wanting it to be over," may have trouble individuating fetus. May have fantasies, dreams, or nightmares about childbirth. Natural fears of labor and birth greater than with older primigravida. Probably has not been in a hospital and may associate this with negative experiences.	Need to assess if preparing for baby by buying supplies and preparing a place in the home. Childbirth education important. Provide hospital tour. Need to assess for discomforts of pregnancy, such as heartburn and constipation. Adolescent may be uncomfortable mentioning these and other problems.

pregnancy as an interruption of the normal process of development. The middle and late adolescent would respond differently, reflecting their maturational progress through the developmental tasks. In addition to her maturational level, the amount of nurturing the pregnant adolescent receives is also a critical factor in the way in which she handles pregnancy and motherhood.

The Adolescent Father

The adolescent father must complete the developmental tasks of his age group and is no better prepared psychologically to deal with the consequences of pregnancy than his female counterpart. Consequently, the adolescent who attempts to assume his responsibility as a father faces many of the same psychologic and sociologic risks as the adolescent mother.

Because he is not yet mature, his level of cognitive development and decision-making skills influence whether he remains supportive of the mother of the child or flees the situation. His educational and career goals may be threatened as he anticipates marrying or quitting school to support the young woman and his child. Data indicate that high school dropout rates are higher for adolescents who acknowledge their role in fathering the forthcoming child than for other youths. However, it is not clear if dropping out of school precedes or follows the knowledge of fatherhood (Furstenberg et al 1989). The job skills of the adolescent father, particularly when he quits school, are minimal and unlikely to contribute significantly to the economic support of the pregnant adolescent.

The unwed adolescent father often faces negative reactions from people in his environment, including his own family and the family of the young woman. Feelings of anger, shame, and disappointment may be aimed at him. He may feel isolated and alone, and if the young woman's parents refuse to allow him to see her, his sole source of emotional support may be gone.

The conscientious adolescent father faces a serious situation that may be overwhelming for him. The unresolved stress may lead to a crisis, manifested by abnormal adaptive behavior, marked depression, somatic symptoms, and/or deviant behavior. He has the same concerns about being rejected by family and peers as does the pregnant adolescent female.

Adolescent fathers are usually within three or four years of age of the adolescent mother. The mother and father are generally from similar socioeconomic backgrounds and have similar education. Many are involved in meaningful relationships. Frequently, the fathers are involved in the decision making regarding abortion or adoption. Many fathers are very involved in the pregnancy and in the childrearing.

Adolescent fathers do become sexually active at an earlier age than adolescent mothers, but, somewhat surprisingly, their knowledge of sexuality and reproduction is no greater than that of their nonfather peers (Barret & Robinson 1985).

Psychologic and sociologic risks to the adolescent father are in many ways similar to the adolescent mother's risks. Adolescent fathers tend to achieve less formal education than older fathers, and they enter the labor force earlier with less education. They tend to pursue less prestigious careers and have less job satisfaction. Adolescent fathers often marry at a younger age and have larger families than older fathers. In addition, the divorce rate of adolescent fathers is greater than that of couples who postpone childbearing and marriage (Furstenberg et al 1989; Teti et al 1987).

The lack of responsibility shown by some unwed fathers is a reflection of our cultural and community attitudes. In a model project to support adolescent fathers assuming parental responsibility, it was reported that teenage males attempting to establish paternity were discouraged by both social service agencies as well as legal agencies that were contacted (Sander & Rosen 1987). This attitude may be in the process of changing. Legal paternity gives children access to military and social security benefits and to medical information about their fathers (Smollar & Ooms 1987). In addition, research has indicated that children born to adolescent parents benefit from having regular contact with their father (Furstenberg et al 1987).

In some situations, the pregnant adolescent female may not want to identify or contact the father of the baby, and the male may not readily acknowledge paternity. Those situations include rape, exploitative sexual relations, incest, and casual sexual relations. If health care providers suspect any of the first three causes, further investigation into the situation is important for the well-being of the pregnant adolescent, and referral to other resources should be done as appropriate.

In situations in which the adolescent father wants to assume some responsibility, he should be supported in his behavior by health care providers as appropriate. It is important, however, that the pregnant adolescent have the opportunity to make the decision about whether she wants the father to participate in her health care.

If the adolescents perceive that they have a caring relationship, the adolescent father may want to be supportive and protective but probably does not understand the physical and psychologic changes his female partner is experiencing. The young man will need education regarding pregnancy, childbirth, child care, and parenting. Some clinics have couples attend classes together; others offer special classes just for fathers. In becoming a parent, the adolescent male needs to learn rates of growth and development so he can understand the newborn's potential and does not become frustrated and dissatisfied with the child's behavior because of unrealistic expectations.

Although the adolescent father may have been included in the health care of the young woman throughout the pregnancy, it is not unusual for the female adolescent to want her mother as her primary support person during labor and birth. This is especially true with younger adolescents. It is important to support her wishes, but it is also important that the adolescent father not be ignored.

As a part of counseling, the nurse should assess the young man's stressors, his support systems, his plans for involvement in the pregnancy and childbearing, and his future plans. He should be referred to social services for an opportunity to be counseled regarding his educational and vocational future. When the father is involved in the pregnancy, the young mother feels less deserted, more confident in her decision making, and better able to discuss her future.

Parents' Reactions to Adolescent Pregnancy

Perhaps the first, most intense crisis of the pregnant adolescent is telling her parents that she is pregnant. The young woman may not talk about her pregnancy until it is obvious. Her mother is usually the first to find out and often attempts to protect the young woman's father from discovering his daughter is pregnant. Little research is available on the reactions of these fathers, however.

Parents' initial reactions to the news are usually shock, anger, shame, guilt, and sorrow. The angry mother may accompany her daughter to the clinic. The nurse needs to assess the disharmony that is occurring and explain the process of adaptation that follows.

Mothers frequently feel guilty about their daughters' pregnancies. They wonder what they have done wrong and feel they have been inadequate parents. They are also angry because they are concerned about themselves. Just as their children are growing up and they see a new sense of freedom coming, they now have the responsibility of helping their daughters deal with a crisis. They may also feel angry at "being made a grandmother," perhaps at a young age. Once these reactions are dealt with, a calmer atmosphere generally develops, which supports necessary decision making. The mother may become involved in decision making regarding abortion, adoption, marriage, and dealing with the father-to-be and his family. Family input in these matters is important in the adolescent's decision making. The adolescent's decisions regarding abortion, relinquishing her newborn for adoption, or keeping the infant are influenced by her family's reactions.

As the pregnancy progresses the mother begins to take on the grandmother role. She may begin to buy presents for the newborn and plan for the future. She may participate in prenatal care and classes and can be an excellent support system for her daughter. She should be encouraged to participate if the mother-daughter relationship is positive. The mother should be updated on obstetric practice to clarify any misconceptions she might have. During labor and birth, the mother will be a key figure for her daughter. Drawing

on her own experience, she can offer reassurance and instill confidence in the adolescent.

The last stages of a mother's acceptance occur after her daughter's child is born. As the mother attempts to integrate her role of grandmother, an initial blurring of roles occurs. The grandmother now sees her daughter as a mother, and the daughter begins to identify herself as a mother. Role confusion may develop and sometimes continues for years—the new grandmother may essentially do all the mothering and caretaking activities for the newborn, while her daughter remains only a daughter and becomes a sibling of her newborn. The degree of role confusion is influenced by the age and maturity of the adolescent mother. Until the daughter is able to internalize her role as mother, her own mother will be unable to identify completely as a grandmother.

This new role development is clouded by the adolescent's struggle to complete her tasks of adolescence. The wise mother will gently encourage a balance between helping her daughter parent and allowing her to complete the tasks of adolescence. As her daughter becomes more confident in the role of parent, the mother can gradually encourage more independence for the daughter.

❧ *APPLYING THE NURSING PROCESS* ❧

Nursing Assessment

The nurse needs to establish a data base to plan interventions for the adolescent mother-to-be. Areas of assessment include a history of family and personal physical health, developmental level and impact of pregnancy, and a thorough assessment of emotional and financial support.

Physical Health
As with all pregnant women, it is important prenatally to have information on general physical health. This may be the first time many adolescents have ever provided a health history. The nurse may find it helpful to ask very specific questions and give examples if the young woman appears confused about a question.

The following areas should be assessed:

- Family and personal history
- Medical history
- Menstrual history
- Obstetric history

Developmental Level and the Impact of Pregnancy
An earlier discussion described adolescent behaviors specific to an age range as the female progresses through the developmental tasks of adolescence. Within any age group, however, the maturational level varies from one individual to another. In planning nursing care, it is important to as-

sess the maturational level of each individual. Assessment of the adolescent's developmental level and the impact of pregnancy is reflected in the degree of recognition of the realities and responsibilities involved in teenage pregnancy and parenting (see Table 15–2). The mother's self-concept (including body image), her relationship with the significant adults in her life, her attitude toward her pregnancy, and her coping methods in the situation are just a few of the significant factors that need to be assessed.

Support Systems
As noted previously, early and thorough prenatal care plays a significant role in decreasing physical risks in adolescent pregnancies and promoting healthy outcomes. The socioeconomic status of the pregnant adolescent, however, often places the baby at risk throughout life, beginning with conception. It is essential also to assess emotional and financial support systems. The nursing response to this data base usually requires referral of pregnant teenagers to social service programs and other community support programs for the pregnant teenager. A multidisciplinary team approach is the most effective in dealing with complex problems created by the socioeconomic needs of this age group.

Adolescent life-styles and support systems vary tremendously. It is imperative that the interdisciplinary health team have information regarding the expectant adolescents' feelings and perceptions about themselves, their sexuality, and the coming baby; their knowledge of, attitude toward, and anticipated ability to care for and support the infant; and their maturational level and needs.

Nursing Diagnosis

Nursing diagnoses that may apply to the pregnant adolescent are similar to those identified for any pregnancy and are listed on p 356. Nursing diagnoses are influenced by the adolescent's age, support systems, health, and personal maturity. Certain diagnoses, however, may be especially applicable to the adolescent who is pregnant. These are identified in Key Nursing Diagnoses to Consider—Adolescent Pregnancy.

Nursing Plan and Implementation

Early, thorough prenatal care is the strongest and most critical determinant for reducing risk for the adolescent mother and her newborn. The nurse needs to understand the special needs of the adolescent mother to meet this challenge successfully. (See Nursing Care Plan: Unplanned Adolescent Pregnancy on p 390).

Development of a Trusting Relationship with the Pregnant Adolescent
The nurse needs to be attentive to the special problems of adolescents. The first visit to the clinic or office may be

Key Nursing Diagnoses to Consider
Adolescent Pregnancy

Altered family processes

Altered growth and development

Altered health maintenance

Altered nutrition: less than body requirements

Altered nutrition: more than body requirements

Body image disturbance

Chronic low self-esteem

Decisional conflict

Defensive coping

High risk for altered parenting

Impaired adjustment

Impaired social interaction

Ineffective denial

Ineffective family coping

Ineffective individual coping

Knowledge deficit

Noncompliance

Parental role conflict

Self-esteem disturbance

Situational low self-esteem

Social isolation

fraught with extreme anxiety on the part of the young woman. Not only will she be nervous because of her situation, but also this may well be her first exposure to the health care system since early childhood. Making this first experience as positive as possible will encourage her compliance in returning for follow-up care and ensure a favorable attitude toward the importance of health care whether she chooses to terminate or maintain the pregnancy.

Depending on how young the adolescent is, this may be her first pelvic examination, an anxiety-provoking experience for any woman. A thorough explanation of the procedure is essential. A gentle and thoughtful examination technique will help the young woman to relax. A mirror is helpful in allowing the client to see her cervix, educating her about her anatomy, and giving her a part in the exam. If she is extremely anxious, she may even take part in speculum insertion; she should be told to insert it as she does a tampon.

Developing a trusting relationship with the pregnant adolescent is essential. Honesty and respect for the individual and a caring attitude promote self-esteem. As the nurse

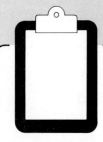

Nursing Care Plan
Unplanned Adolescent Pregnancy

Nursing History:
Note age and subjective symptoms of pregnancy, LMP, gravida, parity, menstrual history. Note client's perception of pregnancy and anxiety level. Identify family structure.

Physical Examination:
Pelvic examination to assess for uterine changes associated with pregnancy.

Diagnostic Studies:
Urine hCG

Nursing Diagnosis/Goals	Nursing Interventions	Rationale	Evaluation
Nursing Diagnosis: Anxiety related to fear of parental reaction secondary to unplanned adolescent pregnancy. *Client Goal:* The adolescent will reduce her anxiety by identifying a support system to help her in her decision-making process. She will understand, however, that the final decision about maintenance of the pregnancy or pregnancy termination should be hers.	Encourage the adolescent to express her own feelings and concerns, including her perception regarding parental response to the pregnancy.	Helps to identify specific areas of concerns where guidance in problem solving is needed. Health care providers must listen carefully, which means previous clarification of own values and beliefs regarding pregnancy termination, and not impose values on client. If unable not to superimpose own values in client, need to refer to more objective counseling source.	The adolescent will begin to realistically identify the potential reactions of her parents to her pregnancy.
	In those states where appropriate, reassure client that decision to share news of pregnancy with parents is hers. Confidentiality of health care providers is required.	Most states do not require parental notification if abortion is chosen. In addition, it is important to investigate the possibility of incest with the young adolescent, especially when adolescent is evasive and uncomfortable about discussing sexual partner.	
	Encourage her to identify a support system in helping her make a decision about how to deal with her unplanned pregnancy.	Important for adolescent to have support from significant individuals in her life in making decision and for follow-up support. This is essential if she plans to maintain the pregnancy.	
	Assess relationship with sexual partner and explore possible consequences in contacting him.	The adolescent may want her sexual partner involved in the decision but may be concerned about parental reaction to his involvement.	

(continued)

Nursing Care Plan (continued)

Nursing Diagnosis/Goals	Nursing Interventions	Rationale	Evaluation
Nursing Diagnosis: Anxiety related to decisional conflict secondary to handling unplanned pregnancy. *Client Goal:* The adolescent will understand the alternatives in dealing with her unplanned pregnancy as she begins to cope effectively with her conflict.	If adolescent accompanied by a parent, important to visit with adolescent initially by herself to assess her concerns without the presence of parents.	May be only way to find out how adolescent feels and any special concerns she has. If under 14, important to explore family relationships since incest is a concern in the early adolescent.	The client will begin to effectively evaluate the consequences in her life of each alternative response to her pregnancy.
	Present the alternatives: terminating pregnancy, maintaining the pregnancy and keeping the baby, maintaining the pregnancy and placing the baby for adoption.	Most adolescents have probably not thought through all the alternatives available in dealing with an unplanned pregnancy.	
	With each alternative, explore with the client her perception of projected consequences as it relates to her situation in life.	It is important to assess the client's perception of projected consequences in her own life in order to help her do more effective problem solving in arriving at a decision most comfortable for her.	
	Identify agency resources for help for each of the alternatives.	Most adolescents are unaware of resources available to support them in the choices they may make, especially if they decide to maintain their pregnancy and give the baby up for adoption.	
Nursing Diagnosis: Knowledge deficit related to induced abortion. *Client Goal:* The adolescent will be able to describe the procedure involved with an induced abortion, and the importance of an early decision if this alternative is chosen.	Assess client's perceptions and knowledge about induced abortion.	Clients frequently have many misconceptions about induced abortions. Important to clarify misconceptions before explaining procedure involved.	The adolescent can describe the abortion process and its consequences. In addition, she understands the importance of an early decision if this option is chosen.
	Explain what to expect with an abortion done in first trimester including procedure, where it is done, what most women experience, etc.	The adolescent is usually unaware of what is actually involved with an abortion, physical consequences, and what to expect regarding the products of conception in first trimester.	
	Discuss how second trimester abortions differ.	Adolescent may not realize that all factors related to induced abortion change as pregnancy progresses.	

(continued)

Nursing Care Plan (continued)

Nursing Diagnosis/Goals	Nursing Interventions	Rationale	Evaluation
	Discuss cost considerations related to an abortion.	Adolescents often have unrealistic ideas about health costs. Cost considerations may be an important factor in the adolescent's decision to share news of pregnancy with parents if parental notification not required by state law.	
	Explain state law requirements related to parental notification with induced abortion.	Most states do not require parental notification, but this may change in the future.	
	Discuss with adolescent the importance of her feeling comfortable with her final decision regarding her pregnancy, recognizing that some ambivalence would be experienced with any of the decisions. In addition, if leaning toward termination of pregnancy, safest when done as early in the pregnancy as possible.	Most adolescents are unaware of the limited timeframe in which a first trimester abortion can be done, especially if they have delayed confirmation of their pregnancy. If delayed too long, procedure for a first-trimester abortion may not be a choice.	
	Encourage her to examine closely her own values and beliefs about abortion.	Important for her to understand examination of her beliefs is important in her comfort with her decision, not the beliefs and values of her parents or peers, which may be in conflict with hers.	

becomes a role model, his or her attitudes about self-care and responsibility affect the adolescent's maturation process.

Promotion of Self-Esteem and Problem-Solving Skills

The nurse assists the adolescent in her decision-making and problem-solving skills so that she may proceed with her developmental tasks and begin to assume responsibility for her life as well as her newborn's life. An overview of what the young woman will experience over the prenatal course, along with thorough explanations and rationale for each procedure as it occurs, will foster the adolescent's understanding and give her some measure of control. Actively involving the young woman in her care will give her a sense of participation and responsibility (Figure 15–1).

Adolescents tend to be egocentric, and even the realization that their health and habits affect the fetus may not be regarded as important by them. It is often helpful to emphasize the effects of these practices on the client herself. Because of their immature cognitive development, adolescents need help in problem solving, in visualizing themselves in the future, and in imagining what the consequences of their actions might be. In addition, the nurse needs to understand that the developmental tasks of preg-

nancy must be met by the adolescent in addition to the stage-related developmental tasks she is already coping with. Table 15–2 identifies the developmental tasks of pregnancy, and the early adolescent's response to pregnancy, with implications for nursing care.

Promotion of Physical Well-Being

Baseline weight and blood pressure measurements will be valuable in assessing weight gain and predisposition to pregnancy-induced hypertension (PIH). The adolescent may be encouraged to take part in her care by measuring and recording her weight. The nurse may use this time as an opportunity for assisting the young woman in problem solving: "Have I gained too much or too little weight?" "What influence does my diet have on my weight?" "How can I change my eating habits?"

Another way to introduce the subject of nutrition is during measurement of baseline and subsequent hemoglobin and hematocrit values. Since the adolescent is at risk for anemia, she will need education regarding the importance of iron in her diet.

The nurse needs to keep in mind that adolescents may fear laboratory tests, which can evoke early childhood memories of being "stuck" with needles or hurt. Explanations help ease nerves, and coordination of services will avoid multiple venous punctures.

A nutritional consultation is indicated for all adolescents. Group classes are helpful because peer pressure is strong among this age group.

Pregnancy-induced hypertension represents the most prevalent medical complication of pregnant adolescents. Blood pressure readings of 140/90 mm Hg are not acceptable as the determinant of PIH in adolescents. Women aged 14 to 20 years without evidence of high blood pressure usually have diastolic readings between 50 and 66 mm Hg. Gradual increases from the prepregnant diastolic readings, along with excessive weight gain, must be evaluated as precursors to PIH. This is one reason why early prenatal care is vital to management of the adolescent.

As mentioned earlier, adolescents have an increased incidence of sexually transmitted diseases (STDs). The initial prenatal examination should include gonococcal and chlamydial cultures and wet prep for *Candida, Trichomonas,* and *Gardnerella.* Tests for syphilis should also be done. Education about STD is important as is careful observation of herpetic lesions or other symptoms throughout the young woman's pregnancy. Research indicates that while today's teens are knowledgeable about AIDS, they know much less about other STDs especially with regard to symptoms and risk reduction (Witwer 1990).

Substance abuse should also be discussed with adolescents. It is important to review the risks associated with the use of tobacco, caffeine, drugs, and alcohol. The young woman should be aware of the effects of these substances on her development as well as on the development of the fetus.

Ongoing care should include the same assessments

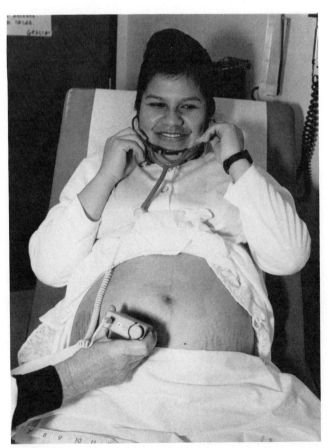

Figure 15–1   The nurse provides this young mother with an opportunity to listen to her baby's heartbeat.

that the older woman receives. Special attention should be paid to evaluating fetal growth by measurement of fundal height, fetal heart tones, quickening, and fetal movement. The corresponding dates of auscultating fetal heart tones with the date of last menstrual period and quickening can be helpful in determining correct estimates of time of birth. If there is a question of size—date discrepancy by 2 cm either way, an ultrasound is warranted to establish fetal age so that instances of IUGR may be diagnosed and treated early.

Promotion of Family Adaptation

It is important for the nurse to assess the family situation during the first prenatal visit. She should find out the level of involvement the adolescent desires from each of her family members as well as her perception of their present support. A sensitive approach to daughter-mother relationships helps motivate their communication. If the mother and daughter agree, the mother should be included in the client's care. Encouraging the mother to become part of the maternity team, to join grandmother crisis support groups, and to obtain counseling aids the mother in adapting to her role and in supporting her daughter.

The nurse should also help the mother assess her daughter's needs and assist her in meeting them. Some adolescents become more dependent during pregnancy, and some become more independent. The mother can ease and encourage her daughter's self-growth by understanding how best to respond and support the adolescent.

The adolescent's relationship with her father will also be affected by the pregnancy. The nurse can provide information to the father and encourage his involvement to the degree that is acceptable for both daughter and father.

Facilitation of Prenatal Education

Prenatal education is crucial in the care of the pregnant adolescent. An important challenge to health professionals is to develop prenatal classes that meet the special needs of this age group (Figure 15–2). Prenatal education programs should include the clinic and the school system.

Many adolescents cite the school as the preferred agency for education during pregnancy and early parenting. School systems are currently attempting to meet this need in a variety of ways. The most effective method appears to be mainstreaming the pregnant adolescent in academic classes with her peers and adding classes appropriate to her needs during pregnancy and initial parenting experiences. Classes about growth and development beginning with the newborn and early infancy can help teenage parents have more realistic expectations of their infants and may help decrease child abuse. Mainstreaming pregnant adolescents in school is also an ideal way to help them complete their education while learning the skills they need to cope with childbearing and parenting. Vocational guidance in this setting is also most beneficial to their future.

Regardless of the sponsorship or setting of prenatal classes for pregnant teenagers and adolescent fathers, the developmental tasks of the adolescent need to be considered. For example, the methods of teaching this age group should be somewhat different from regular prenatal classes. The younger adolescent tends to be a more concrete thinker

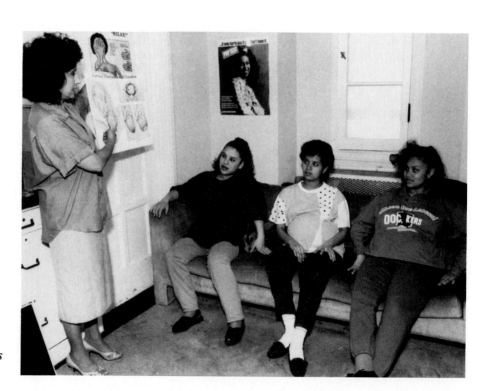

Figure 15–2 Young adolescents may benefit from prenatal classes designed for them.

than the older and more mature pregnant adult. Increased use of audiovisuals that are appropriate to their social situation and age is helpful. More demonstrations may be required, and they need to be simple and direct.

Areas that might be included in prenatal classes are anatomy and physiology, sex education, exercises for pregnancy and postpartum, maternal and infant nutrition, growth and development of the fetus, labor and birth, family planning, and infant development. Adolescents may want to participate in the teaching of these classes and should be encouraged to do so. Peer support and friendships can blossom among these young women, helping them all to mature.

The clinic can offer rap sessions, pamphlets, or films in the waiting room. Giving the clients something to do while they wait for their appointments may encourage them to return and also may help them learn. Decorating the clinic with attractive educational posters and creating an informal atmosphere establishes an environment where adolescents feel free to interact with professionals.

Ideally, prenatal classes for the adolescent are oriented to more than just pregnancy, childbirth, and immediate newborn care (Figure 15–2). The goals of many of these classes are expanding to deal with more complex social issues that result from adolescent pregnancies. A multidisciplinary team approach is important in planning and implementing these classes. Goals for many of these classes now include promoting self-esteem; helping participants identify the problems and conflicts of teenage parenting and how to prepare for them; educating participants about sexuality, relationships, and contraception to deter unwanted pregnancies; teaching participants parenting skills; providing information about community resources and other resources available to teenage parents; and helping participants develop more adaptive coping skills.

Evaluation

Anticipated outcomes of nursing care include the following:

- A trusting relationship is established with the pregnant adolescent.
- The adolescent is able to use her problem-solving abilities to make appropriate choices.
- The adolescent complies with the recommendations of the health care team and receives effective health care throughout her pregnancy and birth and during the postpartum period.
- The adolescent, her partner (if he is involved), and their families are able to cope successfully with the effects of the pregnancy.
- The adolescent is knowledgeable about pregnancy and makes appropriate health care choices.
- The adolescent demonstrates developmental and pregnancy progression within established normal parameters.

- The adolescent develops skill in child care and parenting.

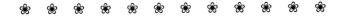

Care of the Expectant Couple Over 35

Today an increasing number of women are choosing to have their first baby after age 35. In fact, the rate of first births to women between the ages of 30 and 39 more than doubled between 1970 and 1986 in the United States. For women between the ages of 40 and 44, the birth rate increased by 50% during the same period (Berkowitz et al 1990; Department of Health and Human Services 1989). Many factors contribute to this trend, including the following:

- Availability of effective birth control methods
- The women's liberation movement and its emphasis on expanded roles for women
- The increased number of women obtaining advanced education, pursuing careers, and delaying pregnancy until they are established professionally
- Increased incidence of later marriage and second marriage
- Higher cost of living, causing some young couples to delay childbearing until they are more secure financially
- Increase in the population of women in this age group

There are advantages to having a first baby after the age of 30. Couples who delay childbearing until they are older tend to be well educated and financially secure. Usually their decision to have a baby was deliberately and thoughtfully made. Given their greater life experiences, they are much more aware of the realities of having a child and what it means to have a baby at their age (Figure 15–3). Many of the women have experienced fulfillment in their careers and feel secure enough to take on the added responsibility of a child. Some women are ready to make a change in their lives, desiring to stay home with a new baby. Those who plan to continue working are able to afford good child care.

Medical Risks

Historically medical professionals considered women who were over 30 at the time of their first pregnancy, and especially those who were 35 or older, at higher risk for maternal or fetal complications than younger women. Recent studies comparing healthy pregnant women over 35 years of age with healthy younger pregnant women, however, do not confirm these beliefs. These studies suggest that preex-

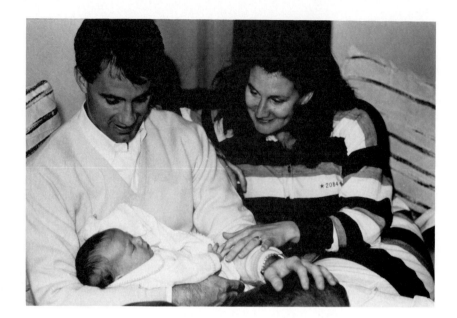

Figure 15–3 For many older couples the decision to have a child may be a very rewarding one.

isting medical problems such as hypertension or diabetes play a more significant role than age in maternal well-being and outcome of pregnancy (Redwine 1988; Mansfield 1986).

A recent study using a sample composed of private clients who were predominantly white, married, and college educated found an increased incidence of pregnancy-induced hypertension (PIH), gestational diabetes, abruptio placentae, gestational bleeding, and placenta previa in women over age 35. Nonetheless, although the older mothers were more likely to have specific complications during the antepartal and intrapartal periods, the rate of poor neonatal outcome was not increased appreciably over that of mothers between ages 20 and 29 (Berkowitz et al 1990).

Fibroid tumors (leiomyoma) occur with greater frequency in women over age 35. Fibroids located inside the uterus may interfere when they increase in size, which can occur as a result of estrogen stimulation during pregnancy. This increased size can lead to malpresentations, premature labor, dystocia, or problems in the third stage of labor (Beischer & MacKay 1986). Fibroid tumors may also increase the incidence of early postpartum hemorrhage if they prevent the uterus from contracting completely after childbirth.

The risk of conceiving a child with Down syndrome does increase with age, especially over age 35 (see Table 5–9). The use of amniocentesis or chorionic villus sampling (CVS) is routinely offered to all women over age 35 to permit the early detection of several chromosomal abnormalities including Down syndrome.

The incidence of cesarean births also rises sharply after the age of 35. Mansfield (1986) suggests that this practice increases because of obstetricians' preset expectations of higher risk with the "elderly primipara" and concern about the increased value of this long-awaited child. Many physicians do not want to take any chances with the outcome of pregnancy in this age group. The research of Berkowitz et al (1990) supports this possibility.

Special Concerns of the Expectant Couple Over 35

No matter what their age, most expectant couples have concerns regarding the well-being of the fetus and their ability to parent. The older couple has additional concerns related to their age, especially the closer they are to 40.

Some couples are concerned about whether they will have enough energy to care for a new baby. Of greater concern is their ability to deal with the needs of the child in ten years when they, too, are ten years older.

The financial concerns of the older couple are usually different from those of the younger couple. The older couple is generally more financially secure than the younger couple. However, when their "baby" is ready for college, the older couple may be close to retirement, when they might not have the means to provide for their child.

While considering their financial future and future retirement, the older couple may be forced to face their own mortality. Certainly this is not uncommon in midlife, but instead of confronting this issue at 40 to 45 years of age or later, the older expectant couple may confront the issue several years earlier as they consider what will happen as their child grows.

The older expectant couple may find themselves somewhat isolated socially. They may feel "different" because they are often the only couple in their peer group expecting their first baby. In fact, many of their peers are likely to be parents of adolescents or young adults and may be grandparents as well.

The response of older couples who already have children to learning that the woman is pregnant may vary greatly depending on whether the pregnancy was planned or unexpected. Other factors influencing their response include the attitudes of their children, family, and friends to the pregnancy; the impact on their life-style; and the financial implications of having another child. Sometimes couples who had previously been married to other mates will choose to have a child together. The concept of **blended family** applies to situations in which "her" children, "his" children, and "their" children come together as a new family group.

Health care professionals may treat the older expectant couple differently than they would a younger couple. Older women may be asked to submit to more medical procedures, such as amniocentesis and ultrasound, than younger women. An older woman may be prevented from using a birthing room or birthing center even if she is healthy because her age is considered to put her at risk.

The woman who has delayed pregnancy may be concerned about the limited amount of time that she has to bear children. When pregnancy does not occur as quickly as she hoped, the older woman may become increasingly anxious as time slips away on her "biological clock." When an older woman becomes pregnant but experiences a spontaneous abortion, her grief for the loss of her unborn child is exacerbated by her anxiety about her ability to conceive again in the time remaining to her.

❀   *APPLYING THE NURSING PROCESS*   ❀

Nursing Assessment

In working with a woman in her thirties or forties who is pregnant, the nurse makes the same assessments as are appropriate in caring for any woman who is pregnant. These include assessment of physical status, the woman's understanding of pregnancy and the changes that accompany it, any health teaching needs that exist, the degree of support the woman has available to her, and her knowledge of infant care. In addition, the nurse explores the woman's and her partner's attitudes about the pregnancy and their expectations of the impact a baby will have on their lives.

Nursing Diagnosis

The diagnoses that are applicable to any woman who is pregnant are identified in Chapter 14. In addition to those diagnoses, the older woman who is pregnant has specific needs that may lead the nurse to formulate additional diagnoses. Key Nursing Diagnoses—The Older Expectant Couple identifies some of these.

℞

Key Nursing Diagnoses to Consider
The Older Expectant Couple

Altered family processes

Decisional conflict

Family coping: potential for growth

Fatigue

High risk for altered parenting

Impaired adjustment

Impaired social interaction

Ineffective family coping

Knowledge deficit

Noncompliance

Ineffective individual coping

Parental role conflict

Nursing Plan and Implementation

Once an older couple has made the decision to have a child, it is the nurse's responsibility to respect and support the couple in this decision. As with any client, risks need to be discussed, concerns need to be identified, and strengths need to be promoted. The woman's age should not be made an issue.

To promote a sense of well-being, the nurse should treat the pregnancy as "normal" unless specific health risks are identified. See Nursing Care Plan: Genetic Counseling for the Older Pregnant Woman.

Promotion of Adaptation to Pregnancy
As the pregnancy continues the nurse should identify and discuss concerns the woman may have related to her age or to specific health problems. The older woman who has made a conscious decision to become pregnant often has carefully thought through potential problems and may actually have fewer concerns than a younger woman or one with an unplanned pregnancy.

Childbirth education classes are important in promoting adaptation to the event of childbirth for expectant couples of any age. However, older expectant couples, who are still in the minority, often feel uncomfortable in classes where the majority of participants are much younger. Because of the differences in age and life experiences, many of the needs of the older couple may not be met in the class. The nurse teaching a childbirth education class should try to anticipate the informational needs of the older couple. At the same time, the nurse should not make the couple feel any more uncomfortable by drawing attention to their age.

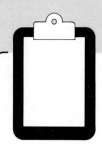

Nursing Care Plan
Genetic Counseling for the
Older Pregnant Woman

Nursing History:
Note age, gravida, parity, religious preference, LMP.

Physical Examination:
Pelvic examination to assess uterine changes associated with pregnancy.

Diagnostic Studies:
Urine hCG

Nursing Diagnosis/Goals	Nursing Interventions	Rationale	Evaluation
Nursing Diagnosis: High risk knowledge deficit related to increase in genetic risks in the older pregnant woman.	Explain increased risks of Down syndrome after age of 35.	Cannot assume that all clients are aware of this risk.	Couple can describe increased risks of Down syndrome with pregnancy over the ages of 35 and 40. In addition, they are able to discuss problems and strengths related to individuals with Down syndrome and implications for their decision making.
Goal: The couple will be able to identify genetic risks associated with pregnancy and the woman who is over the age of 35.	Share statistics that demonstrate incidence of problem in different age groups and how incidence increases at 35 and dramatically increases over age 40.	Help client to develop a more realistic perspective of the increased risk with age.	
	Discuss realities of having a Down syndrome baby and life-long prognosis for adults with Down syndrome.	Recent media attention to problem may not reflect a comprehensive perspective. Important for couples to understand life-long implications and variations in severity of problems.	
	Assess for concerns and questions. Clarify as appropriate.	Help to clarify any misunderstandings or questions the couple may still have.	
Nursing Diagnosis: Knowledge deficit related to amniocentesis.	Assess couple's knowledge and/or preconceived ideas related to amniocentesis.	Couple may have no knowledge about amniocentesis or may have misconceptions that increase their anxieties and fears about the procedure.	The couple will understand the process involved with amniocentesis as demonstrated through their questions and discussion.
Goal: The couple will have accurate information related to amniocentesis.	Clarify misconceptions about procedures with factual information.	Difficult for couple to listen if concerns and misconceptions are not addressed initially.	
	Explain each step of procedure and effect on mother and fetus.	Most couples do not know what to expect and have fears about risks to mother and fetus.	
	Assess for further questions or concerns.	New questions and concerns may arise as procedure is explained.	

As the number of expectant older couples increases, the nurse may find it useful to offer an "over 30" childbirth education class to accommodate the specific needs of older couples. Such classes are being developed in some of the larger urban areas.

Couples who are over 30 years of age are often better educated than other health care consumers. These clients frequently know the kind of care and services they want and are assertive in their interactions with the health care system. The nurse should neither be intimidated by these individuals nor assume that anticipatory guidance and support are not needed. Instead the nurse should support the couple's strengths and be sensitive to their individual needs.

Support of Couple if Amniocentesis Is Advised

In working with older expectant couples, the nurse needs to be sensitive to their special needs. A particularly difficult issue these couples face is the possibility of bearing an unhealthy child. Because of the risk of Down syndrome in these families, amniocentesis is encouraged. Chorionic villus sampling (CVS) may also be suggested if available in the area. The decision to have amniocentesis can be difficult to make merely on the basis of its possible risks to the fetus. But that becomes almost a minor concern when the couple thinks of the implications of the possible findings of Down syndrome or other chromosomal abnormalities. The finding of abnormalities means that the couple may be faced with an even more difficult decision about continuing the pregnancy.

A couple's decision to have amniocentesis is usually related to their beliefs and attitudes about abortion. Amniocentesis is usually not even considered by couples who are strongly opposed to abortion for any reason. Health professionals must respect their decision and take a nonjudgmental approach to their continued care.

Other couples may be opposed to abortion but also concerned about their ability to care for a seriously limited child as times passes. How will they care for this child when he or she becomes an adult and they are elderly? What will happen to this child when they die? Such questions may cause the couple to permit amniocentesis to be performed. The results of the procedure may force the couple to make the painful decision to terminate the pregnancy.

The decision to have an abortion is a painful one even when couples are not opposed to abortion on political or philosophic grounds. Even though the couple may believe that terminating a high-risk pregnancy is right for their family, they may feel a great deal of ambivalence about amniocentesis. If the results are such that the couple elects to have an abortion, they will feel much grief for their loss.

Many health professionals assume that the couple who agrees to amniocentesis will also elect to have an abortion if Down syndrome or another condition is diagnosed. This is not necessarily the case. Some couples choose not to have an abortion after being informed that their unborn child has genetic abnormalities.

For the couple who agrees to amniocentesis, the first few months of pregnancy are a difficult time. Amniocentesis cannot be done until 14 weeks of pregnancy and the chromosomal studies take roughly two weeks to complete. For almost 16 weeks, until the woman is in her second trimester, the couple is "on hold," not knowing if their unborn child is healthy or not. Their fear that the fetus is at risk may delay the successful completion of the psychologic tasks of early pregnancy.

The nurse can support couples who decide to have amniocentesis in several ways:

1. The nurse should make sure that the couple is aware of the risks of amniocentesis and why it is being performed.

2. The nurse who is present during the amniocentesis procedure can offer comfort and emotional support to the expectant woman. The nurse can also provide information about the procedure as it is being performed.

3. The nurse can facilitate a support group for women during the difficult waiting period between the procedure and the results.

4. If the results indicate that the fetus has Down syndrome or another genetic abnormality, the nurse can ensure that the couple has complete information about the condition, its range of possible manifestations, and its developmental implications.

5. The nurse can support the couple in their decision about continuing or terminating the pregnancy. It is essential that the nurse and other health professionals involved with the couple not impose their philosophic or political beliefs about abortion on the couple. The decision is the couple's, and it should be based on their belief system and a nonbiased presentation of risks and choices from care givers.

Evaluation

Anticipated outcomes of nursing care include the following:

● The woman and her partner are knowledgeable about the pregnancy and make appropriate health care choices.

● The expectant couple (and their children) are able to cope successfully with the pregnancy and its implications for the future.

● The woman receives effective health care throughout her pregnancy and during birth and the postpartum period.

● The woman and her partner develop skills in child care and parenting as necessary.

❀ ❀

KEY CONCEPTS

Many factors contribute to the increase in the teenage pregnancy rate, including earlier onset of menarche, earlier age of first sexual intercourse, lack of knowledge related to conception, lack of easy access to contraception, and lessened stigma associated with adolescent pregnancy in some populations.

Factors affecting an adolescent's response to pregnancy includes her degree of achievement of the developmental tasks of adolescence (which can be closely associated with age), as well as cultural, religious, and socioeconomic factors.

The adolescent father who wants to be involved is often overlooked by health care providers. If he assumes accountability, however, he is also at increased risk for social and economic problems.

Often the adolescent has little understanding of pregnancy, childbirth, or parenting. Consequently, education is a primary responsibility of the nurse.

Childbirth among women over 30 is becoming increasingly common. It poses fewer health risks than previously believed and offers definite advantages for the woman or couple who make the choice.

A major risk for the older expectant couple relates to the increased incidence of Down's syndrome in children born to women over age 35 or 40. Amniocentesis can provide information as to whether the fetus has Down's syndrome. The couple can then decide whether they wish to continue the pregnancy.

❀ ❀

References

Adams BN: Adolescent health care: Needs, priorities, and services. *Nurs Clin North Am* June 1983; 18:237.

Beischer NA, MacKay EV: *Obstetrics and the Newborn,* 2nd ed. Sydney: Saunders, 1986.

Berkowitz GS et al: Delayed childbearing and the outcome of pregnancy. *N Engl J Med* March 1990; 322:659.

Brucke MC, Mueller M: Nurse-midwifery care of adolescents *J Nurse-Midwifery* September/October 1985; 30:277.

Corbett MA, Meyer JH: *The Adolescent and Pregnancy.* Boston: Blackwell Scientific Publications, 1987.

Crooks R, Baur K: *Our Sexuality.* Menlo Park, CA: Benjamin/Cummings, 1990.

Department of Health and Human Services, Public Health Service, Centers for Disease Control, National Center for Health Statistics: Trends and variations in first births to older women. Vital and health statistics, Series 21, No. 47. Washington, DC: Government Printing Office, 1989, p 89.

Duany L, Pittman K: *Latino Youths at a Crossroads.* Children's Defense Fund. An Adolescent Pregnancy Prevention Clearinghouse Report (ISSN: 0899–5591) January/February 1990.

Edelman MW: Preventing adolescent pregnancy: A role for social work services. *Urban Education* January 1988; 22:496.

Flanigan B et al: Alcohol use as a situational influence on young women's pregnancy risk-taking behaviors. *Adolescence* Spring 1990; 25:205.

Furstenberg FF et al: Teenaged pregnancy and childbearing. *Am Psychol* February 1989; 44:313.

Furstenburg FF et al: *Adolescent Mothers in Later Life.* Cambridge, MA: Cambridge University Press, 1987.

Hays CD (editor): *Risking the Future: Adolescent Sexuality, Pregnancy, and Childbearing,* Vol. 1. Washington, DC: National Academy Press, 1987.

Hofferth S, Hayes CD (editors): *Risking the Future: Adolescent Sexuality, Pregnancy, and Childbearing,* Vol. 2. Washington, DC: National Academy Press, 1987.

Howard M, McCabe JB: Helping teenagers postpone sexual involvement. *Fam Plann Perspect* January/February 1990; 22:21.

Jones EF et al: Teenage pregnancy in developed countries: Determinants and policy implications. *Fam Plann Perspect* March/April 1985; 17:53.

Korenbrot CC et al: Birth weight outcomes in a teenage pregnancy case management project. *J Adolesc Health Care* March 1989; 10:97.

Mansfield PK: *Pregnancy for Older Women.* New York: Praeger Publications 1986.

McAnarney ER, Hendee WR: Adolescent pregnancy and its consequences. *JAMA* July 1989; 262:74.

Orr DP et al: Pubertal maturation and cognitive maturity in adolescents. *J Adolesc Health Care* July 1988; 9:273.

Osofsky HJ: Mitigating the adverse effects of early parenthood. *Contemp OB/GYN* January 1985; 25:57.

Palmore SV, Shannan, MD: Risk factors for adolescent pregnancy in students. *Pediatr Nurs* May/June 1988; 14:241.

Pete JM, DeSantis L: Sexual decision-making in young black adolescent females. *Adolescence* Spring 1990; 25(97):145.

Piechnik SL, Corbertt MA: Reducing low birth weight among socioeconomically high-risk adolescent pregnancies: Successful intervention with certified nurse-midwife-managed care and a multidisciplinary team. *J Nurse-Midwifery* March/April 1985; 30:88.

Redwine FO: Pregnancy in women over 35. *Female Patient* May 1988; 135:30.

Rhodes AM: Options and issues for pregnant adolescents. *MCN* November/December 1988; 13:427.

Sander JH, Rosen JL: Teenage fathers: Working with the neglected partner in adolescent childbearing. *Fam Plann Perspect* May/June 1987; 19:107.

Smollar J, Ooms T: *Young Unwed Fathers: Research Review, Policy Dilemmas and Options.* U.S. Department of Health and Human Services, 1987.

Spellacy WN et al: Pregnancy after 40 years of age. *Obstet Gynecol* October 1986; 68:452.

Trussell J: Teenage Pregnancy in the United States. *Fam Plann Perspect* November/December 1988; 20:262.

Wallace HM, Vienonen M: Teenage pregnancy in Sweden and Finland: Implications for the United States. *J Adolesc Health Care* May 1989, 10:236.

Wallis C: Children having children: Teen pregnancy in America. *Time* December 1985; 126:78.

Witwer M: Survey finds teenagers know more about AIDS than about other STDs. *Fam Plann Perspect* May/June 1990; 22:138.

Additional Readings

Casper LM: Does family interaction prevent adolescent pregnancy? *Fam Plann Perspect* May/June 1990; 22:109.

Degenhart-Leskosky SM: Health education needs of adolescent and nonadolescent mothers. *JOGNN* May/June 1989; 18:238.

Duncan GJ, Hoffman SD: Teenage welfare receipt and subsequent dependence among black adolescent mothers. *Fam Plann Perspect* January/February 1990; 22:16.

Furstenberg FF et al: The children of teenage mothers: Patterns of early childbearing in two generations. *Fam Plann Perspect* March/April 1990; 22:54.

McAnarney ER, Hendee WR: The prevention of adolescent pregnancy. *JAMA* July 1989; 262:78.

Moore ML: Recurrent teen pregnancy: Making it less desirable. *MCN* March/April 1989; 14:104.

Nachtigall RD: Assessing fecundity after age 40. *Contemp OB/GYN* March 1991; 36:11.

Reedy NJ: The very young pregnant adolescent. *NAACOG's Clin Issues Perinatal Women's Health Nurs* 1991; 2(2):209.

CHAPTER 16

Maternal Nutrition

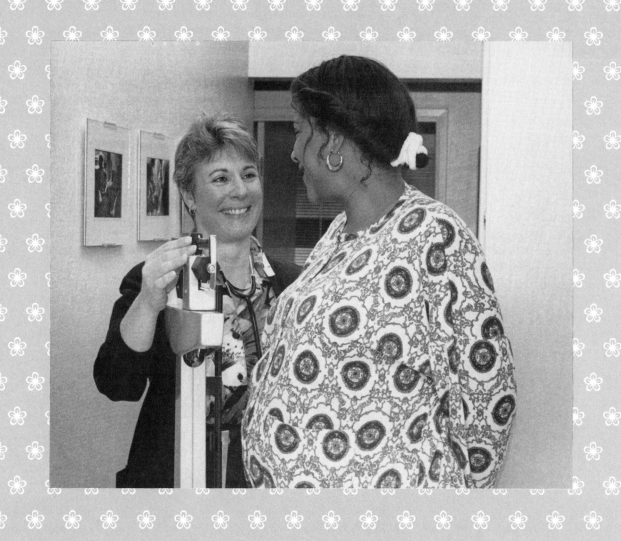

OBJECTIVES

Identify the role of specific nutrients in the diet of the pregnant woman.

Compare nutritional needs during pregnancy, postpartum, and lactation with nonpregnant requirements.

Discuss effects of maternal nutrition on fetal outcomes.

Evaluate adequacy and pattern of weight gain during different stages of pregnancy.

Plan adequate prenatal vegetarian diets based on nutritional requirements of pregnancy.

Describe ways in which various physical, psychosocial, and cultural factors can affect nutritional intake and status.

Compare recommendations for weight gain and nutrient intakes in the pregnant adolescent with those for the mature pregnant adult.

Describe basic factors a nurse should consider when offering nutritional counseling to a pregnant adolescent.

Compare nutritional counseling issues for nursing and nonnursing mothers.

Formulate a nutritional care plan for pregnant women based on a diagnosis of nutritional problems.

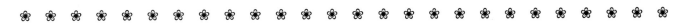

I'm trying to be very careful about what I eat. I've had more salads and fresh fruit than I can remember. Sometimes, though, I get a "cookie attack" and indulge myself. My husband said I should eat oatmeal cookies so I could feel that my cravings were nutritionally sound!

A woman's nutritional status prior to and during pregnancy can significantly influence her health and that of her unborn child. In most prenatal clinics and offices, nurses provide nutritional counseling directly or work closely with nutritionists in providing necessary nutritional assessment and teaching.

This chapter focuses on the nutritional needs of a normal pregnant woman. Special sections consider the nutritional needs of the pregnant adolescent and the woman after birth.

Good prenatal nutrition is the result of proper eating for a lifetime, not just during pregnancy, although pregnancy may motivate a woman to improve poor eating habits. Many factors influence the ability of a woman to achieve good prenatal nutrition.

- *General nutritional status prior to pregnancy.* Nutritional deficits at the time of conception and the early prenatal period may influence the outcome of the pregnancy.

- *Maternal age.* An expectant adolescent must meet her own growth needs in addition to the nutritional needs of pregnancy. This may be especially difficult because teenagers often have nutritional deficiencies. Such deficiencies may be due to a variety of causes such as chronic dieting, frequent intake of fast foods, attempts to conceal pregnancy, and so forth.

- *Maternal parity.* The mother's nutritional needs and the outcome of the pregnancy are influenced by the number of pregnancies she has had and the interval between them.

A mother's nutritional status does affect her fetus. Factors influencing fetal well-being are interrelated, but research suggests that nutrient deficiency can produce measurable effects on cell and organ growth of the developing fetus.

Fetal growth occurs in three overlapping stages: (1) growth by increase in cell number, (2) growth by increase in cell number and cell size, and (3) growth by increase in cell size alone. It is now thought that the nutritional problems that interfere with cell division may have permanent consequences. If the nutritional insult occurs when cells are mainly enlarging, the changes are reversible when normal nutrition resumes.

Growth of fetal and maternal tissues requires increased quantities of essential dietary components. Typically these have been listed as percentage increases in the **recommended dietary allowances (RDA)** over those for nonpregnant women. However, the 10th edition of the Recommended Dietary Allowances now provides absolute, specific figure allowances for pregnant and lactating women (Table 16–1). In addition, "RDAs during lactation are now provided for the first and second 6-month periods to reflect the differences in the amount of milk produced (750 mL and 600 mL, respectively)" (RDA 1989, p 3).

Most of the recommended nutrients can be obtained by eating a well-balanced diet each day. The basic food groups and recommended amounts during pregnancy and lactation are presented in Table 16–2.

Table 16–1 Food and Nutrition Board, National Academy of Sciences—National Research Council Recommended Dietary Allowances (RDAs), for Nonpregnant, Pregnant, and Lactating Females*

Age (years) and Sex Group	Weight‡ kg	lb	Height‡ cm	in.	protein g	Vitamin A μgR§	Vitamin D μg‖	Vitamin E mg α-TE#	Vitamin K μg	Vitamin C	Thiamine	Riboflavin	Niacin mg NE††	Vitamin B₆	Folate	Vitamin B₁₂	Calcium	Phosphorous	Magnesium	Iron	Zinc	Iodine	Selenium
						Fat-soluble Vitamins				Water-soluble Vitamins							Minerals						
										←— mg —→				mg	←μg→		←———— mg ————→					←μg→	
females																							
11–14	46	101	157	62	46	800	10	8	45	50	1.1	1.3	15	1.4	150	2.0	1200	1200	280	15	12	150	45
15–18	55	120	163	64	44	800	10	8	55	60	1.1	1.3	15	1.5	180	2.0	1200	1200	300	15	12	150	50
19–24	58	128	164	65	46	800	10	8	60	60	1.1	1.3	15	1.6	180	2.0	1200	1200	280	15	12	150	55
25–50	63	138	163	64	50	800	5	8	65	60	1.1	1.3	15	1.6	180	2.0	800	800	280	15	12	150	55
51+	65	143	160	63	50	800	5	8	65	60	1.0	1.2	13	1.6	180	2.0	800	800	280	10	12	150	55
pregnant					60	800	10	10	65	70	1.5	1.6	17	2.2	400	2.2	1200	1200	320	30	15	175	65
lactating																							
1st 6 months					65	1300	10	12	65	95	1.6	1.8	20	2.1	280	2.6	1200	1200	355	15	19	200	75
2nd 6 months					62	1200	10	11	65	90	1.6	1.7	20	2.1	260	2.6	1200	1200	340	15	16	200	75

† *The allowances, expressed as average daily intakes over time, are intended to provide for individual variations among most normal persons as they live in the United States under usual environmental stresses. Diets should be based on a variety of common foods in order to provide other nutrients for which human requirements have been less well defined.*

‡ *Weights and heights of Reference Adults are actual medians for the U.S. population of the designated age, as reported by NHANES II. The median weights and heights of those under 19 years of age were taken from Hamill PVV, Drizd TA, Johnson CL, et al: Physical growth. National Center for Health Statistics Percentiles. Am J Clin Nutr 1979; 32:607. The use of these figures does not imply that the height-to-weight ratios are ideal.*

§ *Retinol equivalents. 1 retinol equivalent = 1 μg retinol or 6 μg β-carotene.*

‖ *As cholecalciferol. 10 μg cholecalciferol = 400 IU of vitamin D.*

α-Tocopherol equivalents. 1 mg d-α tocopherol = 1 α-TE.

†† *1 NE (niacin equivalent) is equal to 1 mg of niacin or 60 mg of dietary tryptophan.*

* *Recommended Dietary Allowances. 1980 National Academy of Sciences, National Research Council, Washington, D.C.*

Maternal Weight Gain

The best assurance of an adequate caloric intake during pregnancy is a satisfactory weight gain over time. The optimal weight gain depends on the woman's height, bone structure, and prepregnant nutritional state. The average weight gain during pregnancy is 25 to 30 lb (11 to 13.6 kg). Currently, researchers suggest that weight gain should be considered in terms of optimum ranges. Based on prepregnant weight, the following ranges provide general guidelines for weight gain (Williams 1989; Brown 1984):

- Underweight woman: 28 to 36 lb (13 to 16.5 kg)
- Normal weight woman: 24 to 32 lb (10 to 14.5 kg)
- Overweight woman: 16 to 24 lb (7.3 to 11 kg)

The American College of Obstetricians and Gynecologists (ACOG) recommends a weight gain of 26 to 35 lb, regardless of prepregnant weight (ACOG Newsletter 1986), although some authorities feel this range may be too high (Cunningham et al 1989).

The pattern of weight gain is also important. The ideal pattern of weight gain during pregnancy consists of a gain of 2 to 5 lb (1 to 2.3 kg) during the first trimester, followed by an average gain of slightly less than 1 lb (0.5 kg) per week during the last two trimesters. During the second trimester, most of the weight gain reflects an increase in blood volume; enlargement of breasts, uterus, and associated tissue and fluid; and deposit of maternal fat. In the last trimester, the weight gain is mainly that of the conceptus (fetus, placenta, and amniotic fluid).

The average weight gain is distributed as follows:

11 lb (5 kg)	Fetus, placenta, amniotic fluid
2 lb (0.9 kg)	Uterus
4 lb (1.8 kg)	Increased blood volume
3 lb (1.4 kg)	Breast tissue
5 to 10 lb (2.3. to 4.5 kg)	Maternal stores

Inadequate gains (less than 2.2 lb [1.0 kg] per month during the second and third trimesters of pregnancy) or excessive gains (more than 6.6 lb [3 kg] per month) should be evaluted and the need for nutritional counseling considered. Inadequate weight gain has been associated with low-birth-weight infants. Moreover, "infant birth weight is the variable known to be most closely related to infant mortality" (Brown 1989, p 631). Sudden sharp increases (weight gains of 1.4 to 2.3 kg [3 to 5 lb] in a week) result from fluid retention and require further evaluation because they may indicate that the woman is developing pregnancy-induced hypertension (PIH).

Table 16-2 Daily Food Plan for Pregnancy and Lactation*

Food group	Nutrients provided	Food source	Recommended daily amount during pregnancy	Recommended daily amount during lactation
Dairy products	Protein; riboflavin; vitamins A, D, and others; calcium; phosphorous; zinc; magnesium	Milk—whole, 2%, skim, dry, buttermilk Cheeses—hard, semisoft, cottage Yogurt—plain, low-fat Soybean milk—canned, dry	Four 8-oz cups (five for teenagers) used plain or with flavoring, in shakes, soups, puddings, custards, cocoa Calcium in 1 c milk equivalent to 1½ c cottage cheese, 1½ oz hard or semisoft cheese, 1 c yogurt, 1½ c ice cream (high in fat and sugar)	Four 8-oz cups (five for teenagers); equivalent amount of cheese, yogurt, etc.
Meat group	Protein; iron; thiamine, niacin, and other vitamins; minerals	Beef, pork, veal, lamb, poultry, animal organ meats, fish eggs; legumes; nuts, seeds, peanut butter, grains in proper vegetarian combination (vitamin B$_{12}$ supplement needed)	Three servings (one serving = 2 oz) Combination in amounts necessary for same nutrient equivalent (varies greatly)	Two servings
Grain products, whole grain or enriched	B vitamins; iron; whole grain also has zinc, magnesium, and other trace elements; provides fiber	Breads and bread products such as cornbread, muffins, waffles, hot cakes, biscuits, dumplings, cereals, pastas, rice	Four servings daily: one serving = one slice bread, ¾ c or 1 oz dry cereal, ½ c rice or pasta	Four servings
Fruits and fruit juices	Vitamins A and C; minerals; raw fruits for roughage	Citrus fruits and juices, melons, berries, all other fruits and juices	Two to three servings (one serving for vitamin C): one serving = one medium fruit, ½–1 c fruit, 4 oz orange or grapefruit juice	Same as for pregnancy
Vegetables and vegetable juices	Vitamins A and C; minerals; provides roughage	Leafy green vegetables; deep yellow or orange vegetables such as carrots, sweet potatoes, squash, tomatoes; green vegetables such as peas, green beans, broccoli; other vegetables such as beets, cabbage, potatoes, corn, lima beans	Two to three servings (one serving of dark green or deep yellow vegetable for vitamin A): one serving = ½–1 c vegetable, two tomatoes, one medium potato	Same as for pregnancy
Fats	Vitamins A and D; linoleic acid	Butter, cream cheese, fortified table spreads; cream, whipped cream, whipped toppings; avocado, mayonnaise, oil, nuts	As desired in moderation (high in calories): one serving = 1 Tbsp butter or enriched margarine	Same as for pregnancy
Sugar and sweets		Sugar, brown sugar, honey, molasses	Occasionally, if desired	Same as for pregnancy
Desserts		Nutritious desserts such as puddings, custards, fruit whips, and crisps; other rich, sweet desserts and pastries	Occasionally, if desired (high in calories)	Same as for pregnancy
Beverages		Coffee, decaffeinated beverages, tea, bouillon, carbonated drinks	As desired, in moderation	Same as for pregnancy
Miscellaneous		Iodized salt, herbs, spices, condiments	As desired	Same as for pregnancy

*The pregnant woman should eat regularly, three meals a day, with nutritious snacks of fruit, cheese, milk, or other foods between meals if desired. (More frequent but smaller meals are also recommended.) Four to six (8-oz) glasses of water and a total of eight to ten (8-oz) cups total fluid should be consumed daily. Water is an essential nutrient.

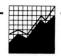

Research Note

Clinical Application of Research

In an effort to determine the relationship between nutrition and weight gain of pregnancy, Lauren Aaronson and Carol Macnee (1989) interviewed 529 women. Questions about a 24-hour recall of food and drink were incorporated as part of a larger study. Nutrition information from the 24-hour recall was used to establish four categories of nutritional quality, with each category having a numeric range. The categories were based on intake of six food groups (milk and dairy products; protein; vitamin A fruits and vegetables; vitamin C fruits and vegetables; other fruits and vegetables; and breads and grains) as well as on consumption of the required number of servings for each group. Other variables, which were obtained from postpartum chart review, included mother's weight gain, baby's birth weight, length of gestation compared to expected date of birth (EDB), body mass index (mother's prepregnant weight in grams divided by reported height in centimeters), and edema.

Although the study showed a weak relationship between nutrition and weight gain, stronger relationships developed between weight gain and edema and weight gain and length of gestation. Weight gain in this study was not associated with either smoking or health care provider recommendations. Weight gain, but not nutrition, related significantly to the baby's weight.

Critical Thinking Applied to Research

Strengths: Graphs comparing weight gain to baby's weight and nutrition to baby's weight visually corroborate statistical results. The reliability and validity issues associated with obtaining quantified symptoms of edema from a chart review, as well as other limitations, were noted.

Concerns: Use of recalled information rather than recorded or observed data can result in bias because the participant wants to please the researcher or does not remember correctly.

Aaronson L, Macnee C: The relationship between weight gain and nutrition in pregnancy. *Nurs Res* 1989; 38(4): 223.

Because of the association between inadequate weight gain and low-birth-weight infants, most care givers pay particular attention to weight gain during pregnancy. A woman should generally gain 10 to 13 lb by 20 weeks' gestation. Failure to do so puts the woman at risk for intrauterine growth retardation and requires further evaluation and possible nutritional counseling.

Monitoring the weight gain of the obese woman (one who weighs 20% or more above her recommended pre-pregnant weight) during pregnancy may be difficult. Obese women, even if not diabetic, have an increased risk of having a large baby. They also have an increased risk of chronic hypertension and PIH (Wolfe & Gross 1988). Obese women may have diets that are high in energy (from carbohydrates and fats) but low in protein, vitamins, and minerals. Thus weight gain alone does not guarantee adequate nutrition. Pregnancy is not a time for dieting, and severe weight restriction during pregnancy can result in maternal ketosis, a threat to fetal well-being. Counseling for the obese pregnant woman usually focuses on encouraging her to eat according to the RDA for pregnancy. Less emphasis is placed on the amount of weight gain and more emphasis is placed on the quality of her intake (Anderson 1986).

Women who are 10% or more below their recommended weight prior to conception have an increased risk of giving birth to a low-weight infant and may have an increased risk of developing PIH as well (Pitkin 1986). Merely advocating the traditional weight gain is not adequate counseling for the underweight woman who is pregnant. The nurse first assesses why the woman is underweight. Once the cause is determined, intervention can be planned with the woman. The underweight woman is usually advised to increase her caloric intake by 500 kilocalories (kcal) above the nonpregnant RDA (as opposed to the 300 kcal usual increase). She should also consume 20 g additional protein. This is often difficult for the underweight woman, especially if she has a small appetite, and she will require support and encouragement from family and health care providers.

Nutritional Requirements

CRITICAL THINKING

In counseling a pregnant woman about nutrition, what role do the new RDAs play?

The RDA for almost all nutrients increases during pregnancy, although the amount of increase varies with each nutrient. In some cases, as with folate and magnesium, the recommended increase during pregnancy has been lowered somewhat in the new guidelines (Table 16–1).

Calories

The term **calorie** (cal) stands for the amount of heat required to raise the temperature of 1 g of water 1C. The **kilocalorie** (kcal) is equivalent to 1000 cal and is the unit used to express the energy value of food.

The RDA for energy is no caloric increase during the first trimester, and a daily increase of 300 kcal during the second and third trimesters. Thus, for example, a moderately active pregnant female, age 22, has a caloric requirement of 2500 kcal (2200 kcal [the RDA for energy for a woman aged 19–24 years] + 300 kcal).

For this reason, weight gains should be monitored regularly, and diets should be individualized for caloric needs. Prepregnant weight, height, maternal age, activity, and health status all affect caloric needs.

The Teaching Guide—Helping the Pregnant Woman Add 300 kcal to Her Diet offers suggestions for providing basic nutritional information to pregnant women.

Protein

During pregnancy protein is needed in increased amounts to provide amino acids for fetal development, blood volume expansion, and growth of other maternal tissues such as breasts and uterus. Protein also contributes to the body's overall energy metabolism. The RDA for protein during pregnancy is 60 g, an increase of about 14 g (Table 16–1).

An important source of protein is milk. A quart of milk supplies 32 g of protein, almost half the average daily protein requirement. (See Table 16–3). Milk can be incorporated into the diet in a variety of dishes, including soups, puddings, custards, sauces, and yogurt. Beverages such as hot chocolate and milk-and-fruit drinks can also be included, but they are high in calories. Various kinds of hard and soft cheeses and cottage cheese are excellent protein sources; although cream cheese is categorized as a fat source only. Table 16–3 provides information on the protein content of commonly used foods.

Women who have allergies to milk (lactose intolerance) or who practice vegetarianism may find dried or canned soy milk acceptable. It can be used in cooked dishes or as a beverage. Tofu, or soybean curd, can replace cottage cheese. Those who are allergic to cow's milk can sometimes tolerate goat's milk and cheese. Frequently, cooked milk can also be tolerated.

Meat, poultry, fish, eggs, and legumes are good sources of protein. Small amounts of complete animal protein can be combined with partially complete plant protein for an excellent, easily used supply of protein. Several examples of complementary proteins are eggs and toast, tuna and rice, cereal and milk, spaghetti and meat sauce, macaroni and cheese, and peanut butter and bread. Except in unusual medical situations, dietary protein should be obtained through natural foods, and the use of protein supplements should be avoided (Johnstone 1984).

Fat

Fats are valuable sources of energy for the body. Fats are more completely absorbed during pregnancy, resulting in a marked increase in serum lipids, lipoproteins, and cholesterol and decreased elimination of fat through the bowel. Fat deposits in the fetus increase from about 2% at midpregnancy to almost 12% at term. The RDA for fat is less than 30% of daily caloric intake, of which less than 10% should be saturated fat.

Carbohydrates

Carbohydrates provide protective substances, bulk, and energy. Carbohydrates contribute to the total caloric intake required. If the total caloric intake is not adequate, the body uses protein for energy. Protein then becomes unavailable for growth needs. In addition, protein breakdown leads to ketosis. Ketosis can be a problem, especially in diabetic women, due to glycosuria, reduced alkaline reserves, and lipidemia.

The carbohydrate and caloric needs of the pregnant woman increase, especially during the last two trimesters. Carbohydrate intake promotes weight gain and growth of the fetus, placenta, and other maternal tissues. Milk, fruits, vegetables, and whole-grain cereals and breads all contain carbohydrates and other important nutrients.

Minerals

Increased minerals needed for the growth of new tissue during pregnancy are obtained by improved mineral absorption and an increase in mineral allowances.

Calcium and Phosphorus

Calcium and phosphorus are involved in mineralization of fetal bones and teeth, energy and cell production, and acid-base buffering. Calcium is absorbed and used more efficiently during pregnancy. Some calcium and phosphorus are required early in pregnancy, but most of the fetus' bone calcification occurs during the last two or three months.

Table 16–3	Amount of Protein in Commonly Used Foods	
Food		**Grams protein**
Milk		
Milk, 8 oz		8
Cheese, cheddar, Swiss, etc, 1 oz		7
Cottage cheese, ¼ c		7
Meat Group		
Meat, fish, poultry, 1 oz		7
Egg, 1		7
Cooked dry beans & peas, ½ c		7
Cooked soybeans, ½ c		11
Peanut butter, 2 Tbsp		7
Peanuts (3 Tbsp), cashews/almonds (5 Tbsp)		7
Breads and Cereals		
Bread, 1 slice		2
Buns, biscuits, muffins, 1		2
Cooked cereals & grain, ½ c		2
Breakfast cereal, 1 oz		2
Vegetables and Fruits		
Vegetables, ½ c		0.5–1
Fruits & juices, ½ c		0.5

TEACHING GUIDE

Helping the Pregnant Woman Add 300 kcal to Her Diet

Assessment: The nurse recognizes that the notion of "eating for two" may cause a woman to overestimate the amount of food she should consume during pregnancy. The nurse assesses the pregnant woman's knowledge of basic nutrition, including the use of the basic four food groups, and assesses her awareness of the best way to increase the nutrients in her diet.

Nursing Diagnosis: The key nursing diagnosis will probably be: Knowledge deficit related to nutritional needs during pregnancy.

Nursing Plan and Implementation: The teaching plan focuses on providing information about the basic four food groups and about the most effective way to use the additional 300 kcal that a woman needs daily during pregnancy.

Client Goals: At the completion of the teaching the woman will:

1. Identify the four basic food group categories and the foods included in each.
2. Cite the increase in kcal indicated during pregnancy.
3. Discuss the most nutritionally sound way to use the additional calories.
4. Use the information she has gained to plan a nutritionally sound sample menu.

Teaching Plan

Content:

The four basic food groups include the following:

Dairy: adult needs two servings (one serving = 1 c milk or yogurt, 1.5 oz hard cheese, 2 c cottage cheese, 1 c pudding made with milk)

Grains: adult needs four servings (one serving = one slice bread, ½ hamburger roll, 1 oz dry cereal, 1 tortilla, ½ c pasta, rice, grits)

Fruits/vegetables: adult needs four servings, one should be a good source of vitamin C (one serving = 1 medium-sized piece of fruit, ½ c cooked vegetable, 1 c raw vegetables, ½ c juice, 1 c green leafy vegetable)

Meats and alternates: adult needs at least two servings (one serving = 2 oz cooked lean meat, poultry, or fish; 2 eggs; ½ c cottage cheese; 1 c cooked legumes [kidney, lima, garbanzo, or soy beans, split peas, etc]; 6 oz tofu; 2 oz nuts or seeds; 4 Tbsp peanut butter)

Not all foods that are nutritionally equivalent have the same number of calories; it is important to consider that in making food choices.

Limited extras are foods that have less nutrient value and should be eaten as limited supplements. Examples include sugary foods such as cake, doughnuts, candy; high-fat foods such as mayonnaise, potato chips, butter, etc.

Emphasize that a woman only has to add 300 kcal/day during pregnancy. This can be achieved by adding two milk servings and one meat or alternate. Because of the varying caloric value a woman needs to consider the advisability of using lowfat milk, lean cuts of meat, or fish broiled or baked instead of fried, etc.

Teaching Method: Ask woman if she has received nutritional information using this approach before. Discuss her understanding of it. Use that information to plan the amount of detail you will use.

Use a chart or colorful handout to explain the basic food groups and to give examples of equivalent foods.

Use a calorie counting guide to compare the calories in a variety of foods that are equivalent, such as 2 oz beef and 2 oz fish, or 1 c lowfat milk and 1 c whole milk.

Use a similar approach to evaluate the calories in the limited extras, but also evaluate their nutrient content, especially levels of vitamin C, iron, etc.

In planning the woman's diet to get optimum nutrition without too many additional calories, it is often helpful to ask her to plan and evaluate a sample menu.

(continued)

TEACHING GUIDE (continued)

Teaching Plan

Foods can be combined. For example, 1 c spaghetti with a 2-oz meatball would count as 1 serving meat, ¾ c spaghetti = 1 grain, and ¼ c tomato sauce = ½ serving vegetable.

Evaluation: Teaching has been effective if all the identified goals are achieved and if the woman seems comfortable planning her diet to provide for the best nutrition possible.

Provide handouts on which the woman can list the foods she has eaten and check off the corresponding nutrient categories. Have her bring her completed handouts to a subsequent visit.

Teeth begin to form at about eight weeks' gestation and are formed by birth. The six-year molars begin to calcify just before birth. This means that calcium is particularly important as a structural element. Additional calcium is stored in the maternal skeleton as a reserve for lactation.

The RDA for calcium for the pregnant or lactating woman, regardless of age, is 1200 mg/day. If calcium intakes are low, fetal needs will be met at the mother's expense by demineralization of maternal bone.

A diet that includes 4 cups of milk or an equivalent dairy alternate (see Table 16–2) will provide sufficient calcium. Smaller amounts of calcium are supplied by legumes, nuts, dried fruits, and dark green leafy vegetables (such as kale, cabbage, collards, and turnip greens). It is important to remember that some of the calcium in beet greens, spinach, and chard is bound with oxalic acid, which makes it unavailable to the body.

The RDA for phosphorus is the same as the RDA for calcium: 1200 mg/day for the pregnant or lactating woman. Phosphorus is readily supplied through calcium- and protein-rich foods, especially milk, eggs, and meat.

As phosphorus is so widely available in foods, the dietary intake of phosphorus frequently exceeds calcium intake. An excess of phosphorus can result in a disturbance of the calcium-phosphorus ratio in the body, decreased calcium absorption, and increased excretion of calcium. Excess phosphorus can be reduced by avoiding the snack foods, processed meats, and cola drinks in which it abounds. However, if vitamin D and magnesium are adequate, most adults can tolerate relatively wide variations in dietary calcium-phosphorus ratios.

Iodine

Inorganic iodine is excreted in the urine during pregnancy. Enlargement of the thyroid gland may occur if iodine is not replaced by adequate dietary intake or additional supplement. Moreover, cretinism may occur in the infant if the mother has a severe iodine deficiency.

The iodine allowance of 175 μg/day can be met by using iodized salt. When sodium is restricted, the physician may prescribe an iodine supplement.

Sodium

The sodium ion is essential for proper metabolism. Sodium intake in the form of salt is never entirely curtailed during pregnancy, even when hypertension or PIH is present. Food may be seasoned to taste during cooking but the use of extra salt at the table should be avoided. Salty foods such as potato chips, ham, sausages, and sodium-based seasonings can be eliminated to avoid excessive intake.

Zinc

Zinc was recognized as a nutrient factor affecting growth in 1974. The RDA during pregnancy is 15 mg. Sources include milk, liver, shellfish, and wheat bran. Zinc deficiency during pregnancy may contribute to developmental disorders in the child (RDA 1989).

Magnesium

Magnesium is essential for cellular metabolism and structural growth. The RDA for pregnancy has been lowered considerably in the new recommendations and is now 320 mg. Sources include milk, whole grains, beet greens, nuts, legumes, and tea.

Iron

Anemia in pregnancy is mainly caused by low iron stores, although it may also be caused by inadequate intake of other nutrients, such as vitamins B_6 and B_{12}, folic acid, ascorbic acid, copper, and zinc. Women with poor diet histories, frequent conceptions, or records of prior iron depletion are particularly at risk.

Anemia is generally defined as a decrease in the oxygen-carrying capacity of the blood. This significantly reduces the hemoglobin per decaliter of blood, the volume of packed red cells per decaliter of blood (hematocrit), or the number of erythrocytes.

The normal hematocrit in the nonpregnant woman is 38% to 47%. In the pregnant woman, the level may drop as low as 34%, even when nutrition is adequate. This condition is called the *physiologic anemia of pregnancy* (see Chapter 12).

Fetal demands for iron further contribute to symptoms of anemia in the pregnant woman. The fetal liver stores iron, especially during the third trimester. The infant needs this stored iron during the first four months of life to compensate for the normally inadequate levels of iron in breast milk and non–iron-fortified formulas.

To prevent anemia, the woman must balance iron requirements and intake. Doing so is a problem for nonpregnant women and a greater one for pregnant women. By carefully selecting foods high in iron, the woman can increase her daily iron intake considerably. Lean meats, dark green leafy vegetables, eggs, and whole-grain and enriched breads and cereals are the foods usually depended on for their iron content. Other iron sources include dried fruits, legumes, shellfish, and molasses.

Iron absorption is generally higher for animal products than for vegetable products. However, absorption of iron from nonmeat sources may be enhanced by combining them with meat or a good vitamin C source.

The most iron that can reasonably be obtained from the diet is about 15 to 18 mg per day. However, the RDA for iron during pregnancy is 30 mg. Thus, during pregnancy a supplement of simple iron salt, such as ferrous gluconate, ferrous fumarate, or ferrous sulfate (30 to 60 mg daily) is needed. Supplements are not usually given during the first trimester because the increased demand is still minimal, and iron may increase the woman's nausea.

Vitamins

Vitamins are organic substances necessary for life and growth. They are found in small amounts in specific foods and generally cannot be synthesized by the body.

Vitamins are grouped according to solubility. Those vitamins that dissolve in fat are A, D, E, and K; those soluble in water include C and the B complex. An adequate intake of all vitamins is essential during pregnancy; however, several are required in larger then normal amounts to fulfill specific needs.

A balanced diet generally provides necessary vitamins without the need for supplementation. Despite this, many food faddists and people who are concerned about nutrition have become involved in the practice of taking exceptionally large doses—megadoses—of vitamins. However, in vitamin therapy more is not necessarily better. Megadoses of vitamins, especially vitamins A, D, C, and B_6, have had a negative effect on the fetus. Furthermore, excessive intake of one vitamin may interfere with the body's use of another vitamin. For example, excessive intake of vitamin C may block the body's use of vitamin

B_{12}, while the body's use of vitamin B_2 (riboflavin) may be altered by megadoses of vitamin B_6 (Luke 1985). Consequently, while it is important to meet the RDA of vitamins during pregnancy, megadoses are best avoided.

Fat-Soluble Vitamins

The fat-soluble vitamins A, D, E, and K are stored in the liver and thus are available should the dietary intake become inadequate. The major complication related to these vitamins is not deficiency but toxicity due to overdose because excess amounts of A, D, E, and K are not excreted in the urine. Symptoms of vitamin toxicity include nausea, gastrointestinal upset, dryness and cracking of the skin, and loss of hair.

Vitamin A is involved in the growth of epithelial cells, which line the entire gastrointestinal tract and compose the skin. Vitamin A plays a role in the metabolism of carbohydrates and fats. The body cannot synthesize glycogen in the absence of vitamin A, and the body's ability to handle cholesterol is also affected. The protective layer of tissue surrounding nerve fibers does not form properly if vitamin A is lacking.

Probably the best-known function of vitamin A is its effect on vision in dim light. A person's ability to see in the dark depends on the eye's supply of retinol, a form of vitamin A. In this manner, vitamin A prevents night blindness. Vitamin A is associated with the formation and development of healthy eyes in the fetus.

If maternal stores of vitamin A are adequate, the overall effects of pregnancy on the woman's vitamin A requirements are not remarkable. The blood serum level of vitamin A decreases slightly in early pregnancy, rises in late pregnancy, and falls before the onset of labor. Thus the RDA for vitamin A does not increase during pregnancy.

Excessive intake of preformed vitamin A is toxic to both children and adults. There are indications that excessive intake of vitamin A in the fetus can cause eye, ear, and bone malformations, cleft palate, possible renal anomalies, and central nervous system damage (Luke 1985).

Rich plant sources of vitamin A include deep green and yellow vegetables, and some fruits; animal sources include liver, liver oil, kidney, egg yolk, cream, butter, and fortified margarine.

Vitamin D is best known for its role in the absorption and utilization of calcium and phosphorus in skeletal development. To supply the needs of the developing fetus, the pregnant woman should have a vitamin D intake of 10 μg/day.

A deficiency of vitamin D results in rickets, a condition caused by improper calcification of the bones. It is treated with relatively large doses of vitamin D under a physician's direction.

Main food sources of vitamin D include fortified milk, margarine, butter, liver, and egg yolks. Drinking a quart of milk daily provides the vitamin D needed during pregnancy.

Excessive intake of vitamin D is not usually a result of eating but of taking high-potency vitamin preparations.

Overdoses during pregnancy can cause hypercalcemia or high blood calcium levels due to withdrawal of calcium from the skeletal tissue. In the fetus, cardiac defects, especially aortic stenosis, may occur (Luke 1985). Continued overdose can also cause hypercalcemia and eventually death, especially in young children. Symptoms of toxicity are excessive thirst, loss of appetite, vomiting, weight loss, irritability, and high blood calcium levels.

The major function of *vitamin E,* or tocopherol, is as an antioxidant. Vitamin E takes on oxygen, thus preventing another substance from undergoing chemical change. For example, vitamin E helps spare vitamin A by preventing its oxidation in the intestinal tract and the tissues. It decreases the oxidation of polyunsaturated fats, thus helping to retain the flexibility and health of the cell membrane. In protecting the cell membrane, vitamin E affects the health of all cells in the body. Its role during pregnancy is not known.

Vitamin E is also involved in certain enzymatic and metabolic reactions. It is an essential nutrient for the synthesis of nucleic acids required in the formation of red blood cells in the bone marrow. Vitamin E is beneficial in treating certain types of muscular pain and intermittent claudication, in surface healing of wounds and burns, and in protecting lung tissue from the damaging effects of smog. These functions may help explain the abundant claims and cures attributed to vitamin E, many of which have not been scientifically proved.

The newborn's need for vitamin E has been widely recognized. Human milk provides adequate vitamin E, whereas cow's milk is lower in E content. Deficiency symptoms of vitamin E are related to long-term inability to absorb fats. In humans, malabsorption problems exist in cases of cystic fibrosis, liver cirrhosis, postgastrectomy, obstructive jaundice, pancreatic problems, and sprue.

The recommended intake of vitamin E increases from 8 IU for nonpregnant females to 10 IU for pregnant women. The vitamin E requirement varies with the polyunsaturated fat content of the diet. Vitamin E is widely distributed in foodstuffs, especially vegetable fats and oils, whole grains, greens, and eggs.

Some pregnant women use vitamin E oil on the abdominal skin to make it supple and possibly prevent permanent stretch marks. It is questionable whether taking high doses internally will accomplish this goal or satisfy any other claims related to vitamin E's role in reproduction or virility. In addition, excessive intake of vitamin E has been associated with abnormal coagulation in the newborn.

Vitamin K, or menadione as used synthetically in medicine, is an essential factor for the synthesis of prothrombin; its function is thus related to normal blood clotting. Synthesis occurs in the intestinal tract by the *Escherichia coli* bacteria normally inhabiting the large intestine. However, the body's need for vitamin K is not totally met through synthesis (Suttie et al, 1988). Green leafy vegetables are an excellent source. The RDA for vitamin K does not increase during pregnancy. Newborn infants, having a sterile intestinal tract and receiving sterile feeding, lack vitamin K. Thus newborns often receive a dose of menadione as a protective measure.

Intake of vitamin K is usually adequate in a well-balanced prenatal diet. Secondary problems may rise if an illness is present that results in malabsorption of fats or if antibiotics are used for an extended period, which would inhibit vitamin K synthesis.

Water-Soluble Vitamins

Water-soluble vitamins are excreted in the urine. Only small amounts are stored, so there is little protection from dietary inadequacies. Thus, adequate amounts must be ingested daily. During pregnancy, the concentration of water-soluble vitamins in the maternal serum falls, whereas high concentrations are found in the fetus.

The requirement for *vitamin C* (ascorbic acid) is increased in pregnancy from 60 to 70 mg. The major function of vitamin C is to aid the formation and development of connective tissue and the vascular system. Ascorbic acid is essential to the formation of collagen. Collagen is like a cement that binds cells together, just as mortar holds bricks together. If the collagen begins to disintegrate due to lack of ascorbic acid, cell functioning is disturbed and cell structure breaks down, causing muscular weakness, capillary hemorrhage, and eventual death. These are symptoms of scurvy, the disease caused by vitamin C deficiency. Infants fed mainly cow's milk become deficient in vitamin C. Surprisingly, newborns of women who have taken megadoses of vitamin C may experience a rebound form of scurvy (Anderson 1986).

Maternal plasma levels of vitamin C progressively decline throughout pregnancy, with values at term being about half those at midpregnancy. It appears that ascorbic acid concentrates in the placenta; levels in the fetus are 50% or more above maternal levels.

A nutritious diet should meet the pregnant woman's needs for vitamin C without additional supplementation. Common food sources of vitamin C include citrus fruit, tomatoes, cantaloupe, strawberries, potatoes, broccoli, and other leafy greens. Ascorbic acid is readily destroyed by oxidation. Therefore, foods containing vitamin C must be stored and cooked properly.

The *B vitamins* include thiamine (B_1), riboflavin (B_2), niacin, folic acid, pantothenic acid, vitamin B_6, and vitamin B_{12}. These vitamins serve as vital coenzyme factors in many reactions, such as cell respiration, glucose oxidation, and energy metabolism. The quantities needed, therefore, invariably increase as caloric intake increases to meet the metabolic and growth needs of the pregnant woman.

The *thiamine* requirement increases from the prepregnant level of 1.1 mg/day to 1.5 mg/day. Sources include pork, liver, milk, potatoes, enriched breads, and cereals.

Riboflavin deficiency is manifested by cheilosis and other skin lesions. During pregnancy, women may excrete less riboflavin and still require more, because of increased energy and protein needs. An additional 0.3 mg/day is recommended. Sources include milk, liver, eggs, enriched breads, and cereals.

An increase of 2 mg daily in *niacin* intake is recommended during pregnancy and 5 mg during lactation. Sources of niacin include meat, fish, poultry, liver, whole grains, enriched breads, cereals, and peanuts.

Folic acid promotes adequate fetal growth and prevents the macrocytic, megaloblastic anemia of pregnancy. Folic acid is directly related to the outcome of pregnancy and to maternal and fetal health. Folate deficiency has been associated with abortion, fetal malformation, abruptio placentae, and other late bleeding complications. Severe maternal folate deficiency may have other unrecognized effects on the fetus and newborn. Hemorrhagic anemia in the newborn is attributed to this deficiency.

Megaloblastic anemia due to folate deficiency is rarely found in the United States, but those caring for pregnant women must be aware that it does occur. Folate deficiency can also be present in the absence of overt anemia.

The RDA for folic acid increases during pregnancy. However, the specific requirements have been lowered significantly in the latest recommendations. The RDA during pregnancy is 400 µg. "This level can be met by a well-selected diet without food fortification or oral supplementation" (RDA 1989, p 154). Due to the risks associated with deficiency during pregnancy, folic acid supplementation of 300 µg is indicated for women with low folate stores or a diet low in folate (RDA 1989).

Women on phenytoin (Dilantin) for the control of seizures and women carrying twins are also especially susceptible to folic acid deficiency. Daily supplements of 0.8 to 1.0 mg folic acid are indicated for these women (Cruikshank 1986).

The best food sources of folates are fresh green leafy vegetables, kidney, liver, food yeasts, and peanuts. Many foods contain small amounts of folic acid. Cow's milk contains a small amount of folic acid, but goat's milk contains none. Therefore, infants and children who are given goat's milk must receive a folate supplement to prevent a deficiency.

Folic acid content of foods can be altered by preparation methods. Since folic acid is a water-soluble nutrient, care must be taken in cooking. Loss of the vitamin from vegetables and meats can be considerable when they are cooked in large amounts of water or simply overcooked.

No allowance has been set for *pantothenic acid* in pregnancy, but 5 mg/day is considered a safe, adequate intake. Sources include meats, egg yolk, legumes, and whole-grain cereals and breads.

Vitamin B_6 (pyridoxine) has long been associated biochemically with pregnancy. The RDA for vitamin B_6 during pregnancy is 2.2 mg, an increase of 0.6 mg over the allowance for nonpregnant women. Since pyridoxine is associated with amino acid metabolism, a higher-than-average protein intake requires increased pyridoxine intake. The slightly increased need can generally be supplied by dietary sources, which include wheat germ, yeast, fish, liver, pork, potatoes, and lentils.

Vitamin B_{12}, or cobalamin, is the cobalt-containing vitamin found only in animal sources. Rarely is B_{12} deficiency found in women of reproductive age. Vegetarians can develop a deficiency, however, so it is essential that their dietary intake be supplemented with this vitamin. Occasionally vitamin B_{12} levels decrease during pregnancy but increase again after birth. The RDA during pregnancy is 2.2 µg/day, an increase of 0.2 µg. This RDA is one-third to one-half lower than the RDA cited in the previous recommendations.

A deficiency may be due to inability to absorb vitamin B_{12} resulting in pernicious anemia; infertility is a complication of this type of anemia.

Folic acid and iron are the only nutritional supplements generally recommended during pregnancy. The increased need for other vitamins and minerals can usually be met with an adequate diet. To avoid possible deficiencies, however, many health care professionals still recommend a daily vitamin supplement. As the new recommendations become more well known, this practice may change.

Fluid

Water is essential for life and is found in all body tissues. It is necessary for many biochemical reactions. It also serves as a lubricant, acts as a medium of transport for carrying substances in and out of the body, and aids in temperature control. A pregnant woman should consume at least eight to ten (8-oz) glasses of fluid each day, of which four to six glasses should be water. Because of their sodium content, diet sodas should be consumed in moderation. Caffeinated beverages have a diuretic effect, which may be counterproductive to increasing fluid intake.

Vegetarianism

Vegetarianism is the dietary choice of many people, for religious (Seventh-Day Adventists), health, and ethical reasons. There are several types of vegetarians. **Lacto-ovo-vegetarians** include milk, dairy products, and eggs in their diet. Occasionally fish, poultry, and liver are consumed. *Lactovegetarians* include dairy products but no eggs in their diet. *Vegans* are "pure" vegetarians who will not eat any food from animal sources.

In their position statement on vegetarian diets, the American Dietetic Association stated that "vegetarian diets are healthful and nutritionally adequate when appropriately planned" (ADA 1988). People following vegetarian diets tend to have lower blood pressure, have a lower incidence of coronary artery disease, osteoporosis, gallstones, kidney stones, and diverticulitis, and have weights closer to desirable levels than do nonvegetarians (ADA Technical Support Paper 1988).

The expectant woman who is vegetarian must eat the proper combination of foods to obtain adequate nutrients. If her diet allows, a woman can obtain ample and complete proteins from dairy products and eggs. Plant protein quality may be improved if consumed with these animal proteins. If the diet contains less than four servings of milk and milk products, calcium supplementation may be necessary.

If a "pure" vegetarian diet is followed, careful planning is necessary to obtain sufficient calories and complete proteins. Obtaining sufficient calories to achieve adequate weight gains can be difficult because vegan diets tend to be higher in bulk and, therefore, filling. Low prepregnancy weight and optimum pregnancy weight gains are often a problem. Supplementation with energy-dense foods helps provide increased energy intake to prevent the body from using protein for caloric needs.

If energy needs are adequate, protein needs can usually be met if recommendations for complementing proteins are followed. An adequate pure vegetarian diet contains protein from unrefined grains (brown rice and whole wheat), legumes (beans, split peas, lentils), nuts in large quantities, and a variety of cooked and fresh vegetables and fruits. Complete protein may be obtained by eating different types of complementary proteins, such as legumes and whole-grain cereals, nuts and whole-grain cereals, or nuts and legumes, over the course of a day (ADA 1988). Seeds may be used in the vegetarian diet if the quantity is large enough.

Because vegans use no animal products, a daily supplement of 4 μg of vitamin B$_{12}$ is necessary. If soy milk is used, only partial supplementation may be needed. If no soy milk is taken, daily supplements of 1200 mg of calcium and 10 μg of vitamin D are needed.

As the best sources of iron and zinc are found in animal products, strict vegetarian diets are also low in these minerals. In addition, a high fiber intake may reduce mineral (calcium, iron, and zinc) bioavailability. Emphasis should be placed on use of foods containing these nutrients.

Sample vegetarian menus that meet the requirements of good prenatal nutrition are given in Table 16–4.

Factors Influencing Nutrition

Besides having knowledge of nutritional needs and food sources, the nurse needs to be aware of other factors that affect a client's nutrition. What are the age, life-style, dietary practices, and culture of the pregnant woman? What food beliefs and habits does she have? What a person eats is determined by availability, economics, and symbolism. These factors and others influence the expectant mother's acceptance of the nurse's intervention.

Lactose Intolerance

Some individuals have difficulty digesting milk and milk products. This condition, known as **lactose intolerance**, results from an inadequate amount of the enzyme lactase, which breaks down the milk sugar lactose into smaller digestible substances.

Lactose intolerance is found in many blacks, Mexican Americans, Native Americans, Ashkenazic Jews, and Asians. People who are not affected are mainly of Northern European heritage. Symptoms include abdominal distention, discomfort, nausea, vomiting, loose stools, and cramps.

In counseling pregnant women who might be intolerant of milk and milk products, the nurse should be aware of the following:

- Even one glass of milk can produce symptoms. Tolerances vary with the individual.
- Milk is sometimes tolerated in cooked form, such as in custards.
- Cultured or fermented dairy products, such as buttermilk, cheese and yogurt, are sometimes tolerated.
- In some instances, the enzyme lactase may be used to alleviate the problem. It is available in several forms: as a tablet to be chewed before ingesting milk or milk products and as a liquid to add to milk itself. Lactase-treated milk is also available commercially in some grocery stores, although it may be more expensive than regular milk.

Pica

Pica is the persistent eating of substances that are not ordinarily considered edible or to have nutritive value. Most women who practice pica in pregnancy eat such substances only during that time.

Pica is most commonly practiced in poverty-stricken areas, where diets tend to be inadequate, but may also be found at other socioeconomic levels. The substances most commonly ingested in this country are dirt, clay, starch, ice, and freezer frost. Less commonly, items such as cardboard or burnt matchsticks may be ingested (Callinan et al 1988). Iron-deficiency anemia is the most common concern in pica. Studies indicate that ingestion of laundry starch or certain types of clay may contribute to iron deficiency by interfering with iron absorption. The ingestion of large quantities of clay could fill the intestine and cause fecal impaction, while the ingestion of starch may be associated with excessive weight gain (Cunningham et al 1989).

Nurses should be aware of pica and its implications for the woman and her fetus. Often pica is part of the tradition of certain communities or families. Assessment for pica is an important part of the nutritional history. However, women may be embarrassed about their cravings or reluctant to discuss them for fear of criticism. It is helpful if the nurse uses a nonjudgmental approach. Reeducation of

Table 16-4 Suggested Menus for Adequate Prenatal Vegetarian Diets

Meal pattern	Mixed diet	Lacto-ovovegetarian	Lactovegetarian	Seventh-Day Adventist	Vegan
Breakfast					
Fruit	¾ c orange juice	Same as mixed diet	Same	Same	Same
Grains	½ c granola, 1 slice whole-wheat toast				1 c granola, 1 slice whole-grain toast
Meat group	1 scrambled egg with cheese		1 oz cheese melted over toast (no egg)		
Fat	1 tsp butter		Same		1 tsp sesame butter
Milk	½ c milk				1 c soy milk
Midmorning					
Milk	1 c hot chocolate				1 c protein drink*
Lunch					
Meat group/vegetable	1 c lentil chowder[†] (made with ground beef)	1 c lentil chowder[†] (no ground beef)	1 c lentil chowder[†] (no ground beef)	1 c lentil chowder[†] (made with vegeburger)[‡]	1½ c lentil chowder[†] (1 Tbsp torula yeast, wheat germ added)
Grains	1 corn muffin	Same	Same	Same	2 corn muffins[§]
Fat	1 tsp butter, honey				2 tsp margarine, honey
Fruit/dessert	½ peach, ½ c cottage cheese salad				½ peach, ½ c tofu salad
Tea	1 c tea			Decaffeinated or herbal tea	Same as Seventh-Day Adventist
Midafternoon					
Milk	¾ c vanilla pudding			Same	1 c pudding (soy milk)
Fruit	¼ c sliced banana				½ banana
Grain	1 graham cracker				1 graham cracker with peanut butter
Dinner					
Meat group/vegetable	¾ c meat sauce (onion, celery, carrot, tomato, mushroom in sauce), parmesan cheese	¾ c tomato sauce (same vegetables as in mixed diet), ¼ c cheese	Same as lacto-ovo-vegetarian	Same (add vegeburger[‡] to tomato sauce)	Same (use tofu instead of cheese)
Grains	¾ c spaghetti, bread	1 c whole-wheat spaghetti, 1 slice French bread			
Vegetable	Mixed vegetable salad	Mixed vegetable salad with ¼ c sprouts, ½ egg, ½ oz cheese, ¼ c kidney beans added	(No egg in salad)		(Add tofu; no egg in salad)
Fat	Oil-vinegar dressing, ½ tsp butter	Same as mixed diet	Same		1 tsp margarine
Fruit	Fresh pear or baked pear half				Same as mixed diet
Tea	1 c tea			Decaffeinated or herbal tea	Same as Seventh-Day Adventist
Bedtime					
Milk	1 c milk			Same	
Meat group/vegetable	2 tsp peanut butter on celery or on wheat crackers				1 c protein drink*
Grain					Corn muffins[§]

[†] *Lentil chowder is made from lentils, celery, carrots, potatoes, onion, and tomatoes.*
[‡] *Vegeburger is made from meat analogues.*
[§] *Wheat germ and soy flour are added to corn muffin mixture.*

---

* *Protein drink recipe is: 3 c cow's or goat's milk, ½ c nonfat soy milk powder, 2 Tbsp wheat germ, 2 Tbsp brewer's yeast, fruit, and vanilla. Vegans may make the drink with soy milk in place of cow's or goat's milk.*
© *the American Dietetic Association. J of the American Dietetic Assn., Vol 38:240, 1961.*

the expectant woman is important in helping her to decrease or eliminate this practice.

Cultural, Ethnic, and Religious Influences

Cultural, ethnic, and occasionally religious background determines one's experiences with food and influences food preferences and habits (Figure 16–1). People of different nationalities are accustomed to eating different foods because of the kinds of foodstuffs available in their countries of origin. The way food is prepared varies, depending on the customs and traditions of the ethnic and cultural group. In addition, the laws of certain religions sanction particular foods, prohibit others, and direct the preparation and serving of meals.

In each culture, certain foods have symbolic significance. Generally, these symbolic foods are related to major life experiences such as birth, death, or developmental milestones. (General food practices of different cultural and ethnic groups are presented in Table 16–5. Sample daily menus that meet minimal nutritional requirements for differing cultural groups during pregnancy are pre-

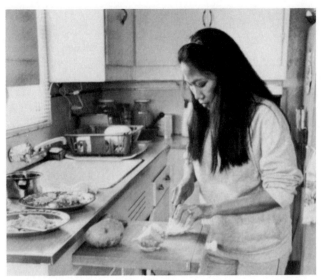

Figure 16–1   Food preferences and habits are affected by cultural factors.

Table 16–5   Food Practices of Various Ethnic and Religious Groups

Cultural group	Staple foods	Prohibitions or foods not used	Food preparation
Jewish Orthodox	Meat: Forequarter of cattle, sheep, goat, deer Poultry: chicken, pheasant, turkey, goose, duck	No blood may be eaten in any form No pork or pork products	Animal slaughter must follow certain rules, including minimal pain to animal and maximal blood drainage
	Dairy products	Combining milk and meat at meal not allowed; milk and cheese may be eaten before meal, but must not be eaten for 6 hours after meal containing meat	Two sets of dishes are used: one for meat, one for milk meals
	Fish with fins and scales No restrictions on cereals, fruits, or vegetables	No shellfish or eels	
Mexican American	Main vegetables: corn (source of calcium) and chili peppers (source of vitamin C); pinto beans or calice beans; potatoes Coffee and eggs Grain products: corn is basic grain; tortillas from enriched flour made daily	Milk rarely used	Chief cooking fat is lard Usually beans are served with every meal
Asian	Rice is staple grain and used at most meals Traditional beverage is tea Most meats are used, but in limited amounts Fruits are usually eaten fresh	Milk and cheese rarely used Meat considered difficult to chew, so may be eliminated from child's diet	Foods are kept short time and are cooked quickly at high temperature so that natural flavors are enhanced and texture and color maintained Chief cooking fat is lard or peanut oil.
Japanese	Seafood (raw fish) eaten frequently Most meats; large variety of vegetables and fresh fruits Rice is staple grain, but corn and oats also used	Milk and cheese rarely used	Chief cooking fat is soybean oil

Table 16–6 Sample Menus for Adequate Prenatal Diet for Various Cultural Groups*

Caucasian	Mexican-American	Southern U.S.	Jewish Orthodox	Italian
Breakfast				
Peaches	Peaches	Peaches	Peaches	Peaches
Oatmeal/milk	Oatmeal/milk	Oatmeal/milk	Oatmeal/milk	Oatmeal/milk
Toast with peanut butter	Corn tortilla	Cornbread with molasses	Bagel with un-salted butter	Bread with butter
Milk	Refried beans	Milk	Milk	Cheese
	Milk			Coffee/milk
Midmorning				
Fruit/juice	Fruit/juice	Fruit	Fruit	Fruit/juice
Lunch				
Cheese omelet and vegetables	1 fried egg	1 fried egg	Cheese omelet	Cheese omelet
Whole-grain muffin with butter	Refried beans with cheese	Black-eyed peas and salt pork	Brown rice	Zucchini, green salad
Lettuce and tomato salad	Corn tortilla	Cornbread with molasses	Lettuce and tomato salad	Grapes/cheese
Raw apple	Fresh tomato and chilies	Turnip greens	Ice cream	Milk
Milk	Banana	Ice cream	Milk	
	Milk			
Midafternoon				
Fruit	Fruit	Fruit	Fruit	Fruit
Cottage cheese	Cottage cheese			Cheese
Dinner				
Roast beef and gravy	Refried beans with cheese	Beef stew with vegetables (car-rots, greens)	Steamed fish with vegetables	Spaghetti and meat-balls with tomato sauce
Whole-grain roll with butter	Fried macaroni	Dumplings	Barley pilaf	Italian bread with butter
Parsley, carrots, cabbage slaw	Tortilla	Steamed potato, cabbage slaw	Cooked cabbage	Sauteed eggplant, cabbage, salad
Banana cream pie	Carrots, steamed tomato, chilies	Corn pudding	Unsalted butter	Fruit
Tea	Corn pudding		Coffeecake	Coffee/milk
	Milk		Fruit/juice	
Bedtime				
Milk	Milk	Milk	Honey cookie	Ice cream
Wheat crackers	Tortilla with beans	Corn pudding		
1 oz cheese	Cheese			

Modified from American Dietetic Association. *Cultural Food Patterns in the U.S.A.* © *The American Dietetic Association.*

sented in Table 16–6.) For example, Navajo women believe that eating raisins will cause brown spots on the mother or baby. Many black Americans believe that craving one food excessively can cause the baby to be "marked"; some say the shape of the birthmark echoes the shape of the food the mother craved during pregnancy. This belief is also held by some Mexican-American women. Some Mexican Americans believe drinking milk makes their babies too big, thereby causing difficult births.

The traditional Chinese classify food as either hot or cold, and these classifications are related to the balance of forces for good health. Since childbirth is considered a cold condition, it must be treated with hot foods, such as chicken, squash, and broccoli.

The relationship of food to pregnancy is reflected in some common beliefs or sayings. Nurses frequently hear that the pregnant woman must eat for two or that the fetus takes from the mother all the nutrients it needs.

Psychosocial Factors

Sharing food has long been a symbol of friendliness, warmth, and social acceptance in many cultures. Food is also symbolic of motherliness; that is, taking care of the family and feeding them well is a part of the traditional mothering role. The mother influences her children's likes and dislikes by what she prepares and by her attitude about foods. Certain foods are assigned positive or negative values, as reflected in the statements "Milk helps you grow" and "Coffee stunts your growth."

Some foods and food-related practices are associated with status. Some foods are prepared "just for company."

Other foods are served only on special occasions—for example, holidays such as Thanksgiving.

Socioeconomic Factors

Socioeconomic level may be a determinant of nutritional status. Poverty-level families are unable to afford the same foods that higher-income families can. Thus, pregnant women with low incomes are frequently at risk for poor nutrition.

Education

Knowledge about the basic components of a balanced diet is essential. Often educational level is related to economic status, but even people on very limited incomes can prepare well-balanced meals if their knowledge of nutrition is adequate.

Psychologic Factors

Emotions affect nutritional well-being directly. For example, anorexia nervosa, a psychologic disorder that occurs primarily in adolescent girls, is due chiefly to self-inflicted starvation, resulting in malnutrition and ultimately death if not treated. Loss of appetite is also a common symptom of serious depression.

The expectant woman's attitudes and feelings about her pregnancy influence her nutritional status. The woman who is depressed or who does not wish to be pregnant may manifest these feelings by loss of appetite or by improper food practices, such as overindulgence in sweets or alcohol.

The Pregnant Adolescent

Nutritional care of the pregnant adolescent is of particular concern to health care professionals. Many adolescents are nutritionally at risk due to a variety of complex and inter-related emotional, social, and economic factors that may adversely affect dietary intake.

Nutritional Concerns

General Concerns

In their position statement, the ADA stated that, "pregnant adolescents as a group are nutritionally at risk and require nutritional intervention early and throughout the duration of their pregnancies" (ADA 1989, p 104). Nutritional status is an important, modifiable variable in any pregnancy, but especially adolescent pregnancy, because teens are more likely than older women to be underweight at the onset of pregnancy and to gain less weight during pregnancy. Studies suggest that good maternal weight gain during adolescent pregnancy significantly improves fetal growth and reduces mortality without increasing overall risk of cesarean birth or complications (Scholl et al 1988; ADA 1989).

Important nutrition-related factors to assess in pregnant adolescents include low prepregnant weight, low weight gain during pregnancy, younger age with regard to menarche, smoking, excessive prepregnant weight, anemia, unhealthy life-style (drugs, alcohol use), chronic disease, and history of an eating disorder (ADA 1989).

In determining nutrient needs for pregnant adolescents, it is important to consider the number of years that have passed since menstruation began. Adolescent females generally are considered physiologically mature about four years after menarche, as linear growth is usually completed by this time. Their nutritional needs would be similar to other "adult" women.

Adolescents who became pregnant less than 4 years after menarche, however, are at a high biologic risk due to their physiologic and anatomic immaturity. Nutritional needs for these young women (who are most likely to be growing) will be higher than for those whose growth has been completed.

Very little information is currently available on the nutritional needs of adolescents. Estimates are usually obtained by using the RDA for nonpregnant teenagers (age 11 to 14 or 15 to 18) and adding nutrient amounts recommended for all pregnant women (see Table 16–1). Although the RDA are based on chronologic age, they are probably the best available figures to use if the pregnant female is still growing. If mature, the pregnant adolescent's nutritional needs would approach those reported for pregnant adults. However, young adolescents (13 to 15 years) need to gain more weight than older adolescents (16 years or older) to produce babies of equal size. Thus, in determining the optimum weight gain for a pregnant adolescent, it is important to consider the following:

- Recommended weight gain for a normal pregnancy
- Amount of weight gain expected during the postmenarcheal year during which the pregnancy occurs

The issue of recommended weight gains during pregnancy was addressed earlier in this chapter (see the section entitled Maternal Weight Gain). Frisch (1976) defined the amount of expected weight gain due to growth according to the number of years postmenarche. These weight gains are reported in Table 16–7.

The weight gain for a normal pregnancy and the expected weight gain due to growth would be added together to obtain a recommended weight gain for the pregnant adolescent. If the teenager is underweight, additional weight gain is recommended to bring her to a normal weight for her height.

Optimum weight gain for the obese adolescent whose prepregnant weight is 135% or more of her ideal weight is not definitely known. Currently, the ADA recommends a weight gain of approximately 20 lb (ADA Technical Support Paper 1989).

Table 16–7 Expected Weight Gain Due to Growth After Menarche

Postmenarcheal year	Pounds gained each year
1	10.12
2	6.16
3	2.42
4 and 5	1.76

Source: *Frisch RE: Fatness of girls from menarche to age 18 years, with a nomogram.* Hum Biol *1976; 48:353.*

Specific Nutrient Concerns

Caloric needs of pregnant adolescents vary widely. Major factors in determining calorie needs include whether growth has been completed and the amount of physical activity. Figures as high as 50 kcal per kg have been suggested for young, growing teens who are very active physically. A satisfactory weight gain will confirm adequacy of caloric intake in most cases.

Inadequate iron intake is a main concern with the adolescent diet. Estimates suggest that 20% of the adolescent population is at risk of iron deficiency anemia (Mellendick 1983). Iron needs are high for the pregnant teen due to the requirement for iron by the enlarging muscle mass and blood volume. Iron supplements—providing between 30 to 60 mg of elemental iron—are definitely indicated.

Calcium is another nutrient that demands special attention from pregnant adolescents. Inadequate intake of calcium is frequently a problem in this age group. Adequate calcium intake is needed to support normal growth and development of the fetus as well as growth and maintenance of calcium stores in the adolescent. To provide for these needs, an intake of 1200 mg/day of calcium is recommended (see Table 16–2). Calcium supplementation is indicated for teens with an aversion to or intolerance of milk, unless other dairy products or significant calcium sources are consumed in sufficient quantities.

As folic acid plays a role in cell reproduction, it is also an important nutrient for pregnant teens. As previously indicated, a supplement is often suggested for pregnant females, whether adult or teenager.

Other nutrients and vitamins must be considered when evaluating the overall nutritional quality of the teenager's diet. Nutrients that have frequently been found to be deficient in this age group include zinc and vitamins A, D, and B_6. Inclusion of a wide variety of foods—especially fresh and lightly processed foods—is helpful in obtaining adequate amounts of trace minerals, fiber, and other vitamins.

Dietary Patterns

Healthy adolescents often have irregular eating patterns. Many skip breakfast, and most tend to be frequent snackers. Teens rarely follow the traditional three-meals-a-day pattern; their day-to-day intake often varies drastically; and they eat food combinations that may seem bizarre to adults. Despite this, adolescents usually achieve a better nutritional balance than most adults would expect.

In assessing the diet of the pregnant adolescent, the nurse should consider the eating pattern over time, not simply a single day's intake. This pattern is critical because of the irregularity of most adolescent eating patterns. Once the pattern is identified, counseling can be directed toward correcting deficiencies.

Counseling Issues

> **CRITICAL THINKING**
>
> *In counseling a pregnant adolescent, what approaches might be most effective in helping the teenager develop a more nutritionally sound eating pattern?*

A positive approach to nutritional counseling for the pregnant adolescent is more effective than a negative one. The nurse must be ready to suggest valuable foods that pregnant teens can choose in many places and at any time. If the adolescent's mother does most of the meal preparation, it may be useful to include her in the discussion if the adolescent agrees. Involving the expectant father in counseling may be beneficial. If the teen is remaining in school, cooperation can also be sought from school lunch personnel (ADA Technical Support Paper 1989).

The pregnant teenager will soon become a parent, and her understanding of nutrition will influence not only her well-being but also that of her child. However, teens tend to live in the present, and counseling that stresses long-term changes may be less effective than more concrete approaches. In many cases, group classes are effective, especially those with other teens. In a group atmosphere, adolescents often work together to plan adequate meals including foods that are special favorites.

Postpartum Nutrition

Nutritional needs will change following the birth. Nutrient requirements will vary depending on whether the mother decides to breast-feed. An assessment of postpartal nutritional status is necessary before nutritional guidance is given.

Postpartal Nutritional Status

Determination of postpartal nutritional status is based primarily on the new mother's weight, hemoglobin and hematocrit levels, clinical signs, and dietary history.

As previously discussed, an ideal weight gain for the

normal-weight woman during pregnancy is between 24 and 32 lb. After birth, there is a weight loss of approximately 10 to 12 lb. Additional weight loss will be most rapid during the first few weeks after birth, as the uterus returns to normal size, tissue fluids are released, and blood volume returns to normal. The mother's weight will then begin to stabilize. Some women reach their prepregnancy weight several weeks after birth; some reach this weight after several months. If excessive weight was gained during pregnancy, returning to prepregnancy weight will take longer.

It is important to evaluate the mother's current weight, ideal weight for her height, weight before pregnancy, and weight before the birth. Women who are interested in weight reduction should be referred to a dietitian. Different guidelines for weight loss are used for nursing mothers and nonnursing mothers.

Hemoglobin and erythrocyte values vary after birth, but they should return to normal levels within two to six weeks. Hematocrit levels should rise gradually due to hemoconcentration as extracellular fluid is excreted. The hematocrit is usually checked at the postpartum visit to detect any anemia. Mothers can be encouraged to eat a diet high in iron. Iron supplements are generally prescribed for two to three months following birth to replenish supplies depleted by pregnancy.

Clinical symptoms the new mother may be experiencing are assessed. Food cravings and aversions typically drop significantly during the postpartal period and are not usually problematic (Worthington-Roberts 1989). However, constipation is a common problem following birth. The nurse can encourage the woman to maintain a high fluid intake to keep the stool soft. Dietary sources of fiber, such as whole grains, fruits, and vegetables, are also helpful in preventing constipation.

Specific information on diet and eating habits is obtained directly from the woman. Visiting the mother during mealtimes provides an opportunity for unobtrusive nutritional assessment. Which foods has a woman selected? Has she avoided fruits and vegetables? Is her diet nutritionally sound? A comment focusing on a positive aspect of her meal selection may initiate a discussion of nutrition.

The dietitian should be informed about any woman whose cultural or religious beliefs require specific foods. Appropriate meals can then be prepared for her. The nurse may also refer women with unusual eating habits or numerous questions about good nutrition to a dietitian. In all cases, the nurse should provide literature on nutrition so that the woman will have a source of appropriate information at home.

Nutritional Care of Nonnursing Mothers

After birth, the nonnursing mother's dietary requirements return to prepregnancy levels (see Table 16–1). If the mother has a good understanding of nutritional principles, it is sufficient to advise her to reduce her daily caloric intake by about 300 kcal and to return to prepregnancy levels for other nutrients.

If the mother has a poor understanding of nutrition, now is the time to teach her the basic principles and the importance of a well-balanced diet. Her eating habits and dietary practices will eventually be reflected in the diet of her child.

If the mother has gained excessive weight during pregnancy (or perhaps was overweight before pregnancy), referral to a dietitian is appropriate. The dietitian can design weight-reduction diets to meet nutritional needs and food preferences. Weight loss goals of 1 to 2 lb/week are usually suggested.

In addition to meeting her own nutritional needs, the new mother will be interested in learning how to provide for her infant's nutritional needs. A discussion on infant feeding, which includes topics such as selecting infant formulas, formula preparation, and vitamin/mineral supplementation, is appropriate and generally well accepted.

Nutritional Care of Nursing Mothers

Nutrient Needs

Nutrient needs are increased during breast-feeding. Table 16–1 lists the RDA during breast-feeding for specific nutrients. Table 16–2 provides a sample daily food guide for lactating women. A few key nutrients need further discussion.

Calories One of the most important factors in the diet while breast-feeding is calories. An inadequate caloric intake can reduce milk volume. However, milk quality generally remains unaffected.

The nursing mother should increase her caloric intake by 200 kcal over the pregnancy requirement (that is, a 500 kcal increase from her prepregnancy requirement). This results in a total of about 2500 to 2700 kcal per day for most women.

A good tool for the nursing mother to use in assessing the adequacy of her caloric intake is her weight. After weight stabilizes several weeks following childbirth, weight loss should not exceed more than 1 lb/week for nursing mothers.

Protein As protein is an important ingredient in breast milk, an adequate intake while breast-feeding is essential. An intake of 65 g/day during the first six months of breast-feeding and 62 g/day during the second six months is recommended. As in pregnancy, it is important to consume adequate nonprotein calories in order to prevent the use of protein as an energy source.

Calcium Calcium is also an important ingredient in milk production, and increases over nonpregnancy needs are expected. Requirements during breast-feeding remain the same as requirements during pregnancy: 1200 mg/day. An inadequate intake of calcium from food sources necessitates the use of calcium supplements.

Iron As iron is not a principal mineral component of milk, needs during lactation are not substantially different from those of nonpregnant women. However, as previously mentioned, continued supplementation of the mother for two to three months after parturition is advisable in order to replenish stores depleted by pregnancy.

Fluids Liquids are especially important during lactation, since inadequate fluid intake may decrease milk volume. Fluid recommendations while breast-feeding are 8 to 10 8-oz. glasses daily, including water, juice, milk, soups, etc.

Counseling Issues

In addition to counseling nursing mothers on how to meet their increased nutrient needs during breast-feeding, it is important to discuss a few issues related to infant feeding.

For example, many mothers are concerned about how specific foods they eat will affect their babies during breast-feeding. Generally there are no foods the nursing mother must avoid except those to which she might be allergic. Occasionally, however, some nursing mothers find that their babies are affected by certain foods. Onions, turnips, cabbage, chocolate, spices, and seasonings are commonly listed as offenders. The best advice to give the nursing mother is to avoid those foods she suspects cause distress in her infant. For the most part, however, she should be able to eat any nourishing food she wants without fear that her baby will be affected. For further discussion of successful infant feeding see Chapter 30.

✿ *APPLYING THE NURSING PROCESS* ✿

Nursing Assessment

Assessment of nutritional status is necessary in order to plan an optimal diet with each woman. Data may be gathered from the woman's chart and by interviewing her. Information is obtained about (1) the woman's height and weight and her weight gain during pregnancy; (2) pertinent laboratory values, especially hemoglobin and hematocrit; (3) clinical signs that have possible nutritional implications, such as constipation, anorexia, or heartburn; and (4) diet history to determine the woman's views on nutrition as well as her specific nutrient intake.

A diet history may be obtained by asking the woman to complete a 24-hour diet recall, in which she lists everything consumed in the previous 24 hours, including foods, fluids, and any supplements. Diet may also be evaluated using a food summary. The woman is given a list of common categories of foods and asked how frequently she consumes foods from the list in a day (or week). Common categories include: vegetables, fruits, milk or cheese, meat or poultry, fish, desserts or sweets, coffee or tea, alcoholic

beverages, etc. This method may be less reliable because it requires the individual to be accurate in generalizing about her intake.

In some instances the nurse will ask the woman to keep a food record or diary of everything she eats for a specified period of time (such as a week). This provides a clearer picture of nutritional patterns and may prompt the woman to make changes if the diary reveals areas of deficiency or excess.

During the data-gathering process the nurse has an opportunity to discuss important aspects of nutrition in the context of the family's needs and life-style. The nurse also seeks information about psychologic, cultural, and socioeconomic factors that may influence food intake.

The nurse can use a nutritional questionnaire such as the one shown in Figure 16–2 to gather and record important facts. This information provides a data base the nurse can use to develop an intervention plan to fit the woman's individual needs. The sample questionnaire has been filled in to demonstrate this process.

Nursing Diagnosis

Once the data are obtained, the nurse begins to analyze the information, formulate appropriate nursing diagnoses, and develop client goals. For a woman during the first trimester, for example, the diagnosis may be "Altered nutrition: less than body requirements related to nausea and vomiting." In many cases the diagnosis may be related to excessive weight gain. In such cases the diagnosis might be "Altered nutrition: more than body requirements related to excessive intake of calories." Although these diagnoses are broad, the nurse must be specific in addressing issues such as inadequate intake of nutrients such as iron, calcium, or folic acid; problems with nutrition due to a limited food budget; problems related to physiologic alterations such as anorexia, heartburn, or nausea; and behavioral problems related to excessive dieting, anorexia nervosa, bulimia, etc. In some instances the category "knowledge deficit" may seem most appropriate. Key Nursing Diagnoses to Consider identifies diagnoses that may apply to the nutritional health of the pregnant woman.

Nursing Plan and Implementation

After the nursing diagnosis is made, the nurse can plan an approach to correct any nutritional deficiencies or improve the overall quality of the diet. In counseling the pregnant woman, it is important to avoid "talking down to" her or "preaching" to her. Information should be presented in a clear, logical way, using appropriate language but avoiding jargon. Examples are often helpful in clarifying material. All questions should be answered appropriately and clearly.

When a person requires nutritional counseling, it usually indicates that a dietary change is necessary. Change is often difficult for people, however. Counseling will be

NUTRITIONAL QUESTIONNAIRE

Name Susan Longmont   **Date** 12-16-87

Age 20

Ethnic group white middle class

Religion Protestant

Gravida 1̇   **Para** 0̇   **EDC** 7-7-88

Age of youngest child? NA

Birth weights of previous children? NA

Usual nonpregnant weight 115   **Present weight** 125

Weight gain during last pregnancy? NA

Vitamin supplements? none

Current medications? aspirin for headache

Do you smoke? yes   **How much per day?** 1–1½ packs

Eating patterns:

1. How many meals per day? 2 **when** 12:30 pm 6:30 pm

2. How many snacks per day? 3 **when** 10:30 am 4:00 pm 10:00 pm

3. What other foods are important to your usual diet? chocolate and candy bars

4. Amount per day 4 bars/week

5. Do you have any different food preferences now? no

6. Do you eat nonfoods such as:

		Amount
laundry starch	no	NA
ice	yes	10 cubes/day
other (name)	no	NA

7. What foods do you dislike or do not eat? spinach and dried beans

8. For added information complete a typical daily intake (24 hour recall is suggested).

Do you have special problems in food preparation such as:

1. Physical disability   yes _____ no ✓   Explain _____

2. Cooking appliances   yes _____ no ✓   Explain _____

3. Refrigeration of food   yes _____ no ✓   Explain _____

Who does the meal planning? I do.   shopping? We both do.

cooking? I do most of the time but my husband likes to help.

Are there transportation problems? We have only one car but we go in the evening.

Financial situation: My husband is working and going to school. I am not working.   **Foodstamps** yes   **w/c** no

Do you have any previous nutritional problems? No. I have never paid much attention to food before, but now I have a lot of questions.

Are there any problems with this pregnancy? Nausea Yes, in the morning.

Constipation No   Other NA

Assessment by the nurse following the completion of the questionnaire.

Basic estimated nutrient and caloric value of typical daily intake.

Please circle one of the following:

Protein intake was	low	(adequate) high
Caloric intake was	low	adequate (high)
Calcium intake was	(low)	adequate high
Iron intake was	(low)	adequate high
Vitamin C intake was	low	(adequate) high

Figure 16–2 Sample nutritional questionnaire used in nursing management of a pregnant woman

---

Dx

Key Nursing Diagnoses to Consider
Nutrition for
the Pregnant Woman

Constipation
Diarrhea
Fluid volume excess
Fluid volume deficit
High Risk fluid volume deficit
Altered health maintenance
Knowledge deficit
Noncompliance
Altered nutrition: Less than body requirements
Altered nutrition: More than body requirements
Altered nutrition: High risk for more than body requirements
Body image disturbance

---

more effective if the nurse understands the client's values and provides explanation for the needed change in a way that is meaningful to the client. Since it is the pregnant woman who must follow the plan, it should be developed in cooperation with her; it should be suitable for her financial level and background and be based on reasonable, achievable goals.

The following example demonstrates one way in which a nurse can plan with a client based on the nursing diagnosis.

Diagnosis: Altered nutrition: less than body requirements related to low intake of calcium.
Client goal: The woman will increase her intake of calcium to RDA levels.
Implementation:

1. Plan with the woman additional milk or dairy products that can reasonably be added to the diet (specify amounts).

2. Encourage the use of other calcium sources such as leafy greens and legumes.

3. Plan for the addition of powdered milk in cooking and baking.

4. If none of the above are realistic or acceptable, consider the use of calcium supplements.

Counseling Families About Good Nutrition

Food is a significant portion of a family's budget, and meeting nutritional needs may be a challenge for families on limited incomes. Some families qualify for special assistance to meet their nutritional needs. The *Food Stamp Program* provides stamps or coupons for participating households whose net monthy income is below a specified level.

These stamps can be used to purchase food for the household each month.

The *Special Supplemental Food Program for Women, Infants, and Children (WIC)* is designed to provide nutritious food for pregnant or breast-feeding women with low incomes and for their children under five years of age. The food distributed, including eggs, cheese, milk, fortified cereals, juice, and infant formula, is designed to provide good sources of iron, protein, and certain vitamins for individuals with an inadequate diet. The WIC program is credited with helping reduce the incidence of low birth weight in infants and in decreasing the incidence of anemia in the infants and young children of low-income families (Williams 1989).

Most families can benefit from guidance about food purchasing and preparation. Women should be advised to plan food purchases thoughtfully by preparing general menus and a list before shopping. It is also helpful to advise clients to monitor sales, compare brands, and be cautious when purchasing "convenience" foods, which tend to be expensive. Other techniques for keeping food costs down without jeopardizing quality include buying food in season, using bulk foods when appropriate, using whole-grain or enriched products, buying lower-grade eggs (grading has no relation to the egg's nutritional value but indicates color of the shell, delicacy of flavor, etc), and avoiding fancy grades of food and foods in elaborate packaging.

Evaluation

Once a plan has been developed and implemented, the nurse and client may wish to identify ways of evaluating its effectiveness. Evaluation may involve keeping a food journal, writing out weekly menus, returning for weekly weigh-ins, and the like. If anemia is a special problem, periodic hematocrit assessments are also indicated.

Women with serious nutritional deficiencies are referred to a nutritionist. The nurse can then work closely with the nutritionist and the client to improve the pregnant woman's health by modifying her diet.

❀ ❀ ❀ ❀ ❀ ❀ ❀ ❀ ❀ ❀ ❀ ❀

Case Study

Mrs Jennifer Snow, age 26, is a slender and well-groomed woman. The Snows have been married for eight months. Mrs Snow is employed as a postal clerk in her hometown.

Mrs Snow is weight conscious and has attempted many fad diets to lose weight. She describes herself as having a small appetite at mealtime. She does not drink milk. Breakfast usually consists of a glass of orange juice and a piece of toast. At noon she eats a slice of cheese or hard-cooked egg plus a piece of fresh fruit. However, after work she is famished and snacks on soda pop and cookies. Mrs Snow eats a late dinner of meat, potatoes, vegetable, and a green salad. Portions are small. Before retiring for the evening, the Snows snack on potato chips, pretzels, and soda pop.

Recently, Mrs Snow has felt queasy in the morning before breakfast. After she missed her menstrual period, a pregnancy test confirmed she was two months pregnant.

The medical history and physical examination were unremarkable. A year ago, she weighed 50 kg (110 lbs). Currently she is 46 kg (101 lbs) and 164 cm (65 in.) tall. Laboratory test results were: hemoglobin, 12 g/100 mL; hematocrit, 36%; and albumin 3.1 g/100 mL. There was no evidence of glucose, protein, or ketones in her urine.

The nurse noted a concern about Mrs Snow's weight and history of weight loss attempts. She talked with Mrs Snow about the importance of a well-balanced diet during pregnancy. Mrs Snow was given a prescription for a vitamin and iron supplement and a pamphlet on nutrition and pregnancy. An appointment was scheduled for one month later. Mrs Snow was asked to bring the nurse a three-day food record.

During the consultation one month later, the nurse learned that Mrs Snow had not followed the diet described in the pamphlet. Her intake was approximately 1200 calories. Mrs Snow feared she would gain too much weight and lose her figure. She had gained 1/2 lb and reported continued nausea.

The nurse recognized that her client's concerns about weight gain were interfering with her ability to make appropriate nutritional choices. The nurse consulted with the staff dietitian who had had some experience working with this type of client. Together they met with Mrs Snow to express their concerns and to plan a nutritional approach that would accomplish the following:

1. Develop a diet that was higher in calories, protein, and essential nutrients such as calcium, while limiting fat.

2. Arrange for ongoing nutrition education and counseling for Mrs Snow, especially involving topics of interest to her.

To accomplish these goals, the nutritionist agreed to work closely with Mrs Snow following childbirth to assist her in losing any remaining weight. Mrs Snow agreed to keep a food diary and to practice evaluating the nutritional content of the food she consumed. In addition to her prenatal vitamin and iron supplements, Mrs Snow began taking a calcium supplement. The nurse and dietitian discussed with Mrs Snow several approaches to relieve her nausea.

It was very difficult for Mrs Snow to change her eating habits, but she was eager to do what she could for her unborn child. She made a conscious effort to improve the nutritional quality of the foods she chose and to avoid an excessive intake of fatty convenience snack foods.

The nurse did not want Mrs Snow to begin feeling that her eating was the entire focus of each visit, so she made certain that all aspects of good prenatal care were discussed. She encouraged Mrs Snow to attend childbirth preparation classes with her husband. At one of the classes a nursing mother spoke about breast-feeding. This mother was fit and slender. Mrs Snow was able to relate to the woman and accept her advice about the importance of an adequate diet and sufficient fluid intake for successful breast-feeding.

Although it was difficult at times, Mrs Snow did improve her eating habits. She rode her bicycle several times a week and did prenatal exercises to keep toned. At term she had gained 26 1/4 lb. Her baby, a son, weighed 6 lb 14 oz and did well after birth. In the weeks following the birth, Mrs Snow followed the guidelines for intake for a nursing mother. To help with weight loss she also attended postpartum exercise classes. With the advice of the nurse and dietitian and the support of her husband, Mrs Snow stabilized her weight at 112 lb. Both the Snows agreed that although they occasionally "splurged on junk food," they were far more conscious about nutrition and planned to remain so to set a good example for their young son.

❀ ❀

KEY CONCEPTS

Maternal weight gains averaging 24 to 32 lb for a normal-weight woman are associated with the best reproductive outcomes.

If the diet is adequate, folic acid and iron are the only supplements generally recommended during pregnancy.

Caloric restriction to reduce weight should not be undertaken during pregnancy.

Pregnant women should be encouraged to eat regularly and to eat a wide variety of foods, especially fresh and lightly processed foods.

Taking megadoses of vitamins during pregnancy is unnecessary and potentially dangerous.

In vegetarian diets, special emphasis should be placed on obtaining ample complete proteins, calories, calcium, iron, vitamin D, vitamin B$_{12}$, and zinc through food sources or supplementation if necessary.

Evaluation of physical, psychosocial, and cultural factors that affect food intake is essential before nutritional status can be determined and nutritional counseling planned.

Adolescents who become pregnant less than 4 years after menarche have higher nutritional needs and are considered to be at a high biologic risk.

Weight gains during adolescent pregnancy must accommodate recommended gains for a normal pregnancy plus necessary gains due to growth.

After childbirth, the nonnursing mother's dietary requirements return to prepregnancy levels.

Nursing mothers require an adequte caloric and fluid intake to maintain ample milk volume.

❀ ❀

References

American College of Obstetricians and Gynecologists: ACOG Newsletter 30:9, 1986.

American Dietetic Association: Nutrition management of adolescent pregnancy: technical support paper. *J Am Diet Assoc* January 1989; 89:105.

American Dietetic Association: Position of the American Dietetic Association: Nutrition management of adolescent pregnancy. *J Am Diet Assoc* January 1989, 89:104.

American Dietetic Association: Position of the American Dietetic Association: Vegetarian diets. *J Am Diet Assoc* March 1988; 88:351.

American Dietetic Association: Position of the American Dietetic Association: Vegetarian Diets—technical support paper. *J Am Diet Assoc* March 1988; 88:352.

Anderson GD: Nutrition in pregnancy. In: *Gynecology and Obstetrics.* Vol. 2 Sciarri JJ (editor). Philadelphia: Harper & Row, 1986.

Brown JE: Improving pregnancy outcomes in the United States: The importance of preventive nutrition services. *J Am Diet Assoc* May 1989; 89:631.

Brown JE: Nutrition services for pregnant women, infants, children, and adolescents. *Clin Nutr* May/June 1984; 3:100.

Callinan V, O'Hare JA: Cardboard chewing: Cause and effect of iron-deficiency anemia. *Am J Med* September 1988; 85:449.

Cruikshank DP: Don't overdo nutritional supplements during pregnancy. *Contemp OB/GYN* February 1986; 27:101.

Cunningham FG et al: *Williams' Obstetrics,* 18th ed. Norwalk, CT: Appleton & Lange, 1989.

Curda LR: What about pica? *J Nurse-Midwifery* Spring 1977; 23:8.

Luke B: Megavitamins and pregnancy: A dangerous combination. *MCN* January/February 1985; 10:18.

Mellendick GJ: Nutritional issues in adolescence. In: *Adolescent Medicine.* Hofmann AD (editor). Menlo Park, CA: Addison-Wesley, 1983.

National Research Council: *Recommended Dietary Allowances,* 10th ed. Washington, DC: National Academy Press, 1989.

Pitkin RL: Nutrition in obstetrics and gynecology. In: *Obstetrics and Gynecology,* 5th ed. Danforth DN, Scott JR (editors). Philadelphia: Lippincott, 1986.

Scholl TO et al: Weight gain during adolescent pregnancy. *J Adolesc Health Care* July 1988; 9:286.

Suttie JW et al: Vitamin K deficiency from dietary vitamin K restriction in humans. *Am J Clin Nutr* 1988; 47:475.

Williams SR; *Nutrition and Diet Therapy,* 6th ed. St. Louis: Times Mirror/Mosby, 1989.

Wolfe HM, Gross TL: Obesity: Counseling before and during pregnancy. *Comtemp OB/GYN* January 1988; 31:45.

Worthington-Roberts B et al: Dietary cravings and aversions in the postpartum period. *J Am Diet Assoc* May 1989; 89:647.

Additional Readings

Abrams B, Parker JD: Maternal weight gain in women with good pregnancy outcome. *Obstet Gynecol* July 1990; 76:1.

Behrman CA et al: Nausea and vomiting during teenage pregnancy: Effects on birth weight. *J Adolesc Health Care* September 1990; 11:418.

Chez RA: Obesity in pregnancy. *Female Patient* October 1989; 14:23.

Haste FM et al: Nutrient intakes during pregnancy: Observations on the influence of smoking and social class. *Am J Clin Nutr* 1990; 51:29.

Mitchell MC: Weight gain and pregnancy outcome in underweight and normal weight women. *J Am Diet Assoc* May 1989; 89:634.

Naeye RL: Maternal body weight and pregnancy outcome. *Am J Clin Nutr* 1990; 52:273.

Scholl TO et al: Maternal growth during pregnancy and decreased infant birth weight. *Am J Clin Nutr* 1990; 51:790.

Symposium: Advising pregnant women about nutrition. *Contemp Ob/Gyn* January 1991; 36:80.

CHAPTER 17

Preparation for Childbirth

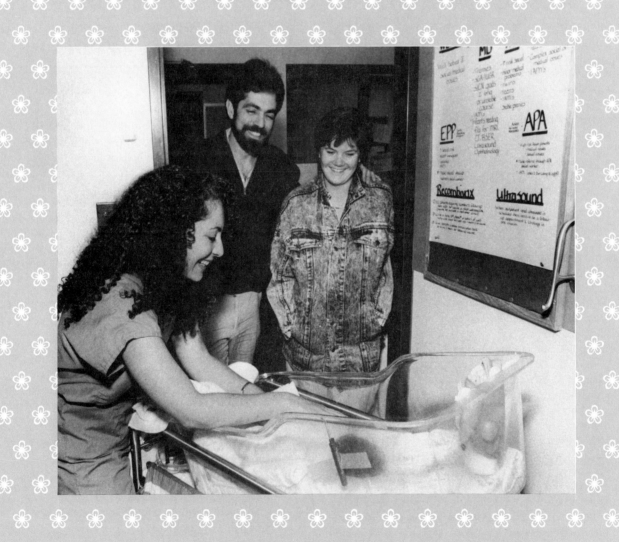

OBJECTIVES

Identify the various issues related to pregnancy, labor, and birth that require decision making by the parents.

Discuss the basic goals of childbirth education.

Describe the types of antepartal education programs available to expectant couples and their families.

Discuss ways of making group teaching effective for maternity clients.

Compare methods of childbirth preparation.

❀ ❀

Choices are important. They determine how you experience giving birth and how your baby enters the world. They must be made in the present and lived with in the future. (Pregnant Feelings)

A person's preparation for parenthood begins with his or her own birth into a family. An individual's attitudes, feelings, and fears about parenthood are molded by the relationship that he or she had with his or her parents as well as observations of and encounters with other children and parents.

A person's experiences with parenting or children may have been pleasant or uncomfortable. The information an individual has about parenthood and related areas may or may not be accurate. Since people bring their beliefs and fears with them to the childbearing period, the nurse can do much to correct misconceptions and calm fears regarding pregnancy, childbirth, and parenthood in general.

One way that a couple can cope with feelings about impending parenthood is to assume an active, participatory role during the antepartal, intrapartal, and postpartal periods. An active role involves the parents-to-be. It enables them to be involved in many of the decisions regarding the conduct of the birth. It offers them a degree of control over what could be an overwhelming experience.

Some of the decisions that the childbearing family must consider are presented in this chapter. The chapter addresses issues such as the choice of care provider, type of childbirth preparation, place of birth, activities during the birth, method of infant feeding, and choices surrounding treatment of the newborn. It also considers the role of the nurse, who provides information that enables the couple to make informed decisions.

❀ *USING THE NURSING PROCESS WITH* ❀

Couples Preparing for Parenthood

Nursing Assessment

The nurse assesses the couple's information base and need for additional information. Cultural factors and developmental needs are also assessed so that the nursing plan of care can deal with the couple holistically. In preparing for childbirth, parents have many decisions to make. The nurse needs to assess the parents' knowledge about selecting a health care provider, where the baby is to be born, who will be at the birth, and which classes would benefit them the most. The nurse should also ascertain the mother's preferences regarding use of analgesia, enema, perineal preparation, stirrups, position for birth, and method of feeding her newborn.

Nursing Diagnosis

After analysis of the learning needs of the couple or family, the nurse establishes appropriate nursing diagnoses. The nurse knows that the childbearing couple's knowledge base will affect the many decisions that they face. Nursing diagnoses that may apply to couples preparing for childbirth and parenthood are as follows:

- Knowledge deficit related to information needs during pregnancy and childbirth
- Knowledge deficit related to self-care measures during childbirth
- Ineffective individual coping related to unknown childbirth environment

Nursing Plan and Implementation

The nurse devises a plan to clarify learning needs and factors that may affect the learning process. The nurse assists the couple in identifying learning goals and helps the fam-

Research Note

Clinical Application of Research

Josephine Green and her associates (1990) ascertained relationships between the prenatal and postnatal expectations, experiences, and feelings of women in England. The first prenatal questionnaire included demographic information and the second surveyed the attitudes, knowledge, and expectations of women about anticipated chidlbirth. The postnatal questionnaire determined actual happenings and assessed psychologic outcomes. Psychologic outcome measures entailed fulfillment, satisfaction with birth, emotional well-being, and description of baby.

Statistical analysis of relationships between prenatal variables and psychologic outcomes showed that primipara mothers were less satisfied with birth and more negative about their babies. Mothers who were negative about their pregnancy were less fulfilled and had low postnatal emotional well-being. Other prenatal variables associated with low emotional well-being in the postnatal period included not cheerful about pregnancy, very worried about labor pain, and not given right amount of information.

Several intrapartal factors had an impact on the psychologic outcomes. One variable of control regarding the mother's own behavior resulted in the mother feeling more fulfilled and more satisfied, having higher emotional well-being, and being more positive about her baby if the mother was a multipara. Additionally, while mothers with a high satisfaction with birth tended to have high emotional well-being scores, low satisfaction scores did not correlate with low emotional well-being.

Critical Thinking Applied to Research

Strengths: Thorough description of sample recruitment. Excellent rate of return on questionnaires with low mortality or loss of subjects who did not complete the study.

Concerns: No psychometric properties of validity or reliability were reported on tools used to measure variables; however, factor analysis was used to determine emotional well-being as well as to separate sources of satisfaction.

Green J, Coupland V, Kitzinger J: Expectations, experiences, and psychological outcomes of childbirth: A prospective study of 825 women. *Birth* 1990; 17(1): 15.

---

ily gather information so that the decisions they make during this time are based on thorough, accurate information.

Another important nursing action is to be an advocate for the childbearing couple. As parent advocates and supporters, nurses need to provide information that reflects respect for the dignity and rights of the couple and promotes the safety of the mother and fetus. The health care information given should focus on:

- The right of the woman to know her own personal health status and the health status of her baby
- The parents' options
- Their participation in decision making
- Responsibilities for self-care
- Treatments and their rationale
- Maintenance of family support systems
- Consideration and respect for each individual's needs

Finally, the nurse needs to operate from a sound knowledge base in order to be able to assist the parents in gaining desired information. Parent education literature and conversations with parents help the nurse stay abreast of parental concerns and trends in childbearing.

Evaluation

In the evaluation process the nurse assesses not only the success of specific teaching situations but also the adequacy of the overall nursing diagnosis. Does the couple have the knowledge base that they need? Have unknown factors interfered with the learning process? Does the couple feel confident in making the needed decisions during pregnancy, childbirth, and newborn care?

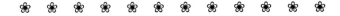

Childbearing Decisions

When a man and woman decide to have a child or learn that she is pregnant, they are faced with many decisions. For instance, they must make decisions about who will provide health care, where their child will be born, who will attend the birth, and whether to attend prepregnancy or prenatal classes (Figure 17–1). The woman must also make decisions about whether to allow analgesia, perineal preparation, an enema, or the use of stirrups; what position to use during labor and birth; and whether to breast-feed her child.

Some parents deal with the numerous decisions regarding childbirth by devising a **birth plan**. In this plan they identify aspects of the childbearing experience that are most important to them. The birth plan helps identify

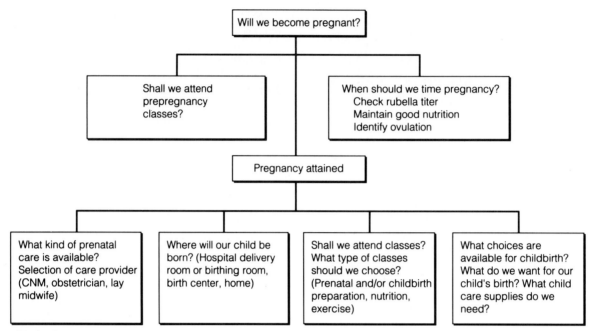

Figure 17–1   Pregnancy decision tree

options that may be available, and it becomes a tool for communication between the couple, the health care providers, and the birth setting. The plan helps the couple set priorities for activities that they want. A sample birth plan is presented in Figure 17–2. Once the couple has used the plan to identify their priorities, the birth plan can be shared with health care providers and can also be taken to the birth setting. (Perez 1990).

The birth plan identifies many factors associated with childbirth. One of the first decisions that the woman or couple needs to make is the type of care provider to use and how to choose that health care provider. The choice of care provider and place of birth frequently go hand in hand.

As the couple seeks information, nurses can assist in the decision-making process. The nurse can discuss various types of care providers so that the couple knows what to expect from each type. The couple needs to know the differences between the educational preparation, skill level, and general philosophy of certified nurse-midwives, obstetricians, family practice physicians, and lay midwives. The nurse also provides information about different types of birth settings and assists the couple in obtaining further information through tours of facilities and reading. Questions regarding the care provider's credentials, basic and special education and training, fee schedule, and availability for new patients can be answered by telephoning a receptionist in the office. As the couple prepares to interview different care providers, they may want to develop a list of questions so that they will learn the desired informa-

tion during the interview process. Sample questions may include:

- Who is in practice with you, or who covers for you when you are off?
- How do your partners' philosophies compare to yours?
- What are your feelings about my partner (or other children) coming to the prenatal visits?
- What weight gain do you recommend and why?
- How many of your parents attend prenatal and/or childbirth preparation classes, and what type do they choose?
- What are your feelings about (add in special desires for the birth event, such as, different positions during labor, episiotomy, induction of labor, other people being present during birth, breast-feeding immediately after birth, no separation of infant and parents following birth, and so on).
- If a cesarean is necessary could my partner be present?

The couple will also need to discuss the qualities that they want in a care provider for their newborn. They will probably want to visit with care providers prior to birth in order to select one who meets their needs.

Choosing a care provider is just one of the myriad of choices and decisions with which the couple is faced (see

Choice	I would like to have		Available	
	Yes	No	Yes	No
Care provider				
Certified nurse-midwife	___	___	___	___
Obstetrician	___	___	___	___
Lay midwife	___	___	___	___
Birth setting	___	___	___	___
Hospital:				
Birthing room	___	___	___	___
Delivery room	___	___	___	___
Birth center	___	___	___	___
Home	___	___	___	___
Partner present	___	___	___	___
During labor	___	___	___	___
During birth	___	___	___	___
During cesarean	___	___	___	___
During whole postpartum period	___	___	___	___
During labor				
Ambulate as desired	___	___	___	___
Shower if desired	___	___	___	___
Wear own clothes	___	___	___	___
Use hot tub	___	___	___	___
Use own rocking chair	___	___	___	___
Have perineal prep	___	___	___	___
Have enema	___	___	___	___
Water birth	___	___	___	___
Electronic fetal monitor	___	___	___	___
Membranes:				
Rupture naturally	___	___	___	___
Amniotomy if needed	___	___	___	___
Labor stimulation if needed	___	___	___	___
Medication:				
Identify type desired	___	___	___	___
Fluids or ice as desired	___	___	___	___
Music during labor and birth	___	___	___	___
During birth				
Position:				
On side	___	___	___	___
Hands and knees	___	___	___	___
Kneeling	___	___	___	___
Squatting	___	___	___	___
Birthing chair	___	___	___	___
Birthing bed	___	___	___	___
Other:	___	___	___	___
Family present (sibs)	___	___	___	___
Filming of birth	___	___	___	___
Leboyer	___	___	___	___
Episiotomy	___	___	___	___
No sterile drapes	___	___	___	___
Partner to cut umbilical cord	___	___	___	___
Hold baby immediately after birth	___	___	___	___
Breast-feed immediately after birth	___	___	___	___
No separation after birth	___	___	___	___
Save the placenta	___	___	___	___
Newborn care:				
Eye treatment for the baby	___	___	___	___
Vitamin K injection	___	___	___	___
Breast-feeding	___	___	___	___
Formula feeding	___	___	___	___
Glucose water	___	___	___	___
Circumcision	___	___	___	___
Feeding on demand	___	___	___	___
Postpartum care:				
Rooming-in	___	___	___	___
Short stay	___	___	___	___
Sibling visitation	___	___	___	___
Infant care classes	___	___	___	___
Self-care classes	___	___	___	___
Other:				

Table 17–1). Another area of decision making is demonstrated in the following situation.

One Couple's Story: Preparation for Parenthood

Mr and Mrs Cline were discussing newborn care with Ms Gayle, the clinic nurse, during one of their prenatal appointments. The Clines had been gathering information about the clothes needed for a newborn and about infant feeding but had not yet considered whether to use (cloth) reuseable or single-use (disposable) diapers. They wanted some help in getting information. Ms Gayle suggested that they collect information from a variety of sources. Together they devised a plan to obtain information regarding cost, convenience, and any implications for their baby. They called a number of stores to determine the prices for cloth and single-use diapers. They investigated the cost of diaper service, as well as the cost of laundering their own diapers. They found that laundering their own diapers was the least expensive, but having a diaper service was only about a dollar more a week, and the convenience was important because of the work schedule that both the Clines would have to keep even after the baby was born. Single-use were the most expensive and were approximately 50% higher than for a diaper service and 66% higher than laundering their own reuseable diapers (Lehrburger, Mullen, Jones 1991). They had seen coupons for single-use and knew that that would affect the price, but they anticipated having a storage problem with the boxes if they purchased many at once.

The Clines were surprised at the amount of information they were gathering. They considered ecologic issues and the implications of a natural product (cotton cloth diapers) versus the use of natural resources (trees) to create the single-use diapers, and they read about the problems associated with disposal of the diapers. Currently in the United States, 16,000,000,000 (sixteen billion) single-use diapers are purchased every year (Primono et al 1990). The disposal of these diapers is heaping more than two million used single-use diapers (12,300 tons of waste) in our landfills every day at a cost of almost $1,000,000 (one million dollars) a day (Primono et al 1990), and it takes about 500 years (approximately 20 generations of one family) for the single-use diapers to decompose (Brink 1990). The Clines also discovered that the disposal of human excrement in a landfill, as opposed to a sewage system, may present health hazards for sanitation workers and every citizen if groundwater around landfills is contaminated. They also discovered that some states and cities are passing legislation about the use and disposal of single-use diapers (Update on Diapers 1990).

Figure 17–2 Birth plan for childbirth choices

Table 17–1 Some Consumer Decisions During Pregnancy, Labor, and Birth

Issue	Benefits	Risks
Breast-feeding	No additional expense Contains maternal antibodies Decreases incidence of infant otitis media, vomiting, and diarrhea Easier to digest than formula Immediately after birth, promotes uterine contractions and decreases incidence of postpartum hemorrhage	Transmission of pollutants to newborn Irregular ovulation and menses can cause false sense of security and nonuse of contraceptives. Increased nutritional requirement in mother
Perineal prep	May decrease risk of infection Facilitates episiotomy repair	Nicks can be portal for bacteria Discomfort as hair grows back
Enema	May facilitate labor Increases space for infant in pelvis May increase strength of contractions May prevent contamination of sterile field	Increases discomfort and anxiety
Ambulation during labor	Comfort for laboring woman May assist in labor progression by: a. Stimulating contractions b. Allowing gravity to help descent of fetus c. Giving sense of independence and control	Cord prolapse with ruptured membranes unless engagement has occurred Delivery of infant in undesirable situations
Electronic fetal monitoring	Helps evaluate fetal well-being Helps diagnose fetal distress Useful in diagnostic testing Helps evaluate labor progress	Supine postural hypotension Intrauterine perforation (with internal monitoring) Infection (with internal monitoring) Decreases personal interaction with mother because of attention paid to the machine Mother is unable to ambulate or change her position freely
Oxytocin	Decreases incidence of cesarean birth with augmentation of labor Restimulates labor in cases of slowing contractions resulting from epidural blocks or uterine atony	Hyperstimulated contractions interfere with oxygenation of fetus Uterine rupture Early placental separation
Analgesia	Maternal relaxation facilitates labor	All drugs reach the fetus in varying degrees and with varying effects
Delivery position (lithotomy) (see Chapter 23 for further discussion of positions)	Ease of visualization of perineum by birth attendant Facilitates elective operative intervention, if necessary	Increases need for episiotomy May decrease normal intensity of contractions
Stirrups	Assist in positioning for pushing (can be used in side-lying position) Comfortable for some women Convenient for the person delivering the baby	Supine postural hypotension Uncomfortable for some women Leg cramping and/or palsy Increased chance of tearing the perineum Thrombophlebitis Prolonged 2nd stage due to ineffective positioning for pushing
Episiotomy	Decreases irregular tearing of perineum May decrease stretch and loss of sexual pleasure after pregnancy	Painful healing May spasm during sexual intercourse due to poor repair Permanent scarring with certain episiotomies Infection

Sources: *Burst H: The influence of consumers on the birthing movement.* Topics Clin Nurs *1983;5(October):42, Hotchner T:* Pregnancy and Childbirth: A Complete Guide for a New Life. *New York: Avon Books, 1979.*

The Clines studied all the information and—based on cost, convenience, identified concerns for their baby, and ecologic concerns—decided to use a diaper service. They shared their information with Ms Gayle and put together a packet for other parents to review if they wanted to. The Clines felt they had investigated the questions thoroughly and were able to make an informed decision.

Although most birth experiences are very close to the desired experience, at times the expectations cannot be met. This may be due to unavailability of some choices in the couple's community or the presence of unexpected problems during pregnancy or birth. It is important for nurses to help expectant parents keep sight of what is realistic and possible and to help them understand that when choices are made, alternatives may be needed.

Birthing Environments: Choices

The maternity nurse needs to be aware of all birthing settings and their similarities and differences. Until recently the most prevalent setting for labor and birth was a hospital labor unit, composed of separate labor rooms, birthing rooms, and recovery area, and a different unit for the remaining hospital stay. This type of unit is still available in some hospitals. However, many hospitals have changed their labor and birth units to reflect the philosophy of family-centered care. In the newer units, the woman is not moved from room to room during labor and birth.

Couples in some communities also have the option of using a free-standing birth center. These facilities have been created in answer to consumer demand for a more homelike, natural setting for their childbearing experience. The childbearing consumer wants to know what is happening, to maintain a sense of dignity, and to maintain control over what the childbearing experience will be.

For the small number of couples who feel that even the family-centered hospital setting or a free-standing birth center do not offer them enough control, home birth is another possibility (Figure 17–3).

The Hospital Setting

Hospitals now offer a wide variety of settings. Some hospitals offer the more traditional maternity service with a separate labor and birth area, newborn nursery, and postpartum area. The nursing staff remains constant in one area, and a physician or certified nurse-midwife may be involved with the birth. This type of birth setting tends to be a large metropolitan hospital with many births per year.

Many other hospitals have incorporated a more relaxed, family atmosphere and are using the term "birth center" to reflect the change in philosophy. The birth center room is usually decorated in a homelike manner with drapes, wall paper, and wooden furniture. The laboring woman is admitted into the birthing room and remains there during labor, birth, and the recovery period, and the newborn remains in the room with the mother. In many centers, she also remains in this room throughout the postpartum stay. The nursing community calls these rooms, "single purpose" and may refer to them as LDR (labor, delivery, and recovery room), LDB (labor, delivery, and birth room) or LDRPP (labor, delivery, recovery, and postpartum room).

In contrast with the traditional labor and delivery unit, in which health care professionals wear sterile gowns, masks, and caps for the birth and the woman is not free to choose alternative birth positions, the birthing center of a less traditional hospital is much more relaxed. The personnel typically wear bright-colored scrub suits, the individual choices of the birthing couple are encouraged, the woman may assume a variety of positions for labor and birth, and the couple are permitted to invite whomever they wish for the birth. The newborn remains with the mother for a time after birth, and breast-feeding is encouraged immediately after birth. The emphasis is placed on family unity and family desires.

The expectant couple may choose this environment because it offers the more homelike setting while also offering high-risk care and the availability of emergency assistance.

Free-Standing Birth Centers

Care in free-standing birth centers is given by certified nurse-midwives, labor and birth nurses, nurse practitioners, physicians, nonmedical assistants, public health nurses, families themselves, or any combination of these. *Birth centers* require families to take more responsibility for the birth experience than usual while at the same time providing a more flexible and less costly way to give birth.

Birth centers strive for a warm, homelike atmosphere, with birthing rooms similar to typical bedrooms. The room is generally furnished with a bed, in which the woman labors and gives birth, comfortable chairs for the father and other relatives or friends, a cradle, and private bath and/or shower. Some free-standing centers also have play rooms for siblings, kitchens where families may keep food or beverages, and other amenities. Most free-standing centers encourage children to participate to whatever extent they choose. Many hospital-based centers are somewhat more reluctant to allow total participation by siblings.

Birth centers meet criteria for maintaining safety in out-of-hospital births. These criteria include: attendance by qualified health care professionals, screening and transfer criteria, a transport system immediately available, and a readily accessible backup physician and hospital facility.

In keeping with the concept of birth as a normal event, most birth center settings are set up for nurse-midwife management of labor and birth rather than for obstetric technology and treatment. Therefore, these centers are not appropriate for high-risk birth. Couples intending to use the centers are screened during pregnancy for high-risk factors (see Chapters 18 and 19). The presence of any one factor does not automatically exclude the woman from giving birth in a birth center, but it does mean that careful and continuous assessment is needed.

. . . what I've seen time and again is that the technology of the hospital overwhelms patients' natural instincts; they are intimi-

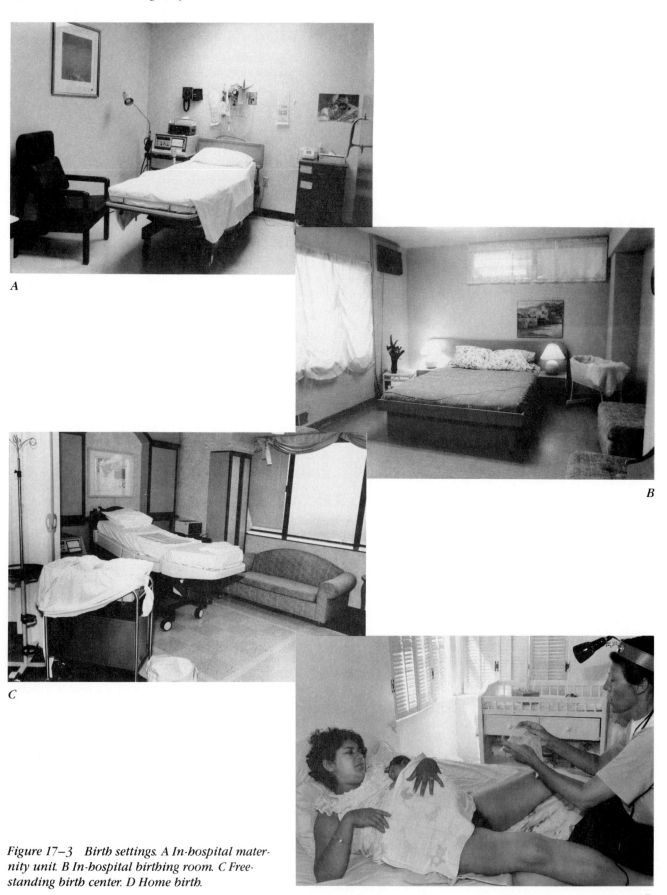

Figure 17–3   Birth settings. A In-hospital mater-nity unit. B In-hospital birthing room. C Free-standing birth center. D Home birth.

dated, afraid of appearing stupid or clumsy or sentimental in a surrounding that seems too efficient and immaculate and intelligent. (A Midwife's Story)

Each center also has policies about various circumstances that would require the woman to be transferred to a hospital birth setting. These may include, but are not limited to, the following:

- An increase in maternal temperature to over 100.4F (37.8C)
- A significant change in blood pressure
- Meconium-stained amniotic fluid
- Prolonged true labor
- Significant vaginal bleeding
- Prolonged second stage of labor (more than two hours for a nullipara and more than one hour for a multipara)
- Indications of fetal distress

The couple is usually required to attend prenatal classes to prepare for childbirth. They are also encouraged to meet birthing center personnel and to discuss their desires and preferences.

Traditional obstetric procedures are frequently not used. Episiotomies are not routine, forceps are not used, and in many centers the woman may give birth in the position of her choice. After the birth, physical contact between the parents and newborn is encouraged. The mother may breast-feed immediately. Siblings and accompanying support persons are also encouraged to interact with the newborn as they choose.

In most instances, rooming-in is immediate, and healthy newborns and their families are never separated. The initial pediatric examination is frequently conducted in the presence of the family. The mother and newborn are monitored for 2 to 24 hours after birth and then discharged.

Birth center personnel usually perform a home visit after discharge. The home visit provides an opportunity to see the family in their home setting, to make assessments of the mother and newborn, to answer questions, and to provide information and support.

Home Births

Another alternative to the traditional hospital birth is home birth. Couples who choose home birth generally have strong beliefs about their rights to make their own birth choices. Couples choosing home births believe that the responsibility for the birth outcome is theirs. Furthermore, they do not believe the hospital is necessarily the safest place to give birth, and they see standard medical practice as frequently involving unnecessary trauma and intervention. Some women may feel that hospital routines and expectations will not allow them to conform to their cultural norms for childbearing behavior.

In making the choice between home and hospital birth, medical risk is only one issue. The effect on the family unit is another issue. Parents who take responsibility for a home birth feel that it is a warm, close, loving experience under their control. The newborn is immediately incorporated into the family, and the continuous contact between the newborn and the family helps to bond the family as a unit. Siblings present during the birth are able to welcome the newborn into the family and are participants in an exciting and beautiful experience.

The safety of any home birth is maximized by thorough planning, careful prenatal care and screening, skilled physicians or nurse-midwives, and an organized and tested transport system to a facility where accepting care givers are available. However, adequate medical backup care is frequently unobtainable. Obstetricians as a group are particularly vocal opponents of home birth. Their opposition is often based on memories of serious emergencies they have witnessed at the time of birth. Therefore, they usually view home birth as a backward step in maternal child care. For the small number of physicians who would participate in home births, the increase in malpractice insurance is prohibitive.

An unfortunate side-effect of physician opposition has been that home births, when they do occur, may be even less safe. Physicians may refuse to supervise the prenatal care of a couple planning a home birth or may refuse to attend one. Many physicians also refuse to act as backup care givers for home births. Hospital personnel in general also tend to oppose home birth. They may manifest this disapproval through punishing attitudes when couples unable to complete birth at home come to the hospital. Despite the opposition, however, the trend toward home births seems to be growing rather than slowing.

Home births may be attended by a certifed nurse-midwife (contingent upon the laws of respective states) or physician, but most often the birth attendant is a lay midwife. Certified nurse-midwives are well-educated, skilled practitioners whose scope of practice is closely regulated by state nurse practice acts, but CNM attendance at home birth is a controversial issue even within the profession. Lay midwives may or may not have formal education; some states have a program of certification, and others consider their practice unlawful.

Choosing the Birth Setting

Information regarding the birth setting can be obtained from tours of the facilities and from talking with nurses and recent parents. Expectant couples may ask recent parents the following questions:

- What kind of support did you receive during labor? Was it what you wanted?

- If the setting has both labor and delivery rooms and birthing rooms, was a birthing room available when you wanted it?
- Were you encouraged to be mobile during labor or to do what you wanted to do (walking, sitting in a rocking chair, remaining in bed, sitting in a hot tub, standing in a shower, and so on)?
- Was your labor partner or coach treated well?
- Was your birth plan respected? Did you share it with the facility before the birth? If something didn't work, why do you think there were problems?
- How were medications handled during labor? Were you comfortable with it?
- Were siblings welcomed in the birth setting? After the birth?
- Was the nursing staff helpful after the baby was born? Did you receive self-care and infant care information? Was it in a usable form? Did you have a choice about what information you got? Did they let you decide what information you needed?

The prospective parents have many choices of birth settings available to them. It is important to ascertain the care providers' philosophy early in the pregnancy as it may affect the possibility of using some birth settings.

Siblings at Birth

More couples are choosing to extend the family-centered concept beyond mother, father, and newborn by including their other children in the birth experience. Many hospitals have yet to develop programs that allow siblings to visit the baby; having siblings attend a birth is an even rarer option. However, families who strongly wish their children to attend will probably find a way, even if they must create their own birthing situation.

The decision to have children present at birth is a personal and individual one. Children who will attend a birth can be prepared through books, audiovisual materials, models, and parental discussion. Nurses can assist parents with sibling preparation by helping them understand the stresses a child may experience. For example, the child may feel left out when there is a new child to love, or a brother may come when a sister was expected.

It is highly recommended that the child have his or her own support person or coach whose sole responsibility is tending to the needs of the child. The support person should be well known to the child, warm, sensitive, flexible, knowledgeable about the birth process, and comfortable with sexuality and birth. This person must be prepared to interpret what is happening to the child and intervene when necessary.

The child should be given the option of relating to the birth in whatever manner he or she chooses as long as it is not disruptive. Children should understand that it is their own choice to be there and that they may stay or leave the room as they choose. To help the child meet his or her goal, the nurse may wish to elicit from the child exactly what he or she expects from the experience. The child needs to feel free to ask questions and express feelings.

In general, the presence of siblings at birth engenders feelings of interest and the desire to nurture "our" baby, as opposed to jealousy and rivalry directed at "Mom's" baby. (DelGiudice 1986). The mother does not disappear mysteriously to the hospital and return with a demanding outsider. Instead, the family attending birth together finds a new opportunity for closeness and growth by sharing in the birth of a new member. Parents view the children's presence as positive, feel it added to family unity, and would have the children present again (Krutsky 1985). Another group of parents who had siblings present at birth felt that sharing the birth experience brought the family closer together. In addition, the parents thought that the event was a good learning experience and taught the child that birth was normal. Finally, the parents felt that the presence of siblings made the baby feel welcome and provided memories that the family could share for many years (Clark 1986).

Classes for Family Members During Pregnancy

Prenatal Education

Antepartal educational programs vary in their goals, content, leadership techniques, and method of teaching. The content of a class is generally dictated by its goals. For example, if the goal of a class is to prepare the couple for childbirth, it does not address the discomforts of pregnancy and the care of the newborn. Other classes may focus only on pregnancy, not labor and birth. Special classes are also available for couples who know that the woman will be having a cesarean birth. Nurses should be aware of couples' goals before directing them to specific classes.

Group Teaching
Group discussion is a useful teaching method. In group teaching, the nurse assesses the needs of the group instead of the needs of an individual. Skill in dealing with groups is essential. Skill in teaching groups can be developed in several ways, including professional reading on the subject, attendance at workshops or courses, and ongoing practice. The following guidelines identify some basic principles of effective group teaching:

- Groups of couples should contain no more than 20 individuals.
- Groups of mothers only should be smaller.

● The environment should be informal and friendly.

● Members should be encouraged to attend consistently, and other activities should be encouraged to increase group cohesiveness.

Helping the group to set an agenda at the initial session is one way of assessing members' needs. The individuals in the group must become comfortable with each other so that they feel free to share concerns, questions, and information.

Nursing intervention during group discussion takes many forms and frequently overlaps with assessment and evaluation as specific interests and concerns are clarified. The nurse may need to draw other members into the discussion or to clarify information. However, most prenatal classes are not purely discussion groups but include films, tours of maternity wards, demonstrations, and lengthy explanations. In classes concerned with selected methods of childbirth preparation, many group members may have read extensively on the subject and can contribute considerably to the discussion. Other members may know nothing about the topic and thus require more explanations and demonstrations by the nurse. In situations where group members know little about the method, a more structured approach to discussion and exercises may be useful.

Evaluation of the teaching-learning process is continuous and difficult. For example, checking each individual's performance after demonstration of an exercise is the most concrete way to evaluate learning. Evaluating members' changes in attitude or misconceptions is more difficult. A general evaluation of the series may be conducted in the last class, or the nurse can give group members evaluation forms to return by mail (Whitley 1985).

Class Content

Childbirth preparation classes usually contain information regarding changes in the woman and the developing baby (Table 17–2).

From the expectant parents' point of view, class content is best presented in chronology with the pregnancy. While both parents expect to learn breathing and relaxation techniques and infant care, fathers usually expect facts and mothers expect coping strategies (Maloney 1985). It is important that the classes begin by finding out what each parent wants to learn (Shearer 1990).

At times prenatal classes are divided into early and late classes.

Early Classes: First Trimester

Early prenatal classes should include both couples in early pregnancy and prepregnant couples. The classes contain information regarding early gestational changes, self-care during pregnancy, fetal development and environmental dangers for the fetus, sexuality in pregnancy, birth settings

Table 17–2 Possible Content for Preparation for Childbirth Classes

Early Classes (First Trimester)

Early gestational changes

Self-care during pregnancy

Fetal development, environmental dangers for the fetus

Sexuality in pregnancy

Birth settings and types of care providers

Nutrition, rest, and exercise suggestions

Relief measures for common discomforts of pregnancy

Psychologic changes in pregnancy

Information for getting pregnancy off to a good start

Later Classes (Second and Third Trimesters)

Preparation for birth process

Postpartum self-care

Birth choices (episiotomy, medications, fetal monitoring, perineal prep, enema, etc)

Newborn safety issues, ie, car seats

Adolescent Preparation Classes

How to be a good parent

Newborn care

Health dangers for the baby

Healthy diet during pregnancy

How to recognize when baby is ill

Baby care: physical and emotional

Breast-Feeding Programs

Advantages and disadvantages

Techniques of breast-feeding

Methods of breast preparation

Involvement of fathers in feeding process

Sibling Preparation

Grandparents' Classes

Preparation for Cesarean Birth

Preparation for Vaginal Birth After Cesarean Birth (VBAC)

and types of care providers, nutrition, rest and exercise suggestions, common discomforts of pregnancy and relief measures, psychologic changes in pregnancy for the woman and man, and information needed to get the pregnancy off to a good start. Early classes should provide information about factors that place the woman at risk for preterm labor and recognition of possible signs and symptoms of preterm labor. Early classes should also include information on advantages and disadvantages of breast- and bottle feeding. Studies indicate that the majority of women (50% to 80%) have made their infant feeding decision before the sixth month of pregnancy, so information in an early prenatal class would be helpful (Aberman & Kirchoff 1985).

Later Classes: Second and Third Trimesters

The later classes focus on preparation for the birth, infant care and feeding, postpartum self-care, birth choices (episiotomy, medications, fetal monitoring, perineal prep, enema, and so forth). Safety issues regarding the newborn should also be included. One of the first issues the new parents encounter is use of a car seat. Since many parents purchase the car seat prior to birth, later classes should include information regarding how car seats work, the importance of car seats, and how to select an approved car seat (Davis 1985).

Adolescent Parenting Classes

Adolescents have special content learning needs during pregnancy. In a survey by Levenson, Smith, and Morrow (1986), teens identified informational needs according to priority. The most important areas of concern were: how to be a good parent, how to care for the new baby, health dangers to the baby, and healthy foods to eat during pregnancy. The teens stated that the need for information about these areas continues after the birth of the baby. Howard and Sater (1985) found that teens identified the highest priority information needs as: how to recognize when the baby is sick, take care of the baby, protect the baby from accidents, and make the baby feel happy and loved. Smoke and Grace (1988) noted that adolescents who participated in prenatal education had fewer complications during pregnancy and birth. In addition, the adolescents who participated in their study had higher hematocrits (reflecting good nutrition and use of vitamins during pregnancy), requested less medication during labor, and had fewer extra infant hospital days following birth.

Breast-Feeding Programs

Programs offering prenatal and postpartal information on breast-feeding are increasing. For many years, the primary source of information has been **La Leche League**. Information can also be obtained from birthing centers, hospitals, health clinics, and individuals such as lactation consultants (Edwards 1985). Content includes advantages and disadvantages of breast-feeding techniques, and methods of breast preparation. The father is being included in educational programs more frequently, as his support and encouragement are vital, and it is important to include him in decision making. Some fathers may feel negative and resentful about breast-feeding and need opportunities in the prenatal period for discussion and sharing of information (Jordan 1986).

Prepared Sibling Programs

The birth of a new sibling is a significant event in a child's life. It may be associated with negative behavior toward the newborn, withdrawal, and sleep problems. More positively, the child seems to increase in developmental maturity after the birth of a sibling (Marecki et al 1985). With increased emphasis on family-centered birth, siblings are now being included in the birthing process. Their involvement may include visiting during labor, being present at birth, and/or visiting in the postpartal period.

The classes usually involve a tour of the maternity ward where the children will visit their mothers. Children generally show interest in such items as television sets, electric beds, and telephones the mothers will use to call them. The youngsters can climb on footstools at the nursery window to see the new babies. Most tours involve a visit to a birthing room. After the tour, the children have an opportunity to see and hear more about what happens to the parents and newborn in the hospital, how babies are born, and what babies are like. This teaching usually involves a combination of books, audiovisual materials, models, parental discussion, formal classes, and play experiences. They also have the opportunity to discuss their feelings about having a new baby in the family (Honig 1986). Discussion sessions may be divided into two age groups if the ages of the children attending vary greatly (Figure 17–4).

After the class, parents usually receive additional resources that tell how to prepare children for a baby in the family. Some programs award certificates to the children who attend, offer refreshments to the children and their parents, and give gift packets with articles similar to those new mothers receive (lotion, diapers for the new baby).

Classes that prepare children for attendance at birth vary. It is important that the children be at least familiar with what to expect during labor and birth: how the parents will act, especially the sounds and faces the mother may make; what they will see, including the messiness, blood, and equipment; and how the baby will look and act at birth. In addition, parents are encouraged to involve the child early in the pregnancy, including taking the child on a prenatal visit to see the CNM/physician and listen to the fetal heart beat. Most advocates feel the child also needs to be comfortable with seeing the mother without clothes prior to seeing her during labor and birth.

Classes for Grandparents

Grandparents are an important source of support and information for prospective and new parents. They are now being included in the birthing process more frequently. Prenatal programs for grandparents can be an important source of information regarding current beliefs and practices in childbearing. The most useful content may include changes in birthing and parenting practices and helpful tips

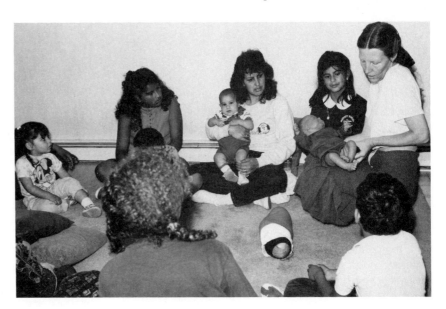

Figure 17–4 It is especially important that siblings be well-prepared when they are going to be present for the birth. But all siblings can benefit from information about birth and the new baby ahead of time.

for being a supportive grandparent. Some grandparents are integral members of the labor and birth experience and also need information on being a coach (Horn & Manion 1985).

Education of the Family Having Cesarean Birth

Preparation for Cesarean Birth

Cesarean birth is an alternative method of childbirth. Since one out of every four births is a cesarean, preparation for this possibility should be an integral part of every childbirth education curriculum. The instructor should treat cesarean birth as a normal event and present factual information that will allow a couple to make choices and participate in their birth experience. The instructor can emphasize the similarities between cesarean and vaginal births to minimize undertones of "normal" versus "abnormal" birth (Affonso 1981). This will diminish feelings of anger, loss, and grief that often accompany cesarean births.

Cesarean birth classes should cover what happens during a cesarean birth, what the parents will feel, and what the parents can do. Fawcett and Burritt (1985) used a pamphlet to give this information. The pamphlet was followed by a home visit or telephone call to emphasize the information and provide time for questions. Their findings indicated that parents found the program very helpful and useful.

All couples should be encouraged to discuss with their physician or nurse-midwife what the approach would be in the event of a cesarean. They can also discuss their needs and desires. Their preferences may include the following:

- Participating in the choice of anesthetic
- Father (or significant other) being present during the procedures and/or birth

Preparation for Repeat Cesarean Birth

When a couple is anticipating a repeat cesarean birth, they have time to analyze the experience, synthesize information, and prepare for some of the specifics. Many hospitals or local groups (such as C-Sec, Inc.) provide preparation classes for cesarean birth. Couples who have had previous negative experiences need an opportunity to discuss issues that contributed to their negative feelings. They should be encouraged to identify what they would like to change and to list interventions that would make the experience more positive. Those who have had positive experiences need reassurance that their needs and desires will be met in the same manner. In addition, an opportunity should be given to discuss any fears or anxieties.

A specific concern of the woman facing a repeat cesarean is anticipation of the pain. She needs reassurance that subsequent cesareans are often less painful than the first. If her first cesarean was preceded by a long or strenuous labor, she will not experience the same fatigue. Giving this information will help her cope more effectively with stressful stimuli, including pain. The nurse can remind the client that she has already had experience with how to prevent, cope with, and alleviate painful stimuli.

Preparation for Couples Desiring Vaginal Birth After Cesarean Birth (VBAC)

Couples who have had a cesarean birth and are now anticipating a vaginal birth have different needs from other couples. Because they may have unresolved questions and concerns about the last birth, it is helpful to begin the series of classes with an informational session. During this session, couples can ask questions, share experiences, and begin to form bonds with each other. The nurse can supply information regarding the criteria necessary to attempt a trial of labor and identify decisions regarding the birth experience. Some childbirth educators find it is helpful to have the couples prepare two birth plans: one for vaginal birth and one for cesarean birth. The preparation of the birth plans seems to assist the couple in taking more control of the birth experience and tends to increase the positive aspects of the experience (Austin 1986).

After an informational session, the classes may be divided depending on the needs of the couple. Those with recent coached childbirth experiences may only need refresher classes, while other couples may need complete training. Some couples may choose to attend regular classes after obtaining the beginning information in the informational session.

Selected Methods of Childbirth Preparation

Various methods of childbirth preparation are taught in North America. Some antepartal classes are more specifically oriented to preparation for labor and birth, have a name indicating a theory of pain reduction in childbirth, and teach specific exercises to reduce pain. The most common methods of this type are the Read (natural childbirth), the Lamaze (psychoprophylactic), the Kitzinger (sensory-memory method), and the Bradley (partner-coached childbirth) methods. Hypnosis is also discussed here because it is sometimes used to help the expectant mother reduce or even eliminate pain in labor and birth. See Table 17–3 for differentiating characteristics of each method.

Each of these methods is designed to provide the woman with self-help measures so that her pregnancy and birth are healthy and happy events in which she participates.

Expectant parents are taught that childbirth exercises and preparation for childbirth do not exclude the use of analgesics but that they often reduce the amount necessary. Some women will not require medication. Unfortunately, some groups teach that childbirth without pain relief medication is the desired goal. This feeling can be extremely destructive to the woman's self-concept at a time when she needs positive reinforcement in her abilities to achieve and perform competently. Fortunately, current thinking recognizes that individuals vary in their responses to stress, that the character of individual labors differs, and

Table 17–3 Summary of Selected Childbirth Preparation Methods

Method	Characteristics	Breathing technique
Lamaze	See narrative discussion.	
Read	First of the "natural" childbirth methods. Method utilizes information on progressive relaxation techniques and on abdominal breathing.	Primarily abdominal. Woman concentrates on forcing the abdominal muscles to rise. Works on slowing number of respirations per minute so that she can take one breath/minute (30 sec inhalation and 30 sec exhalation). Slow abdominal breathing used during first stage. Rapid chest breathing used toward end of labor if abdominal breathing not sufficient; panting is used to prevent pushing until needed.
Bradley	Frequently referred to as partner- or husband-coached natural childbirth. The exercises used to accomplish relaxation and slow controlled breathing are basically those used in the Read method.	Primarily abdominal as in Read method.
Kitzinger	Uses sensory memory to help the woman understand and work with her body in preparation for birth. Incorporates the Stanislavsky method of acting as a way to teach relaxation.	Uses chest breathing in conjunction with abdominal relaxation.
Hypnosis	Basic technique of hypnosis used in obstetrics is called hypnoreflexogenous method and is a combination of hypnosis and conditioned reflexes. Specific techniques of producing anesthesia and analgesia are not taught, but they are believed to be by-products of the method.	Normal breathing pattern.

that pain medication used judiciously may enhance the woman's ability to use relaxation techniques. (Lowe 1989, Crowe 1990).

The programs in prepared childbirth have some similarities. All have an educational component to help eliminate fear. The classes vary in the amount of coverage of various subjects related to the maternity cycle, but they all teach relaxation techniques and they all prepare the participants for what to expect during labor and birth. Except for hypnosis, these methods also feature exercises to condition muscles and breathing patterns used in labor. The greatest differences among the methods lie in the thories of why they work and in the relaxation techniques and breathing patterns they teach.

The advantages of these methods of childbirth preparation are several. The most important is that the baby may be healthier because of the reduced need for analgesics and anesthetics. Another advantage is the satisfaction of the couples for whom childbirth becomes a shared and profound emotional experience. In addition, proponents of each method claim that they shorten the labor process, a claim that has been clinically validated.

All maternity nurses need to know how these methods differ so that they can support each couple in their chosen method. It is important for the nurse to assess the couple's emotional resources and their expectations so that she or he can help them achieve their goals more effectively.

The maternal-newborn nurse may also assist the expectant couple in locating a childbirth education class that best meets their needs. Expectant parents need to know that the qualifications of childbirth educators vary. The oldest nationally accredited certification program in Lamaze childbirth is offered through the American Society for Psychoprophylaxis in Obstetrics, Inc. Lamaze childbirth educators participate in rigorous training and maintain ongoing continuing education. Other educators have a variety of preparation and requirements. In choosing a childbirth education class, Bing (1988) suggests that the expectant parents consider asking the following questions: (a) What is the education and training of the childbirth educator? What education did the educator receive? What credentials does the educator hold?; (b) What will the class size be? (A small class provides opportunities for more individual attention); (c) How will techniques be practiced? Will there be sufficient class time allotted?; (d) What content will be covered?; and (e) How open is the educator to answering questions and adding content based on your requests?

Psychoprophylactic (Lamaze) Method

The terms **psychoprophylactic** and *Lamaze* are used interchangeably. Psychoprophylactic means "mind preven-

tion," and Dr Fernand Lamaze, a French obstetrician, was the first person to introduce this method of childbirth preparation to the Western world. Psychoprophylaxis actually originated in Russia and is based on Pavlov's research with conditioned reflexes. Pavlov found that the cortical centers of the brain can respond to only one set of signals at a time and that they accept only the strongest signal; the weaker signals are inhibited. Pavlov's research also demonstrated that verbal representation of a stimulus can create a response. When the real stimulus is substituted, the conditioned response continues to be produced.

The two components of Lamaze classes are education and training. Class content originally was confined to exercises, relaxation, breathing techniques, and the normal labor and birth experience. Childbirth educators have added information on prenatal nutrition, infant feeding, cesarean birth, and other variations from usual labor as well as discussions concerning sexuality, early parenting, and coping skills for the postpartum period.

Instructors teaching the method in this country have modified many of the original exercises, but the basic theory of conditioned reflex remains the same. Women are taught to substitute favorable conditioned responses for unfavorable ones. Rather than restlessness and loss of control in labor, the woman learns to respond to contractions with conditioned relaxation of the uninvolved muscles and a learned respiratory pattern. Exercises taught in these classes include proper body mechanics and body conditioning, breathing techniques for labor, and relaxation.

Another major modification in the Lamaze method involves the goals of expectant couples. Couples using this method are encouraged to set their own goals for success. Lamaze childbirth education in this country supplies them with the tools to accomplish these goals. The couple is encouraged to discuss their goals with the obstetrician and maternity nursing personnel in labor and birth. The nursing staff who knows the couple's goals and resources is able to offer effective support.

Toning Exercises

Some of the body conditioning exercises, such as the pelvic tilt, pelvic rock, and Kegel's exercises, are taught in childbirth preparation classes. Other exercises strengthen the abdominal muscles for the expulsive phase of labor. (See Chapter 14 for a description of recommended exercises.)

Relaxation Exercises

Relaxation during labor allows the woman to conserve energy and allows the uterine muscles to work more efficiently. Without practice it is very difficult to relax the whole body in the midst of intense uterine contractions. Many people are familiar with **progressive relaxation** exercises such as those taught to aid relaxation and induce sleep. One example follows:

Lie down on your back or side. (The left side position is best for pregnant women.) Tighten your muscles in both feet. Hold the tightness for a few seconds and then relax the muscles completely, letting all the tension drain out. Tighten your lower legs, hold for a few seconds, and then relax the muscles letting all the tension drain out. Continue tensing and relaxing parts of your body, moving up the body as you do so.

Another type of relaxation exercise called **Touch Relaxation** requires cooperation between the woman and her coach. It is particularly useful in learning how to work together during labor. See Table 17–4.

An additional exercise specific to Lamaze is **disassociation relaxation**. This pattern of active relaxation is in contrast to the Read method of passive relaxation. The woman is taught to become familiar with the sensation of contracting and relaxing the voluntary muscle groups throughout her body. She then learns to contract a specific muscle group and relax the rest of her body. This process of isolating the action of one group of voluntary muscles from the rest of the body is called *neuromuscular disassociation* and is basic to the psychoprophylaxis method of prepared childbirth. The exercise conditions the woman to relax uninvolved muscles while the uterus contracts. See Table 17–5.

In order to practice the relaxation exercises in a more realistic setting, the coach may use two methods to induce some discomfort:

1. The coach places both hands in a grasping position firmly on the upper arm and turns them in opposite directions to create a burning sensation. This is begun slowly and gently and increased at the direction of the woman as she continues to practice relaxation and/or practices the breathing techniques (Figure 17–5).

2. The coach places a hand on the woman's inner thigh just above the knee and pinches the area.

Table 17–4 Touch Relaxation

Practice is vital to the following exercises, which require that the pregnant woman and her partner work very closely together. Tell the woman, "With practice you will train yourself to release not only in response to your partner's touch but also to the touch of doctors or nurses as they examine you. This technique will also help you to be more comfortable with your own body."

Goals:

(For her) To recognize and release tension in response to partner's touch; to be able to do this automatically and spontaneously.
(For partner) To recognize her tension in its very early stages; to learn how to touch in a firm yet sensitive way; to concentrate on her problem areas.

Tools:

(For her) Conscious relaxation, comfortable positioning, and trust.
(For him) Sensitivity, patience, and warm hands!

Procedure:

She tenses.
Partner touches.
She immediately releases toward touch.
Partner strokes, "drawing" tension from her.
She releases all residual tension.

Sequence:

- Contract muscles of the scalp and raise eyebrows. Partner cups hands on either side of the scalp. Immediately release tension in response to the pressure of your partner's touch. Then release any residual tension as your partner strokes your head.

- Frown, wrinkle nose, and squeeze eyes shut. Partner rests hands on brow and then strokes down over temples. Release.

- Grit teeth and clench jaw. Partner rests hands on either side of jaw. Release.

- Press shoulder blades back. Partner rests hands on front of shoulders. Release.

- Pull abdominal wall toward spine. Partner rests hands on sides of abdomen and then strokes down over hips. Partner might also stroke the lower curve of abdomen across pubic symphysis. Release.

- Press thighs together. Partner touches outside of each leg. Relax and let legs move apart. Partner strokes firmly down outside of leg with light strokes up on inner thigh.

- Press legs outward, still flexed but forcing thighs apart. Partner rests hands with fingers pointing downward, on inner thighs. Firmly stroke down to knees, then lightly stroke upward on outside of leg. Release.

- Tense arm muscles. Partner places hands on the upper arm and shoulder area, one on the inside and one on the outside of the arm. Stroke down to the elbow and then down forearm to wrist, and over fingertips. Release. Repeat with other arm.

- Tighten leg muscles, being careful not to cramp them. Partner touches foot around the instep, firmly without tickling. Release whole leg. Partner moves hands up, placing one on either side of the thigh, stroking down to the knee then down the calf to the foot and over the toes. Release. Repeat with other leg.

- Change to the Sims lateral or side-lying position. Raise chin, contracting the muscles at the back of the neck. Partner rests hand on nape of neck and massages. Release.

- Curl into fetal position, drawing shoulders forward. Partner applies pressure to back of shoulders. Stroke upper back. Release.

- Hollow the small of back by arching back. Partner rests hands against either side of spine and follows with stroking down over buttocks. Release.

- Press buttocks together. Partner rests one hand on each buttock. After initial release, stroke down toward thighs.

Source: *O'Halloran S: Pregnant and Prepared: A Guide to Preparing for Childbirth. Wayne, NJ, Avery, 1984, pp 43–44. Courtesy of NACE: The Nashua Association for Childbirth Education.*

Table 17–5 Disassociation Relaxation

The uterus, an involuntary muscle over which you have no control, will work most efficiently and effectively when the rest of your body is free from tension. The following exercises will give you further practice in conscious release. They will also give you and your partner a way to evaluate your progress.

Goals:

During pregnancy, disassociation relaxation will teach you consciously to release certain sets of muscles, while contracting others, and to disassociate yourself from voluntary tension.

During labor, this technique will release all voluntary muscles of your body at will, while the uterus contracts. This conserves energy and fights fatigue.

Tools:

Body awareness, touch release, and concentration.

Procedure:

Partner gives consistent suggestions.
Partner checks relaxation using touching.

Example:

Partner: "Contraction begins."
Mother: Relaxation breath (following with a comfortable rate of breathing).
Partner: See suggested patterns below.
Mother: Relaxation breath.

Sequence:

"Contract right arm. Hold. Release."
"Contract left arm. Hold. Release."
"Contract right leg. Hold. Release."
"Contract left leg. Hold. Release."
"Contract both arms. Hold. Release."
"Contract both legs. Hold. Release."
"Contract right side (arm and leg). Hold. Release."
"Contract left side (arm and leg). Hold. Release."
"Contract right arm and left leg. Hold. Release."
"Contract left arm and right leg. Hold. Release."

For Variety:

● Contract right arm and left leg.

● Release left leg. Contract right leg. Release right arm. Contract left arm.

● Release.

Source: *O'Halloran S: Pregnant and Prepared: A Guide to Preparing for Childbirth. Wayne, NJ, Avery, 1984, pp 45–46. Courtesy of NACE: The Nashua Association for Childbirth Education.*

While practicing, the coach checks the woman's neck, shoulders, arms, and legs for relaxation. As tense areas are found, the coach encourages the woman to relax that particular body part. The woman learns to respond to her own perceptions of tense muscles and also to the suggestion from others. The suggestion can come verbally or from touch. The exercises are usually practiced each day so that they become comfortable and easy to do.

A specific type of cutaneous stimulation used prior to the transitional phase of labor is known as *abdominal effleurage* (Figure 17–6). This light abdominal stroking is used in the Lamaze method of childbirth preparation. It

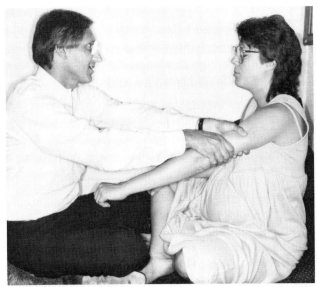
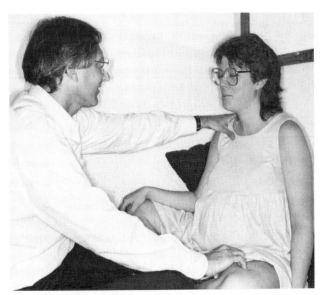

Figure 17–5   To practice relaxing in the presence of discomfort, the coach can induce discomfort by "twisting" the skin of the woman's upper arm or by pinching her inner thigh.

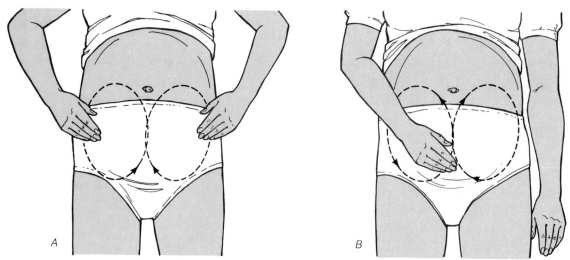

Figure 17–6   Effleurage is light stroking of the abdomen with the fingertips. A Starting at the symphysis, the woman lightly moves her fingertips up and around in a circular pattern. B An alternative approach involves the use of one hand in a figure-eight pattern.

effectively relieves mild to moderate pain, but not intense pain. Deep pressure over the sacrum is more effective for relieving back pain. In addition to the measures just described, the nurse can promote relaxation by encouraging and supporting the client's controlled breathing.

Other methods that may be used to enhance relaxation are guided imagery and meditation.

Breathing Techniques

The patterned-paced breathing techniques use three levels of chest breathing. Proponents of the Lamaze method believe that the variety of chest breathing patterns helps keep the pressure of the diaphragm off the contracting uterus. The patterns of breathing taught in different classes vary. The woman is taught to use one pattern until it is no longer effective rather than in conjunction with the phases of labor.

Regardless of the level of breathing used, a cleansing breath begins and ends each pattern. A cleansing breath involves only the chest. It consists of inhaling through the nose and exhaling through pursed lips (as if blowing on a spoonful of hot food).

First Level   This pattern may also be called slow, deep breathing or slow-paced breathing. During the breathing movements only the chest is moved. The woman inhales slowly through her nose. She lifts her chest up and out during the inhalation. She exhales through pursed lips. The breathing rate is six to nine breaths a minute (or two breaths every 15 seconds). When the first level is no longer effective, the second level is used (see Figure 17–7).

Second Level   This pattern may also be called shallow breathing or modified paced breathing. The woman begins with a cleansing breath and at the end of the cleansing breath she pushes out a short breath. She then inhales and exhales through the mouth at a rate of about four breaths every five seconds. She keeps her jaw relaxed and her mouth slightly open. The air should move in and out smoothly and silently, and the breathing should be mouth centered.

This pattern can be altered into a more rapid rate that does not exceed 2 to 2 1/2 breaths every second. During the second level it is important for the whole body to be relaxed. It may help for the woman to count silently to pace the breathing (eg, count "one and two and three and. . . ." Inhalations occur on the *number* and exhalations on the *and*). Slow and rapid shallow breathing may be combined during the contraction. The more rapid rate is usually used at the height of the contraction.

Third Level   This is also called pant-blow or pattern-paced breathing. This pattern is very similar to the rapid shallow breathing except the breathing is punctuated every few breaths by a forceful exhalation through pursed lips. A variation of this pattern consists of drawing the lips back to the teeth and making a "Hee" sound with the exhalations. The forceful exhalation is through more pursed lips making a "Hoo" sound (Green & Naab 1985).

A pattern of 4 breaths may be used to begin. All breaths are kept equal and rhythmic. As the contraction becomes more intense, the pattern may be changed to 3:1, 2:1, and finally 1:1 as it is important for the woman to adjust the pattern as needed. Thus the pattern evolves as Hee-

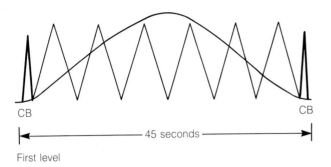

CB   CB

|◄──────── 45 seconds ────────►|

First level

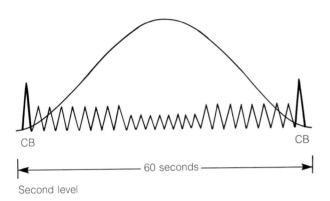

CB   CB

|◄──────── 60 seconds ────────►|

Second level

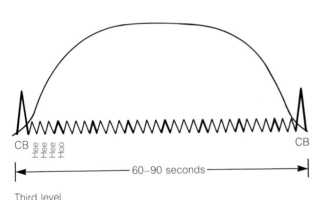

CB Hee Hee Hee Hoo   CB

|◄──────── 60–90 seconds ────────►|

Third level

Figure 17–7 *Lamaze breathing patterns. Each diagram represents a different breathing pattern. The curved line represents the uterine contraction. The peaked lines represent the breaths taken during the contraction. Each pattern begins and ends with a cleansing breath.*

Hee-Hee-Hoo (3:1), Hee-Hee-Hoo (2:1), or Hee-Hoo, depending on the count used.

Slow-paced breathing is the basic breathing skill that provides the most effective way of enhancing relaxation. Modified and pattern-paced breathing are used to assist the women to concentrate and work with the contractions.

Table 17–6 Breathing Techniques Goals
Provide adequate oxygenation of mother and baby, open maternal airways, and avoid inefficient use of muscles.
Increase physical and mental relaxation.
Decrease pain and anxiety.
Provide a means of focusing attention.
Control inadequate ventilation patterns that are related to pain and stress.

Once the desired effect is obtained, a return to slow-paced breathing is desirable. All three breathing patterns are valuable without reference to any specific phase of labor. The decision of how best to use the breathing pattern is in the hands of the expectant parents (Table 17–6).

In the second stage of labor, the woman may assume any comfortable physiologic position (a 35° semisitting, squatting, or side-lying position), take several deep breaths, then hold her breath, bulge abdominal muscles, relax the perineum, and push out through the vagina. The woman lets a little air out of her mouth with each breath. This pushing effort is repeated throughout the contraction, timed and coached by the partner.

A variation to the Lamaze breathing method is for the woman to take a cleansing breath then hold her breath for no longer than five to six seconds. She then exhales forcefully with pushing. The woman vocalizes during her pushing efforts, grunting with an open glottis at will. Between contractions she rests and uses chest breathing. (See Teaching Guide: Labor Breathing Techniques.)

Nurses involved in childbirth education need to include the concept of individuality when providing information to expectant parents about the process of childbirth and their own pattern of coping. Controversy exists over the use of ritualistic breathing techniques in childbirth. The wave of the future in childbirth education is to encourage women to incorporate their natural responses into coping with the pain of labor and birth. Self-care activities that may be used include the following:

- Vocalization or "sounding" to relieve tension in pregnancy and labor
- Massage (light touch) to facilitate relaxation
- Use of warm water for showers or bathing during labor
- Visualization (imagery)
- Relaxing music and subdued lighting

TEACHING GUIDE
Labor Breathing Techniques

Assessment: The nurse focuses on the parents' knowledge and former use of any breathing techniques during a previous labor or during stress reduction programs. Assessment of the parents' educational level and ability to understand is also important information in planning the teaching session. Couples with no prior preparation will benefit from a simple, straightforward approach.

Nursing Diagnosis: The key nursing diagnosis will probably be: Knowledge deficit related to breathing techniques for labor and birth.

Nursing Plan and Implementation: The teaching plan focuses on breathing techniques to be used during labor. Based on information learned during the assessment, the nurse will either build on previous knowledge or teaches a quick method, which is useful for an unprepared woman in active labor. Because of the important role the support person (coach) plays, he or she should be included in the plan.

Client Goals: At the completion of the teaching the woman and her partner will be able to do the following:

1. Identify the value of breathing techniques during labor.
2. Demonstrate Lamaze breathing patterns (or a variation).
3. Describe and implement methods of supporting the woman during the breathing patterns.

Teaching Plan

Content Discuss the benefits of using a patterned breathing technique during labor.

Discuss Lamaze breathing patterns

First-Level Breathing

Pattern begins and ends with a cleansing breath (in through the nose and out through pursed lips as if cooling a spoonful of hot food). While inhaling through the nose and exhaling through pursed lips, slow breaths are taken moving only the chest. The rate should be approximately 6–9/minute or 2 breaths/15 seconds. The coach or nurse may assist by reminding the woman to take a cleansing breath and then the breaths could be counted out if needed to maintain pacing. The woman inhales as someone counts "one one thousand, two one thousand, three one thousand, four one thousand." Exhalation begins and continues through the same count.

First-level breathing pattern for use during uterine contractions. The pattern begins and ends with a cleansing breath (CB).

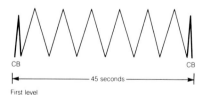

CB   CB

|← ——— 45 seconds ——— →|

First level

Teaching Method Focus on open discussion. It will help to create an environment in which the parents feel free to ask questions.

Demonstrate the breathing method after it is explained.

Use audiovisuals that depict the method.

Teach one level at a time to allow mastery before moving to next level.

Have couple practice each level and provide feedback.

If breathing techniques are being taught as part of a class, encourage couple to practice between classes. Provide handout to take home for review.

(continued)

TEACHING GUIDE (continued)

Teaching Plan

Second-Level Breathing

Pattern begins and ends with a cleansing breath. Breaths are then taken in and out silently through the mouth at approximately 4 breaths/5 seconds. The jaw and entire body needs to be relaxed. The rate can be accelerated to 2–2½ breaths/second. The rhythm for the breaths can be counted out as "one and two and one and two and . . ." with the woman exhaling on the numbers and inhaling on *and.*

Second-level breathing pattern.

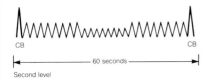

Third-Level Breathing

Pattern begins and ends with a cleansing breath. All breaths are rhythmic, in and out through the mouth. Exhalations are accompanied by a "Hee" or "Hoo" sound in a varying pattern, which begins as 3:1 (Hee Hee Hee Hoo) and can change to 2:1 (Hee Hee Hoo) or 1:1 (Hee Hoo) as the intensity of the contraction changes. The rate should not be more rapid than 2–2½/second. The rhythm of the breaths would match a "one and two and . . ." count.

Demonstrate how a stop watch can be used to time the breaths.

Third-level breathing pattern. Darkened "spike" represents Hoo.

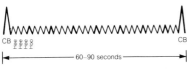

Discuss abdominal breathing. The abdomen moves outward during inhalation and downward during exhalation. The rate remains slow with approximately 6–9 breaths/minute.

Have the woman place her hand on her abdomen so that the movement can be felt.

Breathing sequence for abdominal breathing.

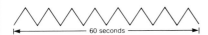

(continued)

TEACHING GUIDE (continued)

Teaching Plan

Quick method

When the woman has not learned a particular method and is in active phase of labor, the nurse may teach her a combination of two patterns. Abdominal breathing may be used until labor is more advanced. Then a more rapid pattern can be used consisting of two short blows from the mouth followed by a longer blow. (This pattern is called "pant pant blow" even though all exhalations are a blowing motion.)

Pant-pant-blow breathing pattern.

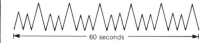

Discuss ways the coach may assist the woman including the following:

1. Providing a verbal cue during the practice session such as "The contraction is beginning"; "The contraction is half over"; "The contraction is ending."

2. Using manual pressure on the woman's arm or thigh to simulate a contraction. This provides an opportunity for the woman to practice with a deterrent present.

3. Using a stop watch or watch with a second hand to call out 10-second intervals so that the woman can pace her breathing.

4. Encouraging the woman to check for tenseness and tightness in her body during the breathing pattern.

5. Providing encouragement by prompting her in the breathing method. The coach may count out loud or verbally describe the breathing level.

6. Trying effleurage during the simulated contraction.

When the couple practices each day, suggest that they practice together. The session could begin with a relaxation exercise.

Evaluation The nurse may evaluate learning by having the woman and her partner explain the types of breathing and demonstrate the technique that they have chosen.

The woman in active labor may feel frightened and unprepared. Explain the value of breathing techniques and teach the quick method.

Encourage the woman and her partner to practice together. Breathe with them if necessary.

❀ ❀

KEY CONCEPTS

Antepartal education programs vary in their goals, content, leadership techniques, and method of teaching.

Antepartal classes may be offered early and/or late in the gestational period. The class content varies depending on the type of class and the individual offering it. Expectant parents tend to want information in chronologic sequence with the pregnancy. Adolescents have special content learning needs.

Breast-feeding programs are offered in the prenatal period. Siblings are now being included in the whole birthing process, and classes for them are available from many sources.

Grandparents have unique needs for information in grandparents' classes.

Information regarding cesarean birth is included in antepartal classes to help prepare parents.

The major types of childbirth preparation methods are Bradley, Read, Kitzinger, hypnosis, and Lamaze.

Lamaze is a type of psychoprophylactic method. The classes include information on toning exercises, relaxation exercises and techniques, and breathing methods for labor.

❀ ❀

References

Aberman S, Kirchoff KT: Infant-feeding practices: Mothers' decision making. *JOGNN* September/October 1985; 14:394.

Affonso DD: *Impact of Cesarean Childbirth*. Philadelphia: Davis, 1981.

Austin SEJ: Childbirth classes for couples desiring VBAC. *MCN* 1986; 11:250.

Bing E: *Six Practical Lessons for an Easier Childbirth*. New York: Bantam Books, 1967.

Bing E: Why Prepare? *Lamaze* 1988, p 13.

Brink S: Cloth diapers help hospital to soften the bottom line. *The Boston Herald*, Wednesday, July 11, 1990.

Center for Policy Alternatives: Update on diapers. September 1990. (Report available from 2000 Florida Avenue, NW, Washington, DC 20009).

Clark L: When children watch their mothers deliver. *Contemp OB/GYN* August 1986; 28:69.

Crowe K, von Baeyer C: Predictors of a positive childbirth experience. *Birth* June 1989; 16:59.

Davis DJ: Infant care safety: The role of perinatal caregivers. *Birth Suppl* Fall 1985; 12:21.

DelGiudice GT: The relationship between sibling jealousy and presence at a sibling's birth. *Birth* December 1986; 13:250.

Edwards M: The lactation consultant: A new profession. *Birth Suppl* Fall 1985; 12:9.

Fawcett J, Burritt J: An exploratory study of antenatal preparations for cesarean birth. *JOGNN* May/June 1985; 14:224.

Honig JC: Preparing preschool-aged children to be siblings. *MCN* January/February 1986; 11:37.

Horn M, Manion J: Creative grandparenting: Bonding the generations. *JOGNN* May/June 1985; 14:233.

Howard JS, Sater J: Adolescent mothers: Self-perceived health education needs. *JOGNN* September/October 1985; 14:399.

Jordan PL: Breast-feeding as a risk factor for fathers, the marital relationship, breast-feeding success and father-infant attachment. *JOGNN* March/April 1986; 15:94.

Karmel M: *Thank You, Dr. Lamaze*. New York: Doubleday, 1965.

Krutsky CD: Siblings at birth: Impact on parents. *J Nurse-Midwifery* September/October 1985; 30:269.

Lehrburger C, Mullen J, Jones CV: Diapers: Environmental impacts and lifecycle analysis. A Report to The National Association of Diaper Services. January 1991. (Report available from Carl Lehrburger, PO Box 998, Great Barrington, MA 01230.

Levenson PM, Smith PB, Morrow JR: A comparison of physician-patient views of teen prenatal information needs. *J Adolesc Health Care* 1986; 7:6.

Lowe NK: Explaining the pain of active labor: the importance of maternal confidence. *Res Nurs Health* 1989; 12:237.

Maloney R: Childbirth education classes: Expectant parents' expectations. *JOGNN* May/June 1985; 14:245.

Marecki M et al: Early sibling attachment period. *JOGNN* September/October 1985; 14:418.

Neifert M: *Dr. Mom: A Guide to Baby and Child Care*. New York: Signet Books, 1986.

Nichols FH, Humenick SS: *Childbirth Education: Practice, Research and Theory*. Philadelphia: Saunders, 1988.

Perez PG: Making Choices for Childbirth. *Lamaze* 1990 p. 46.

Primono J, Bruck AM, Greenstreet PK et al: The high environmental cost of disposable diapers. *MCN* September/October 1990; 15:279.

Shearer M: Effects of prenatal education depend on the attitudes and practices of obstetric caregivers. *Birth* June 1990; 17:73.

Smoke J, Grace MC: Effectiveness of prenatal care and education for pregnant adolescents. *J Nurse-Midwifery* July/August 1988; 33:178.

Whitley N: *Clinical Obstetrics*. Philadelphia: Lippincott, 1985.

Additional Readings

Cahill JM, Mathis DM: Pretesting a childbirth handbook. *Birth* March 1990; 17:39.

Carlton TO, Poole DL: Trends in maternal and child health care: Implications for research and issues for social work practice. *Soc Work Health Care* 1990; Vol 15 no. 1 p. 45.

Chapman L: Searching: Expectant fathers experiences during labor and birth. *J Perinat Neonatal Nurs* March 1991; Vol 44 p. 21

Fortier JC et al: Adjustment to a newborn sibling preparation makes a difference. *JOGNN* Jan/Feb 1991; 20:73.

Green JM, Coupland VA, Kitzinger JV: Expectations, experiences, and psychological outcomes of childbirth: A prospective study of 825 women. *Birth* March 1990; 17:15.

Harmon TM, Hynan MT, Tyre TE: Improved obstetric outcomes using hypnotic analgesia and skill mastery combined with childbirth education. *J Consult Clin Psychol* Oct 1990; 58:525.

Heatherington SE: A controlled study of the effect of prepared childbirth classes on obstetric outcomes. *Birth* June 1990; 17:86.

Oakley A, Rajan L, Robertson P: A comparison of different sources of information about pregnancy and childbirth. *J Biosoc Sci* October 1990; 22:477.

Sturrock WA, Johnson JA: The relationship between childbirth education classes and obstetric outcome. *Birth* June 1990; 17:82.

CHAPTER 18

Pregnancy at Risk:
Pregestational Problems

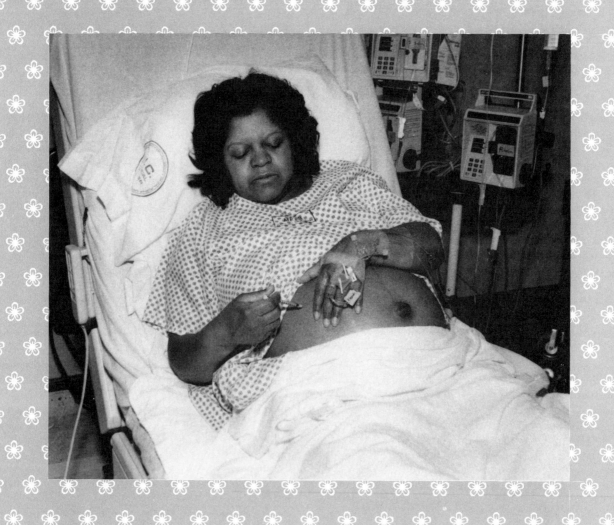

OBJECTIVES

Describe the effects of various heart disorders on pregnancy, including their implications for nursing care.

Discuss the pathology, treatment, and nursing care of pregnant women with diabetes.

Discriminate among the four major types of anemia associated with pregnancy with regard to signs, treatment, and implications for pregnancy.

Discuss Acquired Immunodeficiency Syndrome (AIDS), including care of the pregnant woman with AIDS, neonatal implications, and ramifications for the childbearing family.

Summarize the effects of alcohol and illicit drugs on the childbearing woman and her fetus/newborn.

Compare the effects of selected pregestational medical conditions on pregnancy.

❁ ❁

I've been a nurse for 25 years now and I've never seen anything change nursing practice more than AIDS has. Nursing students today will take universal precautions for granted because they won't know any other way, but I can remember when we could touch more freely. I remember drying a newly born infant and stroking him—my hands warm against his skin. I remember a time when people didn't think twice before trying to stop bleeding or give other first aid at an accident scene. I know this way is safer, but a part of me mourns what we have lost.

Even though it is a normal process, pregnancy is biologically, physiologically, and psychologically stressful. For some women, pregnancy may even be a life-threatening event. Prenatal care is aimed toward identification, assessment, and management of women whose pregnancies are at risk because of potential or existing complications.

Disruptive conditions that arise during the gestational period are the result of many high-risk factors, such as age, blood type, socioeconomic status, parity, psychologic well-being, and predisposing chronic illnesses. The major thrust of prenatal nursing care should be toward screening women for these complications and developing supportive therapies that will promote optimal health for mother and fetus.

This chapter focuses on women with pregestational medical disorders and the possible effects of these disorders on the outcome of pregnancy.

❁ *USING THE NURSING PROCESS WITH* ❁

Pregnant Women at Risk

Nursing Assessment

In some cases a woman enters a pregnancy with a preexisting condition such as heart disease or diabetes. In these cases the nurse assesses the course of the pregnancy, the impact of the condition on the pregnancy, and the effects of pregnancy on the existing condition. In all cases the nurse assesses the woman's physical condition and her psychosocial response, taking a holistic view of the woman and her family.

Nursing Diagnosis

Once the nurse has assessed the woman, it is necessary to analyze the data, draw some conclusions, and formulate nursing diagnoses. For example, for a woman with preexisting heart disease who has had no limitation of activity prior to pregnancy, a possible nursing diagnosis might be "Noncompliance with rest schedule due to lack of understanding of the strain pregnancy places on the heart."

Nursing Plan and Implementation

The nursing plan and its implementation should follow logically from assessment, analysis, and nursing diagnosis. The plan reflects the nurse's understanding of the woman's pregestational medical condition, the impact of pregnancy on the condition, and the impact of the condition on the pregnancy. The plan also reflects the nurse's awareness of the woman's needs, personal preferences, and cultural beliefs and practices.

Evaluation

Evaluation requires that the nurse critically review the plan and its implementation to determine whether it was effective. If the plan was effective, the nurse determines whether it can continue or if changes in the woman's situation require modifications. If it was not effective, the nurse must try to determine why. The nurse then makes necessary additional assessments and modifies the plan accordingly. The goal in all cases is to provide effective nursing care.

❁ ❁ ❁ ❁ ❁ ❁ ❁ ❁ ❁ ❁ ❁ ❁

Care of the Woman with Heart Disease

A healthy woman with a normal heart has adequate cardiac reserve to adjust to the demands of pregnancy with little difficulty. The woman with heart disease however, has decreased cardiac reserve, making it more difficult for her heart to accommodate the higher workload of pregnancy.

Approximately 0.5% to 1.0% of pregnant women are at risk because of pregestational heart disease (Cruikshank 1990). Heart disease ranks fourth after hypertension, hemorrhage, and infection as a cause of maternal mortality. While rheumatic heart disease used to predominate, its prevalence is now equal to congenital heart defects in the United States and Canada (Shime 1989). Other less common causes of heart disease in pregnancy include Marfan syndrome, peripartum cardiomyopathy, and Eisenmenger syndrome. All can cause significant maternal mortality. Mitral valve prolapse is usually asymptomatic but is addressed here because of its frequent occurrence during pregnancy.

Rheumatic heart has declined rapidly in the last four decades, primarily because of prompt identification of pharyngeal infections caused by group A beta-hemolytic streptococcus and the availability of penicillin for treatment. Rheumatic fever, which may develop in untreated streptococcal infections, is an inflammatory connective tissue disease that can involve the heart, joints, central nervous system, skin, and subcutaneous tissue. When the heart is affected, mitral valve stenosis is the most common and serious lesion. Aortic valve involvement, manifested by aortic insufficiency, is the second most common problem. The tricuspid and pulmonic valves are rarely affected.

Recurrent acute inflammation from bouts of rheumatic fever causes scar tissue formation on the valves. The scarring results in stenosis (narrowing) of the mitral valve, which may be accompanied by mitral regurgitation. Obstructed blood flow across the narrowed valve from the left atrium to the left ventricle can lead to elevated left atrial pressure and elevated pulmonary venous and capillary pressures.

The increased blood volume of pregnancy, coupled with the pregnant woman's need for increased cardiac output, stresses the heart of a woman with mitral valve stenosis. She may develop dyspnea, orthopnea, and pulmonary edema and is at increased risk for congestive heart failure (CHF). Even the woman who has no symptoms at the onset of her pregnancy is at increased risk for CHF.

When the aortic valve is involved, the scarring usually leaves the valve unable to close completely (aortic incompetence or insufficiency) during diastole. Blood then regurgitates back into the left ventricle, leading to volume overload of the left ventricle and inadequate perfusion of the coronary arteries. Occasionally there is both aortic stenosis and regurgitation.

With mild aortic insufficiency the woman may be asymptomatic. But if the valve dysfunction worsens, she may experience dyspnea and even chest pain (due to inadequate blood flow to the heart muscle) with exertion.

Congenital heart defects have become a more common finding in pregnant women as improved surgical techniques enable females born with heart defects to live to childbearing age. The exact pathology depends on the specific defect. Congenital defects most often seen in pregnant women include tetralogy of Fallot, atrial septal defect, ventricular septal defect, patent ductus arteriosus, and coarctation of the aorta. When surgical repair can be accomplished with no remaining evidence of organic heart disease, pregnancy may be undertaken with confidence. In such cases antibiotic prophylaxis is recommended to prevent subacute bacterial endocarditis at the time of birth. When congenital heart disease is associated with cyanosis, whether the defect was originally uncorrected or whether the correction failed to relieve the cyanosis, the woman should be counseled to avoid pregnancy because the risk to both her and the fetus would be high. She also needs to know that there is a 2% to 5% chance of the baby inheriting the disorder, since most congenital heart defects are believed to be polygenetic and multifactorial in origin.

Marfan syndrome is an autosomal dominant disorder of connective tissue in which there may be serious cardiovascular involvement—usually dissection or rupture of the aorta (Ramin et al 1989). A pregnant woman with Marfan syndrome needs very careful cardiovascular assessment and counseling regarding her prognosis for a successful pregnancy. Because of the inheritance pattern of the disease, there is a 50% chance of its being passed on to offspring.

Mitral valve prolapse (MVP) is usually an asymptomatic condition that is found in about 6% to 10% of women of childbearing age (Cruikshank 1990). The condition is more common in women than in men and seems to run in families. In MVP the mitral valve leaflets tend to prolapse into the left atrium during ventricular systole because the chordae tendineae that support them are long and thin. As a result, some mitral regurgitation may occur. On auscultation, a midsystolic click and a late systolic murmur are heard.

Women with MVP usually tolerate pregnancy well, and the prognosis is excellent. Most women require assurance that they can continue with normal activities. A few women experience symptoms—primarily palpitations, chest pain, and dyspnea—which are usually due to arrhythmias. They are often treated with propranolol hydrochloride (Inderal). Limiting caffeine intake also helps decrease palpitations. Antibiotics are given prophylactically at the time of childbirth to prevent bacterial endocarditis.

Peripartum cardiomyopathy is a dysfunction of the left ventricle that occurs in the last month of pregnancy or the first five months postpartum in a woman with no previous history of heart disease. The symptoms are related to congestive heart failure: dyspnea, orthopnea, chest pain, palpitations, weakness, and edema. The cause is unknown. Treatment includes digitalis, diuretics, anticoagulants, and bed rest. The condition may resolve with bed rest as the heart gradually returns to normal size. Subsequent pregnancy is strongly discouraged because the disease tends to recur during pregnancy.

Eisenmenger syndrome exists when pulmonary hypertension develops following right-to-left shunting through a septal defect or a patent ductus. This condition cannot be corrected surgically and is associated with a high maternal mortality rate (Degani et al 1989).

Medical Therapy

The primary goal of medical management is early diagnosis and ongoing treatment of the woman with cardiac disease. Echocardiogram, chest x ray, electrocardiogram, auscultation of heart sounds, and sometimes cardiac catheterization are essential for establishing the type and severity of the heart disease. The severity of heart disease can also be determined by the individual's ability to perform ordinary physical activity. The following classification of functional capacity has been standardized by the Criteria Committee of the New York Heart Association (1955):

- Class I. No limitation of physical activity. Ordinary physical activity causes no discomfort; anginal pain is not present.

- Class II. Slight limitation of physical activity. Ordinary physical activity causes fatigue, dyspnea, palpitation, or anginal pain.

- Class III. Moderate to marked limitation of physical activity. During less than ordinary physical activity, the person experiences excessive fatigue, dyspnea, palpitation, or anginal pain.

- Class IV. Inability to carry on any physical activity without experiencing discomforts. Even at rest, the person experiences symptoms of cardiac insufficiency or anginal pain.

Women in classes I and II usually experience a normal pregnancy and have few complications, whereas those in classes III and IV are at risk for more severe complications.

Drug Therapy

Besides the iron and vitamin supplements prescribed during pregnancy, the pregnant woman with heart disease may need additional drug therapy to maintain health. Antibiotics, usually penicillin if not contraindicated by allergy, are used during pregnancy to prevent recurrent bouts of rheumatic fever and subsequent heart valve damage. Antibiotics are also recommended during labor and the early postpartum period for either acquired or congenital disease, to prevent bacterial endocarditis. If the woman develops coagulation problems, the anticoagulant heparin may be used. Heparin offers the greatest safety to the fetus because it does not cross the placenta. The thiazide diuretics and furosemide (Lasix) may be used to treat congestive heart failure if it develops. Digitalis glycosides and common antiarrhythmic drugs may be used to treat cardiac failure and arrhythmias. These agents do cross the placenta but have no reported teratogenic effect; however, they have not been adequately studied to establish their safety in pregnancy (Little & Gilstrap 1989).

Labor

Spontaneous natural labor with adequate pain relief is usually recommended for clients in classes I and II. Those in classes III and IV may need to be hospitalized prior to onset of labor for cardiovascular stabilization (Brady 1989). They may also require invasive cardiac monitoring during labor (Gianopolous 1989).

Childbirth

Use of low forceps provides the safest method of birth, with lumbar epidural anesthesia to reduce the stress of pushing. Cesarean is used only if fetal or obstetric indications exist, not on the basis of heart disease alone.

❀   *APPLYING THE NURSING PROCESS*   ❀

Nursing Assessment

CRITICAL THINKING

What specific information does the nurse need to help the pregnant woman with heart disease plan her schedule to avoid stress and allow sufficient time for rest?

The stress of pregnancy on the functional capacity of the heart is assessed during every antepartal visit. The nurse notes the category of functional capacity assigned to the woman, takes the woman's pulse, respirations, and blood pressure, and compares them to the normal values expected during pregnancy and to the woman's previous values. The nurse then determines the woman's activity level, including rest, and any changes in the pulse and respirations that have occurred since previous visits. The nurse also identifies and evaluates other factors that would increase strain on the heart. These might include anemia, infection, anxiety, lack of support system, and household demands.

The following symptoms, if they are progressive, are indicative of congestive heart failure, the heart's signal of its decreased ability to meet the demands of pregnancy.

- Cough (frequent, with or without hemoptysis)
- Dyspnea (progressive, upon exertion)
- Edema (progressive, generalized, including extremities, face, eyelids)
- Heart murmurs (heard on auscultation)
- Palpitations
- Rales (auscultated in lung bases)

It should be noted that this cycle is *progressive*, because some of these same behaviors are seen to a minor degree in a pregnancy without cardiac problems.

Nursing Diagnosis

Nursing diagnoses that might apply to the pregnant woman with heart disease include the following:

- Decreased cardiac output: easy fatigability
- Impaired gas exchange related to pulmonary edema secondary to cardiac decompensation
- Knowledge deficit related to the cardiac condition and requirement to alter self-care activities
- Fear related to the effects of the maternal cardiac condition on fetal well-being

Nursing Plan and Implementation

Nursing care is directed toward maintaining a balance between cardiac reserve and cardiac workload.

Antepartal Nursing Care

Nursing actions are designed to meet the physiologic and psychosocial needs of the pregnant woman with heart disease. The priority of nursing action varies based on the severity of the disease process and the individual needs of the woman as determined by the nursing assessment.

The woman and her family should thoroughly understand her condition and its management and should recognize signs of potential complications. This will increase their understanding and decrease anxiety. When the nurse provides thorough explanations, uses printed material, and provides frequent opportunities to ask questions and discuss concerns, the woman is better able to meet her own health care needs and seek assistance appropriately.

As part of health teaching, the nurse explains the purposes of the dietary and activity changes that are required. A diet is instituted that is high in iron, protein, and essential nutrients but low in sodium, with adequate calories to ensure normal weight gain. Such a diet best meets the nutrition needs of the client with cardiac disease. To help preserve her cardiac reserves, the woman may need to restrict her activities. In addition, 8–10 hours of sleep, with frequent daily rest periods, is essential. Because upper respiratory infections may tax the heart and lead to decompensation, the woman must avoid contact with sources of infection.

During the first half of pregnancy the woman is seen approximately every two weeks to assess cardiac status. During the second half of pregnancy the woman is seen weekly. These assessments are especially important between weeks 28 and 30 when the blood volume reaches maximum amounts. If symptoms of cardiac decompensa-

tion occur, prompt medical intervention is indicated to correct the cardiac problem.

Intrapartal Nursing Care

Labor and birth exert tremendous stress on the woman and her fetus. This stress could be fatal to the fetus of a woman with cardiac disease because the fetus may be receiving a decreased oxygen and blood supply. Thus, the intrapartal care of a woman with cardiac disease is aimed at reducing the amount of physical exertion and accompanying fatigue.

The nurse evaluates maternal vital signs frequently to determine the woman's response to labor. A pulse rate greater than 100 beats per minute or respirations greater than 25 per minute may indicate beginning cardiac decompensation and require further evaluation. The nurse also auscultates the woman's lungs frequently for evidence of rales and carefully observes for other signs of developing decompensation.

To ensure cardiac emptying and adequate oxygenation, the nurse encourages the laboring woman to assume either a semi-Fowler's or side-lying position with her head and shoulders elevated. Oxygen by mask, diuretics to reduce fluid retention, sedatives and analgesics, prophylactic antibiotics, and digitalis may also be used as indicated by the woman's status.

The nurse remains with the woman to support her. It is essential that the nurse keep the woman and her family informed of labor progress and management plans, collaborating with them to fulfill their wishes for the birth experience as much as possible. The nurse needs to maintain an atmosphere of calm to lessen the anxiety of the woman and her family.

Continuous electronic fetal monitoring is used to provide ongoing assessment of the fetus' response to labor. To prevent overexertion and the accompanying fatigue, the nurse encourages the woman to sleep and relax between contractions and provides her with emotional support and encouragement. During pushing the nurse encourages the woman to use shorter, more moderate open glottis pushing (See Chapter 23), with complete relaxation between pushes. Vital signs are monitored closely during the second stage.

Postpartal Nursing Care

The postpartal period is a significant time for the woman with cardiac disease. After birth, the intraabdominal pressure and the venous pressure are reduced, the splanchnic vessels engorge, and blood flow to the heart increases. As extravascular fluid returns to the bloodstream for excretion, cardiac output and blood volume increase. This physiologic adaptation places great strain on the heart and may lead to decompensation, especially in the first 48 hours postpartum.

So that the health team can detect any possible problems, the woman remains in the hospital for approximately one week to rest and recover. Her vital signs are monitored frequently and she is assessed for signs of decompensation.

She stays in the semi-Fowler's or side-lying position, with her head and shoulders elevated, and begins a gradual, progressive activity program. Appropriate diet and stool softeners facilitate bowel movement without undue strain.

The postpartum nurse gives the woman opportunities to discuss her birth experience and helps her deal with any feelings or concerns that cause her distress. The nurse also encourages maternal-infant attachment by providing frequent opportunities for the mother to interact with her child.

Because there is no evidence that cardiac output is compromised during lactation, the only concern about breast-feeding for women with cardiovascular disease is related to medications that the mother may be taking (Lawrence 1989). These must be evaluated for their ability to pass into the milk and for any effect of the drug on lactation. The nurse can assist the breast-feeding mother to a comfortable side-lying position with her head moderately elevated or to a semi-Fowler's position. To conserve the mother's energy the nurse should position the newborn at the breast and be available to burp the baby and reposition him or her at the other breast.

In addition to providing the normal postpartum discharge teaching, the nurse should ensure that the woman and her family understand the signs of possible problems resulting from her heart disease or from other postpartal complications. The nurse determines what assistance the woman will receive to care for herself and her baby and then helps the woman make realistic home care plans. The nurse also plans with the woman an activity schedule that is gradual, progressive, and appropriate to her needs and home environment. The nurse provides appropriate health teaching, including information about resumption of sexual activity and contraception. Visiting nurse or homemaker assistance referrals may be necessary, depending on the woman's status.

Evaluation

Anticipated outcomes of nursing care include the following:

- The woman clearly understands her condition and its possible impact on pregnancy, labor and birth, and the postpartal period.
- The woman participates in developing an appropriate health care regimen and follows it throughout her pregnancy.
- The woman gives birth to a healthy infant.
- The woman avoids congestive heart failure.
- The woman is able to identify signs and symptoms of possible complications postpartally.
- The woman is comfortable caring for her newborn infant.

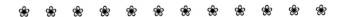

Care of the Woman with Diabetes Mellitus

Diabetes mellitus is an endocrine disorder of carbohydrate metabolism that results from inadequate production or utilization of insulin. Insulin is a powerful hypoglycemic agent, normally produced by the beta cells of the islets of Langerhans in the pancreas. It lowers blood glucose levels by enabling the glucose to move from the blood into muscle and adipose tissue cells.

Carbohydrate Metabolism in Pregnancy

The changes in carbohydrate, protein, and fat metabolism in normal pregnancy are profound. Carbohydrate metabolism is affected early in pregnancy by a rise in serum levels of estrogen, progesterone, and other hormones. These hormones stimulate increased insulin production by the maternal pancreatic beta cells and increased tissue response to insulin early in pregnancy. Therefore an anabolic (building up) state exists during the first half of pregnancy with storage of glycogen in the liver and other tissues.

The second half of pregnancy is characterized by increased resistance to insulin, which appears to be due to secretion of human placental lactogen (hPL) and elevated levels of estrogen, progesterone, and other hormones (Barss 1989a). This diminished effectiveness of insulin results in a catabolic state during fasting periods (eg, during the night and after meal absorption). Because increasing amounts of circulating maternal glucose and amino acids are being diverted to the fetus, maternal fat is metabolized during fasting periods much more readily than in a nonpregnant person. This process is called *accelerated starvation*. Ketones may be present in the urine as a result of lipolysis (maternal metabolism of fat).

A rise in the glomerular filtration rate in the kidneys in conjunction with decreased tubular glucose reabsorption results in glycosuria. A decrease in the normal fasting blood glucose occurs in pregnancy, but free fatty acids and ketones are increased. The fed state is also altered by a more pronounced and prolonged elevation in plasma glucose (Winn & Reece 1989).

In summary, the delicate system of checks and balances that exist between glucose production and glucose utilization is stressed by the growing fetus, who derives energy from glucose taken solely from maternal stores. This stress is referred to as the *diabetogenic effect* of pregnancy. Thus any preexisting disruption in carbohydrate metabolism is augmented by pregnancy, and any diabetic potential may precipitate **gestational diabetes mellitus**.

Pathophysiology of Diabetes Mellitus

In diabetes mellitus, the pancreas does not produce sufficient amounts of insulin to allow necessary carbohydrate metabolism. With inadequate amounts of insulin, glucose cannot enter the cells but remains outside in the blood. The body cells become energy depleted, while the blood glucose level remains elevated. Fats and proteins in the body tissues are then oxidized by the cells as a source of energy. This results in wasting of fat and muscle tissue of the body, negative nitrogen balance due to protein breakdown, and ketosis due to fat metabolism. The strong osmotic force of the glucose concentration in the blood pulls water from the cells into the blood, which results in cellular dehydration. The high level of glucose in the blood eventually spills over into the urine, producing glycosuria. Osmotic pressure of the glucose in the urine prevents reabsorption of water into the kidney tubules, causing extracellular dehydration.

These pathologic developments cause the four cardinal signs and symptoms of diabetes mellitus: polyuria, polydipsia, weight loss, and polyphagia. *Polyuria* (frequent urination) results because water is not reabsorbed by the renal tubules due to the osmotic activity of glucose. *Polydipsia* (excessive thirst) is caused by dehydration from polyuria. *Weight loss* (seen in insulin-dependent diabetes, also called type I diabetes) is due to the use of fat and muscle tissue for energy. *Polyphagia* (excessive hunger) is caused by tissue loss and a state of starvation, which results from the inability of the cells to utilize the blood glucose. Diagnosis of diabetes is based on the presence of clinical symptoms and laboratory tests showing elevated glucose levels in the blood.

Classification of Diabetes Mellitus

States of altered carbohydrate metabolism have been classified several different ways. Table 18–1 shows the current accepted classification, a result of the 1979 report of a special committee of the National Institutes of Health (National Diabetes Data Group 1979). This classification contains

Table 18–1 Classification of Diabetes Mellitus (DM) and Other Categories of Glucose Intolerance

1. Diabetes mellitus
   a. Type I, insulin-dependent (IDDM)
   b. Type II, noninsulin-dependent (NIDDM)
      (1) Nonobese NIDDM
      (2) Obese NIDDM
   c. Secondary diabetes
2. Impaired glucose tolerance (IGT)
3. Gestational diabetes (GDM)

Source: *National Diabetes Data Group of National Institutes of Health, 1979.* Diabetes *1979; 28:1039. Adapted with permission from the American Diabetes Association Inc.*

Table 18–2 White's Classification of Diabetes in Pregnancy

Class	Criterion
A	Chemical diabetes
B	Maturity onset (age over 20 years), duration under 10 years, no vascular lesions
C_1	Age 10 to 19 years at onset
C_2	10 to 19 years' duration
D_1	Under 10 years at onset
D_2	Over 20 years' duration
D_3	Benign retinopathy
D_4	Calcified vessels of legs
D_5	Hypertension
E	No longer sought
F	Nephropathy
G	Many failures
H	Cardiopathy
R	Proliferating retinopathy
T	Renal transplant (added by Tagatz and colleagues of the University of Minnesota)

Source: *From White P: Classification of obstetric diabetes.* Am J Obstet Gynecol *1978; 130:228. C. V. Mosby Co. Used with permission.*

three main categories: diabetes mellitus (DM), impaired glucose tolerance (IGT), and gestational diabetes mellitus (GDM).

In GDM, the diabetes has its onset or is first diagnosed during pregnancy. Except for an impaired tolerance to glucose, the woman may remain asymptomatic or may have a mild form of the disease. Diagnosis of GDM is very important, however, because even mild diabetes causes increased risk for perinatal morbidity and mortality. After pregnancy, women with GDM do have a higher risk of developing type I or type II diabetes later in life.

Table 18–2 shows White's classification of diabetes in pregnancy. This classification is useful for describing the extent of the disease.

Influence of Pregnancy on Diabetes

Pregnancy can affect diabetes significantly. First, the physiologic changes of pregnancy can drastically alter insulin requirements. Second, pregnancy may accelerate the progress of vascular disease secondary to diabetes.

The disease may be more difficult to control during pregnancy because insulin requirements are changeable. Insulin need frequently decreases early in the first trimester. Levels of hPL, an insulin antagonist, are low, energy demands of the embryo are minimal, and the woman may be consuming less food due to nausea and vomiting. Nausea and vomiting may also cause dietary fluctuations, which can increase the risk of hypoglycemia or insulin shock. Insulin requirements usually begin to rise late in the first trimester as glucose use and glycogen storage by the woman and fetus are increased. As a result of placental maturation and production of hPL and other hormones, insulin requirements may double or quadruple by the end of pregnancy.

Increased energy needs during labor may require more insulin to balance intravenous glucose. After delivery of the placenta, insulin requirements usually decrease abruptly with loss of hPL in the maternal circulation.

Other factors contribute to the difficulty in controlling the disease. As pregnancy progresses, the renal threshold for glucose decreases. There is also an increased risk of ketoacidosis, which may occur at lower serum glucose levels in the pregnant woman with diabetes than in the nonpregnant diabetic. The vascular disease that accompanies diabetes may progress during pregnancy. Hypertension may occur. Nephropathy may result from renal impairment, and retinopathy may also occur.

The primary concern for the pregnant woman who has diabetes is control of circulating blood glucose levels. If control can be achieved and maintained, diabetes generally does not worsen during pregnancy. The woman's health status may even improve due to close medical supervision.

Influence of Diabetes on Pregnancy Outcome

The discovery of insulin in 1922 allowed women with diabetes to survive to adulthood and bear children. Since then maternal mortality from diabetes has been minimal. However, the pregnancy of a woman who has diabetes carries a higher risk of complications, especially perinatal mortality and congenital anomalies. The risk of perinatal mortality has been reduced by the recent recognition of the importance of tight metabolic control (blood glucose between 70 mg/dL and 120 mg/dL). New techniques for monitoring blood glucose, delivering insulin, and monitoring the fetus have also reduced perinatal mortality.

Maternal Risks

Maternal health problems in diabetic pregnancy have been greatly reduced with the team approach to early prenatal care and emphasis on maintaining control of blood glucose levels. The prognosis for the pregnant woman with gestational, type I, or type II diabetes that has not resulted in significant vascular damage is positive. However, diabetic pregnancy still carries higher risks for complications than normal pregnancy.

Hydramnios, or an increase in the volume of amniotic fluid, occurs in 10% to 20% of pregnant diabetics (Spellacy 1990). The exact mechanism causing the increase is unknown. Premature rupture of membranes and onset of labor may result, but only occasionally does this pose a threat.

Pregnancy-induced hypertension (PIH) occurs more often in diabetic pregnancies, especially when diabetes-related vascular changes already exist.

Hyperglycemia due to insufficient amounts of insulin can lead to *ketoacidosis* as a result of the increase in ketone bodies (which are acidic) in the blood released when fatty acids are metabolized. Ketoacidosis usually develops slowly, but it may develop more rapidly in the pregnant woman because of the hyperketonemia associated with accelerated starvation in the nonfed state. The tendency for higher postprandial glucose levels because of decreased gastric motility and the contrainsulin effects of hPL also predispose the woman to ketoacidosis. If the ketoacidosis is not treated, it can lead to coma and death of both mother and fetus.

In pregnancy, particularly in the presence of prolonged vomiting, carbohydrate deficiency may lead to ketosis as fat cells are metabolized for energy needs. Measurement of blood glucose levels will easily differentiate starvation ketosis (a hypoglycemic state treated with glucose solution) from diabetic ketoacidosis (a hyperglycemic state treated with insulin).

Another risk to the pregnant woman with diabetes is *dystocia,* caused by feto-pelvic disproportion if fetal macrosomia exists. *Anemia* may develop as a result of vascular involvement and poor nutritional intake. The pregnant woman with diabetes is at increased risk for monilial vaginitis and urinary tract infections because of increased glycosuria, which contributes to a favorable environment for bacterial growth. If untreated, asymptomatic bacteriuria can lead to pyelonephritis, a serious kidney infection.

During pregnancy, about 15% of diabetic women will have some increase in retinopathy. Severe proliferative retinopathy can lead to blindness if not treated with laser coagulation (Spellacy 1990).

Fetal-Neonatal Risks

Maintaining maternal glucose in the normal range has resulted not only in decreased perinatal mortality but also in reduced perinatal morbidity. It is now clear that many of the problems of the neonate result directly from high maternal plasma glucose levels (Sheldon 1988). In the presence of severe maternal ketoacidosis, the risk of fetal death increases to 50% (Spellacy 1990). Fetal enzymes systems cease functioning in an acidic environment.

Macrosomia and *hypoglycemia* in the neonate are due to high levels of fetal production of insulin, stimulated by the high levels of glucose crossing the placenta from the mother. Sustained fetal hyperinsulinism and hyperglycemia ultimately lead to excessive growth and deposition of fat. After birth the umbilical cord is severed, and thus the generous maternal blood glucose supply is eliminated. However, continued islet cell hyperactivity leads to excessive insulin levels and depleted blood glucose (hypoglycemia) in 2 to 4 hours. Macrosomia can be significantly reduced by tight maternal blood glucose control.

Infants of diabetic mothers with vascular involvement may demonstrate intrauterine growth retardation (IUGR).

This occurs because vascular changes in the mother decrease the efficiency of placental perfusion and the fetus is not as well sustained in utero.

Respiratory distress syndrome appears to result from inhibition, by high levels of fetal insulin, of some fetal enzymes necessary for surfactant production. *Polycythemia* in the neonate is due primarily to the diminished ability of glycosylated hemoglobin in the mother's blood to release oxygen. *Hyperbilirubinemia* is a direct result of the inability of immature liver enzymes to metabolize the increased bilirubin resulting from the polycythemia.

The incidence of congenital anomalies in diabetic pregnancies is 3 to 4 times higher than the 2% to 3% incidence found in the general population (Gabbe 1990). The anomalies often involve the heart, central nervous system, and skeletal system. One anomaly, sacral agenesis, appears only in infants of diabetic mothers. Research suggests that the incidence of congenital anomalies is related to high glucose levels in early pregnancy (weeks 3 to 6) (Spellacy 1990). To prevent congenital anomalies, there is a clear need for diabetic control before conception.

Medical Therapy

Detection and Diagnosis of Gestational Diabetes

Gestational diabetes is more common than pregestational diabetes. It is estimated to occur in 3% to 6% of pregnancies (Kaufman 1989). Therefore, screening for the detection of diabetes is a standard part of prenatal care. If the possibility of diabetes is suspected, further testing is undertaken for diagnosis.

Three screening tests are commonly administered to pregnant women:

1. *Urine testing.* The pregnant woman's urine is tested for glucose at her first prenatal visit and again on subsequent visits. Glycosuria is not diagnostic of diabetes mellitus, but the presence of glycosuria is indication for glucose tolerance testing. In the nonpregnant adult, glucose is not generally spilled into the urine until the blood sugar level is 180 mg/dL or greater. During pregnancy the renal threshold is lower, and glucose may spill into the urine when blood glucose levels are 130 mg/dL.

   Tes-Tape and Diastix are methods of choice in urine testing. They are specific for glucose and do not show positive readings in the presence of lactose or fructose. Single-specimen urine tests are used in routine screening at each antenatal visit.

   Urine is also tested for ketones using Ketostix or Acetest. Both are simple tests for detecting ketones in the urine and are usually done routinely for type I (ketosis-prone) diabetes.

2. *50 g, 1-hour diabetes screening test.* It has become common practice to screen all asymptomatic pregnant women for gestational diabetes between 24 and 28 weeks' gestation. Women who have demonstrated glycosuria or have a history of large infants or gestational diabetes in a previous pregnancy should be screened earlier in pregnancy (Kaufman 1989). To do this test, the woman ingests 50 g of an oral glucose solution. One hour later a blood sample is obtained. If the plasma glucose level exceeds 140 mg/dL, a diagnostic glucose tolerance test (GTT) is necessary. The 50 g screen test is convenient because the woman does not need to be fasting, and the test does not need to be done following a meal (Sacks 1989).

3. *Serum fructosamine screening.* This test is an alternative to the one-hour glucose tolerance as a screening tool (Lucas et al 1989). A single blood specimen is drawn and the client does not have to wait an hour. The test is not influenced by diet or activity, nor does it show daily fluctuations in plasma glucose level. Instead it reflects glucose control over the previous 1 to 3 weeks. The test measures serum fructosamines, proteins to which glucose molecules have attached. It differs from Hemoglobin A_{1c} (see p 457) in that it reflects short-term control (1 to 3 weeks) and is less expensive. Some researchers believe that it compares favorably with the one-hour glucose in sensitivity (Kaufman 1990), while others do not (Roberts et al 1990). However, it has not yet been tested on large populations.

During pregnancy, gestational diabetes mellitus is diagnosed using a *100 g oral glucose tolerance test.* To do this test the woman eats a high-carbohydrate (greater than 200 g carbohydrate daily) diet for two days prior to her scheduled test. She then fasts from midnight on the day of the test. A fasting plasma glucose level is obtained, and the woman ingests 100 g of an oral glucose solution. Plasma glucose levels are determined at one, two, and three hours. Gestational diabetes is diagnosed if two or more of the following values are equaled or exceeded (Kaufman 1989; Hare 1989a):

Fasting	105 mg/dL
1 hr	190 mg/dL
2 hr	165 mg/dL
3 hr	145 mg/dL

If the woman presents with any of the following, the screen is omitted and she is given a three-hour glucose tolerance test:

- The cardinal signs of DM (polyuria, polydipsia, polyphagia, weight loss)
- Obesity

- Family history of DM
- Obstetric history that includes a large-for-gestational-age (LGA) neonate, hydramnios, unexplained stillbirth, or congenital anomalies.

Laboratory Assessment of Long-Term Glucose Control

There are two tests now in use for measuring glucose control over a period of time.

Glycosylated Hemoglobin   This test reflects glucose control over the previous 4 to 12 weeks. It measures the percentage in the blood of glycohemoglobin (HbA$_{1c}$, hemoglobin to which a glucose molecule is attached). Because glycosylation is a rather slow and essentially irreversible process, the level of HbA$_{1c}$ gives an indication of previous average serum glucose concentrations.

Normally 6% to 8% of hemoglobin is glycosylated. An elevation of glycohemoglobin in pregnancy over 10% is associated with increased incidence of congenital anomalies; spontaneous abortions increase with glycosylated hemoglobin concentrations over 9% (Lucas et al 1989). Neonatal macrosomia and hyperbilirubinemia are associated with maternal levels over 7%. For a woman who is a known diabetic, this test should be done at preconception counseling, again at the first prenatal visit, and once each succeeding trimester.

Management of Diabetes During Pregnancy

The major goals of medical care for a pregnant woman with diabetes—whether gestational or pregestational—are: (a) to maintain a physiologic equilibrium of insulin availability and glucose utilization during pregnancy, and (b) to deliver an optimally healthy mother and newborn. To achieve these goals, good prenatal care using a team approach is a top priority. The team consists of an obstetrician, an endocrinologist, a perinatologist, a nurse-diabetes educator, a perinatal nurse, a nutritionist, a social worker, and, most importantly, the diabetic woman and her partner. Education of the couple and their active involvement in managing her care are essential for a good outcome.

For the woman with gestational diabetes the diagnosis may be a shock, leaving her frightened and anxious (Chez 1989). She needs clear explanation and teaching to enlist her participation in ensuring a good outcome. The diabetes nurse educator plays a major role in this counseling. The woman with pregestational diabetes needs to understand changes she can expect during pregnancy; thus, she should receive such teaching in preconception counseling.

Antepartal Period   At the initial prenatal visit a careful history and physical are done, with special attention given to dating the pregnancy, and laboratory data are obtained. The diabetes is classified using White's criteria, and a careful funduscopic examination is done to detect any retinopathy. In some cases, the woman may be referred to an ophthalmologist for further evaluation.

Ongoing medical therapy during the antepartal period focuses on the following:

- *Dietary regulation.* The calorie needs of pregnant women are not altered by diabetes (Barss 1989a). In general, women need approximately 30 kcal/kg of ideal body weight (IBW) during the first trimester and 35 to 36 kcal/kg IBW during the second and third trimesters. If ketonuria develops or the woman complains of hunger, the number of calories may be increased. Dietary guidelines are similar for women with gestational and pregestational diabetes. Approximately 50% to 60% of the calories should come from complex carbohydrates with adequate fiber to slow down absorption, about 12% to 20% of calories (or 1.5 g/kg body weight) should be protein, and 20% to 30% should be fat (Holman 1989). This caloric intake is divided among three meals and three snacks. The prebedtime snack is the most important and must include both protein and complex carbohydrates to prevent hypoglycemia at night. Because it is so important that the pregnant woman follow these guidelines, a nutritionist works out meal plans based on the woman's life-style, culture, and food preferences and teaches her food exchanges so she can vary and plan her own meals. Cookbooks for diabetics are available and can be a great help.

- *Glucose monitoring.* Glucose monitoring is an essential part of diabetes management for determining the need for insulin and assessing glucose control. Many physicians have the woman come in for weekly assessment of her fasting glucose levels and one or two postprandial levels (Chez 1989). Other physicians recommend home monitoring for most of their clients. In some centers home monitoring of blood glucose levels has become a standard and routine part of pregnancy management for both gestational and pregestational diabetes.

Home blood glucose monitoring should be taught at the first visit after the diagnosis of gestational diabetes has been established. The woman with pregestational diabetes may already be monitoring her own blood sugar.

It is usually recommended that monitoring be done at least four times per day, a fasting blood sugar before breakfast, then a postprandial test two hours after each meal (Ghiloni 1989). Women are encouraged to maintain blood sugars in the normal ranges as follows: fasting (before eating or taking insulin), 60 to 100 mg/dL; 2 hours after each meal, 100 to 140 mg/dL (Ghiloni 1989). Some recommend more rigid control of blood glucose, with the goal of fasting blood sugar of 70 to 95 mg/dL, and 2-hour postprandial blood sugar of less than 120 mg/dL, if this can be done without frequent hypoglycemic reactions (Barss 1989a).

- *Insulin administration.* Whether or not the woman with gestational diabetes needs additional insulin (over her own body production) depends on how well her blood glucose levels can be maintained by diet alone. Individuals with pregestational diabetes usually have Type I diabetes, requiring insulin administration. Whether the client has gestational or pregestational diabetes, the type of insulin used should be human (Barss 1989a; Hare 1989a). Human insulin is the least likely to cause an allergic response. If the woman has previously used bovine or porcine insulin, she may require smaller doses of human insulin to achieve the same pharmacologic effect (Engel 1989). She is instructed to take an initial glucose reading at 2 AM to avoid nocturnal or early morning hypoglycemic episodes.

  The insulin program should be kept as simple as possible while still achieving the goals of normal fasting and postprandial blood glucose levels. A single dose of intermediate (NPH or Lente) insulin in the morning may be sufficient (Hare 1989a). Most women will need a mixture of intermediate and regular insulin twice daily (Barss 1989a). Often two-thirds of the total insulin dose is taken with breakfast in a ratio of intermediate to regular of 2:1. The remaining third is taken with the evening meal in a 1:1 ratio. It is important to remember that the amount of insulin needed usually increases during each trimester of pregnancy.

  Insulin pumps, providing continuous subcutaneous insulin infusion, are not as widely used during pregnancy as it was thought they might be when they were first introduced. These pumps are effective in improving glucose control, but the woman must be guarded against recurrent hypoglycemia and the possibility of the pump becoming dislodged. With experience, these problems are lessened. However, conventional insulin administration seems to produce similar glucose outcomes (Sheldon 1988).

  Oral hypoglycemics are never used during pregnancy because they cross the placenta, may be teratogenic, and stimulate fetal insulin production (Hare 1989a).

- *Evaluation of fetal status.* Information about the well-being, maturation, and size of the fetus is important for planning the course of the pregnancy and the timing of birth. Because pregnancies complicated by diabetes are at increased risk of neural tube defects, maternal *serum α-fetoprotein (AFP)* screening is done during weeks 16 to 18 of gestation (see Chapter 20).

  Daily maternal evaluation of *fetal activity,* begun at about 28 weeks, is effective and simple to perform. The woman is taught a particular method for counting fetal movement (see Chapter 14), records the results on a special card, and brings the card to each subsequent office visit.

- *Nonstress testing* is usually begun weekly at about 28 weeks, increasing to twice a week at 32 weeks (Gabbe 1990). If evidence of intrauterine growth retardation (IUGR), PIH, oligohydramnios, or poorly controlled blood glucose exists, testing may begin as early as 26 weeks and may be done more often (Barss 1989b). If the woman requires hospitalization (for example, to control glycemia or for complications), nonstress testing may be done daily.

- *Ultrasound* at 18 weeks establishes gestational age and diagnoses multiple pregnancy or congenital anomalies. It is repeated at 28 weeks to monitor fetal growth for IUGR or macrosomia. Some agencies do *biophysical profiles* (ultrasound evaluation of fetal well-being in which fetal breathing movements; fetal activity, reactivity, and muscle tone; and amniotic fluid volume are assessed) as part of an ongoing evaluation of fetal status.

- *Contraction stress testing* is used primarily if there is a nonreactive nonstress test (NST) or if some variable decelerations are seen on the tracing (see Chapter 20).

Intrapartal Period During the intrapartal period, medical therapy includes the following:

- *Timing of birth.* In most diabetic pregnancies, pregnancy is allowed to go to term, with spontaneous labor, thereby decreasing the risk of respiratory distress in the neonate. In pregnancies in which there is evidence of fetal macrosomia, fetal compromise, or elevated maternal HbA_{1c}, amniocentesis is done for lecithin/sphingomyelin (L/S) ratio and the concentration of saturated phosphatidylcholine (SPC). Whereas levels of 2:1 ratio for the L/S ratio and >500 µg/dL of SPC indicate fetal lung maturity in the non-diabetic pregnancy, levels of up to 3.5:1 L/S ratio for the ratio and >1000 µg/dL of SPC have been found necessary at some centers before low risk of respiratory distress syndrome (RDS) is achieved (Barss 1989b). The presence of phosphatidylglycerol (PG) seems to enhance lecithin activity, and its presence is considered favorable for lung maturity. Fetal lung maturity must be weighed against other considerations when deciding time of childbirth.

- *Labor management.* The degree of prenatal maintenance of normal maternal glucose levels (euglycemia) and the maintenance of maternal euglycemia during labor are important in preventing neonatal hypoglycemia. Maternal insulin requirements often decrease dramatically during labor (Hare 1989b). Consequently, maternal glucose levels are measured hourly to determine insulin need. Often two intravenous lines are used, one with a 5% dextrose solution, and one with a saline solution. The saline solution is then available if a bolus is needed or for piggybacking insulin. Insulin clings to the plastic intravenous bag and tubing. To ensure that the woman receives the desired dose, the intravenous tubing must be flushed with insulin before the prescribed amount is added. During the second stage of labor and the immediate postpartum period, the woman may not need additional insulin. The intravenous insulin is discontinued with the completion of the third stage of labor.

Postpartal Period Postpartally maternal insulin requirements fall significantly. This occurs because the levels of hPL, progesterone, and estrogen fall after placental separation and their anti-insulin effect ceases, resulting in decreased blood glucose levels. The diabetic mother may require no insulin for the first 24 hours or only one-fourth to one-half her previous dose. Then reestablishment of insulin needs based on blood sugar testing is necessary. Diet and exercise levels must also be redetermined.

Diabetic control and the establishment of parent-child relationships in light of neonatal needs are the priorities of this period. If her newborn must be cared for in a special care nursery, the mother needs support and information about the baby's condition. Every effort must be made to provide as much contact as possible between the parents and their newborn.

Other components of postpartal care include:

- *Breast-feeding.* Breast-feeding is encouraged as beneficial to both mother and baby. The composition of breast milk is not altered by diabetes, and infants of mothers with diabetes gain weight appropriately. The lactating mother with diabetes often has a sense of well-being and diminished insulin needs even while increasing caloric intake (Lawrence 1989). Blood glucose levels may be lower because glucose is transferred from serum to breast to be converted to lactose, and energy is expended in milk production. Calorie needs increase during lactation to 500 to 800 kcal above prepregnant requirements. Insulin must be adjusted according to individual needs. Home blood glucose monitoring should continue for the insulin-dependent diabetic.

  Initial breast-feeding should take place soon after birth, as with all breast-feeding mothers. The mother and infant should not be separated if at all possible, as this interferes with the establishment of normal lactation. If the baby cannot nurse right away, the mother can be taught to express her milk, with a pump or manually, to prevent engorgement.

- *Contraception.* Barrier methods of contraception (diaphragm and condom) used with spermicide are safe, effective, and inexpensive. They are recommended for the client with diabetes (Barss 1989a). The use of oral contraceptives by diabetic women is controversial. There is some evidence that women with diabetes who take oral contraceptives have a higher risk of cardiovascular disease (Barss 1989a).

Many physicians only prescribe lower-dose pills to women with diabetes and they may restrict their use to women who have no vascular disease and who do not smoke. The progesterone-only pill has a higher failure rate but is otherwise safer. Elective sterilization is chosen by many couples who have completed their families.

❀ *APPLYING THE NURSING PROCESS* ❀

Nursing Assessment

Whether diabetes (usually type I) has been diagnosed before pregnancy occurs or the diagnosis is made during pregnancy (GDM), careful assessment of the disease process and the woman's understanding of diabetes is important. Thorough physical examination, including assessment for vascular complications of the disease, any signs of infectious conditions, and urine and blood testing for glucose, is essential on the first prenatal visit. Follow-up visits are usually scheduled twice a month during the first two trimesters and once a week during the last trimester.

Assessment is also needed to yield information about the woman's ability to cope with the combined stress of pregnancy and diabetes and her ability to follow a recommended regimen of care. Determination of the woman's knowledge about diabetes and self-care is needed before formulating a teaching plan.

Nursing Diagnosis

Nursing diagnoses that may apply are listed in Key Nursing Diagnoses to Consider: Diabetes Mellitus in the nursing care plan beginning on p 460.

Dx

Key Nursing Diagnoses to Consider
Diabetes Mellitus

Activity intolerance: High risk
Ineffective family coping
Ineffective individual coping
Altered family processes
Injury: High risk
Knowledge deficit
Noncompliance
Altered nutrition: Less than body requirements
Altered nutrition: More than body requirements
Altered parenting: High risk
Body image disturbance
Self-esteem disturbance
Altered tissue perfusion
Defensive coping
Ineffective denial
Skin integrity, Impaired: High risk

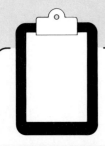

Nursing Care Plan
Diabetes Mellitus

Nursing History

1. Complete assessment: client and family
2. Identification of client's predisposition to diabetes
   a. Recurrent PIH
   b. Previous LGA infants ($\geq$ 4000 g)
   c. Hydramnios
   d. Unexplained fetal death
   e. Obesity
   f. Family history of diabetes

Physical Examination

1. Length of gestation
2. Complaints of thirst and hunger
3. Recurrent monilial vaginitis or urinary tract infection (UTI)
4. Frequent urination beyond first trimester and prior to third trimester
5. Fundal height greater than expected for gestation
6. Obesity
7. Funduscopic examination to detect any vascular changes

Diagnostic Studies

1. Fasting plasma glucose (FPG)
2. 3-hour GTT
3. Urine test for glucose, ketones
4. Ultrasound to evaluate fetal growth and detect hydramnios
5. If woman has IDDM, glycosylated hemoglobin level (HbA_{1c}) determined
6. Serum fructosamine screening is now used in some centers
7. Maternal serum α-fetoprotein (AFP) screen

Third Trimester—Fetal Assessment

1. Serial NSTs
2. CST as necessary
3. Serial ultrasound
4. Biophysical profile to determine fetal maturity
5. Amniocentesis and L/S ratio as necessary

Nursing Diagnosis	Nursing Interventions	Rationale	Evaluation
Altered nutrition: High risk for more than body requirements related to imbalance between intake and available insulin.	Discuss importance of strict dietary control. Work with nutritionist and client to plan an individualized diet.	Dietary management is designed to ensure optimum fetal growth and normalize blood glucose levels. The greatest success occurs when a dietary plan is individualized to meet client needs and preferences.	Woman understands her prescribed diet, follows it carefully, and gains the optimum amount of weight for her prepregnant size.
Client Goal: The woman will understand and follow her prescribed diet as evidenced by weight gain within desired range, ability to discuss diet and plan menus, glycosylated hemoglobin (HbA_{1c}) levels in normal range.	Recommended intake 30–35% kcal/kg body wt 12–20% protein 50–60% carbohydrate 20–30% fat Sodium intake may be restricted somewhat.	Recommended intake is designed to permit the following weight gain (Kitzmiller 1988): underweight 30+ lb desirable wt 24–30 lb overweight 20–24 lb very overweight 15–20 lb	

(continued)

Nursing Care Plan (continued)

Nursing Diagnosis	Nursing Interventions	Rationale	Evaluation
Injury: High risk related to possible complications secondary to hypoglycemia or hyperglycemia	Determine insulin needs: 1. Check lab results of FPG and 2-hour postprandial. 2. Test blood four times daily using Dextrostix.	Sufficient insulin must be present to enable proper carbohydrate metabolism to take place; pregnancy requires a marked increase in circulating insulin to maintain normal blood glucose.	Woman avoids episodes of hyperglycemia or hypoglycemia, or, if they occur, they are detected early and treated successfully. Insulin requirements become stabilized.
Client Goal: Woman will avoid injury associated with hypoglycemia or hyperglycemia as evidenced by absence of signs or symptoms, blood glucose readings in normal range, and stabilization of insulin requirements.	Teach use of home blood glucose monitoring device; determine amount of insulin based on sliding scale. Administer regular or NPH insulin, or combination, as ordered.	Fasting glucose level tends to be lower than nonpregnant value. Effectiveness of insulin may be reduced by presence of hPL.	
	Teach early signs of hypoglycemia, including sweating, periodic tingling, disorientation, shakiness, pallor, clammy skin, irritability, hunger, headache, blurred vision, and, if untreated, coma or convulsions.	Insulin requirements fluctuate widely during pregnancy because of factors mentioned in text and because of lowered glucose tolerance, especially in second half of pregnancy, and fluctuate during intrapartal period because of depletion of glycogen stores during labor; fluctuations during puerperium are a result of involuntary process; in addition, conversion of blood glucose into lactose during lactation may cause marked changes in glucose tolerance and/or hypoglycemia. Client needs to understand appropriate interventions because self-care at home in the event of hypoglycemia may save her life. Rapid treatment of hypoglycemia is essential to prevent brain damage because the brain requires glucose to function (skeletal and heart muscles can derive energy from ketones and free fatty acids).	

(continued)

Nursing Care Plan (continued)

Nursing Diagnosis	Nursing Interventions	Rationale	Evaluation
	Treat within minutes of onset		
	a. Obtain immediate blood glucose level. If < 60 mg/dL, have client drink 8 oz milk (some agencies prefer to use ½ glass orange juice) and notify physician.	Provides baseline information on glucose levels. Liquids are absorbed from the GI tract faster than solids.	
	b. If woman is not alert enough to swallow give 1 mg glucagon subcutaneously or intramuscularly; notify physician.	Glucagon triggers the conversion of glycogen stored in the liver to glucose.	
	c. If woman is in labor with intravenous lines in place, 10–20 mL of 50% dextrose may be given IV. Standing order should be available; notify physician.		
	Teach woman early signs of hyperglycemia and treatment.	Woman can recognize signs and administer self-treatment. Woman can also report any symptoms that may occur.	
	Observe for signs of hyperglycemia such as polyuria, polydipsia, dry mouth, increased appetite, fatigue, nausea, hot flushed skin, rapid deep breathing, abdominal cramps, acetone breath, headache, drowsiness, depressed reflexes, oliguria or anuria, stupor, coma.		
	Administer treatment; notify physician.	Administer insulin to restore body's normal metabolism of carbohydrate, protein, and fat.	
	a. Obtain frequent measurement of blood glucose; measure urine acetone.	Need to establish a baseline and to determine additional insulin dosage and prevent overtreatment; urine acetone indicates development of ketoacidosis.	
	b. Administer prescribed amount regular insulin subcutaneously or intravenously, or combination of routes.	Regular insulin is used because it acts immediately and is of short duration.	

(continued)

Nursing Care Plan (continued)

Nursing Diagnosis	Nursing Interventions	Rationale	Evaluation
	c. Replace fluids IV, orally, or both.	Fluids are depleted in the process of ketoacidosis; hypotension can result from decreased blood volume due to dehydration.	
	d. Measure intake and output.	Polyuria is an early sign of hyperglycemia; oliguria develops with hypotension and decreased bloodflow to kidneys.	
	e. Observe for symptoms of circulatory collapse; monitor BP and pulse.	Circulatory collapse can result from hypotension.	
Injury: High risk related to signs of UTI secondary to glycosuria	Review preventive measures such as voiding frequently, voiding following intercourse, wiping from front to back, wearing cotton crotch underpants, drinking cranberry juice.	Preventive measures are designed to remove bacteria from the bladder, avoid contamination from the rectal area or outside sources, facilitate air flow in the perineal area, and acidify the urine.	Woman implements self-care measures to avoid UTI. If UTI develops, treatment is effective and complications are avoided.
Client Goal: Woman will be able to identify signs of developing UTI and appropriate self-care measures to help prevent UTI. If signs of UTI do develop, therapy will be effective in preventing injury from complications.	Teach signs of developing UTI, including urgency, frequency, dysuria, and hematuria; low back pain with kidney involvement. Obtain clean-catch urine for culture and sensitivity.	Incidence of UTI is increased in diabetes, possibly because the existence of glycosuria provides rich medium for bacterial growth.	
	Administer prescribed antibiotics.	Antibiotic prescribed is specific to causative organism.	
	Encourage fluids to 2000–3000 mL/day. Measure intake and output.	Increased fluid intake promotes urinary removal of organisms.	
Knowledge deficit related to the disease, its treatment, its implications for the woman, her unborn child, and the birth process	Provide teaching as indicated based on individualized assessment of couple's knowledge level: 1. Explain procedures. 2. Allow them to ask questions. 3. Develop a teaching plan to discuss and provide opportunities to practice administering insulin. Provide written information. Include partner so he can administer insulin if necessary.	Decreasing fear and increasing knowledge will make the client a more effective member of the antepartal-intrapartal health team. Anticipatory guidance helps the couple prepare for the upcoming experience.	Woman is able to discuss her condition and its implications, follows the recommendations of her care givers, and correctly carries out self-care activities related to her diabetes.
Client Goal: Woman and her partner will understand the diabetes and its possible implications for her pregnancy as evidenced by their ability to administer insulin, to identify signs of hypo- or hyperglycemia, to discuss basic information about birth and anticipated therapy measures.			

(continued)

Nursing Care Plan (continued)

Nursing Diagnosis	Nursing Interventions	Rationale	Evaluation
	4. Assess their level of knowledge of childbirth and use this to teach about what is happening. **5.** Provide information about possible changes to expect during labor and birth due to DM. Explain about IV insulin, continuous monitoring of fetal status. Stress unchanged aspects of the experience.		
Injury: High risk to fetus related to the effects of diabetes on uteroplacental functioning and fetal growth *Client Goal:* Woman will be able to discuss rationale for fetal monitoring and testing, and will cooperate with fetal testing and assessment schedule.	Explain purpose of all scheduled tests and procedures: **1.** Ultrasound as ordered to provide periodic assessment of fetal size. **2.** Fetal activity diary **3.** Serial NSTs **4.** CST if indicated. **5.** Measurement of L/S ratio and PG levels to determine fetal lung maturity. **6.** Biophysical profile	Compliance is increased when client understands purpose of tests. Information about fetal growth and activity helps care givers evaluate placental functioning, anticipate the need for cesarean birth, determine fetal maturity, and decide on best time for birth.	Woman cooperates with fetal testing schedule. Fetus responds well to tests and shows evidence of normal growth and placental functioning.
Altered family processes related to client's DM and the need for hospitalization. *Client Goal:* Family will deal successfully with the woman's illness, plan for changes necessary following discharge, and share their thoughts, feelings, and concerns with each other.	Encourage visits from family members and older siblings. Discuss with client and family changes that are necessary following discharge with regard to insulin, diet, exercise, and so forth. Assist family to make specific plans. Arrange for social services to visit or for homemaker assistance if necessary following discharge. Give the family members information about the frustration that can occur when a family member is ill. Provide opportunities for them to discuss their feelings. Offer suggestions for coping.	Illness in one family member impacts the entire family. Sometimes outside support is necessary to help the family deal with feelings and identify ways of dealing with the illness of a member.	Woman and family cope successfully with illness, make necessary plans for managing following discharge, and discuss their feelings in an open caring way.

	CONCEPTION 0	4 WEEKS 1	8 WEEKS 2	12 WEEKS 3	16 WEEKS 4

FETAL DEVELOPMENT

The sperm fertilizes the ovum, which then divides and burrows into the uterus.

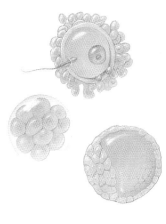

From the embryonic disk (ectoderm, entoderm, mesoderm), the first body segments appear that will eventually become the spine, brain, and spinal cord. Heart, blood circulation, and digestive tract take shape. Embryo is less than a quarter-inch long.

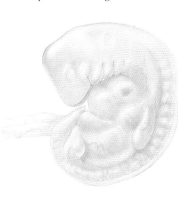

Development is rapid; heart begins to pump blood; limb buds are well developed. Facial features and major divisions of the brain are discernible. Ears develop from skin folds; tiny bones and muscles are formed beneath the thin skin.

Embryo becomes a fetus, its beating heart discernible by ultrasound. Assumes a more human shape as lower body develops. At week 12, first movements begin. Sex is determinable. Kidneys produce urine.

Musculoskeletal system has matured; nervous system begins to exert control. Blood vessels rapidly develop. Fetal hands can grasp; legs kick actively. All organs begin to mature and grow. Fetus weighs about 7 oz (½ lb). FHT discernible with Doppler. Pancreas produces insulin.

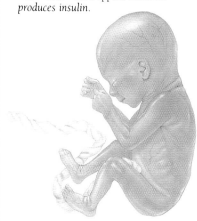

MATERNAL CHANGES

Mother misses first period; breasts become tender, may enlarge. Chronic fatigue and urinary frequency begin, may persist for three or more months. hCG in urine and serum 9 days after conception.

Morning sickness, may persist to 12 weeks. Uterus changes from pear to globular shape. Hegar's, Goodell's and Piskacek's signs appear. Cervix flexes; leukorrhea increases. Surprise and ambivalence about pregnancy may occur. No noticeable weight gain.

Chadwick's sign appears. Uterus rises above pelvic brim by 12 weeks. Braxton Hicks contractions may begin and continue throughout pregnancy. Potential for urinary tract infection (UTI) increases and exists throughout pregnancy. Weight gain of about 2½ to 4 lb during first trimester.

Placenta now fully functioning and producing hormones.

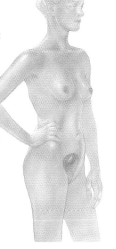

Fundus halfway between symphysis and umbilicus. Woman gains slightly less than 1 lb per wk for remainder of pregnancy. May feel more energetic. BPD measurement on ultrasound. Vaginal secretions increase. Itching, irritation, malodor suggest infection. Woman may begin wearing maternity clothes. Pressure on bladder lessens and urinary frequency decreases.

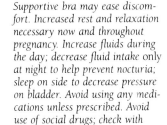

CLIENT TEACHING/ ANTICIPATORY GUIDANCE

Supportive bra may ease discomfort. Increased rest and relaxation necessary now and throughout pregnancy. Increase fluids during the day; decrease fluid intake only at night to help prevent nocturia; sleep on side to decrease pressure on bladder. Avoid using any medications unless prescribed. Avoid use of social drugs; check with caregiver before using any OTC preparations.

Eat dry crackers before arising; try frequent small, dry, low-fat meals with fluids taken between meals. Avoid use of hot tubs, saunas, and steam rooms throughout pregnancy.

Discuss attitudes toward pregnancy. Discuss value of early pregnancy classes that focus on what to expect during pregnancy. Provide information about childbirth preparation classes.

Adequate fluid intake and frequent voiding (every 2 hr while awake) help prevent UTI. Also helpful to void following intercourse. Wipe from front to rear.

Discuss nutrition and appropriate weight gain. Stress value of regular physical exercise, especially nonweightbearing activities or walking. Discuss possible effects of pregnancy on sexual relationship.

Daily shower or bath and thorough drying of vulva helpful; avoid douching during pregnancy. Consult caregiver if infection suspected; use only prescribed medications.

Review danger signs of pregnancy. Discuss infant feeding options; provide information on the value of breastfeeding. Provide information about clothing, shoes.

...ernix protects the body; fine hair (lanugo) covers the body and keeps the ...il on the skin. Eyebrows, eyelashes, ...nd head hair develop. Fetus develops ...a regular schedule of sleeping, sucking ...nd kicking.

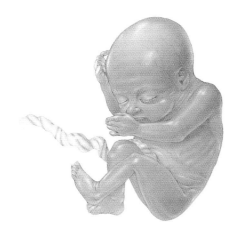

Skeleton develops rapidly as bone-forming cells increase activity. Respiratory movements begin. Fetus weighs about 1 lb, 10 oz.

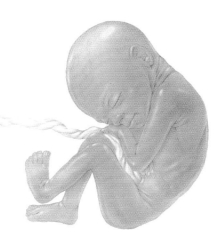

Fetus can breathe, swallow, regulate temperature. Surfactant forms in lungs. Eyes begin to open and close. Baby is ⅔ the size it will be at birth.

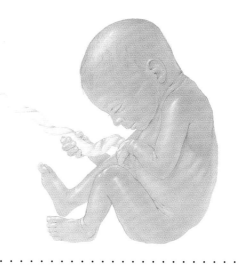

Brown fat deposits are developing beneath the skin to insulate the baby following birth. Baby has grown to about 15–17 in. Begins storing iron, calcium, and phosphorus.

The entire uterus is occupied by the baby, thus restricting its activity. Maternal antibodies are transferred to the baby. This provides immunity for about 6 months until the infant's own immune system can take over.

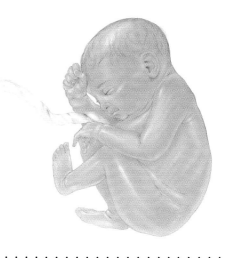

...undus reaches level ...f umbilicus. Breasts ...egin secreting co-...strum. Amniotic ...ac holds about ...00mL fluid. ...aintness and diz-...ness may occur, ...specially with sud-...en position changes. ...aricose veins may ...egin to develop. ...oman experiences ...tal movement, and ...regnancy may sud-...enly seem more ...eal." Areola ...arken. Nasal stuff-...ess may develop. ...eg cramps may ...egin to occur. Con-...ipation may ...evelop.

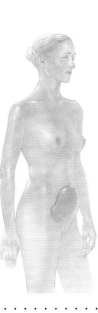

Fundus above umbilicus. Backache and leg cramps may begin. Skin changes can include striae gravidarum, chloasma, linea negra, acne, redness on palms of hands and soles of feet. Nosebleeds can occur. May experience abdominal itching as uterus enlarges; will continue until end of pregnancy.

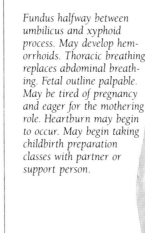

Fundus halfway between umbilicus and xyphoid process. May develop hemorrhoids. Thoracic breathing replaces abdominal breathing. Fetal outline palpable. May be tired of pregnancy and eager for the mothering role. Heartburn may begin to occur. May begin taking childbirth preparation classes with partner or support person.

Fundus reaches xyphoid process; breasts full and tender. Urinary frequency may return. Swollen ankles and sleeping problems may develop. Dyspnea may develop.

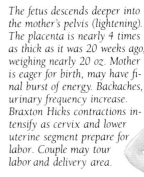

The fetus descends deeper into the mother's pelvis (lightening). The placenta is nearly 4 times as thick as it was 20 weeks ago, weighing nearly 20 oz. Mother is eager for birth, may have final burst of energy. Backaches, urinary frequency increase. Braxton Hicks contractions intensify as cervix and lower uterine segment prepare for labor. Couple may tour labor and delivery area.

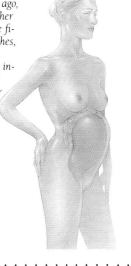

...t with feet elevated when possible; ...se slowly and carefully. Avoid pres-...re on lower thighs. Support stockings ...ay be helpful. Cool-air vaporizer ...ay help. Eat foods containing fiber, ...ch as raw fruits, vegetables, cereals ...ith bran; drink liquids and exercise ...equently.

...iscuss breast care. Discuss dorsiflex-...n of foot to relieve cramps; heat to ...fected muscle.

Assure woman that skin changes generally subside soon after birth. Discuss specific exercises such as pelvic tilt to help strengthen back and abdominal muscles, and stress importance of good body mechanics. Reiterate importance of avoiding medications, caffeine, alcohol and smoking.

Woman may choose to apply petroleum jelly in nostrils to relieve nosebleeds. Cool vaporizer may also help. Lanolin-based cream can relieve itching. Mild soap can remove excess oil associated with acne.

Avoid constipation; use sitz baths, gentle reinsertion of hemorrhoids with a fingertip as necessary. Topical anesthetic agents may offer relief of hemorrhoids. Stool softeners may be prescribed by caregiver. Elevate legs and assume sidelying position when resting. Eat small, more frequent meals; avoid fatty foods, lying down after eating. Maalox or mylanta may be helpful; Avoid sodium bicarbonate. Discuss expectations about labor and delivery, caring for an infant.

Wear well-fitting supportive bra. Elevate legs once or twice daily for an hour or so. Sleep on left side if possible. Use naturally occurring diuretics such as 2 tbsp lemon juice in 1 cup water or a generous serving of watermelon if available. Avoid most diuretics unless specifically prescribed. Maintain proper posture; use extra pillows at night for severe dyspnea. Following culture and personal preference, may begin preparing nursery now.

Review signs of labor. Discuss plans for other children (if any), transportation to agency.

Continue pelvic tilt exercises. Wear low-heeled shoes or flats. Avoid heavy lifting. Sleep on side to relieve bladder pressure. Urinate frequently. Avoid all analgesics except acetaminophen. Pack suitcase for delivery.

Discuss postpartum period including decisions such as circumcision, rooming-in. Discuss common postpartum discomforts; mention postpartum blues. Discuss family planning methods, infant care. Stress need for adequate rest postpartally. Provide support, especially if baby is overdue.

© 1987 Addison-Wesley Publishing Company
Illustrations by Charles W. Hoffman, MA, AMI
Design by Rudy Zehntner, The Belmont Studio
From Olds et al., **Maternal-Newborn Nursing,** Third Edition

ADDISON-WESLEY PUBLISHING COMPANY
Health Sciences Division, Menlo Park, California
Reading, Massachusetts • Menlo Park, California • New York
Don Mills, Ontario • Wokingham, England • Amsterdam • Bonn
Sydney • Singapore • Tokyo • Madrid • Bogota • Santiago • San Juan

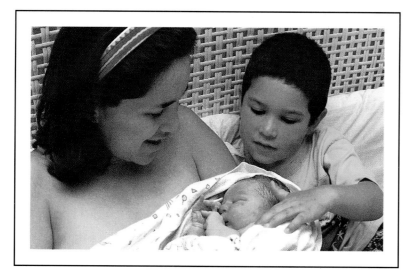

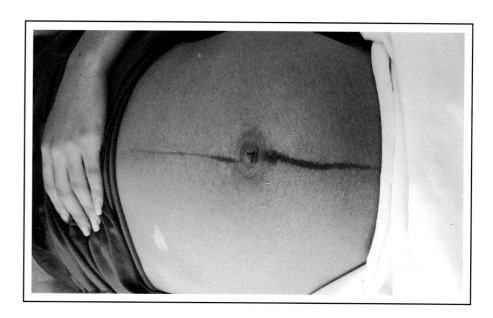

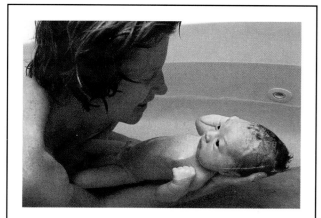

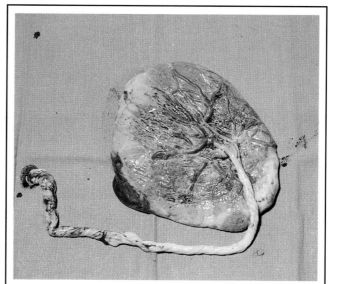

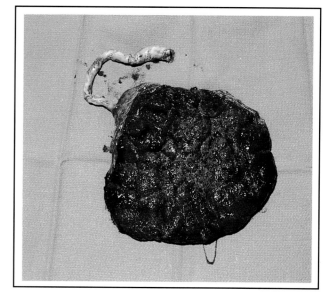

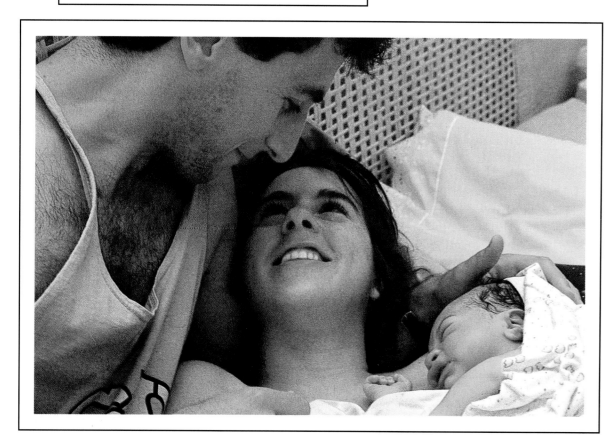

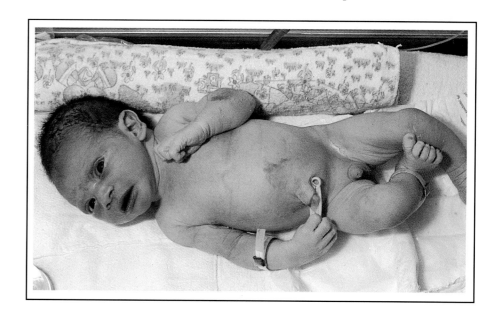

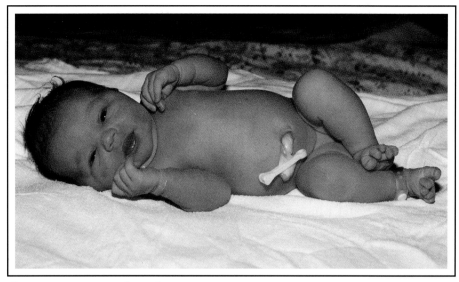

Plate VI   Normal newborn

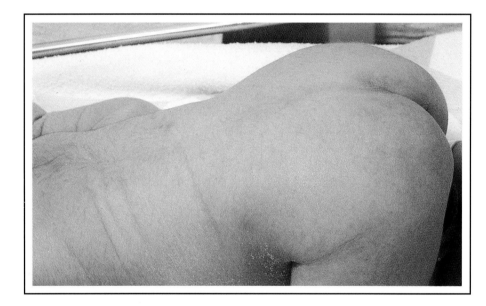

Plate VII   Mongolian spots

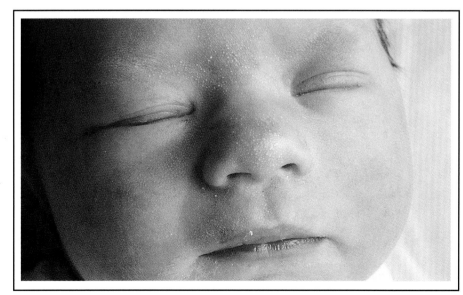

Plate VIII   Facial milia

Plate IX   Stork bites

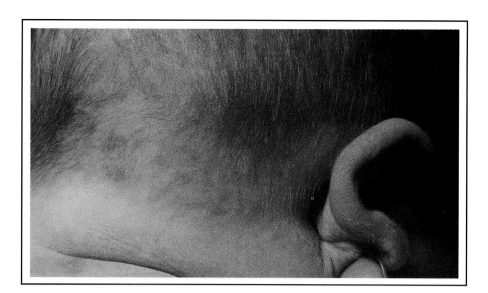

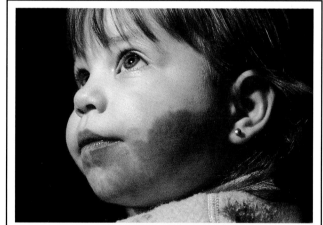

Plate X   Portwine stain

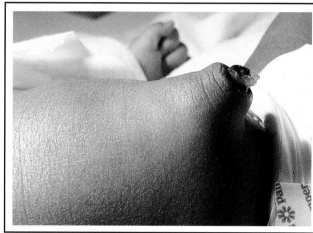

Plate XI   Umbilical hernia

Plate XII   Erythema toxicum

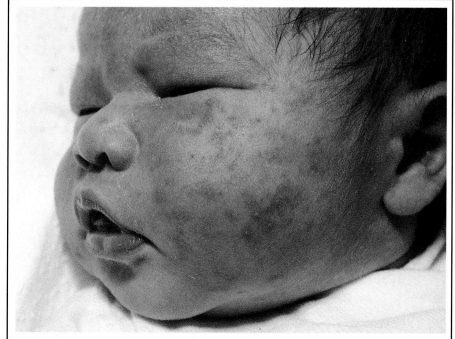

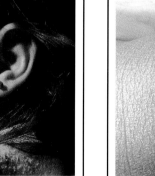

Nursing Plan and Implementation

Provision of Prepregnancy Counseling

This counseling may be provided by a nurse and a physician, using a team approach.

Ideally the couple is seen prior to pregnancy so that the diabetes can be assessed by ophthalmologic evaluation, electrocardiographic study, and a 24-hour urine collection for creatinine clearance and protein excretion. This will determine the woman's suitability for pregnancy (Gabbe 1985). If the diabetes is of recent onset without vascular complications, the outcome of pregnancy should be good if glucose levels can be controlled.

Promotion of Effective Home Blood Glucose Monitoring

The nurse-diabetes educator teaches the client how and when to monitor her blood sugar, the desired range of blood sugar levels, and the importance of good control (Figure 18–1). The woman may opt for either a visual method of blood testing or the use of a glucose meter. With either method the client is taught to follow the manufacturer's directions exactly, to wash hands thoroughly before puncture, and to touch the blood droplet, not her finger, to the test pad on the strip. With the visual method, she waits the prescribed time and then compares the color on the strip with a color chart provided on the strip bottle. The test strips must be stored as directed, and unused strips should be discarded after their expiration date.

If the client is using a blood glucose meter, an electronic eye measures the blood sugar and a digital reading is given. The blood droplet should cover the test pad, as uncovered portions are read as low sugar. The glucose meter is a portable pocket-sized device that is more accurate than the visual, color comparison method. Some meters are able to store and recall a specified number of readings.

The nurse may offer the client the following tips regarding finger puncture: (a) various spring-loaded devices are available that make puncturing easier; (b) hanging the arm down for thirty seconds increases blood flow to the fingers; and (c) the sides of fingers should be punctured instead of the ends because ends contain more pain-sensitive nerves.

Diabetic clients need to keep a record of each blood sugar reading as a guide for management. Specific record sheets are available for this purpose. The woman is instructed to bring the record sheet with her for each visit.

Promotion of Effective Insulin Use

The nurse ensures that the couple understands the purpose of the insulin, the types of insulin the woman is to use, and the correct procedure for its administration. The woman's partner is also instructed about insulin administration in case it should be necessary for him to give it.

For some highly motivated women whose glucose levels are not well controlled with multiple injections, the continuous insulin infusion pump may improve glucose control. A needle is secured in the subcutaneous tissue of the anterior abdominal wall and connected by cannula to a syringe filled with regular insulin. A pump that automatically resets to the basal infusion rate after giving the preprandial bolus is important for preventing problems of hypoglycemia. The woman needs to learn to use the insulin pump and become confident in coordinating the dosages with her glucose readings to achieve euglycemia. The nurse-diabetes educator works with her to achieve these goals.

Promotion of a Planned Exercise Program

Exercise is encouraged for the woman's overall well-being. If she is used to a regular exercise program she is encouraged to continue. She is advised to exercise after meals when blood sugar levels are high, to wear diabetic identification, to carry a simple sugar such as hard candy, to monitor her blood glucose levels regularly, and to avoid injecting insulin into an extremity that will soon be used during exercise.

If she has not been following a regular exercise plan she is encouraged to begin gradually. Due to alterations in metabolism with exercise, the woman's blood glucose should be well controlled before she begins an exercise program.

Education for Self-Care

Using the information gained during the nursing assessment of the pregnant woman with diabetes, the nurse provides appropriate teaching to the woman and her family so

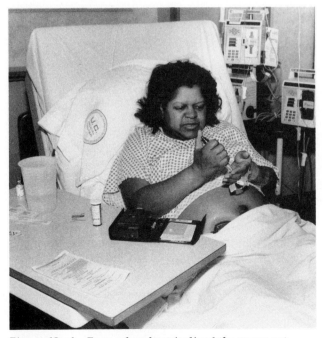

Figure 18–1 Even when hospitalized the pregnant woman with diabetes mellitus can do glucose monitoring.

Table 18–3 Comparison of Hypoglycemia and Hyperglycemia

	Hypoglycemia	Hyperglycemia
Causes	Too much insulin Too little food Increased exercise without increased food	Too little insulin Too much food (especially carbohydrate) Emotional stress Infection
Onset	Usually sudden (minutes to half-hour)	Slow (days)
Symptoms in general order of appearance	Nervousness Shakiness Weakness Hunger Sweatiness Cool clammy skin Pallor Blurred or double vision Headache Disorientation Shallow respirations Irritability Convulsions Coma	Polyuria Polydipsia Dry mouth Increased appetite Tiredness Nausea Hot flushed skin Abdominal cramps Abdominal rigidity Rapid deep breathing Acetone breath Paralysis Headache Soft eyeballs Drowsiness Oliguria or anuria Depressed reflexes Stupor Coma
Laboratory findings: Urine	Glucose—negative Acetone—usually negative	Glucose—positive Acetone—positive
Blood	Glucose—60 mg/dL or lower Acetone—negative	Glucose—±250 mg/dL Acetone—usually positive

Treatment: See Nursing Care Plan for Diabetes Mellitus

Other comas: Hyperosmolar coma is most often seen in persons over 60 years of age with type II diabetes. Lactic acidosis coma occurs in advanced stages of diabetes, especially in persons with uremia, arteriosclerotic heart disease, pneumonia, acute pancreatitis, chronic alcoholism, and bacterial infection.

Adapted from Guthrie DW, Guthrie RA: Nursing Management of Diabetes Mellitus, *2nd ed. St. Louis: Mosby, 1982. Used with permission.*

that the woman can meet her own health care needs as much as possible.

- *Symptoms of hypoglycemia and ketoacidosis.* The pregnant woman with diabetes must recognize symptoms of changing glucose levels (Table 18–3) and take appropriate action by immediately checking her capillary blood glucose level. If it is less than 60 mg/dL she is advised to drink 8 oz of milk and recheck in 15 minutes. Milk is used when possible to avoid a rebound hyperglycemia (Kitzmiller 1988). The woman should carry a snack at all times and should have other fast sources of glucose (simple carbohydrates) at hand so that she can treat an insulin reaction when milk is not available. Family members are also taught how to inject glucagon in the event that food does not work or is not feasible, for instance, in the presence of severe morning sickness.

- *Smoking.* Smoking has harmful effects on both the maternal vascular system and the developing fe-

tus and is contraindicated for both pregnancy and diabetes.

- *Travel.* Insulin can be kept at room temperature while traveling. Insulin supplies should be kept with the traveler and not packed in the baggage. Special meals can be arranged by notifying most airlines a few days before departure. A diabetic identification bracelet or necklace should be worn. In addition, the woman should check with her physician for any instructions or advice before leaving.

- *Hospitalization.* Hospitalization may become necessary during the pregnancy to evaluate blood glucose levels and adjust insulin dosages.

- *Support groups.* Many communities have diabetes support groups or education classes, which can be most helpful to women with newly diagnosed diabetes.

- *Cesarean birth.* Chances for a cesarean birth are increased if the pregnant woman is diabetic. This possibility should be anticipated—enrollment in cesarean birth preparation classes may be suggested. Many hospitals offer classes, and information is available through organizations such as Cesarean/ Support Education and Concern (C/Sec, Inc); Cesarean Birth Council; or the Cesarean Association for Research, Education, Support and Satisfaction in Birthing (Caress). The couple may prefer simply to discuss cesarean birth with the nurse and their obstetrician and read some books on the topic.

Evaluation

Anticipated outcomes of nursing care include the following:

- The woman clearly understands her condition and its possible impact on her pregnancy, labor and birth, and postpartal period.
- The woman cooperates and participates in developing a health care regimen to meet her needs and follows it throughout her pregnancy.
- The woman gives birth to a healthy newborn.
- The woman avoids developing hypoglycemia or hyperglycemia.
- The woman is able to care for her newborn.

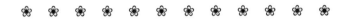

Care of the Woman with Anemia

Anemia indicates inadequate levels of hemoglobin (Hb) in the blood. During pregnancy, anemia exists if the hemoglobin is less than 10 g/dL or the hematocrit is less than 30% (Cruikshank 1990). The common anemias of pregnancy are due either to insufficient hemoglobin production related to nutritional deficiency in iron or folic acid during pregnancy, or to hemoglobin destruction in inherited disorders, specifically sickle-cell anemia and thalassemia.

Iron Deficiency Anemia

Dietary iron is needed to synthesize hemoglobin. Since hemoglobin is necessary for the transport of oxygen, a deficiency of iron leads to a decrease in hemoglobin and may affect the body's transport of oxygen.

Iron deficiency anemia is the most common medical complication of pregnancy. About 15% to 30% of Western women of childbearing age are iron deficient. Of pregnant women not taking iron supplements, 84% are iron deficient at term (Kelton & Cruickshank 1988). Approximately 200 mg of iron will be conserved due to the functional amenorrhea of pregnancy, but a pregnant woman needs approximately 1000 mg more iron intake during the pregnancy. Between 300 and 400 mg of iron is transferred to the fetus; 500 mg is needed for the increased red blood cell

mass in the woman's own increased circulating blood volume; another 100 mg is needed for the placenta; and about 280 mg is needed to replace the 1 mg of iron lost daily through feces, urine, and sweat.

The greatest need for increased iron intake is in the second half of pregnancy. When the iron needs of pregnancy are not met, maternal hemoglobin falls below 11 g/dL. Serum ferritin levels, indicating iron stores, are below 12 μg/L.

Many women begin pregnancy in a slightly anemic state. In pregnancy mild anemia can rapidly become more severe; therefore, it needs immediate treatment.

Maternal Risks

The woman with iron deficiency anemia may be asymptomatic, but she is more susceptible to infection, may tire easily, has an increased chance of PIH and postpartal hemorrhage, and tolerates poorly even minimal blood loss during birth. Healing of an episiotomy or an incision may be delayed. If the anemia is severe (Hb less than 6 g/dL), cardiac failure may ensue.

Fetal-Neonatal Risks

There is evidence of increased risk of low birth weight, prematurity, stillbirth, and neonatal death in infants of women with severe iron deficiency (maternal Hb less than 6 g/dL) (Bhargava M et al 1989; Dallman 1989). The infant is not iron deficient at birth due to active transport of iron across the placenta, even when maternal iron stores are low. However, these babies do have lower iron stores and are at increased risk for developing iron deficiency during infancy (Bhargava M et al 1989; Kelton & Cruickshank 1988).

Medical Therapy

The first goal of health care is to prevent iron deficiency anemia. If it occurs, the goal is to return low iron and hemoglobin levels to normal.

Iron supplements are essential during pregnancy because dietary sources cannot meet the extra requirements. Oral doses of ferrous salt such as ferrous sulfate 300 mg (60 mg of elemental iron) are taken daily to prevent anemia. The dose is increased to three times daily to treat deficiency and restore hemoglobin to 12 g/dL. With a twin pregnancy a larger dose is needed. If a large dose of oral iron causes vomiting, diarrhea, or constipation, or if the anemia is discovered late in pregnancy, parenteral iron may be needed.

❀ *APPLYING THE NURSING PROCESS* ❀

Nursing Assessment

The main presenting symptom of iron deficiency anemia may be fatigue. Nutritional history usually gives evidence of poor dietary intake of iron. Physical examination reveals pallor of skin and conjunctiva. Laboratory studies show Hb values below 11 mg/dL, serum ferritin levels below 12 μ/L, and possibly microcytic and hypochromic red blood cells (a late finding).

Nursing Diagnosis

Nursing diagnoses that might apply to a pregnant woman with iron deficiency anemia include the following:

- Altered nutrition: less than body requirements related to inadequate intake of iron-containing foods
- Constipation related to daily intake of iron supplements

Nursing Plan and Implementation

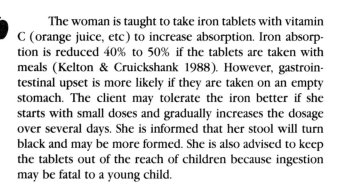

CRITICAL THINKING

In addition to iron supplements, what other sources of iron can the nurse recommend to a woman with iron deficiency anemia?

The woman is taught to take iron tablets with vitamin C (orange juice, etc) to increase absorption. Iron absorption is reduced 40% to 50% if the tablets are taken with meals (Kelton & Cruickshank 1988). However, gastrointestinal upset is more likely if they are taken on an empty stomach. The client may tolerate the iron better if she starts with small doses and gradually increases the dosage over several days. She is informed that her stool will turn black and may be more formed. She is also advised to keep the tablets out of the reach of children because ingestion may be fatal to a young child.

Evaluation

Anticipated outcomes of nursing care include the following:

- The woman is able to identify the risks associated with iron deficiency anemia during pregnancy.
- The woman takes her iron supplements as recommended.
- The woman's hemoglobin levels remain normal or return to normal levels during her pregnancy.

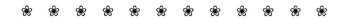

Folic Acid Deficiency Anemia

Folate deficiency is the most common cause of megaloblastic anemia during pregnancy, affecting between 1% and 4% of pregnant women in the United States. It is more prevalent with twin pregnancies.

Folic acid is needed for DNA and RNA synthesis and cell duplication. In its absence, immature red blood cells fail to divide, become enlarged (megaloblastic), and are fewer in number. With the tremendous cell multiplication

that occurs in pregnancy an adequate amount of folic acid is crucial. However, increased urinary excretion of folic acid and fetal uptake can rapidly result in folic acid deficiency. It is usually diagnosed late in pregnancy or the early puerperium. Hemoglobin levels as low as 3 to 5 g/dL may be found.

Medical Therapy

Diagnosis of folic acid deficiency anemia may be difficult. Serum folate levels typically fall as pregnancy progresses. Even though folate levels are lower with deficiency, they will fluctuate with diet. Measurement of erythrocyte folate status is more reliable but indicates folate status of several weeks previously (Fischbach 1988). Bone marrow biopsy is diagnostic but rarely used due to the discomfort it causes the woman.

Folic acid deficiency during pregnancy is prevented by a daily supplement of 0.4 mg of folate. Treatment of deficiency consists of 1 mg folic acid supplement. Iron deficiency anemia almost always coexists with folic acid deficiency, and therefore the woman would also need iron supplements.

Nursing Care

The nurse can help the pregnant woman avoid folate deficiency by teaching her food sources of folic acid and cooking methods for preserving folic acid. The best sources are fresh leafy green vegetables, red meats, fish, poultry, and legumes. As much as 50% to 90% of folic acid can be lost by cooking in large volumes of water. Microwave cooking destroys more folic acid than conventional cooking.

Sickle Cell Anemia

Sickle cell anemia is a recessive autosomal disorder in which hemoglobin A is abnormally formed. The anemia is characterized by acute, recurring, painful episodes. Individuals manifesting the disorder are homozygous for the sickle cell gene. They inherit from each parent an allele causing an amino acid substitution in the two beta protein chains in the hemoglobin molecule. This abnormal hemoglobin is called hemoglobin S (HbS). Heterozygous individuals are carriers for sickle cell anemia but are usually asymptomatic. This condition is called sickle cell trait. One of the beta protein chains formed in their hemoglobin is normal; the other has the amino acid substitution. This is called hemoglobin HbAS. Sickle cell trait is carried by 6% to 13% of black Americans, while approximately 0.2% have sickle cell anemia (Kelton & Cruickshank 1988).

Hemoglobin S causes the red blood cells to be sickle or crescent shaped. Whereas normal hemoglobin is in solution, in conditions of low oxygenation HbS becomes semisolid and distorts the red blood cell shape. These erythrocytes easily interlock and clog capillaries, particularly in organs characterized by slow flow and high oxygen extraction, such as the spleen, bone marrow, and placenta. This phenomenon is called *sickling,* and varies in frequency by the amount of the S hemoglobin in the red blood cells (there is seldom a crisis with levels below 40%) and other hemoglobin factors. Diagnosis is confirmed by hemoglobin electrophoresis or a test to induce sickling in a blood sample.

Maternal Risks

Women with sickle cell trait have a good prognosis for pregnancy if they have adequate nutrition and prenatal care. They are, however, at increased risk for nephritis, bacteriuria, and hematuria, and they tend to become anemic (Kelton & Cruickshank 1988).

Women with sickle cell anemia have considerably more risk during pregnancy. Low oxygen pressure—caused by high temperature, dehydration, infection, or acidosis, for example—may precipitate a vasoocclusive crisis. The crisis produces sudden attacks of pain that may be general or localized in bones or joints, lungs, abdominal organs, or the spinal cord. The pain is due to ischemia in the tissues from occluded capillaries. Vasoocclusive crises are more apt to occur in the second half of pregnancy.

The woman with sickle cell anemia has increased susceptibility to certain infections due to impaired immune functioning. Congestive heart failure or acute renal failure may also occur. The maternal mortality rate has been reduced to about 2% with improved antepartal care (Kelton & Cruickshank 1988).

Fetal-Neonatal Risks

The incidence of fetal death during and immediately following an attack has decreased greatly in recent years but is still high. Prematurity and intrauterine growth retardation (IUGR) are also associated with sickle cell anemia. Fetal loss is believed to be due to sickling attacks in the placenta.

Medical Therapy

Vasoocclusive crisis is best treated by a perinatal team in a medical center. Partial exchange transfusion of HbA (normal adult hemoglobin) for HbS red cells is most important. With erythrocytophoresis, the woman's blood is removed, the HbS is separated out, and the woman's plasma and other blood factors are returned to her through another vein. The crisis and pain subsides more quickly with this technique.

Rehydration with intravenous fluids, administration of antibiotics and analgesics, and fetal heart rate monitoring are also important aspects of therapy. Antiembolism stockings are used postpartally.

If vasoocclusive crisis occurs during labor the previous therapies are instituted. The woman is also given oxygen and kept in a left lateral position. Oxytocics may be used if needed. Episiotomy and outlet forceps are recommended to shorten the second stage.

Several antisickling agents are being extensively researched, and in the future sickle cell crisis may be prevented.

❀ *APPLYING THE NURSING PROCESS* ❀

Nursing Assessment

The woman with sickle cell anemia usually relates a history of frequent illnesses and recurrent abdominal and joint pains and is found to be extremely anemic. The woman may appear undernourished and have long, thin extremities. Ulcers are often present on ankles. Anemia may be severe.

A diagnosis of sickle cell anemia is confirmed by hemoglobin electrophoresis, or a test to induce sickling in a blood sample. The woman should be assessed for infection, which is associated with one-third of sickle cell crises in adults. Those most commonly seen during pregnancy or postpartum are pneumonia, urinary tract infections, puerperal endomyometritis, and osteomyelitis.

Fetal status is assessed during a crisis by electronic fetal monitoring. During labor the woman's vital signs and the FHR are assessed frequently. Compatible blood should be available for transfusion. Oxygen is administered if necessary. The woman is assessed for joint pains and other signs of sickle cell crisis.

Nursing Diagnosis

Nursing diagnoses that might apply to the pregnant woman with sickle cell anemia include the following:

- Acute pain related to the effects of a sickle cell crisis
- Knowledge deficit related to the need to avoid exposure to infection secondary to the risk of a sickle cell crisis

Nursing Plan and Implementation

Education for Self-Care

The nursing goal when working with a pregnant woman with sickle cell disease is to provide effective health teaching to help prevent a sickle cell attack (crisis), improve the anemia, and prevent infection. The woman is taught to increase hydration, use good hygiene practices, avoid people with infections, seek immediate treatment for infection, and take folic acid supplements. Folic acid is important because of its role in red blood cell production. The woman with sickle cell anemia maintains her hemoglobin levels by intense erythropoiesis and thus requires folic acid supplements. Bed rest is sometimes recommended to decrease the chance of preterm labor. Other nursing interventions are aimed at facilitating the medical therapy and alleviating anxiety through support and education.

Genetic counseling is recommended when both parents have the disease or are known carriers.

Evaluation

Anticipated outcomes of nursing care include the following:

- The woman is able to describe her condition and identify its possible impact on her pregnancy, labor and childbirth, and postpartal period.

- The woman takes appropriate health care measures to avoid a sickle cell crisis.

- The woman gives birth to a healthy infant.

- The woman and her care givers quickly identify and successfully manage any complications that arise.

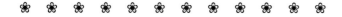

Thalassemia

The thalassemias are a group of autosomal recessive disorders characterized by a defect in the synthesis of the α or β chains in the hemoglobin molecule. The one most frequently encountered in the United States is β-thalassemia. Symptoms are caused by the shortened life span of the red blood cells resulting in active erythropoiesis in the liver, spleen, and bones. This produces hepatosplenomegaly and sometimes bony malformations. The thalassemias are seen most often in persons from Greece, Italy, or southern China and are also known as Mediterranean anemia and Cooley's anemia.

If the woman is heterozygous for β-thalassemia, half of the β chains are formed normally. This is β-thalassemia minor or β-thalassemia trait. Mild anemia is usually the only symptom.

Persons born homozygous for the disease have β-thalassemia major, with severe anemia that appears several months after birth. Newborns have fetal hemoglobin (HbF), which does not have β chains; therefore, there is a delay in onset of the anemia. Once they start producing adult type hemoglobin (HbA), such infants are dependent on transfusions, from which they eventually develop iron overload. Iron chelation therapy must be instituted soon after chronic transfusions are begun (Earles 1986), since excess iron damages the liver and heart. Without chelation therapy these infants do not live past the second or third decade, and those who reach puberty are often amenorrheic and infertile (Kelton & Cruickshank 1988).

Maternal/Fetal-Neonatal Risks

The woman with β-thalassemia minor has mild anemia with small (microcytic) red cells. This mild anemia must be distinguished from iron deficiency anemia, because a woman with β-thalassemia minor should not receive iron therapy. The pregnancy is otherwise uncomplicated by the disease.

β-Thalassemia major increases the woman's risk for PIH and other complications. The risk of fetal loss and the incidence of low birth weight are also increased.

Medical Therapy

Women with thalassemia may need folic acid supplements. Those with thalassemia major may need transfusion and chelation therapy. They should avoid exposure to infections and seek treatment promptly if an infection develops. Amniocentesis to determine the presence of the disease in the fetus is offered to the woman.

Nursing Care

The woman with thalassemia needs to understand her disease, the possibility of transmitting it to her offspring, and the amniocentesis procedure. These clients have lived with thalassemia since childhood but may have questions regarding its effect on pregnancy outcome and their own prognosis.

Care of the Woman with Acquired Immunodeficiency Syndrome (AIDS)

Acquired immunodeficiency syndrome (AIDS), caused by the human immunodeficiency virus (HIV), is one of today's major health concerns. During 1989, for example, 35,238 cases (14.0 per 100,000 population) were reported. This number represents an increase of 9% with the highest rates of infection reported among blacks and Hispanics (MMWR 1990).

The human immunodeficiency virus enters the body through blood, blood products, and other bodily fluids such as semen, vaginal fluid, and urine. The virus is also found in tears and saliva, but the concentration of the virus in these fluids is so low that exposure to them is not considered to be a risk. HIV affects specific T cells, thereby decreasing the body's immune responses. The affected person thus becomes susceptible to opportunistic organisms such as cytomegalovirus, herpes simplex, herpes zoster, *Candida*, *Pneumocystis carinii*, and *Toxoplasma gondii*. Opportunistic infections are the most common cause of death from AIDS; Kaposi's sarcoma, a rare skin cancer, is less commonly the direct cause of death.

Individuals generally develop antibodies and test positive for HIV within 2 to 12 weeks after exposure, although some people will take up to six months to develop antibodies. These people, categorized as HIV-positive, are usually asymptomatic and may remain so for 5 to 7 years or more. **AIDS-related complex (ARC)** is an intermittent stage characterized by the onset of a specific group of symptoms such as fatigue, lymphadenopathy, weight loss, fever, night sweats, and so forth. AIDS is diagnosed when the individual develops a severe infection, usually Kaposi's

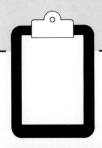

Nursing Care Plan
Care of the Woman with AIDS

Nursing History

1. Present pregnancy course
2. Estimated gestational age
3. Sensitivity to medications
4. History of infections

Physical Examination

1. Fetal size, fetal status (FHR), and fetal maturity
2. Observe for signs of fatigue and weakness, recurrent diarrhea, pallor, night sweats
3. Lymphadenopathy
4. Present weight and amount of weight gain or weight loss
5. Presence of nonproductive cough, fever, sore throat, chills, shortness of breath (*Pneumocystis carinii* pneumonia)
6. Dark purplish marks or lesions, especially on the lower extremities (Kaposi's sarcoma)
7. Oral, gingival lesions

Diagnostic Studies

1. Ultrasound
2. Fetal maturity studies (L/S ratio, PG, creatinine)
3. Hemoglobin and hematocrit
4. WBC
5. Testing for HIV-1 virus
6. T4 lymphocyte count (absolute T4)
7. ESR
8. Differential
9. Platelet count

Nursing Diagnosis	Nursing Interventions	Rationale	Evaluation
Altered nutrition: less than body requirements related to decrease appetite *Client Goal:* The woman will maintain current body weight or gain weight.	Weigh woman. Obtain food history. Plan high-protein, high-calorie diet. Provide teaching regarding nutritional needs.	Establishes baseline weight. Identifying food likes and dislikes will assist in meal planning. Diet must take woman's needs and pregnancy needs into account. Nutritional education and support may assist the woman in planning her daily diet.	The woman maintains current weight or gains weight.
Fear related to outcome of disease *Client Goal:* The woman will have opportunities to talk with nursing staff and other persons she identifies as supportive.	Establish rapport. Provide opportunities to talk without interruption. Provide support and counseling. Refer to community resources.	Establishment of rapport helps create a therapeutic relationship.	The woman has opportunities to talk with staff and contacts other sources of support.

(continued)

Nursing Care Plan (continued)

Nursing Diagnosis	Nursing Interventions	Rationale	Evaluation
Knowledge deficit related to appropriate precautions to prevent transmission of HIV infection *Client goal:* Woman will be able to identify necessary precautions to prevent spread of HIV infection.	Provide information on transmission of HIV and measures to prevent infection. Discuss household safety issues (acceptable to use same dishes, safe to sleep in same bed, safe to use same bathroom, can hold and hug children. Sexual abstinence is safest; if not latex condoms should be used. Avoid sharing razors, toothbrushes. Use 10% bleach solution to clean spills, disinfect bathroom. Use gloves to handle body fluids and so forth).	Information regarding the ways in which the HIV virus is spread is an important basis for medical asepsis. As the woman understands more about the disease, she will be able to take precautions to protect against the spread of the HIV virus.	The woman is able to identify appropriate actions to prevent transmission of HIV and implements the actions as identified.
	Discuss the implications of breast-feeding her infant.	Current information suggests that the virus may be spread in breast milk.	
Exchanging Infection: High risk related to suppressed immune status *Client Goal:* The woman will not develop infections during the hospital stay.	Monitor for signs of infection (fever, cough, sore throat, night sweats, etc).	Any pathogen may be able to establish itself in an immunosuppressed body. *Pneumocystis carinii* pneumonia is an infection frequently associated with AIDS.	The woman does not develop a superimposed infectious disease.
	Maintain universal precautions.	Universal precautions with body secretions are advised for all clients who are hospitalized. In this case, the nurse and others will be protected from exposure to the woman's body secretions. In addition, the woman needs to be protected from other infectious agents.	

sarcoma or *Pneumocystis carinii* pneumonia. AIDS dementia complex (ADC) is a disabling neurologic syndrome that develops in people with AIDS.

Currently the categorization ARC is being used less frequently. Some experts are using the label *HIV disease* to cover the gamut of the illness, others are favoring a six-category classification developed at Walter Reed Army Hospital.

Persons at highest risk for developing AIDS are homosexual or bisexual men, heterosexual partners of persons with AIDS, intravenous (IV) drug users, recipients of drug transfusions prior to 1985, hemophiliacs, and fetuses of mothers at risk or HIV positive. In the United States, the vast majority of pediatric AIDS cases have resulted from perinatal transmission from mother to child. Most infants and children who acquired HIV perinatally live in urban areas with a high incidence of drug abuse. In central and eastern Africa, on the other hand, 5% to 10% of women of childbearing age test positive for HIV (Pizzo 1990).

Today health care providers are emphasizing high-risk behaviors rather than high-risk groups. Even individuals in relatively "safe" groups may engage in risky behavior. High-risk behaviors include unprotected oral, anal, or vaginal intercourse, sharing IV drug needles that have not been bleached and rinsed, or any exchange of body fluids.

As the incidence of AIDS increases, a growing number of health care providers have begun questioning their ethical responsibilities with regard to clients who test HIV positive. Some physicians have refused to provide care to people with AIDS. The Committee on Ethics of the American College of Obstetricians and Gynecologists has formulated a position statement on physicians' responsibilities. It states " . . . it is unethical for an obstetrician-gynecologist to refuse to accept or continue to care for persons solely because they are or are thought to be seropositive for HIV. To avoid or delay treatment of a seropositive person is ethically equivalent to refusal of care" (Committee on Ethics 1990, p 1043).

Maternal Risks

Research suggests that the progress of clinical symptoms in HIV-positive, asymptomatic women may be accelerated by pregnancy, perhaps because of the immune alterations that occur during pregnancy (Landers & Sweet 1990).

Fetal-Neonatal Risks

While AIDS may develop in the infants of mothers who are seropositive, transmission does not always occur. Currently the risk to infants born to women with a positive HIV titer is estimated to be from 30% to 75%. Professionals estimate the actual rate of transmission from mother to child at about 40% to 50% (McMahon 1988). Often infants will have a positive antibody titer, which reflects the passive transfer of maternal antibodies. Infected infants are usually asymptomatic at birth. The infection may not be-

come evident until the child is 12 to 18 months old, although the median age for onset of symptoms is 9 months. Fifty percent of infants can be diagnosed by 12 months and 82% before the age of 3 years (Pizzo 1990). However, some children have been known to be asymptomatic for up to 10 years.

The signs of AIDS in infants may include failure to thrive, hepatosplenomegaly, interstitial lymphocytic pneumonia, recurrent infections, cell-mediated immunodeficiency, evidence of Epstein-Barr virus, and neurologic abnormalities. Recurrent bacterial infections are common in children with AIDS; Kaposi's sarcoma is rare. Encephalopathy, characterized by delayed developmental milestones or the loss of acquired skills including cognitive abilities, is found in 50% to 90% of children with AIDS (Pizzo 1990). These infants are also likely to be small-for-gestational-age (SGA) at birth.

Apparently infection can occur early in fetal development. Facial characteristics that may indicate that the infant has been infected with the AIDS virus include microcephaly; patulous lips; prominent, boxlike forehead; increased distance between the inner canthus of the eyes; a flattened nasal bridge; and a mild obliquity of the eyes. The mortality rate for these infants is especially high.

Medical Therapy

Currently there is no definitive treatment for AIDS although azidothymidine (AZT) has shown promise clinically. However, its safety during pregnancy is not known. The goal for antenatal care is identification of the pregnant woman at risk and education of the public about the transmission of AIDS to decrease its potential spread. Following recommended techniques to decrease nosocomial transmission of AIDS in a hospital setting can decrease the potential risk to health workers. It is very important to decrease exposure to contaminated blood and body fluids, which may harbor potential infectious agents, especially during labor and birth.

Women at risk for AIDS who are pregnant or planning a pregnancy should be offered HIV antibody testing. Testing is done using enzyme-linked immunosorbent assay (ELISA). The Western blot test is used to confirm the diagnosis with positive ELISA results. Women who test positive should be counseled about the implications of the diagnosis for themselves and their fetus, and they may be offered therapeutic abortion. A woman who continues her pregnancy needs excellent prenatal care with special attention to her psychosocial and teaching needs (Landers & Sweet 1990).

❀ *APPLYING THE NURSING PROCESS* ❀

Nursing Assessment

Based on the recommendations of the Centers for Disease Control, the following women should be screened for a positive HIV (MMWR, June 23, 1989):

- Women who have engaged in prostitution
- Women who have a history of sexually transmitted infection
- Women who use drugs intravenously
- Women whose current or previous sexual partners have been bisexual, abused intravenous drugs, have hemophilia, or test positive for HIV

A woman who already has AIDS may present with any of the following signs or symptoms: malaise, progressive weight loss, lymphadenopathy, diarrhea, fever, neurologic dysfunction, cell-mediated immunodeficiency, or evidence of Kaposi's sarcoma (purplish, reddish brown lesions either internally or externally).

Nursing Diagnosis

Examples of nursing diagnoses that might apply for a pregnant woman who tests HIV positive include the following:

- Knowledge deficit related to AIDS and its long-term implications for the woman and her unborn child
- Infection: High-risk related to altered immunity secondary to AIDS
- Ineffective family coping related to the implications of a positive HIV test in one of the family members

Nursing Plan and Implementation

Provision of Anticipatory Guidance

Nurses need to help women understand that AIDS is a fatal disease. The incidence of AIDS is increasing so significantly that if trends continue, it will soon be one of the five leading causes of death for women of childbearing age (Bishop 1990). AIDS can be avoided if women avoid sharing IV drug needles and practice safe sex, including insisting that their sex partners wear a latex condom for each act of intercourse.

Women at risk for AIDS should be offered premarital and prepregnancy screening for HIV antibodies (Kurth 1989). They should be given clear information about the implications of a diagnosis of HIV, including societal attitudes. Access to information about the disease and about the test results empowers women by enabling them to make informed decisions about their sexual activities and about becoming pregnant.

A detailed drug and sexual history of each prenatal client is the first step in perinatal AIDS prevention. Women at risk for AIDS should be offered HIV counseling. The following are counseling and education guidelines for HIV testing:

- HIV testing discussion should be incorporated into the normal prenatal assessment.
- The woman should be assured of confidentiality (the difference between anonymity and confidentiality should be explained).
- An educational environment that is private, comfortable, and nonjudgmental should be provided.
- The woman should be given information about AIDS, including pathophysiology, mode of transmission of HIV, high-risk behaviors, and methods of decreasing transmission, such as practicing safer sex and not sharing needles.
- If the woman chooses to have an antibody test for HIV (ELISA, Western Blot), written consent should be obtained.
- Posttest counseling should be provided. A negative test means that no HIV antibodies were found. It does not ensure that the woman has not been infected with the virus, since antibodies may not be detected for 6 weeks to 6 months after exposure (McMahon 1988).
- If test results are positive, supportive follow-up is necessary. This includes an explanation of the implications for the woman and her unborn child, recommended medical therapy, follow-up of sex partners, transmission prevention, discussion of immediate posttest plans, and referral to appropriate psychologic and educational services.

This information can be overwhelming to the woman who is HIV positive and should be provided orally and in writing. She will need more than one counseling session to absorb the information. The initial reaction may be one of shock or denial, so it is important to allow her a little time to think and to give her empathy and support. The nurse needs to stress that being HIV positive does not mean that the woman has AIDS but that she can transmit the virus to others by sexual contact, sharing IV drug needles, donating blood, and to her fetus during pregnancy. Most people do develop AIDS within 10 years, but it is impossible to predict who will develop the disease or how to prevent it from developing in a person who is HIV positive.

Monitoring the Asymptomatic Pregnant Woman

In monitoring the asymptomatic pregnant woman who is HIV positive, the nurse should be alert for nonspecific symptoms such as fever, weight loss, fatigue, persistent candidiasis, diarrhea, cough, skin lesions, and behavior changes. These may be signs of developing ARC. Laboratory findings such as decreased hemoglobin, hematocrit, and T4 lymphocytes; elevated erythrocyte sedimentation rate (ESR); and abnormal complete blood count, differential, and platelets may indicate complications such as infection or progression of the disease.

Education about optimal nutrition and maintenance

of wellness are important and should be reviewed frequently with the woman.

Reducing the Risk of Transmission

The nurse is faced with the important task of taking the precautions necessary to protect staff, other clients, and families from exposure to AIDS while meeting the needs of the childbearing woman with AIDS.

In 1987 the Centers for Disease Control (CDC) stated that the increasing prevalence of AIDS and the risk of exposure faced by health care workers is significant enough that *precautions should be taken with all clients* (not only those with known HIV infection), especially in dealing with blood and body fluids (MMWR Supplement 1987). These precautions are now called *universal precautions.*

Nurses who deal with childbearing families are exposed frequently to blood and body fluids and should pay careful attention to the CDC guidelines, including the following (Wiley & Grohar 1988):

1. Care givers should wear disposable latex gloves when having contact with a client's mucous membranes, nonintact skin, body fluids, or blood. Contact includes, for example, changing chux pads, peripads, diapers, or dressings; starting or discontinuing intravenous fluids; and drawing blood.

2. After giving care to a client, gloves should be removed and hands should be washed before caring for another client.

3. In addition to gloves, protective coverings such as a plastic apron, gown, mask, and eye or face shield should be worn during any procedures that frequently result in contamination from splashing of body fluids. These include amniotomy, vaginal examination, vaginal or cesarean birth, suctioning, and care of the newborn until after the initial bath has been done. (Note: full-size glasses are considered sufficient eye protection. While agencies are required to provide eye shields, nurses may choose to purchase their own eye goggles and clean them with soap and water.)

4. At birth, the newborn should be suctioned with a disposable bulb syringe or mucus extractor attached to wall suction at a low setting. DeLee mucus traps with mouth suction are not used because of the risk of inadvertently ingesting secretions.

5. Similar care should be taken during any resuscitation procedures. To avoid the need for mouth-to-mouth resuscitation, sufficient mouthpieces and ventilation equipment should be available. Disposable resuscitation masks are recommended.

6. Care should be taken when handling syringes and needles. They are disposed of in a special container. Needles are not broken, bent, or even returned to their protective cap because of the risk of an inadvertent puncture.

7. In the event that a glove is torn, it should be removed, the hands should be cleansed, and new gloves should be applied.

8. Gloves and protective coverings should also be worn during any cleaning procedures.

Provision of Emotional Support

The psychologic implications of AIDS for the childbearing family are staggering. The woman is faced with the knowledge that she and her newborn have decreased chances for survival. She may have feelings of fear, helplessness, anger, and isolation. If she shares her diagnosis with others, she may face rejection and condemnation. The couple must deal with the impact of the illness on the partner, who may or may not be infected, and on other children. Dealing with the tasks and responsibilities of a newborn may be especially difficult if the woman is physically depleted or if she is trying to come to grips with the long-term implications of her condition.

The nonjudgmental, supportive nurse plays an essential role in preserving confidentiality and the client's right to privacy. In addition, the nurse can help ensure that the woman receives complete, accurate information about her condition and ways she might cope. This usually involves a referral to social services for follow-up care. The hospitalized woman will often welcome the opportunity to talk with someone about her fears and desires.

Evaluation

Anticipated outcomes of nursing care include the following:

*   The woman is able to discuss the implications of her positive HIV antibody screen (or diagnosis of AIDS), its implications for her unborn child and for herself, the method of transmission, and treatment options.
*   The woman has information regarding social services (or other agency) referral for follow-up assistance and counseling.
*   The woman is able to begin to verbalize her feelings about her condition and its implications in an atmosphere she finds supportive.
*   The woman implements health-focused self-care practices.

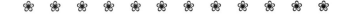

Care of the Woman Practicing Substance Abuse

Substance abuse occurs when an individual experiences difficulties with work, family, social relations, and health as a result of alcohol or drug use. Indiscriminate use of drugs during pregnancy, particularly in the first trimester, may adversely affect the health of the woman and the growth and

Research Note

Clinical Application of Research

Mothers who drink alcohol while they are pregnant may give birth to children with either fetal alcohol syndrome (FAS) or fetal alcohol effects (FAE). Children with FAS experience growth and central nervous system problems. Children with FAE may have maladaptive behaviors, learning disabilities, and other subtle social, learning, or emotional problems. Brenda Barbour (1990) designed a study which examined the drinking patterns of pregnant women and the awareness of these women about the association between adverse outcomes of pregnancy and less than excessive alcohol ingestion.

Results of the study showed that although a downward trend in the consumption of alcohol existed, 40% of the 20 women interviewed continued to drink. Factors that affected continued alcohol use encompassed prior habit, knowledge and beliefs about the impact of alcohol on the fetus, benefits from drinking versus risks, social pressures, and role of significant other. Additionally, 60% of the expectant mothers had been given information, either in writing or verbally during childbirth classes, that an occasional drink was not likely to be harmful.

Questions about the sources of information about alcohol revealed that the majority of the women obtained their information from reading. Only two stated that a health care provider initiated information about alcohol consumption and pregnancy.

Critical Thinking Applied to Research

Strengths: Excellent problem statement and development of significance of the problem to be studied.

Concerns: Although the author described the study as a qualitative study, it is not clear that the categories emerged from the data and that the researcher did not have preconceived ideas about the possible results.

Barbour B: Alcohol and pregnancy. *J Nurse-Midwifery* 1990; 35(2):78.

---

development of her fetus. Drugs that are commonly misused include alcohol, cocaine, crack, marijuana, amphetamines, barbiturates, hallucinogens, heroin, and other narcotics. Table 18–4 identifies common addictive drugs and their effects on the fetus and newborn. Abuse of these drugs poses a major threat to the successful completion of pregnancy.

The term *teratogen* is used to describe drugs that adversely affect fetal growth and development. Originally it was believed that the placenta acted as a protective barrier to keep the drugs ingested by the woman from reaching the fetal system. This is not true. The degree to which a drug is passed to the fetus depends on the drug's chemical properties, including molecular weight, and on whether it is administered alone or in combination with other drugs.

Drug use during pregnancy may be the most frequently missed diagnosis in all of maternity care. The reported incidence of drug use in pregnancy is related to the thoroughness of the prenatal assessments done by health care professionals (Chashoff & Griffith 1989). Unfortunately, substance abusers often wait until late in pregnancy to seek health care. Approximately 50% of addicted women receive no prenatal care (MacGregor & Keith 1989).

The substance abusing woman who seeks prenatal care may not voluntarily reveal her addiction, so care givers should be alert for a history or physical signs that suggest substance abuse (Table 18–5). Since substance abuse has increased rapidly in the past decade, it is helpful to discuss the specific substances that are abused to increase understanding of this serious problem.

Substances Commonly Abused During Pregnancy

Alcohol

Alcohol abuse has increased dramatically among women in the United States. The incidence is highest among women 20–40 years old; alcoholism is also seen in teenagers. Chronic abuse of alcohol can undermine maternal health by causing malnutrition (especially folic acid and thiamine deficiencies), bone marrow suppression, increased incidence of infections, and liver disease. As a result of alcohol dependence, the woman may have withdrawal seizures in the intrapartal period as early as 12–48 hours after she stops drinking. Delirium tremens may occur in the postpartal period, and the neonate may suffer a withdrawal syndrome.

The effects of alcohol on the fetus may result in a group of signs referred to as *fetal alcohol syndrome (FAS)*. The syndrome has characteristic physical and mental abnormalities that vary in severity and combination. (The abnormalities and the care of these infants are discussed in Chapter 31.)

There is no definitive answer to how much alcohol a woman can safely consume during pregnancy. The expectant woman should "play it safe" by avoiding alcohol completely during the early weeks of pregnancy when organogenesis is occurring. During the remainder of pregnancy, she may have an occasional drink, although none at all is safest.

The nursing staff in the maternity unit must be aware of the manifestations of alcohol abuse so that they can prepare for the client's special needs. The care regimen includes sedation to decrease irritability and tremors, seizure precautions, intravenous fluid therapy for hydration, and preparation for an addicted neonate. Although high doses of

Table 18–4 Possible Effects of Selected Drugs of Abuse/Addiction on Fetus and Neonate

Maternal drug	Effect on fetus/neonate
I. Depressants	
A. Alcohol	Cardiac anomalies, IUGR, potential teratogenic effects, FAS, FAE
B. Narcotics	
1. Heroin	Withdrawal symptoms, convulsions, death, IUGR, respiratory alkalosis, hyperbilirubinemia
2. Methadone	Fetal distress, meconium aspiration; with abrupt termination of the drug, severe withdrawal symptoms, neonatal death
C. Barbiturates	Neonatal depression, increased anomalies; teratogenic effect(?); withdrawal symptoms, convulsions, hyperactivity, hyperreflexia, vasomotor instability
1. Phenobarbital	Bleeding (with excessive doses)
D. "T's and Blues" (combination of the following)	
1. Talwin (narcotic)	Safe for use in pregnancy; depresses respiration if taken close to time of birth
2. Amytal (barbiturate)	See barbiturates
E. Tranquilizers	
1. Phenothiazine derivatives	Withdrawal, extrapyramidal dysfunction, delayed respiratory onset, hyperbilirubinemia, hypotonia or hyperactivity, decreased platelet count
2. Diazepam (Valium)	Hypotonia, hypothermia, low Apgar score, respiratory depression, poor sucking reflex, possible cleft lip
F. Antianxiety drugs	
1. Lithium	Congenital anomalies; lethargy and cyanosis in the newborn
II. Stimulants	
A. Amphetamines	
1. Amphetamine sulfate (Benzedrine)	Generalized arthritis, learning disabilities, poor motor coordination, transposition of the great vessels, cleft palate
2. Dextroamphetamine sulfate (dexedrine sulfate)	Congenital heart defects, hyperbilirubinemia
B. Cocaine	Learning disabilities, poor state organization, decreased interactive behavior, CNS anomalies, cardiac anomalies, genitourinary anomalies, SIDS
C. Caffeine (more than 600 mg/day)	Spontaneous abortion, IUGR, increased incidence of cleft palate; other anomalies suspected
D. Nicotine (half to one pack cigarettes/day)	Increased rate of spontaneous abortion, increased incidence placental abruption, SGA, small head circumference, decreased length, SIDS
III. Psychotropics	
A. PCP ("angel dust")	Flaccid appearance, poor head control, impaired neurologic development
B. LSD	Chromosomal breakage?
C. Marijuana	IUGR, potential impaired immunologic mechanisms

Table 18–5 Factors Associated with the Substance Abuser*

Appearance and Physical Signs

Pupils dilated or constricted
Marked fatigue or exhaustion
Abscesses, track marks, or edema of arms and legs
Inflamed nasal mucosa
Inappropriate or disoriented behavior

Medical History

HIV positive
Cirrhosis
Endocarditis
Sexually transmitted disease
Hepatitis
Pancreatitis
Pneumonia
Cellulitis

Maternity History (Previous Pregnancies)

Abruptio placentae
Low-birth-weight infant
Sudden infant death syndrome
Fetal death
Preterm birth
Spontaneous abortion

Current Pregnancy

Abruptio placentae
Sexually transmitted disease
Vaginal spotting or bleeding
IUGR
Low weight gain
Fetal bradycardia
Fetal hyperactivity

*Adapted from MacGregor SN, Keith LG: Substance abuse in pregnancy: A practical management plan. Female Patient January 1989; 14:49; Chashoff IJ: Perinatal effects of cocaine. Contemp OB/GYN 1987; 29:163.

sedatives and analgesics may be necessary for the woman, caution is advised because these can cause fetal depression.

Breast-feeding generally is not contraindicated, although alcohol is excreted in breast milk. Excessive alcohol consumption may intoxicate the infant and inhibit maternal let-down reflex. Discharge planning for the alcohol-addicted mother and newborn should be correlated with the social service department of the hospital.

Cocaine/Crack

Cocaine use is one of the most serious epidemics affecting the childbearing family. Approximately 1 in 10 pregnant women is believed to use cocaine, with even higher rates reported in urban areas (Lynch & McKeon 1990). Cocaine acts at the nerve terminals to prevent the reuptake of dopamine and norepinephrine, which in turn results in vasoconstriction, tachycardia, and hypertension. Placental vasoconstriction decreases blood flow to the fetus.

Cocaine is usually taken in three ways: snorting, smoking, and intravenous injection. **Crack** is a form of freebase cocaine that is made up of baking soda, water, and cocaine mixed into a paste and microwaved to form a rock. The rock can then be smoked. Many women, especially those in low-income areas, favor this form of the drug over other forms because it is readily available and cheaper. In addition, smoking crack leads to a quicker, more intense high because the drug is absorbed through the large surface area of the lungs (Modica 1990).

The onset of effects of cocaine occurs rapidly, but the euphoria lasts only about 30 minutes. This profound euphoria and excitement is usually followed by irritability, depression, pessimism, fatigue, and a strong desire for more cocaine. This pattern often leads the user to take repeated doses to sustain the effect. Cocaine metabolites may be present in the urine of a pregnant woman for up to 4 to 7 days following use.

The cocaine user is difficult to identify prenatally. Because cocaine is an illegal substance, many women are reluctant to volunteer information about their drug use. The nurse who is familiar with the woman may recognize subtle signs of cocaine use, including mood swings and appetite changes, and withdrawal symptoms such as depression, irritability, nausea, lack of motivation, and psychomotor changes.

Major adverse maternal effects of cocaine use include seizures and hallucinations, pulmonary edema, respiratory failure, and cardiac problems (Livesay 1989). Women who use cocaine have an increased incidence of spontaneous first-trimester abortion, abruptio placentae, IUGR, preterm birth, and stillbirth.

Exposure of the fetus to cocaine in utero increases the risk of IUGR, small head circumference, shorter body length, altered brain development, malformations of the genitourinary tract, and lower Apgar scores. Newborns who were exposed to cocaine in utero may have neurobehavioral disturbances, marked irritability, an exaggerated startle reflex, labile emotions, and an increased risk of sudden infant death syndrome (SIDS). These newborns have poor interactive behaviors, have difficulty responding appropriately to voices, and fail to respond well to consoling behaviors (Lynch & McKeon 1990). These complications may interfere with maternal-infant attachment and increase the infant's risk of abuse and neglect.

Cocaine does cross into the breast milk and may cause symptoms in the breast-feeding infant such as extreme irritability, vomiting, diarrhea, dilated pupils, and apnea. Thus, women who continue to use cocaine following childbirth should avoid nursing.

Marijuana

Approximately 15% of pregnant women use marijuana (Abel & Sokol 1988), often in conjunction with alcohol and tobacco. Men who smoke marijuana may have decreased sperm counts and may develop gynecomastia; women may experience menstrual cycle irregularities. To date, however, there is no evidence that marijuana has any teratogenic effects (Niebyl 1990). One study has reported an increase in precipitous labors (less than 3 hours) in heavy marijuana users (Fried 1989), but these results have not been confirmed. The impact of heavy marijuana use on pregnancy is difficult to evaluate because of the variety of social factors that may influence the results.

Infants exposed to marijuana in utero have been reported to have increased fine tremors, prolonged startles, irritability, and poor habituation to visual stimuli, but these symptoms were not present in follow-up at 12 and 24 months of age (Fried 1989).

Phencyclidine (PCP)

Phencyclidine (PCP) is a popular hallucinogen that can be smoked, taken orally, or injected intravenously. The onset of effects occurs in 2 to 4 minutes and lasts about 4 to 6 hours, with no withdrawal state. The drug causes confusion, delirium, and hallucinations and may produce feelings of euphoria. Signs of PCP use include constricted pupils, ataxia, nystagmus, double vision (diplopia), dizziness, and diaphoresis. The greatest risk for the pregnant woman is overdose or a psychotic response. Signs of overdose include hypertension, hyperthermia, diaphoresis, and possible coma, which may jeopardize fetal well-being.

PCP has been associated with facial abnormalities in the newborn (Cunningham et al 1989) and neurobehavioral problems including wild behavior states, flaccid appearance, and poor head control.

Heroin

Heroin is an illicit CNS depressant narcotic that alters perception and produces euphoria. It is an addictive drug that is generally administered intravenously, although a snortable form of heroin called Karachi is available. Pregnancy in women who use heroin is considered high-risk because of the increased incidence in these women of poor nutrition, iron deficiency anemia, and PIH. There is also an increased rate of breech position, abnormal placental implantation, abruptio placentae, preterm labor, premature rupture of the membranes (PROM), and meconium staining. These women also have a higher incidence of sexually transmitted infection because many rely on prostitution to support their drug habit.

The fetus of a heroin-addicted woman is at increased risk for IUGR, meconium aspiration, and hypoxia. The newborn frequently shows signs of heroin addiction such as restlessness; shrill, high-pitched cry; irritability; fist sucking; vomiting; and seizures. Signs of withdrawal usually appear within 72 hours and may last for several days. The newborn may exhibit poor consolability for 3 months or more. These behaviors may interfere with successful maternal-infant attachment and increase the potential for parenting problems in an already high-risk mother.

Methadone

Methadone is the most commonly used drug in the treatment of women who are dependent on opioids such as heroin. Methadone blocks withdrawal symptoms and the craving for street drugs. Dosage should be individualized at the lowest possible therapeutic level. Methadone does cross the placenta and has been associated with problems such as PIH, hepatitis, placental problems, and abnormal fetal presentation (Hans 1989).

Prenatal exposure to methadone may result in reduced head circumference, poor motor coordination, increased body tension, and delayed achievement of motor skills. The neonate may experience withdrawal symptoms that are more severe than those associated with heroin.

Medical Therapy

Antepartal care of the pregnant addict involves medical, socioeconomic, and legal considerations. The use of a team approach allows for the comprehensive management necessary to provide safe labor and childbirth for woman and fetus.

The management of drug addiction may include hospitalization as necessary to initiate detoxification. "Cold turkey" withdrawal is not advisable during pregnancy because of potential risk to the fetus. Maintenance and support therapy are given during weekly prenatal visits.

Urine screening is also done regularly throughout pregnancy if the woman is a known or suspected substance abuser. This testing is helpful in identifying the type and amount of drug being abused.

❋ *APPLYING THE NURSING PROCESS* ❋

Nursing Assessment

> **CRITICAL THINKING**
>
> *What psychosocial factors contribute to the onset of substance abuse?*

The nurse should be alert for clues in the history or appearance of the woman that suggest substance abuse (Table

18–5). If abuse is suspected the nurse needs to ask direct questions, beginning with less threatening questions about use of tobacco, caffeine, and over-the-counter medications. The nurse can then progress to questions about alcohol consumption and finally questions focusing on past and current use of illicit drugs. The nurse who is matter-of-fact and nonjudgmental in approach is more likely to elicit honest responses (Lynch & McKeon 1990).

Nursing assessment of the woman who is a known substance abuser focuses on the woman's general health status, with specific attention to nutritional status, susceptibility to infections, and evaluation of all body systems. The nurse also assesses the woman's understanding of the impact of substance abuse on herself and her pregnancy. Some women are reluctant to discuss their substance abuse, while others are quite open about it. Once the nurse establishes a relationship of trust, he or she can gain information that can be used to plan the woman's ongoing care.

Nursing Diagnosis

Nursing diagnoses that may apply are listed in Key Nursing Diagnoses to Consider: Substance Abuse.

Nursing Plan and Implementation

Prevention of substance abuse during pregnancy is the ideal nursing goal and is best accomplished through client education. Unfortunately, many women who are substance abusers do not receive regular health care and may not seek care until they are far along in pregnancy.

Dx

Key Nursing Diagnoses to Consider
Substance Abuse

Altered growth and development
Altered nutrition: Less than body requirements
Altered parenting
Altered family processes
Altered role performance
Fear
Impaired social interaction
Ineffective individual coping
Knowledge deficit
Noncompliance
Infection: High risk
Injury: High risk
Poisoning: High risk
Trauma: High risk
Altered parenting: High risk
Self-esteem disturbance
Sexual dysfunction
Situational low self-esteem
Social isolation

The nurse's role in providing prenatal care for the woman who is a substance abuser focuses on ongoing assessment and client teaching. The nurse can provide information about the relationship between substance abuse and existing health problems and the implications for the woman's unborn child. By establishing a relationship of trust and support, the nurse may be effective in ensuring the woman's cooperation.

Preparation for labor and birth should be part of the prenatal planning. Relief of fear, tension, or discomfort may be achieved through nonnarcotic psychologic support and careful explanation of the labor process. If pain medication is necessary, it should not be withheld, however, because the notion that it will contribute to further addiction is mistaken (Lynch & McKeon 1990). Preferred methods of pain relief include the use of psychoprophylaxis and regional or local anesthetics such as pudendal block and local infiltration. These techniques are preferred to decrease risk of additional fetal respiratory depression. Immediate intensive care should be available for the newborn, who will probably be depressed, SGA, and premature. For care of the addicted newborn, see Chapter 31.

Evaluation

Anticipated outcomes of nursing care include the following:

- The woman is able to describe the impact of her substance abuse on herself and her unborn child.
- The woman successfully participates in a drug therapy program.
- The woman successfully gives birth to a healthy infant.
- Care givers detect potential complications early and institute appropriate therapy.
- The woman agrees to cooperate with a referral to social services (or another appropriate community agency) for follow-up care after discharge.

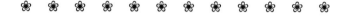

Other Medical Conditions and Pregnancy

A woman with a preexisting medical condition should be aware of the possible impact of pregnancy on her condition, as well as the impact of her condition on the successful outcome of her pregnancy. Table 18–6 discusses some of the less common medical conditions vis-à-vis pregnancy.

Table 18–6 Less Common Medical Conditions and Pregnancy

Condition	Brief description	Maternal implications	Fetal-neonatal implications
Rheumatoid arthritis	Chronic inflammatory disease believed to be caused by a genetically influenced antigen-antibody reaction. Symptoms include fatigue, low-grade fever, pain and swelling of joints, morning stiffness, pain on movement. Treated with salicylates, physical therapy, and rest. Corticosteroids used cautiously if not responsive to above.	Usually there is remission of rheumatoid arthritis symptoms during pregnancy, often with a relapse postpartum. Anemia may be present due to blood loss from salicylate therapy. Mother needs extra rest, particularly to relieve weight-bearing joints, but needs to continue range-of-motion exercises. If in remission, may stop medication during pregnancy. Oral contraception acceptable.	Possibility of prolonged gestation and longer labor with heavy salicylate use. Possible teratogenic effects of salicylates.
Epilepsy	Chronic disorder characterized by seizures; may be idiopathic or secondary to other conditions, such as head injury, metabolic and nutritional disorders such as PKU or vitamin B_6 deficiency, encephalitis, neoplasms, or circulatory interferences. Treated with anticonvulsants.	Seizure frequency often increases during pregnancy, with slightly higher incidence of hyperemesis gravidarum, preeclampsia, and vaginal hemorrhage. A woman who has been seizure free for a year should be withdrawn from medication prior to conception; a woman who requires medication has a 90% chance of having a normal child; women who seek advice after the first trimester should be maintained on their medication. Folic acid, iron, and vitamin D therapy needed during pregnancy (Meadow 1989).	Three times higher incidence of congenital anomalies (10 times higher for cleft lip and palate, 4 times higher for septal heart defects) if mother on anticonvulsive medications. (Meadow 1989).

(continued)

Table 18–6 (*continued*)

Condition	Brief description	Maternal implications	Fetal-neonatal implications
Hepatitis B	Hepatitis B is caused by the hepatitis B virus (HBV). Although HBV can theoretically be transmitted by all body fluids, it is primarily blood-borne or sexually transmitted. Groups at risk include women from areas with a high incidence (primarily developing countries), illegal IV drug users, prostitutes, and women with multiple sexual partners. Symptoms range from none to mild flulike symptoms to fulminating illness. No specific treatment is available. Supportive care is indicated. A vaccine is available for women in high-risk groups and for health care workers.	Hepatitis B does not usually affect the course of pregnancy. Pregnant women have no higher incidence of complications than the general population (Shaw & Maynard 1986). Women in the high-risk groups should be screened for hepatitis antibodies antepartally but close to the EDB. A woman who is negative may be given hepatitis vaccine. If she is positive the infant should receive prophylactic treatment.	The incidence of fetal malformation is not influenced by maternal infection with hepatitis. Infected newborns have 80% to 90% risk of becoming carriers and may remain infected indefinitely. The newborn who becomes a carrier faces a 1 in 4 risk of dying from liver-related disease (Shaw & Maynard 1986). The infant born to a woman with hepatitis can be treated prophylactically with a dose of hepatitis B immunoglobulin given within the first 12 hours after birth, followed by a series of injections of vaccine, the first during the first week of life, the second at one month, and the third at six months.
Hyperthyroidism (thyrotoxicosis)	Enlarged, overactive thyroid gland; increased T4:TBG ratio and increased BMR. Symptoms include muscle wasting, tachycardia, excessive sweating, and exophthalmos. Treatment by antithyroid drug propylthiouracil (PTU) while monitoring free T4 levels. Surgery used only if drug intolerance exists.	Mild hyperthyroidism is not dangerous. Increased incidence of PIH and postpartum hemorrhage if not well controlled. Serious risk related to thyroid storm characterized by high fever, tachycardia, sweating, and congestive heart failure. Now occurs rarely. When diagnosed during pregnancy may be transient or permanent.	Neonatal thyrotoxicosis is rare. Even low doses of antithyroid drug in mother may produce a mild fetal-neonatal hypothyroidism; higher dose may produce a goiter or mental deficiencies. Fetal loss not increased in euthyroid women. If untreated, rates of abortion, intrauterine death, and stillbirth increase. Breast-feeding contraindicated for women on antithyroid medication because it is excreted in the milk (may be tried by woman on low dose if neonatal T4 levels are monitored).
Hypothyroidism	Characterized by inadequate thyroid secretions (decreased T4:TBG ration), elevated TSH, lowered BMR, and enlarged thyroid gland (goiter). Symptoms include lack of energy, excessive weight gain, cold intolerance, dry skin, and constipation. Treated by thyroxine replacement therapy.	Long-term replacement therapy usually continues at same dosage during pregnancy as before. Weekly NST after 35 weeks' gestation.	If mother untreated, fetal loss 50%; high risk of congenital goiter or true cretinism. Therefore newborns are screened for T4 level. Mild TSH elevations present little risk since it does not cross the placenta.
Maternal phenylketonuria (PKU) (hyperphenylalaninemia)	Inherited recessive single gene anomaly causing a deficiency of the liver enzyme needed to convert the amino acid phenylalanine to tyrosine resulting in high serum levels of phenylalanine. Brain damage and mental retardation occur if not treated early.	Low phenylalanine diet is mandatory prior to conception and during pregnancy. The woman should be counseled that her children will either inherit the disease or be carriers depending on the zygosity of the father for the disease. Treatment at a PKU center is recommended.	Risk to fetus if maternal treatment not begun preconception. In untreated women, increased incidence of fetal mental retardation, microcephaly, congenital heart defects, and growth retardation. Fetal phenylalanine levels are approximately 50% higher than maternal levels.
Multiple sclerosis	Neurologic disorder characterized by destruction of the myelin sheath of nerve fibers. The condition occurs primarily in young adults, is marked by periods of remission, progresses to marked physical disability in 10 to 20 years.	Associated with remission during pregnancy, but with 50% relapse rate postpartum (Birk & Rudick 1989). Rest is important; help with child care should be planned. Uterine contraction strength is not diminished, but because sensation is frequently lessened labor may be almost painless.	Increased evidence of a genetic causal effect (Birk & Rudick 1989). Therefore reproductive counseling is recommended.

(continued)

Table 18–6 (*continued*)

Condition	Brief description	Maternal implications	Fetal-neonatal implications
Systemic lupus erythematosus (SLE)	Chronic autoimmune collagen disease, characterized by exacerbations and remissions; symptoms range from characteristic rash to inflammation and pain in joints, fever, nephritis, depression, cranial nerve disorders, and peripheral neuropathies.	Mild cases—little risk to mother or fetus. Severe cases—because of extra burden on the kidneys, therapeutic abortion may be indicated. Woman must be careful to avoid fatigue, infection, and strong sunlight.	Increased incidence of spontaneous abortion, stillbirth, prematurity, and SGA neonates. Infants with neonatal lupus syndrome without cardiac involvement respond well to supportive therapy, and the condition resolves during the first year of life (Dombroski 1989). The prognosis for those with heart lesions (about 25%) depends on their severity but may be guarded (Dombroski 1989).
Tuberculosis (TB)	Infection caused by *Mycobacterium tuberculosis;* inflammatory process causes destruction of lung tissue, increased sputum, and coughing. Associated primarily with poverty and malnutrition and may be found among refugees from countries were TB is prevalent. Treated with isoniazid and either ethambutol or rifampin or both.	If TB inactive due to prior treatment, relapse rate no greater than for nonpregnant women. When isoniazid is used during pregnancy, the woman should take supplemental pyridoxine (vitamin B_6). Extra rest and limited contact with others is required until disease becomes inactive.	If maternal TB is inactive, mother may breast-feed and care for her infant. If TB is active, neonate should not have direct contact with mother until she is noninfectious. Isoniazid crosses the placenta, but most studies show no teratogenic effects. Rifampin crosses the placenta. Possibility of harmful effects still being studied.

❀ ❀

KEY CONCEPTS

The diagnosis of high-risk pregnancy can shock an expectant couple. Providing emotional support, teaching about the condition and prognosis, and educating for self-care are important nursing measures that help the client cope.

Cardiac disease during pregnancy requires careful assessment, limitation of activity, and knowing and reporting signs of impending cardiac decompensation by both client and nurse.

The key point in the care of the pregnant woman with diabetes is scrupulous maternal plasma glucose control. This is best achieved by home blood glucose monitoring, multiple daily insulin injections, and a careful diet. To reduce incidence of congenital anomalies and other problems in the neonate, the woman should be euglycemic prior to conception and throughout the pregnancy. Diabetic clients more than most other clients need to be educated about their condition and involved with their own care.

Almost any health problem that a person can have when not pregnant can coexist with pregnancy. Some problems, such as anemias, may be exacerbated by pregnancy. Others, such as collagen disease, may go into temporary remission with pregnancy. Regardless of the health problem, careful health care is needed throughout pregnancy to improve the outcome for mother and fetus.

Substance abuse (either drugs or alcohol) not only is detrimental to the mother's health but also may have profound lasting effects on the fetus.

❀ ❀

References

Barbour BG: Alcohol and Pregnancy. *J Nurse-Midwifery* 1990; 35(2):78.

Barss VA: Diabetes in pregnancy. *Med Clin North Am* May 1989a; 73:685.

Barss VA: Obstetrical management. In *Diabetes Complicating Pregnancy.* Hare JW (editor). New York: Alan R. Liss, 1989b.

Bhargava M et al: Effect of maternal anaemia and iron depletion on foetal iron stores, birthweight and gestation. *Acta Paediatr Scand* 1989; 78:321.

Birk KA, Rudick RA: Caring for the ob patient who has multiple sclerosis. *Contemp OB/GYN* July 1989; 34:58.

Bishop, JE: AIDS set to be a leading killer of women in '91. *Wall Street Journal,* July 11, 1990, p 134.

Brady K, Duff P: Rheumatic heart disease in pregnancy. *Clin Obstet Gynecol* March 1989; 32:21.

Chashoff IJ: Perinatal effects of cocaine. *Contemp OB/GYN* 1987; 29:163.

Chashoff IJ, Griffith DR: Cocaine: Clinical studies of pregnancy and the newborn. *Ann NY Acad Sci* 1989; 262:265.

Chez RA: Meeting the challenge of gestational diabetes. *Contemp OB/GYN* September 1989; 34:120.

Committee on Ethics, The American College of Obstetricians and Gynecologists: Human immunodeficiency virus infection: Physicians' responsibilities. *Obstet Gynecol* June 1990; 75(6):1043.

Criteria Committee of the New York Heart Association Inc: *Nomenclature and Criteria for Diagnosis of Diseases of the Heart and Blood Vessels,* 5th ed. New York: New York Heart Association, 1955.

Cruikshank DP: Cardiovascular, pulmonary, renal, and hematologic diseases in pregnancy. In: *Danforth's Obstetrics and Gynecology,* 6th ed. Scott JR et al (editors). Philadelphia: Lippincott, 1990.

Cunningham FG et al: *Williams Obstetrics,* 18th ed. Norwalk CT: Appleton & Lange, 1989.

Dallman PR: Iron deficiency: Does it matter? *J Internal Med* 1989; 226:367.

Degani S et al: Mitral valve prolapse and pregnancy: A review. *Obstet Gynecol Surv* February 1989; 44:96.

Dombrowski MP, Sokol RJ: Cocaine and abruption. *Contemp OB/GYN* April 1990; 35:13.

Dombrowski RA: Autoimmune disease in pregnancy. *Med Clin North Am* May 1989; 73:605.

Earles A: The role of the nurse in sickle cell anemia and thalassemia major. In: *Proceedings of the National Conference on Nursing Practice in Clinical Genetics: Prospects for the 21st Century.* Felton G (editor). Iowa City: University of Iowa College of Nursing, 1986.

Engel NS: Insulin therapy in pregnancy. *MCN* January/February 1989; 14:19.

Fischbach FT: *A Manual of Laboratory Diagnostic Tests.* Philadelphia: Lippincott, 1988.

Fried PA: Postnatal consequences of maternal marijuana use in humans. *Ann NY Acad Sci* 1989; 562:123.

Ghiloni SZ: Home management. In: *Diabetes Complicating Pregnancy.* Hare JW (editor). New York: Alan R. Liss, 1989.

Gabbe SG: Management of diabetes mellitus in pregnancy. *Am J Obstet Gynecol* December 1985; 153:824.

Gabbe SG: Diabetes mellitus: Ways of individualizing care. *Contemp OB/GYN* July 1990; 35:68.

Gianopoulos JG: Cardiac disease in pregnancy. *Med Clin North Am* May 1989; 73:639.

Hans SL: Developmental consequences of prenatal exposure to methadone. *Ann NY Acad Sci* 1989; 562:195.

Hare JW: Gestational diabetes. In: *Diabetes Complicating Pregnancy.* Hare JW (editor). New York: Alan R. Liss, 1989a.

Hare JW: Pathophysiology. In: *Diabetes Complicating Pregnancy.* Hare JW (editor). New York: Alan R. Liss, 1989b.

Janke JR: Prenatal cocaine use: Effects on perinatal outcome. *J Nurse-Midwifery* 1990; 35(2):75.

Kaufman HW: Screening for gestational diabetes mellitus. *Am Fam Physician* December 1989; 40:109.

Kelton JG, Cruickshank M: Hematologic disorders of pregnancy. In: *Medical Complications During Pregnancy.* Burrows GN, Ferris TH (editors). Philadelphia: Saunders, 1988.

Kitzmiller JL et al: Managing diabetes and pregnancy. *Curr Probl Obstet Gynecol Fertil* July/August 1988; 11:125.

Kurth A, Hutchison M: A contact for HIV testing in pregnancy. *J Nurse-Midwifery* 1989; 34(5):259.

Landers DV, Sweet RL: Perinatal infections. In: *Danforth's Obstetrics and Gynecology,* 6th ed. Scott JR et al (editors). Philadelphia: Lippincott, 1990.

Lawrence RA: Breastfeeding and medical disease. *Med Clin North Am* May 1989; 73:583.

Little BB, Gilstrap LC: Cardiovascular drugs during pregnancy. *Clin Obstet Gynecol* March 1989; 32:13.

Livesay S et al: Cocaine and Pregnancy: Maternal and infant outcome. *Ann NY Acad Sci* 1989; 562:358.

Lucas MJ et al: Early pregnancy glycoslated hemoglobin, severity of diabetes, and fetal malformations. *Am J Obstet Gynecol* August 1989; 161:426.

Lynch M, McKeon VA: Cocaine use during pregnancy. *JOGNN* July/August 1990; 19:285.

MacGregor SN et al: Cocaine abuse during pregnancy: Correlation between prenatal outcomes. *Obstet Gynecol* 1989; 74(6):882.

MacGregor SN, Keith LG: Substance abuse in pregnancy: A practical management plan. *Female Patient* January 1989; 14:49.

McMahon KM: The integration of HIV testing and counseling into nursing practice. *Nurs Clin North Am* 1988; 23(4):803.

Meadow SR: Epilepsy in pregnancy: What are the hazards? *Contemp OB/GYN* November 1989; 34:51.

Mello NK et al: Neuroendocrine consequences of alcohol abuse in women. *Ann NY Acad Sci* 1989; 562:211.

Morbidity and Mortality Weekly Report: Update: Heterosexual transmission of acquired immunodeficiency syndrome and human immunodeficiency virus infection—United States. June 23, 1989; 38(24):423.

Morbidity and Mortality Weekly Report: Publicly funded HIV counseling and testing—United States 1985–1989: 1990; 39(9):137.

Morbidity and Mortality Weekly Report: Estimates of HIV prevalance and projected AIDS cases: Summary of a workshop, October 31-November 1989. 1989; 39(7):110.

Morbidity and Mortality Weekly Report: Supplement. Recommendations for prevention of HIV transmission in health care settings. August 21, 1987; 36(25):2.

Modica MM: Maternal Drug Abuse: Working with mothers and babies. Workshop sponsored by American Healthcare Institute March 12, 1990.

Niebyl JR: Teratology and drugs in pregnancy and lactation. In: *Danforth's Obstetrics and Gynecology,* 6th ed. Scott JR et al (editors). Philadelphia: Lippincott, 1990.

Norlander E et al: Factors influencing neonatal morbidity in gestational diabetic pregnancy. *Br J Obstet Gynecol* June 1989; 96:671.

Petitti DBK, Coleman C: Cocaine and the risk of low birth weight. *Am J Public Health* 1990; 80(1):25.

Pizzo PA: Pediatric AIDS: Problems within problems. *J Infect Dis* 1990; 161:316.

Ramin SM et al: Congenital heart disease. *Clin Obstet Gynecol* March 1989; 32:41.

Roberts AB et al: Fructosamine compared with a glucose load as a screening test for gestational diabetes. *Obstet Gynecol* November 1990; 76:773.

Sacks DA et al: How reliable is the fifty-gram, one-hour glucose screening test? *Am J Obstet Gynecol* September 1989; 161:642.

Shaw Fe, Maynard JE: Hepatitis B: Still a concern for you and your patients. *Contemp OB/GYN* March 1986; 27:27.

Sheldon GW: Diabetes in pregnancy. *Obstet Gynecol Clin North Am* June 1988; 15:379.

Shime J et al: Congenital heart disease in pregnancy: Short- and long-term implications. *Am J Obstet Gynecol* 1987; 156:313. Cited in Ramin SM et al: Congenital heart disease. *Clin Obstet Gynecol* March 1989; 32:41.

Spellacy WN: Diabetes mellitus and pregnancy. In: *Danforth's Obstetrics and Gynecology,* 6th ed. Scott JR et al (editors). Philadelphia: Lippincott, 1990.

White WBK: Management of hypertension during lactation. *Hypertension* 1984; 6:297. Cited in Lawrence RA: Breastfeeding and medical disease. *Med Clin North Am* May 1989; 73:583.

Wiley K, Grohar J: Human immunodeficiency virus and precautions for obstetric, gynecologic, and neonatal nurses. *JOGNN* May/June 1988; 17:165.

Winn HN, Reece EA: Integrating management of diabetic pregnancies. *Contemp OB/GYN* January 1989; 33:91.

Additional Readings

House MA: Cocaine. *Am J Nurs* April 1990; 90:40.

Krutsky C, Wiener J: Integrating HIV/AIDS risk assessment into a nurse-midwifery practice. *J Nurse-Midwifery* 1989; 34(5):275.

Larson E, Ropka ME: An update on nursing research and AIDS infection. *Image* Spring 1991; 23:4.

Leff EW et al: Type I diabetes in pregnancy . . . are we hearing women's concerns? *MCN* March/April 1991; 16:83.

Margolis HS: The case for universal screening of pregnant women for hepatitis B infection. *Contemp OB/GYN* April 15, 1990; 35(S):16.

Reveille JD: Systemic lupus erythematosus Part I: A clinical and diagnostic challenge. *Female Patient* April 1990; 15:41.

Sumser J et al: Are nurse practitioners prepared for the AIDS epidemic? *Nurse Pract* April 1990; 15:48.

Woods JR, Plessinger MS: Pregnancy increases cardiovascular toxicity to cocaine. *Am J Obstet Gynecol* 1990; 162:529.

CHAPTER 19

Pregnancy at Risk:

Gestational Onset

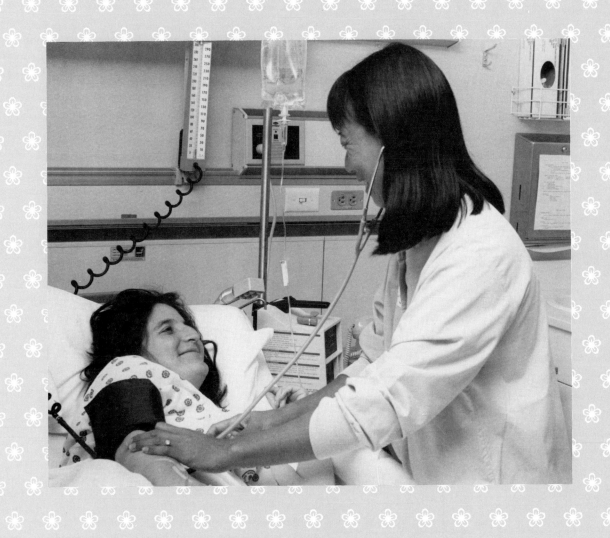

OBJECTIVES

Discuss hyperemesis gravidarum.

Contrast the etiology, medical therapy, and nursing interventions for the various bleeding problems associated with pregnancy.

Delineate the nursing care needs of a woman experiencing premature rupture of the membranes or preterm labor.

Describe the development and course of hypertensive disorders associated with pregnancy.

Explain the cause and prevention of hemolytic disease of the newborn secondary to Rh incompatibility.

Summarize the effects of surgical procedures on pregnancy and explain ways in which pregnancy may complicate diagnosis.

Describe the effects of infections on the pregnant woman and her unborn child.

❀ ❀

A short while ago, my husband and I happily found out that we were expecting our second child, and although we had experienced it before, we anxiously looked forward to each exciting step along the way. On my second routine prenatal visit, however, we were informed that no heartbeat was evident and that I appeared to be no where near my then estimated 14 weeks. An ultrasound verified what my doctor had suspected; there was no viable pregnancy—I had miscarried. I was suddenly overwhelmed with a feeling of great loss. But after my D&C, that feeling of loss turned to one of fear and uncertainty as my doctor informed me that no fetal development had existed; I had had a molar pregnancy.

As my doctor told me about the disease, he stressed the importance of regular follow-up, to be certain that the mole had been removed completely and that there was no cancerous development. As he explained the potential risks, it occurred to me that the possibility existed that I might never have another child. Suddenly, my healthy, happy toddler became the most important element in my life—how blessed I was to have her!

Although some anxiety still exists, I now approach my weekly follow-up visits with a renewed sense of being. It will be at least another year before my husband and I might again rejoice in the anticipation of a second child; but for now, we rejoice more fully in the precious one we have.

Pregnancy is usually a normal, uncomplicated experience. In some cases, however, problems arise during the pregnancy that place the woman and her unborn child at risk.

Regular prenatal care serves to detect these potential complications quickly so that effective care can be provided.

This chapter focuses on problems that primarily occur during pregnancy, those with a gestational onset.

❀ *USING THE NURSING PROCESS WITH* ❀

The Woman at Risk for Gestational Problems

As discussed in Chapter 18, the nursing process forms the basis for nursing actions. This logical approach to problem solving is especially valuable when providing care to women when complications develop during pregnancy. The nurse completes a systematic assessment, analyzes the data, and develops appropriate nursing diagnoses and client goals that will help guide the subsequent interventions. Evaluation provides information on the effectiveness of the plan, leads to further collection of data, and allows possible changes in interventions.

❀ ❀ ❀ ❀ ❀ ❀ ❀ ❀ ❀ ❀ ❀ ❀

Care of the Woman with Hyperemesis Gravidarum

Hyperemesis gravidarum, a relatively rare condition, is excessive vomiting during pregnancy. Hyperemesis can progress to a point at which the woman not only vomits everything she swallows but retches between meals. Dehydration, starvation, and, eventually, death are the result of untreated hyperemesis.

The cause of hyperemesis during pregnancy is still unclear but may be related to increased estrogen levels

(Vanagunas & Sparberg 1989) or to trophoblastic activity and gonadotropin production. It may sometimes be stimulated or exaggerated by psychologic factors. In severe cases the pathology of hyperemesis begins with dehydration. This leads to fluid-electrolyte imbalance and alkalosis from the loss of hydrochloric acid. More prolonged vomiting can result in loss of predominantly alkaline intestinal the juices and the occurrence of acidosis. Hypovolemia from dehydration leads to hypotension and increased pulse rate, with increased hematocrit and blood urea nitrogen levels and decreased urine output. Severe potassium loss (hypokalemia) interferes with the ability of the kidneys to concentrate urine and disrupts cardiac functioning. Starvation causes muscle wasting and severe protein and vitamin deficiencies.

Characteristic symptoms include jaundice and hemorrhage due to deficiencies of vitamin C and B-complex vitamins and bleeding from mucosal areas due to hypothrombinemia. Fetal or embryonic death may result, and the woman may suffer irreversible metabolic changes or death.

The differential diagnosis may involve infectious diseases such as encephalitis or viral hepatitis, intestinal obstruction, hydatidiform mole, or peptic ulcer.

Medical Therapy

The goals of treatment include control of vomiting, correction of dehydration, restoration of electrolyte balance, and maintenance of adequate nutrition. Initially, the woman is given nothing orally, with administration of intravenous fluids of at least 3000 mL in the first 24 hours. This therapy provides fluid, glucose, vitamin (B-complex, C, A, and D), and electrolyte replacement. Desired urine output is a minimum of 1000 mL/24 hours. Use of promethazine (Phenergan) parenterally in a continuous low dose may be helpful in controlling nausea and vomiting, although antiemetic drugs have not been approved for use during pregnancy (Vanagunas & Sparberg 1989).

Usually nothing is given by mouth for 48 hours. IV therapy is continued until all vomiting ceases. If the woman's condition does not respond to this management, total parenteral nutrition may be needed.

When the woman's condition has improved, oral feedings can be given. Six small dry feedings followed by clear liquids is one suggested treatment. Another method is 1 oz of water offered each hour, followed as tolerated by clear, then nourishing liquids, progressing on succeeding days to low-fat soft and regular diets.

❀ *APPLYING THE NURSING PROCESS* ❀

Nursing Assessment

When a woman is hospitalized for control of vomiting, the nurse must regularly assess the amount and character of further emesis, intake and output, fetal heart rate, evidence of jaundice or bleeding, and the woman's emotional state.

Nursing Diagnosis

Nursing diagnoses that may apply to the woman with hyperemesis gravidarum include the following:

- Altered nutrition: less than body requirements related to persistent vomiting secondary to hyperemesis
- Fear related to the effects of hyperemesis on fetal well-being

Nursing Plan and Implementation

Nursing care should be supportive and directed at maintaining a relaxed, quiet environment away from food odors or offensive smells. Once oral feedings are started, food should be attractively served. Oral hygiene is important as the mouth is dry and may be irritated from vomitus. Because emotional factors have been found to play a major role in this condition, psychotherapy may be recommended. With proper treatment, prognosis is favorable.

Evaluation

Anticipated outcomes of nursing care include the following:

- The woman is able to explain hyperemesis gravidarum, its therapy, and its possible effects on her pregnancy.
- The woman's condition is corrected and possible complications are avoided.

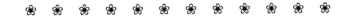

Care of the Woman with a Bleeding Disorder

During the first and second trimesters of pregnancy, the major cause of bleeding is **abortion**. This is the expulsion of the fetus prior to viability, which is considered 20 weeks' gestation. Abortions are either *spontaneous*, occurring naturally, or *induced*, occurring as a result of artificial or mechanical interruption. **Miscarriage** is a lay term applied to spontaneous abortion.

Other complications that can cause bleeding in the first half of pregnancy are ectopic pregnancy and gestational trophoblastic disease. In the second half of pregnancy, particularly in the third trimester, the two major causes of bleeding are placenta previa and abruptio placentae.

General Principles of Nursing Intervention

Spotting is relatively common during pregnancy and can occur following sexual intercourse or exercise due to trauma to the highly vascular cervix. However, the woman is advised to report any spotting or bleeding that occurs during pregnancy so that it can be evaluated.

It is often the nurse's responsibility to make the initial assessment of bleeding. In general, the following nursing measures should be implemented for pregnant women being treated for bleeding disorders:

- Monitor blood pressure and pulse frequently.
- Observe woman for behaviors indicative of shock, such as pallor, clammy skin, perspiration, dyspnea, or restlessness.
- Count pads to assess amount of bleeding over a given time period; save any tissue or clots expelled.
- If pregnancy is of 12 weeks' gestation or beyond, assess fetal heart tones with a Doppler.
- Prepare for intravenous therapy. There may be standing orders to start IV therapy on bleeding clients.
- Prepare equipment for examination.
- Have oxygen therapy available.
- Collect and organize all data, including antepartal history, onset of bleeding episode, laboratory studies (hemoglobin, hematocrit, and hormonal assays).
- Assess coping mechanisms of woman in crisis. Give emotional support to enhance her coping abilities by continuous, sustained presence, by clear explanation of procedures, and by communicating her status to her family. Most importantly, prepare the woman for possible fetal loss. Assess her expressions of anger, denial, silence, guilt, depression, or self-blame.

Spontaneous Abortion

Many pregnancies end in the first trimester as a result of spontaneous abortion. Statistics are inaccurate because some women may have aborted without being aware that they were pregnant during the early weeks of gestation (through week 6), when the bleeding may be seen as a heavy menstrual period. However, the actual incidence of spontaneous abortion is 20% to 62% with an average rate of 43% (Cunningham et al 1989).

When a spontaneous abortion occurs, the woman and her family may search for a cause so that they may plan knowledgeably for future family expansion. However, even with current technology and medical advances, a direct cause cannot always be determined.

About 50% of first trimester spontaneous abortions are related to chromosomal abnormalities (Simpson 1990). Other causes include teratogenic drugs, faulty implantation due to abnormalities of the female reproductive tract, a weakened cervix, placental abnormalities, chronic maternal diseases, endocrine imbalances, and maternal infections from the TORCH group (see p 531). It is believed by some that psychic trauma and accidents are a primary cause of abortion, but statistics do not support this belief.

The pathophysiology of spontaneous abortion differs according to the cause. In most cases embryonic death occurs, which results in loss of hCG and decreased progesterone and estrogen levels. The uterine decidua is then sloughed off (vaginal bleeding) and the uterus becomes irritable, contracts, and usually expels the embryo/fetus. In late spontaneous abortion the cause is usually a maternal factor, for example, incompetent cervix or maternal disease, and fetal death may not precede the onset of abortion.

Spontaneous abortion can be extremely distressing to the couple desiring a child. Chances for carrying the next pregnancy to term after one spontaneous abortion are as good as they are for the general population. Thereafter, however, chances of successful pregnancy decrease with each succeeding spontaneous abortion.

Classification

Spontaneous abortions are subdivided into the following categories so that they can be differentiated clinically:

1. *Threatened abortion.* The fetus is jeopardized by unexplained bleeding, cramping, and backache. Bleeding may persist for days. The cervix is closed. It may be followed by partial or complete expulsion of pregnancy (Figure 19–1).

2. *Imminent abortion.* Bleeding and cramping increase. The internal cervical os dilates. Membranes may rupture. The term *inevitable abortion* also applies.

3. *Complete abortion.* All the products of conception are expelled.

4. *Incomplete abortion.* Part of the products of conception are retained, most often the placenta. The internal cervical os is dilated and will admit one finger.

5. *Missed abortion.* The fetus dies in utero but is not expelled. Uterine growth ceases, breast changes regress, and the woman may report a brownish vaginal discharge. The cervix is closed. Diagnosis is made based on history, pelvic examination, and a negative pregnancy test and may be confirmed by ultrasound if necessary. If the fetus is retained beyond six weeks, fetal autolysis results in the release of thromboplastin and disseminated intravascular coagulation (DIC) may develop.

6. *Habitual abortion.* Abortion occurs consecutively in three or more pregnancies.

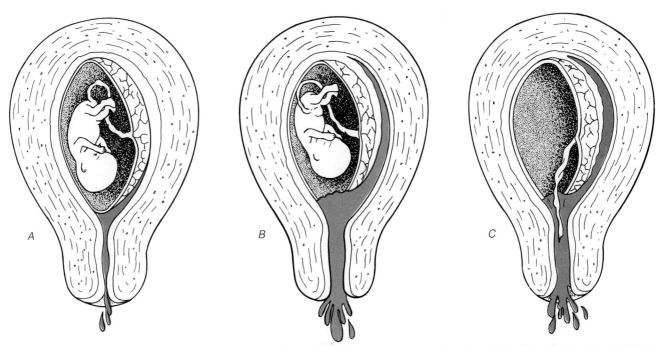

Figure 19–1 Types of spontaneous abortion. A Threatened. The cervix is not dilated and the placenta is still attached to the uterine wall, but some bleeding occurs. B Imminent. The placenta has separated from the uterine wall, the cervix has dilated, and the amount of bleeding has increased. C Incomplete. The embryo/fetus has passed out of the uterus; however the placenta remains.

Medical Therapy

Because 20% to 25% of pregnant women have episodes of spotting or bleeding during early pregnancy, it is important to determine whether vaginal bleeding is related to spontaneous abortion or other factors (Abbott 1989). One of the more reliable indicators is the presence of pelvic cramping and backache. These symptoms are usually absent in bleeding caused by polyps, ruptured cervical blood vessels, or cervical erosion.

Laboratory evaluations to help determine the cause of vaginal bleeding include ultrasound scanning, for presence of gestational sac, and hCG level. The latter can confirm a pregnancy, but because hCG level falls slowly after fetal death, it cannot confirm a live embryo/fetus. Hemoglobin and hematocrit levels are obtained to assess blood loss. Blood is typed and cross-matched for possible replacement needs.

The therapy prescribed for the pregnant woman with bleeding is bed rest, abstinence from coitus, and perhaps sedation. If bleeding persists and abortion is imminent or incomplete, the woman may be hospitalized, intravenous therapy or blood transfusions may be started to replace fluid, and dilation and curettage or suction evacuation is performed to remove the remainder of the products of conception. If the woman is Rh negative and not sensitized, Rh_o (D) immune globulin (RhoGAM) is given within 72 hours.

In missed abortions, the products of conception eventually are expelled spontaneously. If this does not occur within one month to six weeks after fetal death, hospitalization is necessary. Suction evacuation or dilation and curettage is done if the pregnancy is in the first trimester. Beyond 12 weeks' gestation, induction of labor by intravenous oxytocin and prostaglandins may be used to expel the dead fetus.

CRITICAL THINKING

What questions should a nurse ask a woman in her first trimester who calls to report that she is experiencing a small amount of vaginal bleeding? What recommendation should the nurse make to the woman?

✤ *APPLYING THE NURSING PROCESS* ✤

Nursing Assessment

The nurse assesses the amount and appearance of any vaginal bleeding and monitors the woman's vital signs and degree of discomfort. The nurse also assesses the responses of the woman and her family to this crisis and evaluates their coping mechanisms and ability to comfort each other.

Nursing Diagnosis

Nursing diagnoses that may apply include the following:

- Fear related to possible pregnancy loss
- Pain related to abdominal cramping secondary to threatened abortion
- Anticipatory grieving related to expected loss of unborn child.

Nursing Plan and Implementation

Provision of Psychologic Support

Providing emotional support is an important task for nurses caring for women who have spontaneously aborted because the attachment process already begun is disrupted. Feelings of shock or disbelief are normal at first. Couples who approached the pregnancy with feelings of joy and a sense of expectancy now feel grief, sadness, and possibly anger.

Since many women, even with planned pregnancies, feel some ambivalence initially, guilt is a common emotion. These feelings may be even stronger for women who were negative about their pregnancies. The woman may harbor negative feelings about herself, ranging from lowered self-esteem, resulting from a belief that she is lacking or abnormal in some way, to a notion that the abortion may be a punishment for some wrongdoing.

The nurse can offer invaluable psychologic support to the woman and her family by encouraging them to verbalize their feelings, allowing them the privacy to grieve, and listening sympathetically to their concerns about this pregnancy and future ones. The nurse can aid in decreasing any feelings of guilt or blame by supplying the woman and her family with information regarding the causes of spontaneous abortion and possibly referring them to clergy or other health care professionals for additional help, such as a genetic counselor if there is a history of habitual abortions.

The grieving period following a spontaneous abortion usually lasts 6 to 24 months. Many couples can be helped during this period by an organization or support group established for parents who have lost a fetus or newborn.

We lost our baby together. I know, you could say I never really had a baby, except during those few hours when it was already over and done with, but I guess these things aren't entirely logical. I loved my baby. . . . Absorbed in pain and self-pity, still I was flooded with adoration for this tiny, not yet shaped baby who had lived in me. (A Midwife's Story)

Promotion of Physical Well-Being

The physical pain of the cramps and the amount of bleeding may be more severe than a couple anticipates, even when they are prepared for the possibility of an abortion. Nurses need to be aware that couples feel unprepared for their first experience of spontaneous abortion. Nurses should offer support in dealing with the physical experience by explaining why the discomfort is occurring and by offering analgesics for pain relief.

Client Education

The pregnant woman is informed that she should report all episodes of bleeding to her health care provider. The woman hospitalized for spontaneous abortion may require information about possible causes of the loss and the chances of recurrence with a future pregnancy. She may also require information about the grief process so she is prepared for it when she goes home. She should also receive information about available resources if needed.

Evaluation

Anticipated outcomes of nursing care include the following:

- The woman is able to explain spontaneous abortion, the treatment measures employed in her care, and long-term implications for future pregnancies.
- The woman suffers no complications.
- The woman and her partner are able to begin verbalizing their grief and recognize that the grieving process usually lasts several months.

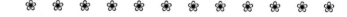

Ectopic Pregnancy

Ectopic pregnancy is an implantation of the blastocyst in a site other than the endometrial lining of the uterus. It may result from a number of different causes, including tubal damage caused by pelvic inflammatory disease, previous pelvic or tubal surgery, endometriosis, hormonal factors that impede ovum transport and mechanically stop the forward motion of the egg in the fallopian tube, congenital anomalies of the tube, and blighted conceptus. Smoking may also be a causative factor in the development of ectopic pregnancy (Handler et al 1989).

The incidence of ectopic pregnancy has increased dramatically in the past several years. In 1970 the rate was 5 per 1000 reported pregnancies. By 1989 the rate had more than quadrupled (Handler et al 1989; Ory 1989). This increased incidence may be related to improved diagnostic technology and to a parallel increase in the incidence of pelvic inflammatory disease (Dorfman 1987). Because maternal mortality from other causes is declining, ectopic pregnancy is now the primary cause of maternal mortality in the first trimester of pregnancy (Handler et al 1989).

The actual pathogenesis of ectopic pregnancy occurs when the fertilized ovum is prevented or slowed in its progress down the tube. The fertilized ovum either implants in the fallopian tube or in the ovary, peritoneal cavity, cervix, or uterine cornua (see Figure 19–2). The most common location for implantation of an ectopic pregnancy is the ampulla of the tube.

Initially the normal symptoms of pregnancy may be present, specifically amenorrhea, breast tenderness, and nausea. The hormone hCG is present in the blood and urine. The chorionic villi grow into the wall of the tube or site of implantation and a blood supply is established.

In the tube the implanted ovum quickly ruptures out of the tiny tubal lumen and grows in the connective tissues between layers of the tube. Bleeding occurs out of this space into the abdominal cavity. In some instances, spontaneous abortion and resolution of the ectopic pregnancy occurs (Leach & Ory 1990). However, if the embryo continues to develop and outgrows the space, the tube ruptures and there is further bleeding into the abdominal cavity. This irritates the peritoneum, causing the characteristic symptoms of sharp, one-sided pain, syncope, and referred shoulder pain as the abdomen fills with blood. The woman may also experience lower abdominal pain and faintness. Vaginal bleeding, a common finding with ectopic pregnancy, occurs with the death of the embryo and sloughing off of the uterine decidua, which has built up in response to the normal hormones of pregnancy.

In many instances, the symptoms are not obvious. One-fourth of ectopic pregnancies may involve uterine enlargement. Physical examination usually reveals adnexal tenderness; an adnexal mass is palpable in approximately one-half of the cases.

If internal hemorrhage is profuse, the woman rapidly develops signs of hypovolemic shock. More commonly the bleeding is slow (chronic), and the abdomen gradually becomes rigid and very tender. If bleeding into the pelvic cavity has been extensive, vaginal examination causes extreme pain and a mass of blood may be palpated in the cul-de-sac of Douglas.

Laboratory tests may reveal low hemoglobin and hematocrit levels and rising leukocyte levels. The hCG titers are lower than in intrauterine pregnancy.

Medical Therapy

It is important to differentiate an ectopic pregnancy from other disorders with similar clinical presenting pictures. Consideration must be given to possible spontaneous abortion, ruptured corpus luteum cyst, appendicitis, salpingitis, torsion of the ovary, ovarian cysts, and urinary tract infection.

The following measures are used to establish the diagnosis of ectopic pregnancy and assess the woman's status:

- A careful assessment of menstrual history, particularly the LMP.
- Careful pelvic exam to identify any abnormal pelvic masses and tenderness.
- Culdocentesis. The woman is positioned with her legs in stirrups, and a needle is inserted through the posterior vaginal vault into the cul-de-sac of Douglas. If nonclotting blood (blood that was clotted and then fibrinolysed) is aspirated, it is indicative of ectopic pregnancy.

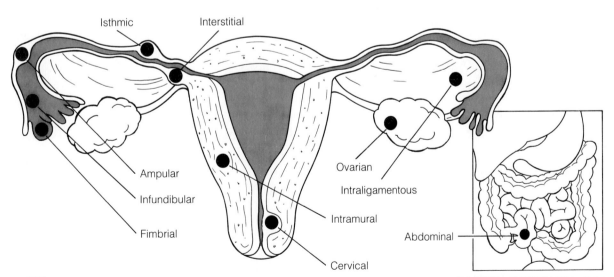

Figure 19–2   Various implantation sites in ectopic pregnancy. The most common site is within the fallopian tube, hence the name "tubal pregnancy."

- Laparoscopy, which may reveal an extrauterine pregnancy and is especially helpful in diagnosing an unruptured tubal pregnancy. If culdocentesis reveals free abdominal blood, laparoscopy is not necessary.
- Ultrasound, which may be useful in identifying a gestational sac in an unruptured tubal pregnancy. Its most common value is in confirming an intrauterine pregnancy, which usually rules out an ectopic one.
- Laparotomy, which will give a confirmed diagnosis and allow opportunity for immediate treatment.

Once the diagnosis of ectopic pregnancy has been made, surgery is usually done. Conservative management by linear salpingostomy is the treatment of choice when this is possible. Using this method, a linear incision is made in the tube and the products of conception are gently removed, usually by washing. The surgical incision in the tube is left open and allowed to close by secondary intention (Droegemueller 1986). If the tube is badly damaged, a total salpingectomy is performed, leaving the ovary in place unless it is damaged. If massive infection is found, a complete removal of uterus, tubes, and ovaries may be necessary.

Intravenous therapy and blood transfusion are used to replace fluid loss. During surgery the most important risk to be considered is potential hemorrhage. Bleeding must be controlled and replacement therapy should be on hand. The Rh-negative nonsensitized woman is given $Rh_o(D)$ immune globulin to prevent sensitization.

Recently, drug therapy to induce dissolution of the ectopic pregnancy has been attempted with some success. The drug used is usually methotrexate, a folinic acid antagonist, which acts by inhibiting cell division. The drug, which is given intramuscularly or intravenously, has the advantage over surgery of being less expensive when done on an outpatient basis. Tubal healing is improved, and there is a greater chance of maintaining fertility (Leach & Ory 1990). Research on this treatment option is ongoing.

✤ *APPLYING THE NURSING PROCESS* ✤

Nursing Assessment

When the woman with a suspected ectopic pregnancy is admitted to the hospital, the nurse assesses the appearance and amount of vaginal bleeding. The nurse monitors vital signs, particularly blood pressure and pulse, for evidence of developing shock.

It is also the nurse's responsibility to assess the woman's emotional status and coping abilities and to evaluate the couple's informational needs.

If surgery is necessary, the nurse performs the ongoing assessments appropriate for any client postoperatively.

Nursing Diagnosis

Nursing diagnoses that may apply for a woman with an ectopic pregnancy include the following:

- Anticipatory grieving related to the loss of the pregnancy
- Pain related to abdominal bleeding secondary to tubal rupture
- Knowledge deficit related to treatment of ectopic pregnancy and its long-term implications

Nursing Plan and Implementation

Once a diagnosis of ectopic pregnancy is made and surgery is scheduled, the nurse starts an IV as ordered and begins preoperative teaching. Signs of developing shock should be reported immediately. If the woman is experiencing severe abdominal pain, the nurse can administer appropriate analgesics and evaluate their effectiveness.

Teaching is an important part of the nursing care. The woman may want her condition and various procedures explained. She may need instruction regarding measures to prevent infection, symptoms to report (pain, bleeding, fever), and her follow-up visit.

The woman and her family will need emotional support during this difficult time. Their feelings and responses to this crisis will probably be similar to those that occur in cases of spontaneous abortion. As a result, similar nursing actions are required.

Evaluation

Anticipated outcomes of nursing care include the following:

- The woman is able to explain ectopic pregnancy, treatment alternatives, and implications for future childbearing.
- The woman and her care givers detect possible complications of therapy early and manage them successfully.
- The woman and her partner are able to begin verbalizing their loss and recognize that the grieving process usually lasts several months.

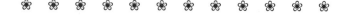

Gestational Trophoblastic Disease

Gestational trophoblastic disease (GTD) includes hydatidiform mole, invasive mole (chorioadenoma destruens), and choriocarcinoma (Soper & Hammond 1990).

Hydatidiform mole (molar pregnancy) is a disease in which (1) the chorioni villi of the placenta become swollen, fluid-filled (hydropic) grapelike clusters (Figure 19–3), while a central fluid-filled space forms in the placenta (central cistern formation); and (2) the trophoblastic tissue proliferates. The significance of this disease for the woman who has it is the loss of the pregnancy and the possibility, though remote, of developing choriocarcinoma from the trophoblastic tissue.

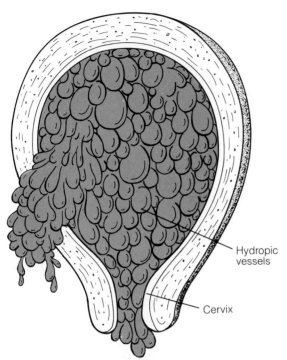

Figure 19–3   Hydatidiform mole. Vaginal bleeding, often brownish (the characteristic "prune juice" appearance) but sometimes bright red, is a common sign. In this figure some of the hydropic vesicles are being passed. This occurrence is diagnostic for hydatidiform mole.

Molar pregnancies are classified into two types, complete and partial, both of which meet the above criteria. Little is known about the cause of either type, but some of the pathophysiology has been clarified. The **complete mole** develops from an ovum that contains no maternal genetic material, an "empty" egg. How the maternal chromosomes are lost is not known. In most cases a haploid sperm, 23X, fertilizes the egg and duplicates before the first cell division. The conceptus then contains in its cells a 46XX chromosomal set of totally paternal origin (Szulman 1988). The embryo dies very early, when just a few millimeters long and before embryo-placental circulation has been established. Therefore, the villous hydropic vesicles are avascular in the complete mole. No embryonic-fetal tissue or membranes are found. The vesicular swelling is of all the villi. Choriocarcinoma seems to be associated primarily with the complete mole.

The *partial mole* has a triploid karyotype; ie, 69 chromosomes. Most often a normal ovum with 23 chromosomes is fertilized by two sperm (dispermy) or by a sperm that has failed to undergo the first meiosis and therefore contains 46 chromosomes. In about one-fifth of the cases the ovum did not undergo reduction division, so it contains 46 chromosomes and is fertilized by a normal sperm (Szulman 1988).

In partial molar pregnancy the villi are often vascularized and may be hydropic only in sections of the placenta rather than universally as with a complete mole. Often partial moles are only recognized after spontaneous abortion, and they may go unnoticed. Unlike the complete mole, the fetus usually survives to 8 or 9 weeks' gestation and occasionally longer. Twin pregnancies in which a normal fetus coexists with a molar pregnancy have been reported (Deaton et al 1989).

The incidence of GTD varies significantly worldwide. In the United States hydatidiform mole occurs in about one in 1500 to 2000 pregnancies. In Southeast Asia and the Far East, however, the incidence is five to 25 times higher (Soper & Hammond 1990). The incidence of molar pregnancy increases with advanced maternal age and has a familial tendency. Although a repeat molar pregnancy is rare, the chances are increased after the first one (Rice et al 1989).

Invasive mole (chorioadenoma destruens) is similar to a complete mole but involves the uterine myometrium. Treatment is the same as for a complete mole.

Medical Therapy

Diagnosis of hydatidiform mole is often suspected in the presence of the following signs:

- Vaginal bleeding is almost universal with molar pregnancies and may occur as early as the fourth week or as late as the second trimester. It is often brownish "like prune juice" due to liquefaction of the uterine clot, but it may be bright red.

- Anemia occurs frequently due to the loss of blood.

- Hydropic vesicles may be passed and if so are diagnostic (Figure 19–3). With a partial mole the vesicles are often smaller and may not be noticed by the woman.

- Uterine enlargement greater than expected for gestational age is a classic sign, present in about 50% of cases. In the remainder, the uterus is appropriate or small for the gestational stage. Enlargement is due to the proliferating trophoblastic tissue and to a large amount of clotted blood.

- Absence of fetal heart sounds in the presence of other signs of pregnancy is a classic sign of molar pregnancy. (Only rarely has a viable fetus been born in a partial molar pregnancy.)

- Elevated serum hCG due to continued secretion by the proliferating trophoblastic tissue may be present.

- Hyperemesis gravidarum may occur, probably as a result of the high levels of hCG.

- Pregnancy-induced hypertension (PIH) may be seen, especially if the molar pregnancy continues into the second trimester. Since PIH is a disease of late pregnancy, if symptoms occur in the first half of pregnancy molar pregnancy must be considered as the first diagnosis (Cunningham et al 1989).

Ultrasound is the primary means of diagnosing a molar pregnancy, usually after six to eight weeks, when the vesicular enlargement of the villi can be identified.

Therapy begins with evacuation of the mole and curettage of the uterus to remove all fragments of the placenta. Early evacuation decreases the possibility of other complications. If the woman is older and has completed her childbearing, or if there is excessive bleeding, hysterectomy may be the treatment of choice to reduce the incidence of malignant sequelae (Soper & Hammond 1990).

Complications associated with hydatidiform mole that require medical recognition and therapy include the following:

- Anemia
- Hyperthyroidism
- Infection, usually seen with late diagnosis and spontaneous abortion of the mole
- Disseminated intravascular coagulation
- Trophoblastic embolization of the lung, usually seen after molar evacuation of a significantly enlarged uterus (this creates a cardiorespiratory emergency)
- Theca-lutein ovarian cysts, which may be small or large enough to displace the uterus.

Malignant GTD, usually choriocarcinoma, can develop following evacuation of a mole. To detect this serious problem early and initiate treatment, follow-up care is essential. Follow-up consists of baseline chest x-ray exam to detect metastasis, physical examination including pelvic exam, and regular measurements of serum hCG levels. Initially, hCG levels are monitored weekly until they return to normal; they are rechecked two to four weeks later to ensure that they have remained normal; they are then monitored every one to two months for six to 12 more months (Soper & Hammond 1990).

Effective contraception is necessary during this time to prevent pregnancy and the resulting confusion about the cause of changes in hCG levels. In addition, pregnancy could mask an hCG rise associated with malignant GTD.

Continued high or rising hCG levels are found in 2% to 3% of women who have had molar pregnancy and indicate malignant GTD (choriocarcinoma). Treatment at a center specializing in GTD is advised. Once pregnancy has been ruled out, full physical examination, chest x-ray exam, abdominopelvic CT scan, and brain CT scan are done to rule out metastatic spread. Chemotherapy is then begun using methotrexate alone or in combination with other chemotherapy agents (Soper & Hammond 1990).

After treatment, careful follow-up monitoring of hCG levels is important. Malignant GTD is curable if diagnosed early and treated appropriately.

❀ *APPLYING THE NURSING PROCESS* ❀

Nursing Assessment

It is important for nurses involved in antepartal care to be aware of symptoms of hydatidiform mole and observe for these at each antepartal visit. The classic symptoms used to diagnose molar pregnancy are found more frequently with the complete than with the partial mole. The partial mole may be difficult to distinguish from a missed abortion prior to evacuation.

When the woman is hospitalized for evacuation of the mole, the nurse should monitor vital signs and vaginal bleeding for evidence of hemorrhage. In addition, the nurse determines whether abdominal pain is present and assesses the woman's emotional state and coping ability.

Nursing Diagnosis

Nursing diagnoses that may apply to a woman with a hydatidiform mole include the following:

- Fear related to the possible development of choriocarcinoma
- Knowledge deficit related to a lack of understanding of the need for regular monitoring of hCG levels

Nursing Plan and Implementation

When molar pregnancy is suspected, the woman needs support. The nurse can relieve some of the woman's anxiety by answering questions about the disease process and explaining what ultrasound and other diagnostic procedures will entail. If a molar pregnancy is diagnosed, the nurse supports the childbearing family as they deal with their grief about the lost pregnancy. Health care counselors, the hospital chaplain, or their own clergy may be of assistance in helping them deal with this loss.

When the woman is hospitalized for evacuation of the mole, explanation of the curettage procedure is necessary. Although the physician is responsible for providing this explanation, the woman and her partner may have many questions and concerns that the nurse can discuss with them. The nurse may also clarify areas of confusion or misunderstanding.

Typed and cross-matched blood must be available for surgery because of previous blood loss and the potential for hemorrhage. Oxytocin is administered to keep the uterus contracted and prevent hemorrhage.

Following surgery the nurse carefully observes the woman's urinary output because of the antidiuretic effects of oxytocin. The nurse also watches for further bleeding and for any signs of infection. If the woman is Rh negative and not sensitized, she is given $Rh_o(D)$ immune globulin to prevent antibody formation (See discussion on p 525).

The woman needs to know the importance of the follow-up visits. She is advised to use contraception to delay becoming pregnant again until after the follow-up program is completed.

Evaluation

Anticipated outcomes of nursing care include the following:

- The woman has a smooth recovery following successful evacuation of the mole.
- The woman is able to explain GTD, its treatment, follow-up, and long-term implications for pregnancy.
- The woman and her partner are able to begin verbalizing their grief at the loss of their anticipated child.
- The woman understands the importance of follow-up assessment and indicates her willingness to co-operate with the regimen.

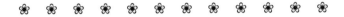

Placenta Previa

In placenta previa, the placenta is improperly implanted in the lower uterine segment, perhaps on a portion of the lower segment or over the internal os. As the lower uterine segment contracts and the cervix dilates in the later weeks of pregnancy, the placental villi are torn from the uterine wall, thus exposing the uterine sinuses at the placental site. Bleeding begins, but because its amount depends on the number of sinuses exposed, it may initially be either scanty or profuse. The classic symptom is painless vaginal bleeding usually occurring after 20 weeks' gestation. See Chapter 25 for an in-depth discussion of placenta previa.

Abruptio Placentae

Abruptio placentae is the premature separation of the placenta from the uterine wall. It occurs prior to birth, usually during the labor process. See Chapter 25 for an in-depth description of abruptio placentae.

Care of the Woman with an Incompetent Cervix

Incompetent cervix (sometimes called **dysfunctional cervix**) refers to the premature dilatation of the cervix, usually about the fourth or fifth month of pregnancy. It is associated with repeated second trimester spontaneous abortion and occurs in about 0.1% to 1.0% of pregnancies (Niebyl 1990). Congenital causes include cervical struc-

tural defects, uterine anomalies, and abnormal cervical development due to maternal exposure to diethylstilbestrol (DES). Acquired defects include previous traumatic birth or trauma to the cervix during D & C (dilatation and curettage), cervical conization, or cauterization (Scott 1990c).

A positive history of repeated, painless, and bloodless second trimester abortion is significant. Serial pelvic examinations early in the second trimester reveal progressive effacement and dilatation of the cervix and bulging of the membranes through the os with a characteristic hourglass appearance. If incompetent cervix is suspected, serial ultrasound provides information on dilatation of the internal cervical os before a dilated external os is detected (Niebyl 1990).

Incompetent cervix has been managed by a variety of surgical, mechanical, and medical methods, including bed rest in the Trendelenburg position, but none of these methods is ideal (Shortle & Jewelewicz 1989). The treatment most commonly used is the Shirodkar-Barter operation (cerclage), or a modification of it by McDonald, which reinforces the weakened cervix by encircling it at the level of the internal os with suture material. A purse-string suture is placed in the cervix between 14 and 18 weeks of gestation. The procedure should not be done if any of the following conditions exists: The diagnosis is in doubt, membranes are ruptured, vaginal bleeding and cramping exists, or the cervix is dilated beyond 3 cm. Once the suture is in place, a cesarean birth may be planned (to prevent repeating the procedure in subsequent pregnancies), or the suture may be released at term and vaginal birth permitted. The woman must understand the importance of contacting her physician immediately if her membranes rupture or labor begins. The physician can remove the suture to prevent possible complications. The success rate for carrying the pregnancy to term is 80% to 90%.

Care of the Woman with Premature Rupture of Membranes

Technically, **premature rupture of the membranes (PROM)** is defined as the spontaneous rupture of membranes prior to the onset of labor irrespective of the gestational age (Creasy & Resnik 1989). Premature rupture of the membranes may be further divided into the latent and interval periods. The latent period is the time from rupture of membranes to the onset of labor. The interval period is the time from rupture of membranes to birth of the fetus (Creasy & Resnik 1989). Some authorities categorize rupture of the membranes occurring before 38 weeks' gestation as *preterm rupture of the membranes* (Cunningham et al 1989).

Although the cause of PROM is unknown, a variety of

contributing factors are correlated with its occurrence. An incompetent cervix may be the cause of second trimester PROM. Infection (UTI), hydramnios, trauma, multiple pregnancy, and maternal genital tract anomalies may also result in PROM.

PROM occurs in 3% to 18.5% of all births, with a significantly higher incidence in association with preterm births (Creasy & Resnik 1989). In 80% to 90% of women at term, the onset of regular uterine contractions occurs within 24 hours after membranes rupture. The latent period exceeds 24 hours in 20% of women at term and exceeds 48 hours in about 10% (Creasy & Resnik 1989).

Maternal Risks

Maternal risk is related to infection, specifically chorioamnionitis (intra-amniotic infection resulting from bacterial invasion and inflammation of the membranes before birth) and endometritis (infection of the endometrium postpartally that may be related to chorioamnionitis or occur independently) (Garite 1990).

Fetal-Neonatal Risks

The most common neonatal complication in pregnancies involving PROM before 37 weeks' gestation is respiratory distress syndrome (RDS) (see Chapter 32), which occurs in 10% to 40% of neonates. Culture-confirmed sepsis is documented in less than 10% of neonates. The preterm fetus is further jeopardized by the associated risks of malpresentation (especially breech) and prolapse of the umbilical cord (see Chapter 25). Perinatal mortality largely depends on gestational age (Creasy & Resnik 1989).

Some research has suggested that a long latent period following preterm rupture of the membranes may stimulate pulmonary maturity in the preterm infant and thereby reduce the rate of RDS. The acceleration of the maturation of the lung is thought to occur because of the stress-producing situation. In contrast, other reports have noted no significant effect on the preterm newborn (Creasy & Resnik 1989).

Medical Therapy

After confirming with nitrazine paper and a microscopic examination (ferning test) that the membranes have ruptured, the gestational age of the fetus is calculated. Single or combination methods of calculation may be used, including Nagele's rule, fundal height, ultrasound to measure the fetal biparietal diameter, and amniocentesis to identify lung maturity (Chapter 20). The gestational age of the fetus and the presence or absence of infection determine the direction of medical treatment for PROM (See Table 19–1). If the fetus is preterm or if infection is present, more drastic medical therapy is necessary to prevent complications

---

Table 19–1 Currently Used Plans for Women with Premature Rupture of Membranes*

Preterm

Observation (expectancy); childbirth when labor or clinical infection develops.

Determination of fetal pulmonary status by testing of amniotic fluid; birth if fetus mature.

Determination of risk of infection by amniotic fluid stains, C-reactive protein, or ultrasound; birth if evidence of infection develops.

Administration of corticosteroids, with or without birth in 24 to 28 hours; tocolytics as needed.

Birth after an arbitrary latent period—for example, 16 to 72 hours.

Detection of group B streptococci (or *Neisseria gonorrhoeae*); selective treatment if positive.

Combinations of the above.

Term

Induction if spontaneous labor does not ensue in approximately 12 hours or if there are other complications (eg, toxemia) or if cervix is ripe.

Expectant management for women with uncomplicated pregnancies and cervix unfavorable for induction.

Adapted from Creasy RK, Resnik R: Maternal-Fetal Medicine, 2nd ed. Philadelphia: W. B. Saunders, 1989. Table 36-1, p. 660.

that are potentially detrimental to the mother and fetus/newborn.

If maternal signs and symptoms of infection are evident, antibiotic therapy (usually intravenously) is begun immediately and the fetus is born vaginally or by cesarean, regardless of the gestational age. Upon admission to the nursery the newborn is assessed for sepsis and started on antibiotics. Chapter 32 provides further information about the newborn with sepsis.

Management of PROM in the absence of infection and gestation of less than 37 weeks is usually conservative. The woman is hospitalized on bed rest. An admission CBC and urinalysis are obtained. Continuous electronic fetal monitoring may be ordered at the beginning of treatment but usually is discontinued after a few hours, unless the fetus is estimated to be very low birth weight (VLBW). Daily prolonged nonstress test (NST) and regular biophysical profiles are used to monitor fetal well-being until labor begins or cesarean birth becomes necessary (Anderson & Merkatz 1990). Maternal B/P, pulse, and temperature and FHR are assessed every four hours. A WBC is ordered daily. Vaginal exams are avoided to decrease the chance of infection. As the gestation approaches 34 weeks, an amniocentesis may be done weekly to evaluate lecithin/sphingomyelin (L/S ratio) and phosphotidylglycerol (PG) (see Chapter 20). After initial treatment and observation, some women may be followed at home. The woman is advised to continue bed rest (with bathroom privileges), monitor her temperature four times a day; avoid intercourse, douches, or tampons; and have a WBC every other day (Oxorn

1986). The woman is advised to contact her physician and return to the hospital if she has fever, uterine tenderness and/or contractions, increased leakage of fluid, or a foul vaginal discharge.

Opinions as to the value of administering glucocorticoids (betamethasone or dexamethasone) prophylactically for PROM are sharply divided (Creasy & Resnik 1989; Avery et al 1986). When gestation is between 34 and 36 weeks, medical practice has been to delay birth for 24 hours to allow natural elevation of maternal-fetal blood glucocorticoids, thereby contributing to fetal lung maturity. If gestation is between 28 and 32 weeks and labor can be delayed for 24 to 48 hours, betamethasone (Celestone) is frequently given. Glucocorticoids are not administered in the presence of uterine infection. (See Drug Guide-Betamethasone.) A large number of studies of the use of gluco-

---

DRUG GUIDE
Betamethasone (Celestone Solupan®)

Overview of Maternal-Fetal Action

"Betamethasone is a glucocorticoid which acts to accelerate fetal lung maturation and prevent hyaline membrane disease by inhibiting cell mitosis, increasing cell differentiation, promoting selected enzymatic actions, and participating in the storage and secretion of surfactant" (Bishop 1981). The best results are obtained when the fetus is between 30 and 32 weeks' gestation. It may be used as early as 26 weeks and as late as 34 weeks (Briggs et al 1986).

To obtain optimal results, birth should be delayed for at least 24 hours after the end of treatment. If birth does not occur, the effect of the drug disappears in about one week. A female fetus seems more likely than a male to obtain the most prophylactic effect (Briggs et al 1986).

Route, Dosage, Frequency

Prenatal maternal intramuscular administration of 12 mg of betamethasone is given once a day for 2 days. Repeated treatment will be needed on a weekly basis until 34 weeks of gestation (unless birth occurs).

Contraindications

Inability to delay birth for 24 to 48 hours

Adequate L:S ratio

Presence of a condition that necessitates immediate delivery (eg, maternal bleeding)

Presence of maternal infection, diabetes mellitus, hypertension

Concomitant use of tocolytic agents, which may increase risk of maternal pulmonary edema (Bishop 1981)

Gestational age greater than 34 completed weeks.

Maternal Side Effects

Bishop (1981) reports that suspected maternal risks include (a) initiation of lactation; (b) increased risk of infection; (c) augmentation of placental insufficiency in hypertensive women; (d) gastrointestinal bleeding; (e) inability to use estriol levels to assess fetal status; (f) pulmonary edema when used concurrently with tocolytics (such as ritodrine)

May cause Na^+ retention, K^+ loss, weight gain, edema, indigestion

Increased risk of infection if PROM present (Briggs et al 1986).

Effects of Fetus/Neonate

Lowered cortisol levels between 1 and 8 days following childbirth (Giacoia & Yaffe 1982)

Possible suppression of aldosterone levels up to 2 weeks following birth (Giacoia & Yaffe 1982)

Hypoglycemia

Increased risk of neonatal sepsis (Briggs et al 1986)

Animal studies have shown serious fetal side effects such as reduced head circumference, reduced weight of the fetal adrenal and thymus glands, and decreased placental weight (Briggs et al 1986). Human studies have not shown these effects, however.

Nursing Considerations

Assess for presence of contraindications.

Provide education regarding possible side effects.

Administer deep into gluteal muscle, avoid injection into deltoid (high incidence of local atrophy).

Periodically evaluate BP, pulse, weight, and edema.

Assess lab data for electrolytes.

corticoids with preterm PROM have not shown a reduction in the rate or severity of neonatal RDS in treated women. Meta-analysis of all research suggests that there is a modest decrease in RDS when corticosteroids are given and a slightly increased risk of maternal infection (Anderson & Merkatz 1990).

❀ *APPLYING THE NURSING PROCESS* ❀

Nursing Assessment

Determining the duration of the rupture of the membranes is a significant component of the antepartal assessment. The nurse asks the woman when her membranes ruptured and when contractions began, because the risk of infection may be directly related to the time involved. Gestational age is determined to prepare for the possibility of a preterm birth. The nurse observes the mother for signs and symptoms of infection, especially by reviewing her WBC, temperature, and pulse rate and the character of her amniotic fluid. If the mother has a fever, hydration status should be checked. When a preterm or cesarean birth is anticipated, the nurse evaluates the childbirth preparation and coping abilities of the woman and her partner.

Nursing Diagnosis

Nursing diagnoses that may be used with PROM include the following:

- Infection: High risk related to premature rupture of membranes

- Impaired gas exchange in the fetus related to compression of the umbilical cord secondary to prolapse of the cord

- Ineffective individual coping: High risk related to unknown outcome of the pregnancy

Nursing Plan and Implementation

Nursing actions should focus on the woman, her partner, and the fetus. The time her membranes ruptured and the time of labor onset are recorded. The nurse observes the woman for signs and symptoms of infection by frequently monitoring her vital signs (especially temperature and pulse), describing the character of the amniotic fluid, and reporting elevated WBC to the physician/nurse-midwife. Uterine activity and fetal response to the labor are evaluated, but vaginal exams are not done unless absolutely necessary. The woman is encouraged to rest on her left side to promote optimal uteroplacental perfusion. Comfort measures may help promote rest and relaxation. The nurse must also ensure that hydration is maintained, particularly if the woman's temperature is elevated.

Provision of education is another important aspect of nursing care. The couple needs to understand the implications of PROM and all treatment methods. It is important to address side effects and alternative treatments. The couple needs to know that although the membranes are ruptured, amniotic fluid continues to be produced.

Providing psychologic support for the couple is critical. The nurse may reduce anxiety by listening empathetically, relaying accurate information, and providing explanations of procedures. Preparing the couple for a cesarean birth, a preterm neonate, and the possibility of fetal or neonatal demise may be necessary.

Evaluation

Anticipated outcomes of nursing care include the following:

- The woman's risk of infection and cord prolapse are decreased.

- The couple understands the implications of PROM and all treatments and alternative treatments.

- The pregnancy is maintained without trauma to the mother or her baby.

❀ ❀ ❀ ❀ ❀ ❀ ❀ ❀ ❀ ❀ ❀ ❀

Care of the Woman at Risk Due to Preterm Labor

Labor that occurs between 20 and 37 completed weeks of pregnancy is referred to as **preterm labor** (Creasy & Resnik 1989). Prematurity continues to be the number one perinatal and neonatal problem in the United States today—it is estimated that 6% to 8% of all live births occur prematurely, or prior to 37 completed weeks of gestation (Herron 1988). The causes may be maternal, fetal, or placental factors. Premature rupture of the membranes occurs in one-third of the cases of preterm births. In the other two-thirds of cases, no known cause has been identified (Anderson & Merkatz 1990). Maternal factors include cardiovascular or renal disease, diabetes, PIH, abdominal surgery during pregnancy, a blow to the abdomen, uterine anomalies, cervical incompetence, DES exposure, history of cone biopsy, and maternal infection. Fetal factors include multiple pregnancy, hydramnios, and fetal infection. Placental factors include placenta previa and abruption of the placenta (Creasy & Resnik 1989).

Other cases reveal a strong correlation between preterm birth and low socioeconomic status (education, income, occupation) and/or history of preterm births.

Risk-scoring tools help identify a large proportion of pregnant women who are at risk for preterm birth. Table

Table 19–2 Major and Minor Risk Factors in Prediction of Spontaneous Preterm Labor[†]

Major

Multiple gestation	Previous preterm birth
DES exposure	Previous preterm labor term birth
Hydramnios	Abdominal surgery during pregnancy
Uterine anomaly	History of cone biopsy
Cervix dilated > 1 cm at 32 weeks	Cervical shortening < 1 cm at 32 weeks
Second trimester abortion ×2	Uterine irritability

Minor

Febrile illness	Cigarettes—more than 10/day
Bleeding after 12 weeks	Second-trimester abortion ×1
History of pyelonephritis	More than 2 first-trimester abortions

[†]*Presence of one or more major factors and/or two or more minor factors places patient in high risk group.*

(Adapted from Creasy RK, Resnik R: Maternal-Fetal Medicine, 2nd ed. Philadelphia: W. B. Saunders, 1989. Table 28-5, p. 481.)

19–2 presents one system for determining the risk of spontaneous preterm birth. If this type of tool is used, it is important to reassess the risks and observe cervical changes as the pregnancy progresses.

Maternal Risks

The major risks for the woman involve psychologic stress factors related to her concern for her unborn child. Physiologic maternal risks are related to possible medical treatments for preterm labor such as tocolytic therapy and prolonged bed rest.

Fetal-Neonatal Risks

Mortality increases for neonates born before 37 weeks' gestation. Although the preterm infant is faced with many maturational deficiencies (fat storage, heat regulation, immaturity of organ systems), the most critical factor is the lack of development of the respiratory system—to the extent that life cannot be supported. In some instances, such as severe maternal diabetes or serious isoimmunization, continuation of the pregnancy may be more life-threatening to the fetus than the hazards of prematurity. See Chapter 32 for in-depth consideration of the preterm neonate.

Medical Therapy

The goal of medical therapy is to prevent preterm labor from advancing to a point that no longer responds to medical treatment. If the cervix is dilated more than 3 to 4 cm and more than 50% effaced, the effects of tocolytics on labor is reduced. If labor cannot be arrested, the priority becomes successful preterm birth and its psychologic effect on the woman and her partner.

Due to the often subtle symptoms of preterm labor, the mother who is at risk for preterm labor may benefit from participating in a preterm birth prevention program. These programs, which have become increasingly popular, generally focus on three areas: (1) early identification of women at high risk for preterm birth; (2) education of these women about the often subtle signs and symptoms of preterm labor; and (3) appropriate and effective management by health care providers during prenatal visits and in the event that preterm labor occurs (Morrison 1990).

Ambulatory home monitoring programs, when coupled with skilled nursing care, have been very successful in early detection of preterm labor. Women at high risk are instructed to use a home uterine activity monitor to record and transmit uterine contractile activity once or twice daily to a nurse specially trained in the signs and symptoms of preterm labor (Figure 19–4). The nurse then uses the uterine contraction frequency data and the woman's reports of symptoms to assess the risk of preterm labor on a daily basis. If uterine activity is excessive or if symptoms are reported, the woman is referred to her physician for prompt evaluation. If preterm labor is diagnosed, intervention is begun immediately. Research indicates that women on daily monitoring who also have regular contact with a perinatal nurse have an increased incidence of early detection of preterm labor (2 cm or less dilatation), successful use of tocolytic drugs, and continuance of pregnancy to term (Hill 1990; Watson et al 1990).

If preterm labor is suspected, the diagnosis should be confirmed before therapy is begun. Common criteria used for diagnosis are found in Table 19–3. Any medical condition that may contribute to preterm labor should also be treated, and maternal or fetal contraindications to inhibiting labor should be identified. Tocolysis is the use of therapeutic interventions to attempt to stop labor, while tocolytic agents are drugs that are used to stop labor.

Creasy and Resnik (1989) specify the following contraindications to interrupting labor. Absolute contraindications include presence of severe PIH, fetal anomalies incompatible with life, chorioamnionitis, hemorrhage, fetal death, severe abruptio placentae, or severe fetal growth retardation. Relative contraindications include cervical dilatation of 5 cm or more, mild chronic hypertension, stable placenta previa, uncontrolled diabetes mellitus, maternal cardiac disease, mild abruptio placentae, hyperthyroidism, fetal distress, fetal anomaly, or mild fetal growth retardation.

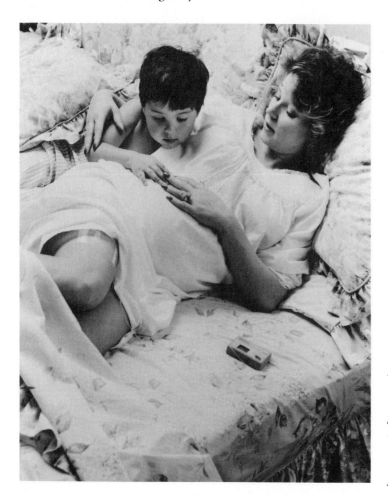

*Figure 19–4   A pregnant woman at risk for pre-
term labor does home uterine activity monitoring.
The monitor is worn on her abdomen under her
gown. She will record activity for about one hour
and then transmit the information to the nurse
via a phone hook-up. Note that the woman is lying
on her left side to promote optimum placental
perfusion.*

Drugs currently used to arrest preterm labor include
beta-adrenergic agonists and magnesium sulfate (MgSO₄).
The beta-adrenergic agonists currently are the most widely
used tocolytics. Ritodrine (Yutopar) is FDA-approved (see
Drug Guide-Ritodrine on p 501). While it is not FDA-
approved for use in preterm labor, terbutaline sulfate
(Brethine) has been used with increasing frequency to inhibit preterm labor because the drug is effective and less
expensive than ritodrine (Lam 1989). Although these drugs
suppress contractions and allow prolongation of pregnancy, they do cause maternal side effects; the most serious
is pulmonary edema. Reduction of dose and duration of
therapy is sometimes used to decrease side effects (Spatling 1989).

Currently, diagnosed preterm labor is treated with IV
tocolytics. Once uterine activity is stopped, the woman is
placed on oral beta-adrenergic agonists (ritodrine or terbutaline) for long-term maintenance. However, studies report
that this regimen is associated with a 40% to 50% incidence of recurrence of preterm labor. Potential causes of
tocolytic failure include lack of client cooperation, drug
side effects, infection, PROM, and drug tolerance (Lam et al
1989).

In response to these potential problems with long-
term oral beta-adrenergic agonist treatment, investigators
have begun using a subcutaneous terbutaline pump for
long-term tocolysis (Lam et al 1988). This pump permits
both low-dose (basal), continuous infusions and intermittent, high-dose boluses. Continuous low doses of medication help to decrease side effects as well as to prevent de-
sensitization of myometrial beta-adrenergic receptor sites.

Table 19–3   Criteria for Diagnosis of Preterm Labor*

Gestation 20–37 weeks
and
Documented uterine contractions
(4/20 min., 8/60 min.)
and

Ruptured membranes	*or*	intact membranes
		and
		documented cervical change
		or
		cervical effacement of 80%
		or
		cervical dilatation 2 cm

*From Creasy RK, Resnik R: Maternal-Fetal Medicine, 2nd ed. Phila-
delphia: W. B. Saunders, 1989. Table 28-9, p. 448.*

DRUG GUIDE
Ritodrine (Yutopar)

Overview of Obstetric Action

Ritodrine is a sympathomimetic β_2-adrenergic agonist which is FDA approved for use in treatment of preterm labor. It exerts its effect on beta$_2$ receptors, which are found in uterine smooth muscle, bronchioles, and diaphragm. Stimulation of beta$_2$ receptors results in uterine relaxation, bronchodilation, vasodilation, and muscle glycogenolysis. As muscles in the vessel walls relax, hypotension is induced. The body compensates by increasing maternal heart rate and pulse pressure.

Ritodrine causes a potassium shift, which may cause hypokalemia but not total body potassium depletion. There may also be an increase in blood glucose and plasma insulin levels and stimulation of glycogen release from muscles and the liver (NAACOG 1984).

Route, Dosage, Frequency

Add 150 mg of ritodrine to 500 mL IV fluid and administer as a piggyback to a primary IV. The resulting dilution is 0.3 mg/mL. Note: Some authorities recommend a saline solution and others believe a dextrose solution reduces the incidence of pulmonary edema (Niebyl et al 1986). The initial dose is 0.1 mg/min (20 mL/hr on an adult infusion pump). The dose is increased 0.05 mg/min (10 mL/hr on an adult infusion pump) every 10 minutes until contractions cease. Maximum dosage is 0.35 mg/min (70 mL/hr on an adult infusion pump). When contractions cease, the infusion rate may be decreased by 0.5 mg/min (10 mL/hr on an adult infusion pump). The infusion may be maintained at a low rate for a period of hours to assure that contractions do not begin again. Before the intravenous infusion is discontinued, PO administration is begun (Pauerstein, 1987).

Gonik and Creasy (1986) recommend administration of oral ritodrine 30 minutes before ending IV ritodrine. The initial PO dose is 10–20 mg every 2 hours, and the time between doses may be increased to 3–4 hours based on uterine response and maternal pulse. The maternal pulse is maintained in the 90–100 BPM range.

This dosage can be administered safely to a maximum of 120 mg over 24 hours. The length of therapy varies.

Current research is directed toward the use of a single injection of ritodrine for other obstetric problems. Rapid relaxation of the uterus may be needed in the presence of tetanic contractions and cord prolapse (Ingemarsson et al 1985b). It has also been suggested for use with fetal bradycardia to improve the heart rate (Ingemarsson et al 1985a) and to inhibit labor in order to manage fetal distress (Caritis et al 1985).

Maternal Contraindications

Preterm labor accompanied by cervical dilatation greater than 4 cm, chorioamniotitis, severe preeclampsia-eclampsia, severe bleeding, fetal death, significant IUGR contraindicate use of ritodrine, as do any of the following:

Hypovolemia, uncontrolled hypertension

Pulmonary hypertension

Cardiac disease, arrhythmias

Diabetes mellitus (use with caution)

Concurrent therapy with glucocorticoids (use with caution)

Gestation less than 20 weeks

Hyperthyroidism (Givens 1988)

Chronic hepatic or renal disease

Maternal Side Effects

Tachycardia, occasionally premature ventricular contractions (PVCs), increased stroke volume, slight increase in systolic and decrease in diastolic pressure, palpitations, tremors, nervousness, nausea and vomiting, headache, erythema, hypotension, shortness of breath (Bealle et al 1985)

Decreased peripheral vascular resistance, which lowers diastolic pressure → widening of pulse pressure

Hyperglycemia (usually peaks within 3 hours after initiation of therapy) (Pauerstein 1987)

Metabolic acidosis

Hypokalemia (causes internal redistribution)

Pulmonary edema in women treated concurrently with glucocorticoids, and who have fluid overload (Skidmore-Roth 1989).

Increased concentration of lactate and free fatty acids ST segment depression, T wave flattening, prolongation of QT interval (Hendricks et al 1986)

Increase in plasma volume as indicated by decreases in hemoglobin, hematocrit, and serum albumin levels (Philipsen 1981)

Possible neutropenia with long-term IV therapy (Wang & Davidson 1986)

(continued)

Effects on Fetus/Neonate

Fetal tachycardia, cardiac dysrhythmias

Increased serum glucose concentration

Fetal acidosis

Fetal hypoxia

Neonatal hypoglycemia, hypocalcemia, ↑ WBC

Neonatal paralytic ileus, irritability, tremors

Neonatal hypotension at birth

May decrease incidence of neonatal respiratory distress syndrome (Lipshitz 1981)

Nursing Considerations

Position woman in left side-lying position to increase placental perfusion and decrease incidence of hypotension.

Complete a history and assessment to identify possible presence of infection and maternal-fetal contraindications to treatment.

Explain procedure, which will include electronic fetal monitor, IV, frequent assessments, possible use of cardiac monitor, blood samples, intake and output, and daily weight, and potential for development of side effects, especially increase in pulse and fetal heart rate.

Monitor uterine activity and fetal heart rate by electronic fetal monitor.

Assess maternal BP and pulse every 10 minutes while dosage is being increased and while woman is being stabilized (Givens 1988). As long as dosage is being increased, some agency protocols recommend taking maternal BP and pulse prior to dose increase. Notify physician if maternal pulse > 120 bpm. (Note: Expect increase of 20–40 bpm. Maternal pulse may exceed 120 bpm for a brief period of time (Pauerstein 1987).

Assess respiratory rate and auscultate breath sounds with maternal vital signs. Note signs of pulmonary edema (rales and rhonchi). When oral therapy is begun, maternal BP, pulse, and respirations may be taken with each PO dose.

Monitor FHR with maternal assessments (Note: Expect increase of approximately 10 bpm. The rate should not exceed 180 bpm. Notify physician of rate > 180 bpm).

Apply antiembolism stockings to prevent pooling of blood in extremities.

Encourage passive range of motion in legs every 1–2 hours.

Assess hydration status by evaluating intake/output, skin turgor, mucous membranes, and urine concentration.

Maintain intake and output records. Intake is usually limited to between 1500 and 2500 mL/day (Pauerstein 1987) and 90–100 mL/hr (Shortridge 1983).

Intake and output are assessed hourly during initial IV therapy and every 4 hours during maintenance therapy (Givens 1988).

Weigh daily at same time after woman has emptied bladder, using same scale and same clothing.

Observe woman closely for problems associated with hypokalemia (muscle weakness, cardiac arrhythmia) and pulmonary edema (dyspnea, wheezing, coughing, rales or rhonchi, or tachypnea). Discontinue therapy if pulmonary edema or cardiac problems develop.

Assess lab data regarding electrolytes, glucose, and WBC (Givens 1988).

Have beta blocking agent available as antidote for betasympathomimetic therapy. Propranolol (Inderal) 0.25 mg IV is usually used (Shortridge 1983). It should be given by a physician and injected over at least 1 minute to reduce the potential for lowering the blood pressure and precipitating cardiac standstill. Cardiac monitoring should be continuous.

Provide psychosocial support. The threat of preterm labor produces anxiety. Provide information and counseling for the woman and partner, and encourage questions. Assist them in making life-style changes such as more frequent rest periods, cessation of employment, and possible changes in sexual activity. If woman is discharged on oral therapy, teach her to take medications on time to ensure optimum effect, to observe for signs of preterm labor, and to assess her pulse with each dose. The woman needs to report pulse above 120, palpitations, tremors, agitation, nervousness, chest pain, and any difficulty breathing.

If birth occurs when woman is on ritodrine therapy, assess newborn for presence of side effects (NAACOG 1984).

It is recommended to discontinue ritodrine in the presence of any of the following: Maternal heart rate above 140 bpm or fetal heart rate above 200 bpm, more than 6 maternal or fetal premature ventricular contractions/min, maternal systolic pressure above 180 mm Hg or diastolic below 40 mm Hg, chest pain, shortness of breath (Bealle et al 1985).

The combined basal and bolus methods of administration allow the woman to sleep at night because she does not have to get up to take medication and corresponds closely with the circadian patterns of contractions seen in preterm labor (Lam et al 1989).

Magnesium sulfate has long been used in the treatment of PIH and has been gaining favor in the treatment of preterm labor because it is effective and has fewer side effects than beta-adrenergic agonists. The usual recommended loading dose is 4 to 6 g IV over 20 to 30 minutes. The constant dose is then 1 to 3 g/hr. The dose may be increased by 0.5 g/hr every 30 minutes until contractions cease or a dose of 3 g/hr is reached. The therapy is maintained for 12 to 24 hours at the lowest rate to maintain cessation of contractions. The maternal serum level that is important for tocolysis seems to be 5 to 8 mg/dL (Creasy & Resnik 1989). Side effects with the loading dose may include flushing, a feeling of warmth, headache, nystagmus, nausea, and dizziness. Other side effects include lethargy and sluggishness and a 2% risk of pulmonary edema if the woman has predisposing conditions such as multiple gestation or hydramnios (Wilkins et al 1986). Side effects are more likely to occur in the presence of serum magnesium levels between 7 to 10 mg/dL (Givens 1988). See Drug Guide-Magnesium Sulfate on page 504 for other side effects. Fetal side effects may include hypotonia that persists for one or two days following birth (Wilkins et al 1986).

In comparison with IV ritodrine, magnesium sulfate has less effect on systolic or diastolic blood pressure (mean blood pressure and uteroplacental perfusion are maintained), no alteration of maternal heart rate (though it may cause a slight decrease in the fetal heart rate), no effect on cardiac output, and only a slight increase in placental blood flow.

Long-term oral therapy may be accomplished with magnesium oxide, magnesium chloride, or magnesium gluconate. The therapeutic dose is usually 250 to 450 mg every 3 hr. This dose maintains a maternal serum level of 2 to 2.5 mg, which is usually sufficient to prevent uterine contractions (Niebyl 1990).

In some centers prostaglandin synthesis inhibitors (PSI) such as indomethacin (Indocin) are being investigated and used in selected instances. However, potential fetal side effects, such as premature closure of the ductus arteriosus, have been reported. Research is also being conducted on the use of calcium channel blockers such as nitrendipine and nifedipine to inhibit preterm labor (Anderson & Merkatz 1990).

❀ *APPLYING THE NURSING PROCESS* ❀

Nursing Assessment

During the antepartal period, the nurse identifies the woman at risk for preterm labor by noting the presence of predisposing factors. During the intrapartal period, the nurse assesses the progress of labor and the physiologic impact of

Table 19–4	Key Nursing Assessments During Ritodrine Therapy
Time interval	**Assessment**
During initial IV therapy and increases in infusion rate	
Every 10 minutes	FHR and maternal BP, pulse, and R. Auscultate lung sounds for rales and rhonchi. Be alert for complaints of dyspnea, chest tightness. Uterine activity.
Every hour	Assess output (should be over 30 mL/hr or match intake). Assess intake (should not exceed 90–100 mL/hr).
During maintenance IV therapy	
Every 30 minutes	Maternal BP, pulse, and R; FHR; lung sounds; uterine activity.
Every 4 hours	Intake and output.
During PO therapy	
Before each dose	Maternal BP, pulse, and R; FHR; lung sounds.
Every 4–8 hours	Intake and output.

Whenever lab work results are available, evaluate K^+ (for hypokalemia), hemoglobin, and hematocrit (for signs of hemodilution, which, together with hypokalemia, may be associated with pulmonary edema).

labor on the mother and fetus. The key nursing assessments during ritodrine therapy are listed in Table 19–4.

Nursing Diagnosis

Nursing diagnoses that may apply to the woman with preterm labor include the following:

- Knowledge deficit related to causes, identification, and treatment of preterm labor
- Fear related to early labor and birth
- Ineffective individual coping related to need for constant attention to pregnancy

Nursing Plan and Implementation

Client Education

Once the woman at risk for preterm labor has been identified, she needs to be taught about the importance of preventing the onset of labor. Increasing the woman's awareness of the subtle symptoms of preterm labor is one of the most important teaching objectives of the nurse. The signs and symptoms of preterm labor include the following:

- Uterine contractions that occur every ten minutes or less.
- Mild menstrual-like cramps felt low in the abdomen.
- Feelings of pelvic pressure that may feel like the baby pressing down. The pressure may feel constant or intermittent.

DRUG GUIDE
Magnesium Sulfate (MgSO$_4$)

Overview of Obstetric Action

MgSO$_4$ acts as a CNS depressant by decreasing the quantity of acetylcholine released by motor nerve impulses and thereby blocking neuromuscular transmission. This action reduces the possibility of convulsion, which is why MgSO$_4$ is used in the treatment of preeclampsia. Because magnesium sulfate secondarily relaxes smooth muscle, it may decrease the blood pressure, although it is not considered an antihypertensive, and may also decrease the frequency and intensity of uterine contractions.

Route, Dosage, Frequency

MgSO$_4$ is generally given intravenously to control dosage more accurately and prevent overdosage. An occasional physician still prescribes intramuscular administration. However it is painful and irritating to the tissues and does not permit the close control that IV administration does.

IV: The intravenous route allows for immediate onset of action and avoids the discomfort associated with IM administration. It must be given by infusion pump for accurate dosage.

Loading Dose: 4 g MgSO$_4$ as a 20% solution is administered over a 3–5 minute period (Scott & Worley 1990; Cunningham et al 1989). (One authority recommends a loading dose of 6 g MgSO$_4$ in 100 mL D$_5$W infused over a 15–20 minute period [Sibai 1990].)

Maintenance Dose: Based on serum magnesium levels and deep tendon reflexes, 2 g/hr is administered.

Maternal Contraindications

Extreme care is necessary in administration to women with impaired renal function because the drug is eliminated by the kidneys and toxic magnesium levels may develop quickly.

Maternal Side Effects

Most maternal side effects are related to magnesium toxicity. Sweating, a feeling of warmth, flushing, nausea, slurred speech, depression or absence of reflexes, muscular weakness, hypothermia, oliguria, confusion, circulatory collapse, and respiratory paralysis are all possible side effects. Rapid administration of large doses may cause cardiac arrest.

Effects on Fetus/Neonate

The drug readily crosses the placenta. Some authorities suggest that transient decrease in FHR variability may occur, while others report that no change occurred. Similarly some report low Apgar scores, hypotonia, and respiratory depression in the newborn, while others report no ill effects. Sibai (1987) suggests that the majority of ill effects observed in the newborn may actually be related to fetal growth retardation, prematurity, or perinatal asphyxia.

Nursing Considerations

1. Monitor the blood pressure closely during administration.
2. Monitor respirations closely. If the rate is less than 14–16/min, magnesium toxicity may be developing, and further assessments are indicated. Many protocols require stopping the medication if the respiratory rate falls below 12/min.
3. Assess knee jerk (patellar tendon reflex) for evidence of diminished or absent reflexes. Loss of reflexes is often the first sign of developing toxicity (Sibai 1990).
4. Determine urinary output. Output less than 100 mL during the preceding 4-hour period may result in the accumulation of toxic levels of magnesium.
5. If the respirations or urinary output fall below specified levels or if the reflexes are diminished or absent, no further magnesium should be administered until these factors return to normal.
6. The antagonist of magnesium sulfate is calcium. Consequently an ampule of calcium gluconate should be available at the bedside. The usual dose is 1 g given IV over a period of about 3 minutes.
7. Monitor fetal heart tones continuously with IV administration.
8. Continue MgSO$_4$ infusion for approximately 24 hours after delivery as prophylaxis against postpartum seizures.

Note: Protocols for magnesium sulfate administration may vary somewhat according to agency policy. Consequently individuals are referred to their own agency protocols for specific guidelines.

TEACHING GUIDE
Preterm Labor

Assessment: During the antepartal period the woman generally is screened for factors that place her at risk for preterm labor. The nurse then spends time with the woman and assesses her understanding of the danger of preterm labor, signs of preterm labor, and actions she can take to prevent it. If she is on a home monitoring program, the nurse assesses the woman's understanding of the purpose and rationale for the program.

Nursing Diagnosis: The key nursing diagnosis will probably be: Knowledge deficit related to the risks of preterm labor and self-care measures to prevent it.

Nursing Plan and Implementation: Teaching will focus on the risks of preterm labor, the functions of and procedures for home monitoring, and self-care activities to decrease the risk of preterm labor.

Client Goals: At the completion of the teaching, the woman will be able to do the following:

1. Discuss the risks of preterm labor.
2. Describe the purpose of home monitoring.
3. Demonstrate the correct procedures for doing home monitoring.
4. Explain self-care measures that help decrease the risk of preterm labor.

Teaching Plan

Content: Describe the dangers of preterm labor, especially the risk of prematurity in the infant, and all the potential problems.

Stress the value of home monitoring in evaluating uterine activity on a regular basis. Emphasize that many of the early symptoms of labor such as backache and increased bloody show may be subtle initially. Home monitoring can often detect increased uterine activity in the early stages before cervical changes progress to the point where it is impossible to stop labor.

If the woman is to be part of a home monitoring program, the monitoring nurse will usually do the initial teaching. Be prepared to reinforce the information provided and answer questions that may arise.

Summarize self-care measures such as excellent fluid intake (2 to 3 quarts daily), voiding q 2 hr, avoiding lifting and overexertion, avoiding nipple stimulation, limiting sexual activity, and cooperating with activity restrictions and bed rest requirements.

Evaluation: At the end of the teaching session the woman will be able to discuss the risks of preterm labor, demonstrate home monitoring techniques and explain their rationale, and implement self-care activities to decrease the risks of preterm labor.

Teaching Method: Discuss the risks specifically. Many people understand in a general way that prematurity can be dangerous, but they fail to understand how the baby is affected.

Use handouts during the discussion. Help the woman clearly understand the value of the program because, to be successful, it requires a real commitment on her part.

Do a demonstration and ask for a return demonstration.

Use a handout during the discussion. Provide opportunities for discussion. If the woman has concerns about certain recommendations, try to modify the approach to best meet her needs.

- Low, dull back ache, which may be constant or intermittent.
- Sudden increase in vaginal discharge (an increase in amount or a change to more clear and watery or a pinkish tinge).
- Abdominal cramping with or without diarrhea.

The woman is also taught to evaluate contraction activity once or twice a day. She does so by lying down tilted to one side with a pillow behind her back for support. The woman places her fingertips on the fundus of the uterus, which is above the umbilicus (navel). She checks for contractions (hardening or tightening in the uterus) for about one hour. It is important for the pregnant woman to know that uterine contractions occur occasionally throughout the pregnancy. If they occur every ten minutes for one hour, however, the cervix could begin to dilate and labor could continue.

The nurse ensures that the woman knows when to report signs and symptoms. If contractions occur every ten minutes (or less) for one hour, if any of the other signs and symptoms are present for one hour, or if clear fluid begins leaking from the vagina, she should telephone her physician/nurse-midwife, clinic, or hospital birthing unit and make arrangements to be checked for ongoing labor.

If the woman experiences any preterm labor symptoms for more than 15 minutes while physically active, she should be instructed to do the following:

- Empty her bladder
- Lie down tilted toward her side
- Drink 3 to 4 8-oz cups of fluid
- Palpate for uterine contractions
- Rest for 30 minutes after the symptoms have subsided and gradually resume activity
- Call her health provider if symptoms persist, even if uterine contractions are not palpable (Herron 1988)

Care givers need to be aware that the woman is knowledgeable and attuned to changes in her body, and her call must be taken seriously. When a woman is at risk for preterm labor, she may have many episodes of contractions and other signs or symptoms. If she is treated positively, she will feel freer to report problems as they arise.

Other preventive measures the woman could follow are presented in Table 19–5.

Promotion of Maternal-Fetal Physical Well-Being During Labor

Provision of supportive nursing care to the woman in preterm labor is important during hospitalization. This care consists of promoting bed rest, monitoring vital signs (especially blood pressure and respirations), measuring intake and output, and continuous monitoring of FHR and uterine contractions. Placing the woman on her left side facilitates maternal-fetal circulation. Vaginal examinations are kept to a minimum. If tocolytic agents are being administered, the mother and fetus are monitored closely for any adverse effects.

Provision of Emotional Support to the Family

Whether preterm labor is arrested or proceeds, the woman and her partner experience intense psychologic stress. Decreasing the anxiety associated with the unknown and the risk of a preterm neonate is a primary aim of the nurse. The nurse also recognizes the stress of prolonged bed rest and of lack of sexual contact and helps the couple find satisfactory ways of dealing with these stresses.

Providing emotional support for the woman and her

Table 19–5	Self-Care Measures to Prevent Preterm Labor

Rest two or three times a day lying on your left side.

Drink 2 to 3 quarts of water or fruit juice each day. Avoid caffeine drinks. Filling a quart container and drinking from it will eliminate the need to keep track of numerous glasses of fluid.

Empty your bladder at least every two hours during waking hours.

Avoid lifting heavy objects. If other small children are in the home, work out alternatives for picking them up, such as sitting on a chair and having them climb on your lap.

Avoid prenatal breast preparation such as nipple rolling or rubbing nipples with a towel. This is not meant to discourage breast feeding but to avoid the potential increase in uterine irritability.

Pace necessary activities to avoid overexertion.

Sexual activity may need to be curtailed or eliminated.

Find pleasurable ways to help compensate for limitations of activities and boost the spirits.

Try to focus on one day or one week at a time rather than on longer periods of time.

If on bed rest, get dressed each day and rest on a couch rather than becoming isolated in the bedroom.

Prepared in consultation with Susan Bennett, RN, ACCE, Coordinator of the Prematurity Prevention Program.

partner during preterm labor and birth is also important. Common behavioral responses include feelings of anxiety and guilt about the possibility that the pregnancy will terminate early. With empathetic communication, the nurse can facilitate the expression of these feelings, thereby helping the couple identify and implement coping mechanisms. The nurse also keeps the couple informed about the labor progress, the treatment regimen, and the status of the fetus so that their full cooperation can be elicited. In the event of imminent vaginal or cesarean birth, the couple should be offered brief but ongoing explanations to prepare them for the actual birth process and the events following the birth.

Evaluation

Anticipated outcomes of nursing care include the following:

- The woman understands the cause, identification, and treatment of preterm labor.
- The woman's fears about early labor and birth are lessened.
- The woman feels comfortable in her ability to cope with her situation and has resources to call on.
- The woman understands self-care measures and can identify characteristics that need to be reported to her care giver.
- The woman and her baby have a safe labor and birth.

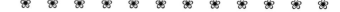

Care of the Woman with a Hypertensive Disorder

A number of hypertensive disorders can occur during pregnancy. Various attempts have been made to classify these disorders. The following classification is recommended by the American College of Obstetricians and Gynecologists (Silver 1989):

1. Pregnancy-induced hypertension (preeclampsia-eclampsia)
2. Chronic hypertension
3. Chronic hypertension with superimposed preeclampsia
4. Late or transient hypertension

Pregnancy-Induced Hypertension

Pregnancy-induced hypertension (PIH) is the most common hypertensive disorder in pregnancy, comprising up to two-thirds of the cases. It is characterized by the development of hypertension, proteinuria, and edema. Because only hypertension may be present early in the disease process, that finding is therefore the basis for diagnosis.

The definition of PIH is an increase in systolic blood pressure of 30 mm Hg and/or of diastolic of 15 mm Hg over baseline. These blood pressure changes must be noted on at least two occasions six hours or more apart for the diagnosis to be made (Sibai 1989). However, many young primigravidas have baseline blood pressures of 80 or 90 mm Hg during the second and early third trimesters of pregnancy. For these women, a blood pressure of 120/75 is relative hypertension (Sibai 1989). In the absence of baseline values, a blood pressure of 140/90 has been accepted as hypertension.

The cause of PIH remains unknown, despite much research over many decades. It has been called "the disease of theories" because so many theories have been proposed for its etiology. The condition's former name, "toxemia of pregnancy," was based on a theory that a toxin produced in a pregnant woman's body caused the disease. The term is no longer applicable, however, because the theory has not been substantiated.

Preeclampsia and eclampsia are types of PIH. **Preeclampsia** indicates that this is a progressive disease unless there is intervention to control it. **Eclampsia** means "convulsion." If a woman has a convulsion she is considered "eclamptic." Most often PIH is seen in the last ten weeks of gestation, during labor, or in the first 48 hours after childbirth. Although birth of the fetus is the only known cure for PIH, it can be controlled with early diagnosis and careful management.

PIH occurs in 6% to 7% of all pregnancies in the United States (Sibai 1989). Among black primigravidas the incidence is 15% to 20%, and in young primigravidas with twin pregnancies it is 30% (Sibai 1989). It is seen more often in primigravidas; teenagers of lower socioeconomic class; and women over 35, especially if they are primigravidas. Women with a family history of PIH are at higher risk for it, as are women with a large placental mass associated with multiple gestation, hydatidiform mole, Rh incompatibility, and diabetes mellitus.

Today PIH seldom progresses to the eclamptic state due to early diagnosis and careful management. Eclampsia is, however, the leading cause of maternal death in the United States (Gavette 1987).

Normal Physiologic Changes in Pregnancy

The following are physiologic changes that occur normally, allowing for a healthy adaptation to pregnancy.

Blood volume increases 30% to 50%. Peripheral vascular resistance decreases, and pregnancy-induced arterial dilation occurs.

The increased blood volume is necessary to perfuse the placenta and the increased tissue mass of the uterus and breasts. The higher blood volume also helps protect the fetus from impaired circulation due to maternal supine position, and it compensates for blood loss during childbirth.

The lowered peripheral vascular resistance results in lower blood pressure from the middle of the first trimester through the second trimester. Whether blood pressure should slowly return to the woman's normal in the third trimester or remain slightly below normal is still unsettled.

Pregnancy stimulates the increased production of various hormones and enzymes, which have varying and sometimes opposing effects. Plasma levels of the enzyme renin are elevated three to four times over nonpregnant levels. Renin is involved in the formation of angiotensin I, which is converted to angiotensin II. The plasma level of angiotensin II, an active vasoconstrictor, which stimulates a rise in blood pressure, is therefore also elevated. But blood pressure does not rise in normal pregnancy, because the pregnant woman develops a resistance to the pressor effects of angiotensin II by ten weeks' gestation that lasts throughout the pregnancy. This resistance is thought to be due to vasodilator prostaglandins, particularly prostacyclin, which increases during pregnancy.

Aldosterone, a potent mineralocorticoid hormone secreted by the adrenal cortex, stimulates the kidney tubules to reabsorb sodium and water. Progesterone blocks the effect of aldosterone. Progesterone levels are elevated early in pregnancy and remain so until term. The result is sodium loss by the renal tubules.

The glomerular filtration rate increases 50%. This results in faster clearance and decreased plasma levels of creatinine, urea, and uric acid and increased urine levels of these chemicals. Thus values that are considered normal for nonpregnant women may be pathologic in pregnancy.

Physiologic edema, located primarily in the ankles, is a normal occurrence during pregnancy. It is caused by the

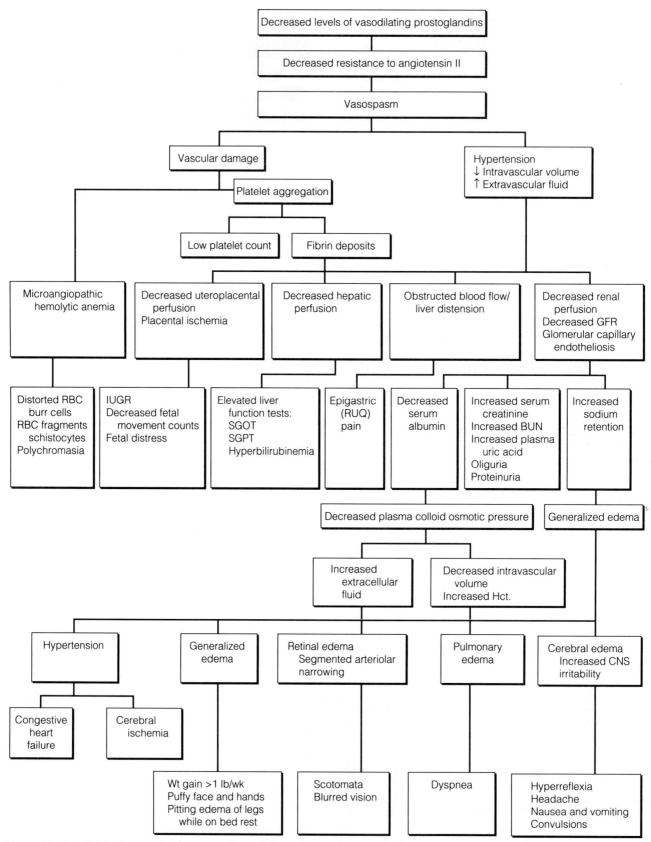

Figure 19–5   Clinical manifestations and possible pathophysiology of PIH

increased movement of fluid out of the intravascular hemo-diluted blood, with its decreased colloid osmotic pressure, into extracellular spaces. This movement is aided by increased hydrostatic pressure in the venous capillaries of the dependent limbs, due to pressure of the gravid uterus on the inferior vena cava.

Clotting factors show some change with normal pregnancy. Platelets remain in the normal range of 150,000/μL to 400,000/μL. Fibrinogen is increased, as are most other clotting factors. However, factor XIII (fibrin stabilizing factor) is decreased due to placental enzymes, which prevents an otherwise hypercoagulable state in pregnancy.

Pathophysiology of PIH

The following pathophysiologic changes are associated with PIH (see also Figure 19–5).

Blood pressure begins to rise after 20 weeks of pregnancy, probably due to a gradual loss of the normal pregnancy resistance to angiotensin II.

A finding that is probably related is that synthesis of the prostaglandin PGE$_2$ and prostacyclin (PGI$_2$) is decreased in women with PIH. The cause of this deficiency is being carefully investigated. Both PGE$_2$ and PGI$_2$ are potent vasodilators. It may be that decreases in these factors are responsible for increased sensitivity to angiotensin II and thereby responsible for most or all of the pathology associated with PIH.

The loss of normal vasodilation of uterine arterioles results in decreased placental perfusion (Figure 19–6). Fibrin deposits and ischemic areas may also be found in the placenta. The effect on the fetus may be growth retardation, decrease in fetal movement, and chronic hypoxia or fetal distress.

Decreased renal perfusion is associated with PIH. With a reduction in GFR, serum levels of creatinine, BUN, and uric acid begin to rise from normal pregnant levels, while urine output diminishes. For each 50% decrease in GFR, serum creatinine and BUN plasma levels double, while sodium is retained in increased amounts. Sodium retention results in increased extracellular volume and increased sensitivity to angiotensin II. The typical kidney lesion of PIH is swollen glomerular capillary endothelial cells containing fibrin deposits. Stretching of the capillary walls allows the large protein molecules, primarily albumin, to escape into the urine, decreasing serum albumin.

Edema is usually more profound in PIH than in normal pregnancy. Its pathologic basis is twofold:

1. The higher salt retention draws out intravascular fluid.
2. Plasma colloid osmotic pressure decreases, which causes fluid movement to extracellular spaces, due to decreased serum albumin.

The decreased intravascular volume causes increased viscosity of the blood and a corresponding rise in hematocrit.

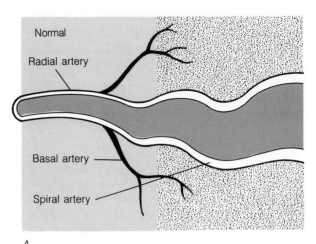

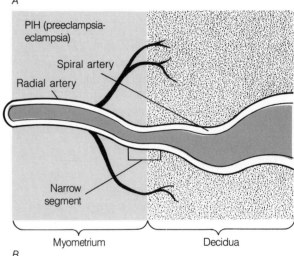

Figure 19–6 A In normal pregnancy the passive quality of the spiral arteries permits increased blood flow to the placenta. B In PIH vasoconstriction of the myometrial segment of the spiral arteries occurs.

HELLP Syndrome A syndrome called **HELLP** (*h*emolysis, *e*levated *l*iver enzymes, and *l*ow *p*latelet count) is sometimes associated with severe preeclampsia. Women who experience this multiple organ failure syndrome and their offspring have high morbidity and mortality rates (Martin et al 1990).

The hemolysis that occurs is termed *microangiopathic hemolytic anemia*. It is thought that red blood cells are distorted or fragmented during passage through small, damaged blood vessels. Elevated liver enzymes occur from blood flow that is obstructed due to fibrin deposits. Hyperbilirubinemia and jaundice may also be seen. Liver distension causes epigastric pain. Thrombocytopenia is a frequent finding in PIH. Vascular damage is associated with vasospasm, and platelets aggregate at sites of damage, resulting in low platelet count (less than 100,000).

Women with HELLP syndrome are best cared for in a tertiary care center. Initially the mother's condition should be assessed and stabilized, especially if her platelets are very low. Platelet transfusions are indicated for platelet counts below 20,000 mm³. The fetus is also assessed using a nonstress test and biophysical profile. All women with true HELLP syndrome should give birth regardless of gestational age. Labor may be induced with oxytocin in women at 32 weeks' gestation or more. At less than 32 weeks' gestation, cesarean birth is indicated (Sibai 1990).

Maternal Risks

Increased intraocular pressure due to PIH can cause retinal detachment, but spontaneous reattachment usually occurs with reduction in blood pressure and diuresis.

Central nervous system changes associated with PIH are hyperreflexia, headache, and convulsions. Hyperreflexia may be due to increased intracellular sodium and decreased intracellular potassium levels. Headaches are usually frontal and occipital, may be constant, and are caused by cerebral vasospasm. Cerebral edema and vasoconstriction are responsible for convulsions, while cerebral hemorrhage—either petechial or related to a large hematoma—is the most common cause of death following eclampsia.

Women who have preeclampsia complicated by HELLP syndrome do tend to have a somewhat longer clinical and hematologic recovery time than those who do not develop HELLP (Martin et al 1990).

Fetal-Neonatal Risks

Infants of women with hypertension during pregnancy tend to be small-for-gestational-age (SGA). The cause is related specifically to maternal vasospasm and hypovolemia, which result in fetal hypoxia and malnutrition. In addition, the newborn may be premature because of the necessity for early birth.

Perinatal mortality associated with preeclampsia is approximately 10%, and that associated with eclampsia is 20%. When preeclampsia is superimposed on chronic hypertension perinatal mortality may be higher.

At birth, the neonate may be oversedated because of medications administered to the woman. The newborn may also have hypermagnesemia due to treatment of the woman with large doses of magnesium sulfate.

Medical Therapy

The goals of medical management are prompt diagnosis of the disease; prevention of cerebral hemorrhage convulsion, hematologic complications, and renal and hepatic diseases; and birth of an uncompromised newborn as close to term as possible. Reduction of elevated blood pressure is essential in accomplishing these goals.

Clinical Manifestations and Diagnosis

Mild Preeclampsia The diagnosis of mild preeclampsia is made based on the following blood pressure findings: a rise in systolic blood pressure of 30 mm Hg or more, and/or a rise in diastolic blood pressure of 15 mm Hg or more above the baseline on two occasions at least six hours

---

Contemporary Issue
How Small Is Too Small?

Advances in medical technology and obstetric/perinatal care have influenced our perception of when a fetus is considered viable. In the past, many infants born prior to 28 weeks' gestation were considered nonviable. With aggressive perinatal management, the limits of birth weight have been progressively lowered. Now fetuses born weighing 750 to 1000 g (approximately 24 to 26 weeks' gestation) are surviving in increasing numbers. The greatest strides have been made with infants weighing over 1000 g, whose survival has doubled in the last 15 years. Many states now consider a live-born fetus viable if it is at least 20 weeks' gestation or weighs 500 g or more. This change in the definition of viability raises many questions regarding obstetric management of premature labor and delivery, decisions regarding initiation of resuscitation and provision of life support treatments, and long-term care needs. The long-term physiologic and psychologic implications for these tiny infants and their families are not known.

This dilemma has produced many philosophic, ethical, legal, and economic questions, such as the following:

- What is a reasonable definition of viability?

- Is there a need for a consensus on the lower limits of birth weight at which efforts at resuscitation will not be made?

- Should the parameters used as a guide for critical decisions involving preterm viability be gestational age or birth weight?

- Who is to be involved in the decision regarding the course of action for "nonviable" fetuses, and when is the decision to be made?

- What are the legal, ethical, social, and economic implications of the current concept of fetal viability?

apart. Blood pressure between 120/80 and 140/90 forms the lower range for mild preeclampsia. A blood pressure of 150/100 is sometimes designated as moderate preeclampsia. Generalized edema, seen as puffy face, hands, and dependent areas such as the ankles and lower legs, may be present. Edema is identified by a weight gain of more than 1.5 kg/month in the second trimester or more than 0.5 kg/week in the third trimester. Edema is assessed on a 1+ to 4+ scale. Proteinuria is often a late sign of preeclampsia. It may not be present until the disease has progressed to the severe or eclamptic stage. If proteinuria is present with mild preeclampsia, protein is generally between 300 mg/L (1+ dipstick) and 1 g/L (2+ dipstick). This is measured in a midstream clean-catch or catheter-derived urine specimen. Over a 24-hour period less than 5 g of protein would be lost in the urine.

Severe Preeclampsia   Severe preeclampsia may develop suddenly. The following clinical signs are often present:

- Blood pressure of 160/110 or higher on two occasions at least six hours apart while the woman is on bed rest
- Proteinuria ≥5 g/24 hours
- Oliguria: urine output ≤400 mL/24 hours
- Changes in laboratory values associated with severe preeclampsia. See Figure 19–4.

Other signs or symptoms that may be present include headache, blurred vision or scotomata (spots before the eyes), narrowed segments on the retinal arterioles when examined with an ophthalmoscope, retinal edema (retinas appear wet and glistening) on funduscopy, dyspnea due to pulmonary edema, moist breath sounds on auscultation, pitting edema of lower extremities while on bed rest, epigastric pain, hyperreflexia, nausea and vomiting, irritability, and emotional tension.

Eclampsia   The grand mal seizure of eclampsia may be preceded by an elevated temperature as high as 38.4C (101.0F), or the temperature may remain normal. If the temperature spikes as high as 39.4C to 40.0C (103F to 104F), it is a very serious sign. The seizure begins with facial twitching. The woman's cyes are usually wide open and staring, with dilated pupils. The convulsion has three phases. The first phase is a tonic phase. All the woman's muscles contract, her back arches, her arms and legs stiffen, and her jaw snaps shut, sometimes causing her to bite her tongue. Her respirations cease due to thoracic muscles held in contraction, and she becomes cyanotic. The tonic phase lasts 15 to 20 seconds, then the woman enters the clonic phase. Alternating forceful contraction and relaxation of all muscles causes the woman to thrash about wildly. She may remain apneic or inhale and exhale irregularly as thoracic muscles contract and relax. Saliva and blood collected in her mouth may foam out. She remains cyanotic.

Incontinence of urine and feces may occur. After about a minute the convulsive movements gradually cease and she slips into the third phase, a motionless coma that may last for less than an hour or for several hours. Respirations increase up to 50/min, and may be noisy and forceful. If the woman is not treated, the coma phase may be quite brief, and convulsions may recur in a few minutes.

Some women experience only one convulsion, especially if it occurs late in labor or during the postpartal period. Others may have from 2 to 20 or more. Unless they occur extremely frequently, the woman often regains consciousness between convulsions.

Antepartal Management   The medical therapy for PIH depends on the severity of the disease.

Mild Preeclampsia   The woman is placed on bed rest, primarily in the left lateral recumbent position, to decrease pressure on the vena cava, thereby increasing venous return, circulatory volume, and placental and renal perfusion. Improved renal blood flow helps decrease angiotensin II levels, promotes diuresis, and lowers blood pressure.

Diet should be well balanced and moderate to high in protein (80 to 100 g/day, or 1.5 g/kg/day) to replace protein lost in the urine. Sodium intake should be moderate, not to exceed 6 g/day. Excessively salty foods should be avoided, but strict sodium restriction and diuretics are no longer used in treating PIH.

Physicians are often wary about managing even mild preeclampsia on an outpatient basis because it can rapidly progress to severe preeclampsia. The woman whose blood pressure is at the lower end of the range for mild preeclampsia and who has no proteinuria may try home management. The woman and her family must understand the importance of bed rest. In such cases the woman is generally seen every one to two weeks and is carefully instructed about signs that her condition is worsening.

Tests to evaluate fetal status are done more frequently as a pregnant woman's PIH progresses. Monitoring fetal well-being is essential to achieving a safe outcome for the fetus. The following tests are used:

- Fetal movement record
- Nonstress test
- Ultrasonography for serial determination of growth
- Contraction stress test
- Serum creatinine determinations
- Amniocentesis to determine fetal lung maturity

These tests are described in detail in Chapter 20.

Severe Preeclampsia   If the uterine environment is considered detrimental to fetal growth and maturation, birth may be the treatment of choice for both mother and fetus even if the fetus is immature.

Other medical therapies for severe preeclampsia include the following:

- *Bed rest.* Bed rest must be complete. Stimuli that may bring on a convulsion should be reduced.

- *Diet.* A high-protein, moderate-sodium diet is given as long as the woman is alert and has no nausea or indication of impending convulsion.

- *Anticonvulsants.* Magnesium sulfate is the treatment of choice for convulsions. Its CNS-depressant action reduces possibility of convulsion. Blood levels of $MgSO_4$ should be maintained at therapeutic levels (levels vary according to laboratory). Excessive blood levels may produce respiratory paralysis and/or cardiac arrest. (See Drug Guide—Magnesium Sulfate.)

- *Fluid and electrolyte replacement.* The goal of fluid intake is to achieve a balance between correcting hypovolemia and preventing circulatory overload. Fluid intake may be oral or supplemented with intravenous therapy. Intravenous fluids may be started "to keep lines open" in case they are needed for drug therapy even when oral intake is adequate. Criteria vary for determining appropriate fluid intake. Electrolytes are replaced as indicated by daily serum electrolyte levels.

- *Medication.* A sedative, such as diazepam (Valium) or phenobarbital is sometimes given to encourage quiet bed rest.

- *Antihypertensives.* The vasodilator hydralazine (Apresoline) is the antihypertensive most widely used in the treatment of preeclampsia in the United States (Silver 1989). It effectively lowers blood pressure without adverse fetal effects. Hydralazine is generally given when the diastolic pressure is higher than 110 mm Hg. It may be administered either by slow intravenous push or drip methods. Hydralazine produces tachycardia; therefore the woman's pulse must be monitored with her blood pressure when she is receiving this drug. Blood pressure is measured every two to three minutes after the initial dose, and then every five to ten minutes thereafter. The diastolic pressure reading is maintained at 90 to 100 mm Hg to ensure adequate uteroplacental flow. The fetal heart tones are monitored continuously during hydralazine therapy. Hydralazine is not intended for long-term use.

Eclampsia An eclamptic seizure is an emergency situation that requires immediate, effective treatment. Therapy is aimed at controlling the convulsions, correcting any hypoxia and acidosis, lowering the blood pressure, and accomplishing birth once the mother is stabilized.

Magnesium sulfate is given intravenously to control the convulsions. Sedatives such as diazepam or amobarbital sodium are used only if the convulsions are not controlled by the magnesium sulfate. Because of their depressant effect on the fetus, they should not be given if birth is expected within an hour or two.

The lungs are auscultated for pulmonary edema. The woman is watched for circulatory and renal failure and for signs of cerebral hemorrhage. Furosemide (Lasix) may be given for pulmonary edema; digitalis for circulatory failure. Urinary output is monitored. The woman is observed for signs of placental separation (see Chapter 25). She should be checked every 15 minutes for vaginal bleeding, which may or may not be present with abruptio placentae. The abdomen is palpated for uterine rigidity. While she is still unconscious, the woman should be observed for onset of labor. Convulsions increase uterine irritability and labor may ensue. While the woman is comatose, she is kept on her side with the side rails up.

Often the woman is cared for in an intensive care unit until labor begins or is induced. Invasive hemodynamic monitoring of either central venous pressure (CVP) or pulmonary artery wedge pressure (PAWP) may be instituted using a Swan-Ganz catheter. Both these procedures carry risk to the woman and the decision to use them should be made judiciously.

When the woman's vital signs have stabilized, urinary output is good, and the maternal and fetal hypoxic and acidotic state alleviated, birth of the fetus should be considered. Birth is the only known cure for PIH. If the neonate will be preterm, it may be necessary to transfer the woman to a perinatal center for childbirth. The woman and her partner deserve careful explanation about the status of the fetus and woman, and the treatment they are receiving. Plans for childbirth and further treatment must be discussed with them.

Intrapartal Management If PIH was previously diagnosed, the labor may be induced by intravenous oxytocin when there is evidence of fetal maturity and cervical readiness. In very severe cases, cesarean birth may be necessary regardless of fetal maturity.

The woman may receive both intravenous oxytocin and $MgSO_4$ simultaneously. The woman in labor who develops a blood pressure higher than 160/110 may be given $MgSO_4$ intravenously. Because $MgSO_4$ has depressant action on smooth muscle, uterine contractions may diminish and labor may be augmented with oxytocin. Another method of inducing labor in the woman with PIH is to administer oxytocin intravenously and then during the course of labor give intravenous $MgSO_4$. Equipment and intravenous lines for both fluids must be checked frequently to ensure that they are being administered at the proper rate. Infusion pumps should be used to guarantee accuracy. Bags and tubings must be labeled carefully.

Meperidine (Demerol) or fentanyl may be given intravenously for labor. A pudendal block is often used for childbirth. An epidural block may be used if it is administered by a skilled anesthesiologist who is knowledgeable about PIH.

Childbirth in the Sims's or semi-sitting position should be considered. If the lithotomy position is used, a wedge should be placed under the right buttock to displace the uterus. The wedge should also be used if birth is by cesarean. Oxygen is administered to the woman during labor if need is indicated by fetal response to the contractions.

A pediatrician or neonatal nurse practitioner must be available to care for the newborn at birth. This care giver must be aware of all amounts and times of medication the woman has received during labor.

Postpartum Management The woman with PIH usually improves rapidly after childbirth, although seizures can still occur during the first 48 hours postpartum. For this reason, when the hypertension is severe the woman may continue to receive hydralazine or magnesium sulfate postpartally.

❀ *APPLYING THE NURSING PROCESS* ❀

Nursing Assessment

An essential part of nursing assessment is to obtain a baseline blood pressure early in pregnancy. Arterial blood pressure varies with position, being highest when the woman is sitting, intermediate when she is supine, and lowest when she is in the left lateral recumbent position. Therefore it is important that the woman be in the same position each visit when the blood pressure is measured.

Blood pressure is taken and recorded each antepartal visit. If the blood pressure rises or even if the normal slight decrease in blood pressure expected between 8 and 28 weeks of pregnancy does not occur, the woman should be followed closely.

When blood pressure and other signs indicate that the PIH has become severe, hospitalization is necessary to monitor the woman's condition closely. The nurse then assesses the following:

- *Blood pressure.* Blood pressure should be determined every two to four hours, more frequently if indicated by medication or other changes in the woman's status.

- *Temperature.* Temperature should be determined every 4 hours; every 2 hours if elevated.

- *Pulse and respirations.* Pulse rate and respiration should be determined along with blood pressure.

- *Fetal heart rate.* The fetal heart rate should be determined with the blood pressure or monitored continuously with the electronic fetal monitor if the situation indicates.

- *Urinary output.* Every voiding should be measured. Frequently, the woman will have an indwelling catheter. In this case, hourly urine output can be assessed. Output should be 700 mL or greater in 24 hours or at least 30 mL per hour.

- *Urine protein.* Urinary protein is determined hourly if an indwelling catheter is in place or with each voiding. Readings of 3+ or 4+ indicate loss of 5 g or more of protein in 24 hours.

- *Urine specific gravity.* Specific gravity of the urine should be determined hourly or with each voiding. Readings over 1.040 correlate with oliguria and proteinuria.

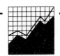

Research Note

Clinical Application of Research

In an effort to elaborate the pathway from self-diagnosis of pregnancy to enrollment in prenatal care, Ellen Patterson and her associates (1990) formulated a qualitative study. Themes that emerged from the data included different approaches to the utilization of care during pregnancy and labor and birth.

One theme to arise from the data was that of safe passage. After a period of "letting it (being pregnant) sink in," attention became focused on maintaining the health of the baby and the mother. The degree of concern paid to safe passage depended on the mother's assessment of either her degree of vulnerability or that of her child.

Searching for prenatal care, a second theme, incorporated consulting and possibly transferring. Consulting consisted of gathering information about prenatal care providers from others, such as spouse, friend, relative, or stranger. Transferring to different sources of prenatal care occurred when expectations of prenatal care were not met.

Criteria for care, another theme, encompassed financial and insurance considerations, reputation of provider or agency, quality of care, and existing relationships.

Waiting occurred before searching for care and between episodes of searching for prenatal care. This decision was an active one, with the assumption that prenatal care would be sought in the future.

Contingency planning followed a self-diagnosis of pregnancy and involved the decision not to utilize care until either initiation of labor or self-detection of a potential threat to mother or baby. This choice included self-monitoring for various deviations in health status.

Critical Thinking Applied to Research
Strengths: Interviews that were guided by the participants. Use of constant comparison to derive categories.
Concerns: Identification of seeking safe passage as the core variable or core category of the study is not clear to the reader.

Patterson E, Freese M, Goldenberg R. Seeking safe passage: Utilizing health care during pregnancy. *Image: Nurs Scholar* 1990; 22(1):27.

- *Edema.* The face (especially eyelids and cheekbone area), fingers, hands, arms (ulnar surface and wrist), legs (tibial surface), ankles, feet, and sacral area are inspected and palpated for edema. The degree of pitting is determined by pressing over bony areas.

- *Weight.* The woman is weighed daily at the same time, wearing the same robe or gown and slippers. Weighing may be omitted if the woman is to maintain strict bed rest or a bed scale may be used.
- *Pulmonary edema.* The woman is observed for coughing. The lungs are auscultated for moist respirations.
- *Deep tendon reflexes.* The woman is assessed for evidence of hyperreflexia in the brachial, wrist, patellar, or Achilles tendons (Table 19–6). The patellar reflex is the easiest to assess (Procedure 19–1). Clonus should also be assessed by vigorously dorsiflexing the foot while the knee is held in a fixed position. Normally no clonus is present. If it is present it is measured as one to four beats and is recorded as such.
- *Placental separation.* The woman should be assessed hourly for vaginal bleeding and/or uterine rigidity.
- *Headache.* The woman should be questioned about the existence and location of any headache.

Table 19–6   Deep Tendon Reflex Rating Scale

Rating	Assessment
4+	Hyperactive; very brisk, jerky, or clonic response; abnormal
3+	Brisker than average; may not be abnormal
2+	Average response; normal
1+	Diminished response; low normal
0	No response; abnormal

- *Visual disturbance.* The woman should be questioned about any visual blurring or changes, or scotomata. The results of the daily funduscopic exam should be recorded on the chart.
- *Epigastric pain.* The woman should be asked about any epigastric pain. It is important to differentiate it from

---

PROCEDURE 19–1
Assessing Deep Tendon Reflexes and Clonus

Nursing Action	**Rationale**
Objective: Assemble and prepare equipment.	
Obtain a percussion hammer. If one is not available, the side of the hand is also useful in assessing DTRs.	A percussion hammer permits accurate delivery of a brisk tap.
Objective: Prepare woman.	
Explain the procedure, indications for the procedure, and information that will be obtained. At a minimum the patellar reflex should be checked. Most nurses check a second reflex such as the biceps, triceps, or brachioradialis.	Explanation decreases anxiety and increases cooperation. Deep tendon reflexes (DTRs) are assessed to gain information about CNS status and to assess the effects of MgSO₄ if the woman is receiving it.
Objective: Elicit reflexes.	
Biceps reflex. The woman's arm is flexed at the elbow with the nurse's thumb placed on the biceps tendon. The nurse's thumb is struck in a slightly downward motion and response is assessed. Normal response is flexion of the arm.	Correct positioning and technique is essential to elicit the reflex. The correct position causes the muscle to be slightly stretched. Then when the tendon is stretched with the tap, the muscle should contract.
Patellar reflex. The woman is positioned with her legs hanging over the edge of the bed (feet should not be touching the floor). She may also lie supine with her knees slightly flexed and supported by the nurse (Figure 19-7). The nurse briskly strikes the patellar tendon, which is located just below the patella. Normal response is extension or a thrusting forward of the foot.	
Objective: Grade reflexes.	
Reflexes are graded on a scale of 1+ to 4+. See Table 19–6.	Normally reflexes are 1+ or 2+. With CNS irritation hyperreflexia may be present; with high magnesium levels reflexes may be diminished or absent.

(continued)

Nursing Action

Rationale

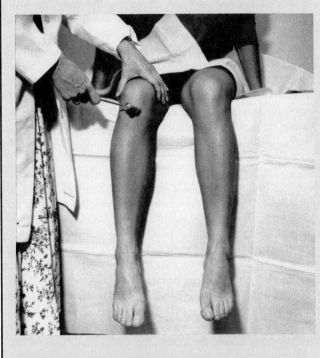

Figure 19–7   Correct position for eliciting patellar reflex. Sitting.

Objective: Assess for clonus.

With the knee flexed and the leg supported, vigorously dorsiflex the foot, maintain the dorsiflexion momentarily and then release. (Figure 19–8).

Clonus indicates more pronounced hyperreflexia and is indicative of CNS irritability.

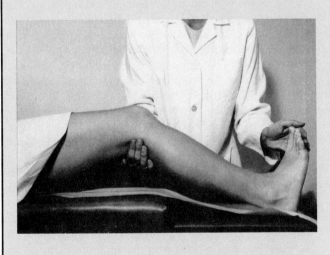

Figure 19–8   To elicit clonus, sharply dorsiflex the foot.

Normal response: The foot returns to its normal position of plantar flexion. Clonus is present if the foot "jerks" or taps against the examiner's hand. If so, the number of taps or beats of clonus is recorded.

Objective: Report and record findings.

For example: DTRs 2+, no clonus or DTRs 4+, 2 beats clonus.

Provides a permanent record.

simple heartburn, which tends to be familiar and less intense.

- *Laboratory blood tests.* Daily tests of hematocrit to measure hemoconcentration; blood urea nitrogen, creatinine, and uric acid levels to assess kidney function; clotting studies for any indication of thrombocytopenia or DIC; liver enzymes; and electrolyte levels for deficiencies are all indicated.

- *Level of consciousness.* The woman is observed for alertness, mood changes, and any signs of impending convulsion or coma.

- *Emotional response and level of understanding.* The woman's emotional response should be carefully assessed, so that support and teaching can be planned accordingly.

In addition, the nurse continues to assess the effects of any medications administered. Since the administration of prescribed medications is an important aspect of care, the nurse is, of course, familiar with the more commonly used medications, their purpose, implications, and associated untoward or toxic effects.

Nursing Diagnosis

Examples of nursing diagnoses that may apply are listed in the Key Nursing Diagnoses to Consider: Pregnancy-Induced Hypertension on p 516, and the Nursing Care Plan: Pregnancy-Induced Hypertension (PIH) beginning on p 517.

Dₓ

Key Nursing Diagnoses to Consider
Pregnancy-Induced Hypertension

Potential activity intolerance
Anxiety
Ineffective family coping
Ineffective individual coping
Diversional activity deficit
Altered family processes
Fear
Fluid volume excess (actual or potential)
Injury: High risk
Knowledge deficit
Impaired physical mobility
Noncompliance
Sexual dysfunction
Altered tissue perfusion
Self-esteem disturbance
Defensive coping
Ineffective denial
Altered role performance

Nursing Plan and Implementation

Provision of Support and Teaching A woman with PIH has several major concerns. She may fear losing the fetus. She may worry about her personal relationship with her other children and her personal and sexual relationship with her partner. She may be concerned about finances—health insurance does not always cover all the tests, prolonged hospitalization, and so on that may be associated with complications during pregnancy. Finally, the woman may be depressed or resentful about being left alone or may feel bored. If she has small children she may have difficulty providing for their care. The woman who does not have children may worry that she never will.

The nurse should identify and discuss each of these areas with the couple. It is necessary to explain to them the reasons for bed rest. A woman with mild preeclampsia may feel very well and be unable to see the need for resting even a few hours a day. The nurse can refer them to many community resources such as homemaking services, a support group for the partner, or a hot-line. Arrangements may be made for the partner to attend childbirth classes if both are not able to, or a nurse may be found to teach the classes privately.

The woman needs to know which symptoms are significant and should be reported at once. Usually the woman with mild preeclampsia is seen every one to two weeks, but she may need to come in earlier if symptoms indicate the condition is progressing. She must understand her diet plan, which must match her culture, finances, and life-style.

The development of severe preeclampsia is a cause for increased concern to the woman and her family. The woman's and her partner's most immediate concerns usually are about the prognosis for herself and the fetus. The nurse can offer honest and hopeful information. She can explain the plan of therapy and the reasons for procedures to the extent that the woman or her partner are interested. The nurse should keep the couple informed on the fetal status and should also take the time to discuss other concerns the couple may express. The nurse provides as much information as possible and seeks other sources of information or aid for the family as needed. Nurses can offer to contact a minister or hospital chaplain for additional support if the couple so chooses.

Prevention of Convulsion The nurse should maintain a quiet, low-stimulus environment for the woman. The woman should be placed in a private room in a quiet location where she can be watched closely. Visitors are limited to close family or main support persons. The woman should maintain the left lateral recumbent position most of the time, with side rails up for her protection. Unlimited phone calls are avoided because the phone ringing unexpectedly may be too jarring. To avoid a sense of isolation, however, some women find it preferable to limit calls to a certain time of the day.

(Text continues on p. 522.)

Nursing Care Plan
Pregnancy-Induced Hypertension (PIH)
(Preeclampsia-Eclampsia)

Nursing History

1. Identification of predisposing factors in client history:
   a. Primigravida
   b. Presence of diabetes mellitus
   c. Multiple pregnancy
   d. Hydramnios
   e. Gestational trophoblastic disease
   f. Preexisting vascular or renal disease
   g. Adolescent or older maternal age

Physical Examination

1. Blood pressure elevated (compared with baseline if possible)
2. Presence of edema as indicated by weight gain, puffy hands and feet; requires ongoing assessment for development of periorbital or facial edema
3. Presence of hyperreflexia and clonus
4. Presence of headache, visual disturbances, drowsiness, epigastric pain
5. Observe any vaginal bleeding, abdominal tenderness, or signs of labor

Diagnostic Studies

1. Evaluate urinary output for quantity and specific gravity.
2. Urine for urinary protein: 1 g protein/24 hr = 1–2+; 5 g protein/24 hr = 3–4+.
3. Hematocrit: Elevation of hematocrit implies hemoconcentration, which occurs as fluid leaves the intravascular space and enters the extravascular space.
4. BUN: Not usually elevated except in women with cardiovascular or renal disease.
5. Blood uric acid appears to correlate well with the severity of the preeclampsia-eclampsia (Note: Thiazide diuretics can cause significant increases in uric acid levels).

Nursing Diagnosis	Nursing Interventions	Rationale	Evaluation
Nursing Diagnosis: Fluid volume deficit related to fluid shift from intravascular to extravascular space secondary to vasospasm *Client Goal:* Fluid volume deficit will be controlled and intravascular volume will be maintained as evidenced by decreased edema, adequate urine output, normal specific gravity, decreased proteinuria, and improved hematocrit.	Assess BP every 1–4 hr, using same arm, with woman in same position. Weigh daily; gain of 1 kg/wk or more in second trimester or ½ kg/wk or more in third trimester is suggestive of PIH. Assess edema: +(1+) Minimal; slight edema of pedal and pretibial areas ++(2+) Marked edema of lower extremities	Blood pressure can fluctuate hourly; BP increases as a result of increased peripheral resistance due to peripheral vasoconstriction and arteriolar spasm. Weight gain and edema are due to sodium and water retention. Decreased plasma colloid osmotic pressure causes movement of fluid from the intravascular to extravascular space.	Woman's edema decreases, urine output remains normal, proteinuria decreases, and hematocrit is within normal limits.

(continued)

Nursing Care Plan (continued)

Nursing Diagnosis	Nursing Interventions	Rationale	Evaluation
	+++(3+) Edema of hands, face, lower abdominal wall, and sacrum ++++(4+) Anasarca with ascites		
	Maintain on bed rest. Encourage left lateral recumbent position.	Bed rest produces an increase in GFR.	
	Maintain normal salt intake (4–6 g/24 hr)	Normal salt intake is now advised, but excessive salt intake may make the condition worse.	
	Report urine output < 30 mL/hr or urine specific gravity > 1.040.	Renal plasma flow and glomerular filtration are decreased in PIH. Increasing oliguria indicates a worsening condition.	
	Test urine for protein hourly or as ordered. Maintain in-dwelling catheter.	Proteinuria results from swelling of the endothelium of the glomerular capillaries.	
	Evaluate hematocrit levels regularly.	Decreased intravascular fluid volume leads to increased hematocrit level because of change in proportion of RBCs to volume of fluid.	
	Provide adequate protein: 1.5 g/kg/24 hr for incipient and mild preeclampsia.	Plasma proteins affect movement of intravascular and extravascular fluids.	
Nursing Diagnosis: Knowledge deficit related to PIH, its treatment, and the implications for her and her unborn child *Client Goal:* Woman will clearly understand her condition and its implications as evidenced by her ability to discuss PIH and its therapy and her cooperation with the treatment regimen.	Discuss PIH, its implications for client and fetus/neonate. Explain purpose and importance of treatment measures. Work with woman and support person to plan ways for the family to deal with the woman's hospitalization.	Illness and hospitalization during pregnancy is usually unanticipated and may cause a major disruption in a couple's life. With thorough information they are better able to understand the condition and its implications.	Woman is able to discuss PIH, its therapy and implications, and she cooperates with the care regimen.

(continued)

Nursing Care Plan (continued)

Nursing Diagnosis	Nursing Interventions	Rationale	Evaluation
Nursing Diagnosis: Injury: High risk related to possibility of convulsion secondary to cerebral vasospasm or edema. *Client Goal:* Woman will not develop seizures, and signs that her condition is worsening will not develop.	Monitor knee, ankle, and biceps reflexes and clonus. Promote bed rest. Encourage woman to rest quietly in a darkened, quiet room. Limit visitors. Administer magnesium sulfate per physician order: 1. IV dose: 4 g loading dose MgSO₄ followed by continuous infusion at a rate of 2 g/hr. 2. IM dose: 10 g of 50% MgSO₄ injected deep IM (½ in the upper outer quadrants of each buttock) using a 20-gauge, 3-inch needle. (1.0 mL of 2% lidocaine may be added to the syringe to decrease the discomfort.) Monitor magnesium levels frequently to prevent overdose (either 2 hours after beginning infusion or prior to next IM dose). Before administering subsequent doses of magnesium sulfate, check reflexes (knee, ankle, biceps), respirations and urine output. Do not give magnesium sulfate if: 1. Reflexes are absent. 2. Respirations are < 12/min 3. < 100 mL urine output in past four hours Have calcium gluconate available. Maintain seizure precautions: 1. Keep room quiet, darkened.	Hyperreflexia indicates central nervous system (CNS) irritability. Rest reduces external stimuli. Magnesium sulfate is a cerebral depressant; it also reduces neuromuscular irritability and causes vasodilation and drop in BP. Therapeutic blood level is 4–7 mEq/L. Knee jerk disappears when magnesium sulfate blood levels are 7 to 10 mEq/L. Toxic signs and symptoms develop with increased blood levels; respiratory arrest can be associated with blood levels of 10 to 15 mEq/L. Cardiac arrest can occur if blood levels are 30 mEq/L. Kidneys are only route for excretion of magnesium sulfate. Calcium gluconate is antidote for magnesium sulfate. Quiet reduces stimuli.	No seizures develop; client's condition improves.

(continued)

Nursing Care Plan (continued)

Nursing Diagnosis	Nursing Interventions	Rationale	Evaluation
	2. Have emergency equipment available—O$_2$, suction, padded tongue blade.		
	3. Pad side rails.	Padding protects client.	
	4. Educate other care givers regarding the possibility of convulsions and appropriate actions.		
	Provide supportive care during convulsion:		
	1. Place tongue blade or airway in patient's mouth, if can be done without force.	Acts to maintain airway and to prevent patient from biting tongue	
	2. Suction nasopharynx as necessary.	Removes mucus and secretions	
	3. Administer oxygen.	Promotes oxygenation	
	4. Note type of seizure and length of time it lasts.	Precipitous labor may start during seizures.	
	After seizure, assess for uterine contractions.		
	Assess fetal status.	Continuous fetal monitoring is necessary to identify fetal stress.	
Nursing Diagnosis: Injury: High risk to fetus related to inadequate placental perfusion secondary to vasospasm or possible abruptio placentae.	Encourage mother to assume a side-lying position.	Side-lying position avoids pressure on vena cava and promotes optimum placental perfusion.	Fetus develops normally and IUGR is avoided. Fetus tolerates stress of labor well.
Client Goal: Fetus will tolerate the stress of maternal condition without injury as evidenced by normal intrauterine growth, reactive NST, and/or negative CST.	Evaluate results of serial fetal assessments such as NST, CST, ultrasound, biophysical profile.	Fetal assessment determines fetal status and ability to withstand stress of labor, as well as fetal maturity.	
	Report any signs of abruptio placentae such as uterine tenderness, vaginal bleeding, change in fetal activity, change in fetal heart rate, sustained abdominal pain.	Vasospasm and high blood pressure of PIH increase the risk of abruptio placentae.	

(continued)

Nursing Care Plan (continued)

Nursing Diagnosis	Nursing Interventions	Rationale	Evaluation
	If labor begins, monitor fetus closely with electronic fetal monitor. Report evidence of late decelerations.	Because of decreased placental perfusion due to vasospasm, fetus may have difficulty tolerating the stress of labor and cesarean birth may be necessary.	
Nursing Diagnosis: Injury: High risk related to development of hematologic and hepatic abnormalities secondary to the HELLP syndrome	1. Obtain blood samples as ordered to evaluate hemoglobin and hematocrit, SGOT, SGPT, and platelet count.	HELLP syndrome refers to hemolysis of RBCs (causing signs of anemia), elevated liver enzymes because of liver damage (causing jaundice, etc) and low platelet count related to severe vasospasm and developing DIC.	Woman does not develop signs of hematologic and hepatic complications.
Client Goal: Woman will not develop injury from the development of complications, as evidenced by normal hemoglobin levels, absence of signs of anemia, normal liver function tests, and adequate platelet count.	2. Monitor test results and report abnormal findings. 3. Report signs of hemolytic anemia including pallor, fatigue, anorexia, and dyspnea. 4. Report signs of liver dysfunction including nausea and vomiting, right upper quadrant pain, jaundice, and malaise. 5. Report signs of developing DIC immediately. Signs include epistaxis, hematuria, petechiae, bleeding gums, GI tract bleeding, and retinal or conjunctival hemorrhages.		

Provision of Effective Care and Support if Eclampsia Develops The occurrence of a convulsion is frightening to any family members who may be present, although the woman will not be able to recall it when she becomes conscious. Therefore, offering explanations to family members, and to the woman herself later, is essential.

When the tonic phase of the contraction begins, the woman should be turned to her side (if she is not already in that position) to aid circulation to the placenta. Her head should be turned face down to allow saliva to drain from her mouth. Attempting to insert a padded tongue blade has been questioned, but if it can be done without force, injury may be prevented to the woman's mouth. The side rails should be padded, or a pillow put between the woman and each side rail.

After 15 to 20 seconds the clonic phase starts. When the thrashing subsides, intensive monitoring and therapy begin. An oral airway is inserted, the woman's nasopharynx is suctioned, and oxygen administration is begun by nasal catheter. Fetal heart tones are monitored continuously. Maternal vital signs are monitored every 5 minutes until they are stable, then every 15 minutes.

Promotion of Maternal-Fetal Well-Being During Labor and Birth The plan of care for the woman with PIH in labor depends on both maternal and fetal condition. The woman may have mild or severe preeclampsia, may become eclamptic during labor, or may have been eclamptic before onset of labor. Therefore, careful monitoring of blood pressure and checking for edema and proteinuria are necessary for all women in labor. The prenatal record should be obtained so that current blood pressure readings may be compared with the baseline reading.

The laboring woman with PIH must receive all the care and precautions needed for normal labor as well as those required for managing PIH.

The woman with PIH in labor is kept positioned on her left side as much as possible. Both woman and fetus are monitored carefully throughout labor. Signs of progressing labor are noted. In addition, the nurse must be alert for indications of worsening PIH, placental separation, pulmonary edema, circulatory renal failure, and fetal distress.

During the second stage of labor the woman is encouraged to push while lying on her side. If she is unable to do so comfortably or effectively, she can be helped to a semisitting position for pushing and to resume the lateral position between each contraction. Birth is in the side-lying position if possible. If the lithotomy position is used, a wedge is placed under the woman's hip.

Promotion of Maternal Psychologic Well-Being During Labor and Birth A family member is encouraged to stay with the woman as long as possible throughout labor and childbirth. This is especially needed if the woman has been transferred to a high-risk center from another facility. The woman in labor and the family member or support person should be oriented to the new surroundings and kept informed of progress and plan of care. The woman should be cared for by the same nurses throughout her hospital stay.

Promotion of Maternal Well-Being During the Postpartal Period The amount of vaginal bleeding should be noted carefully. Because the woman with PIH is hypovolemic, even normal blood loss can be serious. Rising pulse rate and falling urine output are indications of excessive blood loss. The uterus should be palpated frequently and massaged when needed to keep it contracted.

Blood pressure and pulse are checked every 4 hours for 48 hours. Hematocrit may be measured daily. The woman is instructed to report any headache or visual disturbance. No ergot preparations such as methergine are given, as they have a hypertensive effect. Intake and output recordings are continued for 48 hours postpartum. Increased urinary output within 48 hours after birth is a highly favorable sign. With the diuresis, edema recedes and blood pressure returns to normal.

Postpartal depression can develop after the long ordeal of the difficult pregnancy. Family members are urged to visit, and as much mother-infant contact as possible should be allowed. There may be fears about a future pregnancy. The couple needs information about the chance of PIH occurring again. They also should be given family planning information. Oral contraceptives may be used if the woman's blood pressure has returned to normal by the time they are prescribed (usually four to six weeks postpartum).

Evaluation

Anticipated outcomes of nursing care include the following:

- The woman is able to explain PIH, its implications for her pregnancy, the treatment regimen, and possible complications.

- The woman suffers no eclamptic convulsions.

- The woman and her care givers detect evidence of increasing severity of the PIH or possible complications early so that appropriate treatment measures can be instituted.

- The woman gives birth to a healthy newborn.

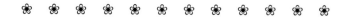

Chronic Hypertensive Disease

Chronic hypertension exists when the blood pressure is 140/90 or higher before pregnancy, or before the twentieth week of gestation or persists indefinitely following childbirth (Scott & Worley 1990). If the diastolic blood pressure is greater than 80 mm Hg during the second trimester, chronic hypertension should be suspected (Zuspan 1984). The cause of chronic hypertension has not been determined. For the majority of chronic hypertensive women the disease is mild. The goal of medical therapy is to prevent the development of preeclampsia and to ensure normal growth of the fetus. When a woman with known hypertension becomes pregnant, she should start prenatal care as soon as possible. She will need to visit her health care provider at least every two weeks during pregnancy. During the woman's initial visit the usual prenatal assessment and laboratory tests are done. Additional laboratory tests include baseline serum creatinine, BUN, serum electrolytes, urine protein, and urine culture. If the hypertension is significant, an ECG and chest x ray are done to obtain baseline values.

Ultrasound is done at 10 to 14 weeks to date the pregnancy as accurately as possible. It is done again between 20 and 26 weeks, and at 32 weeks to diagnose IUGR. Creatinine clearance is determined early in pregnancy and repeated every two months if renal disease is suspected.

In addition to these ongoing assessments, the following interventions are usually instituted:

- *Bed rest.* The woman rests for two one-hour periods, one at midday and one in the late afternoon. Bed rest, primarily in the left lateral recumbent position, is the single most important part of management of the chronic hypertensive woman during pregnancy (Zuspan 1984).
- *Diet.* Protein intake of 1.5 g/kg body weight/day is recommended if proteinuria is significant. Moderate salt intake is acceptable.
- *Medication control.* Diuretic medication is gradually eliminated if the woman was on it prior to pregnancy. Antihypertensive medication may be continued, primarily to prevent maternal complications in women with severe chronic hypertension (blood pressure > 150/110). The drug of choice is methyldopa (Aldomet) (Cunningham et al 1989).
- *Blood pressure.* The woman or her partner can monitor her blood pressure regularly and maintain a record. Home monitoring is often more accurate because the woman is more relaxed and in a familiar environment.

The primary nursing goal is to provide sufficient information so that the woman is able to meet her self-care needs. She is given information about her diet, the importance of regular rest, her medications, and the need for blood pressure control. She is taught to assess fetal movement daily during rest periods.

Chronic Hypertension with Superimposed PIH

Preeclampsia may develop in a woman previously found to have chronic hypertension. When elevations of systolic blood pressure 30 mm Hg above the baseline or of diastolic blood pressure 15 to 20 mm Hg above the baseline are discovered on two occasions at least 6 hours apart, protein-uria develops, or edema occurs in the upper half of the body, the woman needs close monitoring and careful management. Her condition often progresses quickly to eclampsia, sometimes before 30 weeks of pregnancy.

Late or Transient Hypertension

Late hypertension exists when transient elevation of blood pressure occurs during labor or in the early postpartal period, returning to normal within 10 days postpartum.

Care of the Woman at Risk for Rh Sensitization

Rh sensitization results from an antigen-antibody immunologic reaction within the body. Sensitization most commonly occurs when an Rh negative woman carries an Rh positive fetus, either to term or terminated by spontaneous or induced abortion. It can also occur if an Rh negative nonpregnant woman receives an Rh positive blood transfusion.

The red blood cells from the fetus invade the maternal circulation, thereby stimulating the production of Rh antibodies in the mother. Because this usually occurs at birth, the first offspring is not affected by these antibodies. However, in a subsequent pregnancy the mother's Rh antibodies cross the placenta and enter the fetal circulation, causing severe hemolysis. The destruction of fetal red blood cells causing anemia in the fetus is proportional to the extent of maternal sensitization (Figure 19–9).

Several forms of Rh antigen exist. The factors implicated in pathogenesis, in order of antigenic potential, are D, C, E, c, e, and, hypothetically, d (d has never been demonstrated but is thought to exist). There are many genetic combinations (genotypes) possible, such as CDE, cDe, Cde, and so forth. The D antigen is most significant clinically in that it provides the strongest stimulus to antibody formation in Rh negative people. Therefore, individuals who are homozygous for the D antigen (DD) or heterozygous (Dd) are Rh positive because the D antigen is dominant; those whose genotype is dd homozygous for the recessive antigen are Rh negative.

Approximately 87% of white Americans, 92% to 93% of black Americans, and 99% of Asian populations are Rh positive (Cunningham et al 1989). An Rh negative woman who delivers an Rh positive, ABO compatible infant has a 16% risk of becoming sensitized as a result of her pregnancy (Bowman 1985).

Fetal-Neonatal Risks

CRITICAL THINKING

Would problems arise for a fetus if the mother is Rh positive and the father is Rh negative?

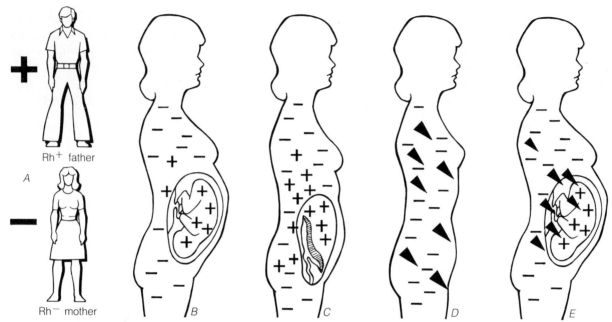

Figure 19–9   Rh isoimmunization sequence. A Rh positive father and Rh negative mother. B Pregnancy with Rh posi-tive fetus. Some Rh positive blood enters the mother's blood. C As the placenta separates, the mother is further exposed to the Rh positive blood. D The mother is sensitized to Rh positive blood; anti-Rh positive antibodies (triangles) are formed. E In subsequent pregnancies with an Rh positive fetus, Rh positive red blood cells are attacked by the anti-Rh positive maternal antibodies, causing hemolysis of red blood cells in the fetus.

Although maternal sensitization can now be pre-vented by appropriate administration of Rh immune globu-lin (RhIgG), infants still die of hemolytic disease secondary to Rh incompatibility. In the fetus, red blood cell destruc-tion leads to hyperbilirubinemia and anemia. If treatment is not initiated, this anemia can cause marked fetal edema, called **hydrops fetalis.** Congestive heart failure may re-sult, as well as marked jaundice (called *icterus gravis*), which can lead to neurologic damage (kernicterus). This severe hemolytic syndrome is known as *erythroblastosis fetalis.*

The possibility also exists that an Rh negative female fetus carried by an Rh positive mother, may become sen-sitized in utero. This female would not demonstrate signs of hemolytic disease, but since she would be sensitized be-fore even becoming pregnant she would have a positive in-direct Coombs' test when receiving prenatal care with her first Rh positive fetus.

Rh sensitization and the resultant hemolytic disease of the newborn are less common today because of the development of Rh immune globulin (RhIgG). See Chap-ter 32 for treatment of the neonate affected by Rh sensitization.

Screening for Rh Incompatibility and Sensitization

At the first prenatal visit (1) a history is taken of previous sensitization, abortions, blood transfusions, or children who developed jaundice or anemia during the neonatal pe-riod; (2) maternal blood type (ABO) and Rh factor are determined and a routine Rh antibody screen is done; and (3) presence of other medical complications such as diabe-tes, infections, or hypertension are identified.

If the woman is Rh negative (dd), the father of the unborn child is asked to come into the clinic or physician's office to be assessed for his Rh factor and blood type. If he is homozygous for Rh positive (DD), all his offspring will be Rh positive. If he is heterozygous (Dd), 50% of his off-spring can be Rh negative and 50% heterozygous for Rh positive. If the father is Rh negative, all their children will be Rh negative, and no Rh incompatibility with the mother will occur. If the father is Rh positive or the mother is known to have previously carried an Rh positive fetus, fur-ther testing and careful management are needed.

When assessment has identified the Rh negative woman who may be pregnant with an Rh positive fetus, an antibody screen (indirect Coombs' test) is done to deter-mine if the woman is sensitized (has developed isoimmu-nity) to the Rh antigen. The indirect Coombs' test mea-sures the number of antibodies in the maternal blood.

Titers should be determined monthly during the first and second trimesters, biweekly during the third trimester, and the week before the due date. If the test shows a mater-nal antibody titer of 1:16 or greater early in pregnancy, a Delta optical density (ΔOD) analysis of the amniotic fluid is performed at 26 weeks. If the titer is 1:16 or less late in pregnancy, birth at 38 weeks or spontaneous labor at term can be anticipated.

Negative antibody titers can consistently identify the fetus *not* at risk. However, the titers cannot reliably point out the fetus in danger, since the level of the titer does not correlate with the severity of the disease. For instance, in a severely sensitized woman, antibody titers may be moderately high and remain at the same level although the fetus is being more and more severely affected. Conversely, a woman sensitized by previous Rh positive fetuses may show a high fixed antibody titer during a pregnancy in which the fetus is Rh negative. Fetal assessment includes amniocentesis, amniotic fluid analysis and ultrasound.

Ultrasound should be done at 14 to 16 weeks to determine gestational age. Then serial ultrasounds and amniotic fluid analysis should be done to follow fetal progress. The presence of ascites and subcutaneous edema are signs of severe fetal involvement (Scott 1990). Other indicators of the fetal condition include an increase in fetal heart size, hydramnios, placental size and texture.

A valuable indicator of fetal status is the ΔOD analysis. The concentration of bilirubin pigments in the amniotic fluid declines during normal pregnancy. Hemolysis would result in a higher ΔOD level, which is constant or rising. Amniotic fluid, obtained by transabdominal amniocentesis, is separated from its cellular components by centrifuge. The amount of pigment from the degradation of red blood cells can be measured in the amniotic fluid. The fluid is subjected to spectrophotometric studies to determine the severity of the fetal hemolytic process. The ΔOD value and gestational age determine the plan of obstetric-pediatric management.

If the spectrophotometric readings are in zone I (A) ΔOD at 450 nm, a normal or mildly anemic neonate may be anticipated and birth at term may be permitted. Prognosis for this newborn is good, but phototherapy or exchange transfusion may be necessary. A reading in zone II (B) ΔOD at 450 nm indicates a moderately anemic fetus who may be hydropic or stillborn if born at term. Once the fetus reaches viability, induced vaginal or cesarean birth is indicated. A fair prognosis and possible need for exchange transfusion are anticipated. Readings within zone III (C) ΔOD at 450 nm indicate a severely affected fetus who may require intrauterine transfusion every 1 to 2 weeks between weeks 26 and 32 until viability is reached, followed by birth, usually by cesarean. Neonatal exchange transfusion is anticipated. Prognosis is guarded.

Fetal monitoring may identify the very ill fetus since less movement or lack of movement could be documented. The appearance of sinusoidal pattern suggests a deteriorating fetal condition (Scott 1990) (see Chapter 22).

Medical Therapy

The goal of medical management is the birth of a mature fetus who has not developed severe hemolysis in utero. This requires early identification and treatment of maternal conditions that predispose to hemolytic disease, identification and evaluation of the Rh-sensitized woman, coordinated obstetric-pediatric treatment for the seriously affected neonate, and prevention of Rh sensitization if none is present.

Antepartal Management

Two primary interventions are used by the physician to aid the fetus whose blood cells are being destroyed by maternal antibodies: early birth of the fetus and intrauterine transfusion, both of which carry risks. Ideally, birth should be delayed until fetal pulmonary maturity is confirmed at about 36 to 37 weeks. This is possible for most pregnancies with spectrophotometric readings in zones I and II (A and B).

Intrauterine transfusion is done to correct the anemia produced by the red blood cell hemolysis. The woman is admitted to the hospital, sedated, and taken to the x-ray department. The location of the placenta and the fetal position are determined by ultrasound. With the woman under local anesthesia and using fluoroscopy, a plastic catheter (threaded through a 15-gauge, 18-cm, Touhy needle) is introduced through the abdomen and the intrauterine space into the fetal peritoneal cavity. A small air bubble is injected to verify that the needle is in the fetal abdomen. About 100 mL of type O, Rh negative, packed red blood cells, which have been cross-matched against the mother's serum, is transfused into the fetus. Diaphragmatic lymphatics absorb the red blood cells into the fetal circulation. Repeat transfusions can be scheduled as necessary until the fetus is sufficiently mature to tolerate birth.

About 80% to 90% of transfused fetuses survive. The procedure is hazardous to the fetus, however (Scott 1990). In addition to the 8% to 20% possibility of fetal death, direct trauma to the fetus with the needles and catheter is possible. Maternal complications are few; those that occur are usually due to bleeding or infection. Birth is delayed until at least 32 weeks' gestation if possible. Premature newborns are generally more susceptible to damage from hemolytic disease. They often require exchange transfusion and usually require intensive nursery care.

Only fetuses between 23 and 32 weeks with a prognosis of death as indicated by the Delta optical density amniotic readings should be given intrauterine transfusion (Cunningham et al 1989). The procedure should be done before hydrops develops because the red blood cells injected into the fetal peritoneal cavity will be absorbed more slowly by the hydropic fetus. However, if ascites has already developed, the fetus should still be transfused since it has a better chance of survival with the transfusion than without it.

Postpartal Management

The goals of postpartal care are to prevent sensitization in the as-yet-unsensitized pregnant woman and to treat the isoimmune hemolytic disease in the newborn.

The Rh negative mother who has no titer (indirect Coombs' negative, nonsensitized) and who has given birth to an Rh positive fetus (direct Coombs' negative) is given an intramuscular injection of 300 μg RhIgG globulin (**Rho-**

GAM®, Hyp Rho-D®, Win Rho®) within 72 hours so that she does not have time to produce antibodies to fetal cells that entered her bloodstream when the placenta separated. RhIgG works to destroy the fetal cells in the maternal circulation before sensitization occurs, thereby blocking maternal antibody production. This provides temporary passive immunity for the mother, which prevents the development of permanent active immunity (antibody formation).

The normal dose of RhIgG should suppress the immune response to approximately 30 mL Rh positive whole blood. However, if a larger fetomaternal bleed may have occurred, a Betke-Kleihauer test can be performed. This test is used to obtain an estimate of the size of a fetomaternal bleed. Based on the findings, an additional 300 μg of RhIgG is given for every 25 mL of fetal blood in the woman's circulation. Thus a 300 μg dose should be given every 12 hours until the total necessary dose is given (Scott 1990).

When the woman is Rh negative and not sensitized and the father is Rh positive or unknown, RhIgG is also given after each abortion, ectopic pregnancy, or amniocentesis. If abortion or ectopic pregnancy occurs in the first trimester, a smaller (50 μg) dose of RhIgG (MICRhoGAM® or Mini-Gamulin Rh®) is used. A full dose is used following second trimester amniocentesis. Since transplacental hemorrhage is possible during pregnancy, RhIgG is generally administered prophylactically at 28 weeks' gestation to prevent sensitization. RhIgG is not given to the neonate or the father. It is not effective for and should not be given to a previously sensitized woman. However, sometimes after childbirth or an abortion, the results of the blood test do not clearly show whether or not the mother is already sensitized to the Rh antigen. In such cases, RhIgG should be given, as it will cause no harm. Table 19–7 summarizes the major considerations in caring for an Rh negative woman. The treatment of the newborn with isoimmune hemolytic disease is discussed in Chapter 32.

✣ *APPLYING THE NURSING PROCESS* ✣

Nursing Assessment

As part of the initial prenatal history the nurse asks the mother if she knows her blood type and Rh factor. Many women are aware that they are Rh negative and that this status has implications for pregnancy. If the woman knows she is Rh negative, the nurse can assess the woman's knowledge of what that means. The nurse can also ask the woman if she ever received RhIgG, if she has had any previous pregnancies and their outcome, and if she knows her partner's Rh factor. Should the partner be Rh negative, there is no risk to the fetus, who will also be Rh negative.

If the woman does not know what Rh type she is, intervention cannot begin until the initial laboratory data are obtained. Once that is done, the nurse plans interventions based on the findings.

If the woman becomes sensitized during her pregnancy, nursing assessment focuses on the knowledge level

---

Table 19–7 Rh Sensitization

When trying to work through Rh problems, the nurse should remember the following:

- A potential problem exists when an Rh⁻ mother and an Rh⁺ father conceive a child that is Rh⁺.

- In this situation, the mother may become sensitized or produce antibodies to her fetus' Rh⁺ blood.

The following tests are used to detect sensitization:

- Indirect Coombs' tests—done on the mother's blood to measure the number of Rh⁺ antibodies.

- Direct Coombs' test—done on the infant's blood to detect antibody-coated Rh⁺ RBCs.

Based on the results of these tests, the following may be done:

- If the mother's indirect Coombs' test is negative and the infant's direct Coombs' test is negative, the mother is given RhIgG within 72 hours of birth.

- If the mother's indirect Coombs' test is positive and her Rh⁺ infant has a positive direct Coombs' test, RhIgG is *not* given; in this case, the infant is carefully monitored for hemolytic disease.

- It is recommended that RhIgG be given at 28 weeks antenatally to decrease possible transplacental bleeding concerns.

- RhIgG is also administered after each abortion (spontaneous or therapeutic), ectopic pregnancy, or amniocentesis.

---

and coping skills of the woman and her family. The nurse also provides ongoing assessment during procedures to evaluate fetal well-being, such as ultrasound and amniocentesis.

Postpartally, the nurse reviews data about the Rh type of the fetus. If the fetus is Rh positive, the mother is Rh negative, and no sensitization has occurred, nursing assessment reveals the need to administer RhIgG.

Nursing Diagnosis

Nursing diagnoses that might apply include the following:

- Knowledge deficit related to a lack of understanding of the need to receive RhIgG and when it should be administered

- Ineffective individual coping related to depression secondary to the development of indications of the need for fetal exchange transfusion

Nursing Plan and Implementation

During the antepartal period the nurse explains the mechanisms involved in isoimmunization and answers any questions the woman and her partner may have. It is imperative that the woman understand the importance of receiving RhIgG after every spontaneous or therapeutic abortion or ectopic pregnancy if she is not already sensitized. The nurse also explains the purpose of the RhIgG administered at 28 weeks if the woman is not sensitized.

If the woman is sensitized to the Rh factor, it poses a threat to any Rh positive fetus she carries. The nurse provides emotional support to the family to help them deal with their grief and any feelings of guilt about the infant's condition. Should an intrauterine transfusion become necessary, the nurse continues to provide emotional support while also assuming his or her responsibilities as part of the health care team.

During labor the nurse caring for an Rh negative woman who has not been sensitized ensures that the woman's blood is assessed for any antibodies and also has been cross-matched for RhIgG. On the postpartum unit the nurse generally is responsible for administering the RhIgG (see Procedure 19–2).

Evaluation

Anticipated outcomes of nursing care include the following:

- The woman is able to explain the process of Rh sensitization and its implications for her unborn child and for subsequent pregnancies.

- If the woman has not been sensitized, she is able to explain the importance of receiving RhIgG when necessary and cooperates with the recommended dosage schedule.

- The woman gives birth to a healthy newborn.

- If complications develop for the fetus (or newborn) they are detected quickly and therapy is instituted.

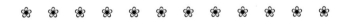

Care of the Woman at Risk Due to ABO Incompatibility

ABO incompatibility is rather common (occurring in 12% of pregnancies) but rarely causes significant hemolysis. In most cases ABO incompatibility is limited to type O mothers with a type A or B fetus. The group B fetus of an A mother and the group A fetus of a B mother are only occasionally affected. Group O infants, because they have no antigenic sites on the red blood cells, are never affected regardless of the mother's blood type. The incompatibility occurs as a result of the maternal antibodies present in her serum and interaction between the antigen sites on the fetal red blood cells.

Anti-A and anti-B antibodies are naturally occurring; that is, women are naturally exposed to the A and B antigens through the foods they eat and through exposure to infection by gram-negative bacteria. As a result, some women have high serum anti-A and anti-B titers before they become pregnant. Once the woman becomes pregnant, the maternal serum anti-A and anti-B antibodies cross the placenta and produce hemolysis of the fetal red blood cells.

With ABO incompatibility the first infant is frequently involved, and no relationship exists between the appearance of the disease and repeated sensitization from one pregnancy to the next.

Unlike in Rh incompatibility, treatment is never warranted antepartally. As part of the initial assessment, however, the nurse should note whether the potential for an ABO incompatibility exists. This alerts care givers so that following birth the newborn can be assessed carefully for the development of hyperbilirubinemia (see Chapter 32).

Care of the Woman Requiring Surgery During Pregnancy

While elective surgery should be delayed until the postpartal period, essential surgery can generally be undertaken during pregnancy. Surgery does pose some risks. The incidence of spontaneous abortion is increased for women who have surgery in the first trimester. There is also an increased incidence of fetal mortality and of low-birth-weight (less than 2500 gm) infants. Finally, when pelvic surgery is necessary the incidence of premature labor and intrauterine growth retardation increases (Mazze & Källén 1989).

Medical Therapy

Although general preoperative and postoperative care is similar for gravid and nongravid women, special considerations must be kept in mind whenever the surgical client is pregnant. The early second trimester is the best time to operate because there is less risk of causing spontaneous abortion or early labor, and the uterus is not so large as to impinge on the abdominal field.

The preoperative chest radiograph and electrocardiogram, which are routine for persons over age 40, should be done on the same basis for the pregnant woman. If a chest radiograph is done, the fetus should be shielded from the radiation. Because of decreased intestinal motility and decreased free gastric acid secretion during pregnancy, stomach emptying time is delayed, which increases risk of vomiting during induction of anesthesia and during the postoperative period. Therefore, a nasogastric tube is recommended prior to major surgery. An indwelling urinary catheter prevents bladder distention, decreases risk of injury to the bladder, and promotes ease of monitoring output. Support stockings during and after surgery help prevent venous stasis and the development of thrombophlebitis. Fetal heart tones must be monitored before, during, and after surgery.

Pregnancy causes increased secretions of the respiratory tract and engorgement of the nasal mucous membrane, often making breathing through the nose difficult. Because of this pregnant women often need an endotracheal tube for respiratory support during surgery. Care

Administration of RhIgG
(RhoGAM, HypRho-D, Win Rho)

Nursing Action	Rationale
Objective: Confirm that RhIgG immune globulin is indicated.	
Confirm that mother is Rh negative by checking her prenatal or intrapartal record. Then confirm that sensitization has not occurred—maternal indirect Coombs' negative.	Sensitization occurs when an Rh negative woman is exposed to Rh positive blood. She develops antibodies to the Rh positive blood. These antibodies can attack the fetal red blood cells causing profound anemia. If both the direct and indirect Coombs' tests are negative, sensitization has not occurred and RhIgG immune globulin (RhIgG is indicated.
Confirm that infant is Rh positive. (A sample of the infant's cord blood is generally sent to the lab immediately after birth for typing and cross-matching.) If infant is Rh positive, confirm that sensitization has not occurred—direct Coombs' negative.	
Objective: Confirm that the woman does not have a history of allergy to immune globulin preparations.	
Review entries on medication allergies in client chart and ask woman specifically whether she has had any allergic reactions to medications, globulins, or blood products.	RhIgG immune globulin is made from the plasma portion of blood. Allergic reactions are possible.
Objective: Explain purpose and procedure. Have consent signed.	
Many agencies require informed consent before administering RhIgG immune globulin.	The woman should clearly understand the purpose of the procedure, its rationale, and the procedure itself, including any risks. Generally the primary side effects are erythema and tenderness at the injection site and allergic responses.
Objective: Obtain correct medication.	
RhIgG is available from the blood bank or pharmacy according to agency policy. Lot numbers for the drug and the cross match should be the same.	Because blood products are involved in the preparation careful verification is essential.
Objective: Confirm client identity and administer medication in deltoid muscle.	
Medication is administered intramuscularly within 72 hours of childbirth. The normal dose of 300 mg provides passive immunity following exposure of up to 15 mL of transfused RBCs. If a larger bleed is suspected (as in cases of severe abruptio placentae) additional doses may be administered at one time using multiple sites, or at regular intervals, as long as all doses are given within 72 hours of childbirth.	The medication causes passive immunity to occur and "tricks" the body into believing that it is not necessary to develop antibodies. Immunization is indicated any time there is a potential for maternal exposure to Rh positive blood. It is given prophylactically at 28 weeks' gestation, within 72 hours after the birth of an Rh positive Coombs' negative child, and following any spontaneous or therapeutic abortion, ectopic pregnancy, or amniocentesis.
Objective: Complete education for self-care.	
Provide opportunities for the woman to ask questions and express concerns.	Many women, especially primigravidas, are not aware of the risks for an Rh positive fetus of a sensitized Rh negative mother. They must understand the importance of receiving medication for each pregnancy to ensure continued protection.
Objective: Complete client record.	
Chart according to agency procedure. Most agencies chart lot number, route, dose, client education.	Provides a permanent record.

givers must guard against maternal hypoxia during surgery as uterine circulation will be decreased and fetal oxygenation can decline very quickly. During surgery and the recovery period the woman is positioned to allow optimal utero-placental-fetal circulation. A wedge is placed under her hip to tip the uterus and thereby avoid pressure by the fetus on the maternal vena cava.

Spinal or epidural anesthesia may produce hypotension and respiratory apnea in the pregnant woman. The frequency and degree of the hypotension increase with higher anesthetic levels. This can be prevented in many cases with a preanesthetic infusion of 900 to 1000 mL of fluid.

Blood loss during surgery is monitored carefully. Measurement of fetal heart tones gives the best indication of blood loss. Because of the normal increased blood volume of pregnancy, uterine blood flow may be reduced significantly before the maternal blood pressure begins to fall. Fluid replacement should be done with balanced electrolyte solution and, if needed, with whole blood.

❀ *APPLYING THE NURSING PROCESS* ❀

Nursing Assessment

During the preoperative period the nurse assesses the pregnant woman's health status in the same way that any preoperative client is assessed. Is there any sign of respiratory infection, fever, urinary tract infection, or anemia? Are laboratory values all within normal limits for surgery (except in the case of emergency surgery, which may, of necessity, be done even with abnormal laboratory values)? Do the woman and her family understand the surgical procedure? Do they know what to expect postoperatively? Do they have any questions or concerns?

The nurse also considers the impact of surgery on the woman's pregnancy. Is the fetal heart rate normal? Does the woman understand the implications of surgery with regard to her pregnancy? How is she coping?

Postoperatively the nurse completes all necessary postoperative assessments and also continues to assess fetal status, primarily by monitoring the fetal heart rate.

Nursing Diagnosis

Nursing diagnoses that might apply to the pregnant woman who requires surgery include the following:

- Altered tissue perfusion (fetal) related to the effects of general anesthesia on fetal oxygenation
- Anxiety related to lack of knowledge of preoperative and postoperative procedures

Nursing Plan and Implementation

Much of the nurse's care during the preoperative period is directed toward the educational needs of the woman and her family. The nurse plans time to review the procedure and answer any questions the family may have. The nurse recognizes that the need for surgery during the woman's pregnancy is probably very distressing for the family. The nurse works to help decrease their anxiety by providing information and emotional support.

Postoperatively the nurse is caring for two clients: the mother and her unborn child. In addition to monitoring the status of both, the nurse considers both in providing care. If surgery is done in the first trimester, the nurse should be aware of the potential teratogenic effect of any medications prescribed and should discuss the implications with the surgeon and obstetrician. During the third trimester the nurse, recognizing the potential for vena caval syndrome if the woman lies flat on her back, helps the woman maintain a side-lying position. To avoid inadequate oxygenation the nurse also encourages the woman to turn, breathe deeply, and cough regularly and also to use any ventilation therapy, such as incentive spirometry, to avoid developing pneumonia. The pregnant woman is also at increased risk for thrombophlebitis, so the nurse applies antiembolism stockings, encourages leg exercises while the woman is confined to bed, and begins ambulation as soon as possible. The nurse also encourages the woman to maintain or resume an adequate diet as soon as possible. If cultural factors influence the woman's dietary practices, the nurse and dietitian should work together to meet the woman's needs.

Discharge teaching is especially important. The woman and her family should have a clear understanding of what to expect regarding activity level, discomfort, diet, medications, and any special considerations. In addition they should know any warning signs that they should report to their physician immediately.

Evaluation

Anticipated outcomes of nursing care include the following:

- The woman is able to explain the surgical procedure, its risks and benefits, and its implications for her pregnancy.
- Care givers maintain adequate oxygenation throughout surgery and postoperatively.
- Potential complications are avoided or detected early and treated successfully.
- The woman is able to describe any necessary post-discharge activities, limitations, and follow-up and agrees to cooperate with the recommended regimen.
- The woman maintains her pregnancy successfully.

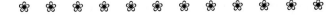

Care of the Woman Suffering Trauma from an Accident

Accidents and injury are not uncommon during pregnancy. Accidental injury may complicate 8% of all pregnancies (Goodwin & Breen 1990). In early pregnancy body changes increase the potential for injury through fatigue, fainting spells, and hyperventilation. Late in pregnancy the woman has less balance and coordination and may fall. Her protruding abdomen is vulnerable to a variety of minor injuries. The fetus is usually well protected by the amniotic fluid, which distributes the force of a blow equally in all directions, and by the muscle layers of the uterus and abdominal wall. In early pregnancy, while the uterus is still in the pelvis it is shielded from blows by the surrounding pelvic organs, muscles, and bony structures. Trauma that causes concern includes blunt trauma, from an automobile accident, for example; penetrating abdominal injuries, such as knife and gunshot wounds; and the complications of maternal shock, premature labor, and spontaneous abortion.

Maternal mortality most often occurs from head trauma or hemorrhage. Uterine rupture may result from strong deceleration forces in an automobile accident with or without seat belts. However, seat belts worn low under the abdomen are recommended. Traumatic separation of the placenta can occur; it results in a high rate of fetal mortality. Premature labor is another serious hazard to the fetus, often following rupture of membranes during an accident. Premature labor can ensue even if the woman is not injured.

Maternal fractures, even of the pelvis, are tolerated well. However, ruptured bladder, retroperitoneal hemorrhage, and shock are complications to watch for with a fractured pelvis.

Complications caused by trauma are more common after assault than after motor vehicle accidents. Fetal or placental injury occurs in 89% of gunshot wounds to the abdomen, with a 66% chance of perinatal mortality. Stab wounds tend to cause less damage than bullet wounds.

Medical Therapy

The goal of medical therapy is to stabilize the injury and promote well-being for both mother and fetus. Thus medical therapy initially focuses on ensuring airway adequacy, maintaining ventilation and adequate circulatory volume, controlling acute bleeding, and splinting fractures to prevent vascular or tissue injury.

Care must be taken at the scene of the injury to avoid the development of supine hypotensive syndrome. A wedge is generally placed under the woman's right hip. A neck brace is used if a neck injury is suspected, or the woman is placed on a backboard and the entire board is tilted to displace the uterus. Prompt treatment of maternal hypotension or hypovolemia also averts poor fetal oxygenation.

Obstetric consultation is necessary to ensure that the needs of both mother and fetus are met. The woman should undergo fetal monitoring for a minimum of 30 minutes. RhIgG should be given to Rh negative mothers. If the woman has bleeding, uterine contractions or uterine tenderness, a 24-hour observation is recommended because there is a 20% possibility of adverse effects on the pregnancy (Goodwin & Breen 1990). If the mother does not survive, and the fetus is at more than 28 weeks' gestation, a rapid cesarean may result in a live child.

❧ *APPLYING THE NURSING PROCESS* ❧

Nursing Assessment

Each individual must be assessed according to the type and extent of her injuries. As with all trauma victims, initial assessments focus on adequacy of the airway, evidence of breathing, existence of cardiovascular stability, and extent of injury. When an injured woman is pregnant, it is necessary to assess fetal status as well in order to avoid fetal hypoxia. Frequent maternal blood gas determinations are indicated if respiratory function is compromised.

Assessment should include a review of the specific history of past and present pregnancies to avoid incorrect interpretation of vital signs. Care givers do diagnostic tests as necessary, avoiding radiology in favor of ultrasonography whenever possible.

Ongoing assessments include evaluation of intake and output and other indicators of shock, determination of neurologic status, and assessment of mental outlook and anxiety level.

Nursing Diagnosis

Nursing diagnoses that might apply include the following:

- Pain related to the effects of the trauma experienced
- Constipation related to immobility secondary to the effects of the accident
- Fear related to the effects of the trauma on fetal well-being

Nursing Plan and Implementation

As a member of the health care team the nurse is actively involved in the ongoing assessment of the status of the woman and fetus. The nurse also has a primary responsibility to assess the childbearing woman's emotional state. The trauma victim must be oriented to her situation and receive explanation and reinforcement as necessary to help her understand any interventions. Family members should be involved as appropriate. The nurse also gives the pregnant woman an opportunity to discuss her feelings and concerns.

Evaluation

Anticipated outcomes of nursing care include the following:

- The woman and her family are able to understand the effects of the trauma on her and on her unborn child.
- Adequate oxygenation is maintained to promote fetal well-being.
- The woman's pain is adequately relieved and her trauma is treated.
- Potential complications are quickly identified and appropriate interventions are instituted.
- The woman gives birth to a healthy newborn.
- If the trauma results in fetal demise, the woman is able to verbalize her feelings and begin working through the grief process.

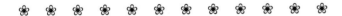

Care of the Battered Pregnant Woman

Domestic violence is an "overwhelming moral, economic, and public health burden" according to former Surgeon General C. Everett Koop (ACOG 1989). Such violence often begins or increases during pregnancy. It may result in loss of pregnancy, preterm labor, low-birth-weight infants, injury to the fetus, and fetal death (Bohn 1990). The first step toward helping the battered woman is to identify her. She needs support, confidence in her decision making, and the recognition that she can help herself.

Chronic psychosomatic symptoms can be an indicator of abuse. The woman may have nonspecific or vague complaints. It is important to assess old scars around the head, chest, arms, abdomen, and genitalia. Any bruising or evidence of pain is also evaluated. Other indicators include a decrease in eye contact, silence when the partner is in the room, and a history of nervousness, insomnia, drug overdose, or alcohol problems. Frequent visits to the emergency room and a history of accidents without understandable causes are possible indicators of abuse.

The goals of treatment are to identify the woman at risk, increase her decision-making abilities to decrease the potential for further abuse, and provide a safe environment for the pregnant woman and her unborn child.

It is important to provide an environment that is private, accepting, and nonjudgmental so the woman can express her concerns. She needs to be aware of community resources available to her, such as emergency shelters; police, legal, and social services; and counseling (Bohn 1990). Nurses need to recognize that, ultimately, it is the woman's decision to either seek assistance or return to old patterns. Sometimes it is difficult for nurses to avoid feeling angry or personally rejected if a woman returns to an abusive situation.

Care of the Woman with a TORCH Infection

The TORCH group of infectious diseases are those identified as causing serious harm to the embryo-fetus. These are: toxoplasmosis (*TO*), rubella (*R*), cytomegalovirus (*C*), and herpesvirus type 2 (*H*). (Some sources identify the *O* as "other infections.") The TORCH identification assists health team members to assess quickly the potential risk to each woman in pregnancy.

The importance of understanding what these infections are and identifying risk factors cannot be overemphasized. Exposure of the woman during the first 12 weeks of gestation may cause developmental anomalies. The three major viral infections are rubella, cytomegalovirus, and herpesvirus type 2. Toxoplasmosis is a protozoal infection.

Toxoplasmosis

Toxoplasmosis is caused by the protozoan *Toxoplasma gondii*. It is innocuous in adults, but when contracted in pregnancy, it can profoundly affect the fetus. The pregnant woman may contract the organism by eating raw or poorly cooked meat or by contact with the feces of infected cats, either through the cat litter box or by gardening in areas frequented by cats. The percentage of childbearing women in North America who are seropositive for toxoplasmosis varies, but in some areas 85% are at risk of infection. In Canada, serologic surveys have shown rates in pregnant women to be about 40% (McDonald et al 1990).

Fetal-Neonatal Risks

The incidence of abortion, prematurity, stillbirths, neonatal deaths, and severe congenital anomalies is increased in the affected fetus and neonate. In very mild cases, retinochoroiditis may be the only recognizable damage, and it and other manifestations may not appear until adolescence or young adulthood. Severe neonatal disorders associated with congenital infection include convulsions, coma, microcephaly, and hydrocephalus. The infant with a severe infection may die soon after birth. Survivors are often blind, deaf, and severely retarded.

Medical Therapy

The goal of medical treatment is to identify the woman at risk for toxoplasmosis and to treat the disease promptly if diagnosed. Diagnosis can be made by serologic testing, including the IgM fluorescent antibody test. Elevated titers peak one month after infection and are usually present for four to eight months, although they may persist for a year.

Other tests include the Sabin-Feldman dye test and the indirect fluorescent antibody test.

If diagnosis can be established by physical findings, history, and positive serologic results, the woman may be treated with sulfadiazine, pyrimethamine, and spiramycin. If toxoplasmosis is diagnosed before 20 weeks' gestation, therapeutic abortion should be considered because damage to the fetus is generally more severe than if the disease is acquired later in the pregnancy.

❀ *APPLYING THE NURSING PROCESS* ❀

Nursing Assessment

The incubation period for the disease is ten days. The woman with acute toxoplasmosis may be asymptomatic, or she may develop myalgia, malaise, rash, splenomegaly, and enlarged posterior cervical lymph nodes. Symptoms usually disappear in a few days or weeks.

Nursing Diagnosis

Nursing diagnoses that might apply to the pregnant woman with toxoplasmosis include the following:

- Altered health maintenance: High risk related to lack of knowledge about ways in which a pregnant woman can contract toxoplasmosis
- Grieving related to potential effects on infant of maternal toxoplasmosis

Nursing Plan and Implementation

The nurse caring for women during the antepartal period has the primary opportunity to discuss methods of prevention of toxoplasmosis with the childbearing woman. The woman must understand the importance of avoiding poorly cooked or raw meat, especially pork, beef, lamb, and, in the arctic region, caribou. Fruits and vegetables should be washed. She should avoid contact with the cat litter box by having someone else clean it. In addition, since it takes approximately 48 hours for the cat's feces to become infectious, the litter should be cleaned frequently. The nurse should also discuss the importance of wearing gloves when gardening and of avoiding garden areas frequented by cats.

Evaluation

Anticipated outcomes of nursing care include the following:

- The woman is able to discuss toxoplasmosis, its methods of transmission, the implications for her fetus, and measures she can take to avoid contracting it.
- The woman implements health measures to avoid contracting toxoplasmosis.
- The woman gives birth to a healthy newborn.

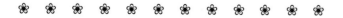

Rubella

The effects of rubella (German measles) are no more severe, nor are there greater complications in pregnant women than in nonpregnant women of comparable age. But the effects of this infection on the fetus and neonate are great, because rubella causes a chronic infection that begins in the first trimester of pregnancy and may persist for months after birth.

An assessment of risk factors (Kaplan et al 1990) showed that first-time mothers were at highest risk of infection, while 39% of women giving birth to infants with congenital rubella syndrome (CRS) had had at least one previous live birth. Young, black and Hispanic first-time mothers are at higher risk for bearing an infant with CRS. Therefore nurses need to be aware of the importance of postpartum immunization to decrease unnecessary perinatal transmission. These figures also emphasize the need for routine immunization programs in the total population, targeting the high-risk populations (young, black, Hispanic, and immigrants from Southeast Asia).

Fetal-Neonatal Risks

The period of greatest risk for the teratogenic effects of rubella on the fetus is during the first trimester. If infection occurs during the first 4 weeks of pregnancy, damage or death occurs in 50% of the affected embryos. In the second month, 25% of affected fetuses may have serious defects, and if infection occurs in the third month, 15% of fetuses are affected (Cunningham et al 1989). If infection occurs early in the second trimester, the resultant fetal effect is most often permanent hearing impairment.

Clinical signs of congenital infection are congenital heart disease, IUGR, and cataracts. Cardiac involvements most often seen are patent ductus arteriosus and narrowing of peripheral pulmonary arteries. Cataracts may be unilateral or bilateral and may be present at birth or develop in the neonatal period. A petechial rash is seen in some infants, and hepatosplenomegaly and hyperbilirubinemia are frequently seen. Other abnormalities, such as mental retardation or cerebral palsy, may become evident in infancy. Diagnosis in the neonate can be conclusively made in the presence of these conditions and with an elevated rubella IgM antibody titer at birth.

Infants born with congenital rubella syndrome are infectious and should be isolated. These infants may continue to shed the virus for months.

The expanded rubella syndrome relates to effects that may develop for years after the infection. These include an increased incidence of insulin-dependent diabetes mellitus; sudden hearing loss; glaucoma; and a slow, progressive form of encephalitis.

Medical Therapy

The best therapy for rubella is prevention. Live attenuated vaccine is available and should be given to all children. Women of childbearing age should be tested for immunity and vaccinated if susceptible and if it is established that they are not pregnant. Health counseling in high school and in premarital clinic visits can emphasize the importance of screening prior to planning a pregnancy.

As part of the prenatal laboratory screen the woman is evaluated for rubella using hemagglutination inhibition (HAI), a serology test. The presence of a 1:16 titer or greater is evidence of immunity. A titer less than 1:8 indicates susceptibility to rubella.

Because the vaccine is made with attenuated virus, pregnant women are not vaccinated. However, it is considered safe for newly vaccinated children to have contact with pregnant women.

If a woman who is pregnant becomes infected during the first trimester, therapeutic abortion is an alternative.

❀   *APPLYING THE NURSING PROCESS*   ❀

Nursing Assessment

A woman who develops rubella during pregnancy may be asymptomatic or may show signs of a mild infection including a maculopapular rash, lymphadenopathy, muscular achiness, and joint pain. The presence of IgM antirubella antibody is diagnostic of a recent infection. These titers remain elevated for approximately one month following infection.

Nursing Diagnosis

Nursing diagnoses that may apply to the woman who develops rubella early in her pregnancy include the following:

- Ineffective family coping due to an inability to accept the possibility of fetal anomalies secondary to maternal rubella exposure
- Altered health maintenance: High risk related to lack of knowledge about the importance of rubella immunization prior to becoming pregnant

Nursing Plan and Implementation

Provision of Information and Emotional Support

Nursing support and understanding are vital for the couple contemplating abortion due to a diagnosis of rubella. Such a decision may initiate a crisis for the couple who have planned their pregnancy. They need objective data to understand the possible effects on their unborn fetus and the prognosis for the offspring.

Evaluation

Anticipated outcomes of nursing care include the following:

- The woman is able to describe the implications of rubella exposure during the first trimester of pregnancy.

- If exposure occurs in a woman who is not immune, she is able to identify her options and make a decision about continuing her pregnancy that is acceptable to her and her partner.
- The nonimmune woman receives the rubella vaccine during the early postpartal period.
- The woman gives birth to a healthy infant.

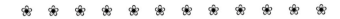

Cytomegalovirus

Cytomegalovirus (CMV) belongs to the herpesvirus group and causes both congenital and acquired infections referred to as *cytomegalic inclusion disease* (CID). The significance of this virus in pregnancy is related to its ability to be transmitted by asymptomatic women across the placenta to the fetus or by the cervical route during birth.

CID is probably the most prevalent infection in the TORCH group. Nearly half of adults have antibodies for the virus. The virus can be found in urine, saliva, cervical mucus, semen, and breast milk. It can be passed between humans by any close contact such as kissing, breast-feeding, and sexual intercourse. Asymptomatic CMV infection is particularly common in children and gravid women. It is a chronic, persistent infection in that the individual may shed the virus continually over many years. The cervix can harbor the virus, and an ascending infection can develop after birth. While the virus is usually innocuous in adults and children, it may be fatal to the fetus.

Accurate diagnosis in the pregnant woman depends on the presence of CMV in the urine, a rise in IgM levels, and identification of the CMV antibodies within the serum IgM fraction. At present, no treatment exists for maternal CMV or for the congenital disease in the neonate.

Fetal-Neonatal Risks

The cytomegalovirus is the most frequent agent of viral infection in the human fetus. It infects 0.5% to 2.0% of neonates, and of these about 10% develop serious manifestations (Britt & Vugler 1990). Subclinical infections in the newborn are capable of producing mental retardation and auditory deficits, sometimes not recognized for several months, or learning disabilities not seen until childhood. CMV may be the most common cause of mental retardation.

For the fetus, this infection can result in extensive intrauterine tissue damage that leads to fetal death; in survival with microcephaly, hydrocephaly, cerebral palsy, or mental retardation; or in survival with no damage at all.

The infected neonate is often SGA. The principal tissues and organs affected are the blood, brain, and liver. However, virtually all organs are potentially at risk. Hemolysis leads to anemia and hyperbilirubinemia. Thrombocytopenia and hepatosplenomegaly may also develop.

Herpes Genitalis (Herpes Simplex Virus Type 2)

Herpes simplex virus type 2 (HSV-2) is a viral infection that can cause painful lesions in the genital area. Lesions may also develop on the cervix. This condition and its implications for nonpregnant women are discussed in Chapter 8. However, because the presence of herpes lesions in the genital tract may profoundly affect the fetus, herpes infection as it relates to a pregnant woman is discussed here as part of the TORCH complex of infections.

Fetal-Neonatal Risks

The risk of transmission to the neonate is highest among women who contract their first herpes infection near the time of birth. It is lower among women with recurrent herpes (CDC 1989). Transmission of HSV-2 to the fetus almost always occurs after the membranes rupture, as the virus ascends from active lesions. It also occurs during vaginal birth, when the fetus comes in contact with genital lesions. Transplacental infection is rare.

If active HSV-2 infection occurs during the first trimester there is a 20% to 50% rate of spontaneous abortion or stillbirth (Stagno & Whitley 1985). Infection after 20 weeks of gestation is associated with an increased risk of preterm labor.

Approximately 54% of all infants who are born vaginally when the mother is shedding HSV-2 in her vagina or cervix develop some form of herpes infection. Of these infants, approximately 70% will die if untreated, while 83% of the survivors will have permanent brain damage (Harger 1985). Asymptomatic women may also harbor the virus. In a recent long-term study, over one-half of infants who developed neonatal herpes infection were born to women with no known history of the infection (Harger 1990).

The infected infant is often asymptomatic at birth but after an incubation period of 2 to 12 days develops symptoms of fever (or hypothermia), jaundice, seizures, and poor feeding. Approximately one-half of infected infants develop the characteristic vesicular skin lesions. Vidarabine has been useful in decreasing serious effects from neonatal herpes, but no definitive treatment exists as yet. Some experts treat asymptomatic infants who were exposed to herpes simplex virus during birth with acyclovir. Positive herpes cultures taken 24 to 48 hours after birth should be obtained before treatment (CDC 1989).

Medical Therapy

Although the vesicular lesions of herpes have a characteristic appearance, they rupture easily. Thus definitive diagnosis is made by culturing active lesions. Because cultures are expensive and not always available, many care givers obtain a discharge from the lesion and prepare a slide as for a Pap test. The presence of multinucleated giant cells indicates herpes.

Treatment is directed first toward relieving the woman's vulvar pain. If the attack is severe, walking, sitting, and even wearing clothing may be painful. The woman may be most comfortable in bed during the peak of the infection. Sitz baths three to four times daily, followed by drying of the vulva with a hair dryer or light bulb, may promote healing and help prevent secondary infection. Cotton underwear helps keep the genital area dry.

Although acyclovir (Zovirax) does not cure the infection or prevent recurrence, it does reduce healing time of the initial attack and shortens the time that the live virus is in the lesions, thereby reducing the infectious period. Currently it is not recommended for use during pregnancy.

HSV-2 has not been found in breast milk. Present experience shows that breast-feeding is acceptable if the mother washes her hands well to prevent any direct transfer of the virus.

Because most infants become infected when they pass through a birth canal containing herpes virus, it was the practice to do serial cervical cultures. Recently, the Infectious Disease Society for Obstetrics and Gynecology issued new guidelines for the management of HSV-2 in pregnancy. They recommend that a history of HSV infection in the woman or her partner should be obtained and recorded at the first prenatal visit. Weekly cultures are not recommended for women with a history of HSV but with no visible lesions. For women with no visible lesions at the time of labor (or rupture of the membranes) vaginal birth should be attempted. For women with visible lesions, cesarean birth is indicated to reduce the risk of neonatal infection. Cesarean birth is best attempted within 4 to 6 hours of rupture of membranes to decrease the risk of ascending infection. However, cesarean birth is still recommended regardless of the time elapsed in women with visible lesions. Cultures every three to five days are indicated for women who have visible lesions at or near term but before the onset of labor. The cultures are useful in documenting the absence of virus and thereby increasing the possibility of vaginal birth (Landers & Sweet 1990).

❀ *APPLYING THE NURSING PROCESS* ❀

Nursing Assessment

During the initial prenatal visit it is important to learn whether the woman or her partner have had previous herpes infections. If so, ongoing assessment is indicated as pregnancy progresses.

Nursing Diagnosis

Nursing diagnoses that may apply to the pregnant woman with HSV-2 include the following:

- Sexual dysfunction related to unwillingness to engage in sexual intercourse secondary to the presence of active herpes lesions

- Ineffective individual coping related to depression secondary to the risk to the fetus if herpes lesions are present at birth

Nursing Plan and Implementation

Nurses need to be particularly concerned with client education about this fast-spreading disease. Women should be informed of the association of genital herpes with spontaneous abortion, neonatal mortality and morbidity, and the possibility of cesarean birth. A woman needs to inform her future health care providers of her infection. She also should know of the possible association of genital herpes with cervical cancer and the importance of a yearly Pap smear.

The woman who acquired HSV-2 as an adolescent may be devastated as a mature young adult who wants to have a family. Clients may be helped by counseling that allows expression of the anger, shame, and depression so often experienced by the herpes victim. Literature may be helpful and is available from Planned Parenthood and many public health agencies. The American Social Health Association has established the HELP program to provide information and the latest research results on genital herpes. The Association has a quarterly journal, *The Helper,* for nurses and herpes clients.

Evaluation

Anticipated outcomes of nursing include the following:

- The woman is able to describe her infection with regard to its method of spread, therapy and comfort measures, implications for her pregnancy, and long-term implications.
- The woman has appropriate cultures done as recommended throughout her pregnancy.
- The woman gives birth to a healthy infant.

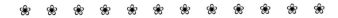

Other Infections in Pregnancy

In addition to the TORCH infections, other infections contribute to risk during pregnancy. Spontaneous abortion is frequently the result of a severe maternal infection. Evidence exists that links infection and prematurity. In addition, if the pregnancy is carried to term in the presence of infection, the risk of maternal and fetal morbidity and mortality increases. Thus it is essential to maternal and fetal health that infection be diagnosed and treated promptly.

Urinary tract, vaginal, and sexually transmitted infections are discussed in detail in Chapter 8. Table 19–8 provides a summary of these infections and their implications for pregnancy.

Table 19–8 Infections That Put Pregnancy at Risk

Condition and causative organism	Signs and symptoms	Treatment	Implications for pregnancy
Urinary Tract Infections			
Asymptomatic bacteriuria (ASB): *E coli, Klebsiella, Proteus* most common.	Bacteria present in urine on culture with no accompanying symptoms.	Oral sulfonamides early in pregnancy, ampicillin and nitrofurantoin (Furadantin) in late pregnancy.	Women with ASB in early pregnancy may go on to develop cystitis or acute pyelonephritis by third trimester if not treated. Oral sulfonamides taken in the last few weeks of pregnancy may lead to neonatal hyperbilirubinemia and kernicterus.
Cystitis (Lower UTI): Causative organisms same as ASB.	Dysuria, urgency, frequency; low-grade fever and hematuria may occur. Urine culture (clean catch) show ↑ leukocytes. Presence of 10^5 (100,000) or more colonies bacteria per mL urine.	Same.	If not treated, infection may ascend and lead to acute pyelonephritis.
Acute pyelonephritis: Causative organisms same as ASB.	Sudden onset. Chills, high fever, flank pain. Nausea, vomiting, malaise. May have decreased urine output, severe colicky pain, dehydration. Increased diastolic BP, positive FA-test, low creatinine clearance. Marked bacteremia in urine culture, pyuria, WBC casts.	Hospitalization; IV antibiotic therapy. Other antibiotics safe during pregnancy include carbenicillin, methenamine, cephalosporins. Catheterization if output is ↓. Supportive therapy for comfort. Follow-up urine cultures are necessary.	Increased risk of premature delivery and IUGR. These antibiotics interfere with urinary estriol levels and can cause false interpretations of estriol levels during pregnancy.

(continued)

Table 19–8 (*continued*)

Condition and causative organism	Signs and symptoms	Treatment	Implications for pregnancy
Vaginal Infections			
Monilial (yeast infection): *Candida albicans.*	Often thick, white, curdy discharge, severe itching, dysuria, dyspareunia. Diagnosis based on presence of hyphae and spores in a wet mount preparation of vaginal secretions.	Intravaginal insertion of miconazole or clotrimazole suppositories at bedtime for 1 week. Cream may be prescribed for topical application to the vulva if necessary.	If the infection is present at birth and the fetus is born vaginally, the fetus may contract thrush.
Bacterial vaginosis: *Gardnerella vaginalis*	Thin, watery, yellow-gray discharge with foul odor often described as "fishy." Wet mount preparation reveals "clue cells." Application of KOH (potassium hydroxide) to a specimen of vaginal secretions produces a pronounced fishy odor.	Nonpregnant women treated with metronidazole (Flagyl). Pregnant women treated with clindamycin (CDC 1989).	Metronidazole has potential teratogenic effects. Possible ↑ risk of PROM and preterm birth. Confirmatory studies needed (CDC 1989).
Trichomoniasis: *Trichomonas vaginalis*	Occasionally asymptomatic. May have frothy greenish gray vaginal discharge, pruritus, urinary symptoms. Strawberry patches may be visible on vaginal walls or cervix. Wet mount preparation of vaginal secretions shows motile flagellated trichomonads.	During early pregnancy symptoms may be controlled with clotrimazole vaginal suppositories. Both partners are treated, but no adequate treatment exists. After first trimester, a single 2-g dose of metronidazole may be used (CDC 1989).	Metronidazole has potential teratogenic effects.
Sexually Transmitted Infections			
Chlamydial infection: *Chlamydia trachomatis*	Women are often asymptomatic. Symptoms may include thin or purulent discharge, burning and frequency with urination, or lower abdominal pain. Lab test available to detect monoclonal antibodies specific for *Chlamydia.*	Although nonpregnant women are treated with tetracycline, it may permanently discolor fetal teeth. Thus, pregnant women are treated with erythromycin ethyl succinate.	Infant of woman with untreated chlamydial infection may develop newborn conjunctivitis, which can be treated with erythromycin eye ointment (but not silver nitrate). Infant may also develop chlamydial pneumonia. May be responsible for premature labor and fetal death.
Syphilis: *Treponema pallidum,* a spirochete	Primary stage: chancre, slight fever, malaise. Chancre lasts about 4 weeks, then disappears. Secondary stage: occurs 6 weeks to 6 months after infection. Skin eruptions (condyloma lata); also symptoms of acute arthritis, liver enlargement, iritis, chronic sore throat with hoarseness. Diagnosed by blood tests such as VDRL, RPR, FTA-ABS. Dark-field examination for spirochetes may also be done.	For syphilis less than 1 year in duration: 2.4 million U benzathine penicillin G IM. For syphilis of more than 1 year's duration: 2.4 million U benzathine penicillin G once a week for 3 weeks. Sexual partners should also be screened and treated.	Syphilis can be passed transplacentally to the fetus. If untreated, one of the following can occur: second trimester abortion, stillborn infant at term, congenitally infected infant, uninfected live infant.
Gonorrhea: *Neisseria gonorrhoeae*	Majority of women asymptomatic; disease often diagnosed during routine prenatal cervical culture. If symptoms are present they may include purulent vaginal discharge, dysuria, urinary frequency, inflammation and swelling of the vulva. Cervix may appear eroded.	Nonpregnant women are treated with ceftriaxone plus doxycycline. Pregnant women are treated with ceftriaxone plus erythromycin (CDC 1989). If the woman is allergic to ceftriaxone, spectinomycin is used. All sexual partners are also treated.	Infection at time of birth may cause ophthalmia neonatorum in the newborn.
Condyloma acuminata: caused by a papovavirus	Soft, grayish-pink lesions on the vulva, vagina, cervix, or anus.	Podophyllin not used during pregnancy. Trichloroacetic acid, liquid nitrogen, or cryotherapy CO_2 laser therapy done under colposcopy is also successful (Lucas 1988)	Possible teratogenic effect of podophyllin. Large doses have been associated with fetal death.

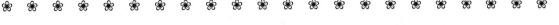

KEY CONCEPTS

Hyperemesis gravidarum, excessive vomiting during pregnancy, may cause fluid and electrolyte imbalance, dehydration, and signs of starvation in the mother, and, if severe enough, death of the fetus. Treatment is aimed at controlling the vomiting, correcting fluid and electrolyte imbalance, correcting dehydration, and improving nutritional status.

Several health problems associated with bleeding arise from the pregnancy itself, such as spontaneous abortion, ectopic pregnancy, and gestational trophoblastic disease. The nurse needs to be alert to early signs of these situations, to guard the woman against heavy bleeding and shock, to facilitate the medical treatment, and to provide educational and emotional support.

Hypertension may exist prior to pregnancy or, more often, may develop during pregnancy. Pregnancy-induced hypertension can lead to growth retardation for the fetus, and if untreated may lead to convulsions (eclampsia) and even death for the mother and fetus. A woman's understanding of the disease process helps motivate her to maintain the required rest periods in the left lateral position. Antihypertensive or anticonvulsive drugs may be part of the therapy.

Rh incompatibility can exist when an Rh⁻ woman and an Rh⁺ partner conceive a child that is Rh⁺. The use of RhIgG has greatly decreased the incidence of severe sequelae due to Rh because the drug "tricks" the body into thinking antibodies have been produced in response to the Rh antigen.

The impact of surgery, trauma, or battering on the pregnant woman and her fetus is related to timing in the pregnancy, seriousness of the situation, and other factors influencing the situation.

Urinary tract infections are a common problem in pregnancy. If untreated the infection may ascend, causing more serious illness for the mother. Urinary tract infections are also associated with an increased risk of premature labor.

TORCH is an acronym standing for toxoplasmosis, rubella, cytomegalovirus, and herpes, all of which pose a grave threat to the fetus.

Sexually transmitted diseases pose less of a threat to the fetus if detected and treated as soon as possible.

References

Abbott JT: Vaginal bleeding: Matching the cause and the cure. *Emerg Med* May 1989; 21:84.

American College of Obstetricians and Gynecologists: Doctors announce campaign to combat domestic violence. ACOG News Release, January 3, 1989.

Anderson HF, Merkatz IR: Preterm Labor. In: *Danforth's Obstetrics and Gynecology,* 6th ed. Scott JR et al (editors). Philadelphia: Lippincott, 1990.

Berkowitz RS, Goldstein DP: Diagnosis and management of the primary hydatidiform mole. *Obstet Gynecol Clin North Am* September 1988; 15:491.

Bishop EH: Acceleration of fetal pulmonary maturity. *Obstet Gynecol* 1981; 58(Suppl):48.

Bohn DK: Domestic violence and pregnancy: Implications for practice. *J Nurse-Midwifery* March/April 1990; 35:86.

Bowman JM: Controversies of Rh prophylaxis: Who needs Rh immunoglobulin and when should it be given? *Am J Obstet Gynecol* 1985; 151(3):289.

Briggs GC et al: *Drugs in Pregnancy and Lactation.* 2nd ed. Baltimore: Williams and Wilkins, 1986.

Britt WJ, Vugler LG: Antiviral antibody response in mothers and their newborns with clinical cytomegalovirus infections. *J Infect Dis* 1990; 161:214.

Caritas SN et al: Evaluation of the pharmacodynamics and pharmacokinetics of ritodrine when administered as a loading dose. *Am J Obstet Gynecol* 1985; 152:1026.

Centers for Disease Control: 1989 Sexually transmitted disease treatment guidelines. *Mortality and Morbidity Weekly Report* September 1, 1989; 38(S-8):1.

Creasy RK, Resnik R: *Maternal-Fetal Medicine: Principles and Practices.* Philadelphia: Saunders, 1989.

Deaton JL et al: Molar pregnancy coexisting with a normal fetus: A case report. *Gynecol Oncol* March 1989; 32:394.

Garite TJ: Premature rupture of membranes. In: *Danforth's Obstetrics and Gynecology,* 6th ed. Scott JR et al (editors) Philadelphia: Lippincott, 1990.

Gavette L, Roberts J: Use of mean arterial pressure (MAP-2) to predict pregnancy-induced hypertension in adolescents. *J Nurse-Midwifery* November/ December 1987; 32:357.

Givens SR: Update on tocolytic therapy in the management of preterm labor. *J Perinatal Neonatal Nurs* 1988; 2:1.

Gonik B et al: Intramuscular versus intravenous ritodrine hydrochloride for preterm labor management. *Am J Obstet Gynecol* 1988; 159:323.

Goodwin TM, Breen MT: Pregnancy outcome and fetomaternal hemorrhage after noncatastrophic trauma. *Am J Obstet Gynecol* 1990; 162:665.

Hammond CB: Gestational trophoblastic neoplasms: History of the current understanding. *Obstet Gynecol Clin North Am* September 1988; 15:435.

Handler A et al: The relationship of smoking and ectopic pregnancy. *Am J Public Health* September 1989; 79:1239.

Harger JH: Improving the care of pregnant women with genital herpes. *Contemp OB/GYN* 1985; 26(4):85.

Harger JH: Infection protocols: Genital herpes. *Contemp OB/GYN* May 1990; 35:83.

Hatjis CG et al: Efficacy of combined administration of magnesium sulfate and ritodrine in the treatment of preterm labor. *Obstet Gynecol* 1987; 69:317.

Hendricks SK et al: Electrocardiographic changes associated with ritodrine-induced maternal tachycardia and hypokalemia. *Am J Obstet Gynecol* 1986; 154:921.

Herron MA: One approach to preventing preterm birth. *J Perinatal Neonatal Nurs* 1988; 2:1.

Iams JD et al: A prospective random trial of home uterine activity monitoring in pregnancies at increased risk of preterm labor. *Am J Obstet Gynecol* 1988; 159:595.

Kaplan KM et al: A profile of mothers giving birth to infants with congenital rubella syndrome: An assessment of risk factors. *Am J Dis Child* 1990; 144:118.

Lam F et al: Use of the subcutaneous terbutaline pump for long-term tocolysis. *Obstet Gynecol* 1988; 72:810.

Lam F et al: Miniature pump infusion of terbutaline: An option in preterm labor. *Contemp OB/GYN* January 1989; 34:133.

Landers DV, Sweet RL: Perinatal infections. In: *Danforth's Obstetrics and Gynecology,* 6th ed. Scott JR et al (editors). Philadelphia: Lippincott, 1990.

Leach RE, Ory SJ: Ectopics: Treating the problem pregnancy without surgery. *Contemp OB/GYN* April 15, 1990; 35(special issue):149.

Lipshitz J: Beta-adrenergic agonists. *Semin Perinatol* July 1981; 5:252.

Lucas VA: Human papilloma virus infections: A potentially carcinogenic sexually transmitted disease. *Nurs Clin North Am* 1988; 23(4):917.

Martin JN et al: Pregnancy complicated by preeclampsia-eclampsia with the syndrome of hemolysis, elevated liver enzymes, and low platelet count: How rapid is postpartum recovery? *Obstet Gynecol* November 1990; 76:737.

Mazze RI, Källén B: Reproductive outcome after anesthesia and operation of 5405 cases. *Am J Obstet Gynecol* 1989; 161:1178.

McDonald JC et al: An outbreak of toxoplasmosis in pregnant women in northern Quebec. *J Infect Dis* 1990; 161:769.

Morbidity and Mortality Weekly Report: Congenital syphilis—New York City 1986–88. December 8, 1989; 38:835.

Morbidity and Mortality Weekly Report: Progress toward achieving the 1990 objectives for the nation for sexually transmitted diseases. February 2, 1990; 39:52.

Morrison JC: Preterm birth: A puzzle worth solving. *Obstet Gynecol* July 1990; 76(1S):5S.

NAACOG: Preterm labor and tocolytics. *OGN Nurs Practice Resource* September 1984; 10.

Niebyl JR: Detecting incompetent cervix. *Contemp OB/GYN* October 1990; 35:37.

Ory SJ: Ectopic pregnancy: Current evaluation and treatment. *Mayo Clin Proc* July 1989; 64:874.

Pauerstein CJ: *Clinical Obstetrics.* New York: Wiley, 1987.

Philipsen T et al: Pulmonary edema following ritodrine cases with prolonged bradycardia. *Am J Obstet Gynecol* 1985; 153:859.

Pisani RS, Rosenow EC: Pulmonary edema associated with tocolytic therapy. *Obstet Gynecol Surv* 1990; 45:1.

Ricci JM et al: Congenital syphilis: The University of Miami/Jackson Memorial Medical Center experience, 1986–88. *Obstet Gynecol* 1989; 74:687.

Rice LW et al: Repetitive complete and partial hydatidiform mole. *Obstet Gynecol* August 1989; 74:217.

Romero R: Can antimicrobials prevent preterm delivery? *Contemp OB/GYN* November 1989; 34:81.

Romero R et al: Mechanisms at work when infection triggers preterm labor. *Contemp OB/GYN* January 1989; 34:133.

Scott JR: Ectopic pregnancy. In: *Danforth's Obstetrics and Gynecology,* 6th ed. Scott JR et al (editors). Philadelphia: Lippincott, 1990a.

Scott JR: Immunologic disorders in pregnancy. In: *Danforth's Obstetrics and Gynecology,* 6th ed. Scott JR et al (editors). Philadelphia: Lippincott, 1990b.

Scott JR: Spontaneous abortion. In: *Danforth's Obstetrics and Gynecology,* 6th ed. Scott JR et al (editors). Philadelphia: Lippincott, 1990c.

Scott JR, Worley RJ: Hypertensive disorders of pregnancy. In: *Danforth's Obstetrics and Gynecology,* 6th ed. Scott JR et al (editors). Philadelphia: Lippincott, 1990.

Shortle B, Jewelewicz R: Cervical incompetence. *Fertil Steril* August 1989; 52:181.

Sibai BM: Preeclampsia-eclampsia. In: *Gynecology and Obstetrics.* Vol. 2. Sciarra JJ (editor). Philadelphia: Lippincott, 1989.

Sibai BM: Preeclampsia-eclampsia: Valid treatment approaches. *Contemp OB/GYN* August 1990; 35:84.

Silver HM: Acute hypertensive crisis in pregnancy. *Med Clin North Am* May 1989; 73:623.

Simpson JL: Genetic causes of spontaneous abortion. *Contemp OB/GYN* September 1990; 35:25.

Skidmore-Roth, L: *Mosby's 1989 Nursing Drug Reference.* St. Louis: CV Mosby, 1989.

Soper JT, Hammond CB: Nonmetastatic gestational trophoblastic disease. *Obstet Gynecol Clin North Am* September 1988; 15:505.

Spatling L et al: Bolus tocolysis: Treatment of preterm labor with pulsatile administration of a β-adrenergic agonist. *Am J Obstet Gynecol* 1989; 160:713.

Stagno S, Whitley RJ: Herpesvirus infections of pregnancy. Part II: Herpes simplex virus and varicella-zoster virus infections. *N Engl J. Med* 1985; 313(21):1327.

Szulman AE: Trophoblastic disease: Clinical pathology of hydatidiform moles. *Obstet Gynecol Clin North Am* September 1988; 15:443.

Thorpe JM et al: Fetal death from chlamydial infection across intact amniotic membranes. *Am J Obstet Gynecol* 1989; 161:245.

Vanagunas A, Sparberg M: Gastrointestinal complications of pregnancy. In: *Gynecology and Obstetrics.* Vol. 3. Sciarra JJ (editor). Philadelphia: Lippincott, 1989.

Wang R, Davidson BJ: Ritodrine-induced neutropenia. *Am J Obstet Gynecol* 1986; 154:924.

Watson DL et al: Management of preterm labor patients at home: Does daily uterine activity monitoring and nursing support make a difference? *Obstet Gynecol* July 1990; 76(1S):32S.

Wilkins IA et al: Long-term use of magnesium sulfate as a tocolytic agent. *Obstet Gynecol* 1986; 67:385.

Zuspan FP: Chronic hypertension in pregnancy. *Clin Obstet Gynecol* December 1984; 27:854.

Additional Readings

Catlin AJ, Wetzle WS: Ectopic pregnancy: Clinical evaluation, diagnostic measures and prevention. *NPract* January 1991; 1638.

Cohen DA et al: The effects of case definition in maternal screening and reporting criteria on rates of congenital syphilis. *Am J Public Health* 1990; 80:316.

Davies K: Genital herpes: An overview. *JOGNN* 1990; 19:401.

Drost TF et al: Major trauma in pregnant women: Maternal/fetal outcome. *J Trauma* May 1990; 30:574.

Gjerdingen DK et al: A causal model describing the relationship of women's postpartum health to social support, length of leave, and complications of childbirth. *Women's Health* 1990; 16(2):71.

Odendaal HJ et al: Aggressive or expectant management for patients with severe preeclampsia between 28–34 weeks' gestation: A randomized controlled trial. *Obstet Gynecol* December 1990; 76:1070.

Smith JF; The clinical management of eclampsia. *Female Patient* March 1991; 16:37.

Swindells HE et al: Blood pressure telemetry from home. *Midwife Health Visit Community Nurse* March 1990; 26:88.

White S, Larson B: Measles in pregnancy. *Contemp OB/GYN* September 1990; 35:57.

CHAPTER 20

Diagnostic Assessment of Fetal Status

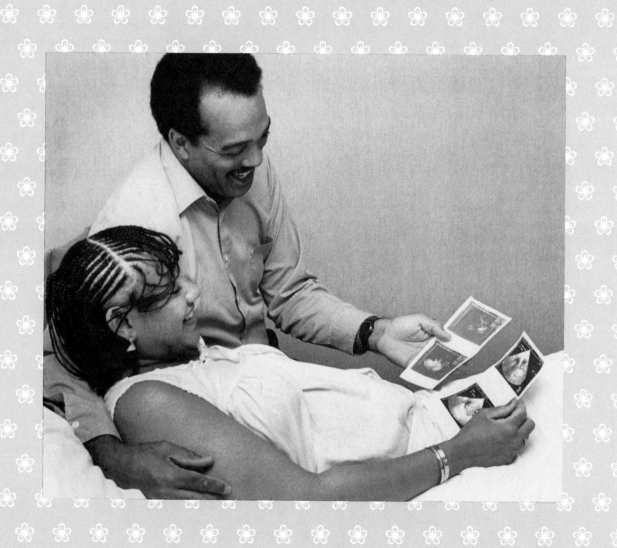

List indications for ultrasonic examination and the information that can be obtained from this procedure.

Outline pertinent information to be discussed with the woman regarding her assessment of fetal activity.

Identify criteria for the evaluation of fetal well-being by biophysical profile assessment.

Discuss the nurse's role in teaching the woman the nipple stimulation contraction stress test and important factors to assess in evaluation of fetal heart rate response.

Contrast amniocentesis and chorionic villus sampling.

Compare the procedures for the nonstress test and contraction stress test, including the indications, contraindications, and predictive value of each.

Discuss counseling regarding alpha-fetoprotein screening and implications of abnormal values.

Discuss implications of prenatal testing with regard to high-risk pregnancy management.

❈ ❈

My first pregnancy was so tenuous that I didn't know from one moment to the next how it would end. I hoped for our baby's safety, but in the end the baby died. When I became pregnant the next time I was very nervous. Being able to see the baby on ultrasound helped me so much. I knew then that our baby was alive and growing.

During the past two decades, increasing interest has been focused on the problems of the at-risk pregnant woman, for health management, and conditions that may affect her unborn child. It is now known that high-risk women and infants have a significantly greater chance of morbidity or mortality before or after childbirth. Perinatal morbidity and mortality can be considerably reduced by early, skillful diagnosis and highly intensive antepartal care of the pregnant woman.

A variety of tests of fetal status are of value in monitoring the well-being of the fetus. These tests include ultrasound, computerized tomography, magnetic resonance imaging, fetoscopy, percutaneous umbilical blood sampling, chorionic villus sampling, measurements of specific hormones and enzymes in maternal blood and urine, amniocentesis, and fetal stress tests. Although the tests have been made as safe as possible, these procedures can always involve some risk. Fetal morbidity, mortality, and health status must be considered before suggesting the diagnostic procedures. In addition, the risks must be acceptable to the pregnant woman. Health care professionals may think the risks are minimal, but they are not the ones who will suffer the consequences of an untoward outcome should it occur.

Not all high-risk pregnancies require the same procedures. One must be certain that the advantages outweigh the potential risks and added expense. Each of these tests has its limitations in terms of screening, diagnostic accu-

racy, and applicability. No one test should be used to determine fetal status in the management of high-risk women. (For a summary of tests, see Table 20–1.)

Nursing Process During Diagnostic Testing

Because many of the diagnostic tests are completed on an outpatient basis, the nurse has only brief contact with the woman and her support person. The nurse uses the nursing process to guide nursing care during these interactions.

❈ *APPLYING THE NURSING PROCESS* ❈

Nursing Assessment

The nursing assessment begins with a history regarding the prenatal course and identification of possible indications for the particular diagnostic testing. The nurse assesses the information that the woman and her support person have regarding the test, the questions and concerns that they have, and the presence of any particular factors that may influence the teaching process. During the test, the nurse completes needed assessments to monitor the status of the woman and her unborn child.

Analysis and Nursing Diagnosis

The primary nursing diagnoses are directed toward providing information regarding the diagnostic test and minimizing any risks to the woman and her unborn child. The woman may also be fearful of the outcome of the tests, and nurses can play an important role in providing education, support, and counseling. Examples of nursing diagnoses that may be applicable include the following:

Table 20–1 Summary of Screening and Diagnostic Tests

Goal	Test	When test may be done
To validate the pregnancy	Ultrasound for gestational sac volume	5 and 6 weeks after LMP
To determine how advanced the pregnancy is	Ultrasound: Crown–rump length Ultrasound: Biparietal diameter and femur length	7 to 10 weeks' gestation 13 to 40 weeks' gestation
To identify normal growth of the fetus	Ultrasound: Biparietal diameter Ultrasound: Head–abdomen ratio Ultrasound: Estimated fetal weight	Most useful from 20 to 30 weeks' gestation 13 to 40 weeks' gestation About 28 to 40 weeks' gestation
To detect congenital anomalies and problems	Ultrasound Chorionic villus sampling Fetoscopy Percutaneous blood sampling	18 to 40 weeks' gestation 8 to 12 weeks' gestation 18 weeks' gestation 2nd and 3rd trimesters
To localize the placenta	Ultrasound	Usually in 3rd trimester or before amniocentesis
To assess fetal status	Biophysical profile Maternal assessment of fetal activity Estriols Magnetic resonance imaging Nonstress test Contraction stress test	Approximately 28 weeks to birth About 28 weeks to birth During the 2nd and 3rd trimesters During the 2nd and 3rd trimesters Approximately 30 weeks to birth After 28 weeks
To diagnose cardiac problems	Fetal echocardiography	2nd and 3rd trimesters

To assess fetal lung maturity	Amniocentesis
	   L/S ratio
	   Phosphatidylglycerol
	   Phosphatidylcholine
	   Shake test
		33 to 40 weeks
		 33 weeks to birth
		 33 weeks to birth
		 33 weeks to birth
		 33 weeks to birth

To obtain more information about breech presentation	Computerized tomography X ray	Just before labor is anticipated or during labor

- Knowledge deficit related to insufficient information about the fetal assessment test, purpose, benefits, risks, and alternatives
- Fear related to the specific test and/or possible unfavorable test results

Nursing Plan and Implementation

The nursing plan of care will be directed toward each specific nursing diagnosis. The nurse generally plays a vital role in providing information about the diagnostic test. The nurse assesses the woman's knowledge of the test and then provides information as needed. Some of the tests require written informed consent, and in these cases the physician, or nurse-midwife is responsible for informing the woman about all aspects of the test. In this instance the nurse can reinforce information and clarify information that is not fully understood (Table 20–2).

Contact with the expectant woman may be very brief. The nurse therefore uses all her or his basic knowledge of communication, developmental psychology, and cultural factors to quickly establish rapport with the woman and her support person.

Table 20–2 Sample Nursing Approaches to Pretest Teaching

Assess whether the woman knows the reason the screening or diagnostic test is being recommended.
Example:
"Has your doctor/nurse-midwife told you why this test is necessary?"
"Sometimes tests are done for many different reasons. Can you tell me why you are having this test?"
"What is your understanding about what the test will show?"

Provide an opportunity for questions.
Example:
"Do you have any questions about the test?"
"Is there anything that is not clear to you?"

Explain the test procedure paying particular attention to any preparation the woman needs to do prior to the test.
Example:
"The test that has been ordered for you is designed to . . ." (add specific information about the particular test. Give the explanation in simple language).

Validate the woman's understanding of the preparation.
Example:
"Tell me what you will have to do to get ready for this test."

Give permission for woman to continue to ask questions if needed.
Example:
"I'll be with you during the test. If you have any questions at any time, please don't hesitate to ask."

The nurse also functions as an advocate for the expectant woman by helping her clarify question areas and obtain needed information. The nurse frequently knows the areas for which most women have questions and can anticipate many of their fears. When the woman is not able to verbalize questions, the nurse can assist by bringing up questions that other women have had.

During the testing sessions, the nurse addresses the woman's fear by providing support and comfort measures. The presence of the nurse reassures the woman and helps her cope with the tests.

Evaluation

The expected outcomes for the woman who is having diagnostic testing are that she understands the reasons for the test and the test results and has had support during the tests. In addition, the tests have been done without complication and the safety of the mother and her unborn child has been maintained.

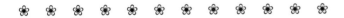

Indications for Diagnostic Testing

Women who are considered to be at risk and for whom the physician/nurse-midwife may order assessments of fetal well-being include women with the following complications:

- Chronic hypertension
- Pregnancy-induced hypertension
- Diabetes mellitus
- History of preterm labor or birth, or risk of preterm labor with this pregnancy
- Pregnancy beyond 41 1/2 to 42 weeks
- Rh isoimmunization
- History of unexplained stillborn or intrapartal fetal death
- Hemoglobinopathies
- Suspected intrauterine growth retardation
- Maternal cyanotic heart disease
- Bleeding complications accompanying the pregnancy, such as abruptio placentae or placenta previa
- Hydramnios or oligohydramnios
- Infections, immunodeficiencies
- Previous history of chromosomal or inherited biochemical disorders.

Each of the listed complications may increase the risk to the expectant woman and her fetus. The list is not complete; other preexisting medical diseases may place the woman at risk and necessitate diagnostic assessment of the fetus.

Ultrasound

The introduction of ultrasound in the 1950s was a major advance in the practice of obstetrics. The first machines were crude compared to those in use today, but as the technology has improved ultrasound has become an integral part of the assessment of fetal age, health, and growth and has led to radical changes in the practice of perinatal medicine (Figure 20–1).

With ultrasound it is now possible to determine gestational age, diagnose fetal growth patterns, recognize fetal congenital anomalies, assess placental location and maturity, assess the effect of disease processes on the fetus, and ascertain fetal responses to the intrauterine environment. Ultrasound is also used to assist diagnostic and therapeutic measures such as amniocentesis, fetoscopy, chorionic villus sampling, and intrauterine fetal transfusion.

Ultrasound scanning is now performed using real-time or a combination of real-time and static scanners. Continuous images are produced by transmission of sound waves via a transducer applied to the woman's abdomen or an endovaginal transducer inserted into the woman's vagina (Figure 20–2). Echoes (from the sound waves) are then reflected from tissues of varying densities (or thickness) back to the crystals in the transducer and converted to electrical signals, which are then amplified and displayed on an oscilloscope (similar to a television screen). Real-

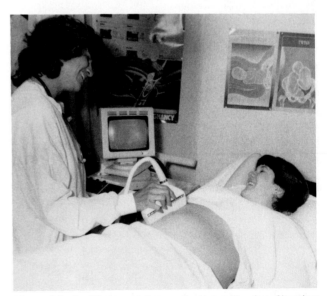

Figure 20–1   Ultrasound scanning permits visualization of the fetus in utero.

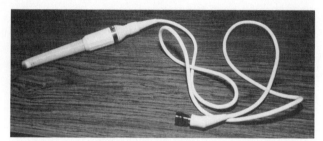

Figure 20–2 Endovaginal ultrasound transducer.

time imaging gives the impression of motion because of the continuous rapid, fixed images produced and permits a visual image of the fetus as it functions in its environment. Such functions as fetal breathing, tone, movement, urination, eye movement, and cardiac activity may all be assessed by means of ultrasound imaging (Figure 20–3).

Ultrasound scanning is categorized as either level I or level II. A level I ultrasound may be performed by minimally trained individuals to assess gestational age, number of fetuses, fetal death, and the status of the placenta. A level II scan must be performed by a highly trained ultrasound clinician who is knowledgeable about assessment of specific congenital anomalies and abnormalities.

Diagnostic ultrasound has several advantages. It is painless, nonradiating to both the woman and fetus, and has no known harmful effects to either (Crane 1990). Serial studies (several ultrasound tests done over a span of time)

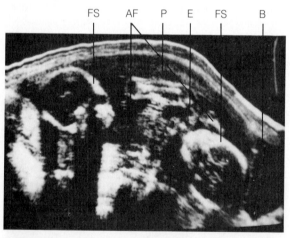

FS AF P E FS B

Figure 20–3 Ultrasound. Longitudinal scan demonstrating twin gestation, anterior placenta, fetal extremity. Both biparietal diameters (BPD) are at approximately 25 to 26 weeks' gestation. (AF = amniotic fluid; FS = fetal skull; E = extremity; B = woman's urinary bladder; P = placenta) (Courtesy Section of Diagnostic Ultrasound, Department of Diagnostic Radiology, Kansas University Medical Center.)

may be done for assessment and comparison. Soft-tissue masses can be differentiated. The practitioner obtains results immediately.

Although ultrasound testing can be beneficial, the National Institutes of Health (NIH) Consensus Development Conference on Ultrasound Imaging in Pregnancy recommended in 1984 that it not be routinely used on all pregnant women because its long-term effects are not fully known (Kremkau 1984; Queenan 1984) (Table 20–3). However, the usefulness of antepartum obstetric ultrasound examinations are currently being studied, and it is predicted that the American Institute of Ultrasound in Medicine (AIUM) will recommend routine ultrasound examinations by 1995 (Hadlock 1990a).

Procedures

There are two methods of ultrasound scanning: transabdominal scanning and endovaginal scanning.

Transabdominal Ultrasound

The woman is usually scanned with a full bladder except when ultrasound is used to localize the placenta prior to amniocentesis. When the bladder is full, the examiner can then assess other structures, especially the vagina and cervix, in relation to the bladder. This is particularly important when vaginal bleeding is noted and placenta previa is the suspected cause. The woman is advised to drink 1 to 1 1/2 quarts of water approximately 2 hours before the examination, and she is asked to refrain from emptying her bladder. If the bladder is not sufficiently filled, she is asked to drink three to four 8-oz glasses of water and is rescanned 30 to 45 minutes later.

Mineral oil or a transmission gel is generously spread over the woman's abdomen, and the sonographer slowly moves a transducer over the abdomen to obtain a picture of the contents of the uterus. Ultrasound testing takes 20 to 30 minutes. The woman may feel discomfort due to pressure applied over a full bladder. In addition, the woman lies on her back during the test; this position may cause shortness of breath, which may be relieved by elevating her upper body during the test.

Endovaginal Ultrasound

Ultrasound may also be performed using a small lightweight endovaginal transducer, which is inserted into the woman's vagina (see Figure 20–2). Endovaginal ultrasound is useful for assessment of early embryonic development, fetal heartbeat, and enhanced visualization of intrapelvic structures. Advantages of this method include enhanced visualization (because the sound waves do not have to pass through as many tissues), closer placement to the tissues being evaluated, and no need for the woman to have a full bladder (Cacciatore 1989).

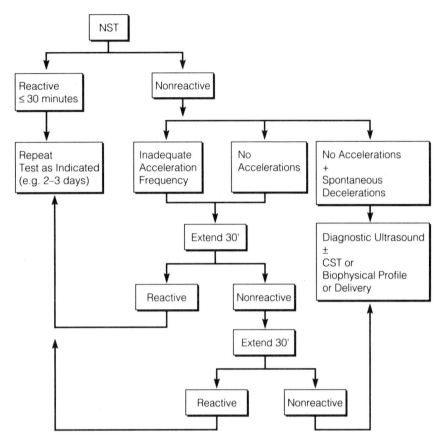

Table 20–3   Ultrasound Can Be of Benefit in the Following Circumstances

Estimation of gestational age for clients (1) with uncertain clinical dates, (2) verification of dates of clients who are to undergo scheduled elective repeat cesarean birth, induction of labor, or for other elective termination of pregnancy. Ultrasound confirmation of dating permits proper timing of cesarean birth or labor induction to avoid premature birth.

Evaluation of fetal growth (eg, when the client has an identified etiology for uteroplacental insufficiency, such as severe preeclampsia, chronic hypertension, chronic renal disease, severe diabetes mellitus, or for other medical complications of pregnancy where fetal malnutrition, ie, IUGR or macrosomia, is suspected). Following fetal growth permits assessment of the impact of a complicating condition on the fetus and guides pregnancy management.

Vaginal bleeding of undetermined etiology in pregnancy. Ultrasound often allows determination of the source of bleeding and status of the fetus.

Determination of fetal presentation when the presenting part cannot be adequately determined in labor or the fetal presentation is variable in late pregnancy. Accurate knowledge of presentation guides management of child birth.

Suspected multiple gestation based upon detection of more than one fetal heartbeat pattern, or fundal height larger than expected for dates, and/or prior use of fertility drugs. Pregnancy management may be altered in multiple gestation.

Adjunct to amniocentesis. Ultrasound permits guidance of the needle to avoid the placenta and fetus, to increase the chance of obtaining amniotic fluid, and to decrease the chance of fetal loss.

Significant uterine size/clinical dates discrepancy. Ultrasound permits accurate dating and detection of such conditions as oligohydramnios and polyhydramnios, as well as multiple gestation, IUGR, and anomalies.

Pelvic mass detected clinically. Ultrasound can detect the location and nature of the mass and aid in diagnosis.

Suspected hydatidiform mole on the basis of clinical signs of hypertension, proteinuria, and/or the presence of ovarian cysts felt on pelvic examination or failure to detect fetal heart tones with a Doppler ultrasound device after 12 weeks. Ultrasound permits accurate diagnosis and differentiation of this malignancy from fetal death.

Adjunct to cervical cerclage placement. Ultrasound aids in timing and proper placement of the cerclage for patients with incompetent cervix.

Suspected ectopic pregnancy or when pregnancy occurs after tuboplasty or prior ectopic gestation. Ultrasound is a valuable diagnostic aid for this complication.

Adjunct to special procedures, such as fetoscopy, intrauterine transfusion, shunt placement, in vitro fertilization, embryo transfer, or chorionic villi sampling. Ultrasound aids instrument guidance that increases safety of these procedures.

Suspected fetal death. Rapid diagnosis enhances optimal management.

Suspected uterine abnormality (eg, clinically significant leiomyomata, or congenital structural abnormalities, such as bicornate uterus or uterus didelphys, etc). Serial surveillance of fetal growth and state enhances fetal outcome.

Intrauterine contraceptive device localization. Ultrasound guidance facilitates removal, reducing chances of IUD-related complications.

Ovarian follicle development surveillance. This facilitates treatment of infertility.

Biophysical evaluation for fetal well-being after 28 weeks of gestation. Assessment of amniotic fluid, fetal tone, body movements, breathing movements, and heart rate patterns assists in the management of high-risk pregnancies.

Observation of intrapartum events (eg, version/extraction of second twin, manual removal of placenta, etc). These procedures may be done more safely with the visualization provided by ultrasound.

Suspected hydramnios or oligohydramnios. Confirmation of the diagnosis is permitted, as well as identification of the cause of the condition in certain pregnancies.

Suspected abruptio placentae. Confirmation of diagnosis and extent assists in clinical management.

Adjunct to external version from breech to vertex presentation. The visualization provided by ultrasound facilitates performance of this procedure.

Estimation of fetal weight and/or presentation in premature rupture of membranes and/or premature labor. Information provided by ultrasound guides management decisions on timing and method of birth.

Abnormal serum alpha-fetoprotein value for clinical gestational age when drawn. Ultrasound provides an accurate assessment of gestational age for the AFP comparison standard and indicates several conditions (eg, twins, anencephaly) that may cause elevated AFP values.

Follow-up observation of identified fetal anomaly. Ultrasound assessment of progression or lack of change assists in clinical decision making.

History of previous congenital anomaly. Detection of recurrence may be permitted, or psychologic benefit to patients may result from reassurance of no recurrence.

Serial evaluation of fetal growth in multiple gestation. Ultrasound permits recognition of discordant growth, guiding client management, and timing of birth.

Evaluation of fetal condition in late registrants for prenatal care. Accurate knowledge of gestational age assists in pregnancy management decisions of this group.

Source: *Shearer MH: Revelations: A summary and analysis of the NIH consensus development conference on ultrasound imaging in pregnancy.* Birth *1984 11(1):27.*

Nursing Care

It is important for the nurse to ascertain whether the woman understands the reason the ultrasound is being suggested. The nurse can provide an opportunity for the woman to ask questions and can act as an advocate if there are questions or concerns that need to be addressed prior to the ultrasound examination. The nurse explains the preparation needed and ensures that adequate preparation is done. After the test is completed, the nurse can assist with clarifying or interpreting test results to the woman.

In some instances, with additional education, the nurse may actually perform the ultrasound exam. This is especially true in a birth setting with real-time ultrasound.

Clinical Application

Currently there are many uses for ultrasound in pregnancy (see Table 20–3). We will discuss some of the uses in more detail in the following sections.

The AIUM have provided guidelines regarding the content of ultrasound examinations during pregnancy. They suggest that ultrasound exams be completed in all pregnancies and that the sonography should include the following areas:

First trimester:

1. Location of gestational sac and crown–rump length (CRL)
2. Presence or absence of fetal life
3. Documentation of fetal number
4. Evaluation of the uterus and adnexal structures

Second and third trimesters:

1. Documentation of fetal life, number of fetuses, and presentation(s)
2. Estimate of the amount of amniotic fluid
3. Location of placenta
4. Assessment of gestational age using biparietal diameter (BPD), femur length (FL), head circumference (HC), abdominal circumference (AC)
5. Evaluation of the uterus and adnexal structures

The images should be labeled with the examination date, patient identification, and image orientation, and a written report of the ultrasound findings should be kept with the client's chart (Hadlock 1990b).

Early Pregnancy Detection

Pregnancy may be detected by diagnostic ultrasound as early as the fourth week following the LMP (called menstrual weeks) with a vaginal probe. A small collection of ringlike echoes may be seen within the uterus; this is called the gestational sac. Gestational sac volume may be used to determine gestational age if performed before eight weeks. The error is ± 5 days (Hadlock 1990b).

Clinical Measurements

Measurement of Crown–Rump Length During the first trimester, measurement of the CRL of the fetus is most useful for accurate dating of a pregnancy. The CRL is the longest length of the fetus (excluding the fetal limbs) and is the most accurate sonographic measurement used to establish gestational age in the first trimester (Figure

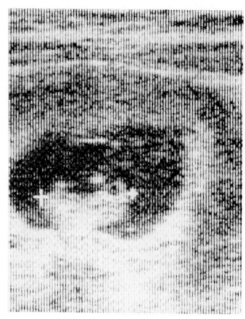

Figure 20–4 Measurement of crown–rump length (CRL). The CRL is measured from the top of the fetal head to the rump (excluding the legs). (From Jeanty P, Romero R: Obstetrical Ultrasound. *New York: McGraw-Hill, 1984, p 53)*

20–4). Because the curvature of the fetus becomes more pronounced after 12 weeks. CRL is not used after this time. Between 7 to 10 weeks CRL can predict gestational age within ± 5 days (Hadlock 1990b).

Measurement of Biparietal Diameter of Fetal Head By far the most important and frequently used application of ultrasound is in the measurement of the biparietal diameter (BPD) of the fetal head. The BPD is the widest diameter of the fetal skull measured at the level of the thalamus and is perpendicular to the fetal midline echo (Figure 20–5). Measurement of the BPD provides the care giver with a useful tool for following fetal development.

Tables correlating the BPD with fetal gestation vary somewhat from one institution to the next, undoubtedly because of socioeconomic and geographic factors inherent in the populations for which the tables were derived. Nevertheless, serial determinations on the same fetus using the same tables can be used as a gross measure of the progress of fetal development. If growth of the fetal head follows a normal curve as gestation advances, one can be assured that the fetus is growing at a normal rate. However, if the curve begins to flatten, the physician must be on the alert for IUGR and must consider this a high-risk pregnancy. The fetus is evaluated by additional means, such as estriol determinations, nonstress tests, and possibly contraction stress tests.

The BPD measurements can be obtained beginning at

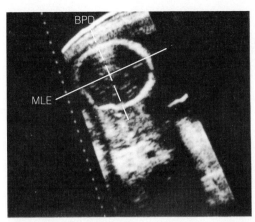

Figure 20–5 Transverse scan of fetal skull at 25 to 26 weeks. The BPD is measured perpendicular to midline echo (MLE). (Section of Diagnostic Ultrasound, courtesy Department of Diagnostic Radiology. Kansas University Medical Center.)

11 weeks of gestation, but the BPD is too small for nomograms to be reliable until about 13 weeks. Detection of IUGR and an accurate prediction of fetal age can be most reliably achieved between 20 and 30 weeks of gestation, when the most rapid growth in the BPD occurs. After 40 weeks' gestation the BPD shows a growth of less than 1 mm/week; thus sonograms obtained at this point are of no value. The BPD measurement generally correlates closely with gestational age, especially if serial determinations were obtained from early in the pregnancy. If only one determination is made late in pregnancy, the gestational age is less accurate and may vary by four weeks either way.

After 28 weeks the BPD alone should not be relied on to determine gestational age. The *cephalic index* (ratio of BPD to occipito-frontal [OF] diameter) should be evaluated to determine normality of the shape of the head. Normally, the fetal head is oval, but molding deformities can be produced by pressure. If the occipito frontal (OF) of the head is shortened and the biparietal (BPD) diameter is elongated, a deformity called brachycephaly exists; if the OF diameter is elongated and the BPD is shortened it is called dolichocephaly. The cephalic index is most useful in assessing the gestational age of the fetus in breech (fetal head crowded under maternal ribs) or vertex (head descended into pelvis) presentations. If the cephalic index is abnormal, gestational age should be determined by other parameters, and abnormalities of the head should be considered and further assessed.

Measurement of Femur Length
Measurement of femur length is done in the second and third trimesters. The femur length appears consistent in all races but will be shortened in the presence of a fetus with osteogenesis imperfecta, or dwarfism (Hadlock 1990b).

Abdominal Measurements
Measurement of the abdominal circumference (measurement at the level of the fetal liver) provides data to aid in the detection of abnormal growth patterns. In IUGR, fetal abdominal girth ceases to increase due to the depletion of glycogen in the fetal liver and also to diminished accumulation of subcutaneous tissue overlying the fetal abdomen. Abdominal circumference measurements alone are meaningless unless the gestational age of the fetus has been defined by CRL or serial BPDs and other measurements, such as estimated fetal weight (EFW), are also used (Watson & Seeds 1990). It appears to be most useful between 34 and 36 weeks' gestation in differentiating normal fetuses from those at risk for IUGR.

CRITICAL THINKING

How would you incorporate the information on fetal development in Chapter 11 with the measurements obtained by ultrasound?

Head-to-Abdomen Ratio
The head circumference (H) to abdomen circumference (A) ratio is used to assess disproportion between the fetal head and body. Disproportion may be observed in asymmetric IUGR and congenital anomalies such as microcephaly. The H:A ratio may also be used to estimate fetal weight (Hadlock 1990b).

Detection of Congenital Anomalies
The role of ultrasound in the detection of structural and functional congenital anomalies is significant since these conditions contribute to 25% to 30% of all perinatal deaths and account for more than 65% of all deaths in high-risk gestations beyond 26 weeks (Manning 1985). Improvement in ultrasound resolution permits earlier and more accurate diagnosis of such conditions as hydrocephaly, anencephaly, meningomyelocele, encephalocele, and meningocele; thoracopulmonary, genitourinary, and musculoskeletal-cutaneous anomalies; and amniotic fluid, umbilical cord, and placental abnormalities. The use of real-time ultrasound now permits detection of these types of anomalies and has had great impact on perinatal morbidity as a result of subsequent in utero therapy or early birth and surgical correction of defects. Fetal anomalies are frequently associated with oligohydramnios or hydramnios, and the clinician should look for anomalies when these conditions are present.

Fetal Growth Determination
One of the most difficult problems facing the clinician is assessment of fetal growth. Ultrasound offers a valuable means of assessing intrauterine growth since the fetus can be measured serially.

Intrauterine growth retardation (IUGR) is classified as symmetric (primary) or asymmetric (secondary). In symmetric IUGR, all organs are reduced in size with equal reduction in body weight and head size. At birth all measurements fall below the tenth percentile. This growth retardation is noted in the first half of the second trimester. It is associated with intrauterine viral infections, chromosomal disorders, major congenital malformations, and maternal malnutrition (Korones 1985).

In asymmetric IUGR the head and brain are normal but there is a reduction in body size, apparently caused by a compromise in the uteroplacental blood flow. The decreased blood flow is associated with PIH, chronic hypertension, and chronic renal disease. This type of IUGR occurs in the majority of cases and is usually not evident prior to the third trimester. Fetuses with asymmetric IUGR are particularly at risk for perinatal asphyxia, hypocalcemia, polycythemia, and hypoglycemia in the neonatal period. Birth weight will be reduced to the 10th percentile, whereas cephalic size may be between the 25th and 30th percentile (Korones 1985).

Second to preterm birth, IUGR is the greatest cause of perinatal mortality. Between 3% and 7% of all pregnancies are complicated by IUGR (Pernoll et al 1986).

The earlier the gestational age is accurately assessed, the more accurate the prediction of IUGR. If a growth-retarded fetus is suspected, serial ultrasounds should be done every two to three weeks.

On first examination, the estimated fetal weight (EFW) is figured as a percentile for that fetus. If the percentile is low, serial sonograms are warranted. If on repeat scan the fetus is at the same percentile, no abnormal growth has occurred. If the percentile increases, growth of the fetus has improved. If the fetus is at a lower percentile, fetal growth is slowing, and this fetus should be further assessed with other means of antenatal surveillance. Serial BPDs will closely assess the type of IUGR, and fetuses can be evaluated further with abdominal-chest measurements, non-stress and contraction stress tests, and biophysical profile. The additional assessments will help determine the optimal timing for birth.

The timing of childbirth with growth-retarded infants is still undecided. Some physicians, in light of pulmonary maturity, effect birth of these infants by 37 to 38 weeks' gestation in hope of preventing long-term CNS deficits. Others choose to wait until other assessment parameters indicate fetal jeopardy (for example, a positive contraction stress test or an abnormal biophysical profile).

Localization of Placenta/Amniotic Fluid Pool

Ultrasound is valuable in localizing the placenta for amniocentesis and in detecting placenta previa. By visualizing its location, the physician can avoid puncturing the placenta during amniocentesis. Ultrasound is used to locate a pool of amniotic fluid, thereby showing the physician exactly where and how deep to insert the needle for amniocentesis (Figure 20–6).

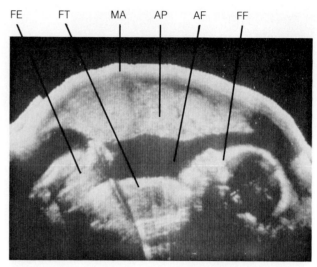

Figure 20–6   Ultrasound scan showing maternal abdomen (MA), anterior placenta (AP), profile of fetal face (FF), adequate amount of amniotic fluid (AF), fetal thorax (FT), and fetal extremities (FE). (From Hobbins JC, Winsberg F, Berkowitz RL: Ultrasonography in Obstetrics and Gynecology, *2nd ed. Baltimore: Williams & Wilkins, 1983, p 123)*

Placental Grading

Grannum, Berkowitz, and Hobbins (1979) noted that throughout gestation the placenta undergoes maturational changes that may be visualized by ultrasound. These morphologic changes in the basal layer, chorionic plate, and intervening placental substance have been classified in terms of grades (0 to III), with increasing changes occurring from 12 weeks' gestation until term. The grade is described according to the presence of echogenic areas in the placental substance, basal layer, and chorionic plate. The reason for these changes is not clear, but they seem to correlate with advancing placental maturity.

Any given placenta may contain more than one grade, but the most mature grade should be used when total assessment is made. Grade I placentas may be noted at any time during gestation (after 12 weeks) and grade III placentas are rarely observed before the 36th week except in women with hypertension, those with growth-retarded fetuses (Hobbins et al 1983), and those who smoke. Pinette et al (1989) found a greater incidence of grade II placentas from 22 to 35 weeks' gestation and a greater incidence of grade III placentas after 25 weeks in women who smoke cigarettes.

Biophysical Profile (BPP)

The **biophysical profile** (BPP), also called fetal biophysical profile (FBPP), is an assessment of five biophysical variables: breathing movement, body movement, tone, amniotic fluid volume, and FHR reactivity. The BPP is used to

Table 20–4 Biophysical Profile Scoring: Technique and Interpretation

Biophysical variable	Normal (score = 2)	Abnormal (score = 0)
1. Fetal breathing movements	≥1 episode of ≥30 sec in 30 min	Absent or no episode of ≥30 sec in 30 min
2. Gross body movements	≥3 discrete body/limb movements in 30 min (episodes of active continuous movement considered as single movement)	≤2 episodes of body/limb movements in 30 min
3. Fetal tone	≥1 episode of active extension with return to flexion of fetal limb(s) or trunk. Opening and closing of hand considered normal tone	Either slow extension with return to partial flexion or movement of limb in full extension or absent fetal movement
4. Reactive fetal heart rate	≥2 episodes of acceleration of ≤15 bpm and of ≥15 sec associated with fetal movement in 20 min	<2 episodes of acceleration of fetal heart rate or acceleration of <15 bpm in 20 min
5. Qualitative amniotic fluid volume	≥1 pocket of fluid measuring ≥1 cm in two perpendicular planes	Either no pockets or a pocket <1 cm in two perpendicular planes

Source: *Manning FA et al: Fetal assessment based on fetal biophysical profile scoring: Experience in 12,620 referred high-risk pregnancies.* Am J Obstet Gynecol *1985; 151(3):344. C. V. Mosby Co.*

assess the fetus at risk for intrauterine compromise. The first four variables are assessed by ultrasound scanning; FHR reactivity is assessed with the nonstress test. By combining these five assessments, the BPP helps to identify the compromised fetus and confirm the healthy fetus.

Specific criteria for normal and abnormal assessments are delineated in Table 20–4 with a score of 2 being assigned to each normal finding and 0 to each abnormal one for a maximum score of 10. The absence of a specific activity is difficult to interpret since it may be indicative of CNS depression or simply the resting state of a healthy fetus. Scores of 8 to 10 are considered normal (Manning 1990). Such scores seem to have the least chance of being associated with a compromised fetus unless a decrease in the amount of amniotic fluid is noted, in which case the infant's birth is indicated (Manning 1990).

A large prospective study of 12,620 high-risk pregnancies (26,257 tests) reported that the gross perinatal mortality rate was 7.4 per 1000. More importantly, the perinatal mortality rate for both the low-risk and high-risk women in the study group has fallen by more than 30% (Manning 1990).

As noted by Vintzileos et al (1987a), increasing use of the BPP has led to recognition of errors in interpretation and subsequent use of this assessment technique. These authors encourage management that is not based solely on BPP score but that includes evaluation of specific biophysical components of the test in order to decrease false-positive and false-negative tests. The biophysical activities of the fetus that develop first are the last to disappear when all activities are arrested due to asphyxia; those that are the last to develop are the most sensitive to hypoxia and their disappearance can be noted first. Therefore, the authors in this study feel that the presence of specific activities should be used to assess the level of fetal compromise at the time

of testing rather than only the BPP score. Fetal tone (exhibited by flexion of the extremities) is the first to function and the last activity to cease during asphyxia. Other activities in the normal developmental sequence are fetal movement, followed by fetal breathing, and then reactivity of the FHR. Therefore, FHR reactivity is the most sensitive to hypoxia. One of the first indications of fetal compromise is a nonreactive nonstress test (NST).

Indications for BPP include those situations in which the NST and CST would be done. Assessment of these fetal biophysical activities is most useful in the evaluation of women who experience decreased fetal movement (who might subsequently have a nonreactive NST) and in the management of IUGR, preterm, diabetic, and postterm pregnancies, and premature rupture of the membranes (PROM). The BPP differentiates the uncompromised fetus from the compromised one in postterm pregnancies (Johnson et al 1986) and, when used in the management of these pregnancies, can allow for a rational approach to client management when lack of cervical ripening does not suggest success with possible induction. Since perinatal mortality increases significantly for each week after 42 weeks of gestation, the BPP allows for continuation of the pregnancy until the cervix is ripe enough for induction or possible fetal jeopardy indicates immediate obstetric intervention.

A management protocol regarding BPP is outlined in Table 20–5 but to date there is no strong consensus of opinion regarding management based on abnormal BPP findings. The BPP has been shown to be more accurate than any other test in being able to identify the compromised fetus (Vintzileos et al 1987b).

Fetal Echocardiography

Ultrasound is now also being used in some select centers to examine fetal cardiac structures. Through the use of

Table 20–5 Interpretation of fetal biophysical profile score results and recommended clinical management based on these results

Test score	Interpretation	Perinatal mortality within 1 week without intervention	Management
10/10 8/10 (normal fluid) 8/8 (NST not done)	Risk of fetal asphyxia extremely rare	< 1/1000	Intervention only for obstetric and maternal factors. No indication for intervention for fetal disease.
8/10 (abnormal fluid)	Probable chronic fetal compromise	89/1000[†]	Determine that there is functioning renal tissue and intact membranes—if so, birth is indicated for fetal indications.
6/10 (normal fluid)	Equivocal test, possible fetal asphyxia	Variable	If the fetus is mature, birth is indicated. In the immature fetus, repeat test within 24 h—if < 6/10, then birth is indicated.
6/10 (abnormal fluid)	Probable fetal asphyxia	89/1000[†]	Birth indicated for fetal indications
4/10	High probability of fetal asphyxia	91/1000[*]	Birth indicated for fetal indications
2/10	Fetal asphyxia almost certain	125/1000[*]	Birth indicated for fetal indications
0/10	Fetal asphyxia certain	600/1000[*]	Birth indicated for fetal indications

From Manning FA: The Biophysical Profile: Contemporary Use. Tenth International Symposium on Perinatal Medicine and Obstetrical Ultrasound. April 9–12, 1990, Las Vegas, Nevada.

echocardiography, treatment of fetal arrhythmias has become possible prior to birth, and many cases of congenital heart disease have been diagnosed prenatally and managed accordingly.

Fetal echocardiography is primarily used for high-risk patients who are suspected of carrying fetuses with congenital anomalies, cardiac arrhythmias, and congestive heart failure. The advantage of being able to obtain information prenatally is that parents, as well as the medical and nursing staff, can be alerted for possible problems that may occur at birth or shortly thereafter and can thus plan appropriate interventions. Fetuses with diagnosed problems are serially evaluated to provide ongoing assessment. When cardiac malformations are diagnosed, level II ultrasound is performed to assess other fetal structures. Genetic amniocentesis may be recommended if cardiac malformations are noted, since the risk of chromosomal abnormalities in these fetuses is about 5%.

Doppler Blood Flow Studies (Umbilical Velocimetry)

Recent advantages in ultrasound technology have made it possible to noninvasively study blood flow changes that occur in maternal and fetal circulations to assess placental function. An ultrasound beam, like that provided by the pocket Doppler (a hand-held ultrasound device) is directed at the umbilical artery (in some cases a maternal vessel such as the arcuate can also be used). The signal is reflected off the red blood cells (RBCs) moving within the vessels, and the subsequent "picture" (waveform) that is received looks like a series of waves. The highest velocity peak of the waves is the systolic measurement and the lowest point is the diastolic velocity. The umbilical artery waveform can then be analyzed to provide information regarding total blood flow in the vessel. In normal pregnancy, maternal and fetal blood flow rates change with advancing fetal gestational age.

A decrease in fetal cardiac output or an increase in resistance of placental vessels will reduce umbilical artery blood flow. Clinical applications of Doppler flow analysis have included situations of fetal growth retardation associated with maternal hypertension. It has been noted that hypertensive or preeclamptic mothers giving birth to growth-retarded infants have abnormal arcuate flow velocity waveforms. In most cases, decreased maternal blood flow has been shown to precede a decrease in fetal blood flow.

Doppler blood flow studies are also helpful in the assessment and management of multiple gestation, diabetes, prolonged pregnancy, growth-retarded fetuses, sickle cell disease, and twin-to-twin transfusion. Umbilical velocimetry has been used to complement the NST, CST, and BPP. Some investigators have suggested that abnormal umbilical velocimetry may precede abnormal findings noted by these other tests (Trudinger 1987). Brar et al (1989) noted that umbilical velocimetry may play an adjunctive role in distinguishing between false-positive and true-positive antepartum and intrapartum late decelerations of fetal heart rate. Tyrrell et al (1989) found that abnormal Doppler umbilical artery waveforms were strongly associated with acidosis, hypoxia, IUGR, and poor perinatal outcome.

Investigators are currently studying other fetal arteries, such as internal carotid, descending aortic, intracerebral, renal, internal iliac and femoral arteries, and the umbilical vein in an attempt to improve the sensitivity of Doppler blood flow study (Reed 1990).

Maternal Assessment of Fetal Activity

Assessment of fetal movement patterns has been used as a screening procedure in the evaluation of fetal status since 1971 when the clinical significance of various types of fetal activity was first described (Sadovsky 1985b). Clinicians now generally agree that vigorous fetal activity provides reassurance of fetal well-being and that marked decrease in activity or cessation of movement may indicate possible fetal compromise requiring immediate follow-up evaluation. Fetal movements are usually assessed by the woman but may also be assessed by FBPP or NST.

Sadovsky (1985a) noted that although there is con-

?

Contemporary Issue
How to Help Couples Make Informed Decisions Regarding Fetal Assessment Techniques

Diagnostic assessment and testing techniques increase in number and complexity with every passing year. Certainly the availability of these techniques has changed the outlook for pregnancies at risk or pregnancies with special problems. Using the new technology, the presence of the fetus can be confirmed and some congenital problems can be identified very early in the pregnancy. Indeed, fetal well-being can be assessed at various times throughout the pregnancy in order to identify problems and make treatment decisions. Because of these advantages, tests are used ever more frequently.

The childbearing couple needs to have as much information as possible in order to make informed decisions when faced with the array of new assessment technologies. Parents need to be clear about the purpose of the proposed test, the information that may be obtained, the risks and benefits for both the mother and the baby, and the alternatives that are available.

Although the majority of the diagnostic tests currently used are administered by physicians, nurses have an integral role in this arena as client educators and advocates. The nurse assesses the informational needs of the couple, provides the information, and ensures that the couple understands the diagnostic technique being used. The nurse does this in preparation for each test, even though the physician will still need to provide required information when obtaining a signed informed consent.

The provision of information and the securing of informed consent are essential, but occasionally problems can get in the way:

- To ensure that the couple has a real choice about having the diagnostic test, the pertinent information needs to be provided ahead of time. It is difficult for parents to make other decisions or to refuse the test once they are in the actual test setting.

- It is often a challenge for nurses to obtain complete information regarding each new technique, and this may stand in the way of comprehensive and accurate teaching.

- Some nurses are unaware of the value they can bring to couples faced with diagnostic testing, and thus they ignore potential educational and advocacy roles.

- Often tests are done without any explanation to the couple. In some instances only the sketchiest information is provided. This makes it difficult for the couple to understand the situation and does not enable them to participate in their own care.

- Some physicians prefer that the couple not have much information, because this may cause them to worry unnecessarily. This approach can quickly lead to conflict when unanticipated problems arise and the couple feel they were not made aware of the potential risks.

siderable variation among individuals, the average number of daily movements rises from about 200 at 20 weeks to a maximum of 575 at 32 weeks and gradually decreases to an average of 282 at term. In women with a multiple gestation, daily fetal movements are significantly higher. Although women report periods of markedly decreased fetal movement, this has been found to be associated with periods of fetal sleep, medications, smoking, and other factors. It has also been noted that some women are not as aware of fetal activity and that more fetal movements are usually noted on ultrasound assessment than by the woman herself. Although there are various types of fetal movements, women at high risk for fetal hypoxia have noted a reduction in or disappearance of fetal movements or changes in the type of fetal activity with a predominance of only weak movements prior to fetal death.

Daily fetal movement assessment by the woman can be done in a variety of ways. The Cardiff-Count-to-Ten or Modified Cardiff count may be used from 28 weeks of gestation (Broussard 1990). See Teaching Guide: What to Tell the Pregnant Woman About Assessing Fetal Activity in Chapter 14 for further information.

It has been observed that sudden, strong, vigorous movements followed by cessation are characteristic signs of acute fetal distress and impending death, often caused by cord compression or sudden abruption (Sadovsky 1985a). Women should immediately notify their physician if they note this type of fetal activity.

Although maternal assessment of fetal activity is a subjective means of evaluating fetal status, it has been found to be an excellent screening test for diagnosing chronic fetal distress. Furthermore, it is simple for the woman to perform, does not interfere with her normal routines, costs nothing, and provides reassurance. Pregnant women need to understand that fetal movements are significant, that fetal activity changes during pregnancy, and that when movements weaken or cease they should contact their care giver for further evaluation.

As discussed in Chapter 14, women should be reassured that there are fetal rest-sleep states during which minimal or no movement may occur. Gross fetal movements may be absent for at least an hour as the fetus rests. Thus fetal movements may be a sign of fetal well-being, but episodic absence of movement is also characteristic of normal fetuses.

Nursing Care

The nurse assists in teaching the technique for DFMR. The nurse can also help the woman devise a daily record in which she can report fetal movements. The nurse is available for questions and to clarify areas of concern.

Nonstress Test (NST)

The **nonstress test** (NST) has become a widely accepted method of evaluating fetal status. The test involves observation of acceleration of the fetal heart rate (FHR) with fetal movement. The test is based on the knowledge that the fetus is normally active throughout pregnancy and that good fetal activity will result in acceleration of the fetal heart rate when the normal fetus moves. Accelerations of

Research Note

Clinical Application of Research

Obstetric nurses, self-identified as having a primary clinical area of either labor and delivery or antepartum, interpreted 5 nonstress test (NST) strips in a study designed by Bonnie Chez and her associates (1990). The 3 purposes of the study were to determine if nurses could correctly interpret NST strips, to determine whether or not demographic variables correlated with the accuracy of interpretation, and to compare the responses of obstetric nurses to those of obstetricians regarding the same strips.

From 84% to 98% of the nurses agreed on the same answer for each of the 5 strips. No association was found between any of the demographic variables and the degree of accuracy of strip interpretation. The demographic variables included educational degree, number of years of experience in obstetrics and reading NSTs, formal course in NSTs, and self-evaluation of ability. Comparison between the nurses and the obstetricians revealed similar interpretations by both groups. "The outcome was that nurses as a group performed in a manner equivalent to physicians as a group in correctly labeling and interpreting nonreassuring findings" (Chez et al 1990, p 230).

Critical Thinking Applied to Research

Strengths: Large sample of 1000 selected for survey with a 41% return rate. Excellent description of sample demographic characteristics. Limitations of study clearly identified.

Concerns: The two groups, nurses and physicians, interpreted the strips at different times for different studies. Comparison of these two groups creates some problems related to internal validity of the study such as history and maturation of subjects. For example, the physician study was several years old at the time of comparison, and the level of physician performance might have changed in the time since the study.

Chez B, Skurnick J, Chez R et al: Interpretations of nonstress tests by obstetric nurses. *JOGNN* 1990; 19(3):227.

the FHR imply an intact central and autonomic nervous system that is not being affected by intrauterine hypoxia.

The advantages of the NST are that it is relatively quick, inexpensive, and easy to interpret; it can be done in an outpatient setting; and there are no known side effects. The disadvantages are that it is sometimes difficult to obtain a suitable tracing, the woman has to sit or lie relatively still for 20 to 30 minutes, and the fetus may be in a sleep cycle at the time the test is performed.

The NST can be used as early as the 27th week of gestation. The NST can be used as an assessment tool in any pregnancy but is especially useful in the presence of diabetes, pregnancy-induced hypertension, intrauterine growth retardation, spontaneous rupture of membranes, multiple gestation, and other high-risk pregnancy problems. Testing intervals may vary depending on the condition of the mother and baby and recommendations of various experts. Clark (1990) recommends twice weekly testing for diabetes, postdates, asymmetric IUGR, and multiple gestation; a daily NST for spontaneous rupture of membranes; and weekly testing for other conditions.

Currently, a *modified NST* may also be used. In this test, a device which sends sound into the fetus (called fetal acoustical stimulation [FAST]) is used after five minutes of testing. If there is no acceleration of the fetal heart rate, the sound stimulus is used again (see next section for further discussion of FAST).

The fairly high false-positive rate with the NST may be related to inadequate testing time, hypotension in the mother during the testing session, or maternal medications such as narcotics, magnesium sulfate, barbiturates, methadone, or antihypertensive medications (Sacks & Sokol 1989).

NST Procedure

The NST is usually scheduled during the day-time hours and the woman is asked to eat approximately two hours prior to the test (Devoe 1989). The woman is positioned in a semi-Fowler's position with a small pillow or blanket under the right hip to displace the uterus to the left. Many facilities use a recliner chair, which permits a semi-Fowler's position while providing a leg and foot rest. An electronic fetal monitor is applied (see discussion on p 628). The examiner applies two belts around the woman's abdomen. One belt holds a device that detects uterine or fetal movement. The other belt holds a device that detects the FHR.

Recordings of the FHR are obtained for approximately 30 to 40 minutes (minimum of 20 minutes and maximum of 90 minutes [Sacks & Sokol 1989]). The woman or nurse notes each fetal movement as it is recorded. If no fetal movements occur after 30 or 40 minutes of observation, the woman is given orange or other fruit juice or a light meal. Fetal movements often increase due to distension of the maternal stomach and elevation in blood glucose. Other stimulation of the fetus may involve the use of FAST or asking the mother to place her hands on her abdomen and gently push on her baby.

Interpretation of NST

The results of the NST are interpreted as follows:

- *Reactive test.* A reactive NST shows at least two accelerations of FHR with fetal movements, of 15 beats per minute, lasting 15 seconds or more, over 20 minutes (Figure 20–7).

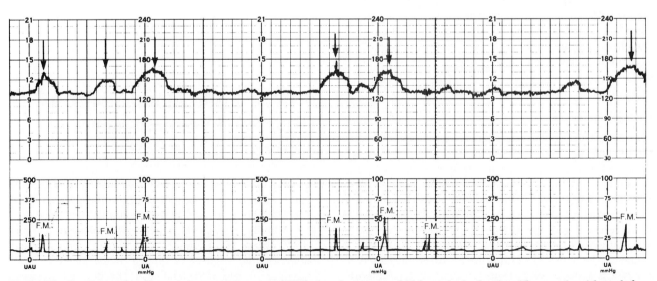

Figure 20–7   Example of a reactive nonstress test (NST). Accelerations of 15 beats/min, lasting 15 seconds with each fetal movement (FM). (Top of strip = fetal heart rate; bottom of strip = uterine activity tracing.) Note that FHR increases (above baseline) at least 15 beats and remains at that rate for at least 15 seconds before returning to the former baseline.

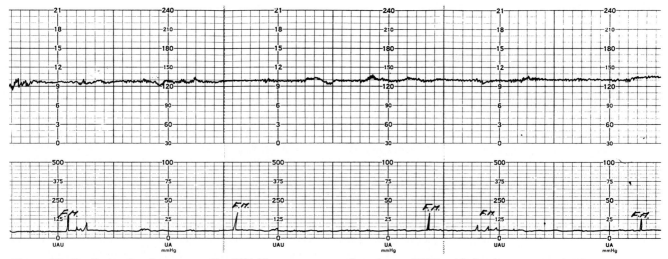

Figure 20–8 Example of a nonreactive NST. There are no accelerations of FHR with fetal movement (FM). Baseline FHR = 130 beats/min; tracing of uterine activity is on the bottom of the strip.

- *Nonreactive test.* In a nonreactive test, the reactive criteria are not met. For example, the accelerations are not as much as 15 beats per minute, or do not last 15 seconds, and so on (Figure 20–8).
- *Unsatisfactory test.* An unsatisfactory NST has data that cannot be interpreted, or inadequate fetal activity.

Note that criteria for the NST appear to vary somewhat from one author to another. Some require two accelerations of FHR in 20 minutes; others require two in 10 minutes.

It is particularly important that anyone who performs the NST also understand the significance of any decelerations of the FHR during testing. If decelerations are noted, the physician/nurse-midwife should be notified for further evaluation of fetal status.

Management

The clinical management may vary somewhat between different clinicians. Devoe (1989) recommends the following: If the NST is reactive in less than 30 minutes the test is concluded and rescheduled as indicated by the condition that is present; if nonreactive, the test time is extended for 30 minutes at a time until the results are reactive, and then the test is rescheduled as indicated—or, if the fetal heart rate is still nonreactive, additional testing such as diagnostic ultrasound and FBPP or CST or immediate birth is considered; if the NST is nonreactive and spontaneous decelerations are present, diagnostic ultrasound and FBPP are recommended. (See Figure 20–9.)

Nursing Care

The nurse ascertains the woman's understanding of the NST, including FAST and the vibroacoustic stimulation test (VST) (see next section) and the possible results. The reasons for the NST, the equipment being used, and the procedure are reviewed prior to beginning the test. The nurse positions the woman and applies the electronic fetal monitor. Maternal blood pressure is monitored during the NST to determine whether hypotension is present. The nurse administers the NST, interprets the results, and reports the findings to the physician/nurse-midwife and the expectant woman.

Fetal Acoustic Stimulation Test (FAST) and Vibroacoustic Stimulation Test (VST)

Use of acoustic (sound) and vibroacoustic (vibration and sound) stimulation of the fetus is becoming more common as an adjunct to the NST. Several methods have been used (for example, loud speakers, bells, artificial larynx). Figure 20–10 shows one example. A hand-held, self-contained, battery-operated device is applied to the maternal abdomen over the area of the fetal head. This device generates a low-frequency vibration and a buzzing sound which are intended to induce accelerations of FHR in response to

```
                          ┌─────────┐
                          │   NST   │
                          └─────────┘
              ┌───────────────┴───────────────┐
              ▼                               ▼
      ┌──────────────┐              ┌──────────────┐
      │ Reactive     │              │ Nonreactive  │
      │ ≤ 30 minutes │              └──────────────┘
      └──────────────┘       ┌──────────┼──────────────────────┐
              ▼              ▼          ▼                      ▼
    ┌──────────────────┐ ┌────────────┐ ┌────────────┐ ┌────────────────┐
    │ Repeat           │ │ Inadequate │ │ No         │ │ No Accelerations│
    │ Test as Indicated│ │ Acceleration│ │ Accelerations│ │ +             │
    │ (e.g. 2–3 days)  │ │ Frequency  │ └────────────┘ │ Spontaneous    │
    └──────────────────┘ └────────────┘                │ Decelerations  │
                                 │         │            └────────────────┘
                                 ▼─────────┘                    │
                           ┌────────────┐              ┌────────────────────┐
                           │ Extend 30' │              │ Diagnostic Ultrasound│
                           └────────────┘              │ ±                  │
                          ┌──────┴──────┐              │ CST or             │
                          ▼             ▼              │ Biophysical Profile │
                   ┌────────────┐ ┌────────────┐       │ or Delivery        │
                   │ Reactive   │ │ Nonreactive│       └────────────────────┘
                   └────────────┘ └────────────┘
                                        ▼
                                  ┌────────────┐
                                  │ Extend 30' │
                                  └────────────┘
                                 ┌──────┴──────┐
                                 ▼             ▼
                          ┌────────────┐ ┌────────────┐
                          │ Reactive   │ │ Nonreactive│
                          └────────────┘ └────────────┘
```

Figure 20–9   NST management scheme. (From Devoe LD: Nonstress and contraction stress testing. In: Gynecology and Obstetrics. Vol. 3. Depp R, Eschenbach DA, Sciarri JJ [editors]: Philadelphia. Lippincott, 1989, Ch 78, figure 5, page 9)

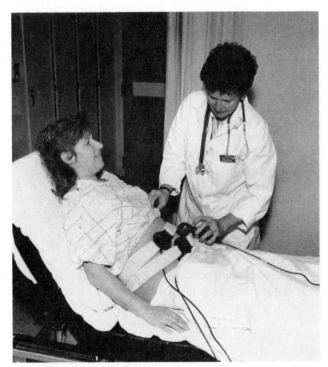

Figure 20–10   Fetal acoustic stimulation testing using a fetal acoustic stimulator.

movement in those fetuses who demonstrate nonreactivity during the NST. This device may be connected to the electronic fetal monitor for automatic documentation on electronic fetal monitoring tracing paper or can be used without the monitor as a stimulus to evoke fetal movement for evaluation of maternal perception of fetal activity. Advantages of FAST or VST are that they are noninvasive techniques, results are rapidly available, time for the NST is shortened, and the test is easy to perform. Whether the fetus responds more to the vibration or to the sound is not known.

Contraction Stress Test (CST)

The **contraction stress test** (CST) is a means of evaluating the respiratory function (oxygen and carbon dioxide exchange) of the placenta. It enables the health care team to identify the fetus at risk for intrauterine asphyxia by observing the response of the FHR to the stress of uterine contractions (spontaneous or induced). During contractions, intrauterine pressure increases. Blood flow to the intervillous space of the placenta is reduced momentarily, thereby decreasing oxygen transport to the fetus. A healthy fetus usually tolerates this reduction well. If the placental reserve is insufficient, fetal hypoxia, depression of the myocardium, and a decrease in FHR occur.

Indications and Contraindications

The CST is indicated for pregnancies at risk for placental insufficiency or fetal compromise because of the following:

- IUGR
- Diabetes mellitus
- Postdates (42 or more weeks' gestation
- Nonreactive NST
- Abnormal or suspicious biophysical profile

Contraindications for the CST are the following:

- Third-trimester bleeding (placenta previa or marginal abruptio placentae)
- Previous cesarean birth with classical uterine incision
- Instances in which the risk of possible preterm labor outweighs the advantage of the CST include:
  1. Premature rupture of the membranes
  2. Incompetent cervix or Shirodkar-Barter operation (cerclage—surgical procedure in which an incompetent cervix is encircled with suture to prevent it from dilating before term)
  3. Multiple gestation

CST Procedure

A necessary component of the CST is the presence of uterine contractions that occur three times in ten minutes. The contractions may occur spontaneously, or they may be induced by oxytocin or nipple stimulation. The most common method of stimulating uterine contractions for a CST has been intravenous administration of oxytocin (Pitocin). This kind of CST is called the *oxytocin challenge test* (OCT). Many facilities now use the *nipple stimulation contraction stress test* (NSCST). The development of this method is based on the knowledge that endogenous oxytocin is produced in response to stimulation of the breasts or nipples.

The CST is performed on an outpatient basis by qualified obstetric nurses well acquainted with fetal monitoring and the interpretation of various FHR patterns. Most facilities require the tests be administered in or near the labor and birth unit, in the event that adverse reactions to oxytocin stimulation occur. In many settings the physician/nurse-midwife must be present. The procedure, reasons for administering the test, equipment, and normal variations in monitoring that occur during the test should be clearly explained prior to the test to alleviate the woman's apprehension. A consent form may be signed. The woman should empty her bladder prior to beginning the CST, because she may be confined to bed for 1 1/2 to 2 hours.

During the test, the woman assumes a semi-Fowler's or side-lying position to avoid supine hypotension. After the area of clearest fetoscopic heart tones is noted, the ultrasonic transducer (from the electronic fetal monitor) is placed on the woman's abdomen over the area of the fetal back or chest so that the FHR may be accurately recorded on the monitoring strip. (See Chapter 22 for further discussion of fetal monitoring.) To record uterine contractions, the tocodynamometer (pressure transducer) is placed over the area of the uterine fundus. For the first 15 minutes the nurse records baseline measurements, including blood pressure, fetal activity, variations of the FHR during fetal movement, and spontaneous contractions. In addition, pertinent medical and obstetric information may be obtained from the woman to aid in her further management.

After a 15-minute baseline recording, a nipple stimulation contraction stress test or intravenous oxytocin contraction stress test is done. In the event that three spontaneous contractions of good quality lasting 40 to 60 seconds have occurred in a 10-minute period, the results are evaluated and the test is concluded.

Nipple Stimulation Contraction Stress Test (NSCST)

In 1982 Garite and Freeman suggested manual stimulation of the mother's nipples to induce contractions sufficient for the CST. The test is also called breast self-stimulation test (BSST) or breast stimulation test (BST).

The exact mechanism by which nipple stimulation works and whether subsequent contractions are similar to those that occur in spontaneous labor or by the OCT have yet to be determined. With nipple stimulation, sensory nerve impulses are related to the neural cells of the hypothalamus where oxytocin is synthesized. These impulses cause the release of endogenous oxytocin from the neural cells, with subsequent transport to nerve terminals in the posterior pituitary gland into the bloodstream. The result is contractions similar to those caused by suckling stimulation during lactation.

Nipple stimulation has been found to be effective in inducing contractions sufficient for the CST. Most women have achieved satisfactory contractions within 15 to 30 minutes. Although the test seems simple to perform and no adverse fetal outcomes have been reported, the possibility of hyperstimulation and exaggerated uterine activity have been noted, occasionally with prolonged FHR decelerations (Figure 20–11). Hyperstimulation is defined as contractions lasting more than 90 seconds or occurring more frequently than every two minutes.

Because pregnancies with compromised placental function are among those evaluated by the NSCST, exaggerated uterine activity and hyperstimulation could be potentially harmful to the fetus. It is suggested that this test be performed in or near a childbirth unit where emergency fetal resuscitation, the administration of tocolytics, or immediate cesarean birth can be performed if hyperstimulation and/or prolonged deceleration of the FHR occurs.

NSCST Procedure

The nurse begins the NSCST by explaining the procedure to the woman. She is positioned in a sitting or side-lying

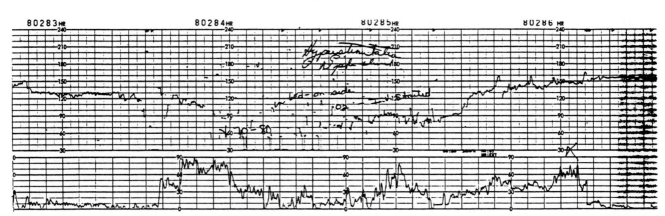

Figure 20–11   Hyperstimulation during nipple stimulation. The onset of contractions is shown two minutes following nipple stimulation. Panels 80284-80286 reveal hyperstimulation of more than 90 seconds and three contractions within an 8 1/2-minute period with accompanying FHR deceleration to 70 to 80 beats per minute lasting 6 1/2 minutes. (From J Perinatol 1985; 5 [summer]:56)

position to maintain optimum uteroplacental circulation and to enhance the quality of the uterine contractions as they occur. The woman's privacy should be protected, yet the nurse needs to stay with the woman during the entire procedure to remind her to cease stimulation at the appropriate time and to complete nursing assessments.

An electronic fetal monitor is applied, and a 15- to 20-minute strip is obtained to get a baseline and to determine uterine status. The FHR is evaluated for reactivity (NST). Nipple stimulation begins with the woman brushing her palm across one nipple through her shirt or gown for 2 to 3 minutes. Nipple stimulation should stop if a uterine contraction begins. The nipple stimulation continues after a 5-minute rest period. The process is continued until 40 minutes have elapsed or uterine contractions of at least 40 seconds in length occur at least three times in ten minutes (Marshall 1986). In some settings, if no contractions occur after 15 to 20 minutes, the other nipple is stimulated in the same manner (Murray et al 1986). Bilateral stimulation should not be instituted unless unilateral stimulation fails to induce contractions; in these cases stimulation should be performed with caution to avoid hyperstimulation. The woman's blood pressure is assessed every 10 minutes throughout the procedure. The FHR is assessed for reactivity and the presence of decelerations. If a deceleration occurs, nipple stimulation is discontinued, the left lateral position is maintained, oxygen is begun per mask at 6 to 8 L/min, and the physician/nurse-midwife is notified (Marshall 1986). If contractions occur more frequently than every two minutes and/or last more than 90 seconds, the nipple stimulation should be discontinued, the side-lying position maintained, the FHR carefully observed, and the physician/nurse-midwife notified (Marshall 1986). Oxygen may be administered. The woman's blood pressure and pulse should be assessed. In the presence of a hyperstimulation pattern the nurse should also be prepared to administer tocolytics or prepare for emergency childbirth in the event of unresolved fetal distress.

The NSCST has been shown to be successful in terms of performance time and adequate contraction frequency. The same criteria that are used for the OCT are used for the NSCST. Embarrassment is rare if the procedure is thoroughly explained to the woman and is performed in a comfortable, relaxed, private environment. Since maternal anxiety may be related to onset of contractions, it is important that the nurse thoroughly explain the procedure and rationale for performance of it and ensure the woman's privacy.

Since this test involves the induction of contractions by release of endogenous oxytocin, only knowledgeable nurses should be responsible for monitoring it.

The NSCST is equivalent to the administration of intravenous oxytocin but takes less time to perform, is less expensive, and causes less discomfort because no IV is used.

Intravenous Oxytocin Contraction Stress Test

A CST can also be done by using intravenous oxytocin. This test is also called an oxytocin challenge test (OCT). In this test an electrolyte solution such as lactated Ringer's solution is started as a primary infusion. A piggyback infusion of oxytocin in a similar solution is attached. An infusion pump is used so that the amount of oxytocin being infused can be measured accurately. The administration procedure is the same as for inducing labor through oxytocin administration. See Chapter 26 for further discussion. Oxytocin is administered until three uterine contractions lasting 40 to 60 seconds occur in a 10-minute period. If late decelerations are repetitive or occur more than three times, the oxytocin infusion should be discontinued and the physician notified immediately.

Interpretation and Management

A CST is usually not done prior to 28 weeks' gestation primarily for two reasons:

Table 20–6 Interpretation of the Contraction Stress Test

Result	Interpretation
Negative	No late decelerations occur with a minimum of three uterine contractions (lasting 40–60 seconds) in 10-minute period.
Positive	Late decelerations occur with 50% or more of the uterine contractions.
Equivocal	
Suspicious	Late decelerations occur with less than 50% of the uterine contractions once an adequate contraction pattern has been established.
Hyperstimulation	Late decelerations occur with excessive uterine activity (contractions closer than every 2 minutes, lasting for longer than 90 seconds, or a persistent increase in uterine tone).
Unsatisfactory	Uterine contraction pattern is inadequate or FHR tracing is too poor to interpret.

From Sacks AJ, Sokol RJ: Clinical use of antepartum fetal monitoring techniques. In: Gynecology and Obstetrics. Vol. 2. Dilts PV, Sciarra JJ (editors). Philadelphia: Lippincott, 1989, Ch 58, table 1, p 4.

1. In light of a positive test, birth and extrauterine survival would be questionable at such an early gestational age.

2. Sufficient research has not been done to determine whether the same test results apply to a fetus of this gestation.

CSTs are usually begun at 32 to 34 weeks' gestation and are repeated once or twice a week until the woman gives birth. Should the woman's condition deteriorate, the CST should be repeated as soon as possible.

A *negative CST* (Table 20–6 and Figure 20–12) is rarely associated with intrauterine fetal death (2.2 per 1000), so the test is usually repeated in seven days (Sacks & Sokol 1989).

A *positive CST* (Table 20–6 and Figure 20–13) may indicate the possibility of insufficient placental respiratory reserve (Devoe 1989), and the fetus that is at higher risk for increased perinatal morbidity and mortality (75 to 100 per 1000) (Sacks & Sokol 1989). The fetus also has an increased risk of fetal distress, low 5-minute Apgar scores after birth, and IUGR (Devoe 1989). Less than 10% of CSTs in high-risk populations are positive (Devoe 1989).

The positive CST is associated with a 20% to 50% false-positive rate and this is attributed to aortocaval compression during uterine contractions, increased uterine tone during intravenous oxytocin-induced contractions, and the lack of any standardization of the "stress" that is produced by the uterine contractions (Sacks & Sokol 1989). Additional information may be obtained by performing an NST and assessing the variability of the FHR. When a reactive NST is present and the FHR has average variability, the outcome of the fetus during labor and birth is usually good. If a nonreactive NST and decreased variability are present, the obstetrician may consider a trial induction of labor or cesarean birth.

An *equivocal* (suspicious) test result may be managed by continuing the CST until the results are either negative or positive or by rescheduling the test for after one to two hours of rest or for the next day. Approximately 7% of CST results are equivocal.

A *hyperstimulation* pattern occurs in less than 3% of CSTs. This pattern is not reassuring in terms of providing information about the fetus, nor is the result useful (Devoe 1989). Repeat testing may be done after a period of rest, or another fetal assessment test may be done (Devoe 1989).

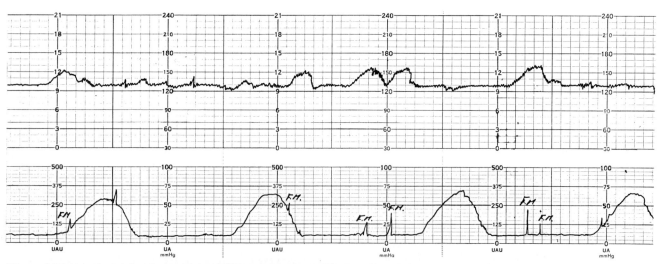

Figure 20–12   Example of a negative CST (and reactive NST). Baseline FHR = 130 beats/minute with acceleration of FHR of at least 15 beats/min lasting 15 seconds with each fetal movement (FM). Uterine contractions recorded on bottom half of strip indicate three contractions in 8 minutes (with paper speed at 3 cm/min).

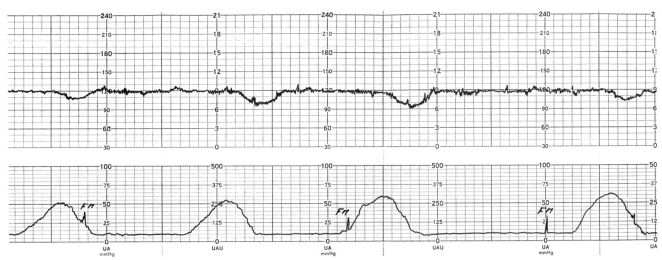

Figure 20–13 Example of a positive contraction stress test (CST). Repetitive late decelerations occur with each contraction. Note that there are no accelerations of FHR with three fetal movements (FM): Baseline FHR = 120 beats/min. Uterine contractions (bottom half of strip) occurred three times in 8 minutes.

Regardless of the test result, if variable decelerations occur, ultrasound examination for amniotic fluid volume and localization of the umbilical cord is recommended (Devoe 1989).

Nursing Care

The nurse ascertains the woman's understanding of the CST and the possible results. The reasons for the CST and the procedure are reviewed before beginning the test. Written consent is required in some settings. In this case, the physician/nurse-midwife is responsible for fully informing the woman about the test. The nurse administers the CST, interprets the results, and reports the findings to the physician/nurse-midwife and the expectant woman. The nurse is available to clarify any further treatment ordered by the physician/nurse-midwife.

Amniocentesis

One of the most valuable studies available for the management of the pregnant woman is analysis of the amniotic fluid, which is obtained by a technique known as amniocentesis.

Determinations that can be made by amniocentesis early in the pregnancy include chromosome and biochemical (enzyme analysis; alpha-feto protein measurement for neural tube defects); and delineation of abnormalities detected by ultrasound. Later in the pregnancy, amniocentesis may be done for lung maturity studies such as L/S ratio and the presence of phosphatidylglycerol and phosphatidylcholine. This procedure is also used to determine the pres-

ence or absence of intrauterine infection with premature rupture of the membrances in preterm labor before tocolytic therapy is considered.

Amniotic fluid may be obtained by either transabdominal or suprapubic amniocentesis. The fetus, umbilical cord, or placenta may be punctured inadvertently, causing injuries ranging from minor scratches of fetal parts to intrauterine hemorrhage, leading to fetal distress and intrauterine fetal death. Placental perforation could result in hemorrhage from the fetal circulation, which could lead to fetal anemia or to increased sensitization of an Rh negative mother. Intra-amniotic infection and induction of preterm labor are also hazards. Complications are rare (0.5% to 1%), but the woman does need to be informed of them. A consent form is generally signed for this procedure.

Procedure

Amniocentesis is done on an outpatient basis but needs to be performed near a birthing area in case acute fetal distress is encountered. The woman should empty her bladder prior to the amniocentesis so that the bladder is not entered instead of the uterus. Amniotic fluid and urine may look similar, and if there is a possibility that urine was obtained during a suprapubic tap, the fluid should be checked for pH and protein content with a dipstick. Amniotic fluid has a high protein content, which is not a normal finding in urine unless the woman has been spilling protein in her urine as a result of PIH or renal disease.

The abdomen is scanned by ultrasound to locate the placenta, fetus, and an adequate pocket of fluid. The amniocentesis, or "tap," is done immediately, before the fetus has the opportunity to move. The needle insertion site is of the utmost importance since the fetus, placenta, umbilical cord, bladder, and uterine arteries must all be avoided. The impor-

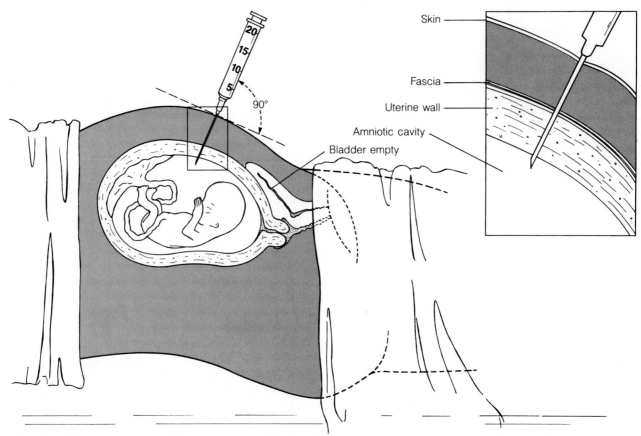

Skin

Fascia

Uterine wall

Amniotic cavity

Bladder empty

90°

Figure 20–14   Amniocentesis. The woman is usually scanned by ultrasound to determine the placental site and to lo-cate a pocket of amniotic fluid. As the needle is inserted, three levels of resistance are felt when the needle penetrates the skin, fascia, and uterine wall. When the needle is placed within the uterine cavity, amniotic fluid is withdrawn.

tance of locating the placenta cannot be stressed enough, especially in cases of Rh isoimmunization, in which trauma to the placenta increases fetal-maternal transfusion and worsens the immunization. In addition, if the placenta is anterior a suprapubic tap may be required to avoid puncturing the placenta. Except for very late in pregnancy, the fetal head can be displaced upward and the amniocentesis done suprapubically (Figure 20–14). If the fetal head cannot be displaced upward, the needle can be inserted from the side of the uterus. In the last few weeks of pregnancy, the fetus may occupy what appears to be all the available space in the uterus. There may be a decrease in the amount of available amniotic fluid. With the aid of ultrasound, fluid can usually be located, although in some cases it is impossible.

After the abdomen is scanned, the skin of the maternal abdomen is cleansed with povidone-iodine (Betadine). A 22-gauge spinal needle is inserted into the uterine cavity. Generally, fluid immediately flows into the needle. The first few drops are discarded, and then a syringe is attached to the needle and the fluid is aspirated (Figure 20–15). From 15 to 20 mL of amniotic fluid are withdrawn, placed in test tubes covered with tape (to shield the fluid from light to prevent breakdown of bilirubin and other pigments), and

sent to the laboratory for analysis. The needle is withdrawn, and the FHR is assessed for approximately 15 minutes. If the woman's vital signs and the FHR are normal, she is allowed to leave. (See Procedure 20–1.)

If the amniotic fluid becomes contaminated with blood, the fluid should be centrifuged immediately. The woman is observed closely for 30 to 40 minutes for alterations in the FHR. The blood should be tested to determine whether it is maternal or fetal.

Rh negative women are given Rh immune globulin after amniocentesis, provided that they are not already sensitized. If the amniotic fluid from these women is contaminated with blood, the sample should be tested to identify fetal cells. In this situation, a larger dose of immune globulin is required.

Nursing Care

The nurse assists the physician during the amniocentesis. Nursing responsibilities are listed in Procedure 20–1. In addition, the nurse supports the woman undergoing amnio-

Nursing Responsibilities During Amniocentesis

Nursing action	Rationale
Objective: Prepare woman.	
Explain procedure.	Information will decrease anxiety.
Reassure woman.	
Have woman sign consent form.	Signing indicates woman's awareness of risks and consent to procedure.
Have woman empty bladder.	Emptying bladder decreases risk of bladder perforation.
Objective: Prepare equipment.	
Collect supplies: 22-gauge spinal needle with stylet 10-mL syringe 20-mL syringe Three 10-mL test tubes with tops (amber-colored or covered with tape)	Amniotic fluid must be shielded from light to prevent breakdown of bilirubin.
Objective: Monitor vital signs.	
Obtain baseline data on maternal BP, pulse, respiration, and FHR. Monitor every 15 minutes.	Status of woman and fetus is assessed.
Objective: Locate fetus and placenta.	
Provide assistance as physician palpates for fetal position. Assist with real-time ultrasound.	Real-time ultrasound is used to identify fetal parts and placenta and locate pockets of amniotic fluid. Amniocentesis is usually performed laterally in the area of fetal small parts where pockets of amniotic fluid are usually seen.
Objective: Cleanse abdomen.	
Prep abdomen with Betadine or other cleansing agent.	Incidence of infection is decreased.
Objective: Collect specimen of amniotic fluid.	
Obtain test tubes from physician; provide correct identification; send to lab with appropriate lab slips.	
Objective: Reassess vital signs.	
Determine woman's BP, pulse, respirations, and FHR; palpate fundus to assess fetal and uterine activity; monitor woman with external fetal monitor for 20–30 minutes after amniocentesis. Have woman rest on left side.	Fetus may have been inadvertently punctured. Uterine contractions may ensue following procedure; treatment course should be determined to counteract any supine hypotension and to increase venous return and cardiac output.
Objective: Complete client record.	
Record type of procedure done, date, time, name of physician performing test, maternal-fetal response, and disposition of specimen.	Client records will be complete and current.
Objective: Educate woman.	
Reassure woman; instruct her to report any of the following side effects:	Client will know how to recognize side effects or conditions that warrant further treatment.

1. Unusual fetal hyperactivity or lack of movement
2. Vaginal discharge—clear drainage or bleeding
3. Uterine contractions or abdominal pain
4. Fever or chills

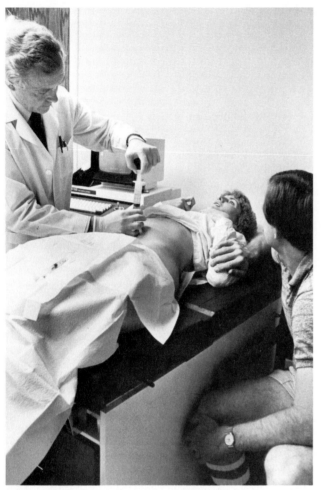

Figure 20–15   During the amniocentesis, amniotic fluid is aspirated into a syringe.

centesis. Women are usually apprehensive about what is about to happen as well as about the information that will be obtained by amniocentesis. The physician explains the procedure before the woman signs the consent form. As it is being performed, the woman may need additional emotional support. She may become anxious during the procedure. She may also become lightheaded, nauseated, and diaphoretic from lying on her back with a gravid uterus compressing the abdominal vessels. The nurse can provide support to the woman by further clarifying the physician's instructions or explanations, by relieving the woman's physical discomfort when possible, and by responding verbally and physically to the woman's need for reassurance.

Amniotic Fluid Tests

Alpha-Fetoprotein (AFP) Screening

Alpha-fetoprotein (AFP) is a fetal serum protein produced in the yolk sac for the first six weeks and then by the fetal gastrointestinal tract and liver in the second trimester. The level of AFP in fetal plasma reaches a peak between 10 to 13 weeks and then declines until term, being excreted in fetal urine and subsequently into the amniotic fluid (Davis et al 1985). The AFP is found in the fetal circulation, amniotic fluid, and maternal serum. Elevated levels in amniotic fluid (AFAFP) or maternal serum (MSAFP) have been found to reflect open neural tube defects (NTD) such as spina bifida and anencephaly. Elevated levels have also been found in women with multiple gestation, incorrect gestational age, a dead fetus, abdominal wall defects (eg, gastroschisis and omphalocele), teratomas, Rh-sensitization, fetal distress, and normal fetuses (Simpson & Elias 1989).

The exact mechanism by which fetal AFP reaches the maternal circulation is unclear. Some authors state that it enters through the fetal kidneys and diffuses across the placenta to the maternal circulation (Jeanty & Romero 1984); others say it leaks through the meninges of the incomplete closure of the neural tube (spinal defect) (Hobbins et al 1985). Still others report that transfer cannot be explained on the basis of simple diffusion from the amniotic fluid to the maternal circulation, since they found no relationship between AFAFP and MSAFP levels (Barford et al 1985).

Maternal serum is assessed for AFP between 15 and 18 weeks of gestation. If the value is elevated and the gestational age is less than 18 weeks, a second sample is drawn one week after the initial test. If the value is still elevated, a level II ultrasound is performed to rule out fetal abnormalities, multiple gestation, or fetal demise. Some centers do an ultrasound after the first elevated AFP finding and do not redraw a second sample. Simpson and Elias (1989) report that this protocol identifies about 90% of fetuses with anencephaly and 80% of fetuses with spina bifida.

The incidence of NTD in the United States is 1 or 2:1000 (Simpson & Elias 1989). The number of false-positive results depends on the cutoff level, but the higher the cutoff level, the greater the number of women who will be suspected of having an abnormal fetus requiring additional testing. Therefore, routine screening and cutoff level depend on the population area at high risk for NTD. There is controversy regarding the necessity for mass screening due to expense of testing, problems related to assay and interpretation of results, the number of false-positive results, and the need for counseling. In any given population the cost-benefit ratio of this expensive screening test must be taken into consideration. Those women who may choose to be tested include those with a history of a child with a NTD, a strong family history of NTD, pregnant women with diabetes, and those residing in areas where NTD is prevalent (Queenan 1985).

Decreased levels of AFP in maternal serum have been found to be associated with fetal chromosome abnormalities such as trisomy 13, trisomy 18, trisomy 21, and others. As noted by Drugan et al (1989, p 273), "genetic counseling for low MSAFP values, as for advanced maternal age, should emphasize the incidence of all aneuploidy and not only the Down syndrome risks."

Specific cutoff values for any given set of maternal and gestational age groups are determined by the population being screened. Evaluation of any specific value is generally determined by the genetics department of the testing facility. Recommendations for follow-up assessment are then referred to the attending clinician responsible for the woman's prenatal course.

Currently there is no consensus regarding how to monitor pregnancies with abnormal MSAFP levels and subsequent normal AFAFP levels even though the chance of adverse pregnancy outcome remains at 22% (Robinson 1989). Women with these findings should be followed with ultrasound to watch for IUGR, and fetal monitoring testing should be initiated early in the pregnancy.

Evaluation of Rh-Sensitized Pregnancies

The first studies of amniotic fluid were done in the early 1950s for the evaluation of bilirubin pigment in the amniotic fluid of Rh-sensitized mothers. The analyst could determine the degree to which the fetus was affected by looking at the optical density of the fluid. Liley (1961) produced a graph that is now universally used in determining the severity of hemolytic disease in the fetus (Figure 20–16).

If a sensitized Rh negative woman produces an incompatible Rh positive fetus, antibodies cross the placenta and cause hemolytic anemia in the fetus. Concentrations of bilirubin and other breakdown products from destroyed red blood cells can be detected in amniotic fluid by spectrophotometry. By plotting their concentration or optical density at ΔOD 450 mu on a Liley curve, the physician can ascertain the degree to which the fetus is affected and the need for intervention or intrauterine transfusion. (See Chapter 19.)

Liley categorized the degree of hemolytic disease in three zones. If the optical density falls in zone I (low zone) at 28 to 31 weeks' gestation, the fetus will either be unaffected or have only mild hemolytic disease. Amniocentesis should be repeated in two or three weeks. When the optical density falls in zone II (midzone), amniocentesis is repeated frequently so that the trend can be determined. The age of the fetus and the trend in optical density indicate the necessity for fetal transfusion via percutaneous umbilical blood sampling (PUBS) or preterm birth. Optical densities falling in zone III (high zone) indicate that the fetus is severely affected and death is a possibility. Today, fetal anemia may be directly assessed through percutaneous umbilical blood sampling and blood transfused directly into the fetal circulation rather than into the fetal peritoneal space as was done with intrauterine transfusion. Exact degrees of hemolysis can be determined by this method, earlier transfusion is possible, and complete reversal of hydrops fetalis has been reported after direct intravascular transfusion (Seeds 1988). The decision concerning birth or fetal transfusion depends on the gestational age of the fetus. If the fetal lungs are not mature, packed red blood cells compatible with the mother's serum are transfused into the fetus through the umbilical artery. Fetal transfusions are re-

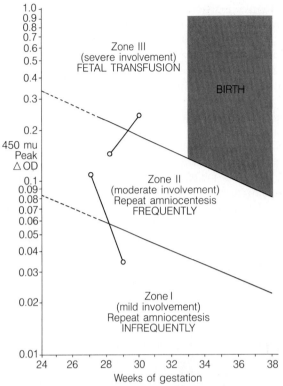

Figure 20–16   The density of amniotic fluid can be useful in determining the severity of erythroblastosis fetalis. There are three zones of optical density, which are correlated with the degree to which the fetus is affected by this condition. In this graph, management of the Rh-sensitized pregnancy is related to the condition of the fetus and gestational age. (Modified from Liley AW: Liquor amnii analysis in the management of the pregnancy complicated by rhesus sensitization. Am J Obstet Gynecol *1961; 32:1359)*

peated whenever the fetal hematocrit falls below 30%. After about 32 or 33 weeks of gestation, early birth and extrauterine treatment are probably preferred to performing fetal transfusion.

Evaluation of Fetal Maturity

In managing the woman and fetus at risk, the physician is constantly faced with the possibility of having to induce the birth of an infant prior to term and before the onset of labor. There are many indications for early termination of pregnancy, including repeat cesarean birth, premature rupture of the membranes, diabetes, hypertensive conditions in the pregnant woman, and placental insufficiency. Unfortunately, the most common cause of perinatal mortality is prematurity, especially in infants weighing 1500 g or less, and complications arising from pulmonary immaturity (Pernoll et al 1986); birth of an infant with immature pulmonary function frequently results in respiratory distress syndrome (RDS), also known as hyaline membrane disease (see Chapter 27).

Because gestational age, birth weight, and the rate of development of organ systems do not necessarily correspond, it may be necessary to determine the lung maturation of the fetus by amniotic fluid analysis before elective delivery. Concentrations of certain substances in the amniotic fluid reflect the pulmonary condition of the fetus (see below). In many cases, birth of the infant can be delayed until the lungs show maturity.

L/S Ratio   The alveoli of the lungs are lined by a substance called *surfactant*, which is composed of phospholipids. Surfactant lowers the surface tension of the alveoli during extrauterine respiratory exhalation. By lowering the alveolar surface tension, surfactant stabilizes the alveoli, and a certain amount of air always remains in the alveoli during expiration. When a newborn with mature pulmonary function takes its first breath, a tremendously high pressure is needed to open the lungs. Upon breathing out, the lungs do not collapse and about half the air in the alveoli is retained. An infant born too early in his or her development, when synthesis of surfactant is incomplete, is unable to maintain lung stability, resulting in underinflation of the lungs and development of RDS.

Fetal lung maturity can be assessed by determining the ratio of two components of surfactant—lecithin and sphingomyelin. Early in pregnancy the sphingomyelin concentration in amniotic fluid is more than that of lecithin (0.5:1 at 20 weeks) resulting in a low **lecithin/sphingomyelin (L/S) ratio**. At about 30 to 32 weeks' gestation, the amounts of the two substances become equal (1:1). The concentration of lecithin begins to exceed that of sphingomyelin, and at 35 weeks the L/S ratio is 2:1. When at least two times as much lecithin as sphingomyelin is found in the amniotic fluid, respiratory distress syndrome is very unlikely. Infants of diabetic mothers are an exception to this finding and have a high incidence of false-positive results; the L/S ratio of 2:1 may not indicate lung maturity in these infants. Delayed maturation is often seen in infants of diabetic mothers because the high blood sugars interfere with biochemical development.

Some types of chronic intrauterine fetal stress cause an acceleration of lung maturation in the fetus. Prolonged rupture of membranes (over 24 hours) results in acceleration of lung maturation by approximately one week and therefore exerts a protective effect. Amnionitis and vaginal bleeding more than 24 hours before birth also have a protective effect for the fetus (White et al 1986).

Although the L/S ratio is the most universally used assay in evaluating pulmonary maturity, the results of L/S ratio are not accurate when blood contaminates the amniotic fluid, and the normal ratio of 2:1 may not indicate lung maturity if the mother is a diabetic.

Phosphatidylglycerol   While lecithin is the most prevalent phospholipid in surfactant, **phosphatidylglycerol (PG)** is the second most abundant phospholipid. Phosphatidylglycerol appears at about 36 weeks of gestation and increases in amount until term. In instances of diabetes complicated by premature rupture of the membranes, vascular disease, or severe PIH, phosphatidylglycerol may be present before 35 weeks' gestation. Phosphatidylglycerol is not measured in specific amounts; rather, the mere presence of this substance is associated with very low risk of RDS while the absence of PG is associated with the development of RDS.

Phosphatidylglycerol determination is also useful in blood-contaminated specimens. Since PG is not present in blood or vaginal fluids, its presence is reliable in predicting lung maturity (Jobe 1989).

In recent years, lung maturity has been most frequently assessed by a combination of L/S ratio and PG. It appears that lung maturity can be confirmed in most pregnancies if PG is present in conjunction with an L/S ratio of 2:1.

Creatinine Level   Amniotic creatinine progressively increases as pregnancy advances. This may be due to excretion of fetal urine, which reflects fetal kidney function, or to muscle mass. The use of this value alone to assess maturity is not advisable since a high creatinine value may be a reflection of muscle mass in a particular fetus and not necessarily indicate kidney maturity. For example, the macrosomic fetus of a diabetic woman may have high creatinine levels due to increased muscle mass, or the small, growth-retarded infant of the hypertensive may demonstrate a low level of creatinine due to decreased muscle mass; in these cases creatinine values can be misleading if used without other data. Nevertheless, when fetal growth (muscle mass) and kidney maturity are at odds, the creatinine is still more indicative of fetal kidney maturity. Creatinine levels of 2 mg/dL of amniotic fluid seem to correlate closely with a pregnancy of 37 weeks or more (Varney 1987).

As long as the maternal serum creatinine is not elevated, measurement of creatinine level has a certain degree of reliability when used in conjunction with other maturity studies. An elevated maternal serum creatinine results in increased amniotic fluid levels. The woman's serum creatinine levels should be determined if the creatinine in the amniotic fluid is not what would normally be expected for a particular gestational age.

Identification of Meconium Staining

Any episode of hypoxia in utero may result in an increased fetal peristalsis, relaxation of the anal sphincter, and passage of meconium into the amniotic fluid. The amniotic fluid is normally clear, but the presence of meconium makes the fluid greenish.

Meconium staining may also be observed when amniocentesis is done. After the membranes have ruptured, meconium staining may be observed in the drainage from the vagina.

Once meconium staining is identified, more assessments must be made to determine if the fetus is suffering ongoing episodes of hypoxia.

Other Diagnostic Techniques

Chorionic Villus Sampling

Chorionic villus sampling (CVS) is performed in some medical centers throughout the country for first trimester prenatal diagnosis of genetic disorders. In a study comparing cytogenic results obtained by CVS and analysis of amniotic fluid cells by amniocentesis, Wright et al (1989) found that although the number of cases demonstrating uncertainty regarding cytogenetic diagnosis was slightly greater with CVS, the difference between the two procedures was not significant. These authors believe that CVS results should be considered of equal value to those obtained by amniocentesis. It is anticipated that CVS will replace amniocentesis for prenatal diagnosis, except for diagnosis of neural tube defects (Ward 1985a). Because CVS makes possible earlier diagnosis of congenital defects, first-trimester therapeutic abortion is possible if indicated and desired.

Villi in the chorion frondosum, present from 8 to 12 weeks, are believed to reflect fetal chromosome, enzyme, and DNA content, thereby permitting earlier diagnosis than can be obtained by amniocentesis. Various equipment has been used to aspirate chorionic villi from the placenta and three transcervical approaches have been used: "sampling by a flexible aspiration catheter under ultrasound guidance, by biopsy forceps under direct endoscopic vision, or by rigid biopsy forceps guided by ultrasound" (Brambati & Oldrini 1985, p 94).

After counseling regarding diagnosis and procedure technique, preliminary blood work is obtained. The morning of the procedure the woman is asked to fill her bladder, since displacement of an anteverted uterus may aid in positioning the uterus for catheter insertion. A high-resolution linear-array or sector ultrasound is used to determine uterine position, cervical position, size of the gestational sac, and CRL measurement and to identify the area of placental formation and cord insertion. The woman is then placed in lithotomy position; the vulva is cleansed with povidone-iodine solution (Betadine); and a sterile speculum is inserted into the vagina. The vaginal vault and cervix are cleansed with the same solution to decrease contamination from the vagina into the uterus. The anterior lip of the cervix is sometimes grasped with a tenaculum to aid in straightening anteflexion of the uterus. The catheter (or cannula) is slowly inserted under ultrasound guidance through the endocervix to the sampling site at the extra-amniotic placental edge (outside the gestational sac) (Figure 20–17). The obturator is withdrawn from the catheter. A 30-mL syringe, containing 3 to 4 mL of Hank's solution with heparin, is attached and a sample of villi is aspirated by using a pressure of 5 to 10 mL (Brambati & Oldrini 1985). The contents of the syringe are flushed into a petri dish containing nutrient medium, and the villi are inspected microscopically and prepared for cell culture.

Risks of CVS include failure to obtain tissue, rupture of membranes or leakage of amniotic fluid, bleeding, in-

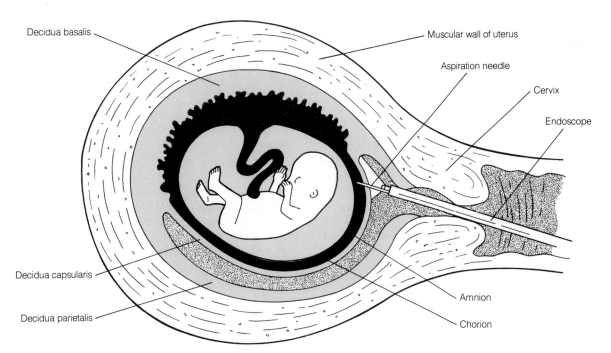

Figure 20–17   Diagram of eight-week pregnancy showing endoscopic needle aspiration of extraplacental villi. (From Rodeck CH, Morsman JM: First trimester chorion biopsy. In Early Prenatal Diagnosis. Ferguson-Smith MA [editor]. New York: Churchill Livingstone, 1983, p 338)

trauterine infection, spontaneous abortion, maternal tissue contamination of the specimen, and Rh isoimmunization. Rh negative women are given Rh_o immune globulin to cover the risk of immunization from the procedure (Hogge et al 1986).

Fetal karyotype, diagnosis of hemoglobinopathies (eg, sickle cell anemia, alpha and some beta thalassemias), phenylketonuria, alpha antitrypsin deficiency, Down syndrome, Duchenne muscular dystrophy, and factor IX deficiency can be detected by this technique. Rapid sex determination can be made so that pregnancies with a male fetus who would be affected in X-linked conditions can be identified early.

One of the greatest advantages to a mother undergoing this procedure is earlier diagnosis and decreased waiting time for results. Whereas amniocentesis is not done until at least 16 weeks' gestation, CVS is performed between 8 and 12 weeks. The CVS results are obtained in one to two weeks as compared to two to four weeks for amniocentesis. Earlier diagnosis may relieve many of the personal, social, and psychologic concerns of families, particularly if therapeutic abortion is being considered. There may be less emotional stress involved with having an abortion at an earlier stage of gestation. First-trimester abortions are also easier to perform, require less time, and are less costly.

Although the incidence of fetal loss is about 5%, births that have occurred following this procedure have resulted in no neonatal malformations (Brambati & Oldrini 1985; Ward 1985b). Follow-up ultrasound and lab evaluation of each pregnancy must be done after performance of this procedure to evaluate fetal status; further neonatal follow-up studies are necessary to evaluate the long-term effects of this experimental technique.

Nursing Care

The nurse ascertains the woman's understanding of the CVS and the possible results. The reasons for the CVS and the procedure can be reviewed before the scheduled test. The nurse provides opportunities for questions and acts as an advocate when additional questions or concerns are raised. The nurse completes assessments following the procedure.

The nurse plays an important supportive role in helping the couple express their feelings and fears regarding the procedure and also regarding the decision-making process if abortion is being considered. That supportive role continues if abortion is selected and chosen, even though the nurse may not be present for the procedure. It is important that support be provided following the procedure by the nurse who established a relationship with the couple previously.

Fetoscopy

Fetoscopy, developed in 1972 but performed in only a few medical centers throughout the world, is a procedure for directly observing the fetus and obtaining a sample of blood or skin. It enables the physician to diagnose such conditions as fetal hemoglobinopathies, immunodeficient diseases, coagulation and metabolic disorders, chromosome abnormalities, Rh isoimmunization, and serious skin defects (Hobbins 1985). It is also used in fetal therapy (eg, ventricular shunts for hydrocephalus and bladder shunts for obstruction). The associated risks include spontaneous abortion (5%), preterm birth (9%), amniotic fluid leakage (1%) (Hobbins et al 1983), and intrauterine fetal death (Antsaklis et al 1985).

Prior to fetoscopy, women at risk for abnormalities are counseled by the genetic team. Indications, risks, and limitations of the procedure are thoroughly explained and a consent form is signed for the procedure, which is done at approximately 18 weeks' gestation. At this time vessels of the placental surface are of adequate size, and fetal parts are readily identifiable, yet therapeutic abortion would not be as hazardous at this time as it would be if done at a later date.

Ultrasound is performed prior to and during fetoscopy to determine the gestational age, fetal position, placental location and thickness, location of umbilical cord insertion into the placenta, pockets of amniotic fluid, position of the part of the fetus or tissue to be viewed or sampled, and placement of the cannula (Antsaklis et al 1985). Following rapid intravenous sedation of the woman to decrease fetal activity, the abdomen is cleansed with povidone-iodine solution (Betadine), a local anesthetic solution may be injected into the maternal abdomen, and a 0.5-cm incision is made through the abdomen to the peritoneum.

A cannula containing a trochar is inserted through the incision into the uterus and the amniotic cavity to the site previously determined by ultrasound. The trochar is removed and amniotic fluid is withdrawn for genetic cell analysis and AFP level. A light source is connected to a 15-cm fiber-optic endoscope, which is about the diameter of a 16-gauge needle, and introduced through the cannula to visualize the fetus. The lens of the endoscope allows magnification up to 30 times, depending on the distance from the structure being visualized to the lens, and allows for a 55° field of vision (Rodeck & Nicolaides 1983).

If fetal blood sampling is to be performed, a 26- to 27-gauge needle is inserted through the side channel of the cannula and advanced until the vessel in the umbilical cord is pierced and a sample of blood is obtained (Figure 20–18).

The numerous indications for fetal blood sampling include suspicion of problems with hemoglobin or coagulation factors and need to assess for rubella, toxoplasmosis, and cytomegalovirus. In those facilities where PUBS is performed, fetoscopy is rarely performed for this purpose. During fetoscopy, blood samples can be taken from vessels in that portion of the cord that is a few centimeters from the placental insertion site. This is usually difficult, however, so a sample (approximately 0.5 mL) is collected from blood that leaks into the amniotic cavity after the needle is withdrawn from the vessel. Because blood aspirated by this method is mixed with amniotic fluid and diagnosis of various inherited diseases requires a pure fetal blood sample, in questionable situations blood is aspirated from a cord vessel at the placental insertion site.

Mother and fetus are monitored for several hours following the procedure for alterations in blood pressure and pulse, FHR abnormalities, uterine activity, vaginal bleeding, and loss of amniotic fluid. The woman is hospitalized until care givers are sure that no immediate complications have arisen. Rh negative mothers are given Rh_o immune globulin unless the fetal blood is found to be Rh negative; antibiotics and tocolytics may or may not be given prophylactically. The following day, prior to discharge, a repeat ultrasound is performed to confirm the adequacy of amniotic fluid and fetal viability. Women are advised to avoid strenuous activity for one to two weeks following fetoscopy and to report any pain, bleeding, leakage of amniotic fluid, or fever.

Although amniocentesis permits the prenatal diagnosis of many sex-linked diseases, chromosome defects, and metabolic disturbances, the majority of fetal cells obtained by this procedure are not found to be viable, culture is difficult and lengthy, and many severe congenital abnormalities may only be diagnosed by direct visualization of the fetus or by analyzing fetal blood or skin tissue. Fetoscopy has been used to view the extremities, spine, genitalia, and face in situations where the fetus is at risk for development of external abnormalities—such as limb and digital deformities, cleft lip and palate, and hereditary skin disorders—and genetic diseases affecting these structures.

As genetic amniocentesis, ultrasound, magnetic resonance imaging (MRI), chorionic villus sampling (CVS), and percutaneous umbilical blood sampling (PUBS) techniques become more sophisticated and conclusive of fetal conditions and more widely used, the need for fetoscopy will decrease except in unusual situations, such as tissue biopsy for diagnosis of genetic skin disorders not detectable by biochemical means, or as a back-up measure when other procedures are inadequate.

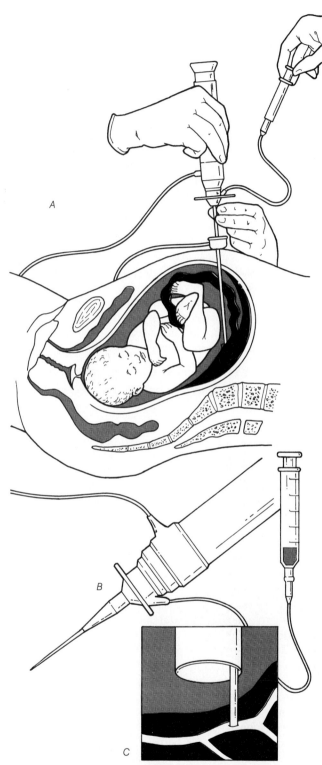

Figure 20–18   A schematic diagram of fetoscopy for fetal blood sampling. B Detail of aspiration apparatus. C Detail of needle puncturing fetal blood vessel. (From McCormack MD. Amniocentesis for detection of sickle cell anemia and the thalassemia disorders using recombinant DNA methodologies. In: Human Prenatal Diagnosis. Filkins K, Russo JF [editors]. New York: Marcel Dekker, 1985, p 142)

Nursing Care

The nurse clarifies the woman's understanding of fetoscopy, providing time for questions and acting as an advocate when additional areas of concern are raised. Following the test, the nurse completes assessments and continues to provide support.

Percutaneous Umbilical Blood Sampling

Since there is an approximately 5% risk of fetal loss associated with fetoscopy (Hobbins 1985), a technique for obtaining pure fetal blood for prenatal diagnosis, called **percutaneous umbilical blood sampling** (PUBS) or cordocentesis, has been developed (Daffos et al 1985). This procedure is beginning to replace fetoscopy in major centers and has been used for diagnosis of hemophilias, hemoglobinopathies, fetal infections, chromosome abnormalities, assessment of fetal distress in labor, level of maternal drugs in the fetus, nonimmune hydrops, isoimmune hemolytic disorders, immunodeficiencies, and assessment of fetal hemoglobin and hematocrit for calculation of transfusion requirements in the second and third trimesters (Hogge et al 1988). PUBS may also be used to assess acid-base abnormalities in growth-retarded fetuses (due to utero-placental insufficiency) (Weiner 1989) and fetal status during labor when scalp sampling is not feasible.

The woman is scanned with a linear-array ultrasound transducer placed in a sterile glove, and a 25-gauge spinal needle is inserted into her abdomen through the skin alongside the transducer and into the fetal umbilical vein approximately 1 to 2 cm from the insertion of the cord into the placenta. The stylet is removed from the needle, and fetal blood is aspirated into a syringe containing an anticoagulant. Red blood cell size is determined to distinguish fetal from maternal cells. A paralytic agent, such as pancuronium bromide (Pavulon), may be given to prevent fetal movement during the procedure.

Risks include transient fetal bradycardia and maternal infection. No evidence of fetal bleeding during or following needle insertion was noted in one study (Hobbins et al 1985) and FHR monitoring following the procedure revealed no abnormal FHR patterns. Another report of over 400 cases (Daffos et al 1985) noted no fetal problems as a result of this procedure except for a transient fetal bradycardia in seven cases.

Although still undergoing considerable research, this procedure appears to be a safe and simple way of obtaining fetal blood for prenatal diagnosis and therapy.

Nursing Care

The nurse plays an important role in helping women who are contemplating PUBS. Although a genetic counselor explains the risks for genetic defects and chromosome disorders, many women and their partners need to be helped to understand the procedure itself and the risks of the procedure. They may need anticipatory guidance to help lessen their anxiety, as well as emotional support, follow-up evaluation and testing, and coordination of financial and social service resources. The nurse can help promote relaxation during the procedure by instructing the woman in breath-

ing techniques, completing assessments during and immediately following the procedure, and, in some cases, performing the NST following the procedure.

Magnetic Resonance Imaging (MRI)

The most recent advance in maternal-fetal assessment has been magnetic resonance imaging (MRI). A major advantage of MRI is its ability to reveal previously inaccessible areas of the body without invasive techniques or risk of ionizing radiation. In addition, MRI can accurately distinguish between normal and impaired or diseased tissues and between fetal and maternal anatomy. Although used in only a few selected regional perinatal centers and still undergoing considerable research for use during pregnancy, this new imaging technology is very promising as a complementary or alternative procedure to ultrasound imaging.

This type of imaging is similar to computerized tomography (CT) and ultrasound scanning. However, its advantages include the following:

- An image can be obtained in different planes.
- Fat and soft tissues can be differentiated easily.
- Assessment does not require the woman to have a distended bladder.
- The entire fetus can be imaged in one scan.

Disadvantages of MRI are its extreme expense to the woman, equipment expense, incapacity for real-time imaging, necessity of having a radiologist interpret findings, unavailability of imaging in the labor and birth unit, longer performance time than ultrasound, difficulty in scanning when the fetus is moving a great deal, and occasional claustrophobia or intolerance by the woman of the confines of the magnetic unit for the extended periods of time required for scanning (45 to 60 minutes).

The woman is placed supine on a sliding table, which moves into a huge cylindrical unit. The outer layers of the cylinder contain coils of wires, which create a magnetic field when electricity is passed through them. The inner layers also contain coils of wires, which act like radio antennae, transmitting and receiving radio waves (energy) to and from the woman by creating a magnetic field and subsequently providing images of the part of the body being scanned (Johnson et al 1984).

Currently MRI can be used for confirmation of fetal abnormalities suggested by ultrasound examination, for pelvimetry, and for assessment of placental localization and size. In the future MRI may be used to assess fetal blood flow, nutritional status (IUGR), and intracranial anatomy.

No harmful effects have been reported in the literature, and clinical evidence to date indicates that MRI is safe. Even so, informed consent is required prior to performance of this procedure.

Psychologic Reactions to Diagnostic Testing

Little is written regarding the impact of antepartum diagnostic testing on women's anxiety levels; however, the need for testing usually provokes fear.

Ultrasound use during pregnancy has become almost routine and many women view this antepartum test as an expected part of the prenatal care. They approach the ultrasound with anticipation because it may provide confirmation of the pregnancy through visualization of the gestational sac or may even identify the sex of the fetus. However, when more invasive testing is recommended it may evoke fear and anxiety in the woman and her partner as they consider the reason for the test, the risk to the fetus and woman during the test, and the implications of the test results.

In one study (Campbell et al 1982), it was noted that being able to see the fetus early in the pregnancy through the use of ultrasound led to more positive attitudes toward the ultrasound procedure and decreased feelings of stress related to the ultrasound. The women who were able to view their fetus on the monitor screen displayed more positive health behavior changes after the ultrasound than those women who were not allowed to view the fetus when the ultrasound was performed. Reading and Platt (1985) studied the reactions of women who had ultrasound examinations for decreased fetal movement. All women approached the ultrasound with anxiety; however, the women who were allowed to view their fetus on the ultrasound screen had a reduction in their anxiety level over other women in the study who were given only verbal communication that their fetus was "okay." This study confirmed that prenatal testing does influence anxiety level (Reading and Platt 1985, p 910) and provides information for care givers regarding the importance of the test for the woman. The findings also emphasize the importance of providing visual feedback during ultrasound examinations.

CRITICAL THINKING

Take a few moments and think about what your reaction would be to seeing your fetus by ultrasound. Would it make you feel anxious, or more comfortable?

❀ ❀

KEY CONCEPTS

Diagnostic ultrasound is advantageous because it is noninvasive and painless, allows the physician to study the gestation serially, is nonradiating to both the woman and her fetus, and to date has no known harmful effects.

The gestational sac may be detected as early as five or six weeks after the LMP.

Measurement of the CRL in early pregnancy is most useful for accurate dating of a pregnancy.

The most important and frequently used ultrasound measurements are BPD and femur length.

Ultrasound offers a valuable means of assessing intrauterine fetal growth because the growth can be followed over a period of time.

A fetal biophysical (FBPP) profile includes five variables (fetal breathing movement, body movement, tone, amniotic fluid volume, and FHR reactivity) to assess the fetus at risk for intrauterine compromise.

Maternal assessment of fetal activity is very useful as a screening procedure in evaluation of fetal status.

A nonstress test (NST) is based on the knowledge that the heart rate normally increases in response to fetal activity. The desired result is a reactive test.

A contraction stress test (CST) provides a method for observing the response of the fetal heart rate to the stress of uterine contractions. The desired result is a negative test.

Amniocentesis can be used to obtain amniotic fluid for testing. A variety of tests are available to evaluate the presence of disease, genetic conditions, and fetal maturity.

The L/S ratio can be used to assess fetal lung maturity. The presence of PG may also provide information about fetal lung maturity.

Chorionic villus sampling is a procedure that permits earlier diagnosis than is now available by amniocentesis.

Fetoscopy is a procedure for observing the fetus directly and obtaining a sample of blood or skin.

Percutaneous umbilical blood sampling (PUBS) is a technique used in the second and third trimester for prenatal diagnosis, assessment, diagnosis, and therapy.

Alpha-fetoprotein (AFP) screening of maternal serum provides information about the possibility of open neural tube defects (NTDs) in the fetus.

Magnetic resonance imaging (MRI) can be used to assess previously inaccessible areas of the body via a non-

invasive process without the risk of ionizing radiation. This procedure can accurately distinguish between normal and impaired or diseased tissues and between fetal and maternal anatomy and pathology.

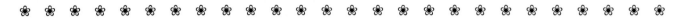

References

Antsaklis AJ, Benzie RJ, Hughes RM: Fetoscopy: Fetal visualization and blood sampling in prenatal diagnosis. In: *Human Prenatal Diagnosis.* Filkins K, Russo JF (editors). New York: Marcel Dekker, 1985, p 109.

Barford DA, Dickerman LH, Johnson WE: α-Fetoprotein: Relationship between maternal serum and alphafetoprotein levels. *Am J Obstet Gynecol* 1985; 151(8):1038.

Brambati B, Oldrini A: CVS for first-trimester fetal diagnosis. *Contemp OB/GYN* 1985; 25:94.

Brar HS et al: Fetal umbilical blood flow velocity waveforms using doppler ultrasonography in patients with late decelerations. *Obstet Gynecol* 1989; 73:363.

Broussard P: Antepartum surveillance: What tests to use, how to do the test. Tenth International Symposium on Perinatal Medicine and Obstetrical Ultrasound. April 9–12, 1990. Las Vegas, Nevada.

Cacciatore B et al: Comparison of abdominal and vaginal sonography in suspected ectopic pregnancy. *Obstet Gynecol* 1989; 73:770.

Campbell S et al: Ultrasound scanning in pregnancy: The short term psychological effects of early realtime scans. *J Psychosom Obstet Gynecol* 1982; 1:57.

Clark SL: Antepartum fetal surveillance: Choice of tests. Tenth International Symposium on Perinatal Medicine and Obstetrical Ultrasound. April 9–12, 1990. Las Vegas, Nevada.

Crane JP: Routine obstetrical ultrasound: Should all pregnancies be screened? Tenth International Symposium on Perinatal Medicine and Obstetrical Ultrasound. April 9–12, 1990. Las Vegas, Nevada.

Daffos F, Capella-Pavlovsky M, Forestier F: Fetal blood sampling during pregnancy with use of a needle guided by ultrasound: A study of 606 consecutive cases. *Am J Obstet Gynecol* 1985; 153(6):655.

Davis RO et al: Decreased levels of amniotic fluid α-fetoprotein associated with Down Syndrome. *Am J Obstet Gynecol* 1985; 153(5):541.

Devoe LD: Nonstress and contraction stress testing. In: Depp R, Eschenbach DA, Sciarra JJ (editors): *Gynecology and Obstetrics.* Vol. 3. Philadelphia: Harper & Row, 1989, Ch 78.

Drugan A et al: Counseling for low maternal serum alphafetoprotein should emphasize all chromosome anomalies, not just Down syndrome! *Obstet Gynecol* 1989; 73:271.

Garite TJ, Freeman RK: EFM today: Nipple-stimulation for antepartum testing. *Contemp OB/GYN* 1982; 203:39.

Grannum PAT, Berkowitz RL, Hobbins JC: The ultrasonic changes in the maturing placenta and their relation to fetal pulmonic maturity. *Am J Obstet Gynecol* 1979; 133:915.

Hadlock FP: Ultrasound: Content of the basic U/S examination. Tenth International Symposium on Perinatal Medicine and Obstetrical Ultrasound. April 9–12, 1990a. Las Vegas, Nevada.

Hadlock FP: Evaluation of fetal growth and size. Tenth International Symposium on Perinatal Medicine and Obstetrical Ultrasound. April 9–12, 1990b. Las Vegas, Nevada.

Hobbins JC: Fetoscopy. In *Management of High-Risk Pregnancy,* 2nd ed. Queenan JT (editor). Oradell, NJ: Medical Economics Books, 1985, p 231.

Hobbins JC, Winsberg F, Berkowitz RL: Normal and abnormal fetal anatomy. In: *Ultrasonography in Obstetrics and Gynecology,* 2nd ed. Baltimore, Williams & Wilkins, 1983, p 113.

Hobbins JC et al: Percutaneous umbilical blood sampling. *Am J Obstet Gynecol* 1985; 152(1):1.

Hogge WA et al: Fetal evaluation by percutaneous blood sampling *Am J Obstet Gynecol* 1988; 158:132.

Hogge JS, Hogge WA, Golbus MS: Chorionic villus sampling. *JOGNN* 1986; 15:24.

Jeanty P, Romero R: *Obstetrical Ultrasound.* New York: McGraw-Hill, 1984.

Jobe A: Amniotic fluid tests of fetal lung maturity. In: *Maternal-Fetal Medicine: Principles and Practice,* 2nd ed. Creasy RK, Resnick R (editors). Philadelphia: Saunders, 1989.

Johnson JM et al: Biophysical profile scoring in the management of the postterm pregnancy: An analysis of 307 patients. *Am J Obstet Gynecol* 1986; 154(2):269.

Kochenour NK: Estrogen assay during pregnancy. *Clin Obstet Gynecol* December 1982; 25:659.

Korones SB: The normal neonate. In: *Gynecology and Obstetrics.* Vol. 2. Sciarri JJ (editor). Philadelphia: Harper & Row, 1985, Ch 97.

Kremkau FW: Safety and long-term effects of ultrasound: What to tell your patients. *Clin Obstet Gynecol* 1984; 27:269.

Liley AW: Liquor amnii analysis in the management of the pregnancy complicated by rhesus sensitization. *Am J Obstet Gynecol* 1961; 32:1359.

Manning FA: The biophysical profile: Contemporary use. Tenth International Symposium on Perinatal Medicine and Obstetrical Ultrasound. April 9–12, 1990. Las Vegas, Nevada.

Manning FA et al: Fetal assessment based on fetal biophysical profile scoring: Experience in 12,620 referred high-risk pregnancies. *Am J Obstet Gynecol* 1985; 151(3):343.

Marshall C: The nipple stimulation contraction stress test. *JOGNN* 1986; 15:459.

McCluggage NA: Nipple stimulation contraction stress test. *J Perinatol* Summer 1985; 5:56.

Murray ML, Canfield S, Harmon J: Nipple stimulation-contraction stress test for the high-risk patient. *MCN* 1986; 11:331.

Pernoll ML, Benda GI, Babson SG: *Diagnosis and Management of the Fetus and Neonate at Risk.* St. Louis: Mosby, 1986.

Pinette MG et al: Maternal smoking and accelerated placental maturation. *Obstet Gynecol* 1989; 73:379.

Queenan JT: Maternal serum α-fetoprotein screening. In: *Management of High-Risk Pregnancy,* 2nd ed. Queenan JT (editor). Oradell, NJ: Medical Economics Books, 1985, p 57.

Queenan JT: The NIH consensus report: A closer look. *Contemp OB/GYN* May 1984; 23:164.

Ray DA, Yeast JD, Freeman RK: The current role of daily serum estriol monitoring in the insulin-dependent pregnant diabetic woman. *Am J Obstet Gynecol* 1986; 154:1257.

Reading AE et al: Health beliefs and health care behavior in pregnancy *Psych Med* 1982; 12:379.

Reading AE, Platt LD: Impact of fetal testing on maternal anxiety. *J Reprod Med* December 1985; 30:907.

Reed K: Ultrasound: Doppler flow, where does it fit in? Tenth International Symposium on Perinatal Medicine and Obstetrical Ultrasound. April 9–12, 1990. Las Vegas, Nevada.

Robinson L et al: Pregnancy outcomes after increasing maternal alpha-feto protein levels. *Obstet Gynecol* 1989; 74:17.

Rodeck CH, Nicolaides KH: Fetoscopy and fetal tissue sampling. In: *Early Prenatal Diagnosis.* Ferguson-Smith MA (editor). New York: Churchill Livingstone, 1983, p 332.

Sacks AJ, Sokol RJ: Clinical use of antepartum fetal monitoring techniques. In: *Gynecology and Obstetrics.* Vol. 2. Dilts PV, Sciarra JJ (editors). Philadelphia: Harper & Row, 1989, Ch 58.

Sadovsky E: Fetal movement. In: *Management of High-Risk Pregnancy,* 2nd ed. Queenan JT (editor). Oradell, NJ: Medical Economics Books, 1985a, pp 183–193.

Sadovsky E: Monitoring fetal movement: A useful screening test. *Contemp OB/GYN* April 1985b; 25:123.

Seeds JW: PUBS: Important new aid for prenatal diagnosis. *Contemp OB/GYN* February 1988; 31:117.

Simpson JL, Elias S: Prenatal diagnosis of genetic disorders. In: *Maternal-Fetal Medicine: Principles and Practice,* 2nd ed. Creasy RK, Resnik R (editors). Philadelphia: Saunders, 1989.

Trudinger BJ et al: Umbilical artery flow velocity waveforms in high-risk pregnancy. Randomized controlled trial. *Lancet* 1987; 1:188.

Tyrrell S et al: Umbilical artery doppler velocimetry as a predictor of fetal hypoxia and acidosis at birth. *Obstet Gynecol* 1989; 74:332.

Varney H: *Nurse-Midwifery,* 2nd ed. Boston: Blackwell Scientific Publications, 1987.

Vintzileos AM et al: The fetal biophysical profile in patients with premature rupture of the membranes: An early predictor of fetal infection. *Am J Obstet Gynecol* 1985; 152:510.

Vintzileos AM et al: The use of fetal biophysical profile improves pregnancy outcome in premature rupture of the membranes. *Am J Obstet Gynecol* 1987a; 157:236.

Vintzileos AM: The use and misuse of the fetal biophysical profile. *Am J Obstet Gynecol* 1987b; 157:527.

Ward H: Symposium: Chorionic villus sampling: Something new in prenatal diagnosis. *Contemp OB/GYN,* May 1985a; 118.

Ward H: Symposium: NST or CST? What's best for spotting the high-risk fetus? *Contemp OB/GYN* April 1985b; 19:92.

Watson WJ, Seeds JW: Diagnostic obstetric imaging. In: *Gynecology and Obstetrics.* Vol. 2. Dilts PV, Sciarra JJ (editors). Philadelphia: Harper & Row, 1990, Ch 57.

Weiner CP, Williamson RA: Evaluation of severe growth retardation using cordocentesis: Hematologic and metabolic alterations by etiology. *Obstet Gynecol* 1989; 73:225.

White E, Shy KK, Benedetti TJ: Chronic fetal stress and the risk of infant respiratory distress syndrome. *Obstet Gynecol* 1986; 67:57.

Wright DJ et al: Interpretation of chorionic villus sampling laboratory results is just as reliable as amniocentesis. *Obstet Gynecol* 1989; 74:739.

Additional Readings

Arulkymaran S et al: Evaluation of maternal perception of sound-provoked fetal movement as a test of antenatal fetal health. *Obstet Gynecol* 1989; 73:182.

Carlan SJ; O'Brien WF: The affect of magnesium sulfate on the biophysical profile of normal term fetuses. *Obstet Gynecol*; May 1991; 77:681.

Fleming AD, Salafia CM, Vintzileos AM et al: The relationship among umbilical artery velocimetry, fetal biophysical profile, and placental inflammation in preterm premature rupture of the membranes. *Am J Obstet Gynecol* 1991; 164(1):38.

Gudmundsson S, Huhta JC, Wood DC et al: Venous doppler ultrasonography in the fetus with nonimmune hydrops. *Am J Obstet Gynecol* 1991; 164(1):33.

Katz BL, Chescheir NC, Cefalo RC: Unexplained elevations of maternal serum alpha-fetoprotein. *Obstet Gynecol Surv* 1990; 45(11):719.

Keenan KL, Basso D, Goldkrand J et al: Low level of maternal serum α-fetoprotein: Its associated anxiety and the effects of genetic counseling. *Am J Obstet Gynecol* 1991; 164(1):54.

Kisilevsky BF et al: Maternal and ultrasound measurements of elicited fetal movements: A methodological consideration. *Obstet Gynecol*; June 1991; 77:889.

Tahilramaney MP, Platt LD, Golde SH: Use of femur length measured by ultrasonography to predict fetal maturity. *J Perinatal* June 1991: 157.

PART FIVE

Birth

CHAPTER 21

Processes and Stages of Labor and Birth

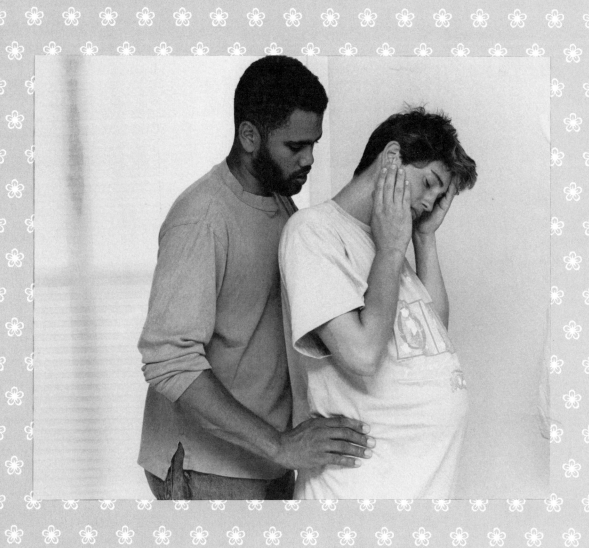

Relate the significance of each type of pelvis to the birth process.

Examine the factors that influence labor and the physiology of the mechanisms of labor.

Describe the fetal positional changes that constitute the mechanisms of labor.

Explain the probable causes of labor onset and the premonitory signs of labor.

Differentiate between false and true labor.

Summarize the physiologic and psychologic changes occurring in each of the stages of labor.

❀ ❀

Birth usually feels like a steamy kitchen—similar to holiday preparations, except that the smells are different. The smell of sweat is more acrid, there are some fetid odors, there is the smell and steam rising from blood. The air is thick, pungent, fertile. It is hard not to be reminded of fresh straw and night stars. There is near and heady promise. (A Midwife's Story)

During the weeks of gestation, the fetus and the expectant woman prepare themselves for birth. The fetus progresses through various stages of growth and development in readiness for the independence of extrauterine life. The expectant woman undergoes various physiologic and psychologic adaptations during pregnancy that gradually prepare her for childbirth and the role of mother. The onset of labor marks a significant change in the relationship between the woman and the fetus.

Critical Factors in Labor

Four factors are important in the process of labor and birth: the maternal pelvis, the fetus, the uterine contractions, and the woman's psychologic state. Within these four areas the following factors are significant:

1. Maternal Pelvis
    a. Size of the pelvis (diameters of the pelvic inlet, midpelvis, and outlet)
    b. Type of pelvis (gynecoid, android, anthropoid, platypelloid, or a combination)
    c. Ability of the cervix to dilate and efface, and ability of the vaginal canal and the external opening of the vagina (the *introitus*) to distend
2. Fetus
    a. Fetal head (size and presence of molding)
    b. Fetal attitude (flexion or extension of the fetal body and extremities)
    c. Fetal lie

    d. Fetal presentation (the part of the fetal body entering the pelvis in a single or multiple pregnancy)
    e. Fetal position (relationship of the presenting part to one of the four quadrants of the maternal pelvis)
    f. Placenta (implantation site)
3. Uterine Contractions
    a. The frequency, duration, and intensity of uterine contractions as the passenger moves through the passage
    b. The effectiveness of pushing effort
    c. The duration of labor
4. Psychologic State
    a. Physical preparation for childbirth
    b. Sociocultural heritage
    c. Previous childbirth experience
    d. Support from significant others
    e. Emotional integrity

The progress of labor is critically dependent on the complementary relationship of these four factors. Abnormalities in the maternal pelvis, the fetus, the uterine contractions, or the woman's psychologic state can alter the outcome of labor and jeopardize both the pregnant woman and her fetus. Complications during labor and birth are discussed in Chapter 25.

The Maternal Pelvis

The true pelvis, which forms the bony canal through which the baby must pass, is divided into three sections: the inlet, the pelvic cavity (midpelvis), and the outlet. (Note: See Chapter 4 for discussion of each part of the pelvis and Chapter 13 for assessment techniques of the pelvis.)

Pelvic Types

The Caldwell-Maloy classification of pelvic types is based on pertinent characteristics of both male and female pelves (Caldwell & Maloy 1933). Although it is common for a particular pelvis to have characteristics of more than one type of pelvis, the four classic types are gynecoid, android, anthropoid, and platypelloid.

The *gynecoid* pelvis is often referred to as the "female" pelvis. Approximately 50% of women have this type of pelvis. All diameters of the gynecoid are adequate for childbirth.

The *android* pelvis is often referred to as the "male" pelvis. Approximately 20% of women have this type of pelvis. The diameters of the android pelvis are usually not adequate for vaginal birth.

The *anthropoid* pelvis is narrowed from side to side and widened from front to back. The diameters are usually adequate for vaginal birth.

The *platypelloid* pelvis is flattened (narrowed) from front to back and widened from side to side. Diameters are usually not adequate for vaginal birth (Table 21–1).

The maternal pelvis is affected by relaxin, a hormone released by the placenta. The presence of this hormone relaxes the pelvis and slightly increases the size of the pelvic diameters. During labor the pelvic diameters may be increased when the woman is in a squatting position or in a lateral Sims' position.

The Fetus

Fetal Head

The fetal head is composed of bony parts that can either hinder childbirth or make it easier. Once the head (the least compressible and largest part of the fetus) has passed through the vaginal opening, the birth of the rest of the body is rarely delayed.

The fetal skull has three major parts: the face, the base of the skull (cranium), and the vault of the cranium

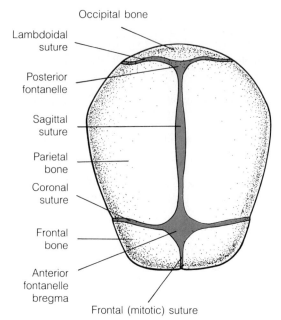

Figure 21–1   Superior view of the fetal skull

(roof). The bones of the face and cranial base are well fused and are basically fixed. The base of the cranium is composed of the two temporal bones, each with a sphenoid and ethmoid bone. The bones composing the vault are the two frontal bones, the two parietal bones, and the occipital bone (Figure 21–1). These bones are not fused, allowing this portion of the head to adjust in shape as the presenting part of the fetus passes through the narrow portions of the pelvis. The cranial bones overlap under pressure of the powers of labor and the demands of the unyielding pelvis. This overlapping is called **molding.**

The **sutures** of the fetal skull are membranous spaces between the cranial bones. The intersections of the cranial

Pelvic type	Pertinent characteristics	Implications for birth
Gynecoid	Inlet rounded with all inlet diameters adequate Midpelvis adequate with parallel side walls Outlet adequate	Favorable for vaginal birth
Android	Inlet heart shaped with short posterior sagittal diameter Midpelvis diameters reduced Outlet capacity reduced	Not favorable for vaginal birth Descent into pelvis is slow Fetal head enters pelvis in transverse or posterior with arrest of labor frequent
Anthropoid	Inlet oval with long anteroposterior diameter Midpelvis diameters adequate Outlet adequate	Favorable for vaginal birth
Platypelloid	Inlet oval with long transverse diameters Midpelvis diameters reduced Outlet capacity inadequate	Not favorable for vaginal birth Fetal head engages in transverse Difficult descent through midpelvis Frequent delay of progress at outlet of pelvis

Table 21–1   Implications of Pelvic Type for Labor and Birth

Note: Description of pelvic shape is exaggerated for easier comprehension.

sutures are called **fontanelles.** These sutures allow for molding of the fetal head and help the examiner to identify the position of the fetal head during vaginal examination. The important sutures of the fetal skull are as follows (see Figure 21–1):

- *Mitotic suture:* Located between the two frontal bones; becomes the anterior continuation of the sagittal suture
- *Sagittal suture:* Located between the parietal bones; divides the skull into left and right halves; runs anteroposteriorly, connecting the two fontanelles
- *Coronal sutures:* Located between the frontal and parietal bones; extend transversely left and right from the anterior fontanelle
- *Lambdoidal suture:* Located between the two parietal bones and the occipital bone; extends transversely left and right from the posterior fontanelle

The anterior and posterior fontanelles are clinically useful in identifying the position of the fetal head in the pelvis and in assessing the status of the newborn after birth. The anterior fontanelle is diamond-shaped and measures 2 × 3 cm. It permits growth of the brain by remaining unossified for as long as 18 months. The posterior fontanelle is much smaller and closes within 8 to 12 weeks after birth. It is shaped like a small triangle and marks the meeting point of the sagittal suture and the lambdoidal suture.

Following are several important landmarks of the fetal skull (Figure 21–2):

- *Sinciput:* The anterior area known as the brow
- *Bregma:* The large diamond-shaped anterior fontanelle
- *Vertex:* The area between the anterior and posterior fontanelles
- *Posterior fontanelle:* The intersection between posterior cranial sutures
- *Occiput:* The area of the fetal skull occupied by the occipital bone, beneath the posterior fontanelle
- *Mentum:* The fetal chin

The diameters of the fetal skull vary considerably within normal limits. Some diameters shorten and others lengthen as the head is molded during labor. Fetal head diameters are measured between the various landmarks on the skull (Figure 21–3). The compound words used to designate the various diameters allow one to identify which measurement is actually being reported. For example, the suboccipitobregmatic diameter is the distance from the undersurface of the occiput to the center of the bregma, or anterior fontanelle. Fetal skull measurements are given in Figure 21–3.

Much can be learned about the degree of extension or flexion of the fetal head from these diameters. Extension of the head results in a larger diameter presenting to the maternal pelvis than if the head is strongly flexed. Altera-

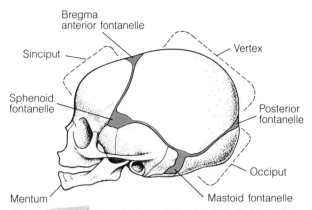

Figure 21–2 Lateral view of the fetal skull identifying the landmarks that have significance during birth

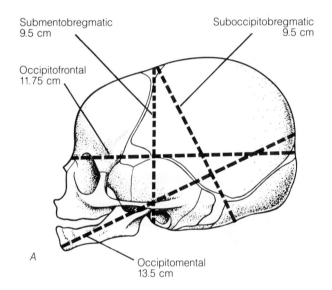

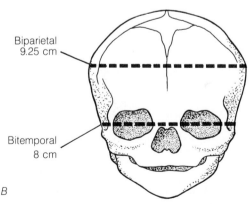

Figure 21–3 A Anteroposterior diameters of the fetal skull. When the vertex of the fetus presents and the fetal head is flexed with the chin on the chest, the smallest anteroposterior diameter (suboccipitobregmatic) enters the birth canal. B Transverse diameters of the fetal skull.

tions in flexion of the fetal head can cause problems during the process of labor. The fetus tries to accommodate its smallest head diameters to the limited measurements of the bony pelvis.

Fetal Attitude

Fetal attitude refers to the relation of the fetal parts to one another. The normal attitude of the fetus is one of moderate flexion of the head, flexion of the arms onto the chest, and flexion of the legs onto the abdomen.

Changes in fetal attitude, particularly in the position of the head, cause the fetus to present larger diameters of the fetal head to the maternal pelvis. These deviations from a normal fetal attitude often contribute to difficult labor (Figure 21–4).

Fetal Lie

Fetal lie refers to the relationship of the cephalocaudal axis of the fetus to the cephalocaudal axis of the woman. The fetus may assume either a longitudinal or a transverse lie. A *longitudinal lie* occurs when the cephalocaudal axis of the fetus (the fetal spine) is parallel to the woman's spine. A *transverse lie* occurs when the cephalocaudal axis of the fetus is at right angles to the woman's spine.

Fetal Presentation

Fetal presentation is determined by fetal lie and by the body part of the fetus that enters the maternal pelvis first. This portion of the fetus is referred to as the **presenting part.** Fetal presentation may be either cephalic, breech, or shoulder (Table 21–2).

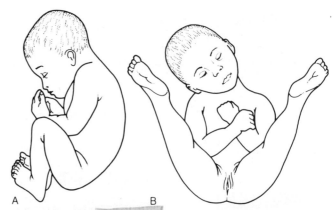

Figure 21–4   Fetal attitude. A The attitude (or relationship of body parts) of this fetus is normal. The head is flexed forward with the chin almost resting on the chest. The arms and legs are flexed. B In this view the head is tilted to the right. Although the arms are flexed, the legs are extended.

The most common presentation is cephalic. When this presentation occurs, labor and birth are more likely to proceed normally. Breech and shoulder presentations are associated with difficulties during labor and do not proceed as normal; therefore, they are called **malpresentations.** (See Chapter 25 for discussion of malpresentations.)

Cephalic Presentation

The fetal head presents itself to the passage in approximately 97% of term births. The cephalic presentation can be further classified according to the degree of flexion or extension of the fetal head (attitude).

Table 21–2   Relationship of Fetus to Maternal Pelvis

Presentation	Attitude	Presenting part	Landmark
Longitudinal lie (99.5%)			
Cephalic (96% to 97%)	Flexion of fetal head onto chest	Vertex (posterior part—occiput)	Occiput (O)
	Military (no flexion, no extension)	Vertex (median part)	Occiput (O)
	Partial extension	Brow	Forehead (frontum) (Fr)
	Complete extension of the head	Face	Chin (mentum) (M)
Breech (3% to 4%)			
Complete	Flexed hips and knees	Buttocks	Sacrum (S)
Frank	Flexed hips, extended knees	Buttocks	Sacrum (S)
Footling: single, double	Extended hips and knees	Feet	Sacrum (S)
Kneeling: single, double	Extended hips; flexed knees	Knees	Sacrum (S)
Transverse or oblique lie (0.5%)			
Shoulder	Variable	Shoulder, arm, trunk	Scapula (Sc or A)

*Adapted from Oxorn H: Human Labor and Birth, **5th ed.** Norwalk, CT: Appleton and Lange, 1986, p 54.*

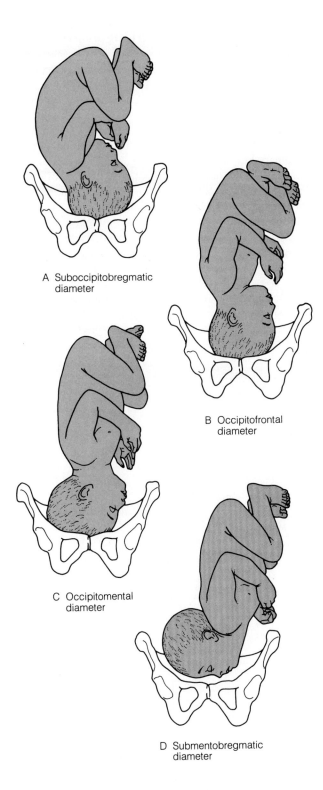

A Suboccipitobregmatic diameter

B Occipitofrontal diameter

C Occipitomental diameter

D Submentobregmatic diameter

Figure 21–5   Cephalic presentations. A Vertex presentation. Complete flexion of the head allows the suboccipitobregmatic diameter to present to the pelvis. B Military (median vertex) presentation, with no flexion or extension. The occipitofrontal diameter presents to the pelvis. C Brow presentation. The fetal head is in partial (halfway) extension. The occipitomental diameter, which is the largest diameter of the fetal head, presents to the pelvis. D Face presentation. The fetal head is in complete extension and the submentobregmatic diameter presents to the pelvis.

occipitofrontal diameter is presented (Figure 21–5*B*). A *brow presentation* occurs when the fetal head is partially extended and the occipitomental diameter, the largest anteroposterior diameter, is presented to the maternal pelvis (Figure 21–5*C*). The most extreme cephalic presentation is the *face presentation* in which the head is hyperextended (complete extension) and the submentobregmatic diameter presents to the maternal pelvis (Figure 21–5*D*).

Breech Presentations

Breech or pelvic presentations occur in 3% of term births. These presentations are classified according to the attitude of the fetal hips and knees. A *complete breech* occurs when the fetal knees and hips are both flexed, placing the thighs on the abdomen and the calves on the posterior aspect of the thighs. On vaginal examination both buttocks and feet can be palpated. Flexion of the hips and extension of the knees changes a complete breech to a *frank breech*. This presentation causes the fetal legs to extend onto the abdomen and chest, presenting the buttocks alone to the pelvis. The buttocks and genitals are palpable on vaginal examination when the fetus assumes a frank breech presentation. A *footling breech* presentation occurs when there is extension both at the knees and at the hips. A *single footling breech* presentation occurs if only one foot is presenting; a *double footling breech* occurs if both feet enter the pelvis first. In all variations of the breech presentation the sacrum is the landmark to be noted. See Chapter 25 for further discussion of the implications of the breech presentations for labor and birth.

Shoulder Presentation

A *shoulder presentation*, usually referred to as a *transverse lie*, is assumed by the fetus when its cephalocaudal axis lies perpendicular to the maternal spine (see Chapter 25, p 749). The fetus appears to lie crosswise in the uterus. Most frequently the shoulder is the presenting part in a transverse lie. In this case the acromion process of the scapula is the landmark to be noted. However, the fetal arm, back, abdomen, or side may present in a transverse lie. Unless the fetus rotates during labor to a longitudinal lie, cesarean birth is necessary. See Chapter 25 for further discussion of the transverse lie and other malpresentations and their effects on the labor and birth processes.

There are four types of cephalic presentation. *Vertex presentation,* in which the head is completely flexed on the chest, is the most common cephalic presentation; the smallest diameter of the fetal head (suboccipitobregmatic) enters the maternal pelvis in this presentation (Figure 21–5*A*). *Military (median vertex) presentation* occurs when the fetal head is neither flexed nor extended and the

Functional Relationships of Presenting Part and Maternal Pelvis

Engagement

Engagement of the presenting part occurs when the largest diameter of the presenting part reaches or passes through the pelvic inlet (Figure 21–6). The biparietal diameter is the largest dimension of the fetal skull to pass through the pelvis in a cephalic presentation. The intertrochanteric diameter is the largest to pass through the inlet in a breech presentation. Once the criteria for engagement have been met, the bony prominences of the presenting part are usually descending into the midpelvis and in most instances have reached the level of the ischial spines.

A vaginal examination determines whether engagement has occurred. In primigravidas, engagement usually occurs two weeks before term. Multiparas, however, may experience engagement several weeks before the onset of labor or during the process of labor. If engagement has occurred, it means the adequacy of the pelvic inlet has been validated. Engagement does not suggest that the midpelvis and outlet are also adequate, however.

The presenting part is said to be *floating* (or ballottable) when it is freely movable above the inlet. When the presenting part begins to descend into the inlet, before engagement has truly occurred, it is said to be *dipping* into the pelvis (Figure 21–6).

Station

Station refers to the relationship of the presenting part to an imaginary line drawn between the ischial spines of the maternal pelvis. In a normal pelvis, the ischial spines mark the narrowest diameter through which the fetus must pass. These spines are not sharp protrusions that harm the fetus but rather blunted prominences at the midpelvis. The ischial spines as a landmark have been designated as zero station (Figure 21–7). If the presenting part is higher than the ischial spines, a negative number is assigned, noting centimeters above zero station. Station −5 is at the inlet, and station +4 is at the outlet. If the presenting part can be seen at the woman's perineum, birth is imminent. During labor, the presenting part should move progressively from the negative stations to the midpelvis at zero station and into the positive stations. Failure of the presenting part to descend in the presence of strong contractions may be due

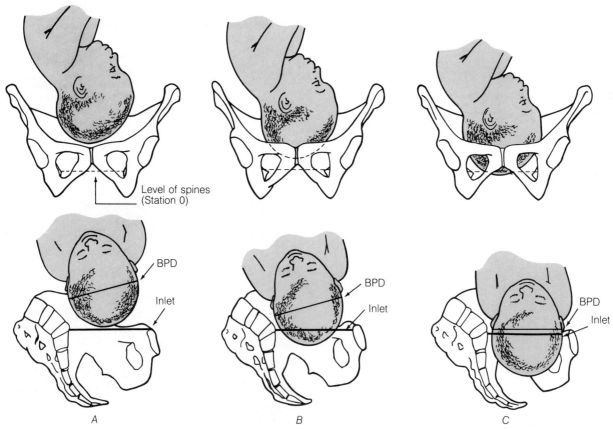

Figure 21–6   Process of engagement in cephalic presentation. A Floating: The fetal head is directed down toward the pelvis but can still easily move away from the inlet. B Dipping: The fetal head dips into the inlet but can be moved away by exerting pressure on the fetus. C Engaged: The biparietal diameter (BPD) of the fetal head is in the inlet of the pelvis. In most instances the presenting part (occiput) will be at the level of the ischial spines (zero station).

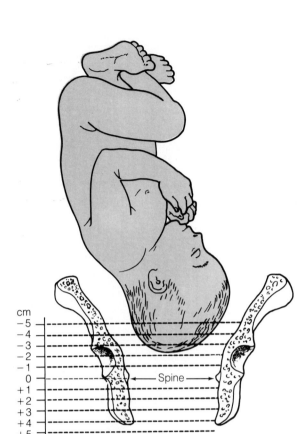

Figure 21–7 Measuring station of the fetal head while it is descending. In this view the station is −2/−3.

to disproportion between the maternal pelvis and fetal presenting part or to a short and/or entangled umbilical cord.

Fetal Position

Fetal position refers to the relationship of the landmark on the presenting fetal part to the front, sides, or back of the maternal pelvis. The landmark on the fetal presenting part is related to four imaginary quadrants of the pelvis: left anterior, right anterior, left posterior, and right posterior. These quadrants designate whether the presenting part is directed toward the front, back, left, or right of the maternal pelvis. The landmark chosen for vertex presentations is the occiput, and the landmark for face presentations is the mentum. In breech presentations, the sacrum is the designated landmark, and the acromion process on the scapula is the landmark in shoulder presentations. If the landmark is directed toward the center of the side of the pelvis, fetal position is designated as *transverse,* rather than anterior or posterior.

Three notations are used to describe the fetal position:

1. Right (R) or left (L) side of the maternal pelvis
2. The landmark of the fetal presenting part: occiput (O), mentum (M), sacrum (S), or acromion process (A)
3. Anterior (A), posterior (P), or transverse (T), depending on whether the landmark is in the front, back, or side of the pelvis.

The abbreviations of these notations help the health care team communicate the fetal position. Thus, when the fetal occiput is directed toward the back and to the left of the passage, the abbreviation used is LOP (left-occiput-posterior). The term *dorsal* (D) is used when denoting the fetal position in a transverse lie; it refers to the fetal back. Thus the abbreviation RADA indicates that the acromion process of the scapula is directed toward the woman's right and the fetus' back is anterior.

Following is a list of the positions for various fetal presentations, some of which are illustrated in Figure 21–8.

Positions in vertex presentation:
ROA   Right-occiput-anterior
ROT   Right-occiput-transverse
ROP   Right-occiput-posterior
LOA   Left-occiput-anterior
LOT   Left-occiput-transverse
LOP   Left-occiput-posterior

Positions in face presentation:
RMA   Right-mentum-anterior
RMT   Right-mentum-transverse
RMP   Right-mentum-posterior
LMA   Left-mentum-anterior
LMT   Left-mentum-transverse
LMP   Left-mentum-posterior

Positions in breech presentation:
RSA   Right-sacrum-anterior
RST   Right-sacrum-transverse
RSP   Right-sacrum-posterior
LSA   Left-sacrum-anterior
LST   Left-sacrum-transverse
LSP   Left-sacrum-posterior

Positions in shoulder presentation:
RADA   Right-acromion-dorsal-anterior
RADP   Right-acromion-dorsal-posterior
LADA   Left-acromion-dorsal-anterior
LADP   Left-acromion-dorsal-posterior

The fetal position influences labor and birth. For example, in a posterior position the fetal head presents a larger diameter than in an anterior position. A posterior position increases the pressure on the maternal sacral nerves, causing the laboring woman backache and pelvic pressure and perhaps encouraging her to bear down or push earlier than normal. The most common fetal position is occiput anterior. When this position occurs the labor and birth is more likely to proceed normally. Positions other than occiput anterior are more frequently associated with problems during labor; therefore they are called **malpositions.** (See Chapter 25 for discussion of malpositions and their management.)

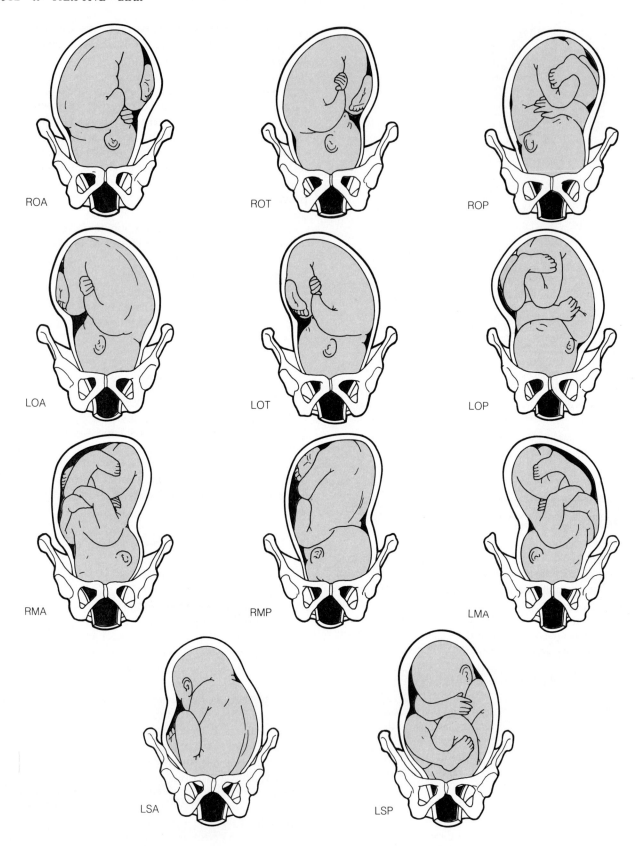

Figure 21–8 Categories of presentation (Courtesy Ross laboratories, Columbus, Ohio)

Assessment techniques to determine fetal position include inspection and palpation of the maternal abdomen, and vaginal examination (see Chapter 22 for further discussion of assessment of fetal position).

Uterine Contractions

Primary and secondary powers work together to deliver the fetus, the fetal membranes, and the placenta from the uterus into the external environment. The *primary power* is uterine muscular contractions, which cause the changes of the first stage of labor—complete effacement and dilatation of the cervix. The *secondary power* is the use of abdominal muscles to push during the second stage of labor. The pushing adds to the primary power after full dilatation has occurred.

In labor, uterine contractions are rhythmic but intermittent. Between contractions is a period of relaxation. This period of relaxation allows uterine muscles to rest and provides respite for the laboring woman. It also restores uteroplacental circulation, which is important to fetal oxygenation and adequate circulation in the uterine blood vessels.

Each contraction has three phases: (a) *increment*, the "building up" of the contraction (the longest phase); (b) *acme*, or the peak of the contraction; and (c) *decrement*, or the "letting up" of the contraction. When describing uterine contractions during labor, care givers use the terms *frequency, duration,* and *intensity.* **Frequency** refers to the time between the beginning of one contraction and the beginning of the next contraction.

The **duration** of each contraction is measured from the beginning of the increment to the completion of decrement (Figure 21–9). In beginning labor, the duration is about 30 seconds. As labor continues, duration increases to an average of 60 seconds with a range of 45 to 90 seconds (Varney 1987).

Intensity refers to the strength of the uterine contraction during acme. In most instances, the intensity is estimated by palpating the contraction but it may be measured directly with an intrauterine catheter. When estimating intensity by palpation, the nurse determines whether it is mild, moderate, or strong by judging the amount of indentability of the uterine wall during the acme of a contraction. If the uterine wall can be indented easily, the contraction is considered mild. Strong intensity exists when the uterine wall cannot be indented. Moderate intensity falls between these two ranges. When intensity is measured with an intrauterine catheter, the normal resting tonus (between contractions) is about 10 to 15 mm Hg of pressure. During acme, the intensity ranges from 30 to 55 mm Hg of pressure (Cibils 1981) (or 20 to 30 mm Hg above the resting tonus) (Zlatnik 1990). (See Chapter 22 for further discussions of assessment techniques.)

At the beginning of labor, the contractions are usually mild, of short duration, and relatively infrequent. As labor progresses, duration of contractions lengthens, the intensity increases, and the frequency is every two to three minutes. Because the contractions are involuntary, the laboring woman cannot control their duration, frequency, or intensity.

Psychologic State

Rubin (1984, p 52) notes that childbearing "requires an exchange of a known self in a known world for an unknown self in an unknown world. This is an act of courage." And no part of the childbearing period brings this more to light than labor. Every woman is uncertain about what her labor will be like: A woman anticipating her first labor faces a totally new experience, and even multiparas cannot be certain what each new labor will bring. The woman does not know whether she will live up to her expectations for herself in relation to her friends and relatives, whether she will be physically injured through laceration, episiotomy, or cesarean incision, or whether significant others will be as supportive as she hopes (Mercer 1985). The woman faces an irrevocable event—the birth of a new family member—and, consequently, disruption of life-style, relationships, and self-image. Finally, the woman must deal with

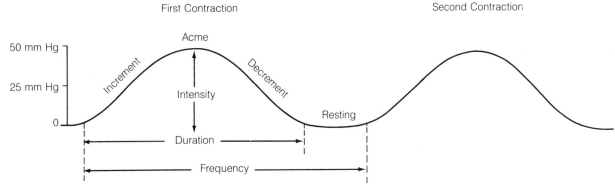

Figure 21–9   Characteristics of uterine contractions

Table 21–3	Factors Associated with a Positive Birth Experience

Motivation for the pregnancy

Attendance at childbirth education classes

A sense of competence or mastery

Self-confidence and self-esteem

Positive relationship with mate

Maintaining control during labor

Support from mate or other person during labor

Not being left alone in labor

Trust in the medical/nursing staff

concerns about her loss of control of bodily functions, emotional responses to an unfamiliar situation, and reactions to the pain associated with labor.

Various factors influence a woman's reaction to the physical and emotional crisis of labor (Table 21-3). Her accomplishment of the tasks of pregnancy, usual coping mechanisms in response to stressful life events, support system, preparation for childbirth, and cultural influences are all significant factors.

Preparation for Labor

In her study of the psychosocial adaptations of pregnancy Lederman (1984) found that certain psychosocial factors of pregnancy were predictive of progress in labor. One such factor was related to a woman's psychologic preparation for labor. Lederman found that expectant women prepared for labor through actions and through imaginary rehearsal. The actions frequently consisted of "nesting behavior" and a "psyching up" for the labor, which seemed to vary depending on the woman's sense of self-confidence, self-esteem, and previous experiences with stress. Specific actions to prepare for labor are usually focused on becoming better informed and prepared. Many women attended prenatal classes to learn about labor and to share the birth experience with their husbands. Others hoped that learning specific techniques of relaxation and breathing would allow them more control during labor so they could take a more active part. Additional information was gained through viewing films, reading books, and talking to other women.

An important developmental step for expectant women is to anticipate the labor in fantasy. Just as a woman "tries on" the maternal role during pregnancy, fantasizing about labor seems to help the woman understand and become more prepared for labor. Her fantasies about the excitement of the baby's birth and the sharing of the experience involve her in constructive preparation even though she may still have some fears of labor. Women who have a great deal of apprehension about becoming a mother or a high fear of pain during labor are not able to fantasize the labor in positive ways and instead have many disturbing thoughts (Lederman 1984).

Positive fantasies seem to involve many areas. The woman thinks about the contractions and the work and pain that will be involved, and this seems to provide a stimulus to becoming more prepared for labor. Lederman (1984) found that women who were able to visualize themselves as active participants in labor were usually well prepared and had positive self-images. Fantasy and thoughts about labor help the woman to have realistic ideas about the work, pain, and risks involved and to develop a sense of confidence in her ability to cope.

Many women fear the pain of contractions. They not only see the pain as threatening but also associate it with a loss of control over their bodies and emotions. Our society seems to value control and cooperation with established routines in health care settings. When a woman is facing labor, especially for the first time, she may worry about her ability to withstand the pain of labor and maintain control over herself. Women are afraid of becoming fatigued and unable to relax because they may then act in a way that is undesirable or may induce bodily injury. In Lederman's study the women who were confident of their abilities usually had less fear than women who doubted their ability to maintain control of themselves.

The laboring woman's support system may also influence the course of labor and birth. For some women the presence of the father and other significant persons, including the nurse, tends to have a positive effect. Other women may prefer not to have a support person or family with them.

Preparation for childbirth is another factor that influences a woman's reaction to childbirth. Much attention has been focused on preparation during pregnancy as a way of increasing the woman's ability to cope during childbirth, decreasing her stress, anxiety, and pain, and imparting satisfaction with the childbearing experience. Although opinions vary concerning whether the amount of pain or discomfort is actually decreased, there is agreement that preparation tends to increase perceived satisfaction. Nichols and Humenick (1987) suggest that *mastery*, or control, of the childbearing experience is the key factor in perceived satisfaction. Childbirth education helps to increase positive reactions to the birth experience because education gives the laboring woman and her support persons greater opportunities to control the experience of labor.

How the woman views the childbirth experience after the birth may have implications for mothering behaviors. Mercer (1985) found a significant relationship between the birth experience and mothering behaviors. It appears that any activities—by the expectant woman or by maternal–child health care providers—that enhance the birth experience will be beneficial as the woman prepares for labor, experiences labor, and begins her new role as a mother.

Physiology of Labor

Possible Causes of Labor Onset

For some reason, usually at the appropriate time for the uterus and the fetus, the process of labor begins. Although medical researchers have been conducting numerous studies to determine the exact cause, it still is not clearly understood. The relationship of some factors is presented in Figure 21–10. Some of the more widely accepted theories are discussed in the following sections.

Oxytocin Stimulation Theory

Throughout the course of pregnancy there is a slow increase in the amount of oxytocin in maternal circulating blood. The level increases more dramatically during labor and peaks in the second stage (Chard 1989). The concentration of oxytocin receptors in the myometrium and decidua also increases and peaks during labor. Due to both of these factors, the uterus is increasingly responsive and reactive to oxytocin as the pregnancy approaches term (38 to 40 weeks) (Garfield & Beier 1989). However, there is

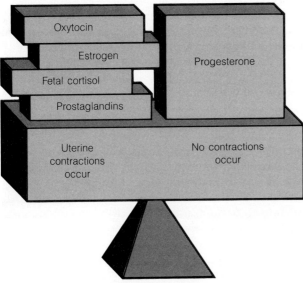

Figure 21–10 Factors affecting initiation of labor. The factors listed on the left have all been identified as providing stimulus to the beginning of labor. Progesterone exerts a relaxing effect, and a balance between all of the factors keeps the uterus quiet, without contraction. When the relationship of factors changes, the balance is tipped and uterine labor begins.

no convincing evidence that maternal or fetal oxytocin initiates labor. Oxytocin does have an effect on the permeability of sodium in the myometrium and raises the intracellular calcium levels that are needed for muscle contraction (Hariharan et al 1986). Some researchers suggest that oxytocin has a dual action on two types of receptors in the uterus, with one leading to myometrial contractions and the other to stimulation of prostaglandin release (Hariharan et al 1986).

Progesterone Withdrawal Theory

Progesterone has been reported to inhibit the estrogen effect of increased contractility by raising the resting membrane potential in the myometrial cells. It may stabilize the myometrial membrane-bound pools of calcium, thereby limiting uterine contractility (Hariharan et al 1986). Although some researchers feel there is insufficient evidence to show that progesterone levels in the maternal blood supply fall before labor (Cunningham et al 1989), others report that progesterone metabolism in the fetal membranes is marked by decreases near term. The decrease in progesterone metabolism may be due to a progesterone-binding protein, which is present near term in the chorion and amnion. The decrease may facilitate prostaglandin synthesis in the chorioamnion, which increases uterine contractility. Although no general agreement exists regarding a decrease in progesterone metabolism, many researchers support the theory that a rising estrogen and decreasing progesterone ratio is important in raising levels of uterine contractility (Hariharan et al 1986).

Estrogen Stimulation Theory

Estrogen causes irritability of the myometrium, perhaps through an increase in concentrations of actin and myosin (contractile proteins in muscle tissue) and adenosine triphosphate (ATP). which is the energy source for contractions. In addition, estrogen may promote prostaglandin synthesis in the decidua and fetal membranes. This enhances myometrial muscle contraction. Once the muscle cell is irritable and contracts, the presence of estrogen also enhances the propagation of impulses over the uterine muscle (Hariharan et al 1986).

Fetal Cortisol Theory

Liggins (1973) found that the removal of a fetal lamb's pituitary gland and adrenal cortex delays the onset of labor. Thus he has postulated that the fetus may play an important role in the initiation of labor. He also has reported premature labor in sheep that were infused with cortisol or ACTH. This phenomenon has not been confirmed in humans. However, a decrease in estrogen in both maternal and fetal plasma can be observed following maternal administration of corticosteroids. Research continues; there is a possibility that cortisol affects the biochemistry of the fetal membrane (Hariharan et al 1986).

Fetal Membrane Phospholipid–Arachidonic Acid–Prostaglandin Theory

According to the theory of fetal membrane phospholipid–arachidonic acid–prostaglandin interaction, estrogen promotes storage of esterified arachidonic acid in the fetal membranes. Withdrawal of progesterone activates phospholipase A_2, which is an enzymatic liberator. Phospholipase A_2 hydrolyzes phospholipids to liberate arachidonic acid in a nonesterified form. The arachidonic acid acts on PGE_2, $F_{2\alpha}$, or both in the decidual membranes. Prostaglandin stimulates the smooth muscle to contract, especially in the myometrium. Prostaglandin is present in increased quantities in the blood and amniotic fluid just prior to and during labor (Hariharan et al 1986). It has been suggested that the key to initiation of labor may be increased synthesis of PGE_2 in the amnion (Cunningham et al 1989).

Biochemical Interaction

The contraction wave of the uterus begins in the fundus, which contains the greatest concentration of myometrial cells, and moves downward throughout the entire myometrium. Because the contraction wave moves quickly, the myometrium appears to contract as a unit. Myometrial contraction efficiency depends on the presence of five factors:

1. Gap junctions must be present. Gap junctions of the myometrium are cell-to-cell contacts that promote synchronous contractions of smooth muscle cells and increase the effectiveness of the contractions. Gap junctions are prevalent at term and increase in number and size during labor. They begin to disappear within 24 hours after birth. Gap junctions are present in premature labor. It is thought that estrogen, PGE_2, and $PGF_{2\alpha}$ promote formation of gap junctions and progesterone prevents them (Hariharan et al 1986; Sokol & Brindley 1990).

2. The contractile substances actin and myosin are essential for muscle contraction to occur.

3. A source of energy (ATP) must be available.

4. Cellular electrolyte exchange of calcium, sodium, and potassium is essential for muscle contraction.

5. The presence of an endocrine stimulus is necessary for conduction of the muscle contraction. During labor oxytocin, $PGF_{2\alpha}$, and acetylcholine are present.

All these factors work together to produce the uterine contractions of labor.

Myometrial Activity

Stretching of the cervix causes an increase in endogenous oxytocin, which increases myometrial activity. This is known as the *Ferguson reflex*. Pressures exerted by the contracting uterus vary from 20 to 60 mm Hg, with an average of 40 mm Hg.

In true labor the uterus divides into two portions. This division is known as the *physiologic retraction ring*. The upper portion, which is the contractile segment, becomes progressively thicker as labor advances. The lower portion, which includes the lower uterine segment and cervix, is passive. As labor continues, the lower uterine segment expands and thins out.

With each contraction the musculature of the upper uterine segment shortens and exerts a longitudinal traction on the cervix, causing effacement. **Effacement** is the taking up of the internal os and the cervical canal into the uterine side walls. The cervix changes progressively from a long, thick structure to a structure that is tissue-paper thin (Figure 21–11). In primigravidas, effacement usually precedes dilatation. The uterine musculature remains shorter and thicker and does not return to its original length. This phenomenon is known as brachystasis. The space in the uterine cavity decreases as a result of brachystasis and this places downward pressure on the fetus.

The uterus elongates with each contraction, decreasing the horizontal diameter. This elongation causes a straightening of the fetal body, pressing the part of the fetus in the upper portion of the uterus against the fundus and thrusting the presenting part down toward the lower uterine segment and the cervix. The pressure exerted by the fetus is called fetal axis pressure. As the uterus elongates, the longitudinal muscle fibers are pulled upward over the presenting part. This action, plus the hydrostatic pressure of the fetal membranes, causes **cervical dilatation.** The cervical os and cervical canal widen from less than a centimeter to approximately 10 cm, allowing birth of the fetus. When the cervix is completely dilated and retracted up into the lower uterine segment, it can no longer be palpated.

The round ligament contracts with the uterus, pulling the fundus forward, thus aligning the fetus with the maternal bony pelvis.

Intraabdominal Pressure

After the cervix is completely dilated, the maternal abdominal musculature contracts as the woman pushes. This pushing is called *bearing down*. The pushing aids in the expulsion of the fetus and the placenta. If the cervix is not completely dilated, bearing down can cause cervical edema, which retards dilatation.

Musculature Changes in the Pelvic Floor

The levator ani muscle and fascia of the pelvic floor draw the rectum and vagina upward and forward with each contraction, along the curve of the pelvic floor. As the fetal head descends to the pelvic floor, the pressure of the presenting part causes the perineal structure, which was once 5 cm in thickness, to change to a structure less than a centimeter thick. Thus a normal physiologic anesthesia is produced as a result of the decreased blood supply to the area.

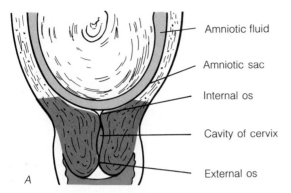

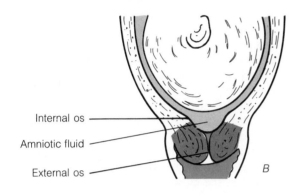

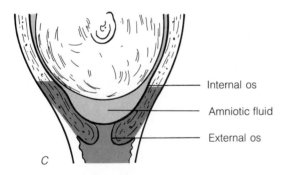

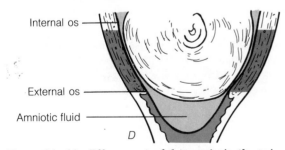

Figure 21–11 Effacement of the cervix in the pri-migravida. A At the beginning of labor there is no cervical effacement or dilatation. The fetal head is cushioned by amniotic fluid. B Beginning cervical effacement. As the cervix begins to efface more amniotic fluid collects below the fetal head. C Cervix is about one-half effaced and slightly dilated. The increasing amount of amniotic fluid exerts hydrostatic pressure. D Complete effacement and dilatation.

The anus everts, exposing the interior rectal wall as the fetal head descends forward (Cunningham et al 1989).

Maternal Systemic Response to Labor

Cardiovascular System

A strong contraction greatly diminishes or completely stops the blood flow in the branches of the uterine artery that supplies the intervillous space. This leads to a redistribution of the blood flow to the peripheral circulation and an increase in peripheral resistance, resulting in an increase of the systolic and diastolic blood pressure and a slowing of the pulse rate. The amount of change in maternal blood pressure and pulse is also dependent on the maternal position. If the woman is in a lateral recumbent position, blood pressure rises slightly, pulse rate decreases about 1%, cardiac output increases 7.6%, stroke volume increases 7.7%, and pulse pressure rises 6%. When the woman is in a supine position, blood pressure rises more significantly, pulse rate decreases 15%, cardiac output increases 25%, stroke volume increases 33%, and pulse pressure increases more than 26% (Ueland & Ferguson 1990).

There is an additional effect on hemodynamics during the bearing down efforts in the second stage. When the laboring woman holds her breath and pushes against a closed glottis (Valsalva maneuver), intrathoracic pressure rises. As intrathoracic pressure increases, the venous return is interrupted, which leads to a rise in the venous pressure. In addition, the blood in the lungs is forced into the left atrium, which leads to a transient increase in cardiac output, blood pressure, and pulse pressure and causes bradycardia. As venous return to the lungs continues to be diminished while the breath is held, a decrease in blood pressure, pulse pressure, and cardiac output occurs.

When the next breath is taken (Valsalva maneuver is interrupted), the intrathoracic pressure is decreased. Venous return increases, which leads to refilling of the pulmonary bed and results in recovery of the cardiac output and stroke volume. This process is repeated with each pushing effort.

Immediately after birth, cardiac output peaks with an 80% increase over prelabor values, and then in the first 10 minutes decreases 20% to 25%. Cardiac output further decreases 20% to 25% in the first hour after the birth (Albright et al 1986). However, these decreases still leave the woman with an elevated cardiac output for at least 24 hours after the birth (Robson et al 1989).

Blood Pressure

As a result of increased cardiac output, systolic blood pressure rises during uterine contractions. Between contractions, the blood pressure returns to its prelabor level. In the immediate postpartal period, the arterial pressure remains essentially normal even though the cardiac output increases due to peripheral vasodilation.

Blood pressure may drop precipitously when the woman lies in a supine position and experiences supine hypotensive syndrome. In addition to hypotension, there is an increase in the pulse rate, diaphoresis, nausea, weakness, and air hunger. These changes are attributed to the decreased cardiac output and a subsequent drop in stroke volume. Some researchers have suggested that in addition to venal caval compression from the weight of the pregnant uterus, there is also aortocaval compression (Bottoms & Scott 1990).

Women with the highest risk of developing supine hypotensive syndrome are women in their first pregnancy with strong abdominal muscles and tightly drawn abdominal skin, women with hydramnios and/or multiple pregnancy, and obese women. Other predisposing factors include hypovolemia; dehydration; hemorrhage; metabolic acidosis; administration of narcotics (which results in vasodilation and inhibits compensatory mechanisms), and administration of regional anesthetics that results in *sympathetic blockade* (blocking of the sympathetic nervous system, which results in vasodilation and hypotension). A sympathetic blockade may occur with an epidural or a spinal block.

Fluid and Electrolyte Balance

Profuse perspiration (diaphoresis) occurs during labor. Hyperventilation also occurs, altering electrolyte and fluid balance from insensible water loss. The muscle activity elevates the body temperature, which increases sweating and evaporation from the skin. As the woman responds to the work of labor the rise in the respiratory rate increases the evaporative water volume, since each breath of air must be warmed to the body temperature and humidified. With the increased evaporative water volume, giving parenteral fluids during labor to ensure adequate hydration becomes increasingly important.

Gastrointestinal System

During labor, gastric motility and absorption of solid food are reduced. Gastric emptying time is prolonged. It is not uncommon for a laboring woman to vomit food she ate up to 12 hours earlier.

Respiratory System

Oxygen consumption, which increased approximately 20% during pregnancy, is further increased during labor. During the early first stage of labor, oxygen consumption increases 40%, with a further increase to 100% during the second stage.

Minute ventilation increases to 20 to 25 L/min (normal 10 L/min), and in the unprepared and unmedicated woman it may reach 35 L/min or more. This hyperventila-

tion results in a rise in the maternal pH in early labor, followed by a return to normal toward the end of the first stage (Albright et al 1986).

Hemopoietic System

Leukocyte levels may increase to $25,000/mm^3$ or more during labor. Although the precise cause of the leukocytosis is unknown, it may be due to the strenuous exercise and stress response of labor (Cunningham et al 1989). It has been found that the longer a woman is in labor, the greater the elevation in leukocyte count (Acker et al 1985). In the absence of ruptured membranes or any signs of infection, this elevation seems to be a normal physiologic reaction.

Plasma fibrinogen increases, and blood coagulation time decreases. Blood glucose levels may decrease due to the increased activity of uterine and skeletal muscles (Varney 1987).

Marked changes in clotting factors VII, II, and X have occurred during pregnancy and continue through the birth. The most dramatic change occurs in factor VII. There is growing speculation that the increase is a phospholipid complex that is affected by trophoblastic tissue. By 40 weeks' gestation, the mean activity of factor VII is 248% above nonpregnant values, and the increase remains during birth. There is a dramatic decrease during the first 30 minutes after expulsion of the placenta. The decrease continues over the next few weeks of the postpartum period. Factor II increases to a mean activity factor of 136%. Factor X increases to 171 percent. These changes help protect against hemorrhage during birth but in addition, they place the woman at higher risk for thrombophlebitis (Dalaker 1986).

Renal System

The base of the bladder is pushed forward and upward when engagement occurs. The pressure from the presenting part may lead to edema of the tissues due to impaired drainage of blood and lymph from the base of the bladder (Cunningham et al 1989).

Approximately one-third to one-half of all laboring women have slight proteinuria (trace) as a result of muscle breakdown from exercise. An increase to 2+ or above is indicative of pathology (Varney 1987).

Pain

Theories of Pain

According to the *gate-control theory* pain results from activity in several interacting specialized neural systems. The gate-control theory proposes that a mechanism in the dorsal horn of the spinal column serves as a valve or gate that increases or decreases the flow of nerve impulses from the periphery to the central nervous system. The gate mechanism is influenced by the size of the transmitting fibers and by the nerve impulses that descend from the brain. Psychologic processes such as past experiences, attention, and emotion may influence pain perception and response by activating the gate mechanism. The gates may be opened or closed by central nervous system activities, such as anxiety or excitement, or through selective localized activity.

The gate-control theory has two important implications for childbirth: Pain may be controlled by tactile stimulation and can be modified by activities controlled by the central nervous system. These include back rub, sacral pressure, effleurage, suggestion, distraction, and conditioning.

Pain During Labor

The pain associated with the first stage of labor is unique in that it accompanies a normal physiologic process. Even though perception of the pain of childbirth is greatly determined by cultural patterning, there is a physiologic basis for discomfort during labor. Pain during the first stage of labor arises from (a) dilatation of the cervix, (b) hypoxia of the uterine muscle cells during contraction, (c) stretching of the lower uterine segment, and (d) pressure on adjacent structures. The primary source of pain is dilatation or stretching of the cervix. Nerve impulses travel through the uterine plexus, inferior hypogastric (pelvic) plexus, middle hypogastric plexus, superior hypogastric plexus, and the lumbar sympathetic and lower thoracic chain and enter the spinal cord through the posterior roots of the 12th, 11th, and 10th thoracic and 1st lumbar nerves (Figure 21–12). As with other visceral pain, pain from the uterus is referred to the dermatomes supplied by the 12th, 11th, and 10th thoracic nerves. The areas of referred pain include the lower abdominal wall and the areas over the lower lumbar region and the upper sacrum (Figure 21–13).

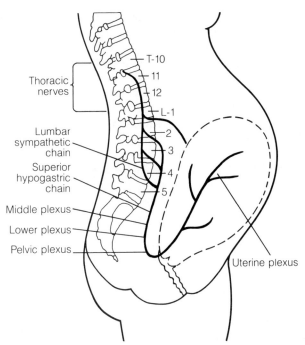

Figure 21–12 Pain pathway from uterus to spinal cord. Nerve impulses travel through the uterine plexus, pelvic plexus, inferior hypogastric plexus, middle and superior hypogastric, and the lumbar sympathetic chain and enter the spinal cord through the 12th, 11th, and 10th thoracic nerves. (Modified from Bonica JJ: Principles and Practice of Obstetric Analgesia and Anesthesia. Philadelphia: FA Davis 1972, p 492)

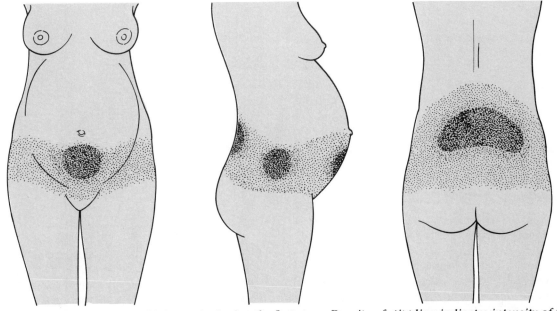

Figure 21–13 Area of reference of labor pain during the first stage. Density of stippling indicates intensity of pain. (From Bonica FF: Principles and Practice of Obstetric Analgesia and Anesthesia. Philadelphia: FA Davis, 1972, p 108)

During the second stage of labor, discomfort is due to (a) hypoxia of the contracting uterine muscle cells, (b) distention of the vagina and perineum, and (c) pressure on adjacent structures. The nerve impulses from the vagina and perineum are transmitted by way of the pudendal nerve plexus and enter the spinal cord through the posterior roots of the second, third, and fourth sacral nerves. The area of pain increases as shown in Figure 21–14.

Pain during the third stage results from uterine contractions and cervical dilatation as the placenta is expelled (Figure 21–15). The mechanism for the transmission of nerve impulses is the same as for the first stage of labor. The third stage of labor is short, and after this phase of labor, anesthesia is needed primarily for episiotomy repair.

Factors Affecting Response to Pain

Many factors affect the individual's perception of pain impulses. Some psychologic and environmental influences particularly appropriate to labor are discussed here.

Effect of Childbirth Education Preparation for childbirth has been shown to reduce the need for analgesia and the subjective experience of tension and stress that occurs during labor. Crowe and Baeyer (1989) reported that women who demonstrated greater knowledge of childbirth and indicated they felt higher confidence after completing the classes reported a less painful childbirth.

Cultural Background Medical and nursing professionals have their own health care culture expectations of the woman in labor. She is expected to use a breathing technique and relaxation methods. Value is placed on maintaining self-control and knowing what to expect during labor and birth. It is important to know that the health care professional will interpret pain according to the health care culture norms while various other cultures have other ways of responding to pain (Bates 1987). The absence of crying and moaning does not necessarily mean that pain is absent, nor does the presence of crying and moaning necessarily mean that pain relief is desired at that moment. Some cultures believe it is natural to communicate the pain experience, no matter how mild. Members of some cultures stoically accept pain out of fear or because it is expected of them.

An Asian woman may not outwardly express pain for fear of shaming herself and her family. Asian women may be anxious about losing face by their behavior (Engel 1989). Black women may also appear stoic in an effort to avoid showing weakness or calling undue attention to themselves (Kay 1982). Mexican women are taught to keep

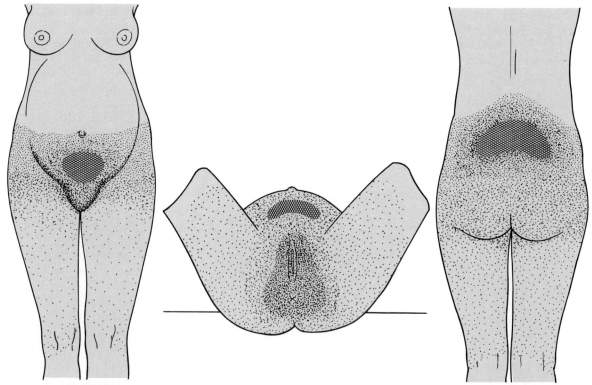

Figure 21–14 Distribution of labor pain during the later phase of the first stage and early phase of the second stage. Crosshatched areas indicate location of the most intense pain; dense stippling, moderate pain; and light stippling, mild pain. Note that the uterine contractions, which at this stage are very strong, produce intense pain. (From Bonica JJ: Principles and Practice of Obstetric Analgesia and Anesthesia. Philadelphia: FL Davis, 1972, p 109)

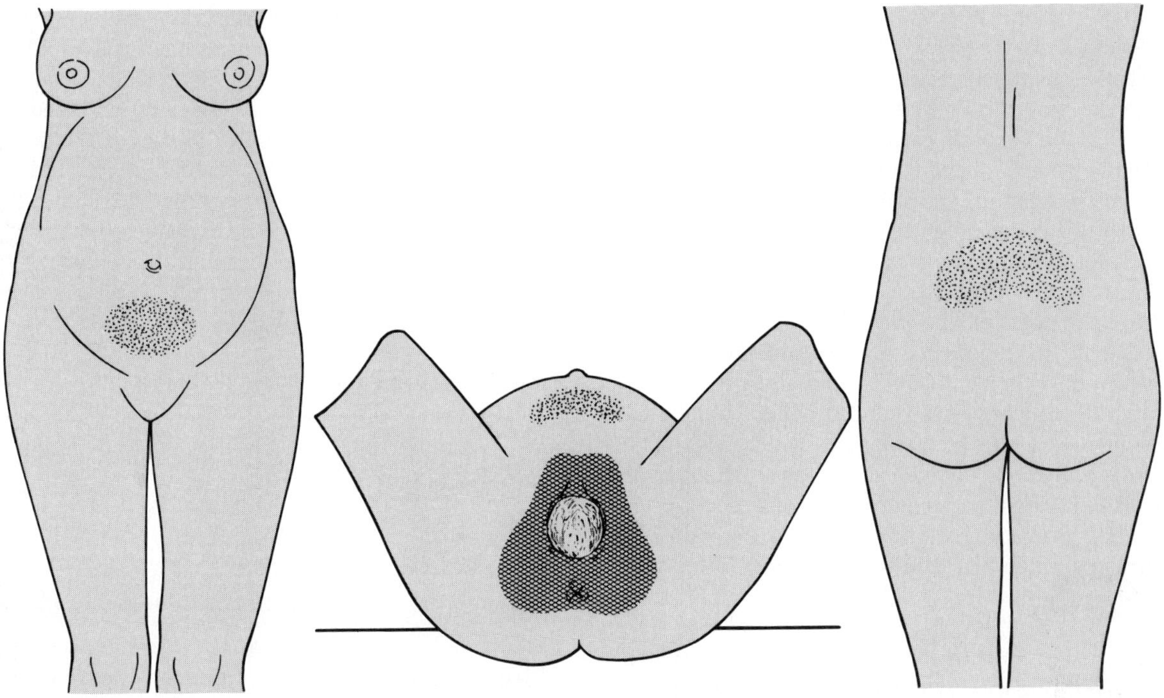

Figure 21–15   Distribution of labor pain during the later phase of the second stage and actual birth. The perineal component is the primary cause of discomfort. Uterine contractions contribute much less. (From Bonica JJ: Principles and Practice of Obstetric Analgesia and Anesthesia. *Philadelphia: FA Davis, 1972, p 109)*

their mouths closed during labor and to avoid breathing in air that may cause the uterus to rise up. They cry out only during exhalation (Kay 1982). Navajo women traditionally keep quiet to preserve the secrecy of the process (Kay 1982). The outward expression of the perceived pain may be difficult to interpret. Navajo women may be willing to receive pain medication but be hesitant to request it (Kay 1982). In a study by Senden et al (1988), it was noted that Dutch women both expected and received less pain medication than their American counterparts. In a different comparison, Middle-Eastern women with little education exhibited more pain behavior than those with higher education (Weisenberg & Caspi 1989). Interestingly, Senden et al (1988) and Weisenberg and Caspi (1989) found that all of the women expressed high satisfaction with their birth experience, which suggests that receiving the type of assistance (physical, medical) that the woman desired was more of an influence on her satisfaction than the pain actually experienced or expressed.

The health care culture may use touching and the support of others to decrease pain during labor. Various other cultural groups may or may not value the same comfort measures. The traditional Native American may want a female with her rather than her husband, and the Japanese woman may feel "ashamed" to be seen by her husband (Kay 1982). Hmong women usually prefer that their husbands remain with them in labor and be involved in comfort measures (Morrow 1986).

It is important, however, to avoid stereotyping women because of their ethnic backgrounds, since exposure to North American culture and expectations may modify the behavioral response to pain. Nurses who are providing support during labor must recognize that there are ways of reacting to pain that are different from the nurse's own personal views of appropriate behavior. Nurses need to be familiar with the cultural beliefs of those they are likely to assist during labor and use this knowledge along with assessment skills to verify the type of support that is needed.

Fatigue and Sleep Deprivation   Exhaustion may be so great that a laboring woman's attention wanders from the physical stimuli of childbirth, or it may have the opposite effect, lowering the powers of resistance and self-control to produce an exaggerated response. Fatigue from sleep deprivation affects an individual's response to pain in several ways. The fatigued person has less energy and a decreased ability to use such strategies as distraction or imagination as coping mechanisms in dealing with pain. The fatigued woman in labor may choose a less demanding alternative, such as analgesia (McCaffery 1972). This is particularly important for a laboring woman who has a prolonged prodromal period, which may interfere with sleep. A woman may begin the active phase of labor in an exhausted state and have difficulty coping with the discomfort of frequent contractions.

Personal Significance of Pain The significance of pain is closely related to the woman's self-concept as well as to cultural expectations. She may view labor as a fearful event, one she has dreaded throughout pregnancy, or she may view it as the happiest event of her life. Pain may be interpreted by some women as punishment for perceived sins, such as engaging in premarital intercourse or feeling ambivalent toward the pregnancy. Others who have had preparation for childbirth may consider the pain a test of their ability to cope with a challenging event. If such women do not handle the pain of labor according to their expectations, they tend to experience a sense of failure, which threatens not only their self-concept but also their ability to mother. Consequently, it is vital that childbirth instructors and nurses stress to each woman that the reaction to childbirth is varied and individual. A woman should not feel a sense of failure if she requires analgesia to assist her in coping. The primary goal of childbirth preparation is a childbirth experience that is satisfying to both father and mother.

Previous Experience One's previous experience with pain affects one's ability to manage current and future pain. Particularly painful experiences can condition one to expect the same degree of pain in a similar situation. All persons, with very few exceptions, have experienced pain. It appears likely that those who have had more experience with pain are more sensitive to painful stimuli.

Anxiety Anxiety related to pain must be approached on two levels, that associated with anticipation of pain and that associated with the presence of pain. While a moderate degree of anxiety about impending pain is necessary for the person to handle the pain experience, anxiety during the pain experience should be reduced as much as possible by nursing intervention. Anxiety during labor produces tension, which increases the intensity of the pain.

Anxieties unrelated to the pain can also intensify the pain experience. For many young women, admission for labor and birth is their first hospitalization. Routine procedures, rules and regulations, equipment, and the general environment are unfamiliar and anxiety-provoking. For many women the spontaneous onset of labor has an element of surprise. Although the event is expected and even anticipated, few women are totally prepared for the actual onset of labor and hospitalization. Last-minute details must be completed. Arrangement for the care of other children have usually been made but now must actually be carried out. Having to leave young children for a few days is accompanied by varying degrees of anxiety for any mother.

Attention and Distraction Both attention and distraction have an influence on the perception of pain. When pain sensation is the focus of attention, the perceived intensity is greater. The classic example is the football player who is unaware of an injury until the game is over and only then experiences painful sensations.

A sensory stimulus can serve as a distraction because the person's attention is focused on the stimulus rather than the pain, for example, providing a client with a back rub. Cutaneous sensations are carried by large-diameter afferent fibers, which can inhibit the pain sensation carried by small-diameter fibers. This is a component of the gate-control theory of pain discussed earlier. Cutaneous stimulation to relieve pain may also be explained by the theory of extinction or perceptual dominance. This theory suggests that sensory input may extinguish pain or raise its threshold.

Fetal Response to Labor

When the fetus is normal, the mechanical and hemodynamic changes of normal labor have no adverse effects.

Heart Rate Changes

Fetal heart rate decelerations can occur with intracranial pressures of 40 to 55 mm Hg. The currently accepted explanation of this early deceleration is hypoxic depression of the central nervous system, which is under vagal control. The absence of these head compression decelerations (early decelerations) in some fetuses during labor is explained by the existence of a threshold that is reached more gradually in the presence of intact membranes and lack of maternal resistance. Early decelerations are harmless in the normal fetus.

Acid-Base Status in Labor

The first stage of labor is associated with a slow decrease in the fetal pH. As the second stage begins, there is a more rapid decrease due to an increase in uterine contractility and bearing down efforts of the laboring woman. There is also an increase in fetal base deficit and in P_{CO_2} and a drop in fetal oxygen saturation of about 10% (Creasy & Resnik 1989).

Fetal Movements

When the fetus is between 35 and 40 weeks, episodes of fetal breathing movements increase in the second and third hour following the mother's meals. There is also a marked increase during the night while the mother is asleep, which is thought to be part of a circadian rhythm in fetal breathing activity. In the healthy term fetus there are periods of no breathing movements that last up to two hours. It has been noted that the incidence of fetal breathing movements slows markedly and may cease about three days before the onset of spontaneous labor (Creasy & Resnik 1989). It has been suggested that the absence of fetal breathing movements might be used to differentiate between true and false labor (Boyland et al 1985).

Gross fetal body movements occur at a rate of about

20 to 50 per hour in the term fetus. The number of movements do not normally increase prior to or during labor (Creasy & Resnik 1989).

Behavior States

The human fetus develops behavioral states between 36 and 38 weeks of gestation (Mulder & Visser 1989). The behavioral states seem to continue during labor even in the presence of uterine contractions. Two sleep states (quiet and active) were most prevalent, although quiet and active awake states were occasionally observed. A decrease in fetal heart rate variability accompanies the quiet sleep state, and there is also a decrease in fetal breathing movements and other general body activity. The quiet sleep state lasted less than 40 minutes. Broussard (1990) suggests that as long as other fetal heart rate parameters are within normal limits, a decrease in variability will usually indicate a normal behavioral sleep state.

Hemodynamic Changes

The adequate exchange of nutrients and gases in the fetal capillaries and intervillous spaces depends in part on the fetal blood pressure. Fetal blood pressure is a protective mechanism for the normal fetus during the anoxic periods caused by the contracting uterus during labor. The fetal

and placental reserve is enough to see the fetus through these anoxic periods unharmed (Creasy & Resnik 1989).

Positional Changes

For the fetus to pass through the birth canal, the fetal head and body must adjust to the maternal pelvis by certain positional changes. These changes, called **cardinal movements** or *mechanisms of labor,* are described in the order in which they occur (Figure 21–16).

Descent
Descent is thought to occur because of four forces: (a) pressure of the amniotic fluid, (b) direct pressure of the fundus of the uterus on the breech of the fetus, (c) contraction of the abdominal muscles, and (d) extension and straightening of the fetal body. The head enters the inlet in the occiput transverse or oblique position because the pelvic inlet is widest from side to side. The sagittal suture is an equal distance from the maternal symphysis pubis and sacral promontory.

Flexion
Flexion occurs as the fetal head descends and meets resistance from the soft tissues of the pelvis, the musculature of the pelvic floor, and the cervix.

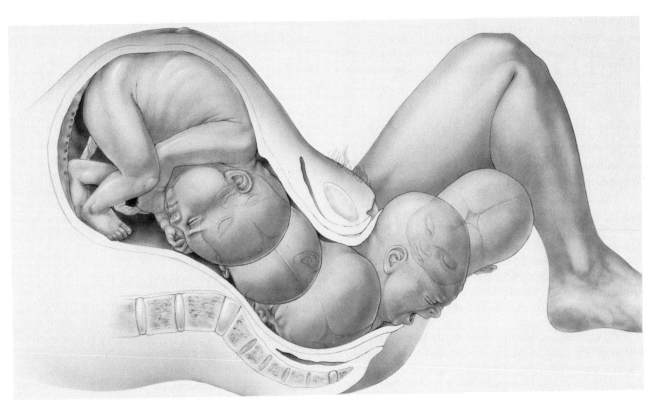

Figure 21–16   Mechanisms of labor: A, B Descent. C Internal rotation. D Extension. E External rotation.

Internal Rotation

The fetal head must rotate to fit the diameter of the pelvic cavity, which is widest in the anteroposterior diameter. As the occiput of the fetal head meets resistance from the levator ani muscles and their fascia, the occiput rotates from left to right and the sagittal suture aligns in the anteroposterior pelvic diameter.

Extension

The resistance of the pelvic floor and the mechanical movement of the vulva opening anteriorly and forward assist with extension of the fetal head as it passes under the symphysis pubis. With this positional change, the occiput, then brow and face, emerge from the vagina.

Restitution

The shoulders of the infant enter the pelvis obliquely and remain oblique when the head rotates to the anteroposterior diameter through internal rotation. Because of this rotation the neck becomes twisted. Once the head emerges and is free of pelvic resistance, the neck untwists, turning the head to one side (restitution), and aligns with the position of the back in the birth canal.

External Rotation

As the shoulders rotate to the anteroposterior position in the pelvis, the head is turned farther to one side (external rotation).

Expulsion

After the external rotation and through expulsive efforts of the laboring woman, the anterior shoulder meets the under surface of the symphysis pubis, slips under it, and as lateral flexion of the shoulder and head occurs, the anterior shoulder is born before the posterior shoulder. The body follows quickly. The adaptations of the newborn to extrauterine life are discussed in Chapter 27.

Premonitory Signs of Labor

Most primigravidas and many multiparas experience signs and symptoms of impending labor.

Lightening

The majority of primigravidas experience the phenomenon of *lightening* about two to three weeks before the onset of labor. This feeling occurs because the fetus begins to settle into the pelvic inlet. With its descent, engagement occurs, the uterus moves downward, and the fundus no longer presses on the diaphragm.

The woman can breathe more easily after lightening. With increased downward pressure of the presenting part, however, the woman may notice leg cramps or pains due to pressure on the nerves that course through the obturator foramen in the pelvis, increased pressure on urinary bladder, increased pelvic pressure, and increased venous stasis leading to dependent edema. Vaginal secretions increase due to congestion of the vaginal mucous membranes. In theory, primigravidas experience lightening because of increased intensity of Braxton Hicks contractions and the bracing action of abdominal muscles of good tone.

Braxton Hicks Contractions

Prior to the onset of labor, Braxton Hicks contractions, the irregular, intermittent contractions that have been occurring throughout the pregnancy, may become uncomfortable. The pain seems to be in the abdomen and groin but may feel like the "drawing" sensations experienced by some with dysmenorrhea. When these contractions are strong enough for the woman to believe she is in labor, she is said to be in false labor. *False labor* is uncomfortable and may be exhausting as the woman wonders if "this is it." Since the contractions can be fairly regular, she has no way of knowing if they are the beginning of true labor. She may come to the hospital for a vaginal examination to determine if cervical dilatation is occurring. Frequent episodes of false labor and trips back and forth to the physician's or nurse-midwife's office or hospital may frustrate or embarrass the woman, who feels that she should know when she is really in labor. Reassurance by nursing staff can ease embarrassment.

Cervical Changes

A few days before the onset of labor, the cervix becomes soft (also called *ripening*) and begins to efface and dilate slightly. The mechanism for this ripening is biochemical and is the result of changes in the connective tissue of the cervix.

Bloody Show

The mucous plug is the accumulated cervical secretions that have closed off the opening of the uterine cavity. With softening and effacement of the cervix, the mucous plug is often expelled, resulting in a small amount of blood loss from the exposed cervical capillaries. The resulting pink-tinged secretions are called **bloody show**.

Bloody show is considered a sign of imminent labor, which usually begins within 24 to 48 hours. Vaginal examination with manipulation of the cervix may also result in a blood-tinged discharge, which may be confused with bloody show.

Rupture of Membranes

In approximately 12% of women, the amniotic membranes rupture before the onset of labor. This is called **rupture of membranes (ROM)**. After membranes rupture, 80% of women will experience spontaneous labor within 24 hours. If membranes rupture and labor does not begin spontaneously within 12 to 24 hours, labor may be induced to avoid infection. An induction of labor is done only if the pregnancy is near term.

When the membranes rupture, the amniotic fluid may be expelled in large amounts. If engagement has not occurred, the danger of the umbilical cord washing out with the fluid (called *prolapsed cord*) exists. In addition, the open pathway into the uterus causes danger of infection. Because of these threats, the woman is advised to notify her physician or nurse-midwife and proceed to the hospital/birthing center. In some instances, the fluid is expelled in small amounts and may be confused with episodes of urinary incontinence associated with urinary urgency, coughing, or sneezing. The discharge should be checked to ascertain its source and to determine further action. (See Chapter 22 for assessment techniques.)

Sudden Burst of Energy

Some women report a sudden burst of energy approximately 24 to 48 hours before labor. They may do their spring housecleaning or rearrange all the furniture; these activities are often referred to as the *nesting instinct*. The cause of the energy spurt is unknown. The nurse in prenatal teaching should warn prospective mothers not to overexert themselves at this time so that they will not be excessively tired when labor begins.

Other Signs

Additional premonitory signs may include a loss of 1 to 3 pounds resulting from fluid loss and electrolyte shifts produced by changes in estrogen and progesterone levels, and increased backache and sacroiliac pressure from the influence of relaxin hormone on the pelvic joints. Some women report diarrhea, indigestion, or nausea and vomiting just prior to the onset of labor. The causes are unknown.

Differences Between True and False Labor

The contractions of true labor produce progressive dilatation and effacement of the cervix. They occur regularly and increase in frequency, duration, and intensity. The discomfort of true labor contractions usually starts in the back and radiates around to the abdomen. The pain is not relieved by ambulation (in fact, walking may intensify the pain).

The contractions of false labor do not produce progressive cervical effacement and dilatation. Classically, they are irregular and do not increase in frequency, duration, and intensity. The contractions may be perceived as a hardening or "balling up" without discomfort, or discomfort may occur mainly in the lower abdomen and groin. The discomfort may be relieved by ambulation.

The woman will find it helpful to know the characteristics of true labor contractions as well as the premonitory signs of ensuing labor. However, many times the only way to differentiate accurately between true and false labor is to assess dilatation. The woman must feel free to come in for accurate assessment of labor and should never be al-

Table 21–4 Comparison of True and False Labor

True labor	False labor
Contractions are at regular intervals.	Contractions are irregular.
Intervals between contractions gradually shorten.	Usually no change.
Contractions increase in duration and intensity.	Usually no change.
Discomfort begins in back and radiates around to abdomen.	Discomfort is usually in abdomen.
Intensity usually increases with walking.	Walking has no effect or lessens contractions.
Cervical dilatation and effacement are progressive.	No change.

lowed to feel foolish if the labor is false. The nurse must reassure the woman that false labor is common and that it often cannot be distinguished from true labor except by vaginal examination. (See Table 21–4.)

Stages of Labor and Birth

There are three stages of labor. The *first stage* begins with the beginning of true labor and ends when the cervix is completely dilated at 10 cm. The *second stage* begins with complete dilatation and ends with the birth of the infant. The *third stage* begins with the expulsion of the infant and ends with the expulsion of the placenta.

Some clinicians identify a *fourth stage* of labor. During this stage, which lasts 1 to 4 hours after expulsion of the placenta, the uterus effectively contracts to control bleeding at the placental site.

In this section we discuss the physiologic events and psychologic changes that occur during labor and birth. The care of the laboring woman is discussed in Chapter 23.

First Stage

The first stage of labor is divided into the *latent, active,* and *transition* phases. Each phase of labor is characterized by physical and psychologic changes.

Latent Phase

The *latent phase* begins with the onset of regular contractions. As the cervix begins to dilate, it also effaces, although little or no fetal descent is evident. For a woman in her first labor (nullipara), the latent phase averages 8.6 hours but should not exceed 20 hours. The latent phase in multiparas averages 5.3 hours but should not exceed 14 hours.

Uterine contractions become established during the latent phase and increase in frequency, duration, and intensity. They may start as mild contractions lasting 15 to 20 seconds with a frequency of 10 to 20 minutes and progress to moderate ones lasting 30 to 40 seconds with a frequency of five to seven minutes. They average 40 mm Hg during acme from a baseline tonus of 10 mm Hg (Varney 1987).

In the early or latent phase of the first stage of labor, contractions are usually mild. The woman feels able to cope with the discomfort. She may be relieved that labor has finally started. Although she may be anxious, she is able to recognize and express those feelings of anxiety. The woman is often talkative and smiling and is eager to talk about herself and answer questions. Excitement is high, and her partner or other support person is often as elated as she is.

Active Phase

During the *active phase,* the cervix dilates from about 3 or 4 cm to 8 cm. Fetal descent is progressive. The cervical dilatation should be at least 1.2 cm/hr in nulliparas and 1.5 cm/hr in multiparas (Cunningham et al 1989).

Transition Phase

The *transition phase* is the last part of the first stage. Cervical dilatation slows as it progresses from 8 to 10 cm and the rate of fetal descent increases. The average rate of descent is at least 1 cm/hr in nulliparas and 2 cm/hr in multiparas. The transition phase should not be longer than three hours for nulliparas and one hour for multiparas (Cunningham et al 1989). The total duration of the first stage may be increased by approximately 2 hours if epidural anesthesia is used (Kilpatrick & Laros 1989).

During the active and transition phases, contractions become more frequent, are longer in duration, and in-

crease in intensity. At the beginning of the active phase the contractions have a frequency of two to three minutes, a duration of 60 seconds, and are strong in intensity. During transition, contractions have a frequency of 1½ to 2 minutes, a duration of 60 to 90 seconds, and are strong in intensity (Varney 1987).

When the woman enters the early active phase, her anxiety tends to increase as she senses the fairly constant intensification of contractions and pain. She begins to fear a loss of control and may use coping mechanisms to maintain control. Some women exhibit decreased ability to cope and a sense of helplessness. Women who have support persons available, particularly fathers, experience greater satisfaction and less anxiety throughout the birth process than those without these supports (Doering et al 1980).

When the woman enters the transition phase, she may demonstrate significant anxiety. She becomes acutely aware of the increasing force and intensity of the contractions. She may become restless, frequently changing position. Because the most commonly expressed fear at this time is that of abandonment, it is crucial that the nurse be available as backup and relief for the support person. By the time the woman enters the transition phase, she is inner-directed and, often, tired. At the same time, the support person may be feeling the need for a break. The woman should be reassured that she will not be left alone. Not only does the woman not want to be left alone but also she may not want anyone to talk to or touch her. However, with the next contraction, she may ask for verbal and physical support. Other characteristics that may accompany this phase

Research Note

Clinical Application of Research

Because research has shown that the recumbent position for labor has some significant risks for the woman in labor and her fetus and is primarily found only in the Western culture, Claire Andrews and Maureen Chrzanowski (1990) designed a study to determine if women who labor in an upright position are more comfortable and have a shorter phase maximum slope in their labor than women who labor in a recumbent position. The maximum slope of labor is the most active phase of labor when the cervix rapidly dilates from 4 cm to 9 cm.

The study found that when a woman labored in an upright position, she had a significantly shorter labor (t(38) = 3.2, p = .003). There were positive correlations between the length of the phase of maximum slope and age and race, with younger, black women having shorter phases. There was no difference in comfort score between the two groups (t(38) = 1.42,

p = .163). Also, women who labored in the recumbent position had external fetal monitoring more often than the women who labored upright. Since no medical conditions existed in the recumbent group that were not also present in the upright group, the author theorized that the recumbent group was more available to be monitored.

Critical Thinking Applied to Research

Strengths: Interesting descriptive statistics, which support prior research. Inclusion of the maternal comfort assessment scale.

Concerns: A new scale developed for this study only had interrater reliability reported. With no other psychometric properties reported, both reliability and validity of the scale are suspect.

Andrews C, Chrzanowski M: Maternal position, labor and comfort. *Appl Nurs Res* 1990; 3(1):7.

are hyperventilation as the woman increases her breathing rate, restlessness, difficulty understanding directions, a sense of bewilderment and anger at the contractions, statements that she "cannot take it anymore," requests for medication, hiccupping, belching, nausea, vomiting, beads of perspiration on upper lip, and increasing rectal pressure.

The woman may also fear that she will be "torn open" or "split apart" by the force of the contractions. Many clients experience a sensation of pressure so great with the peak of a contraction that it seems to them that their abdomens will burst open with the force. The woman should be informed that this is a normal sensation and reassured that such bursting will not happen.

The woman in this phase is anxious to "get it over with." Her support persons may start to feel helpless and may turn to the nurse for increased participation as their efforts at alleviating the woman's discomfort seem less effective.

As dilatation approaches completion, increased rectal pressure and uncontrollable desire to bear down, increased amount of bloody show, and rupture of membranes may occur.

Amniotic Membranes

At the beginning of labor the amniotic membranes bulge through the cervix in the shape of a cone. They may rupture before labor or any time during labor. Rupture of membranes (ROM) generally occurs at the height of an intense contraction with a gush of the amniotic fluid out the vagina. The average amount of amniotic fluid at term is 777 mL (Brace & Wolf 1989).

Second Stage

The second stage of labor begins when the cervix is completely dilated (10 cm) and ends with birth of the infant.

The second stage should be completed within an hour after the cervix becomes fully dilated for primigravidas (multiparas average 15 minutes). The use of conduction anesthesia may extend the duration of the second stage an additional 20 to 30 minutes (Kilpatrick & Laros 1989). Contractions continue with a frequency of 1½ to 2 minutes, a duration of 60 to 90 seconds, and strong intensity (Varney 1987). Descent of the fetal presenting part continues until it reaches the perineal floor.

As the fetal head descends, the woman has the urge to push because of pressure of the fetal head on the sacral and obturator nerves. As she pushes, intra-abdominal pressure is exerted from contraction of the maternal abdominal muscles. As the fetal head continues its descent, the perineum begins to bulge, flatten, and move anteriorly. The amount of bloody show may increase. The labia begin to part with each contraction. Between contractions the fetal head appears to recede. With succeeding contractions and maternal pushing effort, the fetal head descends farther. **Crowning** occurs when the fetal head is encircled by the external opening of the vagina (introitus) and means birth is imminent.

Usually, a childbirth-prepared woman feels relieved that the acute pain she felt during the transition phase is over (see Table 21–5). She also may be relieved that the birth is near and she can now push. Some women feel a sense of control now that they can be actively involved. Others, particularly those without childbirth preparation, may become frightened. They tend to fight each contraction and any attempt of others to persuade them to push with contractions. Such behavior may be frightening and disconcerting to her support persons. The woman may feel she has lost control and become embarrassed and apologetic or she may demonstrate extreme irritability toward the staff or her supporters in an attempt to regain control over external forces against which she feels helpless. Some

---

Table 21–5   Characteristics of Labor

| | First stage | | | |
	Latent phase	Active phase	Transition phase	Second stage
Nullipara	8½ hours	6 hours		1 hour
Multipara	5 hours	4½ hours		15 minutes
Cervical Dilatation	0 to 3–4 cm	4 to 8 cm	8–10 cm	
Contractions Frequency	Every 10–20 minutes at the beginning and progressing to every 5–7 minutes	Every 2–3 minutes	Every 1½–2 minutes	Every 1½–2 minutes
Duration	15–20 seconds progressing to 30–40 seconds	60 seconds	60–90 seconds	60–90 seconds
Intensity	Begin as mild and progress to moderate	Begin as moderate and progress to strong	Strong	Strong

women feel acute, increasingly severe pain and a burning sensation as the perineum distends.

Spontaneous Birth (Vertex Presentation)

As the head distends the vulva with each contraction, the perineum becomes extremely thin and the anus stretches and protrudes.

As extension occurs under the symphysis pubis, the head is born. When the anterior shoulder meets the underside of the symphis pubis, a gentle push by the mother aids in birth of the shoulders. The body then follows (Figure 21–17).

Birth of infants in other than vertex presentations is discussed in Chapter 25.

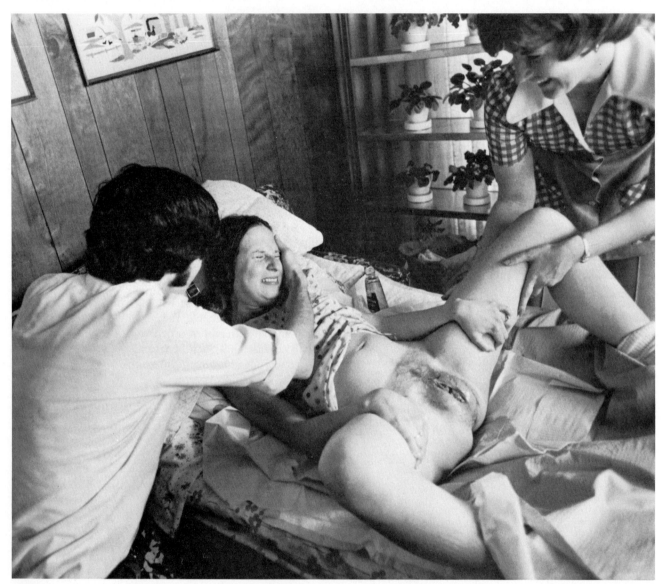

Figure 21–17   The birth sequence. A, B As labor begins, the fetal head settles down firmly on the cervix and engagement occurs. This view demonstrates an LOP position. The occiput is in the left posterior quadrant of the maternal pelvis. The cervix is long and thick with no dilatation. C, D As the fetal head descends, flexion of the head occurs, and the occiput becomes the presenting part. Note the difference in the positions of the suture lines and anterior fontanelle (diamond shape) in views B and D. The cervix has begun to efface and dilate. D, F As the fetal head enters the bony pelvis, internal rotation takes place. In this view the fetal position is changing to occiput anterior. If the membranes are still intact, they precede the fetal head, the fluid acting as a cushion for the head during contractions. Note that the suture line in view F is almost vertical. G, H, I, J Extension begins as the fetal head comes under the maternal symphysis pubis. K, L, M, N In this view extension has occurred. The photos illustrate crowning, the birth of the head, and the beginning of external rotation. O, P, Q External rotation is complete; the shoulders move into the widest part of the maternal pelvis.

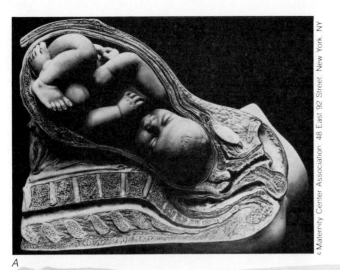
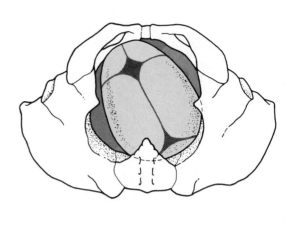

A B

A, B. As labor begins, the fetal head settles down firmly on the cervix and engagement occurs. This view demonstrates an LOP position. The occiput is in the left posterior quadrant of the maternal pelvis. The cervix is long and thick with no dilatation.

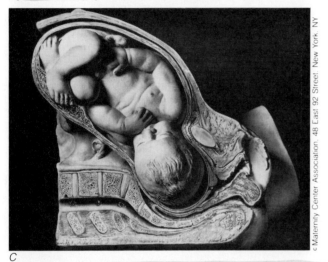
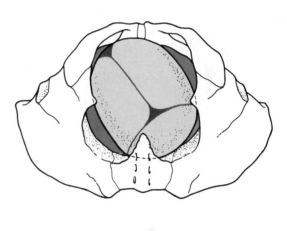

C D

C, D. As the fetal head descends, flexion of the head occurs, and the occiput becomes the presenting part. Note the difference in the positions of the suture lines and anterior fontanelle (diamond shape) in views B and D. The cervix has begun to efface and dilate.

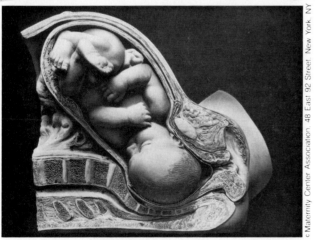
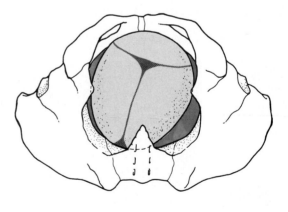

E F

E, F. As the fetal head enters the bony pelvis, internal rotation takes place. In this view the fetal position is changing to occiput anterior. If the membranes are still intact, they precede the fetal head, the fluid acting as a cushion for the head during contractions. Note that the suture line in view F is almost vertical. (Views A, C, E, G, K, O cast molds from Birth Atlas, Maternity Center Association, New York.)

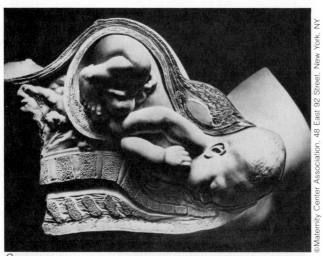

G

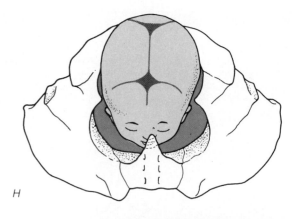

H

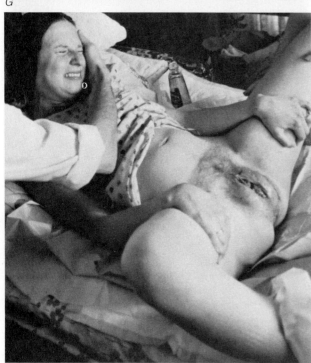

I

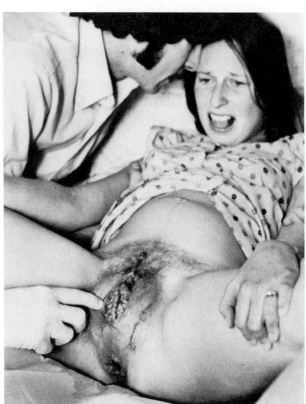

J

G, H, I, J. Extension begins as the fetal head comes under the maternal symphysis pubis.

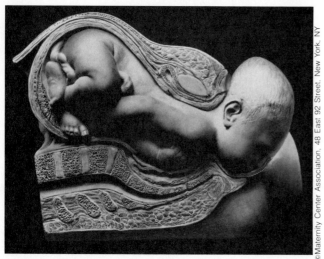

K

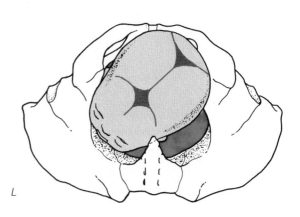

L

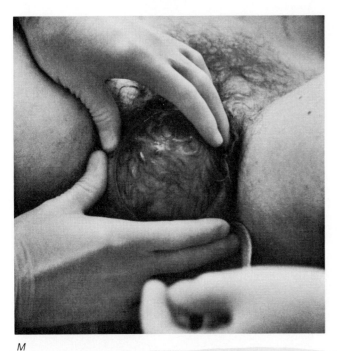
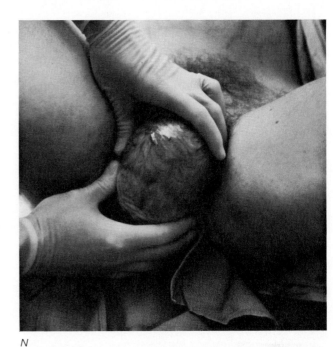

M   N

K, L, M, N. *In this view extension has occurred. The photos illustrate crowning, the birth of the head, and the beginning of external rotation.*

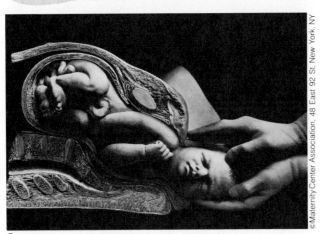

©Maternity Center Association, 48 East 92 St. New York, NY

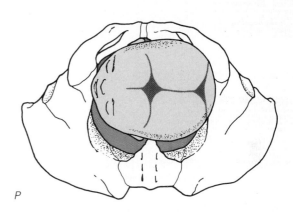

P

O

O, P, Q. *External rotation is complete; the shoulders move into the widest part of the maternal pelvis.*

Third Stage

Placental Separation

After the infant is born, the uterus contracts firmly, diminishing its capacity and the surface area of placental attachment. The placenta begins to separate because of this decrease in surface area. As this separation occurs, bleeding results in the formation of a hematoma between the placental tissue and the remaining decidua. This hematoma accelerates the separation process. The membranes are the last to separate. They are peeled off the uterine wall as the placenta descends into the vagina.

Signs of placental separation usually appear around five minutes after birth of the infant. These signs are (a) a globular-shaped uterus, (b) a rise of the fundus in the abdomen, (c) a sudden gush or trickle of blood, and (d) further protrusion of the umbilical cord out of the vagina.

Placental Expulsion

When the signs of placental separation appear, the woman may bear down to aid in placental expulsion. If this fails and the clinician has ascertained that the fundus is firm, gentle traction may be applied to the cord while pressure is exerted on the fundus. The weight of the placenta as it is guided into the placental pan aids in the removal of the membranes from the uterine wall. A placenta is considered to be *retained* if 30 minutes have elapsed from completion of the second stage of labor.

If the placenta separates from the inside to the outer margins, it is expelled with the fetal or shiny side present-

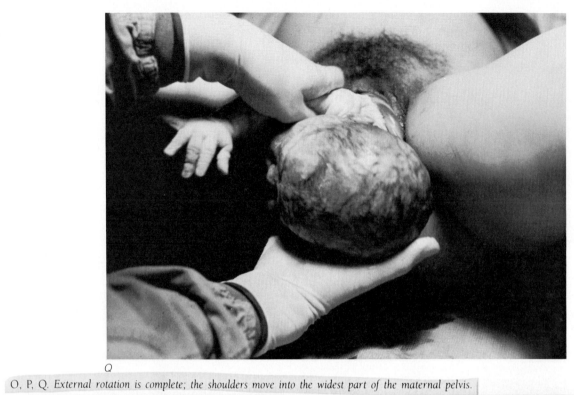

Q

O, P, Q. *External rotation is complete; the shoulders move into the widest part of the maternal pelvis.*

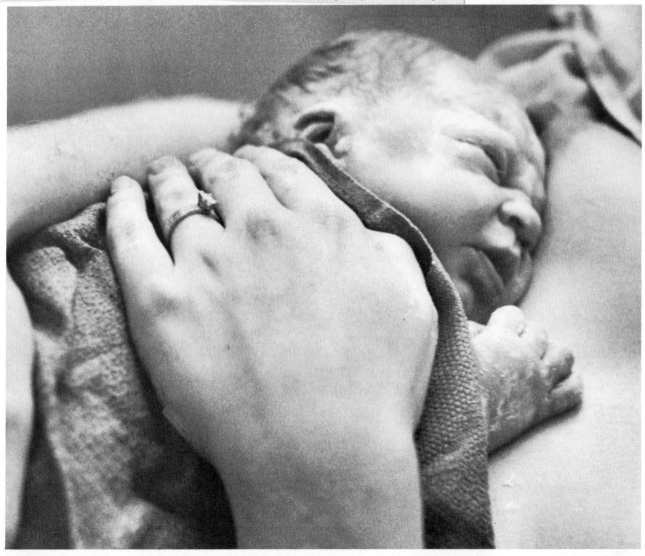

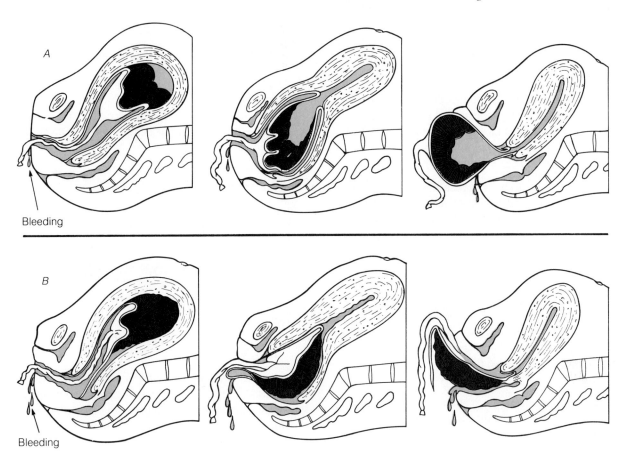

Bleeding

Bleeding

Figure 21–18   Placental separation and expulsion. A Schultze mechanism. B Duncan mechanism.

ing (Figure 21–18). This is known as the *Schultze mechanism* of placental delivery, or more commonly *shiny Schultze*. If the placenta separates from the outer margins inward, it will roll up and present sideways with the maternal surface delivering first. This is known as the *Duncan mechanism* of placental delivery and is commonly called *dirty Duncan* because the placental surface is rough.

Nursing and medical interventions during the third stage of labor are discussed in detail in Chapter 23.

Fourth Stage

The fourth stage of labor is the time from one to four hours after birth, in which physiologic readjustment of the mother's body begins. With the birth, hemodynamic changes occur. Blood loss at birth ranges from 250 to 500 mL. With this blood loss and the weight of the pregnant uterus off of the surrounding vessels, blood is redistributed into venous beds. This results in a moderate drop in both systolic and diastolic blood pressure, increased pulse pressure, and moderate tachycardia (Albright et al 1986).

The cerebrospinal fluid pressure, which increased during labor, now drops and rapidly returns to normal values (Albright et al 1986).

The uterus remains contracted and is in the midline of the abdomen. The fundus is usually midway between the symphysis pubis and umbilicus. Its contracted state constricts the vessels at the site of placental implantation. Immediately after birth of the placenta, the cervix is widely spread and thick.

Nausea and vomiting usually cease. The woman may be thirsty and hungry. She may experience a shaking chill, which is thought to be associated with the ending of the physical exertion of labor. The bladder is often hypotonic due to trauma during the second stage and/or the administration of anesthetics that may decrease sensations. Hypotonic bladder leads to urinary retention. Nursing care of this stage is discussed in Chapter 23.

❀ ❀

KEY CONCEPTS

Four factors that continually interact during the process of labor and birth are the maternal pelvis, the fetus, the uterine contractions and pushing efforts of the laboring woman, and the emotional components the woman brings to the birth setting.

Four types of pelvises have been identified and each has a different effect on labor. The gynecoid and anthropoid are favorable to labor and childbirth. The android and platypelloid are associated with difficult labor because of diminished diameters.

Important parts of the maternal pelvis include the pelvic inlet, pelvic cavity, and pelvic outlet.

The fetus accommodates itself to the maternal pelvis in a series of movements called the cardinal movements of labor, which include descent, flexion, internal rotation, extension, external rotation, expulsion, and restitution.

The fetal head contains bones that are not fused. This allows for some overlapping and molding to facilitate birth.

Fetal *attitude* refers to the relation of the fetal parts to one another.

Fetal *lie* refers to the relationship of the cephalocaudal axis of the fetus to the maternal spine. The fetal lie is either longitudinal or transverse.

Fetal *presentation* is determined by the body part lying closest to the maternal pelvis. Fetal presentations are cephalic, breech, or shoulder.

Engagement of the presenting part takes place when the largest diameter of the presenting part reaches or passes through the pelvic inlet.

Station refers to the relationship of the presenting part to an imaginary line drawn between the ischial spines of the maternal pelvis.

Fetal *position* is the relationship of the landmark on the presenting fetal part to the front, sides, or back of the maternal pelvis.

Each uterine contraction has an increment, acme, and decrement. Contraction frequency is the time from the beginning of one contraction to the beginning of the next contraction.

Duration of contractions refers to the period of time from the beginning to the end of one contraction.

Intensity of contractions refers to the strength of the contraction during acme. Intensity of contractions is termed as mild, moderate, or strong.

Labor stresses the coping skills of women. Women with prenatal education about childbirth usually report more positive responses to labor.

Possible causes of labor include oxytocin stimulation, progesterone withdrawal, estrogen stimulation, fetal cortisol, and prostaglandin theory.

Factors that affect the response to labor pain include education, cultural beliefs, fatigue and sleep deprivation, personal significance of pain, previous experience, anxiety, and the availability of coping techniques.

Premonitory signs of labor include lightening, Braxton Hicks contractions, cervical softening and effacement, bloody show, sudden burst of energy, weight loss, and sometimes rupture of membranes.

There are four stages of labor and birth. The first stage is from beginning of true labor to complete dilatation of the cervix. Second stage is from complete dilatation of the cervix to birth. Third stage is from birth to expulsion of the placenta. Fourth stage is from expulsion of the placenta to a period of one to four hours after.

Placental separation is indicated by lengthening of the umbilical cord, a small spurt of blood, change in uterine shape, and a rise of the fundus in the abdomen.

The placenta is expelled by Schultze or Duncan mechanism. This is determined by the way it separates from the uterine wall.

❀ ❀

References

Acker DB et al: The leukocyte count in labor. *Am J Obstet Gynecol* 1985; 153(7):737.

Albright GA et al: *Anesthesia in Obstetrics: Maternal, Fetal and Neonatal Aspects,* 2nd ed. Boston: Butterworths, 1986.

Bates MS: Ethnicity and pain: A biocultural model. *Soc Sci Med* 1987; 24(1):47.

Bottoms SF, Scott JR: Transfusion and shock. In: *Danforth's Obstetrics and Gynecology,* 6th ed. Scott JR, DiSaia PJ, Hammond CB et al (editors). Philadelphia: Lippincott, 1990, Ch 32.

Boyland PK, O'Donovan P, Owens OJ: Fetal breathing movements and the diagnosis of labor: A prospective analysis of 100 cases. *Obstet Gynecol* 1985; 66(4):517.

Brace RA, Wolf EF: Normal amniotic fluid volume changes throughout pregnancy. *Am J Obstet Gynecol* 1989; 161:382.

Broussard P: Antepartum surveillance: What tests to use, how to do the test. Tenth International Symposium in Perinatal Medicine and Obstetrical Ultrasound. April 9–12, 1990. Las Vegas, Nevada.

Caldwell WE, Maloy HC: Anatomical variations in the female pelvis and their effect on labor with a suggested classification. *Am J Obstet Gynecol* 1933; 26:479.

Chard R: Fetal and maternal oxytocin in human parturition. *Am J Perinatol* April 1989; 6(2):145.

Cibils LA: *Electronic Fetal-Neonatal Monitoring.* Boston: PSG, 1981.

Creasy RK, Resnik R: *Maternal-Fetal Medicine.* Philadelphia: Saunders, 1984.

Crowe K, Baeyer C. Predictors of a positive childbirth experience. *Birth* June 1989; 16:2.

Cunningham FG, MacDonald PC, Gant NF: *Williams Obstetrics,* 18th ed. Norwalk, CT: Appleton & Lange, 1989.

Dalaker K: Clotting factor VII during pregnancy, delivery and puerperium. *Br J Obstet Gynaecol* 1986; 93:17.

Deckardt R, Fembacher PM, Schneider KT et al: Maternal arterial oxygen saturation during labor and delivery: Pain-dependent alterations and effects on the newborn. *Obstet Gynecol* 1989; 70:21.

Engel NS: An American experience of pregnancy and childbirth in Japan. *Birth* June 1989; 16:81.

Garfield RE, Beier S: Increased myometrial responsiveness to oxytocin during term and preterm labor. *Am J Obstet Gynecol* 1989; 161:454.

Hariharan S, Takahashi K, Burd L: Initiation of labor. In: *Gynecology and Obstetrics.* Sciarri JJ (editor). Philadelphia: Saunders, 1986, Ch 86.

Kay MA: *Anthropology of human birth.* Philadelphia: Davis, 1982.

Kilpatrick SJ, Laros RK: Characteristics of normal labor. *Obstet Gynecol* 1989; 74:85.

Lederman RP: *Psychosocial Adaptation in Pregnancy: Assessment of Seven Dimensions of Maternal Development.* Englewood Cliffs, NJ: Prentice Hall, 1984.

Liggins GC: Fetal influences on myometrial contractility. *Clin Obstet Gynecol* 1973; 16:148.

McCaffery M: *Nursing Management of the Patient with Pain* Philadelphia: Lippincott, 1972.

Mercer RT: Relationship of the birth experience to later mothering behaviors. *J Nurse-Midwifery* 1985; 30:204.

Morrow K: Transcultural midwifery: Adapting to Hmong birthing customs in California. *J Nurse-Midwifery* 1986; 31:285.

Nichols FH, Humenick SS: *Childbirth Education: Practice, Research, and Theory.* Philadelphia: Saunders, 1988.

Robson SC, Boys RJ, Hunter S et al: Maternal hemodynamics after normal delivery and delivery complicated by postpartum hemorrhage. *Obstet Gynecol* 1989; 74:234.

Rubin R: *Maternal Identity and the Maternal Experience.* New York: Springer, 1984.

Senden IPM, Wetering MD, Eskes TK et al: Labor pain: A comparison of parturients in a Dutch and an American teaching hospital. *Obstet Gynecol* April 1988; 71:541.

Sokol RJ, Brindley BA: Practical diagnosis and management of abnormal labor. In: *Danforth's Obstetrics and Gynecology,* 6th ed. Scott JR, DiSaia PJ, Hammond CB et al (editors). Philadelphia: Lippincott, 1990.

Ueland K, Ferguson JE: Cardiorespiratory physiology of pregnancy. In: *Gynecology and Obstetrics.* Vol. 3. Depp R, Eschenbach DA, Sciarra JJ (editors). Philadelphia: Lippincott, 1990.

Varney H: *Nurse Midwifery.* Boston: Blackwell Scientific Publications, 1987.

Zlatnik FJ: Normal labor and delivery and its conduct. In: *Danforth's Obstetrics and Gynecology,* 6th ed. Scott JR, DiSaia DJ, Hammond CB et al (editors).

Weisenberg M, Caspi Z: Cultural and educational influences on pain of childbirth. *J Pain Symptom Mgmt* March 1989; 4:13.

Additional Readings

Carlan SJ et al: Fetal head molding; Diagnosis by ultrasound and a review of the literature. *J Perinatol* June 1991; 11:105.

Combs CA, Laros RK: Prolonged third stage of labor: Morbidity and risk factors. *Obstet Gynecol* June 1991; 77:863.

Dennis J, Johnson A, Mutch L et al: Acid-base status at birth and neurodevelopmental outcome at four and one-half years. *Am J Obstet Gynecol* 1989; 161:213.

Grace JT: Development of maternal-fetal attachment during pregnancy: *Nurs Res* July/August 1989; 38:228.

Roemer FJ, Rowland DY, Nuamah IS: Retrospective study of fetal effects of prolonged labor before cesarean delivery. *Obstet Gynecol* May 1991; 77:653.

Thomas VJ, Rose FD: Ethnic differences in the experience of pain. *Soc Sci Med* 1991; 32:9:1063.

Varrassi G: Effects of physical activity on maternal plasma B-endorphin levels and perception of labor pain. *Am J Obstet Gynecol* 1989; 160:707.

Yeomans ER, Hankins GD: Cardiovascular physiology and invasive cardiac monitoring. *Clin Obstet Gynecol* March 1989; 32:2.

CHAPTER 22

Intrapartal Nursing Assessment

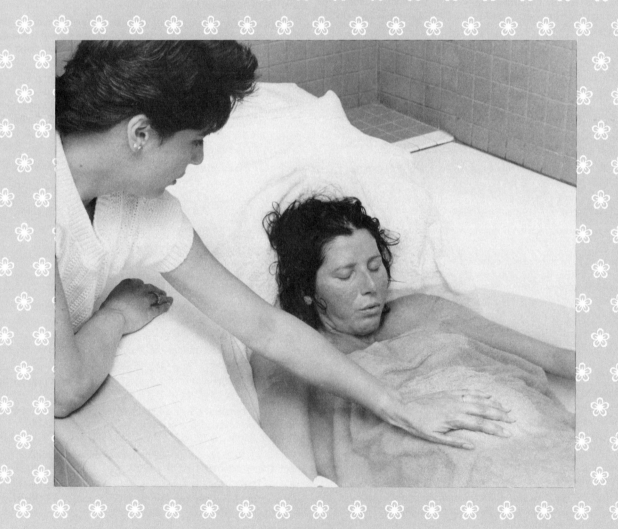

Summarize intrapartal physical and psychosocial assessments necessary for optimum maternal-fetal outcome.

Define and identify the outer limits of normal progress of each of the phases and stages of labor.

Compare the various methods of monitoring FHR and contractions, giving advantages and disadvantages of each.

Differentiate between baseline and periodic changes in the FHR, and describe the criteria and significance of each.

Outline the steps to be performed in the systematic evaluation of FHR tracings, and list factors to consider in evaluation of abnormal findings.

Identify nonreassuring FHR patterns and the interventions that should be carried out in the management of each.

Discuss the indications for fetal blood sampling and guidelines for management of labor for related pH values.

Discuss information to be taught when EFM is used, and provide rationale for teaching.

Discuss psychologic reactions to EFM and the role of the nurse.

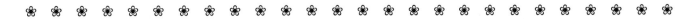

The physiologic events that occur during labor call for many adaptations by the mother and fetus. Accurate and frequent assessment is crucial because the changes are rapid and involve two individuals, mother and child.

The nurse in the birth setting uses a wide variety of assessment skills to provide care to the mother and her child. The skills of observation, palpation, and auscultation are still important as the nurse watches for subtle clues that may indicate a problem is developing. The nurse's presence with the laboring woman provides an opportunity for ongoing assessment, even as the nurse quietly provides comfort measures and assists the woman's coach in offering support.

In current practice, the "hands-on" techniques are enhanced by the use of ultrasound and electronic monitoring. These new techniques can be used to gather additional data and to validate the hands-on assessments. As with any new technological development, it is tempting to let the machine become an important focus of care. In the birth setting where the contact between the couple and the nurse is so intense, "high-tech" assessments are easily meshed with "high-touch" assessments.

This chapter presents the assessments that are important in the birth setting.

Maternal Assessment

History

The woman's history may be obtained in an abbreviated format when the woman is admitted to the labor and birth area. Each agency has its own admission form, but similar information is usually obtained. Relevant data include the following:

- Name and age
- Attending physician or certified nurse-midwife (CNM)
- Personal data: blood type, Rh factor, results of serology testing, prepregnant and present weight, allergies to medications, foods, or substances
- History of previous illness, such as TB, heart disease, diabetes, convulsive disorders, thyroid disorders
- Problems in the prenatal course, for example, elevated blood pressure, bleeding problems, recurrent urinary tract infection
- Pregnancy data: gravida, para, abortions, term and preterm infants, number of living children, neonatal deaths
- The method chosen for infant feeding
- Type of prenatal education
- Requests regarding labor and birth (no enema, no analgesic or anesthetic, father and/or other support persons in attendance, and so on)
- History of special tests such as NST or ultrasound, and reasons for test administration
- History of any preterm labor requiring tocolytic therapy
- Pediatrician

Intrapartal High-Risk Screening

As part of the history and assessment, the nurse should consider intrapartal factors that would increase the risk for the woman and her baby. Intrapartal high-risk factors are shown in Table 22–1. The table includes maternal and fetal or neonatal implications. The factors are presented prior to

(Text continues on p 617)

Table 22–1 Intrapartal High-Risk Factors

Factor	Maternal implication	Fetal-neonatal implication
Abnormal presentation	↑ Incidence of cesarean birth ↑ Incidence of prolonged labor ↑ Hypertension risk ↑ Nausea-vomiting	↑ Incidence of placenta previa Prematurity ↑ Risk of congenital abnormality Neonatal physical trauma ↑ Risk of IUGR
Multiple gestation	↑ Uterine distention → ↑ risk of postpartum hemorrhage ↑ Risk of cesarean birth ↑ Risk of preterm labor	Low birth weight Prematurity ↑ Risk of congenital anomalies Feto-fetal transfusion
Hydramnios	↑ Discomfort ↑ Dyspnea Edema of lower extremities	↑ Risk of esophageal or other high alimentary tract atresias ↑ Risk of CNS anomalies (myelocele)
Oligohydramnios	Maternal fear of "dry birth"	↑ Incidence of congenital anomalies ↑ Incidence of renal lesions ↑ Risk of IUGR ↑ Risk of fetal acidosis Postmaturity
Meconium staining of amniotic fluid	↑ Psychologic stress due to fear for baby	↑ Risk of fetal asphyxia ↑ Risk of meconium aspiration ↑ Risk of pneumonia due to aspiration of meconium
Premature rupture of membranes	↑ Risk of infection (chorioamnionitis) ↑ Risk of preterm labor ↑ Anxiety Fear for the baby Prolonged hospitalization ↑ Incidence of tocolytic therapy	↑ Perinatal morbidity Prematurity ↓ Birth weight ↑ Risk of respiratory distress syndrome Prolonged hospitalization
Induction of labor	↑ Risk of hypercontractility of uterus ↑ Risk of uterine rupture ↑ Length of labor if cervix not ready ↑ Anxiety	Prematurity if gestational age not assessed correctly Hypoxia if hyperstimulation occurs
Abruptio placentae-placenta previa	Hemorrhage Uterine atony	Fetal hypoxia/acidosis Fetal exsanguination ↑ Perinatal mortality
Failure to progress in labor	Maternal exhaustion ↑ Incidence of augmentation of labor ↑ Incidence of cesarean birth	Fetal hypoxia/acidosis Intracranial birth injury
Precipitous labor (< 3 hours)	Perineal, vaginal, cervical lacerations ↑ Risk of PP hemorrhage	Tentorial tears
Prolapse of umbilical cord	↑ Fear for baby Cesarean birth	Acute fetal hypoxia/acidosis
Fetal heart aberrations	↑ Fear for baby ↑ Risk of cesarean birth, forceps, vacuum Continuous electronic monitoring and intervention in labor	Tachycardia, chronic asphyxic insult, bradycardia, acute asphyxic insult Chronic hypoxia Congenital heart block
Uterine rupture	Hemorrhage Cesarean birth for hysterectomy ↑ Risk of death	Fetal anoxia Fetal hemorrhage ↑ Neonatal morbidity and mortality
Postdates (> 42 weeks)	↑ Anxiety ↑ Incidence of induction of labor ↑ Incidence of cesarean birth ↑ Use of technology to monitor fetus ↑ Risk of shoulder dystocia	Postmaturity syndrome ↑ Risk of fetal-neonatal mortality & morbidity ↑ Risk of antepartum fetal death ↑ Incidence/risk of large baby

Intrapartal Assessment Guide: First Stage of Labor
Physical Assessment

Assess/Normal Findings	Alterations and Possible Causes of Alterations*	Nursing Responses to Data Base†
Vital Signs		
Blood pressure: 90–140/60–90 or no more than 15–20 mm Hg rise over baseline BP during early pregnancy	High blood pressure (essential hypertension, PIH, renal disease, apprehension or anxiety)	Evaluate history of preexisting disorders and check for presence of other signs of PIH.
	Low blood pressure (supine hypotension)	Turn woman on her side and recheck blood pressure.
		Do not assess during contractions; implement measures to decrease anxiety and then reassess.
Pulse: 60–90 beats/min	Increased pulse rate (excitement or anxiety, cardiac disorders)	Evaluate cause, reassess to see if rate continues; report to physician.
Respirations: 16–24/min (or pulse rate divided by 4)	Marked tachypnea (respiratory disease)	Assess between contractions; if marked tachypnea continues, assess for signs of respiratory disease.
	Hyperventilation (anxiety)	Encourage slow breaths if woman is hyperventilating.
Temperature: 36.2–37.6C (98–99.6F)	Elevated temperature (infection, dehydration)	Assess for other signs of infection or dehydration.
Weight		
25–30 lb greater than prepregnant weight	Weight gain > 30 lb (fluid retention, obesity, large infant, PIH)	Assess for signs of edema.
Lungs		
Normal breath sounds (see irregular breath sounds)	Rales, rhonchi, friction rub (infection)	Reassess; refer to physician.
Heart		
Normal heart sounds; grade II/VI systolic ejection murmur is normally found in pregnant women due to extra blood volume passing through heart valves	Murmurs	Refer to physician.
Fundus		
At 40 weeks' gestation, located just below xyphoid process	Uterine size not compatible with estimated birth time (SGA, hydramnios, multiple pregnancy)	Reevaluate history regarding pregnancy dating. Refer to physician for additional assessment.

*Possible causes of alterations are placed in parentheses.
†This column provides guidelines for further assessment and initial nursing interventions.

(continued)

Intrapartal Assessment Guide: First Stage of Labor (continued)
Physical Assessment

Assess/Normal Findings	Alterations and Possible Causes of Alterations*	Nursing Responses to Data Base†
Edema		
Slight amount of dependent edema	Pitting edema of face, legs, abdomen (PIH)	Check deep tendon reflexes for hyperactivity, check for clonus; refer to physician.
Hydration		
Normal skin turgor	Poor skin turgor—delayed over 30 seconds of maintained tent shape (dehydration)	Assess skin turgor; refer to physician for deviations.
Perineum		
Tissues smooth, pink color (see Prenatal Initial Physical Assessment Guide, Chapter 13)	Varicose veins of vulva	Exercise care while doing a perineal prep; note on client record need for follow-up in postpartal period; reassess after birth.
Clear mucus	Profuse, purulent drainage	Suspect gonorrhea; report to physician; initiate care to newborn's eyes; notify neonatal nursing staff and pediatrician.
Presence of small amount of bloody show that gradually increases with further cervical dilatation	Hemorrhage	Assess BP and pulse, pallor, diaphoresis; report any marked changes. (Note: Gaping of vagina and/or anus and bulging of perineum are suggestive signs of second stage of labor.)
Energy Status		
Sufficient energy to complete the work of labor	Exhaustion, acetone in urine (deficiency in metabolism of glucose and/or fat, decreasing uterine activity in long labor)	Provide ice chips or hard candy in early labor, IV with dextrose in late labor. Dipstick urine. Assess quality of contractions. Refer to physician.
Labor Status		
Uterine contractions: Regular pattern	Failure to establish a regular pattern, prolonged latent phase Hypertonicity Hypotonicity	Evaluate whether woman is in true labor; ambulate if in early labor. Evaluate woman's status and contractile pattern.
Cervical dilatation: Progressive cervical dilatation from size of fingertip to 10 cm (Procedure 22–1, p 614)	Rigidity of cervix (frequent cervical infections, scar tissue, failure of presenting part to descend)	Evaluate contractions, fetal engagement, position, and cervical dilatation. Inform woman of progress.

*Possible causes of alterations are placed in parentheses.
†This column provides guidelines for further assessment and initial nursing interventions.

(continued)

Intrapartal Assessment Guide: First Stage of Labor (continued)
Physical Assessment

Assess/Normal Findings	Alterations and Possible Causes of Alterations*	Nursing Responses to Data Base†
Cervical effacement: Progressive thinning of cervix (Procedure 22–1)	Failure to efface (rigidity of cervix, failure of presenting part to engage); cervical edema (pushing effort by woman before cervix is fully dilated and effaced, trapped cervix)	Evaluate contractions, fetal engagement, and position. Notify physician/nurse-midwife if cervix is becoming edematous; work with woman to prevent pushing until cervix is completely dilated.
Fetal descent: Progressive descent of fetal presenting part from station −5 to +5	Failure of descent (abnormal fetal position or presentation, macrosomic fetus, inadequate pelvic measurement)	Evaluate fetal position, presentation, and size. Evaluate maternal pelvic measurements.
Membranes: May rupture before or during labor	Rupture of membranes more than 12–24 hours before initiation of labor (infection)	Assess for ruptured membranes using Nitrazine test tape before doing vaginal exam. Instruct women with ruptured membranes to remain on bed rest if presenting part is not engaged. Keep vaginal exams to a minimum to prevent infection.

Findings on Nitrazine test tape:
Membranes probably intact
  yellow   pH 5.0
  olive   pH 5.5
  olive green pH 6.0
Membranes probably ruptured
  blue-green pH 6.5
  blue-gray   pH 7.0
  deep blue   pH 7.5
	False-positive results possible if large amount of bloody show is present or if previous vaginal examination has been done using lubricant	Assess fluid for consistency, amount, odor; assess FHR frequently. Assess fluid at regular intervals for presence of meconium staining.

Amniotic fluid clear, no odor	Greenish amniotic fluid (fetal distress)	Assess FHR; do vaginal exam to evaluate for prolapsed cord; apply fetal monitor for continuous data; report to physician.
	Strong odor (amnionitis)	Take woman's temperature and report to physician.
Fetal Status FHR: 120–160 beats/min	<120 or >160 beats/min (fetal distress); abnormal patterns on fetal monitor: decreased variability, late decelerations, variable decelerations (p 636)	Initiate interventions based on particular FHR pattern (p 629)

*Possible causes of alterations are placed in parentheses.
†This column provides guidelines for further assessment and initial nursing interventions.

(continued)

Intrapartal Assessment Guide: First Stage of Labor (continued)
Physical Assessment

Assess/Normal Findings	Alterations and Possible Causes of Alterations*	Nursing Responses to Data Base†
Presentation: Cephalic, 97% Breech, 3%	Face or brow presentation	Report to physician; after presentation is confirmed as face or brow, woman may be prepared for cesarean birth
Position: LOA most common	Persistent occipital-posterior position; transverse arrest	Carefully monitor maternal and fetal status.
Activity: Fetal movement	Hyperactivity (may precede fetal hypoxia)	Carefully evaluate FHR; may apply fetal monitor.
	Complete lack of movement (fetal distress or fetal demise)	Carfully evaluate FHR; may apply fetal monitor.
Laboratory Evaluation		
Hematologic tests Hemoglobin: 12–16 g/dL	< 12g (anemia, hemorrhage)	Evaluate woman for problems due to decreased oxygen-carrying capacity caused by lowered hemoglobin.

CBC
  Hematocrit: 38%–47%
  RBC: 4.2–5.4 million/μL
  WBC: 4,500–11,000/μL
  although leukocytosis to
  20,000/μL is not unusual
	Presence of infection or blood dyscrasias	Evaluate for other signs of infection or for petechia, bruising, or unusual bleeding.

Serologic tests STS or VDRL test: Nonreactive	Positive reaction (see Chapter 13, Initial Prenatal Physical Assessment Guide)	For reactive test, notify newborn nursery and pediatrician.
Urinalysis Glucose: Negative	Glycosuria (low renal threshold for glucose, diabetes mellitus)	Assess blood glucose; test urine for ketones; ketonuria and glycosuria require further assessment of blood sugars.‡
Ketones: Negative	Ketonuria (starvation ketosis)	
Protein: Negative	Proteinuria (urine specimen contaminated with vaginal secretions, fever, kidney disease); proteinuria of 2+ or greater found in uncontaminated urine may be a sign of ensuing PIH	Instruct woman in collection technique; incidence of contamination from vaginal discharge is common.
Red blood cells: Negative	Blood in urine (calculi, cystitis, glomerulonephritis, neoplasm)	Assess collection technique.
White blood cells: Negative	Presence of white blood cells (infection in genitourinary tract)	Assess for signs of urinary tract infection.
Casts: None	Presence of casts (nephrotic syndrome)	Inform clinician of finding.

*Possible causes of alterations are placed in parentheses.
†This column provides guidelines for further assessment and initial nursing interventions.
‡Glycosuria should not be discounted. The presence of glycosuria necessitates follow-up.

(continued)

Intrapartal Assessment Guide: First Stage of Labor (continued)
Psychologic/Sociocultural Assessment

Assess/Normal Findings	Alterations and Possible Causes of Alterations*	Nursing Responses to Data Base†
Support System		
Physical intimacy of mother-father (or support person): Caretaking activities such as soothing conversation, touching	Limited physical contact or continual clinging together (may reflect normal pattern for this couple or their attempt to cope with this situation)	Encourage caretaking activities that appear to comfort the woman; encourage support to the woman; if support is limited, the nurse may take a more active role.
Support person in close proximity	Maintaining a distance from woman for prolonged periods (may be normal pattern for this couple or may indicate strained relationship or anxiety due to labor)	Encourage support person to stay close (if this seems appropriate).
Relationship of mother-father (or support person): Involved interaction	Limited interaction (may reflect normal interaction pattern or strained relationship)	Support interactions; if interaction is limited, the nurse may provide more information and support.
Anxiety		
Some anxiety and apprehension is within normal limits	Rapid breathing, nervous tremors, frowning, grimacing or clenching of teeth, thrashing movements, crying, increased pulse and blood pressure (anxiety, apprehension)	Provide support and encouragement.
Preparation for Childbirth		
The woman has some information regarding process of normal labor and birth.	Insufficient information	Add to present information base.
Woman has breathing and/or relaxation techniques to use during labor	No breathing or relaxation techniques (insufficient information)	Support breathing and relaxation techniques that the woman is using; provide information if needed.
Response to Labor		
Latent phase: relaxed, excited, anxious for labor to be well established Active phase: becomes more intense, begins to tire	Inability to cope with contractions (fear, anxiety, lack of education)	Provide support and encouragement: establish trusting relationship.
Transitional phase: feels tired, may feel unable to cope, needs frequent coaching to maintain breathing patterns		Provide support and coaching if needed.
Coping mechanisms: Ability to cope with labor through use of support system, breathing, relaxation techniques	Marked anxiety, apprehension (insufficient coping mechanisms)	Support coping mechanisms if they are working for the woman; provide information and support if she is exhibiting anxiety or needs additional alternatives to present coping methods.

*Possible causes of alterations are placed in parentheses.
†This column provides guidelines for further assessment and initial nursing interventions.

PROCEDURE 22–1
Intrapartal Vaginal Examination

Nursing Action	Rationale
Objective: Assemble and prepare equipment.	
Have following equipment easily accessible:	Examination is facilitated and can be done quickly.
• Sterile disposable gloves	
• Lubricant	
• Nitrazine test tape prior to first examination	
Objective: Prepare woman.	
Explain procedure, indications for carrying out procedure, and information being obtained.	Explanation of procedure decreases anxiety and increases relaxation.
Position woman with thighs flexed and abducted; instruct her to put heels of feet together.	Prevents contamination of area during examination and allows for visualization of external signs of labor progress.
Drape so that only the perineum is exposed. Encourage woman to relax her muscles and legs during procedure.	Provides as much privacy as possible.
Objective: Use aseptic technique during examination.	
If leakage of fluid has been noted or if woman reports leakage of fluid, use Nitrazine test tape before doing vaginal exam.	Nitrazine test tape registers a change in pH if amniotic fluid is present (unless a lubricant has already been used).
Put on both gloves; using thumb and forefinger of left hand, spread labia widely, insert well-lubricated second and index fingers of right hand into vagina until they touch the cervix.	Avoid contaminating hand by contact with anus; positioning of hand with wrist straight and elbow tilted downward allows fingertips to point toward umbilicus and find cervix.
Objective: Determine status of fetal membranes.	
Palpate for movable bulging sac through the cervix; observe for expression of amniotic fluid during exam.	If intact, bag of waters feels like a bulge.
Objective: Determine status of labor progress during and after contractions.	
Carry out vaginal examination during and between contractions (Figure 22–1).	Examination varies. Assessment of dilatation is more accurate during contractions.
Objective: Identify degree of cervical dilatation.	
Palpate for opening or what appears as a depression in the cervix.	Estimation of the diameter of the depression identifies degree of dilatation.
Estimate diameter of cervical opening in centimeters (0–10 cm).	One finger represents approximately 1.5–2 cm cervical dilatation.
Objective: Identify degree of cervical effacement.	
Palpate the shortening of the surrounding circular ridge of tissue: estimate degree of shortening in percentages (Figure 22–2).	Effacement results from the lengthening of muscle fibers around the internal os as they are taken up into the lower uterine segment. The endocervix becomes part of the lower uterine segment (Varney 1987).

(continued)

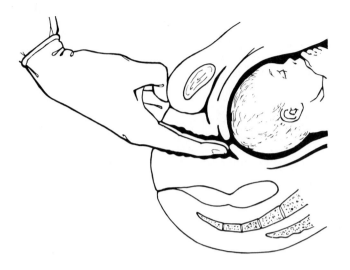

Figure 22–1 *To determine cervical dilatation, the nurse places her index and middle fingers against the cervix and determines the size of the opening. Before labor begins, the cervix is long (approximately 2.5 cm), the sides feel thick, and the cervical canal is closed, so that an examining finger cannot be inserted. During labor, the cervix begins to dilate (open up), and the size of the opening progresses from 1 cm to 10 cm in diameter.*

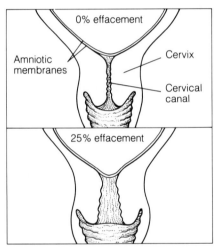

A. Cervix near the end of pregnancy but before labor. Top, primigravida; bottom, multipara.

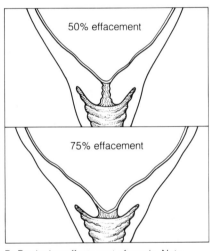

B. Beginning effacement of cervix. Note dilation of internal os and funnel-shaped cervical canal. Top, primigravida; bottom, multipara.

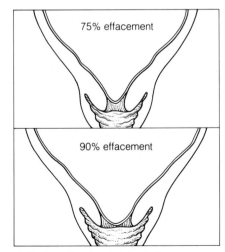

C. Further effacement of cervix. Top, primigravida; bottom, multipara.

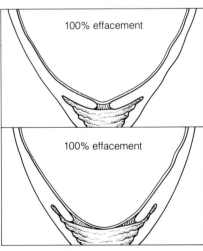

D. Cervical canal obliterated, i.e., the cervix is completely effaced. Top, primigravida; bottom, multipara.

Figure 22–2 *Cervical effacement. A Cervix near the end of pregnancy but before labor. Top, primigravida (0% effacement); bottom, multipara. B Beginning effacement of cervix. Note dilatation of internal os and funnel-shaped cervical canal. Top, primigravida (about 50% effaced); bottom, multipara. C Further effacement of cervix. Top, primigravida (about 75% effaced); bottom, multipara. D Cervical canal obliterated; ie, the cervix is completely effaced. Top, primigravida (100% effaced); bottom, multipara. (From Cunningham FG, MacDonald PC, Gant NF: Williams Obstetrics, 18th ed. Norwalk, CT: Appleton & Lange, 1989. F 10-17, p 217; f 10-18, 10-19, 10-20, p 218)*

PROCEDURE 22–1 (continued)

Nursing Action	Rationale
Objective: Determine presentation and position of presenting part.	
As cervix opens, palpate for presenting part and identify its relationship to the maternal pelvis. (Figures 22–3, 22–4).	Presenting part is easier to palpate through a dilated cervix, and differentiation of landmarks is easier.
Objective: Determine station.	
Locate lowest portion of presenting part (excluding caput) (−5 to +15).	Identification of station provides information as to degree of descent.
Objective: Inform woman about progress in labor.	
Discuss findings of the vaginal examination and correlate them to woman's progress in labor.	Assists in identifying progress and reinforces need for frequency of procedure.
	Information is reassuring and supportive for woman and family.
Objective: Record information on client's record.	
Record on labor record, eg, 4 cm 50% or 8 cm. complete.	Nurse's entry documents progress of labor.

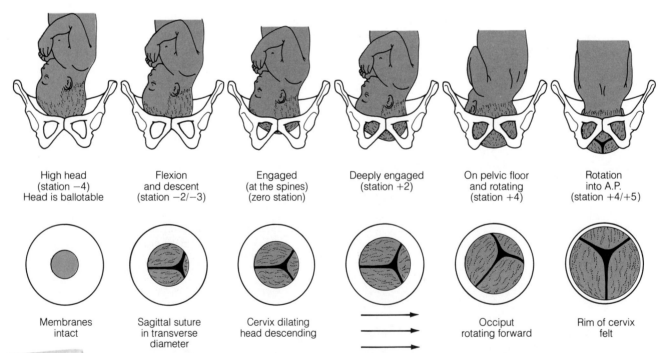

High head (station −4) Head is ballotable	Flexion and descent (station −2/−3)	Engaged (at the spines) (zero station)	Deeply engaged (station +2)	On pelvic floor and rotating (station +4)	Rotation into A.P. (station +4/+5)
Membranes intact	Sagittal suture in transverse diameter	Cervix dilating head descending		Occiput rotating forward	Rim of cervix felt

Figure 22–3 Top, the fetal head progressing through the pelvis. Bottom, the changes that the nurse will detect on palpation of the occiput through the cervix while doing a vaginal examination. (Adapted from Bennett VR, Brown LK (editors): Myles, MF Textbook for Midwives, 11th ed. Edinburgh, Scotland: Churchill Livingstone, 1989, f 11.16 p 158.)

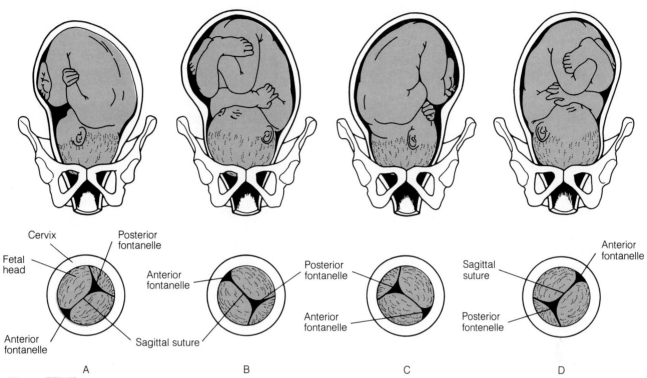

Figure 22–4   Palpation of presenting part. A Left occiput anterior (LOA). The posterior fontanelle (triangular-shaped) is in the upper left quadrant of the maternal pelvis. B Left occiput posterior (LOP). The posterior fontanelle is in the lower left quadrant of the maternal pelvis. C Right occiput anterior. The posterior fontanelle is in the upper right quadrant of the maternal pelvis. D Right occiput posterior. The posterior fontanelle is in the lower right quadrant of the maternal pelvis.

the intrapartal physical assessment guide so that they can be kept in mind during the assessment.

Intrapartal Assessment

Physical Assessment

A physical examination is included as part of the admission procedure and as part of the ongoing care of the woman. The assessment becomes the basis for initiating nursing interventions.

The intrapartal physical assessment is not as complete and thorough as the initial prenatal physical examination (Chapter 13), but it does involve assessment of some body systems and of the actual labor process. The accompanying Intrapartal Assessment Guide provides a framework for the maternity nurse's examination of the laboring woman.

The guide includes assessments performed immediately upon admission and continued as an ongoing assessment. Others may be assessed only once. Critical admission assessments include vital signs, labor status, fetal status, and laboratory and psychologic evaluation. These assessments will be continued throughout the labor process. Assessments that are done only once as part of the admission data, if time permits, include evaluation of weight, breasts, lungs, and heart (in many institutions assessments of breasts, lungs, and heart are omitted).

Psychologic/Sociocultural Assessment

Assessment of the laboring woman's psychologic status is an important part of the total assessment. The woman brings to labor previous ideas, knowledge, and fears that can affect the labor and birth.

Assessment of psychologic parameters requires caring and skill. An atmosphere of rapport and support is essential for evaluating an area that is primarily subjective and allows great latitude in interpretation of responses and behavior. Information is gathered throughout all interactions with the laboring woman, and the observations and assessments are continuously analyzed and evaluated. For instance:

1.   Do the woman's words and actions match?

Mrs Ames is admitted to the birthing unit. She appears unsure and hesitant during the admission process. With support and encouragement she begins to ask questions about the unit and is able to communicate her requests for the labor and birth process. Although Mrs Ames was initially unsure and hesitant, her actions and words were congruent.

Mrs Martin is admitted in active labor. She smiles frequently and states through clenched teeth that she is "just fine." The nurse notes that her hands are tightly clenching the bed rails and her knuckles are white. Mrs Martin's words and actions are not congruent.

2. What coping behaviors are observed and are they effective?

3. What communication patterns are present and are they effective?

Assessment of the woman's psychologic status enables the nurse to meet the laboring woman's needs for information and support. The nurse can support the woman and her partner, or in the absence of a partner, the nurse may become the support person. See the accompanying Intrapartal Psychologic Assessment Guide.

Methods of Evaluating Labor Progress

Contraction Assessment

Uterine contractions may be assessed by palpation and/or continuous electronic monitoring.

Palpation   Contractions are assessed for frequency, duration, and intensity by placing one hand on the uterine fundus. To determine duration of the contraction, the time is noted when hardening of the fundus is first felt (beginning of the contraction) and relaxation occurs (end of the contraction). During the acme (peak) of the contraction, intensity can be evaluated by estimating the indentability of the fundus. At least three successive contractions should be assessed to provide enough data to determine the contraction pattern. Since frequency is determined by noting the time from the beginning of one contraction to the beginning of the next, if contractions began at 7:00, 7:04, and 7:08, the frequency would be every four minutes.

Electronic Monitoring with External Tocodynamometer   Electronic monitoring of the uterine contractions provides continuous data. In many facilities, it may be routinely done for all high-risk women and all women who are having oxytocin-induced labor. An indirect method of monitoring uterine activity is by use of the tocodynamometer (or "toco"), which contains a flexible disk that responds to pressure. This disk is placed against the fundus of the uterus (the area of greatest contractility) and is held in place by an elastic belt. As the uterus contracts, pressure is exerted against the toco, transmitted to the monitor and recorded on graph paper (Figure 22–5). Uterine contractions can be assessed for frequency and duration but not for intensity. The intensity (as displayed on the graph paper) is a reflection of how tightly the belt is applied around the maternal abdomen. When the belt is tight enough, the nurse should be able to note the beginning of contractions on the monitor just before or at the same time the woman begins to feel them. The advantages to this method are that

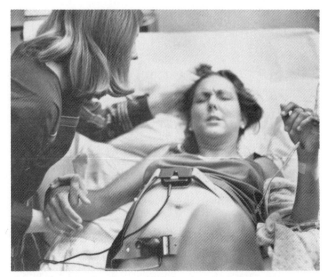

Figure 22–5   Woman in labor with external monitor applied. The "toco" that is placed on the uterine fundus is recording the uterine contractions. The lower belt holds the ultrasonic device that monitors the fetal heart rate. The fetus is probably in a right occiput anterior position. The belts can be adjusted for comfort. This woman is in a semi-Fowler's position. It is important for the woman to be in a semi-Fowler's position or a side-lying position in order to enhance maternal–placental–fetal circulation.

(a) it may be used prior to rupture of membranes antepartally and intrapartally and (b) it provides a continuous recording of the duration and frequency of contractions. The major disadvantage of this method is that it cannot assess the intensity of contractions (because the obtained tracing is influenced by how snugly the elastic belt is applied). Another disadvantage is that sometimes the belt bothers the woman, because it must be snug to monitor uterine contractions accurately—the belt may require frequent readjustment as she changes position, or the woman may feel she needs to remain in one position as not to disturb the belt.

Recently, a beltless tocodynamometer has been developed. This system consists of an adhesive transducer that is applied to the most prominent part of the woman's abdomen with a double-sided adhesive film (Figure 22–6). In a preliminary study, it was noted that this method functioned better than the belted system, particularly with women in early labor. Advantages included a positive patient acceptance due to increased freedom of movement and not having to wear a belt around the abdomen, easy application, infrequent readjustment, and convenience (Fukushima et al 1989).

Electronic Monitoring by Internal Means   In addition to providing information regarding uterine contraction frequency and duration, the intrauterine catheter

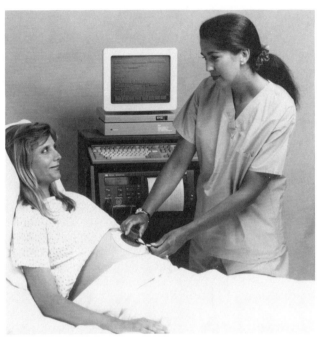

Figure 22–6   Beltless tocodynamometer system with adhesive transducer support-plate and pressure transducer unit (Courtesy of Corometrics Medical Systems, Inc, Wallingford, CT.

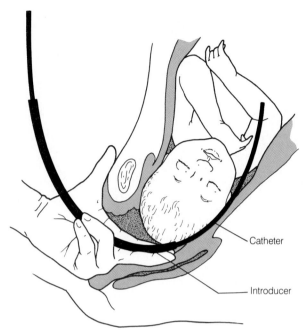

Figure 22–7   Technique of uterine catheter insertion. Note that the introducer (catheter guide) is inserted no farther than beyond the fingertips. (From Perez RH: Fetal monitoring. In Protocols for Perinatal Nursing Practice. St. Louis: Mosby, 1981, p 180.)

method also assesses intensity. One type of intrauterine catheter consists of small polyethylene tubing that is inserted directly into the uterine cavity. The guide tube encasing the catheter is advanced as far as the internal cervical os, and then the tubing is slowly threaded into the uterine cavity, usually in the area where fetal small parts are located. It is advanced only as far as the black marking indicated on the catheter, which should be visualized at the opening to the vagina (Figure 22–7). The catheter and strain gauge are filled with sterile water (not saline as this will corrode the transducer). The gauge is then connected to the monitor. For measurement of accurate baseline resting tone of the uterus, the strain gauge should be adjusted to the height of the maternal xiphoid process. With the woman in the supine position, this will approximate the level of the tip of the intrauterine catheter. By this means, a closed pressure system is maintained so that increases in intrauterine pressure with uterine contractions or hypertonus may be visualized.

The catheter is periodically flushed with sterile water to ensure patency and accurate resting tone. If the catheter becomes clogged with vernix or meconium, it will show an increase in baseline resting tone. If the woman changes position, the catheter should be flushed, the strain gauge readjusted, and the system recalibrated.

An intrauterine pressure catheter by INTRAN that functions without being fluid-filled is now available. IN-

TRAN I is a disposable catheter that has a micropressure transducer (electronic sensor) located at the tip of the catheter. The catheter is inserted into the uterine cavity and then connected by a cable to the electronic fetal monitor. This catheter has several advantages: It does not require flushing to prevent obstruction by blood or meconium in the amniotic fluid; it is simple to equilibrate and easy to insert without assistance; it provides good quality recordings; and thus far it has shown no catheter-associated morbidity. However, the INTRAN I also has several disadvantages: It cannot be re-zeroed without removal (as would be required if the monitor needed to be changed for any reason); it does not allow for amnioinfusion (infusion of warmed saline solution into the uterine cavity); the catheter is stiff and might slightly increase the chance of uterine perforation; it is more expensive than the traditional fluid-filled catheter; and there is occasionally some patient discomfort with insertion because of the size of the IUP device tip.

Recently, the INTRAN II IUP system was introduced with many apparent improvements over INTRAN I (Figure 22–8). This system has incorporated a port for amnioinfusion into the distal end of the catheter, thus permitting fluid infusion while at the same time providing accurate monitoring of intrauterine pressure. In addition to the advantage of providing a method of amnioinfusion, this catheter can be re-zeroed at any time. The effectiveness of this new sys-

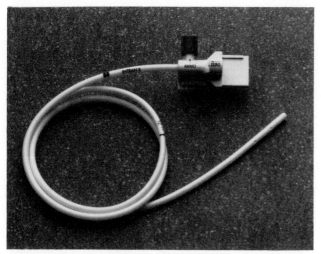

Figure 22–8 INTRAN intrauterine pressure catheter. Note microressure transducer (electronic sensor) located at tip of catheter. There is a port for amnioinfusion at the distal end of the catheter. (Courtesy of Utah Medical Products, Inc., Midvale, Utah 84047-1048. F 22-8)

tem is still being evaluated, and whether it will replace the traditional system remains to be seen.

In many institutions the intrauterine catheter is used only during oxytocin augmentation, induction, or vaginal birth after cesarean. It is particularly important to quantitate the intensity and frequency of contractions to avoid hyperstimulation and possible uterine rupture due to over-administration of oxytocin. If the woman's labor is prolonged, internal monitoring should be instituted to accurately assess the frequency and strength of contractions and resultant FHR pattern response. A slightly increased incidence of maternal infection (approximately 1%) may be noted following use of the intrauterine catheter, but this seems to depend on the duration of ruptured membranes and length of labor.

It is of particular importance that the nurse evaluate the woman's labor status by means other than the fetal monitor. As with any type of technology, no machine is flawless, and the monitor cannot fill the role of the nurse. One should never rely solely on data recorded by a machine. Technology is only useful as an adjunct to good nursing assessment. All too often women are in active labor with adequate contractions that are regarded as being of "poor quality" because the monitor is not functioning properly. The nurse should routinely palpate the intensity of the contractions and compare the assessment with that of data recorded by the monitor.

Trying to figure out if I was in labor was quite a task. Here I was, a labor and delivery nurse, and I couldn't decide if my contractions were the real thing. I timed them, and about the time I

decided this was It, they would slow down. How exasperating not to be able to really know! It was hard on me, because I felt surely a labor and delivery nurse should know for herself. But now I see that all women are in this spot. They want so much to be right, and we often treat them as if they should be able to know absolutely when it's the real thing. I'd like labor and delivery nurses to remember this.

Cervical Assessment

Cervical dilatation and effacement are evaluated directly by sterile vaginal examination (see Procedure 22–1, Intrapartal Vaginal Examination, p 614). The vaginal examination can also provide information regarding membrane status, fetal position, and station of the presenting part.

Evaluation of Labor Progress

Friedman Graph Evaluation of the intensity, frequency, and duration of contractions does not present the entire labor picture: Nurses can evaluate labor progress objectively by plotting cervical dilatation and station of the presenting part on a Friedman graph.

To use the Friedman graph, one needs a graph and skill in determining cervical dilatation and fetal descent. The numbers at the bottom of the graph in Figure 22–9 are

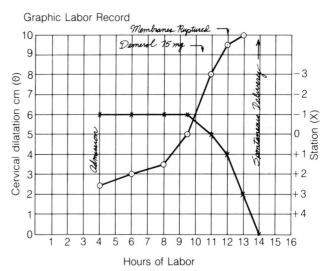

Figure 22–9 Example of charting labor progress on a Friedman graph. Cervical dilatation is on the left (and is indicated by using an 'O') and station is on the right (indicated by using an 'X') On admission, the cervix was dilated 2–3 centimeters and the station was −1, and the woman had been in true labor for four hours. (Modified from Friedman EA: An objective method of evaluating labor. Hosp Pract July 1970; 5:87.)

hours of labor from 1 to 16. Vertically, at the left, cervical dilatation is measured from 0 to 10 cm. The vertical line on the right indicates fetal station in centimeters, from −5 to +5 (Friedman 1970). When one plots cervical dilatation and descent on the basic graph, a characteristic pattern emerges: an S curve represents dilatation and an inverse S curve represents descent.

When the laboring woman enters the hospital or birth center, she is asked at what time regular contractions began. A sterile vaginal examination determines cervical dilatation and the station of the presenting part of the fetus. This information is plotted on the graph. To determine the appropriate point to begin plotting data, the nurse must know how many hours the woman has been having regular contractions. In the example shown in Figure 22−9, on admission the cervix was dilated 2 to 3 cm after 4 hours of labor, and the station was −1. Later examinations are noted on the graph. When the woman was in the eleventh hour of labor, the graph indicates that cervical dilatation was 8 cm and the station was zero. At 14 hours of labor, the graph indicates spontaneous birth.

When utilizing the Friedman graph, the following method may be used to calculate the progress in centimeters of cervical dilatation per hour. Divide the difference between two consecutive observations by the intervening time interval to obtain the value for the slope in centimeters per hour. For example, in the case illustrated in Figure 22−9, at 9 1/2 hours of labor, the cervix is dilated 5 cm. At 11 hours of labor, the cervix is dilated 8 cm. Divide the difference by the intervening time interval, which is 1 1/2 hours: 3 cm ÷ 1 1/2 = 2 cm/hr. (See Table 22−2.)

CRITICAL THINKING

Using Figure 22−9, draw in the labor curve for a woman who dilated 2 cm an hour. Compare the two tracings.

Table 22−2 Contraction and Labor Progress Characteristics*

Contraction Characteristics

Latent phase:	Every 10−20 min × 15−20 seconds; mild, progressing to Every 5−7 min × 30−40 seconds; moderate
Active phase:	Every 2−3 min × 60 seconds; moderate to strong
Transition phase:	Every 2 min × 60−90 seconds; strong

Labor Progress Characteristics

Primipara:	1.2 cm/hr dilatation 1 cm/hr descent < 2 hr in second stage
Multipara:	1.5 cm/hr dilatation 2 cm/hr descent < 1 hr in second stage

Evaluation of the woman's labor progress through use of the Friedman graph will assist in identifying normal or abnormal labor patterns.

Fetal Assessment

Determination of Fetal Position and Presentation

Fetal position is determined by a combination of factors, using various senses and technology. Assessment of the maternal abdomen for fetal positon may be done by inspection, palpation, auscultation of fetal heart tones, determination of presenting part by vaginal examination, and utilization of ultrasound.

Inspection

The nurse should observe the woman's abdomen for size and shape. Attention should be given to the lie of the fetus by assessing whether the shape of the uterus projects up and down (longitudinal lie) or left and right (transverse lie).

Palpation

Use of Leopold's maneuvers provides a systematic evaluation of the maternal abdomen. Frequent practice with these maneuvers increases the proficiency of the examiner in determining fetal position by palpation. Difficulty may be encountered in performing these techniques on an obese woman or on a woman who has excessive amniotic fluid (hydramnios).

Leopold's maneuvers should be performed before listening to the fetal heart tones (FHT). Auscultation of the FHT is facilitated by locating the fetal back, because the sound of the heart tones is carried with more intensity through the fetal back and the uterine wall; it becomes diffused as it passes through the amniotic fluid.

Care should be taken to ensure the woman's comfort during Leopold's maneuvers. The woman should have recently emptied her bladder and should lie on her back with her abdomen uncovered. To aid in relaxation of the abdominal wall, the shoulders should be raised slightly on a pillow and the knees drawn up a little. The procedure should be completed between contractions. The examiner's hands should be warm (Figure 22−10).

Consideration should be given to several questions while inspecting and palpating the maternal abdomen:

- Is the fetal lie longitudinal or transverse?
- What is in the fundus? Am I feeling buttocks or head?
- Where is the fetal back?
- Where are the small parts or extremities?
- What is in the inlet? Does it confirm what I found in the fundus?

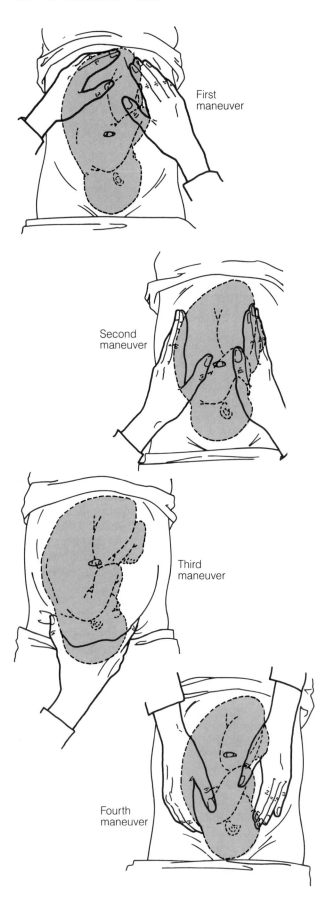

First maneuver

Second maneuver

Third maneuver

Fourth maneuver

- Is the presenting part engaged, floating, or dipping into the inlet?
- Is there fetal movement?
- How large is the fetus? (Appropriate, large, or small for gestational age?)
- Is there one fetus or more than one?
- Is fundal height proportionate to the estimated gestational age?

First Maneuver While facing the woman, the nurse palpates the upper abdomen with both hands (Figure 22–10). The nurse determines the shape, size, consistency, and mobility of the form that is found. The fetal head is firm, hard, and round and moves independently of the trunk. The breech feels softer and symmetrical and has small bony prominences; it moves with the trunk.

Second Maneuver After ascertaining whether the head or the buttocks occupies the fundus, the nurse tries to determine the location of the fetal back and notes whether it is on the right or left side of the maternal abdomen. Still facing the woman, the nurse palpates the abdomen with deep but gentle pressure, using her palms (Figure 22–10). The right hand should be steady while the left hand explores the right side of the uterus. The maneuver is then repeated, probing with the right hand and steadying the uterus with the left hand. The fetal back should feel firm and smooth and should connect what was found in the fundus with a mass in the inlet. Once the back is located, the nurse validates the finding by palpating the fetal extremities (small irregularities and protrusions) on the opposite side of the abdomen.

Third Maneuver Next the nurse should determine what fetal part is lying above the inlet by gently grasping the lower portion of the abdomen just above the symphysis pubis with the thumb and fingers of the right hand (Figure 22–10). This maneuver yields the opposite information from what was found in the fundus and validates the presenting part. If the head is presenting and is not engaged, it may be gently pushed back and forth.

Fourth Maneuver For this portion of the examination, the nurse faces the woman's feet and attempts to locate the cephalic prominence or brow. Location of this landmark assists in assessing the descent of the presenting part into the pelvis. The fingers of both hands are moved gently down the sides of the uterus toward the pubis (Figure 22–10). The cephalic prominence (brow) is located

Figure 22–10 Leopold's maneuvers for determination of fetal position, presentation, and lie. Note: Many nurses do the fourth maneuver first, in order to identify what part of the fetus is in the pelvic inlet.

PROCEDURE 22 – 2

Auscultation of Fetal Heart Rate

Nursing Action	Rationale

Nursing Action

Objective: Assemble equipment.

Obtain a fetoscope or Doppler.

Objective: Prepare woman.

Explain the procedure, indications for the procedure, and the information that will be obtained.

Objective: Auscultate FHR.

Perform Leopold's maneuver to identify the fetal presentation and position.

Uncover the woman's abdomen.

If using a fetoscope, place the metal band on your head; the diaphragm should extend out from your forehead.

If using a Doppler, place ultrasonic gel on the diaphragm. Note: some Dopplers have a plastic cap over the diaphragm that will need to be removed to expose the diaphragm.

Place the bell of the fetoscope or the Doppler diaphragm on the maternal abdomen, about half-way between the umbilicus and symphysis pubis and in the midline. If the FHR is not heard, move the fetoscope out about an inch, in an ever-widening circle until the FHR is heard. When using the Doppler, you may need to tilt the diaphragm slightly in order to hear the FHR. If tilting the diaphragm does not locate the FHR, move the fetoscope in the same manner as described above.

Objective: Differentiate maternal pulse from fetal heart rate.

Place your index finger over the woman's radial pulse to differentiate maternal heart rate from fetal heart rate.

Count the FHR. Note that the FHR has a double rhythm and just one sound is counted. Palpate for uterine contractions while you are auscultating FHR.

Count FHR during a uterine contraction and continue for an additional 30 seconds to identify FHR response.

Determine FHR baseline by counting FHR for 30 to 60 seconds between uterine contractions to identify average baseline rate. Note if the rate is regular or irregular. If the rate changes (abruptly or gradually) recount for a brief period (5 or 10 seconds) to correctly identify an increasing or slowing rate.

Tell the parents what the FHR is; offer to help them listen if they would like to.

Rationale

Fetoscope is a special type of stethoscope that amplifies sound.
Doppler uses ultrasound.

Explanation of the procedure decreases anxiety and increases relaxation.

Assists in locating the fetal back where FHR is most likely to be heard.

It is more difficult to auscultate through cloth.

The metal band conducts sound.

The gel is used to maintain contact with the maternal abdomen and to enhance conduction of ultrasound.

The FHR is most likely to be heard over the fetal back. In LOA or ROA, the fetal back will be located in this portion of the maternal abdomen.

Ensures that the FHR, not the woman's pulse, is being heard.

The FHR has the same "Lub dup" sound of adult heart sounds. The response of the FHR to uterine contractions is important in evaluating FHR changes.

Counting during and just after the contraction evaluates fetal response to the contraction.

The FHR baseline is the rate between contractions.

Increases or decreases in the FHR need to be described as accurately as possible.

(continued)

PROCEDURE 22–2 (continued)

Nursing Action	Rationale
Objective: Provide systematic evaluation.	
Auscultate between, during and for 30 seconds following a uterine contraction. For low-risk women, NAACOG 1990 recommends an auscultation frequency of every 1 hour in latent phase, every 30 minutes in active phase, and every 15 minutes in the second stage. For high-risk women, the recommended frequency is every 30 minutes in latent phase, every 15 minutes in active phase, and every 5 minutes in the second stage.	Evaluation provides the opportunity to assess the fetal status and response to the labor process.
Objective: Record information on client record.	
Document FHR data (rate and rhythm), characteristics of uterine activity, and any actions taken as a result of the FHR.	Complete documentation is mandatory.
Sample nurse's entry:	
1/1/92 FHR 140 by auscultation, regular rhythm. Maternal 0700 pulse 78. UC q 3 min × 60 sec, strong. No increase or decrease in FHR noted during or following UC. J. Smith RN	Nurse's entry documents FHR rate, rhythm, and response to UC.
Sample Nurse's entry for baseline and slowing of FHR after uterine contraction.	
1/1/92 FHR 136 by auscultation with slowing noted during the acme of UC and for 10 seconds following 0800 the UC. Client turned to left side. Maternal pulse 80. FHR 140, regular rhythm with no decrease during or following the next two UC. UC q 3 × 60 sec, strong. J. Smith RN	Nurse's entry documents FHR rate, response to UC, nursing intervention, and fetal response.

---

on the side where there is greatest resistance to the descent of the fingers toward the pubis. It is located on the opposite side from the fetal back if the head is well flexed. However, when the fetal head is extended, the occiput is the first cephalic prominence felt, and it is located on the same side as the back. Therefore, when completing the fourth maneuver, if the first cephalic prominence palpated is on the same side as the back, the head is not flexed. If the first prominence found is opposite the back, the head is well flexed.

CRITICAL THINKING

The fetus in Figure 22–10 is in ROA position. Describe what you would feel during Leopold's Maneuvers if the fetus was LOA.

Vaginal Examination

The vaginal examination reveals information regarding the fetus such as presentation, position, station, degree of flexion of the fetal head, and any swelling that might be present on the fetal scalp (caput succedaneum).

Ultrasound

Real-time ultrasound is frequently available in the birth setting and may be used to obtain specific information regarding the fetus. A real-time ultrasound may be done at this time to assess fetal lie, presentation, and position; obtain measurements of biparietal diameter to estimate gestational age; assess for anomalies when a vaginal examination reveals suspicious findings; and sometimes to confirm the presence of more than one fetus.(See Chapter 20 for further discussion of the use of ultrasound for fetal assessment.)

Evaluation of Fetal Status During Labor

Auscultation of Fetal Heart Rate

The fetoscope is essentially a special stethoscope that is used to listen to the fetal heart rate (FHR). The fetoscope has two designs; One consists of a stethoscope attached to a metal band that goes over the nurse's head and conducts sound, enhancing the ability to hear the fetal heart; a second type is a stethoscope attached to a cone-shaped weighted bell approximately 3 inches in diameter, which is placed on the maternal abdomen and the other end is placed over the nurse's ear. Fetal heart rate may also be auscultated with a hand-held ultrasound device (Figure 22–11).

Before listening to the FHR the first time, some nurses complete Leopold's maneuvers to assist in identifying the fetal presentation and position. The fetus is generally in a head-down (cephalic) presentation with its back to the mother's left side. Thus the nurse could anticipate that the fetal heart rate will be found in the lower quadrant of the maternal abdomen. As the presenting part descends and rotates through the pelvis during labor, the location of the FHR tends to descend and move toward the midline. The FHR can be heard most clearly at the fetal back (Figure 22–12).

After FHR is located, it is counted for 15 seconds and multiplied by 4 to obtain the number of beats per minute. The nurse should occasionally listen for a full minute

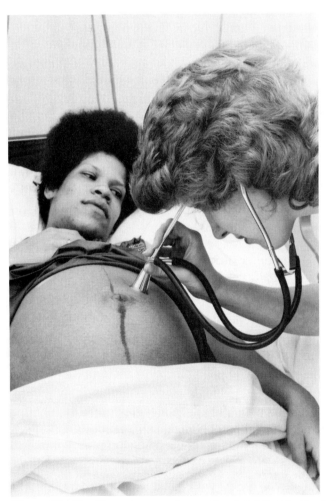

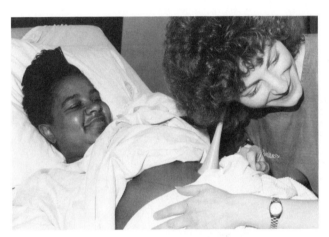

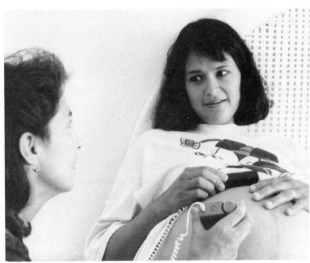

Figure 22–11   Three means of assessing fetal heart rate. A Fetoscope. The nurse holds the fetoscope as she places it against the maternal abdomen and then removes her fingers from the fetoscope while counting the fetal heart rate. B The Penar fetoscope. This type of fetoscope can be easily used in outpatient or community settings. C This ultrasound device is powered by a battery. When the fetal heart rate is picked up by the Doppler, the sound of the heart rate can be heard by all persons in the room.

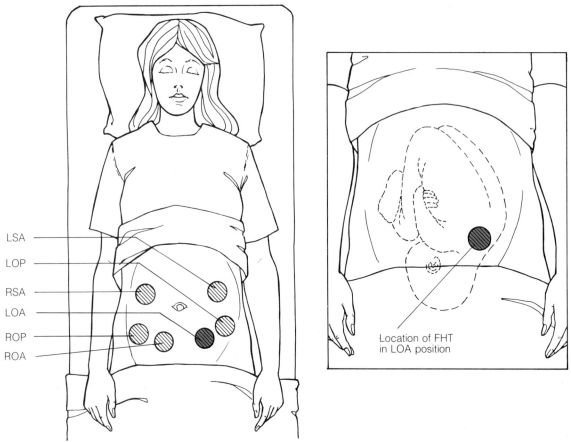

Figure 22–12   Location of FHR in relation to the more commonly seen fetal positions. The fetal heart rate is heard more clearly over the fetal back.

through a contraction to detect any abnormal heart rate especially if tachycardia, bradycardia, or irregular beats are heard. If the FHR is irregular or has changed markedly from the last assessment, the nurse should listen for a full minute. The FHR should be auscultated frequently (see Table 22–3). It is especially important to listen during and after the contraction to detect any deceleration that might occur. It is also important to listen immediately after each contraction when the woman is pushing during second stage since fetal bradycardia frequently occurs as pressure is exerted on the fetal head during descent.

If decelerations (see p 636) are noted, the woman should be electronically monitored to rule out abnormalities in the FHR.

Only gross changes in FHR may be detected with the fetoscope. Subtle changes that occur in response to contractions may not be heard because it is difficult to hear the FHR during the peak of a contraction. Consequently, transient accelerations or decelerations in the FHR may be missed. In addition, occasional counting errors are inevitable. The auscultated FHR is an average measurement.

In current maternity care practice, a fetoscope, handheld Doppler device, or electronic fetal monitoring may be used to assess the FHR during labor and birth.

Electronic Fetal Monitoring

There are two methods of assessing FHR during labor: indirect (external) and direct (internal). The indirect method may be accomplished using a fetoscope, fetal electrocardiography, and Doppler ultrasound (intermittent or continuous). Direct monitoring provides continuous information about the FHR from a scalp electrode.

When the FHR is monitored electronically, the interval between two successive fetal heart beats is measured and the rate is displayed as if the beats occurred at the same interval for 60 seconds. For example, if the interval between two beats is 0.5 second, the rate for one full minute would be 120 beats per minute.

Electronic fetal monitoring (EFM) has major advantages over auscultation with the fetoscope. Electronic monitoring is an objective means of evaluating fetal well-being. Fetal distress can be detected by observing the continuous

Table 22–3	Frequency of Auscultation: Assessment and Documentation*

Low-Risk Patients

First Stage of Labor:
q 1 hr in latent phase
q 30 min in active phase

Second Stage of Labor:
q 15 min

High-Risk Patients

First Stage of Labor:
q 30 min in latent phase
q 15 min in active phase

Second Stage of Labor:
q 5 min

Labor Events

Assess FHR prior to:
initiation of labor-enhancing procedures (eg, artificial rupture of membranes)
periods of ambulation
administration of medications
administration or initiation of analgesia/anesthesia

Assess FHR following:
rupture of membranes
recognition of abnormal uterine activity patterns, such as increased basal tone or tachysystole
evaluation of oxytocin (maintenance, increase, or decrease of dosage)
administration of medications (at time of peak action)
expulsion of enema
urinary catheterization
vaginal examination
periods of ambulation
evaluation of analgesia and/or anesthesia (maintenance, increase, or decrease of dosage)

From NAACOGOGN Nursing Practice Resource, Fetal Heart Rate Auscultation, March 1990. Washington, DC: NAACOG p 5.

Table 22–4	Indications for Electronic Monitoring

Fetal factors

Decreased fetal movement

Abnormal auscultory FHR

Meconium passage

Abnormal presentations/positions

IUGR or SGA fetus

Postdates (>41–42 weeks)

Multiple gestation

Maternal factors

Fever

Infections

PIH

Disease conditions (eg, hypertension, diabetes)

Anemia

Rh isoimmunization

Previous perinatal death

Grand multiparity

Previous cesarean birth

Borderline/contracted pelvis

Uterine factors

Dysfunctional labor

Failure to progress in labor

Oxytocin induction/augmentation

Uterine anomalies

Complications of pregnancy

Prolonged rupture of membranes

Premature rupture of membranes

Preterm labor

Marginal abruptio placentae

Partial placenta previa

Occult/frank polapse of cord

Amnionitis

Regional anesthesia

Elective monitoring

FHR and the periodic changes that occur during and after uterine contractions. Interventions can be timely and thus more effective.

Indications for Electronic Fetal Monitoring Any woman with previous history of medical or obstetric problems that might affect labor or the health of the fetus should be monitored by continuous electronic fetal monitoring. Some physicians advocate monitoring only those women considered to be at risk or at high risk, while many feel the procedure is mandatory for all women in labor. Specific indications for monitoring are listed in Table 22–4.

External Monitoring *External monitoring* of the fetus is usually accomplished by the use of ultrasound. A transducer, which emits continuous sound waves, is placed on the maternal abdomen. A water-soluble gel is applied to the underside of the transducer to aid in conduction of fetal heart sounds. When placed correctly, the sound waves bounce off the fetal heart and are picked up by the electronic monitor. The actual moment-by-moment FHR is displayed simultaneously on a screen and on graph paper (Figure 22–13).

The transducer may inadvertently be directed toward a pulsating maternal vessel. In this case, there will be a soft swooshing sound (uterine souffle) and the rate will be the same as the maternal pulse.

Disadvantages of monitoring fetal heart rate by external means are similar to those of external uterine contraction monitoring. In addition, a poor quality tracing may be obtained if the fetus is quite active, if more than a normal amount of amniotic fluid is present, or if the woman is obese.

PROCEDURE 22–3

Electronic Fetal Monitoring

Nursing Action

Objective: Prepare woman.

Explain the procedure, the indications for the EFM, and the information that will be obtained. Explain the monitor so that parents will know what they are seeing and hearing.

Place the external fetal monitor. Turn on the monitor. Place two elastic belts around the woman's abdomen. Place the "toco" over the uterine fundus in the midline and secure it with a belt so that it fits snugly. Note the UC tracing. The resting tone tracing (without uterine contraction) should be recording on the 10 or 15 mm Hg pressure line.

Apply ultrasonic gel to the diaphragm of the ultrasound transducer. Place the diaphragm on the maternal abdomen between the umbilicus and symphysis pubis, in the midline. Listen for the FHR (which will have a "whip-like" sound). When FHR is located, attach the elastic belt snugly.

Objective: Identify the tracing.

Place the following information on the beginning of the fetal monitor paper: date, time, client name, gravida, para, membrane status, physician name. (Note: Each birthing area may have specific guidelines regarding additional information that is to be included.)

Objective: Evaluate EFM tracing.

For high-risk women, NAACOG (1988) recommends evaluating the EFM tracing every 15 minutes in the first stage, and every 5 minutes in the second stage. For low-risk women specific time intervals have not been recommended by NAACOG. However, evaluation every 15–30 minutes in the first stage, and every 5–15 minutes in the second stage (as long as FHR has reassuring characteristics) is frequently done. The time interval for evaluation needs to be shortened if any nonreassuring characteristics occur.

Objective: Record information on client record.

Sample nurse's entry:
1/1/92 FHR BL 135–140. STV and LTV present. Two accelerations of 20 bpm × 20 sec with fetal movement in 10 minutes. UC q 3 min × 50–60 sec of moderate intensity by palpation. No decelerations noted.

Sample nurse's entry if slowing is noted.
0730 FHR BL 135–144. STV and LTV present. Late deceleration noted with decrease of FHR to 130 bpm for 20 sec. UC q 3 min × 50–60 sec of moderate intensity by palpation. Client turned to left side. No further deceleration with three subsequent UC. Two accelerations of 20 bpm × 20 sec noted with fetal movement. Client instructed to remain on left side.

Rationale

Explanation of the procedure decreases anxiety and increases relaxation.

The uterine fundus is the area of greatest contractility.

If the tracing is on the 0 line, there may be a constant grinding noise.

Ultrasonic gel is used to maintain contact with the maternal abdomen. The ultrasonic beam is directed toward the fetal heart.

Firm contact is necessary to maintain a continuous tracing.

Assures accurate identification.

Evaluation provides the opportunity to assess the fetal status and response to the labor process. Presence of reassuring characteristics is associated with good fetal outcome. Rapid identification of nonreassuring characteristics allows interventions to be initiated and then to determine the fetal response to the interventions.

Nurse's entry documents reassuring FHR characteristics and response to UCs.

Nurse's entry documents FHR rate, presence of variability, response of FHR to UC, the intervention used and subsequent positive fetal response to the intervention.

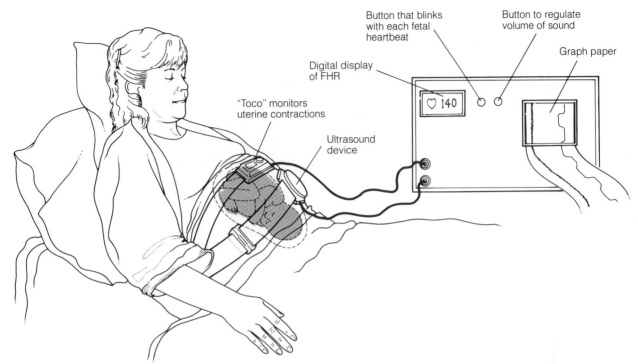

Figure 22–13 Tocodynamometer and ultrasonic technique to monitor maternal and fetal status during labor (From Hon E: An Introduction to Fetal Heart Monitoring. Los Angeles: University of California School of Medicine, 1972, p 65.)

Internal Monitoring Internal monitoring is accomplished through use of an internal spiral electrode, which is attached to the skin of the fetal head or buttocks (Figure 22–14). To insert the spiral electrode, the cervix must be dilated at least 2 cm, the presenting fetal part accessible by vaginal examination, and the membranes ruptured. Even though it is not possible to apply the electrode and catheter under strict sterile conditions, the procedure should be performed as aseptically as possible. The perineum should be cleaned with povidone-iodine solution (Betadine) or another cleansing agent. After determining fetal position by vaginal examination, the examiner (physician or nurse) inserts the electrode, which is encased in a plastic guide, to the level of the internal cervical os and attaches it to the presenting part, being careful not to apply it to the face, suture lines, fontanelles, or perineum if the fetus is in a breech presentation. The electrode is rotated clockwise until it is attached to the presenting part and is then disengaged from the guide tube. The guide tube is removed, and the end wires are connected to a leg plate that is attached to the woman's thigh. The cable from the leg plate is connected to the monitor.

The spiral electrode provides an instantaneous and continuous recording of FHR that is clearer than data provided by external monitoring.

The FHR tracing at the top of Figure 22–15 was obtained by internal monitoring and the uterine contraction tracing at the bottom of the figure by external monitoring.

Note the FHR is variable (the tracing moves up and down instead of in a straight line), and the tracing stays close to the line numbered 150. If the graph paper moves through the monitor at 3 cm per minute, each vertical dark line represents 1 minute. The frequency of the uterine contractions is every 2 1/2 to 3 minutes. The duration of the contractions is 50 to 60 seconds.

Telemetry Fetal heart rate and uterine activity may also be monitored by a telemetry system. Ultrasound, or fetal ECG, and external uterine pressure transducers are connected to a small battery-operated transducer. Signals are transmitted to a receiver connected to the monitor. The monitor displays FHR and uterine activity data on the oscilloscope and prints it out on graph paper to provide documentation. This system, which can be worn by means of a shoulder strap, allows the woman to ambulate, helping her to feel more comfortable and less confined during labor, yet provides for continuous monitoring. Telemetry provides for direct as well as indirect monitoring of FHR, indirect monitoring of uterine pressure, and dual FHR monitoring of twins. (See a comparison of different methods in Table 22–5.)

Fetal Heart Rate Patterns

Fetal heart rate is evaluated by assessing both baseline and periodic changes. Normal FHR ranges from 120 to 160 beats per minute. More important than FHR are the peri-

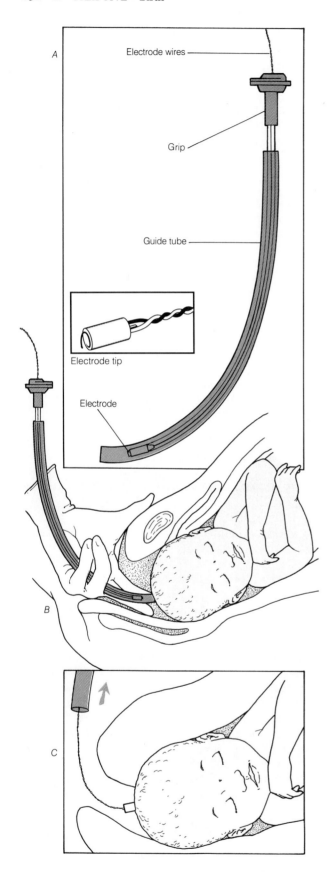

A *Electrode wires*

Grip

Guide tube

Electrode tip

Electrode

B

C

odic changes that occur in response to the intermittent stress of uterine contractions and the baseline beat-to-beat variability of the fetal heart rate. A compromised fetus may have a normal heart rate but demonstrate slight periodic changes and decreased variability indicative of intrauterine hypoxia.

Baseline Rate   The baseline refers to the range of FHR observed between contractions, during a ten-minute period of monitoring. The range does not include the rate present during decelerations.

Baseline Changes   Baseline changes in FHR are defined in terms of ten-minute periods of time. These changes are tachycardia, bradycardia, and variability of the heart rate.

Tachycardia   Tachycardia is defined as a rate of 160 beats per minute or more for a ten-minute segment of time. Moderate tachycardia has rates of 160 to 179 beats per minute. Severe tachycardia is defined as 180 beats per minute or more. Although tachycardia may occur without apparent reason, possible causes include the following:

- Extreme prematurity
- Maternal fever
- Fetal asphyxia
- Fetal infection
- Fetal anemia
- Beta-sympathomimetic drugs given to the pregnant woman
- Maternal anxiety
- Fetal tachyarrhythmias
- Maternal thyrotoxicosis
- Maternal hyperthyroidism
- Drugs, eg, isoxsuprine, atropine, ritodrine, terbutaline
- Excessive fetal activity

Bradycardia   Fetal bradycardia is defined as a rate of less than 120 beats per minute for a ten-minute segment of time. Mild bradycardia ranges from 100 to 119 beats per minute and is considered benign. Moderate bradycardia is a fetal heart rate less than 100 beats per minute. Severe bradycardia is an FHR less than 70 beats per minute and is as-

Figure 22–14 Technique for internal, direct fetal monitoring. A Spiral electrode. B Attaching spiral electrode to scalp. C. Attached spiral electrode with guide tube removed.

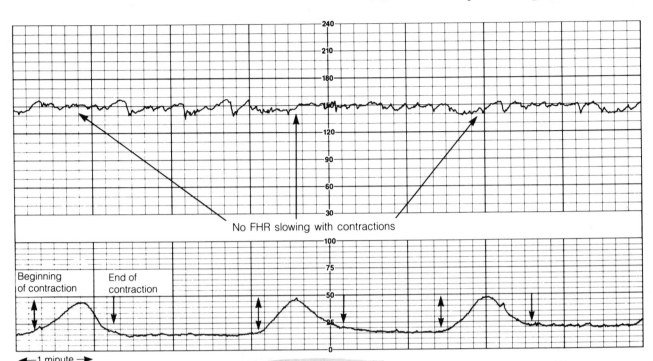

Figure 22–15   Normal FHR range is from 120 to 160 beats per minute. The FHR tracing in the upper portion of the graph indicates FHR range of 140 to 155 beats per minute. The bottom portion depicts uterine contractions. Each dark vertical line marks one minute, and each small rectangle is 10 seconds. The contraction frequency is about every three minutes, and the duration of the contractions is 50 to 60 seconds.

sociated with a rapidly occurring fetal acidosis. Causes of fetal bradycardia include the following:

- Fetal asphyxia (late sign)
- Fetal arrhythmias as seen with congenital heart block
- Drugs (eg, anesthetic agents used as paracervical and epidural blocks)
- Prolapse or prolonged compression of umbilical cord
- Hypothermia
- Initial response to acute asphyxia associated with maternal seizure, excessive uterine contractions, acute maternal hypotension, abruptio placentae, or fetal hemorrhage (due to rupture of anomalous fetal-placental vessel or torn vasa previa)
- End-stage bradycardia (due to continuous pressure on the fetal head during descent in the late second stage)
- Idiopathic sinus bradycardia
- Maternal systemic lupus erythematosus

Baseline Variability   One of the most important parameters of fetal well-being is noted in the variability of the FHR. The term *variability* refers to the irregularity of the FHR as noted on the graph paper. A healthy fetus normally demonstrates an irregular FHR baseline, which is caused by an interplay of the sympathetic and parasympathetic nervous systems. Variability consists of two components—long-term and short-term variability—both of significance in evaluating fetal status (Figure 22–16).

- *Long-term variability* (LTV) refers to the larger rhythmic fluctuations of the FHR that occur from two to six times per minute with a normal range of six to ten beats per minute. The range refers to the difference between the lowest FHR and the highest FHR within one minute (Figure 22–17). Long-term variability is increased by fetal movement and decreased or absent when the fetus is in a sleep cycle. Long-term variability has been classified as follows (Hon 1976):

No variability	0–2 beats/min
Minimal variability	3–5 beats/min
Average variability	6–10 beats/min
Moderate variability	11–25 beats/min
Marked variability (*saltatory*)	>25 beats/min

Table 22–5 Advantages and Disadvantages of Various Monitoring Methods

Method	Advantages	Disadvantages
Fetoscope	Inexpensive Noninvasive Easy to use Easily transported	Intermittent information Gives no information regarding contractions Cannot assess variability or periodic changes in FHR unless moderate to severe Cannot hear FHT until 17–20 weeks' gestation
Doppler (pocket-sized ultrasound)	Inexpensive Noninvasive Easily transported Can hear FHT as early as 10–12 weeks	Gives no information regarding contractions Cannot assess variability Cannot assess periodic changes in FHR unless moderate to severe Intermittent information
External monitoring	Continuous information Noninvasive Uses: antepartal testing, and during labor Gives permanent record Can assess relative frequency of contractions Can assess decreased variability and periodic changes Useful for client teaching	Equipment is expensive Subject to artifact Cannot assess variability unless decreased and then must confirm with internal monitoring Cannot quantitate contractions Belts uncomfortable to some women Subject to double- and half-counting
Internal monitoring	Accurate, continuous information Monitors fetal ECG Not subject to artifact Client more mobile in bed, chair Can quantitate contractions Can assess short-term and long-term variability Accurate assessment of periodic changes Useful for client teaching	Will measure maternal heart rate if fetus is dead Equipment is expensive Need qualified and knowledgeable personnel to interpret Presenting part must be accessible, membranes must be ruptured, and cervix must be dilated enough for application of scalp electrode Requires knowledgeable personnel to apply equipment Client confined to bed or chair Slight increased risk of maternal or fetal infection Subject to double- and half-counting Invasive
Telemetry	Accurate, continuous information Client can be mobile (out of bed or in hall) Same advantages as internal monitoring	Equipment is expensive Invasive Not widely used at the present time Same disadvantages as internal monitoring

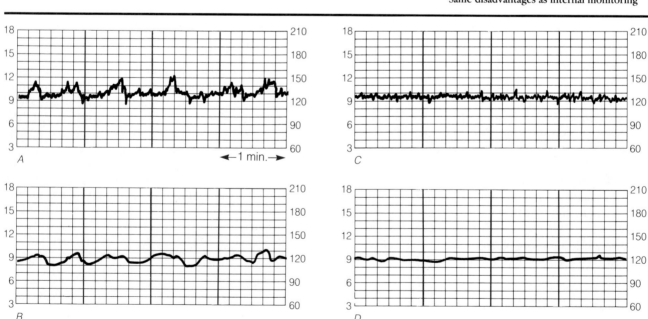

Figure 22–16 Short- and long-term variability. A Increased LTV; STV present. B Average LTV; STV absent. C Absent LTV; STV present. D Absent LTV; STV absent.

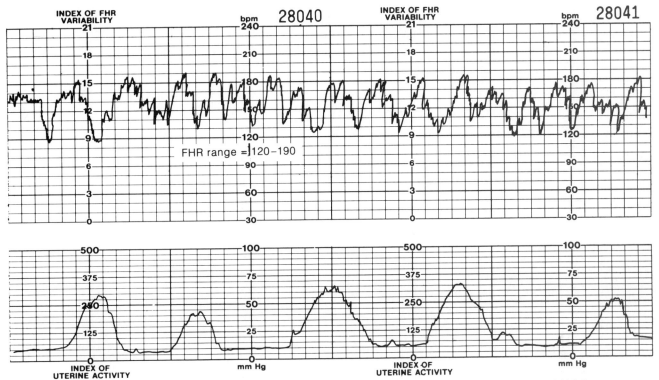

Figure 22–17   Saltatory pattern. Note pattern of marked LTV. FHR varies markedly between 120 and 190 beats per minute. With this type of pattern, it is not possible to determine an average baseline FHR because of the wide, marked variations. STV is present.

The **saltatory pattern** of marked or excessive variability is characterized by rapid variations in FHR that have a bizarre appearance. LTV occurs with a cycle frequency of three to six per minute, and the amplitude is greater than 25 beats per minute (Figure 22–18). The etiology of this pattern is uncertain.

An unusual pattern referred to as **sinusoidal** is occasionally seen. It is characterized by an undulant sine wave that is equally distributed above and below the baseline. The FHR usually ranges between 120 and 160 beats per minute. This wavelike baseline FHR usually has an amplitude of 5 to 15 beats per minute and appears to oscillate in a regular, uniform pattern of 2 to 6 cycles per minute; there are differences of opinion about whether this is LTV. Fetal activity may be minimal or absent and FHR accelerations are lacking. There is no beat-to-beat short-term variability (Figure 22–19).

The sinusoidal pattern is associated with Rh isoimmunization, severe anemia, and occasionally, asphyxiation (Parer 1989). The administration of nalbuphine hydrochloride (Nubain) has also been associated with sinusoidal patterns (Feinstein et al 1986). Hatjis and Meiss (1986) noted in one study that the administration of intravenous butorphanol tartrate (Stadol) has also been noted to cause a sinusoidal pattern approximately 75% of the time it is given.

In the absence of analgesia-related occurrences, true sinusoidal FHR patterns noted intrapartally suggest fetal anemia or severe asphyxia. If noted by external monitoring, internal fetal monitoring should be instituted, and cesarean birth should be considered if the pattern is confirmed. Fetal blood sampling for determination of pH and hematocrit, ultrasound scan for signs of congestive heart failure and hydrops, and biophysical profile may aid in assessment, evaluation, and management of the fetus with this FHR pattern (Schneider & Tropper 1986).

Short-term variability (STV) refers to the differences between successive heart beats as measured by the R–R wave interval of the QRS cardiac cycle and therefore represents actual beat-to-beat fluctuations in FHR. STV refers to the tiny fluctuations in FHR noted within the 10-second intervals of the electronic fetal monitoring tracing. These fluctuations average two to three beats per minute. Short-term variability is classified as either present or absent.

Rather then counting specific beats, with practice one can usually become skillful in "eyeballing" the FHR variability. When decreased LTV is noted, one must suspect some compromise of these mechanisms. Increased variability has not been as well defined, and the causes are unknown. The most important aspect of variability is that even in the presence of abnormal or questionable FHR patterns, if the ST variability is normal, the fetus is not suffer-

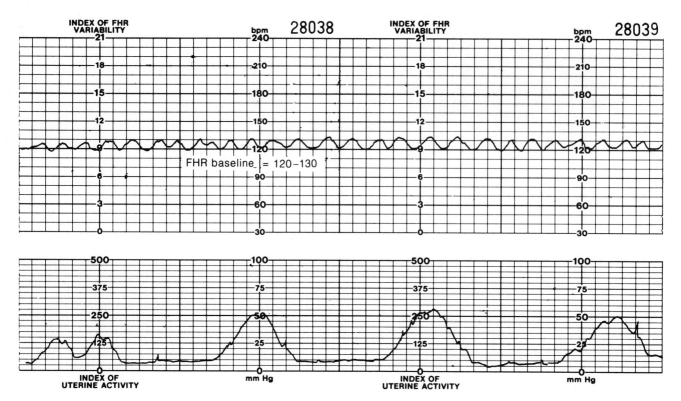

Figure 22–18 Sinusoidal pattern. Note undulating waveform evenly distributed between 120 and 130 beats per minute baseline. There is no STV; no accelerations or decelerations are present.

ing from cerebral asphyxia (Parer 1989). During prolonged bradycardia or severe periodic changes (eg, late or severe variable decelerations, see p 637), the fetus may decompensate and suffer cerebral and myocardial asphyxia and consequently demonstrate a decrease or loss of variability. If loss of ST variability accompanies tachycardia, fetal prognosis is usually poor (Parer 1989), and immediate birth of the fetus should be considered if fetal blood acid-base determination is not feasible.

The nurse needs to keep in mind that STV can be evaluated only by internal monitoring. The external monitor may demonstrate "normal" variability due to the presence of artifact, when in fact it is decreased. An appearance of decreased variability warrants application of an internal electrode. Decreased variability may be seen with the following conditions:

- Administration of drugs (hypnotics, analgesics, and parasympathetic blocking agents to the mother)
- Anesthesia and deep fetal sleep
- Absence of fetal cortex (anencephaly)
- Premature fetus

- Fetal hypoxia, acidosis and asphyxia
- Tachycardia
- Fetal anatomic brain damage, cardiac or CNS anomalies
- Arrhythmias

Stimuli such as maternal activity, abdominal palpation, fetal activity, and myometrial contractions may increase variability because the baby moves. Complete loss of variability may occur with complete heart block.

Periodic Changes Periodic changes are transient decelerations or accelerations of the FHR from the baseline that occur in response to contractions and fetal movement.

Accelerations are transient increases in the FHR normally caused by fetal movement. As the fetus moves in utero, the heart rate increases as it does in adults when they exercise. When the fetus quiets down, the heart rate returns to normal. Acceleration often accompanies contractions, usually as a result of fetal movement in response

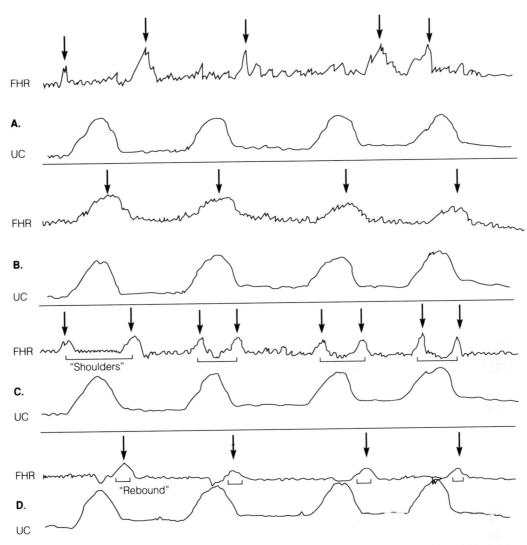

Figure 22–19   Types of accelerations. A Spontaneous accelerations. B Uniform accelerations. C Variable acceleration ("shoulders"). D Rebound accelerations ("overshoot").

to pressure of the contracting uterine musculature. Accelerations of this type are thought to be a sign of fetal well-being and adequate oxygen reserve.

Spontaneous accelerations are symmetric, uniform increases in FHR. They are benign, represent an intact CNS response to fetal movement or stimulation, and are not associated with contractions or decelerations. This type of acceleration serves as the criterion for a reactive NST (Figure 22–20*A*). *Uniform accelerations* are symmetric, occur with contractions, and reflect the shape of the contraction. They are frequently seen in early labor before the membranes have ruptured, are commonly seen with non-

vertex presentations, and are apparently benign (Figure 22–20*B*)

Variable accelerations are of variable shape and do not reflect the shape of contractions. They may be noted as short periods of increased variability that appear at the beginning and the end of a uterine contraction. The shape of the increased variability appears like "shoulders" around the contraction. These accelerations may also occur before and after variable decelerations and are associated with normal baseline variability. They are apparently benign (Figure 22–20*C*).

Rebound Accelerations ("Overshoot") are uniform

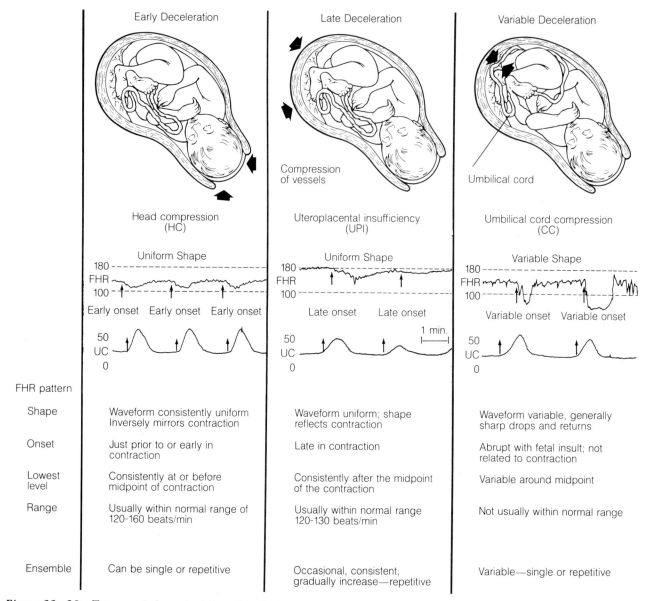

Figure 22–20   Types and characteristics of early, late, and variable decelerations (From Hon E: An Introduction to Fetal Heart Rate Monitoring, *2nd ed. Los Angeles: University of Southern California School of Medicine, 1972, p 65.)*

in shape, immediately follow variable decelerations, and are accompanied by absent baseline variability. Tachycardia is frequently noted with "overshoot." This type of acceleration suggests autonomic nervous system imbalance or exhaustion of fetal compensatory mechanisms. It may be seen in asphyxiated or premature fetuses. Except in the case of prematurity, rebound accelerations should be considered an ominous sign with a deteriorating fetus (Figure 22–19) (Shifrin 1985).

Decelerations are periodic decreases in FHR from the normal baseline. Hon and Quilligan (1967) categorized them as early, late, and variable, according to when they

occur in the contraction cycle and to their waveform (Figure 22–20).

Early decelerations are due to pressure on the fetal head as it progresses down the birth canal. They have a uniform, smooth waveform that inversely mirrors that of the corresponding contraction. Beginning at the onset of the contraction and ending as the contraction ends, the nadir (lowest point) occurs at the peak of the contraction. The nadir is usually within the normal fetal heart rate range (Figure 22–21).

Early decelerations are generally benign and seen late in labor when the fetal head is on the perineum. In-

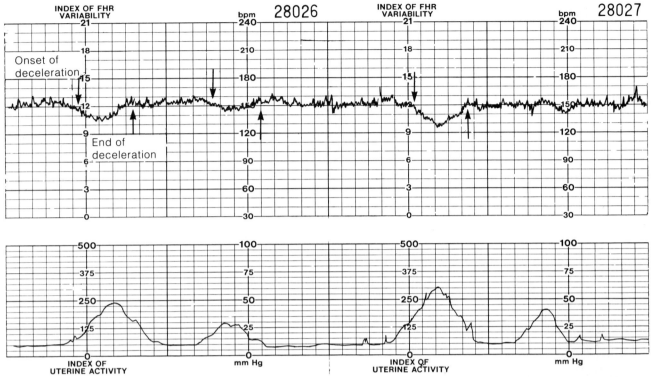

Figure 22–21   Early decelerations. Baseline FHR is 150 to 155 beats per minute. Nadir (the lowest point) of decelerations is 130–145. LTV is absent; STV is present.

creased intracranial pressure results in local changes in cerebral blood flow, which in turn results in stimulation of vagal centers and produces a slowing of heart rate through the vagus nerve (Figure 22–22). If this pattern occurs early in labor, it may be due to head compression from cephalopelvic disproportion. A nurse must take great care in differentiating this type of deceleration from late decelerations: They look identical yet differ in time of onset.

Early decelerations are not associated with loss of variability, tachycardia, or other FHR changes nor are they associated with fetal hypoxia, acidosis, or low Apgar scores. Early decelerations are viewed as a reassuring FHR pattern unless seen in early labor or with lack of descent of the fetal head.

Late decelerations are due to uteroplacental insufficiency as the result of decreased blood flow and oxygen transfer to the fetus through the intervillous space during uterine contractions causing hypoxemia (Figure 22–23). They have a smooth, uniform shape that inversely mirrors the contraction (as do early decelerations) but are late in their onset and recovery. They begin at or within a few seconds after the peak of the contraction; the nadir is noted near the end of the contraction. They tend to occur with every contraction. When uteroplacental reserve is adequate, the fetus normally tolerates the transient stress of re-

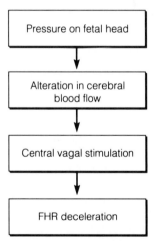

Figure 22–22   Mechanism of early deceleration (head compression) (Adapted from Freeman RK, Garite TJ: The physiologic basis of fetal monitoring. In Fetal Heart Rate Monitoring. Baltimore, MD: Williams & Wilkins, 1981, ch 2, p 13.)

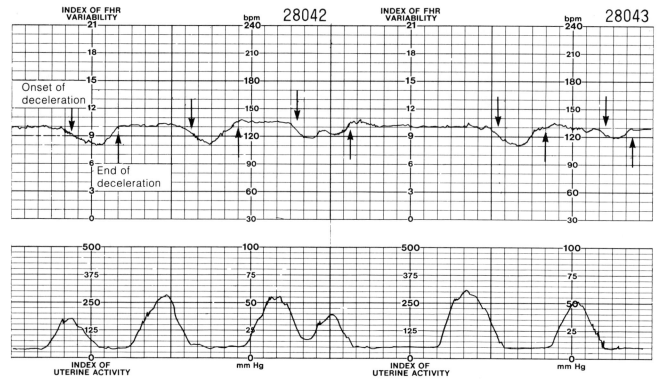

Figure 22–23   *Late decelerations. Baseline FHR is 130 to 148 beats per minute. Nadir (lowest point) of decelerations is 110–120. LTV and STV are absent.*

petitive contractions. If fetal hypoxia occurs because of a decrease in uteroplacental blood flow (for example, from maternal hypotension or excessive uterine activity), late decelerations generally occur (Figure 22–24).

This pattern is always considered an ominous sign but does not necessarily require immediate birth of the fetus. If late decelerations do not appear to be worsening and the variability of the FHR is normal, birth may be delayed although the fetus warrants constant observation. Should decelerations worsen, tachycardia occur, or variability decrease, fetal blood sampling for pH determination is indicated to evaluate the acid-base status of the fetus.

Sometimes, late decelerations are found to be due to the supine position of the laboring woman. In this case, decreased uterine blood flow to the fetus may be alleviated by raising the woman's upper trunk or turning her to the side to displace pressure of the gravid uterus on the inferior vena cava. If the woman remains flat on her back, the fetus will continue to have decelerations due to oxygen compromise.

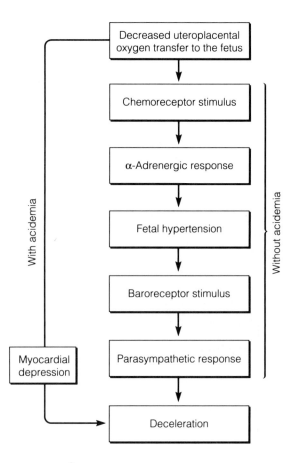

Figure 22–24   *Mechanism of late deceleration (From Freeman RK, Garite TJ: The physiologic basis of fetal monitoring. In* Fetal Heart Rate Monitoring. *Baltimore, MD: Williams & Wilkins, 1981, ch 2, p 15.)*

Late decelerations normally occur within the normal heart rate range (120–160 beats/min) and may be quite obvious or very subtle and almost indistinguishable. Some fetuses at highest risk demonstrate a flat FHR baseline with late decelerations that are barely noticeable. It must be kept in mind that the depth of the deceleration does not indicate the severity of the insult.

Chronic uteroplacental insufficiency during pregnancy results in intrauterine growth retardation and, if severe enough, antenatal death. When uteroplacental insufficiency is acute due to factors occurring during labor, fetal distress may ensue. If not properly treated intrapartal fetal death may occur.

Variable decelerations are appropriately named in that they vary in their onset, occurrence, and waveform. They are thought to be due to umbilical cord occlusion, which decreases the amount of blood flow (therefore oxygen supply) to the fetus (Figure 22–25). Either the fetus squeezes the cord or rolls over onto it, transient pressure is exerted on the cord from compression, or the cord is around the neck of the fetus (Figure 22–26). An occasional or isolated variable deceleration is usually benign. Variable decelerations that are repetitive and begin to worsen during the course of labor are a cause for concern. Variable decelerations usually fall outside the normal FHR range and are classified as mild, moderate, and severe. They are acute in onset, vary in duration and intensity, and

abruptly disappear when the insult of cord com relieved (Figure 22–26).

With repetitive decelerations, one should su chal cord (umbilical cord around the neck) short occult prolapse of the cord. If this pattern becomes early in labor, variable decelerations may subsequently onstrate a slow return to baseline due to repetitive s Acid-base status of the fetus should be assessed since sarean birth, forceps birth, or vacuum extraction might indicated.

Decelerations that seem to deviate more from the baseline and widen are ominous and warrant further investigation. When they are prolonged and severe, a significant oxygen deficit develops from myocardial depression, resulting in hypoxemia and subsequent fetal metabolic acidosis (Freeman & Garite 1981). If hypoxia and acidosis are allowed to continue, fetal death may result.

With progressively worsening variable decelerations, an "overshoot" may occur. This is a blunt, smooth acceleration following the contraction and may be due to an attempt of the fetus to compensate for hypoxemia through sympathetic and adrenal mechanisms (Martin & Gingerich 1976).

Criteria for evaluation of variable decelerations vary from one author to another, and the very nature of these periodic changes can pose considerable anxiety regarding management. Dr. Robert Goodlin's "rule of the 60s" (in

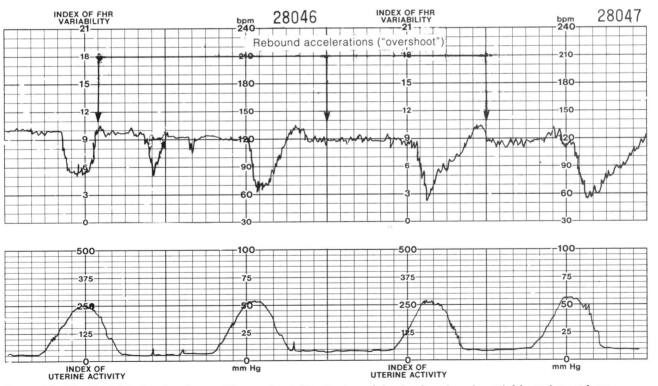

Figure 22–25   Variable decelerations with overshoot. The timing of the decelerations is variable and most have a sharp decline. A rebound acceleration (overshoot) occurs after most of the deceleration. Baseline FHR is 115 to 130 beats per minute. Nadir (lowest point) of decelerations is 55–80. LTV is absent; STV is present.

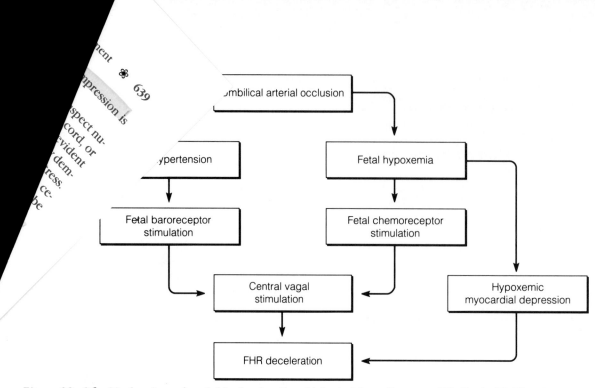

Figure 22–26 Mechanism of variable deceleration (Adapted from Freeman RK, Garite TJ: The physiologic basis of fetal monitoring, in Fetal Heart Rate Monitoring. Baltimore, MD: Williams & Wilkins, 1981, ch 2, p 15.)

Parer, 1984b, p 285) describes severe variable decelerations as having the following characteristics: variable decelerations below 60 beats per minute, 60 beats per minute below baseline FHR, or variable decelerations lasting more than 60 seconds in duration. These criteria seem to be the easiest to remember and perhaps the most practical.

Variable decelerations are frequently seen in labor when the membranes are ruptured. This decreases protection to the cord especially as the fetus descends down the birth canal. Variable decelerations usually do not warrant immediate birth unless a rising baseline, loss of variability, and other ominous signs accompany them. Repositioning the woman often corrects this type of pattern. If it does not, the clinician may attempt to alleviate this pattern by insertion of sterile saline via intrauterine catheter (amnioinfusion) to help take pressure off the umbilical cord.

Krebs et al (1983) describe various "atypical variable decelerations," noting that variable decelerations are probably innocuous unless these features are present (Figure 22–27). They noted that the presence of these atypical decelerations should be regarded as signs of fetal hypoxia. The nurse should be cognizant of pattern interpretation and be able to recognize severe and "atypical" variables. A point to remember, however, is that in the presence of normal variability of the FHR, these variables have not been found to be associated with fetal acidosis and poor outcome.

Prolonged decelerations are those in which the FHR decreases from the baseline for two or more minutes (Figure 22–28). They may occur suddenly, and if the pattern is promptly corrected, FHR variability will remain good. Rebound tachycardia is an ominous sign implying that a state of hypoxia has occurred. Prolonged decelerations are

frequently seen following paracervical or epidural block. These decelerations are thought to be due to fetal toxicity from fetal absorption of the drug through the uterine arteries or spasm of the uterine arteries resulting in decreased blood flow and hypoxia and reflex slowing of the FHR. Prolonged decelerations may often be seen with sudden occult or frank prolapse of the umbilical cord. When decelerations occur following administration of regional anesthesia, the woman should be turned on her side, evaluated for hypotension, and given a bolus of intravenous fluid (500 to 600 mL) to fill the dilated vascular space. This situation can usually be avoided by administering an IV bolus (800 to 900 mL) of lactated Ringer's or normal saline solution to the woman prior to administering regional anesthesia. Solutions containing dextrose should not be given, since they may cause fetal hyperglycemia.

Combined decelerations may be seen occasionally when two different deceleration patterns occur together. The specific types of patterns must then be ascertained. For instance, variable decelerations with a slow return to baseline should be differentiated from a combined pattern of variable and late decelerations. The former is a sign that the compression of the umbilical cord is worsening; the latter is an indication of cord compression *plus* utero-placental insufficiency. Initial management should be aimed at treatment of the most ominous pattern first (Shifrin 1985).

Sporadic decelerations usually have the appearance of variable decelerations, are unrelated to contractions, and are usually short-lived. They usually appear with reassuring FHR patterns and are apparently of little clinical significance (Shifrin 1985).

Unclassified decelerations are uniform, often re-

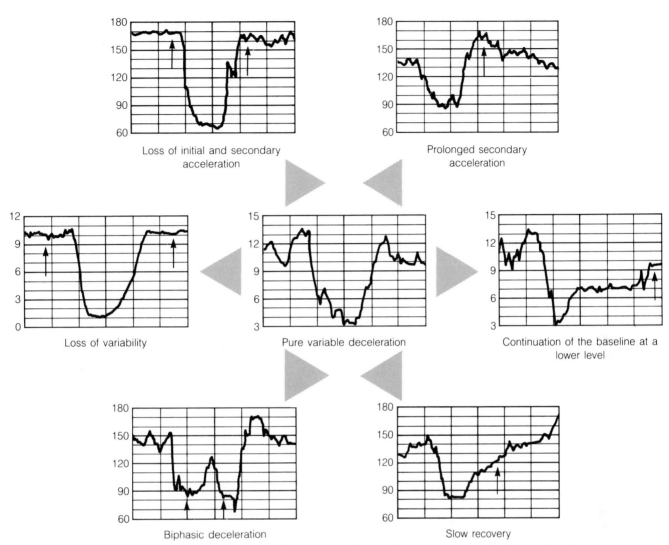

Figure 22–27 Atypical variable decelerations. The presence of any of these types of variable decelerations is very suggestive of fetal hypoxia, especially when variability is decreased. (From Krebs HB, Petrie RE, Dunn LJ: Atypical variable decelerations. Am J Obstet Gynecol 1983; 145:3:298.)

semble late or early decelerations, may be preceded by accelerations, and are not usually repetitive or in proportion to the amplitude or duration of contractions. Treatment is unnecessary if the variability is normal. Scalp sampling should be considered if variability is poor, and the possibility of a fetus with a congenital anomaly should be considered (Shifrin 1985).

Value of Electronic Fetal Monitoring

Despite several years of experience with fetal monitoring, the benefits in the normal labor are not yet conclusive. Certainly electronic monitoring has identified problems during labor that otherwise would have been undetected, and intervention has meant the survival of many infants who might otherwise have died during labor. In 1979 the Task Force of the National Institutes of Health recommended

that electronic fetal monitors be considered in the management of high-risk clients "whenever the potential benefits of the technique exceed the known risks."

High-risk women, who account for approximately 25% of the obstetric population, account for only about one-half of the perinatal morbidity and mortality. The remainder of the perinatal casualties come from the low-risk group (75% of the obstetric population) (Wilson & Schifrin 1980). Obviously, classification of women according to risk prior to labor is not predictive of whether or not pregnancy outcome will be positive or not.

Only seven randomized controlled clinical trial studies have compared auscultation to electronic fetal monitoring. Many clinicians believe these seven studies are insufficient to support the monitoring of all laboring women. They conclude that in a well-screened population the value of electronic monitoring over careful auscultation is of

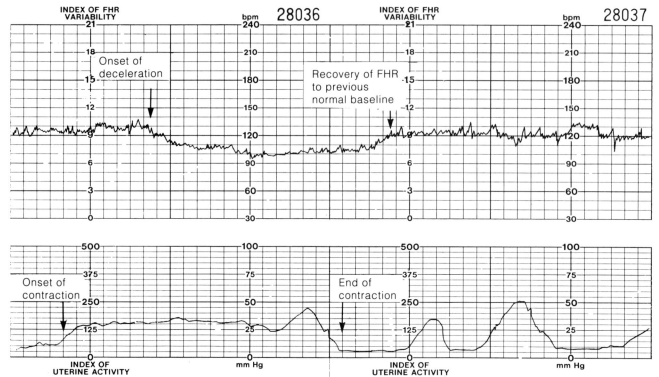

Figure 22–28   *The prolonged deceleration depicted lasts approximately 160 seconds. Note the prolonged contraction of 120 seconds. The deceleration begins after 80 seconds of uterine contraction. Note the beginning return of FHR 30 seconds after uterine tone returns to normal resting tone (contraction ends). An important aspect of this tracing is that STV is present despite the prolonged deceleration.*

little or no increased benefit. Others, however, prefer to use electronic fetal monitoring because it gives an indication of reassuring FHR patterns (normality) and an early indication of subtle FHR changes that might not be detected by auscultation by even the most experienced clinicians and nurses. In a study of almost 35,000 women, the authors concluded that "not all pregnancies, and particularly not those considered at low risk of perinatal complications, need continuous electronic fetal monitoring during labor" (Leveno et al 1986, p 33).

Thacker (1987), in a report regarding the efficacy of electronic fetal monitoring, reviewed the valuable information that can be gleaned from the pooled seven studies regarding clinical practice and research but stated that the seven studies were designed to assess the effectiveness of electronic monitoring with regard to reduction of specific outcomes. He further stated that although electronic fetal monitoring "might better identify an abnormal fetus" (p 29), outcomes may not be improved by intervention.

Although the seven trials failed to support the idea of improved perinatal outcome, Larson et al (1989), in a study comparing effectiveness of EFM with periodic auscultation, found that more accurate predictions about 5-minute Apgar scores were made with EFM than with auscultation, suggesting that "EFM may provide better information about neonatal well-being than does periodic auscultation"

(p 584). If these findings can be generalized, then one of the benefits of EFM may be its "ability to enable clinicians to make better predictions and judgment" (p 589) regarding neonatal well-being.

Psychologic Reactions to Electronic Monitoring

Many women have no knowledge of monitoring unless they have attended a prenatal class that dealt with this subject and even then the type of prenatal class may affect the perception of fetal heart rate monitoring. Hansen et al (1985) found that women who attended classes provided by medical or nursing staff preferred EFM, while women who attended nonmedical classes preferred auscultation (Syndal 1988).

Studies regarding reactions of women to electronic FHR monitoring reveal a variety of perceived advantages and disadvantages. Hansen et al (1985) found that women who had had a previous stillbirth or were currently in a high-risk pregnancy preferred EFM. While being monitored, women noted they felt constant reassurance that their baby was healthy and that problems would be identified quickly. Some women felt that use of the monitor helped them cope with contractions and even provided a diversion during labor. The monitor also provided a feeling of closeness to their baby and a sense of security. When questioned in the postpartum period, women noted that EFM promoted more involvement of the father during labor and birth (Syndal 1988).

Disadvantages of EFM were also experienced. Restricted mobility and discomfort caused by the belts were the most common complaints. In a study by Butani and Hodnett (1980) a mother noted: "The belts bothered me when I had a contraction—it's like laboring with a girdle on." Other women felt that the EFM increased their anxiety because of the monitor's frequent beeping and buzzing and a lack of understanding of how the monitor worked. The monitor became the focus of attention for many staff members and some women felt that they had less attention from the nursing staff because a monitor was in place (Syndal 1988).

Nurses should examine their own feelings about monitoring and give women the opportunity to talk about feelings regarding use of it. Nurses have influence in modifying attitudes and providing information. The nurse's attitudes influence the type of nursing care provided. If nurses express negativism or lack of confidence in the equipment they may not be able to incorporate this technology into their nursing assessment and therefore may give inadequate care and support to the woman.

The emphasis in maternity nursing is directed toward meeting the physical, emotional, and psychosocial needs of the woman while also being concerned for the fetus. Use of the monitor enhances maternal and fetal surveillance, but the nurse must not lose sight of the woman's needs and overrely on the monitor.

Role of the Nurse

Prior to application of the monitor, the nurse should fully explain to the woman the reason for it and the information that can be derived from its use. The nurse explains how the monitor can help identify the beginning of contractions and thus aid in breathing during the various phases of labor. An explanation alleviates apprehensions about equipment that may be totally unfamiliar to the woman. During labor it is advantageous to provide education regarding the use of the internal equipment, as the care giver may quickly decide to convert to this method as a result of examination findings. Women who are informed about the possibility of internal monitoring are better prepared if a quick decision must be made to apply an electrode or catheter.

After the monitor is applied, basic information should be recorded on the monitor strip. The data included are the date, time, woman's name, physician, hospital or agency number, age, gravida, para, estimated date of birth, membrane status, maternal vital signs, and current medical problems. As the monitor strip continues to run and care is provided, it is important that documentation of occurrences during labor be recorded not only in the nurse's notes on the woman's hospital record, but also on the fetal

Research Note

Clinical Application of Research

"When a nurse tells the patient that she is 'doing fine,' for all her good intentions, she [the nurse] may really be telling the patient that her viewpoint is not the one that counts" (Beaton 1990, p 406). In her study about nurse-patient interactions during labor, Janet Beaton found that patients and nurses communicated from two different centers of experience which seldom overlapped.

Recorded interactions between nurse and patient were analyzed for form (explicit or superficial message) and intent (more covert communication). Each interaction was also examined for three role dimensions: attentiveness, acquiescence, and presumptuousness. In the study, attentiveness pertains to using verbal modes to ascertain information about another person's experience. Acquiescence refers to allowing the other person's frame of reference to guide the course of the conversation. Presumptuousness involves the speaker's assumption of knowledge about the other person's experience.

In the role dimension of attentiveness, nurses and patients used verbal modes pertaining to their own experiences, not that of the other. However, the nurse was more apt to be attentive to the laboring woman's experience during noninstrumental care. Neither the patient nor the nurse acquiesced to the other's point of view, particularly in the area of coaching. The nurse was directive and did not acknowledge the woman's comments. Nurses were more presumptuous than patients, in both form and intent, during the labor experience. The nurse presumed to know the labor experience of the patient, and the patient accepted this presumption.

Critical Thinking Applied to Research
Strengths: Description of theoretical assumptions and methodology. Inclusion of interpretable tables and concise, clear explication of findings.
Concerns: The section on coding is complex and requires more than one reading to identify the structure of data analysis.

Beaton J: Dimensions of nurse patient roles in labor. *Health Care Women Internat* 1990; 11: 393.

monitor tracing. The following information should be included on the tracing:

1. Vaginal examinations (dilatation, effacement, station, and position)

2. Amniotomy, spontaneous rupture of membranes, presence and consistency of meconium

3. Maternal vital signs
4. Maternal position changes
5. Application of spiral electrode and intrauterine pressure catheter
6. Medications, oxygen (route and flow rate), IV fluids, regional blocks
7. Maternal behaviors (emesis, coughing, hiccups)
8. Fetal blood sampling, amnioinfusion
9. Voiding or catheterization
10. Time of birth, method, Apgar scores, cord blood gases

This information is helpful in subsequent evaluation of maternal and fetal status. The tracing is considered to be a legal part of the medical record and is submissible in court. All pertinent information should be appropriately documented.

Interpretation of FHR Tracing

As in interpreting ECG tracings, a systematic approach is required in evaluating FHR tracings to avoid misinterpretation of findings on the basis of inadequate or erroneous data. (See Table 22–6 for a method of systematic evaluation.) Developing a systematic approach to evaluation allows the nurse to make a more accurate and rapid assess-

---

PROCEDURE 22–4
Assessing for Amniotic Fluid

Nursing Action	**Rationale**
Objective: Assemble equipment.	
Gather Nitrazine test tape and a pair of disposable gloves.	Nitrazine test tape reacts to alkaline fluids and confirms presence of amniotic fluid.
May need microscope and glass slide if determining ferning of obtained fluid.	Microscope is used to detect ferning pattern.
Objective: Prepare woman.	
Explain the procedure, indications for the procedure, and information that may be obtained. Determine whether she has noted the escape of any clear fluid from the vagina.	Explanation of the procedure decreases anxiety and increases relaxation.
Objective: Test fluid.	
Prior to doing a vaginal exam that uses lubricant, put on gloves. With one gloved hand, spread the labia, and with the other hand place a small section (approx. 2 inches long) against the vaginal opening. You may also place the test tape against any clothing or pads that have been soaked with possible amniotic fluid.	Contamination of the Nitrazine test tape with lubricant can make the test unreliable.
Compare the color on the test tape to the guide on the back of the Nitrazine test tape container to determine the test results.	Enough fluid needs to be placed on the test tape to make it wet. Amniotic fluid is alkaline, and an alkaline fluid turns the Nitrazine Test Tape a dark blue. If the test tape remains a beige color, the test is negative for amniotic fluid.
Amniotic fluid may also be obtained by speculum exam. Some labor and birth nurses are using this technique.	
If fluid is present in sufficient amount to draw some into a syringe, a small amount of fluid can be placed on a glass slide, allowed to dry, and then looked at under a microscope. A ferning pattern confirms the presence of amniotic fluid. See Figure 5–4 for an example of ferning.	Obtaining a specimen by speculum exam reduces the contamination of the fluid with other substances such as blood.
Objective: Record information on client's record.	
Record on labor record, eg, SROM, Nitrazine positive	Nurse documents status of membranes, intact or ruptured.

Table 22–6 Evaluating FHR Tracings

Evaluation of the electronic monitor tracing begins by looking at the uterine contractions. Characteristics of the fetal heart rate are then evaluated.

Evaluate the uterine contraction pattern.

1. Determine the uterine resting tone.

2. Assess the contractions.

   What is the frequency?
   What is the duration?
   What is the intensity?

Evaluate the fetal heart rate tracing.

1. Determine the baseline.

   Is the baseline within normal range?
   Is there evidence of tachycardia?
   Is there evidence of bradycardia?

2. Determine FHR variability.

   Is short-term variability present or absent?
   Is long-term variability average? Minimal to absent? Moderate to marked?

3. Is a sinusoidal pattern present?

4. Assess for periodic changes

   Are accelerations present? Type?
   Do they meet the criteria for reactive NST?
   Are decelerations present?
   Are they uniform in shape? If so determine if they are early or late decelerations.
   Are they nonuniform in shape? If so determine if they are variable decelerations. Do they have a late component? Are they prolonged?

ment and to feel confident in communicating data to physicians and staff.

As a result of evaluation of the FHR tracing, the nurse makes decisions regarding care and the need for further assessment. The assumption is that labor and the response of the fetus to uterine contractions will be within normal parameters. When possible problems are identified, the nurse responds with needed interventions (see Tables 22–7 and 22–8). The nurse also needs to be constantly aware of changes in the maternal-fetal condition and how the change might affect the FHR tracing. A sound knowledge base regarding the cause of various FHR patterns is necessary so that appropriate assessments may be made and interventions carried out as needed.

All nurses who provide care to women in labor should be skilled in application of electronic monitoring equipment and assessment of baseline and periodic changes.

Since electronic fetal monitoring has become a "standard" in hospital care (if only intermittently used) and the nomenclature and criteria for classification of periodic changes has been established. The nurse should know these criteria and use appropriate terminology if interpretation, evaluation, documentation, and communication with other health team members. For example, if the FHR begins to decrease from the baseline at or after the peak of the contraction, inversely mirrors the contraction, has a uniform and smooth waveform, and returns to the baseline as the contraction wanes, the nurse can appropriately document and communicate to others that late decelerations are occurring. This is not a medical diagnosis but a recognition and documentation of an accepted standard of classification of FHR periodic change. Knowledge of EFM is necessary in order to attempt to correct nonreassuring patterns, document assessments correctly, communicate assessments to physicians, and provide follow-up management and evaluation to ensure optimum fetal outcome. (See Table 22–9.)

Additional Assessment Techniques

Scalp Stimulation Test

The scalp stimulation test is based on the knowledge that when the fetus is aroused or stimulated, there is an acceler-

Table 22–7 General Guidelines for Management of FHR Baseline Changes

FHR baseline	Nursing management
Normal	Evaluate maternal vital signs.
	Follow labor by means of vaginal examination at appropriate intervals.
	Assess and evaluate the quality of labor and FHR patterns.
	Document data and assessment of findings.
	Assure adequate hydration.
	Assist with maternal position changes.
Tachycardia	Report findings to physician/CNM.
	Assess maternal temperature.
	Assure adequate hydration.
	Reconfirm EDB.
	Monitor for changes in FHR pattern.
	Assist physician with fetal blood sampling if indicated (especially if decreased variability is present).
Bradycardia	Report findings to physician/CNM.
	Monitor for changes in FHR pattern (especially decreased variability).
	Assist physician with fetal blood sampling if indicated (especially with bradycardia on initial tracing).

Table 22−8 Guidelines for Management of Deceleration Patterns

Pattern	Nursing interventions
Early decelerations	Monitor for changes in FHR pattern. Evaluate for possible cephalopelvic disproportion if decelerations occur in early labor.

Variable decelerations
  Isolated or occasional
  Moderate
	Report findings to physician/CNM and document in chart.
	Provide explanation to woman and partner.
	Change maternal position to one in which FHR pattern is most improved.
	Discontinue oxytocin if it is being administered.
	Perform vaginal examination to assess for prolapsed cord or change in labor progress.
	Monitor FHR continuously to assess current status and for further changes in FHR pattern.

If variable decelerations are severe and uncorrectable and woman is in First stage	Report findings to physician/CNM and document in chart. Provide explanation to woman and partner. Prepare for probable cesarean birth.
Second stage labor	Prepare for vaginal birth unless baseline variability is decreasing and/or FHR is progressively rising, then cesarean, forceps, or vacuum birth if indicated. Assist physician with fetal scalp sampling if ordered Prepare for cesarean birth if scalp pH shows acidosis or downward trend.
Late decelerations	Report findings to physician/CNM and document in chart. Provide explanation to woman and partner. Monitor for further FHR changes. Maintain maternal position on left side. Maintain good hydration with IV fluids (normal saline or lactated Ringer's). Discontinue oxytocin if it is being administered. Administer oxygen by face mask at 7 to 10 L/min. Monitor maternal blood pressure and pulse for signs of hypotension; possibly increase flow rate of IV fluids to treat hypotension. Follow physician's orders for treatment for hypotension if present. Increase IV fluids to maintain volume and hydration (normal saline or lactated Ringer's). Assess labor progress (dilatation and station). Assist physician with fetal blood sampling: If pH stays above 7.25, physician will continue monitoring and resample; if pH shows downward trend (between 7.25 and 7.20) or is below 7.20, prepare for birth by most expeditious means.
Late decelerations with tachycardia and/or decreasing variability	Report findings to physician/CNM and document in chart. Maintain maternal position on left side. Administer oxygen by face mask at 7−10 L/min. Discontinue oxytocin if it is being administered. Assess maternal blood pressure and pulse. Increase IV fluids (normal saline or lactated Ringer's). Assess labor progress (dilatation and station). Prepare for immediate cesarean birth. Explain plan of treatment to woman and partner. Assist physician with fetal blood sampling (if ordered).
Prolonged decelerations	Perform vaginal examination to rule out prolapsed cord or to determine progress in labor status. Change maternal position as needed to try to alleviate decelerations. Discontinue oxytocin if it is being administered. Notify physician/CNM of findings/initial interventions and document in chart. Provide explanation to woman and partner. Increase IV fluids (normal saline or lactated Ringer's). Administer tocolytic if hypertonus noted and ordered by physician/CNM. Anticipate normal FHR recovery following deceleration if FHR previously normal. Anticipate intervention if FHR previously abnormal or deceleration lasts >3 minutes.

Table 22–8 (*continued*)

Pattern	Nursing interventions
Combined decelerations	See management guidelines for individual patterns and manage according to most ominous pattern first. Report findings to physician/CNM and document in chart.
Sporadic/Unclassified decelerations with average variability	Report findings to physician/CNM and document in chart. No treatment necessary.
with poor variability	Assist physician with scalp sampling if ordered. Administer oxygen by face mask at 7–10 L/min. Provide explanation to woman and partner. Consider possibility of birth of baby with congenital anomalies and notify pediatrician.

ation of the FHR if the fetus is not compromised in some way. The scalp stimulation test (SST) may be used when there is a nonreassuring FHR pattern present. To perform the test, the nurse, CNM, or obstetrician stimulates the fetal head while performing a sterile vaginal examination. This pressure usually precipitates a fetal heart rate acceleration if the fetus is not compromised. The SST requires that the fetal head be firmly pressing on the cervix and that there be sufficient dilatation of the cervix to apply pressure on the fetal head.

Monitoring of Fetal Acid-Base Status

Fetal Scalp Sampling When nonreassuring or confusing FHR patterns are noted, it becomes necessary to seek additional information regarding the acid-base status of the fetus. This is accomplished by means of fetal blood sampling, which is usually done from the fetal scalp but may be performed on the fetus in the breech position (Brady et al 1989).

Boylan and Parisi (1989) suggest that fetal blood sampling may be of benefit in the following situations:

Presence of thick meconium in the amniotic fluid (Thick meconium may be associated with fetal hypoxia, and the development of meconium aspiration syndrome is associated with the presence of acidosis at birth.)

Absent short-term variability

Decreased short-term variability that is present when the fetus is first monitored or that develops in the absence of administration of CNS depressants to the mother

Later decelerations that persist for more than 10 minutes and do not respond to treatment measures

Variable decelerations with decreased or absent short-term variability

FHR patterns that are difficult to interpret

Table 22–9 Classification of Fetal Heart Rate Patterns*

	Baseline features	Periodic features
Reassuring	Average variability Stable baseline rate	Absent decelerations Early decelerations "Mild" variable decelerations Uniform accelerations
Nonreassuring Suspicious	Tachycardia (>150) Bradycardia Decreased variability	Decelerations absent
Threatening	Average variability Stable baseline rate Rising baseline rate	Late decelerations Variable decelerations
Ominous	Absent variability Unstable baseline rate Bradycardia Tachycardia	Late decelerations Variable decelerations with overshoot
Chronic	Absent variability Tachycardia (>150)	Variable decelerations with overshoot

* *Source: Shifrin BS:* Exercises in Fetal Monitoring. *Vol 1. Los Angeles:bpm inc., 1985, p 3 with permission of CV Mosby Co.*

Fetal Blood Sampling Procedure Equipment needed for fetal blood sampling is available in sterile disposable trays. Items included are: heparinized capillary tubes; a short capillary tube holder; a 2 mm blade on long handle; a conical beveled endoscope; clay sealant; silicone gel; long sponge swabs. An extra light source is needed. The woman's vulva and perineum should be thoroughly cleansed with povidone-iodine solution (Betadine) and sterile drapes arranged. A conical vaginal endoscope is inserted into the vagina and through the cervix to visualize the fetal site to be sampled (Figure 22–29). Working through the endoscope, the physician cleanses the site to remove vernix, blood, and amniotic fluid. Silicone gel is then applied to the site to provide a surface for the formation of a globule of blood. The site is punctured with a 2 × 2 mm

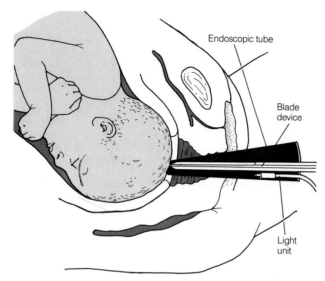

Figure 22–29 Technique of obtaining fetal blood from scalp during labor (From Creasy RK, Parer JT: Prenatal care and diagnosis. In Rudolph AM [editor]: Pediatrics, 16th ed. Englewood Cliffs, NJ: Appleton-Century-Crofts, 1977.)

microscalpel. A small amount (0.25 mL) of blood is then collected in a long heparinized capillary tube and immediately assessed for pH and base deficit values. Two or three samples should be collected during each procedure to confirm reliability of values. pH and base deficit determinations should be readily available in 10 to 15 minutes for this procedure to be of value.

The clotting mechanism is compromised when pH is lowered; therefore oozing at the site may occur for a period of time. Because loss of even minimal amounts of blood may be disastrous to the fetus, pressure is applied to the puncture site throughout two maternal contractions, then the site is observed through a third contraction. After the procedure the woman is observed for vaginal bleeding to assure that what may appear to be heavy bloody show is not a fetal hemorrhage from the puncture site.

The major fetal problem that may occur with fetal blood sampling is hemorrhage, especially if the fetus has blood dyscrasia such as hemophilia or von Willebrand's disease. In addition, the use of a vacuum extractor to assist in vaginal birth following numerous punctures may be associated with bleeding problems. Infection of the scalp may occur about 1% of the time (Boylan & Parisi 1989).

Fetal Blood Sample Results Normal pH values during labor are at or above 7.25, with 7.20 to 7.24 considered preacidotic. Values below 7.20 indicate serious acidosis. Most clinicians consider a pH value of 7.25 or more as normal and reassuring and resample only as indicated by FHR variability or periodic pattern. Values between 7.20 and 7.25 are evaluated on the basis of several factors and sampling is usually repeated within 15 to 20 minutes (Depp

1990) to observe the trend in pH and base deficit. When a low pH is present, it is important to distinguish between respiratory and metabolic acidosis because management of each situation is different. Respiratory acidosis is indicated by a pH below 7.25 and a base deficit less than −6. Respiratory acidosis is associated with cord compression or uterine hyperstimulation, and the fetus may benefit from intrauterine resuscitation. Metabolic acidosis is indicated by a pH less than 7.25 and a base deficit of greater than −6. Metabolic acidosis is more frequently associated with a chronic condition of the fetus and indicates the need for immediate birth (Boylan & Parisi 1989). Values below 7.20 are considered acidotic and warrant immediate birth (Depp 1990; Goyert et al 1989).

Associated Factors Some FHR patterns seem to be associated with abnormal fetal acid-base status. Short-term and long-term variability correlate better with fetal pH than deceleration patterns do. If STV and LTV are present, the pH will be in the normal range. If STV is present, the fetal pH is usually normal even in the presence of late decelerations. If STV is absent, however, the risk of acidosis increases. When STV is absent and variable decelerations occurring, the pH will be in the preacidotic range. If late decelerations occur with no STV present, the pH will probably be in the acidotic range (Campbell et al 1986).

These findings are of particular significance when nonreassuring FHR patterns are observed and fetal acid-base determination is not feasible. One can be reassured that the fetus is not acidotic in almost 100% of cases if the variability remains normal (Parer 1984a). A pH above 7.25 predicts that the fetus will be vigorous in about 90% of cases; a pH below 7.15 predicts a depressed fetus with only 80% reliability (Parer 1984a). Fetal blood sampling seems unnecessary when variability is normal, since the fetus will be vigorous despite the pH value.

Although not universally used at present, it is possible to monitor fetal pH continuously by a pH electrode attached to the fetal scalp tissue. This electrode does not measure fetal blood pH level per se but rather the subcutaneous tissue pH level. In hypoxia, an increase in alpha-adrenergic activity occurs initially with accompanying fetal hypertension, causing acidosis to occur in peripheral tissue more rapidly than in the central circulation. Conversely, as hypoxia is corrected, there may be a recovery lag of about 5 minutes in the pH value in the peripheral tissue (Boyland & Paris 1989).

Considerable skill is required for both continuous and intermittent fetal blood sampling. As yet, even intermittent sampling is not widely done due to the difficulty of the procedure and the scarcity of blood gas microanalyzers on or near the birth unit to obtain immediate results.

Percutaneous Umbilical Blood Sampling In this new fetal assessment technique, fetal blood is obtained from the umbilical cord by means of a needle inserted into the maternal abdomen. The procedure can be performed at the bedside to assess fetal acid-base status during labor when fetal blood sampling may not be feasible and FHR patterns are confusing or worrisome (Hobbins et al 1985). See Chapter 20 for a description of the procedure. The procedure is also most helpful in the management of women with idiopathic thrombocytopenic purpura. Early assessment of fetal platelet count using this procedure may allow these women to give birth vaginally rather than by cesarean when the fetus cannot be assessed by fetal blood sampling because of inadequate dilatation of the cervix.

Cord Blood Analysis at Birth   In cases where there have been significant abnormal FHR patterns noted prior to birth, meconium-stained amniotic fluid, or a depressed infant at birth, analysis of umbilical cord blood may be done immediately after birth to assess the infants' respiratory status. The cord is usually clamped before the infant takes its first breath to provide evaluation of blood gas status before the infant interacts with the extrauterine environ-ment, since values can change after only a few seconds of neonatal breathing.

An 8- to 10-inch segment of the umbilical cord is double-clamped and cut, and a small amount of blood is aspirated from one of the umbilical arteries (arterial blood seems to provide the most reliable indication of blood gas status and fetal tissue pH). Blood is collected in a heparinized syringe unless it is to be analyzed immediately; it should not be allowed to remain in the segment of cord longer than 30 minutes. As noted by Depp (Chez & Depp 1987), the only reason for not doing routine cord blood analysis is the added expense. Other clinicians may collect a segment of cord and only send samples if the Apgar score is below 7 at 5 minutes. In this instance, values might be used to clarify the cause for a low Apgar score while minimizing any medicolegal exposure and expense. Determination of pH and base deficit values can differentiate whether fetal acidemia is due to hypoperfusion of the placenta or cord compression.

❀ ❀

KEY CONCEPTS

Intrapartal assessment includes attention to both physical and psychologic parameters of the laboring woman, assessment of the fetus, and ongoing assessment for conditions that place the woman and her fetus at increased risk.

A sterile vaginal examination determines status of fetal membranes, cervical dilatation and effacement, and fetal presentation, position, and station.

Uterine contractions may be assessed by palpation or by electronic monitoring.

Labor progress may be objectively evaluated using a Friedman graph, which plots cervical dilatation and fetal descent.

Leopold's maneuvers provide a systematic evaluation of fetal presentation, position, and lie.

The fetal heart rate may be assessed by auscultation (with a fetoscope) or electronic monitoring.

Electronic fetal monitoring is accomplished by indirect ultrasound or by direct methods that require the placement of a spiral electrode on the fetal presenting part.

Indications for electronic monitoring include fetal, maternal, and uterine factors; presence of pregnancy complications; regional anesthesia; and elective monitoring.

Baseline FHR refers to the range of FHR observed between contractions during a ten-minute period of monitoring.

The normal baseline range of FHR is 120 to 160 beats per minute.

Baseline changes of the FHR include tachycardia, bradycardia, and variability.

Tachycardia is defined as a rate of 160 beats per minute or more for a ten-minute segment of time.

Bradycardia is defined as a rate of less than 120 beats per minute for a ten-minute segment of time.

❀ ❀

References

Boesel RR et al: Umbilical cord blood studies help assess fetal respiratory status. *Contemp OB/GYN* November 1986; 28: (Medical Economics Co. reprint, p 1).

Boylan PC, Parisi VM: Acid-Base Physiology in the Fetus. In Creasy RK, Resnik R (editors): *Maternal-Fetal Medicine: Principles and Practice,* 2nd ed. Philadelphia: Saunders, 1989.

Brady K et al: Reliability of fetal buttock blood sampling in assessing the acid-base balance of the breech fetus. *Obstet Gynecol* 1989; 74:886.

Butani P, Hodnett E: Mothers' perceptions of their labor experiences. *Matern Child Nurs J* 1980; 9(2):72.

Campbell WA, Vintzileos AM, Nochimson DJ: Intrauterine versus extrauterine management/resuscitation of the fetus/neonate. *Clin Obstet Gynecol* 1986; 29(1):33.

Chez RA, Depp R: What cord blood analysis tells you. (Clinical dialogue). *Comtemp OB/GYN* November 1987; 30:43.

Depp R: Clinical evaluation of fetal status. In Scott JR et al: *Danforth's Obstetrics and Gynecology.* Philadelphia: Lippincott, 1990.

Devoe LD et al: Monitoring intrauterine pressure during active labor. *J Reprod Med* October 1989; 34:811.

Feinstein, SJ et al: Sinusodial fetal heart rate pattern after administration of nalbuphine hydrochloride: A case report. *Am J Obstet Gynecol* 1986; 154(1):159.

Freeman RK, Garite TJ: *Fetal Heart Rate Monitoring.* Baltimore: Williams & Wilkins, 1981.

Friedman EA: An objective method of evaluating labor. *Hosp Pract* 1970; 5:82.

Fukushima T et al: A beltless tocodynamometer: A preliminary report. *Obstet Gynecol* May 1989; 73:823.

Goyert GL, Sokol RJ, D'Angelo LJ: Practical fetal monitoring during labor. In Dilts PV, Sciarri JJ (editors): *Gynecology and Obstetrics.* Vol 2. 1989.

Hansen PK et al: Maternal attitudes to fetal monitoring. *Eur J Obstet Gynecol Reprod Biol* 1985; 20:43.

Hatjis CG, Meis PJ: Sinusoidal fetal heart rate pattern associated with butorphanol administration. *Obstet Gynecol* 1986; 67(3):377.

Hobbins JC et al: Percutaneous umbilical blood sampling. *Am J Obstet Gynecol* 1985; 152(1):1.

Hon EH: *An Introduction to Fetal Heart Rate Monitoring* 2nd ed. Los Angeles: University of Southern California School of Medicine, 1976.

Hon EH, Quilligan EJ: The classification of fetal heart rate: II. A revised working classification. *Conn Med* 1967; 31:779.

Krebs HB, Petrie RE, Dunn LJ: Atypical variable deceleration. *Am J Obstet Gynecol* 1983; 142:297.

Larson EB, et al: Fetal monitoring and predictions by clinicians: Observations during a randomized clinical trial in very low birth weight infants. *Obstet Gynecol* October 1989; 74:584.

Martin CB, Gingerich B: Factors affecting the fetal heart rate: Genesis of FHR patterns. *JOGNN* 1976; 5(suppl):305s.

NAACOG Statement. Nursing Responsibilities in Implementing Intrapartum Fetal Heart Rate Monitoring. October 1988.

NAACOG: *Fetal Heart Rate Auscultation.* OGN Nursing Practice Resource. March 1990.

Parer JT: Fetal acid-base balance. In Creasy RK, Resnik R (editors): *Maternal-Fetal Medicine.* Philadelphia, Saunders, 1984a, pp. 321.

Parer JT: Fetal Heart Rate. In Creasy RK, Resnik R (editors): *Maternal-Fetal Medicine: Principles and Practice.* Philadelphia, Saunders, 1989.

Parer JT: Fetal Heart Rate. In Creasy RK, Resnik R (editors): *Maternal-Fetal Medicine.* Philadelphia: Saunders, 1984b. p 285.

Schneider EP, Tropper PJ: The variable deceleration, prolonged deceleration, and sinusoidal fetal heart rate. *Clin Obstet Gynecol* 1986; 29(1):64.

Shifrin BS: *Exercises in Fetal Monitoring.* Vol 1. Los Angeles; bpm inc, 1985.

Strong TH, Paul RH: Intrapartum evaluation of an intrauterine pressure transducer. *Obstet Gynecol* March 1989; 73:432.

Syndal SH: Responses of laboring women to fetal heart rate monitoring. *J Nurse-Midwifery* September/October 1988; 33:208.

Thacker SB: The efficacy of intrapartum electronic fetal monitoring. *Am J Obstet Gynecol* November 1987; 156:4.

Wilson RW, Shifrin BS: Is any pregnancy low risk? *Obstet Gynecol* 1980; 55:653.

Additional Readings

Chez RA: Effective labor on intelligence of the offspring. *Obstet Gynecol* 1991; 77:5:777.

Foley MR et al: Development and initial experience with a manually controlled spring wire device ("Cordostat") to aid in difficult funipuncture. *Obstet Gynecol* March 1991; 77:471.

Fukushima T et al: An improved spiral electrode applicator system for fetal heart rate monitoring *Obstet Gynecol* March 1991; 77:475.

Lawson A: Whose side are we on now? Ethical issues in social research and medical practice. *Soc Sci Med* 1991; 32:5:591.

Miller-Slade D et al: Acoustic stimulation–induced fetal response compared to traditional nonstress testing. *JOGNN* March/April 1991; 20:160.

Naidoo DP et al: Continuous electrocardiographic monitoring in hypertensive crisis in pregnancy. *Am J Obstet Gynecol* February 1991; 164:530.

Parer JT, Livingston EG: What is fetal distress? *Am J Obstet Gynecol* 1990; 162:1421.

Sherer DM et al: Fetal panting: Yet another response of the external vibratory acoustic stimulation test. *Am J Obstet Gynecol* February 1991; 164:591.

CHAPTER 23

The Family in Childbirth:

Needs and Care

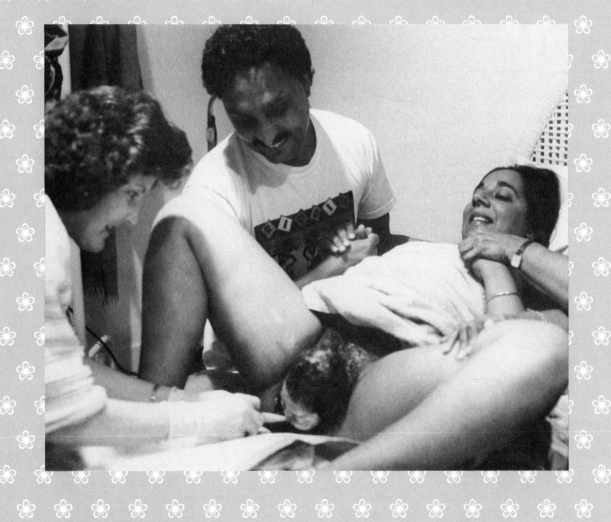

OBJECTIVES

Compare the advantages and disadvantages of alternative settings for labor and birth.

Identify options that women and their families have during the intrapartal period.

Identify the data base to be obtained when a woman is admitted to a birthing unit and the associated nursing care.

Discuss nursing interventions to meet the psychologic and physiologic needs of the woman during each stage of labor and birth.

Integrate knowledge of nursing care of the healthy woman and baby in the intrapartal period through use of the nursing process.

Summarize immediate nursing care of the newborn following birth.

Discuss management of birth in less-than-optimal situations.

❀ ❀

Maybe shock more than fear. All that preparation, but then you have to do it. This is not pretend. (Harriette Hartigan, Women in Birth)

It is time for a child to be born. The waiting is over, labor has begun. The dreams and wishes of the past months fade as the expectant parents face the reality of the tasks of childbearing and childrearing that are ahead.

The couple is about to undergo one of the most meaningful and stressful events in their life together. The adequacy of their preparation for childbirth will now be tested, as will the coping mechanisms, communication, and support systems that they have established as a couple. In particular, the childbearing woman may feel that her psychologic and physical limits are about to be challenged.

Throughout the pregnancy, the couple has been involved in collecting information and making decisions about their childbearing experience. Many expectant parents are well-informed health care consumers who request alternatives to traditional maternity care. As a result, many hospitals now offer a variety of birthing experiences.

Maternity nurses have kept pace with the changing philosophy of childbirth and continue to bring personal caring and comfort to an increasingly high technology area (Hodnett & Osborn 1989). Today's maternity nurse in the birth setting uses the full spectrum of nursing skills in working with childbearing families. Maternity nurses assess clients; gather information; provide information and teaching so that couples can make informed choices; function as a client advocate; collaborate with other health care professionals; ensure that they function within current nursing standards of care; and communicate with physicians and certified nurse-midwives. Maternity nurses have become an integral part of family-centered care as they provide support, encouragement, and safe, caring nursing management.

Childbirth is usually joyous, but sometimes it is a time of grief and sadness. The needs of the childbearing couple in the event of crisis during or after labor and birth are discussed in later chapters. This chapter describes the needs and nursing care of the family during normal labor and birth.

During the Intrapartal Period

Maternity nurses will find that using the nursing process enhances their ability to provide individualized family-centered care during the intrapartal period. By applying the nursing process, nursing skills and theory, and their knowledge about childbirth, maternity nurses can function in a variety of birthing settings.

❀ *APPLYING THE NURSING PROCESS* ❀

Nursing Assessment

When the laboring woman is admitted to the birthing unit, the first member of the health care team that she and her partner encounter is usually the nurse. The accuracy of the nurse's admission assessment of the woman's physical and psychologic status is significant in determining the quality of the childbearing experience the couple will have. The nursing assessment is the basis for determining initial management of care by other members of the health care team.

The initial nursing assessment usually focuses on the imminence of birth and the well-being of the fetus. Careful assessment of labor progress will help the nurse determine the priorities of care that must follow. After the safety of the mother and fetus have been assured, the nursing assessment focuses on the woman's coping mechanisms and her support system. The nurse also determines the goals the couple have established for their birth experience.

During labor, the nurse continually reassesses maternal and fetal physical status and the couple's coping mechanisms in order to intervene appropriately.

Nursing Diagnosis

Nursing diagnoses are based on physical and psychosocial assessments of the childbearing woman. Common nursing diagnoses in the intrapartal period include the following:

- Pain related to the birth process
- High risk for ineffective individual coping related to ineffective labor coping strategies and/or unanticipated events
- Knowledge deficit related to breathing techniques and measures to increase comfort during labor and birth

Nursing Plan and Implementation

Once nursing diagnoses are formulated, the nurse must determine which are most significant to the woman's well-being. Priorities of care differ for every woman admitted to the birthing unit. While physiologic alterations usually form the basis for priorities of care when labor is progressing rapidly or high-risk factors are identified, this may not be the situation with a healthy woman admitted in early labor. After the safety of the mother and fetus have been assured, important factors that must be considered in developing the nursing plan of care include the woman's goals for her birth experience, her coping mechanisms, and the strength of her support systems. For example, the 16-year-old single nullipara who has had no prenatal care and comes to the hospital alone has different needs from the couple who planned the pregnancy and attended prepared childbirth classes. Nursing diagnoses and priorities for the plan of care will be quite different in these two situations. The nurse may be the 16-year-old girl's only support, but the couple may have only minimal need for the nurse's support.

A major challenge for the nurse is helping laboring women to achieve realistic goals for their birth experience. Each woman is admitted to the birthing unit at a different phase in the laboring process and with a different level of wellness. The nurse may not have time to assess the choice of birthing options of a multipara who is about to give birth on admission or to support the goal of unmedicated labor in a primigravida who develops severe PIH during her labor. Regardless of the individual factors each woman or couple brings to the labor, the nurse and the woman or couple work together to achieve a safe labor and birth.

To be effective, the nurse must use many types of interventions during labor and birth. These include technical interventions; interventions that ensure that the birth setting is safe and comfortable for the woman and her baby; communication techniques for use with the laboring woman, her support person(s), and other members of the health team; and teaching techniques.

Evaluation

Evaluation of the effectiveness of nursing intervention is ongoing as the nurse continually reassesses the woman. Evaluation results in a constant cycle of nursing process application.

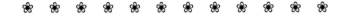

Care of the Woman and Her Partner Upon Admission to the Birthing Unit

The woman is instructed during her prenatal visits to come to the birthing unit if any of the following occur:

- Rupture of the amniotic membranes
- Regular, frequent uterine contractions (nulliparas, 5 to 10 minutes apart for one hour; multiparas, 10 to 15 minutes apart for one hour)
- Any vaginal bleeding

Early admission means less discomfort for the laboring woman when traveling to the birth setting and more time to prepare for the birth. Sometimes the labor is advanced and birth is imminent, but usually the woman is in early labor at admission.

The earlier the woman is admitted to the birth setting, however, the longer the labor seems to both her and her care givers. This may increase the likelihood that interventions (such as augmentation of labor) will ultimately be used.

Special Nursing Considerations

Informed Consent

When the woman enters the health care facility, she may be facing a number of unfamiliar procedures that health care providers tend to take for granted as routine practice. It is important to remember that all women have the right to determine what happens to their bodies. *The client's informed consent should be obtained prior to any procedure that involves touching her body.* Informed consent requires that the woman be given information about the procedure or care, its reasons, potential benefits and risks, and possible alternatives. In most instances involving the nurse as the care giver, the informed consent may be verbal. Each nurse needs to be aware of the requirements of the state and the individual hospital (Geiser & Fraley 1989). (See Chapter 1 for additional discussion.)

To give informed consent, whether verbal or written, the woman should be considered a rational adult and should not be under the influence of any medication that may affect her ability to make decisions. Furthermore, the laboring woman should be considered as a "special subject" with regard to the informed consent process, as she is particularly likely to be distracted (by pain) or to feel obligated to comply, either by a hope that an experimental procedure will reduce her pain or improve her progress in labor, or by a fear of compromising her own care or the care of her baby if she does not agree to participate (van Lier & Roberts 1986).

Admission Environment

The manner in which the woman and her partner are greeted by the maternity nurse influences the course of the woman's stay. It should be remembered that the sudden environment change and sometimes impersonal technical aspects of the admission procedures can produce additional sources of stress.

"When I realized I was in labor, I cried for fear of hurting, fear of the unknown, fear of the end of my childhood." (Harriette Hartigan, Women in Birth)

If a woman is greeted in a brusque, harried manner, her anxiety usually increases, and she is less likely to look to the nurse for support. A calm, pleasant manner promotes calmness in the woman and indicates to her that what she has to say is important. It helps instill in the couple a sense of confidence in the staff's ability to provide quality care during this critical time.

❦ *APPLYING THE NURSING PROCESS* ❦

Initial Nursing Assessments

Following the initial greeting, the woman is taken into the labor or birthing room. Some couples prefer to remain together during the admission process, and others prefer to have the partner wait outside. As the nurse helps the woman undress and get into a hospital gown or her own personal gown, the nurse can begin conversing with her to develop rapport and establish the nursing data base.

Assessment of Labor Status

The nurse immediately assesses the status of the woman's labor to develop nursing diagnoses and priorities of care in the admission process. Information that the nurse must obtain includes the following:

- Gravidity, parity
- Time of onset of true labor (generally defined as when contractions began to be five minutes apart)

- Frequency and duration of contractions on admission
- Status of membranes
- Presence of bloody show versus bleeding
- Estimated date of birth (EDB)
- Any significant prenatal history
- Present coping behaviors with contractions

See Table 23–1 for indicators of normal labor process.

On admission the woman and her support person are intensely focused on the changes occurring in her body and are eager and relieved to share this information with the nurse. They frequently share essential information about the status of the woman's labor before the nurse has an opportunity to ask specific questions about it. In many birthing settings the nursing staff has access to the woman's prenatal records and will know her gravidity, parity, EDB, and any significant prenatal history before she arrives on the unit. With the couple's cooperation, the nurse can collect a seemingly overwhelming amount of data very quickly without appearing rushed.

Assessment of Fetal and Maternal Vital Signs

After the laboring woman has changed into a gown, she is helped into bed for completion of the admission assessment. From the time the woman enters the birth setting, it is critical to remember that two people must be monitored; the laboring woman and the unborn baby. One of the vital signs to assess immediately after the laboring woman is in bed is the fetal heart rate (FHR). (Detailed information on monitoring the fetal heart rate is presented in Chapter 22). If her membranes have ruptured prior to admission, a description of the color of the amniotic fluid is also important in determining the well-being of the fetus.

Fluid that is stained dark green due to the presence of meconium and has a thick consistency (like pea soup) due to a decreased volume of amniotic fluid is associated

Table 23–1	Indicators of Normal Labor Process on Admission
Indicator	**Normal characteristics**
Uterine contractions	Frequency of not less than 2 minutes Duration of less than 75 seconds Uterine relaxation between contractions Most intense discomfort occurs only with contractions. (Some women, especially those with occiput posterior position, complain of less intense lower abdominal and/or back pain between contractions.)
Fetal heart rate	Rate 120 to 160 with average variability Absence of variable or late decelerations
Maternal vital signs	B/P below 140/90 or less than +30/+15 above prepregnancy readings Pulse 60 to 100 Temperature between 97.8 and 99.6F
If membranes ruptured	Fluid clear without odor

TEACHING GUIDE

What to Expect During Labor

Assessment As each woman is admitted into the birthing area, the nurse assesses the woman's knowledge regarding the childbirth experience. The woman's knowledge base will be affected by previous births, attendance at childbirth education classes, and the amount of information she has been able to gather during her pregnancy by asking questions or reading. The nurse also assesses the factors that affect communication and anxiety level. Labor process is assessed so that decisions regarding what to teach and the time available for teaching can be ascertained. If the woman is in early labor and she needs additional information, the nurse proceeds with teaching.

Nursing Diagnosis The key nursing diagnosis probably will be: Knowledge deficit related to nursing care during labor.

Nursing Plan and Implementation The teaching focuses on information regarding the assessments and support the woman will receive during labor.

Client Goals At the completion of the teaching the woman will be able to do the following:

1. Verbalize the assessments the nurse will complete during labor.
2. Discuss the support/comfort measures that are available.

Teaching Plan

Content Aspects of the admission process include the following:

- Abbreviated history
- Physical assessment (maternal vital signs [VS], fetal heart rate [FHR], contraction status, status of membranes)
- Assessment of uterine contractions (frequency, duration, intensity)
- Orientation to surroundings
- Introductions to other staff that will be assisting her

Present aspects of ongoing physical care, such as when to expect assessment of maternal VS, FHR, and contractions.

If electronic fetal monitor is used, orient the woman to how it works and the information that it provides. Orient woman to the sights and sounds of the monitor. Explain what the "normal" data will look like and what characteristics are being watched for.

Be sure to note that the assessments will increase as the labor progresses; about the time that the woman would like to be left alone (transition phase), the assessments increase in order to help keep the mother and baby safe by noting any changes from the normal course.

Explain the vaginal examination and what information can be obtained.

Review comfort techniques that may be used in labor. First ascertain what the woman thinks will be effective in promoting comfort.

Teaching Method Provide information on the basic assessment and care activities. Allow time for questions and discussion as labor progress permits.

Bring a fetal monitor into the birthing room and demonstrate how it works.

Use a cervical dilatation chart to illustrate the amount of dilatation.

Discussion

(continued)

TEACHING GUIDE (continued)

Teaching Plan

Review the breathing techniques that the woman has learned so the nurse will be able to support her technique.	Ask woman to demonstrate technique.
Review comfort/support measures such as positioning, back rub, effleurage, touch, distraction techniques, ambulation, etc.	Discussion
If the woman is in early labor, offer to give her a tour of the birthing area.	Provide a tour of birthing area, explaining equipment and routines. Include partner.
Evaluation: At the end of this teaching session the woman will be able to verbalize the assessments that will occur during her labor and will be able to discuss comfort/support measures that may be used.	

---

with meconium aspiration syndrome in those infants who have such fluid and who also become acidotic during labor (Boylan 1990). Consequently, these infants must be watched with special care during labor.

Assessment of the fetus helps determine whether the rest of the admission process can proceed at a more leisurely pace or whether additional interventions have higher priority. For example, FHR of 90 beats per minute on auscultation or meconium-stained amniotic fluid are assessments indicating that a fetal monitor should be applied promptly to obtain additional data. The admission process will continue after these assessments are completed.

Throughout the admission it is important to have the woman indicate when a contraction is beginning; thus, contraction frequency, duration, and intensity are assessed as other data are gathered. The nurse needs to be aware that contractions may decrease in frequency with the trip to the birth unit. The contractions will resume when the woman is comfortable and relaxed again. The status of uterine contractions on admission helps the nurse determine the priorities of care. Contractions that are more than four minutes apart, with a duration of less than 40 seconds, are usually associated with early labor, and the admission process can usually progress in a leisurely manner. If the contractions are three minutes apart or less, with a duration of more than 45 seconds, and there have been previous labors, the admission needs to proceed more quickly.

Additional vital signs to assess are the woman's blood pressure, pulse, respiration, and oral temperature.

Assessment of the Couple's Preparation for Labor

Other necessary admission data require assessment of the woman's coping mechanisms, support system, and goals and expectations for her birthing experience. Examples of information collected from these assessments include the following:

- Attendance at childbirth education classes and if so, what kind (Lamaze, Bradley, etc)
- Name of support person
- Any expectations for the labor and birth experience that the woman discussed with her physician/nurse-midwife, such as no prep or enema, siblings in attendance, etc.

Some childbirth education classes and physician/nurse-midwives offer couples a checklist of options about their birthing experience. Couples who use the checklists are encouraged to share their choices with the nurse on admission (see Figure 17–2).

Vaginal Examinations

If the contraction pattern and behavioral response of the woman have not indicated rapid progress of labor, the vaginal exam can be delayed until this time. (If there are signs of excessive bleeding or if the woman has reported episodes of bleeding in the last trimester, a vaginal exam should not be done.) Before the sterile vaginal examination, the nurse informs the woman about the procedure and its purpose. Afterward the nurse tells the woman about the findings. Sterile vaginal exams should be kept at a minimum to reduce risks of infection whether membranes are ruptured or not.

Indications for vaginal exams during a normal labor are based on a need to know the woman's status in order to make management decisions, such as what position(s) to recommend and when to call the certified nurse-midwife/physician.

Nursing Diagnosis

The nurse can anticipate that for many women with a low-risk pregnancy, certain nursing diagnoses will be used more frequently than others. This will of course vary from woman to woman according to the individual labor experience. Many of the more commonly used nursing diagnoses are identified in the box Key Nursing Diagnoses to Consider—During the Birth Process.

Nursing Plan and Implementation During Admission

After the nurse completes the admission assessment, her responsibilities focus on readying the laboring woman for birth. Nursing actions include collecting a urine specimen, performing a prep and administering an enema if ordered, facilitating laboratory tests, and notifying the physician/certified nurse-midwife. In many hospitals the nursing admission interventions include requesting the woman to sign a birth permit, fingerprinting the woman for the infant records, and fastening an identification bracelet to her wrist.

Collection of Urine Specimen

After admission data are obtained, a clean voided midstream urine specimen is collected. The woman with intact membranes may walk to the bathroom. If the membranes are ruptured and the presenting part is not engaged, the woman is generally asked to remain in bed to avoid prolapse of the umbilical cord. The advisability of ambulation when membranes are ruptured depends on the woman's desires, the requests of the certified nurse-midwife/physician, and agency policy.

The nurse can test the woman's urine for the presence of protein, ketones, and glucose by using a dipstick. This procedure is especially important if edema or elevated blood pressure is noted on admission. Proteinuria may be a sign of impending PIH if it is 2+ or more and the urine is not contaminated with blood or amniotic fluid. Ketonuria is a good index of starvation ketosis. Glycosuria is found frequently in pregnant women because of the increased glomerular filtration rate in the proximal tubules and the inability of these tubules to increase reabsorption of glucose. However. it may also be associated with latent diabetes and should not be discounted.

Prep and Enema Procedures

While the woman is collecting the urine specimen, the nurse can prepare the equipment for shaving the pubic area (the shaving is referred to as the *prep*) and for the enema if one is to be given. Prep orders vary, but many physicians/certified nurse-midwives leave standing orders for prep measures. Complete preps, which involve the removal of all pubic, perineal, and rectal hair, were formerly done. A prep now is usually the removal of perineal hair below the vaginal orifice where an episiotomy or repair of a laceration would be done. The area can be shaved or clipped with a pair of sterile scissors. A miniprep is usually considered the removal of perineal hair from the labia parallel to the upper aspect of the vaginal orifice and downward to the rectum.

The use of preps is controversial. Some physicians/certified nurse midwives believe that this form of skin preparation facilitates their work during the birth, makes perineal repair easier and prevents infection (Garforth & Garcia 1989). Others believe that a prep is unnecessary, since hair is minimal between the vagina and rectum, and that shaving may actually increase the risk of infection. Many women question the need for a prep and request that it be omitted. The nurse needs to ascertain the woman's wishes in this matter. Women who do not want a prep probably have already discussed it with the certified nurse-midwife/physician during the prenatal period. If the woman has not discussed her desire not to have a prep, the nurse acts as the woman's advocate in communicating the woman's wishes to the physician/certified nurse-midwife.

When a prep is to be done, the nurse explains the procedure to the woman. Most women feel embarrassed and vulnerable during this procedure, so the nurse needs to exercise great care to provide privacy and support.

The nurse performing a prep washes hands, dons disposable gloves, and positions the woman as for a vaginal examination. The nurse places a towel under the woman's buttocks and adjusts the lighting so that the perineal area can be well visualized. The woman is questioned about the presence of any moles or warts while the nurse is applying the soap solution with a gauze square or sponge provided in the prep set. The (right-handed) nurse holds the skin taut with the left hand and shaves in short strokes, holding the razor in the right hand and working downward to the vagina. When the perineum has been shaved, the woman is asked to turn to her left side and to assume the lateral Sims' position. The nurse pulls the upper buttock upward to expose the rectal area. After sudsing, the area around the

---

Dx

Key Nursing Diagnoses to Consider During the Birth Process

Coping, Ineffective individual
Fear
Fluid volume deficit: High risk
Injury: High risk
Pain [Acute]
Skin integrity, Impaired: High risk
Sleep pattern disturbance
Trauma: High risk
Urinary incontinence, Total
Urinary retention

rectum is shaved. The nurse must take care to prevent contaminants from the rectal area from entering the vaginal area.

Administration of an enema is also controversial. Proponents say the purposes of an enema are to (a) evacuate the lower bowel so that labor will not be impeded, (b) stimulate uterine contractions, (c) avoid embarrassment if bowel contents are expelled during pushing efforts, and (d) prevent contamination of the sterile field during birth. Those who question the routine use of an enema on admission suggest that labor is impeded only by a severe bowel impaction, question whether labor is stimulated, and find that feces may still be expelled during pushing efforts. They also note that the enema is usually uncomfortable.

After determining the woman's wishes regarding an enema, the nurse notifies the certified nurse-midwife/physician. Some factors contraindicate the enema. They are vaginal bleeding, unengaged presenting part, rapid labor progress, and imminent birth. These factors need to be identified. If an enema is to be given, the reasons and the procedure are explained to the woman. The enema is administered while she is on her left side.

If the membranes are intact and labor is not far advanced, the woman may expel the enema in the bathroom. Otherwise she is positioned on a bedpan in the bed. The side rails of the bed should be raised for safety.

Before leaving the birthing area, the nurse must be sure that the woman knows how to operate the call system so that she can obtain help if she needs it. After the enema is expelled, the nurse monitors the FHR again to assess any changes. If the woman's partner has been out of the labor/birthing room, the couple is reunited as soon as possible.

Laboratory Tests

Laboratory tests may also be carried out during admission. Hemoglobin and hematocrit values help determine the oxygen-carrying capacity of the circulatory system and the ability of the woman to withstand blood loss during the birth. Elevation of the hematocrit indicates hemoconcentration of blood, which occurs with edema, (PIH) or dehydration. A low hemoglobin, in the absence of other evidence of bleeding, suggests anemia. Blood may be typed and crossmatched if the woman is in a high-risk category. A serology test for syphilis is obtained if one has not been done in the last three months or if an antepartal serology result was positive.

Notification of the Physician/Nurse-Midwife

Depending on how rapidly labor is progressing, the nurse notifies the certified nurse-midwife/physician before or after completing the admission procedures. The report should include the following information: cervical dilatation and effacement, station, presenting part, status of the membranes, contraction pattern, FHR, vital signs that are not in the normal range, gestational age, pregnancy complications, the woman's wishes, and her reaction to labor.

Evaluation

Anticipated outcomes of nursing care include the following:

- The woman and her support person feel comfortable in the birth setting.
- The woman and her support person are able to request care based on individual wishes.
- The woman has been admitted in a caring, competent manner.

❀ ❀ ❀ ❀ ❀ ❀ ❀ ❀ ❀ ❀ ❀ ❀

Nursing Care of the Woman and Her Partner During the First Stage of Labor

❀ *APPLYING THE NURSING PROCESS* ❀

Nursing Assessment

Assessment during the first stage will focus on physiologic and psychologic stresses to the woman and the fetus. The maternal-fetal response to labor and the woman's ability to cope with the labor are also important areas to assess.

Nursing Diagnosis

Nursing diagnoses during the first stage of labor will probably focus first on knowledge deficit and anxiety and then on comfort. The following are examples of nursing diagnoses:

- Knowledge deficit related to birth setting and procedures
- Anxiety related to unknown course of the labor and personal ability to cope with labor and birth
- Pain related to uterine contractions and cervical dilatation

Additional nursing diagnoses are presented in the box Key Nursing Diagnoses to Consider—During the First Stage.

Nursing Plan and Implementation

Integration of Cultural Beliefs Influencing the Childbirth Experience

Knowledge of values, customs, and practices of different cultures is as important during labor as it is in the prenatal period. Without this knowledge, a nurse is less likely to understand a woman's behavior and may impose personal values and beliefs on her. As cultural sensitivity increases, so does the likelihood of providing high quality care. As cultural sensitivity increases, the nurse develops insights into both the woman's culture and his or her own. This understanding between the woman and her nurse begins a

Dx

Key Nursing Diagnoses to Consider During the First Stage

Pain
Altered family processes
Anxiety
Impaired physical mobility
Ineffective breathing pattern
Increased cardiac output
Fatigue
Fluid volume deficit
Infection: High risk
Urinary retention, acute

spiral of "mutuality and cooperation" that makes the relationship more positive for both of them (Dobson 1989).

As with many other critical events, a woman's experience of childbirth is strongly influenced by her cultural background. The variations due to culture are notable in the following behaviors.

Pain Expression   Understanding pain behavior helps lead to a more accurate assessment of the woman's condition. Nonverbal communication becomes vital. In working with women of another culture, language is often a barrier (Windsor-Richards & Gillies 1988). If possible, an interpreter should be used. A female interpreter is usually preferred, since in many cultures such as the Khmer of Cambodia, it would be indecent for a man to talk of the intimate aspects of childbirth in the presence of a woman (Sargent & Marcucci 1988). It is also important to be aware of communication differences, so that a nurse does not inadvertently indicate hostility toward, rejection of, or lack of interest in a woman (Morse & Park 1988).

In assessing a woman's pain, it is beneficial for the nurse to assess her own views of physical and psychologic distress. One study of nurses in six different cultures found that nurses' beliefs regarding suffering reflected their cultural backgrounds (Davitz et al 1976). For example, it was found that most Americans believe that Asians feel less pain because their behavior does not appear to reflect pain. On the other hand, a nurse with a cultural background that dictates stoic behavior may have difficulty in understanding a woman who has learned to express pain freely. Awareness of one's own values helps to achieve greater acceptance of another's behavior.

Modesty   In most cultures, modesty during childbirth is important. For example, Asians, Native Americans, Mexican Americans, and Australian Aboriginals view pregnancy as "female business" (Barclay et al 1989; Chung 1977). Some

Asian woman are not accustomed to male physicians and attendants and may prefer female physicians and attendants. Modesty is of great concern, and exposure of as little of the woman's body as possible is strongly recommended (Calhoun 1986). Orthodox Jewish women usually require long-sleeved hospital gowns so that their elbows and knees are covered; some even require caps, because they believe that the hair is also a "private part" (Lutwak et al 1988). On

Research Note

Clinical Application of Research

Susan McKay and Joyce Roberts (1990) identified maternal vocalizations as the core variable in their grounded theory study about maternal sounds during the second stage of labor. The data for the study developed from the responses of both experienced care givers and laboring mothers, either during the second stage of labor or from responses after viewing video tapes of the labor experience.

Five categories or states arose from the analysis of the data. Each category incorporated typical sounds and had designated significance for the care giver. The category of work/effort, designated as adaptive and effective, included guttural, low-pitched animalistic sounds. These sounds denoted an expression of effort and efficient use of abdominal muscles. The category of coping was adaptive and self-soothing and contained low-pitched sounds of sighing, moaning, and groaning. The significance to the care giver was that of an expression of tension and relief. The category of childlike was interpreted as nonadaptive, with emotions predominating. The sounds included high-pitched cries, whimpers, or whines and signified pain or distress. The mother who was out of control manifested nonadaptation, with emotions predominating, and her sounds were overbreathing or very high-pitched hollering or yelling. These sounds denoted extreme pain or distress. The last category of epidural anesthesia indicated a mind/body split because the sounds of the mother, normal conversation, were incongruous with her body changes and gave the care givers no cues about the physiologic state of her labor. Each category also had identified care giver responses.

Critical Thinking Applied to Research

Strengths: Incorporation of participants' verbalizations to support category development. Integration of the findings with existing literature.

McKay S, Roberts J: Obstetrics by ear: Maternal and caregiver perceptions of the meaning of maternal sounds during the second stage of labor. *J Nurse-Midwifery* 1990; 35(5): 266.

the other hand, many American women desire to remove all clothing during birth if privacy is provided, and this should also be accepted.

Role of the Father   In some cultures the husband or father attends the birth. In other groups the man is not present. In some Native American tribes, a midwife and female relatives traditionally assist the woman giving birth. In the traditional Navajo tribe, all family members view the birth process (Farris 1978). The Hmong father frequently remains with his wife during labor (Morrow 1986), but Khmer, Vietnamese and other Asian fathers do not participate in childbirth since it is considered "woman's work" (Sargent & Marcucci 1988). An orthodox Jewish husband may not touch his wife during labor and childbirth or postpartum because of her vaginal discharge. Historically, black women provided emotional support to a woman during childbirth. Today many black women prefer to have their mothers present instead of the newborn's father (Carrington 1978).

Who participates in the birth process is an important consideration for nurses. The participation of the father should not be assumed: His participation varies among cultures. A nurse's sensitivity to these different values alleviates stress for the family. Nurses should be aware that fathers often do perform definite functions even though they may not participate in the actual childbirth (Briesemeister & Haines 1988). In this case they are still viewed as active participants. They may adhere to certain taboos, perform certain rituals, experience couvade, or even simulate labor (Heggenhougen 1980), or they may assist with newborn care.

Cultural Beliefs: Some Examples   A culture often assigns certain superstitions, taboos, and beliefs regarding spirits to significant events such as the birth of a child. This activity is often a mechanism for dealing with anxiety. For example, in a rural Cambodian home, a laboring woman often lies on a bed with a fire beneath it to drive away evil spirits (Hollingsworth et al 1980). As soon as a baby is born to a Mexican-American woman, she places her legs together to prevent air from entering the womb (Kay 1978).

It is also common to prescribe certain activities for the relief of pain during childbirth. In other Native American tribes, the medicine man may be called to give a special potion to the woman and to offer prayers for her. A badger claw is often given to a laboring Keresian woman, since it is believed that badgers are good at "digging out" (Higgins & Wayland 1981). During labor, the Laguna Pueblo woman often holds onto a belt that has been blessed (Farris 1978).

In looking at specific practices on position, food, and drink during labor, obvious differences between cultures are apparent. In most non-European societies uninfluenced by Westernization, women assume an upright position in childbirth. For example, Hmong women who have emigrated from Laos to the United States report that squatting during childbirth is common in their culture (LaDu 1985).

Some traditional Native American women give birth in upright positions. For example, the Pueblo woman gives birth on her knees, the Zuni woman kneels or squats while a midwife kneads her abdomen, and in some tribes teas made of juniper twigs may be given to relax the woman (Higgins & Wayland 1981). The Khmer emphasize "cold" foods and balancing the "wind," although each woman determines her specific diet herself (Sargent & Marcucci 1988; Giger & David-Hizor 1991).

Hmong women have special customs regarding childbirth. The beginning of labor signifies the beginning of a transition and entails certain dietary restrictions. The woman may want to be active and may be able to move about during labor. The husband is frequently present and actively involved in providing comfort. During labor the woman usually prefers only "hot" foods (such as chicken, eggs, fried foods) and warm water to drink. Traditionally the woman prefers that the amniotic membranes not rupture until just before birth. It is thought that the escape of fluid at this time makes the birth easier. As soon as the baby is born, an egg needs to be soft-boiled and given to the mother to eat to restore her energy. During the postpartum period the mother prefers "warm" foods such as chicken prepared with warm water and warm rice (Morrow 1986).

Vietnamese women also follow prescribed customs during pregnancy and birth (Calhoun 1986). While in labor, the woman usually maintains self-control and may smile throughout the labor. She may prefer to walk about during labor and to deliver in a squatting position. She may avoid drinking cold water and prefer fluids at room temperature. The newborn is protected from praise to prevent jealousy.

In working with women from another culture, an awareness of historical beliefs and practices helps the nurse understand their behavior. In many cases, certain traditional practices are retained either in part or in full. An awareness of cultural values is also necessary, since they often dictate specific behavior.

CRITICAL THINKING

What cultural beliefs do you bring to the birthing area? How have your beliefs been influenced by your family and friends?

Promotion of Maternal and Fetal Physical Well-being

Latent Phase   After the admission process is completed, the nurse can help the laboring woman and her partner to become comfortable with the surroundings. The nurse can also assess their individual needs and plans for this experience. As long as there are no contraindications (such as vaginal bleeding or rupture of membranes [ROM] with the fetus unengaged), the woman may be encouraged to ambulate (Figure 23–1). Many women feel much more at ease

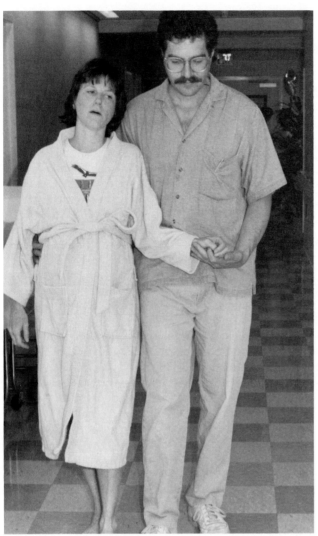

Figure 23–1   If there are no contraindications, the woman in early labor can be encouraged to walk around the birth facility.

and comfortable if they can move around and do not have to remain in bed. In addition, ambulation may decrease the need for analgesics, shorten labor, and decrease the incidence of FHR abnormalities (Roberts 1989).

The nurse will need to monitor the physical parameters of the woman and her fetus (Table 23–2). Maternal temperature is obtained every four hours unless the temperature is over 37.5C (99.6F) or the membranes are ruptured. In this case the temperature is taken every hour. Blood pressure, pulse, and respirations are evaluated every hour. If the woman's blood pressure is greater than 140/90, or elevated by 30/15 mm Hg over her baseline pressure, or if her pulse is more than 100, the physician or nurse-midwife must be notified. The blood pressure and pulse are then reevaluated more frequently. Uterine contractions are monitored for frequency, intensity, and duration every 60 minutes. In low-risk women, the FHR is auscultated every 60 minutes as long as it remains between 120 and 160 beats per minute with good long-term variability, short-term variability, and no variable or late decelerations. FHR is assessed every 30 minutes in high-risk women (NAACOG 1990).

The FHR should be auscultated throughout one contraction and for about 30 seconds after the contraction to ensure that there are no decelerations. If the FHR is not in the 120 to 160 range and/or decelerations are heard, continuous electronic monitoring is recommended. In some institutions, the external monitor is routinely attached for at least 15 minutes to assess fetal status. If no problems are noted, it is removed.

The laboring woman may be feeling some discomfort during contractions. The nurse can assist by providing diversions, encouraging ambulation, or by repositioning the woman on her left or right side. The woman may begin to use her breathing method during contractions (see the following discussion of management of pain).

If the laboring woman has not had childbirth education classes, the latent phase is a time when the nurse can

Table 23–2	Nursing Assessments in the First Stage	
Phase	**Mother**	**Fetus**
Latent	Blood pressure, respirations q 1 hr if in normal range Temperature q 4 hr unless over 37.5C (99.6F) or membranes ruptured, then q 1 hr Uterine contraction q 30 minutes	FHR every 60 minutes for low-risk women and every 30 minutes for high-risk women if normal characteristics present (average variability, baseline in the 120–160 BPM range, without late or variable decelerations) (NAACOG 1990). Note fetal activity. If electronic fetal monitor in place assess for reactive NST.
Active	Blood pressure, pulse, respirations q 1 hr if in normal range Uterine contractions q 30 min	FHR every 30 minutes for low-risk women and every 15 minutes for high-risk women if normal characteristics are present (NAACOG 1990).
Transition	Blood pressure, pulse, respiration q 30 min	FHR every 30 minutes for low-risk women and every 15 minutes for high-risk women if normal characteristics are present (NAACOG 1990).

do much teaching and anticipatory guidance. Most women are not too uncomfortable with contractions at this time and are responsive to teaching about breathing techniques they can use with contractions as labor progresses. In fact many women in the latent phase seek information about what to expect. The unprepared woman may hesitate to ask questions and thus can benefit even more from anticipatory guidance from the nurse. If the laboring woman's membranes are intact, a tour of the birthing facility can help decrease anxiety and distract her from her discomfort.

The nurse should offer fluids in the form of clear liquids and/or ice chips at frequent intervals. Because gastric-emptying time is prolonged during labor, solid foods are usually avoided.

Active Phase During this phase, the contractions have a frequency of 3 to 5 minutes, a duration of 30 to 60 seconds, and a moderate intensity. Contractions need to be evaluated every 15 to 30 minutes. As the contractions become more frequent and intense, vaginal exams should be done judiciously, as they are invasive and can be uncomfortable. During the active phase, the cervix dilates from 4 to 7 cm, and vaginal discharge and bloody show increase. Maternal blood pressure, pulse, and respirations should be monitored every 30 to 60 minutes. The FHR is assessed every 30 minutes for low-risk women and every 15 minutes for high-risk women. (NAACOG 1990).

During this phase, the laboring woman begins to withdraw from social interaction and focuses more on coping with her contractions; however, she does not want to be left alone. As she progresses into this phase, support in her breathing pattern with contractions becomes important. (See Procedure 23–1.)

A woman who has been ambulatory up to this point may now wish to sit in a chair or on a bed. If the woman wants to lie on the bed, she is encouraged to assume a side-lying position to avoid the vena caval syndrome. The quality of contractions is often better in this position. A supine position should be avoided for another, more important reason: When the woman is supine, the weight of the uterus and fetus lie on the vena cava and obstruct venous return from the extremities. Reduction of blood volume results in fetal distress, which may initially be assessed only by observation of late decelerations on a fetal monitor strip. Severe fetal distress, which can be assessed by intermittent auscultation and the fetal monitor, may be accompanied by symptoms of shock in the mother. These symptoms can occur suddenly and include a drop in blood pressure, increased pulse, air hunger, pallor, and moist clammy skin. Turning the woman to a left lateral position and starting oxygen by face mask can relieve maternal and fetal symptoms rapidly.

It is important, therefore, for the nurse to assist the woman into a position of safety and comfort. When a lateral position is assumed, pillows can be placed between the woman's legs to support the joints. Pillows behind her back help support her body and remind her to remain in the lateral position. To increase comfort, the nurse can encourage the support person to give back rubs or effleurage or place a cool cloth on the woman's forehead or across her neck. If the laboring woman is alone, the nurse implements these comfort measures.

Because vaginal discharge increases, the nurse needs to change the absorbent pads (Chux) frequently. Washing the perineum with warm soap and water removes secretions and increases comfort.

Pharmacologic support may be administered at this time if the woman has a well-established contraction pattern and she is not expected to give birth within the next hour or two. If an analgesic is given, the woman must remain in bed to promote her safety. If no one can be at the bedside with her, the side rails should be up.

For the woman experiencing slow progress of labor, an intravenous electrolyte solution may be started to provide energy and prevent dehydration (Newton et al 1988; Keppler 1988). If this occurs, it becomes even more important to encourage voiding every one or two hours to prevent bladder distention.

If the amniotic membranes have not ruptured previously, they may during this phase. When the membranes rupture, the nurse notes the color, amount, and odor of the amniotic fluid and the time of the rupture and immediately auscultates the FHR. The fluid should be clear with no odor. Although the amount varies, the perineum usually remains damp with almost constant spotting of fluid on the absorbent pad.

Fetal stress leads to intestinal and anal sphincter relaxation, and meconium may be released into the amniotic fluid. Meconium turns the fluid greenish-brown. Whenever the nurse notes meconium-stained fluid, an electronic monitor is applied to assess the FHR continuously (see Chapter 22).

The time of rupture is noted. Some clinicians suggest that birth should occur within 24 hours of ROM. Others suggest that emphasis should be placed on monitoring for signs of infection and that all invasive procedures (for example, sterile vaginal exams) be kept to a minimum. An additional concern is prolapse of the umbilical cord, which may occur when membranes rupture before the fetus is engaged. The concern is that amniotic fluid coming through the cervix will propel the umbilical cord downward into the pelvic cavity ahead of the presenting part. As the fetus descends, increased pressure against the umbilical cord would occur, cutting off the oxygen supply to the fetus. In the more extreme situation, the umbilical cord could prolapse through the cervix with the rupture of membranes. The FHR is auscultated immediately because a drop in the rate might indicate an undetected prolapsed cord. Immediate intervention is necessary to remove pressure on a prolapsed umbilical cord (see Chapter 19). See Table 23–3 for additional deviations from normal.

Transition During transition, the contraction frequency is every 2 to 3 minutes, duration is 45 to 90 seconds, and

Table 23–3   Deviations from Normal Labor Process Requiring Immediate Intervention

Problem	Immediate action
Woman admitted with vaginal bleeding or history of painless vaginal bleeding	1. Do not perform vaginal examination. 2. Assess FHR. 3. Evaluate amount of blood loss. 4. Evaluate labor pattern. 5. Notify physician/CNM immediately.
Presence of greenish or brownish amniotic fluid	1. Continuously monitor FHR. 2. Evaluate dilatation status of cervix and determine whether umbilical cord is prolapsed. 3. Evaluate presentation (vertex or breech). 4. Maintain woman on complete bed rest on left side. 5. Notify physician/CNM immediately.
Absence of FHR and fetal movement	1. Notify physician/CNM. 2. Provide truthful information and emotional support to laboring couple. 3. Remain with the couple.
Prolapse of umbilical cord	1. Relieve pressure on cord manually. 2. Continuously monitor FHR; watch for changes in FHR pattern. 3. Notify physician/CNM. 4. Assist woman into knee-chest position. 5. Administer oxygen.

Woman admitted in advanced labor; birth imminent	1. Prepare for immediate birth.
	2. Obtain critical information:
	  a. EDB
	  b. History of bleeding problems
	  c. History of medical or obstetric problems
	  d. Past and/or present use/abuse of prescription/otc/illicit drugs
	  e. Problems with this pregnancy
	  f. FHR and maternal vital signs if possible
	  g. Whether membranes are ruptured and how long since rupture
	  h. Blood type and Rh
	3. Direct another person to contact.
	  Do not leave woman alone.
	4. Provide support to couple.
	5. Put on gloves.

intensity is strong. Cervical dilatation increases from 8 to 10 cm, effacement is complete (100%), and there is usually a heavy amount of bloody show. Contractions are assessed at least every 15 minutes. Auscultated every 30 minutes for low-risk women and every 15 minutes for high-risk women. The nurse should be alert for the signs of rapid progress that characterize the transition phase, including behavioral changes (such as increasing irritability) as well as physical changes (for example, onset of spontaneous bearing-down efforts). Here again, vaginal examinations should be used sparingly.

A common sign that a woman has entered transition is a decrease in coping mechanisms. A woman who has coped well with her labor through the active phase may now have difficulty in breathing effectively with contractions and may fear loss of control. This change is obviously a response to the change in contraction patterns. Even if she has not received an analgesic, the laboring woman in the transition phase often appears to doze between contractions. The woman who received an analgesic in the active phase will get better rest between contractions. The nurse can awaken the woman in either situation just before another contraction begins so she can begin her breathing pattern. Breathing with the woman during each contraction helps guide her in maintaining effective coping mechanisms.

As the fetal presenting part moves down the birth canal and complete dilatation approaches, the woman begins to feel increased rectal pressure. The woman indicates this by verbalizing the need to have a bowel movement or the urge to push, or by actually pushing by holding her breath with a contraction. A vaginal exam may be done to verify complete dilatation, although an exam is usually not necessary in the presence of clear evidence of descent, such as bulging of the perineum. In general, women are discouraged from pushing (by using rapid, shallow breathing instead of bearing-down) before complete dilatation is confirmed. However, indulgence of an overwhelming urge to push when the woman is almost completely dilated is rarely associated with cervical lacerations or edema (Sleep et al 1989). Conversely, some women have a period of time between the time of complete dilatation and the onset of the urge to push (Aderhold 1989; Simkin 1984). These women may be encouraged to rest until reflexive bearing-down efforts begin.

Promotion of Comfort

A labor nurse is in the unique position of assisting during one of the most profound experiences of human existence. The nurse has the privilege of sharing in each couple's personal miracle. But it is sometimes difficult for the nurse, who may be admitting a seventh woman toward the end of a busy shift, to share her enthusiasm and excitement. Nurses who care for women in labor face a challenge. They must integrate sophisticated technical skills with sensitivity and an awareness of the influence of the nurse's attitude and behavior on the laboring woman's perceptions. A warm and supportive nurse helps set the stage for a satisfying childbirth experience.

Behavioral Responses to Labor   The woman's response to labor changes with each phase as labor progresses. This does not mean that each woman in labor responds in the same way. It does mean that regardless of a woman's coping mechanisms, her response to labor changes as contractions increase in frequency, duration, and intensity. In some women, the progress from the latent to the active phase may be more subtle than it is for others. Progress from the active phase to transition is usually more obvious. Awareness and sensitivity to even subtle changes are significant in assessing the progress of normal labor. Identification of behavioral changes can reduce considerably the need for excessive vaginal examinations. Behavioral changes also signal the need for increased monitoring of indicators of maternal and fetal well-being, such as contraction patterns, FHR, and maternal blood pressure.

Although every woman's behavior changes as labor progresses, individual responses vary considerably due to many factors. In addition to uterine contractions, these factors include previous childbearing experiences, previous orientation to coping with pain, support systems, acceptance of pregnancy, childbirth education classes, physical variables, culture, the response of nurses and other members of the health team, level of wellness, and developmental level if the woman is an adolescent. Most of these factors cannot be changed by the nurse once the woman is admitted in labor. It is important, however, that the nurse recognize the significant influence of these factors and work with the woman to enhance her ability to cope with labor.

Comfort Measures   A decrease in the intensity of discomfort is one of the goals of nursing support during labor.

Ensuring General Comfort   General comfort measures are of utmost importance throughout labor. By relieving minor discomforts the nurse helps the woman use her coping mechanisms to deal with pain.

The woman should be encouraged to assume any position that she finds the most comfortable (Figure 23–2). A side-lying position on the left side is generally the most advantageous for the laboring woman, although frequent position changes seem to achieve more efficient contractions (Roberts 1989). Care should be taken that all the body parts are supported, with the joints slightly flexed. If the woman is more comfortable on her back, the head of the bed should be elevated to relieve the pressure of the uterus on the vena cava. Back rubs and frequent change of position contribute to comfort and relaxation.

Diaphoresis and the constant leaking of amniotic fluid can dampen the woman's gown and bed linen. Fresh, smooth, dry bed linen promotes comfort. To avoid having to change the bottom sheet following rupture of the membranes, the nurse may replace absorbent pads at frequent intervals. The perineal area should be kept as clean and dry

as possible to promote comfort as well as to prevent infection. A full bladder adds to the discomfort during a contraction and may prolong labor by interfering with the descent of the fetus. The bladder should be kept as empty as possible by having the woman void every one to two hours. Even though the woman is voiding, urine may be retained because of the pressure of the fetal presenting part. A full bladder can be detected by palpation directly over the symphysis pubis. Some of the regional procedures for analgesia during labor contribute to the inability to void, and catheterization may be necessary.

The woman may experience dryness of the oral mucous membranes. Popsicles, ice chips, or a wet 4-by-4 sponge may relieve the discomfort. Some prepared childbirth programs advise the woman to bring suckers to help combat the dryness that occurs with some of the breathing patterns.

Decreasing Anxiety   The anxiety experienced by women entering labor is related to a combination of factors inherent to the process. A moderate amount of anxiety about the pain enhances the woman's ability to deal with the pain. An excessive degree of anxiety decreases her ability to cope with the pain and leads to increased tension, which causes increased pain and anxiety.

Anxiety not directly related to pain can be decreased in a number of ways. Anxiety is decreased as the nurse shares information, which eases fear of the unknown, and establishes rapport with the couple, which helps them preserve their personal integrity. In addition to being a good listener, the nurse must demonstrate genuine concern for the laboring woman. Remaining with the woman as much as possible conveys a caring attitude and dispels fears of abandonment. Praise for correct breathing, relaxation efforts, and pushing efforts not only encourages repetition of the behavior but also decreases anxiety about the ability to cope with labor.

A nurse's attitude of confidence in the woman's ability to handle the labor is very important. Even a frightened laboring woman seems to sense the nurse's confidence in her, and it gives her strength and courage to carry on.

Education for Self–Care   Providing information about the nature of the discomfort that will occur during labor is important. Stressing the intermittent nature and maximum duration of the contractions can be most helpful. The woman can cope with pain better when she knows that a period of relief will follow. Describing the type of discomfort and specific sensations that will occur as labor progresses helps the woman recognize these sensations as normal and expected when she does experience them.

During the second stage, the woman may interpret rectal pressure as a need to move her bowels. The instinctive response is to tighten muscles rather than bear down (push). A sensation of splitting apart also occurs in the latter part of the second stage, and the woman may be afraid to bear down. The woman who expects these sensa-

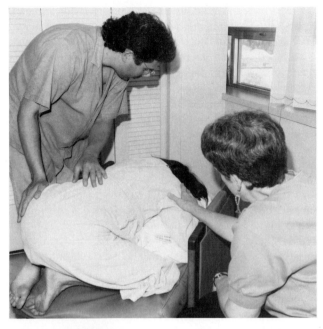

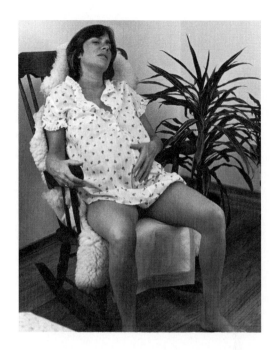

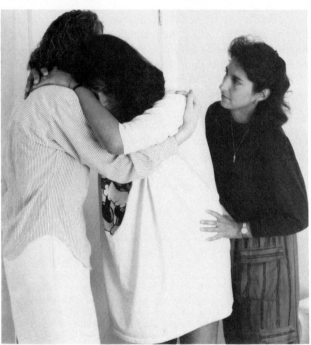

Figure 23–2   The laboring woman is encouraged to choose a position of comfort. The nurse modifies assessments and interventions as necessary.

tions and understands that bearing down contributes to progress at this stage is more likely to do so.

Descriptions of sensations should be accompanied with information on specific comfort measures. Some women experience the urge to push during transition when the cervix is not fully dilated and effaced. Usually, this sen-

sation can be controlled by panting, and instructions should be given prior to the time that panting is required.

A thorough explanation of surroundings, procedures, and equipment being used also decreases anxiety, thereby reducing pain. Attachment to an electronic monitor can produce fear, because equipment of this type is associated with critically ill patients. The beeps, clicks, and other strange noises should be explained, and a simplified explanation of the monitor strip should be given. The nurse can emphasize that the use of the monitor provides a more accurate way to assess the well-being of the fetus during the course of labor. In addition, the nurse can show the woman and her coach how the monitor can help them use controlled breathing techniques to relieve pain. The monitor may indicate the beginning of a contraction just seconds before the woman feels it. The woman and coach can learn how to read the tracing to identify the beginning of the contraction. The disadvantages and possible risks also need to be discussed. Some women decrease their movements out of fear of disturbing the monitor equipment, thereby unnecessarily causing themselves increased discomfort and anxiety. The nurse can relieve such concerns by advocating positioning for comfort and displaying a willingness to adjust the monitor if necessary (Snydal 1988).

Supportive Relaxation Techniques   Tense muscles increase resistance to the descent of the fetus and contribute to maternal fatigue. This fatigue increases pain perception and decreases the woman's ability to cope with the pain. Comfort measures, massage, techniques for decreasing anxiety, and client teaching can contribute to relaxation, as can adequate sleep and rest. The laboring woman needs to be encouraged to use the periods between con-

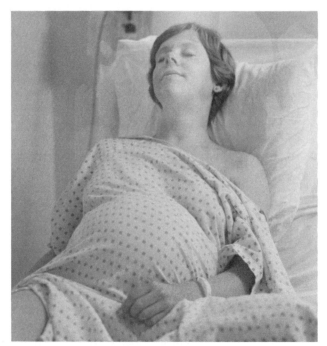

Figure 23–3 It is important for the laboring woman to conserve her energy and to reduce fatigue by relaxing between contractions.

tractions for rest and relaxation (Figure 23–3). A prolonged prodromal phase of labor may have prohibited sleeping. An aura of excitement naturally accompanies the onset of labor, making it difficult for the woman to sleep although the contractions are mild and infrequent.

Distraction is another method of increasing relaxation and coping with discomfort. During early labor, conversation or activities, such as light reading, cards, or other games, serve as distractions. Ambulation is an effective distraction and also helps stimulate labor. One technique that is effective for relieving moderate pain is to have the woman concentrate on a pleasant experience she has had in the past. This helps enhance relaxation between contractions and provides a focus point as she breathes with each contraction. As labor progresses the breathing pattern with contractions may be the main source of distraction. Another form of distraction is called visualization (Geden et al 1989). With this technique the woman visualizes her body or her perineum relaxing. It is probably most beneficial to begin practicing this technique early in pregnancy. However, even the woman in early labor can be taught this technique fairly quickly (see Table 23–4).

Touch is another type of distraction. Although some women regard touching as an invasion of privacy or threat to their independence, others want to touch and be touched during a painful experience.

The support person who has attended childbirth education classes is aware of various types of touch during labor, such as sacral pressure, a backrub, a light stroking of the arms, or hand holding. Those who have not attended can be taught about the importance of touch and shown what can be helpful. Most couples spontaneously use touch as part of their ongoing relationship. If the support person is not involved, and it appears that he wants to be, it is important for the nurse to encourage involvement. The nurse can model behaviors such as reaching out to touch the woman's hand or placing her hand at the woman's side within reach. The nurse can suggest the support person "take over" and perhaps sit beside the bed with one hand on the bed within reach. The woman who needs touch will reach out for contact. At other times the nurse can demonstrate how to do a back rub or provide sacral pressure. If no support person is present, the nurse provides this important comfort measure.

Effleurage, a light abdominal stroking, may be used at this time to maintain abdominal muscle relaxation. The technique is believed to work by providing stimulation to large-diameter fibers, which inhibits pain impulses carried by small-diameter fibers. Effleurage is effective for mild-to-moderate pain but is not very effective for intense pain (see Figure 17–5.)

Finally, there is the technique called "therapeutic touch," which is used to help a person in distress by altering the energy fields around that person. This technique is not widely practiced, as some formal training is required for its proper use. However, it is anticipated that this technique will become more commonly used in the future (Simkin 1989).

A shower or whirlpool bath may also be used as a comfort measure. The laboring woman may sit on a stool or chair in the shower with warm water directed onto her abdomen. In some birthing units the woman can sit in a whirlpool bath for prolonged periods, or she can recline in

---

Table 23–4 Simple Visualization Method

Direct a visualization by saying something like the following: "Think about a place you have been that has pleasant memories and feelings around it. A place that was relaxing, where all your stress disappeared. As you think about this place, take in a breath and remember the smells around it. If it was outside, feel the warmth of the sun or the way the breeze felt on your face. In your mind, sit in that place again. Let all your tension and tiredness leave your body as you feel the warmth and breezes."

Give the woman a few moments to think about her special place. Ask if she would like to share information about the setting. If the woman chooses to do this add the information to help her with the visualization (for example, "think about the mountain cabin and the warmth of the sun on your face as you sit in the rocking chair on the front porch," etc).

After the woman has a visualization set up, suggest thinking about it during contractions as a means of increasing relaxation and focusing concentration. You could say: "As each contraction begins, think about this special place for a moment and let your body relax. Keep a picture of your place in your mind as you breathe with the contraction. When the contraction is over, let your body stay relaxed. Feel the comfort of this room and support of those around you."

a bathtub of warm water. The nurse can continue her assessments but needs to be alert for the rupture of membranes, which may be more difficult to detect while the woman is in water.

Back pain associated with labor may be relieved by firm pressure on the lower back or sacral area. The nurse can show the support person how to place the palm of the hand in the small of the woman's back and provide slow and firm massage. Since much force is usually needed for sacral pressure to be effective, the nurse can offer to relieve the support person for short periods.

In addition to the measures just described, the nurse can enhance the woman's relaxation by providing encouragement and support for her controlled breathing techniques. The support person who has attended childbirth education classes with the woman is usually the most effective in helping the woman with her chosen breathing technique.

Controlled Breathing Controlled breathing is helpful to the laboring woman. Used correctly, it increases the woman's pain threshold, permits relaxation, enhances the woman's ability to cope with the uterine contractions, and allows the uterus to function more efficiently.

Women usually learn Lamaze breathing in prenatal classes and practice it a number of weeks before childbirth. If the woman has not learned Lamaze or another controlled breathing technique, teaching her may be difficult when she is admitted in active labor. In this instance, the nurse can teach slow, deep abdominal and pant-pant-blow breathing. In abdominal breathing, the woman moves the abdominal wall upward as she inhales and downward as she exhales. This method tends to lift the abdominal wall off the contracting uterus and thus may provide some pain relief. The breathing is deep and rhythmic. As transition approaches, the woman may feel the need to breathe more rapidly.

As the woman uses her breathing technique, the nurse can assess and support the interaction between the woman and her coach or support person. In the absence of a coach, the nurse assists the laboring woman by helping to identify the beginning of each contraction and encouraging her as she breathes through each contraction. Continued encouragement and support with each contraction throughout labor have immeasurable benefits (see Figure 23–4).

Hyperventilation is related to uneven breathing patterns, which occur most often with uncontrolled breathing during a contraction. Hyperventilation may also occur when a woman breathes very rapidly over a prolonged period. Hyperventilation is the result of an imbalance of oxygen and carbon dioxide (that is, too much carbon dioxide is exhaled, and too much oxygen remains in the body). The signs and symptoms of hyperventilation are tingling or numbness in the tip of the nose or the lips, fingers or toes; dizziness; spots before the eyes; or spasms of the hands or feet (carpal-pedal spasms). If hyperventilation occurs, the woman should be encouraged to slow her breathing rate

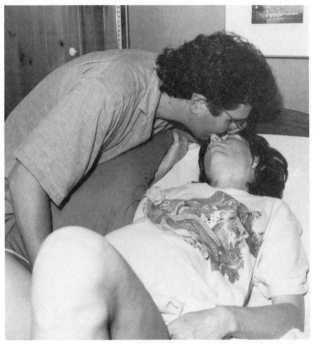

Figure 23–4 The woman's partner provides support and encouragement during labor.

and to take shallow breaths. With instruction and encouragement, many women are able to change their breathing to correct the problem. Encouraging the woman to relax and counting out loud for her so she can pace her breathing during contractions are also helpful. If the signs and symptoms continue or become more severe (that is, if they progress from numbness to spasms), the woman can breath into a paper surgical mask, her hands cupped in front of her face, or a paper bag until symptoms abate. Breathing into a mask or bag causes rebreathing of carbon dioxide. The nurse should remain with the woman to reassure her.

In some instances, analgesics and/or regional anesthetic blocks may be used to enhance comfort and relaxation during labor. See Chapter 24 for a discussion of analgesia and anesthesia. Table 23–5 summarizes labor progress, possible responses of the laboring woman, and support measures.

Evaluation

Anticipated outcomes of nursing care include the following:

- The woman progresses through the first stage without difficulty.

- The woman has increased comfort through the use of self-comfort measures and nursing support.

- The fetus shows no sign of distress and has a reassuring FHR.

- The woman's intake and output and fluid and electrolyte status is within normal limits.

Table 23–5 Normal Progress, Psychologic Characteristics, and Nursing Support During First and Second Stages of Labor

Phase	Cervical dilatation	Uterine contractions	Woman's response	Support measures
Latent phase	1–4 cm	Every 15–30 min, 15–30 sec duration Mild intensity	Usually happy, talkative, and eager to be in labor Exhibits need for independence by taking care of own bodily needs and seeking information	Establish rapport on admission and continue to build during care. Assess information base and learning needs. Be available to consult regarding breathing technique if needed; teach breathing technique if needed and in early labor. Orient family to room, equipment, monitors, and procedures. Encourage woman and partner to participate in care as desired. Provide needed information. Assist woman into position of comfort; encourage frequent change of position; and encourage ambulation during early labor. Offer fluids/ice chips. Keep couple informed of progress. Encourage woman to void every one to two hours. Assess need for and interest in using visualization to enhance relaxation and teach if appropriate.
Active phase	4–7 cm	Every 3–5 min, 30–60 sec duration Moderate intensity	May experience feelings of helplessness; exhibits increased fatigue and may begin to feel restless and anxious as contractions become stronger; expresses fear of abandonment Becomes more dependent as she is less able to meet her needs	Encourage woman to maintain breathing patterns; provide quiet environment to reduce external stimuli. Provide reassurance, encouragement, support; keep couple informed of progress. Promote comfort by giving back rubs, sacral pressure, cool cloth on forehead, assistance with position changes, support with pillows, effleurage. Provide ice chips, ointment for dry mouth and lips. Encourage to void every one to two hours. Offer shower/jacuzzi/warm bath if available.
Transition	8–10 cm	Every 2–3 min, 45–90 sec duration Strong intensity	Tires and may exhibit increased restlessness and irritability; may feel she cannot keep up with labor process and is out of control Physical discomforts Fear of being left alone May fear tearing open or splitting apart with contractions	Encourage woman to rest between contractions; if she sleeps between contractions, wake her at beginning of contraction so she can begin breathing pattern (increases feeling of control). Provide support, encouragement, and praise for efforts. Keep couple informed of progress; encourage continued participation of support persons. Promote comfort as listed above but recognize many women do not want to be touched when in transition. Provide privacy. Provide ice chips, ointment for lips. Encourage to void every one to two hours.
Stage 2	Complete	Every 1½ to 2 minutes	May feel out of control, helpless, panicky	Assist woman in pushing efforts. Encourage woman to assume position of comfort. Provide encouragement and praise for efforts. Keep couple informed of progress. Provide ice chips. Maintain privacy as woman desires.

- The woman has sufficient energy to manage the pushing efforts of the second stage.

❀ ❀ ❀ ❀ ❀ ❀ ❀ ❀ ❀ ❀ ❀ ❀ ❀

Care of the Woman and Her Partner During the Second Stage of Labor

The second stage of labor begins when the cervix is completely dilated and is completed when the baby is born.

❀ *APPLYING THE NURSING PROCESS* ❀

Nursing Assessment

Assessment during the second stage focuses on the physiologic stresses during the pushing efforts and the descent and birth of the baby. The contraction status, maternal physical status, energy requirements for effective pushing, and fetal response to descent are closely assessed.

Nursing Diagnosis

Nursing diagoses during the second stage of labor will probably focus on fatigue and increasing comfort and decreasing anxiety in order for the second stage to progress smoothly. The following are examples of nursing diagnoses:

- Fatigue related to inability to rest during labor and the pushing efforts of the second stage.
- Anxiety related to unknown outcome of the labor process.
- Pain related to descent of the fetus and stretching of vaginal and perineal tissues.

Additional nursing diagnoses are presented in the box Key Nursing Diagnoses to Consider—During the Second Stage.

Nursing Plan and Implementation

Promotion of Comfort

Most of the comfort measures that have been used during the first stage of labor remain appropriate at this time. Cool

Key Nursing Diagnoses to Consider During the Second Stage

Fatigue
Fear
Pain
Increased cardiac output
Tissue perfusion (for mother and fetus)
Infection: High risk

Table 23–6 Nursing Assessments in the Second Stage	
Mother	**Fetus**
Blood pressure, pulse, respirations q 5–15 min.	FHR every 15 minutes for low-risk women and every 5 minutes for high-risk women (NAACOG 1990).
Uterine contraction palpated continuously.	

cloths applied to the face and forehead may help keep the woman cool during the intense physical exertion of pushing. The woman may feel hot and want to remove some of the covers. Care still needs to be taken to provide privacy even though covers are removed. The woman can be encouraged to rest and let all muscles relax during the period between contractions. The nurse and support person(s) can assist the woman into a pushing position with each contraction to further conserve energy. Sips of fluids or ice chips may be used to provide moisture and relieve dryness of the mouth.

Assisting the Woman in Her Pushing Efforts

During the second stage of labor, the cervix is completely dilated (10 cm). The uterine contractions continue as in the transition phase. Maternal pulse, blood pressure, and FHR are assessed every 5 to 15 minutes; some protocols recommend assessment after each contraction (Table 23–6). The woman usually feels an uncontrollable urge to push (bear down). The nurse can help by encouraging her and by assisting with positioning (see Figure 23–5). The woman can be propped up with pillows to a semireclining position.

I knew when I was completely dilated. I knew when to push and I did it without tearing. My body told me to listen. I knew what to do. (Harriette Hartigan, Women in Birth)

The wisdom of using the sustained, strenuous (Valsalva maneuver) style of pushing against a closed glottis is now being questioned, as there is increasing evidence that it compromises maternal-fetal gas exchange (Sleep, et al 1989). Instead, studies now support the use of spontaneous bearing-down efforts (pushes). These efforts are made with an open or partially open glottis. Typically, the laboring woman will make three to five such efforts within a contraction, each lasting 4 to 6 seconds, although the number of bearing-down efforts per contraction increases as the second stage progresses (Roberts et al 1987). While there is some reason to believe that these less vigorous bearing-down efforts contribute to a slightly longer second stage (Perlis 1988; Sleep et al 1989), the fetal outcomes are generally good.

The woman is encouraged to rest between contractions. Although the laboring woman may appear exhausted at this time, most experience relief at being able to push with contractions. Perspiration increases with the pushing

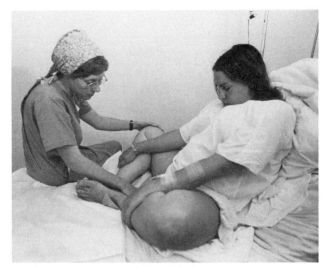

Figure 23–5 Long and strenuous bearing-down efforts (such as the one illustrated here) are the most common style of pushing used in the United States today. However, recent research suggests that shorter, less forceful pushes may be better for both mother and baby.

efforts, and a cold washcloth for forehead and face is most soothing.

When I began pushing, I felt in control because I could do something. . . . I could push the baby out. I knew he was ready to be born. (Harriette Hartigan, Women in Birth)

Maternal positions such as standing, squatting while leaning back on a partner, lying in a lateral or Sims' position, and crouching on hands and knees may increase comfort and effectiveness of pushing. Some women feel that sitting on a toilet seat is a comfortable position that assists their pushing efforts. This position usually causes anxiety in the care givers, however, for fear that the birth may occur quickly in this most inopportune place.

Additional comfort measures may be used during this stage. Hot perineal, abdominal, and back compresses may be used to increase muscle relaxation. Perineal massage and stretching with a lubricant (Lubafax) may relieve the tearing and burning sensation as the perineal tissue distends. (At this time, perineal stretching is done by the CNM and not other nursing staff.)

Visualization techniques may be helpful (Simkin 1989). The woman can be encouraged to envision the infant descending the birth canal. Phrases such as "Open to your baby" and "Let the baby come; don't try to hold back" can be useful and calming.

Nurses frequently have learned one way for assisting the woman during pushing efforts and may hesitate to encourage unique positions. It is important to support the

woman's needs and to encourage a change in position if anticipated progress is not made.

A woman in labor for the first time (nullipara) is usually prepared for birth when perineal bulging is noted. A multipara usually progresses much more quickly, so she may be prepared for birth when the cervix is dilated 7 to 8 cm.

Preparations in the Birthing Room

Couples often choose the birthing room for labor and birth because of its more relaxed atmosphere. Not having to transfer a woman from the room where she has labored to a different room for the birth contributes tremendously to a relaxed atmosphere for both the woman and the nursing staff. It also avoids an uncomfortable transfer from one bed to another just before the birth. The needed equipment and supplies are brought to the birthing room when the birth is imminent (see Table 23–7).

Birthing rooms usually have birthing beds that can be adapted for giving birth by removing a small section near the foot. Stirrups are available if needed or desired. In settings where birth is managed by nurse-midwives, an ordinary double bed is often found, which prevents the use of stirrups.

Many other factors facilitate the relaxed, nonmedical atmosphere in the birthing room. Other family members may be in attendance in addition to the support person. They are not usually required to change into scrub attire. Good handwashing technique is required of all staff, but they often do not wear caps and masks. Sterile gloves for the birth attendant and sterile equipment are still common and all health care personnel wear sterile or disposable

---

Table 23–7 Birthing Room Equipment and Supplies

Equipment for Birth

Disposable pack containing drapes, towels, and gown

Instruments (scissors, clamps, etc)

Sterile gloves

Sterile, warmed baby blankets

Prep set for perineal scrub prior to birth

Warmed sterile water

Equipment for the Newborn

Radiant-heated infant care unit

Bulb syringe

Device for assessing newborn's temperature

Oxygen

Suction equipment

Suction catheters (size 10, 12, and 14 French and sizes 8, 10, 12, and 14 French disposable plastic catheters with finger control)

Laryngoscope with a working light, Miller size 0 premature and size 1 blade

Endotrachael tubes size 2.5–4 mm or size 10, 12, and 14 and stylets for insertion if desired

Bag resuscitation set capable of delivering 100% oxygen

gloves and eye glasses or goggles to observe universal precautions and body substance isolation. The birth attendant wears a plastic apron to protect clothing from contamination with amniotic fluid. Even medical interventions for a normal birth seem minimized in a birthing room in contrast to the birthing room setting.

Preparations in the Delivery Room

When it is time for the laboring woman to be moved to the delivery room, safety in transfer is a priority. Side rails must be used.

Another priority is to provide privacy and preserve modesty for the laboring woman as she is pushed from her room to the delivery room. The woman is usually involved in her pushing efforts and may throw the covers off. Although she may be unaware of others at this time, after the birth she may be embarrassed that others were able to see her.

After being wheeled into the delivery room, the labor bed or transfer cart must be carefully supported against the delivery bed. This ensures the woman's safety during the transfer.

It is important that the woman move from one bed to another between contractions. If birth seems imminent, it is safer for the woman to give birth in her labor bed. Transfer to the delivery bed is then delayed until after the baby has been born and the cord has been clamped and cut.

During transfer and preparation of the woman for the birth, the woman's partner or support person is also preparing for birth. In most facilities, the support person is required to put on a scrub suit, disposable boots, and perhaps cap and mask before entering the delivery room.

Since the birth is usually conducted under strict sterile precautions, all those who enter the delivery room wear scrub apparel and wash their hands. Caps and masks may be optional.

Assisting the Couple and Physician/Nurse-Midwife During Birth

Maternal Birthing Positions The woman is usually positioned for the birth on a bed, birthing chair, or delivery table. The position that the woman assumes is determined not only by her individual wishes but also by the physician/nurse-midwife.

Stirrups, if used, are padded to alleviate pressure, and both legs should be lifted simultaneously to avoid strain on abdominal, back, and perineal muscles. The stirrups should be adjusted to fit the woman's legs. The feet are supported in the stirrup holders. The height and angle of the stirrups are adjusted so there is no pressure on the back of the knees or the calf, which might cause discomfort and postpartal vascular problems. The birthing table or bed is elevated 30° to 60° to help the woman bear down, and handles are provided so she may pull back on them.

The upright posture for labor and birth was considered normal in most societies until modern times. Squatting, kneeling, standing, and sitting were variously selected for birth by women. Only within the last two hundred years has the recumbent position become more usual in the Western world. Its use in this century has been reinforced because of the convenience it offers in applying new technology. The lithotomy position has thus become the conventional manner in which North American women give birth in hospitals. In searching for alternative positions, consumers and professionals alike are refocusing on the comfort of the laboring woman rather than on the convenience to the birth attendant (see Figure 23–6 and Table 23–8).

Traditional Recumbent Position The traditional lithotomy position for birth enhances the maintenance of asepsis, assessment of FHR, and performance of episiotomy and repair. In contrast, when the comfort and well-being of the woman and fetus are considered, the following disadvantages have been noted:

1. There is a decrease of as much as 30% in the blood pressure of 10% of women.
2. Many women experience difficulty breathing because of pressure of the uterus on the diaphragm.

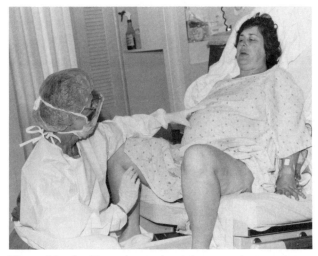

Figure 23–6 Observing universal precautions and body substance isolation at the time of birth involves using a number of articles. In this high risk situation, the nurse wears disposable gloves, disposable paper gown that ties in the back and is either impervious to fluids or has a plastic splash apron on it, a disposable mask and eyeglasses or goggles to avoid splashes in the face and eyes at the time of birth to meet recommendations of both universal precautions and body substance isolation. This nurse has also donned a disposable hat which is not required for universal or BSI precautions. The nurse must work hard to avoid the distancing that the mask and other garb may create. This nurse continues to maintain eye contact, to use touch and provide encouragement and support to the laboring woman.

Table 23–8 Comparison of Birthing Positions

Position	Advantages	Disadvantages	Nursing implications
Sitting in birthing chair	Gravity aids descent and expulsion of infant. Does not compromise venous return from lower extremities. Chair can be tilted to various degrees. Woman can view birth process.	If woman is short, sitting with legs spread may increase tension on perineum, which may lead to lacerations. Position of body, legs, and feet cannot be altered. Potential for increased blood loss (Sleep, et al, 1989)	Encourage woman to tilt the chair to increase her comfort. Assess for pressure points on legs.
Semi-Fowler's	Does not compromise venous return from lower extremities. Woman can view birth process.	If legs are positioned wide apart, relaxation of perineal tissues is decreased.	Assess that upper torso is evenly supported. Increase support of body by changing position of bed or using pillows as props.
Left lateral Sims'	Does not compromise venous return from lower extremities. Increased perineal relaxation and decreased need for episiotomy. Appears to prevent rapid descent.	It is difficult for the woman to see the birth if she desires.	Adjust position so that the upper leg lies on the bed (scissor fashion) or is supported by the partner or on pillows.
Squatting	Size of pelvic outlet is increased. Gravity aids descent and expulsion of newborn. Second stage may be shortened (Sleep, et al, 1989).	May be difficult to maintain balance while squatting.	Help woman maintain balance. Use a squatting bar if available.
Sitting in birthing bed	Gravity aids descent and expulsion of the fetus. Does not compromise venous return from lower extremities. Woman can view the birth process. Leg position may be changed at will.		Ensure that legs and feet have adequate support.

3. The uterine axis is directed toward the symphysis pubis instead of the pelvic inlet.
4. Aspiration of vomitus is more likely.
5. The woman may feel resentment at being forced to assume an "embarrassing" position.
6. Tightening of the vagina and perineum as the thighs are flexed may increase the need for an episiotomy.
7. The position may interfere with the frequency and intensity of contractions.
8. Stirrups cause excessive pressure on the legs.
9. The woman works against gravity.

These disadvantages may be lessened slightly if the woman is in a lithotomy position with her back elevated 30° to 40° (Sleep, et al 1989).

Left Lateral Sims' An alternative position favored by some women and birth attendants is the left lateral Sims' (Figure 23–7). In assuming this position for birth, the woman lies on her left side with her left leg extended and her right knee drawn against her abdomen or flexed by her side or with both legs bent at the knees. Those who favor this position find it increases overall comfort, does not compromise venous return from the lower extremities, and diminishes the chances of aspiration should vomiting occur. Women also perceive the lateral Sims' as a more natural and comfortable position and less intrusive with no stirrups or overhead lights required. Birth attendants have found the position has a positive effect on the management of fetal shoulder dystocias. Fewer episiotomies are required in this position since the perineum tends to be more relaxed (Lehrman 1985). The disadvantages cited relate to the difficulty of cutting and repairing large episiotomies, and problems with difficult forceps births (Gardosi et al 1989).

Squatting The squatting position is favored by some women primarily for the positive use it makes of gravity. Squatting is thought to facilitate the entrance of the presenting part into the pelvic inlet, thus hastening engagement. A squatting bar may be used across a bed or on the floor to increase the woman's balance and provide some support (Figure 23–8). During the second stage of labor, squatting increases the size of the pelvic outlet and helps in the woman's pushing efforts. Some birth attendants object to this position because the perineum is relatively inac-

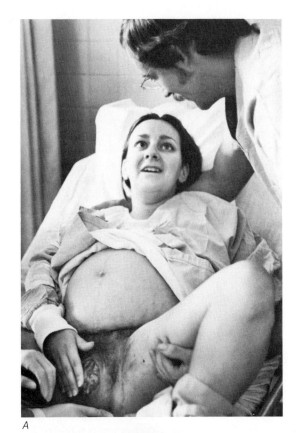

A

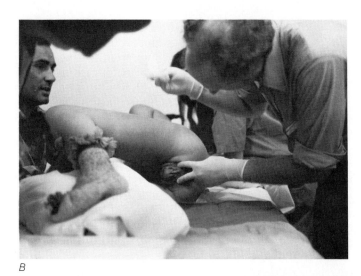

B

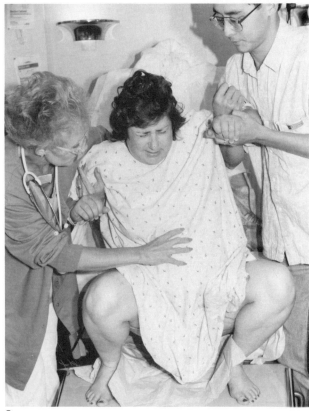

C

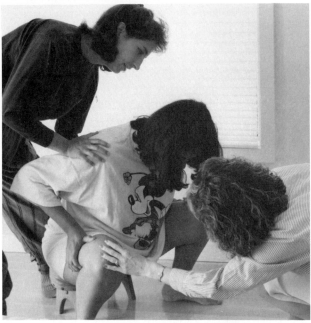

D

Figure 23–7   Birthing positions (clockwise from upper left). A Lithomy position with the woman's back elevated. B Side-lying position. C Supported squatting position used in the second stage of labor. D Using a birthing stool.

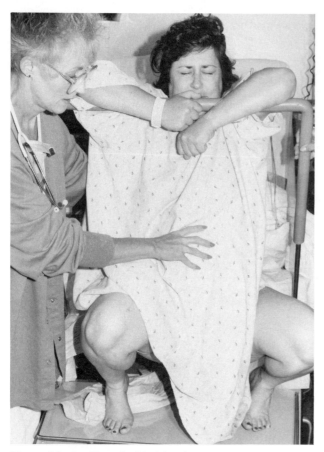

Figure 23–8   Use of a birthing bar.

cessible and it is difficult for them to control the birth process. Squatting also increases the difficulty of administering analgesia, using instruments, and monitoring fetal status.

Semi-Fowler's Position   A semi-Fowler's position is advocated by some as an appropriate middle ground between the recumbent and upright positions. This position enhances the effectiveness of the abdominal muscle efforts while the woman is pushing and thereby shortens the second stage of labor. Raising and supporting the torso helps the woman view the birth process. At the same time, the birth attendant has access to the perineum. Many older delivery room tables cannot be adjusted to a semi-Fowler's position. A large foam wedge placed under the woman's head and shoulders will approximate the elevation of a semi-Fowler's position. Supporting a woman in this position is not difficult with most birthing beds.

Sitting   The sitting position is becoming an option for more women with the increased availability of birthing chairs. The use of birthing chairs or stools can be traced back to ancient Egypt and was broadly used in ancient Greek, Roman, and Incan civilizations. In the wake of the nineteenth century battle against puerperal fever, birthing chairs began to vanish on hygienic grounds. Birthing chairs

are being used again during the second stage of labor and are perceived by some women who use them as a positive way to participate in the birth process. A supported sitting position may also be achieved in many of the newer birthing beds.

The upright sitting position offers advantages similar to squatting. It has been postulated that the weight of a term fetus is sufficient force in itself to supply much of what is needed to bring the newborn into the world. Proponents of the birthing chair state that it makes possible spontaneous births that would have required operative assistance in the recumbent position. Women experiencing severe back pain have found use of the chair can diminish or eliminate the pain. The woman can curl forward and grasp her knees or ankles during pushing efforts. She can usually see the birth without aid of mirrors and following birth she can lift the baby up toward her face.

Duration of second stage and fetal outcome is not significantly affected by use of the birthing chair. However, a potential for increased blood loss may exist.

CRITICAL THINKING

What factors might influence the birthing position that a woman chooses?

Cleansing the Perineum   After being positioned for the birth, the woman's vulvar and perineal area is cleansed to increase her comfort and to remove the bloody discharge that is present prior to the actual birth. An aseptic technique such as the one that follows is recommended.

After a thorough hand washing, the nurse opens the sterile prep tray, dons sterile gloves, and cleans the vulva and perineum with the cleansing solution (Figure 23–9). Some agency policy dictates the area be rinsed with sterile water. Beginning with the mons pubis, the area is cleansed up to the lower abdomen. A second sponge is used to clean the inner groin and thigh of one leg, and a third is used to clean the other leg, moving outward to avoid carrying material from surrounding areas to the vaginal outlet. The last three sponges are used to clean the labia and vestibule with one downward sweep each. The used sponges are discarded.

Support of the Couple   The labor coach and/or support person is given a stool to sit on if desired. Both the woman and the coach are kept informed of procedures and progress and are supported throughout the birth. In some birth settings, there is a mirror that can be adjusted so that the couple may watch the birth.

The woman's blood pressure is monitored between contractions, and the contractions are palpated until the birth. FHR is auscultated every 15 minutes for low-risk women and every 5 minutes for high-risk women (NAACOG 1990). The nurse and support person continue to assist the woman in her pushing efforts.

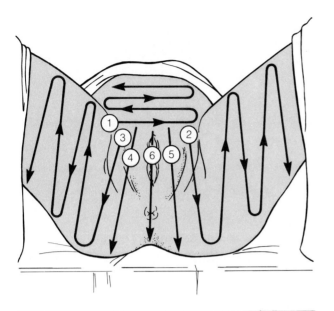

Figure 23–9   Cleansing the perineum prior to birth. The nurse follows the numbered diagram, using a new sponge for each area. The woman in this drawing is in dorsal recumbent position to demonstrate the cleansing. The perineal scrub may be accomplished in any maternal position.

In addition to assisting the woman and her partner, the nurse also assists the physician or nurse-midwife in preparing for the birth.

Physician/Nurse-Midwife Interventions When the fetal head has distended the perineum about 5 cm, the clinician may perform certain hand maneuvers that are believed to prevent undue trauma to the fetal head and maternal soft tissues. The woman may be asked to pant to avoid too rapid a birth of the fetal head.

After the infant's head is born, the clinician palpates the neck for the presence of a cord, which can be slipped over the fetal head if it is loose. If the cord is tight, it is double-clamped and cut.

Restitution and external rotation occur after the head is born. The only assistance needed during this time is support of the maternal perineum. While awaiting completion of external rotation, the clinician suctions the newborn's nose and mouth to remove mucus. When the newborn's shoulder appears at the symphysis pubis, the clinician may use both hands to grasp the newborn's head gently and pull downward for release of the anterior shoulder. Gentle upward traction facilitates release of the posterior shoulder.

Birth of the newborn's body may be controlled by grasping the posterior shoulder with one hand, palm turned toward the perineum. The left hand may be used for this if the newborn is LOA. The right hand then follows along the infant's back, and the feet are grasped as they are expelled. The newborn's head is kept down and to the side as the newborn's feet, legs, and body are tucked under the clinician's left arm in a football hold. The clinician's right hand is then free for further care of the newborn and the newborn is securely held. The nose and mouth are suctioned with a bulb syringe, and respiratory passages are cleared.

There is considerable controversy about when to clamp and cut the cord. If the newborn is held at or below the vagina as cord clamping is delayed, as much as 50 to 100 ml of blood may be shifted from the placenta to the fetus. If the newborn is held 50 to 60 cm above the vagina, a negligible amount of blood is transferred to the newborn even after three minutes. The extra amount of blood added to the newborn's circulation may reduce the frequency of iron deficiency anemia, which can occur later in infancy—or the circulatory overload may produce polycythemia and favor hyperbilirubinemia. Cunningham et al (1989) advocate clamping the cord after clearing the newborn's airway, which takes about 30 seconds. The newborn is not elevated above the vagina.

The cord is usually clamped with two Kelly clamps and cut between them, although some birth attendants may ask that the cord be double-clamped so that a section is available for the collection of cord blood gases. The clamp on the placental side is placed on the mother's abdomen. A plastic cord clamp or umbilical tape may be applied on the newborn's cord about 2 cm from the newborn's abdomen, and then the Kelly clamp on the newborn's side may be removed.

Figure 23–10 on p 676 depict the labor and birthing experience of one family.

The sheer pleasure of the feeling of a born baby on one's thighs is like nothing on earth. (Margaret Drabble, in Ever Since Eve*)*

The Leboyer Method
In 1975 Leboyer introduced a birthing technique directed toward easing the newborn's transition to extrauterine life. Leboyer advocated a more soothing and tender approach to the handling of the newborn at birth. The lights in the birthing area are dimmed, and the noise level is kept to a minimum. As the newborn is born, the physician/nurse-midwife handles the baby gently. Suctioning is not done, and the newborn is placed on his or her stomach on the mother's bare abdomen. The mother is encouraged to gently stroke and touch the newborn. Care is taken to keep the newborn's spine in a curved position similar to its position in utero.

Clamping of the umbilical cord is delayed until all pulsations have ceased. After the umbilical cord is clamped, the newborn is gently and slowly placed in a water bath that has been warmed to 98 to 99F. The newborn remains in the bath until he or she is completely relaxed. Following the bath the infant is carefully and gently dried and wrapped in layers of warm blankets.

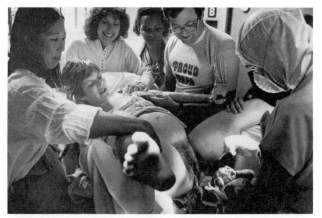

Delivery of the first twin.

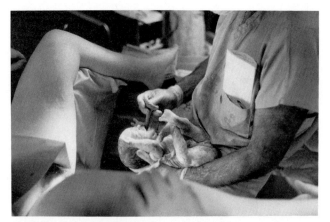

The baby's nose and mouth are suctioned.

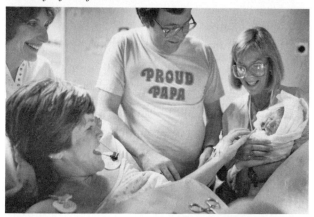

The nurse shows the first baby to Pat and Steve.

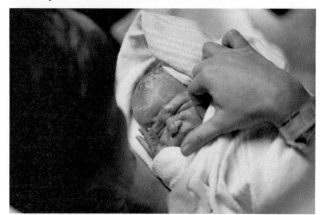

Pat meets the second baby.

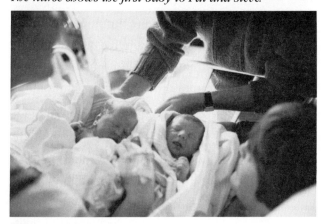

Hilary and Rebecca.

Figure 23–10   A birth story

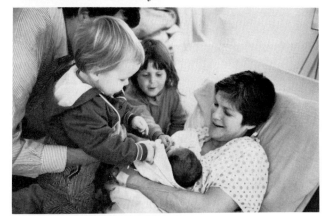

*Amanda and Lloyd meet their sisters
a few hours after birth.*

Evaluation

Anticipated outcomes of nursing care include the following:

- The woman is able to push effectively.
- The woman feels support and comfort from her partner and the nursing personnel.
- The support person has been supported and encouraged.

- The woman's physiologic and psychologic status has been maintained.
- The baby is born without difficulty.
- The couple's wishes for their childbirth experience have been realized if at all possible.

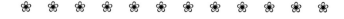

Care of the Woman and Her Partner During the Third Stage

The second stage of labor ends with birth of the newborn and signals the beginning of the third stage. The placenta is expelled during the third stage.

Although care of the newborn is an immediate concern of the nurse, the nurse must keep in mind that physical changes are still occurring in the new mother. The tremendous reduction in uterine surface area causes the rapid process of detachment of the placenta from the uterine wall. The uterus continues to contract and relax rhythmically until the placenta is expelled, completing the third stage of labor. Although the maximum length of the third stage is considered to be 30 minutes, it usually lasts 5 to 10 minutes.

❀ *APPLYING THE NURSING PROCESS* ❀

Nursing Assessment

Assessment during the third stage focuses on the period of time from the birth of the baby to the birth of the placenta. The uterine contractions and maternal vital signs will continue to be assessed. The newborn is assessed during this transition to extrauterine life.

Nursing Diagnosis

Nursing diagnoses during the third stage will probably focus on fatigue, and pain. The following are examples of nursing diagnoses:

- Fatigue related to inability to rest during labor and pushing efforts associated with birth.
- Pain, acute related to pushing efforts, episiotomy, perineal distention, and muscle strain during birth.

Additional nursing diagnoses are presented in the box Key Nursing Diagnoses to Consider—During the Third Stage.

Dₓ Key Nursing Diagnoses to Consider During the Third Stage

Increased cardiac output.
Fatigue
Pain
Impaired skin integrity

Nursing Plan and Implementation

Provision of Immediate Newborn Care

Most immediate care of the newborn can be accomplished while the newborn is in the parent's arms or in the radiant-heated unit, which may be placed by the parents so they can see the baby. The physician/nurse-midwife places the newborn on the mother's abdomen or in the radiant-heated unit.

Since the first priority is to maintain respirations, the newborn is placed in a modified Trendelenburg position to aid drainage of mucus from the nasopharynx and trachea. The newborn is also suctioned with a bulb syringe or De-Lee mucus trap (see Procedure 23–1) as needed.

The second priority is to provide and maintain warmth, so the newborn is dried immediately. Warmth can be maintained by placing warmed blankets over the newborn or placing the newborn in skin-to-skin contact with the mother. If the newborn is in a radiant-heated unit, he or she is dried, placed on a dry blanket, and left uncovered under the radiant heat. Because radiant heat warms the outer surface of objects, a newborn wrapped in blankets will receive no benefit from radiant heat.

Apgar Scoring System The Apgar scoring system (Table 23–9) was designed in 1952 by Dr. Virginia Apgar, an anesthesiologist. The purpose of the *Apgar score* is to evaluate the physical condition of the newborn at birth and the immediate need for resuscitation. The newborn is rated 1 minute after birth and again at 5 minutes and receives a total score ranging from 0 to 10 based on the following criteria:

1. The *heart rate* is auscultated or palpated at the junction of the umbilical cord and skin. This is the most important assessment. A newborn heart rate

Table 23–9 The Apgar Scoring System*

	Score		
Sign	**0**	**1**	**2**
Heart rate	Absent	Slow—below 100	Above 100
Respiratory effort	Absent	Slow—irregular	Good crying
Muscle tone	Flaccid	Some flexion of extremities	Active motion
Reflex irritability	None	Grimace	Vigorous cry
Color	Pale blue	Body pink, blue	Completely

*From Apgar V: The newborn (Apgar) scoring system: Reflections and advice. Pediatr Clin North Am *August 1966; 13:645.*

Nasal Pharyngeal Suctioning

Nursing action

Objective: Clear secretions from newborn's nose and/or oropharynx if respirations are depressed and/or if amniotic fluid was meconium stained.

Tighten the lid on the DeLee mucus trap or other suction device collection bottle (Figure 23–11).

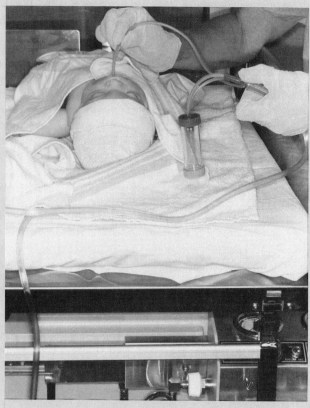

Connect one end of the DeLee tubing to low suction.

Insert other end of tubing in newborn's nose or mouth 3 to 5 inches.

Continue suction as tube is removed.

Continue reinserting tube and providing suction for as long as fluid is aspirated.

Note: Excessive suctioning can cause vagal stimulation, which causes decreased heart rate.

Occasionally the tube may be passed into the newborn's stomach to remove secretions or meconium that was swallowed before birth; if this is necessary, insert tube into newborn's mouth and then into the stomach. Provide suction and continue suction as tube is removed. Be careful not to aspirate the fluid yourself.

Objective: Record information on client's record.

Document completion of procedure and amount and type of secretions obtained.

Rationale

Avoids spillage of secretions and prevents air from leaking out of lid.

Figure 23–11   DeLee mucus trap

Provides suction
Clears nasopharynx

Avoids redepositing secretions in newborn's nasopharynx

Facilitates removal of secretions

If meconium was present in amniotic fluid the baby may have swallowed some.
Secretions and/or meconium aspirate may be removed from newborn's stomach to decrease incidence of aspiration of stomach contents.

Provides documentation of intervention and status at birth

of less than 100 beats per minute indicates the need for immediate resuscitation.

2. The *respiratory effort* is the second most important Apgar assessment. Complete absence of respirations is termed *apnea*. A vigorous cry indicates good respirations.

3. The *muscle tone* is determined by evaluating the degree of flexion and resistance to straightening of the extremities. A normal newborn's elbows and hips are flexed, with the knees positioned up toward the abdomen.

4. The *reflex irritability* is evaluated by flicking the soles of the feet or by inserting a nasal catheter in the nose. A cry merits a full score of 2. A grimace is 1 point, and no response is 0.

5. The *skin color* is inspected for cyanosis and pallor. Newborns generally have blue extremities, and the rest of the body is pink, which merits a score of 1.

This condition is termed *acrocyanosis* and is present in 85% of normal newborns at 1 minute after birth. A completely pink newborn scores a 2 and a totally cyanotic, pale infant is scored 0. Newborns with darker skin pigmentation will not be pink in color. Their skin color is assessed for pallor and acrocyanosis, and a score is selected based on the assessment.

A score of 8 to 10 indicates a newborn in good condition who requires only nasopharyngeal suctioning and perhaps some oxygen near the face. If the Apgar score is below 8, resuscitative measures may need to be instituted. See the discussion in Chapter 32.

Care of the Umbilical Cord   If the physician/nurse-midwife has not placed a cord clamp (Figures 23–12 and 23–13) on the newborn's umbilical cord, it is the responsibility of the nurse to do so. Before applying the cord clamp, the nurse examines the cut end for the presence of two arteries and one vein. The umbilical vein is the largest vessel, and the arteries are seen as smaller vessels. The presence of only one artery in the umbilical cord is associated with genitourinary abnormalities. The number of vessels is recorded on the birth and newborn records. The cord is clamped approximately 1/2 to 1 inch from the abdomen to allow room between the abdomen and clamp as the cord dries. Abdominal skin must not be clamped, as this will cause necrosis of the tissue. The clamp is removed in the

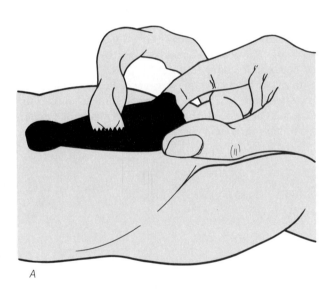

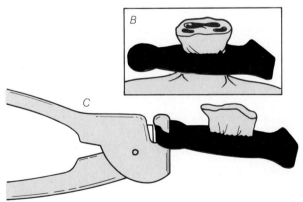

Figure 23–12   Hollister cord clamp. A Clamp is positioned 1/2 to 1 inch from the abdomen and then secured. B Cut cord. C Plastic device for removing clamp after cord has dried.

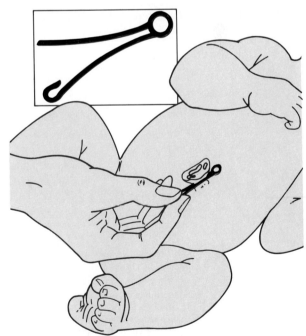

Figure 23–13   Hesseltine cord clamp. Two clamps are often used to reduce the possibility of hemorrhage should one inadvertently open. When the cord has dried, the clamp may be removed manually.

newborn nursery approximately 24 hours after the cord has dried.

Evaluation of the Newborn After Birth

As more newborns remain with their parents in the birth area, the initial evaluation of the newborn becomes even more important. Babies at risk must be identified at once so that stabilization or treatment is initiated quickly in the nursery. Although a full head-to-toe assessment is not necessary at this time, the evaluation must be thorough enough to determine that the newborn will not be compromised by remaining in the birth area. An initial newborn evaluation that identifies critical aspects is presented in Table 23–10.

Additional assessments focus on easily observed congenital anomalies. The head and face are observed for symmetry, and the mouth for an intact palate. The upper and lower extremities are inspected for the correct number of digits. The back is observed for any dimples, tufts of hair over the spine or lower back, and for any openings over the spinal column. At this time the anus may also be observed to determine if there is an opening.

This brief examination reveals any gross abnormalities and permits a quick determination of gestational age. Most of this examination is accomplished by visual assessment. Further neurologic assessment and an in-depth physical examination are performed in the newborn nursery (see Chapter 28).

The newborn may be weighed and measured in the delivery room/birthing room or in the newborn nursery.

Newborn Identification Procedures

To ensure that the parents are given the correct newborn, the mother and baby are tagged with identical bands or bracelets before the newborn is separated from the mother. One bracelet is applied to the mother's wrist, and two bracelets are applied to the newborn—one on each wrist, one on a wrist and one on an ankle, or one on each ankle. The bands must be applied snugly to prevent loss.

Most hospitals footprint the newborn and fingerprint the mother for further identification purposes. When preparing to footprint the newborn, the nurse wipes the soles of both the newborn's feet to remove any vernix caseosa, which interferes with the placement of ink on the foot creases.

Initiation of Attachment

The beginning of the third stage is usually emotional for all involved. For the couple the birth of the healthy newborn is the culmination of the long months of pregnancy and the intense experience of labor. The expulsion of the newborn and the sound of the first cry creates an exhilarating and emotional moment for the new parents. The new mother may be exhausted but is usually elated and eager to see her new baby. The parents' concerns are usually about the well-being and gender of the baby. Given the alertness of newborns immediately after birth and the excitement and curiosity of the parents, it is an ideal time to initiate the attachment process. The baby may remain with the mother, and the nurse may help position the baby so that eye-to-eye

---

Table 23–10 Initial Newborn Evaluation

Assess	Normal findings
Respirations	Rate 30–60, irregular No retractions, no grunting
Apical pulse	Rate 120–160 and somewhat irregular
Temperature	Skin temp above 97.8F (36.5C)
Skin color	Body pink with bluish extremities
Umbilical cord	Two arteries and one vein
Gestational age	Should be 38–42 weeks to remain with parents for extended time
Sole creases	Sole creases that involve the heel

In general expect: scant amount of vernix on upper back, axilla, groin; lanugo only on upper back; ears with incurving of upper ⅔ of pinnae and thin cartilage that springs back from folding; male genitalia—testes palpated in upper or lower scrotum; female genitalia—labia majora larger; clitoris nearly covered

In the following situations, newborns should generally be stabilized rather than remaining with parents in the birth area for an extended period of time:

Apgar is less than 8 at one minute and less than 9 at five minutes, or a baby requires resuscitation measures (other than whiffs of oxygen).
Respirations are below 30 or above 60, with retractions and/or grunting.
Apical pulse is below 120 or above 160 with marked irregularities.
Skin temperature is below 97.8F (36.5C).
Skin color is pale blue, or there is circumoral pallor.
Baby is less than 38 or more than 42 weeks' gestation.
Baby is very small or very large for gestational age.
There are congenital anomalies involving open areas in the skin (meningomyelocele).

contact is possible. The lights of the birthing room may be dimmed so that the baby's eyes open fully. The parents can be encouraged to explore and touch their baby.

I was hungry for the baby as he was born. I wanted to see, hold him. It was hours before I realized or even thought love in relation to him. (Harriette Hartigan, Women in Birth)

Nurse-Midwife/Physician Interventions

After the cord has been clamped and cut, the physician/nurse-midwife observes for the following signs of placental separation:

1. The uterus rises upward in the abdomen because the placenta settles downward into the lower uterine segment.

2. As the placenta proceeds downward, the umbilical cord lengthens.

3. A sudden trickle or spurt of blood appears.

4. The uterus changes from a discoid to a globular shape.

While waiting for these signs, the nurse or birth attendant gently palpates the uterus to check for ballooning of the uterus caused by uterine relaxation and subsequent bleeding into the uterine cavity.

After the placenta has separated, it may be expelled by various techniques such as maternal effort, controlled cord traction, and fundal pressure. Maternal effort allows the placenta to be expelled spontaneously and is best accomplished in an upright position. When the mother is in a dorsal recumbent or lithotomy position, she or the nurse can help the process by splinting or supporting her abdominal muscles. The mother or nurse can place her palms over the lower abdomen, or the mother can flex her thighs over her abdomen. The mother then bears down to expel the placenta.

Controlled cord traction may also be used to deliver the placenta. The physician/nurse-midwife first ensures that separation has occurred and then places one hand above the symphysis with the palm against the anterior surface of the uterus. The uterus is displaced upward and backward as the mother is asked to relax her abdominal muscles and breathe through an open mouth. The elevation of the uterus straightens out the birth canal and facilitates expulsion of the placenta, as well as protecting the uterus from inversion. Gentle traction is exerted on the umbilical cord. During this procedure the nurse encourages the mother to continue breathing through an open mouth and to relax her abdominal muscles.

Fundal pressure is not a method of choice because it is very uncomfortable for the mother and may damage uterine supports. If this method is needed, the mother is asked to relax her abdominal muscles and then the physician's/nurse-midwife's hand is placed behind the uterus with the fingers directed downward toward the maternal spine. With a quick "scooping" motion the contracted uterus is pressed downward in an arc. This motion is different from direct downward pressure, which folds the uterus over the lower segment and does not enhance movement of the placenta. During the procedure the nurse provides continued encouragement to maintain abdominal relaxation. This is very difficult due to the discomfort of the procedure (Long 1986).

After expulsion of the placenta, the physician/nurse-midwife inspects the placental membranes to make sure they are intact and that all cotyledons are present. This inspection is especially important with placentas expelled via the Duncan mechanism. If there is a defect or a part missing from the placenta, a digital uterine examination is done. The vagina and cervix are inspected for lacerations, and any necessary repairs are made. An episiotomy may be repaired now if it has not been done previously. (See further discussion of episiotomy on pp 796–797.) The fundus of the uterus is palpated; normal position is at the midline and below the umbilicus. If the fundus is displaced, it may be because of a full bladder or a collection of blood in the uterus.

The time and mechanism (Schultze or Duncan) of expulsion of the placenta are noted on the birth record.

Use of Oxytocics Some nurse-midwives/physicians advocate the use of oxytocic drugs (Pitocin, Syntocinon) to promote homeostasis by stimulating myometrial contractions after birth and to reduce the incidence of third-stage hemorrhage (Long 1986).

The physician/nurse-midwife may request that 10 units of oxytocin be given intramuscularly when the anterior shoulder of the infant appears. Others question whether this method increases the incidence of neonatal hyperviscosity because an additional bolus of blood may be infused into the fetus when the uterus contracts in response to the oxytocin. At other times, 10 units of oxytocin (Pitocin) may be administered IM, or by slow IV push at the time of placental expulsion. More recently, some physicians are injecting oxytocin into the umbilical vein immediately after the cord is clamped and cut (Reddy & Carey 1989). Both techniques are thought to facilitate expulsion of the placenta. It should be noted that an IV bolus of oxytocin may cause profound hypotension and tachycardia (Prendiville & Elbourne 1989). Some prefer to add 10 units of oxytocin to IV fluids administered over a period of hours. Additional information and associated nursing implications are presented in the Drug Guide–Oxytocin in Chapter 26.

Methylergonovine maleate (Methergine) or prostaglandin F_2 alpha (Douglas et al 1989; Prendiville & Elbourne 1989) may be given IM after expulsion of the placenta to cause contraction of the uterus. Information regarding Methergine and associated nursing implications are presented in the Drug Guide–Methergine in Chapter 34.

Evaluation

Anticipated outcomes of nursing care include the following:

- The woman's placenta is expelled without difficulty.
- The woman's physiologic status remains normal.
- The woman and her partner have an opportunity to be with their baby if they desire.

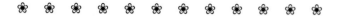

One Family's Story

Allison and Scott Jones are expecting their first child. During the pregnancy, they attended prenatal classes and made special preparations in anticipation of using the birthing room at their local hospital. The pregnancy has proceeded without difficulty or problems.

When labor begins, they go to the hospital and are greeted by Marie Carlson, a nurse in the birthing unit. Ms Carlson helps Allison and Scott get settled and completes the admission process. Allison is having contractions every two to three minutes lasting 45 seconds, and cervical dilation is 5 cm. She is breathing with each contraction and focusing on a picture of their pet sheepdog, Max, as a focal point. Scott provides encouragement while he times contractions. He carefully unpacks their supply bag and they are quickly surrounded by extra pillows, knee socks for Allison, powder to use with effleurage, and suckers. They are both excited that the birth day is at hand.

Ms Carlson works to provide a comfortable, unhurried atmosphere. She is already acquainted with the Joneses because they have attended the prenatal classes that she teaches. She is familiar with their level of knowledge and will now work to support them as labor progresses. She notes that Allison and Scott are working well together in timing contractions and using relaxation techniques and breathing methods. She continues her assessments in a quiet manner and continues to offer support and encouragement to Allison and Scott. She assists Allison in position changes and helps arrange pillows to provide support. When Allison wants a back rub and effleurage, Ms Carlson takes over one of the activities as Scott does the other.

As Allison proceeds into transition, Ms Carlson notes that the Joneses need more encouragement and support, so she stays in constant attendance. She assesses maternal, fetal, and labor status and keeps the Joneses informed of their progress.

Dr Grey comes in to see the Joneses and stays close by because the labor is progressing rapidly. Toward the end of the transition, Ms Carlson prepares the equipment to be used during the birth. She assists Allison in her pushing efforts when the cervix has completely dilated. During the birth, she assists Allison, Scott, and Dr Grey. The birth is managed in the same unhurried manner. Ms Carl-

son assesses the physical parameters and offers continuing support as Allison gives birth to a baby girl of healthy appearance. Ms Carlson assesses the newborn quickly and then places her in her mother's arms.

The post birth recovery period is monitored closely so that any problems can be identified. Allison is recovering without problems and is eager to learn more about her new daughter. Ms Carlson talks to the Joneses to assess their level of knowledge and provides needed information. She does a physical assessment of the newborn and explains the findings to the Joneses. She assists Allison as she breast-feeds her baby for the first time. After the feeding, the nurse assists Scott in giving the baby her first bath. Ms Carlson has found that the bath time provides opportunities to talk and share information.

During the recovery period, Ms Carlson provides quiet time for the new family to be together and get acquainted.

A few hours after the birth, Ms Carlson assists the Joneses as they prepare for discharge. She will be making a visit to the Joneses' home the next morning to assess the mother and newborn and to provide information and continued support.

Care of the Woman and Her Partner During the Fourth Stage

The period immediately following expulsion of the placenta is referred to as the fourth stage of labor and birth. Actually the label is misleading since labor and the birth are completed with delivery of the placenta, and the next few hours are actually the immediate recovery phase. The fourth stage is usually defined as lasting one to four hours after the birth, or until vital signs are stable. Nursing care in this phase involves the basics of postpartum nursing care.

Since the fourth stage begins immediately after the placenta is expelled, repair of an episiotomy or vaginal lacerations is done at this time. The uterus is palpated at frequent intervals to ensure that it remains firmly contracted (medical interventions during this period are described on pp 684–685). If the mother has not held her baby yet, immediate newborn care should be completed at her side and within her reach so that she can touch her baby during this time. As soon as immediate care is completed, the new mother is usually eager to cuddle and explore her baby. If she plans to breast-feed her baby, and the baby is interested, she should be encouraged and helped to do so right after birth while the baby is awake and alert. Care should be taken not to try to force an uninterested baby to breast-feed as it will just lead to frustration for both mother and baby.

Behavioral characteristics of the mother vary depending on such factors as the length of labor and the extent of interruption in normal sleep patterns. After the initial excitement of becoming acquainted with their new baby and notifying others of the birth, many new mothers are very tired and want to rest. Others are wide awake, eager to talk about their labor and satisfy basic body needs, such as hunger and thirst. Although labor is completed, the uterus is sensitive to touch and palpation of the uterus is not appreciated unless the woman understands the importance of the procedure.

❀ *APPLYING THE NURSING PROCESS* ❀

Nursing Assessment

Assessment during the fourth stage focuses on the physiologic status of the mother, which includes maternal vital signs, uterine contractility, lochia, bladder status, and perineal condition.

Nursing Diagnosis

Nursing diagnoses during the fourth stage are directed toward the maternal physiologic status, introduction to the newborn, and the establishment of breast-feeding (if this is the chosen feeding method). Examples of nursing diagnoses are presented in the box Key Nursing Diagnoses—During the Fourth Stage.

Nursing Plan and Implementation

Preparation for the Recovery Period

As soon as the CNM/physician completes her or his tasks, drapes are removed. The nurse washes the perineum with gauze squares and sterile solution and dries the area with a sterile towel. If the woman is to remain in the birthing bed, the nurse helps her get clean and dry by placing clean absorbent pads beneath her and applying maternity pads. A clean gown is also provided if necessary. Linen can be changed later when she first gets up to void.

If the woman gave birth in the birthing room and stirrups were used, her perineum is cleaned and maternity pads applied before her legs are removed from the stirrups. In order to avoid muscle strain, both legs are removed from the stirrups at the same time. The legs may be "bicycled" to promote circulation return. The woman is transferred to a recovery room bed. If the mother has not had a chance to hold her infant, she may do so before she is transferred from the birthing room. The nurse ensures that the mother and father and newborn are given time to begin the attachment process.

Promotion of Maternal Physical Well-Being

The primary goal during the immediate recovery period is to ensure that the mother has minimal bleeding. The most significant source of bleeding is from the site where the placenta was implanted and where uterine vessels previously provided pooling of maternal blood to nourish the fetus. It is critical, therefore, that the fundus stay well-contracted in order to clamp off these uterine vessels and prevent hemorrhage. It is the nurse's responsibility to assess the mother's blood pressure, pulse, firmness and position of fundus, and amount and character of vaginal blood flow every 15 minutes for the first hour or two. Deviations from the normal ranges require more frequent checking (see Table 23–11). Blood pressure should return to the prelabor level, and pulse rate should be slightly lower than it was in labor. The return of the blood pressure is due to an increased volume of blood returning to the maternal circulation from the uteroplacental shunt. Baroreceptors cause a vagal response, which slows the pulse. The physiologic slowing may be offset by excitement, increased temperature, and/or dehydration. A rise in the blood pressure may be a response to oxytocic drugs or may be caused by PIH. Blood loss may be reflected by a lowered blood pressure and a rising pulse rate.

The fundus should be firm at the umbilicus or lower and in the midline. The uterus should be palpated (Figure

---

Key Nursing Diagnoses to Consider
During the Fourth Stage

Breast-feeding, effective
Increased cardiac output
Impaired skin integrity
Fluid volume deficit: High risk
Infection: High risk
Injury: High risk
Knowledge deficit
Pain
Urinary retention, acute

Table 23–11 Maternal Adaptations Following Birth

Characteristic	Normal finding
Blood pressure	Should return to prelabor level.
Pulse	Slightly lower than in labor.
Uterine fundus	In the midline at the umbilicus or 1–2 fingerbreadths below the umbilicus.
Lochia	Red (rubra), small to moderate amount (from spotting on pads to ¼–½ of pad covered in 15 minutes). Should not exceed saturation of one pad in first hour.
Bladder	Nonpalpable.
Perineum	Smooth, pink, without bruising or edema.
Emotional state	Wide variation, including excited, exhilarated, smiling, crying, fatigued, verbal, quiet, pensive, and sleepy.

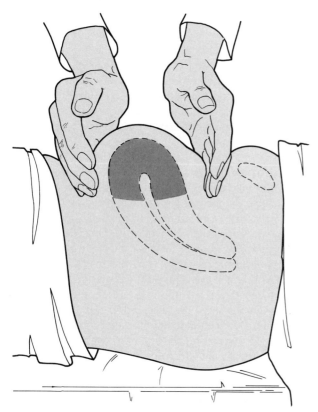

Figure 23–14 Suggested method of palpating the fundus of the uterus during the fourth stage. The left hand is placed just above the symphysis pubis, and gentle downward pressure is exerted. The right hand is cupped around the uterine fundus.

23–14) but not massaged unless boggy (atonic). When a uterus becomes boggy, pooling of blood occurs within the uterus, resulting in the formation of clots. Anything left in the uterus prevents the uterus from contracting effectively. Thus, if it becomes boggy or appears to rise in the abdomen, the fundus should be massaged until firm; then with one hand supporting the uterus at the symphysis, the nurse should attempt to express retained clots.

A boggy uterus feels very soft instead of firm and hard. In some cases the uterus has relaxed so much that it cannot be found when the nurse attempts to palpate it. In this case, the nurse places her hand in the midline of the abdomen about at the level of the umbilicus and begins to make kneading motions. This motion stimulates the uterine fundus to contract, and the nurse will feel the fundus tighten to a firm, hard object.

The nurse inspects the bloody vaginal discharge for amount and charts it as minimal, moderate, or heavy. It should be bright red. A soaked perineal pad contains approximately 100 mL of blood. If the perineal pad becomes soaked in a 15-minute period, or if blood pools under the buttocks, continuous observation is necessary. As long as the woman remains in bed during the first hour, bleeding should not exceed saturation of one pad (Long 1986). Laceration of the vagina, cervix, or an unligated vessel in the episiotomy may be indicated by a continuous trickle of blood even though the fundus remains firm. (See Procedure 23–2.)

If the fundus rises and displaces to the right, the nurse palpates the bladder to determine whether it is distended. All measures should be taken to enable the mother to void. If she is unable to void, catheterization is necessary. Postpartal women have decreased sensations to void as a result of the decreased tone of the bladder due to the trauma imposed on the bladder and urethra during childbirth. The bladder fills rapidly as the body attempts to rid itself of the extra fluid volume returned from the uteroplacental circulation and of intravenous fluid that may have been received during labor and birth. If the mother is unable to void, a warm towel placed across the lower abdomen or warm water poured over the perineum or spirits of peppermint poured into a bedpan may help the urinary sphincter relax and thus facilitate voiding. A distended bladder can cause uterine atony thus increasing postpartal bleeding.

The perineum is inspected for edema and hematoma formation. With an episiotomy or laceration, an ice pack often reduces swelling and alleviates discomfort (Hill 1989; La Foy & Geden 1989).

The following conditions should be reported to the CNM/physician: hypotension, tachycardia, uterine atony, excessive bleeding, or a temperature over 100F or 38C. The nurse should be aware that the blood pressure may not fall rapidly in the presence of dangerous bleeding in postpartal mothers because of the extra systemic volume. However, an increasing pulse rate may be noted before a decrease in blood pressure is detected. A normal blood pressure with the mother in the Fowler's position is a good confirmation of a normotensive woman.

Women frequently have tremors in the immediate postpartal period. It has been proposed that this shivering response is caused by a difference in internal and external body temperatures (higher temperature inside the body than on the outside). Another theory is that the woman is reacting to the fetal cells that have entered the maternal circulation at the placental site. A heated bath blanket placed next to the woman and, perhaps, a warm drink tend to alleviate the problem.

The couple may be tired, hungry, and thirsty. Some hospitals serve the couple a meal. The tired mother will probably drift off into a welcome sleep. The father should also be encouraged to rest, since his supporting role is physically and mentally tiring. The mother is usually transferred from the birthing unit to the postpartal unit after two hours or more depending on agency policy and if the following criteria are met: Stable vital signs; no bleeding; nondistended bladder; firm fundus; sensations fully recovered from any anesthetic agent received during childbirth.

PROCEDURE 23–2

Evaluating Lochia After Birth

Nursing Action	Rationale
Objective: Prepare woman.	
Explain the procedure, the reason for carrying out the procedure, and information that will be obtained.	Explanation of procedure decreases anxiety and increases relaxation
Objective: Obtain and evaluate maternal vital signs.	
Assess maternal temperature, blood pressure, and pulse.	Provides information regarding physiologic status
Objective: Accurately evaluate the amount of lochia after birth.	
Put on disposable gloves prior to the assessment.	Universal precautions and body substance isolation require use of gloves when exposed to body secretions such as lochia.
Lower perineal pad so amount of lochia can be visualized.	Allows nurse to view amount of lochia collected during the assessment
Palpate uterine fundus by placing one hand on the fundus and the other hand just over the symphysis pubis and press downward. With the other hand, palpate the uterine fundus.	The fundus is located in the midline at the umbilicus or 1 to 2 fingerbreadths below the umbilicus. Downward pressure exerted just above the symphysis will prevent excessive downward movement of the uterus during assessment.
Determine firmness of fundus.	The uterus needs to remain firmly contracted to prevent excessive blood loss.
If fundus is boggy, massage by rubbing in circular motion.	Manual pressure stimulates uterine contractions.
Evaluate the color and amount of lochia, and observe for the presence of clots. The following guidelines may be used to evaluate and describe the amount of lochia:	Provides information regarding expected status. After birth, a moderate amount of lochia rubra, without clots, is expected.
Small: smaller than a 4-in. stain on the pad; 10 to 25 mL	
Moderate: smaller than a 6-in. stain; 25 to 50 mL	
Large: larger than 6-in. stain; 50 to 80 mL (Luegenbiehl et al 1990)	
If blood loss exceeds above guidelines, the perineal pads and the chux may be weighed to more accurately estimate blood loss.	An estimate may be obtained by using the equivalent of 1 g of weight equals 1 mL. Weighing the pads and chux can provide important information, as amounts of blood loss may be underestimated due to the expectation that some blood loss is to be expected.

Enhancing Attachment

Evidence indicates that the first few hours and even minutes after birth are a sensitive period for attachment of mother and infant (Klaus & Kennell 1982). Separation during this critical period not only delays attachment but also may affect maternal and child behavior over a much longer period. At one month and one year after childbirth, mothers who were merely shown their infants after birth and had them only briefly for 15- to 20-minute feeding periods demonstrated less eye contact and less soothing behavior during physical examination than did mothers who were allowed to hold their infants for an hour beginning one to two hours after birth and for five hours on each of three succeeding days. The mothers with this extended contact asked twice as many questions about their children and used fewer commands at two years. The results of this and other research indicate that as soon as feasible the newborn needs to be united with his or her parents.

I feel different about my body now . . . feel proud of myself. I can do it again. I did such a great thing. (Harriette Hartigan, Women in Birth)

Klaus and Kennell (1982) believe the bonding experience can be enhanced by at least 30 to 60 minutes of early contact in privacy. If this period of contact can occur during the first hour after birth, the newborn will be in a quiet state and able to interact with parents by looking at them. Newborns also turn their heads in response to a spoken voice. (See Chapter 27 for further discussion of newborn states.)

The first parent–newborn contact may be brief (a few minutes) to be followed by a more extended contact after uncomfortable procedures (expulsion of the placenta and suturing of the episiotomy) are completed. When the newborn is returned to the mother, she can be assisted to begin breast-feeding if she so desires. The nurse can help the mother to a more comfortable position for holding the infant and breast-feeding. Even if the newborn does not actively nurse, he or she can lick, taste, and smell the mother's skin. This activity by the newborn stimulates the maternal release of prolactin, which promotes the onset of lactation.

Darkening the birthing room by turning out most of the lights causes newborns to open their eyes and gaze around. This in turn enhances eye-to-eye contact with the parents. (*Note:* if the physician or nurse-midwife needs a light source, the spotlight can be left on.) Treatment of the newborn's eyes may also be delayed. Many parents who establish eye contact with the newborn are content to gaze quietly at their infant. Others may show more active involvement by touching and/ or inspecting the newborn. Some mothers talk to their babies in a high-pitched voice, which seems to be soothing to newborns. Some couples verbally express amazement and pride when they see they have produced a beautiful, healthy baby. Their verbalization enhances feelings of accomplishment and ecstasy.

Both parents need to be encouraged to do whatever they feel most comfortable doing. Some parents prefer limited contact with the newborn in the delivery room and private time together in a quieter environment, such as the recovery room or postpartal area. In spite of the current zeal for providing immediate attachment opportunities, nursing personnel need to be aware of parents' wishes. The desire to delay interaction with the newborn does not necessarily imply a decreased ability of the parents to bond to their newborn (see Chapter 35 for further discussion of parent–newborn attachment).

Preparing for Early Discharge

More hospitals are offering new mothers—whether they deliver in a conventional labor and birth setting, a birthing room, or an inhospital birth center—the option of discharge within a few hours after the birth. Most institutions have written policies and criteria about the mother and the newborn eligible for early discharge. Criteria for the mother may include any or all of the following:

- No antepartal or intrapartal complications
- Length of labor within normal limits
- A small episiotomy
- A spontaneous or low-forceps birth
- Stable vital signs
- A firm uterine fundus
- Voiding without difficulty
- Ability to ambulate
- Demonstrated understanding of home-care instructions

Early discharge criteria for the newborn may include the following:

- Stable vital signs
- Normal physical examination
- A hematocrit level of 45% to 65% and a Dextrostix result of greater than 45%
- At least one successful feeding

The desired practice is to follow up early discharges with home visits by birthing, postpartum, or public health nurses. The early discharge option offers both financial benefits, by reducing the costs of obstetric care, and psychologic benefits, by reuniting families in their homes more quickly.

Since early discharge programs began in the 1960s, the most frequent neonatal problem requiring readmission to the hospital has been hyperbilirubinemia (Norr & Nacion 1987). However, this is not thought to be a reflection of inadequate or inappropriate care (Norr et al 1988) but may be attributable to the high percentage of breast-feeding mothers who are discharged early, the trend toward late cord clamping in the birth experience of this group, and the thorough newborn assessment by nurses making home visits (Barton et al 1990).

Evaluation

Anticipated outcomes of nursing care include the following:

- The woman's physiologic status is within normal limits as evidenced by normal vital signs, a well-contracted uterus, scant to moderate lochia rubra, a nondistended bladder, and the use of measures to decrease perineal swelling and pain.

- The woman and her partner have had an opportunity to be with the newborn as they desire.

- The woman has been able to initiate breast-feeding if she desires.

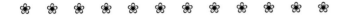

Care of the Adolescent During Labor and Birth

Each adolescent in labor is different. As with any laboring woman, the nurse needs to assess what the adolescent brings to the experience by asking the following questions:

- Has the young woman received prenatal care?

- What are her attitudes and feelings about the pregnancy?

- Who will attend the birth?

- What preparation has she had for the experience?

- What are her expectations and fears regarding birth?

- Does she have certain culturally reinforced beliefs regarding pregnancy?

- What are her usual coping mechanisms?

- Does she plan to keep the newborn?

The primary goals of nursing care for the adolescent during labor and birth are to promote maternal and fetal well-being; and to provide support to the adolescent.

Promotion of Maternal and Fetal Well-Being

Any adolescent who has not had prenatal care requires close observation during labor. Fetal well-being is established by fetal monitoring. Adolescents are among the highest risk populations for problems during labor and birth. However, it is likely that the risk factors that affect adolescents arise primarily from economic and psychosocial problems, rather than from physiological ones (Gale et al 1989).

The nurse should be alert to any physiologic complications of labor in the adolescent. The young woman's prenatal record is carefully reviewed for risks. The adolescent is screened for PIH, CPD, anemia, drugs ingested during pregnancy, sexually transmitted disease, and discrepancies between the size of the fetus and the gestational age.

Support During Labor and Birth

One of the greatest fears of any laboring woman is being left alone. This fear is greater in the adolescent, whether or not she acknowledges it to those around her.

The support role of the nurse depends on the young woman's support system during labor. She may not be accompanied by someone who will stay with her during childbirth. Whether she has a support person or not, it is important for the nurse to establish a trusting relationship with the young woman. In this way, the nurse can help her maintain control and understand what is happening to her. Establishing rapport without recrimination for possible inappropriate behavior is essential. The adolescent who is given positive reinforcement for "work well done" will leave the experience with increased self-esteem, despite the emotional problems that may accompany her situation.

If a support person did accompany the adolescent, that person also needs the nurse's encouragement and support. Whether that person is the father of the baby, a parent, or a friend of the laboring adolescent, establishing rapport with the support person without recrimination is essential in gaining his or her cooperation. Without this sense of acceptance, the support person may isolate himself or herself from the laboring adolescent, thus increasing her anxiety. The nurse must explain changes in the young woman's behavior and show the support person ways to help the young woman cope. If the support person is also an adolescent, the nursing staff should reinforce the adolescent's feelings that he or she is wanted and important.

The adolescent who has taken childbirth education classes is generally better prepared than the adolescent who has had no classes. The nurse must keep in mind, however, that the younger the adolescent, the less she may be able to participate actively in the process.

The very young adolescent (under age 14) has fewer coping mechanisms and less experience to draw on than her older counterparts have. Because her cognitive development is incomplete, the younger adolescent may have fewer problem-solving capabilities. Her ego integrity may be more threatened by the experience, and she may be more vulnerable to stress and discomfort.

The very young woman needs someone to rely on at all times during labor. She may be more childlike and dependent than older teens. The nurse must be sure that instructions and explanations are simple and concrete. During the transition phase, the young teenager may become withdrawn and unable to express her need to be nurtured. Touch, soothing encouragement, and measures to maintain her comfort help her maintain control and meet her needs for dependence. During the second stage of labor, the young adolescent may feel as if she is losing control and may reach out to those around her. By remaining calm and giving directions, the nurse helps her control feelings of helplessness.

The middle adolescent (age 14 to 16 years) often attempts to remain calm and unflinching during labor. If unable to break through the teenager's stoic barrier, the nurse needs to rise above frustration and realize that a caring attitude will still affect the young woman.

Many older adolescents feel that they "know it all," but they may be no more prepared for childbirth than their younger counterparts. The nurse's reinforcement and nonjudgmental manner will help them save face. If the adolescent has not taken classes, she may require preparation and explanations. The older teenager's response to the stresses of labor, however, is similar to that of the adult woman.

If the adolescent is planning to relinquish her newborn, she should be given the option of seeing and holding the infant. She may be reluctant to do this at first, but the grieving process is facilitated if the mother sees the infant. However, seeing or holding the newborn should be the young woman's choice. (See Chapter 34 for further discussion of the relinquishing mother and the adolescent parent.)

Care of the Woman During Precipitous Birth

Occasionally labor progresses so rapidly that the maternity nurse is faced with the task of managing the birth of the baby. This is called a precipitous birth. The attending maternity nurse has the primary responsibility for providing a physically and psychologically safe experience for the woman and her baby.

A woman whose physician or nurse-midwife is not present may feel disappointed, frightened, and abandoned, especially if she is not prepared through childbirth education. Fear is an inhibiting factor in childbirth: therefore, the nurse can support the woman by keeping her informed about the labor progress and assuring her that the nurse will stay with her. If birth is imminent, the nurse must not leave the mother alone. Auxiliary personnel can be directed to contact the attending physician or nurse-midwife, or other physicians/CNMs who are in the facility. The auxiliary personnel should also retrieve the emergency pack ("precip pack"), which should be readily accessible to the labor rooms. A typical pack contains the following items: A small drape that can be placed under the woman's buttocks to provide a sterile field; several 4-by-4 gauze pads for wiping off the newborn's face and removing secretions from the mouth; a bulb syringe to clear mucus from the newborn's mouth; two sterile clamps (Kelly or Rochester) to clamp the umbilical cord before applying a cord clamp; sterile scissors to cut the umbilical cord; a sterile umbilical cord clamp, either Hesseltine or Hollister; a baby blanket to wrap the newborn in after birth; a package of sterile gloves.

As the materials are being gathered, the nurse must remain calm. The woman is reassured by the nurse's composure and feels that the nurse is competent.

The primary goal of nursing care is the safe birth of the fetus whether it is in vertex or breech presentation.

Birth of Infant in Vertex Presentation

The nurse who manages precipitous birth in the hospital conducts it as follows. The woman is encouraged to assume a comfortable position. If time permits, the nurse scrubs her hands with soap and water and puts on sterile gloves. Sterile drapes are placed under the woman's buttocks.

At all times during the birth, the nurse gives clear instructions to the woman, supports her efforts, and provides reassurance. The nurse needs to remain calm and proceed in a slow, confident manner.

When the infant's head crowns, the nurse instructs the woman to pant, which decreases her urge to push. The nurse checks whether the amniotic sac is intact. If it is, the nurse tears the sac with a clamp so the newborn will not breathe in amniotic fluid with the first breath.

The nurse may place an index finger inside the lower portion of the vagina and the thumb on the outer portion of the perineum and *gently* massage the area to aid in stretching of perineal tissues and to help prevent perineal lacerations. This is called "ironing the perineum."

With one hand, the nurse applies gentle pressure against the fetal head to maintain flexion and prevent it from popping out rapidly. *The nurse does not hold the head back forcibly.* Rapid birth of the head may result in tears of the woman's perineal tissues. The rapid change in pressure within the fetal head may cause subdural or dural tears. The nurse supports the perineum with the other hand and allows the head to be delivered between contractions.

As the woman continues to pant, the nurse inserts one or two fingers along the back of the fetal head to check for the umbilical cord. If the cord is around the neck, the nurse bends her fingers like a fish hook, grasps the cord, and pulls it over the baby's head, loosens it, or slips it down over the shoulders. It is important to check that the cord is not wrapped around more than one time. If the cord is tightly looped and cannot be slipped over the baby's head, the nurse places two clamps on the cord, cuts the cord between the clamps, and unwinds the cord.

Immediately after birth of the head, the mouth, throat, and nasal passages are suctioned. The nurse places one hand on each side of the head and instructs the woman to push gently so that the rest of the body can be expelled quickly. The newborn must be supported as it emerges.

The newborn is held at the level of the uterus to facilitate blood flow through the umbilical cord. The combination of amniotic fluid and vernix makes the newborn very slippery, so the nurse must be careful to avoid dropping the newborn. The nose and mouth of the newborn are suctioned again, using a bulb syringe. The nurse then dries the newborn quickly to prevent heat loss.

As soon as the nurse determines that the newborn's respirations are adequate, the infant can be placed on the mother's abdomen. The newborn's head should be slightly lower than the body to aid drainage of fluid and mucus. The weight of the newborn on the mother's abdomen stimulates uterine contractions, which aid in placental separation. The umbilical cord should not be pulled.

The nurse is alert for signs of placental separation. When these signs are present, the nurse places one hand just above the symphysis to guard the uterus and uses the other hand to maintain *gentle* traction on the cord, while the mother is instructed to push so that the placenta can be expelled. In some instances the mother can squat, and this usually helps expel the placenta. The nurse inspects the placenta to determine whether it is intact.

The nurse checks the firmness of the uterus. The fundus may be gently massaged to stimulate contractions and decrease bleeding. Putting the newborn to breast also stimulates uterine contractions through release of oxytocin from the pituitary gland.

The umbilical cord may now be cut. Two sterile clamps are placed approximately 2 to 4 inches from the newborn's abdomen. The cord is cut between them with sterile scissors. A sterile cord clamp (Hollister or Hesseltine) can be placed adjacent to the clamp on the newborn's cord, between the clamp and the newborn's abdomen. The clamp *must not* be placed snugly against the abdomen, because the cord will dry and shrink.

The area under the mother's buttocks is cleaned, and her perineum is inspected for lacerations. Bleeding from lacerations may be controlled by pressing a clean perineal pad against the perineum and instructing the woman to keep her thighs together.

If the physician's/nurse-midwife's arrival is delayed or if the newborn is having respiratory distress, the newborn should be transported immediately to the nursery. *The newborn must be properly identified before he or she leaves the birthing area.*

Record Keeping The following information is noted and placed on a birth record:

1. Position of fetus at birth
2. Presence of cord around neck or shoulder (nuchal cord)
3. Time of birth
4. Apgar scores at one and five minutes after birth
5. Gender of newborn
6. Time of expulsion of placenta
7. Method of placental expulsion
8. Appearance and intactness of placenta
9. Mother's condition
10. Any medications that were given to mother or newborn (per agency protocol)

Postbirth Interventions Postbirth implications are the same as those on p 681.

Birth of Infant in Breech Presentation

A significant factor in a breech birth is that the smallest part of the fetus presents first; succeeding parts are progressively larger. The cervix is not as effectively dilated when the fetus is in breech presentation as it is when the fetus is in the vertex position. Therefore, descent is usually slow and may not occur until the cervix is fully dilated and the membranes rupture.

The primary concern in a breech birth is to prevent the entrapment of the head in the cervix. The nurse is advised to avoid intervening until the buttocks are born. Then, the nurse pulls down a loop of cord (to avoid stress on its point of insertion) and supports the breech in both hands. The infant's body is lifted slightly upward for birth of the posterior shoulder and arm. The newborn may then be lowered, and the anterior shoulder and arm will pass under the symphysis.

Suprapubic pressure should be applied to maintain the normal flexion of the baby's head and should be continued until the baby is born. The nape of the neck pivots under the symphysis, and the rest of the head is born over the perineum by a movement of flexion (Varney 1987).

The remaining birth and postbirth interventions for breech birth are described in the preceding section on precipitous birth of an infant in vertex presentation.

❈ ❈

KEY CONCEPTS

Admission to the birth setting involves assessment of many physiologic and psychologic factors. The information gained helps the nurse establish priorities of care.

Before care is begun it is important to explain what will be done, the reasons, potential benefits and risks, and possible alternatives if appropriate. This helps the woman determine what happens to her body, and is a critical element in the process of obtaining informed consent.

Behavioral responses to labor vary with the phase of labor; the preparation the woman has had; and her previous experience, cultural beliefs, and developmental level.

Each woman's cultural beliefs affect her needs for privacy, expression of discomfort, and expectations for the birth and the role she wishes the father to play in the birth event.

The laboring woman's comfort may be increased by general comfort measures, supportive relaxation techniques, methods of handling anxiety, controlled breathing, and support by a caring person.

The laboring woman fears being alone during labor. Even though there is a support person available, the woman's anxiety may be decreased when the nurse remains with her.

Maternal birthing positions include a wide variety of possibilities from side-lying to sitting, squatting, and lying flat.

Immediate assessments of the newborn include evaluation of the Apgar score and an abbreviated physical assessment. These early assessments help determine the need for resuscitation and whether the newborn's adaptation to extrauterine life is progressing normally. The newborn who is not experiencing problems may remain with the parents for an extended period of time following birth.

Immediate care of the newborn following birth also includes maintenance of respirations, promotion of warmth, prevention of infection, and accurate identification.

The new parents and their baby are given time together as soon as possible after birth.

Nursing assessments continue after the birth and are important to ensure that normal physiologic adaptations are happening after birth.

The adolescent has special needs in the birth setting. Her developmental needs require specialized nursing care.

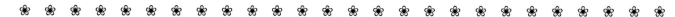

References

Aderhold K: Phases of second stage labor: Four descriptive case studies. Unpublished Master's thesis. University of Colorado Health Sciences Center, Denver, Colorado, 1989.

Apgar V: The newborn (Apgar) scoring system: Reflections and advice. *Pediatr Clin North Am* August 1966; 13:645.

April IF: Mexican-American folk beliefs: How they affect health care. *MCN* May/June 1977; 2:168.

Barclay L, Andre CA, Glover PA: Women's business: The challenge of childbirth. *Midwifery* 1989; 5:122.

Barton J et al: Alternative birthing center: Experience in a teaching obstetric service. *Am J Obstet Gynecol* 1990; 137:377.

Bergstrom L, Roberts J, Seidel J et al: *"You'll Feel Me Touching You, Sweetie": Vaginal Examinations During Second Stage Labor.* Unpublished manuscript. 1990.

Boylan PC: Liquor assessment: Meconium and oligohydramnios. In *Fetal Monitoring: Physiology and Techniques of Antenatal and Intrapartum Assessment.* Spencer JAD (editor). Philadelphia: Davis, 1990.

Briesemeister LH, Haines BA: The interactions of fathers and newborns. In: *Childbirth in America: Anthropological Perspectives.* Michaelson KL (editor). South Hadley, MA: 1988.

Calhoun MA: The Vietnamese woman: Health/illness attitudes and behaviors. In: *Women, Health and Culture.* Stern PN (editor). Washington: Hemisphere, 1986.

Carrington BW: The Afro American. In: *Culture, Childbearing, Health Professionals.* Clark AL (editor). Philadelphia; Davis, 1978.

Chung JJ: Understanding the Oriental maternity patient. *Nurs Clin North Am.* March 1977; 12:67.

Davitz LJ et al: Suffering as viewed in six different cultures. *Am J Nurs* 1976; 76:1296.

Dobson SM: Conceptualizing for transcultural health visiting: The concept of transcultural reciprocity. *J Adv Nurs* 1989; 14:97.

Douglas MJ, Farquharson DF, Ross PL et al: Cardiovascular collapse following an overdose of prostaglandin F2 alpha: A case report. *Can J Anaesth* July 1989; 36:466.

Engel NS: An American experience of pregnancy and childbirth in Japan. *Birth.* June 1989; 16:81.

Farris L: The American Indian. In: *Culture, Childbearing, Health Professionals.* Clark AL (editor). Philadelphia: Davis, 1978.

Gale R, Seidman DS, Dollberg S et al: Is teenage pregnancy a neonatal risk factor? *J Adolesc Health Care* September 1989; 10:404.

Gardosi J, Sylvester S, B-Lynch C: Alternative positions in the second stage of labour: A randomized controlled trial. *Br J Obstet Gynecol* November 1989; 96:1290.

Garforth S, Garcia J: Hospital admission practices. In: *Effective Care in Pregnancy and Childbirth, Vol. 2: Childbirth.* Chalmers I, Enkin M, Keirse MJNC (editors). New York: Oxford University Press, 1989.

Geden EA, Lower M, Beattie S et al: Effects of music and imagery on physiologic and self-report of analogued labor pain. *Nurs Res* January/February 1989; 38:37.

Geiser R, Fraley K: Perinatal outreach: Liability issues. *J Perinatal Neonatal Nurs* January 1989; 2:31

Heggenhougen HK: Father and childbirth: An anthropological perspective. *J Nurse-Midwifery* November/December 1980; 25:21.

Higgins PG, Wayland JR: Labour and delivery in North America. *Nurs Times* September 1981, Midwifery suppl, p. 77.

Hill PD: Effects of heat and cold on the perineum after episiotomy/laceration. *JOGNN* March/April 1989; 18:124.

Hodnett ED, Osborn RN: Effects of continuous intrapartum professional support on childbirth outcomes. *Res Nurs Health* October 1989; 12:289.

Hollingsworth AO et al: The refugees and childbearing: What to expect. *RN* November 1980; 43:45.

Kay MA: *Anthropology of Human Birth.* Philadelphia; Davis, 1982.

Kay MA: The Mexican American. In: *Culture, Childbearing, Health Professionals.* Clark AL (editor). Philadelphia; Davis, 1978.

Keppler AB: The use of intravenous fluids during labor. *Birth* June 1988; 15:75.

Klaus MH, Kennell JH: *Parent-Infant Bonding.* 2nd ed. St. Louis: Mosby, 1982.

LaDu EB: Childbirth care for Hmong families. *MCN* November/December 1985; 10:382.

LaFoy J, Geden EA: Postepisiotomy pain: Warm versus cold sitz bath. *JOGNN* September/October 1989; 18:399.

Leboyer F: *Birth Without Violence.* New York: Knopf, 1976.

Long PJ: Management of the third stage of labor: A review. *J Nurse Midwifery* May/June 1986; 31:135.

Luegenbiehl DL, Brophy GH, Artigue GS et al: Standardized Assessment of blood loss *MCN* July/August 1990; 15:241.

Lutwak RA, Ney AM, White JE: Maternity nursing and Jewish law. *MCN* January/February 1988; 13:44.

McCaffrey M: *Nursing Management of the Patient with Pain,* 2nd ed. Philadelphia: Lippincott, 1979.

Morrow K: Transcultural midwifery: Adapting to Hmong birthing customs in California. *J Nurse Midwifery* November/December 1986; 31:285.

Morse JM, Park C: Differences in cultural expectations of the perceived painfulness of childbirth. In: *Childbirth in America: Anthropological Perspectives.* Michaelson KL (editor). South Hadley, MA: 1988.

Murrillo-Rohde I: Cultural sensitivity in the care of the Hispanic patient. *Wash State J Nurs.* 1979 (special suppl):25.

Murphee AH: A functional analysis of southern folk beliefs concerning birth. *Am J Obstet Gynecol* September 1968; 102:125.

Myles MF: *Textbook for Midwives,* 11th ed. New York: Churchill-Livingstone, 1990.

NAACOG OGN Nursing Practice Resource. Fetal Heart Rate Auscultation. March 1990.

Newton N, Newton M, Broach J: Psychologic, physical, nutritional, and technologic aspects of intravenous infusion during labor. *Birth* June 1988; 15:67.

Norr KF, Nacion KW, Abramson R: Early discharge with home follow-up: Impacts on low-income mothers and infants. *JOGNN* March/April 1988; 18:133.

Norr KF, Nacion K: Outcomes of postpartum early discharge, 1960–1986: A comparative review. *Birth* September 1987; 14:135.

Perlis DW: *The Influence of Bearing Down Technique on the Fetal Heart Rate During the Second Stage of Labor.* Unpublished doctoral dissertation. University of Illinois, Chicago, IL: 1988.

Prendiville W, Ellbourne D: Care during the third stage of labour. In: *Effective Care in Pregnancy and Childbirth, Vol. 2: Childbirth.* Chalmers I, Enkin M, Keirse MJNC (editors). New York: Oxford University Press, 1989.

Reddy VV, Carey JC: Effect of umbilical vein oxytocin on puerperal blood loss and length of the third stage of labor. *Am J Obstet Gynecol* January 1989; 160:206.

Roberts J: Maternal position during the first stage of labour. In: *Effective Care in Pregnancy and Childbirth, Vol. 2: Childbirth.* Chalmers I, Enkin M, Keirse MJNC (editors). New York: Oxford University Press, 1989.

Roberts JE, Goldstein SA, Gruener JS et al: A descriptive analysis of involuntary bearing-down efforts during the expulsive phase of labor. *JOGNN* January/February 1987; 16:48.

Sargent C, Marcucci J: Khmer prenatal health practices and the American clinical experience. In: *Childbirth in America: Anthropological Perspectives.* Michaelson KL (editor). South Hadley, MA: 1988.

Senden IPM, Wetering MD, Eskes TKAB et al: Labor pain: A comparison of parturients in a Dutch and an American teaching hospital. *Obstet Gynecol* April 1988; 71:541.

Simkin P: Non-pharmacological methods of pain relief during labour. In: *Effective Care in Pregnancy and Childbirth, Vol. 2: Childbirth.* Chalmers I, Enkin M, Keirse MJNC (editors). New York: Oxford University Press, 1989.

Simkin P: Active and physiologic management of second stage: A review and hypothesis. In: *Episiotomy and the Second Stage of Labor.* Kitzinger S. Simkin P (editors). Seattle: Pennypress, 1984.

Sleep J, Roberts J, Chalmers I: Care during the second stage of labor. In: *Effective Care in Pregnancy and Childbirth, Vol. 2: Childbirth.* Chalmers I, Enkin M, Keirse MJNC (editors). New York: Oxford University Press, 1989.

Snydal SH: Responses of laboring women to fetal heart rate monitoring: A critical review of the literature. *J Nurse Midwifery* September/October 1988; 33:208.

van Lier DJ, Roberts, JE: Promoting informed consent of women in labor. *JOGNN* September/October, 1986; 15:419.

Varney H: *Nurse-midwifery,* 2nd ed. Boston: Blackwell Scientific Publications, 1987.

Weisenberg M, Caspi Z: Cultural and educational influences on pain of childbirth. *J Pain Symptom Mgmt* March 1989; 4:13.

Williams LM, Harrison-Clark A: Advocacy for healthy births. *Women's Health* 1989; 15:101.

Windsor-Richards K, Gillies PA: Racial grouping and women's experience of giving birth in hospital. *Midwifery* 1988; 4:171.

Zaborowski M: Cultural components in responses to pain. *J Social Issues* 1952; 8:16.

Additional Readings

Brazelton TB, Cramer BG: *The Earliest Relationship: Parents, Infants, and the Drama of Early Attachment.* Reading, MA: Addison-Wesley, 1990.

Eganhouse DJ: Electronic fetal monitoring: Education and quality assurance. *JOGNN* January/February 1991; 20:16.

Fleming N: Can the suturing method make a difference in postpartum perineal pain? *J Nurse-Midwifery* January/February 1990; 35:19.

Greener D: Development and validation of the nurse-midwifery clinical data set. *J Nurse-Midwifery* May/June 1991; 36:168.

Iams JD, Zuspan FP: *Zuspan & Quilligan's Manual of Obstetrics and Gynecology.* St. Louis: Mosby, 1990.

Murray M: *Antepartal and Intrapartal Fetal Monitoring.* Washington, D.C.: NAACOG, 1988.

Seidman DS et al: Apgar scores and cognitive performance at 17 years of age. *Obstet Gynecol* June 1991; 77:875.

Spencer JAD: *Fetal Monitoring: Physiology and Techniques of Antenatal and Intrapartum Assessment.* Philadelphia: Davis, 1990.

Thomas VJ, Rose FD: Ethnic differences in the experience of pain. *Soc Sci Med* 1991; 32:9:1063.

CHAPTER 24

Maternal Analgesia and Anesthesia

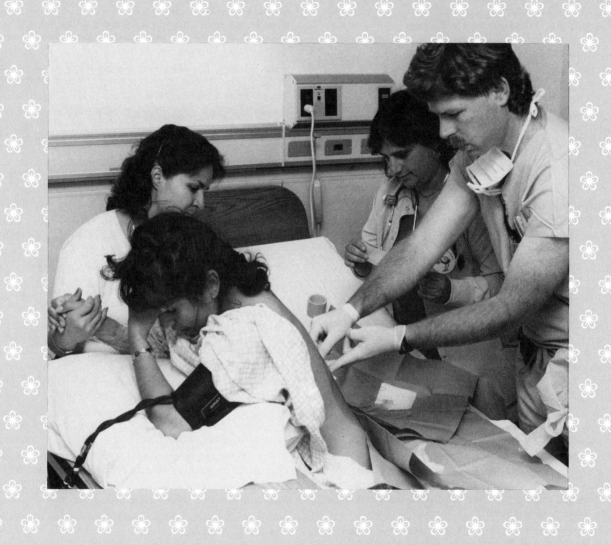

Formulate a nursing care plan to meet the needs of a woman receiving systemic drugs for pain relief during labor.

Differentiate between the major techniques of regional anesthesia.

Develop a nursing care plan to meet the specific needs of a woman receiving regional analgesia or anesthesia for pain relief during labor and/or birth.

Distinguish between the actions of inhalation and intravenous anesthetic agents used to provide general anesthesia for childbirth and describe the nursing implications of both methods.

Discuss the nursing role when complications of regional and general anesthesia occur.

❀ ❀

I kept trying to do my breathing but I just couldn't make it work. At that moment, I would have taken anything from anybody. The epidural my doctor suggested was wonderful. I could still participate but I didn't hurt.

The management of pain during childbirth is an important aspect of maternity health care. The discomfort associated with labor and birth has been a subject of concern and controversy throughout history. Currently, the goal of pain relief in childbirth is to alleviate discomfort in the woman while ensuring the safety of both the woman and the fetus. To date, no method or agent has been discovered that can meet all these criteria. The search for a safe, effective method of pain relief during labor and birth continues.

Methods of Pain Relief

Reduction or relief of pain during labor is achieved by several different methods, including psychoprophylactic methods (discussed in Chapters 17 and 23), systemic drugs, and regional nerve blocks.

The methods are not exclusive. The agents used for regional nerve blocks may enter general circulation and cause unwanted side effects. Systemic drugs such as meperidine (Demerol) may assist the tense laboring woman to regain control and progress to a satisfying childbirth experience. Regional nerve blocks with analgesic doses of anesthetic agents administered during the course of labor are compatible with the goals of prepared childbirth.

Although systemic analgesics and local anesthetic agents affect the fetus, so do the pain and stress experienced by the woman. Altered breathing techniques may lead to hypoventilation or hyperventilation, both of which cause a decrease of oxygen to the fetus (Nicholson 1989). During the pain and stress of labor there is an increase in maternal ventilation and oxygen consumption, which de-

creases the amount of oxygen available to the fetus. Hyperventilation causes a decrease in maternal $Paco_2$ level which increases the $Hco_3/Paco_2$ ratio of the blood and thus elevates the pH. This elevation in blood pH leads to maternal respiratory alkalosis. Fetal hypoxemia and acidosis may result, but a maternal $Paco_2$ level of less than 20 mm Hg needs to be present for this to occur (Miller 1986). Fetal hypoxia and acidosis may be caused by reduced uterine and umbilical blood flow, which would cause maternal hemoglobin to have a greater affinity for oxygen and therefore less placental transfer of oxygen (Cousins et al 1988). Maternal respiratory alkalosis and acidosis tend to be easier to treat than fetal problems because it may require simply increasing or decreasing the maternal respiratory rate.

Plasma epinephrine and norepinephrine levels are higher during labor than in the last trimester of pregnancy. The body's response to the pain and stress of labor causes a release of high levels of catecholamines. Epidural analgesia significantly reduces maternal plasma catecholamine levels during labor (Cousins et al 1988), although it is not clear whether this reduction is due to alleviation of pain. When discussing medication alternatives with a prepared couple a positive approach should be taken to help them understand that maternal discomfort and anxiety may have as much adverse effect on the fetus as the administration of a small amount of an analgesic agent.

Many couples who have had childbirth education approach childbirth confident that the psychoprophylactic techniques they have learned will enable them to cope with the discomforts of labor. There is a good deal of peer pressure on expectant parents to have the "ideal" birth experience. They may plan a natural childbirth with, perhaps, local infiltration anesthesia for episiotomy repair. The necessity for analgesia may elicit a sense of inadequacy and a feeling of guilt. The nurse has a very special role in assisting a woman and her partner to accept alterations in their original plan. Reassurance that accepting analgesia for discomfort is not a failure is important in maintaining the woman's self-esteem. The emphasis should be placed on the goal of a healthy, satisfying outcome for the family.

Research Note

Clinical Application of Research

In order to explore touch from a nursing framework, Donna Weaver (1990) explored the meaning of touch for a group of labor nurses. This qualitative study included participant observation and interviews.

Nurses identified that cues existed for either initiating or avoiding touch and the cues could be initiated by either nurse or client. Touch initiated by the nurse occurred if the patient were alone or if prior touch had been successful. Nurse-initiated touch was an intuitive process and included hand holding, back rubbing, or massage. Touch avoidance by the nurse also involved an intuitive element. Cues regarding touch avoidance related to previous rebuff by the client, caring for another nurse's client, distraction of the client's concentration, or hygiene or communicable disease issues.

Interpretations derived from the study included touch being an essential relational strategy in obstetric nursing, touch being based on experience and sensitivity, and touch being a learned competency. "Nurses share themselves and their feelings with the ones they touch and receive satisfaction in return" (Weaver 1990, p 159).

Critical Thinking Applied to Research

Strengths: Addressed several issues of qualitative rigor such as peer debriefing, member checking, and establishment of an audit trail.

Concerns: It is difficult for the reader to identify how the themes of the study differed from the initial questions identified on the interview schedule.

Weaver D: Nurses' views on the meaning of touch in obstetrical nursing practice. *JOGNN* 1990; 19(2): 157.

Systemic Drugs

The goal of pharmacologic pain relief during labor is to provide maximal analgesia with minimal risk for the woman and fetus. Three factors must be considered in the use of analgesic agents: (1) the effects on the woman, (2) the effects on the labor contractions, and (3) the effects on the fetus.

Maternal drug action is of primary importance because the well-being of the fetus depends on adequate functioning of the maternal cardiopulmonary system. Any alteration of function that disturbs the woman's homeostatic mechanism affects the fetal environment. Maintaining the maternal respiratory rate and blood pressure within normal range is thus of prime importance. The use of electronic fetal monitoring has provided a means of accurately assessing the effects of pharmacologic agents on uterine contractions.

All systemic drugs used for pain relief during labor cross the placental barrier by simple diffusion, with some agents crossing more readily than others. Drug action in the body depends on the rate at which the substance is metabolized by liver enzymes and excreted by the kidneys. The fetal liver enzymes and renal systems are inadequate to metabolize analgesic agents, so high doses remain active in fetal circulation for a prolonged period of time. The fetal brain receives a greater amount of the cardiac output than the neonatal brain. The percentage of blood volume flowing to the brain is increased even further during intrauterine stress, so that the hypoxic fetus receives an even larger amount of a depressant drug. The blood-brain barrier is more permeable at the time of birth, a factor that also increases the amount of drug carried to the central nervous system.

Administration of Analgesic Agents

The optimal time for administering analgesia is determined after making a complete assessment of many factors. In general, an analgesic agent is administered to nulliparas when the cervix has dilated to 5 or 6 cm and to multiparas when the cervix has reached 3 or 4 cm dilatation. This is only a generalization, however, the character of each labor must be taken into account. Analgesia given too early may prolong labor and depress the fetus. Analgesia given too late is of no value to the woman and may cause neonatal respiratory depression. In many institutions the nurse decides when to give the analgesic ordered by the physician/ CNM or certified registered nurse anesthetist. This decision is based on a complete assessment of the woman and the progress of labor.

Currently, a minimal amount of an analgesic agent is given during labor. Oral analgesics are not used because of poor absorption and prolonged gastric-emptying time. The intramuscular and intravenous routes are used instead. When the prescribed route is intramuscular, the needle must be of sufficient length to penetrate the muscle rather than only the subcutaneous fat. The intravenous route is preferred because it results in prompt, smooth, and more predictable action with a smaller total dose than the intramuscular route. When an agent is given intravenously it should be administered by titrating the drug until the desired effect is achieved (see Table 24–1). It has been suggested that the intravenous injection be given with the onset of a contraction, when the blood flow to the uterus and the fetus is decreased. Whatever the route of administration, the power of suggestion on the part of the nurse greatly increases the effectiveness of the agent. The general principles of administering analgesic drugs are listed in Table 24–1.

Narcotic Analgesics

Narcotics that are injected into the circulation have their primary action at sites in the brain. Specifically, a narcotic that diffuses out of cerebral capillaries and reaches the periventricular/periaquaductal grey area of the brain will acti-

---

Table 24-1 General Nursing Principles for Administering Analgesic Drugs

1. The woman should be in an individual labor room.

2. The environment should be free from sensory stimuli, such as bright lights, noise, and irrelevant conversation, to allow the woman to focus on the drug action.

3. An explanation of the effects of the medication should be given, including how long the effects will last and how the drug will make the woman feel.

4. The woman should be encouraged to empty her bladder prior to administration of the drug.

5. The baseline FHR and maternal vital signs should be recorded prior to administration.

6. The physician's/nurse-midwife's/anesthetist's written order should be checked, and the medication prepared and signed out on the narcotic or control sheet.

7. The woman should be asked again if she is allergic to any medication and her arm band should be checked for identification.

8. The drug should be administered by the route ordered, using correct technique.

9. The side rails should be pulled up for safety, and the reasons explained to the woman.

10. The medication, dosage, time, route, and site of administration should be charted on the nurse's notes and on the monitor strip.

11. The FHR should be monitored to assess the effects of the medication on the fetus, and the woman should be evaluated for the effectiveness of the analgesic agent.

12. The woman should not be left alone. If no support person is present and it is necessary for the nurse to leave, the woman should be given a short explanation and assurance that the nurse will return.

13. The woman's blood pressure, pulse, and respirations and the FHR should be rechecked after administration to identify untoward effects.

---

vate the neurons that descend to the spinal cord and inhibit the transmission of pain impulses in the substantia gelatinosa (Paradise 1990). Nausea and vomiting are produced by stimulation of the medullary chemoreceptor trigger zone.

Meperidine (Demerol) Meperidine, a pure agonist, is the most frequently used opioid in obstetric analgesia. It is effective for alleviating pain during the first stage of labor. Meperidine has essentially replaced morphine because meperidine appears to cause less neonatal depression. However, it has an active metabolite, normeperidine, that has been implicated in contributing to neonatal depression (Barash et al 1989).

Effective analgesia with intravenous administration occurs within five to ten minutes and has a duration of about 3 hours. The usual intravenous dose is 25 mg. Intravenous injection of meperidine must be done with caution; it is given as a slow intravenous push over a few minutes in order to assess the effect on the pregnant women and her fetus. Using this administration method allows the nurse to determine if there are untoward effects developing before the full dose has been given. In this instance, the nurse can discontinue the intravenous injection and minimize untoward effects.

Some of the major maternal side effects of meperidine are nausea, vomiting, respiratory depression, and orthostatic hypotension. It also causes neonatal depression, which is reflected in lower Apgar scores. Neonatal depression is related to the dose and the amount of time between administration of the drug and the birth of the infant. Fetal exposure to meperidine is greatest two to three hours after

maternal administration (Cousins et al 1988) (see Drug Guide-Meperidine).

Butorphanol Tartrate (Stadol) is a mixed agonist-antagonist agent. This type of agent can exert an analgesic effect when other more powerful agonists (such as morphine or meperidine) are not present in the body. In the presence of a more powerful agonist, the mixed agonist-antagonist reverses the analgesic effects. This action may precipitate withdrawal in drug-dependent adults.

The recommended dosage in labor is 2 mg intramuscularly or 1 mg intravenously every three to four hours. A titrated intravenous dose should begin with 0.5 mg. The onset is rapid, peaking at 5 minutes intravenously and 30 to 50 minutes intramuscularly, and the duration is two to four hours. It rapidly crosses the placental barrier.

As with the opiates, respiratory depression can occur. Additional adverse reactions include sedation, clamminess, nausea, dizziness, and a "floating feeling." Sedation is the most frequent side effect and occurs in 40% of those receiving the drug (Barash et al 1989).

Nursing Implications The respiratory depression and other effects are additive when butorphanol is administered with other central nervous system depressants such as sedatives, phenothiazides, and other tranquilizers, hypnotics, and general anesthetics. The respiratory and cardiac status of the woman should be evaluated by careful observation of vital signs and pulse oximetry. The maternal level of consciousness should also be checked frequently. Continuous electronic monitoring of the fetal heart rate, pattern, and variability is recommended. Respiratory depres-

DRUG GUIDE
Meperidine Hydrochloride (Demerol)

Overview of Obstetric Action

Meperidine hydrochloride is a narcotic analgesic that interferes with pain impulses at the subcortical level of the brain. In addition, it enhances analgesia by altering the physiologic response to pain, suppressing anxiety and apprehension, and creating a euphoric feeling. Meperidine hydrochloride is used during labor to provide analgesia. Peak analgesia occurs in 40 to 60 minutes with intramuscular and in 5 to 7 minutes with intravenous administration. Duration is 2 to 4 hours. Administration after labor has reached the active phase does not appear to delay labor or decrease uterine contraction frequency or duration. Meperidine HCl crosses the placental barrier and appears in cord blood within 2 minutes and after maternal intravenous injection can be detected in amniotic fluid 30 minutes after IM injection (Briggs et al 1990).

Route, Dosage, Frequency

IM: 50 to 100 mg every 3 to 4 hours

IV: 25 to 50 mg by slow intravenous push every 3 to 4 hours

Maternal Contraindications

Hypersensitivity to meperidine, asthma

CNS depression

Respiratory depression

Fetal distress

Preterm labor if birth is imminent

Hypotension

Respirations <12 per minute

Concurrent use with anticonvulsants may increase depressant effects

Maternal Side Effects

Respiratory depression

Nausea and vomiting, dry mouth

Drowsiness, dizziness, flushing

Transient hypotension

Increased intracranial pressure (Skidmore-Roth 1991)

May precipitate or aggravate seizures in women prone to convulsive activity (Giacoia & Yaffee 1982)

Effect on Fetus/Neonate

Neonatal respiratory depression may occur if birth occurs 60 minutes or longer after administration of the drug to the mother; incidence of respiratory depression peaks at 2 to 3 hours after administration (Briggs et al 1990).

Neonatal hypotonia, lethargy, interference of thermoregulatory response

Neurologic and behavioral alterations for up to 72 hours after birth; presence of meperidine in neonatal urine up to 3 days following birth (Briggs et al 1990).

May have depressed attention and social responsiveness for first 6 weeks of life (Briggs et al 1990)

Nursing Considerations

Assess the woman's history, labor and fetal status, maternal blood pressure and respirations to identify contraindications to administration.

Intramuscular doses should be injected deeply to avoid irritation to subcutaneous tissue.

Intravenous doses should be diluted and administered slowly.

Provide for the woman's safety by instructing her to remain on bed rest and by keeping side rails up and placing call bell within reach.

Evaluate effect of drug.

Observe for maternal side effects.

Assess for respiratory depression, notify physician/CNM if respirations are <12/min (Skidmore-Roth 1991).

Observe newborn for respiratory depression, be prepared to initiate resuscitative measures and administer antagonist naloxone if needed.

---

sion can be reversed by naloxone (Narcan), which is a specific antagonist for this agent. This slightly depressed newborn is not likely to have prolonged drowsiness or sluggishness because the metabolites of butorphanol are inactive.

This agent should not be used for women with a known opiate dependency and should be used with caution if drug dependence is suspected.

Urinary retention following administration of this drug is rare. The nurse should, however, be alert for bladder distention when a woman has received butorphanol for analgesia during labor, has intravenous fluids infusing, and receives regional anesthesia (epidural or subarachnoid block) for the birth. Butorphanol should be protected from light and stored at room temperature. This agent is not federally controlled and has been placed in the nonscheduled category. Hospitals vary in their own control of the drug.

Nalbuphine (Nubain) Nalbuphine is a synthetic agonist-antagonist. It is structurally related to naloxone and oxymorphone but is pharmacologically similar to butorphanol and pentazocine. See the discussion of butorphanol for drug action and nursing implications. The recommended dosage by subcutaneous or intramuscular route is 10 to 20 mg, and the dose can be repeated in three to six hours. The initial dose for intravenous titration should be no greater than 5 mg. It is longer acting than butorphanol, but the respiratory depression apparently is not increased with cumulative doses. It should be used with caution in women giving birth to premature infants (Physicians' Desk Reference 1989).

Oxymorphone (Numorphan) Oxymorphone, a pure agonist, is a potent, semisynthetic substitute for morphine. The recommended dosage is 0.5 to 1.0 mg subcutaneously or intramuscularly, and it may be repeated every four to six hours as necessary. The initial intravenous dose is usually 0.5 mg.

Opiate Antagonists

Naloxone (Narcan) Naloxone is a semisynthetic narcotic antagonist devoid of agonistic (analgesic) properties. It exhibits little pharmacologic activity in the absence of opiates. Naloxone can be used to reverse the mild respiratory depression following small doses of opiates. The drug is useful for respiratory depression caused by fentanyl, alpha-prodine, morphine, and meperidine as well as pentazocine and butorphanol. *Naloxone is the drug of choice when the depressant is unknown because it will cause no further depression.* An initial dose of 0.4 mg to 2.0 mg may be administered intravenously. Neonatal administration is 0.01 mL to reverse depression caused by narcotics (Physicians' Desk Reference 1989). It is best to administer naloxone to the depressed infant directly so that the exact amount of the drug the infant receives is known.

Nursing Implications When naloxone is given, other resuscitative measures and trained personnel should be readily available. The duration of the drug is shorter (minutes to hours) than the analgesic drug it is acting as an antagonist for, so the nurse must be alert to the return of respiratory depression and the need for repeated doses. Naloxone should be given with caution in women with known or suspected opiate dependency because it may precipitate severe withdrawal symptoms in the newborn. For further discussion see Drug Guide—Narcan in Chapter 32.

Sedatives

Sedatives formerly played an important role in the pharmacologic management of labor. However, barbiturates have the disadvantage of producing restlessness in the presence of moderate to severe pain, and they readily cross the placental barrier, causing respiratory depression in the newborn.

The principal use of barbiturates in current obstetric practice is in false labor or in the early stages of prodromal labor. An oral dose of 100 mg of secobarbital (Seconal) or pentobarbital (Nembutal) promotes relaxation and allows the woman to sleep a few hours. If the woman is in false labor, the contractions usually stop. Women in prodromal labor enter the active phase of labor in a more relaxed and rested state.

An increase in fetal depression has been reported when barbiturates are followed with opiate-type agents as labor progresses.

Regional Analgesia and Anesthesia

Regional analgesia and anesthesia are achieved by injecting anesthetic agents (called *local anesthetics*) into an area that will bring the agent into direct contact with nervous tissue. Local agents stabilize the cell membrane, which prevents initiation and transmission of nerve impulses and produces a temporary and reversible loss of sensation called a regional block. The regional blocks most commonly used in childbearing include peridural block (lumbar epidural), subarachnoid block (spinal for cesarean birth, or low spinal for vaginal birth), pudendal block, and local infiltration. The regional blocks may be accomplished by a single injection or continuously by means of an indwelling plastic catheter. Before initiating any regional block, intravenous fluids should be infusing to provide hydration and direct access to the intravascular system in case of adverse effects. Also, oxygen—along with necessary equipment for rapid conversion to a general anesthetic—should be available prior to regional block administration. Regional blocks have gained widespread popularity in recent years and are particularly compatible with the goals of psychoprophylactic preparation for childbirth.

Essential prerequisites for the administration of regional analgesia and anesthesia are knowledge of the anatomy and physiology of pertinent structures, techniques for administration, the pharmacology of local anesthetics, and potential complications. With the exception of nurse anesthetists and nurse-midwives, who may perform procedures for which they have been trained, nurses in the United States may *not* legally administer anesthetic agents. However, the nurse must have an adequate knowledge of all aspects of regional anesthesia to provide support and give appropriate reinforcement of the administrator's explanation to the woman. The nurse who has a thorough understanding of the techniques and agents can also provide more efficient assistance to the administrator. The woman's safety is increased when the nurse recognizes complications and immediately initiates appropriate intervention.

The relief of pain associated with the first stage of labor can be accomplished by blocking the sensory nerves supplying the uterus with the techniques of paracervical, lumbar sympathetic, and peridural (epidural and caudal) blocks. Pain associated with the second stage and with birth can be alleviated with pudendal, peridural, and subarachnoid (spinal and low spinal) blocks (Figure 24–1, Table 24–2).

It is important for the laboring woman to have information regarding the regional block that is to be administered. As with other procedures, the woman needs to know how the block is given, the expected effect on her and the fetus, advantages and disadvantages, and possible complications. Many women discuss possible anesthetic blocks with their care provider at some point in the pregnancy. If they have not, it will be important for them to have an opportunity to ask questions and obtain information prior to receiving the block while in labor.

Anesthetic Agents for Regional Blocks

Local anesthetic agents block the conduction of nerve impulses from the periphery to the central nervous system by preventing the propagation of an action potential from the source of pain (Firestone et al 1988). The types of nerve fibers are differentially sensitive to the various anesthetic agents. In general, the smaller the fiber, the more sensitive it is to local agents. For example, it is possible to block the small C and A delta fibers, which transmit pain and temperature, without blocking the larger A alpha, A beta, and A gamma fibers, which continue to maintain a sense of pressure, muscle tone, position sense, and motor function.

Absorption of local anesthetics depends primarily on the vascularity of the area of injection. The agents also contribute to increased blood flow by causing vasodilation. High concentrations of drugs cause greater vasodilation. Good maternal physical condition or a high metabolic rate aids absorption. Malnutrition, dehydration, electrolyte imbalance, and cardiovascular and pulmonary problems increase the potential for toxic effects. The pH of tissues affects the rate of absorption, which has implications for fetal complications such as acidosis. The addition of vasoconstrictors such as epinephrine delays absorption and prolongs the anesthetic effect. Recent studies have demonstrated that epinephrine decreases uteroplacental blood flow, making it an undesirable additive in many situations. The breakdown of local anesthetics in the body is accomplished by the liver and plasma esterase, and the resulting substance is eliminated by the kidneys.

It is important to use the weakest concentration and the smallest amount necessary to produce the desired results.

Types of Agents

Three types of local anesthetic agents are currently available—esters, amides, and opiates. The ester type includes

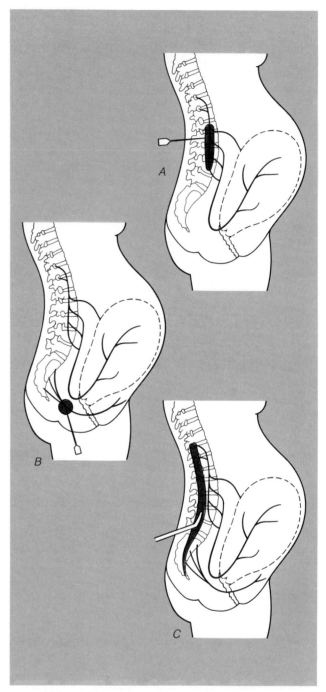

Figure 24–1 Schematic diagram showing pain pathways and sites of interruption. A Lumbar sympathetic block: relief of uterine pain only. B Pudendal block: relief of perineal pain. C Lumbar epidural block: dark area demonstrates peridural (epidural) space and nerves affected, and the white tube represents continuous plastic catheter. (From Bonica JJ: Principles and Practice of Obstetric Analgesia and Anesthesia. Philadelphia: FA Davis, 1972, pp 492, 512, 521, 614)

Table 24-2 Summary of Commonly Used Regional Blocks

Type of block	Area affected	Use during labor and birth	Nursing actions
Lumbar epidural	Vagina and perineum	Given in first stage and second stage of labor	Assess woman's knowledge regarding the block. Act as advocate to help her obtain further information if needed. Monitor maternal blood pressure to detect the major side effect, which is hypotension. Provide support and comfort. See Nursing Care Plan (p 705) for further nursing actions.
Pudendal	Perineum and lower vagina	Given in the second stage just prior to birth to provide anesthesia for episiotomy or for low forceps birth	Assess woman's knowledge regarding the block. Act as advocate to help her obtain further information if needed.
Local infiltration	Perineum	Administered just before birth to provide anesthesia for episiotomy	Assess woman's knowledge regarding the block. Provide information as needed. Provide comfort and support. Observe perineum for bruising or other discoloration in the recovery period.

procaine hydrochloride (Novocain), chloroprocaine hydrochloride (Nesacaine), and tetracaine hydrochloride (Pontocaine). Esters are rapidly metabolized; therefore toxic maternal levels are not as likely to be reached, and placental transfer to the fetus is prevented. Amide types include lidocaine hydrochloride (Xylocaine), mepivacaine hydrochloride (Carbocaine), and bupivacaine hydrochloride (Marcaine). Amide types are more powerful and longer-acting agents. They readily cross the placenta, can be measured in the fetal circulation, and affect the fetus for a prolonged period.

The use of intrathecal and epidural routes for opiate-type agents is relatively new in obstetric analgesia and anesthesia. Some of the agents being used include morphine, fentanyl, and meperidine. The mechanism of action seems to involve specific opiate receptors in the spinal cord (Paradise 1990).

A variety of agents and a wide range of doses have been used for epidural anesthesia with varying results. The most commonly used agents are lidocaine 2% with epinephrine 1:200,000, bupivacaine 0.5%, and 2-chloroprocaine 3%. Each agent provides adequate anesthesia with 15 to 20 ml of the solution but each has been identified with side effects. The pharmacology of each drug must be understood before they are used.

Epidural anesthesia can provide prolonged pain relief by intraspinal injection of an opioid. Some of the opioids used are morphine, butorphanol, hydromorphone, fentanyl, and sufentanil. The woman must be carefully monitored when these drugs are administered. Some of the side effects include pruritus, nausea and vomiting, vertigo, drowsiness, respiratory depression, and urinary retention. The clinical application of spinal opioids in labor remains controversial (Cousins et al 1989).

Adverse Maternal Reactions to Anesthetic Agents

Reactions to local anesthetic agents range from mild symptoms to cardiovascular collapse. Mild reactions include palpitations, vertigo, tinnitus, apprehension, confusion, headache, and a metallic taste in the mouth. Moderate reactions include more severe degrees of mild symptoms plus nausea and vomiting, hypotension, and muscle twitching, which may progress to convulsions and loss of consciousness. The severe reactions are sudden loss of consciousness, coma, severe hypotension, bradycardia, respiratory depression, and cardiac arrest. High concentrations of the agents may also cause local toxic effects on tissues. Anesthetic agents should not be used unless an intravenous line is in place.

Systemic toxic reactions most commonly occur with an excessive dose through too great a concentration or too large a volume. Accidental intravenous injection that suddenly increases the amount of the drug in maternal circulation results in depression of vasomotor, respiratory, and other medullary centers of the brain. It also depresses the heart and peripheral vascular bed. A massive intravascular dose can result in sudden circulatory collapse within one minute. Reactions to subcutaneous and extradural injection occur in 5 to 40 minutes. The short-acting agents can produce toxic reactions in 10 to 15 minutes (procaine), and the long-acting agents (mepivacaine), in 20 to 40 minutes. *It is imperative that the woman be under close supervision by knowledgeable personnel throughout the time that the agent is being used.*

If epinephrine has been added to the anesthetic agent to prolong the anesthesia, it is necessary to differentiate between reaction to the anesthetic agent and to the epinephrine. Reaction to epinephrine is characterized by pallor, perspiration, a greater increase in blood pressure and pulse than occurs with reactions to anesthetic agents, and dyspnea.

Psychogenic reactions can occur, with symptoms similar to systemic toxic reactions. This phenomenon may occur as the procedure is begun and prior to the injection of the anesthetic agent. Regardless of the cause, the symptoms must be treated.

Allergic reactions to anesthetic agents may also occur. The manifestations of the antigen-antibody reaction include urticaria, laryngeal edema, joint pain, swelling of the tongue, and bronchospasm.

Interventions

Treatment of Systemic Toxicity   In the treatment of mild toxicity, the administration of oxygen by mask and intravenous injection of a short-acting barbiturate to decrease anxiety is advocated. Preparation must be made to treat convulsion or cardiovascular collapse. Specific nursing interventions in the treatment of systemic toxicity are included in the nursing care plan for regional anesthesia.

Treatment of Convulsions   The best treatment for convulsions is establishing the airway and administering 100% oxygen (Barash 1989). Thiopental or diazepam may be administered to stop convulsions. Small doses are adequate and help avoid cardiorespiratory depression. Typical intravenous doses are 50 to 100 mg for thiopental and 5 to 10 mg for diazepam.

Treatment of Sudden Cardiovascular Collapse   In sudden collapse an airway must be established as cardiopulmonary resuscitation begins. The airway of choice is an endotracheal tube with 100% oxygen for ventilations. Intravenous fluids are increased and emergency cesarean birth may be started immediately (Barash 1989).

Peridural Block—Lumbar Epidural

Peridural anesthesia can provide pain relief throughout the course of labor. The peridural or *epidural space* is a potential space between the dura mater and the ligamentum flavum extending from the base of the skull to the end of the sacral canal (Figure 24–2). It contains areolar tissue, fat lymphatics, and the internal vertebral venous plexus. Access to the space is through the lumbar area. The technique is most frequently used as a continuous block to provide analgesia and anesthesia from active labor through episiotomy repair.

Considerable skill is required for peridural techniques, and the incidence of success correlates highly with the skill and experience of the administrator. Pain relief is slower than with other methods, and a higher volume of anesthetic agent is required than for spinal anesthesia.

Fewer bony abnormalities occur in the lumbar vertebras than in the sacrum. The administrator must guard against accidental perforation of the dura mater, particularly with the lumbar epidural method, and against the in-

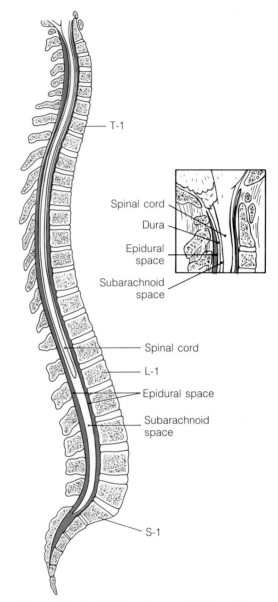

Figure 24–2   Epidural space. Epidural space is between the dura mater and the ligmentum flavum extending from the base of the skull to the end of the sacral canal.

jection of an epidural dose into the spinal canal, with resultant high spinal anesthesia.

Lumbar epidural block, particularly continuous lumbar epidural block, has become the obstetric analgesia and anesthesia of choice in many areas of the United States. It can be initiated as soon as active labor is established and is usually given when a nullipara is 5 to 6 cm dilated, (in some facilities the block may be given at 3 to 4 cm) and a multipara is 3 to 4 cm dilated.

Advantages   The lumbar epidural block produces good analgesia that alters maternal physiologic responses to pain and lowers maternal catecholamine levels (Joseppila 1984; Abboud et al 1984a). The mother is fully awake during labor and childbirth. This continuous technique allows different blocking for each stage of labor so that internal rotation can be accomplished, and many times the reflex urge to bear down is preserved.

Disadvantages   The most common complication of an epidural block is maternal hypotension, and this is generally prevented through intravenous fluid administration. Other disadvantages of the lumbar epidural block are that the onset of analgesia may be delayed 10 to 20 minutes. Epidural block requires skilled personnel for administration and close observation of the woman and fetus. Variability of the fetal heart may decrease, which makes interpretation of the FHR tracing difficult. Epidural analgesia does not prolong and may even shorten the first stage of labor; however, the influence on the second stage of labor remains controversial (Cousins et al 1988).

Contraindications   The absolute contraindications for epidural block are client refusal, infection at the site of puncture, maternal problems with coagulation, allergy to the anesthetic agent, and chronic placental insufficiency. Relative contraindications include mild-to-moderate bleeding, moderate-to-severe fetal distress, prematurity, intrauterine growth retardation, postmaturity, and multiple fetuses (Nicholson et al 1989).

     The use of epidural (or spinal block) for cesarean birth in a woman with herpetic lesions is very controversial. Some feel that the virus may be present on the skin and the skin puncture may allow for dissemination of the virus in the epidural or subarachnoid space. Ravindran (1982) reported no complications with epidural anesthesia in a sample of 30 women with herpetic lesions. Despite the fact that epidurals have been done without viral dissemination, Marx (1986) felt the risk to be too great unless there are significant contraindications to general anesthesia. Gieraerts (1989) felt Herpes Simplex Virus transmission was based on epidural morphine administration and not the epidural block.

Technique for Lumbar Epidural Block   The following steps must be taken in administering a lumbar epidural block:

1. The woman is placed on her left side, shoulders parallel, with her legs slightly flexed. *The spinal column is not kept convex, as it is for a spinal block, because that position reduces the peridural space to a greater degree and stretches the dura mater, making it more susceptible to puncture.* (The epidural space is decreased during pregnancy because of venous engorgement. It is also smaller in obese and short individuals.)

2. The skin is prepared with an antiseptic agent.

3. A skin wheal is made to anesthetize the supraspinous and interspinous ligaments.

4. A short beveled 18-gauge needle with stylet is passed to the ligamentum flavum of the second, third, or fourth lumbar interspace (Figure 24–3). The ligamentum flavum is identified by its resistance to injection of saline or air. A rebound effect takes place.

5. Resistance disappears as the peridural space is entered.

6. Aspiration rules out penetration of a blood vessel.

7. A test dose of 2 to 3 mL of anesthetic agent is injected to make sure the dura mater has not been penetrated.

8. A test period of at least 5 minutes is allowed. During this time, vital signs and levels of anesthesia are checked to make sure that no untoward effects have occurred.

9. After checking again to make sure the dura mater has not been perforated, a single dose of 10 to 12 mL is injected to provide anesthesia for the birth.

Technique for Continuous Lumbar Epidural Block   The procedure of a continuous lumbar epidural block is the same as for a lumbar epidural block through step 6, after which the following steps are taken:

7. A plastic catheter is threaded 3 to 5 cm beyond the tip of the needle. Hyperesthetic response in the leg, hip, or back is sometimes elicited if the soft catheter touches a nerve in the peridural space. The needle is removed. (The plastic catheter is *never* pulled back through the needle. Risk of shearing plastic catheters must be kept in mind.)

8. The catheter is taped in place.

9. A test dose of 2 to 3 mL of anesthetic agent is injected.

10. An analgesic dose of 5 to 6 mL is given for relief of uterine pain during the first stage of labor. Additional injections are made through the catheter as necessary.

11. An anesthetic dose of 10 to 12 mL is given just prior to birth, with the woman sitting in an upright position.

     Many agents have been used for the continuous infusion epidural block. Drugs such as bupivacaine (Marcaine) and chloroprocaine (Nesacaine) have been used with success. However, narcotics are now being used with higher frequency. The narcotics do have maternal side effects and need to be administered with caution. The use of narcotics in continuous epidural infusion is still felt to be controversial by some researchers, however.

     A distressing maternal problem is inadequate block, unilateral block, or block failure. Epidural anesthesia has

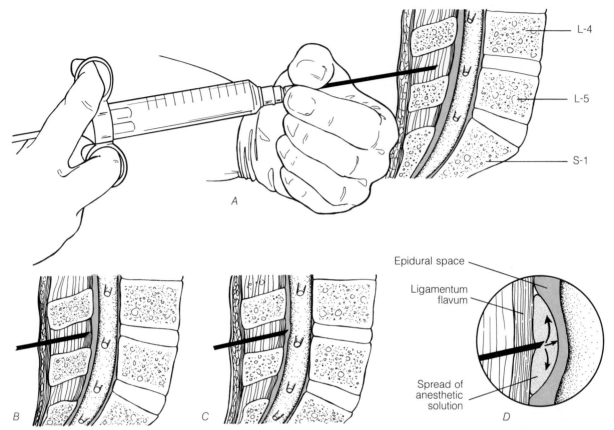

Figure 24–3   Technique of epidural block. A Proper position of insertion. B Needle in the ligamentum flavum. C Tip of needle in epidural space. D Force of injection pushing dura away from tip of needle. (From Bonica JJ: Principles and Practice of Obstetric Analgesia and Anesthesia. Philadelphia: FA Davis, 1972, p 631)

a higher failure rate than spinal anesthesia, because the catheter must be properly placed for adequate analgesia to occur. Fink (1989) cites nerve fiber length along with volume and weak concentration of anesthetics as probable causes of poor analgesia. A one-sided block is fairly common and can be overcome by having the woman lie on the unanesthetized side and injecting more of the agent. A block may be effective except for a "spot" of pain in the inguinal or suprapubic area. The large spinal nerves (L5, S1 and S2) may be more difficult to block because more anesthetic is required to penetrate the large spinal nerves (Nicholson et al 1989).

Adverse Effects   The major side effect of epidural anesthesia is maternal hypotension. This kind of anesthesia creates a sympathetic blockade, which causes a loss of peripheral resistance, a decrease in venous return to the heart, and a subsequent decrease in cardiac output resulting in lowered blood pressure. This problem can be minimized by placing a wedge under the right hip to displace uterine pressure on the vena cava and by hydrating prior to the procedure. From 500 to 1000 mL of fluid should be rapidly infused to increase blood volume and increase cardiac output. It is recommended that dextrose-free solutions be

used because dextrose can cause fetal hyperglycemia with rebound hypoglycemia the first few hours after birth. Systolic pressure below 100 mm Hg or a fall in systolic pressure of greater than 30% of the baseline blood pressure requires treatment (Shnider et al 1983). The treatment of mild-to-moderate hypotension is to place the mother in a left lateral position, increase the rate of intravenous fluids, administer oxygen by mask to help decrease the nausea associated with a drop in blood pressure and increase fetal oxygenation, and provide reassurance to the mother. With severe or prolonged hypotension added treatment includes elevation of the woman's legs for two or three minutes to increase blood return from the extremities and administration of intravenous ephedrine. To avoid fetal compromise, it is essential to detect and treat hypotension as soon as it occurs. Maternal blood pressure and pulse and the FHR must be taken every 1 to 2 minutes for 15 minutes after the injection and every 10 to 15 minutes thereafter. The regimen for initial surveillance should be repeated each time the epidural catheter is reinjected.

Other side effects include urinary retention, shivering, headache, and pyrexia. During epidural block the urge to void is diminished. The bladder must be checked carefully, and the woman should be encouraged to void at frequent intervals to avoid bladder distention. Catheterization may be necessary as most women are unable to void. Shivering may be caused by heat loss from increased peripheral blood flow or alteration of thermal input to the central nervous system when warm but not cold sensations have been suppressed. Reassurance for the woman and application of a warm blanket are the supportive therapies. Headache (of the type with spinal blocks) is not a side effect of epidural anesthesia, because the dura mater of the spinal canal has not been penetrated and there is no leakage of spinal fluid. Pyrexia may be present and it is thought to be the result of vascular and autoregulatory modifications due to epidural anesthesia (Fusi 1989).

Complications   One of the most serious complications of regional anesthesia, systemic toxic reaction, has been discussed in the section on adverse maternal reactions to anesthetic agents. Toxic reactions following a lumbar epidural may be caused by unintentional placement of the drug in the arachnoid or subarachnoid space, excessive amount of the drug in the epidural space (massive epidural), or accidental intravascular injection. Since large quantities of anesthetic agent are used for epidural block, the likelihood of toxic reactions is higher than with some of the other regional procedures. The incidence of drug reactions is relatively low but the possibility is always present. Neurologic sequelae have been reported with all anesthetic agents, but the unintentional injection of chloroprocaine (Nesacaine) into the subarachnoid space has been associated with prolonged neurologic disorders (Shisky & Mallampati 1985). It has been suggested that prolonged sensorimotor disturbances are due to a low pH and the sodium bisulfite additive in chloroprocaine (Gissen & Leith 1985; Wang et al 1984). The addition of sodium bicarbonate to the solution should decrease the possibility of nerve damage if accidental placement occurs.

Nursing Role   The nurse assesses the maternal vital signs and the FHR for a baseline. The procedure and expected results are explained, and the woman's questions are answered. The woman is positioned on her left side with her shoulders parallel and her legs slightly flexed. After the block is given the woman will be returned to a supine or semi-recumbent position. A wedge should be placed under the woman's right hip to help eliminate aortocaval compression. The nurse takes the woman's blood pressure and pulse every one to two minutes during the first 15 minutes after the injection and every 10 to 15 minutes thereafter until they are stable.

If hypotension occurs, the nurse assists with corrective measures such as positioning the woman in a left side-lying position and increasing the flow rate of the intravenous infusion. The FHR should be assessed continuously during any hypotensive episode.

The bladder is assessed at frequent intervals because the epidural block lessens the urge to urinate. It is helpful to provide an opportunity for the woman to void just prior

to the epidural if possible. During the second stage of labor, the woman may also require more assistance with pushing, if she cannot feel her contractions and does not experience the urge to push.

Ambulation should be delayed until the anesthesia has worn off. This may take several hours, depending on the agent and the total dose. Motor control of the legs is weak but not totally absent after birth. Return of complete sensation and the ability to control the legs are essential before ambulation is attempted. The woman must also be able to maintain blood pressure in a sitting or standing position.

Continuous Epidural Infusion Pumps   The newest approach in epidural anesthesia is the use of a continuous infusion pump (Figure 24–4). Some of the potential benefits (Cohen 1990) include the following: good to excellent analgesia; infrequent nausea; minimal sedation; decreased anxiety; earlier mobilization; cough reflex retained; decreased risk of deep vein thrombosis; decreased myocardial oxygen demand; decreased length of hospitalization; and ease of administration.

Obviously, ease of administration does not indicate lack of need for close observation. Malfunctioning equipment with subsequent overdose is always a possibility. Some infusion pumps are specifically designed for use in epidural anesthesia and have safety factors incorporated. At the present time, continuous epidural infusions should be administered with the same precautions used for intermittent injections (Figure 24–5).

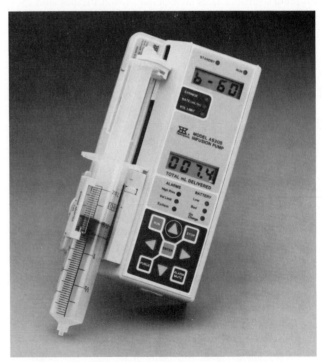

Figure 24–4   Auto syringe infusion pump used as "Epidural Pump" (Baxter Healthcare Corporation. Auto Syringe Division.)

Infusion Technique

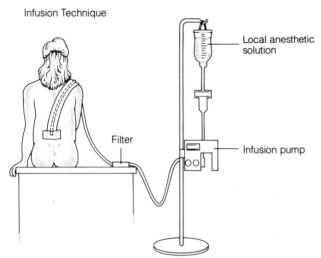

Local anesthetic solution

Filter

Infusion pump

Figure 24–5   Arrangement used for continuous epidural analgesia. Similar arrangement can be used at any other perineural site. (Adapted from Raj PP: Chronic Pain. In: Raj PP (editor) Clinical Practice of Regional Anesthesia. New York: Churchill-Livingstone, 1991, p 489.)

Some of the potential problems of epidural infusions include "breakthrough pain," sedation, nausea and vomiting, pruritis, and hypotension.

Breakthrough pain may occur at any time during the epidural infusion. It usually occurs when the infusion rate of the agent is below the recommended rate for therapeutic dose. It may also occur when the infusion pump rate is altered or the integrity of the epidural line is broken. When breakthrough pain occurs, the nurse should check the integrity of the epidural infusion line and notify the anesthetist. There may be standing orders for treatment of breakthrough pain, but it is best to inform the anesthetist of any problems that do occur.

Sedation may occur from the systemic effect of the narcotic. The epidural agents are absorbed into the circulation and can cause enough general sedation that the respiratory system will be affected. In this situation the treatment is prevention. The respiratory rate, along with the quality of respirations, should be assessed no less than every 15 to 30 minutes. The nurse should notify the anesthetist of any significant decreases in respiratory rate or respiratory pattern change. If respiratory rate decreases below 14 respirations per minute, naloxone may be given to remove the effect of the anesthetic agent; respirations will then return to a normal rate.

Nausea and vomiting can occur at any time during or after epidural infusion. The nurse should give an antiemetic if one is ordered and call the anesthetist. If there are no standing orders for an antiemetic, the nurse can call the anesthetist to get one. The nausea and vomiting can make the woman very uncomfortable, and the infusion rate of the epidural may need to be decreased or terminated to alleviate this discomfort.

Pruritus may occur at any time during the epidural infusion. It usually appears first on the face, neck, or torso and is usually the result of the agent in the epidural infusion. Treatment involves administration of Benadryl. The usual dose is 50 mg given intramuscularly. Should no standing order exist, the nurse should notify the anesthetist and identify the problem. The epidural infusion may need to be terminated or decreased. The nurse should assess the woman for any signs of pruritus at regular intervals or when assessing respirations.

Hypotension may occur from hypovolemia or from the effect of the epidural agent. Treatment involves applying oxygen by mask, administering a bolus of crystalloid (usually 200 to 400 mL), and notifying the anesthetist. Usually there are standing orders for treatment of hypotension that are graded in terms of the degree of hypotension. The epidural infusion may have to be terminated and the woman placed in the Trendelenburg position.

To provide analgesia for approximately 24 hours after the birth, the anesthesiologist may inject morphine, 5.0 mg or 7.5 mg, into the epidural space immediately following the birth. The analgesic effect begins approximately 30 to 60 minutes after the injection. The side effects include pruritus, which occurs in 11% to 90% of clients. Nausea and vomiting affects between 12% and 50% of patients and most commonly occurs between four and seven hours after the morphine injection. Urinary retention occurs in 15% to 90% of clients. The onset seems to occur early and resolves within 14 to 16 hours following the birth. Occasionally, respiratory depression (respirations of less than 12 per minute) may develop as early as one to two hours or as late as 8 to 16 hours after the morphine administration (Inturrisi et al 1988). Specific nursing care is presented in the Nursing Care Plan.

Subarachnoid Block (Spinal or Low Spinal)

In subarachnoid block, a local anesthetic agent is injected directly into the spinal fluid in the spinal canal to provide anesthesia for vaginal or cesarean birth. For vaginal birth, blockade to the T_{10} dermatome is usually effective, whereas cesarean birth requires anesthesia to the T_8 dermatome (Figure 24–6).

The subarachnoid space is the fluid-filled area between the dura and the spinal cord. During pregnancy, the space decreases because of the distention of the epidural veins. Thus a specific dose of anesthetic produces a much higher level of anesthesia in the pregnant woman than in the nonpregnant woman. When a low spinal block is properly administered, failure rate is low.

Advantages   The advantages are immediate onset of anesthesia, relative ease of administration, a smaller drug volume, and maternal compartmentalization of the drug.

(Text continues on p 712)

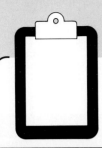

Nursing Care Plan
Regional Anesthesia—Lumbar Epidural

Client Assessment

Nursing History

Maternal information

1. Allergies to drugs (especially anesthetic agents)
2. Psychologic status
   a. What kind of anesthesia does woman want and what kind will she accept?
   b. Does she understand the procedure?
   c. What does she expect it to accomplish?
   d. Is she able to cope with the labor process, and can she follow directions?
3. Prenatal preparation and education
   a. Type of childbirth classes
   b. Degree of involvement in preparation classes
4. Presence of disease states
   a. Cardiovascular disorders
   b. Pulmonary disorders
   c. CNS disorders
   d. Metabolic problems
5. Course of current pregnancy
6. Support person available
7. When did she last eat or take fluids
8. What other drugs has she taken recently

Fetal information

1. Gestational age
   a. Calendar dates
   b. Ultrasound
2. Status of fetus
   a. Stability of FHR
   b. Result of assessments of fetal well-being

Physical Examination

1. Maternal vital signs and FHR to establish baselines
2. Estimation of pregnant uterus (Leopold's maneuver to determine fetal size, presentation, and position)

3. Quality of contractions
   a. Frequency
   b. Duration
   c. Intensity
4. Vaginal examination to determine
   a. Status of cervix
      (1) Dilatation
      (2) Effacement
   b. Maternal-fetal pelvic relationship
      (1) Presentation and position
      (2) Station of presenting part
   c. Rate of progress in labor
5. Determination whether site to be used for injection is free from infection

Diagnostic Studies

1. Screening lab tests for coagulation disorders (Nicholson et al 1990)

TEST	NORMAL VALUE
Bleeding time	1 to 5 minutes
Platelet count	150,000 to 400,000 μL
Thrombin time	16 to 20 seconds
Partial thromboplastin time	24 to 36 seconds
Prothrombin time	11 to 12 seconds

2. Fetal scalp blood samples if fetal distress occurs

Analysis of Nursing Priorities

1. Maintaining a safe environment for the mother and fetus
2. Continuous monitoring of maternal status to detect and treat potential problems
3. Continuous monitoring of fetal status for same reason
4. Promoting thorough understanding of procedure through education of both parents

Nursing Diagnosis	Nursing Interventions	Rationale	Evaluation
Nursing Diagnosis: Knowledge deficit related to regional anesthetic and analgesia	Determine current knowledge level.	Determination of woman's current knowledge level and factors that affect learning allows nurse to provide individualized teaching.	Woman is able to discuss the regional block and has no further questions.

(continued)

Nursing Care Plan (continued)

Nursing Diagnosis	Nursing Interventions	Rationale	Evaluation
Client Goal: Woman will be able to discuss the regional block, as measured by ability to verbalize: • Type of regional block • Expected effect • Possible adverse effects • Alternatives to regional block • Expected nursing care	Evaluate factors related to learning such as primary language spoken, ability to hear and interpret information, and/or presence of anxiety, which may affect ability to process information. Provide information regarding: • Reason for the block • Effect of the block • Possible side effects • Possible alternative pain relief measures • Associated nursing care that may be expected	Understanding of the anticipated effects, side effects, and nursing care will help woman be informed and participate in decision making.	

Nursing Diagnosis: Injury: High risk related to hypotension secondary to vasodilation and pooling of blood in the extremities
 	
Client Goal: Woman will not experience hypotension as measured by:
    Blood pressure (BP) remains above 90/60.
    Pulse remains in 60–80 range.
	Have legal consents signed. Have woman empty bladder. Begin intravenous fluids. Initiate intravenous infusion.
	
	Hydrate the woman receiving an epidural block with 500–1000 mL fluid prior to procedure. Dextrose-free solution is recommended.
	
	Position woman correctly for procedure (see text for proper positioning for individual procedures).
	
	Assess maternal status:
	
	1. Obtain baseline vital signs before any anesthetic agent is given.
		Regional anesthesia interferes with woman's urge to void. Intravenous fluids maintain adequate hydration and provide systemic access in the event of maternal hypotension or other untoward events.
		
		Increased intravenous fluid intake increases blood volume and increases cardiac output to help minimize hypotension. Rapid infusion of fluids containing dextrose causes fetal hyperglycemia with rebound hypoglycemia in the first two hours after birth.
		
		Baseline reading allows more complete evaluation of maternal status.
			Woman remains normotensive. FHR is between 120 and 160; accelerations are present with fetal movement; no variable or late deceleration.

(continued)

Nursing Care Plan (continued)

Nursing Diagnosis	Nursing Interventions	Rationale	Evaluation
	2. Monitor blood pressure every five min for 30 min following administration of anesthetic agent.	Hypotension is a frequent complication of regional anesthesia.	
	3. Monitor pulse and respiration.	Pulse may slow following spinal anesthesia due to decreased venous return, decreased venous pressure, and decreased right heart pressure. Respiratory paralysis is a potential complication of regional anesthesia.	
	Monitor fetal status:		
	1. Use fetal monitoring to establish a baseline reading of FHR. **2.** Monitor FHR continuously.	Maternal hypotension may interfere with fetal oxygenation and is evidenced by fetal bradycardia.	
	Observe, record, and report complications of anesthesia, including hypotension, fetal distress, respiratory paralysis, changes in uterine contractility, decrease in voluntary muscle effort, trauma to extremities, nausea and vomiting, loss of bladder tone, and spinal headache.		
	Observe, record, and report symptoms of hypotension, including systolic pressure <100 mm Hg or a 25% fall in systolic pressure, apprehension, restlessness, dizziness, tinnitus, headache.		
	Institute treatment measures:		
	1. Place woman with head flat and foot of bed elevated.	Gravity increases venous filling of the heart and the pulmonary blood volume; the result is an increase in stroke volume and cardiac output with a rise in blood pressure.	

(continued)

Nursing Care Plan (continued)

Nursing Diagnosis	Nursing Interventions	Rationale	Evaluation
	2. Increase IV fluid rate.	Blood volume increases and circulation improves.	
	3. Administer O₂ by face mask.	Oxygen content of circulating blood increases.	
	4. Administer vasopressors as ordered.	Vasoconstriction occurs; vasopressors are not used in pregnant women unless absolutely necessary because they may further compromise the fetus.	
	Specific interventions for treatment of hypotension following peridural anesthesia:		
	1. Raise knee gatch on bed.		
	2. Manually displace uterus laterally to left.	Increases venous return (vena cava is usually to the right).	
	3. Administer O₂ by face mask at 6–10 L/min.	Face mask is preferred because woman in labor breathes through her mouth.	
	4. Increase rate of IV fluids.		
	5. Keep woman supine for 5–10 min following administration of block to allow drug to diffuse bilaterally; after 5–10 min position woman on side.		
	Specific interventions for hypotension following spinal anesthesia:	BP drops following spinal anesthesia, probably because of paralysis of the sympathetic vasoconstrictor fibers to blood vessels.	
	1. Administer O₂ by face mask at 6–10 L/min.		
	2. Manually displace uterus to left.	Increases venous return.	
	3. Increase rate of IV fluids.		
	4. Place legs in stirrups.		
		Observe, record, and report fetal bradycardia (FHR <120/min) and loss of beat-to-beat variability.	Maternal hypotension causes decreased blood circulation to fetus and results in fetal hypoxia.

(continued)

Nursing Care Plan (continued)

Nursing Diagnosis	Nursing Interventions	Rationale	Evaluation
		Institute treatment measures for maternal hypotension. (Note: Paracervical blocks commonly cause a drop in FHR for a short period.)	Amide group of anesthetic agents (bupivacaine, mepivacaine, and lidocaine) have potential to produce direct fetal myocardial depression; bradycardia may be caused by reduced placental blood flow.
Nursing Diagnosis: Decreased cardiac output related to sympathetic blockade	Monitor uterus for onset of a contraction	Uterine contraction during injection of anesthetic agent may increase upward spread to a higher level than desired.	Woman is normotensive.
Client Goal: Woman remains normotensive as measured by BP in 110/80 to 138/88 range.	Converse with woman during test dose.	Altered sensorium may indicate a complication.	
	Assist with injection and taping of catheter.	Catheter must be securely taped to prevent displacement.	
	Monitor maternal BP, pulse, and respiration every five minutes for 20–30 minutes.	Local anesthetic agent causes sympathetic blockade, may cause other complications. Regimen must also be followed after every reinjection.	
Nursing Diagnosis: Impaired gas exchange in fetus due to anesthetic agent	Observe, record, and report symptoms of hypotension: BP <100 mm Hg or 25% fall in systolic pressure, nausea, and apprehension.	Maternal hypotension will decrease oxygenation of fetus. Early detection and immediate treatment decrease hypoxia in fetus.	FHR remains 120–160, with average variability, and no late or variable decelerations.
Client Goal: FHR is 120–160, with average variability, no late or variable decelerations or accelerations with fetal movement or scalp stimulation.	If hypotension occurs institute treatment measures:		
	1. Place woman with head flat and foot of bed elevated, left lateral position.	Gravity increases venous return to heart, increasing pulmonary blood volume; result is an increase in stroke volume and cardiac output with a rise in BP.	
	2. Increase IV fluid rate.	Blood volume increases and circulation improves.	
	3. Administer O_2 by face mask at 6–10 L/min.	Increases oxygen content of circulating blood.	
	4. Administer vasopressor as ordered.	Vasoconstriction occurs; used only when BP cannot be maintained by other means.	
	Monitor BP and pulse following birth.	Hypotension due to anesthetic agent may be delayed in onset.	

(continued)

Nursing Care Plan (continued)

Nursing Diagnosis	Nursing Interventions	Rationale	Evaluation
	Explain possible delayed effects of anesthetic agents on fetus.	Anesthetic agents may produce neonatal neurobehavioral effects that could interfere with bonding.	
	Assist woman to assume left lateral position.	Left lateral position prevents compression of vena cava, assisting venous return from extremities.	
	Monitor and record BP and pulse every 5 minutes initially and then every 15 minutes.	Early detection and treatment of hypotension can minimize effect on the fetus.	
	Monitor FHR continuously.	Local anesthetic agents may cause loss of variability and late decelerations.	
Nursing Diagnosis: Altered patterns of urinary elimination related to effects of epidural	Assess bladder and encourage woman to void at frequent intervals.	Urinary retention frequently accompanies epidural block; client may be unaware of need to void.	Woman's bladder remains empty, no bladder distention is present.
Client Goal: Woman will have normal urinary elimination as measured by: • Bladder is not distended. • Urination occurs without difficulty. • No urinary retention is present.	Catheterize if necessary.	Client has been overhydrated and distention may (1) impede progress of labor, (2) increase chance of bladder trauma, and (3) cause lack of postpartum bladder tone. Anesthetic agents may decrease frequency of contractions. Return of uncomfortable contractions is an indication of need for reinjection of epidural catheter. Optimal time is prior to the return of painful contractions.	
Nursing Diagnosis: Injury: High risk related to decreased motor control	Assess progress of labor: increase in frequency and duration of contractions, observe for increase in show, perform vaginal examinations.	Woman who chooses epidural wants to experience and participate in labor and birth.	
Client Goal: The woman's extremities will be supported during movement. The woman will verbalize need for assistance as measured by her using the call light to request assistance when ambulating.	Inform woman of progress in labor. Provide reassurance throughout labor. During second stage of labor coordinate woman's pushing effort with increased uterine pressure of contractions.	Loss of sensation may decrease awareness of the urge to push and the ability to push. Pushing without contraction will be ineffective and cause maternal exhaustion.	The woman's extremities are supported during movement. Woman asks for assistance during ambulation in early postpartum period.

(continued)

Nursing Care Plan (continued)

Nursing Diagnosis	Nursing Interventions	Rationale	Evaluation
	Assist with "sitting dose" reinjection for birth.	Additional anesthesia is necessary for perineal relaxation, birth, and episiotomy repair.	
	Support extremities during movement. Position legs securely in stirrups (or on table for cesarean delivery).	Epidural block should not produce motor paralysis but the client may not have full control of extremities.	
	Ensure woman understands need for assistance with ambulation.	Motor control of the legs may be weak following epidural. Ambulation is delayed until complete sensation and ability to control legs has returned.	
Nursing Diagnosis: Injury: High risk related to toxic systemic reaction *Client Goal:* Woman will remain free of signs and symptoms of toxic systemic reaction as measured by no evidence of: • Excitement • Disorientation • Incoherent speech • Nausea • Vomiting • Loss of consciousness • Severe hypotension • Bradycardia • Respiratory or cardiac arrest	Observe for and report symptoms of toxic reaction: excitement, disorientation, incoherent speech, muscle twitching, nausea and vomiting, and convulsions or severe reactions of sudden loss of consciousness, severe hypotension, bradycardia, respiratory depression, and cardiac arrest. Small, more frequent doses of analgesic agent are recommended to avoid severe reactions.	Larger volume of anesthetic agent used with epidural increases likelihood of toxic reaction.	Woman remains free of signs and symptoms.
	Institute treatment immediately: 1. Support ventilation. 2. Increase IV fluids. 3. Administer muscle relaxant for convulsions as ordered. 4. Be prepared for respiratory and cardiac resuscitation.	Immediate treatment will lessen the effects of toxic systemic reactions on fetus.	

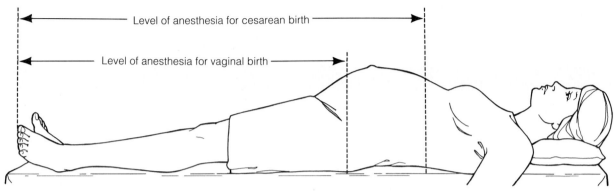

Figure 24–6   Levels of anesthesia for vaginal and cesarean births (From Regional Anesthesia in Obstetrics. *Clinical Education Aid No. 17, Columbus, OH: Ross Laboratories)*

Disadvantages   The primary disadvantage is intense blockade of sympathetic fibers resulting in a high incidence of hypotension. This leads to a greater potential for fetal hypoxia. In addition, uterine tone is maintained, which makes intrauterine manipulation difficult, and the level of spinal blockage is less predictable in laboring women.

Contraindications   Spinal anesthesia is contraindicated for women with severe hypovolemia, regardless of cause; central nervous system disease; infection over the site of puncture; maternal coagulation problems; and allergy to local anesthetic agents. Sepsis and active genital herpes may be considered relative rather than absolute contraindications. It is also contraindicated for women who do not wish to have spinal procedures (Cunningham et al 1989).

Technique   The following steps are followed in administering a subarachnoid block:

1. The woman is placed in a sitting or left lateral position. This may be uncomfortable because the block is not done until the fetal head begins to distend the perineum.
2. Intravenous infusion should be checked for patency.
3. The woman places her arms between her knees, bows her head, and arches her back to widen the intervertebral space.
4. Careful skin preparation is done, maintaining sterility.
5. A skin wheal is made over L3 or L4.
6. A 25-gauge needle with stylet is passed through the wheal into the interspinous ligament, ligamentum flavum, and epidural space into the subarachnoid space (Figure 24–7).
7. Upon removal of the stylet, a drop of fluid can be seen in the hub of the needle if the spinal canal has been entered.
8. The appropriate amount of anesthetic agent is injected slowly, and both needles are removed.
9. With hyperbaric solutions, the woman remains sitting up for 45 seconds.
10. The woman is placed on her back with a pillow under her head. Position changes can alter the dermatome level if done within three to five minutes. After ten minutes, a position change will not affect the level of anesthesia.

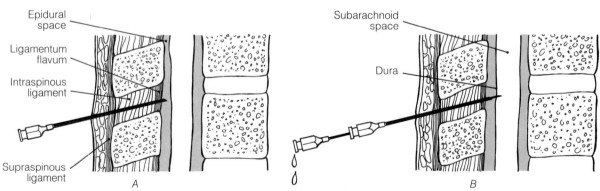

Figure 24–7   Double needle technique for spinal injection. A Large needle in epidural space. B 25- to 26-gauge needle in larger needle entering the spinal canal. (From Bonica JJ: Principles and Practice of Obstetric Analgesia and Anesthesia. *Philadelphia: FA Davis, 1972, p 563)*

11. Blood pressure, pulse, and respiration must be monitored every one to two minutes for the first ten minutes then every five to ten minutes.

A sitting or left lateral position may be used for the administration of spinal (subarachnoid block) anesthesia. Since the procedure is not done until the presenting part is on the perineum, sitting on the edge of the operating room bed may be very difficult for the laboring woman. The nurse helps the woman into position and provides encouragement and support during the procedure. The nurse informs the physician when a contraction is beginning so the anesthetic agent will not be injected at that time.

In the absence of maternal hypotension or toxic reaction there is no direct effect on the fetus with subarachnoid block. The amount of anesthetic used is too small to reach fetal circulation in a quantity that might cause fetal depression. Spinal anesthesia has been shown to be well tolerated by a healthy fetus when a maternal IV fluid load in excess of 1000 mL preceded the administration of the spinal.

Complications The complications of spinal anesthesia include hypotension, drug reaction, total spinal, neurologic sequelae, and spinal headache. The side effects include nausea, shivering, and urinary retention as described in the section on lumbar epidural anesthesia. The hypotension that occurs with spinal anesthesia seems more profound than with epidural anesthesia (Stoelting et al 1988).

Hypotension can be minimized by prehydrating with 500 to 1000 mL of non-dextrose-containing fluids and displacing the uterus to the left. The practice of placing an already hypotensive woman in a sitting position following injection to prevent upward spread of hyperbaric solution is dangerous since it will cause venous pooling in the lower extremities, further decreasing the maternal blood pressure. The normal curve of the thoracic spine prevents cranial spread of an intrathecal agent. A pillow is placed under the woman's head to exaggerate the curve.

Treatment of hypotension is the same as with an epidural: positioning the women in a left lateral, head-down position and rapid infusion of intravenous fluids. The prevention of cardiovascular collapse requires early detection, supplemental oxygen, assisted ventilation, and measures to maintain the blood pressure. The extent to which the fetus is affected relates to the degree of maternal hypotension. When maternal hypotension has been reversed it is best to delay the birth for four to five minutes to allow the fetus to recover. Resuscitative equipment and trained personnel must be available to treat the mother and baby.

A total spinal occurs when there is paralysis of the respiratory muscles. It is a relatively rare but critical event. The symptoms are apnea, dilation of the pupils, loss of consciousness, and absence of blood pressure. The onset of symptoms usually occurs within minutes of the injection but can occur in a span of time ranging from 30 seconds to 45 minutes. Resuscitative treatment, airway control, and support of blood pressure must begin immediately. If this complication occurs, it is important to remember that this

woman is not asleep; although she may be paralyzed, she is aware of everything going on around her. She requires assurance that her respiration is being maintained and will continue to be maintained until she can breathe on her own.

Neurologic complications may occur coincidentally with spinal anesthesia such as with preexisting disease or faulty positioning of the woman. Genuine neurologic sequelae such as paralysis is extremely rare (Albright et al 1986).

Although much less serious than other complications, headache may be an unpleasant aftermath of spinal anesthesia. It is the most frequent complication. Leakage of spinal fluid at the site of dural puncture is thought to be the cause. Several techniques have been suggested to decrease the possibility of headache. The use of a 25- or 26-gauge needle and entering the dura at a shallow angle rather than a right angle help reduce the incidence of leaking spinal fluid (Nicholson et al 1989). The incidence of spinal headache varies from about 70% after puncture with a 16-gauge needle to only about 2% with a 25-gauge spinal needle (Cousins et al 1988). Hyperhydration and keeping the woman flat in bed for 6 to 12 hours after birth have been recommended as preventive measures, but there is no evidence that these procedures are effective.

The postspinal block headache usually begins on the second postpartal day and lasts several days to a week. It may be of varying degrees of severity. The pain occurs or becomes worse when the woman sits or stands and decreases or ceases when she lies down or flexes and extends her head.

Treatment consists primarily of bed rest, increased fluids, and analgesics for the mild or moderate forms. Severe and incapacitating headache has been treated successfully by saline injection. In another technique, a "blood patch" is placed over the site of dural puncture. About 10 to 20 mL of blood is drawn from the woman and immediately injected, via sterile technique, into the epidural space over the site of the perforation; the clot applies pressure and seals off the leak. In many cases, this procedure has dramatically relieved symptoms. The success rate ranges from 89% to 100%.

Nursing Role Prior to the administration of a low spinal block for vaginal birth, intravenous fluids should be infusing and the woman's knowledge about the procedure assessed. The woman should be able to verbalize what she thinks will happen and what is expected of her during the administration. Maternal vital signs and fetal heart rate are taken and recorded as a baseline for determining any deviation from normal during the procedure. The woman is then hydrated with 500 to 1000 mL of dextrose-free solution to maintain blood volume. Amount and time of increased infusion are noted and recorded.

The nurse positions the woman correctly on the operating room table, usually upright with her legs on a stool. The woman places her arms between her knees, bows her head (shoulders should be even with hips), and arches her back to widen the intervertebral spaces. The nurse supports the woman in this position and palpates the uterus to detect the beginning of a contraction. Intrathecal agents are not administered during a contraction because the increased pressure could cause a higher level of anesthesia than desired. After the agent has been administered the woman is asked to sit upright for the length of time determined by the anesthetist and is then assisted to the supine position with a wedge under her right hip to displace the uterus; a pillow is placed under her head. The nurse monitors blood pressure, pulse, and respirations every five minutes until the birth. Some physicians administer oxygen as a prophylactic measure. The woman should be kept informed of everything that is going on in the birthing area, particularly if she is receiving mask oxygen. Placing her legs in stirrups will facilitate venous return from the extremities. Both legs should be raised at the same time to avoid undue tension and possible injury to back muscles.

If hypotension should occur, the intravenous fluids should be increased and the uterus displaced manually to the left. Total spinal rarely occurs but the possibility must always be kept in mind. The woman should be observed for apnea, unconsciousness, pupil dilation, and unobtainable blood pressure. Prompt treatment, which may include the use of a vasopressor (such as ephedrine), may avert a catastrophe for the woman and/or baby. It is essential to establish an airway and give oxygen with positive pressure until the woman can be intubated and other emergency measures instituted.

Following birth the legs should be lowered slowly and simultaneously. A sudden movement of the extremities when vasomotor paralysis is present can precipitate a hypotensive episode. Although the effectiveness of the supine position to avoid headache following a spinal is controversial, the physician's orders may include lying flat for six to eight hours.

The nursing interventions during administration of a spinal for cesarean birth will be the same except for placing the legs in lithotomy position. It is even more important that the woman be kept informed about activities around her and reminded of the fact that she may have sensations but will not have pain. Reassurance and support of the woman are essential in helping her participate in the birth experience.

Pudendal Block

The pudendal block technique provides perineal anesthesia for the second stage of labor, birth, and episiotomy repair. An anesthetic agent is injected below the pudendal plexus, which arises from the anterior division of the second and third sacral nerves and the entire fourth sacral nerve. The pudendal nerve crosses the sacrosciatic notch and passes the tip of the ischial spine, where it divides into the perineal, dorsal, and inferior hemorrhoidal nerves. The perineal nerve, which is the largest branch of the pudendal plexus, supplies the skin of the vulvar area, the perineal muscles, and the urethral sphincter. The dorsal nerve sup-

plies the clitoris, and the inferior hemorrhoidal nerve supplies the skin and muscles of the perianal region as well as the internal anal sphincter. Pudendal block provides relief of pain from perineal distention but does not relieve pain of uterine contractions.

Pudendal block is a relatively simple procedure but requires a thorough knowledge of pelvic anatomy to block the pudendal nerve adequately.

Advantages/Disadvantages The advantages of pudendal block are ease of administration and absence of maternal hypotension. It also allows the use of low forceps for birth.

A moderate dose of anesthetic agent (10 mL per side) has minimal ill effects on the woman and the course of labor. The urge to bear down during the second stage of labor may be decreased, but the woman is able to do so with appropriate coaching. There is usually little effect on the uncompromised fetus unless overly rapid or intravascular injection occurs. The block may be done by a transvaginal or transperineal approach. Transvaginal injection is simpler, safer, and more direct, making it the procedure of choice.

Technique A pudendal block is administered as follows:

1. The woman is placed in a lithotomy or dorsal recumbent position with her knees flexed.
2. A 12.7 to 15.24 cm, 22-gauge needle with guide is used to protect the vaginal wall and control needle depth.
3. The instrument is guided into the vagina until the ischial spine is reached (Figure 24–8).
4. The needle is advanced through the vaginal wall into the space where the pudendal nerve passes.
5. Following aspiration to make sure that the needle is not in a blood vessel, 3 to 5 mL of solution is injected.
6. The needle is advanced 1 cm more, aspiration is repeated, and another 3 to 5 mL of the agent is injected.
7. Injection of the agent into the pudendal nerve on the opposite side follows the same procedure.

Chloroprocaine (Nesacaine), which has a low toxicity, may be used if prompt but brief anesthesia is needed. Lidocaine (Xylocaine) has prompt effect and intermediate action. Other agents used are mepivacaine (Carbocaine) and bupivacaine (Marcaine).

For most women, the pudendal block is compatible with the goals of psychoprophylactic preparation for childbirth. The transvaginal technique must be done before the fetal head has advanced too far in the birth canal. Demonstrable blood levels of anesthetic agents have been documented in the fetus but serious fetal complications are rare.

Complications Systemic toxic reaction can occur from accidental vascular injection. Other possible maternal com-

A disadvantage is that large amounts of solution must be used. Although any local anesthetic may be used, chloroprocaine (Nesacaine), lidocaine (Xylocaine), and mepivacaine (Carbocaine) are the agents of choice in local infiltration because of their capacity for diffusion.

Technique The technique of local anesthesia consists of injecting the agent with a long, beveled 22-gauge needle into the various fascial planes of the perineum (Figure 24–9). The procedure is deceptively simple; however, over-

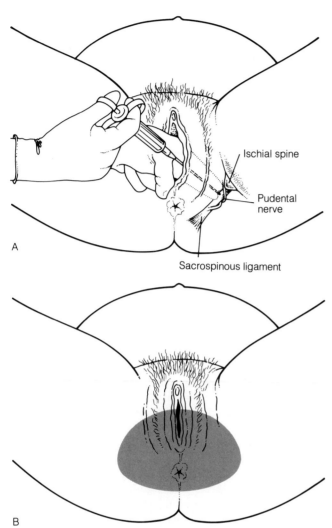

A

Ischial spine

Pudental nerve

Sacrospinous ligament

B

Figure 24–8 A Pudendal block by the transvaginal approach. B Area of perineum affected by pudendal block.

plications specific to pudendal block include broad ligament hematoma, perforation of the rectum, and trauma to the sciatic nerve. Following the birth, neonatal bradycardia, hypoventilation or apnea, hypotonia, tonic seizures, and reduced responsiveness have been reported. These difficulties can usually be attributed to accidental injection of the fetal scalp.

Nursing Role The nurse explains the procedure and the expected effect and answers any questions. Pudendal block does not alter maternal vital signs or FHR, so assessments in addition to the expected ones are not necessary.

Local Anesthesia
Local anesthesia is accomplished by injection of an anesthetic agent into the intracutaneous, subcutaneous, and intramuscular areas of the perineum. It is generally used at the time of birth for episiotomy repair and is especially useful for women giving birth by psychoprophylactic methods of childbirth. The procedure is technically simple and is practically free from complications.

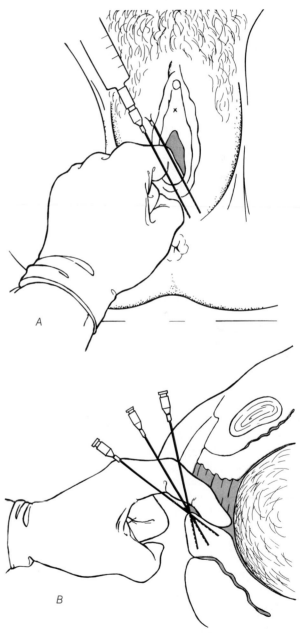

A

B

Figure 24–9 Local anesthesia. A Technique of local infiltration for episiotomy and repair. B Technique of local infiltration showing fan pattern for the fascial planes. (From Bonica JJ: Principles and Practice of Obstetric Analgesia and Anesthesia. Philadelphia: FA Davis, 1972, p 505)

dose may occur if the anesthetist does not wait for the anesthetic to take effect before injecting more solution. An excessive volume or concentration contributes to systemic toxic reactions and local toxic effects.

Nursing Role The nurse explains the procedure and the expected effect and answers any questions. Local anesthetic agents have no effect on maternal vital signs or FHR, so additional assessments are unnecessary.

General Anesthesia

The goal of obstetric anesthesia is to provide maximal pain relief with minimal side effects to the woman and her fetus. Anesthetic techniques and drugs should be selected to meet their needs. A general anesthesia may be needed for cesarean birth and surgical intervention with some obstetric complications. The method used to achieve general anesthesia may be intravenous injection, inhalation of anesthetic agents, or a combination of both methods.

General anesthesia is not without risk, however. The leading cause of obstetric anesthetic death is regurgitation and aspiration of gastric contents. The physiologic changes in the gastrointestinal tract during pregnancy include decreased gastric motility and delayed gastric emptying. The gastric contents are highly acidic and produce chemical pneumonitis if aspirated. Prophylactic antacid therapy to reduce the acidic content of the stomach prior to general anesthesia has become common practice in the past decade. Administration of a nonparticulate oral antacid (such as polycitra or bicitra) may be used. Cimetidine (Tagamet) has been advocated by some anesthesiologists but others criticize its use (Dunn 1990).

The risk of aspiration with the use of mask anesthesia without placement of an endotracheal tube can no longer be justified (Albright et al 1986, Devore 1985). In order to prevent possible regurgitation during intubation, the simplest and most effective method is to apply cricoid pressure. During the process of rapid induction of anesthesia, an assistant applies cricoid pressure as the woman loses consciousness. This is accomplished by depressing the cricoid cartilage 2 to 3 cm posteriorly so that the esophagus is occluded. Figure 24–10 shows the appropriate technique. It is important to note that cricoid pressure is increased if active retching occurs and in any case should not be released until the cuffed endotracheal tube is in place and the cuff is inflated.

Prior to induction of anesthesia, the woman should have a wedge placed under the right hip to displace the uterus and avoid vena caval compression in the supine position. She should also be preoxygenated with three to five minutes of 100% oxygen. Intravenous fluids should be initiated so that access to the intravascular system is immediately available. The woman who has been in prolonged

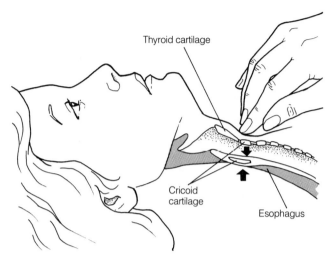

Figure 24–10 Proper position for fingers in applying cricoid pressure

labor may also need to be hydrated if an infusion was not previously in place.

Inhalation anesthetics depress the central nervous system in varying degrees, which correlate to the concentration of the agent in arterial blood entering cerebral circulation. By balancing the amount of a drug entering arterial circulation by way of the lung against the amount returning chemically intact to the lung by way of venous circulation, the anesthesiologist/anesthetist can control the concentration in the brain and keep the woman at the desired level of anesthesia. Inhalation anesthetics are considered to be safer than intravenously administered drugs because the circulating concentrations can be more quickly and better controlled. Once injected, intravenous agents cannot be retrieved and must be metabolized by the body for excretion.

Inhalation Anesthetics

Inhalation general anesthesia is rarely used for vaginal birth. It may be required when time constraints prevent induction of regional anesthesia, as in acute fetal distress (Barash et al 1989).

Nitrous Oxide

Nitrous oxide provides rapid and pleasant induction; it is nonirritating, nonexplosive, and inexpensive; and it provides less disturbance in physiologic functioning than other agents. At a concentration of 40%, it produces excellent analgesia yet permits the laboring woman to cooperate. Little or no fetal depression occurs with this concentration. When used alone, there is no effect on the maternal respiratory center.

Nitrous oxide is generally used in combination with other agents for anesthesia. Although it is a good analgesic, nitrous oxide provides poor muscular relaxation. The main use of nitrous oxide is as an analgesic agent during the second stage of labor, as an induction agent or supplement to more potent inhalation anesthetics, and as a part of balanced anesthesia.

Enflurane (Ethrane)

Enflurane is considered by many to be the ideal inhalation agent since it provides cardiac stability, very good analgesia even at low levels, and a higher oxygen concentration than nitrous oxide. Effects are rapidly reversible, and the substance is rapidly eliminated by the fetus. Although seizure potential has been demonstrated on EEG, there has been no report of seizure activity (Stoelting et al 1988). The low solubility and rapid elimination may account for the lack of nephrotoxicity.

Isoflurane (Forane)

Isoflurane is associated with low incidence of myocardial and ventilatory depression and does not cause seizure potential (Stoelting et al 1988). This agent is a good choice when uterine relaxation is essential. It provides relaxation while maintaining uterine blood flow and maternal blood pressure.

Intravenous Anesthetics

Sodium Thiopental (Pentothal)

Sodium thiopental is an ultrashort-acting barbiturate that produces narcosis within 30 seconds after intravenous administration. Induction and emergence are smooth and pleasant, with little incidence of nausea and vomiting. The woman goes from the first stage of anesthesia to the first plane of the third stage so rapidly that the clinical signs of the levels in between are difficult to detect. Barbiturates are nonirritating to the respiratory tract and are nonexplosive. They differ from the inhalation anesthetics in two major ways: Little or no analgesia occurs, and the method of administration is less controllable.

Sodium thiopental is extremely irritating to tissues, and sloughing may result if infiltration occurs with high concentrations of the agent. Because of this effect, the integrity of the intravenous line must be checked prior to administration. The rapidity of action makes it valuable in convulsive states, particularly those that occur as side effects of local anesthetics. Maternal peak plasma concentration after injection may fall as much as 90% in 1 minute, so injection at the onset of a contraction prevents the fetus from receiving the transient high concentration of the agent. Significant complications include hypotension, vasodilation, and laryngospasm, and muscle relaxation is inadequate.

Sodium thiopental is rarely used alone, because the dosage required for anesthesia (3 to 4 mg/kg) produces profound central nervous system depression. It is most frequently used for induction.

Ketamine Hydrochloride (Ketalar, Ketaject)

The intravenous agent ketamine hydrochloride is a dissociative anesthetic with amnesic and analgesic properties. It is a useful alternative to sodium thiopental for induction of general anesthesia and is most frequently used as a single-dose induction of general anesthesia. Ketamine crosses the placental barrier within 60 to 90 seconds after injection but causes little fetal depression with maternal doses of 0.2 to 0.4 mg/kg or less (Barash et al 1989). Administration of higher doses is associated with neonatal respiratory depression and elevated bilirubin levels (Joyce et al 1986).

The advantages of ketamine are that induction is rapid and pleasant, and recovery from anesthesia is rapid. It is thought to produce less suppression of pharyngeal and laryngeal reflexes, thereby reducing risks of aspiration if vomiting should occur.

The disadvantages include a 10% to 20% increase in blood pressure and heart rate; increased oral secretions, which can be decreased by the administration of atropine; transitory apnea, which is usually associated with rapid intravenous injection, overdose, or prior medication with depressant drugs; skeletal muscle hypertonus, which is usually associated with excessive dosage and can be treated with intravenous succinylcholine; and unpleasant dreams. Use of ketamine may also induce amnesia about events surrounding birth, which is unacceptable to many women.

Complications of General Anesthesia

The primary dangers of general anesthesia include fetal depression, uterine relaxation, and vomiting and aspiration.

Fetal Depression

Most general anesthetic agents reach the fetus in about two minutes. The depression in the fetus is directly proportional to the depth and duration of the anesthesia. The long-term significance of fetal depression in a normal birth has not been determined. The poor fetal metabolism of general anesthetic agents is similar to that of analgesic agents administered during labor. General anesthesia is not advocated in cases in which the fetus is considered to be at high risk, particularly in premature births.

Uterine Relaxation

Most general anesthetic agents cause some degree of uterine relaxation as well as postpartal uterine atony. Following complicated vaginal or cesarean birth, the uterus must be carefully monitored for tone and vaginal flow must be observed frequently.

Vomiting and Aspiration

Prevention of regurgitation has been discussed previously. If the recommended regimen has not been used or has failed, the woman may aspirate gastric contents and develop a pneumonitis called Mendelson syndrome. The onset and severity of symptoms depend on the pH of the aspirate, amount aspirated, and area in lung in contact with the aspirate. Aspiration of solid food will cause coughing, bronchospasm, cyanosis, and shock. Immediate treatment is to place the operating room bed in a 30° headdown position and quickly suction pharynx and larynx or remove the food with a gauze-wrapped finger. *Clearing the airway is the primary concern.* Intubation and 100% oxygen for pulmonary ventilation follow.

If the aspirate is liquid the symptoms range from fine rales in the lungs, to tachypnea, tachycardia, and cyanosis, to pulmonary edema and circulatory failure. The right lung is usually affected because the right bronchus is 25° from the vertical axis of the trachea in the adult, whereas the left bronchus is at a 45° angle. Onset of symptoms ranges from immediately to six to eight hours later.

Neonatal Neurobehavioral Effects of Anesthesia and Analgesia

Recent studies have focused on the neonatal neurobehavioral effects of pharmacologic agents used during labor and birth. The American Academy of Pediatrics has recommended the use of drugs that have been demonstrated to have the least effect during labor. While studies have shown that analgesic and anesthetic agents may alter the behavioral and adaptive function of the neonate, the long range importance of these findings has not been established. Because of the methodological shortcomings in most studies, it is not possible to state whether there is a clear-cut relationship between agents and outcomes. Neurobehavioral testing does not predict long-term outcome for the infant. Most of the agents are safe and effective when administered in the proper dosage, at the proper site, with the proper precautions and with assessments (Cooke & Spielman 1985).

Analgesic and Anesthetic Considerations for the High-Risk Mother and Fetus

Up to this point the discussion of obstetric analgesia and anesthesia has dealt with the healthy woman and healthy fetus. Pain relief for high-risk women during labor and birth requires skill in decision making, close observation, and awareness of potential threats to the woman and fetus. Safety for all involved necessitates the close cooperation of obstetrician, anesthesiologist, pediatrician, and labor nurse. The pathophysiologic changes that accompany maternal disorders have a direct influence on the choice of agent or technique. It is difficult to separate maternal and fetal complications, because whatever alters the woman's response will also affect the fetus. The effects on the woman cannot be considered without the potential effects on the fetus.

Preterm Labor

The preterm fetus has special risks and requirements. An immature fetus is more susceptible to depressant drugs because he or she has less protein available for binding; has a poorly developed blood-brain barrier, which increases the likelihood that pharmacologic agents will attain a higher concentration in the central nervous system; and has a decreased ability to metabolize and excrete drugs after birth. Analgesia during labor should be avoided whenever possible. If it becomes necessary, the smallest dose that will provide relief should be administered. Emotional support will be very valuable to the woman in this situation.

Pregnancy-Induced Hypertension
Pregnancies complicated by PIH are high-risk situations, as indicated in Chapter 19. The potential for chronic placental insufficiency and/or preterm are also present. The woman with mild PIH usually may have the analgesia or anesthesia of choice although the incidence of hypotension with epidural anesthesia is increased. If hypotension occurs with the epidural, it provides further stress on an already compromised cardiovascular system. Hypotension can usually be managed with judicial fluid increase and positioning.

The woman with severe PIH is a real challenge. Regional anesthesia seems to be the preferred method as long as hypotension can be avoided. Raising the central venous pressure by 3 to 4 cm H_2O with intravenous fluids helps avoid hypotension, but it must be remembered that this woman is already threatened with heart failure. The effect of fluid intake can be monitored with a CVP line or pulmonary catheter. It is important to monitor and record the fluid intake and output. Some physicians use vasopressors, while others avoid them because of the possible decrease in uterine blood flow to an already compromised fetus and the threat of a maternal cerebral vascular accident. Spinal anesthesia is rarely used because of the greater potential for hypotension.

With the use of general anesthesia, there is a risk of aggravating maternal hypertension. The safest method for general anesthesia includes intubation, which may cause a hypertensive episode. Administration of antihypertensive therapy during this period will avoid the hypertensive episode (Hood et al 1985). The use of ketamine should be avoided in the induction procedure because of its potential to raise the blood pressure.

Diabetes Mellitus

The fetus may have compromised placental reserve, and hypotension during regional anesthesia can deplete this reserve even further. If labor can be managed without fetal distress, small doses of intravenous narcotics with pudendal block at birth or the continuous epidural technique may be undertaken. If fetal distress occurs, cesarean birth may be necessary. General anesthesia is frequently used, but McDonald (1985) has used the lumbar epidural technique with 3% chloroprocaine (Nesacaine) successfully for cesarean births.

Cardiac Disease

Pregnancy imposes significant risk for the woman with cardiac disease. With mild mitral stenosis the preferred anesthetic is continual epidural anesthesia with low forceps birth. This method avoids the cardiovascular changes associated with contractions and the Valsalva maneuver during bearing down in the second stage of labor. Hypotension can be avoided with carefully controlled intravenous fluids, and measuring CVP to avoid overload. A cesarean birth may be done with epidural or general anesthesia. Ketamine should be avoided because it produces tachycardia.

Bleeding Complications

The current trend is toward scheduled cesarean birth when possible (Cunningham et al 1989). When the maternal cardiovascular system is stable and there is no evidence of fetal distress, an epidural may be given for birth (Gibbs 1985). However, when either of these conditions results in active bleeding, the threat of hypovolemia must be treated immediately. Maternal hypovolemia and shock produce fetal hypoxia, acidosis, and possible fetal death.

Regional blocks are contraindicated during active bleeding because the sympathetic block causes vasodilatation and further reduction of the vascular volume. General anesthesia is recommended for these cases. While sodium thiopental may be used, it is a cardiac depressant and vasodilator and ketamine may be a more appropriate choice for induction (Barash et al 1989). Following birth of the infant and placenta, oxytocin should not be given as an intravenous bolus to contract the uterus because the vasodilatation produced causes a decrease in blood pressure and in total peripheral resistance. Oxytocin should be given as a dilute infusion to gain the oxytocic effect but avoid the incidence of cardiovascular changes (Gibbs 1985).

❀ ❀

KEY CONCEPTS

Pain relief during labor may be enhanced by psychoprophylactic methods and administration of analgesics and regional anesthesia blocks.

The goal of pharmacologic pain relief during labor is to provide maximal analgesia with minimal risk for the woman and fetus.

The optimal time for administering analgesia is determined after making a complete assessment of many factors. An analgesic agent is generally administered to nulliparas when the cervix has dilated 5 to 6 cm and to multiparas when the cervix has reached 3 to 4 cm dilatation.

The most common analgesic agents include meperidine and butorphanol.

Opiate antagonists, such as naloxone, counteract the respiratory depressant effect of the opiate narcotics by acting at specific receptor sites in the CNS.

Regional anesthesia is achieved by injecting local anesthetic agents into an area that will bring the agent into direct contact with nerve tissue. Methods most commonly used in childbearing include peridural block (lumbar epidural), subarachnoid block (spinal, or low spinal), pudendal block, and local infiltration.

Two types of local anesthetic agents used in regional blocks are amide and ester groups. The amides are absorbed quickly and can be found in maternal blood within minutes after administration, while the esters are metabolized more rapidly and have only limited placental transfer.

New agents in use for intrathecal and epidural routes include morphine, fentanyl, meperidine, and sufentanil.

Untoward reactions of the woman to local anesthetic agents range from mild symptoms, such as palpitations, to cardiovascular collapse.

The goal of general anesthesia is to provide maximal pain relief with minimal side effects to the woman and her fetus.

Complications of general anesthesia include fetal depression, uterine relaxation, vomiting, and aspiration.

The choice of analgesia and anesthesia for the high-risk woman and fetus requires careful evaluation.

❀ ❀

References

Abboud TK et al: Continuous infusion epidural anesthesia in parturients receiving bupivacaine, chloroprocaine or lidocaine: Maternal, fetal and neonatal effects. *Anesth Analg* 1984a; 63:421.

Abboud TK et al: Effect of epidural analgesia during labor on fetal plasma catecholamine release. *Anesthesiology* September 1984b; 61:A413.

Abboud TK et al: Lack of adverse neonatal neurobehavioral effects of lidocaine. *Anesth Analg* 1983; 62:473.

Abboud TK et al: Maternal, fetal and neonatal responses after epidural anesthesia with bupivacaine, chloroprocaine or lidocaine. *Anesth Analg* 1982; 61:638.

Abboud TK et al: The neonatal neurobehavioral effects of mepivacaine for epidural anesthesia during labor. *Anesthesiology* September 1985; 63:A449.

Albright BA, Joyce TH, Stevenson DK: *Anesthesia in Obstetrics*, 2nd ed. Boston: Butterworth, 1986.

Barash P et al: Epidural and spinal anesthesia. In: *Clinical Anesthesia*. Covino BG, Lambert DH (editors). Philadelphia: Lippincott, 1989.

Bonica JJ: *Principles of Practice of Obstetric Analgesia and Anesthesia*. Philadelphia: Davis, 1972.

Briggs GG, Freeman RK, Yaffe SJ: *Drugs in Pregnancy and Lactation*, 3rd ed. Baltimore: Williams & Wilkins, 1990.

Cohen M: Continued epidural infusions for acute postoperative pain: Part 1. *Curr Rev Nurs Anesthetists* 1990; 21:171.

Cohen M: Continuous epidural infusions for acute postoperative pain: Part II. *Curr Rev Nurs Anesthetists* 1990; 22:181.

Cooke BC, Spielman FJ: Problems associated with epidural anesthesia in obstetrics. *Obstet Gynecol* June 1985; 65:837.

Cousins M et al: Neural blockade for obstetrics and gynecological surgery. In: *Neural Blockade*, 2nd ed. Philadelphia: Lippincott, 1988.

Cunningham FG, MacDonald PC, Gant NF: *Williams Obstetrics*, 18th ed. Norwalk, CT: Appleton & Lange, 1989.

Dunn LJ: Cesarean section and other obstetric operations. In: *Danforth's Obstetrics and Gynecology*, 6th ed. Scott JR et al (editors). Philadelphia: Lippincott, 1990.

Fink BR: Mechanisms of differential axial blockade in epidural and subarachnoid anesthesia. *Anesthesiology* 1989; 70(5):855.

Firestone L et al: *Clinical Anesthesia Procedures by the Massachusetts General Hospital*, 3rd ed. Boston: Little, Brown, 1988.

Fusi L et al: Maternal pyrexia associated with the usage of epidural analgesia in labour. *Lancet* 1989; 6(1):1250.

Giacoia GP, Yaffee S: Perinatal pharmacology, in Sciarri JJ (ed) *Gynecology and Obstetrics*. Vol 3. Philadelphia: Harper & Row, 1982.

Gibbs CP: Anesthetic management of the high risk mother. In: *Gynecology and Obstetrics*. Vol 3. Sciarra JJ, Depp R, Eschenbach DA (editors). Philadelphia: Harper & Row, 1985, Ch 90.

Gieraerts R et al: Recurrent HSUL and the uses of epidural morphine in obstetrics. *Anesth Analg* 1989; 68(3):418.

Gissen D, Leith DE: Transient decreases in respiratory rate following epidural injections. *Anesthesiology* June 1985; 62:822.

Henrikson ML, Wild LR: A nursing process approach to epidural analgesia. *JOGNN* September/October 1988; 17:316.

Hodgkinson R, Husain FJ: The duration of effect of maternally administrated meperidine on neonatal behavior. *Anesthesiology* 1982; 56:51.

Hood DD et al: Use of nitroglycerine in preventing the hypertensive response to tracheal intubation in severe preeclampsia. *Anesthesiology* August 1985; 63:329.

Inturrisi M, Camenga CF, Rosen M: Epidural morphine for relief of postpartum, postsurgical pain. *JOGNN* July/August 1988; 17:238.

Joseppila R: Maternal and umbilical cord noradrenaline concentrations during labor with and without segmental extradural analgesia and during caesarean section. *B Jr Anaesth* 1984: 56:251.

Kileff ME et al: Neonatal neurobehavioral responses after epidural anesthesia for cesarean section using lidocaine and bupivacaine. *Anesth Analg* 1984; 63:413.

Kuhnert BR et al: Effect of maternal epidural anesthesia on neonatal behavior. *Anesth Analg* 1984; 63:301.

Marx G: Fundamental concerns. In *Anesthesia in Obstetrics*, 2nd ed. Albright GA et al (editors). Boston: Butterworth, 1986, Ch 10, p 251.

McDonald JS: Anesthesia and the high risk fetus. In: *Gynecology and Obstetrics*. Sciarra JJ, Depp R, Eschenbach DA (editors). Philadelphia: Harper & Row, 1985, Ch 91.

Miller R: Obstetric Anesthesia. In: *Anesthesia*, 2nd ed. New York: Churchill-Livingstone, 1986.

Nicholson C et al: Avoiding the pitfalls of epidural anesthesia in obstetrics. *J Am Assoc Nurse Anesthetists* 1989; 57(3):220.

Paradise NF: Personal Communication. Biology Department, University of Akron, Akron, OH, 1990.

Physicians' Desk Reference, 43rd ed. New Jersey: Medical Economics Co., 1989.

Ravindran RS: Epidural analgesia in the presence of herpes simplex virus (type 2) infection. *Anesth Analg* 1982; 61:714.

Shisky MC, Mallampati SR: Prolonged neural blockade following caudal epidural block with chloroprocaine. *Reg Anesth* 1985; 10:28.

Shnider SM et al: Maternal catecholamines decrease during labor after lumbar epidural anesthesia. *Am J Obstet Gynecol* September 1983; 147:13.

Skidmore-Roth L: Mosby's 1991 Nursing Drug Reference. St. Louis: Mosby Year Book, 1991.

Stefani SJ et al: Neonatal neurobehavioral effects of inhalation analgesia for vaginal delivery. *Anesthesiology* 1982; 56:351.

Stoelting R et al: Spinal, epidural, and caudal blocks. In: *Basics of Anesthesia*, 2nd ed. New York: Churchill-Livingstone, 1988.

Wang BC et al: Effects of the anesthetic chloroprocaine on the anti-oxidant sodium bisulfate. *Anesth Analg* April 1984; 63:445.

Additional Readings

Benlabed M, Dreizzen E, Ecoffey C et al: Neonatal patterns of breathing after cesarean section with or without epidural fentanyl. *Anesthesiology* December 1990; 73:1110.

Carrie LE: Extradural, spinal or combined block for obstetric surgical anaesthesia. *Br J Anaesth* August 1990; 65:225.

Eakes M: Economic considerations for epidural anesthesia in childbirth. *Nurs Econ* September/October 1990; 8:329.

Endler GC: The risk of anesthesia in obese parturients. *J Perinatol* June 1990; 10:175.

Gambling DR, McMorland GH, Yu P et al: Comparison of patient-controlled epidural analgesia and conventional intermittent "top-up" injections during labor. *Anesth Analg* March 1990; 70:256.

Katz VL et al: Catecholemine levels in pregnant physicians and nurses: A pilot study of stress and pregnancy. *Obstet Gynecol* March 1991; 77:338.

MacArthur C, Lewis M. Know EG et al: Epidural anaesthesia and long term backache after childbirth. *Br Med J* July 1990; 301(6742):9.

Stampone D: The history of obstetric anesthesia. *J Perinatal Neonatal Nurs* July 1990; 4:1.

Viscomi CM, Eisenach JC: Pain controls epidural anesthesia during labor. *Obstet Gynecol* March 1991; 77:348.

Viscomi CM, Hood DD, Melone PJ et al: Fetal heart rate variability after epidural fentanyl during labor. *Anesth Analg* December 1990; 71:679.

Westmore MD: Epidural opioids in obstetrics—A review. *Anaesth Intensive Care* August 1990; 18:292.

CHAPTER 25

Childbirth at Risk

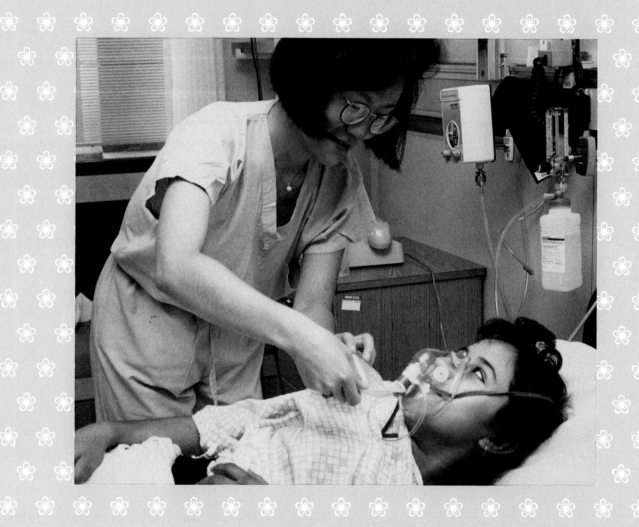

OBJECTIVES

Examine the psychologic factors that may contribute to complications during labor and birth.

Discuss dysfunctional labor patterns.

Relate various types of fetal malposition and malpresentation to possible associated problems.

Describe pathophysiology and subsequent nursing care for clients experiencing abruptio placentae, placenta previa, and associated bleeding problems.

Explain the nursing care that is indicated in the event of fetal distress.

Discuss intrauterine fetal death including etiology, diagnosis, management, and the nurse's role in assisting the family.

Distinguish variations that may occur in the umbilical cord and insertion into the placenta.

Relate the implications of pelvic contractures to the labor and birth process and outcome.

Discuss complications of the third and fourth stages.

Summarize the effects of childbirth complications on the family.

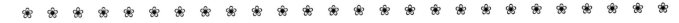

. . . She was smooth-skinned, as if very finely made. I was riveted by the look of peace on her face. And profoundly confused by the umbilical cord knotted so tightly about her neck. . . . It was the absence of life. . . . Usually I felt as if I was helping give life, but here I was unneeded; death had managed for itself. . . . I wrapped the baby in old soft flannel. I covered her and carried her to her parents. (A Midwife's Story)

The successful completion of the 40-week gestational period requires the harmonious functioning of all the components associated with the pregnancy: the fetus, placenta, and amniotic fluid; the maternal pelvis, which includes not only the bony structure but also the vagina and perineal tissues; the contractions and the woman's voluntary pushing effort; and the woman's emotional state and intellectual processes, which are influenced by her feelings about the pregnancy and motherhood. Disruptions in any of these areas may affect the others and cause **dystocia** (abnormal or difficult labor and birth).

❀ *USING THE NURSING PROCESS WITH* ❀

Families at Risk During Childbirth

As with all other conditions that present during childbirth, the nursing process with its component parts forms a basis for the provision of nursing care to the woman and her family when the labor and birth are at risk.

Nursing Assessment

The nurse collects information regarding the woman's history and correlates it with known information regarding predisposing factors. The history helps the nurse identify pertinent assessments that need to be made.

Nursing Diagnosis

The nurse looks for cues that may suggest the woman is at risk for problems during the intrapartal period. Sometimes subtle clues may be the only indication of a developing problem. The nurse operates on her or his knowledge of normal labor and birth and thus is able to identify problems quickly.

The nurse organizes the data and assessment information into nursing diagnoses that are appropriate for a woman and family at risk during childbirth. Nursing diagnoses that may apply include the following:

- Knowledge deficit related to the possible implications and problems associated with intrapartal problems
- Injury to the fetus: High risk related to decreased blood supply, secondary to cord compression, problems during labor, or birth trauma
- Ineffective individual (or family) coping: High risk related to unanticipated problems in labor and/or birth
- Fear related to unknown outcome of the labor and birth

Additional nursing diagnoses are presented in the Key Nursing Diagnoses to Consider: During Complications of Childbirth p 726.

Nursing Plan and Implementation

After nursing diagnoses are identified, the nurse plans nursing interventions to prevent or treat designated client problems. The nurse uses basic nursing skills and special

Dx
Key Nursing Diagnoses to Consider During Complications of Childbirth

Adjustment impaired

Anxiety

Aspiration: High risk

Body temperature, altered: High risk

Breathing pattern, ineffective

Cardiac output, decreased

Coping, individual, ineffective

Decisional conflict

Family coping, compromised

Family processes, altered

Fatigue

Fear

Fluid volume deficit (actual loss)

Gas exchange, impaired

Grieving, anticipatory

Hopelessness

Hyperthermia

Infection: High risk

Injury: High risk

Knowledge deficit

Pain

Parenting, altered

Powerlessness

Role performance, altered

Self-care deficit, bathing/hygiene

Sleep pattern disturbance

Tissue integrity, impaired

Tissue perfusion, altered

Urinary retention, acute

intrapartal interventions to provide nursing care to the family at risk during childbirth.

Evaluation

Evaluation of the woman's response to care and the effectiveness of the nursing interventions is an ongoing process. As a result of evaluation, the nurse may redesign the plan of care or add other nursing interventions.

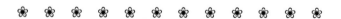

Care of the Woman at Risk Due to Excessive Anxiety and Fear

Stress, anxiety, and fear have a profound effect on labor, particularly when complications occur that imply maternal or fetal jeopardy. A labor process that was initially viewed with confidence and happiness may provoke anxiety and a variety of physiologic and psychologic responses once labor has begun.

Neural and endocrine changes are produced by stress and anxiety. The liver releases glucose to satisfy the body's increased energy needs. The bronchial tree dilates for increased oxygen intake. The anterior pituitary is stimulated, which results in an increase in production of glucocorticoids and mineralocorticoids by the adrenal cortex. These hormones promote the retention of sodium and the excretion of potassium and also stimulate the posterior pituitary to release antidiuretic hormone for the conservation of water. The loss of potassium is believed to assist in the reduction of myometrial activity. The reduction of glucose stores from stress and anxiety decreases the availability of glucose used by a contracting uterus.

The sympathetic nervous system stimulates the adrenal medulla to secrete epinephrine, which increases heart rate, cardiac output, and blood pressure. The sympathetic nervous system also stimulates the adrenals to release norepinephrine, which increases peripheral vasoconstriction and blood flow to the vital organs. This physiologic reaction can adversely affect the contracting uterus. The uterus responds to alpha-excitatory and beta-inhibitory effects of epinephrine. Through baroreceptor stimulation, epinephrine inhibits myometrial activity (beta-receptors), uterine contractility decreases, and labor is prolonged (Lederman 1984).

The anxiety, fear, and pain experienced by the laboring woman may produce a vicious cycle, resulting in increased fear and anxiety because of continued central pain perception. This leads to enhanced catecholamine release, which in turn increases physical distress and may result in myometrial dysfunction and ineffectual labor (Lederman et al 1985) (Figure 25–1).

❀ *APPLYING THE NURSING PROCESS* ❀

Nursing Assessment

Unless birth is imminent or severe complications exist, the nurse begins the assessment by reviewing the woman's background. Factors such as age, parity, marital and socioeconomic status, culture, and knowledge and understanding of the labor process contribute to the woman's psychologic response to labor.

As labor progresses, the nurse is alert for the woman's verbal and nonverbal behavioral responses to the pain and anxiety coexisting with labor. The woman who is agitated and noncompliant, or too quiet and compliant, may require further appraisal for anxiety. Verbal statements such as "Is everything okay?" "I'm really nervous," or "What's going on?" usually indicate some degree of anxiety and concern. Other women may be irritable, require frequent explanations, or repeat the same questions. The nurse further observes for nonverbal cues including a tense posture, clenched hands, or pain out of context to the stage of labor. Recognizing the impact of fatigue on pain and anxiety is another important nursing observation.

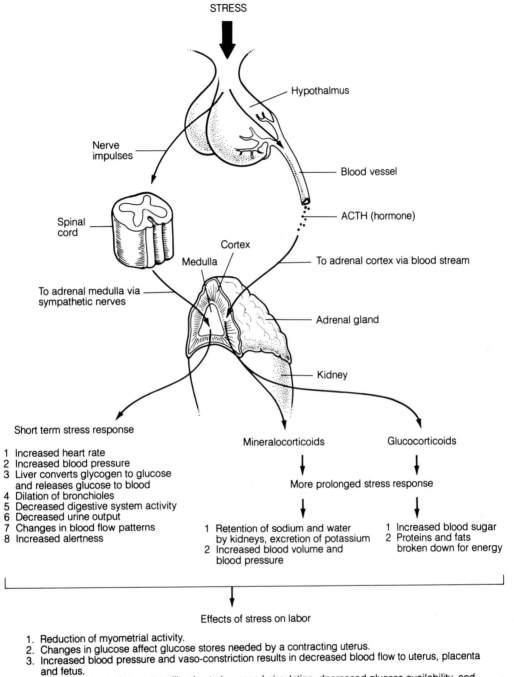

STRESS

Hypothalmus

Nerve impulses

Blood vessel

ACTH (hormone)

Spinal cord

Cortex

Medulla

To adrenal cortex via blood stream

To adrenal medulla via sympathetic nerves

Adrenal gland

Kidney

Short term stress response

1 Increased heart rate
2 Increased blood pressure
3 Liver converts glycogen to glucose and releases glucose to blood
4 Dilation of bronchioles
5 Decreased digestive system activity
6 Decreased urine output
7 Changes in blood flow patterns
8 Increased alertness

Mineralocorticoids

Glucocorticoids

More prolonged stress response

1 Retention of sodium and water by kidneys, excretion of potassium
2 Increased blood volume and blood pressure

1 Increased blood sugar
2 Proteins and fats broken down for energy

Effects of stress on labor

1. Reduction of myometrial activity.
2. Changes in glucose affect glucose stores needed by a contracting uterus.
3. Increased blood pressure and vaso-constriction results in decreased blood flow to uterus, placenta and fetus.
4. Decreases in uterine contractility due to increased circulation, decreased glucose availability, and inhibition of myometrial activity caused by increased amounts of epinephrine.

STRESS

Figure 25–1   Effects of stress on labor. Adapted from Campbell Biology, *2nd ed. Redwood City, CA, Benjamin/ Cummings, 1990.*

Nursing Diagnosis

Nursing diagnoses that may apply to the woman with excessive fear or anxiety include the following:

- Anxiety related to stress of the labor process
- Fear related to unknown outcome of labor
- Ineffective individual coping related to inability to use relaxation techniques during labor

Nursing Plan and Implementation

Anticipatory Education During the Prenatal Period

Prenatal classes provide relevant information about the developmental and psychologic changes that can be expected during childbirth and teach relaxation strategies to reduce the anxiety and pain of labor. Couples learn coping mechanisms in the form of physical and emotional comfort measures, controlled breathing exercises, and relaxation techniques.

Nursing research demonstrates that education is effective in minimizing the stress accompanying labor. Research findings indicate that women who participate in prenatal classes benefit by maintaining more positive attitudes, experiencing feelings of anticipation rather than fear, and developing a heightened awareness that fosters early maternal infant attachment (Lindell 1988). Requiring further study is the relationship between education and the physiologic effectiveness of labor, specifically in terms of the length of labor, the use of ataractics (sedation) and analgesics, and the impact of the labor upon the newborn (Lindell 1988).

Provision of Support During Labor and Birth

Couples who have had prenatal education should be offered support and encouragement by the nurse as they employ the techniques they have learned. If the woman begins to lose control, the nurse can often assist the partner in helping the woman regain control. If anxiety is evident, the nurse should acknowledge and alleviate it, if possible, through comfort measures (see Chapter 23).

Unprepared couples can be taught many of these activities at the time of admission, especially if active labor has not begun. Clear but succinct information about the labor process, medical procedures, the environment, simple breathing exercises, and relaxation techniques can be given, thereby preventing or relieving some apprehension and fear. Even a woman in active labor who has had no prior preparation can achieve a great deal of relaxation from physical comfort measures, touch, constant attention, therapeutic interaction, and, possibly, analgesics.

The nurse's ability to help the woman and her partner cope with the stress of labor is directly related to the rapport established among them. By employing a calm, caring, confident, nonjudgmental approach, the nurse not only is able to acknowledge the anxiety, but also is often able to

identify the source of the distress. Once the causative factors are known, the appropriate interventions, such as information, comfort measures, touch, or therapeutic communication, can be implemented.

Provision of Support During the Postpartal Period

If possible, the nurse should follow up with the mother after the labor and birth to review the intrapartal process. Further explanations and reassurance may be offered as the woman's needs dictate. This is also an opportune time for the woman to share feelings about the labor.

Evaluation

Anticipated outcomes of nursing care include the following:

- The woman experiences a decrease in physiologic signs of stress and an increase in psychologic comfort.
- The woman is able to use effective coping mechanisms to manage her anxiety in labor.
- The woman's and the family's fear is decreased.
- The woman is able to verbalize feelings regarding her labor.

Care of the Woman Experiencing Dysfunctional Labor

The myometrial forces of the contracting uterus depend on one or more contracting muscles stimulating the contraction of one or more adjacent muscles. The resulting wave of contractions then spreads for variable distances over the myometrium. The contractility of the uterus is affected by the following factors: (a) the energy source; (b) the ionic exchange of electrolytes; (c) the contractile proteins; and (d) the endocrine sources (Scott et al 1990). See page 583 for further discussion. These four factors must interact for effective labor to occur. Any disruption in the interaction of these factors may result in ineffective, dysfunctional labor.

Dysfunctional labor includes hypertonic and hypotonic labor patterns, prolonged labor, and precipitous labor. In hypertonic labor patterns, ineffectual contractions of poor quality occur in the latent phase of labor. In hypotonic labor patterns, early labor is well established with effective contractions, but the active phase of labor becomes prolonged or halts. Either type of dysfunctional labor may result in prolonged labor, which has potentially serious implications for the woman and fetus.

Hypertonic Labor Patterns

In **hypertonic** patterns, the resting tone of the myometrium rises more than 15 mm Hg and may rise as much

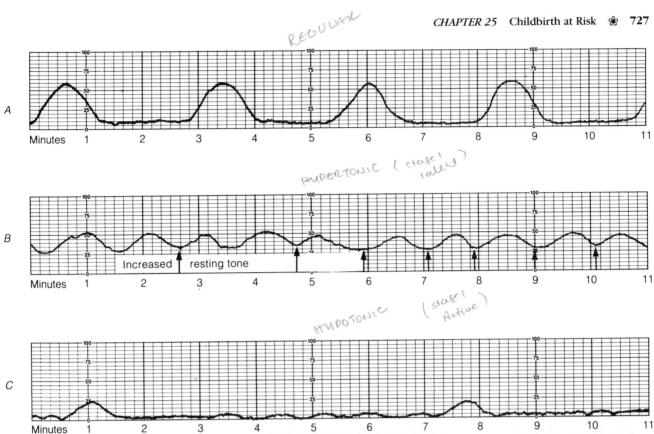

REGULAR

HYPERTONIC (stage 1 latent)

Increased ↑ resting tone

HYPOTONIC   (stage 1 Active)

Figure 25–2   Comparison of labor patterns. A Normal uterine contraction pattern. Note contraction frequency is every 3 minutes, duration is 60 seconds. The baseline resting tone is below 10 mm Hg. B Hypertonic uterine pattern. Note in this example that the contraction frequency is every minute, duration is 50 seconds (which allows only a 10-second rest between contractions), intensity increases approximately 25 mm Hg during the contraction, and the resting tone of the uterus is increased. C Hypotonic uterine contraction pattern. Note in this example that the contraction frequency is every 7 minutes with some uterine activity between contractions, duration is 50 seconds, and intensity increases approximately 25 mm Hg during contractions.

as 50 to 85 mm Hg. The frequency of contractions is usually increased, whereas the intensity may be decreased (Figure 25–2B). The hypertonic pattern usually occurs prior to the cervix reaching a dilatation of 4 cm or more.

Contractions are painful but ineffective in dilating and effacing the cervix, which may lead to a prolonged latent phase. Very anxious nulliparas at term or postterm are most commonly afflicted with hypertonic labor.

Maternal Risks

Hypertonic labor patterns are extremely painful because of uterine muscle cell anoxia. There is an increase in uterine muscle tone but little cervical dilatation and effacement. Because hypertonic labor often occurs in the latent phase of the first stage of labor, when dilatation may be no more than 2 or 3 cm, the woman may be accused of overreacting to her labor. She may be aware of the lack of progress and become anxious and discouraged. A woman who has prepared for her labor and birth may feel frustrated as her coping mechanisms are severely tested.

Fetal-Neonatal Risks

Fetal distress occurs early, because contractions interfere with the uteroplacental exchange. If this distress goes unidentified, the fetus may not survive. In any situation in which pressure on the fetal head is prolonged, cephalhematoma, caput succedaneum, or excessive molding may occur (Figure 25–3).

Medical Therapy

As long as the membranes are intact and there are no indications of fetal distress, the goal of treatment is to arrest uterine activity and establish a more effective labor pattern. This is accomplished by promoting relaxation and reducing pain. Bed rest and sedation are common medical treatments. Oxytocin is not administered to a woman suffering from hypertonic uterine activity, because it is likely to accentuate the abnormal labor pattern (Cunningham et al 1989). If the hypertonic pattern continues and develops into a prolonged latent phase, the physician may use an oxytocin infusion and/or amniotomy as treatment meth-

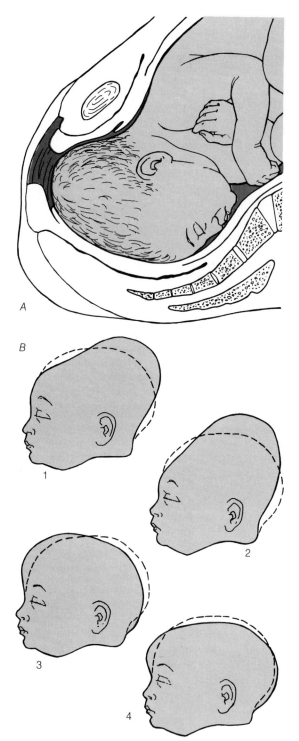

Figure 25–3   Effects of labor on fetal head. A Caput succedaneum formation. The presenting portion of the scalp is encircled by the cervix during labor, which causes swelling of the soft tissue. B Molding of fetal head in cephalic presentations: 1 occiput anterior, 2 occiput posterior, 3 brow, 4 face.

ods. These methods are instituted only after cephalopelvic disproportion (CPD) and fetal malpresentations have been ruled out. If signs of fetal distress become apparent, cesarean birth may be necessary.

❧   *APPLYING THE NURSING PROCESS*   ❧

Nursing Assessment

The relationship between the intensity of pain being experienced and the degree to which the cervix is dilating and effacing should be evaluated as a part of the labor assessment. Whether anxiety is having a deleterious effect on labor progress should also be noted, especially if the woman is a primigravida or is postterm. Evidence of increasing frustration and discouragement on the part of the woman and her partner may become apparent as labor ensues and their birth plan cannot be followed.

Nursing Diagnosis

Nursing diagnoses that may apply to the woman in hypertonic labor include the following:

- Pain related to woman's inability to relax secondary to hypertonic uterine contractions
- Ineffective individual coping: High risk related to ineffectiveness of breathing techniques to relieve discomfort
- Anxiety related to slow labor progress
- Knowledge deficit related to lack of understanding regarding dysfunctional labor patterns

Nursing Plan and Implementation

Provision of Comfort and Support to the Laboring Woman and Her Partner

The woman experiencing a hypertonic labor pattern will probably be very uncomfortable because of the increased force of contractions. Her anxiety level and that of her partner may be high. The nurse attempts to reduce the woman's discomfort and promote a more effective labor pattern by directly acknowledging her anxiety and explaining what will be done for her.

The nurse may wish to suggest ambulation or a change of position for the woman; lateral position may correct the hypertonic pattern. Comfort measures include mouth care, effleurage, back rub, and change of linens. If sedation is ordered, the nurse ensures that the environment is conducive to relaxation. The labor coach may also need assistance in helping the woman cope. A calm understanding approach by the nurse offers the woman and her partner further support. Provision of information about the cause of the hypertonic labor pattern and assurances that the woman is not overreacting to the situation are also important nursing actions.

Promotion of Maternal-Fetal Physical Well-Being

Fluid balance must be maintained through adequate hydration. Urine ketones should be monitored hourly. The couple should be informed of labor progress.

Nursing measures in the event of fetal-neonatal distress are given in the Nursing Care Plan on page 730.

Client Education

The laboring woman needs to have information about the dysfunctional labor pattern and the possible implications for herself and her baby. Information will help relieve anxiety and thereby increase relaxation and comfort. The nurse needs to explain treatment methods and offer opportunities for questions.

Evaluation

Anticipated outcomes of nursing care include following:

- The woman experiences a more effective labor pattern.
- The woman has increased comfort and decreased anxiety.
- The woman and her partner understand the hypertonic labor pattern.

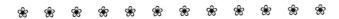

Hypotonic Labor Patterns

In **hypotonic** *dysfunctional labor,* uterine activity in early labor has been within normal limits, but then a hypotonic pattern consisting of infrequent uterine contractions of mild to moderate intensity and a marked slowing or arrest of cervical dilatation and fetal descent occurs. In this pattern the myometrial resting tone is below 8 mm Hg. Fewer than two to three contractions occur in a ten-minute period (see Figure 25–2C). The hypotonic pattern usually occurs after at least 4 cm of cervical dilatation. Hypotonic labor may occur when uterine fibers are overstretched from twins, large singletons, hydramnios, and grandmultiparity. Hypotonic uterine motility also occurs when sedation such as meperidine (Demerol) is given in the latent phase of labor or in the presence of various degrees of CPD. It may also occur with pelvic contraction and fetal malposition. Clinically, hypotonic uterine motility may occur in the latent or active phase, but it is most often seen in the active phase. It is painless and responds to oxytocin if conditions permit its use.

Maternal Risks

If labor is prolonged, intrauterine infection may result, along with maternal exhaustion and psychologic stress. Any woman experiencing a dysfunctional labor pattern is a candidate for postpartal hemorrhage, but the woman with

hypotonic labor is especially threatened. If the hypotonic pattern persists, the uterus may be less likely to contract efficiently after the birth, which can lead to postpartal hemorrhage.

Fetal-Neonatal Risks

Fetal and neonatal distress often accompany the intrauterine infection resulting from a prolonged hypotonic labor (Cunningham et al 1989). Antimicrobial therapy prescribed for the mother during labor appears to have little if any effect on preventing neonatal infection. Fetal tachycardia is observed on the electronic monitor or auscultated by the nurse. The newborn born to a mother with prolonged labor because of uterine hypotonia should be observed closely in the nursery for signs of sepsis.

Medical Therapy

Improving the quality of the uterine contractions while ensuring a safe outcome for the woman and her baby are the goals of therapy.

Prior to initiating treatment for hypotonic labor, the nurse-midwife or physician validates the adequacy of pelvic measurements and completes tests to establish gestational age if there is any question about fetal maturity. After CPD, fetal malpresentation, and fetal immaturity have been ruled out, oxytocin (Pitocin) may be given intravenously via an infusion pump to improve the quality of uterine contractions. Intravenous fluid is useful to maintain adequate hydration and prevent maternal exhaustion. Amniotomy may be done prior to beginning the oxytocin infusion or later in the labor process.

An improvement in the quality of uterine contractions is demonstrated by noticeable progress in the labor process. If the labor pattern does not become effective, or if other complications develop, further interventions, including cesarean birth, may be necessary.

❀ *APPLYING THE NURSING PROCESS* ❀

Nursing Assessment

Assessing contractions (for frequency and intensity), maternal vital signs, and FHR provides the nurse with data to evaluate maternal-fetal status. The nurse is also alert for signs and symptoms of infection and dehydration. Because of the stress associated with a prolonged labor, observing the woman and her partner's degree of success with their coping mechanisms is also important.

Nursing Diagnosis

Possible nursing diagnoses include the following:

- Pain related to inability to cope with uterine contractions secondary to dysfunctional labor
- Knowledge deficit related to lack of information regarding dysfunctional labor

(*Text continues on p 732*)

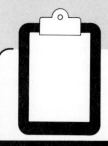

Nursing Care Plan
Fetal Distress

Nursing History

Assess client for presence of predisposing factors:

1. Preexisting maternal diseases
2. Maternal hypotension, bleeding
3. Placental abnormalities

Physical Examination

Asphyxia is suggested when one or more of the following are present:

1. FHR decelerations, decreased variability, tachycardia followed by bradycardia
2. Presence of meconium in amniotic fluid
3. Fetal scalp blood pH determination ≤7.20

Diagnostic Studies

Maternal hemoglobin and hematocrit
Urinalysis

Nursing Diagnosis	Nursing Interventions	Rationale	Evaluation
Nursing Diagnosis: Decreased cardiac output in fetus related to decreased uteroplacental perfusion secondary to maternal hypotension, circulating blood volume, and vasoconstriction associated with PIH	Observe and record the signs of fetal asphyxia:	Fetal asphyxia implies hypoxia (reduction in P_{O_2}), hypercapnia (elevation of P_{CO_2}), and acidosis (lowering of blood pH). Anaerobic glycolysis (breakdown of glycogen) takes place in the presence of hypoxia, and the end product of this process is lactic acid, resulting in metabolic acidosis.	FHR baseline remains in 120–140 range, short-term variability present, average long-term variability, no late or variable decelerations.
Client Goal: The FHR will remain in the range of 120–160 with short-term variability present, average long-term variability, accelerations with fetal movement, and no late or variable decelerations.	1. Presence of meconium in amniotic fluid	Fetal hypoxic episode leads to increased intestinal peristalsis and anal sphincter relaxation resulting in meconium release.	
	2. Decreased variability	Variability of FHR depends on intact sympathetic and parasympathetic nervous systems. When variability decreases, it indicates the fetus is no longer able to react or compensate for changes in the uterine environment.	
	3. Late decelerations in FHR	Vagal stimulation elicited through hypoxic brain tissues causes bradycardia.	
	4. Fetal hyperactivity	Fetus may initially become hyperactive in an attempt to increase circulation.	

(continued)

Nursing Care Plan (continued)

Nursing Diagnosis	Nursing Interventions	Rationale	Evaluation
	Initiate following interventions: 1. Administer O_2 to the woman with tight face mask at 6–10 L/min, per physician order. 2. Change maternal position (lateral, left side preferred).	Administration of O_2 may increase amount of oxygen available for transport to fetus. Tight face mask is used because laboring woman tends to breathe through her mouth. Changed maternal position may relieve compression of the maternal vena cava and the cord, thereby facilitating O_2 exchange.	
	Institute emergency measures for prolapse of cord: 1. Manually exert pressure on the presenting part; this must be done continuously; woman may be maintained in supine position, Trendelenburg position, knee-chest position, or on her side with a pillow to elevate her hips. 2. If occult prolapse is suspected, change maternal position to side-lying position. 3. Notify physician/nurse-midwife immediately.		
Nursing Diagnosis: Fear related to knowledge of fetal distress *Client Goal:* The woman will have opportunity to ask questions and will verbalize whether she receives support.	Inform woman of fetal status. Explain treatment plan. Provide accurate information.	Anxiety is decreased when factual information is provided.	The woman verbalizes understanding of current problem and has no further questions.

Nursing Plan and Implementation

Promotion of Maternal-Fetal Physical Well-Being

Nursing measures include frequent monitoring of contractions, maternal vital signs, and FHR. If meconium is present in the amniotic fluid, observing fetal status closely becomes more critical, and in most instances an internal scalp electrode is placed in order to obtain more accurate data. Maintaining an intake and output record provides a way of determining maternal hydration or dehydration. The woman should be encouraged to void every two hours, and her bladder should be checked for distention. If the bladder is distended and the woman cannot void, catherization will be necessary. Because her labor may be prolonged, the woman must continue to be monitored for signs of infection (elevated temperature, chills, changes in characteristics of amniotic fluid). Vaginal examinations should be kept to a minimum but in this case they are done more often to be sure of dilatory progress, especially when it is suspected that cesarean birth will be necessary. The nursing implications of oxytocin infusion are presented in the Drug Guide–Oxytocin on page 796.

Provision of Psychologic Support

The nurse assists the woman and her partner to cope with the frustration of a lengthy labor process. A warm, caring approach coupled with techniques to reduce anxiety are very important strategies for the nurse to employ.

Providing Client Education

The teaching plan needs to include information regarding the dysfunctional labor process and implications for the woman and baby. Disadvantages and alternatives of treatment also need to be discussed and understood by the woman and her partner.

Evaluation

Anticipated outcomes of nursing care include the following:

- The woman can verbalize the type of labor pattern that is occurring and the treatment plan.
- The risk of infection to the woman and fetus has been reduced.
- The woman maintains comfort during labor.
- The father's role of protector and helper is respected and maintained, and he is included in all planning.

❀　❀　❀　❀　❀　❀　❀　❀　❀　❀　❀

Prolonged Labor

Labor lasting more than 24 hours is termed **prolonged labor.** In these cases usually the first stage is extended and

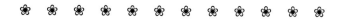

the active and/or latent phase is prolonged. The cervix fails to dilate within a reasonable period of time. Early recognition and treatment are imperative to prevent maternal-fetal complications.

According to Oxorn (1986), the incidence of prolonged labor varies from 1% to 7% and is most common in the nullipara. The principal causes are CPD, malpresentations, malpositions, labor dysfunction, and cervical dystocia. Other influencing factors are excessive use of analgesics, anesthetics, and sedatives in the latent phase of labor; premature rupture of the membranes in the presence of an uneffaced, closed cervix; and reduced pain tolerance associated with high anxiety.

Maternal Risks

Prolonged labor usually has a deleterious effect on the woman. Intense but unproductive pain from labor contractions in the latent phase or a prolonged active phase is likely to result in maternal exhaustion and moderate to severe stress. The woman also becomes a prime candidate for infection and hemorrhage (Combs et al 1991) from uterine atony, uterine rupture, or lacerations of the birth canal. An already stressful situation may be compounded by the necessity to deliver the fetus by forceps or cesarean birth.

Fetal-Neonatal Risks

Fetal distress may occur early or late in labor depending on which phase of labor is prolonged. Uteroplacental perfusion may be impeded by the length of the labor, resulting in fetal asphyxia. Premature rupture of the membranes (PROM) increases the risk of infection for both fetus and neonate. Prolapse of the cord may occur after rupture of the membranes if the presenting part fails to descend and engage. Continuing pressure on the head or a birth by forceps may cause soft tissue edema and bruising, and in some instances, cerebral trauma (see Figure 25–3).

Medical Therapy

Management of prolonged labor begins with identification of any causal and complicating factors. Depending on these factors, the goal of treatment may be to stimulate labor through the administration of oxytocin or by performing an amniotomy.

Hydration is maintained with intravenous fluids, and anxiety is minimized with rest and sedation. In the event of serious maternal-fetal distress, birth is likely to be by forceps or cesarean birth. Further discussion of the management of patterns that may be precursors of prolonged labor is found on page 729.

❀　*APPLYING THE NURSING PROCESS*　❀

Nursing Assessment

Monitoring maternal-fetal status is a primary nursing responsibility. The FHR patterns are assessed for signs of distress, including subtle tachycardia followed by bradycardia, late decelerations, and decreasing variability. Amniotic fluid is observed for meconium staining and signs of infection. The nurse evaluates labor progress by considering the pattern of the contractions, the degree of cervical dilatation and effacement, and descent. Ongoing assessment of maternal hydration occurs throughout labor. If the woman is receiving oxytocin (Pitocin) augmentation, the nurse watches maternal-fetal response to the treatment closely.

Nursing Diagnosis

Possible nursing diagnoses for the woman with prolonged labor include the following:

- Pain related to prolonged time in labor
- Ineffective individual (and family) coping: High risk related to ineffectiveness of breathing techniques to relieve discomfort and anxiety
- Infection: High risk related to increased need for invasive assessments secondary to extended time in labor

Nursing Plan and Implementation

Promotion of Maternal-Fetal Physical Well-Being The nurse uses labor progress as an indicator of maternal-fetal status. If the fetus is in a vertex presentation, the nurse may evaluate the amount of pressure on the fetal head by the presence or absence of a caput succedaneum and/or molding. Calculating fluid intake and output and checking urine for presence of ketones provide the nurse with information about the maternal hydration state. If the woman is receiving oxytocin therapy, the nurse should implement appropriate nursing measures to ensure the safety of the woman and fetus. For further information on the administration of oxytocin, refer to Chapter 26 and Drug Guide–Oxytocin, p 796.

Provision of Psychologic Support Following childbirth the mother should be closely monitored for signs and symptoms of hemorrhage, shock, and infection. The newborn should be observed for signs of sepsis, cerebral trauma, and the appearance of cephalhematoma. Nursing actions for fetal distress are given on page 730.

Assisting the woman and her partner to deal with the anxiety and frustration of a prolonged labor is another important nursing responsibility. Support and encouragement become critical to assist the woman and her partner in coping with the numerous potential and actual problems associated with prolonged labor. The nurse offers information as appropriate. Comfort measures such as a change in position, oral hygiene, skin care, and cool washcloths on the forehead may help the woman relax. Encouraging the involvement of her partner and/or support persons in care of the woman may further reduce anxiety.

Evaluation

Anticipated outcomes of nursing care include following:

- The woman and her partner are able to cope with the prolonged labor.
- The risk of infection to the woman and fetus has been reduced.
- The woman maintains comfort during the labor.

✿ ✿ ✿ ✿ ✿ ✿ ✿ ✿ ✿ ✿ ✿ ✿

Precipitous Labor

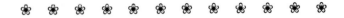

Precipitous labor is extremely rapid labor that lasts for less than three hours. The most common causes are abnormally low resistance in maternal tissues, which allows for rapid cervical dilatation and fetal descent; exceptionally strong uterine contractions; and in rare circumstances a lack of pain sensations associated with unusually strong contractions (Cunningham et al 1989).

Other contributing factors in precipitous labor are multiparity, large pelvis, previous precipitous labor, and a small fetus in a favorable position. Precipitous labor may also be caused by oxytocin overdose, which can occur during induction of labor. In this case, precipitous labor results from medical error.

Precipitous labor and precipitous birth are not the same. A precipitous birth is an unexpected, sudden, and often unattended birth. See page 688 for discussion of precipitous birth.

Maternal Risks
If the cervix is effaced and the maternal soft tissues are not resistant to stretching, maternal complications may be few. However, if the cervix is not ripe (soft) and the maternal soft tissues are resistant, lacerations of the cervix, vagina, perineum, and periurethral area may occur because the tissues do not stretch adequately. There is also a possibility of uterine rupture. When resistance is present, amniotic fluid embolism may occur (see page 774). The woman is also at risk for postpartal hemorrhage due to expanded uterine fibers and may lose control because of the rapidity of the labor process.

Fetal-Neonatal Risks
Rapid labor and birth causes increased pressures on and in the fetal head and may cause cerebral trauma to the newborn. If the birth is unattended and unassisted, the newborn may suffer from lack of care in the first few minutes of life.

Medical Therapy
Any woman with a history of precipitous labor requires close medical monitoring and preparation for an emer-

gency birth to facilitate a safe outcome for the mother and fetus. Drugs such as magnesium sulfate or tocolytic agents (ritodrine or terbutaline) may be used to slow the uterine contractions (Cunningham et al 1989). (See Drug Guide–Magnesium Sulfate and Ritodrine in Chapter 19.)

❀ *APPLYING THE NURSING PROCESS* ❀

Nursing Assessment

Assessments of the woman with precipitous labor will reveal a contraction pattern that is accelerated beyond the normal labor pattern. As this more rapid pattern is identified, the need for more frequent assessments will be apparent. Frequent assessment of the fetal response to the rapid labor is important.

Nursing Diagnoses

Possible nursing diagnosis for the woman with precipitous labor include the following:

- Pain related to rapid labor
- Ineffective individual coping: High risk related to rapid labor pattern and precipitous birth

Nursing Plan and Implementation

Monitoring Labor Progress

If the woman is at risk for precipitous labor, the nurse is particularly attentive to the progress of labor and ensures that an emergency birth pack is close at hand. The physician should be informed of a labor pattern that has rapid cervical dilatation. The nurse should be in constant attendance if at all possible.

To avoid hyperstimulation of the uterus and possible precipitous labor during oxytocin administration, the nurse should be alert to the danger of oxytocin overdosage (see Drug Guide–Oxytocin on page 796). If the woman receiving oxytocin develops an accelerated labor pattern, the oxytocin should be discontinued immediately, and the woman should be turned on her left side to improve uterine perfusion. Oxygen may be started to increase the available oxygen in the maternal circulation; this increases the amount available for exchange at the placental site.

Promotion of Psychologic Well-Being

Comfort and rest may be promoted by assisting the woman to a comfortable position, providing a quiet environment, and administering sedatives as needed. Information and support are given before and after the birth.

Assistance During Labor

An imminent birth may be slowed by having the woman pant or blow with each contraction. It is also helpful for the nurse to breathe with the woman during this time to help the woman pace her breathing. If birth is imminent, the nurse can assist with the birth (Chapter 23). The nurse should never attempt to stop a birth by holding the woman's legs together. This may cause trauma to the newborn's head and separation of the placenta.

Evaluation

Anticipated outcomes of nursing care include following:

- The woman and her baby are closely monitored during labor and a safe birth occurs.
- The woman feels support and enhanced comfort during labor and the birth.

❀ ❀ ❀ ❀ ❀ ❀ ❀ ❀ ❀ ❀ ❀ ❀

Care of the Woman with Postdate Pregnancy

Postdate pregnancy has become recognized as an important problem that affects approximately 3% to 12% of pregnancies (Spellacy 1990). **Postdate** pregnancy is one that extends past 42 weeks of gestation (or exceeds 294 days past the first day of the last menstrual period). While many pregnancies extend beyond the anticipated date of birth (EDB), the true postdate pregnancy is associated with increased perinatal morbidity and mortality.

Maternal Risks

Although postdate pregnancy does not pose any significant risk to the woman during the pregnancy, the labor and birth process may be affected. In many instances labor is induced and frequently the woman's cervix is unripe (cervix is firm, posterior, with minimal effacement and dilatation) which leads to a longer labor. There is an increased incidence of operative birth (use of forceps and need for episiotomy due to macrosomia) and cesarean birth (Cucco et al 1989).

Fetal-Neonatal Risks

True postdate pregnancies are frequently associated with placental changes that cause a decrease in the uterine–placental–fetal circulation. This decrease reduces the blood supply, oxygen, and nutrition for the fetus. Oligohydramnios (decreased amount of amniotic fluid) is frequently present and may increase the risk of umbilical cord compression (because the cord does not have as much fluid to float in). Macrosomia (fetal weight in excess of 4000 g) occurs 3 to 7 times more frequently than in term infants and is more likely to be associated with birth trauma or shoulder dystocia (difficulty or inability to deliver the baby's shoulders) (Rodriguez 1989). During labor, the postdate fetus has a very high incidence of FHR baseline changes such as tachycardia, saltatory changes (marked variability) and variable decelerations (due to cord compression), meconium staining of the amniotic fluid, and neonatal depression at birth (Cucco et al 1989). Perinatal mortality has been reported in some studies as two to three times that of term infants (Sims & Walther 1989).

Medical Therapy

Medical therapy begins in early pregnancy with accurate dating. It is difficult to establish the date of pregnancy accurately when it is far advanced.

Antenatal testing that may be used in postdate pregnancy includes weekly or twice weekly nonstress tests (NST), fetal acoustic stimulation test (FAST), fetal biophysical profile (FBPP), ultrasound examinations, maternal assessment of fetal movement, and in some instances contraction stress tests (CST) (Eden 1989; Gilson et al 1988). (See Chapter 20 for discussion of these tests.)

✤ *APPLYING THE NURSING PROCESS* ✤

Nursing Assessment

When the woman is admitted into the birthing area, it is important to establish the EDB and ascertain the type of antenatal testing that has been completed. During labor, ongoing assessments of the FHR by continuous electronic fetal monitoring are important to identify reassuring characteristics (presence of short-term and long-term variability, accelerations with fetal movement) and to determine the presence of variable decelerations so that corrective actions may be taken. When amniotic membranes rupture, the nurse assesses the fluid for the presence of meconium. Ongoing assessments of labor progress (contractions, progressive cervical dilatation and effacement, and fetal descent) may provide clues to the presence of a macrosomic fetus, as labor may be lengthened.

Nursing Diagnosis

Possible nursing diagnoses for the woman with postdate pregnancy include the following:

- Knowledge deficit related to lack of information regarding postdate pregnancy
- Fear related to the unknown outcome for the baby
- Alteration in individual (or family) coping: High risk related to concern regarding the status of the baby

Nursing Plan and Implementation

Promotion of Fetal Well-Being
The woman may be taught to assess fetal activity each day to become more familiar with fetal movement and to detect any decrease in movement. (See Chapter 20 for further discussion of fetal movement records.)

While in the birth setting, the fetal heart rate is monitored by continuous electronic monitoring. The FHR tracing is evaluated frequently for signs of distress.

Promotion of Maternal Psychologic Support
Women with pregnancies that extend past the due date frequently report that they would like more support from nursing personnel. In one study (Campbell 1986), women reported that they felt increased stress and anxiety and had more difficulty coping. Encouragement, support, and recognition of the woman's anxiety were all identified as helpful strategies by health personnel.

Providing Client Education
The woman needs to have information regarding the postdate pregnancy and the antenatal testing that will be done. The implications and associated risks for the baby need to be addressed as well as possible treatment plans. The woman and her partner need opportunities to ask questions and clarify information.

Evaluation

Anticipated outcomes of nursing care include the following:

- The woman's knowledge regarding the postdate pregnancy is improved.
- The woman and her partner/family feel supported and able to cope with the postdate pregnancy.
- Fetal status is maintained, abnormalities, if any, are quickly identified, and supportive measures are initiated.

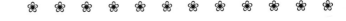

Care of the Woman with a Ruptured Uterus

A **ruptured uterus** involves the tearing of previously intact uterine muscle or of an old uterine scar. Rupture during pregnancy is usually in the upper segment of the uterus. If it occurs during labor, the rupture usually occurs in the lower segment. The incidence of uterine rupture is about 1 in 1230 to 6673 births (Phelan 1990).

Uterine rupture is classified as complete or incomplete. The complete rupture extends through the three muscle layers of the uterus and there is direct communication between the uterine and abdominal cavity (Oxorn 1986). Incomplete rupture involves the whole myometrium, while the peritoneum that overlies the uterus remains intact (Oxorn 1986). A uterine rupture is also classified as spontaneous, which occurs during labor, or traumatic, which is associated with a manipulation or procedure—such as an external version—that puts stress on the uterus. The rupture can be caused by one or more of the following:

- A weakened cesarean scar, usually from a classic incision into the uterus (see Chapter 26)
- Obstetric trauma that may occur with a version or a difficult forceps-assisted birth
- Mismanagement of oxytocin induction or augmentation
- Obstructed labor (as with CPD)
- Trauma or a blow to the uterus
- Vaginal birth after previous cesarean birth

Maternal Risks

Maternal mortality ranges from 3% to 40% (Oxorn 1986). The main causes of death are shock and blood loss. If the rupture is recognized and treatment can be instituted, a hysterectomy is usually done.

Fetal-Neonatal Risks

When the blood supply to the uterus is interrupted, about 80% of fetuses demonstrate fetal distress such as FHR decelerations, developing bradycardia, and loss of variability (Rodriguez et al 1989). In a spontaneous rupture, the fetus may be forced through the rupture into the abdominal cavity, where it quickly dies (Oxorn 1986). Overall, the fetal mortality rate ranges from 3%, in labors that include the use of external EFM or an intrauterine pressure catheter, to 38% in labors with no uterine monitor (Rodriguez et al 1989).

Medical Therapy

Treatment needs to be prompt and appropriate for the woman's condition. Medical management of shock, cardiovascular support and immediate surgery for a laparotomy or hysterectomy is usually needed.

Nursing Care

The nurse should be alert for warning signs of an impending rupture such as fetal distress, abdominal pain, and hemorrhage.

The nurse may be the one to identify the warning signs of impending rupture or maternal hemorrhage if rupture has occurred. In acute rupture, the nurse quickly mobilizes the staff for emergency surgery. The nurse continues to assess the maternal-fetal status and initiates treatments to stabilize the woman during the hemorrhage.

When the physiologic needs of the woman and the fetus are met, the nurse can focus on the emotional needs of the family. The family must have a clear understanding of the procedure and its implications for future childbearing. If fetal death has occurred, the mother and father should also be given an opportunity to grieve and to see their infant if they desire.

Care of the Woman and Fetus at Risk Due to Fetal Malposition

Occiput-Posterior Position

Persistent occiput-posterior position of the fetus is probably one of the most common complications encountered in obstetrics. Although this position may be normal in some races because of a genetically small transverse diameter of the midpelvis, it is considered a malposition because of the maternal and fetal difficulties that may result. It should be remembered that the fetus generally rotates to conform with the orientation of maternal pelvis. For a fetus in an occiput-posterior position to rotate to an occiput-anterior position, it must rotate 135 degrees (ROP to ROT to ROA to OA), and in most cases this rotation is accomplished. In others, however, it is not. Labor progress may cease or the fetus may be born in a posterior position.

Maternal Fetal-Neonatal Risks

The woman may suffer a third- or fourth-degree perineal laceration or extension of a midline episiotomy during the second stage of labor. There is no increased risk of fetal mortality due to the occiput-posterior position unless labor is protracted or an operative birth is performed.

Medical Therapy

Medical treatment focuses on close monitoring of the maternal and fetal status and labor progress to determine whether vaginal or cesarean birth is the safer method. According to Cunningham, MacDonald, and Gant (1989), vaginal birth is possible as follows:

1. Await spontaneous birth
2. Forceps assisted birth with the occiput directly posterior

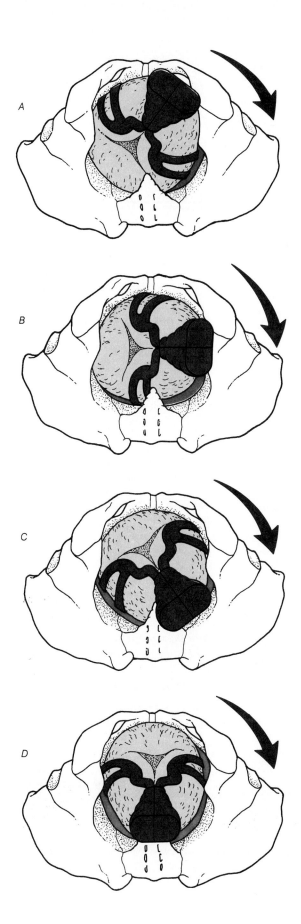

3. Forceps rotation of the occiput to the anterior position and birth (Scanzoni's maneuver; see Figure 25–4).

4. Manual rotation to the anterior position followed by forceps-assisted birth (Figure 25–5).

If the pelvis is roomy and the perineum is relaxed, as found in grandmultiparity, the fetus may have no particular problem emerging spontaneously in the occiput-posterior position. If, however, the perineum is rigid, the second stage of labor may be prolonged. A prolonged second stage is one that lasts over an hour in multiparas and two hours or more in nulliparas. One complication of the fetus emerging in the occiput-posterior position is the possibility of a third- or fourth-degree perineal laceration or extension of a midline episiotomy.

In the event of a prolonged second stage with arrest of descent due to occiput-posterior position, a midforceps or manual rotation may be done if no CPD is present. In cases of CPD, cesarean birth is the preferred treatment.

❀ *APPLYING THE NURSING PROCESS* ❀

Nursing Assessment

The first sign of occiput-posterior position is intense back pain in the first stage labor. The back pain is caused by the fetal occiput compressing the sacral nerves. Other signs and symptoms may include a dysfunctional labor pattern, a prolonged active phase, secondary arrest of dilatation, or arrest of descent. Further assessment may reveal a depression in the maternal abdomen above the symphysis (because the fetal face, rather than the back of its head, is turned up against the symphysis). Fetal heart tones may be heard far laterally on the maternal abdomen, and on vaginal examination the nurse will find the wide diamond-shaped anterior fontanelle in the anterior portion of the pelvis. This fontanelle may be difficult to feel because of molding of the fetal head.

Nursing Diagnosis

Nursing diagnoses that may apply to women with persistent occiput posterior include the following:

Figure 25–4 Scanzoni maneuver; anterior rotation. A Forceps are applied to the fetal head, which is in ROP position. B Fetal head is rotated 45° to ROT. C Fetal head is rotated another 45° to ROA. D Fetal head is rotated another 45° to OA. The fetal position has changed from ROP to ROT to ROA to OA for a rotation of 135°. The forceps are now upside-down, so they are removed and reapplied to provide the traction necessary for a forceps-assisted birth. (From Oxorn H: Human Labor and Birth, 5th ed. Norwalk CT: Appleton & Lange, 1986, p 401)

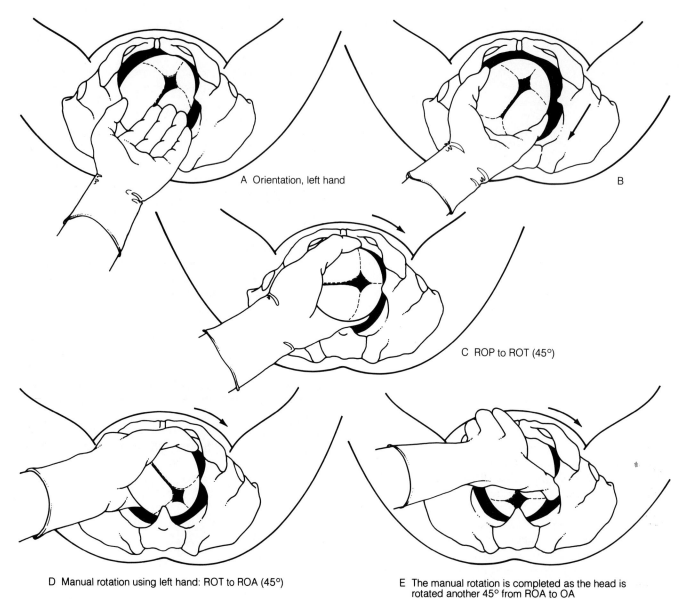

A Orientation, left hand

B

C ROP to ROT (45°)

D Manual rotation using left hand: ROT to ROA (45°)

E The manual rotation is completed as the head is rotated another 45° from ROA to OA

Figure 25–5 Manual rotation of ROP to OA. A The physician's left hand is inserted into the vagina. B The back of the fetal head is grasped. C The head is flexed and then rotated 45 degrees to ROT. D the head is rotated another 45 degrees to ROA. E The manual rotation is completed as the head is rotated another 45 degrees from ROA to OA. During the manual rotation, the physician's other hand is placed on the maternal abdomen and the body is turned in the same direction by applying pressure to the fetal breech or shoulders.

- Pain related to unexpected back discomfort secondary to occiput posterior position
- Ineffective individual coping related to unanticipated discomfort and slow progress in labor

Nursing Plan and Implementation

Facilitation of Fetal Position Change

Changing maternal posture has been used for many years to enhance rotation of OP or OT to OA. The woman may be placed on one side and then asked to move to the other side as the fetus begins to rotate. This side-lying position may promote rotation; it also enables the support persons to apply counterpressure on the sacral area to decrease discomfort. A knee-chest position provides a downward slant to the vaginal canal, directing the fetal head downward on descent. Andrews and Andrews (1983) suggest that a hands-and-knees position is often effective in rotating the fetus. In addition to maintaining a hands-and-knees position on the bed, the woman may do pelvic rocking, and the support person may perform firm stroking motions on the abdomen. The stroking begins over the fetal back and swings around to the other side of the abdomen. After the fetus has rotated, the woman lies in a Sims' position on the side opposite the fetal back. In addition to these positions, the woman may want to sit on the toilet, walk around the room, stand beside the bed and lean forward with her hands on the bed and do the pelvic rock, rest in a jacuzzi, or she may want to lie on her side in the bed.

Evaluation

Anticipated outcomes of nursing care include the following:

- The woman's discomfort is decreased.
- The woman and her partner understand comfort measures and position changes that may assist her.
- The woman's coping abilities are strengthened.
- The woman and her partner feel supported and encouraged.

❁ ❁ ❁ ❁ ❁ ❁ ❁ ❁ ❁ ❁ ❁

Transverse Arrest

In women with hypotonic labor or a diminished anteroposterior pelvic diameter (as seen with the platypelloid pelvis) or diminished transverse diameter (in the android pelvis), an incomplete internal rotation may occur, resulting in a transverse arrest. This may also result in arrest of descent and a prolonged second stage of labor. In cases of severe molding and caput formation, the fetal scalp is visible at the vaginal opening even though the biparietal diameters have not entered the inlet. If labor is effective, spontaneous rotation may occur as labor continues.

Maternal Risks

Manipulation during birth can cause maternal soft tissue damage. Any prolonged pressure by the fetal head in one position may cause the woman later gynecologic problems, such as fistulas resulting from tissue anoxia. Postpartal hemorrhage may result from undetected lacerations or atony if the labor was hypotonic.

Fetal-Neonatal Risks

Unless a protraction or arrest disorder is present or an operative birth is performed, fetal mortality is not increased with transverse position, because most fetuses do rotate spontaneously. Cerebral damage may be caused in cases of undetected CPD. The fetus should be closely observed in utero by the nurse, and at the time of birth a pediatrician should be present if a midforceps-assisted birth is anticipated.

Medical Therapy

The choice of medical treatment depends on the degree of fetal rotation. In the presence of a hypotonic labor pattern and no CPD, dilute oxytocin may be administered while closely monitoring the maternal-fetal response (Cunningham et al 1989). When rotation, uterine activity, and CPD are absent, birth is often accomplished by midforceps, manual rotation, or vacuum extraction. If deep transverse arrest exists, forceps may be applied as long as excessive force is avoided. Cesarean birth is preferred, however.

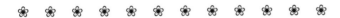

❁ *APPLYING THE NURSING PROCESS* ❁

Nursing Care

After identifying women in whom transverse arrest may occur, the nurse institutes ongoing review of the labor progress. If the labor becomes prolonged or a cesarean birth is necessary, the nurse assesses the coping abilities and knowledge level of the woman and her partner.

The nurse continues efforts to support and comfort the laboring woman. Continuous monitoring of contractions (character and frequency), amount of maternal discomfort, maternal vital signs, and fetal response to labor are important nursing interventions. The nurse notifies the physician/nurse-midwife in case of distress or dysfunctional labor.

The couple is prepared by the nurse for the extreme molding of the infant's head. The nurse remains alert for signs of postpartal hemorrhage.

Care of the Woman and Fetus at Risk Due to Fetal Malpresentation

Three vertex attitudes of the fetus are classified as abnormal presentations: the sinciput (military), brow, and face (Figure 25–6). The fetal body straightens out in these presentations from the classic fetal position to an S-shaped position. The sinciput presentation is probably the least difficult for the woman and fetus. In most cases, as soon as the head reaches the pelvic floor, flexion occurs and a vaginal birth results.

In addition to the vertex malpresentation, the breech, shoulder (transverse lie), and compound presentations can cause significant difficulty during labor. These and the vertex presentations are discussed here.

Brow Presentation

The brow presentation occurs more often in the multipara than in the nullipara and is thought to be due to lax abdom-

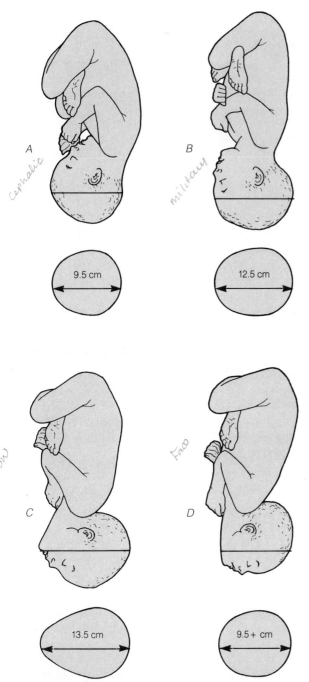

Figure 25–6   Types of cephalic presentation. A The occiput is the presenting part because the head is flexed and the fetal chin is against the chest. The largest AP diameter that presents and passes through the pelvis is approximately 9.5 cm. B Military presentation. The head is neither flexed nor extended. The presenting AP diameter is approximately 12.5 cm. C Brow presentation. The largest diameter of the fetal head (approximately 13.5 cm) presents in this situation. D Face presentation. The AP diameter is 9.5 cm (From Scott JR, DiSaia PJ, Hammond CB et al: Danforth's Obstetrics and Gynecology. *New York: Lippincott/Harper & Row, 1990. Fig 8–9, p 170)*

inal and pelvic musculature. The largest diameter of the fetal head, the occipitomental, presents in this type of presentation. The nullipara whose fetus has a brow presentation commonly has a small infant. Upon descent into the inlet, the brow presentation frequently converts to an occiput position. Some brow presentations convert to face presentations.

Maternal Fetal-Neonatal Risks

Birth should be accomplished by cesarean birth in the presence of CPD or failure of a brow presentation to convert to an occiput or face presentation. With a vaginal birth, perineal lacerations are inevitable and may extend into the rectum or vaginal fornices.

Fetal mortality is increased due to injuries received during the birth and/or infection because of prolonged labor. Trauma during the birth process can include tentorial tears, cerebral and neck compression, and damage to the trachea and larynx.

Medical Therapy

Active medical intervention is not necessary as long as cervical dilatation and fetal descent are occurring. In the presence of labor problems but no CPD, a manual conversion may be attempted. Some medical experts advocate midforceps-assisted birth in the presence of complete dilatation and fetal station at +2. In the presence of failed conversions, CPD, or secondary arrest of labor, cesarean birth is the preferred method of management. Adequate resuscitation equipment and pediatric assistance should be available at the time of birth.

❀   *APPLYING THE NURSING PROCESS*   ❀

Nursing Assessment

Leopold's maneuvers reveal a cephalic prominence on the same side as the fetal back. A brow presentation can be detected on vaginal examination by palpation of the diamond-shaped anterior fontanelle on one side and orbital ridges and root of the nose on the other side (Figure 25–7).

Nursing Diagnosis

Nursing diagnoses that may apply to brow presentation include the following:

- Anxiety/fear related to outcome for fetus
- Knowledge deficit related to the possible maternal-fetal effects of brow presentation
- Injury to the fetus: High risk related to pressure on fetal structures secondary to brow presentation

Nursing Plan and Implementation

Nursing management of abnormal cephalic presentations include close observation of the woman for labor aberra-

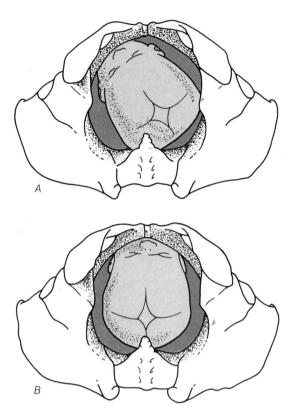

Figure 25–7   Brow presentation. A Descent. B Internal rotation in the pelvic cavity. (From Oxorn H: Human Labor and Birth, *5th ed. Norwalk, CT: Appleton & Lange, 1986, p 211)*

tions and of the fetus for signs of distress. The fetus should be observed closely during labor for signs of hypoxia as evidenced by late decelerations and bradycardia.

The nurse may need to explain the position of the fetus to the laboring couple or to interpret what the physician/nurse-midwife has told them. The nurse should stay close at hand to reassure the couple, inform them of any changes, and assist them with labor-coping techniques.

In face and brow presentation, the appearance of the newborn may be affected. The couple may need help in beginning the attachment process because of the newborn's facial appearance. After the infant is inspected for gross abnormalities, the pediatrician and nurse can assure the couple that the facial edema and excessive molding are only temporary and will subside in three or four days.

Evaluation

Anticipated outcomes of nursing care include the following:

- The woman and her partner understand the implications and associated problems of brow presentation.
- The mother and her baby have a safe labor and birth.

❋ · ❋ · ❋ · ❋ · ❋ · ❋ · ❋ · ❋ · ❋ · ❋ · ❋ · ❋ · ❋

Face Presentation

Face presentation of the fetus occurs most frequently in multiparas, in preterm birth, and in the presence of anencephaly. The head is hyperextended, and the chin is the presenting part.

Maternal/Fetal-Neonatal Risks

The risks of CPD and prolonged labor are increased with face presentation. As with any prolonged labor, the chance of infection is increased.

The fetus may develop caput succedaneum of the face during labor, and after birth the edema gives the newborn a grotesque appearance. As with the brow presentation, the neck and internal structures may swell due to the trauma received during descent. Petechiae and ecchymoses are often seen in the superficial layers of the facial skin because of the birth trauma.

Medical Therapy

If no CPD is present, the chin (mentum) is anterior, and the labor pattern is effective, the objective of medical treatment is a vaginal birth (Figure 25–8). Mentum posteriors can become wedged on the anterior surface of the sacrum (Figure 25–9). In this case as well as in the presence of CPD, cesarean birth is the preferred method of management.

❋   *APPLYING THE NURSING PROCESS*   ❋

Nursing Assessment

When performing Leopold's maneuvers, the nurse finds that the back of the fetus is difficult to outline, and a deep furrow can be palpated between the hard occiput and the fetal back (Figure 25–10). Fetal heart tones can be heard on the side where the fetal feet are palpated. It may be difficult to determine by vaginal examination whether a breech or face is presenting, especially if facial edema is already present. During the vaginal examination, palpation of the saddle of the nose and the gums should be attempted. When assessing engagement, the nurse needs to remember that the face has to be deep within the pelvis before the biparietal diameters have entered the inlet.

Nursing Diagnosis

Nursing diagnoses that may apply to the woman with a fetus in face presentation include the following:

- Fear related to unknown outcome of the labor and appearance of the baby
- Injury to the newborn's face: High risk related to edema secondary to the birth process

Nursing Plan and Implementation

Nursing interventions are the same as for the brow presentation.

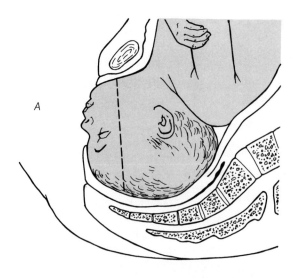

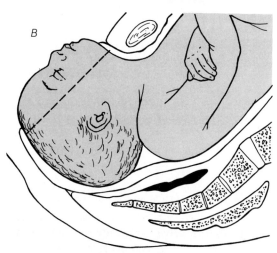

Figure 25–8   *Mechanism of birth in face (mentoanterior position). A The submentobregmatic diameter at the outlet. B The fetal head is born by movement of flexion.*

Evaluation

Anticipated outcomes of nursing care include the following:

- The woman and her partner understand the implications and associated problems of face presentation.
- The mother and her baby have a safe labor and birth.

❀   ❀   ❀   ❀   ❀   ❀   ❀   ❀   ❀   ❀   ❀

Breech Presentations

The incidence of breech presentation varies from 4% of all births to 15% of births of infants weighing less than 2500 g (Figure 25–11). In babies who weigh 1000 to 1499 g the

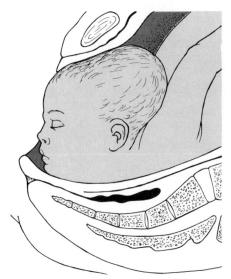

Figure 25–9   *Face presentation. Mechanism of birth in mentoposterior position. Fetal head is unable to extend farther. The face becomes impacted.*

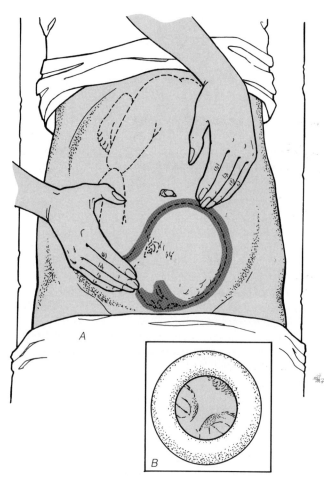

Figure 25–10   *Face presentation. A Palpation of the maternal abdomen with the fetus in RMP. B Vaginal examination may permit palpation of facial features of the fetus.*

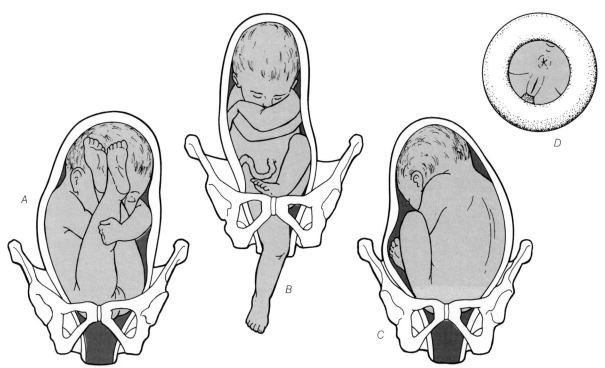

Figure 25–11   Breech presentation. A Frank breech. B Incomplete (footling) breech. C Complete breech in LSA position. D On vaginal examination, the nurse may feel the anal sphincter. The tissue of the fetal buttocks feels soft.

incidence of breech presentation is 30%, and in babies under 1000 g the incidence is 40%. Breech presentation has a fourfold increase in perinatal mortality when compared to term cephalic presentation and a two- to threefold increase in preterm infants. In addition to increased mortality, breech infants have an increased incidence of congenital anomalies (17% in preterm infants and 9% in term infants) (Cruikshank 1990). The incidence of hydrocephalus is 10 times greater than among infants in cephalic presentation. Breech presentation is also more frequently associated with placenta previa, hydramnios, multiple gestation, and grandmultiparity (Cruikshank 1990).

Maternal Risks

Breech presentation may prolong labor because the breech does not exert as much pressure on the cervix as the fetal head. Prolonged labor increases the mother's risk of infection.

Prior to the mid-1970s more than 90% of breeches were born vaginally. Since then, approximately 90% of breeches have been born by cesarean birth (Cruikshank 1990).

Fetal-Neonatal Risks

The fetus is at increased risk for prolapsed cord once the membranes rupture because there is more space around the body as it rests against the cervix.

The most critical problem with a breech presenta-tion during a vaginal birth is that the largest part of the infant (the head) emerges last. In the presence of unrecognized cephalopelvic disproportion, the fetal head may not fit through the maternal pelvis (head entrapment), and the baby may die before any other action can be taken.

The increased incidence of perinatal mortality is associated with trauma to the head regardless of vaginal or cesarean birth, malformation, infection, maternal disease, and asphyxia (Cruikshank 1990).

Medical Therapy

For the mother, a vaginal birth has less risk than a cesarean. Therefore, an increasing number of physicians are performing external version to convert a breech to cephalic presentation so that vaginal birth is possible. If a version is not done or is unsuccessful, birth will most likely be by cesarean. The childbearing woman needs to know the implications of breech presentation and understand the rationale behind the method of childbirth chosen.

To minimize infant mortality and morbidity, medical management includes searching for any evidence of any actual or potential complications that justify cesarean birth. Cunningham et al (1989) list the following criteria for vaginal birth: (1) The pelvis is determined to be adequate when examined by x-ray pelvimetry, (2) the fetus presents as a frank breech with a fetal weight less than 3500 g as estimated by a sonogram or two or more experienced clinicians, (3) the woman is in spontaneous labor as demonstrated by progressive dilatation and effacement of the cervix and fetal descent, and (4) a clinician skilled in breech birth and infant resuscitation is in attendance.

❀ *APPLYING THE NURSING PROCESS* ❀

Nursing Assessment

Frequently it is the nurse who first recognizes a breech presentation. On palpation the hard vertex is felt in the fundus and ballottement of the head can be done independently of the fetal body. The wider sacrum is palpated in the lower part of the abdomen. If the sacrum has not descended, on ballottement the entire fetal body will move. Furthermore, FHTs are usually auscultated above the umbilicus. Passage of meconium from compression of the infant's intestinal tract on descent is common.

CRITICAL THINKING

Try to visualize what your hands would feel if you did Leopold's maneuvers. Compare this to a transverse lie.

The nurse is particularly alert for a prolapsed umbilical cord, especially in incomplete breeches, because space is available between the cervix and presenting part through which the cord can slip. If the infant is small and the membranes rupture, the danger is even greater. This is one reason why any woman admitted to the birthing area with a history of ruptured membranes should not be ambulated until a full assessment, including vaginal examination, is performed.

Nursing Diagnosis

Nursing diagnoses that may apply to breech presentation include the following:

- Impaired gas exchange in the fetus: High risk related to interruption in umbilical blood flow secondary to compression of the cord
- Knowledge deficit related to the implications and associated complications of breech presentation on the mother and fetus

Nursing Plan and Implementation

Promotion of Maternal-Fetal Well-Being

During labor it is important for the nurse to continue to make frequent assessments to evaluate fetal and maternal status. The nurse needs to be aware of the associated problems and look for subtle clues of beginning problems. The nurse provides teaching and information regarding the breech presentation and the nursing care needed.

Assistance During Vaginal Birth

Although many infants in breech presentations are born by cesarean, a few are born vaginally. The nurse should include Piper forceps as a part of the birth table setup. During the birth process, the nurse may have to assist in the support of the infant's body if the physician elects to use forceps. The circulating nurse should monitor the FHR closely during the birth.

If the family and physician elect a cesarean birth, the nurse intervenes as with any cesarean procedure.

Evaluation

Anticipated outcomes of nursing care include the following:

- The woman and her partner understand the implications and associated problems with breech presentation.
- The mother and baby have a safe labor and birth.
- Major complications are recognized early and corrective measures are instituted.

❀ ❀ ❀ ❀ ❀ ❀ ❀ ❀ ❀ ❀ ❀ ❀

Shoulder Presentation (Transverse Lie)

A transverse lie occurs in approximately 1 of every 300 births (Cruikshank 1990). The infant's long axis lies across the woman's abdomen, and on inspection the contour of the maternal abdomen appears widest from side to side (Figure 25–12).

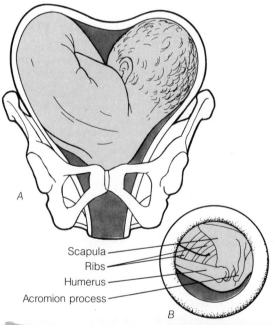

Scapula
Ribs
Humerus
Acromion process

Figure 25–12 A Transverse lie (shoulder presentation). B On vaginal examination the nurse may feel the acromion process as the fetal presenting part.

Maternal conditions associated with a transverse lie are grandmultiparity with lax uterine musculature (the most common cause), obstructions such as bony dystocia, placenta previa, neoplasms, and fetal anomalies; hydramnios; and preterm labor. It is not uncommon in multiple gestations for one or more of the fetuses to be in a transverse lie.

Maternal Risks

Labor can be dysfunctional in the presence of a transverse lie. Uterine rupture can occur. As in any case of prolonged labor, the woman is more prone to infection.

Fetal-Neonatal Risks

One danger of transverse lie is a prolapsed umbilical cord, because there is nothing in the pelvic inlet to serve as a blocking agent. Prolapse of a fetal arm may also occur. If the woman is allowed to labor in the presence of a transverse lie, the fetus may die from asphyxia and trauma.

Medical Therapy

With a viable fetus at term in the transverse lie, the medical goal is cesarean birth. External version for vaginal birth may be attempted if the following criteria are met:

- There is no indication for rapid termination of labor.
- The fetus is highly movable.
- Contractions are not strong and frequent.
- There is no cephalopelvic disproportion.
- The membranes are intact.
- There is an adequate amount of amniotic fluid.
- Placenta previa has been ruled out.

When the required criteria are met, attempts at external version are appropriate prior to the onset of labor or in early labor. (See discussion in Chapter 26.)

❀ *APPLYING THE NURSING PROCESS* ❀

Nursing Assessment

The nurse can identify a transverse lie by inspection and palpation of the abdomen, by auscultation of FHTs in the midline of the abdomen (not conclusive), and by vaginal examination.

On palpation no fetal part is felt in the fundal portion of the uterus or above the symphysis. The head may be palpated on one side and the breech on the other. Fetal heart tones are usually auscultated just below the midline of the umbilicus. On vaginal examination, if a presenting part is palpated, it is the ridged thorax or possibly an arm that is compressed against the chest.

Nursing Diagnosis

Nursing diagnoses that may apply when transverse lie is present include the following:

- Knowledge deficit related to possible implications and problems associated with transverse lie
- Impaired gas exchange in the fetus: High risk related to decrease in blood flow secondary to cord compression associated with prolapsed cord
- Individual/family coping, compromised: High risk related to unknown outcome
- Fear related to unknown outcome of birth

Nursing Plan and Implementation

The primary nursing actions are to assist in the interpretation of the fetal presentation and to provide information and support to the couple. The nurse assesses maternal and fetal status frequently and prepares the woman for an operative birth. The nurse explains to the parents the need for cesarean and the assessments and care surrounding a cesarean. (See Chapter 26 for further information regarding teaching with cesarean birth.)

Evaluations

Anticipated outcomes of nursing care include the following:

- The transverse lie is recognized promptly and crucial assessments are completed.
- The mother and baby have a safe birth.
- The couple understands the implications and associated problems of transverse lie.

❀ ❀ ❀ ❀ ❀ ❀ ❀ ❀ ❀ ❀ ❀ ❀

Compound Presentation

A **compound presentation** is one in which there are two presenting parts. It can occur when the pelvic inlet is not totally occluded by the primary presenting part. If the prolapsed part is a hand, the birth is generally not difficult. Sometimes the hand slips back and occasionally it is born alongside the head; however, this may increase the chance of laceration. If the prolapsed part is left alone, the birth is generally not difficult. Cesarean birth is indicated in the presence of uterine dysfunction or fetal distress (Cunningham et al 1989).

Care of the Woman and Fetus at Risk Due to Developmental Abnormalities

Macrosomia

Fetal macrosomia occurs when a neonate weighs more than 4000 g (8 lb, 14 oz) at birth. The incidence of macrosomia is 43% in insulin-dependent diabetic women and 11.4% in the general population (Berk et al 1989). Overall the incidence of babies weighing over 4500 g (9 lb, 15 oz) is 1% in all births (Tamura & Sabbagha 1990).

Maternal Risks

The pelvis that is adequate for an average-sized fetus may be disproportionately small for an oversized fetus. Distention of the uterus causes overstretching of the myometrial fibers, which may lead to dysfunctional labor and an increased incidence of postpartal hemorrhage. If the oversized fetus acts as an obstruction, the chance of uterine rupture during labor increases. During vaginal birth there is an increased risk of perineal lacerations.

Fetal-Neonatal Risks

Fetal prognosis is guarded. If a macrosomic fetus is unsuspected and labor is allowed to continue in the presence of disproportion, the fetus can receive cerebral trauma from intermittent forceful contact with the maternal bony pelvis. During difficult operative procedures performed at the time of vaginal birth, the fetus may become asphyxiated or experience neurologic damage from pressure exerted on its head.

    Shoulder dystocia, defined as difficulty in the birth of the shoulders, or impaction of the shoulders (Mashburn 1988), may occur in 0.15%% to 2.0% of all births (Gonik et al 1989). If the fetus weighs more than 4500 g, the incidence of shoulder dystocia may be as high as 35.7% (Mashburn 1988). Asphyxia is the most immediate danger to the baby and if birth is not accomplished within a few minutes after the birth of the head, the baby will die (Mashburn 1988). As many as one-third of babies with shoulder dystocia have an Apgar score of 5 or less at one minute (Smeltzer 1986). If correct management of the shoulder dystocia is not accomplished correctly, there may be permanent injury to the baby. Brachial plexus injury (due to improper or excessive traction applied to the fetal head) and fractured clavicles occur in about 20% of shoulder dystocias (Mashburn 1988; Oxorn 1986).

Medical Therapy

The occurrence of the maternal and fetal problems associated with macrosomic infants may be somewhat lessened by identifying macrosomia prior to the onset of labor. If a large fetus is suspected, the maternal pelvis should be evaluated carefully. An estimation of fetal size can be made by palpating the crown–rump length of the fetus in utero, but the greatest errors in estimation occur on both ends of the spectrum—the macrosomic fetus and the very small fetus. Fundal height can give some clue. Ultrasound or x-ray pelvimetry may give further information about fetal size. Whenever the uterus appears excessively large, hydramnios, an oversized fetus, or a multiple pregnancy must be considered.

    Labor may proceed within normal limits or there may be a slowing of fetal descent (change of station) and a prolonged second stage (Gross et al 1987). Even though these problems are present, it is still not possible to anticipate shoulder dystocia that results in trauma to the newborn. If difficulty extracting the shoulders occurs during the birth, the obstetrician/nurse-midwife may direct the woman to sharply flex her thighs up against her abdomen (McRoberts maneuver). This position is thought to change the maternal pelvic angle and therefore reduce the force needed to extract the shoulders and decrease the incidence of brachial plexus stretching and clavicular fracture (Gonik et al 1989). In addition, the physician/nurse-midwife may incorporate other interventions such as checking the placement of the shoulder, enlarging the episiotomy, asking the labor and birth nurse to apply suprapubic pressure, and using the Woods Screw maneuver (consists of rotating the anterior shoulder 180 degrees to the posterior position) (Figure 25–13).

❁ *APPLYING THE NURSING PROCESS* ❁

Nursing Assessment

The nurse assists in identifying factors associated with macrosomic infants, which include: multiparity, maternal obesity, excessive weight gain during this pregnancy, small or borderline pelvis, maternal diabetes, history of a large infant or previous shoulder dystocia, and pregnancy that extends to 42 weeks or beyond (Mashburn 1988). During the intrapartum period, the risk factors include slow descent of the fetus and prolonged second stage. Because women with these risk factors are prime candidates for dystocia and its complications, the nurse frequently assesses the FHR for indications of fetal distress and evaluates the rate of cervical dilatation and fetal descent.

Nursing Diagnosis

Nursing diagnoses that may apply to the woman with a macrosomic fetus include the following:

- Injury to the fetus: High risk related to trauma during the birth process
- Infection: High risk related to traumatized tissue secondary to maternal tissue damage during birth
- Knowledge deficit related to the implications and possible problems associated with birth of a macrosomic baby

Nursing Plan and Implementation

Promotion of Maternal-Fetal Physical Well-Being

The fetal monitor is applied for continuous fetal evaluation. Early decelerations could mean disproportion at the bony inlet of the maternal pelvis. Any sign of labor dysfunction or fetal distress should be reported to the physican/nurse-midwife.

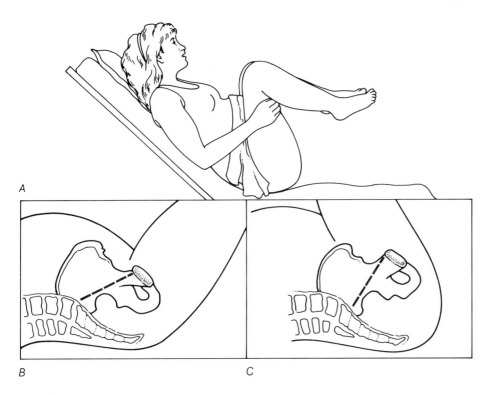

Figure 25–13   McRoberts maneuver. A The woman flexes her thighs up onto her abdomen. B The angle of the maternal pelvis prior to McRoberts maneuver. C The angle of the pelvis with McRoberts maneuver.

After the birth, the nurse inspects the baby for cephalhematoma, Erb palsy (caused by overstretching of the brachial plexus and damage to C5, C6, C7), and fractured clavicles (exhibited by non-movement of one arm) and informs the nursery of any problems. If the nursery staff is aware of a difficult birth, the newborn will be observed more closely for cerebral and neurologic damage.

Postpartally, the nurse checks the uterus for potential atony and the maternal vital signs for deviations suggesting shock.

Providing Emotional Support

The nurse provides support for the laboring woman and her partner and information regarding the implications and possible associated problems. During the birth, the nurse continues to provide support and encouragement to the couple.

Evaluation

Anticipated outcomes of nursing care include the following:

- The woman and her partner understand the implications and some of the possible associated problems.
- The mother and baby have a safe labor and birth.

✤   ✤   ✤   ✤   ✤   ✤   ✤   ✤   ✤   ✤   ✤   ✤

Hydrocephalus

In hydrocephalus, 500 to 1500 mL of cerebrospinal fluid accumulates in the ventricles of the brain. The rate of occurrence, 1 in 2000 fetuses, represents about 12% of the severe malformations found at birth (Cunningham et al 1989). When this condition exists before birth, severe CPD results because of the enlarged cranium of the fetus.

Maternal Risks

Obstruction of labor can occur, and if the uterus is allowed to continue contracting without medical interference, uterine rupture can result.

Fetal-Neonatal Risks

Outlook for the fetus is poor. Frequently, other congenital malformations accompany this condition, such as spina bifida and myelomeningocele. The neonate may be severely brain damaged and often succumbs during birth or afterward in the nursery because of malformations and the presence of infection.

Medical Therapy

Medical intervention is directed toward effecting birth of the fetus by the least traumatic means. It is important to know the degree of hydrocephalus and whether other anomalies or abnormalities are present that would make it very unlikely that the baby could live after the birth. When potentially fatal anomalies are present, the decision regarding the method of birth needs to be discussed between the physician and the parents. A cesarean birth may give the newborn the best chance, but if the predicted chance of survival is very small, or if the fetus is already dead, a cesarean birth unnecessarily increases the risk to the mother. The decisions regarding method of birth are not easy; they are best made by the physician and parents together.

❀ *APPLYING THE NURSING PROCESS* ❀

Nursing Assessment

The nurse performing abdominal palpation discovers the presence of a hard mass just above the symphysis; this is the unengaged head. If the presentation is breech, it is difficult on external palpation to distinguish between the breech and an enlarged head. An ultrasound is indicated in the presence of breech presentations to evaluate the cranium and the size of the maternal pelvis. Vaginal examination with a vertex presentation reveals wide suture lines and a globular cranium.

Additional nursing assessments focus on the information needs of the woman and her partner. It is also important to assess their emotional state in order to provide support.

Nursing Diagnosis

Nursing diagnoses that may apply include the following:

- Anxiety related to unknown outcome for the baby
- Grief related to knowledge of the baby's anomalies
- Knowledge deficit related to the implications of hydrocephalus

Nursing Plan and Implementation

The nurse helps the couple cope with the crisis and to deal with their grief (see discussion on page 781).

The nurse helps prepare the woman and her partner for ultrasound, assists with diagnostic procedures and interprets the findings if the couple has questions after conversations with the physician. The type of assistance at birth will depend on the method chosen.

Evaluation

Anticipated outcomes of nursing care include the following:

- The parents receive accurate information regarding their child and have their questions answered in a supportive and caring manner.
- The parents have support in beginning the grief process and have resources available in the days ahead.

- The parents are able to participate in the selection of the method of birth.
- The parents have their wishes respected in handling the labor and birth and in decisions regarding their baby.

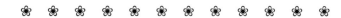

Care of the Woman with a Multiple Pregnancy

Twin Pregnancy

The incidence of twin pregnancy in the United States is 10 per 1000 births (Hollenbach & Hickok 1990). Twins may be either monozygotic or dizygotic. When two fetuses develop from the fertilization of one ovum, the twins are categorized as **monozygotic**. The twins are further classified as diamniotic (two amnions), dichorionic (two chorions), or monochorionic (one chorion), depending on the period in which the division of the ovum occurs (Figure 11–21). Monozygotic twins are identical and thus the same sex (Table 25–1).

Dizygotic twins result from the fertilization of two separate ova. They are diamniotic, dichorionic, and fraternal. They may or may not be the same sex and are not identical.

The incidence of monozygotic twins is largely independent of race, heredity, age, and parity (Hollenbach & Hickok 1990). The incidence of dizygotic twinning is associated with increased maternal age; increased parity; a family history of twins; increased maternal nutrition; increased frequency of coitus, as in the first three months of marriage; and race (black) (Hollenbach & Hickok 1990).

The perinatal morbidity and mortality rates for twins are almost twice that of singleton pregnancies, and the mortality rate for monozygotic twins is three times the rate for fraternal twins. The incidence of preterm birth is 12 times that of single births and only 5% of twins reach 40 weeks of gestation (Hunter 1989).

Maternal Risks

In addition to the normal physiologic changes in pregnancy, the woman with twins has further changes in the cardiovascular system. The blood volume is increased an additional 500 mL. The heart does not enlarge, but cardiac output is increased in the second and third trimesters. The change in cardiac output is accomplished by an increase in heart rate and contractility. These changes probably reduce cardiac reserve so maternal activity and exercise should be tailored to take these physiologic changes into consideration (Veille et al 1986).

Table 25-1 Characteristics of Twin Pregnancy

Type	Time of division	Characteristics	Frequency*	Mortality rate*
Dizygous				
(Double ovum) Fraternal twins	Develop from two ova released at the same time.	Each twin has own placenta, chorion, amnion. Dizygous twins are called fraternal twins. They may be the same or different sex.	75% of all twins are dizygous.	
Monozygous				
(Single ovum) Identical twins Dichorionic-diamniotic twins	Division occurs at blastomere stage, 2 to 3 days past fertilization. Inner cell mass not yet developed.	Each twin has own chorion, amnion, placenta.	30% of monozygous twins	9%
Monochorionic-diamniotic twins	Division occurs at blastocyst stage, 4 to 6 days after fertilization. Inner cell mass divides in two.	Placenta has one chorion and two amnions. Each twin lies in own sac.	68% of monozygous twins	25%
Monochorionic-mono-amniotic twins	Division occurs in primitive germ disc, 7 to 13 days past fertilization.	Twins lie in the same amniotic sac. Increased risk of umbilical cords becoming tangled or knotted.	2% of monozygous twins	>50%

Women with twin gestations have an 83% incidence of antenatal complications as compared to an incidence of 32% in singleton gestations (Kovacs et al 1989). Some of the complications include the following:

- Spontaneous abortions are more common, possibly because of genetic defects or poor placental implantation or development.

- Maternal anemia occurs because the maternal system is nurturing more than one fetus.

- The increased incidence of pregnancy-induced hypertension (PIH) is thought to result from an oversized uterus and increased amounts of placental hormones.

- Third trimester bleeding from placenta previa and abruptio placentae occurs more frequently.

- Hydramnios may be due to increased renal perfusion from cross-vessel anastomosis of monozygotic twins.

Complications during labor include (a) uterine dysfunction due to an overstretched myometrium, (b) abnormal fetal presentations, and (c) preterm labor. With rupture of membranes and hydramnios, abruptio placentae can occur. Danger of placental abruption after the birth of

the first twin also exists because of a decrease in the surface area of the uterus to which the placenta is still attached.

The woman pregnant with twins may experience more physical discomfort during her pregnancy, such as shortness of breath, dyspnea on exertion, backaches, and pedal edema, because of the oversized uterus.

Occasionally multiple pregnancies are not diagnosed until the time of birth; this occurs most often in cases of preterm labor. If the family has physically, psychologically, and financially prepared for one baby, problems can arise when they are suddenly confronted with more than one child. Infants of multiple pregnancies frequently require intensive care, and this may cause financial and emotional stress.

Fetal-Neonatal Risks

Fetal problems in the presence of twin pregnancy are numerous. Congenital anomalies are twice as common (Polin & Frangipane 1986). The fetus is preterm at a rate of five to 10 times that of singletons, and 50% of twins weigh less than 2500 g at birth (Theroux 1989).

Twins with monochorionic placentas may develop artery-to-artery anastomosis, which comprises fetoplacental circulation. One twin is overperfused and is born with polycythemia and hypervolemia and may have hypertension with an enlarged heart. This twin's amniotic sac exhibits hydramnios because of the increased renal perfusion and excessive voiding. The other twin has hypovolemia and exhibits intrauterine growth retardation (IUGR). In the newborn period the neonate with increased perfusion has an increased chance of hyperbilirubinemia as the system tries to rid itself of the extra red blood cells. The other twin is anemic, with all the problems that small-for-gestational-age (SGA) infants exhibit (Danskin & Neilson 1989).

Twins that share the same amniotic sac have some special problems. They have an increased chance of becoming entangled in each other's umbilical cords, and this problem is responsible for a stillborn rate of over 50%. They are also more likely to have developmental problems after birth. Their intelligence quotients are slightly lower than normal until the age of 11, and their physical growth continues to lag behind that of singletons (Theroux 1989).

Conjoined or Siamese twins occur when the division of the embryonic disk is incomplete. The incidence is 1 in 50,000 births and 1 in 400 pairs of monozygotic twins. The stillborn rate is 40% (Sakala 1986).

Medical Therapy

The goals of medical care are the promotion of normal fetal development for both fetuses, preventing the birth of preterm fetuses, and diminishing fetal trauma during labor.

Once the presence of twins has been detected, preventing and treating problems that infringe on the development and birth of normal fetuses is a significant medical activity. Prenatal care is comprehensive. The woman's visits are more frequent than those of the woman with one fetus. The childbearing woman needs to understand nutritional implications, assessment of fetal activity, signs of preterm labor, and danger signs.

Serial ultrasounds are done to assess the growth of each fetus and to provide early recognition of IUGR. A program of restricted activity should begin as early as 20 weeks, and then modified bed rest at home should start at 20 to 24 weeks (Hunter 1989). Some physicians believe that bed rest in the lateral position enhances uterine–placental–fetal blood flow and decreases the risk of preterm labor. Others question the value of bed rest, especially for the prevention of uterine contractions, which seem to precede preterm labor (Hunter 1989).

Testing usually begins at 30 to 34 weeks' gestation and may include NST fetal biophysical profile, and Doppler ultrasound to assess umbilical blood waveforms. A reactive NST is associated with good fetal outcome if birth occurs within one week of the testing. The NST is done every three to seven days until birth or until results become nonreactive (Hunter 1989). The fetal biophysical profile is also accurate in assessing fetal status with twin pregnancies. A biophysical profile of 8 or better for each fetus is considered reassuring, and weekly or biweekly biophysical profiles and NSTs are continued (Hunter 1989).

Intrapartal management and assessment require care-

ful attention to maternal and fetal status. The mother should have an IV in place with a large-bore needle. Anesthesia and cross-matched blood should be readily available. The twins are monitored by dual electonic fetal monitoring. The labor may progress very slowly or very quickly.

The decision regarding method of birth may not be made until labor occurs, and the method depends on a variety of factors. The presence of maternal complications such as placenta previa, abruptio placentae, or severe PIH usually indicate the need for cesarean birth. Fetal factors such as severe IUGR, preterm birth, fetal anomalies, fetal distress, or unfavorable fetal position or presentation also require cesarean birth.

Any combination of presentations and positions can occur with twins (Figure 25–14). Approximately 50% of twins are delivered by cesarean, which is chosen in the hope of reducing complications for the twins, especially birth asphyxia (Jackson 1989).

Vaginal birth is planned when the following factors are present (Polin & Frangipane 1986):

- Gestation is greater than 32 weeks and estimated fetal size is greater than 2000 g each.
- Twin A (the fetus closest to the cervix) is the larger twin.
- Twin A is vertex.
- Twin B is vertex, breech, or transverse and smaller than twin A.
- There is no evidence of fetal distress.
- There is no CPD.

Since most breech presentations are born by cesarean, many physicians choose cesarean birth if either of the twins is breech.

An anesthesiologist should be present during the vaginal birth in case a cesarean needs to be done. One additional obstetrician is usually available to assist in the event that complications occur. The presence of two pediatricians, two nurses to care for the babies, and two labor and delivery nurses is usually recommended.

Since labor is frequently preterm and the labor progress difficult to predict, the mother is usually not given analgesics. An epidural may be used for the last part of labor and birth, or local anesthesia may be given at the time of birth.

The twins are continually monitored by electronic fetal monitoring. After the birth of twin A, twin B is observed by ultrasound to assess position and descent into the pelvis. If twin B is in a transverse lie, the obstetrician converts it to a double footling breech by internal podalic version. The anesthesiologist administers general anesthesia such as halothane to effect good uterine relaxation during this procedure. Some physicians use external version to change the presentation of the second twin (Jackson 1989). If the baby weighs more than 1500 g there does not seem to be increased morbidity (Gocke et al 1989).

In some instances the second twin may need to be born by cesarean. Complications that would require this include profound fetal distress when vaginal birth is not imminent; prolapse of the cord; and contractions of the uterus that trap the second twin (Polin & Frangipane 1986).

Birth in the presence of dysfunctional labor due to overstretched uterine fibers can be managed with cesarean birth or infusion of diluted oxytocin. There is little agreement on the benefits and dangers of the two methods or on the most beneficial type of analgesia and anesthesia to employ for labor and birth. In the presence of an unstable maternal circulatory system, as found with PIH, regional anesthetic agents such as epidurals or caudals can cause hypovolemic shock due to the blocking of the sympathetic nervous system. Large and continuous doses of narcotics can cause neonatal respiratory depression, especially if these infants are premature, as twins frequently are. Cunningham et al (1989) advocate the use of pudendal block paired with the administration of nitrous oxide and oxygen at the time of vaginal birth. Others prefer epidural anesthesia, especially if external version of the second twin is contemplated (Jackson 1989).

The placentas are examined after the birth. If the twins are of the same sex, the placentas are sent to the pathology laboratory for examination to determine whether they are monozygotic or dizygotic twins.

❀   *APPLYING THE NURSING PROCESS*   ❀

Nursing Assessment

When obtaining a maternal history, it is important to identify a family history of twinning. Equally important is a history of medication taken to enhance fertility. These facts should be noted on the antepartal record.

At each antepartal clinic visit, the nurse should measure the fundal height. Any growth, fetal movement, or heart tone auscultation out of proportion to gestational age by dates is indicative of twins. During palpation, many small parts on all sides of the abdomen may be felt (Figure 25–15). If twins are suspected, the nurse should attempt to auscultate two separate heartbeats in different quadrants of the maternal abdomen. Use of the Doppler device may be helpful. Conclusive evidence of twins is found on sonography.

During the prenatal visits, the nurse should determine the family's level of preparation for integrating more than one new member. Although the thought of having twins can be very exciting, the reality of the stress of attaching to two infants and the parental role may be a difficult adjustment (Niefert & Thorpe 1990).

During labor it is important to monitor both twins. An external electronic monitor can be applied to both twins, or if conditions permit, the internal monitor can be applied to twin A and the external monitor to twin B. The heart rates may be auscultated on different quadrants of the maternal abdomen, but continuous monitoring is more beneficial. Signs of distress should be reported to the obstetrician.

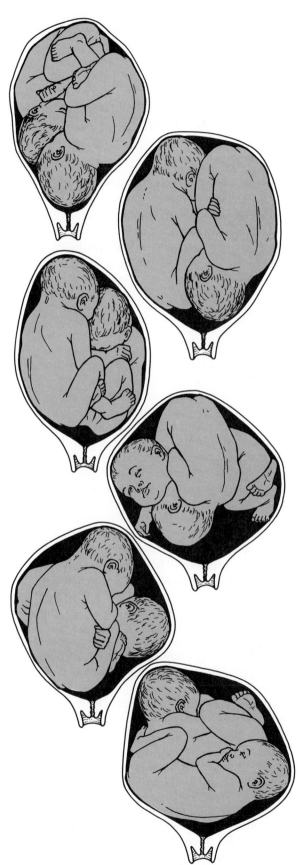

Figure 25–14   Twins may be in any of the above presentations while in utero.

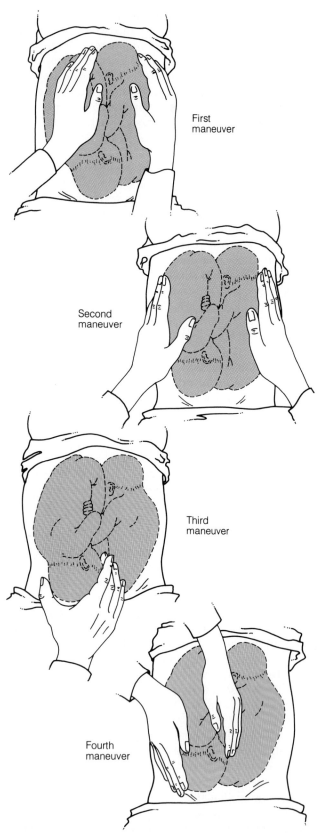

First
maneuver

Second
maneuver

Third
maneuver

Fourth
maneuver

Figure 25–15 Leopold's maneuvers in twin pregnancy. The fetus on the mother's right side is in cephalic presentation and the fetus on the left is in breech presentation.

After a multiple birth, the mother is closely monitored for postpartal hemorrhage.

Nursing Diagnosis

Nursing diagnoses that may apply to a woman with a twin pregnancy include the following:

- Fear related to unknown outcome of the birth process
- Ineffective individual coping related to uncertainty about the labor and birth plan
- Knowledge deficit related to implications and problems associated with twin pregnancy
- Impaired gas exchange in the twins: High risk related to decreased oxygenation secondary to cord compression

Nursing Plan and Implementation

Prenatal Education for Self-Care

Antepartally, the woman may need counseling about diet and daily activities. The nurse can help her plan meals to meet her increased needs. A daily intake of 4000 calories (minimum) and 135 g of protein is recommended for optimal weight gain and fetal growth. A prenatal vitamin and 1 mg of folic acid should also be taken daily. A weight gain of 40 to 60 pounds has been recommended with a 15- to 20-pound weight gain by 20 weeks (Hunter 1989).

Occasionally in multiple pregnancies women exhibit nausea and vomiting past the first trimester. A diet consisting of dry, nongreasy foods may be helpful. Antiemetics may be necessary to provide relief. The woman is more prone to have a feeling of fullness after eating, but this may be alleviated by eating small but frequent meals.

Maternal hypertension is treated with bed rest in the lateral position to increase uterine and kidney perfusion. The nurse can help the woman schedule frequent periods of rest during the day. Family members or friends may be willing to care for the woman's other children periodically to allow her time to get rest. Back discomfort can be alleviated by pelvic rocking, good posture, and good body mechanics.

Teaching regarding prevention and recognition of preterm labor is very important. For further discussion see Chapter 19.

Preparation for Birth

The nurse must prepare to receive two neonates instead of one. This means a duplication of everything, including resuscitation equipment, radiant warmers, and newborn identification papers and bracelets. Two staff members should be available for newborn resuscitation.

If twins are discovered at the time of birth, the nurse must move quickly to prepare for the second newborn. The pediatric team may need to be notified at this time.

While one nurse is monitoring the second twin in utero, the other nurse is caring for the first newborn and preparing to ensure correct identification of the neonates. Special precautions should be observed to ensure correct identification of the neonates. The first born is usually tagged Baby A and the second, Baby B.

Provision of Support to the Family

The nurse determines the woman's or family's need for referral to social welfare agencies, public health clinics, or other community agencies for follow-up care. The family may be unprepared financially and psychologically for the arrival of twins and thus at risk for further difficulties.

Evaluation

Anticipated outcomes of nursing care include the following:

- The woman gains knowledge regarding the implications and problems associated with twin pregnancy.
- The woman feels she is able to cope with the pregnancy and birth.
- The woman understands the treatment plan and how to gain further information.
- The mother and her babies have a safe prenatal course, labor, and birth and a safe postpartal/newborn course.

❈ ❈ ❈ ❈ ❈ ❈ ❈ ❈ ❈ ❈ ❈ ❈ ❈

Three or More Fetuses

When three or more fetuses are present, maternal and fetal problems are increased. The more fetuses conceived, the smaller they tend to be at the time of birth. Birth of three or more fetuses is best accomplished by cesarean because of the risk of fetal insult due to decreased placental perfusion and hemorrhage from the separating placenta during the intrapartal period (Cunningham et al 1989). Complicated obstetric maneuvers such as breech extraction and podalic version, the risk of prolapse of the cord, and an increase in fetal collision provide additional reasons for cesarean birth.

Care of the Woman and Fetus in the Presence of Fetal Distress

When the oxygen supply is insufficient to meet the physiologic demands of the fetus, fetal distress results. The condition may be acute, or chronic, or a combination of both. A variety of factors may contribute to fetal distress. The most common are related to cord compression and uteroplacental insufficiency associated with placental abnormalities and preexisting maternal or fetal disease. If the resultant hypoxia persists and metabolic acidosis follows, the situation is potentially life threatening to the fetus.

The most common initial signs of fetal distress are meconium-stained amniotic fluid (in a vertex presentation) and changes in the FHR The presence of ominous FHR patterns, such as late or severe variable decelerations, decrease or lack of variability, and progressive acceleration in the FHR baseline, are indicative of hypoxia. Fetal scalp blood samples demonstrating a pH value of 7.20 or less provide a more sophisticated indication of fetal problems and are generally obtained when questions about fetal status arise. (For further discussion, see Chapter 22).

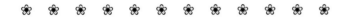

CRITICAL THINKING

Draw an FHR pattern that depicts late decelerations with minimal variability.

Maternal Risks

Indications of fetal distress greatly increase the psychologic stress a laboring woman must face.

Fetal-Neonatal Risks

Prolonged fetal hypoxia may lead to mental retardation or cerebral palsy and ultimately to fetal demise.

Medical Therapy

When there is evidence of possible fetal distress, treatment is centered on relieving the hypoxia and minimizing the effects of anoxia on the fetus. Initial interventions include changing the mother's position and administering oxygen by mask at 6 to 10 L per minute. If electronic fetal monitoring has not yet been used, it is usually instituted at this time. If oxytocin is in use, it should be discontinued. Fetal scalp blood samples are taken.

❈   *APPLYING THE NURSING PROCESS*   ❈

Nursing Assessment

The nurse reviews the woman's prenatal history to anticipate the possibility of fetal distress. When the membranes rupture, it is important to assess FHR and to observe for meconium staining. As labor progresses, the nurse is particularly alert for even subtle changes in the FHR pattern and the fetal scalp pH, if available. Reports by the mother of increased or greatly decreased fetal activity may also be associated with fetal distress. For further discussion of FHR patterns and characteristics, see page 636.

Nursing Diagnosis

Nursing diagnoses that may apply are presented in the Nursing Care Plan on page 730.

Nursing Plan and Implementation

The professional staff may become so involved in assessing fetal status and initiating corrective measures that they fail to give explanations and emotional support to the woman and her partner and other family members. It is imperative to provide both full explanations of the problem and comfort to the couple. In many instances, if birth is not imminent, the woman must undergo cesarean birth. This operation may be a source of fear and frustration for the couple, especially if they were committed to a shared, prepared birth experience.

The nurse stays alert for clues of fetal distress, initiates corrective measures, and answers any questions the couple has. Additional information regarding nursing interventions are presented in the Nursing Care Plan on page 730. Also refer to Chapter 22 for discussion of fetal heart rate patterns.

Evaluation

Anticipated outcomes of nursing care include the following:

- The woman and her family feel supported and able to cope with their situation.
- The fetal distress is identified quickly, and corrective, supportive measures are instituted.
- The fetal heart rate remains in normal range or supportive measures maintain the FHR as normal as possible.

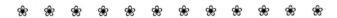

Care of the Family at Risk Due to Intrauterine Fetal Death

Fetal death, often referred to as fetal demise, accounts for one-half of the perinatal mortality after 20 weeks' gestation. Intrauterine fetal death (IUFD) results from unknown causes or a number of physiologic maladaptations including PIH, abruptio placentae, placenta previa, diabetes, infection, congenital anomalies, and isoimmune disease.

Maternal Risks

Prolonged retention of the fetus may lead to the development of **disseminated intravascular coagulation** (DIC)

(also referred to as consumption coagulopathy). After the release of thromboplastin from the degenerating fetal tissues into the maternal bloodstream, the extrinsic clotting system is activated, triggering the formation of multiple tiny blood clots. Fibrinogen and factors V and VII are subsequently depleted, and the woman begins to display symptoms of DIC. Fibrinogen levels begin a linear descent three to four weeks after the death of the fetus and continue to decrease without appropriate medical intervention. An in-depth discussion of DIC is found on page 766.

Medical Therapy

Abdominal x-ray examination may reveal Spalding's sign (an overriding of the fetal cranial bones). In addition, maternal estriol levels fall. Diagnosis of IUFD is confirmed by absence of heart action on real-time ultrasonography.

Most women have spontaneous labor within two weeks of fetal death and if other complications are not present, some physicians wait for labor to begin spontaneously (Cunningham et al 1989).

✤ *APPLYING THE NURSING PROCESS* ✤

Nursing Assessment

Cessation of fetal movement reported by the mother to the nurse is frequently the first indication of fetal death. It is followed by a gradual decrease in the signs and symptoms of pregnancy. Fetal heart tones are absent, and fetal movement is no longer palpable. Once fetal demise is established by the physician, ongoing support and communication will become even more important. Open communication among the mother, her partner, and the health team members contributes to a more realistic understanding of the medical condition and its associated treatments. The nurse may discuss prior experiences the family has had with stress and what they feel were their coping abilities at that time. Determining what social supports and resources the family has is also important.

Birth and death together. It's confusing and frightening enough for adults, but how are young children to understand it? For them the baby never really existed, or lived only briefly. What does this mean for them? Why are the parents so distraught? Too often, children's feelings about these issues are ignored or misunderstood. When parents are struggling to deal with their own feelings, they find it even harder to respond to the emotional needs of their other children. (When Pregnancy Fails)

Nursing Diagnosis

Nursing diagnoses that may apply to the woman experiencing intrauterine fetal death include the following:

- Grieving related to an actual loss
- Alteration in family process related to loss of a family member
- Ineffective individual and family coping related to depression in response to loss of child
- Ineffective family coping related to death of a child
- Anxiety related to death of a child

A friend asked if we had named our stillborn baby. After telling her the name, we both began referring to the baby by her name, Sarah. It felt good to call her a name. (When Pregnancy Fails)

Nursing Plan and Implementation

Provision of Emotional Support to the Family

The parents of a stillborn infant suffer a devastating experience, precipitating an intense emotional trauma. During the pregnancy, the couple has already begun the attachment process, which now must be terminated through the grieving process. The behaviors that couples exhibit while mourning may be associated with the five stages of grieving described by Elizabeth Kübler-Ross (1969). Often the first stage is *denial* of the death of the fetus. Even when the initial health care provider suspects fetal demise, the couple is hoping that a second opinion will be different. Some couples may not be convinced of the death until they view and hold the stillborn infant. The second stage is *anger*, resulting from the feelings of loss, loneliness, and perhaps guilt. The anger may be projected at significant others and health team members, or it may be omitted when the death of the fetus is sudden and unexpected. *Bargaining*, the third stage, may or may not be present depending on the couple's preparation for the death of the fetus. If the death is unanticipated, the couple may have no time for bargaining. In the fourth stage, *depression* is evidenced by preoccupation, weeping, and withdrawal. Physiologic postpartal depression appearing 24 to 48 hours after the stillbirth may compound the depression of grief. The final stage is *acceptance*, which involves the process of resolution. This is a highly individualized process that may take months to complete.

In some facilities, a checklist is used to make sure important aspects of working with the parents are addressed. The checklist becomes a communication tool between staff members to share information particular to this couple (Beckey et al 1985; Carr and Knupp 1985). Such a checklist might include the following items:

- When the fetal death is known before admission, inform the admission department and nursing staff so that inappropriate remarks are not made.
- Allow the woman and her partner to remain together as much as they wish. Provide privacy by assigning them to a private room.
- Stay with the couple and do not leave them alone and isolated.
- As much as possible, have the same nurse provide care to increase the support for the couple. Develop a care plan to provide for continuity of care. Encourage family members to visit support persons.
- Have the most experienced labor and birth nurse auscultate for fetal heart tones. This avoids the searching that a more inexperienced nurse might feel compelled to do. Avoid the temptation to listen again "to make sure."
- Listen to the couple; do not offer explanations. They require solace without minimizing the situation.
- Facilitate the woman and her partner's participation in the labor and birth process. When possible, allow them to make decisions about who will be present and what ritual will occur during the birth process. Allow the woman to make the decision regarding whether to have sedation during labor and birth. Provide a quiet supportive environment; ideally the labor and birth should occur in a labor room or possibly a birthing room rather than the delivery room.
- Give parents accurate information regarding plans for labor and birth.
- Provide ongoing opportunities for the couple to ask questions.
- Arrange for the woman to be assigned to a room that is away from new mothers and babies if she requests it. It is important to let the woman decide if she wants to be on another unit. If early discharge is an option, allow the family to make that selection.
- Encourage the couple to experience the grief that they feel. Accept the weeping and depression. A couple may have intense feelings that they are unable to share with each other. Encourage them to talk together and allow emotions to show freely. Help them understand that they may each experience different feelings. (Cordell and Thomas 1989).
- Give the couple and family an opportunity to see and hold the stillborn infant in a private quiet location. (Advocates of seeing the stillborn believe that viewing assists in dispelling denial and enables the couple to progress to the next step in the grieving process.) If they choose to see their stillborn infant, prepare the couple for what they will see by saying "the baby is cold," "the baby is blue," "the baby is bruised," or other appropriate statements (Furrh & Copley 1989).

- Some families may elect to bathe or dress their still-born; support them in their choice.

- Take a photograph of the infant, and let the family know it is available if they want it now or some time in the future.

- Offer a card with footprints, crib card, ID band, and possibly a lock of hair to the parents. These items may be kept with the photo if the parents do not want them at this time (Beckey et al 1985).

- Prepare the couple for returning home. If there are siblings, each will usually progress through age-appropriate grieving. Provide the parents with information about normal mourning reactions, both psychologic and physiologic.

- Furnish the mother with educational materials that discuss the changes she will experience in returning to the nonpregnant state.

- Provide information about community support groups including group name, contact person if possible, and phone number. Use materials such as the book *When Hello Means Goodbye* by Schwiebert & Kirk (1985).

- Remember it is not so important to "say the right words." The caring support and human contact that a couple receives is important and can be conveyed through silence and your presence.

The nurse experiences many of the same grief reactions as the parents of a stillborn infant. It is important to have support persons and colleagues available for counseling and support.

Evaluation

Anticipated outcomes of nursing care include the following:

- The family members express their feelings about the death of their baby.

- The family participates in decisions regarding whether to see their baby and in other decisions regarding the baby.

- The family has resources available for continued support.

- The family knows the community resources available and has names and phone numbers to use if they choose.

- The family is moving into and through the grieving process.

I knew something was wrong just by the way everyone was scurrying around in the delivery room and by that terrible silence. Then we knew the baby was dead. The doctor's only comment was, "It must be congenital," as if to say it certainly must

be my fault, not his. Then a nurse said: "It would be worse if you had a five-year-old that died." I suppose she was right, but it certainly didn't make me feel any better. Later, the doctor said, "You're young, you'll have lots more kids." I was appalled—I was thirty-three already. Where do they learn all these stupid comments? (When Pregnancy Fails)

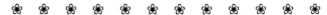

Care of the Woman and Fetus at Risk Due to Placental Problems

Maintenance of placental function is paramount to ensure fetal well-being and continuance of the pregnancy. Because the placenta is so vascular, problems that develop are usually associated with maternal and possible fetal hemorrhage. Causes and sources of hemorrhage are reviewed in Table 25–2.

Table 25–2 Causes and Sources of Hemorrhage

Causes and sources	Signs and symptoms
Antepartal Period	
Abortion	Vaginal bleeding Intermittent uterine contractions Rupture of membranes
Placenta previa	Painless vaginal bleeding after seventh month
Abruptio placentae	
Partial	Vaginal bleeding; no increase in uterine pain
Severe	No vaginal bleeding Extreme tenderness of abdominal area Rigid, boardlike abdomen Increase in size of abdomen
Intrapartal Period	
Placenta previa	Bright red vaginal bleeding
Abruptio placentae	Same signs and symptoms as listed above
Uterine atony in stage III	Bright red vaginal bleeding Ineffectual contractility
Postpartal Period	
Uterine atony	Boggy uterus Dark vaginal bleeding Presence of clots
Retained placental fragments	Boggy uterus Dark vaginal bleeding Presence of clots
Lacerations of cervix or vagina	Firm uterus Bright red blood

Abruptio Placentae

Abruptio placentae is the premature separation of a normally implanted placenta from the uterine wall. Premature separation is considered a catastrophic event because of the severity of the hemorrhage that occurs. The incidence of abruptio placentae is 1 in 75 to 90 births (Lowe & Cunningham 1990) and is more frequent in pregnancies complicated by cocaine abuse (Dombrowski et al 1991). The risk of recurrence is much higher than for the general population. Karegaard and Gennser (1986) report a recurrence risk of tenfold—a one in 25 incidence in subsequent pregnancies.

The cause of abruptio placentae is largely unknown. Theories have been proposed relating its occurrence to decreased blood flow to the placenta through the sinuses during the last trimester. Excessive intrauterine pressure caused by hydramnios or multiple pregnancy, maternal hypertension, cigarette smoking, alcohol ingestion, increased maternal age and parity, trauma, and sudden changes in intrauterine pressure (as with amniotomy) have been suggested as contributing factors.

Pathophysiology

Premature separation of the placenta may be divided into three types (Figure 25–16):

1. *Marginal.* The blood passes between the fetal membranes and the uterine wall and escapes vaginally. Separation begins at the periphery of the placenta; this marginal sinus rupture may or may not become more severe.

2. *Central.* The placenta separates centrally, and the blood is trapped between the placenta and the uterine wall. Entrapment of the blood results in concealed bleeding.

3. *Complete.* Massive vaginal bleeding is seen in the presence of almost total separation.

The signs and symptoms of these three types of placental abruption are given in Table 25–3. In severe cases of central abruptio placentae, a blood clot forms behind the placenta. With no place to escape, the blood invades the myometrial tissues between the muscle fibers. This occurrence accounts for the uterine irritability that is a significant sign of premature separation of the placenta. If hemorrhage continues, eventually the uterus turns en-

(*Text continues on p 763*)

Table 25–3 Differential Diagnosis

	Placenta previa	Abruptio placentae
Onset	Quiet and sneaky	Sudden and stormy
Bleeding	External	External and concealed
Color of blood	Bright red	Dark venous
Anemia	= Blood loss	> Apparent blood loss
Shock	= Blood loss	> Apparent blood loss
Toxemia	Absent	May be present
Pain	Only labor	Severe and steady
Uterine tenderness	Absent	Present
Uterine tone	Soft and relaxed	Firm to stony hard
Uterine contour	Normal	May enlarge and change shape
Fetal heart tones	Usually present	Present or absent
Engagement	Absent	May be present
Presentation	May be abnormal	No relationship

From Oxorn H: Human Labor and Birth, *5th ed. Norwalk, CT: Appleton & Lange, 1986, p 507.*

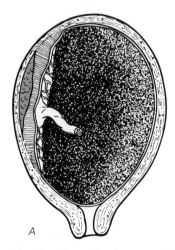 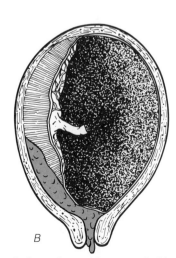 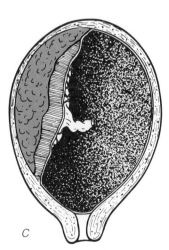

Figure 25–16   Abruptio placentae. A Central abruption with concealed hemorrhage. B Marginal abruption with external hemorrhage. C Complete separation. (From Abnormalities of the Placenta. *Clinical Educational Aid No. 12, Ross Laboratories, Columbus, Ohio)*

Nursing Care Plan
Hemorrhage in Third Trimester and at Birth

Client Assessment

Nursing History

Identify factors predisposing to hemorrhage:

1. Presence of preeclampsia-eclampsia (PIH)
2. Overdistention of the uterus
   a. Multiple pregnancy
   b. Hydramnios
3. Grandmultiparity
4. Advanced age
5. Uterine contractile problems
   a. Hypotonicity
   b. Hypertonicity
6. Painless vaginal bleeding after seventh month
7. Presence of hypertension
8. Presence of diabetes
9. History of previous hemorrhage or bleeding problems, blood coagulation defects, abortions
10. Retained placental fragments
11. Cervical and/or vaginal lacerations

Determine religious preference to establish whether client will permit a blood transfusion.

Physical Examination

Severe abdominal pain (central abruptio placentae)

External or concealed bleeding (see Table 25–3)

Painless vaginal hemorrhage (placenta previa)

Shock symptoms (decreased blood pressure, increased pulse, pallor)

Uterine tetany or uterine atony

Portwine amniotic fluid with abruptio placentae

Degree of hemorrhage

Changes in FHR

Increased resting tone of uterus between contractions

Diagnostic Studies

Hemoglobin and hematocrit

Type and cross-match

Fibrinogen levels

Platelets

Prothrombin time

Activated partial thromboplastin time

Fibrin split products

Nursing Diagnosis	Nursing Interventions	Rationale	Evaluation
Nursing Diagnosis: Altered tissue perfusion (renal, cerebral, and peripheral) secondary to excessive blood loss *Client Goal:* The woman will maintain adequate tissue perfusion as measured by the following: • BP between 110/70 and 138/88 • Pulse rate 60–90 • Urine output > 30 mL/hr • Skin warm and nonclammy	General interventions: Observe, record, and report blood loss. Evaluate woman experiencing decrease in blood volume using following parameters: 1. Monitor rate and quality of respirations frequently. 2. Measure pulse rate.	Monitoring the amount of blood loss aids in determining appropriate interventions. Initially respiratory rate increases as a result of sympathoadrenal stimulation, resulting in increased metabolic rate; pain and anxiety may cause hyperventilation. Increased pulse rate is an effect of increased epinephrine.	Woman maintains normal tissue perfusion; BP remains between 110/70 and 138/88; pulse rate 60–90 beats/min; urine output > 30 mL/hr, urine clear, straw colored; specific gravity 1.010–1.025; skin warm, dry.

(continued)

Nursing Care Plan (continued)

Nursing Diagnosis	Nursing Interventions	Rationale	Evaluation
	3. Assess pulse quality by direct palpation. Determine pulse deficit by comparing apical-radial rates.	Reflects circulatory status. Thready pulse indicates vasoconstriction and reflects decreased cardiac output; peripheral pulses may be absent if vasoconstriction is intense. Bounding pulse may indicate overload.	
	4. Compare present BP with woman's baseline BP; note pulse pressure.	Hypotension indicates loss of large amount of circulatory fluid or lack of compensation in circulatory system. As cardiac output decreases, there is usually a fall in pulse pressure. Peripheral vasoconstriction may make accurate readings difficult.	
	5. Monitor urine output (decrease to less than 30 mL/hr is sign of shock): a. Insert Foley catheter. b. Measure output hourly. c. Measure specific gravity to determine concentration of urine.	Vasoconstrictor effect of norepinephrine decreases blood flow to kidneys, which decreases glomerular filtration rate and the output of urine. Inability to concentrate urine may indicate renal damage from vasoconstriction and decreased blood perfusion.	
	6. Inspect skin for presence of following: a. Pallor and cyanosis: *Pallor* in brown-skinned persons appears yellowish-brown; black-skinned individuals appear ashen gray; generally pallor may be observed in mucous membranes, lips, and nail beds. *Cyanosis* is assessed by inspecting lips, nail beds, conjunctiva, palms, and soles of feet at regular intervals; evaluate capillary refilling by pressing on nail bed and observing return of color; compare by testing your own nail bed.	Skin reflects amount of vasoconstriction. Pallor is determined by intensity of vasoconstriction. Cyanosis occurs when the amount of unoxygenated hemoglobin in the blood is ≤5 g/dL blood.	

(continued)

Nursing Care Plan (continued)

Nursing Diagnosis	Nursing Interventions	Rationale	Evaluation
	b. Coldness c. Clamminess	Produced by slow blood flow.	
	Evaluate state of consciousness frequently.		
	Measure CVP: normal CVP is 5–10 cm H$_2$O.	Caused by sympathetic stimulation of sweat glands. Diminished cerebral blood flow causes restlessness and anxiety; as shock progresses, state of consciousness decreases. Provides estimation of volume of blood returning to heart and ability of both chambers in right heart to propel blood. Low CVP indicates a decrease in the circulating volume of blood (hypovolemia).	
	Assess amount of blood loss: 1. Count pads. 2. Weigh pads and chux (1 g = 1 mL blood approximately). 3. Record amount in a specific amount of time (for example, 50 mL bright red blood on pad in 20 min).	In obstetric clients, blood is replaced according to estimates of actual blood loss, rather than using parameters of increased and decreased BP.	
	Hypovolemia: Relieve decreased blood pressure by administration of whole blood.	Hypotension results from decreased blood volume.	
	While waiting for whole blood to be available, infuse isotonic fluids, plasma, plasma expanders, or serum albumin, per physician order.	Degree of hypovolemia may be assessed by CVP, hemoglobin, and hematocrit.	
	Marginal abruptio placentae: If abruptio placentae is diagnosed, nurse and physician will:		

(continued)

Nursing Care Plan (continued)

Nursing Diagnosis	Nursing Interventions	Rationale	Evaluation
	1. Evaluate blood loss. 2. Assess uterine contractile pattern, tenderness, and height. 3. Start continuous monitoring of uterine contractions by EFM. 4. Monitor maternal vital signs. 5. Assess fetal status per continuous EFM. 6. Assess cervical dilatation and effacement to determine labor progress if uterine contractions are present. 7. Rule out placenta previa. 8. Perform amniotomy and begin oxytocin infusion if labor does not start immediately or is ineffective. 9. Review and evaluate diagnostic lab blood tests (hemoglobin, hematocrit, PT, APPT, fibrin split products, fibrinogen). Central abruptio placentae with severe blood loss: 1. Perform same assessments as for marginal abruptio placentae. 2. Monitor CVP. 3. Replace blood loss. 4. Effect immediate delivery. 5. Observe for signs and symptoms of disseminated intravascular coagulation (DIC).	Provides information on type of abruption and maternal and fetal status.	Bleeding often stops as shock develops but resumes as circulation is restored.

(continued)

Nursing Care Plan (continued)

Nursing Diagnosis	Nursing Interventions	Rationale	Evaluation
Nursing Diagnosis: Altered tissue perfusion: High risk related to blood loss secondary to uterine atony following birth *Client Goal:* The woman's uterus will remain well contracted in the midline and below the umbilicus.	1. Assess contractility of uterus and amount of vaginal bleeding. 2. Postpartally, massage uterus every 15 min for one hour, every 30 min for one hour, every 60 min for two to four hours. Evaluate more frequently if uterus is boggy or not in the midline. Administer oxytocin per protocol or physician/nurse-midwife order.	Muscle fibers that have been overstretched or overused do not contract well; contraction of muscle fibers over open placental site is essential; slight relaxation of uterus muscle fibers leads to continuous oozing of blood.	The woman's uterus remains firm, in the midline, and below the umbilicus.
Nursing Diagnosis: Fear related to concern for own personal status and the baby's safety *Client Goal:* The woman will have opportunities to verbalize concern.	Keep woman informed of present status. Provide accurate information. Provide opportunities for questions. Establish trusting relationship. Encourage woman to participate in decision making if at all possible.	As hemorrhage occurs, the safety of the mother and baby are threatened. Anxiety and fear may be lessened somewhat when the woman is informed, understands what is happening, and has some part in the decision-making process.	The woman verbalizes questions and receives support.
Nursing Diagnosis: Impaired fetal gas exchange: High risk related to decreased blood volume and hypotension *Client Goal:* The FHR will remain within normal limits without signs of stress or distress.	Assess and monitor fetal heart rate (range 120–160 beats/min). Observe for meconium in amniotic fluid. Assist in obtaining fetal blood sample (pH < 7.20 indicates severe jeopardy).	Hemorrhage from woman disrupts blood flow pattern to fetus, possibly compromising fetal status. Hypoxia causes increased motility of fetal intestines and relaxation of abdominal muscles, with release of meconium into amniotic fluid.	Fetal heart rate baseline remains stable between 120–160 beats/min, short-term variability present, long-term variability is average, no late or variable decelerations, fetal scalp blood pH is > 7.25.

tirely blue in color. After birth of the neonate, the uterus contracts only with difficulty. This syndrome is known as a *Couvelaire uterus* and frequently necessitates hysterectomy.

As a result of the damage to the uterine wall and the retroplacental clotting with covert abruption, large amounts of thromboplastin are released into the maternal blood supply, which in turn triggers the development of disseminated intravascular coagulation (DIC) and the resultant hypofibrinogenemia. Fibrinogen levels, which are ordinarily elevated in pregnancy, may drop to incoagulable amounts within a matter of minutes as a result of rapidly developing premature separation of the placenta. Further information on DIC is found on p 766.

Maternal Risks

Maternal mortality is now uncommon, although maternal morbidity is common (Cunningham et al 1989). Problems following the birth depend in large part on the severity of the intrapartal bleeding, coagulation defects (DIC), hypofibrinogenemia, and length of time between separation and the birth. Moderate to severe hemorrhage results in hemorrhagic shock, which ultimately may prove fatal to the mother if not reversed. In the postpartal period, women who have suffered this disorder are at risk for hemorrhage and renal failure due to shock, vascular spasm, intravascular clotting, or a combination of the three. Another cause of renal failure is incompatible emergency blood transfusion. Failure is directly proportional to the number of units transfused.

Fetal-Neonatal Risks

Perinatal mortality associated with abruptio placentae ranges from 20% to 35% (Lowe & Cunningham 1990). In severe cases in which separation is almost complete, infant mortality is 100%. In less severe separation, fetal outcome depends on the level of maturity. The most serious complications in the neonate arise from preterm labor, anemia, and hypoxia. If fetal hypoxia progresses unchecked, irreversible brain damage or fetal demise may result. With thorough assessment and prompt action on the part of the health team, fetal and maternal outcome can be optimized.

Medical Therapy

Because of the risk of DIC, evaluating the results of coagulation tests is imperative. In DIC, fibrinogen levels and platelet counts are usually decreased; prothrombin times and partial thromboplastin times are normal to prolonged. If the values are not markedly abnormal, serial testing may be helpful in establishing an abnormal trend that is indicative of coagulopathy. Another very sensitive test determines fibrin degradation products levels; these values rise with DIC.

After establishing the diagnosis, emphasis is placed on maintaining the cardiovascular status of the mother and developing a plan for effecting the birth of the fetus. Which birth method is selected depends on the condition of the woman and fetus; in many circumstances, cesarean birth may be the safest option.

If the separation is mild and gestation is near term, labor may be induced and the fetus may be born vaginally with as little trauma as possible. If the induction of labor by rupture of membranes and oxytocin infusion by pump does not initiate labor within eight hours, a cesarean birth is usually done. A longer delay would increase the risk of increased hemorrhage, with resulting hypofibrinogenemia. Supportive treatment to decrease risk of DIC includes typing and cross-matching for blood transfusions (at least three units), clotting mechanism evaluation, and intravenous fluids.

In cases of moderate to severe placental separation, a cesarean birth is done after hypofibrinogenemia has been treated by intravenous infusion of cryoprecipitate or plasma. Vaginal birth is impossible in the event of a Couvelaire uterus, because it would not contact properly in labor. Cesarean birth is necessary in the face of severe hemorrhage to allow an immediate hysterectomy to save both woman and fetus.

The hypovolemia that accompanies severe abruptio placentae is life threatening and must be combated with whole blood. If the fetus is alive but in distress, emergency cesarean birth is the method of choice. With a stillborn fetus, vaginal birth is preferable unless shock from hemorrhage is uncontrollable. Intravenous fluids of a balanced salt solution such as lactated Ringer's are given through a 16- or 18-gauge cannula (Cunningham et al 1989). Central venous pressure (CVP) monitoring may be needed to evaluate intravenous fluid replacement. A normal CVP of 10 cm H_2O is the goal. The CVP is evaluated hourly, and results are communicated to the physician. Elevations of CVP may indicate fluid overload and pulmonary edema. The hematocrit is maintained at 30% through the administration of packed red cells and/or whole blood (Cunningham et al 1989).

Laboratory testing is ordered to provide ongoing data regarding hemoglobin, hematocrit, and coagulation status. A clot observation test may be done at the bedside to evaluate coagulation status. A glass tube containing 5 mL of maternal blood is inverted four to five times. If a clot fails to form in six minutes, a fibrinogen level of less than 150 mg/dL is suspected. If a clot is not formed in 30 minutes, the fibrinogen level may well be less than 100 mg/dL. A clot observation test may be completed by a physician or a nurse.

Measures are taken to stimulate labor to effect vaginal birth as indicated by the condition of the mother and fetus. The birth may be hastened by performing an amniotomy and by oxytocin stimulation. Previously, birth within six hours of the diagnosis of severe placental abruption was recommended to reduce maternal mortality and morbidity. Currently, changing medical practice directed to ensuring adequate fluid replacement, especially blood, appears to accomplish the same outcome (Cunningham et al 1989).

❀ *APPLYING THE NURSING PROCESS* ❀

Nursing Assessment

Electronic monitoring of the uterine contractions and resting tone between contractions provides information regarding the labor pattern and effectiveness of the oxytocin induction. Since uterine resting tone is frequently increased with abruptio placentae, it must be evaluated frequently for further increase. Abdominal girth measurements may be ordered hourly and are obtained by placing a tape measure around the maternal abdomen at the level of the umbilicus. Another method of evaluating uterine size, which increases as more bleeding occurs at the site of abruption, is to place a mark at the top of the uterine fundus. The distance from the symphysis pubis to the mark may be evaluated hourly.

Nursing Diagnosis

Nursing diagnoses that may apply to the woman with abruptio placentae are presented in the Nursing Care Plan on page 756.

Nursing Plan and Implementation

The psychologic aspects of nursing care are very important. Maternal apprehension increases as the clinical picture changes. Factual reassurance and an explanation of the procedures and what is happening are essential for the emotional well-being of the expectant couple. The nurse can reinforce positive aspects of the woman's condition, such as normal FHR, normal vital signs, and decreased evidence of bleeding.

Other nursing care measures are addressed in the Nursing Care Plan on page 758.

Evaluation

Anticipated outcomes of nursing care include the following:

- Any signs of fetal distress are recognized promptly and corrective measures are begun.
- The woman and her baby have a safe labor and birth without further complications for the mother or child.
- The woman and family verbalize understanding of reasons for medical therapy and risks.
- The hemorrhage ceases and any hypovolemia is corrected as indicated by normal blood studies and normal vital signs.

❀ ❀ ❀ ❀ ❀ ❀ ❀ ❀ ❀ ❀ ❀ ❀ ❀ ❀

Care of the Woman with Disseminated Intravascular Coagulation

Disseminated intravascular coagulation (DIC) is an abnormal overstimulation of the coagulation process, secondary to an underlying disease. The coagulation process remains essentially the same, but certain medical conditions hasten and intensify the response to the point that hemorrhage may be life threatening as coagulation factors are overconsumed (Figure 25–17).

Sepsis in the childbearing woman may activate the intrinsic coagulation pathway because of damage to the endothelial cells. The extrinsic pathway is activated by the release of thromboplastin from damaged tissues in such conditions as abruptio placentae, PIH, chorioamnionitis, and retained products of conception. The normally high levels of tissue thromboplastin in the placenta and decidua of the uterus may contribute to the occurrence of DIC. Amniotic fluid released into the bloodstream from amniotic fluid emboli and intraamniotic saline infusions activates both pathways. With the initiation of the coagulation process, massive numbers of clots form rapidly. Fibrinogen becomes depleted as it is converted to fibrin. Platelets are entrapped in the clots, leading to a decrease in the number of platelets. The coagulation process also activates plasminogen conversion to plasmin, which can lyse fibrinogen (dissolve clots), and as the fibrin clots are destroyed, fibrin split products having an anticoagulant effect are released. Because of the elevated fibrin split products level, the decrease in the number of platelets, and the reduced fibrinogen level, the outcome is generalized bleeding. Ischemia of the organs follows from the vascular occlusion of the numerous fibrin thrombi. The multisite hemorrhages result in shock and can result in death.

The clinical manifestations of DIC begin subtly and become more overt with severity of the disease. The signs and symptoms are indicators of the degree of bleeding, which ranges from generalized hemorrhage to minor generalized bleeding to localized bleeding in the form of purpura and petechiae.

Medical Therapy

The goals of therapy are early diagnosis and supportive treatment of the woman with DIC. Confirmation of DIC is made with several blood tests. The prothrombin time (PT) test evaluates the extrinsic pathway in clotting. The PT is prolonged in DIC. The intrinsic pathway is evaluated by testing the partial thromboplastin time, which is also prolonged in DIC. Both platelets and fibrinogen levels decrease. Platelet counts below $50,000/\mu L$ result in spontaneous bleeding. Fibrinogen levels may be within normal ranges but will be lower than the initial level. The number

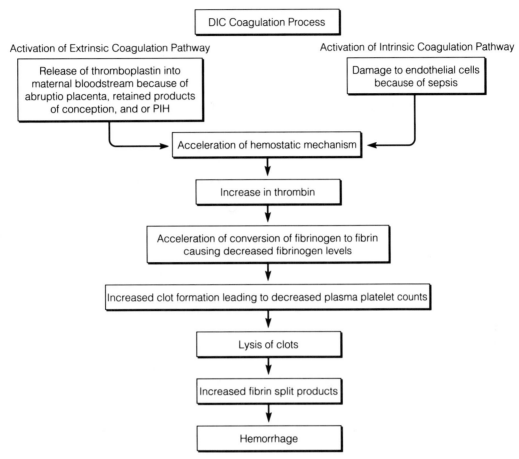

Figure 25–17   DIC coagulation process

of fibrin split products is elevated. The frequency of testing depends on the severity of the disease (Kelton & Cruikshank 1988).

Cases of DIC can frequently be resolved by correcting the underlying cause. In the childbearing woman, terminating the pregnancy removes the causative factor. Until birth can be accomplished, supportive therapy is critical to maintain maternal-fetal status.

Initial treatment includes evaluation of vital signs; assessment of vaginal bleeding, uterine contractility, and resting tone; continuous FHR monitoring; and fetal blood studies. Intravenous infusions of lactated Ringer's are given through a 16- or 18-gauge cannula. An indwelling bladder catheter is used to allow better evaluation of urinary output, which should be maintained at 30 mL per hour to assure adequate renal perfusion. Anemia (hematocrit less than 30%) is treated by giving packed red cells. Each unit generally increases the hematocrit by 3 points and the hemoglobin by 1 to 1.5 g. Fresh frozen plasma may also be used to replace fibrinogen, factors V and VII, and antithrombin III. If fibrinogen levels are very low, cryoprecipitate is used. Each unit of cryoprecipitate provides approximately 250 mg of fibrinogen and raises the fibrinogen level by approximately 5 mg/dL (Cunningham et al 1989).

The administration of heparin is a controversial issue. Heparin is used to decrease thrombin generation and activity. When the causative factor cannot be removed, as with infection or in self-limiting cases in childbearing women, heparin is not used routinely. In some instances the use of heparin may even increase the hemorrhage (Cunningham et al 1989).

Vaginal birth without an episiotomy is the preferred birthing method as it avoids the surgical incision of numerous tissues and further stress on the hemostatic system. Conduction anesthesia should be avoided because of the chance of bleeding from injection puncture sites and the formation of hematomas.

❊   *APPLYING THE NURSING PROCESS*   ❊

Nursing Assessment

The nurse should carefully observe for signs and symptoms of DIC in women who are candidates for this complication.

Bleeding from injection sites, epistaxis, bleeding gums, and the presence of purpura and petechiae on the skin may be signs of developing DIC.

Clinical evidence may also be apparent in the results of laboratory blood tests specific to DIC. As appropriate, the nurse continues to assess maternal-fetal status by checking vital signs, uterine activity, FHR, and urinary output.

The nurse documents and reports signs and symptoms of DIC to the physician as well as any changes in the FHR, maternal vital signs, and uterine activity.

Nursing Diagnosis

Nursing diagnoses that may apply to the woman with DIC include the following:

- Fear related to unknown outcome of the labor and birth
- Impaired gas exchange: High risk related to impaired oxygen-carrying ability of blood secondary to hemorrhage
- Infection: High risk related to decreased hemoglobin.

Nursing Plan and Implementation

In the event of major blood loss, nursing measures are directed toward assessment of maternal-fetal status and corrective or supportive treatment measures. The nurse is also responsible for monitoring administration of blood products.

Protecting the woman from further bleeding involves interventions such as padding the side rails, avoiding IM injections, assessing IV insertion sites, and placing the blood pressure cuff carefully to prevent bruising.

Meeting the woman's psychologic needs is another nursing priority. Accurate, informative explanations should be offered frequently. The nurse who listens and projects warmth and understanding is most likely to help the woman cope with her anxiety and frustration.

Evaluation

Anticipated outcomes of nursing care include the following:

- The woman's circulatory status is restored to normal and blood loss is replaced.
- The mother and baby have a safe labor and birth and further complications are quickly identified and treated.
- The parents understand the complication that occurred and are able to participate in decision making as much as possible.

❀ ❀ ❀ ❀ ❀ ❀ ❀ ❀ ❀ ❀ ❀ ❀

Placenta Previa

In placenta previa, the placenta is improperly implanted in the lower uterine segment. This implantation may be on a portion of the lower segment or over the internal os (Figure 25–18). As the lower uterine segment contracts and dilates in the later weeks of pregnancy, the placental villi are torn from the uterine wall, thus exposing the uterine sinuses at the placental site. Bleeding begins, but because its amount depends on the number of sinuses exposed, it may initially be either scanty or profuse.

The cause of placenta previa is unknown. Statistically it occurs in about 1 of every 250 births. Women with a previous history of placenta previa have a recurrence rate of 4% to 8% (Lavery 1990). Other factors associated with placenta previa are multiparity, increasing age, placenta accreta, defective development of blood vessels in the decidua, and a large placenta (Cunningham et al 1989).

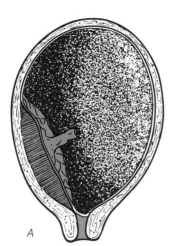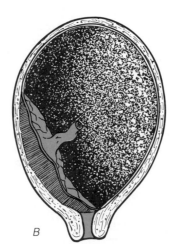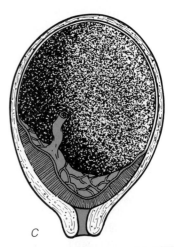

Figure 25–18   Placenta previa. A Low placental implantation. B Partial placenta previa. C Complete placenta previa. (From Abnormalities of the Placenta. *Clinical Educational Aid No. 12, Ross Laboratories, Columbus, Ohio)*

Medical Therapy

The goal of medical care is to identify the cause of bleeding and to provide treatment that will ensure birth of a mature newborn. Indirect diagnosis is made by localizing the placenta through tests that require no vaginal examination. The most commonly employed diagnostic test is the ultrasound scan (Figure 25–19). If placenta previa is ruled out, a vaginal examination can be performed with a speculum to determine the cause of bleeding (such as cervical lesions).

Direct diagnosis of placenta previa can only be made by feeling the placenta inside the cervical os. However, such an examination may cause profuse bleeding due to tearing of tissue in the cotyledons of the placenta. Because of the danger of bleeding, a vaginal examination should be performed only if ultrasound is not available, the pregnancy is near term, and there is profuse vaginal bleeding. The examination may be done using a double setup procedure. In this situation, it must be determined whether the cause of the bleeding is placenta previa or advanced labor with copious bloody show (which is normal). *Double setup* means that the delivery room is set up for the vaginal examination and normal vaginal birth and for a cesarean birth should placenta previa be present and the examination precipitates brisk bleeding. Adequate personnel must be present to respond to treatment decisions.

The differential diagnosis of placental or cervical bleeding takes careful consideration. Partial separation of the placenta may also present with painless bleeding, and a

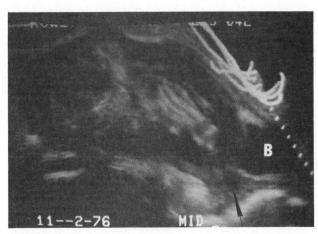

Figure 25–19   Ultrasound of placenta previa. The maternal bladder is indicated by the letter "B." The placenta is indicated by the arrow.

true placenta previa may not demonstrate overt bleeding until labor begins, thus confusing the diagnosis. Another important fact to note is that the causes of slight-to-moderate antepartal bleeding episodes in 20% to 25% of women are never accurately diagnosed.

Care of the women with painless late gestational bleeding depends on (a) the week of gestation during which the first bleeding episode occurs and (b) the amount of bleeding (Figure 25–20). If the pregnancy is less than 37

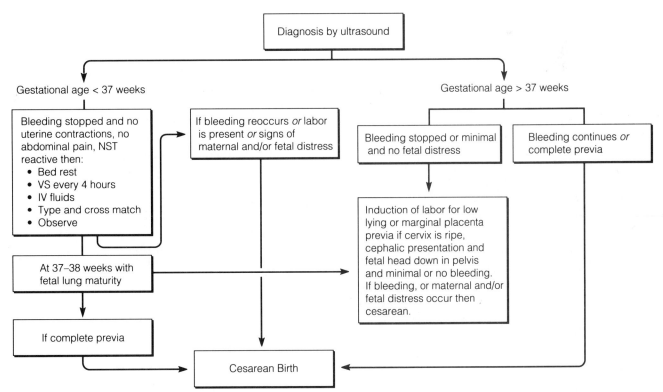

Figure 25–20   Management of placenta previa (Barker RK, Fields DH, Kaufman SA: Quick Reference to OB-GYN Procedures, 3rd Ed. New York: Lippincott/Harper & Row, 1990)

weeks' gestation, expectant management is employed to delay birth until about 37 weeks' gestation to allow the fetus to mature. Expectant management involves stringent regulation of the following:

1. Bed rest with bathroom privileges only as long as the woman is not bleeding
2. Absolutely no rectal or vaginal exams
3. Monitoring of blood loss, pain, and uterine contractility
4. Evaluating FHTs with external monitor
5. Monitoring of vital signs
6. Complete laboratory evaluation: hemoglobin, hematocrit, Rh factor, and urinalysis
7. Intravenous fluid (lactated Ringer's) with drip rate monitored
8. Two units of cross-matched blood available for transfusion

If frequent, recurrent, or profuse bleeding persists, or if fetal well-being appears threatened, a cesarean birth will need to be performed before 37 weeks.

❀ *APPLYING THE NURSING PROCESS* ❀

Nursing Assessment

Assessment of the woman with placenta previa must be ongoing to prevent or treat complications that are potentially lethal to the mother and fetus. Painless, bright red vaginal bleeding is the best diagnostic sign of placenta previa. If this sign should develop during the last three months of a pregnancy, placenta previa should always be considered until ruled out by examination. The first bleeding episode is generally scanty. If no rectal or vaginal examinations are performed, it often subsides spontaneously. However, each subsequent hemorrhage is more profuse.

The uterus remains soft, and if labor begins, it relaxes fully between contractions. The FHR usually remains stable unless profuse hemorrhage and maternal shock occur. As a result of the placement of the placenta, the fetal presenting part is often unengaged, and transverse lie is common.

Blood loss, pain, and uterine contractility are appraised by the nurse from both subjective and objective perspectives. Maternal vital signs and the results of blood and urine tests provide the nurse with additional data about the woman's condition. FHR is evaluated with an external fetal monitor. Another pressing nursing responsibility is observing and verifying the family's ability to cope with the anxiety associated with an unknown outcome.

Nursing Diagnosis

Nursing diagnoses that may apply are presented in the Nursing Care Plan on page 758.

Nursing Plan and Implementation

Preparation for Double Setup Procedure

Before a double setup procedure is performed, the laboring couple should be physiologically and psychologically prepared for possible surgery (Chapter 26). A whole-blood setup should be readied for intravenous infusion and a patent intravenous line established before any intrusive procedures are undertaken. The maternal vital signs should be monitored every 15 minutes in the absence of hemorrhage and every 5 minutes with active hemorrhage. The external tocodynamometer should be connected to the maternal abdomen to monitor uterine activity continuously.

Promotion of Physical Well-Being

The nurse continues to monitor the woman and her fetus to determine the status of the bleeding and to determine the mother's and baby's responses. Vital signs, intake and output, and other pertinent assessments must be made frequently. The nurse evaluates the electronic monitor tracing to evaluate the fetal status.

Provision of Emotional Support to the Family During Expectant Management

Emotional support for the family is an important nursing care goal. When active bleeding is occurring, the assessments and management must be directed toward physical support. However, emotional aspects need to be addressed simultaneously. The nurse can explain the assessments being completed and the treatment measures that need to be done. Time can be provided for questions, and the nurse can act as an advocate in obtaining information for the family. Emotional support can also be offered by staying with the family and by the use of touch.

Promotion of Neonatal Physiologic Adaptation

The newborn's hemoglobin, cell volume, and erythrocyte count should be checked immediately and then monitored closely. The newborn may require oxygen and administration of blood and admission into a neonatal intensive care unit.

Provision of Care to the Woman with Bleeding

Additional information regarding nursing care is addressed in the Nursing Care Plan on page 758.

Evaluation

Anticipated outcomes of nursing care include the following:

- The cause of hemorrhage is recognized promptly and corrective measures are taken.
- The woman's vital signs remain in the normal range.

- The woman and her baby have a safe labor and birth.
- Any other complications are recognized and treated early.
- The family understands what has happened and the implications and associated problems of placenta previa.

❀ ❀ ❀ ❀ ❀ ❀ ❀ ❀ ❀ ❀ ❀ ❀ ❀

Other Placental Problems

Other problems of the placenta can be divided into those that are developmental and those that are degenerative. Developmental problems of the placenta include placental lesions, placenta succenturiata, circumvallate placenta, and battledore placenta (Figure 25–21). Degenerative changes include infarcts and placental calcification.

Succenturiate Placenta

In succenturiate placenta, one or more accessory lobes of fetal villi have developed on the placenta, with vascular connections of fetal origin (Figure 25–21*A*). Vessels from the major to the minor lobe(s) are supported only by the membranes, thus increasing the risk of the minor lobe being retained during the third stage of labor.

The gravest maternal danger is postpartal hemor-rhage if this minor lobe is severed from the placenta and remains in the uterus. All placentas should be examined closely for intactness. If vessels appear to be severed at the margin of the placenta, the uterus should be explored for retained placental tissue. This condition is not usually diagnosed until after the birth of the placenta (Cunningham et al 1989). If the vascular connections rupture between the lobes, life-threatening fetal hemorrhage can result. At birth the infant should be inspected for pallor, cyanosis, retractions, tachypnea, tachycardia, and feeble pulse. The infant's cry will be weak and the muscle tone flaccid.

Circumvallate Placenta

In circumvallate placenta, the fetal surface of the placenta is exposed through a ring opening around the umbilical cord (Figure 25–21*B*). The vessels descend from the cord and end at the margin of the ring instead of coursing through the entire surface area of the placenta. The ring is composed of a double fold of amnion and chorion with some degenerative decidua and fibrin between. The cause of this condition is unknown. Maternal-fetal problems include an increased incidence of late abortion or fetal death, antepartal hemorrhage, prematurity, and abnormal maternal bleeding during or following the third stage of labor, resulting from improper placental separation or shearing of membranes from the placenta.

Battledore Placenta

In the case of battledore placenta, the umbilical cord is inserted at or near the placental margin (Figure 25–21*C*). As a result, all fetal vessels transverse the placental surface in the same direction. The chances of preterm labor are high because of interference with fetal circulation and nutrition. Fetal distress or bleeding during labor is also likely because of cord compression or vessel rupture.

Placental Infarcts and Calcifications

In the aging process the placenta may develop infarcts and calcifications. They become significant if they cover a large enough area to interfere with the uterine–placental–fetal exchange. Altered exchange can also occur with certain maternal disease processes, such as hypertension. Infarcts are most often seen in cases of severe pregnancy-induced hypertension and in women who smoke.

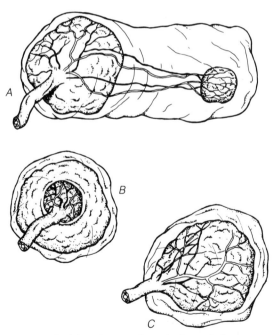

Figure 25–21 Placental variations. A Succenturiate placenta. B Circumvallate placenta. C Battledore placenta. (From Abnormalities of the Placenta. Clinical Educational Aid No. 12, Ross Laboratories, Columbus, Ohio)

Care of the Woman and Fetus at Risk Due to Problems Associated with the Umbilical Cord

Prolapsed Umbilical Cord

Prolapsed cord occurs when the umbilical cord falls or is washed down through the cervix into the vagina. Another

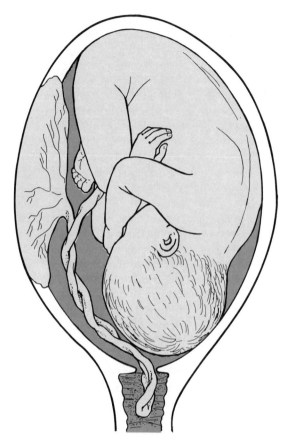

Figure 25-22   Prolapse of the umbilical cord

type of prolapsed cord is called **occult cord prolapse**. In this type the cord lies beside or just ahead of the fetal head. Conditions associated with a prolapsed cord include breech presentation, transverse lies, contracted inlets, small fetus, extra long cord, low-lying placenta, hydramnios, and multiple gestations. Any time the inlet is not occluded and the membranes rupture, the cord can be washed down (Figure 25-22) into the birth canal in front of the presenting part.

Maternal/Fetal-Neonatal Risks

When predisposing factors to cord prolapse exist, the woman should be considered high risk and should be monitored closely. If prolapse occurs prior to complete cervical dilatation, immediate cesarean birth is the preferred method of treatment.

Because with each contraction the umbilical cord becomes compressed between the maternal pelvis and the presenting part, fetal distress is common. If the cord ceases to pulsate, it is generally indicative of fetal demise.

Medical Therapy

Preventing the occurrence of prolapse of the cord is the preferred medical approach. If the prolapse does happen, it is most usually discovered by the nurse, and relieving the compression on the cord is critical to fetal outcome. The

medical and nursing team must work together to facilitate birth.

Bed rest is indicated for all laboring women with a history of ruptured membranes, until engagement with no cord prolapse has been documented. Furthermore, at the time of spontaneous rupture of membranes or amniotomy, the FHR should be auscultated for at least a full minute and again at the end of a contraction and after a few contractions. If fetal bradycardia is detected on the auscultation, the woman should be examined to rule out a cord prolapse. In the presence of cord prolapse, electronic monitor tracings show severe, moderate, or prolonged variable decelerations with baseline bradycardia. If these patterns are found, the woman is examined vaginally.

If a loop of cord is discovered during a sterile vaginal exam by the physician/nurse-midwife or birthing nurse, the gloved fingers are left in the vagina, and attempts are made to lift the fetal head off the cord to relieve compression until the physician arrives (if she/he is not in attendance). This is a life-saving measure. Oxygen is begun, and FHR is monitored to see if the cord compression is adequately relieved.

The force of gravity can be employed to relieve the compression. The woman assumes the knee-chest position or the bed is adjusted to the Trendelenburg position and the woman should be transported to the birthing or operating room in this position. The nurse must remember that the cord may be occultly prolapsed with an actual loop extending into the vagina or lying alongside the presenting part. It may be pulsating strongly or so weakly that it is difficult to determine on palpation of the cord whether the fetus is alive.

Occasionally a cord prolapses out of the vagina. If this condition is identified in a home situation, some of the previously discussed life-saving actions can be implemented by the nurse. The lateral Sims' position may be more feasible for the woman if the position is to be assumed for any extended period of time. The pelvis should be elevated on pillows. Compression on the cord can be relieved in the vagina as in the hospital situation, and wet dressings soaked in a mild salt solution should be wrapped around the protruding cord. The woman should be transported to the hospital immediately. If the cord is pale, limp, and obviously not pulsating, no action is necessary other than transport. At no time should attempts be made to replace the cord into the uterus, because this could cause devastating trauma to the cord and could greatly increase the possibility of intrauterine infection. Vaginal birth (with or without forceps) is possible if the following criteria are met:

- The cervix is completely dilated.
- A vertex is presenting at least at zero station.
- The membranes are ruptured.
- Pelvic measurements are adequate.

If these conditions are not present, cesarean birth is the preferred method. The woman is taken to the birthing room while the nurse vaginally relieves the pressure on the cord until the infant has been born. The medical and nursing team must work together quickly to facilitate birth in this obstetric emergency.

❅ *APPLYING THE NURSING PROCESS* ❅

Nursing Assessment

By reviewing the nursing history, the nurse ascertains whether the woman is at risk for prolapse of the cord. Particularly when the presenting part is not engaged and spontaneous or artificial rupture of the membranes occurs, the nurse observes the perineum and evaluates the FHR for changes that may signify a prolapsed cord. During labor, bradycardia accompanied by variable decelerations may also indicate prolapse.

Nursing Diagnosis

Nursing diagnoses that may apply to the woman with a prolapsed cord include the following:

- Impaired gas exchange in the fetus: High risk related to decreased blood flow secondary to compression of the umbilical cord
- Fear related to unknown outcome

Nursing Plan and Implementation

In addition to monitoring the woman closely for the occurrence of this complication, the nurse must be prepared to intervene instantaneously if the cord prolapses. Relieving the compression of the cord alleviates fetal distress and increases the likelihood that the woman will give birth to a healthy live newborn.

In the event of fetal death, assisting the family to deal with their loss becomes a priority. See discussion on p 754.

Evaluation

Anticipated outcomes of nursing care include the following:

- The FHR remains in normal range with supportive measures.
- The fetus is born safely.
- The woman and her partner feel supported.
- The woman and her partner understand the problem and the corrective measures that are undertaken.

❅ ❅ ❅ ❅ ❅ ❅ ❅ ❅ ❅ ❅ ❅

Umbilical Cord Abnormalities

Umbilical cord abnormalities include congenital absence of an umbilical artery, insertion variations, cord length vari-

ations, and knots and loops of the cord. Insertion variations include velamentous insertion and vasa previa, and cord length problems include long and short cords.

Congenital Absence of Umbilical Artery

Absence of an umbilical artery may have serious fetal implications. The incidence of all types of fetal anomalies is 25% in infants born with two-vessel cords.

Immediately after the umbilical cord is cut, it should be inspected to determine whether the correct number of vessels is present. If an artery is absent, the nurse should examine the newborn more closely for anomalies and gestational age problems.

Insertion Variations

In a *velamentous insertion* condition, the vessels of the umbilical cord divide some distance from the placenta in the placental membranes (Figure 25–23). Velamentous insertions occur more frequently in multiple gestations than in singletons. Other placental anomalies often accompany this condition, such as succenturiate placenta. The velamentous insertion is more easily compressed or kinked during pregnancy or labor because of the lack of Wharton's jelly to protect it. If the vessels become torn during labor, fetal hemorrhage can occur and is signaled by FHR abnormalities accompanied by vaginal bleeding.

When the vessels of a velamentous insertion transverse the internal os and appear in front of the fetus, a *vasa previa* has occurred. Fetal hemorrhage with asphyxia is

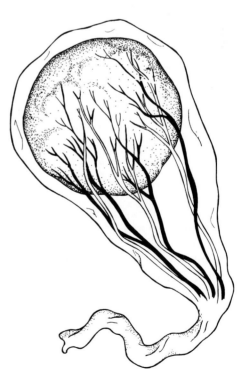

Figure 25–23 Placenta with a velamentous umbilical cord insertion

likely to result because the hemorrhage will probably be diagnosed as maternal.

Cord Length Variations

The average length of the umbilical cord is 55 cm. Although short cords rarely cause complications directly, they have been associated with umbilical hernias in the fetus, abruptio placentae, and cord rupture. Long cords tend to twist and tangle around the fetus, causing transient variable decelerations. A long cord rarely causes fetal death, however, because it is generally not pulled tight until descent at the time of birth. With a long cord and an active fetus, one or more true knots can result. Again, these knots usually are not pulled tight enough to cause fetal distress until the infant has been born, and the cord can then be clamped and cut.

Medical Therapy

Preventing serious fetal complications and examining the newborn for anomalies that coexist with umbilical cord abnormalities are the goals of medical treatment.

In the presence of any vaginal bleeding during labor, continuous monitoring of the fetus is imperative. Monitoring is best done with the aid of the external electronic monitor. Any signs of fetal distress should be reported immediately. In the presence of bleeding, laboratory tests may be used to differentiate fetal from maternal red blood cells. Fetal hemorrhage is resolved by termination of the pregnancy vaginally or through cesarean birth and by correction of neonatal anemia. Expediting the birth, whether vaginally or surgically, is paramount when severe fetal distress is apparent. Following the birth, the pediatric team identifies and/or treats any neonatal complications or anomalies.

❀ *APPLYING THE NURSING PROCESS* ❀

Nursing Assessment

The presence of umbilical abnormalities may not become evident until the birth of the fetus. During labor, the nurse should observe for signs of fetal distress and fetal blood that escapes through the woman's vagina.

Nursing Diagnosis

Nursing diagnoses that may apply include the following:

- Alteration of gas exchange in the fetus: High risk related to decreased blood flow secondary to placental abnormalities
- Knowledge deficit related to lack of information regarding implications and associated problems with placental abnormalities

Nursing Plan and Implementation

The nurse is alert for unusual bleeding during the labor and birth. Following the birth, the placenta is inspected for abnormalities.

Often any mild or moderate variable deceleration can be successfully managed by the nurse. Repositioning of the woman often alleviates pressure on the cord if this is the reason for the deceleration.

Evaluation

Anticipated outcomes of nursing care include the following:

- The mother and baby have a safe labor and birth.
- The woman's bleeding is assessed quickly and corrective measures are taken.
- The family is able to cope successfully with fetal/neonatal anomalies if they exist.

Care of the Woman and Fetus at Risk Due to Amniotic Fluid-Related Complications

Amniotic Fluid Embolism

Amniotic fluid embolism can occur naturally after a tumultuous labor or from oxytocin induction with hypertonic uterine contractions. In the presence of a small tear in the amnion or chorion high in the uterus, the fluid may leak into the chorionic plate and enter the maternal circulation through the gaping venous system. The fluid can also enter at areas of placental separation or cervical tears. Under pressure from the contracting uterus, the fluid is driven into the maternal system. Amniotic fluid embolus occurs more often in multiparas. The incidence is 1 in 15,000 to 20,000 pregnancies, with a mortality rate of 80% (Burrow and Ferris 1988; Chatelain & Quirk 1990).

Maternal Risks

This condition frequently occurs during or after the birth when the woman has had a difficult, rapid labor. Suddenly she experiences respiratory distress, circulatory collapse, acute hemorrhage, and cor pulmonale, as the embolism blocks the vessels of the lungs. The more debris in the amniotic fluid (such as meconium), the greater the maternal problems. The acute hemorrhage is a result of DIC (page 766), which is caused by the thromboplastinlike material found in amniotic fluid, in which factor VII is not essential. It has been demonstrated in vitro and in vivo that mucus, which is also found in amniotic fluid, induces coagulation by activation of factor X.

Maternal mortality is extremely high. In suspected cases in which the women survive, it is difficult to determine whether an amniotic fluid embolism actually occurred.

Fetal-Neonatal Risks

Birth must be facilitated immediately to ensure a live fetus. In many cases the birth has already occurred or the birth can be assisted vaginally with forceps. If labor has been tumultuous, the fetus may suffer problems associated with dysfunctional labor.

Medical Therapy

The goals of medical therapy are to maintain oxygenation, support the cardiovascular system and blood pressure, and assess coagulopathy (Clark 1986).

Any woman exhibiting chest pain, dyspnea, cyanosis, frothy sputum, tachycardia, hypotension, and massive hemorrhage needs the cooperation of every member of the health team if her life is to be saved. Medical and nursing interventions are supportive. Recovery is contingent upon the return of the mother's cardiovascular and respiratory stability. If necessary the birth is assisted to enhance the health of the newborn.

❁ *APPLYING THE NURSING PROCESS* ❁

Nursing Assessment

The nurse must be especially observant for manifestations of amniotic fluid embolism when the labor has been short and difficult. Signs and symptoms of respiratory and circulatory collapse are sudden, acute, and severe and require immediate medical intervention.

Nursing Diagnosis

Nursing diagnoses that may apply in cases of amniotic fluid embolism include the following:

- Alteration of gas exchange: High risk related to anxiety, restlessness, and dyspnea secondary to amniotic fluid embolism
- Fear related to unknown outcome of the complication

Nursing Plan and Implementation

Maintenance of Oxygenation

In the absence of the physician, the nurse administers oxygen under positive pressure until medical help arrives. An intravenous line is quickly established. If respiratory and cardiac arrest occurs, cardiopulmonary resuscitation (CPR) is initiated immediately.

Provision of Cardiovascular Support

The nurse readies the equipment necessary for blood transfusion and for the insertion of the CVP line. As the blood volume is replaced, using fresh blood to provide clotting factors, the CVP is monitored frequently. In the presence of cor pulmonale, fluid overload could easily occur.

When DIC is controlled with fibrinogen replacement, the nurse is responsible for obtaining fibrinogen and other medications needed. Intravenous heparin may be life saving.

Promotion of Fetal-Neonatal Well-Being

As one nurse helps the physician maintain maternal homeostasis, another nurse intervenes as necessary to maintain the well-being of the fetus in utero and the newborn after birth.

Evaluation

Anticipated outcomes of nursing care include the following:

- The woman's signs and symptoms are recognized and corrective measures taken quickly.
- Fetal distress is recognized and corrective measures taken early.
- The mother and her baby are stabilized and no further complications develop.

❁ ❁ ❁ ❁ ❁ ❁ ❁ ❁ ❁ ❁ ❁ ❁

Hydramnios

Hydramnios (also called polyhydramnios) occurs when there is over 2000 mL of amniotic fluid. The exact cause of hydramnios is unknown; however, it often occurs in cases of major congenital anomalies. It is postulated that a major source of amniotic fluid is found in special amnion cells that lie over the placenta (Cunningham et al 1989). During the second half of the pregnancy, the fetus begins to swallow and inspire amniotic fluid and to urinate, which contributes to the amount present. In cases of hydramnios, no pathology has been found in the amniotic epithelium. However, hydramnios is associated with fetal malformations that affect the fetal swallowing mechanism and neurologic disorders in which the fetal meninges are exposed in the amniotic cavity. This condition is also found in cases of anencephaly in which the fetus is thought to urinate excessively due to overstimulation of the cerebrospinal centers. When a monozygotic twin manifests hydramnios, it is possible that the twin with the increased blood volume urinates excessively. The weight of the placenta has been found to be increased in some cases of hydramnios, indicating that increased functioning of the placental tissue may be contributory.

There are two types of hydramnios: chronic and acute. In the chronic type, the fluid volume increases gradually. Most cases are of this variety. In acute cases, the volume increases rapidly over a period of a few days.

Maternal Risks

When the amount of amniotic fluid is over 3000 mL, the woman experiences shortness of breath and edema in the lower extremities from compression of the vena cava. If hydramnios is severe enough, she can experience intense pain. The acute form of hydramnios tends to be more severe. Milder forms of hydramnios occur more frequently and are associated with minimal symptoms. Hydramnios is associated with such maternal disorders as diabetes and Rh sensitization.

Antepartally, if the amniotic fluid is removed too rapidly, abruptio placentae can result from a decreased attachment area. Because of these overstretched fibers, uterine dysfunction can occur intrapartally, and there is increased incidence of postpartal hemorrhage.

Fetal-Neonatal Risks

Fetal malformations and preterm birth are common with hydramnios; thus perinatal mortality is high. Prolapsed cord can occur when the membranes rupture, which adds a further complication for the fetus. The incidence of malpresentations is also increased.

Medical Therapy

Hydramnios is managed with supportive treatment unless the intensity of the woman's distress and symptoms dictate otherwise.

If the accumulation of amniotic fluid is severe enough to cause maternal dyspnea and pain, hospitalization and removal of the excessive fluid are required. This can be done vaginally or by amniocentesis. The dangers of performing the technique vaginally are prolapsed cord and the inability to remove the fluid slowly. If amniocentesis is performed, it should be done with the aid of sonography to prevent inadvertent damage to the fetus and placenta. The fluid should be removed slowly to prevent abruption (Cunningham et al 1989).

When performing amniocentesis it is vital to maintain sterile technique. The nurse can offer support to the couple by explaining the procedure to them. The nurse assists the clinician in interpreting sonographic findings.

❀ *APPLYING THE NURSING PROCESS* ❀

Nursing Assessment

Hydramnios should be suspected when the fundal height increases out of proportion to the gestational age.

CRITICAL THINKING

At only 24 weeks' gestation, what fundal height might indicate hydramnios?

As the amount of fluid increases, the nurse may have difficulty palpating the fetus and auscultating the FHR. In more severe cases, the maternal abdomen appears extremely tense and tight on inspection. On sonography, large spaces can be identified between the fetus and the uterine wall. An anencephalic infant or a dilated fetal stomach resulting from esophageal atresia may also be identified, and multiple gestations may be confirmed. An x-ray fetogram will also show a radiolucent area of space and any fetal skeletal defects.

Nursing Diagnosis

Nursing diagnoses that may apply include the following:

- Alteration in gas exchange: High risk related to pressure on the diaphragm secondary to hydramnios
- Fear related to unknown outcome of the pregnancy

Nursing Plan and Implementation

When amniocentesis is performed, it is vital to maintain sterile technique to prevent infection. The nurse can offer support to the couple by explaining the procedure to them. The nurse assists the clinician in interpreting sonographic findings.

If the fetus has been diagnosed with a congenital defect in utero or is born with the defect, psychologic support is needed to assist the family. Often the nurse collaborates with social services to offer the family this additional help.

Evaluation

Anticipated outcomes of nursing care include the following:

- The woman and her partner understand the procedure, implications, risks, and characteristics that need to be reported to the care giver.

❀ ❀ ❀ ❀ ❀ ❀ ❀ ❀ ❀ ❀ ❀ ❀

Oligohydramnios

Oligohydramnios is defined as a less-than-normal amount (approximately 500 mL is considered normal) of amniotic fluid. Although no exact amount of fluid has been identified, oligohydramnios is diagnosed when, on ultrasound examination, the largest vertical pocket of amniotic fluid is less than 1 cm (Watson & Seeds 1990). Although the cause of oligohydramnios is unknown, it is associated with congenital anomalies (renal agenesis and Potter syndrome), intrauterine growth retardation, early rupture of amniotic membranes (24 to 26 weeks), and postmature syndrome (Watson & Seeds 1990). If oligohydramnios occurs in the first few weeks of pregnancy, there is a danger of fetal adhesions (one part of the fetus may adhere to another part).

Maternal Risks

Labor may be dysfunctional; some women report that labor is more painful.

Fetal-Neonatal Risks

During the gestational period, fetal skin and skeletal abnormalities may occur because fetal movement is impaired as a result of reduced amniotic fluid volume. Because there is less fluid available for the fetus to use during fetal breathing movements, pulmonary hypoplasia may develop. During the labor and birth, the lessened amounts of fluid reduce the cushioning effect for the umbilical cord, and cord compression is more likely to occur.

CRITICAL THINKING

What FHR pattern is associated with cord compression?

Medical Therapy

During the antepartum period oligohydramnios may be suspected when the uterus does not increase in size according to the dates, the fetus is easily palpated and outlined by the examiner, and the fetus is not ballotable. The fetus can be assessed by fetal biophysical profiles, nonstress tests, and serial ultrasound. During labor, the fetus will be monitored by continuous electronic fetal monitoring (EFM) to detect cord compression, which will be indicated by variable decelerations. Some clinicians advocate the use of an amnioinfusion (a transcervical instillation of 200 to 300 mL of sterile saline after membranes have ruptured) to decrease the frequency and severity of variable decelerations in the FHR during labor (Barber et al 1990). The infusion of saline provides more fluid for the umbilical cord to float in and thereby lessens or prevents cord compression.

Nursing Care

Continuous electronic fetal monitoring will be an important part of the assessment during the labor and birth. The nurse will evaluate the EFM tracing for presence of variable decelerations or other nonreassuring signs (such as increasing or decreasing baseline, decreased variability, or presence of late decelerations). If variable decelerations are noted, the woman's position can be changed (to relieve pressure on the umbilical cord) and the physician/nurse-midwife needs to be notified. After the birth, the newborn is evaluated for signs of congenital anomalies, pulmonary hypoplasia and/or postmaturity.

Care of the Woman with Cephalopelvic Disproportion

The birth passage includes the maternal bony pelvis, beginning at the pelvic inlet and ending at the pelvic outlet, and the maternal soft tissues within these anatomic areas. A contracture in any of the described areas can result in cephalopelvic disproportion (CPD). Abnormal fetal pre-

---

Table 25–4 Clues to Contractures of Maternal Pelvis

- Diagonal conjugate <11.5 cm (contracture of inlet), outlet <8 cm (contracture of outlet)
- Unengaged fetal head in early labor in primigravidas (consider contracture of inlet, malpresentation, or malposition)
- Hypotonic uterine contraction pattern (consider contracted pelvis)
- Deflexion of fetal head (fetal head not flexed on fetal chest; may be associated with occiput posterior)
- Uncontrollable pushing prior to complete dilatation of cervix (may be associated with occiput posterior)
- Failure of fetal descent (consider contracture of inlet, midpelvis, or outlet)
- Edema of anterior portion (lip) of cervix (consider obstructed labor at the inlet)

---

sentations and positions occur in CPD as the fetus moves to accommodate to passage through the maternal pelvis.

The gynecoid and anthropoid pelvic types are usually adequate for vertex birth, but the android and platypelloid types predispose to CPD. Certain combinations of types also can result in pelvic diameters inadequate for vertex birth. (See Chapter 13 for a description of the types of pelves and their implications for childbirth.) Clues that may lead to suspicion of contractures of the maternal pelvis are presented in Table 25–4.

Types of Contractures

Contractures of the Inlet

The pelvic inlet is contracted if the shortest anterior-posterior diameter is less than 10 cm or the greatest transverse diameter is less than 12 cm. The anterior-posterior diameter may be approximated by measuring the diagonal conjugate, which in the contracted inlet is less than 11.5 cm. Clinical and x-ray pelvimetry are used to determine the smallest anterior-posterior diameter through which the fetal head must pass. Sonography then can be used to cause transverse arrest of the head, leading to potentially difficult midforceps-assisted birth.

The treatment goal is to allow the natural forces of labor to push the biparietal diameter of the fetal head beyond the potential interspinous obstruction. Although forceps may be used, they cause difficulty because pulling on the head destroys flexion and the space is further diminished. A bulging perineum and crowning indicate that the obstruction has been passed.

Contractures of the Outlet

An interischial tuberous diameter of less than 8 cm constitutes an outlet contracture. Outlet and midpelvic contractures frequently occur simultaneously. Whether vaginal birth can occur depends on the woman's interischial tuberous diameters and the fetal posterosagittal diameter.

Implications of Pelvic Contractures

Maternal Risks

Labor is prolonged and protracted in the presence of CPD, and premature rupture of the membranes (PROM) can result from the force of the unequally distributed contractions being exerted on the fetal membranes. In obstructed labor, uterine rupture can also occur. With protracted (or delayed) descent, necrosis of maternal soft tissues can result from pressure exerted by the fetal head. Eventually necrosis can cause fistulas from the vagina to other nearby structures. Difficult forceps-assisted births can also result in damage to maternal soft tissue.

Fetal-Neonatal Risks

If the membranes rupture and the fetal head has not entered the inlet, there is a grave danger of cord prolapse. Extreme molding of the fetal head can result in skull fracture or intracranial hemorrhage. Traumatic forceps-assisted births can cause damage to the fetal skull and central nervous system.

Medical Therapy

The goal of medical treatment is to assess the maternal pelvis accurately and determine whether CPD is present.

Fetopelvic relationships can be appraised by x-ray pelvimetry when the pregnancy is at term or in early labor. The x-ray pelvimetry provides measurements for the maternal pelvic inlet, midpelvis, outlet, degree of fetal descent, and selected diameters of the fetal head (Figures 25–24, 25–25). When pelvimetry is used in combination with ultrasonography, the mechanisms of labor are even more predictable.

In addition to x-ray pelvimetry, assessment tech-

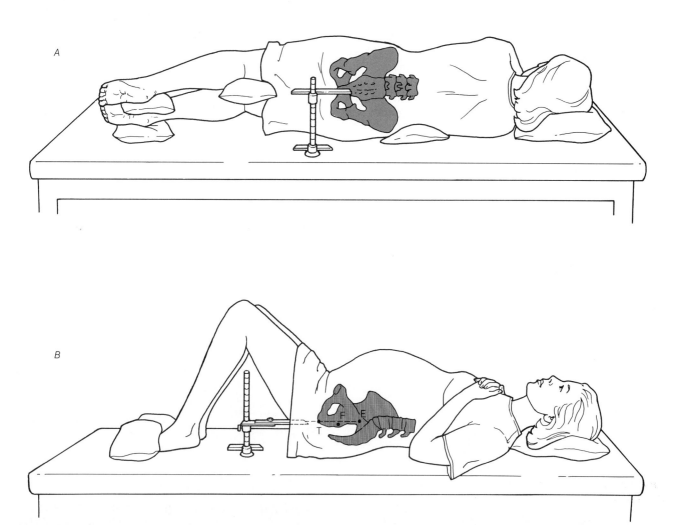

Figure 25–24   Colcher-Sussman method for x-ray pelvimetry. X-ray pelvimetry is obtained by placing a ruler at the level of points to be measured. The markings on the ruler are projected onto the x-ray film and become the known length with which to compare the other measurements. The measurements are recorded on a special chart for interpretation: E = inlet, F = midpelvis, T = outlet. (From Colcher AE, Sussman W: Practical technique for roentgen pelvimetry with new positioning. Am J Roentgenol Ther Nucl Med 1944; 51:207. (c) by American Roentgen Ray Society.)

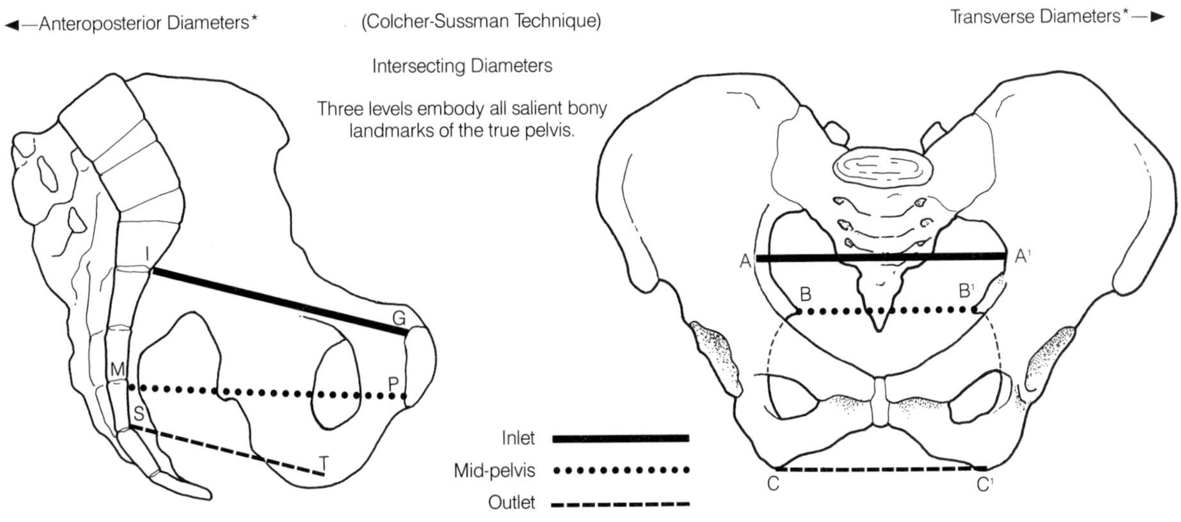

◄—Anteroposterior Diameters*   (Colcher-Sussman Technique)   Transverse Diameters*—►

Intersecting Diameters

Three levels embody all salient bony
landmarks of the true pelvis.

Inlet ▬▬▬▬▬
Mid-pelvis ••••••••••
Outlet ‐‐‐‐‐‐‐‐‐

			Total	Average Normal	Average Total	Low Normal
ACTUAL INLET	Anteroposterior	I to G		12.5	25.5	22.0
	Transverse	A to A¹		13.0		
MID-PELVIS	Anteroposterior	M to P		11.5	22.0	20.0
	Transverse (Bispinous)	B to B¹		10.5		
OUTLET	Anteroposterior (Post. Sagittal)	S to T		7.5	18.0	16.0
	Transverse (Bituberal)	C to C¹		10.5		

FETAL HEAD	Anteroposterior View	Longest Diameter	Shortest Diameter	Average (10cm) . . . .
	Lateral View	Longest Diameter	Shortest Diameter	

Position of Fetal Head: Separation of Symphysis:
Position of Fetal Spine: Coccyx:
Location of Vertex: Sacrum:
Moulding of Fetal Head: Sub-Pubic Angle: (75°)
Remarks:

Shape of inlet

Round ●   Flat ▬●

Oval ●   Heart ♥

Figure 25–25   X-ray pelvimetry chart. The assessed diameters are recorded on the chart. Average normals are identified for the inlet, midpelvis, and outlet. The chart also identifies low normal measurements.

niques, such as careful manual examination of the pelvis and magnetic resonance imaging (MRI) are used to identify inadequate diameters and determine the treatment plan.

When the pelvic diameters are borderline or questionable, a trial of labor (TOL) may be advised. In this process, the woman continues to labor and careful, frequent assessments of cervical dilatation and fetal descent are made by the physician and nurse. As long as there is continued progress, the TOL continues. If progress ceases, the decision for a cesarean birth is made.

❦   *APPLYING THE NURSING PROCESS*   ❦

Nursing Assessment

The adequacy of the maternal pelvis for a vaginal birth should be assessed intrapartally as well as antepartally. Dur-

ing the intrapartal assessment, the size of the fetus and its presentation, position, and lie must also be considered. (See Chapter 22 for intrapartal assessment techniques).

The nurse should suspect CPD when labor is prolonged, cervical dilatation and effacement are slow, and engagement of the presenting part is delayed.

Nursing Diagnosis

Nursing diagnoses that may apply include the following:

- Knowledge deficit related to lack of information regarding implications and associated complications of CPD
- Fear related to unknown outcome of labor

Nursing Plan and Implementation

Promotion of Maternal and Fetal Well-Being

Nursing actions during the TOL are similar to care during any labor with the exception that the assessments of cervical dilatation and fetal descent are more frequent. Contractions should be monitored continuously, and the labor progress may be charted on the Friedman graph. The fetus should also be monitored continuously. Any signs of fetal distress are reported to the physician immediately.

Position Changes to Increase Pelvic Diameters

The woman may be positioned in a variety of ways to increase the pelvic diameters. Sitting or squatting increases the outer diameters and may be effective in instances where there is failure of or slow fetal descent. Changing from one side to the other, and/or maintaining a hands-and-knees position may assist the fetus in occiput-posterior position to change to an occiput-anterior position. The woman may instinctively want to assume one of these positions. If not, the nurse may encourage a change of position.

Provision of Emotional Support

A couple may need support in coping with the stresses of complicated labor. The nurse should keep the couple informed of what is happening and explain the procedures that are being used. This knowledge can reassure the couple that measures are being taken to resolve the problem.

Evaluation

Anticipated outcomes of nursing care include the following:

- The woman's fear is lessened.
- The woman has additional knowledge regarding the problems, implications, and treatment plans.

❀ ❀ ❀ ❀ ❀ ❀ ❀ ❀ ❀ ❀ ❀ ❀

Care of the Woman at Risk Due to Complications of Third and Fourth Stages

Lacerations

Lacerations of the cervix or vagina may be indicated when bright red vaginal bleeding persists in the presence of a well-contracted uterus. The incidence of lacerations is higher when the childbearing woman is young or a nullipara, has an epidural, has forceps-assisted birth and an episiotomy (Bromberg 1986), and has not done perineal massage or preparation during pregnancy (Avery & Burket 1986). Vaginal and perineal lacerations are often categorized in terms of degree, as follows:

- First-degree laceration is limited to the fourchet, perineal skin, and vaginal mucous membrane.
- Second-degree laceration involves the perineal skin, vaginal mucous membrane, underlying fascia, and muscles of the perineal body; it may extend upward on one or both sides of the vagina.
- Third-degree laceration extends through the perineal skin, vaginal mucous membranes, and perineal body and involves the anal sphincter; it may extend up the anterior wall of the rectum.
- Fourth-degree laceration is the same as the third degree but extends through the rectal mucosa to the lumen of the rectum; it may be called a third-degree laceration with a rectal wall extension.

Placenta Accreta

The chronic villi attach directly to the myometrium of the uterus in *placenta accreta*. Two other types of placental adherence are *placenta increta*, in which the myometrium is invaded, and *placenta percreta*, in which the myometrium is penetrated. The adherence itself may be total, partial, or focal, depending on the amount of placental involvement. The incidence of placenta accreta is 1 in 2000 to 3570 births (Zahn & Yeomans 1990). Placenta accreta is the most common type of adherent placenta and accounts for 80%, while 15% of adherent placentas are placenta increta, and 5% are placenta percreta (Zahn & Yeomans 1990).

The primary complication with placenta accreta is maternal hemorrhage and failure of the placenta to separate following birth of the infant. An abdominal hysterectomy may be the necessary treatment, depending on the amount and depth of involvement.

For further discussion of hemorrhage following birth see Chapter 36.

Inversion of Uterus

Uterine inversion occurs when the fundus of the uterus is prolapsed, inside out, through the cervix (Barber et al 1990). The incidence of uterine rupture is approximately 1 in 2500 births (Zahn & Yeomans 1990). It can be caused by a lax uterine wall coupled with undue tension on an umbilical cord when the placenta has not separated. Forceful pressure on the fundus with a dilated cervix and sudden emptying of the uterine contents may be contributing factors. Maternal bleeding occurs in 94% of women, and blood loss ranges from 800 to 1800 mL (Zahn & Yeomans 1990).

Restoration of the uterus to its normal position manually or by surgical intervention is the goal of medical treatment. The uterus is replaced manually by grasping the vaginal mass, spreading the cervical ring with the fingers and thumb, and steadily forcing the fundus upward. The woman is often placed under deep anesthesia for this procedure.

Complicated Childbirth: Effects on the Family and the Role of the Nurse

A complicated pregnancy and difficult labor and birth are crisis situations that can test the coping mechanisms of every individual involved. The family may respond to the crisis in relatively typical ways or may respond dysfunctionally.

During the antepartal period of a normal, low-risk pregnancy, resolution of any ambivalence about the pregnancy usually occurs when fetal movement is felt. With a complicated pregnancy, feelings of ambivalence may continue as the family experiences fear and anxiety about the woman's health and the health and welfare of the fetus. Hostile behaviors and feelings of guilt may be displayed as a woman questions her ability to bear healthy children, a father blames himself for the pregnancy, or the family accuses the health care team of poor management.

If a pregnancy is going well, the parents begin to develop a desire to nurture and love their child as they prepare for their parenting role. With a complicated pregnancy, the uncertainty about the outcome for the fetus inhibits the parents' ability to adapt to the pregnancy and hinders the evolvement of feelings of adequacy as parents.

When an infant is stillborn or dies following birth, the couple must mourn and deal with the pain of detaching themselves. As the parents respond to their loss, they experience the anger, guilt, pain, and sadness associated with the grieving process.

Parents of an ill or deformed infant must not only resolve their feelings of guilt and grief, but they must also prepare themselves to care for that child. This couple may be unable to face the possibility that their infant may not survive. They may doubt their ability to care properly for the child. The great costs of caring for the high-risk child may create financial difficulties for the family. The emotional toll of caring for such a child may also be extreme.

The birth of an ill, abnormal, or stillborn infant presents the couple with the reality that they may have been fearing throughout the pregnancy. It is imperative that the medical and nursing staff respond in supportive ways. Maintaining communication and providing support for the woman and her family is important. At times nurses are reluctant to say anything to the parents because they are searching for the "right words." In reality, it is reassuring to know that any words which are offered in genuine support and with a sense of caring are "right."

When a malformed infant is born, powerful reactions are not unusual even among care givers. Such a child is frequently the focus of a great deal of staff attention in the nursery. After they have seen the newborn, they feel shock and sadness similar to that experienced by the parents. This reaction is especially common for those who have had little experience with congenital anomalies. In an effort to deal with their reactions, they have a tendency to avoid the parents. In such instances it is frequently helpful to provide the staff with occasions to talk through their feelings so that they can be more supportive of the family's grief. In some centers with intensive care nurseries, this practice has been formalized through regular staff meetings and has been of great benefit to staff and, indirectly, to families.

Providing emotional support to the family is a vital nursing role. When a labor is complicated or when the fetus dies, the woman should have consistent support and not be left alone. The partner should be encouraged to remain, and the nurse should be present to observe the woman or couple and to provide support. By attending and

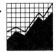

Research Note

Clinical Application of Research

Margaret Kearney and her associates (1990) examined the relationships among type of birth, time of initial breast-feeding, and duration of breast-feeding. Additionally, they studied whether mothers who had given birth by cesarean had more pain and fatigue associated with breast-feeding than mothers who had given birth vaginally.

Results revealed that the group of mothers who had given birth vaginally was significantly different from those who had given birth by cesarean section on the variables of timing of first breast-feeding following the birth and satisfaction with labor and birth. The mean time for first feeding for cesarean mothers was 11 hours compared to 4.5 hours for the other group. Mothers of vaginally born infants were more satisfied with their labor and birth. Multiple regression analysis found no significant relationship between week of weaning in the first 6 months and time of first breast-feeding or type of birth. No significant difference was found between the groups in duration of breast-feeding. Only one time frame, at two months, showed a significant difference between the groups in terms of breast-feeding problems. The researchers concluded that the supportive hospital environment present in this study and maternal commitment to breast-feeding counteracted negative events associated with birth.

Critical Thinking Applied to Research

Strengths: Tested for homogeneity of variance in order not to violate assumptions of statistical test (student t) used for part of the analysis.

Concerns: This study was part of a larger study which required a 6-week commitment to breast-feeding and might have communicated experimenter expectations to the subjects.

Kearney M, Cronenwett L, Reinhardt R: Cesarean delivery and breastfeeding outcomes. *Birth* 1990; 17(2): 97.

responding with empathy, the nurse helps the couple acknowledge their loss and begin their grieving process. Using comfort measures to meet basic needs also demonstrates a caring attitude.

When a malformed infant is born, the couple must deal with their mourning and with the future needs of their child. Attachment may be facilitated by keeping parents and their newborn together as much as possible. The newborn can frequently be returned to the parents after a brief physical assessment in the nursery. The contact between the parents and infant may ultimately be a source of great satisfaction to the parents.

❀ ❀

KEY CONCEPTS

Stress, anxiety, and fear have a profound effect on labor, particularly when complications occur that imply maternal or fetal jeopardy.

A hypertonic labor pattern is characterized by painful contractions that are not effective in effacing and dilating the cervix. It usually leads to a prolonged latent phase.

Hypotonic labor patterns begin normally and then progress to infrequent, less intense contractions. If there are no contraindications, IV oxytocin is used as treatment.

Prolonged labor lasts more than 24 hours.

Precipitous labor is extremely rapid labor that lasts for less than three hours. It is associated with an increased risk to the mother and newborn infant.

The occiput posterior position of the fetus during labor prolongs the labor process, causes severe back discomfort in the laboring woman, and predisposes her to vaginal and perineal trauma and lacerations during birth.

The types of fetal malpresentations include face, brow, breech, and shoulder.

A fetus/newborn weighing more than 4000 g is termed *macrosomic.* Problems may occur during labor, birth, and in the early neonatal period.

Preventing and treating problems that infringe on the development and birth of normal fetuses are significant medical-nursing activities once the presence of twins has been detected.

Intrauterine fetal death poses a major nursing challenge to provide support and caring for the parents.

Major bleeding problems in the intrapartal period are abruptio placentae and placenta previa.

❀ ❀

References

Abdella TN, Sibae BM, Hays JM Jr et al: Perinatal outcome in abruptio placentae. *Obstet Gynecol* 1984; 63:365.

Andrews DB, Sachs BP, Friedman EA: Risk factors for shoulder dystocia. *Obstet Gynecol* 1985; 66:762.

Avery MD, Burket BA: Effect of perineal massage on the incidence of episiotomy and perineal laceration in a nurse-midwifery service. *J Nurse-Midwifery* May/June 1986; 31:128.

Barber KRK, Fields DH, Kaufman SA: *Quick Reference to OB-GYN Procedures,* 3rd ed. Philadelphia: Lippincott, 1990.

Beckey RD et al: Development of a perinatal grief checklist. *JOGNN* May/June 1985; 14:194.

Berk MA, Mimouni F, Miodovnik M et al: Macrosomia in infants of insulin-dependent diabetic mothers. *Pediatrics* June 1989; 83:1029.

Blackburn C, Copley R: One precious moment: what you can offer when a newborn infant dies. Nursing 1989; 19:52.

Bromberg MH: Presumptive maternal benefits of routine episiotomy: A literature review. *J Nurse-Midwifery* May/June 1986; 11:170.

Burrow GN, Ferris TF: *Medical Complications During Pregnancy.* Philadelphia: Saunders, 1988.

Campbell B: Overdue delivery: Its impact on mothers-to-be. *MCN* May/June 1986; 11:170.

Carr D, Knupp SF: Grief and perinatal loss: A community hospital approach to support. *JOGNN* March/April 1985; 14:130.

Chatelain SM, Quirk JG: Amniotic and thromboembolism. *Clin Obstet Gynecol* September 1990; 33:473.

Clark SL et al: Squamous cells in the maternal pulmonary circulation. *Am J Obstet Gynecol* January 1986; 154:104.

Combs CA, Murphy EL, Laros RK: Factors associated with postpartum hemorrhage with vaginal birth. *Obstet Gynecol* January 1991; 77:69.

Cordell AS, Thomas N: Fathers and grieving: Coping with infant death. *J Perinatol* 1989; 10:75.

Cruikshank DP: Malpresentations and umbilical cord complications. In: *Danforth's Obstetrics and Gynecology,* 6th ed. Scott JR, DiSaia PJ, Hammond CB et al (editors). Philadelphia: Lippincott, 1990.

Cucco C, Osborne MA, Cibils LA: Maternal-fetal outcomes in prolonged pregnancy. *Am J Obstet Gynecol* 1989; 161:916.

Cunningham FG, MacDonald PC, Gant NF: *Williams Obstetrics,* 18th ed. Norwalk CT: Appleton & Lange, 1989.

Danskin FH, Neilson JP: Twin-to-twin transfusion syndrome: What are appropriate diagnostic criteria? *Am J Obstet Gynecol* 1989; 161:365.

Eden RD: Postdate pregnancy: Antenatal assessment of fetal well-being. *Clin Obstet Gynecol* June 1989; 32:235.

Furrh CB, Copley R: One precious moment. *Nursing 89* September 1989; 52.

Gilson GJ, O'Brien M, Vera RW et al: Prolonged pregnancy and the biophysical profile: A birthing center perspective. *J Nurse-Midwifery* July/August 1988; 33:171.

Gocke SE, Nageotte MP, Garite T et al: Management of the non-vertex second twin: Primary cesarean section, external version, or primary breech extraction. *Am J Obstet Gynecol* 1989; 161:111.

Gonik B, Allen R, Sorab J: Objective evaluation of the shoulder dystocia phenomenon: Effect of maternal pelvic orientation on force reduction. *Obstet Gynecol* 1989; 74:44.

Gross TL, Sokol RJ, Williams R et al: Shoulder dystocia: A fetal-physician risk. *Am J Obstet Gynecol* June 1987; 156:408.

Hollenbach KA, Hickok DE: Epidemiology and diagnosis of twin gestation. *Clin Obstet Gynecol* March 1990; 33:3.

Hunter LP: Twin gestation: Antepartum management. *J Perinat Neonatal Nurs* 1989; 3:1.

Jackson VM: Delivery of the second twin. *J Perinat Neonatal Nurs* 1989; 3(1):22.

Karegaard M, Gennser G: Incidence and recurrence rate of abruptio placenta in Sweden. *Obstet Gynecol* 1986; 67:523.

Kelton JG, Cruickshank: Hematologic disorders of pregnancy. In *Medical Complications During Pregnancy.* Burrow GN, Ferris TF (editors). Philadelphia: Saunders, 1988.

Kovacs BW, Kirschbaum TH, Paul RH: Twin gestations: I. Antenatal care and complications. *Obstet Gynecol* 1989; 74:313.

Kübler-Ross E: *On Death and Dying.* New York: Macmillan, 1969.

Lavery JP: Placenta previa. *Clinic Obstet Gynecol* September 1990; 33:414.

Lederman RP: *Psycho-Social Adaptation in Pregnancy.* Englewood Cliffs NJ: Prentice Hall, 1984.

Lederman RP, Lederman E, Work B: Anxiety and epinephrine in multiparous women in labor: Relationship to duration of labor and fetal heart rate pattern. *Obstet Gynecol* 1985; 153:870.

Lindell SG: Education for discharge: a time for change. *JOGNN* Mar/Apr 1988; 17(2):108.

Lowe TW, Cunningham FG: Placental abruption. *Clin Obstet Gynecology* September 1990; 33:406.

Mashburn J: Identification and management of shoulder dystocia. J Nurse Midwife Sept/Oct 1988; 33(5):225.

Neifert M, Thorpe J: Twins: Family adjustment, parenting, and infant feeding in the fourth trimester. *Clin Obstet Gynecol* March 1990; 33:102.

Oxorn H: *Oxorn-Foote Human Labor and Birth,* 5th ed. Norwalk, CT: Appleton-Century-Crofts, 1986.

Phelan JP: Uterine rupture. *Clin Obstet Gynecol* September 1990; 33:432.

Phelan JP: Postdatism. *Clin Obstet Gynecol* June 1989; 32:219.

Polin JI, Frangipane WL: Current concepts in management of obstetric problems for pediatricians: II. Modern concepts in the management of multiple gestation. *Pediatr Clin North Am* 1986; 33:649.

Rodriguez H: Ultrasound evaluation of the postdate pregnancy. *Clin Obstet Gynecol* June 1989; 32:257.

Rodriguez MH, Masaki DI, Phelan JP et al: Uterine rupture: Are intrauterine pressure catheters useful in the diagnosis? *Obstet Gynecol* 1989; 161:666.

Sakala EP: Obstetric management of conjoined twins. *Obstet Gynecol* 1986; 67:21S.

Schwiebert P, Kirk P: *When Hello Means Goodbye.* Oregon Health Sciences University, 1985.

Scott JR, DiSaia PJ, Hammond CB et al: *Danforth's Obstetrics and Gynecology,* 6th ed. Philadelphia: Lippincott, 1990.

Sims ME, Walther FJ: Neonatal morbidity and mortality and long-term outcome of postdate infants. *Clin Obstet Gynecol* June 1989; 32:285.

Smeltzer JS: Prevention and management of shoulder dystocia. *Clin Obstet Gynecol* 1986; 29:229.

Spellacy WN: The postdate pregnancy. In: *Danforth's Obstetrics and Gynecology,* 6th ed. Scott JR, DiSaia PJ, Hammond CB et al (editors). Philadelphia: Lippincott, 1990.

Tamura RK, Sabbagha RE: Altered fetal growth. In *Gynecology and Obstetrics.* Vol. 3. Depp R, Eshenbach DA, Sciarra JJ (editors). Philadelphia: Lippincott, 1990.

Theroux R: Multiple birth: A unique parenting experience. *J Perinat Neonatal Nurs* 1989; 3:35.

Veille JC et al: The effect of a calcium channel blocker (nifedipine) in uterine blood flow in the pregnant goat. *Am J Obstet Gynecol* 1986; 154:1160.

Watson WJ, Seeds JW: Diagnostic Obstetric Imaging. In: *Gynecology and Obstetrics.* Dilts PV, Sciarra JJ (editors). Philadelphia: Lippincott, 1990.

Additional Readings

Allen R et al: Risk factors for shoulder dystocia: An engineering study of clinician-applied forces. *Obstet Gynecol* March 1991; 77:352.

Anderson A, Anderson B: Toward a substantive theory of mother-twin attachment. *MCN* November/December 1990; 15:373.

Borlum KG: Third trimester fetal death in triplet pregnancies. *Obstet Gynecol* January 1991; 77:6.

Green NL: Stressful events related to childbearing in African-American women: A pilot study. *J Nurse-Midwifery* July/August 1990; 35:231.

Jones JS, Newman RB, Miller MC: Cross-sectional analysis of triplet birth weight. *Am J Obstet Gynecol* January 1991; 164:135.

Kline-Kaye V, Miller-Slade D: The use of fundal pressure during the second stage of labor. *JOGNN* November/December 1990; 19:511.

Lieberman JR, Fraser D, Kasis A et al: Reduced frequency of hypertensive disorders in placenta previa. *Obstet Gynecol* January 1991; 77:83.

Luegenbiehl DL, Brophy GH, Artigue GS: Standardized assessment of blood loss. *MCN* July/August 1990; 15:241.

Read-Sisti D: A dream dies. *MCN* July/August 1990; 15:258.

CHAPTER 26

Obstetric Procedures:

The Role of the Nurse

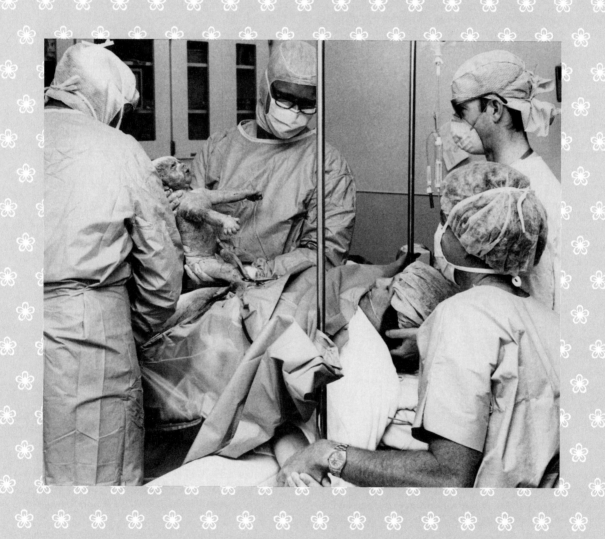

OBJECTIVES

Examine the methods of external and internal version and the related nursing interventions.

Discuss the use of amniotomy in current maternity care.

Compare methods for inducing labor, explaining their advantages and disadvantages.

Describe the types of episiotomies performed, the rationale for each, and the associated nursing interventions.

Describe the indications for forceps-assisted birth and the type of forceps that may be used.

Discuss the use of vacuum extraction, including indications, procedure, complications, and related nursing interventions.

Determine the indications for cesarean birth, the impact on the family unit, preparation and teaching needs, and associated nursing interventions.

Discuss vaginal birth following previous cesarean birth.

❀ ❀

As women in childbirth we bring our complete selves to the experience: body, mind, emotions, habits, past experiences, lessons to be learned . . . a woman births as she lives, expressing this continuity of birth within the rest of a woman's life. (Birthing Normally: A Personal Growth Approach to Childbirth)

Most births occur without the need for operative obstetric intervention. In some instances, however, obstetric procedures are necessary to maintain safety for the woman and the fetus. The most common obstetric procedures are induction of labor, episiotomy, cesarean birth, and vaginal birth following a previous cesarean birth.

Most women are aware of the possible need for an obstetric procedure during their birth; however, some women expect to have a "natural" labor and birth and do not anticipate the need for any medical intervention. This conflict between expectation and the need for intervention presents a challenge to maternity nurses. The nurse can provide information regarding any procedure to make sure the woman and her partner understand what is proposed, the anticipated benefits and possible risks, and any possible alternative treatments.

Care of the Woman During Version

Version, or turning the fetus, is a procedure used to change the fetal presentation by abdominal or intrauterine manipulation. The most common type of version is **external** (or cephalic) version. In an external version the presentation of the fetus is changed from a breech to a cephalic presentation by external manipulation of the maternal abdomen

(Figure 26–1). The other type of version, called **internal** (or podalic) version is used only with the second twin during a vaginal birth. In an internal version the obstetrician places her/his hand inside the uterus and grabs the fetus' feet. The fetus is then turned from a transverse or cephalic to a breech presentation (Figure 26–2).

External Version

If breech or shoulder presentation (transverse lie) is detected in the later weeks of pregnancy, an external version may be attempted. The version is usually done after 37 weeks' gestation because most fetuses still in breech presentation at this time will not spontaneously convert to a vertex presentation. After the version, 75% of fetuses will remain in cephalic presentation. The other 25% spontaneously convert back to a breech presentation (Dyson et al 1986).

The requirements for external version include the following (Cunningham et al 1989):

- The presenting part is not engaged.
- A normal amount of amniotic fluid is present and the amniotic membrane is intact.
- There is a reactive nonstress test (NST) and there are no signs of fetal distress.
- The woman is not obese (obesity makes manipulation of the fetus very difficult).

External Version Procedure

The external version is accomplished in a birthing unit, rather than an outpatient setting, in case further intervention (such as an emergency cesarean birth) is necessary. As the woman is admitted, the nurse begins her assessment by ensuring that no contraindications are present. Contraindications include ruptured membranes, nonreactive

783

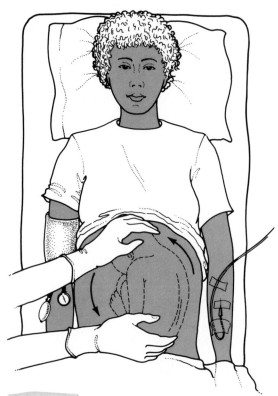

Figure 26–1 *External (or cephalic) version of the fetus. The technique involves pressure on the fetal head and buttocks so that the fetus completes a "backward flip" or a "forward roll."*

stress test, presence of uterine contractions, intrauterine growth retardation (IUGR), placenta previa, or previous cesarean birth. If no contraindications are present the nurse then assesses maternal vital signs and fetal heart rate (FHR) to establish a baseline and an NST is done to ascertain reactivity of the FHR. The fetus is then monitored continuously by electronic fetal monitoring (EFM). An ultrasound exam is completed by the physician just prior to the version to confirm the fetal presentation and locate the placenta. After these initial assessments, intravenous ritodrine or terbutaline is given to achieve uterine relaxation. The obstetrician does the version by rotating the fetus in a backward or forward flip (Figure 26–1) and holds it in the new position as the intravenous infusion is discontinued. The version is discontinued immediately in the presence of severe maternal discomfort or significant fetal bradycardia (less than 90 beats per minute for more than 60 seconds) or if the attempt is unsuccessful after a maximum of 15 minutes (Dyson et al 1986).

Nursing Care

The nurse completes the assessments previously discussed and continues to monitor maternal blood pressure and

pulse about every 5 minutes throughout the version and for about 30 minutes after. Assessment of the maternal-fetal response to the ritodrine or terbutaline are also done (see Drug Guide, page 501). The nurse also provides information for the woman and her partner. The admission period and time when the initial NST is performed are excellent opportunities for client teaching. The woman should be encouraged to express her understanding and expectation of the procedure, verbalize her fears, and ask questions. The possibility of failure of the procedure and need for cesarean birth if the fetus becomes distressed should be discussed. Explaining what will occur in either of these circumstances will better prepare the woman if intervention becomes necessary.

Care of the Woman During an Amniotomy

Amniotomy is the artificial rupture of the amniotic membranes (AROM). It is probably the most common operative procedure in obstetrics. Since the amniotomy requires that an instrument be inserted through the cervix, there needs to be at least 2 cm of cervical dilatation present. The amniotomy may be performed as a method of induction of labor (to stimulate the beginning of labor) or it may be done at any time during the first stage of labor. Amniotomy may also be done during labor to allow access to the fetus to apply an internal fetal heart monitoring electrode to the fetal scalp, to insert an intrauterine pressure catheter, or to obtain a fetal scalp blood sample for acid-base determination.

Amniotomy seems to be a successful method of labor induction. When there is a favorable cervix (some cervical dilatation and effacement), 85% to 90% of women have an onset of labor within 12 hours of AROM (Nugent 1989).

Amniotomy as a method of labor induction has the following advantages:

1. The contractions elicited are similar to those of spontaneous labor.

2. There is usually no risk of hypertonus or rupture of the uterus, as with intravenous oxytocin induction.

3. The woman does not require the same intensive monitoring as with intravenous oxytocin induction.

4. Electronic fetal monitoring is facilitated because once the membranes are ruptured a fetal scalp electrode may be applied, an intrauterine catheter may be inserted, and scalp blood sampling for pH determinations may be done to assist in evaluating a fetal heart rate pattern.

5. The color and composition of amniotic fluid can be evaluated.

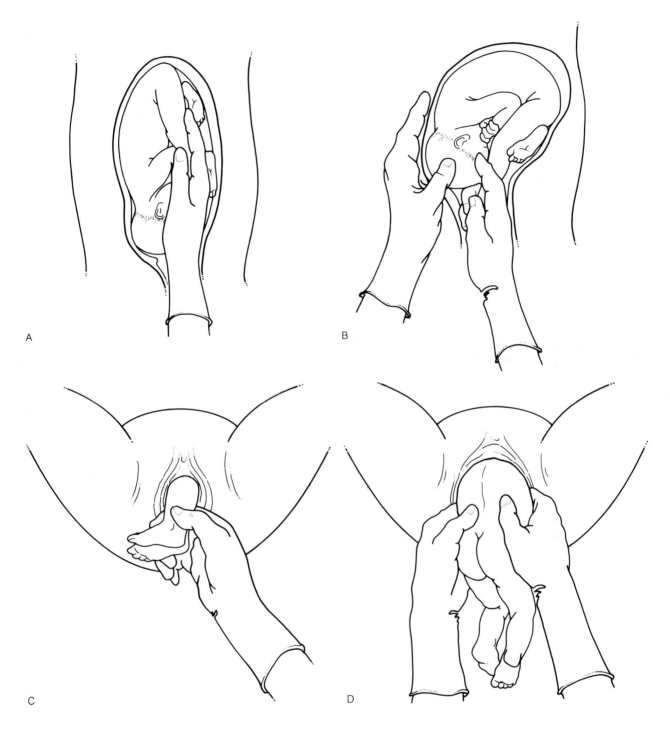

Figure 26–2 **Podalic version and extraction of the fetus is used to assist in the vaginal birth of the second twin.** *A The physician reaches into the uterus and grasps a foot. Although a vertex birth is always preferred, in this instance of assisting in the birth of a second twin, it is not possible to grasp any other fetal part. The fetal head would be too large to grasp and pull downward, and grasping the fetal arm would result in a transverse lie and make vaginal birth impossible. B While applying pressure on the outside of the abdomen to push the baby's head up toward the top of the uterus with one hand, the physician pulls the baby's foot down toward the cervix. C Both feet have been pulled through the cervix and vagina. D The physician now grasps the baby's trunk and continues to pull downward on the baby to assist the birth.*

The disadvantages of amniotomy are as follows:

1. Once an amniotomy is done, birth must occur because microorganisms can now invade the intrauterine cavity and cause amnionitis.

2. The danger of a prolapsed cord is increased once the membranes have ruptured, especially if the fetal presenting part is not firmly pressed down against the cervix.

3. Compression and molding of the fetal head are increased due to loss of the cushioning effect of the amniotic fluid for the fetal head during uterine contractions.

4. Labor may not be successfully induced, necessitating cesarean birth.

AROM Procedure

Before an amniotomy is performed, the fetus is assessed for presentation, position, and station. Unless the fetal head is well engaged in the pelvis, some obstetricians do not advocate an amniotomy because of the danger of prolapsed cord. Other risks are abruptio placentae (due to rapid decompression of the uterus with the rapid loss of amniotic fluid), infection (due to the introduction of organisms into the cervix and intrauterine cavity), and amniotic fluid embolus (due to rapid decompression of the uterus and small amounts of fluid entering the maternal vascular system from under the edge of the placenta).

 While performing a sterile vaginal examination, the physician/certified nurse-midwife introduces an amnihook (or other rupturing device) into the vagina. A small tear is made in the amniotic membrane. Following rupture of the membranes, amniotic fluid is allowed to escape.

Nursing Care

Prior to the procedure the physician/certified nurse-midwife needs to provide the client with information regarding the AROM procedure, its purpose, anticipated benefits, and risks. The nurse can assess client understanding and be available for further discussion or for additional questions. Prior to the AROM it is helpful to explain the sensations that the laboring woman will feel in order to decrease her anxiety. The laboring woman can expect to feel the draining of the amniotic fluid onto her perineum but usually she will not feel discomfort.

It is imperative that the FHR be auscultated before and immediately after the procedure so that any changes from the previous FHR pattern can be noted. If changes are marked at the time of AROM, the physician/certified nurse-midwife should check for prolapse of the cord by vaginal exam. The amniotic fluid should be inspected for amount, color, odor, and presence of meconium or blood. The findings are documented in the chart and on the fetal monitoring strip. If meconium is present, the nurse can inform the woman to expect some special interventions at the birth. The naso-oro-pharynx will be suctioned with a suction device mucus trap as soon as the head is born, and after birth a laryngoscope will be used to visualize the vocal cords. If meconium is present at or below the cords, further deep suctioning is done. These interventions are completed in order to help prevent meconium aspiration syndrome.

Care of the Woman During Prostaglandin Administration

Prostaglandin E_2 (PGE_2) vaginal suppositories are used extensively in the management of intrauterine fetal demise in the second trimester of pregnancy. However, the FDA has not approved the use of prostaglandin induction if the fetus is alive (Dunn 1990). Currently, prostaglandin gel (2 to 5 mg in 10 mL of hydroxycellulose gel) is being used for softening the cervix (called cervical ripening) in preparation for an induction with oxytocin (Dunn 1990). Researchers report that preinduction use of prostaglandin results in a higher success rate for inductions, shorter induction time, and lower cesarean birth rates (Dunn 1990).

There are few maternal contraindications to PGE_2 gel. The presence of a fundal uterine scar is a contraindication because previous studies have documented uterine rupture. Amnionitis is also a contraindication because of the increased uterine irritability that accompanies this infection. Women with cardiac disease have routinely been excluded from PGE_2 studies, although the physiologic rationale for this decision has not been established (Jacobs 1989).

Maternal side effects of prostaglandin administration usually include nausea, vomiting, and diarrhea, which results from stimulation of the gastrointestinal smooth muscle. Most side effects are thought to be dose dependent, so the higher the dose the more likely the woman will have side effects (Jacobs 1989).

Prostaglandin Gel Insertion Procedure

Two common methods are used to insert the PGE_2 gel. The gel may be placed into a diaphragm such as those used for contraceptive purposes. The physician then inserts the diaphragm into the vagina and places it up against the cervix. The other method involves first placing the diaphragm against the cervix. A small catheter is then introduced into the vagina and the tip of the catheter is placed into the diaphragm. The PGE_2 gel is then injected through the catheter. This method ensures placement of the gel in the diaphragm and keeps gel from being dispensed against the vaginal tissues as the diaphragm is inserted.

Nursing Care

In some institutional protocols, the nurse may draw up the gel into the syringe in preparation for the insertion by the physician. After the insertion, the uterus is assessed for the presence of contractions and the FHR is evaluated (by auscultation or EFM) to determine fetal response and condition. The woman is monitored for the development of any side effects.

Care of the Woman During Induction of Labor

The American College of Obstetricians and Gynecologists (ACOG) defines **induction of labor** as the initiation of uterine contractions before the spontaneous onset of labor by medical and/or surgical means for the purpose of accomplishing birth (ACOG 1988a). The procedure may be either elective or indicated.

Elective induction is defined as the initiation of labor for convenience. In general, ACOG guidelines do not recommend elective induction (ACOG 1988a).

Indicated induction may be considered in the presence of a preexisting maternal disease (such as diabetes mellitus, renal disease, chronic obstructive pulmonary disease (COPD), pregnancy-induced hypertension (PIH), premature rupture of the membranes (PROM), chorioamnionitis, fetal demise, postterm gestation, and logistic factors (such as risk of rapid labor or distance from the hospital) (ACOG 1988a). Additional indications include severe fetal hemolytic disease, IUGR and mild abruptio placentae with no fetal distress (Dunn 1990).

The most frequently used methods of induction are amniotomy, intravenous oxytocin (Pitocin) infusion, or both. The use of PGE₂ to induce labor is currently being investigated.

Oxytocin infusion is discussed later in this section. See page 784 for discussion of amniotomy.

Contraindications

All contraindications to spontaneous labor and vaginal birth are contraindications to the induction of labor (Dunn 1990).

Relative maternal contraindications include but are not limited to the following (ACOG 1988):

- Client refusal
- Placenta previa or vasa previa
- Abnormal fetal presentation
- Cord presentation
- Presenting part above the pelvic inlet
- Prior classic uterine incision
- Active genital herpes infection
- Pelvic structural deformities or cephalopelvic disproportion
- Invasive cervical carcinoma

Fetal contraindications are as follows:

- Severe fetal distress or abnormal results of contraction stress test.
- Low-birth-weight or preterm fetus

Before induction is attempted, appropriate assessment must indicate that both the woman and fetus are ready for the onset of labor. This includes evaluation of fetal maturity and cervical readiness.

Labor Readiness

Fetal Maturity

Early diagnosis of pregnancy with adequate recorded data during the early months of pregnancy, including serial sonograms, is helpful in determining the expected date of birth. External abdominal examination of the growing uterus and amniotic fluid studies are also beneficial in assessing fetal maturity.

Cervical Readiness

The findings on vaginal examination will help determine whether cervical changes favorable for induction have occurred. Bishop (1964) developed a prelabor scoring system that is still helpful in predicting the inducibility of women (Table 26–1). Components evaluated are cervical dilatation, effacement, consistency, and position, as well as the station of the fetal presenting part. A score of 0, 1, 2, or 3 is given to each assessed characteristic. The higher the total score for all the criteria, the more likely it is that labor will occur. The lower the total score, the higher the failure rate. A favorable cervix is the most important criterion for a successful induction.

The presence of a cervix that is anterior, soft, 50% effaced, and dilated at least 2 cm, with the fetal head at + 1 station or lower (Bishop score of 9) is favorable for successful induction (Dunn 1990).

Oxytocin Infusion

Intravenous administration of oxytocin is an effective method of initiating uterine contractions to induce labor.

(Text continues on p 793)

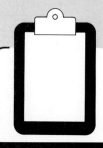

Nursing Care Plan
Induction of Labor

Client Assessment

Nursing History

Previous pregnancies
Present pregnancy course
Childbirth preparation
Estimated gestational age

Physical Examination

1. Examination of pregnant uterus (Leopold's maneuvers to determine fetal size and position)
2. Vaginal examination to evaluate cervical readiness
   a. Ripe cervix: Feels soft to the examining finger, is located in a medial to anterior position, is more than 50% effaced, and is 2–3 cm dilated
   b. Unripe cervix: Feels firm to the examining finger, is long and thick, perhaps in a posterior position, with little or no dilatation
3. Presence of contractions
4. Membranes intact or ruptured
5. Fetal size (Leopold's maneuvers, ultrasound)
6. Fetal readiness
7. CPD evaluation
8. Maternal vital signs and FHR before beginning induction

Diagnostic Studies

Fetal maturity tests (lecithin/sphingomyelin ratio, creatinine concentrations, ultrasonography), NST, CST, FBPP

Maternal blood studies (complete blood cell count [CBC], hemoglobin, hematocrit, blood type, Rh factor)

Urinalysis

Nursing Diagnosis	Nursing Interventions	Rationale	Evaluation
Nursing Diagnosis: Knowledge deficit related to induction procedure. *Client Goal:* The woman will discuss the induction procedure, the benefits, and the potential risks.	Assess the woman's feelings regarding induction. She may ask, "Will this work?" "How long will it take?" "Will it hurt more?"	Woman may be apprehensive about what will happen, or feel a sense of failure that she cannot "go into labor by herself."	The woman is able to discuss the induction procedure, feels comfortable asking questions as they arise, and has no further questions.
	Assess knowledge base regarding the induction process. Provide needed information (for example, when the cervix is ripe, contractions should begin in 30–60 minutes); length of labor depends on a number of factors.	After assessing knowledge base, appropriate information can be given to allay apprehension.	

(continued)

Nursing Care Plan (continued)

Nursing Diagnosis	Nursing Interventions	Rationale	Evaluation
	Assess knowledge of breathing techniques; if woman does not have a method to use, teach breathing techniques before starting oxytocin infusion.	Use of breathing techniques during contractions will help relaxation; although a woman may be apprehensive about induction, teaching a new breathing method will be easier before contractions are present.	
Nursing Diagnosis: Decreased cardiac output related to positional changes and the weight of the uterus on the vena cava *Client Goal:* The woman will maintain vital signs within normal range with no significant increase or decrease.	Position woman on her side; encourage her to avoid supine position. Monitor maternal blood pressure (BP) and pulse and FHR every 15–20 minutes.	Side-lying position maintains optimal blood flow to uterus and placenta.	The woman's vital signs remain within normal limits.
	If she becomes hypotensive: 1. Keep the woman on her side, may change to other side. 2. Discontinue oxytocin infusion. 3. Increase rate of primary IV. 4. Monitor FHR. 5. Notify physician. 6. Assess for cause of hypotension.	Initial hypotension is secondary to peripheral vasodilatation induced by oxytocin, which causes diminished blood supply to placenta and resultant decrease in O$_2$ supply to fetus. Actions are directed toward improving blood flow and oxygenation of tissues.	
Nursing Diagnosis: Altered tissue perfusion (placenta) related to potential hypertonic contraction pattern *Client Goal:* The woman will maintain normal contraction pattern as measured by: • Frequency of 2½–3 minutes • Duration of about 60 seconds • Relaxation of uterus between contractions	Apply monitor to obtain 15 minutes of tracing prior to starting induction.	Establishes baseline data.	The woman's contraction pattern is established with contractions every two to three minutes, lasting about 60–75 seconds with relaxation of the uterus between contractions.
	Administer oxytocin in electrolyte solution.	Oxytocin has slight antidiuretic effect, especially when administered in electrolyte-free solutions.	
	Encourage voiding every 2 hours. Monitor and record fluid intake and output. Monitor for nausea, vomiting, hypotension, tachycardia, cardiac arrhythmias.	Provides information on hydration status. These are signs and symptoms of water intoxication; they must be differentiated from other problems.	

(continued)

Nursing Care Plan (continued)

Nursing Diagnosis	Nursing Interventions	Rationale	Evaluation
	Monitor FHR by continuous electronic fetal monitoring. Obtain 15-minute tracing prior to beginning induction to evaluate fetal status; *do not* start infusion or advance rate (if induction has already begun) if FHR is not in range of 120–160 beats/min, if decelerations are present, or if variability decreases.	Will provide continuous data regarding fetal response to induction.	
	Evaluate maternal BP and pulse before beginning induction and then before each increase in infusion rate; do not advance infusion rate in presence of maternal hypertension or hypotension or radical changes in pulse rate.	To establish baseline data and to assess client response in induction; client status may change rapidly.	
	Evaluate contraction frequency, duration, and intensity prior to each increase in infusion rate.	Evaluates uterine response to induction.	
	Do not increase rate of infusion if contractions are every two to three minutes, lasting 40–60 seconds, with moderate intensity.	Desired effect has been obtained. Further increase in rate may produce hypertonic labor pattern (contractions with frequency of less than two minutes, for example more than five contractions in ten minutes or a duration of longer than 75–90 seconds).	
	Discontinue oxytocin infusion if: 1. Contractions are more frequent than every two minutes. 2. Contraction duration exceeds 75–90 seconds. 3. Uterus does not relax between contractions.	Uterus is being overstimulated and serious complications may develop for woman and fetus. Ruptured uterus or abruptio placentae can result from drug-induced tumultuous labor. (Note: Terms hyperstimulation, hypertonic labor pattern, and tumultuous labor are used interchangeably.) Contractions lasting over 90 seconds with decreased resting tone may result in fetal hypoxia.	

(continued)

Nursing Care Plan (continued)

Nursing Diagnosis	Nursing Interventions	Rationale	Evaluation
	Increase oxytocin IV infusion rate every 20 minutes until adequate contractions are achieved; do *not* exceed an infusion rate of 20–40 mU/min. (Note: protocols directing how often oxytocin is increased may vary from 30–60 minutes. See American College of Obstetrics and Gynecology [ACOG 1988] guidelines and agency protocol.)	Uterine response to oxytocin may be individualized.	
	Check infusion pump to assure oxytocin is infusing; check whether pump is on, chamber refills and empties, level of fluid in IV bottle becomes lower; if problem is found, correct it, and restart infusion at beginning dose. Check main IV site frequently. Check piggy-back connection to primary tubing to assure solution is not leaking	Oxytocin may not be infusing due to pump, mechanical, or human error.	
	Evaluate cervical dilatation by vaginal examination with each oxytocin dosage increase after labor is established.	When cervix responds by stretching or pulling, *do not* increase oxytocin dosage; overdosage may occur, causing rapid labor with possible cervical lacerations and fetal damage; when there is no change in the cervix, additional oxytocin is needed.	
	Monitor FHR continuously (normal range is 120–160/min). In episodes of bradycardia (<120 beats/min) lasting for more than 30 seconds, administer O_2 by face mask at 6–10 L/min. Stop oxytocin infusion. Position woman on left side if quick recovery of FHR does not occur.	O_2 deficiency may occur over a long period of time; in cases of placental insufficiency or cord compression, compensated tachycardia may be evoked.	

(continued)

Nursing Care Plan (continued)

Nursing Diagnosis	Nursing Interventions	Rationale	Evaluation
	Carefully evaluate fetal tachycardia (>160 beats/min). Sustained tachycardia may necessitate discontinuation of oxytocin infusion. Assess for presence of meconium staining. Notify physician/CNM.	Persistent fetal tachycardia causes more prominent O_2 deficiency (hypoxia) and CO_2 increase in fetal blood. Vasoconstriction occurs, with increased fetal blood flow through coronary arteries, brain, and placenta; this increased demand on myocardial performance leads to cardiac decompensation if oxygen exchange is impaired and hypoxia continues. Fetal hypoxia may also cause central vasomotor center to release adrenal catecholamines; at term, this enhances depolarization of cardiac pacemaker cells, which will result in direct bradycardia. Bradycardia or subsequent reflex tachycardia temporarily remedies the O_2 deficiency.	
Nursing Diagnosis: Pain related to uterine contractions *Client Goal:* The woman will maintain her breathing pattern and a relaxed state during contractions.	Provide support to woman as she uses breathing techniques. Encourage use of effluerage, back rub, and other supportive measures. Assess need for analgesia or anesthesia.	Contractions may build up more quickly with oxytocin induction and may be more painful. Techniques help maintain relaxation and thereby decrease pain sensation. After labor is well established, analgesia or epidural anesthesia may be given without delaying progress.	The woman maintains breathing pattern and a sense of control during labor.

Table 26–1 Prelabor Status Evaluation Scoring System*

Factor	Assigned value			
	0	1	2	3
Cervical dilatation	Closed	1–2 cm	3–4 cm	5 cm or more
Cervical effacement	0%–30%	40%–50%	60%–70%	80% or more
Fetal station	–3	–2	–1, 0	+1, or lower
Cervical consistency	Firm	Moderate	Soft	
Cervical position	Posterior	Midposition	Anterior	

Modified from Bishop EH: Pelvic scoring for elective induction. Obstet Gynecol 1964; 24:266.

During administration, the goal is to achieve two to three uterine contractions with a duration of 40 to 60 seconds in ten minutes with good uterine relaxation and return to the baseline tone between contractions (Dunn 1990).

Medical Therapy

Ten units of oxytocin (Pitocin) are added to 1 L of intravenous fluid (usually 5% dextrose in balanced salt solution—for example, 5% dextrose in lactated Ringer's). The resulting mixture will contain 10 mU of oxytocin per milliliter (1 mU/min = 6 mL/hr) and the prescribed dose can be calculated easily. Other dosage concentrations are presented in the Drug Guide on p 794.

A second bottle of intravenous fluid is prepared and used to start and maintain the infusion. This avoids infusing a large dose of oxytocin as the line is begun and provides additional fluids while the oxytocin solution is being kept at a low infusion rate. After the infusion is started, the oxytocin solution is piggybacked into the primary tubing port closest to the catheter insertion. This allows only a small amount of oxytocin to backflow into the tubing and ensures greater dosage accuracy. The oxytocin should be administered with a device that permits precise control of the flow rate. The recommended initial dosage is 0.5 to 1.0 mU/min. The dosage is gradually increased in increments of no more than 1 to 2 mU/min at 30- to 60-minute intervals until the woman experiences a contraction pattern similar to that in normal labor (ACOG 1988).

It is unusual for a woman to require more than 20 to 40 mU of oxytocin per minute to achieve progressive cervical dilatation; 90% of women will respond with 16 mU/min or less (ACOG 1988). Once labor is established and cervical dilatation reaches 5 to 6 cm, oxytocin may be reduced by similar increments (ACOG 1988).

Oxytocin induction is not without some associated risks. Hyperstimulation of the uterus, resulting in uterine contractions that are too frequent (more often than every two minutes), uterine contractions that are too intense, and/or an increased uterine resting tone. Other risks include uterine rupture and water intoxication due to infusion of excessive oxytocin and large volumes of non-electrolyte-containing solutions (ACOG 1988).

❊ *APPLYING THE NURSING PROCESS* ❊

Nursing Assessment

Close observation and accurate assessments are mandatory to provide safe, optimal care for both woman and fetus. Baseline data (maternal temperature, pulse, respiration, blood pressure, and FHR) should be obtained before beginning the infusion. A fetal monitor is used to provide continuous data. Many institutional protocols recommend obtaining a 15- to 20-minute EFM recording and NST before the infusion is started to obtain baseline data on uterine contractions and FHR.

Before each advancement of the infusion rate, assessments of the following should be made: (a) maternal blood pressure and pulse; (b) rate and reactivity of the FHR tracing (any bradycardia or decelerations are noted); and (c) contraction status, frequency, intensity, duration, and resting tone between contractions. During the induction, urinary output is assessed to identify any problems with retention, fluid deficit, and possible development of water intoxication.

As contractions are established, vaginal examinations are done to evaluate cervical dilatation, effacement, and station. The frequency of vaginal examinations primarily depends on the woman's parity and on characteristics of contractions. For example, a nullipara with contractions every five to seven minutes, each lasting 30 seconds, who does not perceive her contractions does not usually require a vaginal examination, but when her contractions are every two to three minutes, lasting 50 to 60 seconds with good intensity, a vaginal examination will be needed to evaluate her status.

When evaluating the need for analgesia, a vaginal examination should be performed to avoid giving the medication too early and increasing the risk of prolonging labor and to identify advanced dilatation and imminent birth.

DRUG GUIDE
Oxytocin (Pitocin)

Overview of Obstetric Action

Oxytocin (Pitocin) exerts a selective stimulatory effect on the smooth muscle of the uterus and blood vessels. Oxytocin affects the myometrial cells of the uterus by increasing the excitability of the muscle cell, increasing the strength of the muscle contraction, and supporting propagation of the contraction (movement of the contraction from one myometrial cell to the next). Its effect on the uterine contraction depends on the dosage used and on the excitability of the myometrial cells. During the first half of gestation, little excitability of the myometrium occurs and the uterus is fairly resistant to the effects of oxytocin. However, from midgestation on, the uterus responds increasingly to exogenous intravenous oxytocin. When at term, cautious use of diluted oxytocin, administered intravenously, results in a slow rise of uterine activity.

The circulatory half-life of oxytocin is 3–4 minutes. It takes approximately 40 minutes for a particular dose of oxytocin to reach a steady-state plasma concentration (Nugent 1989).

The effects of oxytocin on the cardiovascular system can be pronounced. There may be an initial decrease in the blood pressure, but with prolonged administration, a 30% increase in the baseline blood pressure may be noted. Cardiac output and stroke volume are increased. With doses of 20 mU/min or above, the antidiuretic effect of oxytocin results in a decrease of free water exchange in the kidney and a marked decrease in urine output (Marshall 1985).

Oxytocin is used to induce labor at term and to augment uterine contractions in the first and second stages of labor. Oxytocin may also be used immediately after birth to stimulate uterine contraction and thereby control uterine atony.

Oxytocin is not thought to cross the placenta because of its molecular weight and the presence of oxytocinase in the placenta (Giacoia & Yaffe 1982).

Route, Dosage, Frequency

For induction of labor: Add 10 units Pitocin (1 mL) to 1000 mL of intravenous solution. (The resulting concentration is 10 mU oxytocin per 1 mL of intravenous fluid.) Using an infusion pump, administer IV, starting at 0.5 mU/min and increasing the rate stepwise at no less than every 30–60 minutes until good contractions (every 2–3 minutes, each lasting 40–60 seconds) are achieved.

Maternal Contraindications

Severe preeclampsia-eclampsia (PIH)

Predisposition to uterine rupture (in nullipara over 35 years of age, multigravida 4 or more, overdistention of the uterus, previous major surgery of the cervix or uterus)

Cephalopelvic disproportion

Malpresentation or malposition of the fetus, cord prolapse

Preterm infant

Rigid, unripe cervix; total placenta previa

Presence of fetal distress

Maternal Side Effects

Hyperstimulation of the uterus results in hypercontractility, which in turn may cause the following:

Abruptio placentae

Impaired uterine blood flow → fetal hypoxia

Rapid labor → cervical lacerations

Rapid labor and birth → lacerations of cervix, vagina, perineum, uterine atony, fetal trauma

Uterine rupture

Water intoxication (nausea, vomiting, hypotension, tachycardia, cardiac arrhythmia) if oxytocin is given in electrolyte-free solution or at a rate exceeding 20 mU/min. Hypotension with rapid IV bolus administration postpartum.

Effect on Fetus/Neonate

Fetal effects are primarily associated with the presence of hypercontractility of the maternal uterus. Hypercontractility causes a decrease in the oxygen supply to the fetus, which is reflected by irregularities and/or decrease in FHR. Hyperbilirubinemia.

Trauma from rapid birth.

Nursing Considerations

Explain induction or augmentation procedure to client.

Apply fetal monitor and obtain 15- to 20-minute tracing and NST to assess FHR before starting IV oxytocin.

For induction or augmentation of labor, start with primary IV and piggy-back secondary IV with oxytocin.

Ensure continuous fetal and uterine contraction monitoring.

(continued)

The maximum rate is 40 mU/min (ACOG 1988). Decrease oxytocin by similar increments once labor has progressed to 5–6 cm dilatation (ACOG 1988).

0.5 mU/min = 3 mL/hr	8 mU/min = 48 mL/hr
1.0 mU/min = 6 mL/hr	10 mU/min = 60 mL/hr
1.5 mU/min = 9 mL/hr	12 mU/min = 72 mL/hr
2 mU/min = 12 mL/hr	15 mU/min = 90 mL/hr
4 mU/min = 24 mL/hr	18 mU/min = 108 mL/hr
6 mU/min = 36 mL/hr	20 mU/min = 120 mL/hr

Protocols may vary from one agency to another.

For augmentation of labor: Prepare and administer IV Pitocin as for labor induction. Increase rate until labor contractions are of good quality. The flow rate is gradually increased at no less than every 30 minutes to a maximum of 10 mU/min (Cunningham et al 1989). In some settings, or in a situation when only limited fluids may be administered, a more concentrated solution may be used. When 10 U Pitocin is added to 500 mL IV solution the resulting concentration is 1 mU/min = 3 mL/hr. If 10 U Pitocin is added to 250 mL IV solution the concentration is 1 mU/min = 1.5 mL/hr.

For administration after expulsion of placenta: One dose of 10 units Pitocin (1 mL) is given intramuscularly or by slow intravenous push or added to IV fluids for continuous infusion.

Assess FHR, maternal blood pressure, pulse, and uterine contraction frequency, duration, and resting tone before each increase in oxytocin infusion rate.

Record all assessments and IV rate on monitor strip and on client's chart. Record oxytocin infusion rate in mU/min and mL/hour. For example: 0.5 mU/min (3 mL/hr)

Record all client activities (such as change of position, vomiting), procedures done (amniotomy, sterile vaginal examination), and administration of analgesics on monitor strip to allow for interpretation and evaluation of tracing.

Assess cervical dilatation as needed.

Apply nursing comfort measures.

Discontinue IV oxytocin infusion and infuse primary solution when (a) fetal distress is noted (bradycardia, late or variable decelerations; (b) uterine contractions are more frequent than every 2 minutes; (c) duration of contractions exceeds more than 60 seconds; or (d) insufficient relaxation of the uterus between contractions or a steady increase in resting tone are noted (ACOG 1988); in addition to discontinuing IV oxytocin infusion, turn client to side, and if fetal distress is present, administer oxygen by tight face mask at 6–10 L/min; notify physician.

Maintain intake and output record.

Nursing Diagnosis

The nursing diagnoses that may be appropriate for labor induction are presented in the Nursing Care Plan on page 788.

Nursing Plan and Implementation

During the oxytocin infusion, the woman needs to be attended by nurses who are able to identify both maternal and fetal complications. A qualified obstetrician should be readily accessible to manage any complication that may occur (ACOG 1988).

For additional information on nursing interventions, see Drug Guide–Oxytocin on page 794 and Nursing Care Plan: Induction of Labor on page 788.

Intravenous oxytocin may also be given for augmentation of labor; see Drug Guide–Oxytocin for further discussion.

Evaluation

Anticipated outcomes of nursing care include the following:

- The woman's labor is successfully induced.
- The labor and birth process are within normal limits and the woman and her baby do not experience any complications.

❀ ❀ ❀ ❀ ❀ ❀ ❀ ❀ ❀ ❀ ❀ ❀

Care of the Woman During an Episiotomy

An episiotomy is a surgical incision of the perineal body that is done to protect the perineum, sphincter, and rectum from lacerations during the birth and to decrease the length of the second stage of labor (Rockner et al 1989).

An episiotomy is one of the most common procedures in maternal-child care. Researchers estimate the rate of episiotomies in all births is 62.5% and the rate for nulliparas approaches 90% (Rockner et al 1989). Even though the procedure is very common, its routine use has been questioned (Thorp & Bowes 1989). Current research suggests that rather than protecting the perineum from lacerations, the presence of an episiotomy makes it more likely that the woman will have deep perineal tears. Borgatta et al (1989) reported that third- and fourth-degree perineal tears occurred in 27.9% of women who had an episiotomy and used stirrups during birth, as compared to 0.9% of women who gave birth without episiotomy or the use of stirrups. Additional complications associated with an episiotomy may be infection, blood loss, and pain and perineal discomfort that may continue for days or weeks past birth.

Episiotomy Procedure

The episiotomy is performed with sharp scissors that have rounded points, just before birth, when approximately 3 to 4 cm of the fetal head is visible during a contraction (Cunningham et al 1989). There are two types in current practice: midline and mediolateral (Figure 26–3). A midline episiotomy is performed along the median raphe of the perineum. It extends down from the vaginal orifice to the fibers of the rectal sphincter. This type of episiotomy avoids muscle fibers and major blood vessels because it divides the insertions of the superficial perineal muscles. A midline episiotomy is preferred if the perineum is of adequate length and no difficulty is anticipated during the birth, because the blood loss is less and the incision is easy to repair and heals with less discomfort for the mother. The major disadvantage is that a tear of the midline incision may extend through the anal sphincter and rectum.

In the presence of a short perineum or an anticipated difficult birth, a mediolateral episiotomy provides more room and decreases the possibility of a traumatic extension into the rectum. The mediolateral episiotomy begins in the midline of the posterior fourchette (in order to avoid incision into the Bartholin's gland) and extends at a 45° angle downward to the right or left (the direction depending on the handedness of the clinician). The mediolateral episiotomy may be complicated by greater blood loss, a longer healing period, and more postpartal discomfort.

The episiotomy is usually performed with regional or local anesthesia but may be performed without anesthesia in emergency situations. It is generally proposed that as crowning occurs, the distention of the tissues causes numbing. Adequate anesthesia must be given for the repair.

Repair of the episiotomy (episiorrhaphy) and any lacerations is accomplished either during the period between birth of the neonate and before expulsion of the placenta or after expulsion of the placenta.

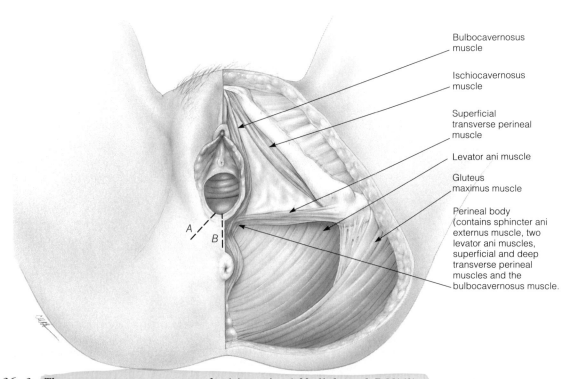

Figure 26–3 *The two most common types of episiotomies: A Mediolateral, B Midline.*

Nursing Care

The woman needs to be supported during the repair as she may feel some pressure sensations. In the absence of adequate anesthesia, she may feel pain. Placing a hand on her shoulder, and talking with her can provide comfort and distraction from the repair process. If the woman is having more discomfort than she can comfortably handle, the nurse needs to act as an advocate in communicating the woman's needs to the physician/nurse-midwife. At all times the woman needs to be the one who decides whether the amount of discomfort is tolerable, and she should never be told "This doesn't hurt." She is the person experiencing the discomfort, and her evaluation needs to be respected. If there are just a few (three to five) stitches left, she may choose to forego more local anesthesia, but she should be given the choice.

The type of episiotomy is recorded on the birth record. This information should also be included in a report to the recovery room, so that adequate assessments can be made and relief measures can be instituted if necessary.

Pain relief measures may begin immediately after birth with application of an ice pack to the perineum. For optimal effect the ice pack should be applied for 20 to 30 minutes and removed for at least 20 minutes before being reapplied because the ice causes vasoconstriction and if left in place more than 30 minutes, vasodilitation and subsequent edema may occur. The perineal tissues should be assessed frequently to prevent injury from the ice pack. After a few hours (8 to 10) warm sitz baths (101F to 105F) are recommended to increase circulation to the area and promote healing. The use of cool sitz baths is currently being investigated, with some women reporting increased pain relief from using a lukewarm sitz bath to which ice chips have been added (Varner 1986; Ramler & Roberts 1986). The episiotomy site should be inspected every 15 minutes during the first hour after the birth and thereafter daily for redness, swelling, tenderness, and hematomas. Mild analgesic sprays and oral analgesics are ordered as needed. The mother will need instruction in perineal hygiene care and may need instructions about use of the analgesic spray. (See Chapter 34 for additional discussion of relief measures.)

Care of the Woman During Forceps-Assisted Birth

Forceps are designed to assist the birth of a fetus by providing traction or by providing the means to rotate the fetal head to an occiput-anterior position. A special type of forceps is designed to be used with a breech presentation, in which the forceps are applied to the aftercoming fetal

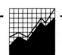

Research Note

Clinical Application of Research

To examine the popular notion that a prophylactic episiotomy decreases postpartum perineal discomfort and preserves or enhances postpartum sexual function, Fleming and Schafer (1989) designed a prospective study with 102 participants who subsequently had either a vaginal or cesarean birth.

Women experiencing vaginal birth had an episiotomy, an intact perineum, an unsutured first-degree laceration, or a sutured laceration. Additionally, the authors questioned 280 women about the perceived tightness or looseness of their vaginal outlet after vaginal delivery.

Women with an intact perineum or an unsutured laceration reported significantly less perineal pain between 24 hours and two weeks. However, by four weeks, all groups described almost no perineal discomfort.

Participants with either intact or unsutured perineum resumed sexual intercourse at a significantly sooner period than the other two groups. Two other outcomes were related to the episiotomy group: significantly more dyspareunia or discomfort with sexual intercourse at 6 months and reported decreases in orgasmic patterns, rather than both increases and decreases in orgasmic patterns as is found in all other groups. Of the 280 subjects who gave birth vaginally, no differences were found in the perceived tightness or looseness of the vaginal outlet, regardless of type of perineal outcome.

Critical Thinking Applied to Research

Strengths: Use of ANOVA with unequal N's, as in this study, requires establishment of homogeneity of variance—as was done by these authors. Identification of the problems of generalization based on the small numbers of this study.

Concerns: Use of t-tests with multiple groups increases the alpha level, or the possibility of incorrectly finding statistical significance where none exists.

Fleming N, Schafer AW: Postpartum perineal pain and sexual function in women with and without episiotomies. In: *The free woman: Women's health in the 1990's.* van Hall E, Everaerd W Park Ridge, NJ: The Parthenon Publishing Group, 1989.

head (called aftercoming because the head is born after the body). In 1988, after years of defining forceps applications as either low/outlet forceps or midforceps, the American College of Obstetricians and Gynecologists reclassified forceps applications into three categories: outlet, low, and midforceps. To meet the criteria for **outlet** application, forceps are applied when the fetal skull has reached the perineum, the scalp is visible between contractions, and the sagittal suture is not more than 45 degrees from the midline. A **low forceps** application is used when the leading edge of the fetal skull is at a station of +2 or more. A **midforcep** application is used when the head is engaged but the leading

edge of the fetal skull is above +2 station. Types of forceps are illustrated in Figure 26-4.

Indications

Indications for the use of forceps include the presence of any condition that threatens the mother or fetus and that

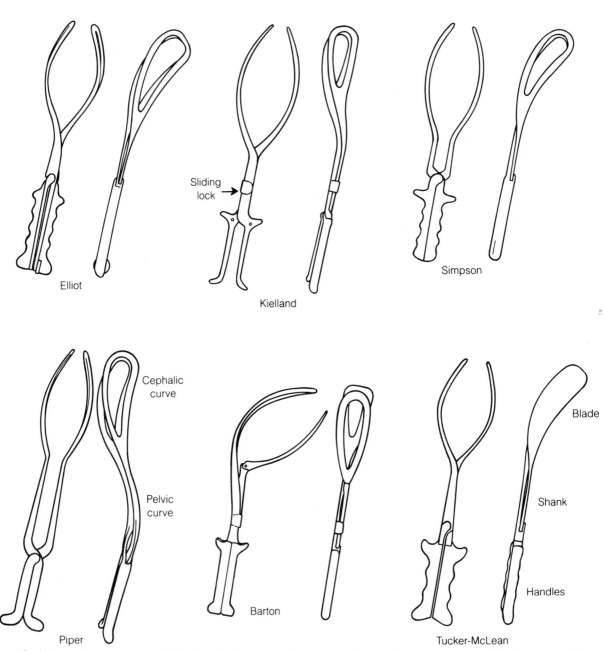

Figure 26-4   Forceps are composed of a blade, shank, and handle and may have a cephalic and pelvic curve. (Note labels on Piper and Tucker-McLean forceps.) The blades may be fenestrated (open) or solid. The front and lateral views of these forceps illustrate differences in blades, open and closed shank, and cephalic and pelvic curves. Elliot, Simpson, and Tucker-McLean forceps are used as outlet forceps. Kielland and Barton forceps are used for midforceps rotations. Piper forceps are used to provide traction and flexion of the aftercoming head (the head comes after the body) of a fetus in breech presentation.

can be relieved by birth. Conditions that put the woman at risk include heart disease, acute pulmonary edema, intrapartal infection, or exhaustion. Fetal conditions include premature placental separation, and fetal distress. Forceps may be used electively to shorten the second stage of labor and spare the woman's pushing effort (when exhaustion and/or heart disease is present), or when regional anesthesia has affected the woman's motor innervation and she cannot push effectively. In the past, outlet forceps have been used to protect the head of a preterm infant during birth, however, the advantages of this practice are now being questioned (Cunningham et al 1989).

Neonatal Risks

Some neonates may develop a small area of ecchymosis and/or edema along the sides of the face as a result of forceps application. Caput succedaneum or cephalhematoma (and subsequent hyperbilirubinemia) may occur as well as transient facial paralysis. Previous studies identified an increased risk of cerebral palsy and brain damage when midforceps were used. However, recent studies do not support these findings (Sokol & Brindley 1990).

Prerequisites for Forceps Application

Use of forceps requires complete dilatation of the cervix and knowledge of the exact position and station of the fetal head. The membranes must be ruptured to allow a firm grasp on the fetal head. The presentation must be vertex or face with the chin anterior. In addition, there must be no disproportion between the fetal head and the maternal pelvis (Cunningham et al 1989).

Trial or Failed Forceps Procedure

In a trial forceps procedure, the physician attempts to use forceps with the knowledge that there is a degree of CPD. A complete setup for immediate cesarean birth needs to be available before the forceps are applied. If a good application cannot be obtained or if no descent occurs with the application, cesarean birth is the method of choice. A failed forceps procedure is an attempt to perform a forceps-assisted birth without success.

Nursing Care

The nurse can explain the procedure briefly to the woman. With adequate regional anesthesia, the woman should feel some pressure but no pain. The nurse encourages her to maintain breathing techniques to prevent her from pushing during application of the forceps (Figure 26–5). The nurse monitors contractions and with each contraction the physician will provide traction as the woman pushes. The FHR

should be monitored after each contraction until the birth. It is not uncommon to observe bradycardia as traction is being applied to the forceps. This bradycardia results from head compression and is transient in nature.

The neonate is assessed for facial edema, bruising, caput succedaneum, cephalhematoma, or any sign of cerebral edema. In the fourth stage, the nurse assesses the woman for perineal swelling and/or bruising, hematoma, and hemorrhage. In the postpartum period, it is important to assess for signs of infection.

Care of the Woman During Vacuum Extraction

Vacuum extraction is an obstetric procedure with widespread use throughout the world, although it has not become as common in the United States (Cunningham et al 1989). The vacuum extractor is composed of a suction cup attached to a suction bottle (pump) by tubing. The suction cup, which comes in various sizes, is placed against the occiput of the fetal head. Care must be taken to ensure that the cervix or vaginal tissue is not trapped under the cup. The pump is used to create negative pressure (suction) and an artificial caput ("chignon") is formed. The physician then applies traction in coordination with uterine contractions and the fetal head is born (Figure 26–6). During the time the physician is using the vacuum extractor, the following clinical guidelines should be followed: traction is exerted with a contraction; maximum time for application of the cup does not exceed 25 minutes; there is a maximum of five traction pulls; there is a maximum of two cup detachments (cup pulls off the fetal head); and the fetal head should descend with the first traction (O'Grady 1988).

The most common indication for use of the vacuum extractor is prolonged second stage labor. The vacuum extractor is preferred to forceps in cases of borderline CPD, when successful passage of the fetal head requires the availability of all potential space inside the vaginal canal. Other indications are the same as for forceps-assisted birth (Cunningham et al 1989). Absolute contraindications for use of the vacuum extractor include the presence of CPD, face, or breech presentation. Relative contraindications include fetal distress, fetal demise, congenital abnormalities of the cranium, and premature infants (less than 37 weeks' gestation) (O'Grady 1988).

The theoretical advantages of the vacuum extractor are a great reduction in intracranial pressure during traction and no pressure on maternal soft tissue. Risks of vacuum extraction may include abrasion of the fetal scalp, cephalhematoma, and intracranial and/or retinal hemorrhage (Cunningham et al 1989).

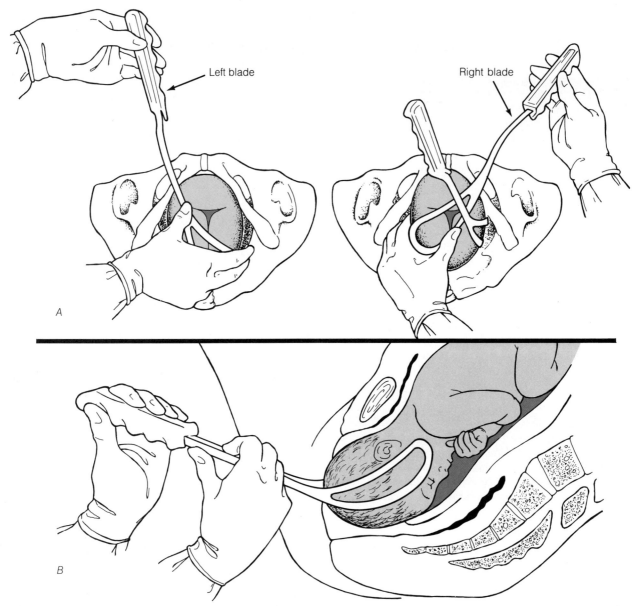

Figure 26–5   Application of forceps in occiput-anterior (OA) position A The left blade is inserted along the left side wall of the pelvis, over the parietal bone. B The right blade is inserted along the right side wall of the pelvis over the parietal bone. C With correct placement of the blades, the handles lock easily. During uterine contractions, traction is applied to the forceps in a downward and outward direction to follow the birth canal.

Nursing Care

There are many different types of vacuum extractors. The nurse should be familiar with the types used within the birthing setting and learn the pressure limits of each type.

The woman should be informed about what is happening during the procedure. If adequate regional anesthesia has been administered, the woman feels only pres-

sure during the procedure. The fetus should be auscultated at least every five minutes or assessed by continuous electronic fetal monitoring. The parents need to be informed that the caput (chignon) on the baby's head will disappear in a few hours.

Assessment of the newborn should include inspection and continued observation for cerebral trauma.

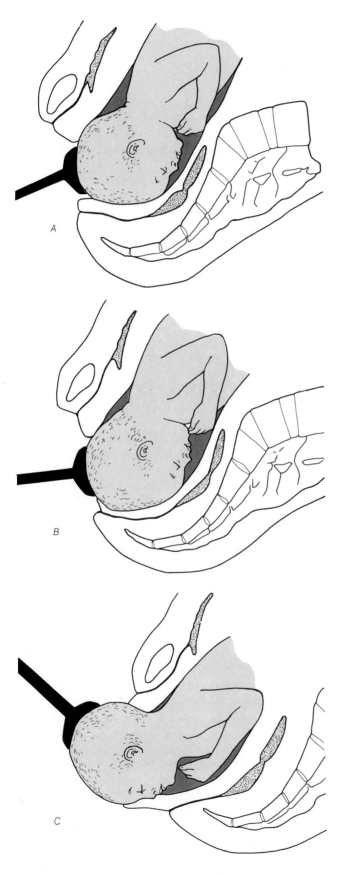

Care of the Family During Cesarean Birth

Cesarean birth is the birth of the infant through an abdominal and uterine incision. The word *cesarean* is derived from the Latin word *caedere,* meaning "to cut." Cesarean birth is one of the oldest surgical procedures known. Until the twentieth century, caesareans were primarily equated with an attempt to salvage the fetus of a dying woman. Currently, the maternal and perinatal morbidity associated with cesarean birth has decreased to the point that cesarean birth is the method of birth for approximately 30% of all women (Freeman 1990). This rate reflects a steady rise from about 5.5% in 1970.

Indications

Cesarean births are performed in the presence of a variety of maternal and fetal conditions. Commonly accepted indications include placenta previa, prolapsed cord, absolute pelvic contracture, active genital herpes, and transverse lie. These indications account for approximately 20% of the total number of cesarean births. The other 80% of cesareans are done in cases of failure to progress due to CPD, breech presentation, fetal distress, and repeat cesarean birth. It is this 80% of cases that some authorities have recently begun to question (Freeman 1990).

Failure to progress is the indication in approximately 30% to 50% of the primary cesarean births done today. The reason for failure to progress is sometimes clearly due to cephalopelvic disproportion; however, in other instances the underlying cause is not clear. Gould et al (1989) noted that socioeconomic factors seem to be related to increased cesarean birth rates. Women of higher socioeconomic rank are more likely to have epidural anesthesia, oxytocin, and cesarean birth. Breech births will continue to be an indication for cesarean birth, especially in a first pregnancy or with a preterm fetus. External version done at 37 weeks has the potential to significantly decrease the need for cesarean birth if the 65% to 85% success rate of version continues (Freeman 1990).

Fetal distress is another category that has been associated with the increased cesarean birth rate. As the use of electronic fetal monitoring (EFM) has increased, the inci-

Figure 26–6 Vacuum extractor traction. A The cup is placed on the fetal occiput and suction is created. Traction is applied in a downward and outward direction. B Traction continues in a downward direction as the fetal head begins to emerge from the vagina. C Traction is maintained to lift the fetal head out of the vagina.

dence of fetal distress has also increased. Some studies have found no relationship between routine EFM and improved fetal outcome (Leveno et al 1986). Some researchers contend that fetal distress is diagnosed more often than it actually exists, resulting in unnecessary cesarean births; others suggest that the factors involved are not clearly understood at this time (Freeman 1990).

Prior cesarean birth still accounts for 30% to 50% of the cesarean birth rate, but this category has the greatest potential for change. In Europe, women with previous low transverse uterine scars were allowed to labor (called vaginal birth after cesarean or VBAC), with a success rate of 50% to 75%. The practice of VBAC is becoming more prevalent in the United States and has great potential to decrease the overall cesarean birth rate in this country. Overall, Petitti (1989) suggests that the cesarean birth rate could be maintained at about 15% if failure to progress were treated more aggressively, if external versions were done, and if VBAC was recommended when possible.

Maternal Mortality and Morbidity

Cesarean births have two to four times the maternal mortality of vaginal births. Although mortality is still low (approximately 1 to 2 deaths per 1000 caesareans as opposed to 0.06 deaths per 1000 live vaginal births), 25% of deaths are due to anesthesia complications (Dunn 1990). Morbidity is associated with a fairly wide variety of complications such as unexplained fever, endometritis, wound infection, urinary tract infection, atelectasis, thrombophlebitis, and pulmonary embolism (Dunn 1990).

Surgical Techniques

Skin Incisions

The skin incision for a cesarean birth is either transverse (Pfannenstiel) or vertical and is not indicative of the type of incision made into the uterus. The transverse incision is made across the lowest and narrowest part of the abdomen. Since the incision is made just below the pubic hair line, it is almost invisible after healing. The limitations of this type of skin incision are that it does not allow for extension of the incision if needed. Since it usually requires more time, this incision is used when time is not of the essence (eg, with failure to progress and no fetal or maternal distress). The vertical (infraumbilical midline) incision is made between the navel and the symphysis pubis. This type of incision is quicker and is therefore preferred in cases of fetal distress when rapid birth is indicated, preterm or macrosomic infants, or when the woman is obese (Cunningham et al 1989). The type of skin incision is determined by time factor, client preference, or physician preference.

Uterine Incisions

The type of uterine incision depends on the need for the cesarean. The choice of incision affects the woman's op-

portunity for a subsequent vaginal birth and her risks of a ruptured uterine scar with a subsequent pregnancy.

The two major types of uterine incisions are in the lower uterine segment or in the upper segment of the uterine corpus.

The lower uterine segment incision that is most commonly used is a transverse incision, although a vertical incision may also be used (Figure 26–7). The transverse incision is preferred for the following reasons (Cunningham et al 1989; Scott et al 1990):

1. The lower segment is the thinnest portion of the uterus and involves less blood loss.
2. It requires only moderate dissection of bladder from underlying myometrium.
3. It is easier to repair.
4. The site is less likely to rupture during subsequent pregnancies.
5. There is a decreased chance of adherence of bowel or omentum to the incision line.

The disadvantages include the following:

1. It takes longer to make and repair a transverse incision.
2. It is limited in size because of the presence of major blood vessels on either side of the uterus.
3. It has a greater tendency to extend laterally into the uterine vessels.
4. The incision may stretch and become a thin window, but it usually does not create problems clinically until subsequent labor ensues.

The lower uterine segment vertical incision is preferred for multiple gestation, abnormal presentation, placenta previa, fetal distress, and preterm and macrosomic fetuses. Disadvantages of this incision are as follows:

1. The incision may extend downward into the cervix.
2. More extensive dissection of the bladder is needed to keep the incision in the lower uterine segment.
3. If it extends upward into the upper segment, hemostasis and closure are more difficult.
4. The chance of rupture with subsequent labor is increased (Cunningham et al 1989; Scott et al 1990).

One other incision, the classic incision, was the method of choice for many years but is used infrequently now. This vertical incision was made into the upper uterine segment. There was more blood loss, and it was more difficult to repair. Most important, there was an increased risk of uterine rupture with subsequent pregnancy, labor, and birth because the upper uterine segment is the most contractile portion of the uterus.

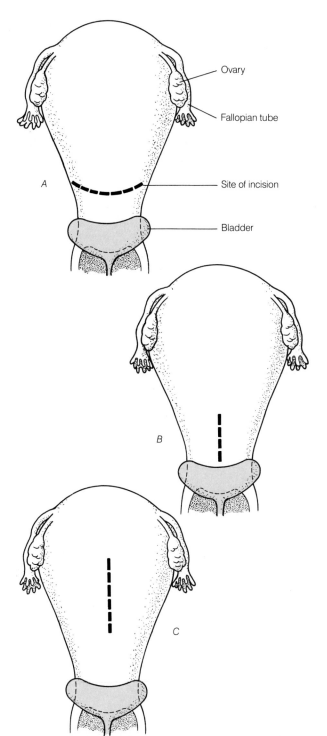

Figure 26–7   Uterine incisions for a cesarean birth. A This transverse incision in the lower uterine segment is called a Kerr incision. B The Sellheim incision is a vertical incision in the lower uterine segment. C This view illustrates the classic uterine incision that is done in the body (corpus) of the uterus. The classic incision was commonly done in the past and is associated with increased risk of uterine rupture in subsequent pregnancies and labor.

Nursing Care

Preparation for Cesarean Birth

Since one out of every three to four births is a cesarean, preparation for this possibility should be an integral part of prenatal education. *All* couples should be encouraged to discuss with their obstetrician what the approach would be in the event of a cesarean. They can also discuss their needs and desires as a couple under those circumstances. Their preferences may include the following:

- Participating in the choice of anesthetic
- Father (or significant other) being present during the procedures and/or birth
- Father (or significant other) being present in the recovery or postpartum room
- Audio recording and/or taking pictures of the birth
- Delayed instillation of eye drops to promote eye contact between parent and infant in the first hours after birth
- Physical contact or holding the newborn while on the operating room table and/or in the recovery room (if the mother cannot hold the newborn the father can hold the baby for her)
- Breast-feeding immediately after birth

Information that couples need about cesarean birth includes the following:

- Preparation that may be done such as abdominal prep, insertion of an indwelling bladder catheter, and starting an intravenous infusion
- Description or viewing of the delivery room
- Types of anesthesia for birth and analgesia available postpartum
- Sensations that may be experienced
- Roles of significant others
- Interaction with neonate
- Immediate recovery phase
- Postpartal phase

The context in which this information is given should be "birth-oriented" rather than surgery-oriented.

Preparation for Repeat Cesarean Birth

When a couple is anticipating a cesarean birth, they have time to analyze and synthesize the information they are given and to prepare for the experience. Many hospitals or local groups (such as C-Sec Inc) provide preparation classes for cesarean birth. The instructor should impart factual information and a feeling of normality, which will allow a couple to make choices and participate in their birth experience. Couples who have had previous negative experiences need an opportunity to describe what they felt con-

(Text continues on p 808)

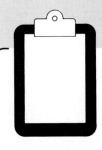

Nursing Care Plan
Cesarean Birth: Preparation and Immediate Recovery Period

Client Assessment

Nursing History

Present pregnancy course
Estimated gestational age
Childbirth preparation
Sensitivity to medications and anesthetic agents
Past bleeding problems
Allergies
Last time woman ate and drank fluids

Physical Examination

1. Fetal size, fetal status (FHR), and fetal maturity
2. Maternal lung and cardiac status
3. Complete physical examination prior to administration of anesthetic

Diagnostic Studies

CBC
Hemoglobin and hematocrit
Type and cross-match for two units whole blood
Rh
Prothrombin time
Testing for syphilis
Urinalysis

Nursing Diagnosis	Nursing Interventions	Rationale	Evaluation
Nursing Diagnosis: Knowledge deficit related to the cesarean birth *Client Goal:* The woman will discuss the cesarean birth procedure as measured by the following: • Reason for cesarean • Preoperative preparation • Postoperative care measures such as turn, cough, deep breathe, and need for frequent monitoring by nursing personnel • Woman will demonstrate deep breathing, coughing, and splinting.	Integrate cesarean birth information into childbirth preparation classes. Emphasize the similarities between vaginal and cesarean birth. Minimize perceptions of "normal" versus "abnormal" birth. Provide factual information. Encourage couple to discuss with obstetrician the approach and birth preferences in the event of a vaginal or cesarean birth. Encourage expression of feelings. Assess reaction to and interpretation of past cesarean birth or other surgical experiences.	Couples may deny the possibility of an unplanned cesarean birth. Preparatory needs are basically the same for all couples anticipating childbirth. A good knowledge base will allow for adaptive coping responses should birth occur. Information enables couples to make choices and participate in their birth experience. Opportunity to discuss needs and desires minimizes unrealistic expectations, disappointment, and/or feelings of loss; promotes understanding of options, beliefs of birth attendant, and hospital policies; and allows couple to do anticipatory problem solving and develop effective coping behaviors. Enables couple to work through fears, ambivalent or unresolved feelings, and potential grief associated with loss of vaginal birth. Identifies need for information and opportunity to work through fears or unresolved feelings.	Woman is able to discuss cesarean birth procedure and associated pre- and postoperative care.

(continued)

Nursing Care Plan (continued)

Nursing Diagnosis	Nursing Interventions	Rationale	Evaluation
	Encourage the development of mutual support by couples sharing their experiences and common concerns.	Decreases sense of being "different" or "alone" by realizing that their fears and concerns are not unique and feelings of anger or guilt are normal.	
	Describe preoperative procedure:	Explanation of pre- and postoperative measures decreases client anxiety and increases the woman's ability to participate in care.	
	• Abdominal prep		
	• Insertion of in-dwelling bladder catheter		
	• Insertion of IV		
	• Administration of preoperative medications		
	Teach postoperative measures:		
	• How to deep breathe and cough		
	• Need for frequent position changes		
	• Frequency of monitoring vital signs		
	Create a safe, nonthreatening environment for couples to work through unresolved negative feelings.	Negative feelings may contribute to distortion of information, impede learning, and affect expectations of upcoming birth experience.	
	Encourage couples to identify events that would make this birth experience more positive.	Allow for anticipatory problem solving, and enhance ability to meet goals and expectations for birth event.	
	Cover most salient points of what to anticipate:	Knowing what to expect increases coping capability.	
	• What is going to happen to the woman's body and how it will feel		
	• What and why specific procedures will be done		
	• How to handle discomfort associated with procedures		
	• What the woman will see and hear during the cesarean		

(continued)

Nursing Care Plan (continued)

Nursing Diagnosis	Nursing Interventions	Rationale	Evaluation
	Provide couple with brief period of privacy.	They need an opportunity to pool their coping strengths to deal with the anxiety of the situation.	
	Inquire if couple has any questions about the decision.	Give opportunity for further clarification.	
	Prepare woman in stages, giving information and rationale for each procedure.	Crisis-altered cognitive grasp leads to information being misinterpreted or not being heard.	
	Avoid silence.	Silence is often interpreted by the client as frightening and/or negative.	
	Employ eye contact and therapeutic touch.	Conveying a feeling of caring and reality orientation provides support.	
Nursing Diagnosis: Impaired gas exchange related to decreased air exchange secondary to shallow breathing with incisional pain and ineffective cough *Client Goal:* The woman will maintain effective respiratory function as measured by: • Respirations between 14 and 20 per minute • Secretions removed from respiratory tract	As a part of preoperative teaching: • Teach deep breathing and coughing. • Teach abdominal splinting while deep breathing and coughing. • Assess lung sounds. Explain that she will be turned every two hours and offer rationale. After surgery: assess respiratory rate	Promotes good air exchange. Provides support and decreases pain. Provides data on respiratory status. Provides aeration of lungs and assists in preventing pulmonary complications. Determines that respiratory rate is in normal range.	Woman's respirations are between 14 and 20 per minute; lung sounds are clear; secretions are removed from respiratory track. The woman is able to discuss the need for position changes and can demonstrate deep breathing and coughing. In the postpartal period she will be able to deep breathe and cough effectively, and her lungs remain clear.
In the Postoperative Period *Nursing Diagnosis:* Pain related to incision, uterine involution, and contractions resulting from oxytocin administration *Client Goal:* The woman will have increased comfort as measured by: • Woman states pain has lessened. • Woman able to relax and rest.	Administer analgesic medications. Provide quiet environment to enhance rest. Provide comfort measures such as the following: • Change position and support body parts. • Back rub. • Therapeutic touch. • Use music. • Modify environment.	Provides relief of pain. Promotes comfort. Identified comfort measures. Use gate control theory.	The woman has decreased pain as evidenced by reporting decreased pain on a 0 to 10 pain scale, is normotensive and eupneic, is able to move in bed and complete deep breathing and coughing with minimal discomfort.

(continued)

Nursing Care Plan (continued)

Nursing Diagnosis	Nursing Interventions	Rationale	Evaluation
Nursing Diagnosis: Altered tissue perfusion related to excessive blood loss secondary to inadequate contraction of the uterus after birth	Evaluate firmness and position of fundus. Palpate fundus after pain medication is administered to promote patient comfort.	Provides opportunity to monitor involution. Palpation of fundus causes discomfort to the woman and is frequently neglected and therefore becomes increasingly important.	
Client Goal: The woman will maintain normal tissue perfusion as measured by: • No excessive blood loss • Uterus remains contracted, in midline and below umbilicus • Skin warm, dry, and nonclammy • Normotensive	Fundus may be palpated from side of abdomen to avoid placing pressure on vertical incision. Administer oxytocin per physician order. Evaluate lochia.	Avoid tenderness at incisional site. Stimulates uterine contractions and thereby prevents bleeding. Lochia progresses from rubra to serosa to alba. Increase in flow indicates inefficient contraction of uterus and/or subinvolution.	The woman remains normotensive, uterus is well contracted in the midline and below the umbilicus, and blood loss is not excessive.
Nursing Diagnosis: Altered parenting	Provide information about the baby as soon as possible.	Interaction may be impaired because of recovery from anesthesia and discomfort in first few hours after birth.	
Client Goal: The parents will have opportunities to interact with their baby and will move into a positive attachment.	Provide opportunities for the parents to be with the baby as soon as possible. Provide opportunities to discuss feelings about the cesarean birth and the woman's self-image as a mother.	Feelings of failure associated with birthing experience can be generalized to ability to assume mothering role.	The woman is interacting with her newborn and engaging in care-taking behaviors.

tributed to these events. They should be encouraged to identify what they would like to have altered and to list interventions that would make the experience more positive. Those who have had positive experiences need reassurance that their needs and desires will be met in the same manner. In addition, an opportunity should be given to discuss any fears or anxieties.

A specific concern of the woman facing a repeat cesarean is anticipation of pain. She needs reassurance that subsequent cesareans are often less painful than the first. She will not experience the extreme fatigue that followed the primary cesarean if it was preceded by a long and/or strenuous labor. Giving this information will enable the woman to cope more effectively with stressful stimuli, including pain. The nurse can remind the woman that she has already had experience with how to prevent, cope with, and alleviate painful stimuli.

Preparation for Emergency Cesarean Birth

Usually a couple is prepared for an emergency cesarean by either the "last minute" or the "mutual decision" approach. All too frequently physicians/nurse-midwives wait until the last minute to inform the woman of the need for a cesarean birth under the guise of "sparing the couple undue anxiety." Ironically, the woman's reaction to this delayed approach is not only excessive anxiety but also anger, shock, and resentment resulting in a state of crisis or panic (Cox & Smith 1982). In contrast, the mutual decision approach between the birth attendants and the woman keeps the family fully informed as developments occur. The physician/nurse-midwife presents all the facts, suggests alternatives, and describes likely outcomes of nonintervention, allowing the expectant parents to participate in the decision making. The opportunity to make choices and have control over their birthing experience is the major factor influencing a couple's positive perception of the event (Cox & Smith 1982).

The period preceding surgery must be used to its greatest advantage. The couple needs some time for privacy to assimilate the information given to them and to gather strength to face this new crisis. It is imperative that care givers use their most effective communication skills. Silence is often interpreted by the woman as indicating danger for her and her fetus and/or care giver anger resulting from her failure to perform (Affonso 1981). The woman may experience panic and/or fear. She may be confused and numb to instructions. It is essential for the nurse to address what the couple may anticipate during the next few hours. Asking the couple "What questions do you have about the decision?" gives the couple an opportunity for further clarification. The nurse can prepare the woman in stages, giving her information and the rationale for each procedure before commencing. Before carrying out a procedure it is essential to tell the woman (a) what is going to happen; (b) why it is being done; and (c) what sensations she may experience. This allows the woman to be informed and to consent to the procedure.

The woman experiences a sense of control and therefore less helplessness and powerlessness.

Preparing the woman for surgery involves more than the procedures of establishing intravenous lines and urinary catheter or doing an abdominal prep. As discussed previously, good communication skills are very influential in helping the woman stay in control. Therapeutic touch and eye contact do much to maintain reality orientation and control. These measures reduce anxiety for the woman during the stressful preparatory period. All women will experience some degree of anxiety and apprehension: behavioral manifestations of anxiety include withdrawal, crying, apologies, or inappropriate laughter. Increased heart rate, blood pressure, body temperature, dilated pupils, pallor, and/or dry mouth are physiologic signs of anxiety. Anxiety also affects senses such as sight, hearing, and cognitive grasp. Severe anxiety often results in distortion of reality. The nurse should continually assess how the woman is perceiving the event and coping with her apprehension.

If the cesarean birth is scheduled and not an emergency, the nurse has ample time for preoperative teaching. The woman needs to practice her turning, coughing, and deep breathing. It is helpful if she is taught to splint her abdominal muscles when she coughs. An informed consent for surgery will need to be signed.

To prepare the woman for the surgery, she is given nothing by mouth. To reduce the likelihood of serious pulmonary damage should aspiration of gastric contents occur, antacids may be administered within 30 minutes of surgery. If epidural anesthesia is used, the nurse may assist with the procedure, monitor the woman's blood pressure and response, and continue EFM if it is used. An abdominal and perineal prep is done (from below the breasts to the pubic region), and an indwelling catheter is inserted to prevent bladder distention. At least two units of whole blood are readied for administration. An intravenous line is started, with a needle of adequate size to permit blood administration, and preoperative medication is ordered. The pediatrician should be notified and adequate preparation made to receive the infant. The nurse should make sure that the infant warmer is functional and that appropriate resuscitation equipment is available. The circulating nurse assists in positioning the woman on the operating table. Fetal heart rate should be ascertained before surgery and during preparation, since fetal hypoxia can result from aortocaval compression. The operating table may be adjusted so it slants slightly to one side, or a wedge (folded blanket or towels) may be placed under the right hip. The uterus should be displaced about 15° from the midline (Bassell 1985). This helps relieve the pressure of the heavy uterus on the vena cava and lessens the incidence of vena caval compression and supine maternal hypotension. The suction should be in working order, and the urine collection bag should be positioned under the operating table to ensure proper urinary drainage. Auscultation or electronic monitoring of the fetal heart rate needs to continue until immediately prior to the surgery. A last-minute check is done to ensure that the fetal scalp electrode has been removed if the fetus was internally monitored.

Birth

Every effort should be made to include the father in the birth experience. Hospital routines can be established to provide for the father's presence in the operating room.

When the father attends the cesarean birth, he must scrub and wear a surgical gown and mask as do others in the operating suite. A stool can be placed beside the woman's head. The father can sit nearby to provide physical touch, visual contact, and verbal reassurance to his partner.

Other measures, such as the following, can be taken to promote the participation of the father who chooses not to be in the delivery room:

1. Allowing the father to be near the delivery/operating room where he can hear the newborn's first cry
2. Encouraging the father to carry or accompany the infant to the nursery for the initial assessment
3. Involving the father in postpartal care in the recovery room

In addition to meeting the emotional and informational needs of the expectant parents, other nursing functions are carried out to ensure physiologic support and safety of the mother and baby. The nurse should stand by to connect the suction when the operating team is ready and should record the actual time the incision is made and the infant is born. An oxytocin preparation is administered intravenously just as the infant is born.

After birth, the nurse assesses the Apgar score and completes the initial assessment and identification procedures as after a vaginal birth. Every effort must be made to assist the parents in bonding with the infant. If the mother is awake, one of the mother's arms should be freed to enable her to touch and stroke the infant. The baby can be given to the father to hold until she or he must be taken to the nursery.

Repeat administration of oxytocin during surgery may be necessary to control uterine bleeding. The circulating nurse assists with the application of the dressing to the incision and, with the aid of other staff, transfers the woman back into bed.

Analgesia and Anesthesia

There is no perfect anesthesia for cesarean birth. Each has its advantages, disadvantages, possible risks, and side effects. Goals for analgesia and anesthesia administration include safety, comfort, and emotional satisfaction for the client. See Chapter 24.

Immediate Postpartal Recovery Period

The postpartal recovery room must be equipped with suction and oxygen to ensure a patent airway and avoid respiratory obstruction resulting from secretions. The nurse caring for the postpartal woman should check the mother's vital signs every 5 minutes until they are stable, then every 15 minutes for an hour, then every 30 minutes until she is discharged to the postpartal floor. The nurse should remain with the woman until she is stable.

The dressing and perineal pad must be checked every 15 minutes for at least an hour, and the fundus should be gently palpated to determine whether it is remaining firm. The fundus may be palpated by placing a hand to support the incision. Intravenous oxytocin is usually administered to promote the contractility of the uterine musculature. If the woman has been under general anesthesia, she should be positioned on her side to facilitate drainage of secretions, turned, and assisted with coughing and deep breathing every 2 hours for at least 24 hours. If she has received a spinal or epidural anesthetic, the level of anesthesia should be checked every 15 minutes until sensation has fully returned. It is important to monitor intake and output and to observe the urine for bloody tinge, which could mean surgical trauma to the bladder. The physician prescribes medication to relieve the mother's pain and nausea, and this should be administered as needed. Some physicians use a single dose of epidural morphine (5 to 7.5 mg) for postsurgical pain relief. Facilitation of parent-infant interaction following birth and postpartal care is discussed in Chapter 35.

Care of the Woman Undergoing Vaginal Birth After Cesarean (VBAC)

There is an increasing trend to have a trial of labor and vaginal birth after a previous cesarean birth in cases of nonrecurring indications (for example, umbilical cord accident, placenta previa, fetal distress). This trend has been influenced by consumer demand and a growing body of evidence that suggests that vaginal birth after a cesarean poses less risk for maternal and neonatal mortality and morbidity than a repeat cesarean birth (Martin et al 1988).

Martin et al (1988) report that resistance to implementing a VBAC program is usually associated with one of four stated concerns. Fear for maternal safety is frequently cited; however, ". . . no maternal death in association with VBAC in a patient with a previous lower-segment incision has been reported for decades in industrialized societies" (Martin et al 1988, p 722). A second fear is for fetal safety. The fetus is not free of risk with either vaginal or cesarean birth; however, paradoxically, there is more risk to the fetus with elective cesarean birth than with a successful VBAC. Fear of legal action is another commonly held fear in the current medical-legal environment. Currently, the recommendations favoring VBAC and the standards of practice are such that failure to suggest VBAC may now be associated with more legal risk than proceeding with an elective cesarean. Lastly, stress, practice, and financial disincentives are concerns for the obstetrician. A trial of labor and VBAC may be more stressful for the obstetrician than a scheduled elective cesarean when busy office hours and the need to stay readily available during labor are considered.

The 1988 ACOG Guidelines state that the following aspects need to be considered for VBAC:

- A woman with one previous cesarean birth and a low transverse uterine incision should be counseled and encouraged to attempt VBAC
- A woman with two or more previous cesareans may attempt VBAC
- A classic uterine incision is a contraindication
- It must be possible to do a cesarean in 30 minutes
- A physician who is able to do a cesarean needs to be available

Success rates for VBAC have been encouraging. Hangsleben et al (1989) report that in a VBAC program in a nurse-midwifery service, 83% of women successfully gave birth vaginally. Martin et al (1988) report a similar success rate of 81%. Although VBAC was once reserved for women of low risk status, now women who need oxytocin augmentation or induction and those who have multiple gestations or a breech presentation with a flexed head are able to attempt VBAC (Martin et al 1988).

Nursing Care

Support of the laboring woman undergoing VBAC is the same as it would be for any laboring woman. Hangsleben et al (1989) report the use of many supportive measures for the laboring woman. Early ambulation, as well as adequate rest, is also encouraged. Warm baths and a variety of alternative positions are used to promote comfort. Many women express fear that the VBAC will not be successful and seem to need frequent reassurance until the birth actually occurs (Hangsleben et al 1989).

❀ ❀

KEY CONCEPTS

An external (or cephalic) version may be done after 37 weeks' gestation to change a breech presentation to a cephalic. The benefits of the version are that a lower-risk vaginal birth may be anticipated. The version is accomplished with the use of tocolytics to relax the uterus. An internal podalic version is used only when needed during the vaginal birth of a second twin.

Amniotomy (AROM) is probably the most common procedure in obstetrics. The risks are prolapse of the umbilical cord and infection.

Indicated induction of labor is done for many reasons. The methods include amniotomy, prostaglandins, and oxytocin infusion.

Nursing responsibilities are heightened during an induced labor.

An episiotomy may be done just prior to birth of the fetus. Although in this country it is very prevalent, it is becoming more controversial.

Forceps-assisted birth can be outlet, low or midforceps. Outlet and low forceps are the most common and are associated with few maternal-fetal complications. Midforceps are associated with more complications but when needed are an important aid to birth.

A vacuum extractor is a soft pliable cup attached to suction that can be applied to the fetal head and used in much the same way as forceps.

At least one in three or four births is now accomplished by cesarean birth. The increase in the cesarean birth rate has been influenced by many factors. The nurse has a vital role in providing information, support, and encouragement to the couple participating in a cesarean birth.

Vaginal birth after cesarean (VBAC) is becoming more popular. Overcoming the old fears of uterine rupture is a high priority for both the parents and the medical community.

❀ ❀

References

Affonso DD: *Impact of Cesarean Childbirth.* Philadelphia: Davis, 1981.

American College of Obstetricians and Gynecologists: *Induction and Augmentation of Labor.* Technical Bulletin No. 110. Washington, DC, 1988.

American College of Obstetricians and Gynecologists: *Guidelines for Vaginal Delivery After a Previous Cesarean Birth.* ACOG Committee Opinion No. 64. Washington DC, October 1988.

Bassel GM: Anesthesia for cesarean section. *Clin Obstet Gynecol* December 1985; 28:722.

Bishop EH: Pelvic scoring for elective inductions. *Obstet Gynecol* 1964; 24:266.

Borgatta L, Piening SL, Cohen WR: Association of episiotomy and delivery position with deep perineal laceration during spontaneous delivery in nulliparous women. *Am J Obstet Gynecol* 1989; 160:294.

Bromberg MH: Presumptive maternal benefits of routine episiotomy: A literature review. *J Nurse-Midwifery* May/June 1986; 31:121.

Cox BE, Smith EC: The mother's self-esteem after a cesarean delivery, *MCN* September/October 1982; 7:309.

Cunningham FG, MacDonald PC, Gant NF: *Williams Obstetrics,* 18th ed. Norwalk, CT: Appleton & Lange, 1989.

Dawood MY: Evolving concepts of oxytocin for induction of labor. *Am J Perinatol* April 1989; 6:167.

Department of Health, Education and Welfare: New restrictions on oxytocin use. Food and Drug Administration Bulletin, Vol. 8, October/November 1978.

Dunn LJ: Cesarean section and other obstetric operations. In: *Danforth's Obstetrics and Gynecology,* 6th ed. Scott JR et al (editors). Philadelphia: Lippincott, 1990, Ch 31.

Dyson DC, Ferguson JE, Hensleigh P: Antepartum external cephalic version under tocolysis. *Obstet Gynecol* January 1986; 67:63.

Freeman RK: Can we lower the cesarean birth rate? Tenth International Symposium on Perinatal Medicine and Obstetrical Ultrasound. April 9–12, 1990. Las Vegas, Nevada.

Giacoia GP, Yaffe S: Perinatal pharmacology. In: *Gynecology and Obstetrics,* Vol. 3. Sciarri JJ (editor). Philadelphia: Harper & Row, 1982, Ch 100.

Gould J, Davey B, Stafford F: Socioeconomic differences in rates of cesarean section. *N Engl J Med* 1989; 321:233.

Hangsleben KL, Taylor MA, Lynn NM: VBAC program in a nurse-midwifery service: Five Years of experience. *J Nurse-Midwifery* July/August 1989; 34:179.

Jacobs MM: Prostaglandins for cervical ripening. In: *Antepartum and Intrapartum Management.* Parer JT (editor). Philadelphia: Lea & Febiger, 1989, Ch 13.

Leveno KJ, Cunningham FG, Nelson S et al: A prospective comparison of selective and universal electronic fetal monitoring in 34,995 pregnancies. *N Engl J Med* 1986; 315:615.

Marshall C: The art of induction/augmentation of labor. *JOGNN* January/February 1985; 14:22.

Martin JN, Morrison JC, Wiser WL: Vaginal birth after cesarean section: The demise of routine repeat abdominal delivery. *Obstet Gynecol Clin North Am* December 1988; 15:719.

NAACOG: The Nurse's Role in the Induction/Augmentation of Labor, January 1988.

Niswander KR: Induction of labor. In: *Gynecology and Obstetrics,* Vol. 2. Sciarri JJ (editor). Hagerstown MD: Harper & Row, 1985, Ch 71.

Nugent CE: Induction of labor. In: *Gynecology and Obstetrics,* Vol. 2. Dilts PV, Sciarri JJ (editors). Philadelphia: Lippincott, 1989, Ch 71.

O'Grady JP: *Modern Instrumental Delivery.* Baltimore: Williams & Wilkins, 1988.

Petitti DB: The ideal cesarean section rate. In *Antepartum and Intrapartum Management.* Parer JT (editor). Philadelphia: Lea & Febiger, 1989, Ch 16.

Ramler D, Roberts J: A comparison of cold and warm sitz baths for relief of postpartum perineal pain. *JOGNN* November/December 1986; 15:471.

Rockner G, Wahlberg V, Olund A: Episiotomy and perineal trauma during childbirth. *J Adv Nurs* 1989; 14:264.

Scott JR, DiSaia PJ, Hammond CB et al (editors): *Danforth's Obstetrics and Gynecology,* 6th ed. Scott JR et al (editors). Philadelphia: Lippincott, 1990.

Sokol RK, Brindley BA: Practical diagnosis and management of abnormal labor. In: *Danforth's Obstetrics and Gynecology,* 6th ed. Scott JR, DiSaia PJ, Hammond CB, et al (editors). Philadelphia: Lippincott, 1990.

Thorp JM, Bowes WA: Episiotomy: Can its routine use be defended? *Am J Obstet Gynecol* 1989; 160:1027.

Varner MW: Episiotomy: Techniques and indications. *Clin Obstet Gynecol* June 1986; 29:309.

Additional Readings

Elster AD et al: Birth weight standards for triplets under modern obstetric care in the United States 1984–1989. *Obstet Gynecol* March 1991; 77:387.

Firian MA et al: The "Allis" test for easy cesarean delivery. *Am J Obstet Gynecol* March 1991; 772.

Hagadorn-Freathy AS et al: Validation of the 1988 ACOG forceps classification system. *Obstet Gynecol* March 1991; 77:356.

Philip AG, Allan WC: Does cesarean section prevent against intraventricular hemorrhage in preterm infants? *J Pernatol* March 1991; 11:3.

Pridjian G et al: Cesarean: Changing the trends. *Obstet Gynecol* February 1991; 77:195.

Rosen MC: Vaginal birth after cesarean: A meta-analysis of morbidity and mortality *Obstet Gynecol* March 1991: 465.

Schifrin BS, Hamilton T: Abnormal labor curve with inappropriate use of forceps *J Perinatol* March 1991; 11:63.

Winkler CL et al: Mid-second trimester labor induction: Concentrated oxytocin compared with prostaglandin E$_2$ vaginal suppositories. *Obstet Gynecol* February 1991; 77:297.

PART SIX

The Newborn

CHAPTER 27

Physiologic Response of the Newborn to Birth

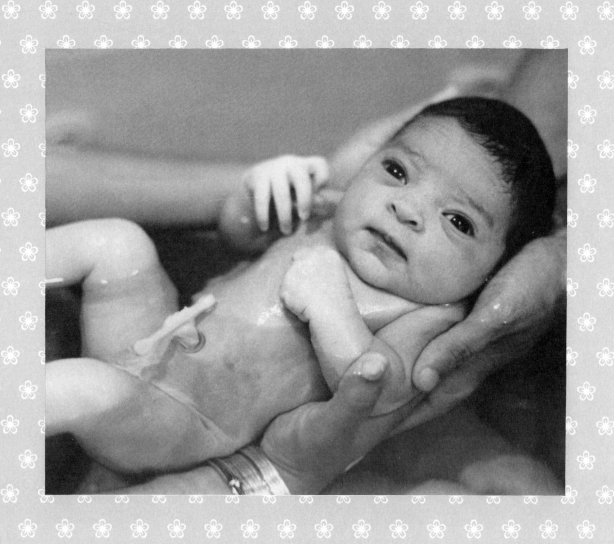

Summarize the cardiovascular and respiratory changes that occur during the transition to extrauterine life.

Summarize the major mechanisms of heat loss in the newborn and how the newborn produces heat.

Describe the functional abilities of the newborn's gastrointestinal tract.

Explain the steps involved in conjugation and excretion of bilirubin in the newborn.

Identify the reasons why the newborn's kidneys have difficulty in maintaining fluid and electrolyte balance.

List the immunologic responses available to the newborn.

Describe how various factors affect the newborn's blood values.

Describe the normal sensory/perceptual abilities present in the newborn period.

❀ ❀

The incredible attributes of the newborn have a major purpose. They prepare the baby for interaction with the family and for life in the world. (The Amazing Newborn)

The newborn period includes the time for birth through the first 28 days of life. During this period, the newborn adjusts from intrauterine to extrauterine life. The nurse needs to be knowledgeable about a newborn's normal biopsychologic adaptations to recognize alterations from it.

To begin life as a separate being, the baby must immediately establish respiratory exchange in conjunction with marked circulatory changes. These radical and rapid changes are crucial to the maintenance of life. All other newborn body systems change their level of functioning or become established over a longer period of time.

Respiratory Adaptations

Although the significant respiratory events occur at birth, certain intrauterine factors also enhance the newborn's ability to breathe.

Intrauterine Factors Supporting Respiratory Function

Fetal Lung Development

The respiratory system is in a continuous state of development during fetal life, and the development continues into the neonatal period. During the first 20 weeks of gestation, development is limited to the differentiation of pulmonary, vascular, and lymphatic structures.

At 20 to 24 weeks alveolar ducts begin to appear, followed by primitive alveoli at 24 to 28 weeks. During this time, the alveolar epithelial cells begin to differentiate into type I cells (structures necessary for respiratory gas exchange) and type II cells (structures that provide for the synthesis and storage of surfactant). **Surfactant** is composed of a group of surface-active phospholipids, of which one component, *lecithin,* is the most critical for alveolar stability.

At 28 to 32 weeks the number of type II cells increases further, and surfactant is produced by a choline pathway within the type II cells. Surfactant production by this pathway peaks at about 35 weeks' gestation and remains high until term, paralleling late fetal lung development. At this time, the lungs are structurally developed enough to permit maintenance of good lung expansion and adequate exchange of gases (Avery 1987).

Clinically, the peak production of surfactant by the choline pathway corresponds closely with the marked decrease in incidence of idiopathic respiratory distress syndrome after 35 weeks' gestation. Production of sphingomyelin remains constant throughout gestation. The neonate born before the lecithin/sphingomyelin (L/S) ratio is 2:1 will have varying degrees of respiratory distress. (See discussion of L/S ratio in Chapters 20, 32.)

Fetal Breathing Movements

The ability of the neonate to breathe air immediately upon exposure to extrauterine life appears to be the consequence of weeks of intrauterine practice. In this respect, breathing can be perceived as a continuation of an intrauterine process as the lungs convert from a fluid to a gas medium. Fetal breathing movements (FBM) occur as early as 11 weeks' gestation (see Chapter 20 for discussion). These breathing movements are essential for development of chest wall muscles (including the diaphragm) and to a lesser extent for regulating lung fluid volume and, therefore, lung growth.

Initiation of Breathing

To maintain life, the lungs must function immediately after birth. The following must occur to establish respiratory function:

1. Extrauterine respiratory movements begin.

2. Air entry overcomes opposing forces so that the lungs expand.

3. Some air remains in the alveoli during expiration, thus preventing lung collapse. (The amount of air remaining is called the functional residual capacity.)

4. Pulmonary blood flow increases, and cardiac output is redistributed.

The first breath of life—the gasp in response to mechanical, chemical, thermal, and sensory and physical changes associated with birth—initiates the serial opening of the alveoli. Thus begins the transition from a fluid-filled environment to an air-breathing, extrauterine life.

Mechanical Events

During the latter half of gestation, the fetal lungs produce fluid continuously. This secretion fills the lungs almost completely, expanding the air spaces. Some of the lung fluid moves up into the trachea and into the amniotic fluid and is then swallowed by the fetus.

Secretion of lung fluid diminishes two to four days before onset of labor (Eden & Boehm 1990). However, approximately 80 to 110 mL of fluid remains in the respiratory passages of a normal term fetus at the time of birth. This fluid must be removed from the lungs to permit adequate movement of air.

The primary mechanical events that initiate respiration involve the removal of fluid from the lungs as the baby passes through the birth canal. As the fetal chest is compressed, thus increasing intrathoracic pressure, approximately one-third of the fluid is squeezed out of the lungs. After the birth of the newborn's trunk, the chest wall recoils. This chest recoil is thought to produce a small, passive inspiration of air (negative intrathoracic pressure sucks air in), which is drawn into the lungs to replace the fluid that was squeezed out. After this first inspiration, the newborn exhales, with crying, against a partially closed glottis, creating a positive intrathoracic pressure. The high positive pressure distributes the inspired air throughout the alveoli and begins the establishment of functional residual capacity (FRC). The increased thoracic pressure also increases absorption of fluid via the capillaries and lymphatic system. On inspiration, the diaphragm descends, creating greater pressure within the alveoli than outside. Fluid flows from the alveoli across the alveolar membranes into the pulmonary interstitial tissue.

With each succeeding breath, the lungs expand, stretching the alveolar walls and enlarging the alveolar pores. The expansion of the pores facilitates movement of the remaining lung fluid into the interstitial tissue. Since the protein concentration is higher in the pulmonary capillaries, the interstitial fluid passes by osmosis into the capillaries and lymphatics. As pulmonary vascular resistance decreases, pulmonary blood flow increases, and more fluid is absorbed into the bloodstream. In the normal term newborn, movement of lung fluid to the interstitial tissue is rapid, but movement into lymph and blood vessels may take several hours. Some of the lung fluid remains to form surfactant bubbles (Eden & Boehm 1990).

Some of the inspired air is also forced into the proximal airways. An air–liquid interface (the surface boundary between these two components) is established in the smaller airways and alveoli. About 70% of the fluid is reabsorbed within 2 hours after birth, and it is completely absorbed within 12 to 24 hours after birth (Korones 1986). Figure 27–1 summarizes the initiation of respiration.

Although the initial expiration should clear the airways of accumulated fluid and permit further inspiration, some clinicians feel it is wise to suction mucus and fluid from the newborn's mouth and oropharynx, especially after cesarean births. They use a DeLee mucus trap attached to suction or a bulb syringe as soon as the newborn's head and shoulders are born and again as the newborn adapts to extrauterine life and stabilizes (see Procedure 23–1 Chapter 23).

Problems associated with lung clearance and/or initiation of respiratory activity may be caused by a variety of factors. The lymphatics may be underdeveloped, thus decreasing the rate at which the fluid is absorbed from the lungs. Complications that occur antenatally or during labor and birth can interfere with adequate lung expansion, resulting in increased pulmonary vascular resistance and decreased blood flow. These complications include inadequate compression of the chest wall in a very small neonate, the absence of chest wall compression in the neonate delivered by cesarean birth, severe asphyxia at birth, or aspiration of amniotic fluid or meconium.

Chemical Stimuli

An important chemical stimulator that contributes to the onset of breathing is transitory asphyxia of the fetus and newborn. Elevation in PCO_2 and decrease in pH and PO_2 are the natural outcomes of normal vaginal birth with cutting of the umbilical cord and cessation of the cord's pulsation and placental gas exchange. These changes, which are present in all newborns to some degree, stimulate the aortic and carotid chemoreceptors, initiating impulses that trigger the medulla's respiratory center. Although brief periods of asphyxia are a significant stimulator, prolonged asphyxia is abnormal and acts as a central nervous system depressant.

Thermal Stimuli

A significant decrease in ambient temperature after birth (from 98.6F to 70–75F or 37C to 21–23.9C) is enough thermal stimulus for initiation breathing. As skin nerve endings are stimulated to transmit impulses to the medullary respiratory control center, the newborn responds with rhythmic respirations. Excessive cooling may result in profound depression and evidence of cold stress, but the nor-

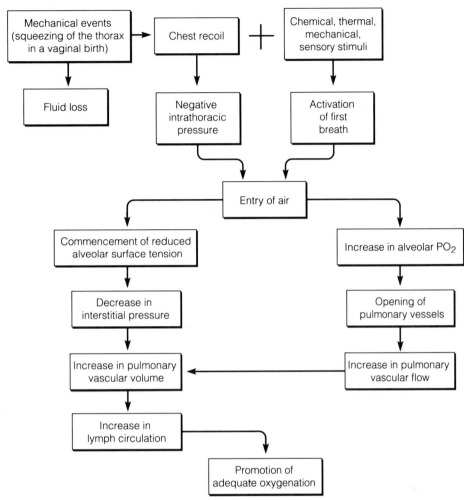

Figure 27–1   Initiation of respiration in the neonate

mal temperature changes that occur at birth are apparently within acceptable physiologic limits (see Chapter 32 for discussion of cold stress).

Sensory/Physical Stimuli

As the fetus moves from a familiar, comfortable environment, a number of sensory and physical influences help initiate respiration. They include the numerous tactile, auditory, and visual stimuli of birth. Historically, vigorous stimulation was provided by slapping the buttocks or heels of the newborn, but today greater emphasis is placed on gentle physical contact. Thoroughly drying the infant provides stimulation in a far more comforting way and also decreases heat loss.

Factors Opposing the First Breath

Three major factors may oppose the initiation of respiratory activity: (1) alveolar surface tension, (2) viscosity of lung fluid within the respiratory tract, and (3) degree of lung compliance.

Because of alveolar surface tension, there is a constant tendency for surfaces to contract. The small airways and alveoli would collapse between each inspiration were it not for the presence of surfactant, which reduces the attracting force between the moist surfaces of the alveoli. Surfactant promotes lung expansion by preventing the alveoli from completely collapsing with each expiration and increases lung *compliance* (the ability of the lung to fill with air easily). When surfactant is decreased, compliance is also decreased and the pressure needed to expand the lungs with air increases. Resistive forces of the fluid-filled (presence of viscous lung fluid) lung combined with the small radii of the respiratory airways require the generation of pressures of 40 to 80 cm of water to initially open the lung. The first breath generally establishes a functional residual capacity that is 30% to 40% of the fully expanded lung volume. The FRC allows alveolar sacs to remain partially expanded on expiration. This remaining air in the lungs after expiration alleviates the need for continuous high pressure for successive breaths. Subsequent breaths require only 6 to 8 cm H_2O pressure to open alveoli during inspiration. Therefore, the first breath of life is usually the most difficult.

Cardiopulmonary Physiology

With the onset of respiration, the functions of the cardiovascular and respiratory systems become interrelated; hence the term **cardiopulmonary adaptation**. As air enters the lungs, PO_2 rises in the alveoli, which stimulates the relaxation of the pulmonary arteries and triggers a decrease in the pulmonary vascular resistance. At the same time, the lowered surface tension decreases interstitial pressure. As pulmonary vascular resistance decreases, the vascular flow in the lung increases to 100% at 24 hours of life. This greater blood volume to the lungs contributes to the conversion from fetal circulation to newborn circulation.

After pulmonary circulation is established, blood is distributed throughout the lung, although the alveoli may or may not be fully open. For adequate oxygenation to occur, sufficient blood must be delivered by the heart to the lungs. It is important to remember that shunting of blood is common in the early newborn period. This bidirectional blood flow, or right-to-left shunting through the ductus arteriosus, may divert a significant amount of blood away from the lungs depending on the pressure changes of respiration, crying, and the cardiac cycle. This shunting in the newborn period is also responsible for the unstable transitional period to neonatal respiratory functions.

Oxygen Transport

The transportation of oxygen to the peripheral tissues depends on the type of hemoglobin in the red blood cell. In the fetus and neonate, a variety of hemoglobins exist, the most significant being fetal hemoglobin (Hb F) and adult hemoglobin (Hb A). Approximately 70% to 90% of hemoglobin in the fetus and neonate is of the fetal variety. The greatest difference between Hb F and Hb A is related to the transport of oxygen.

In the newborn, the greater affinity of Hb F for oxygen causes a shift to the left in the oxygen dissociation curve (Figure 27–2). Since more oxygen is bound to Hb F, the oxygen saturation in the newborn's blood is greater than in the adult's, but the amount of oxygen available to the tissues is less. This is beneficial prenatally, because the fetus must maintain adequate oxygen uptake in the presence of very low oxygen tension (umbilical venous Po_2 cannot exceed the uterine venous Po_2). Because of this phenomenon, hypoxia in the neonate is particularly difficult to recognize because of the high concentration of oxygen in the blood. Clinical manifestations of cyanosis are lacking until low blood levels of oxygen are present. Shifts to the left in the curve also may be caused by alkalosis (increased pH) and hypothermia. Acidosis, hypercarbia, and hyperthermia may cause the oxygen dissociation curve to shift to the right. In summary, a shift to the left results in less oxygen being available to the body tissues, and a shift to the right in the oxygen dissociation curve results in less oxygen bound to the hemoglobin and more oxygen being released to the body tissues.

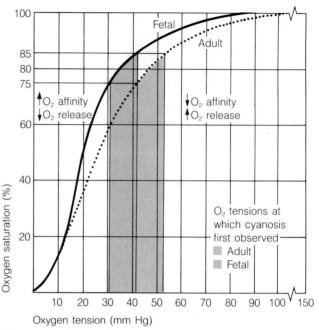

Figure 27–2   Fetal oxygen dissociation curve (Modified from Klaus M, Fanaroff AA: Care of the High Risk Infant 3rd ed. Philadelphia: WB Saunders, 1986, p 234)

Other factors that regulate oxygen supply to the tissues are blood oxygen capacity and cardiac output. Oxygen capacity is the maximum amount of hemoglobin and oxygen that can be bound together and is directly affected by hemoglobin concentration. One gram of hemoglobin is able to combine with 1.34 mL of oxygen. The actual amount of oxygen-bound hemoglobin divided by the oxygen capacity gives a percentage signifying *oxygen saturation.* Oxygen saturation, which is controlled by arterial oxygen tension (PaO_2) and hemoglobin-oxygen affinity, usually has values between 96% and 98% after several hours of life. A significant reduction in the oxygen capacity results in an increased cardiac output to compensate for the decreased oxygen concentration of the hemoglobin.

Maintaining Respiratory Function

The ability of the lung to maintain oxygen (oxygenation) and carbon dioxide exchange (ventilation) is influenced by such factors as lung compliance and airway resistance. Lung compliance is influenced by the elastic recoil of the lung tissue and by anatomic variation. Anatomic differences between the neonate and the adult influence lung compliance. The infant has a relatively large heart and mediastinal structures that reduce available lung space. The large abdomen further encroaches on the high diaphragm to decrease lung space. Anatomically, the neonatal chest is equipped with weak intercostal muscles, a rigid rib cage with horizontal ribs, and a high diaphragm that restricts the space available for lung expansion. Ventilation is also limited by airway resistance, which depends on the radii, length, and number of airways.

Characteristics of Neonatal Respiration

The normal neonatal respiratory rate is 30 to 60 breaths per minute. Initial respirations may be largely diaphragmatic, with shallow and irregular depth and rhythm. They are primarily abdominal and synchronous with the chest movement. Short periods of apnea are to be expected. When the breathing pattern is characterized by pauses lasting 5 to 15 seconds followed by an interval of regular respirations so that the respiratory rate for one minute is within normal limits, then **periodic breathing** is occurring. Periodic breathing is rarely associated with differences in skin color or heart rate changes, and it has no prognostic significance. Tactile or other sensory stimulation increases the inspired oxygen and converts periodic breathing patterns to normal breathing patterns. Neonatal sleep states in particular influence respiratory patterns. The pattern is regular in deep sleep. Periodic breathing occurs with rapid-eye-movement (REM) sleep, and grossly irregular breathing is evident with motor activity, sucking, and crying.

The neonate is an obligatory nose breather, and any obstruction will cause respiratory distress, so it is important to keep the throat and nose clear. If respirations drop below 30 or exceed 60 per minute when the infant is at rest, or if dyspnea, cyanosis, or nasal flaring and expiratory grunting occurs, the physician should be notified. Immediately after birth and for the first few (about 2) hours after birth, respiratory rates of 60 to 70 breaths per minute are normal. Some initial dyspnea, cyanosis, and acrocyanosis is

normal for several hours. Any increased use of the intercostal muscle (retracting) may indicate respiratory distress. (See Chapter 32 and Table 32–3 for signs of respiratory distress.)

Cardiovascular Adaptations

As described on page 818, blood flow to the lungs increases with the first respirations of the normal newborn. This greater blood volume contributes to the conversion from fetal circulation to neonatal circulation.

Fetal-Neonatal Transitional Anatomy and Physiology

During fetal life, blood with higher oxygen content is diverted to the heart and brain. Blood in the descending aorta is less oxygenated and supplies the kidneys and intestinal tract. Limited amounts of blood, pumped from the right ventricle toward the lungs, enters the pulmonary vessels. In the fetus, increased pulmonary resistance forces most of the blood through the ductus arteriosus into the descending aorta (Table 27–1).

Marked changes occur in the cardiovascular system at birth. Expansion of the lungs with the first breath decreases the pulmonary vascular resistance and left artrial pressure, and the clamping of the cord raises systemic vascular resistance. This physiologic mechanism marks the beginning of transition from fetal to neonatal circulation and shows the interplay of the cardiovascular and respiratory systems (Figure 27–3). As the newborn adapts to extrauterine life, there are five major areas of change in circulatory function:

Table 27–1 Fetal and Neonatal Circulation

System	Fetal	Neonatal
Pulmonary blood vessels	Constricted with very little blood flow; lungs not expanded	Vasodilation and increased blood flow; lungs expanded; increased oxygen stimulates vasodilation.
Systemic blood vessels	Dilated with low resistance; blood mostly in placenta	Arterial pressure rises due to loss of placenta; increased systemic blood volume and resistance.
Ductus arteriosus	Large with no tone; blood flow from pulmonary artery to aorta	1. Reversal of blood flow. Now from aorta to pulmonary artery due to increased left atrial pressure. 2. Ductus is sensitive to increased oxygen and body chemicals and begins to constrict.
Foramen ovale	Patent with large blood flow from right atrium to left atrium	Increased pressure in left atrium attempts to reverse blood flow and shuts one-way valve.

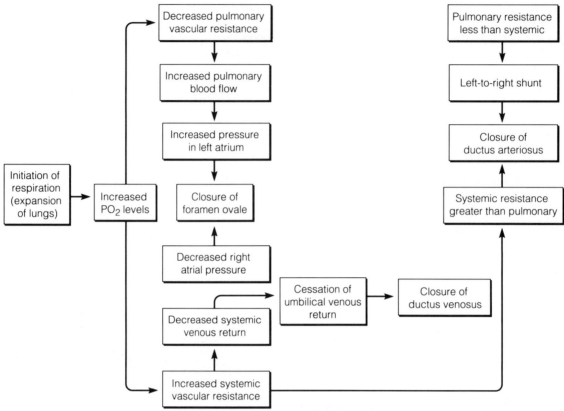

Figure 27–3   Transitional circulation: conversion from fetal to neonatal circulation

1. **Increased aortic pressure and decreased venous pressure.** With cutting of the cord, the placental vascular bed is eliminated and the intravascular space is reduced. Consequently, aortic (systemic) blood pressure is increased. At the same time, when the newborn is separated from the placenta, blood return via the inferior vena cava is decreased, resulting in a small decrease in pressure within the venous circulation.

2. **Increased systemic pressure and decreased pulmonary artery pressure.** With the loss of the low-resistance placenta, pressure increases in the systemic circulation, resulting in greater systemic resistance. At the same time, lung expansion promotes increased pulmonary blood flow, and the increased blood PO_2 associated with initiation of respirations produces vasodilatation of pulmonary blood vessels. The combination of increased pulmonary blood flow and vasodilatation results in decreased pulmonary artery resistance. As a result of opening the vascular beds, the systemic vascular pressure decreases, causing perfusion of the other body systems.

3. **Closure of the foramen ovale.** Closure of the foramen ovale is a function of atrial pressures. In utero, pressure is greater in right atrium, and the foramen ovale is open. Decreased pulmonary

resistance and increased pulmonary blood flow result in increased pulmonary venous return into the left atrium, thereby increasing left atrial pressure slightly. The decreased pulmonary vascular resistance also causes a decrease in right atrial pressure. The pressure gradients are now reversed, left atrial pressure is greater, and the foramen ovale is functionally closed. Although the foramen ovale closes one to two hours after birth, a slight right-to-left shunting may occur in the early neonatal period. Any increase in pulmonary resistance may result in reopening of the foramen ovale, causing a right-to-left shunt. Permanent closer occurs within several months.

4. **Closure of the ductus arteriosus.** Initial elevation of the systemic vascular pressure above the pulmonary vascular pressure increases pulmonary blood flow by causing a reversal of the flow through the ductus arteriosus. Blood now flows from the aorta into the pulmonary artery. Furthermore, although the presence of oxygen causes the pulmonary arterioles to dilate, an increase in blood PO_2 triggers the opposite response in the ductus arteriosus—active constriction.

In utero, the placenta provides prostaglandin E_2 (PGE_2), which causes ductus vasodilatation. With the loss of the placenta and increased pulmonary blood flow, PGE₂ levels drop, leaving the active constriction by PO₂ unopposed. If the lungs fail to expand or if PO₂ levels drop, the ductus remains patent. Fibrosis of the ductus occurs within three weeks after birth, but functional closure is accomplished within 15 hours after birth (Long 1990).

5. *Closure of the ductus venosus.* Although the mechanism of initiating closure of the ductus venosus is not known, it appears to be related to mechanical pressure changes after severing of the cord, redistribution of blood, and cardiac output. Closure of the bypass forces perfusion of the liver. Fibrotic closure occurs within two months (Long 1990) (Figure 27–4).

Characteristics

Heart Rate

Shortly after the first cry and the advent of cardiopulmonary circulation, the newborn heart rate accelerates to 175 to 180 beats per minute. Thereafter the rate follows a fairly uniform course, slowing to 115 beats per minute at 4 to 6 hours of life; then rising and leveling off at approximately 120 beats per minute at 12 to 24 hours of life (Smith & Nelson 1976). The range of the heart rate in the full-term neonate is 100 beats per minute while asleep and 120 to 150 while awake. Resting heart rates are as low as 70 to 90 beats per minute, and rates as high as 180 while crying have been reported as normal. Apical pulse rates should be obtained by auscultation for a full minute, preferably when the neonate is asleep. Peripheral pulses should also be evaluated to detect any lags or unusual characteristics.

Blood Pressure

During the newborn period, the blood pressure tends to be highest immediately after birth, and then it descends to its lowest level about three hours of age. By four to six days of life, the blood pressure rises and plateaus at a level approximately the same as the initial level. Blood pressure is particularly sensitive to the changes in blood volume that occur in the transition to neonatal circulation. Figure 27–5 diagrams this response.

Blood pressure values during the first 12 hours of life vary with the birth weight. In the full-term resting neonate, the average blood pressure is 74/47 mm Hg and 64/39 mm Hg for the preterm newborn. Crying may cause an elevation of 20 mm Hg in both the systolic and diastolic blood pressure; thus, accuracy is more likely in the quiet newborn. The measurement of blood pressure is best accomplished by using the Doppler technique or a 1- to 2-inch cuff and a stethoscope over the brachial artery.

Heart Murmurs

Murmurs are usually produced by turbulent blood flow. Murmurs may be heard when blood flows across an abnormal valve or across a stenosed valve, when there is an atrial septal or ventricular septal defect, or when there is increased flow across a normal valve.

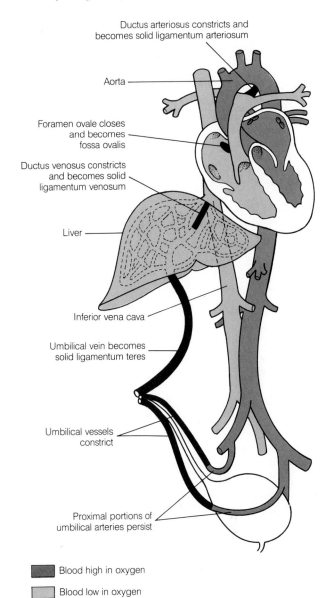

Ductus arteriosus constricts and becomes solid ligamentum arteriosum

Aorta

Foramen ovale closes and becomes fossa ovalis

Ductus venosus constricts and becomes solid ligamentum venosum

Liver

Inferior vena cava

Umbilical vein becomes solid ligamentum teres

Umbilical vessels constrict

Proximal portions of umbilical arteries persist

▓ Blood high in oxygen

▒ Blood low in oxygen

Figure 27–4 Major changes that occur in the newborn's circulatory system (From Hole JW: Human Anatomy and Physiology, 5th ed. Dubuque, IA: William C Brown Publishers, 1990. All Rights Reserved. Reprinted by permission.)

In newborns, 90% of all murmurs are transient and not associated with anomalies. They usually involve incomplete closure of the ductus arteriosus or foramen ovale. Soft murmurs may be heard as the pulmonary branch arteries increase their blood flow from 7% to 50% of combined ventricular output during transition, causing physiologic peripheral pulmonary stenosis. With early discharge, murmurs associated with ventricular septal defect and patent ductus arteriosus are not being picked up until the first well-baby checkup at four to six weeks of age. It should also be noted that murmurs are sometimes absent in seriously malformed hearts. Presence of a split S1 may be re-

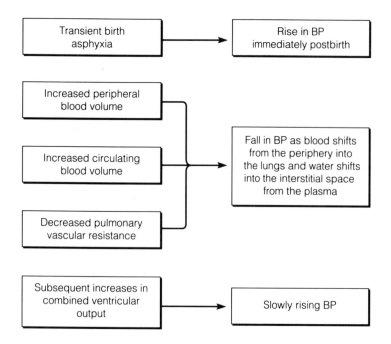

Figure 27–5 Response of BP to neonatal changes in blood volume

assuring whereas a gallop may be an ominous finding. See Chapter 31 for discussion of congenital heart defects.

Cardiac Workload

In the first two hours after birth when the ductus arteriosus remains mostly patent, about one-third of the ventricular output is returned to the pulmonary circulation. Minimal amounts of blood may also shunt from left to right through the foramen ovale. As a result, the left ventricle has a significantly greater volume load than the right ventricle. In the adult, right and left ventricular outputs are equal; in the neonate, right ventricular output equals systemic blood flow, and left ventricular output equals pulmonary blood flow. Systemic blood volume and pulmonary blood volume are *not* equal in the neonate. The newborn's combined cardiac output (left and right ventricular) is greater per unit of body weight than it will be in later childhood.

Prior to birth, the right ventricle does approximately two-thirds of the cardiac work. This workload is seen in the increased size and thickness of the right ventricle at birth and may explain why left-sided heart defects are less tolerable than right-sided lesions after birth. After birth the left ventricle must assume a larger share of the cardiac workload, and it increases in size and thickness.

Hematologic Adaptations

In the fetus, the hemoglobin and erythrocyte counts are high because of the nature of fetal circulation. Fetal blood (umbilical vein) in utero is 50% oxygen saturated; this relative hypoxia causes increased amounts of erythropoietin to be secreted, resulting in active erythropoiesis (an increase in nucleated red blood cells and reticulocytes). After birth (8 to 12 weeks postnatally), erythropoietin is again produced by the kidney. In the first days of life, hemoglobin concentration may rise by 1 to 2 g/dL above fetal levels as a result of placental transfusion, low oral fluid intake, and diminished extracellular fluid volume. By one week postnatally, peripheral hemoglobin is comparable to fetal blood counts. The hemoglobin level declines progressively thereafter during the first three months after birth and then begins to increase slowly (Avery 1987). The initial decline in hemoglobin creates a phenomenon known as **physiologic anemia of infancy.** A factor that influences the degree of physiologic anemia is the nutritional status of the neonate. Supplies of vitamin E, folic acid, and iron may be inadequate given the amount of growth in the later part of the first year of life. Hemoglobin values fall, mainly from a decrease in red cell mass rather than from the dilutional effect of increasing plasma volume. The fact that red cell survival is lower in newborns than in adults, and that red cell production is less, also contribute to this anemia. Neonatal red blood cells have a life span of 80 to 100 days, which is approximately two-thirds of an adult's red blood cell life span.

Leukocytosis is a normal finding because the trauma of birth stimulates increased production of neutrophils during the first week of life. Neurtophils then decrease to 35% of the total leukocyte count by two weeks of age. The thymus provides lymphoblasts to the lymph nodes and other lymphoid tissue, which then play a role in antibody formation. Megakaryocytes appear in the liver and spleen as platelets at about 11 weeks' gestation and approach adult values by 30 weeks. Lymphocytes eventually become the predominant type of leukocyte, and the total white blood count falls.

Blood volume of the term infant is estimated to be 80 to 85 mL/kg of body weight. The true amount of blood volume varies based on the amount of placental transfusion re-

Table 27–2   Normal Term Newborn Blood Values

Laboratory data	Normal range
Hemoglobin	15–20 g/dL
Hematocrit	43%–61%
WBC	10,000–30,000/mm³
Neutrophils	40%–80%
Immature WBC	3%–10%
Platelets	100,000–280,000/mm³
Reticulocytes	3%–6%
Blood volume	82.3 mL/kg (third day after early cord clamping) 92.6 mL/kg (third day after delayed cord clamping)
Sodium mmol/L	124–156
Potassium mmol/L	5.3–7.3
Chloride mmol/L	90–111
Calcium mg/dL	7.3–9.2
Glucose mg/dL	40–97

ceived. The concentration of serum electrolytes in the blood indicates the fluid and electrolyte status of the baby. See Table 27–2 for normal term newborn electrolyte and blood values. Hematologic values in the newborn are affected by several factors, including the following:

The site of the blood sample. Hemoglobin and hematocrit levels taken simultaneously are significantly higher in capillary blood than in venous blood. Sluggish peripheral blood flow creates red blood cell stasis, thereby increasing their concentration in the capillaries. Because of this, blood samples taken from venous blood sites are more accurate.

Delayed cord clamping and the normal shift of plasma to the extravascular spaces. Neonatal hemoglobin and hematocrit values are higher when a placental transfusion occurs postnatally. Placental vessels contain about 100 mL of blood at term, most of which can be transfused into the newborn by holding the newborn below the level of the placenta and by late clamping of the cord (Figure 27–6). Blood volume increases by

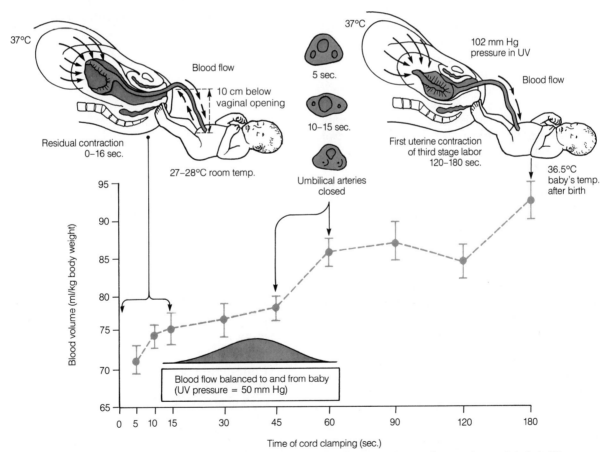

Figure 27–6   Schematic illustration of the mechanisms in placental transfusion (normal term births). The mean neonatal blood volume at 30 minutes is plotted against time of cord clamping after birth (mean + SE, data from 114 full-term infants). Note episodic, stepwise increments in blood volume at 10, 60, and 180 seconds (From: Yao AC, Lind J: Placental Transfusion: A Clinical and Physiological Study. Springfield, IL: Charles C. Thomas, 1982)

40% to 60% with late cord clamping (Korones 1986). The increase is reflected by a rise in hemoglobin level and an increase in the hematocrit to 65% about 48 hours after birth (compared with 48% when the cord is clamped immediately). For greatest accuracy, the initial hemoglobin and hematocrit levels should be measured in the cord blood, although this is not a routine practice.

Gestational age. There appears to be a positive association between increasing gestational age, higher red blood cell numbers, and greater hemoglobin concentration. This means that the gestational age of the newborn influences the values.

Prenatal and/or perinatal hemorrhage. Occurrence of significant prenatal or perinatal bleeding decreases the hematocrit level and causes hypovolemia.

Temperature Regulation

Temperature regulation is the maintenance of thermal balance of the loss of heat to the environment at a rate equal to the production of heat. Newborns are *homeothermic;* they attempt to stabilize their internal (core) body temperatures within a narrow range in spite of significant temperature variations in their environment.

Thermoregulation in the newborn is closely related to the rate of metabolism and oxygen consumption. Within a specific environmental range called the **thermal neutral zone (TNZ)**, the rates of oxygen consumption and metabolism are minimal, and internal body temperature is maintained because of thermal balance (Table 27–3). For an unclothed full-term newborn, the TNZ range is an ambient temperature of 32 to 34C (89.6–93.2F). The limits for an adult are 26 to 28C (78.8–82.4F). Thus, the normal newborn requires higher environmental temperatures to maintain a thermoneutral environment.

Several newborn characteristics affect the establishment of a TNZ. The newborn has decreased subcutaneous fat and a thin epidermis. Blood vessels are closer to the skin than those of an adult. Therefore, the circulating blood is influenced by changes in environmental temperature and in turn influences the hypothalamic temperature-regulating center.

The flexed posture of the term infant decreases the surface area exposed to the environment, thereby reducing heat loss. Other neonatal characteristics such as size and age may also affect the establishing of a TNZ. Preterm small-for-gestational-age (SGA) newborns (due to decreased adipose tissue and hypoflexion) require higher environmental temperatures to achieve a thermal neutral environment while a larger, well-insulated newborn may be able to cope with lower environmental temperature. If the environmental temperature falls below the lower limits of the TNZ, the newborn responds with increased oxygen consumption and raised metabolism, which results in greater heat production. Prolonged exposure to the cold may result in depleted glycogen stores and acidosis. Oxygen consumption also increases if the environmental temperature is above the TNZ.

Heat Loss

A newborn is at a distinct disadvantage in maintaining a normal temperature. With a larger body surface in relation to mass and a limited amount of insulating subcutaneous fat, the full-term newborn loses about four times as much heat as an adult (Cunningham et al 1989). The neonate's poor thermal stability is primarily due to excessive heat loss rather than to impaired heat production. Because of the risk of hypothermia, minimizing heat loss in the newborn after birth is essential (see Chapters 23 and 29 for nursing measures).

Two major routes of heat loss are from the internal core of the body to the body surface, and from the body surface to the environment. Usually the core temperature is 0.5C higher than the skin temperature, resulting in continuous transfer or conduction of heat to the body surface. The greater the difference in temperatures between core and skin, the more rapid the transfer. Heat loss from the body surface to the environment takes place by four avenues—convection, radiation, evaporation, and conduction.

- **Convection** is the loss of heat from the warm body surface to the cooler air currents. Air-conditioned rooms, oxygen by mask, and removal from an incubator for procedures done without an overhead warmer increase convective heat loss of the neonate.

- **Radiation** losses occur when heat transfers from the heated body surface to cooler surfaces and objects not in direct contact with the body. The walls of a room or of an incubator are potential causes of heat loss by radiation, even if the ambient temperature of the isolette is within the thermal neutral range for that infant.

- **Evaporation** is the loss of heat incurred when water is converted to a vapor. The newborn is particularly prone to heat loss by evaporation immediately after birth, when the infant is wet with amniotic fluid, and during baths.

- **Conduction** is the loss of heat to a cooler surface by direct skin contact. Chilled hands, cool scales, cold examination tables, and cold stethoscopes can cause loss of heat by conduction.

After birth, the highest losses of heat generally result from radiation and convection, because of the newborn's large body surface compared with weight, and from thermal conduction because of the marked difference between core temperature and skin temperature. The newborn can

Table 27–3   Neutral Thermal Environmental Temperatures*

Age and weight	Range of temperature (C)[†]	Age and weight	Range of temperature (C)[†]
0–6 Hours		*72–96 Hours*	
Under 1200 g	34.0–35.4	Under 1200 g	34.0–35.0
1200–1500 g	33.9–34.4	1200–1500 g	33.0–34.0
1501–2500 g	32.8–33.8	1501–2500 g	31.1–33.2
Over 2500 (and >36 weeks)	32.0–33.8	Over 2500 (and >36 weeks)	29.8–32.8
6–12 Hours		*4–12 Days*	
Under 1200 g	34.0–35.4	Under 1500 g	33.0–34.0
1200–1500 g	33.5–34.4	1501–2500 g	31.0–33.2
1501–2500 g	32.2–33.8	Over 2500 (and >36 weeks)	
Over 2500 (and >36 weeks)	31.4–33.8	4–5 days	29.5–32.6
12–24 Hours		5–6 days	29.4–32.3
Under 1200 g	34.0–35.4	6–8 days	29.0–32.2
1200–1500 g	33.3–34.3	8–10 days	29.0–31.8
1501–2500 g	31.8–33.8	10–12 days	29.0–31.4
Over 2500 (and >36 weeks)	31.0–33.7	*12–14 Days*	
24–36 Hours		Under 1500 g	32.6–34.0
Under 1200 g	34.0–35.0	1500–2500 g	31.0–33.2
1200–1500 g	33.1–34.2	Over 2500 (and >36 weeks)	29.0–30.8
1501–2500 g	31.6–33.6	*2–3 Weeks*	
Over 2500 (and >36 weeks)	30.7–33.5	Under 1500 g	32.2–34.0
36–48 Hours		1500–2500 g	30.5–33.0
Under 1200 g	34.0–35.0	*3–4 Weeks*	
1200–1500 g	33.0–34.1	Under 1500 g	31.6–33.6
1501–2500 g	31.4–33.5	1500–2500 g	30.0–32.7
Over 2500 (and >36 weeks)	30.5–33.3	*4–5 Weeks*	
48–72 Hours		Under 1500 g	31.2–33.0
Under 1200 g	34.0–35.0	1500–2500 g	29.5–32.2
1200–1500 g	33.0–34.0	*5–6 Weeks*	
1501–2500 g	31.2–33.4	Under 1500 g	30.6–32.3
Over 2500 g (and >36 weeks)	30.1–33.2	1500–2500 g	29.0–31.8

[†] *Generally speaking, the smaller infants in each weight group will require a temperature in the higher portion of the temperature range. Within each time range, the younger the infant, the higher the temperature required.*

*Adapted from Scopes and Ahmed (1966). For his table, Scopes had the walls of the incubator 1–2 degrees warmer than the ambient air temperatures.

From Klaus MH, Fanaroff AA: Care of the High-Risk Neonate, 3rd ed. Philadelphia: WB Saunders, 1986, p 103.

respond to the cooler environmental temperature with adequate peripheral vasoconstriction, but this mechanism is less effective because of the minimal amount of fat insulation present, the large body surface, and ongoing thermal conduction. Because of these factors, minimizing the baby's heat loss and preventing hypothermia are imperative. Nursing measures for preventing hypothermia can be found in Chapter 29.

Heat Production (Thermogenesis)

When exposed to a cool environment, the newborn requires additional heat. Several sources of heat production, or *thermogenesis,* are available, including increased basal metabolic rate, muscular activity, and chemical thermo-

genesis (also referred to as *nonshivering thermogenesis*) mediated through the release of catecholamines such as norepinephrine (Avery & First 1989).

Nonshivering thermogenesis is unique to the newborn and uses the newborn's stores of brown adipose tissue. **Brown adipose tissue (BAT),** also called brown fat, is the primary source of heat in the cold-stressed newborn. It first appears in the fetus at 26 to 30 weeks' gestation and continues to increase until two to five weeks after the birth of a full-term neonate, unless it is depleted by cold stress. Brown fat is deposited in the midscapular area, around the neck, and in the axillas, with deeper placement around the trachea, esophagus, abdominal aorta, kidneys, and adrenal glands (Figure 27–7). BAT constitutes 2% to 6% of the newborn's total body weight. Brown fat receives

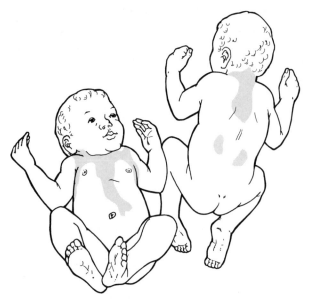

Figure 27–7   The distribution of brown adipose tissue (brown fat) in the neonate (Adapted from Davis V: Structure and function of brown adipose tissue in the neonate. JOGNN November/December, 1980; 9:364)

its name from its dark color, which is due to its enriched blood supply, dense cellular content, and abundant nerve endings.

The large numbers of fat cells facilitate the speed with which triglycerides can be metabolized to produce heat. Energy is provided by the presence of glycogen and large numbers of mitochondria releasing adenosine triphosphate (ATP) for rapid metabolic turnover and production of heat. In addition, brown fat possesses a rich blood supply to enhance distribution of heat throughout the body and a nerve supply for initiation of metabolic activity. The brown fat is metabolized and used within several weeks after birth (Korones 1986).

Nonshivering thermogenesis occurs when skin receptors perceive environmental temperature changes and transmit sensations to the CNS, which in turn stimulates the sympathetic nervous system. Release of norepinephrine by the adrenal gland and at local nerve endings in the brown fat causes the metabolism of the triglycerides to fatty acids, thereby releasing heat to be distributed to the body. Brown fat is a major producer of heat for the cold-stressed neonate because of its greater heat production capacity.

Shivering, a form of muscular activity common in the cold adult, is rarely seen in the newborn, although it has been observed at ambient temperatures of 15C (59F) or less. If shivering does appear, it means the infant's metabolic rate has already doubled and the extra muscular activity does little to produce needed heat.

Thermographic studies of newborns exposed to cold show an increase in the skin heat over the brown fat deposits in the neonate between 1 and 14 days of age. If the

brown fat supply has been depleted, the metabolic response to cold will be limited or lacking. An increase in basal metabolism as a result of hypothermia results in an increase in oxygen consumption. A decrease in the environmental temperature of 2C, from 33C to 31C, is a drop sufficient to double the oxygen consumption of a term newborn (Avery & First 1989).

The normal term neonate is usually able to cope with the increase, but the preterm neonate may be unable to increase ventilation to the necessary level of oxygen consumption. As a consequence, providing the newborn with an optimal thermal environment is absolutely necessary to prevent neonatal cold stress and the resulting metabolic physiologic responses. (See Chapter 32 for discussion of cold stress.)

Hypoxia and the effect of certain drugs such as meperidine (Demerol) may also prevent metabolism of brown fat. Meperidine given to the laboring woman leads to a greater fall in the newborn's body temperature during the neonatal period. It is important to remember that neonatal hypothermia prolongs as well as potentiates the effects of many analgesic and anesthetic drugs in the neonate.

Response to Heat

Sweating is the usual initial response of the newborn to hyperthermia. The neonate has six times as many sweat glands as the adult, but the newborn's activity level is one-third that of the adult. The glands have limited function until after the fourth week of extrauterine life. Dissipation of heat is accomplished by peripheral vasodilatation and evaporation of insensible water loss. Oxygen consumption and metabolic rate also increase in response to hyperthermia. Severe hyperthermia can lead to death or to gross brain damage if the baby survives.

Hepatic Adaptations

In the newborn, the liver is frequently palpable 2 to 3 cm below the right costal margin. It is relatively large and occupies about 40 percent of the abdominal cavity. The neonatal liver plays a significant role in iron storage, carbohydrate metabolism, conjugation of bilirubin, and coagulation.

Iron Storage and Red Blood Cell Production

As red blood cells are destroyed after birth, the iron is stored in the liver until needed for new red blood cell production. Neonatal iron stores are determined by total body hemoglobin content and length of gestation. The term newborn has about 270 mg of iron at birth, and about 140 to 170 mg of this amount is in the hemoglobin (Avery & Taeusch 1984). If the mother's iron intake has been adequate, enough iron will be stored to last until the fifth month of neonatal life. At this time, foods containing iron or iron supplements must be given to prevent anemia in the infant.

Carbohydrate Metabolism

At term, the newborn's cord blood glucose is 70% to 80% of the maternal blood. Neonatal carbohydrate reserves are relatively low. One-third of this reserve is in the form of liver glycogen. Neonatal glycogen stores are twice that of the adult. Blood glucose levels are influenced by a balance between liver glucose output and peripheral uptake, body temperature, insulin concentration, and muscular activity. The newborn enters an energy crunch at the time of birth with the removal of the maternal glucose supply and the increased energy expenditure associated with the birth process and extrauterine life. Fuel sources are consumed at a faster rate because of the work of breathing, loss of heat when exposed to cold, activity, and activation of muscle tone. Glucose is the main source of energy in the first few (four to six) hours after birth. The blood glucose level falls rapidly and then stabilizes at values of 50 to 60 mg/dL for several days; by the third day postnatally, the mean values increase to 60 to 70 mg/dL. Assessment of glucose level using a Chemstrip method is done upon admission and at four hours of age. If the fetus or neonate experiences hypoxia, the glycogen stores are used and may be depleted to meet metabolic requirements. As stores of liver and muscle glycogen and blood glucose decrease, the neonate compensates by changing from a predominantly carbohydrate metabolism to fat metabolism. Energy is derived from fat and protein as well as from carbohydrates. The amount and availability of each of these "fuel substrates" depends on constraints imposed by immature metabolic pathways (lack of specific enzymes or hormones) in the first few days of life.

Conjugation of Bilirubin

Conjugation of bilirubin is the conversion of yellow lipid-soluble pigment into water-soluble pigment. Unconjugated (indirect) bilirubin is a breakdown product derived from hemoglobin that is released from lysed red blood cells and from heme pigments found in cell elements (nonerythrocyte bilirubin). Unconjugated bilirubin is not in excretable form and is a potential toxin. Total serum bilirubin is the sum of direct (conjugated) and indirect bilirubin.

The fetus does not conjugate bilirubin because unconjugated bilirubin can cross the placenta to be excreted. Fetal unconjugated bilirubin is normally excreted by the placenta in utero, so total bilirubin at birth is usually less than 3 mb/dL unless an abnormal hemolytic process has been present. Postnatally, the infant must conjugate bilirubin (convert a lipid-soluble pigment into a water-soluble pigment) in the liver, producing a rise in serum bilirubin in the first few days of life.

Unconjugated albumin-bound bilirubin is taken up by the liver cells. Since albumin does not transfer into the liver cells, the bilirubin must be transferred to two other intracellular binding proteins labeled Y and Z. These determine the amount of bilirubin held in a liver cell for processing and consequently the potential amount of bilirubin uptake into the liver. The clearance and conjugation of bilirubin depend on the glucuronyl transferase enzyme. Activity of this enzyme results in the attachment of unconjugated bilirubin to glucuronic acid (product of liver glycogen), producing conjugated, direct bilirubin. Direct bilirubin is excreted into the tiny bile ducts, then into the common duct and duodenum. The conjugated bilirubin then progresses down the intestines, where bacteria transform it into urobilinogen. This product is not reabsorbed but is excreted as a yellow-brown pigment in the stools.

The newborn liver has relatively less glucuronyl transferase activity at birth and in the first few weeks of life than an adult liver. This reduction in activity predisposes the newborn to decreased conjugation of bilirubin and increased susceptibility to jaundice.

Even after the bilirubin has been conjugated and bound it can be converted back to unconjugated bilirubin by enterohepatic circulation. In the intestines β-glucuronidase enzyme acts to split off (deconjugate) the bilirubin from glucuronic acid if it has not first been reduced by gut bacteria to urobilinogen; the free bilirubin is reabsorbed through the intestinal wall and brought back to the liver via portal vein circulation. This recycling of the bilirubin and decreased ability to clear bilirubin from the system are prevalent in babies who have very high β-glucuronidase activity levels as well as delayed bacterial colonization of the gut (see Figure 27–8).

Physiologic Jaundice—Icterus Neonatorum

Physiologic jaundice is caused by accelerated destruction of fetal RBCs, impaired conjugation of bilirubin, and increased bilirubin reabsorption from the intestinal tract. This condition does not have a pathologic basis, but rather is a normal biologic response of the newborn.

Oski (1984) describes six factors whose interactions may give rise to physiologic jaundice:

1. *Greater bilirubin loads to the liver.* In the neonate, the combination of an increased blood volume, largely due to delayed cord clamping, and accelerated lysis of the fetal red blood cell contributes to an increased bilirubin level in the blood. The neonate has a shorter erythrocyte (RBC) life span (80 to 100 days instead of 120) and a proportionately larger amount of nonerythrocyte bilirubin formed than the adult. Therefore, newborns have two to three times greater production or breakdown of bilirubin.

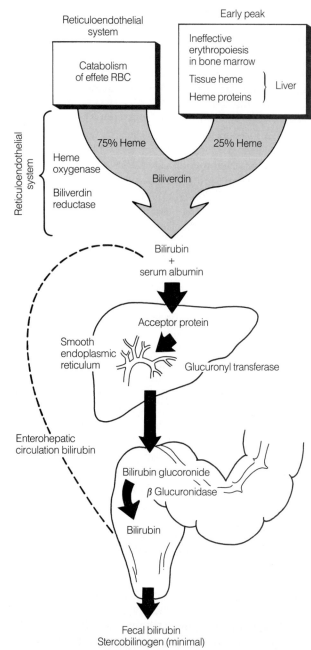

Figure 27–8   Conjugation of bilirubin in newborns (From Avery GB: Neonatology: Pathophysiology and Management of the Newborn, *3rd ed. Philadelphia: Lippincott, 1987, p 541)*

2. *Defective uptake of bilirubin from the plasma.* If the newborn does not ingest adequate calories, the formation of hepatic binding proteins diminishes, resulting in higher bilirubin levels.

3. *Defective conjugation of the bilirubin.* Decreased glucuronyl-transferase activity results in greater bilirubin values. The presence of the enzyme $3\alpha20\beta$

propregnanediol in breast milk is thought to further impede the conjugation of bilirubin.

4. *Defect in bilirubin excretion.* A congenital infection may cause impaired excretion. Delay in introduction of bacterial flora and decreased intestinal mobility can also delay excretion.

5. *Inadequate hepatic circulation.* Decreased oxygen supplies to the liver associated with neonatal hypoxia or congenital heart disease lead to a rise in the bilirubin level.

6. *Increases reabsorption of bilirubin from the intestine.* Reduced bowel motility, intestinal obstruction, or delayed passage of meconium increases the circulation of bilirubin in the enterohepatic pathway, thereby resulting in higher bilirubin values.

About 50% of full-term neonates and 80% of preterm neonates exhibit physiologic jaundice on about the second or third day after birth. The characteristic yellow color results from increased levels of unconjugated bilirubin, which are a normal product of RBC breakdown and reflect a temporary inability of the body to eliminate bilirubin. The signs of physiologic jaundice appear *after* the first 24 hours postnatally. This differentiates physiologic jaundice from pathologic jaundice (Chapter 32), which is clinically seen at birth or within the first 24 hours of postnatal life. Serum levels of bilirubin are about 4 to 6 mg/dL before yellow coloration of the skin and sclera appears.

During the first week, unconjugated bilirubin levels in physiologic jaundice should not exceed 13 mg/dL in the full-term or preterm newborn. Peak bilirubin levels are reached between days 3 and 5 in the full-term infant and between days 5 and 6 in the preterm infant. These values are established for European and American newborns. Chinese, Japanese, Korean, and Native American neonates have considerably higher bilirubin levels that persist for longer periods with no apparent ill effects (Oski 1984).

Nursery or postpartum room environment, including lighting, hinders the early detection of the degree and type of jaundice. Pink walls and artificial lights mask the beginning of jaundice in newborns. Daylight assists the observer in early recognition by eliminating distortions caused by artificial light.

The following nursery or newborn care procedures are designed to decrease the probability of high bilirubin levels:

● The infant's skin temperature is maintained at 36.5C (97.8F) or above, since chilling results in acidosis (Avery & First 1989). This condition in turn decreases available serum albumin–binding sites, weakens albumin–binding powers, and causes elevated unconjugated bilirubin levels.

● Stool is monitored for amount and characteristics. Bilirubin is eliminated in the feces; inadequate stooling may result in reabsorption and recycling of bilirubin. Early breast-feeding is encouraged because the laxative effect of colostrum increases excretion of stool.

● Early feedings are also encouraged to promote intestinal elimination and bacterial colonization and to provide caloric intake necessary for formation of hepatic binding proteins.

If jaundice is suspected, the nurse can quickly assess the neonate's coloring by pressing his or her skin with a finger. As the blanching occurs, the nurse can observe the icterus (yellow coloring). If jaundice becomes apparent, nursing care is directed toward keeping the neonate well hydrated and promoting intestinal elimination. For specific nursing management and therapies, see the Nursing Care Plan on page 1046.

Physiologic jaundice may be very upsetting to parents; they require emotional support and thorough explanation of the condition. Necessary hospitalization of the newborn for a few additional days may also be disturbing to parents. They should be encouraged to provide for the emotional needs of their newborn by continuing to feed, hold, and caress the infant. If the mother is discharged, the parents should be encouraged to return for feedings and feel free to telephone or visit whenever possible. In many instances, the mother, especially if she is breast-feeding, may elect to remain hospitalized with her infant; this decision should be supported. As an alternative to extended hospitalization, some newborns are treated in home phototherapy programs.

Breast-Feeding Jaundice

Breast-feeding is implicated in prolonged jaundice in some newborns. According to Korones (1986) 1% to 5% of newborns being breast-fed will develop breast-feeding jaundice. The breast-fed jaundice newborn's bilirubin level begins to rise about the fourth day after the mother's milk has come in. The level peaks at two to three weeks of age and may reach 20 to 25 mg/dL without intervention (Oski 1984).

It is theorized that some women's breast milk may contain several times the normal concentration of certain free fatty acids. These free fatty acids may inhibit the conjugation of bilirubin or increase lipase activity, which disrupts the red blood cell membrane. Increased lipase activity enhances absorption of bile across the GI tract membrane, thereby increasing the enterohepatic circulation of bilirubin. In the past it was thought that the breast milk of women whose newborns have breast-feeding jaundice contained an enzyme that inhibited glucuronyl transferase.

Newborns with breast milk jaundice appear well, and at present there is an absence of documented neurologic signs with this type of jaundice. Even so it is suggested that traditional guidelines should be followed (Neville & Neifert 1983). Temporary cessation of nursing may be advised if bilirubin reaches presumed toxic levels of approximately 20 mg/dL or if the interruption is necessary to establish the

Table 27–4 Jaundice
Physiologic Jaundice
Physiologic jaundice occurs *after* the first 24 hours of life.
During first week of life, bilirubin should not exceed 13 mg/dL. Some pediatricians allow levels up to 15 mg/dL.
Bilirubin levels peak at three to five days in term infants.
Breast-Milk Jaundice
Bilirubin levels begin to rise about the fourth day after mature breast milk comes in.
Peak of 20–25 mg/dL is reached at two to three weeks of age.
It may be necessary to interrupt nursing for a short period when bilirubin reaches 20 mg/dL.

cause of hyperbilirubinemia (Oski 1984). Within 24 to 36 hours after discontinuing breast-feeding, the newborn's serum bilirubin levels begin to fall dramatically and breast-feeding may be resumed.

Many physicians believe that breast-feeding may be resumed once other causes of jaundice have been ruled out, although the bilirubin concentration may rise 1 to 3 mg/dL with a subsequent decline (Oski 1984). Nursing mothers need encouragement and support in their desire to nurse their infants, assistance and instruction regarding pumping and expressing milk during the interrupted nursing period, and reassurance that nothing is wrong with their milk or mothering abilities (see Table 27–4).

Coagulation

The liver plays an important part in blood coagulation during fetal life and continues this function to some degree during the first few months following birth. Coagulation factors II, VII, IX, X (synthesized in the liver), are activated under the influence of vitamin K and therefore are considered vitamin K-dependent. The absence of normal flora needed to synthesize vitamin K in the newborn gut results in low levels of vitamin K and creates a transient blood coagulation alteration between the second and fifth day of life. From a low point at about two to three days after birth, these coagulation factors rise slowly but do not approach adult levels until nine months of age or later. Other coagulation factors with low cord blood levels are XI, XII, and XIII. Fibrinogen and factors V and VII are near adult ranges (Eden & Boehm 1990).

Although newborn bleeding problems are rare, an injection of vitamin K (AquaMEPHYTON) is given prophylactically on the day of birth to combat potential clinical bleeding problems. (Hemorrhagic disease of the newborn is discussed in more depth in Chapter 31.)

Platelet counts at birth are in the same range as for adults, but newborns may manifest mild transient difficulty in platelet aggregation functioning. This platelet problem is accentuated by phototherapy (Eden & Boehm 1990).

Prenatal maternal therapy with phenytoin sodium (Dilantin) or phenobarbital also causes abnormal clotting studies and neonatal bleeding in the first 24 hours after birth. Infants born to mothers receiving coumarin (warfarin) compounds may bleed because these agents cross the placenta and accentuate existing vitamin K-dependent factor deficiencies.

Gastrointestinal Adaptations

Fetal-Neonatal Transitional Physiology

Full maturity of the gastrointestinal tract is achieved by 36 to 38 weeks' gestation with the presence of enzymatic activity and the ability to transport nutrients. Development of the secretory and absorbing surfaces is greater than that of the supporting musculature. All glandular elements found in the adult mucosa are present at birth, but the fetal structures are more shallow and less functional.

By birth, the neonate has experienced swallowing, gastric emptying, and intestinal propulsion. In utero, swallowing is accompanied by gastric emptying and peristalsis of the fetal intestinal tract. By the end of gestation, peristalsis becomes much more active in preparation for extrauterine life. Fetal peristalsis is also stimulated by anoxia, causing the expulsion of meconium into the amniotic fluid.

Air enters the stomach immediately after birth. The small intestine is filled within 2 to 12 hours and the large bowel within 24 hours. The salivary glands are immature at birth and little saliva is manufactured until the infant is about three months old. The newborn's stomach has a capacity of 50 to 60 mL. It empties intermittently, starting within a few minutes of the beginning of a feeding and ending between two and four hours after feeding.

The cardiac sphincter is immature, as is nervous control of the stomach, so some regurgitation may be noted in the neonatal period. Regurgitation of the first few feedings during the first day or two of life can usually be lessened by avoiding overfeeding and by burping the newborn well during and after the feeding.

When no other signs and symptoms are evident, vomiting is limited and ceases within the first few days of life. Continuous vomiting or regurgitation should be observed closely. If the newborn has swallowed bloody or purulent amniotic fluid, lavage may be indicated to relieve the problem.

Normal term newborns pass meconium within 12 to 48 hours of birth (Avery & Taeusch 1984). **Meconium** is formed in utero from the amniotic fluid and its constituents, together with intestinal secretions and shed mucosal cells. It is recognized by its thick, tarry, dark green appear-

Table 27–5 Physiologic Adaptations to Extrauterine Life

Periodic breathing may be present.

Desired skin temperature 36–36.5 C (96.8–97.7 F), stabilizes four to six hours after birth.

Desired blood glucose level reaches 60–70 mg/dL by third postnatal day.

Stools (progresses from):
   Meconium (thick, tarry, dark green)
   Transitional stools (thin, brown to green)
   Breast-fed infants (yellow gold, soft, or mushy)
   Bottle-fed infants (pale yellow, formed, and pasty)

ance. Transitional (thin brown to green) stools consisting of part meconium and part fecal material are passed for the next day or two, after which the stools become entirely fecal. Generally, the stools of a breast-fed newborn are pale yellow (but may be pasty green); they are more liquid and more frequent than those of formula-fed neonates, whose stools are browner in color. Bowel movement is individualized but ranges from one every two to three days to as many as 10 daily (see Table 27–5).

When the nurse took my first child and put him to my breast his tiny mouth opened and reached for me as if he had known forever what to do. (Leslie Kenton, All I Ever Wanted Was a Baby)

Digestive Function

The term neonate has adequate intestinal and pancreatic enzymes to digest most simple carbohydrates, proteins, and fats. The newborn's gastric acidity is equal to an adult's but becomes less acidic in about a week and remains lower than that of adults for two to three months. The stomach secretes pepsinogen, which is necessary for protein digestion and production of hydrochloric acid. Both pepsinogen and hydrochloric acid are necessary for the digestion of milk prior to its entrance into the small bowel. Digestion and absorption of nutrients are primarily functions of the small bowel, where pancreatic secretions digest starches and proteins. Bile secretions from the gallbladder through the bile duct aid in fat absorption, and duodenal secretions complete this complex process.

Digestion of Carbohydrates, Proteins, and Fats

The carbohydrates requiring digestion in the newborn are usually disaccharides (lactose, maltose, sucrose), which are split into monosaccharides (galactose, fructose, and glucose) by the enzymes of the intestinal mucosa. Lactose is the primary carbohydrate in the breast-feeding newborn and is generally easily digested and well absorbed. The only enzyme lacking at birth is pancreatic amylase, which remains relatively deficient during the first few months of life. Therefore, newborns have trouble digesting starches (changing more complex carbohydrates into maltose).

Although proteins require more digestion than carbohydrates, they are well digested and absorbed from the neonatal intestine.

Fats are digested and absorbed less efficiently by the newborn because of the minimal activity of the pancreatic enzyme lipase. The neonate excretes 10% to 20% of the dietary fat intake, compared with 10% for the adult. The fat in breast milk is absorbed more completely by the newborn than is the fat in straight cow's milk because it consists of more medium-chain triglycerides and contains lipase. (See Chapter 30 for a more detailed discussion of infant nutrition.)

Urinary Adaptations

Kidney Development and Function

Certain physiologic features of the newborn's kidneys are important to consider when looking at the newborn's ability to manage body fluids and excretional function:

1. The term newborn's kidneys have a full complement of functioning nephrons.

2. The glomerular filtration rate of the newborn's kidney is low in comparison with the adult rate. Because of this physiologic inefficiency, the newborn's kidney is unable to dispose of water rapidly when necessary.

3. The juxtamedullary portion of the nephron has limited capacity to reabsorb Na$^+$ and H$^+$ and concentrate urine. The limitation of tubular reabsorption can lead to inappropriate loss of substances present in the glomerular filtrate, such as amino acids and bicarbonate.

Full-term newborns are less able than adults to concentrate urine (reabsorb water back into the blood) because the tubules are short and narrow. There is a greater capacity for glomerular filtration than for tubular reabsorption-secretion. Although feeding practices may affect the osmolarity of the urine, the maximum concentrating ability of the newborn is a specific gravity of 1.025. The inability to concentrate urine is due to the limited excretion of solutes (principally sodium, potassium, chloride, bicarbonate, urea, and phosphate) in the growing newborn. The ability to concentrate urine fully is attained by three months of age.

Since the newborn has difficulty concentrating urine,

the effect of excessive insensible water loss or restricted fluid intake is unpredictable. The newborn kidney is also limited in its dilutional capabilities. Maximal dilution ability is specific gravity of 1.001. Concentrating and dilutional limitations of renal function are important considerations in monitoring fluid therapy to avoid dehydration and overhydration.

Characteristics of Newborn Urinary Function

Many newborns void in the birthing room and it goes unnoticed. Among normal newborns, 92% void by 24 hours after birth and 99% void by 48 hours (Fanaroff & Martin 1987). A newborn who has not voided by 72 hours should be assessed for adequacy of fluid intake, bladder distention, restlessness, and symptoms of pain. Appropriate clinical personnel should be notified if indicated.

The initial bladder volume is 6 to 44 mL of urine. Unless edema is present, normal urinary output is often limited, and the voidings are scanty until fluid intake increases. (The fluid of edema is eliminated by the kidneys, so infants with edema have a much higher urinary output.) The first two days postnatally, the newborn voids two to six times daily, with a urine output of 30 to 60 mL per day. The newborn subsequently voids 5 to 25 times every 24 hours, with a volume of 30 to 50 mL/kg per day.

Following the first voiding, the newborn's urine frequently appears cloudy (due to mucus content) and has a high specific gravity, which decreases as fluid intake increases. Occasionally pink stains ("brick dust spots") appear on the diaper. These are caused by urates and are innocuous. Blood may occasionally be observed on the diapers of female infants. This *pseudomenstruation* is related to the withdrawal of maternal hormones. Males may have bloody spotting from a circumcision. In the absence of apparent causes for bleeding, the physician/CNM/NNP should be notified. Normal urine during early infancy is straw-colored and almost odorless, although odor occurs when certain drugs are given or when infection is present. Table 27–6 contains urinalysis values of the normal newborn.

Table 27–6 Newborn Urinalysis Values
Protein < 5–10 mg/dL
WBC < 2–3
RBC 0
Casts 0
Bacteria 0
Specific gravity 1.001–1.025
Color pale yellow

Immunologic Adaptations

The newborn possesses varying degrees of nonspecific and specific immunity. The nonspecific mechanism of *opsonization*—the process of coating invasive bacteria to ready them for ingestion by phagocytic cells—is impaired. *Immunoglobulins* (specific immunity) are a type of antibody secreted by the lymphocytes and plasma cells into the body fluids. Fetal albumin, globulin, and other immunoglobulins are present throughout the last trimester of gestation.

Of the three major types of immunoglobulins primarily involved in immunity—IgG, IgA, and IgM—only IgG crosses the placenta. The pregnant woman forms antibodies in response to illness or immunization. This process is called **active acquired immunity**. When IgG antibodies are transferred to the fetus in utero, **passive acquired immunity** results, since the fetus does not produce the antibodies itself. IgG is very active against bacterial toxins.

Because the maternal immunoglobin is transferred primarily during the third trimester, preterm infants (especially those born prior to 34 weeks) may be more susceptible to infection. In general, newborns have immunity to tetanus, diphtheria, smallpox, measles, mumps, poliomyelitis, and a variety of other bacterial and viral diseases. The period of resistance varies: Immunity against common viral infections such as measles may last four to eight months, whereas immunity to certain bacteria may disappear within four to eight weeks.

The normal newborn does produce antibodies in response to an antigen, but not as effectively as an older child would. It is customary to begin immunization at two months of age, and then the infant can develop active acquired immunity.

IgM immunoglobulins are produced in response to blood group antigens, gram-negative enteric organisms, and some viruses in the expectant mother. Because IgM does not normally cross the placenta, most or all is produced by the fetus beginning at 10 to 15 weeks' gestation. Elevated levels of IgM at birth may indicate placental leaks, or more commonly, antigenic stimulation in utero. Consequently, elevations suggest that the infant was exposed to an intrauterine infection such as syphilis or a TORCH (toxoplasmosis, rubella, cytomegalovirus, herpes virus hominis type 2) infection. (For in-depth discussion see Table 32–7.) The lack of available maternal IgM in the newborn also accounts for the infant's susceptibility to gram-negative enteric organisms such as *Escherichia coli*.

The functions of IgA immunoglobins are not fully understood. IgA appears to provide protection mainly on secreting surfaces such as the respiratory tract, gastrointestinal tract, and eyes. Serum IgA does not cross the placenta and is not normally produced by the fetus in utero. Unlike the other immunoglobins, IgA is not affected by gastric action. Colostrum, the forerunner of breast milk, is very high in the secretory form of IgA. Consequently, it may be of significance in providing some passive immunity

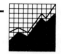

Research Note

Clinical Application of Research

Cranial molding occurs when children born at lower gestational ages are positioned from side to side on a firm mattress. The resultant flattening of both sides of the calvarium (upper part of the skull) should improve within the first two years but may persist into adulthood.

Ginette Budreau (1989) hypothesized that infants with cranial molding may be perceived as less attractive and thus may not elicit the same nurturant reaction as infants without cranial molding. In her study, she asked 42 undergraduate nursing students to rate 21 sets of photographs of infants as to least cute, second cutest, and cutest. Each set of infants consisted of pictures of a full-term infant, a preterm infant, and a preterm infant with cranial molding assigned in random order. Raters also identified the cranial or facial features which had the most impact on their negative perception of least cute.

The three groups were significantly different from each other, with the preterm infants being rated the cutest, the term infants the second cutest, and the preterm infants with cranial molding the least cute.

Critical Thinking Applied to Research

Strengths: Identification of limitations of study.

Concerns: Although the interpretation of the two way ANOVA seems to be logical, the two-way ANOVA as constructed by the author appears to have a built-in interaction; a one-way ANOVA might have provided more clear-cut information.

Budreau G: The perceived attractiveness of preterm infants with cranial molding. *JOGNN* January/February 1990; 18:38.

to the infant of a breast-feeding mother (Eden & Boehm 1990). Newborns begin to produce secretory IgA in their intestinal mucosa at about four weeks after birth.

Neurologic and Sensory/Perceptual Adaptations

The newborn's brain is about one-quarter the size of an adult's, and myelination of nerve fibers is incomplete. Unlike the cardiovascular or respiratory systems, which undergo tremendous changes at birth, the nervous system is minimally influenced by the actual birth process.

Because many biochemical and histologic changes have yet to occur in the newborn's brain, the postnatal period is considered a time of risk to the development of the brain and nervous system. For neurologic development—including development of intellect—to proceed, the brain and other nervous system structures must mature in an orderly, unhampered fashion.

Intrauterine Factors Influencing Newborn Behavior

The newborn responds to and interacts with the environment in a predictable pattern of behavior that is somewhat shaped by his or her intrauterine experience. This intrauterine experience is affected by intrinsic factors such as maternal nutrition and external factors such as the mother's physical environment. Depending on the newborn's intrauterine experience and individual temperaments, neonatal behavioral responses to various stresses vary from dealing quietly with the stimulation, to becoming overreactive and tense, to a combination of the two.

Brazelton (1975, 1977) found a positive association between newborn behavior and nutritional status of the pregnant woman. Newborns with higher birth weight attended and responded to visual and auditory cues and exhibited more mature motor activity than low-birth-weight newborns.

Factors such as exposure to intense auditory stimuli in utero can eventually be manifested in the behavior of the newborn. For example, the fetal heart rate initially increases when the pregnant woman is exposed to an auditory stimuli, but repetition of the stimuli leads to decreased FHR. Thus the newborn who was exposed to intense noise during fetal life is significantly less reactive to loud sounds postnatally.

Characteristics of Newborn Neurologic Function

Partially flexed extremities with the legs near the abdomen is the usual position of the normal newborn. When awake, the newborn may exhibit purposeless, uncoordinated bilateral movements of the extremities. The organization and intensity of the newborn's motor activity are influenced by a number of factors including the following (Brazelton 1984): (a) sleep-wake states; (b) presence of environmental stimuli such as heat, light, cold, and noise; (c) conditions causing a chemical imbalance, such as hypoglycemia; (d) hydration status; (e) state of health; and (f) recovery from the stress of labor and birth.

Eye movements are observable during the first few days of life. An alert neonate is able to fixate on faces and brightly colored objects. If a bright light shines in the newborn's eyes, the blinking response is elicited.

The cry of the newborn should be lusty and vigorous. High-pitched cries, weak cries, or no cries are all causes for concern.

Growth of the newborn's body progresses in a cephalocaudal (head-to-toe), proximal-distal fashion. The newborn is somewhat hypertonic; that is, there is resistance to extending the elbow and knee joints. Muscle tone should be symmetric. Diminished muscle tone and flaccidity may indicate neurologic dysfunction.

Specific symmetric deep tendon reflexes can be elicited in the newborn. The knee jerk is brisk; a normal ankle clonus may involve three or four beats. Plantar flexion is present. Other reflexes, including the Moro, grasping, rooting, Bobinski, and sucking reflexes are characteristic of neurologic integrity.

Performance of complex behavioral patterns reflects the newborn's neurologic maturation and integration. The newborn who can bring a hand to his mouth is demonstrating motor coordination as well as self-quieting technique, thus increasing the complexity of the behavioral response. Neonates also possess complex organized defensive motor patterns as exhibited by the ability to approach and remove an obstruction, such as a cloth across the face.

Behavioral States of the Newborn

The behavior of the newborn can be divided into two categories, the sleep state and the alert state (Brazelton 1984). These postnatal behavioral states are similar to those that have been identified during pregnancy (Tuck 1986). Subcategories are identified under each major category.

Sleep States

The sleep states in the newborn are as follows:

1. *Deep or quiet sleep.* Deep sleep is characterized by closed eyes with no eye movements, regular even breathing, and jerky motion or startles at regular intervals. Behavioral responses to external stimuli are likely to be delayed. Startles are rapidly suppressed, and changes in state are not likely to occur.

2. *Active REM.* Irregular respirations, eyes closed with REM, irregular sucking motions, minimal activity, and irregular but smooth movement of the extremities can be observed in active REM sleep. Environmental and internal stimuli initiate a startle reaction and a change of state.

Sleep cycles in the newborn have been recognized and defined according to duration. The length of the cycle is dependent upon the age of the newborn. At term, REM active sleep and quiet sleep occur in intervals of 45 to 50 minutes. About 45% to 50% of the total sleep of the neonate is active sleep, 35% to 45% is quiet (deep) sleep, and 10% of sleep is transitional between these two periods. It is hypothesized that REM sleep stimulates the growth of the neural system. Over a period of time, the neonate's sleep-wake patterns become diurnal; that is, the infant sleeps at night and stays awake during the day. (See Chapter 28 for in-depth discussion of assessment of neonatal states.)

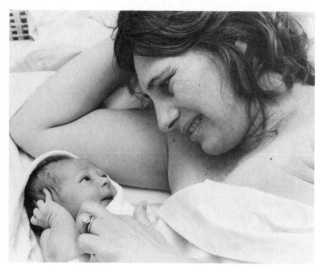

Figure 27–9   Mother and baby gaze at each other. This quiet, alert state is the optimal state for interaction between baby and parents

Alert States

In the first 30 to 60 minutes after birth, many neonates display a quiet alert state, characteristic of the first period of reactivity (Figure 27–9). About 12 to 18 hours after birth, the infant is again alert when the second period of reactivity occurs. (A further description of these two periods of reactivity is found on page 885.) These periods of alertness tend to be short during the first two days after birth to allow the baby to recover from the birth process. Subsequently, alert states are of choice or of necessity (Brazelton 1984). Increasing choice of wakefulness by the newborn indicates a maturing capacity to achieve and maintain consciousness. Heat, cold, and hunger are but a few of the stimuli that can cause wakefulness by necessity. Once the disturbing stimuli are removed, sleep tends to recur.

The following are subcategories of the alert state (Brazelton 1984):

1. *Drowsy or semidozing.* The behaviors common to the drowsy state are open or closed eyes, fluttering eyelids, semidozing appearance, and slow, regular movements of the extremities. Mild startles may be noted from time to time. Although the reaction to a sensory stimulus is delayed, a change of state often results.

2. *Wide awake.* In the wide awake state, the neonate is alert and follows and fixates on attractive objects, faces, or auditory stimuli. Motor activity is minimal, and the response to external stimuli is delayed.

3. *Active awake.* The eyes are open and motor activity is quite intense with thrusting movements of the extremities in the active awake state. Environmental stimuli increase startles or motor activity,

but discrete reactions are difficult to distinguish because of generalized high activity level.

4. *Crying.* Intense crying is accompanied by jerky motor movements. Crying serves several purposes for the newborn. It may be used as a distraction from disturbing stimuli such as hunger and pain. Fussiness often allows the neonate to discharge energy and reorganize behavior. Most important, crying elicits an appropriate response of help from the parents.

Behavioral and Sensory Capacities of the Newborn

Habituation is the newborn's ability to process and respond to complex visual and auditory stimulation. For example, when a bright light is flashed into the newborn's eyes, the initial response is blinking, constriction of the pupil, and perhaps a slight startle reaction. However, with repeated stimulation, the newborn's response repertoire gradually diminishes and disappears. The capacity to ignore repetitious disturbing stimuli is a neonatal defense mechanism readily apparent in the noisy well-lighted nursery.

Orientation is the newborn's ability to be alert to, to follow, and to fixate on complex visual stimuli that have a particular appeal and attraction. The newborn prefers the human face and eyes and bright shiny objects. As the face or object is brought into the line of vision, the neonate responds with bright, wide eyes, still limbs, fixed staring. This intense visual involvement may last several minutes, during which time the neonate is able to follow the stimulus from side to side. Figures 27–9 and 27–10 illustrate these responses. The newborn uses this sensory capacity to become familiar with family, friends, and surroundings.

Self-quieting ability refers to newborns' ability to use their own resources to quiet and comfort themselves. Their repertoire includes hand-to-mouth movements, suck-

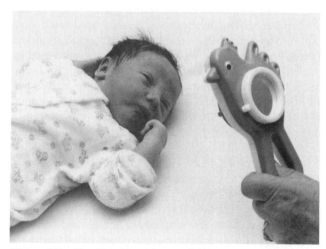

Figure 27–10   Head turning to follow

ing on a fist or tongue, and attending to external stimuli. Neurologically impaired newborns are unable to use self-quieting activities and require more frequent comforting from care givers when stimulated.

Auditory Capacity

The newborn responds to auditory stimulation with a definite, organized behavior repertoire. The stimulus used to assess auditory response should be selected to match the state of the newborn. A rattle is appropriate for light sleep, a voice for an awake state, and a clap for deep sleep. As the neonate hears the sound, the cardiac rate rises, and a minimal startle reflex may be observed. If the sound is appealing, the newborn will become alert and search for the site of the auditory stimulus.

Olfactory Capacity

Neonates are able to distinguish their mother's breast pads from those of other mothers by one week postnatally (Brazelton 1984). Apparently this phenomenon is related to the ability of the neonate to select by smell.

Taste and Sucking

The newborn responds differently to varying tastes. Sugar, for example, increases sucking. Sucking pattern variations also exist in newborns fed cow's milk or human breast milk (Brazelton 1984). When breast-feeding, the neonate sucks in bursts with frequent regular pauses. The bottle-fed newborn tends to suck at a regular rate with infrequent pauses. The pauses in feeding may be used to interject social communication between the mother and neonate, whether at regular or irregular intervals.

When awake and hungry, the neonate displays rapid searching motions in response to the rooting reflex. Once feeding begins, the newborn establishes a sucking pattern according to the method of feeding. Finger sucking is present not only postnatally but also in utero. The neonate frequently uses sucking as a self-quieting activity, which assists in the development of self-regulation.

Tactile Capacity

The neonate is very sensitive to being touched, cuddled, and held. Often a mother's first response to an upset or crying newborn is touching or holding. Swaddling, placing a hand on the abdomen, or holding the arms to prevent a startle reflex are other methods that may soothe the newborn. The settled neonate is then able to attend to and interact with the environment.

❀ ❀

KEY CONCEPTS

The production of surfactant is crucial to keeping the lungs expanded during expiration by reducing alveolar surface tension.

Neonatal respiration is initiated primarily by chemical and mechanical events in association with thermal and sensory stimulation.

The characteristics of newborn respirations differ from those of adult respirations because the newborn is an obligatory nose breather. Respirations move from being primarily shallow, irregular, and diaphragmatic to synchronous, abdominal, and chest breathing.

Periodic breathing is normal, and newborn sleep states affect breathing patterns.

Oxygen transport in the newborn is significantly affected by the presence of greater amounts of HbF (fetal hemoglobin) than HbA (adult hemoglobin), which holds oxygen easier but releases it to the body tissues only at low PO_2 levels.

Blood values in the newborn are modified by several factors such as site of the blood sample, gestational age, prenatal and/or perinatal hemorrhage, and the timing of the clamping of the umbilical cord.

Blood glucose level should reach 60 to 70 mg/dL by the third postnatal day.

The newborn is considered to have established thermoregulation when oxygen consumption and metabolic activity are minimal.

Excessive heat loss occurs from radiation and convection because of the newborn's larger surface area when compared to weight; and from thermal conduction because of the marked difference between core temperature and skin temperature.

The normal newborn possesses the ability to digest and absorb nutrients necessary for neonatal growth and development.

The newborn's stools change from meconium (thick, tarry, dark green) to transitional stools (thin, brown-to-green) and then to the distinct forms for either breast-fed newborns (yellow-gold, soft, or mushy) or bottle-fed newborns (pale yellow, formed, and pasty).

Controversy continues to exist about the relationship of breast-feeding and the development of prolonged jaundice.

The neonatal kidney is characterized by a decreased rate of glomerular flow, limited tubular reabsorption, limited excretion of solutes, and limited ability to concentrate urine. Most newborns void by between 24 and 48 hours of extrauterine life.

The immune system in the newborn is not fully activated until sometime after birth, but the newborn does possess some specific and nonspecific immunologic abilities.

Neurologic and sensory/perceptual functioning in the newborn is evident from the newborn's interaction with the environment, presence of synchronized motor activity, and well-developed sensory capacities.

The behavioral states in the neonate can be divided into sleep states and alert states.

❀ ❀

References

Avery GB: *Neonatology: Pathophysiology and Management of the Newborn,* 3rd ed. Philadelphia: Lippincott, 1987.

Avery ME, First LR: *Pediatric Medicine.* Baltimore: Williams & Wilkins, 1989.

Avery, ME, Taeusch HW (editors): *Schaffer's Diseases of the Newborn,* 5th ed. Philadelphia: Saunders, 1984.

Brazelton TB et al: Biomedical variables and neonatal performance of Guatemalan infants. Presented to American Academy of Cerebral Palsy, New Orleans, 1975.

Brazelton TB et al: The behavior of nutritionally deprived Guatemalan neonates. *Dev Med Child Neurol* 1977; 19:364.

Brazelton TB: Neonatal behavior and its significance. In: *Schaffer's Diseases of the Newborn.* Avery ME, Taeusch HW (editors). Philadelphia: Saunders, 1984.

Cunningham FG, MacDonald PC, Gant NG: *Williams Obstetrics.* Norwalk, CT: Appleton & Lange, 1989.

Eden RD, Boehm FH (editors): *Assessment and Care of the Fetus: Physiological, Clinical, and Medicolegal Principles.* Norwalk, CT: Appleton & Lange, 1990.

Fanaroff AA, Martin RJ: *Neonatal-Perinatal Medicine,* 4th ed. St Louis: Mosby, 1987.

Korones SB: *High Risk Newborn Infants: The Basis for Intensive Care Nursing,* 4th ed. St. Louis: Mosby, 1986.

Long WA: *Fetal and Neonatal Cardiology.* Philadelphia: Saunders, 1990.

Neville MC, Neifert MR: *Lactation: Physiology, Nutrition, and Breastfeeding.* New York: Plenum Press, 1983.

Nijhuis JG et al: Are there behavioral states in the human fetus? *Early Hum Dev* 1982; 6:177.

Oski FA: Physiologic jaundice. In: *Schaffer's Diseases of the Newborn.* Avery ME, Taeusch HW (editors). Philadelphia: Saunders, 1984.

Scopes J, Ahmed I: Range of critical temperatures in sick and premature newborn babies. *Arch Dis Child* 1966; 41:417.

Smith CA, Nelson NM: *The Physiology of the Newborn Infant,* 4th ed. Springfield, IL: Thomas, 1976.

Tuck SM: Ultrasound monitoring of fetal behavior. *Ultrasound Med Biol* April 1986; 12:307.

Additional Readings

Berenson A, Heger A, Andrews S: Appearance of the hymen in newborns. *Pediatrics* 1991; 87(4):458.

Nelson SE, Rogers RR, Ziegler EE, Fomon SJ: Gain in weight and length during early infancy. *Early Human Development* 1989; 19:223.

Teitel DF, Iwamoto HS, Rudolph AM: Changes in the pulmonary circulation during birth-related events. *International Pediatric Research Foundation* 1990; 27:372.

Turner BS: Embryologic and physiologic basis of neonatal respiration. *AACN* 1990; 1(2):389.

Yip R, Li Z, Chong, W-H: Race and birth weight: The Chinese example. *Pediatrics* 1991; 87(5):688.

CHAPTER 28

Nursing Assessment of the Newborn

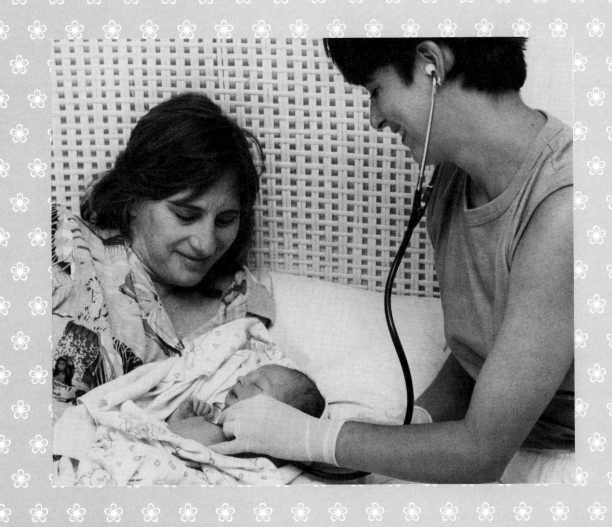

OBJECTIVES

Describe the normal physical and behavioral characteristics of the newborn.

Identify the components of a complete newborn physical exam and the significance of abnormal findings.

Explain the various gestational age assessment criteria.

Describe the reflexes that may be present at birth.

Describe the categories of the neonatal behavioral assessment.

❀ ❀

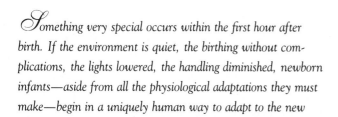

Something very special occurs within the first hour after birth. If the environment is quiet, the birthing without complications, the lights lowered, the handling diminished, newborn infants—aside from all the physiological adaptations they must make—begin in a uniquely human way to adapt to the new experience of being in the world. (The Amazing Newborn)

Unlike adults, newborns communicate needs primarily by behavior. Because nurses are the most consistent observers of the newborn, they must be able to interpret this behavior to gain information about the neonate's condition and to respond with appropriate nursing interventions. This chapter focuses on the assessment of the neonate and interpretation of findings.

Assessment of the newborn is a continuous process used to evaluate development and adjustments to extrauterine life. In the delivery room, Apgar scoring and careful observation of the newborn form the basis of the assessment and are correlated with information such as the following:

- Maternal prenatal care history
- Birthing history
- Maternal analgesia and anesthesia
- Complications of labor or birth
- Treatment instituted in the birthing room, in conjunction with determination of clinical gestational age
- Consideration of the newborn's classification by weight and gestational age and neonatal mortality risk.
- Physical examination of the newborn

The nurse incorporates data from these sources with the assessment findings during the first one to four hours after birth to formulate a plan for nursing intervention.

Timing of Newborn Assessments

The first 24 hours of life are significant because during this period the newborn makes the critical transition from intrauterine to extrauterine life. The risk of mortality and morbidity is statistically high during this period. Assessment of the infant is essential to ensure that the transition is proceeding successfully.

Three major assessments of newborns are completed while they are in the birth facility. The first assessment is done immediately after birth in the delivery room to determine the need for resuscitation or other immediate interventions. The newborn who is stable stays with the parents after birth to initiate early attachment. The newborn who has complications is usually taken to the nursery for further evaluation and intervention.

A second evaluation is done in the first one to four hours after birth as part of the routine admission procedures. During this assessment, the nurse carries out a brief physical examination to evaluate the newborn's adaptation to extrauterine life and to estimate gestational age. Any problems that place the newborn at risk are assessed further during this time.

Prior to discharge, a physician or nurse-practitioner does a complete physical examination to detect any emerging or potential problems. A behavioral assessment is also done at this time.

This chapter presents the procedures for estimating gestational age and performing the complete physical examination and behavioral assessment. Chapter 23 discusses the immediate postbirth assessment. Chapter 29 describes the brief assessment performed during the first four hours of life.

Parental Involvement

The various neonatal assessments and the data obtained from them are only as effective as the degree to which the findings are shared with the parents and incorporated into the interaction between the couple and their infant. Parents must be included in the assessment process from the moment of their child's birth. The Apgar score and its meaning should be explained to them immediately. As soon as possible, the parents should also be a part of the physical and behavioral assessments.

The nurse can encourage the parents to identify the unique behavioral characteristics of their infant and to learn nurturing activities. Attachment is promoted when parents explore their infant in private, identifying individual physical and behavioral characteristics. The nurse's supportive responses to the parents' questions and observations are essential throughout the assessment process. The nurse should emphasize the uniqueness of the infant. With the nurse's help, attachment and the beginning of interactions between family members are established.

Estimation of Gestational Age

The nurse must establish the newborn's gestational age in the first four hours after birth so that careful attention can be given to age-related problems. Traditionally, the gestational age of a neonate was determined from the date of the pregnant woman's last menstrual period. This method was accurate only 75% to 85% of the time. Because of the problems that develop with the newborn who is preterm or whose weight is inappropriate for gestational age, a more accurate system was developed to evaluate the newborn. Once learned, the procedure can be done in a few minutes.

Clinical **gestational age assessment tools** have two components: external physical characteristics and neurologic and/or neuromuscular development evaluations. Physical characteristics generally include sole creases, amount of breast tissue, amount of lanugo, cartilaginous development of the ear, testicular descent, and scrotal rugae or labial development. These objective clinical criteria are not influenced by labor and birth and do not change significantly within the first 24 hours after birth.

During the first 24 hours of life, the newborn's nervous system is unstable; thus, neurologic evaluation findings based on reflexes or assessments dependent on the higher brain centers may not be reliable. If the neurologic findings drastically deviate from the gestational age derived by evaluation of the external characteristics, a second assessment is done in 24 hours.

The neurologic components (excluding reflexes) can aid in assessing neonates of less than 34 weeks' gestation. Between 26 and 34 weeks, neurologic changes are significant, whereas significant physical changes are less evident. The important neurologic changes consist of replacement of extensor tone by flexor tone in a *caudocephalad* (tail to head) progression. Neurologic examination facilitates assessment of functional or physiologic maturation in addition to physical development.

Of the gestational assessment aids, Dubowitz and Dubowitz's tool is the most thoroughly documented and validated way to assess intrauterine growth alterations and preterm neonates. This assessment tool lists physical characteristics and neuromuscular tone components to be assessed on admission to the nursery.

Ballard's *estimation of gestational age* by maturity rating is a simplified version of the Dubowitz tool. The Ballard tool omits some of the neuromuscular tone assessments, such as head lag, ventral suspension (which is difficult to assess in very ill newborns or those on respirators), and leg recoil. The scoring method of Ballard's tool is much like that of the Dubowitz tool; each physical and neuromuscular finding is given a value, and the total score is matched to a gestational age (Figure 28–1). The maximum score on the Ballard's tool is 50, which corresponds to a gestational age of 44 weeks.

For example, upon completing a gestational assessment of a one-hour-old newborn, the nurse gives a score of 3 to all the physical characteristics, for a total of 18, and gives a score of 3 to all the neuromuscular assessments, for a total neurologic score of 18. The physical characteristics score of 18 is added to the neurologic score of 18 for a total score of 36, which correlates with 38+ weeks' gestation. Since all newborns vary slightly in the development of physical characteristics and maturation of neurologic function, scores will usually vary instead of all being 3, as in the example.

The Dubowitz and Ballard tools are less accurate for neonates of less than 28 weeks' or more than 43 weeks' gestation. Some nurseries use the physical characteristics component of Brazie and Lubchenco's "Clinical Estimation of Gestational Age Chart" (Appendix G) as the initial assessment for all newborns admitted to the nursery. In carrying out gestational age assessments, the nurse should keep in mind that maternal conditions such as pregnancy-induced hypertension (PIH) and diabetes and maternal analgesia and anesthesia may affect certain gestational assessment components and warrant further study. Maternal diabetes, although it appears to accelerate fetal physical growth, seems to retard maturation. Maternal hypertensive states, which retard fetal physical growth, seem to speed maturation.

Newborns of women with PIH have a poor correlation with the criteria involving active muscle tone and edema. Maternal analgesia and anesthesia may cause the baby to have respiratory depression. Babies with respiratory distress syndrome (RDS) tend to be flaccid and edematous and to assume a "frog-like" posture. These characteristics affect the scoring of the neuromuscular components of the assessment tool used.

Assessment of Physical Characteristics

The nurse first evaluates observable characteristics without disturbing the baby. Selected physical characteristics common to both gestational assessment tools are presented here in the order in which they might be evaluated most effectively:

**Estimation of Gestational Age
by Maturity Rating**
Symbols: X=First exam   O=Second exam

Neuromuscular Maturity

	0	1	2	3	4	5
Posture						
Square window (wrist)	90°	60°	45°	30°	0°	
Arm recoil	180°		100°-180°	90°-100°	<90°	
Popliteal angle	180°	160°	130°	110°	90°	<90°
Scarf sign						
Heel to ear						

Gestation by dates _____ wks.

Birth date _____ Hour _____ am/pm

APGAR _____ 1 min _____ 5 min

Score	Wks
5	26
10	28
15	30
20	32
25	34
30	36
35	38
40	40
45	42
50	44

Physical Maturity

	0	1	2	3	4	5
Skin	gelatinous red, transparent	smooth pink, visible veins	superficial peeling and/or rash, few veins	cracking pale area, rare veins,	parchment, deep cracking, no vessels	leathery, cracked, wrinkled
Lanugo	none	abundant	thinning	bald areas	mostly bald	
Plantar creases	no crease	faint red marks	anterior transverse crease only	creases anter. 2/3	creases cover entire sole	
Breast	barely perceptible	flat areola, no bud	stippled areola, 1-2 mm bud	raised areola, 3-4 mm bud	full areola, 5-10 mm bud	
Ear	pinna flat, stays folded	sl. curved pinna, soft with slow recoil	well-curv. pinna, soft but ready recoil	formed and firm with instant recoil	thick cartilage, ear stiff	
Genitals (male)	scrotum empty, no rugae		testes decending, few rugae	testes down, good rugae	testes pendulous, deep rugae	
Genitals (female)	prominent clitoris and labia minora		majora and minora equally prominent	majora large, minora small	clitoris and minora completely covered	

Figure 28–1   Newborn maturity rating and classification (Figure adapted from Sweet AY, Fanaroff AA: Care of the High-Risk Infant. *Philadelphia: WB Saunders, 1977, p 47)*

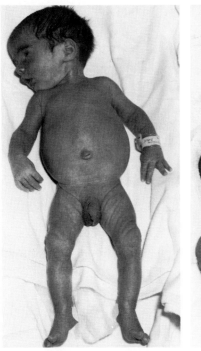
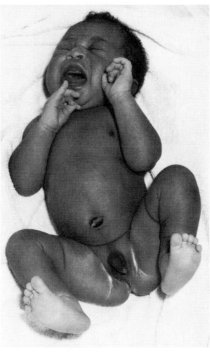
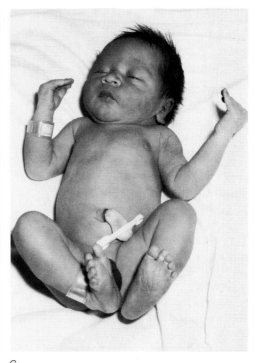

A   B   C

Figure 28–2   Resting posture. A Infant exhibits beginning of flexion of the thigh. The gestational age is approximately 31 weeks. Note the extension of the upper extremities. B Infant exhibits stronger flexion of the arms, hips, and thighs. The gestational age is approximately 35 weeks. C The full-term infant exhibits hypertonic flexion of all extremities. (From Dubowitz L, Dubowitz V: The Gestational Age of the Newborn. *Menlo Park, CA: Addison-Wesley, 1977. Reprinted by permission of V Dubowitz, MD, Hammersmith Hospital, London, England.)*

1. *Resting posture,* although a neuromuscular component, it should be assessed as the baby lies undisturbed on a flat surface (Figure 28–2).

2. *Skin* in the preterm newborn appears thin and transparent, with veins prominent over the abdomen early in gestation. As term approaches, the skin appears opaque because of increased subcutaneous tissue. Disappearance of the protective vernix caseosa promotes skin desquamation and is commonly seen in postmature infants.

3. *Lanugo,* a fine hair covering, decreases as gestational age increases. The amount of lanugo is greatest at 28 to 30 weeks and then disappears, first from the face, then from the trunk and extremities.

4. *Sole (plantar) creases* are reliable indicators of gestational age in the first 12 hours of life. After this, the skin of the foot begins drying, and superficial creases appear. Development of sole creases begins at the top (anterior) portion of the sole and, as gestation progresses, proceeds to the heel (Figure 28–3). Peeling may also occur. Plantar creases vary with race. Black newborns' sole creases may be less developed at term.

5. The *areola* is inspected and the *breast bud tissue* is gently palpated by application of the forefinger and middle finger to the breast area and is mea-

sured in centimeters or millimeters (Figure 28–4). At term gestation, the tissue will measure between 0.5 and 1 cm (5 to 10 mm). During the assessment the nipple should not be grasped because skin and subcutaneous tissue will prevent accurate estimation of size. The nurse may also cause trauma to the breast tissue if this procedure is not done gently. As gestation progresses, the breast tissue mass and areola enlarge. However, a large breast tissue mass can occur as a result of conditions other than advanced gestational age or the effects of maternal hormones on the baby. The infant of a diabetic mother tends to be large for gestational age (LGA) and the accelerated development of breast tissue is a reflection of subcutaneous fat deposits. Small-for-gestational-age (SGA) term or postterm newborns may have used subcutaneous fat (which would have been deposited as breast tissue) to survive in utero; as a result, their lack of breast tissue may indicate a gestational age of 34 to 35 weeks, even though other factors indicate a *term* or *postterm* neonate.

6. *Ear form and cartilage distribution* develop with gestational age. The cartilage gives the ear its shape and substance (Figure 28–5). In a newborn of less than 34 weeks' gestaton the ear is relatively shape-

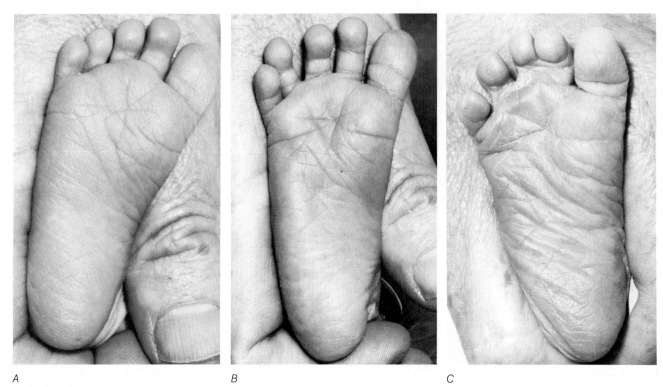

A   B   C

Figure 28–3   Sole creases. A Infant has a few sole creases on the anterior portion of the foot. Note the slick heel. The gestational age is approximately 35 weeks. B Infant has a deeper network of sole creases on the anterior two-thirds of the sole. Note the slick heel. The gestational age is approximately 37 weeks. C The full-term infant has deep sole creases down to and including the heel as the skin loses fluid and dries after birth; sole (plantar) creases can be seen even in preterm newborns. (From Dubowitz L, Dubowitz V: Gestational Age of the Newborn. *Menlo Park, CA: Addison-Wesley, 1977. Reprinted by permission of V Dubowitz, MD, Hammersmith Hospital, London, England.)*

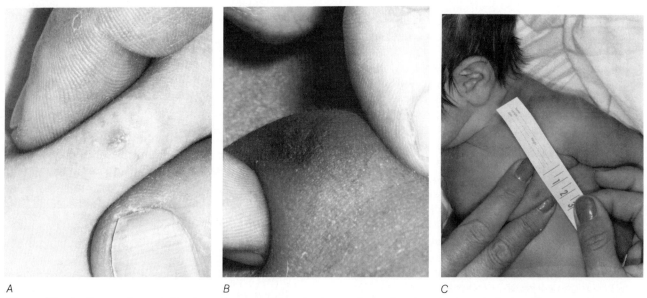

A   B   C

Figure 28–4   Breast tissue. A Newborn has a visible raised area. On palpation the area is 4 mm. The gestational age is 38 weeks. B Newborn has 10 mm breast tissue area. The gestational age is 40 to 44 weeks. C Gently compress the tissue between the middle and index fingers and measure the tissue in centimeters or millimeters. Absence of or decreased breast tissue often indicates premature or SGA newborn. (From Dubowitz L, Dubowitz V: Gestational Age of the Newborn. *Menlo Park, CA: Addison-Wesley, 1977. Reprinted by permission of V Dubowitz, MD, Hammersmith Hospital, London, England.)*

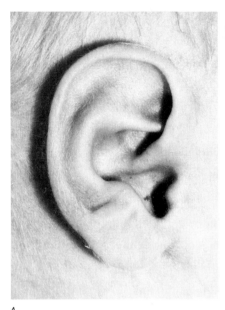
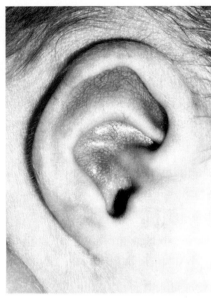
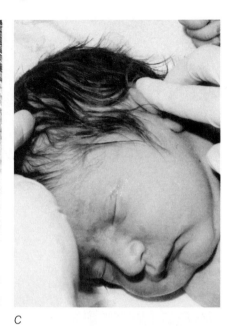

A   B   C

Figure 28–5 Ear form and cartilage. A The ear of the infant at approximately 36 weeks' gestation shows incurving of the upper two-thirds of the pinna. B Infant at term shows well-defined incurving of the entire pinna. C If the auricle stays in the position in which it is pressed, or returns slowly to its original position, it usually means the gestational age is less than 38 weeks. (From Dubowitz L, Dubowitz V: Gestational Age of the Newborn. *Menlo Park, CA: Addison-Wesley, 1977. Reprinted by permission of V Dubowitz, MD, Hammersmith Hospital, London, England.)*

less and flat; it has little cartilage, so the ear folds over on itself and remains folded. By approximately 36 weeks' gestation, some cartilage and slight incurving of the upper pinna are present, and the pinna springs back slowly when folded. (This response is tested by holding the top and bottom of the pinna together with the forefinger and thumb and then releasing it, or by folding the pinna of the ear forward against the side of the head and releasing it, and observing the response.) By term, the newborn's pinna is firm, stands away from the head, and springs back quickly from the folding.

7. *Male genitals* are evaluated for size of the scrotal sac, the presence of rugae, and descent of the testes (Figure 28–6). Prior to 36 weeks, the small scrotum has few rugae, and the testes are palpable in the inguinal canal. By 36 to 38 weeks, the testes are in the upper scrotum, and rugae have developed over the anterior portion of the scrotum. By term, the testes are generally in the lower scrotum, which is pendulous and covered with rugae.

8. The appearance of the *female genitals* depends in part on subcutaneous fat deposition and therefore relates to fetal nutritional status (Figure 28–7). The clitoris varies in size and occasionally is so large that it is difficult to identify the sex of the infant. This may be caused by adrenogenital syn-

drome, which causes the adrenals to secrete excessive amounts of adrogen and other hormones. At 30 to 32 weeks' gestation, the clitoris is prominent, and the labia majora are small and widely separated. As gestational age increases, the labia majora increase in size. At 36 to 40 weeks, they nearly cover the clitoris. At 40 weeks and beyond, the labia majora cover the labia minora and clitoris.

In the full-term female newborn, some tissue may protrude from the floor of the vagina. This tissue, the hymenal tag, is a normal segment of the hymen and disappears in several weeks.

Other physical characteristics assessed by some gestational age scoring tools include the following:

1. *Vernix* covers the preterm newborn. The postterm newborn has no vernix. After noting vernix distribution, the birthing room nurse dries the newborn to prevent evaporative heat loss, thus disturbing the vernix. The birthing area nurse must communicate to the neonatal nurse the amount of vernix and the areas of vernix coverage.

2. *Hair* of the preterm newborn has the consistency of matted wool or fur and lies in bunches rather than in the silky, single strands of the term newborn's hair.

3. *Skull firmness* increases as the fetus matures. In a term newborn the bones are hard, and the sutures

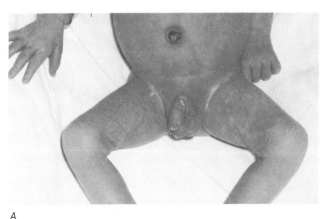
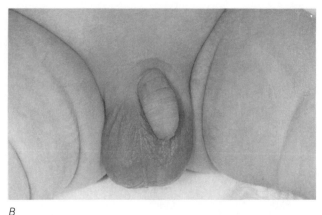

A   B

Figure 28–6   Male genitals. A Preterm infant's testes are not within the scrotum. The scrotal surface has few rugae. B Term infant's testes are generally fully descended. The entire surface of the scrotum is covered by rugae. (From Dubowitz L, Dubowitz V: Gestational Age of the Newborn. *Menlo Park, CA: Addison-Wesley, 1977. Reprinted by permission of V Dubowitz, MD, Hammersmith Hospital, London, England.)*

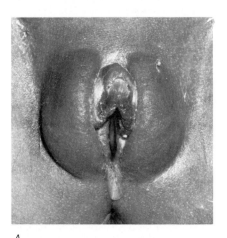
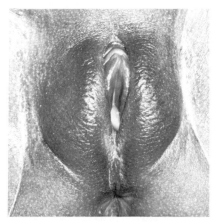
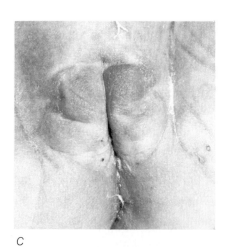

A   B   C

Figure 28–7   Female genitals. A Infant has a prominent clitoris. The labia majora are widely separated, and the labia minora, viewed laterally, would protrude beyond the labia majora. The gestational age is 30 to 36 weeks. B The clitoris is still visible; the labia minora are now covered by the larger labia majora. The gestational age is 36 to 40 weeks. C The term infant has well-developed, large labia majora that cover both clitoris and labia minora (From Dubowitz L, Dubowitz V: Gestational Age of the Newborn. *Menlo Park, CA: Addison-Wesley, 1977. Reprinted by permission of V Dubowitz, MD, Hammersmith Hospital, London, England.)*

are not easily displaced. The nurse should not attempt to displace the sutures forcibly.

4. *Nails* appear and cover the nail bed at about 20 weeks' gestation. Nails extending beyond the fingertips may indicate a postterm newborn.

Assessment of Neuromuscular Maturity Characteristics

The central nervous system of the human fetus matures at a fairly constant rate. Specific neurologic parameters have been correlated with gestational age. Tests have been designed to evaluate neurologic status as manifested by neuromuscular tone. In the fetus, neuromuscular tone develops from the lower to the upper extremities. The neurologic evaluation requires more manipulation and disturbances than the physical evaluation of the newborn.

The neuromuscular evaluation (see Figure 28–1) is best performed when the infant has stabilized. The following characteristics are evaluated:

1. The *square window sign* is elicited by flexing the baby's hand toward the ventral forearm. The angle formed at the wrist is measured (Figure 28–8).

2. *Recoil* is a test of flexion development. Because flexion first develops in the lower extremities, recoil is first tested in the legs. The newborn is placed on his or her back on a flat surface. With a hand on the newborn's knees and while manipulat-

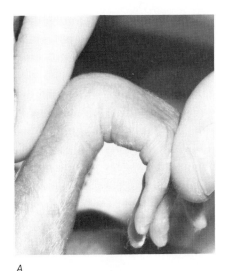
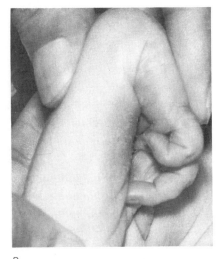
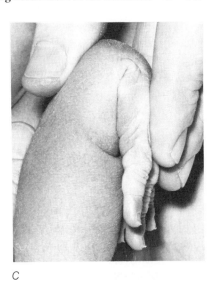

A   B   C

*Figure 28–8   Square window sign. A This angle is 90° and suggests an immature newborn of 28 to 32 weeks' gesta-
tion. B A 30° angle is commonly found from 38 to 40 weeks' gestation. C A 0° angle occurs from 40 to 42 weeks. (From
Dubowitz L, Dubowitz V: Gestational Age of the Newborn. Menlo Park, CA: Addison-Wesley, 1977. Reprinted by permission of V Dubowitz, MD, Hammersmith Hospital, London, England.)*

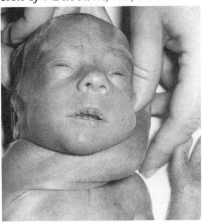
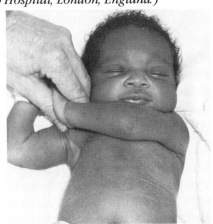
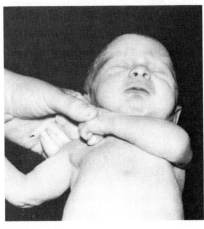

A   B   C

*Figure 28–9   Scarf sign. A No resistance is noted until after 30 weeks' gestation. The elbow can be readily moved past
the midline. B The elbow is at midline at 36 to 40 week's gestation. C Beyond 40 weeks' gestation, the elbow will not
reach the midline. (From Dubowitz L, Dubowitz V: Gestational Age of the Newborn. Menlo Park, CA: Addison-Wesley,
1977. Reprinted by permission of V Dubowitz, MD, Hammersmith Hospital, London, England.)*

ing the hip joint, the nurse places the baby's legs in
flexion, then extends them parallel to each other
and flat on the surface. The response to this maneuver is recoil of the neonate's legs. According to
gestational age, they may not move or they may
return slowly or quickly to the flexed position.

Arm recoil is tested by flexion at the elbow
and extension of the arms at the newborn's side.
While the baby is in the supine position, the nurse
completely flexes both elbows, holds them in this
position for five seconds, extends the arms at the
baby's side, and releases them. Upon release, the
elbows of a full-term newborn form an angle of less
than 90° and rapidly recoil back to flexed position.

The elbows of preterm newborns have slower recoil time and form a less-than-90° angle. Arm recoil
is also slower in healthy but fatigued newborns
after birth; therefore arm recoil is best elicited
after the first hour of birth when the baby has had
time to recover from the stress of birth. Assessment of arm recoil should be bilateral in order to
rule out brachial palsy.

3. The *popliteal angle* (degree of knee flexion) is determined with the newborn supine and flat. The
thigh is flexed on the abdomen/chest, and the
nurse places the index finger of the other hand behind the newborn's ankle to extend the lower leg
until resistance is met. The angle formed is then

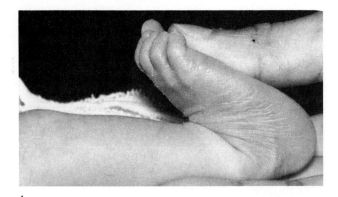
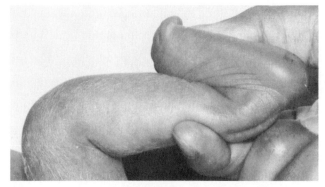

A   B

Figure 28–10　Ankle dorsiflexion. A A 45° angle is indicative of 32 to 36 weeks' gestation. A 20° angle is indicative of 36 to 40 weeks' gestation. B An angle of 0° is common at gestational age of 40 weeks or more. (From Dubowitz L, Dubowitz V: Gestational Age of the Newborn. Menlo Park, CA: Addison-Wesley, 1977. Reprinted by permission of V Dubowitz, MD, Hammersmith Hospital, London, England.)

measured. Results vary from no resistance in the very immature infant to an 80° angle in the term infant.

4. The *scarf sign* is elicited by placing the newborn supine and drawing an arm across the chest toward the infant's opposite shoulder until resistance is met. The location of the elbow is then noted in relation to the midline of the chest (Figure 28–9).

5. The *heel-to-ear maneuver* is performed by placing the baby in a supine position and then gently drawing the foot toward the ear on the same side until resistance is felt. Both the popliteal angle and the proximity of the foot to the ear are assessed.
   In a very preterm newborn, the leg will remain straight and the foot will go to the ear or beyond. Maneuvers involving the lower extremities of newborns who had frank breech presentation should be delayed to allow for resolution of leg positioning (Ballard et al 1979).

6. *Ankle dorsiflexion* is determined by flexing the ankle on the shin. The examiner uses a thumb to push on the sole of the newborn's foot while the fingers support the back of the leg. Then the angle formed by the foot and the interior leg is measured (Figure 28–10). This sign can be influenced by intrauterine position and congenital deformities.

7. *Head lag* (neck flexors) is measured by pulling the baby to a sitting position and noting the degree of head lag. Total lag is common in infants up to 34 weeks' gestation, whereas the postmature newborn (42 + weeks) will hold the head in front of the body line.

8. *Ventral suspension* (horizontal position) is evaluated by holding the newborn prone on the examiner's hand. The position of head and back and degree of flexion in the arms and legs are then noted. Some flexion of arms and legs indicates 36 to 38 weeks' gestation; fully flexed extremities,

with head and back even, are characteristic of a term neonate.

9. *Major reflexes* such as sucking, rooting, grasping, Moro, tonic neck, Babinski, and others are evaluated and scored (see page 861).

A supplementary method for estimating gestational age (done by the physician or NNP) is to view the vascular network of the cornea with an ophthalmoscope. The amount of vascularity present over the surface of the lens correlates with gestational age. In babies of less than 27 weeks' gestation, the cornea is cloudy and the vascular network is not visible; after 34 weeks' gestation, the vascular network has generally disappeared completely.

Determination of gestational age and correlation with birth weight (Figure 28–11) enables the nurse to assess the infant more accurately and to anticipate possible physiologic problems. This information is then used in conjunction with a complete physical examination to determine priorities and to establish a plan of care appropriate to the individual infant.

Physical Assessment

After the initial determination of gestational age and related potential problems, a more extensive physical assessment is done. (The nursing student is expected to be able to do most of the assessments, although she or he may not be required to know all the alterations and possible causes.) The nurse should choose a warm, well-lighted area that is free of drafts. Completing the physical assessment in the presence of the parents provides an opportunity to acquaint them with their unique newborn. The examination is performed in a systematic, head-to-toe manner, and all findings are recorded. When assessing the physical and neurologic status of the newborn, the nurse should first consider general appearance and then proceed to specific areas.

A guide for systematically assessing the newborn ap-

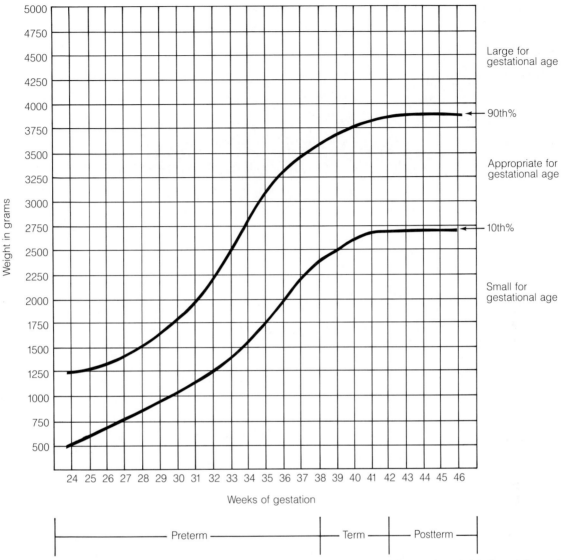

Figure 28–11   Classification of newborns by birth weight and gestational age. The newborn's birth weight and gestational age are placed on the graph. The newborn is then classified as large for gestational age, appropriate for gestational age, or small for gestational age. (From Battaglia FC, Lubchenco LO: A practical classification of newborn infants by weight and gestational age. J Pediatr *1967; 71:161)*

pears on pages 864–878. Normal findings, alterations, and related causes are presented and correlated with suggested nursing responses. The findings are typical for a full-term newborn.

General Appearance

The newborn's head is disproportionately large for the body. The center of the baby's body is the umbilicus rather than the symphysis pubis, as in the adult. The body appears long and the extremities short. The flexed position that the neonate maintains contributes to the short appearance of the extremities. The hands are tightly clenched. The neck looks short because the chin rests on the chest. Newborns have a prominent abdomen, sloping shoulders, narrow

hips, and rounded chests. They tend to stay in a flexed position similar to the one maintained in utero and will offer resistance when the extremities are straightened. After a breech birth, the feet are usually dorsiflexed, and it may take several weeks for the newborn to assume typical newborn posture.

Weight and Measurements

The normal full-term Caucasian newborn has an average birth weight of 3405 g (7 lb, 8 oz), whereas black, Asian, and Native American newborns are usually somewhat smaller. Other factors that influence weight are age and size of parents, health of mother, and interval between pregnancies. After the first week and for the first six months, the

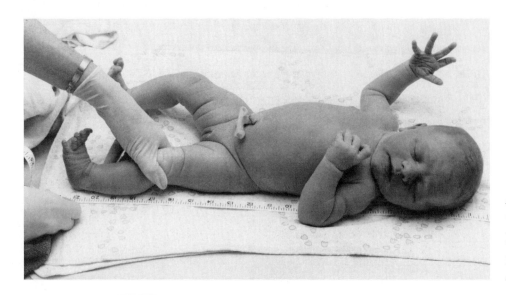

Figure 28–12 Measuring the length of a newborn (From Swearingen PL: The Addison-Wesley Photo-Atlas of Nursing Procedures. Redwood City, CA: Benjamin/Cummings, 1984)

neonate's weight will increase about 198 g (7 oz) weekly.

Approximately 70% to 75% of the neonate's body weight is water. During the initial newborn period (the first three or four days), there is a physiologic weight loss of 5% to 10% for term newborns because of fluid shifts. This weight loss may reach 15% for preterm newborns. Large babies may tend to lose more weight because of greater fluid loss in proportion to birth weight. If weight loss is greater than expected, clinical reappraisal is necessary. Factors contributing to weight loss include small fluid intake resulting from delayed breastfeeding or a slow adjustment to the formula, increased volume of meconium excreted, and urination. Weight loss may be marked in the presence of temperature elevation because of associated dehydration.

The length of the normal newborn is difficult to measure because the legs are flexed and tensed. To measure length, the nurse should place infants flat on their backs with legs extended as much as possible (Figure 28–12). The average length is 50 cm (20 in.), with the range being 45 to 55 cm (18 to 22 in.). The newborn will grow approximately an inch a month for the next six months. This is the period of most rapid growth.

At birth, the newborn's head is one-third the size of an adult's head. The circumference of the newborn's head is 32 to 37 cm (12.5 to 14.5 in.). For accurate measurement, the tape is placed over the most prominent part of the occiput and brought to just above the eyebrows (Figure 28–13A). The circumference of the newborn's head is approximately 2 cm greater than the circumference of the newborn's chest at birth and will remain in this proportion for the next few months. (Factors that alter this measurement are discussed on page 851.)

The average circumference of the chest at birth is 32 cm (12.5 in.). Chest measurements should be taken with the tape measure at the lower edge of the scapulas and brought around anteriorly directly over the nipple line (Figure 28–13B). The abdominal circumference or girth may also be measured at this time by placing the tape around the newborn's abdomen at the level of the umbilicus, with the bottom edge of the tape at the top edge of the umbilicus (see Table 28–1).

Temperature

Initial assessment of the newborn's temperature is critical. In utero, the temperature of the fetus is about the same as or slightly higher than the expectant mother's. When the baby enters the outside world, his or her temperature can suddenly drop as a result of exposure to cold drafts and the skin's heat-loss mechanisms.

If no heat conservation measures are started, the normal term newborn's deep body temperature falls 0.1C (0.2F) per minute; skin temperature lowers 0.3C (0.5F) per minute. Marked decrease in skin temperature occurs within ten minutes after exposure to room air (Korones 1986). The temperature should stabilize within 8 to 12 hours. Temperature should be monitored when the newborn is admitted to the nursery and at four-hour intervals until stable, then once every eight-hour shift (AAP 1988). Many institutions use a continuous probe, or measurements are obtained every 15 to 30 minutes for the first hour, then each hour for four hours. (See Chapter 27 for a discussion of the physiology of temperature regulation.)

Body temperature can be assessed by the rectum, axilla, or skin. Rectal temperature is assumed to be the closest approximation to core temperature, but this depends on the depth of the thermometer insertion. Normal rectal temperature is 36.6C to 37.2C (97.8F to 99F). The rectal route is not recommended as a routine method as it may predispose to rectal mucosal irritation and increase chances of perforation (AAP 1988). If the temperature is taken rectally, the nurse inserts the lubricated thermometer one-half inch into the rectum and continuously holds the thermometer in the rectum for five minutes (Figure 28–14A). Rectal temperatures were previously advocated to detect

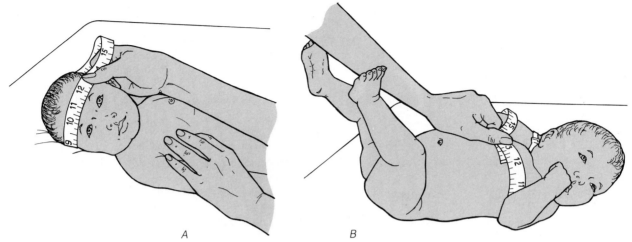

Figure 28–13   A Measuring the head circumference of the newborn. B Measuring the chest circumference of the newborn.

imperforate anus, but nurses can make this assessment by observing the newborn's stools.

Axillary temperature reflects body temperature and the body's compensatory response to the thermal environment. Axillary temperatures are recommended as an alternative to rectal temperatures. Axillary temperatures are reliable as a close estimation of the rectal temperature (Korones 1986). In preterm and term newborns, there is less than 0.1C (0.20F) difference between the two sites. If the axillary method is used, the thermometer must remain in place at least three minutes unless an electronic thermometer is used (Figure 28–14B). Normal axillary temperature ranges from 36.5C to 37C (97.7F to 98.6F). Axillary temperatures can be misleading because the friction caused by apposition of the inner arm skin and upper chest wall and the nearness of brown fat to the probe may elevate the temperature.

Table 28–1   Newborn Measurements

Weight

Average: 3405 g (7 lb, 8 oz)

Range: 2500–4000 g (5 lb, 8 oz–8 lb, 13 oz)

Weight is influenced by racial origin and maternal age and size

Physiologic weight loss: 5%–10% for term infants, up to 15% for preterm infants

Growth: 7 oz (198 g) per week for first six months

Length

Average: 50 cm (20 in.)

Range: 45–55 cm (18–22 in.)

Growth: 1 inch (2.5 cm) per month for first six months.

Head Circumference

32–37 cm (12½–14½ in.)

Approximately 2 cm larger than chest circumference

The best measure of skin temperature is by means of continuous skin probe rather than axillary temperature, especially for small newborns or newborns maintained in incubators or under radiant warmers. Normal skin temperature is 36C to 36.5C (96.8F to 97.7F). Skin temperature assessment allows time for initiation of interventions prior to a more serious fall in core temperatures.

Temperature instability, a deviation of more than 1C (2F) from one reading to the next, or a subnormal temperature may indicate an infection. In contrast with an elevated temperature in older children, an increased temperature in a newborn may indicate reactions to too much covering, too hot a room, or dehydration. Dehydration, which tends to increase body temperature, occurs in newborns whose feedings have been delayed for any reason. Newborns respond to overheating (temperature greater than 37.5C or 99.5F) by increased restlessness and eventually by perspiration. The perspiration is initially seen on the head and face, then on the chest. Normal term newborn temperature is 36.5C to 37.5C (97.7F–99.4F) (Eden & Boehm 1990).

Skin

The skin of the newborn should be pink tinged or ruddy in color and warm to the touch. The ruddy color results from increased concentration of red blood cells in the blood vessels and from limited subcutaneous fat deposits.

Acrocyanosis

Acrocyanosis (bluish discoloration of the hands and feet) may be present in the first two to six hours after birth. This condition is due to poor peripheral circulation, which results in vasomotor instability and capillary stasis, especially when the baby is exposed to cold. If the central circulation is adequate, the blood supply should return quickly to the extremity after the skin is blanched with a finger (Color Plate V).

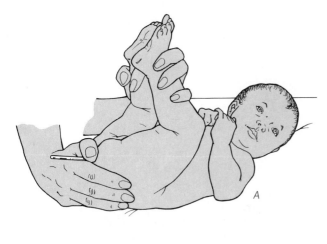

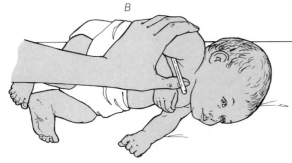

Figure 28–14   A The rectal thermometer must be held in place for 5 minutes and the legs supported. B The axillary temperature should be taken for 3 minutes. The newborn's arm should be tightly but gently pressed against the thermometer and the newborn's side as illustrated.

Mottling (lacy pattern of dilated blood vessels under the skin) occurs as a result of general circulation fluctuations. It may last several hours to several weeks or may come and go periodically.

Harlequin Sign

Harlequin sign (clown) color change is occasionally noted: A deep red color develops over one side of the newborn's body while the other side remains pale, so that the skin resembles a clown's suit. This color change results from a vasomotor disturbance in which blood vessels on one side dilate while the vessels on the other side constrict. It usually lasts from 1 to 20 minutes. Affected neonates may have single or multiple episodes.

Jaundice

Jaundice is first detectable on the face (where skin overlies cartilage) and the mucous membranes of the mouth. It is evaluated by blanching the tip of the nose, the forehead, or the gum line. This procedure must be carried out in appropriate lighting. If jaundice is present, the area will appear yellowish immediately after blanching. Another area to assess for jaundice is the sclera. Evaluation and determina-

tion of the cause of jaundice must be initiated immediately to prevent possibly serious consequences. The jaundice may be related to breast-feeding (small incidence), hematomas, immature liver function, or bruises from forceps, or it may be caused by blood incompatibility, oxytocin (Pitocin) augmentation or induction, or severe hemolytic process. For detailed discussion of causes and assessment of jaundice, see Chapter 32.

Erythema Neonatorum Toxicum

Erythema toxicum is a perifollicular erupton of lesions that are firm, vary in size from 1 to 3 mm, and consist of a white or pale yellow papule or pustule with an erythematous base. The rash may appear suddenly, usually over the trunk and diaper area, and is frequently widespread (Color Plate XII). The lesions do not appear on the palms of the hands or the soles of the feet. The peak incidence is at 24 to 48 hours of life. The cause is unknown and no treatment is necessary. The lesions disappear in a few hours or days. If a maculopapular rash appears and there is a question whether it is erythema toxicum, a smear of the aspirated papule will show numerous eosinophils on staining and no bacteria will be cultured.

Skin Turgor

Skin turgor is assessed to determine hydration status, the need to initiate early feedings, and the presence of any infectious processes. The usual place to assess skin turgor is over the abdomen. Skin should be elastic and should return to its original shape.

Vernix Caseosa and Milia

Vernix caseosa, a whitish cheeselike substance, covers the fetus while in utero and lubricates the skin of the newborn. The skin of the term or postterm newborn has less vernix and is frequently dry and peeling, especially on the hands and feet. **Milia,** which are plugged sebaceous glands, appear as raised white spots on the face, especially across the nose (Color Plate VIII).

Forceps Marks

Forceps marks may be present after a difficult forceps birth. The newborn may have reddened areas over the cheeks and jaws. It is important to reassure the parents that these will disappear, usually within one or two days. Transient facial paralysis resulting from the forceps pressure is a rare complication.

Birthmarks

Telangiectatic nevi, or "**stork bites,**" appear as pale pink or red flat, dilated capillaries and are frequently found on the eyelids, nose, lower occipital bone, and nape of the neck (Color Plate IX). These lesions are common in light-complexioned neonates and are more noticeable during periods of crying. These areas blanch easily, have no clinical significance, and fade during infancy, usually disappearing by the second birthday. In many children, they reappear during crying episodes.

Mongolian spots are macular areas of bluish-black pigmentation found on the dorsal area and the buttocks. They are common in Asian and black infants and newborns of other dark-skinned races (Color Plate VII). They gradually fade during the first or second year of life.

Nevus flammeus, or **port-wine stain**, is a capillary angioma directly below the epidermis. It is a nonelevated, sharply outlined, red-to-purple dense area of capillaries (Color Plate X). The size and shape are variable, but it commonly appears on the face. It does not grow in size, does not fade with time, and does not blanch as a rule. In the black infant, the nevus flammeus appears jet black in color. The birthmark may be concealed by using an opaque cosmetic cream. If convulsions, contralateral hemiplegia, or intracortical calcifications accompany the nevus flammeus, it is suggestive of Sturge-Weber syndrome with involvement of the fifth cranial nerve.

Nevus vasculosus, or "**strawberry mark**," is a capillary hemangioma. It consists of newly formed and enlarged capillaries in the dermal and subdermal layers. It is a raised, clearly delineated, dark red, rough-surfaced birthmark commonly found in the head region. Such marks usually grow (often rapidly) for several months and become fixed in size by eight months. They then begin to shrink and start to resolve spontaneously several weeks to months after peak growth is reached. Except in rare cases, they are completely gone by the time the child is 7 years old. Parents can be told that resolution is heralded by a pale purple or gray spot on the surface of the hemangioma. The best cosmetic effect is achieved when the lesions are allowed to resolve spontaneously.

Birthmarks are frequently a cause of concern for the parents. The mother may be especially anxious, fearing that she is to blame. Guilt feelings are common in the presence of misconceptions about the cause. Birthmarks should be identified and explained to the parents. By providing appropriate information about the cause and course of birthmarks, the nurse frequently relieves the fears and anxieties of the family. The nurse should note any bruises, abrasions, or birthmarks seen upon admission to the nursery.

Head

General Appearance

The newborn's head is large (approximately one-fourth of the body size), with soft, pliable skull bones. The head may appear asymmetrical in the newborn of a vertex delivery. This asymmetry, called **molding**, is caused by overriding of the cranial bones during labor and birth (Figure 28–15). The degree of molding varies with the amount and length of pressure exerted on the head. Within a few days after birth, the overriding usually diminishes and the suture lines become palpable. Because head measurements are affected by molding, a second measurement is indicated a few days after birth. The heads of breech-born newborns and those born by cesarean birth are characteristically round and well shaped since pressure was not exerted on them during birth. Any extreme differences in head size may indicate microcephaly or hydrocephalus. Variations in the shape, size, or appearance of the head measurements may be due to *craniostenosis* (premature closure of the cranial sutures) and *plagiocephaly* (asymmetry caused by pressure on the fetal head during gestation).

Two *fontanelles* ("soft spots") may be palpated on the infant's head. Fontanelles, which are openings at the juncture of the cranial bones, can be measured with the fingers. Accurate measurement necessitates that the examiner's finger be measured in centimeters. The diamond-shaped *anterior fontanelle* is 3 to 4 cm long by 2 to 3 cm wide. It is located at the juncture of the frontal and parietal bones. The *posterior fontanelle*, smaller and triangular, is formed by the parietal bones and the occipital bone. The fontanelles will be smaller immediately after birth than several days later because of molding. The anterior fontanelle closes within 18 months, whereas the posterior fontanelle closes within 8 to 12 weeks.

The fontanelles are a useful indicator of the newborn's condition. The anterior fontanelle may swell when the newborn cries or may pulsate with the heartbeat, which is normal. A bulging fontanelle usually signifies increased intracranial pressure, and a depressed fontanelle indicates dehydration. The sutures between the cranial bones should be palpated for amount of overlapping.

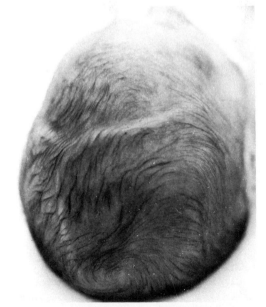

Figure 28–15 Overlapped cranial bones produce a visible ridge in a small, premature infant. Easily visible overlapping does not often occur in term infants. (From Korones SB: High-Risk Newborn Infants, 4th ed. St. Louis: CV Mosby, 1986)

In addition to being inspected for degree of molding and size, the head should be evaluated for soft tissue edema and bruising.

Cephalhematoma

Cephalhematoma is a collection of blood resulting from ruptured blood vessels between the surface of a cranial bone (usually parietal) and the periosteal membrane (Figure 28–16). The scalp in these areas feels loose and slightly edematous. These areas emerge as defined hematomas between the first and second day. Although external pressure may cause the mass to fluctuate, it does not increase in size when the infant cries. Cephalhematomas may be unilateral or bilateral and do not cross suture lines. They are relatively common in vertex births and may disappear within two to three weeks or slowly over subsequent months.

Caput Succedaneum

Caput succedaneum is a localized, easily identifiable soft area of the scalp, generally resulting from a long and difficult labor or vacuum extraction. The sustained pressure of the presenting part against the cervix results in compression of local blood vessels, and venous return is slowed. This causes an increase in tissue fluids, an edematous swelling, and occasional bleeding under the periosteum. The caput may vary from a small area to a severely elongated head. The fluid in the caput is reabsorbed within 12 hours or a few days after birth. Caputs resulting from vacuum extractors are sharply outlined, circular areas up to 2 cm thick. They disappear more slowly than naturally occurring edema. It is possible to distinguish between a cephalhematoma and a caput because the caput overrides suture lines (Figure 28–17), whereas the cephalhematoma, because of its location, never crosses a suture line. See Table 28–2.

Face

The newborn's face is well designed to help the infant suckle. Sucking (fat) pads are located in the cheeks, and a labial tubercle (sucking callus) is frequently found in the center of the upper lip. The chin is recessed, and the nose is flattened. The lips are sensitive to touch, and the sucking reflex is easily initiated.

Symmetry of the eyes, nose, and ears is evaluated. See the Neonatal Physical Assessment Guide in page 867 for deviations in symmetry and variations in size, shape, and spacing of facial features. Facial movement symmetry should be assessed to determine the presence of facial palsy.

Facial paralysis appears when the neonate cries; the affected side is immobile and the palpebral (eyelid) fissure widens (Figure 28–18). Paralysis may result from forceps delivery or pressure on the facial nerve from the maternal pelvis during birth. Facial paralysis usually disappears within a few days to three weeks.

Eyes

The eyes of the Caucasian neonate are a blue or slate blue gray. Scleral color tends to be bluish because of its relative thinness. The infant's eye color is usually established at approximately three months, although it may change any time up to one year. Dark-skinned neonates tend to have dark eyes at birth.

The eyes should be checked for size, equality of pupil size, reaction of pupils to light, blink reflex to light, and edema and inflammation of the eyelids. The eyelids can be edematous during the first few days of life because of the birth and the instillation of silver nitrate drops in the newborn's eyes. **Chemical conjunctivitis** may also appear a

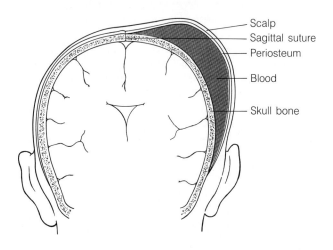

A

B

Figure 28–16 Cephalhematoma is a collection of blood between the surface of a cranial bone and the periosteal membrane. This is a cephalhematoma over the left parietal bone. (Photo reproduced with permission from Potter EL, Craig JM: Pathology of the Fetus and Infant, *3rd ed. Copyright 1975 by Year Book Medical Publishers, Chicago)*

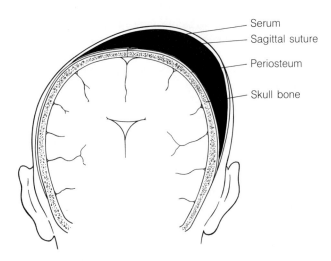

Serum
Sagittal suture
Periosteum
Skull bone

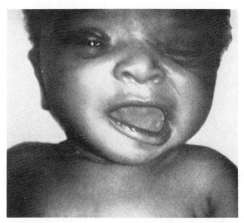

Figure 28–18 Facial paralysis. Paralysis of the right side of the face from injury to right facial nerve. (Courtesy of Dr. Ralph Platow. In: Potter EL, Craig JM: Pathology of the Fetus and Infant, 3rd ed. Copyright 1975 by Year Book Medical Publishers, Chicago)

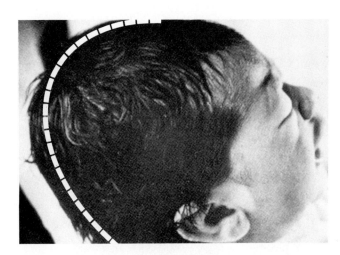

Figure 28–17 Caput succedaneum is a collection of fluid (serum) under the scalp. (Photo courtesy Mead Johnson Laboratories, Evansville, IN)

Table 28–2 Comparison of Cephalhematoma and Caput Succedaneum

Cephalhematoma

Collection of blood between cranial (usually parietal) bone and periosteal membrane

Does not cross suture lines

Does not increase in size with crying

Appears on first and second day

Disappears after two to three weeks or may take months

Caput Succedaneum

Collection of fluid, edematous swelling of the scalp

Crosses suture lines

Present at birth or shortly thereafter

Reabsorbed within 12 hours or a few days after birth

few hours after the instillation of the ophthalmic drops but disappears without treatment in one to two days. If infectious conjunctivitis exists, the newborn has the same purulent (greenish-yellow) discharge as in chemical conjunctivitis. But it is caused by staphylococci or a variety of gram-negative bacteria and requires treatment with ophthalmic antibiotics. Onset is usually after the second day. Edema of the orbits or eyelids may persist for several days until the newborn's kidneys can evacuate the fluid.

Small **subconjunctival hemorrhages** appear in about 10% of newborns and are commonly found on the sclera. These hemorrhages are caused by the changes in vascular tension or ocular pressure during birth. They will remain for a few weeks and are of no pathologic significance. Parents need reassurance that the infant is not bleeding from within the eye and that vision will not be impaired.

The neonate may demonstrate transient strabismus caused by poor neuromuscular control of eye muscles (Figure 28–19). It gradually regresses in three to four months. The "doll's eye" phenomenon is also present for about ten days after birth. As the newborn's head position is changed to the left and then to the right, the eyes move to the opposite direction. This results from underdeveloped integration of head-eye coordination.

The nurse should observe the neonate's pupils for opacities or whiteness and for the absence of a normal red reflex. Red reflex is a red-orange flash of color observed when an ophthalmoscope light reflects off the retina. In dark-colored newborns, the retina may appear more greyish. Absence of red reflex occurs with cataracts. Congenital cataracts should be suspected in infants of mothers with a history of rubella, cytomegalic inclusion disease, or syphilis.

The cry of the newborn is commonly tearless because the lacrimal structures are immature at birth and are not usually fully functional until the second month of life.

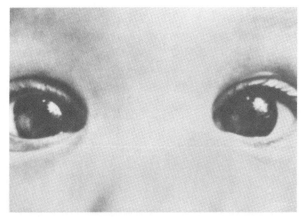

Figure 28–19 Transient strabismus may be present in the newborn due to poor neuromuscular control. (Courtesy Mead Johnson Laboratories, Evansville, IN)

a cleft palate, which can be present even in the absence of a cleft lip. The examiner places a clean index finger along the hard and soft palate to feel for any openings (Figure 28–20).

Occasionally, an examination of the gums will reveal *precocious teeth* on the lower central incisor. If they appear loose, they should be removed to prevent aspiration. Gray-white lesions (*inclusion cysts*) on the gums may be confused with teeth. On the hard palate and gum margins, **Epstein's pearls**, small glistening white specks (keratin-containing cysts) that feel hard to the touch are often present. These usually disappear in a few weeks and are of no significance. **Thrush** may appear as white patches that look like milk curds adhering to the mucous membranes and that cause bleeding when removed. Thrush is caused by *Candida albicans,* often acquired from an infected vaginal tract during birth, and is treated with a preparation of nystatin (Mycostatin).

Some newborns may produce tears during the neonatal period. Poor oculomotor coordination and absence of accommodation limit visual abilities, but the newborn does have peripheral vision and can fixate on near objects (9 to 12 in.) for short periods (Ludington-Hoe 1983). The newborn can perceive faces, shapes, and colors and begins to show visual preferences early. The neonate blinks in response to bright lights, to a tap on the bridge of the nose (glabellar reflex), or to a light touch on the eyelids. Pupillary light reflex is also present. Examination of the eye is best accomplished by rocking the newborn from an upright position to the horizontal a few times or by other methods that will elicit an opened-eye response.

Nose

The newborn's nose is small and narrow. Infants are characteristically nose breathers for the first few months of life. The newborn generally removes obstructions by sneezing. Nasal patency is assured if the baby breathes easily with mouth closed. If respiratory difficulty occurs, the nurse checks for *choanal atresia* (congenital blockage of the passageway between nose and pharynx).

The newborn has the ability to smell after the nasal passages are cleared of amniotic fluid and mucus. This ability is demonstrated by the search for milk. Infants will turn their heads toward the milk source, whether bottle or breast.

Mouth

The lips of the newborn should be pink, and a touch on the lips should produce sucking motions. Saliva is normally scant. The taste buds are developed prior to birth, and the newborn can easily discriminate between sweet and bitter.

The easiest way to examine the mouth completely is to stimulate infants gently to cry by depressing their tongue, thereby causing them to open the mouth fully. It is extremely important to observe the entire mouth to look for

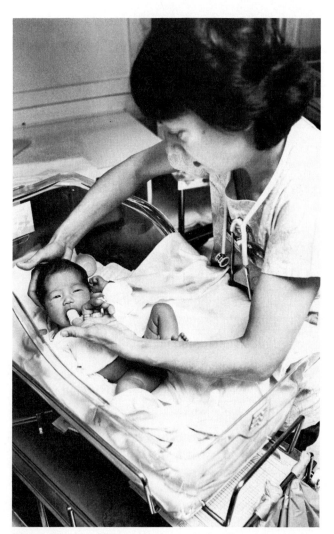

Figure 28–20 The nurse inserts index finger into the newborn's mouth and feels for any openings along the hard and soft palates.

A *tongue-tied* neonate has a ridge of frenulum tissue attached to the underside of the tongue at varying lengths from its base, causing a heart shape at the tip of the tongue. "Clipping the tongue," or cutting the ridge of tissue, is not recommended. This ridge does not affect speech or eating, but cutting does create an entry for infection.

Transient nerve paralysis resulting from birth trauma may be manifested by asymmetric mouth movements when the neonate cries or by difficulty with sucking and feeding.

Ears

The ears of the newborn should be soft and pliable and should recoil readily when folded and released. In the normal newborn, the top of the ear (pinna) should be parallel to the outer and inner canthus of the eye. The ears should be inspected for shape, size, position, and firmness of ear cartilage. *Low-set ears* are characteristic of many syndromes and may indicate chromosomal abnormalities (especially trisomies 13 and 18), mental retardation, and/or internal organ abnormalities, especially bilateral renal agenesis as a result of embryologic developmental deviations (Figure 28–21). A *preauricular skin tag* and dermal sinus may be present just in front of the ear. Preauricular tags are ligated at the base and allowed to slough off.

Visualization of the tympanic membranes is not usually done soon after birth since blood and vernix block the ear canal.

Following the first cry, the newborn's hearing becomes acute as mucus from the middle ear is absorbed and the eustachian tube is aerated. Risk factors (Duara et al 1986) associated with potential hearing loss include the following:

- The presence of hearing loss in any family member prior to the age of 50 years
- Serum bilirubin level greater than 20 mg/dL for the full-term newborn
- Suspected maternal rubella infection during pregnancy, resulting in congenital rubella syndrome
- Congenital defects of the ear, nose, or throat
- Small neonatal size, particularly less than 1500 g at birth
- Perinatal asphyxia

The newborn's hearing is evaluated by response to loud or moderately loud noises unaccompanied by vibrations. The sleeping neonate should stir or awaken in response to the nearby sounds. The newborn can discriminate the individual characteristics of the human voice and is especially sensitive to sound levels within the normal conversation range (Querleu 1989).

Neck

A short neck, creased with skin folds, is characteristic of the normal newborn. Because muscle tone is not well de-

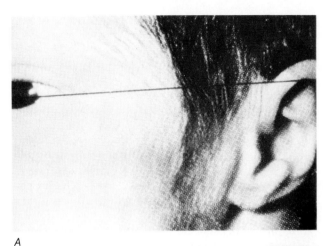

A

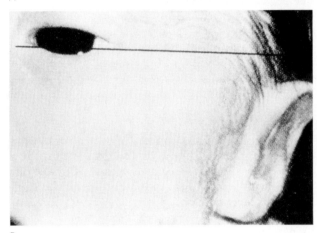

B

Figure 28–21 The position of the external ear may be assessed by drawing a line across the inner and outer canthus of the eye to the insertion of the ear. A Normal position. B True low-set. (Courtesy Mead Johnson Laboratories, Evansville, IN)

veloped, the neck cannot support the full weight of the head, which rotates freely. The head lags considerably when the neonate is pulled from a supine to a sitting position, but the prone newborn is able to raise the head slightly. The neck is palpated for masses and presence of lymph nodes and is inspected for webbing. Adequacy of range of motion and neck muscle function is determined by fully extending the head in all directions. Injury to the sternocleidomastoid muscle (congenital torticollis) must be considered in the presence of neck rigidity.

The clavicles are evaluated for evidence of fractures, which occasionally occur during difficult births or in neonates with broad shoulders. The normal clavicle is straight. If fractured, a lump and a grating sensation during movements may be palpated along the course of the side of the break. The Moro reflex (page 861) is also elicited to evaluate bilateral equal movement of the arms. If the clavicle is fractured, this response will be demonstrated only on the unaffected side.

Chest

The thorax is cylindric at birth, and the ribs are flexible. The general appearance of the chest should be assessed. A protrusion at the lower end of the sternum, called the *xiphoid cartilage,* is frequently seen. It is under the skin and will become less apparent after several weeks as the infant accumulates adipose tissue.

Engorged breasts occur frequently in both male and female newborns. This condition, which occurs by the third day, is a result of maternal hormonal influences and may last up to two weeks (Figure 28–22). The infant's breast should not be massaged or squeezed, because this practice may cause a breast abscess. Extra or *supernumerary nipples* are occasionally noted below and medial to the true nipples. These harmless pink spots vary in size and do not contain glandular tissue. Accessory nipples can be differentiated from a pigmented nevi (mole) by placing the fingertips alongside the accessory nipple and pulling the adjacent tissue laterally. The accessory nipple will appear dimpled. At puberty the accessory nipple may darken.

Cry

The newborn's cry should be strong, lusty, and of medium pitch. A high-pitched, shrill cry is abnormal and may indicate neurologic disorders or hypoglycemia. Cries usually vary in length after consoling measures are used. The baby's cry is an important method of communication and alerts care givers to changes in his or her condition and needs.

Respiration

Normal breathing for a term newborn is 30 to 60 respirations per minute and predominantly diaphragmatic, with

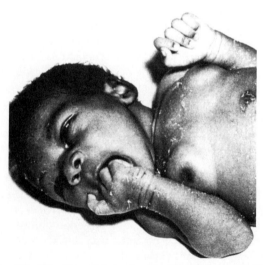

Figure 28–22   Breast hypertrophy (From Korones SB: High-Risk Newborn Infants, 4th ed. St. Louis: CV Mosby, 1986)

associated rising and falling of the abdomen during inspiration and expiration. Any signs of respiratory distress, nasal flaring, intercostal or xiphoid retractions, expiratory grunting or sigh, see-saw respirations, or tachypnea (sustained or greater than 60 respirations per minute) should be noted. Hyperextension (chest appears high) or hypoextension (chest appears low) of the anteroposterior diameter of the chest should also be noted. Both the anterior and posterior chest are auscultated. Some breath sounds are heard better when the neonate is crying, but localization and identification of breath sounds are difficult in the newborn. Upper airway noises and bowel sounds may also be heard over the chest wall and make auscultation difficult. Since sounds may be transmitted from the unaffected lung to the affected lung, the absence of breath sounds may not be diagnosed. Air entry may be noisy in the first couple of hours until lung fluid resolves, especially in cesarean births.

Heart

Heart rates can be as rapid as 180 beats per minute in newborns and fluctuate a great deal. Normal range is 120 to 160 beats per minute. Auscultation provides the nurse with valuable assessment data. The heart is examined for rate and rhythm, position of apical impulse, and heart sound intensity.

The pulse rate is variable and follows the trend of respirations in the neonatal period. The pulse rate is influenced by physical activity, crying, state of wakefulness, and body temperature. Auscultation is performed over the entire heart region (precordium) below the left axilla, and below the scapula. Apical pulse rates are obtained by auscultation for a full minute, preferably when the neonate is asleep.

The placement of the heart in the chest should be determined when the neonate is in a quiet state. The heart is relatively large at birth and is located high in the chest, with its apex somewhere between the fourth and fifth intercostal space.

A shift of heart tones in the mediastinal area to either side may indicate pneumothroax, dextrocardia (heart placement on the right side of the chest), or a diaphragmatic hernia. The experienced nurse can diagnose these and many other problems early with a stethoscope. Normally, the heart beat has a "toc tic" sound. A slur or slushing sound (usually after the first sound) may indicate a *murmur.* Although 90% of all murmurs are transient and are considered normal (Korones 1986), they should be observed closely by a physician.

In newborns, a low-pitched, musical murmur heard just to the right of the apex of the heart is fairly common. Occasionally, significant murmurs will be heard, including the murmur of a patent ductus arteriosus, aortic or pulmonary stenosis, or small ventricular septal defect. However, some significant murmurs may not appear immediately after birth. See Chapter 32 for a discussion of congenital heart defects.

Peripheral pulses (brachial, femoral, pedal) are also evaluated to detect any lags or unusual characteristics. Brachial pulses are palpated bilaterally for equality and compared with the femoral pulses. Femoral pulses are palpated by applying gentle pressure with the middle finger over the femoral canal (Figure 28–23). Decreased or absent femoral pulses indicate coarctation of the aorta and require additional investigation. A wide difference in blood pressure between the upper and lower extremities also indicates coarctation. The measurement of blood pressure is best accomplished by using the Doppler technique or a 1- to 2-inch cuff and a stethoscope over the brachial artery.

Blood pressure is becoming a routine measurement in newborns, especially if they are exhibiting distress, are premature, or are suspected of having a cardiac anomaly. Blood pressure is usually 80–60/45–40 mm Hg at birth, and by the tenth day of life it rises to 100/50 mm Hg. It may be difficult to obtain the diastolic pressure or to hear the blood pressure with a standard sphygmomanometer. If a cardiac anomaly is suspected, the blood pressure is assessed in all four extremities (Table 28–3).

Abdomen

The nurse can learn a great deal about the newborn's abdomen without disturbing the infant. It should be cylindrical and protrude slightly. A certain amount of laxness of the abdominal muscles is normal. A scaphoid appearance suggests the absence of abdominal contents. No cyanosis should be present, and few if any blood vessels should be apparent to the eye. There should be no gross distention or bulging. The more distended the abdomen, the tighter the skin becomes, with engorged vessels appearing. Distention is the first sign of many of the abnormalities found in the gastrointestinal tract.

Prior to palpation of the abdomen, the presence or

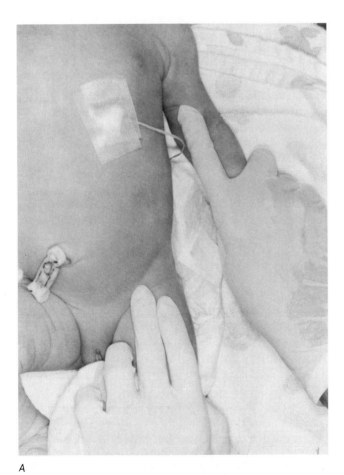

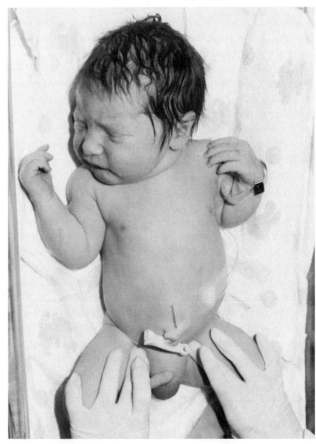

A

B

Figure 28–23   A Bilaterally palpate the femoral arteries for rate and intensity of the pulses. Press fingertip gently at the groin as shown. B Compare the femoral pulses to the brachial pulses by palpating the pulses simultaneously for comparison of rate and intensity.

Table 28–3 Newborn Vital Signs

Pulse

120–160 beats/min

During sleep as low as 100 beats/min; if crying, up to 180 beats/min

Apical pulse is counted for one (1) full minute

Respirations

30–60 respirations/min

Predominantly diaphragmatic but synchronous with abdominal movements

Respirations are counted for one (1) full minute

Blood Pressure

80–60/45–40 mm Hg at birth

100/50 mm Hg at day 10

Temperature

Normal Range: 36.5–37.5 C (97.7–99.4 F)

Axillary: 36.5–37 C (97.7–98.6 F)

Skin: 36–36.5 C (96.8–97.7 F)

Rectal: 36.6–37.2 C (97.8–99 F)

---

absence of bowel sounds should be auscultated for in all four quadrants. Palpation can cause a transient decrease in intensity of the bowel sounds.

Abdominal palpation should be done systematically. The nurse palpates each of the four abdominal quadrants and moves in a clockwise direction until all four quadrants have been palpated for softness, tenderness, and the presence of masses.

When palpating the abdomen, the nurse should feel for the liver. The newborn's liver is large in proportion to the rest of the body and can usually be felt between 1 and 2 cm below the right costal margin. Depending on institutional protocol, palpation of the kidney may be done by the staff nurse. Kidneys are more difficult to feel, but examination is easier if done within four to six hours after birth, before the intestines become distended with air and feedings are initiated. By placing a finger at the posterior flank and pushing upward while pressing downward with the opposite hand, each kidney may be palpated as a firm oval mass between the examiner's finger and hand. The lower pole of the kidney is usually found 1 to 2 cm above the umbilicus. The spleen tip may be palpated in the lateral aspect of the left upper quadrant in the normal newborn.

Umbilical Cord

Initially the umbilical cord is white and gelatinous in appearance, with the two umbilical arteries and one umbilical vein readily apparent. Because a single umbilical artery is frequently associated with congenital anomalies, the vessels should be counted as part of the newborn as-

sessment. The cord begins drying within one or two hours after birth and is shriveled and blackened by the second or third day. Within seven to ten days, it sloughs off, although a granulating area may remain for a few days longer.

Cord bleeding is abnormal and may result because the cord was inadvertently pulled or because the cord clamp was loosened. Foul-smelling drainage is also abnormal and is generally caused by infection. Such infection requires immediate treatment to prevent the development of septicemia. If the neonate has a patent urachus (abnormal connection between the umbilicus and bladder), moistness or draining urine may be apparent at the base of the cord.

Genitals

Female Infants

The labia majora, labia minora, and clitoris are examined, and the nurse notes the size of each as appropriate for gestational age. A vaginal tag or hymenal tag is often evident and will usually disappear in a few weeks. During the first week of life, the neonate may have a vaginal discharge composed of thick whitish mucus. This discharge, which can become tinged with blood, is referred to as **pseudomenstruation** and is caused by the withdrawal of maternal hormones. Smegma, a white cheeselike substance, is often present under the labia.

Male Infants

The penis is inspected to determine whether the urinary orifice is correctly positioned. *Hypospadias* occurs when the urinary meatus is located on the ventral surface of the penis. It occurs most commonly in white infants in the United States. *Phimosis* is a condition commonly occurring in newborn males in which the opening of the prepuce is narrowed and the foreskin cannot be retracted over the glans. This condition may interfere with urination, so the adequacy of the urinary stream should be evaluated.

The scrotum is inspected for size and symmetry and should be palpated to verify the presence of both testes. The testes are palpated separately between the thumb and forefinger, with the thumb and forefinger of the other hand placed together over the inguinal canal. Scrotal edema and discoloration are common in breech births. *Hydrocele* (collection of fluid surrounding the testes in the scrotum) is common in newborns and should be identified.

Anus

The anal area is inspected to verify that it is patent and has no fissure. Imperforate anus and rectal atresia may be ruled out by a digital examination. The passage of the first meconium stool is also noted. Atresia of the gastrointestinal tract or meconium ileus with resultant obstruction must be considered if the newborn does not pass meconium in the first 24 hours of life.

Extremities

Extremities are examined for gross deformities, extra digits or webbing, clubfoot, and range of motion. The normal neonate's extremities appear short, are generally flexible, and move symmetrically.

Arms and Hands

Nails extend beyond the fingertips in term infants. Fingers and toes should be counted. *Polydactyly* is the presence of extra digits on either the hands or feet. Polydactyly is more common in black infants. If the infant has polydactyly and the parents do not, a dominant genetic disorder can be ruled out. *Syndactyly* refers to fusion (webbing) of fingers or toes. Hands should be inspected for normal palmar creases. A single palmar crease, called *simian line* (see Figure 5–21) is frequently present in children with Down syndrome. (See Chapter 5 for further discussion.)

Brachial palsy, which is partial or complete paralysis of portions of the arm, results from trauma to the brachial plexus during a difficult birth. It occurs most commonly when strong traction is exerted on the head of the neonate in an attempt to free a shoulder lodged behind the symphysis pubis in the presence of shoulder dystocia. Brachial palsy may also occur during a breech birth if an arm becomes trapped over the head and traction is exerted.

The portion of the arm affected is determined by the nerves damaged. *Erb-Duchenne paralysis* involves damage to the upper arm (fifth and sixth cervical nerves) and is the most common type. Injury to the eighth cervical and first thoracic nerve roots and the lower portion of the plexus produces the relatively rare *lower arm injury*. The *whole arm type* results from damage to the entire plexus.

With Erb-Duchenne paralysis (Erb palsy) the newborn's arm lies limply at the side (Figure 28–24). The elbow is held in extension, with the forearm pronated. The newborn is unable to elevate the arm, and therefore the Moro reflex cannot be elicited on the affected side. When lower arm injury occurs, paralysis of the hand and wrist results; complete paralysis of the limb occurs with the whole arm type.

Treatment involves passive range-of-motion exercises to prevent muscle contractures and to restore function. The nurse should carefully instruct the parents in the correct method of performing the exercises and supervise practice sessions. In more severe cases, splinting of the arm is indicated until the edema decreases. The arm is held in a position of abduction and external rotation with the elbow flexed 90°. The "Statue of Liberty" splint is commonly used, although similar results are obtained by attaching a strip of muslin to the head of the crib and tying the other end around the wrist, thereby holding the arm up.

Prognosis is related to the degree of nerve damage resulting from trauma and hemorrhage within the nerve sheath. Complete recovery occurs within a few months

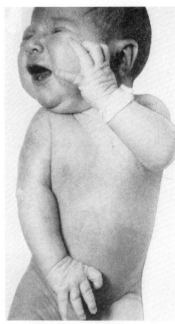

Figure 28–24   Erb palsy resulting from injury to the fifth and sixth cervical roots of brachial plexus (Photo reproduced with permission from Potter EL, Craig JM: Pathology of the Fetus and Infant, 3rd ed. Copyright 1975 by Year Book Medical Publishers, Chicago)

with minimal trauma. Moderate trauma may result in some partial paralysis. Recovery is unlikely with severe trauma, and muscle wasting may develop.

Legs and Feet

The legs of the newborn should be of equal length, with symmetric skin folds. However, they may assume a "fetal posture" secondary to position in utero, and it may take several days for the legs to relax into normal position. *Ortolani's maneuver* is performed to rule out the possibility of congenital hip dysplasia. With the baby supine, the nurse places thumbs on the inner thighs and fingers on the outer aspect of the neonate's leg from the knee to the head of the femur. The legs are flexed, abducted, and pressed downward. If a "clunk" is felt under the index finger and there is resistance to abduction, a dislocation exists (Figure 28–25).

The feet are then examined for evidence of a talipes deformity (clubfoot). Intrauterine position frequently causes the feet to appear to turn inward (Figure 28–26); this is termed a "positional" clubfoot. If the feet can easily be returned to midline by manipulation, no treatment is indicated. Further investigation is indicated when the foot will not turn to a midline position or align readily. This is considered a "true" clubfoot.

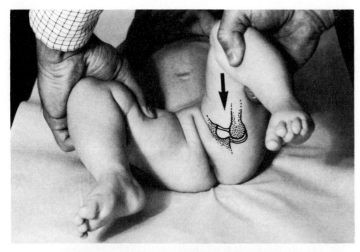

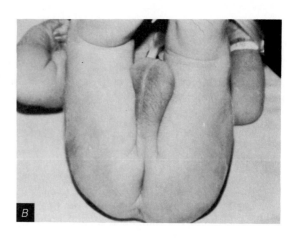

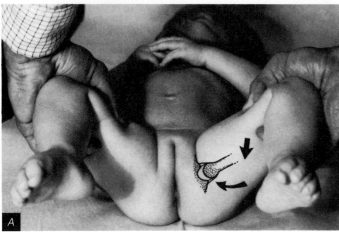

Figure 28–25 Congenital dislocation of the right hip. A Ortolani's maneuver puts downward pressure on the hip and then inward rotation. If the hip is dislocated, this will force the femoral head over the acetabular rim with a noticeable "clunk." B Dislocated right hip in a young infant as seen on gross inspection. (From Smith DW: Recognizable Patterns of Human Deformation. *Philadelphia: WB Saunders, 1981)*

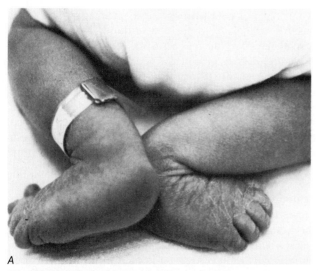

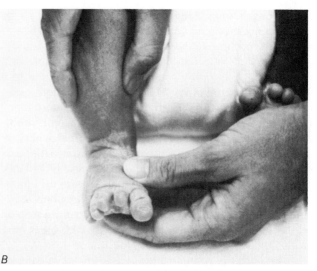

Figure 28–26 Infant with bilateral talipes equinovarus. B To determine the presence of clubfoot, the nurse moves the foot to the midline. Resistance indicates true clubfoot.

Back

With the baby prone, the nurse examines the back. The spine should appear straight and flat, since the lumbar and sacral curves do not develop until the infant begins to sit. The base of the spine is then examined for a dermal sinus. The nevus pilosus ("hairy nevus") is only occasionally found at the base of the spine in newborns, but it is significant because it is frequently associated with spina bifida.

Assessment of Neurologic Status

The neurologic examination assesses the intactness of the neonatal nervous system. It should begin with a period of observation, noting the general physical characteristics and behavior of the newborn. Important behaviors to assess are the state of alertness, resting posture, cry, and quality of muscle tone and motor activity.

The usual position of the newborn is with partially flexed extremities with the legs abducted to the abdomen. When awake, the newborn may exhibit purposeless, uncoordinated bilateral movements of the extremities. If these movements are absent, minimal, or obviously asymmetric, neurologic dysfunction should be suspected. Eye movements are observable during the first few days of life. An alert neonate is able to fixate on faces and brightly colored objects. If a bright light shines in the newborn's eyes, the blinking response is elicited. The cry of the newborn should be lusty and vigorous. High-pitched cries, weak cries, or no cries are all causes for concern.

Muscle tone is evaluated with the head of the neonate in a neutral position as various parts of the body are passively moved. The newborn is somewhat hypertonic; that is, there is resistance to extending the elbow and knee joints. Muscle tone should be symmetric. Diminished muscle tone and flaccidity require further evaluation.

Neonatal tremors are common in the full-term newborn and must be evaluated to differentiate them from a convulsion. A fine jumping of the muscle is likely to be a central nervous system disorder and requires further evaluation. Tremors may also be related to hypoglycemia or hypocalcemia. Neonatal seizures may consist of no more than chewing or swallowing movements, deviations of the eyes, rigidity, or flaccidity, because of central nervous system immaturity.

Specific deep tendon reflexes can be elicited in the neonate but have limited value unless they are obviously asymmetric. The knee jerk is brisk; a normal ankle clonus may involve three or four beats. Plantar flexion is present.

The central nervous system of the newborn is immature and characterized by a variety of reflexes. Because the newborn's movements are uncoordinated, methods of communication are limited, and control of bodily functions is drastically limited, the reflexes serve a variety of purposes. Some are protective (blink, gag, sneeze), some aid in feeding (rooting, sucking), and some stimulate human interaction (grasping). Neonatal reflexes and general neurologic activity should be carefully assessed.

The most common reflexes found in the normal neonate are the following:

- The **tonic neck reflex** *(fencer position)* is elicited when the neonate is supine and the head is turned to one side. In response, the extremities on the same side straighten, whereas on the opposite side they flex (Figure 28–27). This reflex may not be seen during the early neonatal period, but once it appears it persists until about the third month.

- The **grasping reflex** is elicited by stimulating the palm with a finger or object. The neonate will grasp and hold the object or finger firmly enough to be lifted momentarily from the crib (Figure 28–28).

- The **Moro reflex** is elicited when the neonate is startled by a loud noise or is lifted slightly above the crib and then suddenly lowered. In response, the newborn straightens arms and hands outward while the knees flex. Slowly the arms return to the chest, as in an embrace. The fingers spread, forming a C, and the infant may cry (Figure 28–29). This reflex may persist until about 6 months of age.

- The **rooting reflex** is elicited when the side of the neonate's mouth or cheek is touched. In response, the newborn turns toward that side and opens the lips to suck (Figure 28–30).

- When an object is placed in the neonate's mouth or anything touches his/her lips a **sucking reflex** is elicited.

- The **Babinski reflex**, or hyperextension of all toes, occurs when the lateral aspect of the sole is stroked from the heel upward and across the ball of the foot.

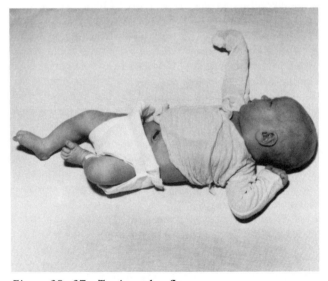

Figure 28–27 Tonic neck reflex

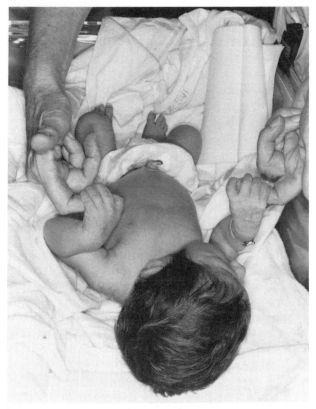

Figure 28–28   Grasping reflex

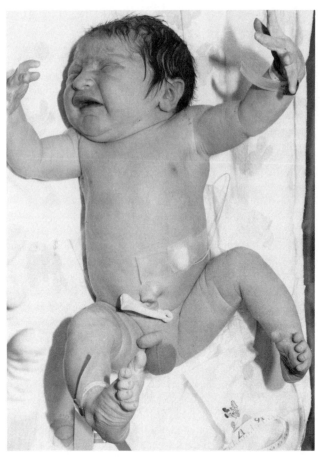

Figure 28–29   Moro reflex

- When the newborn is prone, stroking the spine causes the pelvis to turn to the stimulated side. This is called **trunk incurvation**.

In addition to these reflexes, the newborn can *blink, yawn, cough, sneeze,* and draw back from pain (protective reflexes). Neonates can even move a little on their own. When placed on their stomachs, they push up and try to crawl (*prone crawl*). When he or she is held upright with one foot touching a flat surface, the neonate puts one foot in front of the other and walks (*stepping reflex*) (Figure 28–31). This reflex is most pronounced at birth and is lost at about 4 to 5 months of age. Table 28–4 summarizes the stimulus for and response of the common newborn reflexes.

Brazelton (1984) recommends the following steps as a means of assessing central nervous system integration:

1. Insert a clean finger into the newborn's mouth to elicit a sucking reflex.

2. As soon as the neonate is sucking vigorously, assess hearing and vision responses by noting sucking changes in the presence of a light, rattle, and a voice.

3. The neonate should respond with a brief cessation of sucking followed by continuous sucking with repeated stimulation.

This examination demonstrates auditory and visual integrity as well as the ability for complex behavioral interactions.

Neonatal Physical Assessment

Following is a guide for systematically assessing the newborn. Normal findings, alterations, and related causes are presented, in correlation with suggested nursing responses. The findings are typical for a full-term neonate.

(Text continues on p 879)

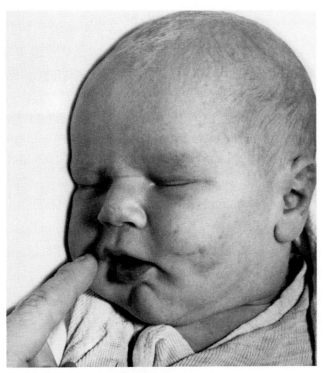

Figure 28–30   Rooting reflex

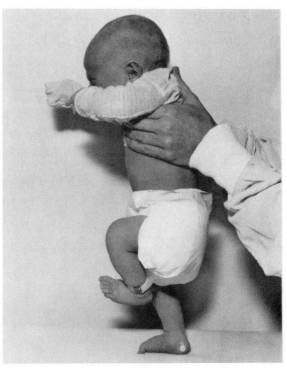

Figure 28–31   The stepping reflex disappears after about one month.

Table 28–4   Common Reflexes of the Neonate

Reflex name	Evoking stimulus	Response
Blinking reflex	Light flash	Eyelids close.
Pupillary reflex	Light flash	Pupil constricts.
Rooting reflex	Light touch of finger on cheek close to mouth	Head rotates toward stimulation: mouth opens and attempts to suck finger. Disappears by about 4 months of age.
Sucking reflex	Finger (or nipple) inserted into mouth	Rhythmic sucking.
Moro reflex	Infant lying on back: slightly raised head suddenly released; infant held horizontally, lowered quickly about 6 in., and stopped abruptly	Arms are extended, head is thrown back, fingers are spread wide; arms are then brought back to center convulsively with hands clenched; spine and lower extremities are extended. Disappears by about 6 months of age.
Startle reflex	Loud noise	Similar to Moro reflex flexion in arms; fists are clenched.
Grasping reflex	Finger placed in palm of hand	Infant's fingers close around and grasp object.
Tonic neck reflex	Head turned to one side while infant lies on back	Arm and leg are extended on the side the infant faces. Opposite arm and leg are flexed.
Abdominal reflex	Tactile stimulation or tickling	Abdominal muscles contract.
Withdrawal reflex	Slight pinprick to the sole of the infant's foot	Leg flexes.
Walking reflex	Infant supported in an upright position with feet lightly touching a flat surface	Rhythmic stepping movement. Disappears at about 4 months of age.
Babinski reflex	Gentle stroking on the sole of each foot	Fanning and extension of the toes (adults respond to this stimulation with flexion of toes.)
Plantar, or toe-grasping, reflex	Pressure applied with the finger against the balls of the infant's feet	A plantar flexion of all toes. Disappears by the end of the first year of life.

Adapted from Mott SR, James SR, Sperhac AM: Nursing Care of Children and Families: A Holistic Approach, 2nd ed. Menlo Park, CA: Addison-Wesley, 1990.

Neonatal Physical Assessment Guide

Assessment and Normal Findings	Alterations and Possible Causes*	Nursing Responses to Data Base†
Vital Signs		
Blood pressure (BP): At birth: 80–60/45–40 mm Hg Day 10: 100/50 mm Hg (may be unable to measure diastolic pressure with standard sphygmomanometer)	Low BP (hypovolemia, shock)	Monitor BP in all cases of distress, prematurity, or suspected anomaly. Low BP; refer to physician immediately so measures to improve circulation are begun.
Pulse: 120–160 beats/min (if asleep 100/min; if crying, up to 180/min)	Weak pulse (decreased cardiac output) Bradycardia (severe asphyxia) Tachycardia (over 160 beats/min at rest) (infection, central nervous system [CNS] problems)	Assess skin perfusion by blanching (capillary refill test). Correlate finding with BP assessments; refer to physician. Carry out neurologic and thermoregulation assessments.
Respirations: 30–60 breaths/min Synchronization of chest and abdominal movements Diaphragmatic and abdominal breathing Transient tachypnea	Tachypnea (pneumonia, respiratory distress syndrome [RDS]) Rapid, shallow breathing (hypermagnesemia due to large doses given to mothers with PIH) Respirations below 30 breaths/min (maternal anesthesia or analgesia) Expiratory grunting, subcostal and substernal retractions; flaring of nares (respiratory distress); apnea (cold stress, respiratory disorder)	Identify sleep-wake state; correlate with respiratory pattern. Evaluate for all signs of respiratory distress; report findings to physician.
Crying: Strong and lusty Moderate tone and pitch Cries vary in length from three to seven minutes after consoling measures are used	High-pitched, shrill (neurologic disorder, hypoglycemia) Weak or absent (CNS disorder, laryngeal problem)	Discuss neonate's use of cry for communication. Assess and record abnormal cries.
Temperature: Axilla 36.5–37 C (97.7–98.6 F) Rectal 36.6–37.2 C (97.8–99 F); 36.8 C (98.8 F) desired Heavier neonates tend to have higher body temperatures	Elevated temperature (room too warm, too much clothing or covers, dehydration, sepsis, brain damage) Subnormal temperature (brain stem involvement, cold) Swings of more than 2 F from one reading to next or subnormal temperature (infection)	Notify physician of elevation or drop. Counsel parents on possible causes of elevated or low temperatures, appropriate home-care measures, when to call physician. Teach parents how to take rectal and/or axillary temperature; assess parents' information regarding use of thermometer; provide teaching as needed.

* Possible causes of alterations are placed in parentheses.
† This column provides guidelines for further assessment and initial nursing interventions.

(continued)

Neonatal Physical Assessment Guide (continued)

Assessment and Normal Findings	Alterations and Possible Causes*	Nursing Responses to Data Base†
Weight: 2500–4000 g (5–8.75 lb)	< 2748 g (< 6 lb) = SGA or preterm infant > 4050 g (> 9 lb) = LGA or infants of diabetic mothers (IDMs)	Plot weight and gestational age to identify high-risk infants. Ascertain body build of parents. Counsel parents regarding appropriate nutritional/fluid intake.
Within first three to four days, normal weight loss of 5%–10% Large babies tend to lose more due to greater fluid loss in proportion to birth weight except IDMs	Loss greater than 15% (small fluid intake, loss of meconium and urine, feeding difficulties)	Notify physician of net losses or gains. Calculate fluid intake and losses from all sources (insensible water loss, radiant warmers, and phototherapy lights).
Length: 45 cm (18 in.) to 55 cm (22 in.) Grows 10 cm (3 in.) during first three months	Less than 45 cm (congenital dwarf) Short/long bones proximally (achondroplasia) Short/long bones distally (Ellis-Van Creveld syndrome)	Assess for other signs of dwarfism. Determine other signs of skeletal system adequacy. Plot progress at subsequent well-baby visits.
Posture Body usually flexed, hands may be tightly clenched, neck appears short as chin rests on chest In breech births, feet are usually dorsiflexed	Only extension noted, inability to move from midline (trauma, hypoxia, immaturity) Constant motion	Record spontaneity of motor activity and symmetry of movements. If parents express concern about neonate's movement patterns, reassure and evaluate further if appropriate.
Skin *Color:* Color consistent with racial background	Pallor of face, conjunctiva (anemia, hypothermia, anoxia)	Discuss with parents common skin color variations to allay fears.
Pink-tinged or ruddy color over face, trunk, extremities	Beefy red (hypoglycemia, immature vasomotor reflexes, polycythemia)	Document extent and time of occurrence of color change.
Common variations: acrocyanosis, circumoral cyanosis, or harlequin color change	Meconium staining (fetal distress) Icterus (hemolytic reaction from blood incompatibility, sepsis)	Obtain hemoglobin and hematocrit values. Assess for respiratory difficulty. Differentiate between physiologic and pathologic jaundice.
Mottled when undressed	Cyanosis (choanal atresia, CNS damage or trauma, respiratory or cardiac problem, cold stress)	Assess degree of (central or peripheral) cyanosis and possible causes; refer to physician.
Minor bruising over buttocks in breech presentation and over eyes and forehead in facial presentations		Discuss with parents cause and course of minor bruising related to labor and birth.

*Possible causes of alterations are placed in parentheses.
†This column provides guidelines for further assessment and initial nursing interventions.

(continued)

Neonatal Physical Assessment Guide (continued)

Assessment and Normal Findings	Alterations and Possible Causes*	Nursing Responses to Data Base†
Texture:		
Smooth, soft, flexible; may have dry, peeling hands and feet	Generalized cracked or peeling skin (SGA or postterm; blood incompatibility; metabolic, kidney dysfunction)	Report to physician.
	Seborrhea-dermatitis (cradle cap) Absence of vernix (postmature) Yellow vernix (bilirubin staining)	Instruct parents to shampoo the scalp and anterior fontanelle area daily with soap; rinse well; avoid use of oil.
Turgor:		
Elastic, returns to normal shape after pinching	Maintains tent shape (dehydration)	Assess for other signs and symptoms of dehydration.
Pigmentation:		
Clear; milia across bridge of nose or forehead will disappear within a few weeks		Advise parents not to pinch or prick these pimplelike areas.
Café-au-lait spots (one or two)	Six or more (neurologic disorder such as Von Recklinghausen disease, cutaneous neurofibromatosis)	
Mongolian spots common in dark-skinned infants over dorsal area and buttocks		Assure parents of normalcy of this pigmentation; it will fade in first year or two.
Erythema toxicum	Impetigo (group A β-hemolytic streptococcus or *Staphylococcus aureus* infection)	If impetigo occurs, instruct parents about hand-washing and linen precautions during home care.
Telangiectatic nevi	Hemangiomas: Nevus flammeus (port-wine stain) Nevus vascularis (strawberry hemangioma) Cavernous hemangiomas	Collaborate with physician. Counsel parents about birthmark's progression to allay misconceptions. Record size and shape of hemangiomas. Refer for follow-up at well-baby clinic.
Rashes	Rashes (infection)	Assess location and type of rash (macular, papular, vesicular). Obtain history of onset, prenatal history, and related signs and symptoms.
Petechiae of head or neck (breech presentation, cord around neck)	Generalized petechiae (clotting abnormalities)	Determine cause; advise parents if further health care is needed.

Head

Assessment and Normal Findings	Alterations and Possible Causes*	Nursing Responses to Data Base†
General appearance, size, movement		
Round, symmetrical, and moves easily from left to right and up and down; soft and pliable	Asymmetrical, flattened occiput on either side of the head (plagiocephaly) Head held at angle (torticollis) Unable to move head side-to-side (neurologic trauma)	Instruct parents to change infant's sleeping positions frequently. Determine adequacy of all neurologic signs.

*Possible causes of alterations are placed in parentheses.
†This column provides guidelines for further assessment and initial nursing interventions.

(continued)

Neonatal Physical Assessment Guide (continued)

Assessment and Normal Findings	Alterations and Possible Causes*	Nursing Responses to Data Base†
Circumference: 32–37 cm (12.5–14.5 in.); 2 cm greater than chest circumference Head one fourth of body size	Extreme differences in size may be: micro-encephaly (Cornelia de Lange syndrome, cytomegalic inclusion disease (CID), rubella, toxoplasmosis, chromosome abnormalities), hydrocephalus (meningomyelocele, achondroplasia), anencephaly (neural tube defect) Head is 3 cm or more larger than chest circumference (preterm, hydrocephalus)	Measure circumference from occiput to frontal area using metal or paper tape. Measure chest circumference using metal or paper tape and compare to head circumference. Record measurements on growth chart. Reevaluate at well-baby visits.
Common variations: Molding Breech and cesarean newborns' heads are round and well shaped	Cephalhematoma (trauma during birth, persists up to three weeks) Caput succedaneum (long labor and birth; disappears in one week)	Reassure parents regarding common manifestations due to birth process and when they should disappear.
Fontanelles: Palpation of juncture of cranial bones Anterior fontanelle; 3–4 cm long by 2–3 cm wide, diamond-shaped	Overlapping of anterior fontanelle (malnourished or preterm infant)	Discuss normal closure times with parents and care of "soft spots" to allay misconceptions.
Posterior fontanelle; 1–2 cm at birth, triangle-shaped	Premature closure of sutures (craniostenosis) Late closure (hydrocephalus)	Refer to physician. Observe for signs and symptoms of hydrocephalus.
Slight pulsation	Moderate to severe pulsation (vascular problems)	Refer to physician.
Moderate bulging noted with crying, stooling, or pulsations with heartbeat	Bulging (increased intracranial pressure, meningitis) Sunken (dehydration)	Evaluate hydration status.
Hair *Texture:* Smooth with fine texture variations (Note: variations dependent on ethnic background)	Coarse, brittle, dry hair (hypothyroidism) White forelock (Waardenburg syndrome)	Instruct parents regarding routine care of hair and scalp.
Distribution: Scalp hair high over eyebrows (Spanish-Mexican hairline begins mid-forehead and extends down back of neck)	Low forehead and posterior hairlines may indicate chromosomal disorders.	Assess for other signs of chromosomal aberrations. Refer to physician.
Face Symmetric movement of all facial features, normal hairline, eyebrows and eyelashes present		Assess and record symmetry of all parts, shape, regularity of features, sameness or differences in features.

*Possible causes of alterations are placed in parentheses.
†This column provides guidelines for further assessment and initial nursing interventions.

(continued)

Neonatal Physical Assessment Guide (continued)

Assessment and Normal Findings	Alterations and Possible Causes*	Nursing Responses to Data Base†
Spacing of features:		
Eyes at same level; nostrils equal size, cheeks full, and sucking pads present	Eyes wide apart—ocular hypertelorism (Apert syndrome, cri-du-chat, Turner syndrome)	Observe for other signs and symptoms indicative of disease states or chromosomal aberrations.
Lips equal on both sides of midline	Abnormal face (Down syndrome, cretinism, gargoylism)	
Chin recedes when compared to other bones of face	Abnormally small jaw—micrognathia (Pierre Robin syndrome, Treacher Collins syndrome)	Maintain airway. Initiate surgical consultation and referral.
Movement:		
Makes facial grimaces	Inability to suck, grimace, and close eyelids (cranial nerve injury)	Initiate neurologic assessment and consultation.
Symmetric when resting and crying	Asymmetry (paralysis of facial cranial nerve)	Assess and record symmetry of all parts, shape, regularity of features, sameness or differences in features.

Eyes

General placement and appearance:		
Bright and clear; even placement; slight nystagmus	Gross nystagmus (damage to third, fourth, and sixth cranial nerves)	
Concomitant strabismus	Constant and fixed strabismus	Reassure parents that strabismus is considered normal up to six months.
Move in all directions		
Blue- or slate-blue gray	Lack of pigmentation (albinism) Brushfield spots (may indicate Down syndrome)	Discuss with parents any necessary eye precautions. Assess for other signs of Down syndrome.
Brown color at birth in dark-skinned infants		Discuss with parents that permanent eye color is usually established by three months of age.
Eyelids:		
Position: above pupils but within iris, no drooping	Elevation or retraction of upper lid (hyperthyroidism)	Assess for signs of hydrocephalus and hyperthyroidism.
	"Setting sun" (hydrocephalus), ptosis (congenital or paralysis of oculomotor muscle)	Evaluate interference with vision in subsequent well-baby visits.
Eyes on parallel plane Epicanthal folds in Asian and 20% of Caucasian newborns	Upward slant in non-Asians (Down syndrome) Epicanthal folds (Down syndrome, cri-du-chat syndrome)	Assess for other signs of Down syndrome.
Movement:		
Blink reflex in response to light stimulus		

*Possible causes of alterations are placed in parentheses.
†This column provides guidelines for further assessment and initial nursing interventions.

(continued)

Neonatal Physical Assessment Guide (continued)

Assessment and Normal Findings	Alterations and Possible Causes *	Nursing Responses to Data Base †
Inspection: Edematous for first few days of life, resulting from birth and instillation of silver nitrate (chemical conjunctivitis); no lumps or redness	Purulent drainage (infection); infectious conjunctivitis (staphylococcus or gram-negative organisms) Marginal blepharitis (lid edges red, crusted, scaly) Any discharge	Initiate good hand washing. Refer to physician. Evaluate infant for seborrheic dermatitis; scales can be removed easily.
Cornea: Clear Corneal reflex present	Ulceration (herpes infection); large cornea or corneas of unequal size (congenital glaucoma) Clouding, opacity of lens (cataract)	Refer to ophthalmologist. Assess for other manifestations of congenital herpes; institute nursing care measures.
Sclera: May appear bluish in newborn, then white; slightly brownish color frequent in blacks	True blue sclera (osteogenesis imperfecta)	Refer to physician.
Pupils: Pupils equal in size, round, and react to light by accommodation	Anisocoria—unequal pupils (CNS damage) Dilation or constriction (intracranial damage, retinoblastoma, glaucoma) Pupils nonreactive to light or accommodation (brain injury)	Refer for neurologic examination.
Slight nystagmus in infant who has not learned to focus Pupil light reflex demonstrated at birth or by three weeks of age	Nystagmus (labyrinthine disturbance, CNS disorder)	
Conjunctiva: Chemical conjunctivitis Subconjunctival hemorrhage	Pale color (anemia)	Obtain hematocrit and hemoglobin. Reassure parents that chemical conjunctivitis will subside in one to two days and subconjunctival hemorrhage disappears in a few weeks.
Palpebral conjunctive (red but not hyperemic)	Inflammation or edema (infection, blocked tear duct)	
Vision: 20/150 Tracks moving object to midline Fixed focus on objects at a distance of about 7 in.; may be difficult to evaluate in newborn Prefers faces, geometric designs, and black and white to colors	Cataracts (congenital infection)	Record any questions about visual acuity and initiate follow-up evaluation at first well-baby checkup.
Lashes and lacrimal glands: Presence of lashes (lashes may be absent in preterm infants)	No lashes on inner two thirds of lid (Treacher Collins syndrome); bushy lashes (Hurler syndrome); long lashes (Cornelia de Lange syndrome)	

*Possible causes of alterations are placed in parentheses.
†This column provides guidelines for further assessment and initial nursing interventions.

(continued)

Neonatal Physical Assessment Guide (continued)

Assessment and Normal Findings	Alterations and Possible Causes*	Nursing Responses to Data Base†
Cry commonly tearless	Excessive tearing (plugged lacrimal duct, natal narcotic withdrawal)	Demonstrate to parents how to milk blocked tear duct. Refer to ophthalmologist if tearing is excessive before third month of life.

Nose

Appearance of external nasal aspects:

Assessment and Normal Findings	Alterations and Possible Causes*	Nursing Responses to Data Base†
May appear flattened as a result of birth process	Continued flat or broad bridge of nose (Down syndrome)	Arrange consultation with specialist.
Small and narrow in midline; even placement in relationship to eyes and mouth	Low bridge of nose; beaklike nose (Apert syndrome, Treacher Collins syndrome) Upturned (Cornelia de Lange syndrome)	Initiate evaluation of chromosomal abnormalities.
Patent nares bilaterally (nose breathers)	Blockage of nares (mucus and/or secretions)	Inspect for obstruction of nares.
Sneezing common to clear nasal passages	Flaring nares (respiratory distress) Choanal atresia	
Identifies odors, appears to smell breast milk	No response to stimulating odors	Inspect for obstruction of nares.

Mouth

Function of facial, hypoglossal, glossopharyngeal, and vagus nerves:

Assessment and Normal Findings	Alterations and Possible Causes*	Nursing Responses to Data Base†
Symmetry of movement and strength	Mouth draws to one side (transient seventh cranial nerve paralysis due to pressure in utero or trauma during birth, congenital paralysis)	Initiate neurologic consultation. Administer eye care if eye on affected side is unable to close.
	Fishlike shape (Treacher Collins syndrome)	
Presence of gag, swallowing, coordinated with sucking reflexes Adequate salivation	Suppressed or absent reflexes	Evaluate other neurologic functions of these nerves.

Palate (soft and hard):

Assessment and Normal Findings	Alterations and Possible Causes*	Nursing Responses to Data Base†
Hard palate dome-shaped Uvula midline with symmetrical movement of soft palate	High-steepled palate (Treacher Collins syndrome)	
Palate intact, sucks well when stimulated Epithelial (Epstein's) pearls appear on mucosa	Clefts in either hard or soft palate (polygenic disorder)	Initiate a surgical consultation referral. Assure parents that these are normal in newborn and will disappear at two or three months of age.
Esophagus patent; some drooling common in newborn	Excessive drooling or bubbling (esophageal atresia)	Test for patency of esophagus.

*Possible causes of alterations are placed in parentheses.
†This column provides guidelines for further assessment and initial nursing interventions.

(continued)

Neonatal Physical Assessment Guide (continued)

Assessment and Normal Findings	Alterations and Possible Causes*	Nursing Responses to Data Base†
Tongue:		
Free-moving in all directions, midline	Lack of movement or asymmetrical movement (neurologic damage) Tongue-tied	Further assess neurologic functions. Test reflex elevation of tongue when depressed with tongue blade.
	Deviations from midline (cranial nerve damage)	Check for signs of weakness or deviation.
Pink color, smooth to rough texture, noncoated	White cheesy coating (thrush) Tongue has deep ridges	Differentiate between thrush and milk curds. Reassure parents that tongue pattern may change from day to day.
Tongue proportional to mouth	Large tongue with short frenulum (cretinism, Down syndrome, other syndromes)	Evaluate in well-baby clinic to assess development delays. Initiate referrals.
Ears		
External ear:		
Without lesions, cysts, or nodules	Nodules, cysts, or sinus tracts in front of ear Adherent earlobes Low-set	Evaluate characteristics of lesions. Counsel parents to clean external ear with washcloth only; discourage use of cotton-tip applicators.
	Preauricular skin tags	Refer to physician for ligation.
Hearing:		
With first cry, eustachian tubes are cleared		
Absence of all risk factors	Presence of one or more risk factors	Assess history of risk factors for hearing loss.
Attends to sounds; sudden or loud noise elicits Moro reflex	No response to sound stimuli (deafness)	Test for Moro reflex.
Neck		
Appearance:		
Short, straight, creased with skin folds	Abnormally short neck (Turner syndrome) Arching or inability to flex neck (meningitis, congenital anomaly)	Report findings to physician.
Posterior neck lacks loose extra folds of skin	Webbing of neck (Turner syndrome, Down syndrome, trisomy 18)	Assess for other signs of the syndromes.
Clavicles:		
Straight and intact	Knot or lump on clavicle (fracture during difficult birth)	Obtain detailed labor and birth history; apply figure-8 bandage.
Moro reflex elicitable	Unilateral Moro reflex response on unaffected side (fracture of clavicle, brachial palsy, Erb-Duchenne paralysis)	Collaborate with physician.
Symmetrical shoulders	Hypoplasia	

*Possible causes of alterations are placed in parentheses.
†This column provides guidelines for further assessment and initial nursing interventions.

(continued)

Neonatal Physical Assessment Guide (continued)

Assessment and Normal Findings	Alterations and Possible Causes*	Nursing Responses to Data Base†
Chest		
Appearance and size:		
Circumference: 32.5 cm, 1–2 cm less than head		Measure at level of nipples after exhalation
Wider than it is long		
Normal shape without depressed or prominent sternum	Funnel chest (congenital or associated with Marfan syndrome)	Determine adequacy of other respiratory and circulatory signs.
Lower end of sternum (xiphoid cartilage) may be protruding; is less apparent after several weeks	Continued protrusion of xiphoid cartilage (Marfan syndrome, "pigeon chest")	Assess for other signs and symptoms of various syndromes.
Sternum 8 cm long.	Barrel chest	
Expansion and retraction:		
Bilateral expansion	Unequal chest expansion (pneumonia, pneumothorax respiratory distress)	Assess respiratory effort regularity, flaring of nares, difficulty on both inspiration and expiration.
No intercostal, subcostal, or supracostal retractions	Retractions (respiratory distress)	Record and consult physician.
Auscultation:		
Breath sounds are louder in infants	Decreased breath sounds (decreased respiratory activity, atelectasis, pneumothorax)	Perform assessment and report to physician any positive findings.
Chest and axilla clear on crying	Increased breath sounds (resolving pneumonia or in cesarean births)	
Bronchial breath sounds (heard where trachea and bronchi closest to chest wall, above sternum and between scapulae):		
Bronchial sounds bilaterally	Adventitious or abnormal sounds (respiratory disease or distress)	
Air entry clear		
Rales may indicate normal newborn atelectasis		
Cough reflex absent at birth, appears in two or more days		
Breasts:		
Flat with symmetrical nipples	Lack of breast tissue (preterm or SGA)	
Breast tissue diameter 5 cm or more at term	Discharge	
	Enlargement	
Distance between nipples 8 cm		
Breast engorgement occurs on third day of life; liquid discharge may be expressed in term infants	Breast abscesses	Reassure parents of normality of breast engorgement.
Nipples	Supernumerary nipples	
	Dark-colored nipples	

*Possible causes of alterations are placed in parentheses.
†This column provides guidelines for further assessment and initial nursing interventions.

(continued)

Neonatal Physical Assessment Guide (continued)

Assessment and Normal Findings	Alterations and Possible Causes*	Nursing Responses to Data Base†
Heart		
Auscultation:		
Location: lies horizontally, with left border extending to left of midclavicle		
Regular rhythm and rate	Arrhythmia (anoxia), tachycardia, bradycardia	Refer all arrhythmia and gallop rhythms.
Determination of point of maximal impulse (PMI)	Malpositioning (enlargement, abnormal placement, pneumothorax, dextrocardia, diaphragmatic hernia)	Initiate cardiac evaluation.
Usually lateral to midclavicular line at third or fourth intercostal space		
Functional murmurs	Location of murmurs (possible congenital cardiac anomaly)	Evaluate murmur: location, timing, and duration; observe for accompanying cardiac pathology symptoms; ascertain family history.
No thrills		
Horizontal groove at diaphragm shows flaring of rib cage to mild degree	Marked rib flaring (vitamin D deficiency) Inadequacy of respiratory movement	Initiate cardiopulmonary evaluation; assess pulses and blood pressures in all four extremities for equality and quality.
Abdomen		
Appearance:		
Cylindrical with some protrusion; appears large in relation to pelvis; some laxness of abdominal muscles	Distention, shiny abdomen with engorged vessels (gastrointestinal abnormalities, infection, congenital megacolon)	Examine abdomen thoroughly for mass or organomegaly. Measure abdominal girth. Report deviations of abdominal size. Assess other signs and symptoms of obstruction.
No cyanosis, few vessels seen Diastasis recti—common in black infants	Scaphoid abdominal appearance (diaphragmatic hernia) Increased or decreased peristalsis (duodenal stenosis, small bowel obstruction) Localized flank bulging (enlarged kidneys, ascites, or absent abdominal muscles)	Refer to physician.
Umbilicus:		
No protrusion of umbilicus (protrusion of umbilicus common in black infants)	Umbilical hernia Patent urachus (congenital malformation) Omphalocele Gastroschisis	Measure umbilical hernia by palpating the opening and record; it should close by one year of age; if not, refer to physician.
Bluish white color Cutis navel (umbilical cord projects); granulation tissue in navel	Redness or exudate around cord (infection) Yellow discoloration (hemolytic disease, meconium staining)	Instruct parents on cord care and hygiene.
Two arteries and one vein apparent	Single umbilical artery (congenital anomalies)	
Begins drying one to two hours after birth No bleeding Auscultation and percussion		

*Possible causes of alterations are placed in parentheses.
†This column provides guidelines for further assessment and initial nursing interventions.

(continued)

Neonatal Physical Assessment Guide (continued)

Assessment and Normal Findings	Alterations and Possible Causes*	Nursing Responses to Data Base†
Soft bowel sounds heard shortly after birth; heard every 10–30 sec	Bowel sounds in chest (diaphragmatic hernia) Absence of bowel sounds	Collaborate with physician.
	Hyperperistalsis (intestinal obstruction)	Assess for other signs of dehydration and/or infection.
Femoral pulses: Palpable, equal, bilateral	Absent or diminished femoral pulses (coarctation of aorta)	Monitor blood pressure in upper and lower extremities.
Inguinal area: No bulges along inguinal area No inguinal lymph nodes felt	Inguinal hernia	Initiate referral. Continue follow-up in well-baby clinic.
Bladder: Percusses 1–4 cm above symphysis	Failure to void within 24–48 hours after birth	Check if baby voided at birth. Consult with clinician; obtain urine specimen if infection is suspected.
Emptied about three hours after birth; if not, at time of birth	Exposure of bladder mucosa (exstrophy of bladder)	
Urine—inoffensive, mild odor	Foul odor (infection)	
Genitals Gender clearly delineated	Ambiguous genitals	Refer for genetic consultation.
Male *Penis:* Slender in appearance, about 2.5 cm long, 1 cm wide at birth Normal urinary orifice, urethral meatus at tip of penis	Micropenis (congenital anomaly) Meatal atresia	Observe and record first voiding.
	Hypospadias, epispadias	Collaborate with physician in presence of abnormality.
Noninflamed urethral opening	Urethritis (infection)	Palpate for enlarged inguinal lymph nodes and record painful urination.
Foreskin adheres to glans; prepuce can be retracted beyond urethral opening	Ulceration of meatal opening (infection, inflammation)	Evaluate whether ulcer is due to diaper rash; counsel regarding care.
Uncircumcised foreskin tight for two to three months	Phimosis—if still tight after three months	Instruct parents on how to care for uncircumcised penis.
Circumcised Erectile tissue present		Teach parents how to care for circumcision.
Scrotum: Skin loose and hanging or tight and small; extensive rugae and normal size	Large scrotum containing fluid (hydrocele) Red, shiny scrotal skin (orchitis)	Shine a light through scrotum (transilluminate) to verify diagnosis.
Normal skin color Scrotal discoloration common in breech		

*Possible causes of alterations are placed in parentheses.
†This column provides guidelines for further assessment and initial nursing interventions.

(continued)

Neonatal Physical Assessment Guide (continued)

Assessment and Normal Findings	Alterations and Possible Causes*	Nursing Responses to Data Base†
Testes:		
Descended by birth; not consistently found in scrotum	Undescended testes (cryptorchidism)	If testes cannot be felt in scrotum, gently palpate femoral, inguinal, perineal, and abdominal areas for presence.
Testes size 1.5–2 cm at birth	Enlarged testes (tumor) Small testes (Klinefelter syndrome or adrenal hyperplasia)	Refer and collaborate with physician for further diagnostic studies.
Female		
Mons:		
Normal skin color; area pigmented in dark-skinned infants		
Labia majora cover labia minora; symmetric size appropriate for gestational age	Hematoma, lesions (trauma)	Evaluate for recent trauma.
Clitoris:		
Normally large in newborn Edema and bruising in breech birth	Hypertrophy (hermaphroditism)	
Vagina:		
Urinary meatus and vaginal orifice visible (0.5 cm circumference)	Inflammation; erythema and discharge (urethritis)	Collect urine specimen for laboratory examination.
Vaginal tag or hymenal tag disappears in a few weeks	Congenital absence of vagina	Refer to physician.
Discharge; smegma under labia	Foul-smelling discharge (infection)	Collect data and further evaluate reason for discharge.
Bloody or mucoid discharge	Excessive vaginal bleeding (blood coagulation defect)	
Buttocks and Anus		
Buttocks symmetric	Pilonidal dimple	Examine for possible sinus. Instruct parents about cleansing this area.
Anus patent and passage of meconium within 24–48 hours after birth	Imperforate anus, rectal atresia (congenital gastrointestinal defect)	Evaluate extent of problems. Initiate surgical consultation. Perform digital examination to ascertain patency, if patency uncertain.
No fissures, tears, or skin tags	Fissures	
Extremities and Trunk		
Short and generally flexed; extremities move symmetrically through range of motion but lack full extension	Unilateral or absence of movement (spinal cord involvement) Fetal position continued or limp (anoxia, CNS problems, hypoglycemia)	Review birth record to assess possible cause.

*Possible causes of alterations are placed in parentheses.
†This column provides guidelines for further assessment and initial nursing interventions.

(continued)

Neonatal Physical Assessment Guide (continued)

Assessment and Normal Findings	Alterations and Possible Causes*	Nursing Responses to Data Base†
All joints move spontaneously; good muscle tone, of flexor type, birth to two months	Spasticity when infant begins using extensors (cerebral palsy, lack of muscle tone, "floppy baby" syndrome) Hypotonia (Down syndrome)	Collaborate with physician.
Arms: Equal in length Bilateral movement Flexed when quiet	Brachial palsy (difficult birth) Erb-Duchenne paralysis Muscle weakness, fractured clavicle Absence of limb or change of size (phocomelia, amelia)	Report to clinician.
Hands: Normal number of fingers	Polydactyly (Ellis-Van Creveld syndrome) Syndactyly—one limb (developmental anomaly) Syndactyly—both limbs (genetic component)	Report to clinician.
Normal palmar crease	Simian line on palm (Down syndrome)	
Normal size hands	Short fingers and broad hand (Hurler syndrome)	
Nails present and extend beyond fingertips in term infant	Cyanosis and clubbing (cardiac anomalies) Nails long (postterm)	
Spine: C-shaped spine Flat and straight when prone Slight lumbar lordosis Easily flexed and intact when palpated At least half of back devoid of lanugo Full-term infant in ventral suspension should hold head at 45° angle, back straight	Spina bifida occulta (nevus pilosus) Dermal sinus Myelomeningocele Head lag, limp, floppy trunk (neurologic problems)	Evaluate extent of neurologic damage; initiate care of spinal opening.
Hips: No sign of instability	Sensation of abnormal movement, jerk, or snap of hip dislocation	Examine all newborn infants for dislocated hip prior to discharge from hospital.
Hips abduct to more than 60°		If this is suspected, refer to orthopedist for further evaluation. Reassess at well-baby visits.
Inguinal and buttock skin creases: Symmetric inguinal and buttock creases	Asymmetry (dislocated hips)	Refer to orthopedist for evaluation, counsel parents regarding symptoms of concern and discuss therapy.
Legs: Legs equal in length Legs shorter than arms at birth	Shortened leg (dislocated hips) Lack of leg movement (fractures, spinal defects)	Refer to orthopedist for evaluation. Counsel parents regarding symptoms of concern and discuss therapy.

*Possible causes of alterations are placed in parentheses.
†This column provides guidelines for further assessment and initial nursing interventions.

(continued)

Neonatal Physical Assessment Guide (continued)

Assessment and Normal Findings	Alterations and Possible Causes*	Nursing Responses to Data Base†
Feet: Foot is in straight line Positional clubfoot—based on position in utero Fat pads and creases on soles of feet	Talipes equinovarus (true clubfoot)	Discuss differences between positional and true clubfoot with parents. Teach parents passive manipulation of foot. Refer to orthopedist if not corrected by three months of age.
Talipes planus (flat feet) normal under three years of age		Reassure parents that flat feet are normal in infant.
Neuromuscular		
Motor function: Symmetric movement and strength in all extremities	Limp, flaccid, or hypertonic (CNS disorders, infection, dehydration, fracture)	Appraise newborn's posture and motor functions by observing activities and motor characteristics.
May be jerky or have brief twitchings	Tremors (hypoglycemia, hypocalcemia, infection, neurologic damage)	Evaluate electrolyte imbalance and neurologic functioning.
Head lag not over 45°	Delayed or abnormal development (preterm, neurologic involvement)	
Neck control adequate to maintain head erect briefly	Asymmetry of tone or strength (neurologic damage)	
Reflexes		
Blink: Stimulated by flash of light, response is closure of eyelids	Damage to cranial nerve	
Pupillary reflex: Stimulated by flash of light, response is constriction of pupil	Damage to cranial nerve	
Moro: Response to sudden movement or loud noise should be one of symmetric extension and abduction of arms with fingers extended; then return to normal relaxed flexion Infant lying on back: slightly raised head suddenly released; infant held horizontally, lowered quickly about 6 in., and stopped abruptly Fingers form a C Present at birth, disappears by six months of age	Asymmetry of body response (fractured clavicle, injury to brachial plexus) Consistent absence (brain damage)	Discuss normality of this reflex in response to loud noises and/or sudden movements.

*Possible causes of alterations placed in parentheses.
†This column provides guidelines for further assessment and initial nursing interventions.

(continued)

Neonatal Physical Assessment Guide (continued)

Assessment and Normal Findings	Alterations and Possible Causes*	Nursing Responses to Data Base†
Rooting and sucking: Turns in direction of stimulus to cheek or mouth; opens mouth and begins to suck rhythmically when finger or nipple is inserted into mouth; difficult to elicit after feeding; disappears by four to seven months of age. Sucking is adequate for nutritional intake and meeting oral stimulation needs; disappears by 12 months	Poor sucking or easily fatigable (preterm; breast-fed infants of barbiturate-addicted mothers). Possible cardiac problem. Absence of response (preterm, neurologic involvement, depressed infants)	Evaluate strength and coordination of sucking. Observe neonate during feeding and counsel parents about mutuality of feeding experience and neonate's responses.
Palmar grasp: Fingers grasp adult finger when palm is stimulated and hold momentarily; lessens at three to four months of age	Asymmetry of response (neurologic problems)	Evaluate other reflexes and general neurologic functioning.
Plantar grasp: Toes curl downward when sole of foot is stimulated; lessens by eight months	Absent (defects of lower spinal column)	
Stepping: When held upright and one foot touching a flat surface, will step alternately; disappears at four to five months of age	Asymmetry of stepping (neurologic abnormality)	Evaluate muscle tone and function on each side of body. Refer to specialist.
Babinski: Fanning and extension of all toes when one side of sole is stroked from heel upward across ball of foot	Absence of response (low spinal cord defects)	Refer for further neurologic evaluation.
Tonic neck: Fencer position—when head is turned to one side, extremities on same side extend and on opposite side flex; this reflex may not be evident during early neonatal period; disappears at three to four months of age. Response often more dominant in leg than in arm	Absent after one month of age or persistent asymmetry (cerebral lesion)	
Prone crawl: While on abdomen, neonate pushes up and tries to crawl	Absence or variance of response (preterm, weak or depressed infants)	Evaluate motor functioning. Refer to specialist.
Trunk incurvation: In prone position, stroking of spine causes pelvis to turn to stimulated side	Failure to rotate to stimulated side (neurologic damage)	

*Possible causes of alterations are placed in parentheses.
†This column provides guidelines for further assessment and initial nursing interventions.

Neonatal Behavioral Assessment

Two conflicting forces influence parents' perceptions of their infant. One is the parents' preconceptions, based on hopes and fears, of what their newborn will be like. The other is their initial reaction to their baby's temperament, behaviors, and physical appearance. Nurses can assist parents in identifying their baby's specific behaviors.

One of the newborn's first responses is to move into a quiet but alert state of consciousness. The baby is still; his body molds to yours; his hands touch your skin; his eyes open wide and are bright and shiny. He looks directly at you.

This special alert state, this innate ability to communicate, may be the initial preparation for becoming attached to other human beings. One feels awed by the intensity and appealing power of this little bud of humanity meeting the world for the first time. (The Amazing Newborn)

Brazelton (1973) developed a tool that has revolutionized our understanding and perception of the newborn's capabilities and responses, permitting us to recognize each infant's individuality. **Brazelton's neonatal behavioral assessment** tool provides valuable guidelines for assessing the newborn's state changes, temperament, and individual behavior patterns. It provides a means by which the health care provider, in conjunction with the parents (primary care givers), can identify and understand the individual newborn's states. Parents learn which responses, interventions, or activities best meet the special needs of their infant, and this understanding fosters positive attachment experiences.

The assessment tool attempts to identify the newborn's repertoire of behavioral responses to the environment and also documents the newborn's neurologic adequacy and capabilities. The examination usually takes 20 to 30 minutes and involves about 30 tests. It should be noted that to administer the complete assessment tool accurately and ensure reliability, the nurse must have completed a training course. The scale includes 27 behavioral items, which are scored on a nine-point scale, and 20 elicited reflexes, which are scored on a three-point scale. Some items are scored according to the newborn's response to specific stimuli. Others, such as consolability and alertness, are scored as a result of continuous behavioral observations throughout the assessment. For a complete discussion of all test items and maneuvers, the student is referred to Brazelton (1973). The entire tool is not routinely done in clinical practice.

Generally the tool is set up so that the midpoint is the norm for most items. The Brazelton assessment tool differs from most in that the newborn's score is determined not on the average performance but on the best. Since the first few days after birth are a period of behavioral disorganization, the complete assessment should be done on the third day after birth. Every effort should be made to elicit the best response. This may be accomplished by repeating tests at different times or by testing during situations that facilitate the best possible response, such as when parents are holding, cuddling, rocking, and singing to their baby.

The assessment of the newborn should be carried out initially in a quiet, dimly or softly lit room, if possible. The newborn's state of consciousness should be determined, because scoring and introduction of the test items are correlated with the sleep or awake state. The newborn's state depends on physiologic variables, such as the amount of time from the last feeding, positioning, environmental temperature, and health status; presence of such external stimuli as noises and bright lights; and the wake-sleep cycle of the infant. An important characteristic of the neonatal period is the *pattern of states*, as well as the transitions from one state to another. The pattern of states is a predictor of the infant's receptivity and ability to respond to stimuli in a cognitive manner. Babies learn best in a quiet, alert state and in an environment that is supportive and protective and that provides appropriate stimuli.

The nurse should observe the newborn's sleep-wake patterns (as discussed in Chapter 27) and the rapidity with which the newborn moves from one state to another, the newborn's ability to be consoled, and the newborn's ability to diminish the impact of disturbing stimuli. The following questions may provide the nurse with a framework for assessment:

- Does the newborn's response style and ability to adapt to stimuli indicate a need for parental interventions that will alert the newborn to the environment so that he or she can grow socially and cognitively?
- Are parental interventions necessary to lessen the outside stimuli, as in the case of the baby who responds to sensory input with intensity?
- Can the baby control the amount of sensory input that he or she must deal with?

The behaviors and the sleep-wake states in which they are assessed are categorized as follows:

Habituation The infant's ability to diminish or shut down innate responses to specific repeated stimuli, such as a rattle, bell, light, or pinprick to heel, is assessed.

Orientation to inanimate and animate visual and auditory assessment stimuli How often and where the newborn attends to auditory and visual stimuli are observed. The infant's orientation to the environment is determined by an ability to respond to cues given by others and by a natural ability to fix on and to follow a visual object horizontally and vertically. This capacity and parental appreciation of it are important for positive communication between infant and parents; the parents' visual (*en face*) and auditory (soft, continuous voice) presence stimulates their infant to orient to them. Inability or lack of response may indicate visual or auditory problems. It is important for parents to know that their infant can turn to voices usually soon after birth or by 3 days of age and can become alert at different times with a varying degree of intensity in response to sounds.

Motor activity Several components are evaluated. Motor tone of the newborn is assessed in the most characteristic state of responsiveness. This summary assessment includes overall use of tone as the neonate responds to being handled—whether during spontaneous activity, prone placement, or horizontal holding—and overall assessment of body tone as the neonate reacts to all stimuli.

Variations Frequency of alert states, state changes, color changes (throughout all states as examination progresses), activity, and peaks of excitement are assessed.

Self-quieting activity Assessment is based on how often, how quickly, and how effectively newborns can use their resources to quiet and console themselves when upset or distressed. Considered in this assessment are such self-consolatory activities as putting hand to mouth, sucking on a fist or the tongue, and attuning to an object or sound. The infant's need for outside consolation must also be considered, for example, seeing a face; being rocked, held, or dressed; using a pacifier; and having extremities restrained.

Cuddliness or social behaviors This area encompasses the infant's need for and response to being held. Also considered is how often the newborn smiles. These behaviors influence the parents' self-esteem and feelings of acceptance or rejection. Cuddling also appears to be an indicator of personality. Cuddlers appear to enjoy, accept, and seek physical contact; are easier to placate; sleep more; and form earlier and more intense attachments. Noncuddlers are active, restless, have accelerated motor development, and are intolerant of physical restraint. Smiling, even as a grimace reflex, greatly influences parent-infant feedback. Parents identify this response as positive.

Research Note

Clinical Application of Research

New mothers have certain perceptions about their ability to care for their new infant. In an attempt to determine the nurse's sensitivity about these maternal perceptions and to further validate an infant care skills tool, Robin Froman and Steven Owen (1990) developed a research study using a framework of self-efficacy. Self-efficacy "stems from four major influences: previous task performance, observation of others' performance, persuasion, and physiological state" (Froman & Owen 1990, p 248). Self-efficacy involves a sense of confidence that one can successfully accomplish a task.

Prior to discharge, new mothers rated themselves using an infant care skills tool (ICS), which encompassed five specific skills: infant feeding, burping, diapering, bathing, and holding ability. The nurse caring for the mother also rated the mother's ability on the five skills. Significant predictor variables for maternal score on the ICS scale included mother's age, number of children, and nurse's rating of skills. Interestingly, first-time mothers felt the least confidence in bathing their infants if those infants were male when they were compared as a group to multiparous mothers and primiparous mothers with female children. Implications for nursing include suggestions incorporating self-efficacy theory into teaching methods for new mothers.

Critical Thinking Applied to Research

Strengths: Use of factor analysis to validate infant self-efficacy scale. Reports of psychometric properties of the tool used to measure efficacy from both prior and current study. Description of treatment of statistical outliers.

Froman R, Owen S: Mothers' and nurses' perceptions of infant care skills. *Res Nurs Health* 1990; 13:247.

❀ ❀

KEY CONCEPTS

A perinatal history, determination of gestational age, physical examination, and behavior assessment form the basis for complete newborn assessment.

The common physical characteristics included in the gestational age assessment are: skin, lanugo, sole (plantar) creases, breast tissue and size, ear form and cartilage, and genitalia.

The neuromuscular components of gestational age scoring tools are usually posture, square window sign, popliteal angle, arm recoil, heel to ear, and scarf sign.

By assessing the physical and neuromuscular components of a gestational age tool, the nurse can determine the gestational age of the newborn.

After determining the gestational age of the baby, the nurse can assess how the newborn will make the transition to extrauterine life and anticipate potential physiologic problems.

In-depth knowledge of normal newborn physical characteristics and common variations is essential for the newborn nurse.

Normal ranges for vital signs assessed in the newborn are: Heart rate—120–160 beats/min; respirations—30–60 respirations/min; axillary temperature—36.5C–37C (97.7F–98.6F), or skin temperature—36C–36.5C (96.8F–97.7F), or rectal temperature—36.6C–37.2C (97.8F–99F); and blood pressure at birth of 80–60/45–40 mm Hg.

Normal newborn measurements include: Weight range 2500–4000 g (5 lb, 8 oz–8 lb, 13 oz), with weight dependent on maternal size and age; length range 45–55 cm (18–22 in.); and head circumference range of 32–37 cm (12.5–14.5 in.)—approximately 2 cm larger than the chest circumference.

Commonly elicited newborn reflexes are tonic neck, Moro, grasping, rooting, sucking, and blink.

An important role of the nurse during the physical and behavioral assessments of the newborn is to teach parents about their newborn and involve them in their baby's care. This facilitates the parents' identification of their newborn's uniqueness and allays their concerns.

❀ ❀

References

AAP Committee on Fetus and Newborn and ACOG Committee on Obstetrics: *Guidelines for Perinatal Care.* Evanston, IL: American Academy of Pediatrics, 1988.

Ballard JL et al: A simplified score for assessment of fetal maturation of newly born infants. *J Pediatr* November 1979; 95:769.

Brazelton T: *The Neonatal Behavioral Assessment Scale.* Philadelphia: Lippincott, 1973.

Brazelton T: Neonatal behavior and its significance. In: *Schaeffer's Diseases of the Newborn.* Avery ME, Taeusch HW (editors). Philadelphia: Saunders, 1984.

Duara S et al: Neonatal screening with auditory brainstem responses: Results of a follow-up audiometry and risk factor evaluation. *J Pediatr* 1986; 108(2):276.

Eden RD, Boehm FH (editors): *Assessment and Care of the Fetus: Physiological, Clinical, and Medicolegal Principles.* Norwalk, CT: Appleton & Lange, 1990.

Korones, SB: *High-Risk Newborn Infants,* 4th ed. St. Louis: Mosby, 1986.

Ludington-Hoe SM: What can newborns really see? *Am J Nurs* 1983; 83:1286.

Querleu D et al: Hearing by the Human Fetus? *Semin Perinatol* October 1989; 13:409.

Additional Readings

Allen MC, Capute AJ: Tone and reflex development before term. *Pediatric* 1990; 85:393.

Brown AM: Development of visual sensitivity to light and color vision in human infants: A critical review. *Vision Res* 1990; 30(8):1159.

Bureau G, Kleiber C: Clinical indicators of infant irritability. *Neonatal Netw* February 1991; 9:23.

Joseph PR, Rosenfeld W: Clavicular fractures in neonates. *AJDC* February 1990; 144:165.

Kenner C: Measuring neonatal assessment. *Neonatal Netw* December 1990; 9:17.

K. C. Leung A, C. H. Ma K, Oswald Siu T, Robson LM: Palpebral fissure length: In Chinese newborn infants. *Clinical Pediatrics* March 1990; 29:172.

Thurston FE, Roberts SL: Environmental noise and fetal hearing. *Journal of the Tennessee Medical Association* January 1991; 84:9.

CHAPTER 29

The Normal Newborn:

Needs and Care

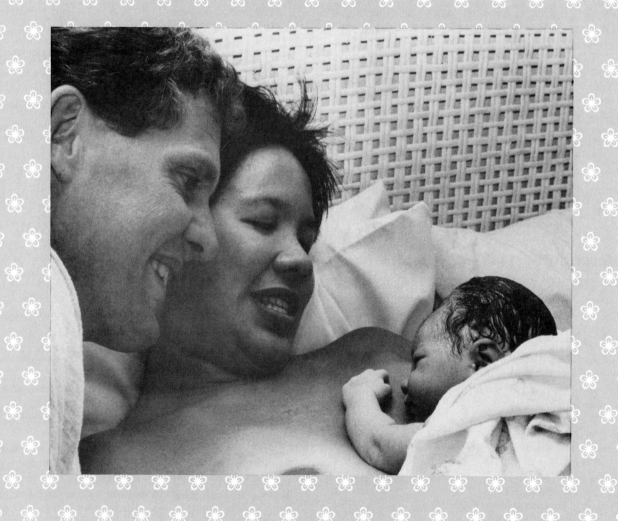

OBJECTIVES

Summarize the essential areas of information to be obtained about a newborn's birth experience and immediate postnatal period.

Explain the physiologic and behavioral responses of newborns during periods of reactivity and possible interventions needed.

Discuss the major nursing considerations and activities to be carried out during the first four hours after birth (admission and transitional period) and subsequent daily care.

Identify the assessments and activities that should be included in a daily care plan for a normal newborn.

Determine common parental concerns regarding their newborns.

Describe the topics and related content to be included in parent education classes on newborn/infant care.

Delineate the information to be included in discharge planning with parents.

❀ ❀

This moment of meeting seemed to be a birthtime for both of us; her first and my second life. Nothing, I knew, could ever be the same again. (Laurie Lee, Two Women)

At the moment of birth, numerous physiologic adaptations begin to take place in the newborn's body. Because of these dramatic changes, the newborn requires close observation to determine how smoothly she or he is making the transition to extrauterine life. The newborn also requires care that enhances her or his chances of making the transition successfully.

The two broad goals of nursing care during this period are to promote the physical well-being of the newborn and to promote the establishment of a well-functioning family unit. The first goal is met by providing comprehensive care to the newborn during the immediate postpartum period. The second goal is met by teaching parents how to care for their new baby and by supporting their parenting efforts so that they feel confident and competent.

❀ *USING THE NURSING PROCESS DURING* ❀

The Normal Newborn Period

Nursing Assessment

Assessment during the neonatal period gives the nurse an opportunity to identify any actual or potential physical problems facing the newborn. Careful assessment of the general characteristics, variations, and responses of the newborn helps the nurse differentiate between normal physiologic adaptations and abnormal findings that require further evaluation. Individual temperament and behavior patterns are also assessed.

During the newborn assessment, the nurse determines the presence of any psychosocial factors that may affect the family's ability to integrate its newest member. The nurse's assessment should reveal the extent of the family's need for information, support, and instruction about child care. Identifying the family's strengths is just as important as identifying problems because these strengths can be incorporated in the care plan. To perform an accurate family assessment, the nurse must be knowledgeable about the characteristics of the expanding family.

The plan of care is based on the findings of the assessment. If the assessment is inadequate, the plan of care will most likely be ineffective as well. The newborn's successful transition to extrauterine life may ultimately depend on the nurse's ability to identify physiologic needs correctly. The family's ability to meet the physical and psychologic needs of the newborn may be affected by the nurse's accuracy in identifying the family's strengths and weaknesses.

Assessment is performed on a daily basis while the newborn is present on the birthing unit. The daily assessment period is an opportune time for parent education. The nurse can explain the newborn's physiologic and behavioral changes and responses as the assessment proceeds.

Nursing Diagnosis

Nursing diagnoses are based on an analysis of findings of the assessment. Physiologic alterations of the newborn form the basis of many nursing diagnoses. The following nursing diagnoses may apply:

● Ineffective airway clearance related to mucus obstruction

● Alteration in nutrition: less than body requirements related to limited nutritional/fluid intake

● Altered patterns of urinary elimination related to circumcision

- Pain related to heelsticks for blood glucose and hematocrit
- Alteration in peripheral tissue perfusion related to decreased thermoregulation

Nursing diagnoses that may apply to family functioning are the following:

- Knowledge deficit related to lack of experience in infant care
- Knowledge deficit related to decision about male circumcision
- Altered family processes related to the need to integrate the newborn into the family unit

Identification, prioritization, and documentation of the nursing diagnoses are essential for developing a thoughtful, systematic plan of care.

Nursing Plan and Implementation

Even though most newborns are healthy, every newborn has physiologic needs that must be met. The family also has needs, which are usually psychologic and educational. To meet these needs in an organized fashion, the neonatal nurse must develop a plan of care based on the assessment findings and nursing diagnoses.

A nursing care plan is important to ensure consistent and comprehensive care. Even though most newborns and their mothers remain in the birthing unit for a brief period, they may have several nurses administering care during their stay. When there is one care plan implemented by all personnel caring for the family, the goals of care are more likely to be achieved. Redundancy or missed interventions are less likely, and parent education can proceed at a steady pace, even though different nurses are teaching.

Evaluation

Through ongoing observations nurses evaluate whether the newborn's body systems are successfully maturing and adapting to extrauterine life. This evaluation is based on knowledge of the expected cardiovascular, pulmonary, renal, and neurologic changes that occur in the days immediately following birth.

To evaluate the daily nursing care given to the newborn, the nurse notes whether complications have developed in the baby. The success of parent education can be evaluated by how well the parents perform infant care measures and how comfortable they feel in caring for their baby.

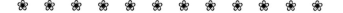

Nursing Assessment During the First Four Hours

After birth, the baby is formally admitted to the health care facility. The admission procedures include an assessment to ensure that the newborn's adaptation to extrauterine life is proceeding normally and several interventions to promote successful adaptation.

If the initial assessment indicates that the newborn is not at risk physiologically, many of the routine admission procedures are performed in the presence of the parents in the maternal recovery area. The care measures indicated by the assessment findings may be performed by the nurse or by the parents under the supervision of the nurse in an effort to educate and support the parents. Other interventions may be delayed until the infant has been transferred to an observational nursery.

Admission Assessment Procedures

As discussed in Chapter 27, the newborn's physiologic adaptations to extrauterine life occur rapidly. All the body systems are affected. Thus the newborn requires close monitoring during the first few hours of life so that any deviation from normal can be identified immediately.

During the assessment in the first four hours after birth, the nurse focuses on the newborn's physiologic adaptations. A complete physical examination is done later by the physician or nurse practitioner, usually within the first 24 hours of life or just prior to discharge (see Chapter 28 and Table 29–1).

CRITICAL THINKING

Which critical perinatal and neonatal assessments have the most significant impact on the newborn's care during the first 4 hours after birth?

If the newborn is transferred to an observational nursery for the first four-hour assessment, the nurse receiving the infant first checks and confirms the newborn's identification. The birth nurse who carries the baby to the nursery communicates via a concise verbal report all significant information regarding the newborn. The essential data to be reported and recorded as part of the newborn's chart include the following:

1. *Condition of the newborn.* Pertinent information includes the newborn's Apgar scores at one and five minutes, resuscitative measures required in the birthing area, vital signs, voidings, and passing of meconium. Complications to be noted are excessive mucus, delayed spontaneous respirations or

Table 29-1 Timing and Types of Newborn Assessments

1. Evaluation immediately after birth by nurse to determine need for resuscitation or if newborn is stable and can remain with parents to initiate attachment.

2. Assessment within first one to four hours after birth:
   - Evaluate adaptation to extrauterine life.
   - Determine gestational age.
   - Evaluate for high-risk problems.

3. Assessment within first 24 hours or prior to discharge:
   - Perform complete physical examination. (Depending on agency protocol, the nurse may complete some components on her own, with a physician or nurse practitioner completing the exam prior to discharge.)
   - Evaluate behavior.

responsiveness, abnormal number of cord vessels, and obvious physical abnormalities.

2. *Labor and birth record.* A copy of the labor and birth record should be placed in the newborn's chart. The record contains all the significant data about the birth, for example, duration, course, and status of mother and fetus throughout labor and birth and any analgesia or anesthesia administered to the mother. Particular care is taken to note any variation or difficulties such as prolonged rupture of membranes, abnormal fetal position, meconium-stained amniotic fluid, signs of fetal distress during labor, nuchal cord (cord around the newborn's neck at birth), precipitous birth, and use of forceps.

3. *Antepartal history.* Any maternal problems that may have compromised the fetus in utero, such as PIH, spotting, illness, recent infections, or a history of maternal substance abuse, are of immediate concern in the assessment of the newborn. Information about maternal age, estimated date of birth (EDB), previous pregnancies, and presence of any congenital anomalies is also included.

4. *Parent-infant interaction information.* Parental interactions with their newborn and their desires regarding care, such as rooming-in, circumcision, and type of feeding, are noted. Information about other children in the home, available support systems, and interactional patterns within each family unit assists in providing comprehensive care.

In the absence of any newborn distress, the nurse continues with the admission assessment by taking the newborn's vital signs. The initial temperature should be taken by the axillary method, which is safer than the rectal method and correlates closely with rectal temperature in the newborn (Mayfield et al 1984). Normal axillary tem-

perature is 36.5C to 37C (97.7F–98.6F). Some hospitals still choose to use a rectal thermometer for the initial temperature, theorizing that rectal patency can be assessed simultaneously. Equally successful alternative methods for assessing anal patency are digital examination or use of a sterile, flexible rubber catheter. Patency can also be assessed by observing the newborn having a bowel movement.

Once the initial temperature assessment is made, the core temperature is monitored either by obtaining an axillary temperature at intervals or by placing a skin sensor on the newborn for continuous reading. The usual skin sensor placement site is on the newborn's abdomen (Figure 29–1), but placement on the upper thigh or arm gives a reading more closely correlated with the mean body temperature. The axillary temperature for the healthy term infant should be monitored at least every four hours until stable, every eight hours until discharged (Neonatal Thermoregulation 1990).

The apical pulse and respirations are assessed every 15 to 30 minutes for one hour and then every one to two hours until stable. The apical pulse is best assessed while the newborn is at rest. The newborn's respirations may be irregular and still be normal. The normal pulse range is 120 to 160 beats per minute, and the normal respiratory range is 30 to 60 respirations per minute.

Blood pressure is assessed by ausculation, palpation, or by Doppler or Dinemapp instrument (Figure 29–2). If a Dinemapp or Doppler device is used, the newborn's extremities must be immobilized during the assessment, and the cuff should cover two-thirds of the upper arm or upper

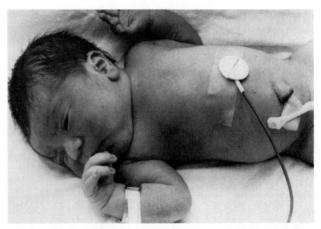

Figure 29–1 Temperature monitoring for the newborn. A skin thermal sensor is placed on the newborn's abdomen, upper thigh, or arm and secured with porous tape or a foil-covered foam pad. (From Swearingen P: The Addison-Wesley Photo-Atlas of Nursing Procedures. Menlo Park, CA: Addison-Wesley, 1984)

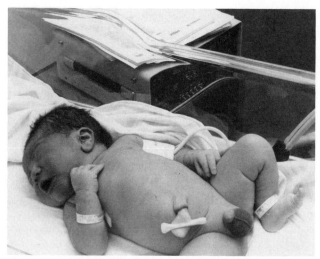

Figure 29–2 Blood pressure measurement using the Dinemapp and Doppler devices. The cuff can be applied to either the neonate's upper arm or thigh.

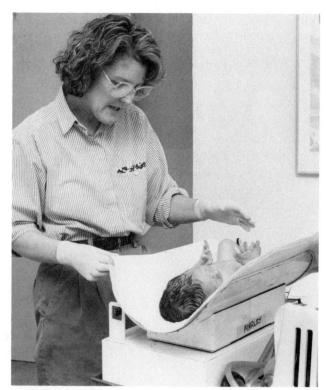

Figure 29–3 Weighing of newborns. The scale is balanced before each weighing, with the protective pad in place. The care giver's hand is poised above the infant as a safety measure.

leg. Movement, crying, and inappropriate cuff size can give inaccurate measurements of the blood pressure.

The newborn is weighed in grams and pounds. Most parents understand pound measurement (Figure 29–3). The scales are covered each time an infant is weighed to prevent cross-infection and heat loss from conduction. The newborn is measured; the measurements are recorded in both centimeters and inches. Three routine measurements are (a) length, (b) circumference of the head, and (c) circumference of the chest (see Chapter 28 and Figures 28–12, 28–13). In some facilities, abdominal girth may also be determined. The nurse rapidly appraises the baby's color, muscle tone, alertness, and general state. Gestational age is estimated and the physical examination is completed (for further discussion, see Chapter 28). A hematocrit and blood glucose evaluation is routinely done on all newborns in many institutions (see Procedure 32–2). This may be done on admission or within the first four hours.

The assessment during the first four hours after birth provides a basis for establishing nursing diagnoses regarding the infant and setting priorities for care and family education needs. In many settings, the father accompanies the newborn to the nursery. This is an excellent opportunity for him to get to know his child while the nurse systematically examines and explains the newborn's responses and characteristics. It is also an excellent opportunity for the astute nurse to take note of the father's bonding process and comfort level with the newborn. The nurse needs to recognize that the father may be overwhelmed by the unfamiliar birthing setting. However, he may benefit from observing and interacting with the nurse who cares for his baby.

The nurse should also assess the newborn's physiologic adaptation and behavior during the transitional periods (Table 29–2). The baby usually shows a predictable pattern of behavior during the first several hours after birth, which is characterized by two **periods of reactivity** separated by a sleep phase.

Table 29–2 Signs of Newborn Transition

Normal findings for the newborn during the first few hours of life include the following:

Pulse: 120–160 beats/min
  During sleep as low as 100 beats/min
  If crying, up to 180 beats/min

Respirations: 30–60 respirations/min
  Predominantly diaphragmatic but synchronous with abdominal movements

Temperature: Axillary: 36.5–37C (97.7–98.6F)
  Skin: 36–36.5C (96.8–97.7F)

Dextrostix: Greater than 45 mg %

Hematocrit: Less than 65%–70% central venous sample

Periods of Reactivity

First Period of Reactivity

This phase lasts approximately 30 minutes after birth. During this phase the newborn is awake and active and may appear hungry and have a strong sucking reflex. This is a natural opportunity to initiate breast-feeding if this is the mother's choice. Bursts of random, diffuse movements may alternate with relative immobility. Respirations are rapid, as high as 80 breaths per minute, and there may be chest retractions, transient flaring of the nares, and grunting. The heart rate is rapid and irregular. Bowel sounds are absent.

Sleep Phase

The newborn's activity gradually diminishes, and the heart rate and respirations decrease as the baby enters the sleep phase. First sleep usually occurs an average of three hours after birth, and may last from a few minutes to two to four hours. During this period, the newborn will be difficult to awaken and will show no interest in sucking. Bowel sounds become audible, and cardiac and respiratory rates return to baseline values.

Second Period of Reactivity

The newborn is again awake and alert. This phase lasts four to six hours in the normal newborn. Physiologic responses are variable during this stage. The heart and respiratory rates increase; however, the nurse must be alert for apneic periods, which may cause a drop in the heart rate. The newborn must be stimulated to continue breathing during such times. the newborn may develop rapid color changes, becoming mildly cyanotic or mottled during these fluctuations. Production of respiratory and gastric mucus increases, and the baby responds by gagging, choking, and regurgitating. Continued close observation and interventions may be necessary to maintain a clear airway during this period of reactivity. The gastrointestinal tract becomes more active. The first meconium stool is frequently passed during this second active stage, and the initial voiding may also occur at this time. The newborn will indicate readiness for feeding by such behaviors as sucking, rooting, and swallowing. If feeding was not initiated in the first period of reactivity, it is done at this time. See page 893 for further discussion of this first feeding.

Nursing Diagnosis

Nursing diagnoses that may apply to the newborn and family during the first four hours of life are presented in the Key Nursing Diagnoses to Consider—The Newborn and Family. Many of these nursing diagnoses and associated interventions must be identified and implemented very quickly during this period.

Key Nursing Diagnoses to Consider
The Newborn and Family

Ineffective airway clearance

Ineffective breathing pattern

Ineffective thermoregulation

Decreased cardiac output

Altered tissue perfusion (peripheral)

Hypothermia

Fluid volume deficit

Pain

Infection: High risk

Injury: High risk

Altered parenting

Knowledge deficit

Nursing Plan and Implementation During Admission and First Four Hours

The nurse evaluates the newborn's need to remain under observation by assessing the newborn's ability to maintain a clear airway, maintain body temperature, maintain stable vital signs, demonstrate normal neurologic status and no observable complications, and tolerate the first feeding. If these criteria are met, it indicates a successful beginning adaptation to extrauterine life. The baby is moved to a regular nursery or to rooming-in. This transfer usually takes place between two and six hours after birth.

Maintenance of a Clear Airway

The nurse positions the newborn on his or her side. If necessary, a bulb syringe (see page 898) or DeLee wall suction (Procedure 23–2, and Figure 23–9) is used to remove mucus from the nasal passages and oral cavity. Another routine but controversial practice in some institutions is use of the DeLee catheter to remove mucus from the stomach to help prevent possible aspiration. This practice can cause vagal nerve stimulation, which can result in bradycardia and apnea in the unstabilized neonate.

PROCEDURE 29–1
Thermoregulation of the Newborn

Nursing Action

Objective: Prepare warming equipment

Prewarm incubator or radiant warmer. Have warmed towels/lightweight blankets available
Maintain birthing room at 22C (71F) with relative humidity of 60% to 65%.

Objective: Establish a stable temperature after birth

Wipe newborn free of blood and excessive vernix, especially from the head, with prewarmed towels.

Place newborn under radiant warmer.

Wrap newborn in prewarmed blanket and transfer to mother.

Place skin-to-skin with mother under warmed blanket.

Objective: Maintain stable infant temperature

Diaper newborn and place hat on head. Place newborn uncovered (except for diaper and hat) under radiant warmer.

Tape servocontrol probe on infant's anterior abdominal wall (metal side next to skin) and cover with aluminum heat deflector patch.

Monitor infant's axillary and skin probe temperature per institution protocol.

Once infant's temperature reaches 98.6F (37C), remove infant from radiant warmer. Dress infant in T-shirt, diaper, and stocking hat then wrap in two blankets (called double wrap). Place in open crib.
Recheck axillary temperature in one hour.

Objective: Rewarm infant gradually if temperature < 97F (36.1C)

Assess temperature frequently
Check axillary temperature per hospital routine usually every 2 to 4 hours.

Place unclothed infant with diaper under radiant warmer with servocontrol probe on abdomen.

Gradually rewarm infant back to normal temperature.

Rationale

Change from warm, moist intrauterine environment to cool, dry, drafty environment stresses the immature thermoregulation mechanisms of newborn.

Prevents loss of body heat from large surface area through evaporation.

Creates a heat-gaining environment.

Reduces convective heat loss
Facilitates immediate maternal-infant contact without compromising infant thermoregulation.

Skin-to-skin contact with mother or father acts to maintain newborn's temperature.

Radiant heat warms outer surface skin so skin needs to be exposed.

Aluminum cover prevents heating of probe directly and overheating of infant.
Turn heater to servocontrol mode with abdominal skin temperature maintained at 36.5C–37C.

Rechecking temperature ensures that it is within desired range. Temperature indicator on the radiant warmer continually displays baby's probe temperature so nurse checks baby's axillary temperature to ensure that the machine accurately reports baby's temperature.

It is important to monitor infant's ability to maintain own thermoregulation.

Early detection of hypothermia, which predisposes infant to cold stress.

Rapid heating leads to hyperthermia.

Hyperthermia caused by too-rapid warming is associated with apnea, increased insensible water loss, and increased metabolic rate.

(continued)

PROCEDURE 29–1 (continued)

Nursing Action

Recheck temperature in 30 minutes, then hourly.

Once infant's temperature reaches 98.6F (37C), remove from heater, dress, double-wrap with hat on, and place in open crib. Recheck temperature in 1 hour.

Objective: Prevent drops in baby's temperature.

Keep infant clothing and bedding dry.
Double-wrap with hat on.
Use heat lamp during procedures.
Reduce exposure to drafts.
Warm objects coming in contact with infant, eg, stethoscopes.
Encourage mother to snuggle with infant under blankets or breast-feed with light cover over infant.

Rationale

Prevents loss of heat by conduction, convection, radiation, and evaporation.

Maintenance of a Neutral Thermal Environment

A neutral thermal environment is essential to minimize the newborn's need to expend calories to maintain body heat in the optimal range of 36.5 to 37.0C (97.7F–98.6F). If the newborn becomes hypothermic, the physiologic response can lead to metabolic acidosis, hypoxia, and shock.

A neutral thermal environment is best achieved by performing the assessment and interventions with the newborn unclothed and under a radiant warmer. The thermostat of the radiant warmer is controlled by the thermal skin sensor taped to the newborn's abdomen, upper thigh, or arm. The sensor indicates when the newborn's temperature exceeds or falls below the acceptable temperature range. The nurse should be aware that leaning over the newborn may block the radiant heat waves from reaching the newborn.

It is common practice in some institutions to cover the neonate's head with a stockinette or knit cap to prevent further heat loss in addition to placing the baby under a radiant warmer. One study (Ruchala 1985) comparing axillary temperatures of neonates whose heads were covered and those remaining uncovered failed to demonstrate a significant difference two hours after birth. More definitive studies are necessary. However, these limited results lead to the question whether heat can more effectively be conserved by using a head covering while the newborn is outside the radiant warmer but not when the newborn is under the radiant warmer (to avoid a barrier effect).

When the newborn's temperature is normal and vital signs are stable (about two to four hours after birth), the baby may be given a sponge bath. However, this admission bath may be postponed for some hours if the newborn's condition dictates or the parents desire it. The admission sponge bath and shampoo are done quickly to minimize heat loss. The bath takes place while the baby is either under the radiant warmer or in the bassinet in the parents' room. The temperature is rechecked after the bath and if it is stable, the newborn is dressed, wrapped, and placed in an open crib at room temperature. If the baby's axillary temperature is below 36.5C (97.7F), the baby is returned to the radiant warmer. The rewarming process should be gradual to prevent possibility of hyperthermia. Slow rewarming is accomplished by maintaining the ambient temperature 1.5C (3F) higher than the infant's current skin temperature (Neonatal Thermoregulation 1990). Once this new skin temperature is reached, the control point of the heater can be set another 1.5C higher until the desired skin temperature is reached. Once the infant is rewarmed, the nurse implements measures to prevent further neonatal heat loss, such as keeping the infant dry, double-wrapped with hat on and avoiding cool surfaces or use of cool instruments. The infant is also protected from drafts, open windows or doors, or air conditioners. Blankets and clothing are stored in a warm place. See discussion on nonshivering thermogenesis and the mechanism of heat loss in Chapter 27 and Procedure 29–1 Thermoregulation of the Newborn.

Prevention of Complications of Hemorrhagic Disease of Newborn

A prophylactic injection of vitamin K is given to prevent hemorrhage, which can occur due to low prothrombin levels in the first few days of life (see the accompanying Drug Guide–Vitamin K₁ phytonadione). The potential for hemorrhage is considered to result from the absence of gut bacterial flora, which influences the production of vitamin K in

DRUG GUIDE
Vitamin K₁ Phytonadione (AquaMEPHYTON)

Overview of Neonatal Action

Phytonadione is used in prophylaxis and treatment of hemorrhagic disease of the newborn. It promotes liver formation of the clotting factors II, VII, IX, and X. At birth the neonate does not have the bacteria in the colon that is necessary for synthesizing fat-soluble vitamin K₁, therefore the newborn may have decreased levels of prothrombin during the first 5–8 days of life reflected by a prolongation of prothrombin time.

Route, Dosage, Frequency

Intramuscular injection is given in the vastus lateralis thigh muscle. A one-time only prophylactic dose of 0.5–1.0 mg is given in the birthing area or upon admission to the newborn nursery. If the mother received anticoagulants during pregnancy, an additional dose may be ordered by the physician and is given at 6–8 hours post first injection.

Neonatal Side Effects

Pain and edema may occur at injection site. Possible allergic reactions such as rash and urticaria.

Nursing Considerations

Observe for bleeding (usually occurs on second or third day). Bleeding may be seen as generalized ecchymoses or bleeding from umbilical cord, circumcision site, nose, or gastrointestinal tract. Results of serial PT and PTT should be assessed.

Observe for jaundice and kernicterus especially in preterm infants.

Observe for signs of local inflammation.

Protect drug from light.

---

the newborn (see Chapter 32 for further discussion). Controversy exists over whether the administration of vitamin K may predispose the newborn to significant hyperbilirubinemia. Cunningham et al 1989 indicate there is no evidence to support this concern as long as a standard dose of 1 mg is given. Some people have questioned the need to give vitamin K to newborns who have had a nontraumatic birth.

A study by Von Kries (1988) looked at replacing parenteral vitamin K with oral vitamin K to avoid injecting the infant. The study demonstrated a considerably higher level of vitamin K present after intramuscular administration than after oral administration Thus, parenteral vitamin K prophylaxis is a safer means of providing infants with high vitamin K load.

The vitamin K injection is given intramuscularly in the middle one-third of the vastus lateralis muscle located in the lateral aspect of the thigh (Figure 29–4). An alternate site is the rectus femoris muscle in the anterior aspect of the thigh. However, this site is near the sciatic nerve and femoral artery and should be used with caution (Figure 29–5).

Prevention of Eye Infection

 The nurse is also responsible for giving the legally required prophylactic eye treatment for *Neisseria gonorrhoea*, which may have infected the newborn of an infected

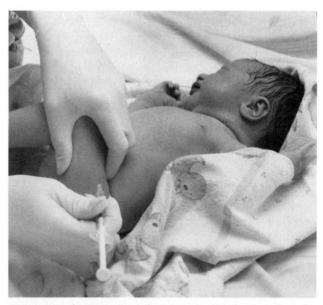

Figure 29–4   Procedure for vitamin K injection. Bunch the tissue of the upper thigh (vastus lateralis muscle) and quickly insert the needle at a 90° angle to the thigh. Aspirate, then slowly inject the solution to distribute the medication evenly and minimize the baby's discomfort. Remove the needle and massage the site with an alcohol swab.

Greater trochanter

Sciatic nerve

Femoral and
deep femoral artery

Femoral and
deep femoral vein

Rectus femoris
muscle

Vastus lateralis
muscle

Patella

mother during the birth process. In the past the drug of choice was 1% silver nitrate solution. Other ophthalmic ointments used instead of silver nitrate are erythromycin (Ilotycin, see the accompanying Drug Guide–Erythromycin), tetracycline, or penicillin. Silver nitrate is not effective against *Chlamydia trachomatis.*

The eyes should be treated within the first few hours after birth. Successful eye prophylaxis requires that the medication be instilled into the lower conjunctival sac (Figure 29–6). The prophylaxis should be done in the nursery rather than the birthing area (Coen & Koeffler 1987). It may be delayed up to a few hours after birth to allow eye contact during parent-infant bonding. (See Procedure 29–2.)

Silver nitrate and the other medications can cause chemical conjunctivitis, and silver nitrate has a higher incidence of this effect. Chemical conjunctivitis causes the newborn some discomfort and may interfere with the

Figure 29–5   Injection sites. The middle third of the vastus lateralis muscle is the preferred site for intramuscular injection in the newborn. The middle third of the rectus femoris is an alternate site, but its proximity to major vessels and the sciatic nerve necessitates caution in using this site.

DRUG GUIDE
Erythromycin (Ilotycin) Ophthalmic Ointment

Overview of Neonatal Action

Erythromycin (Ilotycin) is used as prophylactic treatment of ophthalmia neonatorum, which is caused by the bacteria *Neisseria gonorrhoeae.* Preventive treatment of gonorrhea in the newborn is required by law. Erythromycin is also effective against ophthalmic chlamydial infections. It is either bacteriostatic or bactericidal depending on the organisms involved and the concentration of drug.

Route, Dosage, Frequency

Ophthalmic ointment (0.5%) is instilled as a narrow ribbon or strand, ¼-inch long, along the lower conjunctival surface of each eye, starting at the inner canthus. It is instilled only once in each eye. Administration may be done in the birthing area or later in the nursery so that eye contact is facilitated and the bonding process immediately after birth is not interrupted. After administration, gently close eye and manipulate to ensure spread of ointment (Milan & McFeely 1990; Pawlak & Herfert 1990).

Neonatal Side Effects

Sensitivity reaction; may interfere with ability to focus and may cause edema and inflammation. Side effects usually disappear in 24–48 hours.

Nursing Considerations

Wash hands immediately prior to instillation to prevent introduction of bacteria.

Do not irrigate the eyes after instillation. Use new tube or single-use container for ophthalmic ointment administration shortly after birth.

Observe for hypersensitivity.

Teach parents about need for eye prophylaxis. Educate them regarding side effects and signs that need to be reported to the physician/CNM.

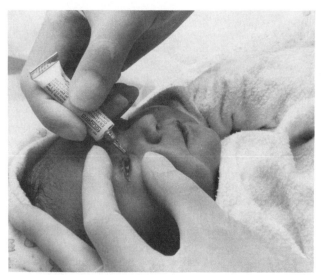

Figure 29–6   Opthalmic eye ointment. Retract lower eyelid outward to instill 1/4-inch long strand of ointment along lower conjunctival surface.

baby's ability to focus on the parents' faces. The resulting edema, inflammation, and discharge may cause concern if the parents have not been given information that the side effects will clear in 24 to 48 hours and that this prophylactic eye treatment is necessary for the newborn's well-being.

Early Assessment of Neonatal Distress

During the first 24 hours of life, the nurse is constantly alert for signs of distress. If the newborn is with his or her parents during this period, extra care must be taken to teach them how to maintain their newborn's temperature, recognize the hallmarks of physiologic distress, and respond immediately to signs of respiratory problems. The parents should be taught to observe the infant for changes in color or activity, rapid breathing with chest retractions, or facial grimacing. Their interventions should include nasal and oral suctioning with bulb syringe, positioning, and vigorous fingertip stroking of the newborn's spine to stimulate respiratory activity if necessary. The nurse also must be available immediately should the baby develop distress (see Table 29–3).

PROCEDURE 29–2
Instillation of Ophthalmic Ilotycin Ointment

Nursing Action	Rationale
Objective: Provide newborn prophylactic eye care	
Wash hands prior to instillation.	Prevents introduction of bacteria.
Clean infant's eyes of any drainage.	Removal of exudate allows instillation of ointment.
Retract lower eyelid outward with forefinger to allow instillation of ¼-inch long strand of ointment along lower conjunctival surface, starting at inner canthus.	Maximizes absorption of ointment.
Repeat process on other eye.	
Instill only a single dose per eye.	Prophylaxis requires only a single dose.
Do not irrigate eyes.	Irrigation will remove ointment.
Assess for sensitivity reaction such as: edema, inflammation, drainage.	May interfere with ability to focus and the bonding process.
Inform parents about rationale for eye prophylaxis, that instillation can be done in the birthing area or admission nursery, it may interfere with newborn's ability to focus on parents' face, and that there may be temporary side effects.	Preventive treatment of gonorrhea and chlamydia infection, which can cause blindness. Required by law. Side effects usually disappear in 24 to 48 hours.
Objective: Record completion of procedure	
Document the instillation of the prophylaxis eye medication	Provides a permanent record to meet the legal requirements.

Table 29-3   Signs of Neonatal Distress
The most common signs of distress in the newborn are the following:
Increased rate (more than 60/min) or difficult respirations
Sternal retractions
Excessive mucus
Facial grimacing
Cyanosis (generalized)
Abdominal distention or mass
Lack of meconium elimination within 24 hours of birth
Inadequate urine elimination
Vomiting of bile-stained material
Unusual jaundice of the skin

Initiation of First Feeding

The timing of the first feeding varies depending on whether the newborn is to be breast-fed or bottle-fed. Mothers who choose to breast-feed their newborns may seek to put their baby to breast while in the birthing area. This practice should be encouraged since successful, long-term breast feeding during infancy appears to be related to beginning breast-feedings in the first few hours of life (Beske & Garvis 1982). Bottle-fed babies usually begin the first feedings by 5 hours of age, during the second period of reactivity, when they awaken and appear hungry.

Signs indicating newborn readiness for the first feeding are: active bowel sounds, absence of abdominal distention, and a lusty cry that quiets with rooting and sucking behaviors when a stimulus is placed near the lips (see page 918).

Facilitation of Parent-Infant Attachment

Eye-to-eye contact between the parents and baby is extremely important during the early hours after birth, when the newborn is in the first period of reactivity. The newborn is alert during this time, the eyes are wide open, and often direct eye contact is made with human faces within optimal range for visual acuity (7 to 8 inches). It is theorized that this eye contact is an important foundation in establishing attachment in human relationships (Klaus & Klaus 1985). Consequently the prophylactic eye medication is often delayed to provide an opportunity for this period of eye contact between parents and their newborn, thus facilitating the attachment process.

Nursing Assessment for Daily Newborn Care

The nurse is responsible for the daily assessment of the health of the newborn and routine daily care. While performing assessment and care tasks, the nurse can encourage the parents to participate, thus strengthening the family unit and enhancing the parents' confidence in their ability to care for their baby. Due to today's changing family structures and lack of extended family, many new parents have had no opportunities to learn about babies. They often look to the nurse for guidance and information. The nurse must have a complete understanding of newborn needs to be able to anticipate and answer questions.

Routine daily assessments vary among birthing facilities. However, the following should be assessed daily while the newborn baby is in the birthing setting.

- *Vital signs.* These are taken once a shift or more, depending on the newborn's status.
- *Weight.* The baby should be weighed at the same time each day for accurate comparisons. A weight loss of up to 10% for term infants is expected during the first week of life. This is the result of limited intake, loss of excess extracellular fluid, and passage of meconium. Parents should be told about the expected weight loss, the reason for it, and the expectations for regaining the birth weight.
- *Skin color.* Changes in skin color may indicate the need for closer assessment of temperature, cardiopulmonary status, hematocrit, and bilirubin levels.
- *Intake/output.* Fluid intake and voiding and stooling patterns are recorded. If 24 hours have passed and the first voiding and passage of stool has not occurred, the nurse continues the normal observation routine while also assessing for abdominal distention, status of bowel sounds, hydration, fluid intake, and temperature stability.
- *Umbilical cord.* The cord is assessed for signs of hemorrhage or infection, such as oozing and foul smell.
- *Circumcision.* The circumcision is assessed for signs of hemorrhage and infection. The first voiding after a circumcision is also a significant assessment in order to evaluate for possible urinary obstruction due to trauma and edema.
- *Newborn nutrition.* Caloric and fluid intake are recorded. The nurse is also responsible for assessing the mother's skill and education needs regarding breast-feeding or bottle-feeding.
- *Parent education.* The nurse assesses the parents knowledge of newborn and infant care. The nurse also assesses whether the parents learning needs can best be met in a group or individual setting.

● *Attachment.* Ongoing attachment between newborn and parents is assessed. Parents may find it difficult to bond with an infant who is hypotonic, noninteractive, or inconsolable or who does not meet their preconceived picture of the ideal infant. Some indications of possible difficulties in attachment are verbalizations indicating disappointment with the newborn and lack of eye contact and physical comforting behaviors. Attachment is promoted by encouraging all family members to be involved with the new member of the family.

Nursing Diagnosis

Nursing diagnoses that may apply to the newborn and family in the provision of daily newborn care are presented in the Key Nursing Diagnoses to Consider—Daily Newborn Care.

Nursing Plan and Implementation of Daily Newborn Care

Maintenance of Cardiopulmonary Function

The newborn should always be placed in a prone or propped, side-lying position when left unattended to prevent aspiration and facilitate drainage of mucus. A bulb syringe is kept within easy reach should the baby need oral-

┌─────────────────────────────────┐

D͓ₓ
Key Nursing Diagnoses to Consider
Daily Newborn Care

Ineffective airway clearance

Hypothermia

Impaired skin integrity

Altered patterns of urinary elimination

Constipation

Infection: High risk

Altered nutrition: less than body requirements

Knowledge deficit

Altered health maintenance

Family coping: Potential for growth

Altered family processes

Altered parenting

└─────────────────────────────────┘

nasal suctioning. If the newborn has respiratory difficulty, the airway is cleared. Vigorous fingertip stroking of the baby's spine will frequently stimulate respiratory activity. A cardiorespiratory monitor can be used on newborns who are not being observed at all times and are at risk for decreased respiratory or cardiac function. Indicators of risk are pallor, cyanosis, a ruddy color, apnea, or other signs of instability.

Maintenance of Neutral Thermal Environment

Every effort is made to maintain the newborn's temperature within the normal range. The nurse must make certain the newborn is undressed and exposed to the air as little as possible. A stockinette or knit head covering should be used for the small newborn who has less subcutaneous fat to act as insulation in maintaining body heat. The ambient temperature of the room where the newborn is kept should be monitored routinely and kept at approximately 37.8C (70F). A newborn whose temperature falls below optimal levels will use calories to maintain body heat rather than for growth. Chilling also decreases the affinity of serum albumin for bilirubin, thereby increasing the likelihood of newborn jaundice.

A newborn who is overheated will increase activity and respiratory rate in an attempt to cool the body. Both measures deplete caloric reserves. In addition the increased respiratory rate leads to increased insensible fluid loss.

Promotion of Adequate Hydration and Nutrition

Infant nutrition is addressed in depth in Chapter 30. Adequate hydration is enhanced by maintaining a neutral thermal environment and by offering early and frequent feedings. Early feedings promote gastric emptying and increase peristalsis, thereby decreasing the potential for hyperbilirubinemia by decreasing the amount of time fecal material is in contact with the enzyme beta-glucuronidase in the small intestine. This enzyme acts to free the bilirubin from the feces, allowing bilirubin to be reabsorbed into the vascular system.

Excessive handling of the newborn can cause an increase in the newborn's metabolic rate and caloric use. The nurse should be alert to the baby's subtle cues of fatigue. These include turning the head away from eye contact, decrease in muscle tension and activity in the extremities and neck, and loss of eye contact, which may be manifested by fluttering or closure of the eyelids. The nurse quickly ceases stimulation when signs of fatigue emerge. The nurse's care should demonstrate to the parents the need for awareness of newborn cues and the use of periods of alertness in the baby for contact and stimulation.

Prevention of Complications and Promotion of Safety

Newborns are at continued risk for the complications of hemorrhage, late-onset cardiac symptoms, and infection.

Pallor may be an early sign of hemorrhage and must be reported to the physician. The newborn may be placed on a cardiorespiratory monitor to permit continuous as-sessment. All newborns are at risk from hemorrhage, but this is especially true following a circumcision procedure (see page 907). Cyanosis that is not relieved by oxygen administration requires emergency intervention, may indicate a congenital cardiac condition or shock, and requires ongoing assessment.

Infection in the nursery is best prevented by requiring that all personnel having direct contact with newborns follow a three-minute scrub procedure at the beginning of each shift. The hands must also be washed well before and after contact with every newborn or after touching any soiled surface such as the floor or one's hair or face. Parents are often instructed to use an antiseptic hand cleaner before touching the baby as well. Anyone with an infection should refrain from working with newborns until the infection has cleared. Some agencies ask fathers, siblings, and grandparents to wear a gown, preferably disposable, over their street clothes and to wash their hands before handling their newborn.

Safety of the newborn is provided through a variety of nursing interventions. It is essential to verify the identity of the newborn, by comparing the numbers and names on the identification bracelets of mother and newborn before giving a baby to a parent. Other safety issues are specifically covered later in the sections on circumcision, positioning and handling, bathing, nail care, and safety considerations.

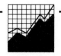

Research Note

Clinical Application of Research

Research does not support the traditional practice of wearing cover gowns in the normal newborn nursery, and the use of cover gowns adds a significant cost to nursery care. Therefore, Janet Rush and her associates (1990) constructed a study to examine the difference in colonization rates of *Staphylococcus aureus* between a group of newborns who received care with gowns and a group receiving care without gowns.

The 32-week study involved a total sample of 452 infants randomly assigned to either the control or experimental group. Infants were not restricted either from rooming-in or in numbers of visitors.

No statistically significant difference in colonization rates was found between the two groups based on gowning procedure. However, further examination of the data did explicate variables that were associated with positive colonization cultures. Statistically significant differences were found when the infants with positive cultures were compared with infants with negative cultures. The significant variables identified included number of vaginal examinations during labor, length of labor in hours, vaginal deliveries, and circumcision. No difference was found between the positive and negative groups with the following variables: use of internal monitor, breast-feeding, gender, length of stay, rooming-in, or number of visitors.

Critical Thinking Applied to Research

Strengths: Used observers to control for possible compensatory equalization of treatments since the care givers were not blind to assigned group (Cook & Campbell 1979). Completed a power analysis to determine number of subjects needed to obtain desired statistical significance.

Cook T, Campbell D: *Quasi-Experimentation: Design & Analysis Issues for Field Settings.* Boston: Houghton-Mifflin, 1979.

Rush J, Fiorino-Chiovitti R, Kaufman K et al: A randomized controlled trial of a nursery ritual: Wearing cover gowns to care for healthy newborns. *Birth* 1990; 17(1): 25.

CRITICAL THINKING

What factors should you consider when providing parents with information about their baby's care needs?

Enhancement of Parent-Infant Attachment

Attachment is promoted by encouraging all family members to be involved with the new member of the family. Specific interventions are examined in depth in Chapter 35, Teaching Guide 35–1.

Enhancement of Parental Knowledge of Infant Care

To meet parent needs for information, the nurse who is responsible for the daily care of the mother and newborn should assume the primary responsibility for education. Nearly every contact with the parents presents an opportunity for sharing information that can facilitate the parents' sense of competence in newborn care. The nurse also needs to recognize and respect the fact that there are many good ways to provide safe baby care. The parents' methods of giving care should be reinforced rather than contradicted unless their care methods are harmful to the newborn.

The information in the following section is provided to increase the nurse's knowledge of infant care and can also be used to meet parents' needs for information.

Opportunities for Parent Teaching

Parents may be familiar with handling and caring for infants, or this may be their first time to interact with a newborn. If they are new parents, the sensitive nurse gently teaches them by example and instructions geared to their needs and previous knowledge about the various aspects of newborn care.

The nurse observes how parents interact with their infant during feeding and caregiving activities. Rooming-in, even for a short time, offers opportunities for the nurse to provide information and evaluate whether the parents are comfortable with changing diapers and wrapping, handling, and feeding their newborn. Do both parents get involved in the infant's care? Is the mother depending on someone else to help her at home? Does the mother give excuses for not wanting to be involved in her baby's care? ("I am too tired," "My stitches hurt," or "I will learn later.") All these considerations need to be taken into account when evaluating the educational needs of the parents.

Several methods may be used to teach parents about newborn care. Daily child care classes are a nonthreatening way to convey general information. Individual instruction is helpful to answer specific questions or to clarify an item that may have been confusing in class (Figure 29–7). See

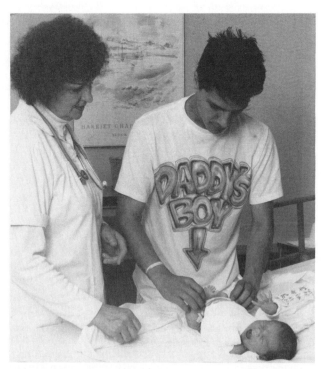

Figure 29–7 Individualizing parent education. Father returns demonstration of diapering his daughter.

Teaching Guide–What to Tell Parents About Daily Infant Care.

Discharge planning is necessary to verify the mother's knowledge when she leaves the hospital. Follow-up calls or visits after discharge lend added support by providing another opportunity for parents to have their questions answered.

With the new life come new rhythms. Or perhaps I should say no rhythms. The day is divided into phone calls, meals eaten on the run, visitors who've come to see the baby, trips from hospital to home to walk the dog.

The new life brings new thoughts, new perceptions of the world.

Why don't men take paternity leaves? Why is time off, if any, basically reserved for women? Why don't we take a month off. In those first few chaotic days, filled with ecstasy and fear, the family needs to be together. Being together in times of joy and sadness is what a family is. A month's distance from the office grind, from the bottom line could not help but create a healthier world. (Dennis Donziger, Daddy)

Positioning and Handling

Methods of positioning and handling the newborn are demonstrated to parents if needed. As the parents provide care, the nurse can enhance parental confidence by giving them positive feedback. If the parents encounter problems, the nurse can express confidence in their abilities to master the new skill or information, suggest alternatives, and serve as a role model.

How to pick up a newborn is one of the first concerns of anyone who has not handled many babies. When the infant is in the side-lying position, he or she is easily picked up by sliding one hand under the baby's neck and shoulders and the other hand under the buttocks or between the legs, then gently lifting the newborn from the crib. This technique provides security and support for the head (which the baby is unable to support until the age of 3 or 4 months).

After the baby is out of the crib, one of three holds may be used (Figure 29–8). The *cradle hold* is frequently used during feeding. It provides a sense of warmth and closeness, permits eye contact, frees one of the nurse's or parent's hands, and provides security because the cradling protects the newborn's body. Extra security is provided by gripping the thigh with the hand while the arm supports the infant's body. The *upright position* provides security and a sense of closeness and is a good position for burping the infant. One hand should support the neck and shoulders, while the other hand holds the buttocks or is placed

TEACHING GUIDE
What to Tell Parents About Daily Infant Care

Assessment The nurse determines parents' prior knowledge and experience with infants and any concerns they may have about caring for their baby.

Nursing Diagnosis The key nursing diagnoses would be: Knowledge deficit related to ongoing newborn daily care needs and Alterations in parenting related to integration of new family member.

Nursing Plan and Implementation The teaching plan will include information about sponge and tub baths, umbilical cord care, care of circumcised and uncircumcised infant, feeding techniques, elimination patterns, use of bulb syringe, signs and symptoms of illness, expected

sleep patterns, comfort measures, and attachment behaviors.

Demonstration of bath, cord care, use of bulb syringe, thermometer, and comfort measures

Parent Goals At the completion of the class the parents will be able to:

1. Demonstrate safe techniques of caring for their infant, especially in use of bulb syringe, thermometer, cord cleaning, and comforting measures.
2. List signs and symptoms of illness.
3. Describe infant's sleep patterns and attachment behaviors.

Teaching Plan

Content Demonstrate bathing techniques of sponge and tub (see p 899) emphasizing safety and timing of cord separation. Demonstrate cord care to be carried out at home—see Teaching Guide, p 901 for specific techniques.

Discuss care required for circumcised and uncircumcised infants (see p 907).

Discuss the signs of illness (see Table 29–5) and demonstrate use of thermometer and bulb syringe.

Discuss normal newborn eating, sleep, elimination patterns and behavioral characteristics.

Demonstrate comfort measures for infants

Evaluation Parents are able to describe general infant care. Parents demonstrate use of bulb syringe, taking temperature, umbilical cord care, and care of circumcision (if appropriate) to primary nurse prior to discharge from birthing center.

Teaching Method Discussion and demonstration. Stress basic useful information that new parents need. Avoid patronizing tone. Provide opportunities for parents to practice.

Demonstration, discussion

Discussion, handouts, pamphlets and posters are helpful, as are videos.

Discussion, demonstration, and return demonstration.

---

between the newborn's legs. The *football hold* frees one of the care giver's hands and permits eye contact. This hold is ideal for shampooing, carrying, or breast-feeding. It frees the parent to talk on the telephone or answer the door at home or do the myriad of tasks that await his or her attention.

The newborn infant is most frequently positioned on the side with a rolled blanket or cloth diaper behind the back for support (Figure 29–9). A side-lying position aids drainage of mucus and allows air to circulate around the cord. It is also more comfortable for the newly circumcised male. After feeding, the newborn is placed on the right side

to prevent aspiration of regurgitated feeding and to aid digestion; this position makes it easier to expel air bubbles from the stomach.

Once the cord is healed, many newborns prefer to lie on their stomachs. Newborns have enough head control to turn their heads from side to side to prevent suffocation.

The baby's position should be changed periodically during the early months of life, because neonatal skull bones are soft, and flattened areas may develop if the newborn consistently lies in one position. The newborn should not be left in a supine position when unattended due to the danger of aspiration.

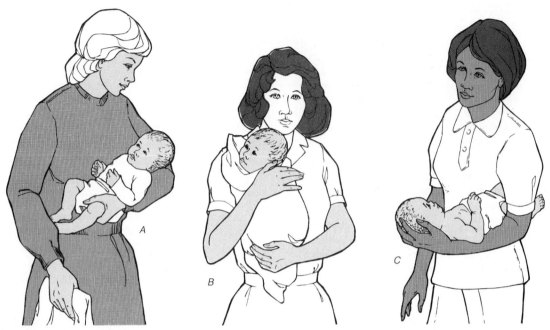

Figure 29–8 Various positions for holding an infant. A Cradle hold. B Upright position. C Football hold.

Nasal and Oral Suctioning

Most babies are obligatory nose breathers for the first months of life. They generally maintain air passage patency by coughing or sneezing. During the first few days of life, however, the newborn has increased mucus, and gentle suctioning with a bulb syringe may be indicated. The nurse can demonstrate the use of the bulb syringe in the nose and mouth and have the parents do a return demonstration. The parents should repeat this demonstration before discharge so they will feel more confident and comfortable with the procedure.

To suction the newborn, the bulb syringe is compressed, then the tip is placed in the nostril, taking care not to occlude the passageway, and the bulb is permitted to re-expand slowly as the nurse or parent releases the compression on the bulb (Figure 29–10). The bulb syringe is removed from the nostril and drainage is then compressed out of the bulb onto a tissue. The bulb syringe may also be used in the mouth if the newborn is spitting up and unable to handle the excess secretions. The bulb is compressed; the tip of the bulb syringe is placed about 1 inch in one side of the infant's mouth; and compression is released. This draws up the excess secretions. The procedure is repeated on the other side of the mouth. The roof of the mouth and back of the throat is avoided because suction in this area might stimulate the gag reflex. The bulb syringe should be washed in warm, soapy water and rinsed in warm water daily. A bulb syringe should always be kept near the newborn. New parents and nurses who are inexperienced with babies may fear that the baby will choke and may be relieved if they know how to take action if such an event occurs. They should be advised to turn the newborn's head to the side or down as soon as there is any indications of gagging or vomiting and to use the bulb syringe as needed.

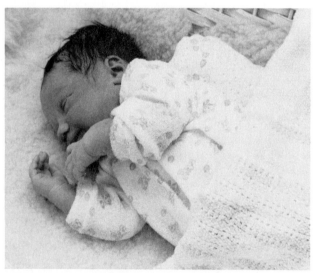

Figure 29–9 The most common sleeping position of the newborn is on the side. A rolled blanket is placed behind the back to provide additional support.

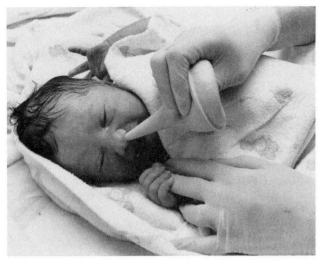

Figure 29–10   Nasal and oral suctioning. The bulb is compressed, then the tip is placed in either the mouth or nose; the bulb is released.

Bathing

An actual bath demonstration is the best way for the nurse to provide information to parents. Because excess bathing and use of soap will dry out the baby's sensitive skin, bathing should be done every other day or twice a week. Sponge baths are recommended for the first two weeks or until the umbilical cord completely falls off and has healed.

Supplies can be kept in a plastic bag or some type of container to avoid hunting for them each time. The mother may want to use a small plastic tub, a clean kitchen or bathroom sink, or a large bowl. Expensive baby tubs are not necessary, but some parents may prefer to purchase them (see Table 29–4).

Before starting, if no one else is at home, the parent may want to take the phone off the hook and put a sign on

Table 29–4   Bath Supplies
Washcloths
Towels
Blanket
Nonperfumed mild soap (eg, Castile, Neutrogena)
Shampoo
Petroleum jelly or A and D ointment
Rubbing alcohol
Cotton balls
Diapers
Clean clothes

the door to prevent being disturbed or decide just to ignore these intrusions. Having someone home during the first few baths will be helpful because that person can get forgotten items and provide moral support. The room should be warm and free of drafts.

Sponge Bath

After the supplies are gathered, the tub (or any of the containers mentioned above) is filled with water that is warm to the touch. The water temperature is tested with an elbow or forearm. Parents may also choose to purchase a thermometer to help them determine when the bath water is at approximately 37.8C (100F) and safe to use. Soap should not be added to the water. The infant should be wrapped in a blanket, with a T-shirt and diaper on. This helps keep the newborn warm and secure.

To start the bath, a washcloth is wrapped around the index finger once. Each of the baby's eyes is gently wiped from inner to outer corner. This direction is the way eyes naturally drain, and wiping in this direction prevents irritation of the eyes. A different portion of the washcloth is used for each eye to prevent cross-contamination. Cotton balls can also be used for this purpose, using a new one for each eye. Some swelling and drainage may be common the first few days after birth.

The ears are washed next by wrapping the washcloth once around an index finger and gently cleaning the external ear and behind the ear. Cotton swabs are never used in the ear canal because it is possible to put the swab too far into the ear and damage the ear drum. In addition, the swab may pack any discharge farther down into the ear canal.

The remainder of the baby's face is then wiped with the soap free washcloth. Many babies start to cry at this point. The face should be washed every day and the mouth and chin wiped off after each feeding.

The neck is washed carefully but thoroughly with the washcloth. Soap may now be used. Castile soap or nonperfumed soap is preferable to a strong deodorant soap, which may irritate sensitive skin. Formula or breast milk and lint collect in the skin folds of the neck, so it may be helpful to sit the baby up, supporting the neck and shoulders with one hand while washing the neck with the other hand.

The baby's T-shirt is now removed and the blanket unwrapped. The chest, back, and arms are wet with the washcloth. The parent may then lather his or her hands with soap and wash the baby's chest, back, and arms. Wetting the cord is avoided, if possible, because it delays drying. Soap is rinsed off with the wet washcloth, and the upper part of the body is dried with a towel or blanket. The baby's upper body is then wrapped with a dry clean blanket to prevent a chill.

Next the infant's legs are unwrapped, wet with the washcloth, lathered, rinsed, and well dried. If the infant has dry skin, a *small* amount of unperfumed lotion or ointment (petroleum jelly or A and D ointment) may be used. Ointments are better than lotions for dry cracked feet and hands. Baby oil is not recommended because it clogs skin pores. Powders aggravate dry skin and should be avoided.

Both baby oil and baby powder can cause serious respiratory problems if inhaled. Parents should be warned of this danger and advised to take measures to prevent these substances from being aspirated by the baby. If parents want to use powder, advise them to select one that is talc free. The powder should be shaken into the parent's hand and then placed on the infant rather than shaking the powder directly over the baby.

The genital area is cleaned daily with soap and water and with water after each wet or dirty diaper. Girls are washed from the *front* of the genital area toward the rectum to avoid fecal contamination of the urethra and thus to the bladder. Newborn girls often have a thick, white mucous discharge or a slight bloody discharge from the vagina. This discharge is normal for the first one to two weeks and should be wiped off gently with a damp cloth at diaper changes.

Parents of uncircumcised newborn boys should clean the small exposed area of the glans daily (King et al 1989). For in-depth discussion of care of uncircumcised boys, see page 907.

Newborn boys who have been circumcised also need daily gentle cleaning. A very wet washcloth is rubbed over a bar of soap. The washcloth is squeezed above the baby's penis, letting the soapy water run over the circumcision site. The area is rinsed off with plain warm water and lightly patted dry. A small amount of petroleum jelly, A and D ointment, or bactericidal ointment may be put on the circumcised area, but excessive amounts may block the meatus and should be avoided. If a Plastibell is in place, no ointment should be put on the penis. The Plastibell usually falls off within five to eight days. If it doesn't, the parents need to call the health care provider.

It is important to cleanse the diaper area with each diaper change in order to prevent diaper rash. Although this cleansing is done on a routine basis, a diaper rash may occasionally occur.

Baby powder (or cornstarch) is not recommended for diaper rash. Baby powder may cake with urine and irritate the infant's perineal area. Cornstarch may promote fungal infection. Ointments that provide a barrier, such as zinc oxide, A and D ointment, or petroleum jelly are more effective for diaper rash. If the ointment does not help the rash, parents using disposable diapers should try another brand of diaper. If cloth diapers are used, a different detergent or fabric softener may alleviate the problem. If the rash persists, parents should discuss the problem with a nurse practitioner or physician because it may be a yeast or fungal infection.

The umbilical cord should be kept clean and dry. The close proximity of the umbilical vessels makes the cord a common portal for infection. Various preparations such as triple dye, alcohol, hexachlorophene, Betadine, and Bacitracin are used for newborn cord care in nurseries to promote drying and provide a bactericidal effect. Triple dye may be used and seems to be a highly effective antistaphylococcal agent (Coen & Koeffler 1987). At discharge, most parents are advised to clean the area around the cord with a cotton ball and alcohol two to three times a day until the cord is completely gone and the stump is healed. The cord stump generally falls off in 7 to 14 days. The diaper should be folded down to allow air to circulate around the cord. The care provider should be consulted if redness appears around the umbilicus, bright red bleeding or pus-like drainage occurs, or if the area remains unhealed two to three days after the cord stump has sloughed off. See Teaching Guide–What to Tell Parents About Home Cord Care.

The last step in bathing is washing the infant's hair (some suggest doing this step first). The newborn is swaddled in a dry blanket, leaving only the head exposed and held in the football hold with the head tilted slightly downward to prevent water running in the eyes. Water should be brought to the head by a cupped hand. The hair is moistened and lathered with a small amount of shampoo. A *very* soft brush may be used to massage the shampoo over the entire head. The brush may be used over the soft spots. Frequently a disposable soapless scrub brush is used because the bristles are soft and pliable. The hair is then rinsed and toweled dry. To assist in preventing cradle cap, the infant's hair should be brushed every day and the hair washed during baths. Oils or lotions are not used on the newborn's head unless there is evidence of cradle cap. Moistening the scaly area with lotion half an hour or more before shampooing softens the crusts or scales and makes it easier to remove them.

Tub Baths

The infant may be put in a tub after the cord has fallen off and the circumcision site is healed (approximately two weeks) (Figure 29–11). Infants usually enjoy a tub bath more than a sponge bath, although some newborns cry during either type.

Only 2 or 3 inches of water are needed in the tub. To prevent slipping, a washcloth is placed in the bottom of the tub or sink, or the baby can be brought into a tub with the parent.

The face is washed in the same manner as for a sponge bath. The parent then places the newborn in the tub using the cradle hold and grasping the distal thigh. The neck is supported by the parent's elbow in the cradle position. An alternative hold is to support the newborn's head and neck with the parent's forearm while grasping the distal shoulder and arm.

Because wet infants are slippery, some parents have found that pulling a cotton sock (with holes cut out for the fingers) over the arm will prevent the baby from slipping.

The body may be washed with a soapy washcloth or hand. To wash the baby's back, the parent places his or her noncradling hand on the infant's chest with the thumb under the infant's arm closest to the parent. Gently tipping the baby forward onto the supporting hand frees the cradling arm to wash the back of the baby. After the bath the

TEACHING GUIDE
What to Tell Parents About Home Umbilical Cord Care

Assessment The nurse focuses on the parents' previous experience with newborns and their understanding of what the umbilical cord is and what naturally happens during the first few weeks after birth.

Nursing Diagnosis The key nursing diagnoses will probably be: Knowledge deficit related to home care of the umbilical cord and Infection High risk related to contamination of umbilical cord.

Nursing Plan and Implementation The teaching plan will include information about the need for daily cleansing, expected changes in the umbilical cord, and demonstration of actual procedure for care of the umbilical cord.

Parent Goals At the completion of the teaching session the parents will be able to:

1. State the normal changes in the umbilical cord.
2. List the signs of infection of the cord.
3. Demonstrate proper cord care.

Teaching Plan

Content Explain the following steps in performing cord care:

1. Clean the cord and skin around base of cord with a cotton ball or cotton-tipped swab. Lift the cord stump and, using a wet cotton ball with 70% isopropyl, wipe around the cord. Start at the top and wipe around halfway; then rotate cotton ball and start at the top again and wipe around the other half of the cord. With a cotton-tipped swab, swab around the base of the cord to clean away any drainage, since bacteria grows on dried drainage. Cord care should be done at least two to three times a day, or it could be done with each diaper change. Baby may cry when the cold alcohol touches the tummy; however, cord care is not painful because there are no nerve ends in the cord. No tub baths until the cord falls off in 7–14 days.

2. Fold diapers below the umbilical cord to air-dry the cord. Wet or soiled diapers slow the drying process and increase the possibility of infection.

3. Check the cord each day for any odor, oozing of yellow puslike material, or reddened areas around the cord. The area around the cord may also be tender. Report any signs of infection to health care provider.

Normal changes in cord: Cord should look dark and dry up, falling off at about 7–14 days after birth. A little drop of blood may appear on the diaper as the cord is about to fall off. Never pull the cord or attempt to loosen it.

Evaluation Teaching has been effective and learning has occurred if the parents are able to identify the signs of infection and normal changes seen in the cord prior to its falling off and can demonstrate proper cord care procedure prior to baby's discharge.

Teaching Method Discussion

Use of poster showing cleaning techniques, position of diapers, and colored pictures of signs of infection.

Demonstration of cord cleaning.

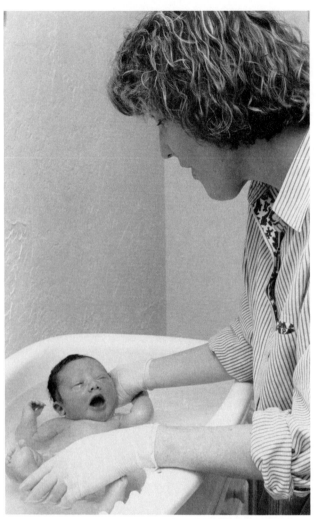

Figure 29–11 Tub bath. When bathing the infant, it is important to support the head.

baby is lifted out of the tub in the cradle position, dried well, and wrapped in a dry blanket. The hair can then be washed in the same way as for a sponge bath.

Nail Care

The nails of the newborn are seldom cut in the birthing unit. During the first days of life, the nails may adhere to the skin of the fingers, and cutting is contraindicated. Within a week the nails separate from the skin and frequently break off. If the nails are long or if infants are scratching themselves, the nails may be trimmed. This is most easily done while babies sleep. Nails should be cut straight across using adult cuticle scissors or blunt-ended infant cuticle scissors.

Wrapping the Newborn

Wrapping (swaddling) helps the newborn maintain body temperature, provides a feeling of closeness and security, and may be effective in quieting a crying baby. When wrap-

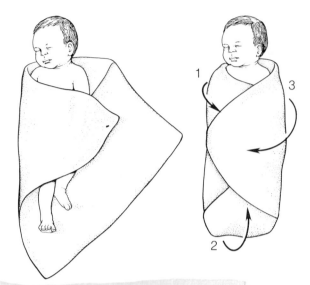

Figure 29–12 Steps used for wrapping a baby

ping, a blanket is placed on the crib (or secure surface) in the shape of a diamond. The top corner of the blanket is folded down slightly, and the baby's body is placed with the head at the upper edge of the blanket. The right corner of the blanket is wrapped around the infant and tucked under the left side (not too tightly—newborns need a little room to move). The bottom corner is then pulled up to the chest, and the left corner is wrapped around the baby's right side (Figure 29–12). This wrapping technique can be shared with a new mother so she will feel more skilled in handling her baby.

Dressing the Newborn

Newborns need to wear a T-shirt, diaper, (diaper cover or plastic pants if using cloth diapers), and a sleeper. On a fairly cool day, they should also be wrapped in a light blanket while being fed.

A good rule of thumb is for the parent to add one more light layer of clothing than the parent is wearing. An infant may be covered with a blanket in air-conditioned buildings. The blanket should be unwrapped or removed when inside a warm building.

At home the amount of clothing the infant wears is determined by the temperature. Families who maintain the home at 60F to 65F should dress the infant more warmly than those who maintain the temperature at 70F to 75F.

Infants should wear head coverings outdoors to protect their sensitive ears from drafts. The blanket can be wrapped around the infant, leaving one corner free to place over the head while outdoors or in crowds for added protection. Parents must also be advised of the ease with which a baby's skin can burn when exposed to the sun. To prevent sunburn the baby should remain shaded, wear a light layer of clothing, or be protected with a sunscreen product.

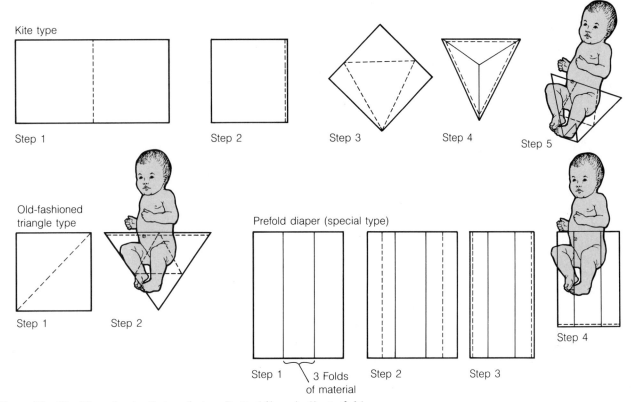

Figure 29–13   Three basic diaper shapes. Dotted lines indicate folds.

Diaper shapes vary and are subject to personal preference (Figure 29–13). Prefolded and disposable diapers are usually rectangular. Cloth diapers may also be triangular or kite-folded. Extra material is placed in front for boys and toward the back for girls to aid in absorbency.

Baby clothing should be laundered separately using a mild soap or detergent. Diapers may be presoaked before washing. All clothing should be rinsed twice to remove soap and residue and to decrease the possibility of rash. Some babies may not tolerate clothing treated with fabric softeners added to the washer or softener sheets added to the dryer.

Temperature Assessment

The nurse demonstrates how to take axillary and rectal temperatures for the parents. A return demonstration is an effective way to evaluate their understanding. The different types of thermometers are discussed with parents. It is important that parents understand the differences and how to select the appropriate one. Other general instructions include how to shake the mercury down (the mercury needs to be below 94F on the thermometer) and how to read the thermometer.

When parents take a rectal temperature, the infant should be supine with the legs held up in one hand, exposing the rectum. The end of the rectal thermometer is lubricated with petroleum jelly, and the thermometer is in-

serted just until the silver bulb is covered, approximately *half an inch*. The thermometer is held in place *five minutes*. A baby is never left alone with a thermometer in place and the adult must maintain a hold on the thermometer at all times. Some pediatricians think that rectal temperatures are more accurate and prefer that parents take temperatures this way; others think rectal temperatures are more dangerous and irritating for the baby. Parents may be more receptive to taking axillary temperatures and should make their preferences known to the care giver.

To take an axillary temperature, the thermometer is placed under one of the infant's arms, making sure that the bulb of the thermometer is underneath the armpit. It is held in place *three to four minutes* (Figure 28–14). It is important to hold the baby's arm still because friction between the arm and chest creates heat and can make the thermometer record an inaccurate temperature.

A parent needs to take the newborn's temperature only when the signs of illness are present. Parents are advised to call their physician or pediatric nurse practitioner immediately if any of the signs listed in Table 29–5 occur. Parents should also check with their clinician for advice about over-the-counter medications they should have in the medicine cabinet. All parents should be advised to avoid giving any form of aspirin to their infants for any illness that may be viral. Use of aspirin in viral illnesses has been linked to Reye syndrome in children under 19 years

Table 29–5 When Parents Should Call Their Health Care Provider

If any of the following signs are present, parents need to call their health provider:

- Temperature above 38.4C (101F) rectally or 38C (100.4F) axillary or below 36.1C (97F) rectally or 36.6C (97.8F) axillary
- Continual rise in temperature
- More than one episode of forceful vomiting or frequent vomiting (over 6 hours).
- Refusal of two feedings in a row
- Lethargy (listlessness), difficulty in wakening baby
- Cyanosis with or without a feeding
- Absence of breathing longer than 15 seconds
- Inconsolable infant (quieting techniques are not effective) or continuous high-pitched cry
- Discharge or bleeding from any opening
- Two consecutive green, watery stools
- No wet diapers for 18 to 24 hours or less than 6 wet diapers per day.

of age. Flu, colds, teething, constipation, diarrhea, and other common ailments and their management should be discussed with the clinician before they occur.

Stools and Urine

The appearance and frequency of the newborn's stools can cause concern for parents. The nurse prepares parents by discussing and showing pictures of meconium stools, transitional stools, and the difference between breast-milk and formula stools.

Although each baby develops his or her own stooling patterns, parents can be given an idea of what to expect. Parents should be told that breast-fed babies may have six to ten small, yellow stools per day by the third or fourth day since milk production is now established unless the mother is having problems with her milk supply. Once breast-feeding is well established, usually by one month, the infant may have only one stool every few days because of the increased digestibility of breast milk. Constipation is unlikely to occur in infants receiving only breast milk. Infrequent stooling in the first few weeks may be indicative of inadequate milk intake (Neifert 1989). Bottle-fed infants may have only one or two stools a day. The stools are more formed and will be yellow or yellow-brown in color. The parents may also be shown pictures of a constipated (small, pelletlike) stool and diarrhea (loose, green ringed with water, or perhaps blood-tinged). Parents should understand that a green color is common in transitional stools so that transitional stools are not confused with diarrhea in the first week of a newborn's life. However, it is important to help parents differentiate a greenish-colored transitional stool and a green diarrheal stool.

Constipation may be an indication that the baby needs additional fluid intake. The parents might try offering

additional water in an attempt to reverse the constipation. Babies normally void six to ten times per day. Fewer than six wet diapers a day may indicate the newborn needs more fluids. Frequency of voiding is easy to assess with cloth diapers. Parents who use the newer super-absorbent disposable diapers may have difficulty determining voiding patterns.

Sleep and Activity

Perhaps nothing is more individual to each baby than the sleep-activity cycle. It is important for the nurse to recognize the individual variations of each newborn and to assist parents as they develop sensitivity to their infant's communication signals and rhythms of activity and sleep. (See Table 29–6)

The newborn demonstrates several different sleep-wake states (see Chapter 27) after the initial periods of reactivity described earlier. It is not uncommon for a baby to sleep almost continuously for the first two to three days following birth, awakening only for feedings every three or four hours. Some newborns bypass this stage of deep sleep and may require only 12 to 16 hours of sleep. The parents need to know that this is normal.

Quiet sleep is characterized by regular breathing and no movement except for sudden body jerks. During this sleep state, normal household noise will not awaken the infant. In the *active sleep state,* the newborn has irregular breathing and fine muscular twitching. The newborn may cry out during sleep, but this does not mean he or she is uncomfortable or awake. Unusual household noise may awaken the infant more easily in this state; however, the newborn will quickly go back to sleep.

Quiet, alert is a state in which newborns are quietly involved with the environment. They watch a moving mobile, smile, and as they become older, discover and play with their hands and feet. When infants become uncomfortable due to wet diapers, hunger, or cold, they enter the *active awake and crying state.* In this state, the cause of the crying should be identified and eliminated. Sometimes parents are frustrated as they try to identify the external or internal stimuli that are causing the angry, hurt crying. Parents need to be told that the baby's state may be changed from crying to quiet alert by moving the baby toward an upright position where scanning and exploration are possible (Klaus & Klaus 1985).

Crying

For the newborn, crying is the only means of expressing needs vocally. Parents and care givers learn to distinguish different tones and qualities of the neonate's cry. The amount of crying is highly individual. Some will cry as little as 15 to 30 minutes in 24 hours or as long as 2 hours every 24 hours. When crying continues after causes such as discomfort or hunger are eliminated, the newborn may be comforted by swaddling or by rocking and other reassuring activities. There is some indication that infants who are held more tend to be calmer and cry less when not being

Table 29–6 Infant State* Chart (Sleep and Awake States)

	Characteristics of state					
Sleep states	Body activity	Eye movements	Facial movements	Breathing pattern	Level of response	Implications for care giving
Deep sleep	Nearly still except for occasional startle or twitch	None	Without facial movements, except for occasional sucking movement at regular intervals	Smooth and regular	Only very intense and disturbing stimuli will arouse infants.	Care givers trying to feed infant in deep sleep will probably find the experience frustrating. Infants will be unresponsive, even if care givers use disturbing stimuli (flicking feet) to arouse infants. Infants may only arouse briefly and then become unresponsive as they return to deep sleep. If care givers wait until infants move to a higher, more responsive state, feeding or care giving will be much more pleasant.
Light sleep	Some body movements	Rapid eye movement (REM): Fluttering of eyes beneath closed eyelids	May smile and make brief fussy or crying sounds	Irregular	More responsive to internal and external stimuli. When these stimuli occur, infants may remain in light sleep or move to drowsy state.	Light sleep makes up the highest proportion of newborn sleep and usually precedes wakening. Due to brief fussy or crying sounds made during this state, care givers who are not aware that these sounds occur normally may think it is time for feeding and may try to feed infants before they are ready to eat.
Drowsy	Activity level variable, with mild startles interspersed from time to time; movements usually smooth	Eyes open and close occasionally; are heavy-lidded with dull, glazed appearance	May have some facial movements; often there are none and the face appears still	Irregular	Infants react to sensory stimuli although responses are delayed. State change after stimulation frequently noted.	From the drowsy state infants may return to sleep or awaken further. In order to wake them care givers can provide something for infants to see, hear, or suck, as this may arouse them to quiet alert state, a more responsive state. Infants left alone without stimuli may return to a sleep state.
Quiet alert	Minimal	Brightening and widening of eyes	Faces have bright, shining, sparkling looks	Regular	Infants attend most to environment, focusing attention on any stimuli that are present.	Infants in this state provide much pleasure and positive feedback for care givers. Providing something for infants to see, hear, or suck will often maintain a quiet alert state in the first few hours after birth. Most newborns commonly experience a period of intense alertness before going into a long sleeping period.
Active alert	Much body activity; may have periods of fussiness	Eyes open with less brightening	Much facial movement; faces not as bright as in alert state	Irregular	Increasingly sensitive to disturbing stimuli (hunger, fatigue, noise, excessive handling).	Care givers may intervene at this stage to console and to bring infants to a lower state.
Crying	Increased motor activity with color changes	Eyes may be tightly closed or open	Grimaces	More irregular	Extremely responsive to unpleasant external or internal stimuli.	Crying is the infant's communication signal. It is a response to unpleasant stimuli from the environment or from within infants (fatigue, hunger, discomfort). Crying tells us infants have been reached. Sometimes infants can console themselves and return to lower states. At other times they need help from care givers.

*State *is a group of characteristics that regularly occur together: body activity, eye movements, facial movements, breathing pattern, and level of response to external stimuli (eg, handling) and internal stimuli (eg, hunger).*

From Blackburn S, Kang R: Early parent-infant relationships. 2nd ed, module 3, series 1. The First Six Hours After Birth. White Plains, NY: March of Dimes Birth Defects Foundation, in press. Reprinted with permission of the copyright holder.

Contemporary Issue
To Circumcise or Not to Circumcise?

Circumcision is the most frequently performed surgical procedure in the United States. Circumcisions are carried out on anywhere from 30% of males born in alternative birth settings to 80% to 90% of those born in traditional hospital settings. This surgical procedure continues in spite of the American Academy of Pediatrics 1989 statement "that newborn circumcision has potential medical benefits and advantages as well as disadvantages and risks. When circumcision is being considered the benefits and risks should be explained to the parents and informed consent obtained." (American Academy of Pediatrics, 1989, p 390)

What then motivates parents to have their male newborns circumcised? Various reasons have been given for the circumcision, including: traditional practice (It's always been done—why question it?); wanting the child to have a similar appearance to the father; rites of passage into manhood (religious and cultural rites); desire to conform to the dominant culture; sexual adequacy and cosmetic appearance; and hygiene. Opponents provide equally strong

rationale and cultural data for not carrying out this procedure. It is important for nurses to identify and acknowledge the sociocultural motivating factors involved in the decision to circumcise or not to circumcise.

The current controversy over the continuation of the practice of circumcision raises important issues and concerns of parents.

- When is the optimal time for providing parents information about the circumcision procedure?
- What information should be provided to facilitate an informed choice?
- How do sociocultural factors influence the continued practice of circumcision?
- How does the health professional's ethnocentrism affect the information provided parents?
- Does the child have a right to freedom from pain (if circumcision is done without anesthesia)?

---

held. Some parents may be afraid that holding the baby may "spoil" the baby and will need reassurance and information. Excessive crying should be noted and assessed, taking other factors into consideration. After the first two or three days, newborns settle into individual patterns.

Circumcision

Circumcision is a surgical procedure in which the prepuce, an epithelial layer covering the penis, is separated from the glans penis and is excised. This permits exposure of the glans for easier cleaning.

The parents make the decision about circumcision for their newborn male child. In most cases the choice is based on cultural, social, and family tradition. To ensure informed consent, parents should be informed about possible long-term medical effects of circumcision and noncircumcision during the prenatal period.

Recommendations regarding circumcision have varied in the past. Prior to about 1980, circumcision was recommended by the American Academy of Pediatrics; then, from 1980 to 1988, it was no longer recommended. Cultural practices, social customs, parental wishes, and sometimes lack of knowledge regarding the procedure results in many parents choosing to have the male child circumcised. In 1988, the American Academy of Pediatrics wrote a position paper again recommending circumcision and cited the following medical reasons: It helps prevent phimosis (ste-

nosis of the preputial space), paraphimosis and balanoposthitis (inflammation of the glans penis and foreskin); the incidence of penile cancer is lower in men in the United States; and there is a decreased incidence of urinary tract infections in infants under 1 year of age (Wiswell 1987). It should still be considered an elective procedure, but the procedure should not be performed if the newborn is premature or compromised, has a known bleeding problem, or is born with a genitourinary defect such as hypospadias or epispadias, which may necessitate the use of the foreskin in future surgical repairs (Cunningham et al 1989; Lund 1990).

Circumcision was originally a religious rite of the Jewish religion and ritual circumcision is also practiced by Moslems (Scharli 1989). The practice gained widespread cultural acceptance in the United States but is done infrequently in many European countries. Many parents choose circumcision because they want the infant to have a similar physical appearance to the father or the majority of other children, or they may feel that it is expected by society (King et al 1989).

Another frequently cited reason for circumcising newborn males is to prevent the need for anesthesia, hospitalization, pain, and trauma should the procedure be needed later in life (Lund 1990). Cunningham et al (1989) noted that only 5% to 10% of males are estimated to be in this category.

Nurse's Role   The nurse plays an essential role in providing parents with current information about circumcision. Nurses can facilitate parental informed consent because of their knowledge of the medical, social, and psychologic aspects of newborn circumcision. A well-versed nurse can allay parents' anxiety by sharing information and allowing them to express their concerns. Parents must be informed about potential risks and outcomes of circumcision. Hemorrhage, infection, difficulty in voiding, separation of the edges of the circumcision, discomfort, and restlessness are early potential problems. Later there is the risk that the glans and urethral meatus can become irritated and inflamed from contact with ammonia from urine. Ulcerations and progressive stenosis may develop. Adhesions, entrapment of the penis, and damage to the urethra are all potential complications that could require surgical correction (King et al 1989).

Parents who are doubtful about their ability to use good hygienic practices in caring for their uncircumcised male infant and child require information from the nurse. They should be told that the foreskin and glans are two similar layers of cells that separate from each other. The separation process begins prenatally and is normally completed at between three and five years of age. Parents need to understand that physiologic preputial nonretractability is the norm for infancy (Lund 1990). In the process of separation, sterile sloughed cells build up between the layers. This buildup looks similar to the smegma secreted after puberty, and it is harmless. Occasionally during the daily bath, the parents can gently test for retraction. If retraction has occurred, daily gentle washing of the glans with soap and water is sufficient to maintain adequate cleanliness (Gibbons 1984). The child should be taught to incorporate this practice into his daily self-care activities.

If circumcision is to be done, the procedure is not usually done until the day before discharge when the newborn is well stabilized and there is less chance of cold stress. The parents may also choose to have the circumcision done after discharge. However, they need to be advised that if the baby is older than 1 month, he will probably be hospitalized, and the procedure will be done in surgery under general anesthesia.

The nurse's responsibilities during a circumcision are to determine if the parents have any further questions about the procedure and to ensure that the circumcision permit is signed. The nurse gathers the equipment and prepares the newborn by removing the diaper and placing him on a circumcision board or some other type of restraint (Figure 29–14). In the Jewish ceremonies, the infant is held by the parent and given wine before the procedure.

There are a variety of techniques for circumcision (Figures 29–15, 29–16), and all produce minimal bleeding. During the procedure, the nurse assesses the newborn's response. One consideration is pain experienced by the newborn. Some physicians use local anesthesia for this procedure. The American Academy of Pediatrics Committee on the Fetus and Newborn and Committee on Drugs (1987) have published a policy statement endorsing the administration of local or systemic anesthesia to infants undergoing surgical procedures. A dorsal penile nerve block (DPNB) using 1% Lidocaine without epinephrine significantly minimizes the pain and the shifts in behavioral

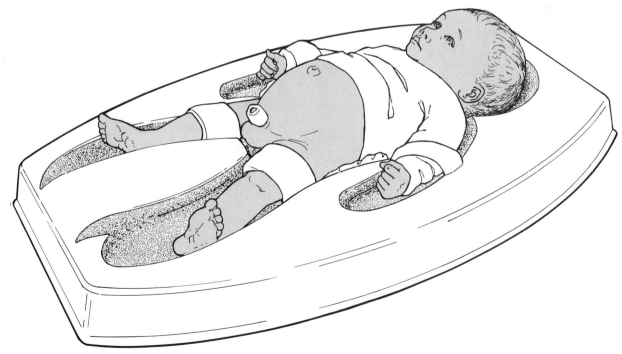

Figure 29–14   Proper positioning of the infant on a circumcision restraining board

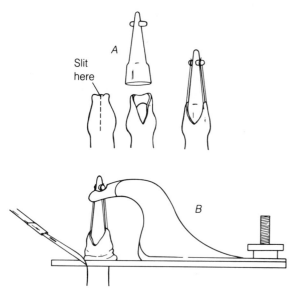

Figure 29–15   When the Yellen or Gumco clamp is used for circumcision, the prepuce is drawn over the cone (A), and the clamp is applied (B). Pressure is maintained for three to five minutes, and then the excess prepuce is cut away.

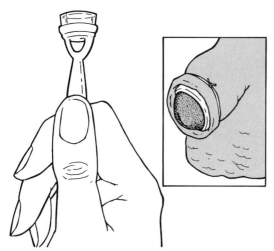

Figure 29–16   Circumcision using the Plastibell. The bell is fitted over the glans. A suture is tied around the bell's rim, and the excess prepuce is cut away. The plastic rim remains in place for three to four days until healing takes place. The bell may be allowed to fall off or may be removed if still in place after eight days.

patterns such as crying, irritability, and erratic sleep cycles (Stang et al 1988; Lund 1990).

The nurse can provide comfort measures such as lightly stroking the baby's head, providing a pacifier, and talking to him. Following the circumcision he should be held and comforted by a parent or the nurse. The nurse must be alert to any cues that these measures are over-

stimulating the newborn instead of comforting him. Such cues are turning away of the head, increased generalized body movement, skin color changes, hyperalertness, and hiccoughing.

After the circumcision, A and D ointment is placed on the penis to keep the diaper from adhering to the site in all procedures except those using the Plastibell. New ointment is applied with each diaper change or at least four to five times a day for at least 24 to 48 hours. Petroleum jelly may be used instead of A and D ointment.

The baby's voiding is assessed for amount, adequacy of stream, and presence of blood. If bleeding does occur, light pressure is applied intermittently to the site with a sterile gauze pad, and the physician is notified. The newborn may cry when he voids after circumcision. He should be positioned on his side with the diaper fastened loosely to prevent undue pressure. He may remain fussy for several hours and be less interested in feedings.

The parents should be instructed to squeeze water gently over the penis and pat it dry after each diaper change. The diaper is loosely fastened for two to three days, because the glans remains tender for this length of time.

Before discharge, the parents should be instructed to observe the penis for bleeding or possible signs of infection. A whitish yellow exudate around the glans is granulation tissue. It is normal and not indicative of an infection. The exudate may be noted for about two or three days and should not be removed.

If the Plastibell is used, parents are informed that it can remain in place for up to eight days and then fall off. If it is still in place after eight days, it may require manual removal by the clinician.

Nursing Diagnosis

Nursing diagnoses that may apply to the newborn and family in preparation for discharge are presented in the Key Nursing Diagnoses to Consider: Newborn Discharge from the Birthing Center.

CRITICAL THINKING

What behaviors would you consider as indicative of new parents being ready for discharge and being ready to integrate the baby into the family?

Nursing Plan and Implementation for Discharge

The nurse can do much to assist parents in feeling comfortable with newborn care before the family is sent home with their new baby. By discussing with parents how to meet their newborn's needs and ensure her or his safety, the

Dx

Key Nursing Diagnoses to Consider
Newborn Discharge from the Birthing Center

Altered family process

Knowledge deficit

Injury: High risk

Altered health maintenance

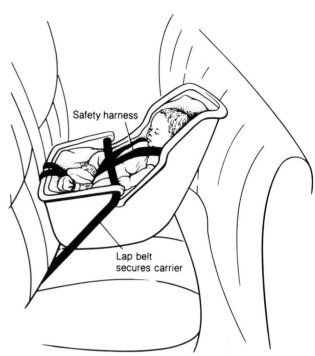

Figure 29–17   Infant car restraint. Infant carrier for use from birth to about 12 months of age. (From Mott Sr, James SB, Sperbac AM: Nursing Care of Children and Families, *2nd ed. Redwood City, CA: Addison-Wesley, 1990, p 530)*

nurse can get the new family off to a good start. The nurse also plays a vital role in fostering parent-infant attachment.

In addition to the information the nurse provides to parents during their stay in the birthing site, the nurse should provide information about safety, the newborn screening program, and follow-up care before the mother and baby are discharged.

Safety Considerations

The nurses can be an excellent role model for parents in the area of safety. Newborns should always be positioned on the stomach or side with a blanket rolled up behind them. Correct use of the bulb syringe must be demonstrated. The baby should never be left alone anywhere but in the crib. The mother is reminded that while she and the newborn are together in the birthing unit, she should never leave the baby alone because newborns spit up frequently the first day or two after birth.

Accidents are the number one cause of death in children, with car accidents causing the most deaths, followed by poisonings. Half the children killed or injured in automobile accidents could have been protected by the use a federally approved car seat. Newborns should go home from the hospital in a car seat (not an infant carrier seat) (Figure 29–17). The seat should be positioned to face the rear of the car until the baby is a year old or weighs 20 pounds. At this time the child's bone structure is adequately mineralized and better able to withstand a forward impact in a five-point harness restraint belt. In many states, the use of car seats for children up to the age of 4 is mandatory.

Newborns do not need pillows or stuffed animals in the crib while they sleep; these items could cause suffocation. Mattresses should fit snugly in a crib to prevent entrapment and suffocation and the crib should be inspected regularly to determine whether it is in safe working order. Crib slats should be no more than 2 3/8 inches apart. Parents can be encouraged to attend infant cardiopulmonary resuscitation (CPR) classes.

Newborn Screening Program

Before the newborn and mother are discharged from the hospital, parents are informed about the normal screening tests for newborns and should be told when to return to the hospital or clinic to have the tests completed. **Newborn screening tests** detect disorders that cause mental retardation, physical handicaps, or death if left undiscovered. Inborn errors of metabolism can usually be detected within one to two weeks after birth and important treatment begun before any damage has occurred. The disorders that can be identified from several drops of blood obtained by a heel stick on the second or third day are galactosemia, homocystinuria, hypothyroidism, maple syrup urine disease, phenylketonuria (PKU), and sickle cell anemia. Parents should be instructed that a second blood specimen will be required after 7 to 14 days (American Academy of Pediatrics: Committee on Genetics 1989). However, it must be clarified that an abnormal test result is not diagnostic. More definitive tests must be performed to verify the results (Seashore 1990).

If additional tests are positive, treatment is initiated. These conditions may be treated by dietary means or by administration of the missing hormones. The inborn conditions cannot be cured, but they can be treated. Although they are not contagious, they may be inherited (Chapter 5).

DATE AND TIME OF BIRTH_____

TOPICS:	TIME & DATE	INT.	COMMENTS:
I. PHYSICIAN INSTRUCTION BOOKLET			
II. INITIAL M/B CONTACT ON MATERNITY			
A. Orient to Mother/Baby			
B. Permits (PKG,Circ)			
C. Diapering & wrapping			
D. Crying			
E. Positioning in crib			
F. Bulb syringe			
G. Regurgitation			
III. BREAST FEEDING			
A. Mechanics & position			
B. Length of feeding			
C. Rooting reflex			
D. New bottle pc			
E. Expression/pump			
F. Burping			
G. Formula & preparation			
IV. BOTTLE FEEDING			
A. Mechanics			
B. Rooting reflex			
C. New bottle each feeding			
D. Propping			
E. Amount & time			
F. Burping			
G. Formula & preparation			
V. NEWBORN CHARACTERISTICS			
A. Rash, Milia			
B. Vag. discharge			
C. Jaundice (Handout)			
D. Molding			
E. Coloring			
F. Vision & hearing			
VI. BATH DEMONSTRATION			
A. Cord care			
B. Genital care			
C. Circumcision care			
D. Support & safety			
VII. DISCHARGE INSTRUCTIONS			
A. Normal void & stool			
B. Constipation			
C. Car seats			
D. When to call Doctor			
E. Choking baby			
F. Use of thermometer			
G. Safety			
F. PKU			

    I. Referral   YES____ NO____

Parent's Signature_____Comments:_____

Witness to Signature_____

Figure 29–18 *Infant Teaching Checklist. Adapted from Memorial Hospital, Colorado Springs, Colorado. Section I & II are completed upon initial contact. Section III & IV are completed by 4 hours from initial contact. Section V is completed by 12 hours from initial contact, and sections VI and VII completed by time of discharge.*

Follow-Up Care

Each newborn will have variations in normal physiologic responses. Parents need to learn how to interpret these changes in their child. To assist parents in caring for their newborn at home, some physicians encourage pediatric prenatal visits so that this contact is established before the birth. Public health nurses have long been involved in newborn care and parent education. Birthing units are now expanding their primary care functions to the new family to include one home visit by the primary nurse who cared for the family in the birthing unit. The birthing unit nursery staff may also make themselves available as a 24-hour telephone resource for the new mother who needs additional support and consultation during the first few days at home with her newborn.

Routine well-baby visits should be scheduled with the clinic, pediatric nurse practitioner, or physician.

Parents should be taught all necessary care-giving methods before discharge. A checklist may be helpful to see if the teaching has been completed. The nurse needs to review all areas for understanding or questions with the mother, without rushing, taking time to answer all queries. The mother should have the physician's/CNM's phone number, address, and any specific instructions. Having the birthing unit or nursery phone number is also reassuring to a new mother. The parents are encouraged to call with questions.

Documentation

The final step of discharge planning is documentation. Any concern of the parents or nurse are noted. The nurse records which demonstrations and/or classes the mother and/or father attended and their expressed understanding of the instructions given to them.

One method of documenting health teaching during the hospital stay is to use a multiple-copy teaching checklist that is dated and initialed by the nurse after completion of each topic. Parents sign the sheet, acknowledging their understanding of the material, and are given a copy upon discharge (Figure 29–18).

Evaluation

Anticipated outcomes of nursing care include the following:

- The newborn baby's adaptation to extrauterine life is supported and complete.
- The baby's physiologic and psychologic integrity is supported.
- The parent-newborn feeding pattern will be satisfactorily established.
- The parents express understanding of bonding process and display attachment behaviors.
- The parents verbalize developmentally appropriate behavioral expectations of and follow-up care for their baby.
- The parents demonstrate safe techniques for caring for their baby.

❀ ❀

KEY CONCEPTS

The overall goal of newborn nursing care is to provide comprehensive care while promoting the establishment of a well-functioning family unit.

The period immediately following birth, during which adaptation to extrauterine life occurs, requires close monitoring to identify any deviations from normal.

The first period of reactivity lasts for 30 minutes after birth. The newborn is alert and hungry at this time, making this a natural opportunity to promote attachment.

The second period of reactivity requires close monitoring by the nurse as apnea, decreased heart rate, gagging, choking, and regurgitation are likely to occur and require nursing intervention.

Nursing goals during the first four hours after birth (admission period) are to: maintain a clear airway, maintain a neutral thermal environment, prevent hemorrhage and infection, initiate oral feedings, and facilitate attachment.

The newborn is routinely given prophylactic vitamin K to prevent possible hemorrhagic disease of the newborn.

Prophylactic eye treatment for *Neisseria gonorrhoea* is legally required for all newborns.

Essential daily care includes assessments of the vital signs, weight, overall color, intake/output, umbilical cord and circumcision, newborn nutrition, parent education, and attachment.

The care giver should be notified if there is evidence of bright red bleeding or puslike drainage near the cord stump or if the umbilicus remains unhealed.

Following a circumcision the newborn must be observed closely for signs of bleeding, inability to void, and signs of infection.

Signs of illness in newborns include: temperature above 38.4C (101F) or below 36.1C (97F), more than one episode of forceful vomiting, refusal of two feedings in a row, lethargy, cyanosis with or without a feeding, and absence of breathing for longer than 15 seconds.

Newborn screening for galactosemia, homocystinuria, hypothyroidism, maple syrup urine disease, phenylketonuria, and sickle cell anemia is done on all newborns in the first one to three days, with a second blood specimen drawn after 7 to 14 days.

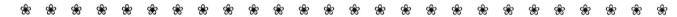

References

American Academy of Pediatrics, Committee on Fetus and Newborn and Committee on Drugs: Neonatal anesthesia. *Pediatrics* 1987; 80:446.

American Academy of Pediatrics, Committee on Pediatrics and Committee on Genetics: Newborn screening fact sheets. *Pediatrics* 1989; 83:449.

American Academy of Pediatrics, Committee on Fetus and Newborn: Report of the ad hoc task force on circumcision. *Pediatrics* 1989; 83:388.

Beske E, Garvis M: Important factors in breast feeding success. *MCN* May/June 1982; 7:174.

Coen RW, Koeffler H: *Primary Care of the Newborn.* Boston: Little, Brown, 1987.

Cunningham FG, MacDonald PC, Gant NG: *Williams Obstetrics.* Norwalk, CT: Appleton & Lange, 1989.

King PA, Caddy GM, Cohen SH et al: Circumcision: Maternal attitudes *Pediatr Surg Int* 1989; 4:222.

Klaus M, Klaus P: *The Amazing Newborn.* Menlo Park, CA: Addison-Wesley, 1985.

Lund MM: Perspectives on Newborn Male Circumcision. *Neonatal Netw* 1990; 9(3):7.

Mayfield S et al: Temperature measurement in term and preterm neonates. *J Pediatr* February 1984; 104:271.

Milan EM, McFeely EJ: *Memory Bank for Neonatal Drugs.* Baltimore: Williams & Wilkins, 1990.

Neonatal Thermoregulation. *NAACOG-OGN Nursing Practice Resource* February 1990.

Niefert M: *Breastfeeding Standards of Care for Low Risk Infants.* Denver: St. Luke's Hospital, 1989.

Pawlak RP, Tabor Herbert LA: *Drug Administration in the NICU: A Handbook for Nurses,* 2nd ed. Petaluma, CA: Neonatal Network, 1990.

Scharli AF: Circumcision, an everlasting discussion. *Pediatr Surg Int* 1989; 4:221.

Seashore MR: Neonatal Screening for Inborn Errors of Metabolism: Update. *Semin Perinatol* 1990; 14:431.

Stang HJ, Gunnar MR, Snellman L et al: Local anesthesia for neonatal circumcision: Effects on distress and cortisol response. *JAMA* 1988; 259:1507.

Von Kries R: Vitamin K Prophylaxis: Oral or Parenteral. *Am J Dis Child* 1988; 142:14.

Wiswell TE et al: Declining frequency of circumcision: Implications for change in the absolute incidence and male to female sex ratio of urinary tract infections in early infancy. *Pediatrics* 1987; 79:338.

Additional Readings

DiFlorio I: Mothers' comprehension of terminology associated with the care of a newborn baby. *Pediatr Nurs* 1991; 17(2):193.

Harrison LL: Patient education in early postpartum discharge programs. *MCN* 1990; 15:39.

Ho E: Early days. *Nursing* 1989; 3:12.

Pascoe JM, French J: Development of positive feelings in primiparous mothers toward their normal newborns: A descriptive study. *Clin Pediatr* 1989; 28:452.

Tiedje LB, Collins C: Combining employment and motherhood. *MCN* January/February 1989; 14:9.

Tomlinson PS: Father involvement with first-born infants: Interpersonal and situational factors. *Pediatr Nurs* March/April 1987; 13:101.

Vaughans B: Early maternal-infant contact and neonatal thermoregulation. *Neonatal Netw* 1990; 8:19.

CHAPTER 30

Newborn Nutrition

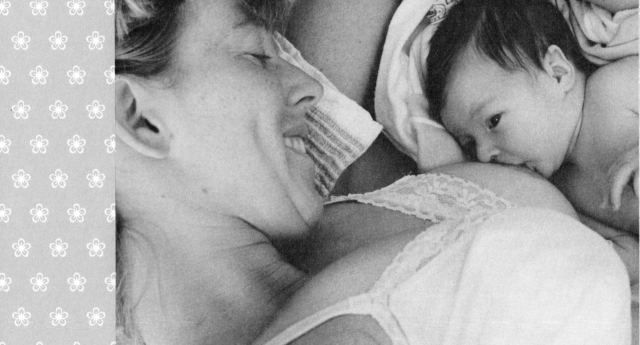

Compare the nutritional value and composition of breast milk and formula preparations.

Identify the benefits of breast-feeding for both mother and infant.

Develop guidelines for helping both breast-feeding and bottle-feeding mothers to feed their infants successfully.

Delineate nursing responsibilities for client education about problems the breast-feeding mother may encounter at home.

Describe an appropriate process for weaning an infant from breast-feeding.

Summarize the advantages and disadvantages of breast-feeding and formula feeding.

❈ ❈

I had been told that most babies ate every three or four hours and slept the rest of the time. Not mine! She wanted to nurse every two hours, and sometimes more often than that. Sometimes she would sleep for an hour, sometimes for fifteen minutes. I loved her, but I also felt consumed by her needs. It was hard to adjust to the fact that I couldn't get anything finished, whether it was an article I was reading or folding the laundry. At the end of the day I would realize I hadn't accomplished anything. Once I accepted the fact that I was not going to function at my old efficient rate (at least for a while) and stopped feeling guilty about what I wasn't getting done, I felt freer to enjoy the time I was spending with my baby. (The New Our Bodies, Ourselves)

Feeding a newborn is an exciting, satisfying, and often worrisome task for parents. Meeting this essential need of their new child helps parents strengthen their attachment to their baby and fosters their self-images as nurturers and providers. Whether a woman chooses to breast-feed or bottle-feed, she can be reassured that she can adequately meet her infant's needs. Questions about feeding may arise, however, and the nurse works with the woman to help her develop skill in her chosen method. The nurse provides information, assists the parent, and answers questions as necessary. In every interaction it is the nurse's responsibility to promote the family's sense of confidence.

Nutritional Needs of the Newborn

The newborn's diet must supply nutrients to meet the rapid rate of physical growth and development. A neonatal diet should provide adequate calories and include protein, carbohydrate, fat, water, vitamins, and minerals. The recommendations in Table 30–1 are based on limited research data but give generalizations about requirements for optimal nutrition for the first year of life.

The calories (50–55 cal/lb/day or 110–120 cal/kg/day) in the newborn's diet are divided among protein, carbohydrate, and fat and should be adjusted according to the infant's weight. Protein is needed for rapid cellular growth and maintenance. Carbohydrates provide energy. The fat portion of the diet provides calories, regulates fluid and electrolyte balance, and is necessary for the development of the neonatal brain and neurologic system.

Water requirements are high (64–73 mL/lb/day or 140–160 mL/kg/day) because of the newborn's inability to concentrate urine. Fluid needs are further increased in illness or hot weather.

The iron needs of the infant will be affected by accumulation of iron stores during the fetal life, and by the mother's iron and other food intake if she is breast-feeding. Ascorbic acid (usually in the form of fruit juices) and meat, poultry, and fish are known to enhance absorption of iron in the mother just as it does later in the infant. Adequate minerals and vitamins are needed by the newborn to prevent deficiency states such as scurvy, cheilosis, and pellagra. See Table 30–2.

Breast Milk

Three types of milk are produced during the establishment of lactation: (a) colostrum, (b) transitional milk, and (c) mature milk. **Colostrum** is a yellowish or creamy-appearing fluid that is thicker than later milk and contains more protein, fat-soluble vitamins, and minerals. It also contains high levels of immunoglobulins (antibodies), which are a source of passive immunity for the newborn. Colostrum production begins early in pregnancy and may last for several days after birth. However, in most cases colostrum is replaced by transitional milk within two to four days after birth. **Transitional milk** is produced from the end of co-

Table 30–1 Nutritional Needs of the Normal Newborn

	At birth
Calories	120/kg/day
Protein	1.9 g/100 kcal*
Fat	30%–55% of total calories
Carbohydrate	35%–55% of total calories
Water	330 mL†
Calcium	388 mg
Phosphate	132 mg
Magnesium	16 mg
Iron	7 mg
Copper	Not established
Zinc	Not established
Vitamins	
A	100–200 IU*
D	0.4 mg/dL*
E	0.4 mg/dL*
K	75 mg/day*
C	10 mg/day*
Thiamine	0.2 mg/100 kcal*

†*Approximately.*

**Estimated to be approximately equivalent to levels in breast milk.*

Adapted from information contained in Eckstein EF: Food, People, and Nutrition. Westport, CT: AVI Publishing, 1980.

lostrum production until approximately two weeks postpartum. This milk contains elevated levels of fat, lactose, water-soluble vitamins, and more calories than colostrum.

The final milk produced, **mature milk**, has a high percentage of water. Although it appears similar to skim milk and may cause mothers to question whether their milk is "rich enough," mature breast milk provides 20 kcal/ounce, as do most prepared formulas. However, the percentage of calories derived from protein is lower in breast milk than in formulas, with a greater proportion of calories being derived from carbohydrates in the form of lactose (Pipes 1989). The nitrogen wastes produced by protein metabolism are, therefore, lessened in the breast-fed newborn, providing a positive effect on the infant's immature renal system.

The American Academy of Pediatrics (1988) recommends breast milk as the optimal food for the first four to six months of life. The advantages that breast-feeding pro-

Table 30–2 Newborn Caloric and Fluid Needs

Caloric intake: 50–55 cal/lb/day or 110–120 cal/kg/day

Fluid requirements: 64–73 mL/lb/day or 140–160 mL/kg/day

Weight gain: First six months—1 oz/day
　　　　　　Second six months—0.5 oz/day

vides to newborns and infants are generally immunologic, nutritional, and psychosocial.

Immunologic Advantages

Immunologic advantages identified by Pipes (1989) include varying degrees of protection from respiratory and gastrointestinal infections, otitis media, meningitis, sepsis, and allergies. This protection has a positive effect on the health of the breast-fed baby into the infant and toddler period (Lawrence 1989). Secretory IgA, an immunoglobulin present in colostrum and breast milk, has antiviral, antibacterial, and antigenic-inhibiting properties. It is theorized that the infant's immature intestine allows antigenic macromolecules, such as those found in cow's milk, to cross the mucosa of the small intestine. Secretory IgA plays a role in decreasing the permeability of the intestine to these macromolecules. Other properties in colostrum and breast milk that act to inhibit the growth of bacteria and/or viruses are *Lactobacillus bifidus,* lysozymes, lactoperoxidase, lactoferrin, transferrin, and various immunoglobulins. Immunoglobulins to the poliomyelitis virus are also present in the breast milk of mothers who have immunity to this virus. Because the presence of these immunoglobulins may inhibit the desired intestinal infection and immune response of the infant, some clinics suggest that breast-feedings be withheld for 30 to 60 minutes following the administration of the Sabin oral polio vaccine. Table 30–3 identifies the factors in breast milk with specific antibacterial and antiviral actions.

In addition to its immunologic properties, breast milk is known to be nonallergenic and is not affected by unsafe water or insect-carried disease (Lawrence 1989).

Nutritional Advantages

Breast milk is composed of lactose, lipids, polyunsaturated fatty acids, and amino acids, especially taurine, and has a whey-to-casein protein ratio that facilitates the digestion, absorption, and full use of breast milk compared to formulas (Worthingon-Roberts & Williams 1989). Some researchers feel the high concentration of cholesterol and the balance of amino acids in breast milk make it the best food for myelination and neurologic development. It is also suggested that high cholesterol levels in breast milk may stimulate the production of enzymes that lead to more efficient metabolism of cholesterol, thereby reducing its long-term harmful effects on the cardiovascular system (Worthington-Roberts & Williams 1989).

Breast milk provides newborns with minerals in more acceptable doses than those provided by formulas (Schanler 1989). The iron found in breast milk, even though much lower in concentration than that of prepared formulas, is much more readily and fully absorbed and appears sufficient to meet the infant's iron needs for the first four to six months (Duncan et al 1985). The American Academy of Pediatrics states that there is generally no need to give supplemental iron to breast-fed newborns before the age of 6 months. Supplemental iron may decrease the ability of

Table 30–3 Antibacterial and Antiviral Factors in Breast Milk

Factor	Shown in vitro to be active against
Antibacterial Factors	
L. bifidus growth factor	Enterobacteriaceae, enteric pathogens
Secretory IgA	*E. coli, E. coli* enterotoxin, *C. tetani, C. diphtheriae, D. pneumoniae, Salmonella, Shigella*
C1–C9	Effect not known
Lactoferrin	*E. coli, C. albicans*
Lactoperoxidase	*Streptococcus, Pseudomonas, E. coli, S. typhimurium*
Lysozyme	*E. coli, Salmonella, M. lysodeikticus*
Lipid (unsaturated fatty acid)	*S. aureus*
Milk cells	By phagocytosis: *E. coli, C. albicans* By sensitized lymphocytes: *E. coli*
Antiviral Factors	
Secretory IgA	Polio types 1,2,3; Coxsackie types A9, B3, B5; ECHO types 6, 9; Semliki Forest virus; Ross River virus; rotavirus
Lipid (unsaturated fatty acids and monoglycerides)	Herpes simplex; Semliki Forest virus, influenza, dengue, Ross River virus, Murine leukemia virus, Japanese B encephalitis virus
Nonimmunoglobulin macromolecules	Herpes simplex; vesicular stomatitis virus
Milk cells	Rotavirus; induced interferon active against Sendai virus; sensitized lymphocytes? phagocytosis

Modified from Welsh JK, May JT: J Pediatr 1979; 94: 1.

breast milk to protect the newborn by interfering with lactoferrin, an iron-binding protein that enhances the absorption of iron and has anti-infective properties.

Another advantage of breast milk is that all its components are delivered to the infant in an unchanged form, and vitamins are not lost through processing and heating. If the breast-feeding mother is taking daily multivitamins and her diet is adequate, the only supplements the infant will need are Vitamin D and fluoride until the age of 6 months (American Academy of Pediatrics Committee on Nutrition 1985). If the mother's diet or vitamin intake is inadequate or questionable, care givers may choose to prescribe additional vitamins for the infant.

Psychosocial Advantages

The psychosocial advantages of breast-feeding are primarily those associated with attachment. Breast-feeding enhances attachment by providing the opportunity for frequent, direct skin contact between the newborn and the mother. The newborn's sense of touch is highly developed at birth and is a primary means of communication. The tactile stimulation associated with breast-feeding can communicate warmth, closeness, and comfort. The increased closeness provides both newborn and mother with the opportunity to learn each other's behavioral cues and needs. The

mother's sense of accomplishment in being able to satisfy her baby's needs for nourishment and comfort is enhanced when the newborn sucks vigorously and is satiated and calmed by the breast-feeding. Some mothers prefer breast-feeding as a means of extending the close, unique, nourishing relationship between mother and baby that existed prior to birth. In the event of a twin birth, breast-feeding not only is possible but also enhances the mother's individualization and attachment to each newborn. The fantasized single baby is replaced more readily with the reality of two individual babies when the mother has close and frequent contact with each (Sollid et al 1989). Other studies have been cited that associate breast-feeding with improved language and cognitive development as well as scholastic ability (Anholm 1986).

Disadvantages

One disadvantage of breast-feeding is that most drugs taken by the mother are transmitted through breast milk and may cause harm to the infant. Jaundice caused by breast milk may be another reason to interrupt breast-feeding. Breast-feeding can normally be resumed after 48 hours without resulting in further hyperbilirubinemia.

A mother's poor nutritional, physical, or mental health

or a personal aversion to breast-feeding may be contraindications to nursing. Difficulty in maintaining milk supply, concern over the adequacy of the breast milk to meet the newborn's needs, sore nipples, resumption of a heavy work schedule, and constant demands on her time are other reasons mothers discontinue breast-feeding. Lack of support and encouragement from health care providers or family may also contribute to a woman's decision to stop breast-feeding.

Opinion varies as to the advisability of continuing breast-feeding in the event of another pregnancy. Some feel the nutritional demands on the pregnant mother are too great and advocate gradual weaning. Others suggest that with adequate rest, a proper diet, and strong emotional support, continued breast-feeding during pregnancy is a valid choice. The practice of nursing one infant throughout pregnancy and then breast-feeding both infants after birth is called *tandem nursing* (Lawrence 1989). When pregnancy occurs, the decision is best made on an individual basis after considering maternal health and motivation and the age of the first child.

Even though many mothers obtain information about breast-feeding from written sources, family and friends, and La Leche League, the nurse needs to be a ready source of information, encouragement, and support as well. The nurse can be helpful during the time when parents are deciding whether to breast-feed, after the birth process when breast-feedings are just being established, and after the family returns home.

Bottle Feeding

Numerous types of commercially prepared lactose formulas adequately meet the nutritional needs of the infant. These milk formulas contain different amounts of amino acids: tyrosine and phenylalanine are more prevalent in formula milk; the taurine present in breast milk is absent in cow's milk formula. Bottle-fed babies do gain weight faster than breast-fed babies because of the higher protein content in commercially prepared formula.

Bottle-fed infants up to 6 months of age may gain as much as 1 ounce per day and tend to regain their birth weight by ten days after birth (Pipes 1989). Healthy breast-fed babies, however, gain approximately 1/2 ounce per day in the first six months of life (Sawley 1989) and tend to regain their birth weight about 14 days after birth. Formula-fed infants generally double their weight within 3 1/2 to 4 months, whereas nursing infants double their weight at about 5 months of age.

Formulas contain mostly saturated fatty acids, whereas breast milk is higher in unsaturated fatty acids. Calcium, sodium, and chloride, which occur in higher concentrations in some commercially made formulas, may be detrimental to the newborn's immature kidneys, which may not be ready to handle such high solute loads. High solute loads may also lead to thirst in the formula-fed infant, causing overfeeding and possible obesity (Mott et al 1990).

Another potential problem with formulas is an allergic reaction in the newborn. The small intestine of the infant is permeable to macromolecules such as those found in cow's milk and milk-based formulas. The introduction of foreign proteins in formula may cause an allergic reaction, with signs such as spitting up and decreased appetite. See Table 30–4.

Clinicians recommend the use of iron-fortified formulas or supplements to mothers who are bottle-feeding, as iron deficiency anemia is still very prevalent. The recommended iron dosage is 7 mg per day. However, the nurse must be aware that too much iron in the form of extra iron-fortified cereal given the infant may interfere with the infant's natural ability to defend against disease (Winick 1989). Parents also need to be informed about the constipation that sometimes results from iron-enriched formula and about various methods of alleviating the constipation. Opinion varies about the use of vitamin supplements for newborns, but it is generally agreed that commercially prepared formulas adequately meet the needs of the healthy newborn and infant.

Many companies make an enriched formula that is similar to breast milk. These formulas all have sufficient levels of carbohydrate, protein, fat, vitamins, and minerals to meet the newborn's nutritional needs.

The American Academy of Pediatrics recommends that infants be given breast milk or formula rather than whole milk until 1 year of age. However, the American Academy of Pediatrics Committee on Nutrition (1989) has indicated that cow's milk could be substituted in the second 6 months of age *only if* (a) the amount of milk calories consumed does not exceed 65% of total calories, and (b) the solid food portion of the diet replaces the iron and vitamins deficient in cow's milk. This method of feeding must meet these guidelines and is not the recommended method for providing infant nutrition. Table 30–5 compares the components of breast milk, unmodified cow's milk, and a commercially standardized formula. Table 30–6 describes some of the commonly prescribed formulas for healthy newborns, infants with milk allergies, and infants with certain metabolic disorders.

Neither unmodified cow's milk nor skim milk is an acceptable alternative for newborn feeding. The protein content in cow's milk is too high (50% to 75% more than human milk), is poorly digested, and may cause bleeding of the gastrointestinal tract. Unmodified cow's milk is also inadequate in vitamins. Skim milk lacks adequate calories, fat content, and essential fatty acids necessary for proper development of the neonate's neurologic system. Nutritionists advise against use of unmodified cow's milk, cow's milk with decreased fat content, or skim milk for children under 2 years of age.

Table 30–4 Pros and Cons of Breast- and Bottle-Feeding

Breast	**Bottle**
Newborn's Health	
Colostrum is rich in antibodies until baby's own immune system is established.	Some babies are allergic to certain formulas. Trial and error may be necessary.
Mother's milk is almost always tolerated by baby. Breast milk proteins are easily digested and fats well absorbed.	Formula is linked to an increased number of GI and respiratory infections.
Baby can't overeat, limits self to natural weight. No need to empty bottle.	More air may be ingested into stomach, causing gas, cramps, and spitting up.
Composition	
Breast milk contains higher levels of lactose, cystine, and cholesterol, which are necessary for brain and nerve growth.	Made to be as close to human milk as possible, but nutrients not as biodegradable. Contains adequate vitamins and minerals.
Perfect balance of proteins, carbohydrates, fats, vitamins, and minerals.	
Purity	
Pure and as free from foreign materials as whatever the mother consumes.	Formula companies comply with federal guidelines for sterility and quality.
No storage, sanitation, or spoilage unless pumped milk is not refrigerated. Frozen milk can be safely kept for at least one month.	Ready-to-drink formula has an expiration date and shelf half-life even if unopened. Once mixed, powdered formula should be used within 24 hours.
Cost	
Costs are minimal, including the cost of two or three nursing bras, cloth or disposable nursing pads used for about first six weeks, breast milk to prevent and/or treat sore and cracked nipples, manual or electric breast pump, and the cost of a well-balanced diet for the mother. No waste with breast milk.	Expenses include cost of bottles or disposable nursers with plastic liners, nipples, nipple caps, and a heat-resistant mixing container. Formula is a major expense, especially when baby takes 24 oz or four bottles a day.
Convenience	
Mother can feed whenever baby needs; milk is at perfect temperature.	Mother has more freedom to come and go rather than timing her trips from home based on baby's feeding schedule.
If baby is only on breast milk, mother is tied down and can't miss too many feedings. She risks decreasing her supply if she supplements.	Requires frequent trips to store or buying formula in large quantities.
Engorgement can cause discomfort. Certain clothes may make nursing discreetly difficult.	Night feedings are more disruptive. Preparation time is about the same as for making iced tea.
Emotional Aspects	
Pleasant way to nurture—skin-to-skin contact enhances closeness. Nursing has calming effect on baby, who hears familiar sound of mother's heartbeat and smells her scent.	Same degree of intimacy as with breast if mother or father holds baby close, smiles, and snuggles during feedings.
Mother may be embarrassed, nervous, or have aversion to breast-feeding, especially in public.	Mother may be more at ease with bottle than with offering breast.
Father is left out of nurturing experience if baby is breast-fed exclusively.	Father equal partner in nurturing and feeding experience.

Source: Adapted from Lesko W, Lesko M: The Maternity Source Book. New York: Warner Books, 1984, pp 284–87.

Newborn Feeding

Initial Feeding

The time when the first feeding is given should be determined by the physiologic and behavioral cues of the newborn. The nurse should assess for active bowel sounds, absence of abdominal distention, and a lusty cry, which quiets and is replaced with rooting and sucking behaviors when a stimulus is placed near the lips. These signs are indicators that the newborn is hungry and physically ready to tolerate the feeding.

Assessment of the newborn's physiologic status is of primary and ongoing concern to the nurse throughout the first feeding. The initial feeding raises from a medical perspective the need to assess the infant for the congenital anomaly of tracheoesophageal fistula or esophageal atresia (see Chapter 32 for in-depth discussion). In cases of esophageal atresia, the feeding is taken well initially, but as the esophageal pouch fills, the feeding is quickly regurgitated unchanged by stomach contents. If a fistula is present, the infant gags, chokes, regurgitates mucus, and may be-

Table 30–5 Composition of Mature Breast Milk, Unmodified Cow's Milk, and a Routine Infant Formula

Composition/dL	Mature breast milk	Cow's milk	Routine formula (20 cal) with iron
Calories	75.0	69.0	67.0
Protein, g	1.1	3.5	1.5
Lactalbumin %	80	18	60
Casein %	20	82	40
Water, mL	87.1	87.3	90
Fat, g	4.5	3.5	3.8
Carbohydrate, g	7.1	4.9	7.0
Ash, g	0.21	0.72	0.34
Minerals			
Na, mg	16.0	50.0	21.0
K, mg	51.0	144.0	69.0
Ca, mg	33.0	118.0	46.0
P, mg	14.0	93.0	32.0
Mg, mg	4.0	13.0	5.3
Fe, mg	0.05	Tr.	1.3
Zn, mg	0.15	0.4	0.42
Vitamins			
A, IU	182.0	140.0	210.0
C, mg	5.0	1.0	5.3
D, IU	2.2	4.2	42.3
E, IU	0.18	0.04	0.83
Thiamine, mg	0.01	0.03	0.04
Riboflavin, mg	0.04	0.17	0.06
Niacin, mg	0.2	0.1	0.7
Curd size	Soft Flocculent	Firm Large	Mod. firm Mod. large
pH	Alkaline	Acid	Acid
Anti-infective properties	+	±	−
Bacterial content	Sterile	Nonsterile	Sterile
Emptying time	More rapid		

From Avery GB: Neonatology, *3rd ed. New York: Lippincott/Harper & Row, Medical Texts, 1987, p. 1192.*

come cyanotic as fluid passes through the fistula into the lungs.

It is the practice in many institutions to offer the newborn who is to be formula-fed a few milliliters of plain sterile water one to four hours after birth. If aspiration should occur, as is often the case with a tracheoesophageal fistula, the water is readily absorbed by the lung tissue. Glucose water and/or formula should not be used, since it will damage the newborn's lung tissue if aspirated (Avery 1987). The sterile water feeding provides an opportunity for the nurse to assess the effectiveness of the newborn's suck, swallow, and gag reflexes. A softer nipple made for preterm infants may be used if the newborn appears to tire easily. Extreme fatigue coupled with rapid respiration, circumoral cyanosis, and diaphoresis of the head and face may indicate cardiovascular complications and should be assessed further. Glucose water or formula is then given after the newborn has successfully taken between 5 and 15 mL

without any signs of distress. Early glucose water substitution provides sugar needed to prevent hypoglycemia.

The mother who plans to breast-feed will ask to nurse her newborn immediately following birth. Throughout the first two hours after birth, the infant is usually alert and eager to suck and is ready for the initial nursing at this time (Huggins 1986). This practice provides stimulation for milk production, aids in maternal-newborn attachment, and enhances the probability that the mother will be successful in her efforts to breast-feed.

Since colostrum is not irritating if aspirated and is readily absorbed by the respiratory system, breast-feeding can usually be done immediately after birth. Only a few contraindications exist to immediate nursing, which are (a) a heavily sedated mother, (b) a baby with a 5-minute Apgar score less than 6, or (c) a premature infant of less than 36 weeks' gestation (Lawrence 1989). With regard to tracheoesophageal fistula, the nurse can assess for this pos-

Table 30–6 Pediatric Formulas

Formula (Company)	Carbohydrate	Protein	Fat	Stool characteristics	Explanation
Enfamil (Mead Johnson)	Lactose	Nonfat milk	Soy, coconut oils	Formed, greenish-brown with very little free water around stool	Can be used with infants with fat intolerance. Appropriate formula for normal infants who have no special nutritional requirements
Similac (Ross)	Lactose	Nonfat milk	Soy, coconut, corn oils	Formed, greenish-brown with very little free water around stool	Iron may be added to any of these formulas to supply a dependable daily intake; for premature infants; for offspring of anemic mothers; for infants of multiple births; for infants with low birth weights and those who grew rapidly; for infants who have lost weight.
SMA (Wyeth)	Lactose	Electrolyzed whey, nonfat milk	Coconut, safflower, soybean oils	Similar to breast milk stools: small volume, pasty yellow, some free water	
Isomil (Ross)	Sucrose, cornstarch, corn syrup solids	Soy protein isolates	Soy, coconut, corn oils	Mushy, yellow-green with more free water than cow's milk stools	Used for children with milk allergies
Neomulsoy (Syntex)	Sucrose	Soy protein isolates	Soy oil		
Nursoy (Wyeth)	Sucrose, corn syrup	Soy protein isolates	Coconut, oleic, safflower, soybean oils, and soy oil		
Prosobee (Mead Johnson)	Sucrose, corn syrup	Soy protein isolates	Soy oil		Metabolic defects, eg, galactosemia
Lofenalac (Mead Johnson)	Corn syrup solids, tapioca starch	Hydrolyzed casein (most of phenylalanine removed)	Corn oil	Similar to cow's milk formula: formed, greenish-brown with very little free water around stool	Used in children with phenylketonuria in whom a low phenylalanine diet is needed

From Mott S, James S, Sperhac AM: Nursing Care of Children and Families, *2nd ed. Redwood City, CA: Addison-Wesley, 1990, p 153.*

sibility by looking for the signs of potential aspiration such as low Apgar score, increased mucus, and maternal polyhydramnios prior to putting the baby to the breast. If these indicators exist, tracheal patency can be determined by passing a tube down to the stomach. If the passage is patent, then the infant may nurse.

The newborn will usually take 15 to 30 mL at the first feeding. For the breast-fed newborn this means that there are signs of being satisfied after 3 to 5 minutes of strong sucking at the breast.

It is not unusual for the newborn to regurgitate some mucus and water following a feeding, even if it was taken without difficulty. Consequently, the newborn is observed closely and positioned on the right side after a feeding to aid drainage and facilitate gastric emptying.

Establishing a Feeding Pattern

In the past it was the practice to establish artificial three- to four-hour time frames for feedings after the initial feeding. This scheduling may present difficulties for the new mother trying to establish lactation, and it fails to recognize and respond to the individual needs of the newborn infant. Breast milk is rapidly digested by the newborn, who may desire to nurse every 1 1/2 to 3 hours initially, with one or two feedings during the night.

Rooming-in permits the mother to feed the infant as needed. When rooming-in is not available, a supportive nursing staff and flexible nursery policies will allow the mother to feed her infant on demand, when the infant is hungry. Nothing is more frustrating to a new mother than attempting to nurse a newborn who is sound asleep because he or she is either not hungry or exhausted from crying. Once lactation is established and the family is home, a feeding pattern agreeable to both mother and child is usually established.

Formula-fed newborns may awaken for feedings every two to five hours but are frequently satisfied with feedings every three to four hours. Because formula is digested more slowly, the bottle-fed infant may go longer between feedings and may begin skipping the night feeding within about six weeks. This is very individualized depending on the size and development of the infant.

Both breast-fed and bottle-fed infants experience growth spurts at certain times and require increased feeding. The mother of a breast-fed infant may meet these increased demands by nursing more frequently to increase her milk supply; however, it will take about 24 hours for the milk supply to increase adequately to meet the new demand (Lawrence 1989). A slight increase in feedings will meet the needs of the formula-fed infant.

Providing nourishment for her newborn is a major concern for the new mother. Her feelings of success or failure may influence her self-concept as she assumes her maternal role. With proper instruction, support, and encouragement from health care providers, feeding becomes a source of pleasure and satisfaction to both parents and infant.

Promotion of Successful Infant Feeding

Parents may see the task of feeding their baby as the center of their relationship with the new family member. Whether the mother has chosen to bottle-feed or breast-feed, the nurse can help the mother have a successful experience while in the hospital and during the early days at home. Feeding and caring for newborns may be routine tasks for the nurse, but the success or nonsuccess that a mother achieves the first few times may determine her feelings about herself as an adequate mother.

The response of the newborn to caring is important as an expression of personality. A parent may interpret the newborn's behavior as rejection, which may alter the progress of parent-child relationships. A parent may also interpret the sleepy infant's refusal to suck or inability to retain formula as evidence of his or her incompetence as a parent. Likewise, the breast-feeding mother may deduce that the newborn does not like her if the baby fails to take her nipple readily. Conversely, infants pick up messages from the muscular tension of those holding them.

A nurse who is sensitive to the needs of the mother can form a relationship with her that permits sharing of knowledge about techniques and emotions connected with the feeding experience. Breast-feeding women frequently express disappointment in the help given to them by hospital nurses, saying they would like more encouragement, support, and practical information about feeding their newborn (Beske & Garvis 1982). This desire and need also applies to nonnursing mothers. Consistency in teaching by nursing personnel is paramount. A new mother becomes very frustrated if she is shown a number of different methods of feeding her newborn.

The decision by the mother about whether to breast-feed or bottle-feed is usually made by the sixth month of pregnancy and often even before conception. The final decision however, may not be made until the mother's admission to the birth center. The decision is frequently based on the influences of relatives—especially the father and maternal grandmother (Lawrence 1989), friends, and social customs rather than on knowledge about the nutritional and psychologic needs of herself and her newborn. With the technologic advances in formula production and the availability of knowledge about breast-feeding techniques, the mother should be confident that the choice she makes will promote normal growth and development of her newborn.

If the mother makes the decision to breast-feed at the time of birth without prenatal preparation or support from her partner or other members of her family, she may encounter difficulty. It is necessary for the nurse to find out before delivery whether the woman really wants to breast-feed or has made the decision based on social or family influences (Lawrence 1989).

The nurse's primary responsibility is to support the feeding method decision and to help the family achieve a positive result. No woman should be made to feel inadequate or superior because of her choice in feeding. There are advantages and disadvantages to breast- and bottle-feeding, but positive bonds in parent-child relationships may be developed with either method.

Immediately before feeding, the mother should be made as comfortable as possible. Preparations may include voiding, washing her hands, and assuming a position of comfort. The woman who has had a cesarean birth needs support so that the infant does not rest on her abdomen for long periods of time. If she is breast-feeding, she may be more comfortable lying on her side with a pillow behind her back and one between her legs. The nurse can position the newborn next to the woman's breast and place a rolled towel or small pillow behind the infant for support. The mother will initially need assistance turning from side to side and burping the newborn. She may prefer to breast-feed sitting up with a pillow on her lap and the infant resting on the pillow rather than directly on her abdomen. It may be helpful to place a rolled pillow under the arm supporting the infant's head.

An alternative position that avoids pressure on the incision while allowing for maximum visualization of the infant's face is the football hold. Bottle-feeding mothers who have undergone cesarean birth frequently use the sitting position also. If incisional pain makes this position difficult, the bottle-feeding mother may also find it helpful to assume the side-lying position. The infant can be positioned in a semisitting position against a pillow close to the mother, who can hold the bottle in her right hand.

Depending on the newborn's level of hunger, the parents may want to use the time before feeding to get acquainted with their infant. The presence of the nurse during part of this time to answer questions and provide reinforcement of parenting skills will be helpful for the family.

For the sleepy baby, a period of playful activity—such as gently rubbing the feet and hands or adjusting clothing and loosening coverings to expose the infant to room air may increase alertness so that, when the feeding is initiated, the infant is ready and sucks eagerly. It may allow the active newborn an opportunity to calm down so that he or she can find and grasp the nipple effectively. After the feeding, when the infant is satisfied and asleep, parents may explore the characteristics unique to their newborn. Hospital routines must be flexible enough to allow this time for the family. Rooming-in offers spontaneous, frequent encounters for the family and provides opportunities to practice handling skills, thereby increasing confidence in care after discharge. It may also allow for demand, rather than scheduled, feeding times, which should be encouraged.

Cultural Considerations in Infant Feeding

Breast-feeding has been the traditional feeding method for most cultures. However, bottle-feeding has become extremely popular much to the chagrin of some older members of a culture. Navajo elders, for instance, believe that breast-feeding ensures respect and obedience because the child remains close to the mother, while the bottle-fed infant will be more disobedient (Clark 1981).

Western practices encourage the new mother to breast-feed as soon as possible, but in many cultures (for example, Mexican American, Navajo, Filipino, and Vietnamese) colostrum is not offered to the newborn. Breast-feeding begins only after the milk flow is established. Interestingly, when a group of Vietnamese mothers who delayed breast-feeding until the third day after birth was studied, it was found they had no difficulty breast-feeding (Ward et al 1981).

In many Asian cultures the newborn is given boiled water until the mother's milk flows. The newborn is fed on demand and cries are responded to immediately. If the crying continues, evil spirits may be blamed and a priest's blessing may be necessary. Although many of the Hmong women of Laos combine breast-feeding with some bottle-feeding, they find it unacceptable to express their milk or pump their breasts. Thus other methods of providing relief should be suggested if breast engorgement develops (LaDu 1985).

In the black-American culture there is much emphasis on feeding. Solid foods are introduced early and may even be added to the infant's formula. For the traditional Mexican American, a fat baby is considered a healthy baby and infants are fed on demand. "Spoiling" is encouraged, and a colicky baby (a baby with unexplained paroxysms of irritability, fussing, and crying for a prolonged period) may be given mint or olive oil for relief.

Breast-Feeding

Lactation

The female breast is divided into 15 to 24 lobes separated from one another by fat and connective tissue. These lobes are subdivided into lobules, composed of small units called *alveoli* where milk is synthesized by the alveolar secretory epithelium. The lobules have a system of lactiferous ductiles that join larger ducts and eventually open onto the nipple surface. During pregnancy increased levels of estrogen stimulate breast duct proliferation and development, and elevated progesterone levels promote the development of lobules and alveoli in preparation for lactation.

Birth results in a rapid drop in estrogen and progesterone with a concomitant increase in the secretion of **prolactin** by the anterior pituitary. This hormone promotes milk production by stimulating the alveolar cells of the breasts. When the newborn sucks on the mother's nipple, **oxytocin** is released from the posterior pituitary. This hormone increases the contractility of the myoepithelial cells lining the walls of the mammary ducts, and a flow of milk results. This is called the **letdown reflex**. Mothers have described the letdown reflex as a prickling or tingling sensation during which they feel the milk coming down. It is not unusual for the breasts to leak some milk prior to feeding.

The letdown reflex can be stimulated by the newborn's sucking, presence, or cry, or even by maternal thoughts about her baby. It may also occur during sexual orgasm because oxytocin is released. Conversely, the mother's lack of self-confidence, fear of, embarrassment about, or pain connected with breast-feeding may prevent the milk from being ejected into the duct system. Milk production is decreased with repeated inhibition of the letdown reflex. Failure to empty the breasts frequently and completely also decreases production, because as milk accumulates and is not withdrawn, the buildup of pressure in the alveoli suppresses secretion.

Once lactation is well established, prolactin production decreases. Oxytocin and sucking continue to be the facilitators of milk production. The release of oxytocin in response to the infant's suckling is beneficial to the new mother. Oxytocin stimulates uterine contraction and thus promotes rapid involution of the uterus.

Client Education for Breast-Feeding

The nurse caring for the breast-feeding mother should help the woman achieve independence and success in her feeding efforts (Figure 30–1). Prepared with a knowledge of the anatomy and physiology of the breast and lactation, the components and positive effects of breast milk, and the techniques of breast-feeding, the nurse can help the woman and her family use their own resources to achieve a successful experience. The objectives involved in breast-feeding are (a) to provide adequate nutrition, (b) to establish an adequate milk supply, and (c) to prevent trauma to the nipples. All instructions are aimed toward these goals.

The newborn who is breast-feeding should be put to the breast as soon as possible, depending on the situation of birth. Some infants are not interested so soon, but for those who are, early breast-feeding affords a soothing experience and has considerable physiologic and psychologic benefit for the mother. Colostrum has sufficient nutrients to satisfy the infant until milk is established in two to four

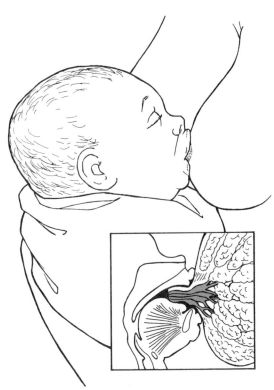

Figure 30–2 To nurse effectively, it is important that the infant's mouth cover the majority of the areola to compress the ducts below. (Courtesy Ross Laboratories, Columbus, Ohio)

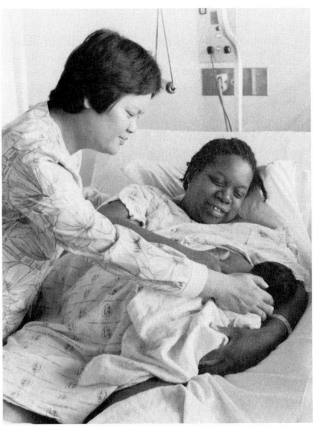

Figure 30–1 For many mothers, the nurse's support and knowledge are instrumental in establishing successful breast-feeding. Breast-feeding is facilitated when the baby is close and lies on his or her side, with the head, neck, and trunk in alignment.

days. Establishment of lactation depends on the strength of the infant's suck and the frequency of nursing.

Positioning of the baby at the breast is a critical factor. The entire body of the infant should be turned toward the mother's breast, with the mouth adjacent to the nipple and the ear, shoulder, and hip in direct alignment. The mother should not have to lift her shoulder or breast to direct the nipple into the infant's mouth. The nipple should be directed straight into the mouth, not toward the palate or tongue, and as much of the areola as possible should be included so that, as the baby sucks, the jaws compress the ducts that are directly beneath the areola (Figure 30–2). To do this, the mother holds her breast with her thumb placed on the upper portion of the breast and the remainder of her fingers cupped under her breast. She then lightly brushes the infant's lips with the nipple. Through the rooting reflex, the infant can locate the nipple. The mother should avoid stimulating both cheeks, which only confuses the hungry infant.

If the mother does not have a prominent nipple or if she has an everted nipple, she may try rolling the nipple between her thumb and forefinger or stretching the nipple by pressing inward and outward around the nipple prior to feeding. Use of the electric breast pump will quickly stimulate the nipple to become more prominent, and when a few drops of colostrum are expressed, the infant is encouraged to latch on more eagerly.

The use of a traditional red rubber nipple shield to correct nipple position may reduce the transfer of milk from the breast to the infant by 58% while increasing the infant's suck rate and resting time. Newer thin latex shields, although they do not affect sucking patterns, still reduce milk transfer by 22% (Lawrence 1989). A shield should be

---

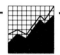

Research Note

Clinical Application of Research

To determine whether a nipple shield would alter milk volume and to discover whether one nipple shield design differed from a second, revised shield design in terms of milk volume, Kathleen Auerbach (1990) designed a study using mothers who had already established breast-feeding with their infants. These mothers were either already pumping their breasts because of employment or planned to start pumping their breasts in preparation for employment.

Every woman served as her own control by having 2 different pumping sessions, one with each breast. All women used the new shield for five minutes, the old shield for five minutes, and no shield for five minutes. The sequential order of shield use or non-use was randomly assigned to each woman at each session. To ensure consistent suction, breast pumps were used at all pumping sessions.

Results of the study demonstrated that, regardless of pumping order, more milk resulted when no shield was used than with either type of shield. Slightly more milk was obtained with the new shield design when compared with the old design.

A limitation of the study, identified by the author, was that a breast pump does not exert the same stimulation for the ejection of milk as the sucking action of the infant. Suggestions for other study designs included pumping one breast while simultaneously putting the baby on the other breast or replicating the design of an earlier study.

Critical Thinking Applied to Research
Strengths: Each participant served as her own control, minimizing a type of error variance—that of statistical difference being due to preexisting differences in the subjects not occurring as a result of the treatment. Strong design to test hypotheses. Ethical considerations when determining a potential sample.

Auerbach K: The effect of nipple shields on maternal milk volume. *JOGNN* 1990; 19(5): 419.

---

used as a last resort and preferably after consultation with a lactation expert. The use of any rubber or other artificial nipple for feeding a nursing baby should be avoided because they are more pliable and thus allow more milk to pass through them per suck than the breast does, and the infant may experience "nipple confusion" and refuse the breast when it is reoffered. Routine sterile water or dextrose and water feedings after nursing should be avoided.

The nipples should be assessed for trauma after each feeding (see the section on nipple soreness and cracked nipples on page 929). A small amount of breast milk expressed and applied to the nipple and areola helps keep the area soft and pliable and has been shown to be successful in treating cracked nipples.

Recent literature suggests that imposing time limits for breast-feeding (five minutes, then seven minutes, etc) is not as helpful in preventing nipple soreness as was previously believed (L'Esperance & Frantz 1985; Neifert 1989). Instead it may simply delay the onset of soreness. Furthermore, since letdown may take up to three minutes to occur (in the first few days at least), artificial time limits may actually interfere with successful feeding. In working to avoid undue nipple trauma it is crucial that the nipple be properly positioned and that the infant's mouth cover a large portion of the areola.

The mother is encouraged to alternate the breast she offers to the infant first at each feeding. A convenient way for the mother to remember which breast to begin with is to fasten a small safety pin to the bra cup on that side. Generally the infant will empty the breasts during a feeding. Another technique, called "switch nursing," is to alternate breasts several times during a single feeding. Once the infant stops sucking nutritively, as evidenced by sucking without swallowing, the mother should break suction gently and switch to the other breast. Once the infant has emptied the second breast, the mother should burp the infant and reoffer the first breast. Alternating breasts allows for an improved or increased number of letdowns and access to hindmilk (milk the baby takes after the first few minutes of feeding), which has higher protein and fat content. The mother may continue alternating breasts until the infant is satisfied. Total feeding time is usually no longer than 10 to 15 minutes at each breast during the feeding. Alternating breasts also prevents constant sucking for prolonged periods, which can be uncomfortable or painful if the nipple is tender.

If a full breast appears to be occluding the infant's nares, the mother should either lift the breast slightly or gently press the breast away from the nares. Pressure must be gentle to avoid inadvertently pulling the breast from the infant's mouth.

The mother is instructed in techniques for breaking suction prior to removing the infant from the breast. By inserting a finger into the infant's mouth beside the nipple, she can break the suction, and the nipple may be removed without trauma. Burping between feedings on each breast and at the end of the feeding continues to be necessary. If the infant has been crying, it is also advisable to burp before beginning feeding.

Initially more milk is produced than is required by the infant. Later the amount of milk will be produced to meet the infant's nutritional needs as manifested through sucking. Milk may tend to leak until supply meets demand. The mother should expect this and use breast pads in her bra to absorb the secretions. She should be cautioned to remove wet pads frequently to avoid irritation to the nipples or infection. The mother may also be taught to apply direct pressure to the breast with her hand or forearm once breast-feeding is well established, usually after the first month. This will often stop the leaking.

The use of supplementary feedings for the breast-feeding infant may weaken or confuse the sucking reflex and may interfere with successful outcome. Often parents are concerned because they have no visual assurance of the amount consumed. The mother may be reassured about adequacy of intake if she listens for sounds of swallowing while the baby is nursing. In addition, if the infant gains weight and has six or more wet diapers a day, he or she is receiving adequate amounts of milk. Activity levels and intervals between feedings may also indicate how satisfied the infant is. Parents should know that, because breast milk is more easily digested than formulas, the breast-fed infant becomes hungry sooner. Thus the frequency of breast-feedings may be greater, particularly after discharge, when fatigue or excitement may decrease milk supply temporarily. Increasing the frequency of feedings alleviates problems during these periods. The parents may also expect the infant to demand more frequent nursing during periods when growth spurts are expected, such as 10 days to 2 weeks, 5 to 6 weeks, 2 1/2 to 3 months, and 4 1/2 to 6 months (Huggin 1986).

Expression of Milk   The mother may be taught to express her milk manually and freeze it for bottle-feeding if she will be absent for a scheduled feeding. Breast milk should be frozen in plastic bottles; if glass bottles are used, the antibodies will adhere to the sides of the bottle and their benefits will be lost. Manual expression to relieve maternal discomfort and to maintain the milk supply is advisable if the mother must go several hours without feeding. The mother's milk supply will decrease unless the breasts are emptied regularly.

Milk may be expressed by hand or by using a breast pump. Expression of milk is used to collect milk for supplemental feedings. It is also used to relieve breast fullness or engorgement and to help build the woman's milk supply. To express her milk manually, the woman first washes her hands and then massages her breast to stimulate letdown. To massage her breast, the woman grasps the breast with both hands at the base of the breast near the chest wall. Using the palms of her hands she then firmly slides her hands toward her nipple. She repeats this process several times. Then she is ready to begin hand expression. The woman generally uses her left hand for her right breast and right hand for her left breast. However, some women find it preferable to use the hand on the same side as the breast (right hand for right breast). The nurse should encourage the woman to use the method she finds most effective. She grasps the areola with her thumb on the top and her first two fingers on the lower portion (Figure 30–3). Without allowing her fingers to slide on her skin, she pushes inward

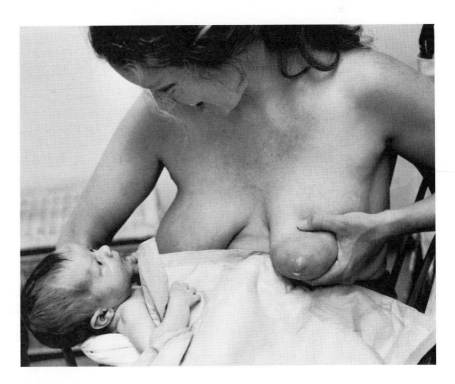

Figure 30–3   Hand position for manual expression of milk

toward the chest and then squeezes her fingers together while pulling forward on the areola. She can use a container to catch any fluid that is squeezed out. She then repositions her hand by rotating it slightly so that she can repeat the process. She continues to reposition her hand and repeat the process to empty all the milk sinuses.

Hand or electric breast pumps are useful for building and maintaining a milk supply when the infant is not able to nurse (premature infant, ill infant, infant with breast-milk jaundice, mother on medications that are excreted in the breast milk) or for the working mother who regularly misses certain feedings. Hand pumps are more portable, can be purchased by the mother, and are less expensive. Electric pumps are more efficient but are bulky and expensive. They may be rented in many areas. Breast pumps work by suction to express the milk. Some have collection systems for easy milk saving. Many agencies have a variety of pumps available and provide instruction on correct methods of pumping the breasts (Figure 30–4). Videotapes or photographs are also useful in demonstrating the process to new mothers. See Procedure 30–1.

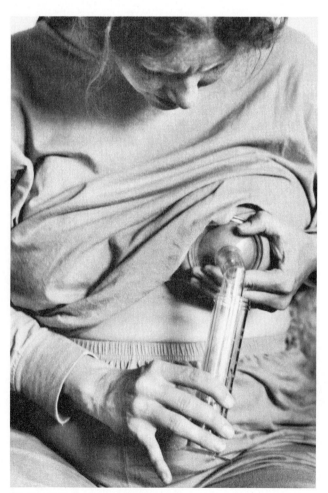

Figure 30–4 Hand-held breast pump

External Supports

La Leche League is an organized group of volunteers who work to provide education about breast-feeding and assistance to women who are breast-feeding their infants. They sponsor activities, have printed material available, have electric breast pumps available for rental, offer one-to-one counseling to mothers with questions or problems, and provide group support to breast-feeding mothers.

Numerous books and pamphlets are also available to help the breast-feeding mother. The mother needs the support of all family members, her physician/nurse-midwife, pediatrician or pediatric nurse practitioner, and all nursing personnel because it is often the attitudes of these people that ultimately lead the woman to success or failure.

Prescription Drugs and Breast-Feeding

It has long been recognized that certain medications taken by the mother may have an effect on her infant. A drug may affect the newborn in one of three ways (Nice 1989):

1. Lactation may be inhibited, thereby decreasing the supply of breast milk.

2. The newborn's physiologic processes may be directly affected by the drug if it crosses into the breast milk.

3. The mother's physical or emotional ability to care for her newborn may be altered.

Certain characteristics of a drug influence whether it passes into the breast milk, including its degree of protein binding. In general, unbound drugs enter the breast milk. Other factors are (a) the degree of ionization (drugs tend to cross in un-ionized form); (b) molecular weight (drugs with a molecular weight greater than 200 will not cross into the breast milk); (c) mechanism of transport (drugs enter breast milk by active transport, simple diffusion, or carrier-mediated diffusion); and (d) solubility of the drug (the alveolar epithelium presents a lipid barrier that tends to be more permeable when colostrum is present). The effects of the drug are also influenced by the infant's ability to absorb the drug from the gastrointestinal tract and by the body's ability to detoxify the drug and excrete it (Lawrence 1989).

Four adjustments should be made to decrease the effects on the infant when administering drugs to a nursing mother (Lawrence 1989):

1. The use of long-acting drug forms, which are usually detoxified in the liver, should be avoided. The infant may have difficulty excreting them and accumulation may be a problem.

2. Absorption rates and peak blood levels should be considered in scheduling the administration of the drugs. Less of the drugs crosses into the milk if the medication is given immediately after the woman has nursed her baby.

3. The infant should be closely observed for any signs

Methods of Breast Pumping and Milk Storage

Breast-Pumping—Manual Expression

Advantages

1. Collection container only equipment needed.
2. Technique easily learned

Disadvantages

1. Time-consuming
2. Less effective than pumping

Procedure

1. Assemble sterilized container and wash hands and breasts.
2. Perform gentle breast massage to stimulate the letdown reflex.
3. Position thumb and index finger about ½ inch behind nipple where milk sinuses are located.
4. Push fingers straight back toward chest and then squeeze them together with a slight rolling motion, lifting nipple outward. Avoid sliding fingers away from original position.
5. Rotate fingers around nipple to empty other milk sinuses. (Helpful hint: Practice technique on one breast while baby is nursing on other breast so infant will stimulate letdown reflex.)
6. Express milk into sterilized container
7. Store as directed (see milk storage section).
8. Switch breasts as soon as flow in each breast decreases.

Breast Pumping—Using Breast Pumps

Advantages

1. Milk has a higher fat content when pumped with a breast pump than when expressed manually because more complete emptying of breasts allows access to hindmilk.
2. Increased volume obtained
3. Less potential for milk contamination

Disadvantages

1. More expensive—cost varies depending on equipment chosen.
2. Increased possibility of nipple trauma due to incorrect use or high pressures.

Procedures

Hand (Cylinder) Pump

1. Collect equipment. All equipment including hand pump, tubing, and collection bottles should be cleaned and/or sterilized between uses.
2. Wash hands and breasts.
3. Apply gentle massage or heat to breasts to stimulate flow of milk.
4. Alternate breasts as soon as flow decreases.
5. Place flange on breast and secure with one hand. If flange is not angled, mother should lean forward.
6. Suction is created by sliding outer cylinder away from breast, starting with short frequent pulls with other hand to initiate milk flow.
7. Empty breast milk into plastic storage container.
8. Repeat on opposite breast.
9. Store milk as directed.

Battery-Operated Pumps

1. Follow steps 1 through 4 as for hand pump method.
2. Place flange on breast.
3. Turn on and regulate suction by depressing button or bar with one hand to achieve gentle, continuous suction.
4. Milk flows gently into storage container.

(continued)

PROCEDURE 30–1 (continued)

5. Repeat on other breast.
6. Store milk as directed.
7. Clean equipment.

Electric Pump

1. Follow steps 1 through 4 as for hand pump method.
2. After assembling pump, place flange over breast. If using double pump with Y connector, overall production is increased and pumping time is decreased by half.
3. Turn machine on with pressure setting on low and gradually increase pressure setting as tolerance permits.
4. Pump creates a rhythmic suck-release pattern closely approximating sucking action of baby.
5. Milk is expressed directly into storage container.
6. Seal and store milk as directed.
7. Clean equipment.

Milk Storage

Procedure

1. Although milk may be stored in small plastic or glass bottles or disposable plastic bottle liners, the most recommended collection container is the rigid polypropylene plastic container, which maintains the stability of all constituents in human milk and is easier and safer to use (Lawrence 1989).
2. Label milk with name, date, and time.
3. Once collected and sealed, milk may be stored in refrigerator for no more than 48 hours, freezer compartment of refrigerator for 2 weeks, or deep freezer for 6 months.
4. Warm refrigerated milk in warm water for 10 to 15 minutes just prior to use. Do not microwave or heat on stove.
5. Discard all unused milk. Breast milk cannot be refrozen.
6. Freshly pumped milk can be added to already frozen milk by chilling it in refrigerator for 30 to 60 minutes prior to adding it to prevent the top layer of frozen breast milk from defrosting.
7. Thaw frozen milk in refrigerator up to 24 hours prior to use or in water just before feeding, gradually increasing temperature from cool to warm. Do not microwave or heat on stove.
8. Frozen breast milk may take on a yellow color which does not indicate spoilage.
9. If pumping and transporting milk, place milk in insulated pouch or cooler with ice to prevent spoilage.

of drug reaction including rash, fussiness, lethargy, or changes in sleeping habits or feeding pattern.

4. Using an appropriate table, whenever possible a drug should be selected that shows the least tendency to pass into breast milk.

The mother should be given information about the potential of most drugs to cross into breast milk. She should also be advised to tell any physician who may prescribe medications for her that she is breast-feeding. Clinicians who do not routinely care for obstetric or pediatric clients may not be familiar with the effects on breast milk of the drugs they prescribe and may need to consult the obstetrician. The positive and negative effects of the medication on the woman and her infant must be considered carefully.

Selected Potential Problems in Breast-feeding

Many women stop nursing because the problems encountered seem to have no solutions. The nurse can offer anticipatory guidance about remedies and solution to such problems. This allows the mother to provide her infant with the nutritional and emotional experience that she has planned for during the pregnancy. Table 30–7 summarizes

---

Table 30–7 Self-Care Measures for the Woman with Breast-Feeding Problems

Abnormal Nipples

Use Hoffman's exercises antepartally to increase protractility (see Chapter 14).

Use special breast shields such as Woolrich or Eschmann.

Use hand to shape nipple when beginning to nurse.

Apply ice for a few minutes prior to feeding to improve nipple erection.

Use electric or hand pump to cause nipple prominence and express a few drops of breast milk, then switch to regular nursing.

Inadequate Letdown

Massage breasts prior to nursing.

Feed in a quiet, private place, away from distraction.

Take a warm shower before nursing to relax and stimulate letdown.

Apply warm pack for 20 minutes before nursing.

Use relaxation techniques and focus on letdown.

Drink water, juice, or noncaffeinated beverages before and during feeding.

Avoid overfatigue by resting when the baby sleeps, feeding while lying down, and having quiet time alone.

Develop a conditioned response by establishing a routine for starting feedings.

Allow the baby sufficient time (at least 10 to 15 minutes per side) to trigger the letdown reflex.

Use breast alternating method (p 924)

If all else fails obtain a prescription for oxytocin nasal spray from the health care provider.

Nipple Soreness

Ensure that infant is correctly positioned at the breast, with ear, shoulder & hip in straight alignment.

Rotate breast-feeding positions.

Use finger to break suction before removing infant from the breast.

Hold baby close when feeding to avoid undue pulling on nipple.

Don't allow baby to sleep with nipple in mouth.

Nurse more frequently.

Begin nursing on less sore breast.

Apply ice to nipples and areola for a few minutes prior to feeding.

Protect nipples to prevent skin breakdown:
—Clean nipple gently with warm water.
—Allow nipples to air dry, or dry nipples with hair dryer set to low heat, or expose nipples to sunlight.

If clothing rubs nipples, use ventilated shields to keep clothing away from skin.

To promote healing, apply a small amount of breast milk to nipple and areola after nursing and allow to dry.

The routine application of ointment to nipple, areola, or breast (eg, lanolin, Massé cream, Eucerin cream, or A&D ointment) should be discouraged.

Apply tea bags soaked in warm water.

Change breast pads frequently.

Nurse long enough to empty breasts completely.

Alternate breasts several times during feeding.

Cracked Nipples

Use interventions discussed under sore nipples.

Inspect nipples carefully for cracks or fissures.

Temporarily stop nursing on the affected breast and hand express milk for a day or two until cracks heal.

Maintain healthy diet. Protein and vitamin C are essential for healing.

Use a mild analgesic such as acetaminophen for discomfort.

Consult health care providers if signs of infection develop (see Chapter 36).

A nipple shield should be tried before the nursing on a breast is stopped, but it should be used only as a last resort. A consultation with a lactation specialist prior to use is advised.

Breast Engorgement

Nurse frequently (every 1½ to 3 hours) around the clock.

Wear a well-fitting supportive bra at all times.

Take a warm shower or apply warm compresses to trigger letdown.

Massage breasts and then hand express some milk to soften the breast so the infant can "latch on."

Breast-feed long enough to empty breast.

Alternate starting breast.

Take a mild analgesic 20 minutes before feeding if discomfort is pronounced.

Plugged Ducts (Caked Breasts)

Nurse frequently and for long enough to empty the breasts completely.

Rotate feeding position.

Massage breasts prior to feeding, in a warm shower when possible.

Maintain good nutrition and adequate fluid intake.

self-care measures the nurse can suggest to a woman with a breast-feeding problem.

Nipple Soreness The mother should be told that some soreness often occurs initially with breast-feeding and that the problem will resolve as soon as the letdown reflex is established. The infant should not be switched to bottle-feeding or have feedings delayed, as these measures will only cause engorgement and more soreness.

Because the area of greatest stress to the nipple is in line with the newborn's chin and nose, nipple soreness may be decreased by encouraging the mother to rotate positions when feeding the infant. Figure 30–5 illustrates the cradle hold, football hold, and maternal side-lying positions. Changing positions alters the focus of greatest stress and promotes more complete breast emptying.

Nipple soreness is usually due to one of two conditions: trauma to the nipple and irritation of the nipple. The traumatized nipple may be blistered, scabbed, or cracked, whereas the irritated nipple is very pink (the irritation may cause a burning sensation). Occasionally, a mother may have both irritated and traumatized nipples.

Nipple soreness may also develop if the infant has faulty sucking habits. Traumatized nipples may have in-

jured tips that are bruised, scabbed, or blistered from the nipple entering the baby's mouth at an upward angle and rubbing against the roof of the mouth, where the tongue does not act as a cushion. Soreness may also develop if the infant falls asleep with the breast in his or her mouth. This continuous negative pressure on the nipple can lead to problems (L'Esperance & Frantz 1985).

Chewed nipples, which result from improper positioning, are cracked or tender at or near the base. In these cases, the baby's jaws close only on the nipple instead of the areola, or the baby's mouth is not opened wide enough, or the infant's mouth has slipped down to the nipple from the areola as a result of engorgement. Soreness on the underside of the nipple is caused by the infant nursing with her or his bottom lip tucked in rather than out, causing a friction burn. Vigorous sucking produces little milk because the milk sinuses under the areola are not compressed. This results in a frustrated infant and marked soreness for the mother. The problem is overcome by positioning the infant with as much areola as possible in his or her mouth.

Nipple soreness is especially pronounced during the first few minutes of the feeding. If the mother is not expecting this, she may become discouraged and quickly stop. The letdown reflex may take a few minutes to activate, and it

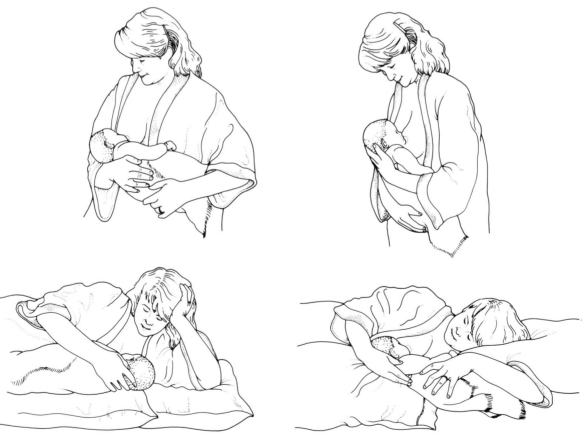

Figure 30–5   Examples of breast-feeding position changes to facilitate thorough breast emptying and prevent nipple soreness

may not occur if the mother stops nursing too quickly. The problem is compounded if the infant is unsatisfied, and the possibility of breast engorgement increases.

Because nipple soreness can also result from an overeager infant, the mother may find it helpful to nurse more frequently. This helps ease the vigorous sucking of a ravenous infant. The woman can also apply ice to her nipples and areola for a few minutes prior to feeding. This promotes nipple erectness and numbs the tissue to ease the initial discomfort. To prevent excoriation and skin breakdown, the nipples and areola should be washed with water and then allowed to dry thoroughly. Drying may be accomplished by leaving the bra flaps down for several minutes after feeding or by exposing the nipples to sunlight or ultraviolet light, for 30 seconds at first and gradually increasing to 3 minutes. Drying the nipples with a hair dryer on low heat setting also facilitates drying and promotes healing, especially if breast milk is allowed to dry on the nipples.

The use of substances such as lanolin, Massé Breast Cream, Eucerin cream, or A and D ointment on the nipples between feedings should be discouraged. These preparations may cause allergic reactions, or irritation may be increased if the substance needs to be washed off prior to nursing. In addition, the substance may be contaminated. Pesticide residue has been found in lanolin, which forms the basis for many breast care products (Rosanove 1987). Most recently, rapid healing has been demonstrated by the application of breast milk, which is then allowed to dry on the nipples (Renfrew, Fisher & Arms 1990). Breast milk is high in fat, fights infection and will not irritate the nipples. An obvious advantage is that it is readily available at no cost to the mother.

If the woman finds that her bra or clothing rubs against her nipples and add to her discomfort, she may insert shields into her bra to prevent this. Both Medela Shells and Woolrich Shields, for example, relieve friction and promote air circulation.

A woman may use breast pads inside her bra to prevent leaking of milk onto her clothes. These pads should be changed frequently so that the nipples remain dry. Breast pads with plastic liners interfere with air circulation; the plastic should be removed before using them.

Older remedies for nipple soreness are receiving renewed acceptance. For instance, tea bags may be moistened in warm water and applied to the nipples. The tannic acid seems to help toughen the nipples, and the warmth is soothing and promotes healing. Irritated nipples or nipple dermatitis, which causes swollen, erythematous, burning nipples, are most commonly caused by thrush or by allergic response to breast cream preparations.

If the nipple soreness has a sudden onset, it may be caused by a thrush infection transmitted from the infant to the mother. White patches or streaks in the infant's mouth indicate a need for treatment of the mouth and nipple infection. If the problem is treated, the mother can usually continue breast-feeding.

Cracked Nipples Nipple soreness is frequently coupled with cracked nipples. Whenever a breast-feeding mother complains of soreness, the nipples must be carefully examined for fissures or cracks, and the mother should be observed during breast-feeding to see whether the infant is correctly positioned at the breast. If the positioning is correct and cracks exist, further interventions are necessary. The mother's first reaction may be to cease nursing on the sore breast, but this may aggravate the problem if engorgement and plugged ducts result. All the interventions described for sore nipples may be used. It may also help the mother to begin nursing on the breast that is less sore. This allows the letdown reflex to occur in the affected breast, and the infant does more vigorous sucking on the less tender breast, which decreases trauma to the cracked nipple.

With severe cases, the temporary use of a nipple shield for nursing may be necessary. For the mother's comfort, analgesics may be taken after nursing.

Breast Engorgement About the time their milk initially comes in, many women complain of feelings of engorgement. Their breasts are hard, painful, warm, and appear taut and shiny. At first this fullness is caused by venous congestion due to the increased vascularity in the breasts. Later the problem may be compounded by the pressure of accumulating milk.

The mother should be encouraged to wear a wellfitting nursing bra 24 hours a day. The bra supports the breasts and prevents further discomfort from tension and pulling on the Cooper's ligament. Frequent nursing is also helpful in preventing or decreasing engorgement. Breastfeeding every 1 1/2 to 3 hours initially keeps the breasts emptied, increases the circulation in the breast, and helps remove the fluid that might lead to engorgement.

Because the engorged breast is quite hard, nursing may be difficult for the infant and painful for the mother. Manual expression of milk or the use of a nontraumatic breast pump to initiate the flow may be helpful, as is the judicious use of analgesics. Warmth is often soothing, and the mother who has problems with engorgement may find a warm shower comforting. It is also useful in stimulating the letdown reflex. The mother may find it helpful to stand in the shower and manually express some milk before feeding. To prevent discomfort, it is advisable to avoid having the spray beat directly on the nipples and breasts. Warm, moist cloths may also be used for relief. Additional relief measures include the use of ice packs between feedings, with hot packs applied 20 minutes prior to a feeding. The engorgement is generally relieved within 12 to 24 hours.

Plugged Ducts Some mothers experience plugging of one or more ducts, especially in conjunction with or following engorgement. This is often referred to as caked breasts. Manifested as an area of tenderness or "lumpiness" in an otherwise well woman, plugging may be relieved by the use of heat and massage. The mother can be encouraged to massage her breasts from her chest wall forward to the nipple while standing in a warm shower or following the application of hot packs to the breast (Riordan 1983). She should then nurse her infant, starting on the unaffected breast if the plugged breast is tender. Frequent nursing will help prevent the problem and fatigue as well. In cases of repeatedly plugged ducts or caked breasts, it may be necessary for the mother to limit her fat intake to polyunsaturated fats and to add lecithin to her diet (Lawrence 1989).

Breast-Feeding and the Working Mother

Often a mother returning to work elects to continue breast-feeding her infant. This decision requires planning on her part and family encouragement and assistance. She will find this easier to accomplish if she has six to eight weeks at home to establish lactation before returning to work. She should use this time to accustom her infant to taking supplemental feedings from a bottle. This permits others to care for the baby while the mother works. A few days before returning to work she can begin manually expressing and freezing her milk for her infant's use while she is gone. At work it will be necessary for her to pump her breasts during lunch or coffee breaks to avoid the discomfort of full breasts. She should attempt to pump her breasts at least every four hours. Because milk production follows the principle of supply and demand, if breasts are not pumped, the milk supply will decrease. Whenever a nursing mother is separated from her infant for more than six hours, a piston electric breast pump and double collection system, if available, is considered the optimal means of milk expression (Neifert 1989).

Sometimes a mother has a flexible schedule and can return home to nurse at lunch time or have the baby brought to her. If this is not possible, the infant may be fed expressed milk or a supplemental bottle of formula. If the mother is expressing milk at work for use the next day, she must be certain to keep it refrigerated and use it within 48 hours. Breast milk can be frozen in plastic bottles or bags and stored for up to six months.

To maintain an adequate milk supply the working mother must pay special attention to her fluid intake. She can ensure an adequate intake by drinking extra fluid at each break whenever possible during the day. In addition, it is helpful to nurse more on weekends, to nurse during the night, to eat a nutritionally sound diet, and to continue manual expression or pumping when not nursing (Neifert 1989).

Night nursing presents a dilemma in that it may help a working mother maintain her milk supply but may also contribute to fatigue. Some women choose to have the infant sleep with them so that breast-feeding is more easily accomplished. Other women find it difficult to sleep soundly when the infant is in the same bed. For the mother who works long hours or has a rigid work schedule, the best alternative may be to limit breast-feeding to morning and evening feedings with supplemental feedings at other times. This choice allows her to maintain a close relationship with

the infant and provides some of the unique benefits of breast milk.

Weaning

The decision to wean the baby from the breast may be made for a variety of reasons including family or cultural pressures, change in the home situation, pressure from the woman's partner, or a personal opinion about when **weaning** should occur. For the woman who is comfortable with breast-feeding and well-informed about the process, the appropriate time to wean her infant will become evident if she is sensitive to the child's cues. Often weaning falls between periods of great developmental activity for the child. Thus weaning commonly occurs at 8 to 9 months, 12 to 14 months, 18 months, 2 years, and 3 years of age. Within our society, however, weaning commonly occurs before the child is 9 months old, although it may occur any time from soon after birth to 4 years of age (Williams & Morse 1989).

If weaning is timed to respond to the child's cues, and if the mother is comfortable with the timing, it can be accomplished with less difficulty than if the process is begun before both mother and child are ready emotionally. Nevertheless, weaning is a time of emotional separation for mother and baby; it may be difficult for them to give up the closeness of their nursing sessions. The nurse who is understanding about this possibility can help the mother see that her infant is growing up and plan other comforting, consoling, and play activities to replace breast-feeding. A gradual approach is the easiest and most comforting way to wean the child from breast-feedings. Other activities can enhance the parent-infant attachment process.

During weaning, the mother should substitute one cup-feeding or bottle-feeding for one breast-feeding session over several days to a week so that her breasts gradually produce less milk. Eliminating the breast-feedings associated with meals first facilitates the mother's ability to wean the infant as satiation with food lessens the desire for milk (Bishop 1985). Over a period of several weeks she should substitute more cup-feedings or bottle-feedings for breast-feedings. Many mothers continue to nurse once a day in the early morning or late evening for several months until the milk supply is gone. The slow method of weaning prevents breast engorgement and allows infants to alter their eating methods at their own rates and also allows time for psychologic adjustment.

Client Education for Bottle-Feeding

Most women cradle their infants in the crook of the arm close to the body, which provides the intimacy and cuddling so essential to an infant and provides the same benefits as the closeness of breast-feeding. With the great emphasis placed on successful breast-feeding, the teaching needs of the bottle-feeding new mother may be overlooked. If she has had only limited experience in feeding infants, she may need some guidelines to feed her newborn successfully. The following important principles should be included in the teaching provided:

1. Bottles should always be held, not propped. Positional otitis media may develop when the infant is fed horizontally, because milk and nasal mucus may occlude the eustachian tube. Holding the infant provides a rest for the feeder, social and close physical contact for the baby, and an opportunity for parent-child interaction and bonding. Once feeding is initiated, the infant should be held securely to provide physical closeness and facilitate eye contact (Figure 30–6).

2. The nipple should have a hole big enough to allow milk to flow in drops when the bottle is inverted. Too large an opening may cause overfeeding or regurgitation because of rapid feeding. If feeding is too fast, the nipple should be changed and the infant should be helped to eat more slowly by stopping the feeding frequently for burping and cuddling.

3. The nipple should be pointed directly into the mouth, not toward the palate or tongue, and should be on top of the tongue. The nipple should be full of liquid at all times to avoid ingestion of extra amounts of air, which decreases the amount of feeding and increases discomfort.

4. The infant should be burped at intervals, preferably at the middle and end of the feeding. The infant who seems to swallow a great deal of air while sucking may need more frequent burping. In addition, if the infant has cried before being fed, air may have been swallowed, and the infant should be burped before beginning to feed or after taking just enough to calm down. Burping is done by holding the infant upright on the shoulder or by holding the infant in a sitting position on the feeder's lap with chin and chest supported on one hand. The back is then gently patted or stroked with the other hand. Too-frequent burping may confuse a newborn who is attempting to coordinate sucking, swallowing, and breathing simultaneously.

5. Newborns frequently regurgitate small amounts of feedings. This may look like a large amount to the inexperienced parent, however, and she or he may require reassurance that this is normal. Initially it may be due to excessive mucus and gastric irritation from foreign substances in the stomach from birth. Later, regurgitation may result when the infant feeds too rapidly and swallows air. It may also occur when the infant is overfed and the cardiac sphincter allows the excess to be regurgitated. Because this is such a common occurrence, experienced parents and nurses generally keep a "burp cloth" available. Although regurgitation is normal, vomiting or a forceful expulsion of fluid is not. When forceful expulsion occurs, further evaluation may be indicated, especially if other symptoms are present.

6. A fat baby is not necessarily a healthy one. Parents should be encouraged to avoid overfeeding or feeding infants every time they cry. Infants should be encouraged but not forced to feed and should be allowed to set their own pace once feedings are established. Parents sometimes set artificial goals— "The baby must take all five ounces"—and tend to keep feeding the child until those goals are met, even though the infant may not be hungry. Overfeeding results in infant obesity. During early feedings, however, the infant may need simple tactile stimulation—such as gently rubbing feet and hands, adjusting clothing, and loosening coverings—to maintain adequate sucking for a sufficient time to complete a full feeding.

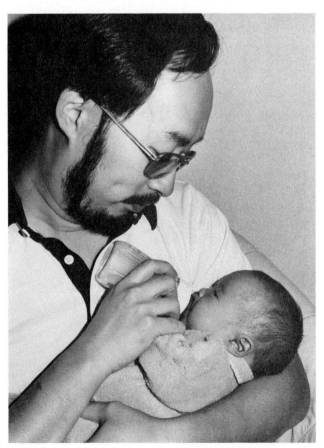

Figure 30–6 An infant is supported comfortably during bottle-feeding.

Formula preparation and sterilization techniques are always important to discuss with families. Cleanliness remains an essential component but sterilization is necessary only if the water source is questionable. (Procedure 30–2 describes methods of sterilization.) Bottles may be effec-

PROCEDURE 30–2
Methods of Bottle Sterilization

Terminal sterilization

Advantages

1. Safest, most efficient method
2. More easily learned

Disadvantages

1. Prolonged cooling period (1 hr)
2. Not suitable for disposable bottles

Procedure

1. Assemble equipment and wash hands.
2. Thoroughly wash bottles, caps, and nipples in warm soapy water; squeeze some water through holes to rid them of accumulated milk; rinse well.
3. Wash the lid of the formula can (if using a liquid) and prepare formula according to directions.
4. Fill the bottles with the desired amount of formula and loosely apply the nipples and caps; one or two bottles of water may be prepared at the same time.
5. Place the prepared bottles in a large kettle or bottle sterilizer and add the appropriate amount of water (as specified on the sterilizer or 2–3 in. if a kettle is used).
6. Cover the sterilizer, bring the water to a gentle boil, and boil for 25 min. at 212F.
7. Remove from heat but let the bottles remain in the sterilizer with the lid on until the sides of the pan are cool to the touch.
8. Remove the bottles, tighten the lids, and refrigerate until needed.

Aseptic method of sterilization

Advantages

1. May be modified for use with disposable bottles

Disadvantages

1. Difficult to learn, contamination more likely

Procedure

1. Same as steps 1 and 2 of terminal method.
2. Place all equipment needed (bottles, nipples, caps, can opener, tongs, measuring pitcher, and spoon) in a large kettle or sterilizer; cover with water, and boil for 5 min.
3. In another pan boil the amount of water necessary to make the formula (boil for 5 min).
4. Drain the water from the sterilizer pan and let the equipment cool 1 hour.
5. Remove the measuring pitcher, being certain to touch only the handle.
6. Use the sterilized can opener to open a can of formula after first washing the lid with soapy water and rinsing well; pour the formula into the prepared measuring pitcher, and add the correct amount of boiled water; mix with the prepared spoon.
7. Use tongs to remove the bottles from the sterilizer and fill them with the desired amount of formula; (one or two bottles of water may also be prepared by boiling enough additional water).
8. Use the tongs to set the nipples on the bottles; then apply the caps, touching only the edges.

(continued)

PROCEDURE 30–2 *(continued)*

9. Refrigerate until needed.

To modify for disposable bottles:

Complete all steps as directed except *do not boil the bottles* with the other equipment and allow the water to cool for 15–20 min before preparing the formula (the plastic bag may melt if the formula is too hot).

Dishwasher Sterilization

Advantages

1. Easy

Disadvantages

1. May not have access to dishwasher
2. Hot water tank needs to be set at 120F or medium heat setting.

Procedure

1. Place bottles, caps into dishwasher rack.
2. Wash on hot water cycle then machine dry.
3. Spoon dry formula powder into bottles, cap with nipples, invert, and store at room temperature. Add tap water at time of feeding.
4. If liquid formula is used, add unboiled tap water to the liquid formula after dishwasher sterilization of bottles; refrigerate filled, capped bottles until needed.
5. Clean nipples separately with hot, soapy water; rinse thoroughly; then boil for 5 minutes. Cool for one hour. Nipples become softened if sterilized in dishwasher.
6. Sterilize disposable bottles in the top rack of dishwasher; clean nipples as in step 5 above.

---

tively prepared in dishwashers (nipples may be weakened by the temperature of dishwashers and therefore should be washed thoroughly by hand with soap and water and rinsed well) or washed thoroughly in warm soapy water and rinsed well. Tap water, if from an uncontaminated source, may be used for mixing powdered formulas, which are less expensive than the concentrated or ready-to-use prepared formulas. Honey should not be used as a "sugar source" because of the danger of infant botulism (Mott et al 1990).

Bottles may be prepared individually, or up to one day's supply of formula may be prepared at one time. Extra bottles are stored in the refrigerator and should be warmed slightly before feeding. Ready-to-use disposable bottles of formula are very convenient but are also expensive.

Nutritional Assessment of the Infant

During the early months of life, the food offered to and consumed by infants will be instrumental in their proper growth and development. At each well-baby visit the nurse assesses the nutritional status of the newborn. Assessment should include four components:

- Nutritional history from the parent
- Weight gain since the last visit
- Growth chart percentiles
- Physical examination

The nutritional history reports the type, amount, and frequency of milk and supplemental foods being given to the infant on a daily basis. The healthy formula-fed infant should generally gain 1 ounce per day for the first six months of life and 0.5 ounce per day for the second six months. Healthy breast-fed babies may fall within these weight-gain parameters but may also be normal while gaining 0.5 ounce per day for the first six months. Individual charts show the infant's growth with respect to height, weight, and head circumference. The important consideration is that infants continue to grow at their own individual rates.

For the breast-feeding mother who is concerned about whether her infant is getting adequate nutrition, the nurse can recommend looking for an appearance of weight gain and counting the number of wet diapers in a 24-hour period. Six wet diapers or more in a day indicates adequate nutrition is being attained in the totally breast-fed infant. If additional water is ingested, this count is low. The presence of urine can most accurately be assessed when the diaper is free of feces. This is most likely prior to feedings. The gastrocolic reflex often stimulates stooling following a feeding. For the anxious parent, another means of reassurance of adequate intake and output is to keep a record of the frequency and duration of feedings and the exact number of wet and/or soiled diapers. Keeping a record tends to give the worried parent a sense of control and a tangible indication on which to rule out or base concern.

The physical examination will assist in identifying any nutritional disorders. Iron deficiency should be suspected in a pale, diaphoretic, irritable infant who is obese and consumes more than 35 to 40 ounces of formula per day.

By calculating the nutritional needs of infants, the nurse can recommend a diet that supplies appropriate nutrition for infant growth and development. The assessment is especially helpful in counseling mothers of infants under 6 months of age in view of the tendency to add too many supplemental foods or offer too much formula to infants of this age. Clinicians generally advise that an infant should not be given more than 32 ounces of formula in one day. If additional calories are needed, supplemental foods should be added to the diet. Conversely, if the caloric intake is adequate or excessive, formula alone gives the infant enough calories and introduction of solid foods can be delayed until later.

When an infant's caloric intake and weight gain is found to be excessive, clinicians do not advise putting the infant on a weight reduction diet because tissue growth is rapid during this period and must be supported. The appropriate advice is to provide a maintenance caloric intake as a means of allowing the infant to maintain weight while growing in length and age.

Identification of appropriate nutritional intake can be done by comparing the infant's dietary intake with the desired caloric intake, weight, age, and the number of calories needed by the infant. Most commercial formulas prescribed for the normal healthy newborn contain 20 calories per ounce. If the infant is eating solids, the caloric value of those foods must be determined and included in the calculation of nutritional intake. With knowledge of the amount of calories needed by the infant according to weight (55 calories/lb) the nurse can counsel the parents about how many ounces per day the child needs to meet caloric requirements. The following case study shows the effectiveness of these assessments.

Case Study: Age 1 Week

Jamie, age 1 week, is visited at home by the nurse associated with a health maintenance organization (HMO). Jamie is Mrs Adams' first child, and Mrs Adams is con-cerned about whether Jamie is getting adequate nourishment. Jamie weighed 7 pounds at birth and has regained her birth weight after an 11-ounce (10%) loss. Mrs Adams reports that Jamie takes 3 ounces of formula at each of eight feedings during a 24-hour period, does not spit up any formula, and has eight to ten wet diapers a day with one to two soft bowel movements per day. Jamie is a contented baby who sleeps between feedings.

❀   *APPLYING THE NURSING PROCESS*   ❀

Nursing Assessment

Based on requirements of 55 calories/lb, the nurse calculates 1-week-old Jamie's dietary needs as follows:

Jamie's weight = 7 lb

Jamie's 24-hour caloric need = 7 lb x 55 cal/lb = 385 cal/lb

Needed formula (20 cal/oz) for 24 hours = 19 oz

Jamie's 24-hour intake = 24 oz (20 cal/oz) = 480 cal

Nursing Diagnosis

- Alteration in nutrition: more than body requirement related to formula intake that is greater than necessary to meet Jamie's growth needs
- Knowledge deficit related to assessing adequacy of food intake

Nursing Plan and Implementation

Encourage Mrs Adams to offer Jamie 2 3/4 ounces of formula at each of the seven feedings a day. The amount per feeding may vary depending on Jamie's needs, but the total per 24 hours should not exceed 19 ounces.

Teach Mrs Adams not to offer the bottle immediately when Jamie awakes crying between feedings but to comfort her by changing her diaper, rocking her, giving her a pacifier, or putting her in a swing. Jamie's need to suck may be interpreted by her mother as a hunger signal rather than a normal reflex. True hunger behavior will be demonstrated by intense crying with fisted hands and tense body.

Teach Mrs Adams to observe appropriate feeding behaviors that include an active rooting reflex with coordinated suck and swallow pattern, tongue thrust and retraction, active gag reflex, and need to burp. Mrs Adams should be instructed to observe the bubbling pattern in the formula bottle while Jamie is sucking vigorously. A decrease in the bubbling indicates that Jamie needs to be burped, usually every 1 to 2 ounces.

Discuss with Mrs Adams the behaviors that indicate satiation. These include minimal sucking with release of the nipple and falling asleep with hands and body relaxed. She should not attempt to force the remaining milk, if any, but should discard it because of the potential for bacterial growth even if refrigerated.

Formula amounts can be increased gradually to meet Jamie's changing caloric needs and growth without excessive caloric intake. Once Jamie is ingesting 32 ounces a day, the addition of solid foods can be considered after discussion with the health provider.

Explore alternative methods for providing comfort to a newborn.

Evaluation

On a follow-up well-baby visit, Jamie is weighed and is gaining 1 ounce per day. Jamie continues to have eight to ten wet diapers a day and is alert and responsive.

❀ ❀

KEY CONCEPTS

The newborn needs 50 to 55 cal/lb/day and 2 to 2 1/2 oz of water/lb/day.

Signs indicating newborn readiness for the first feeding are: active bowel sounds, absence of abdominal distention, and a lusty cry that quiets, with rooting and sucking behaviors when a stimulus is placed near the lips.

Breast milk is the optimal food for the first four to six months of life.

Mature breast milk and commercially prepared formulas (unless otherwise noted) provide 20 cal/ounce.

Breast-fed infants need supplements of vitamin D and fluoride. However, there is no need to give supplemental iron to breast-fed infants before 6 months of age.

Breast-fed infants are getting adequate nutrition if they are gaining weight and have at least six wet diapers a day when not receiving additional water supplements.

Breast-feeding mothers should be encouraged to ensure that the infant is correctly positioned at the breast, with a large portion of the areola in his or her mouth. The mother is advised to rotate position to ensure that all ducts are emptied.

To prevent sore nipples the nurse can encourage the breast-feeding mother to allow her breasts to air dry after feeding.

A disadvantage of breast-feeding is that most drugs taken by the mother are transmitted through breast milk.

Formula-fed infants regain their birth weight by 10 days of age and gain 1 ounce/day for the first six months and 0.5 ounce/day for the second six months; birthweight is doubled at 3.5 to 4 months of age. Healthy breast-fed babies gain approximately 0.5 ounce/day in the first six months of life, regain their birth weight by about 14 days of age, and double their birth weight at approximately 5 months of age.

Formula-fed infants need no vitamin or mineral supplements other than iron, if it is not already in the formula, and fluoride if it is not obtained in the water system.

The bottle-feeding mother may require assistance with feeding and burping her infant. She will also benefit from information about feeding schedules and types of formula.

The use of skim milk, cow's milk with lowered fat content, or unmodified cow's milk is not recommended for children under 2 years old.

Nutritional assessment of the infant includes: nutritional history from parent, weight gain, growth chart percentiles, and physical examination.

❀ ❀

References

American Academy of Pediatrics, Committee on Fetus and Newborn: *Guidelines for Perinatal Care,* 2nd ed. Elk Grove Village, Il: AAP, 1988.

American Academy of Pediatrics, Committee on Nutrition: *Pediatric Nutrition Handbook,* 2nd ed. Elk Grove Village, IL: AAP, 1985.

American Academy of Pediatrics, Committee on Nutrition: Follow-up or weaning formulas. *Pediatrics* 1989, 83: 1067.

Anholm P: Breast feeding: A preventive approach to health care in infancy. *Issues Comp Pediatr Nurs* 1986; 9:1.

Avery G: *Neonatology,* 3rd ed. Philadelphia: Lippincott, 1987.

Beske JE, Garvis M: Important factors in breastfeeding success. *MCN* May/June 1982; 7:174.

Clark AL: *Culture and Childrearing.* Philadelphia: Davis, 1981.

Duncan B, Schifman RB, Corrigan JJ et al: Iron and the exclusively breastfed infant from birth to six months, *J Pediatr Gastroenterol* 1985; 4:421.

Huggins K: *The Nursing Mother's Companion.* Boston: The Harvard Common Press, 1986.

LaDu EB: Childbirth care for Hmong families. *MCN* November/December 1985; 10:382.

Lawrence RA: *Breastfeeding: A Guide for the Medical Profession,* 3rd ed. St. Louis: Mosby, 1989.

L'Esperance C, Frantz K: Time limitation for early breast feeding. *JOGNN,* March/April 1985; 14:114.

Mott SR, James SR, Sperhac AM: *Nursing Care of Children and Families,* 2nd ed. Menlo Park, CA: Addison-Wesley, 1990.

Neifert M: *Breastfeeding Standards of Care for Low Risk Infants.* Denver: St. Luke's Hospital, 1989.

Nice FJ: Can a breastfeeding mother take medication without harming her infant? *MCN* 1989; 14:27.

Pipes P: *Nutrition in Infancy and Childhood,* 4th ed. St. Louis: Mosby, 1989.

Renfrew M, Fisher C, Arms S: *Breastfeeding: Getting Breastfeeding Right for You.* Berkeley: Celestial Arts, 1990.

Riordan J: *A Practical Guide to Breastfeeding.* St. Louis: Mosby, 1983.

Rosanove. R. *Dangers of the application of lanolin* (letter). Med. J. Aust. 146:232, Feb. 16, 1987.

Sawley L: Infant feeding. *Nursing* 1989; 39:18.

Schanler R: Human milk for preterm infants: Nutritional and immune factors. *Semin Perinatol* 1989; 13:69.

Sollid, DT, et al: Breastfeeding Multiples. *J. Perinatal Neonatal Nursing,* 1989:3(1):46.

Ward BG, et al: Vietnamese refugees in Adelaide: An obstetric analysis. *Med J Aust* 1981; 1:72.

Williams KM, Morse JM: Weaning patterns of first time mothers. *MCN* 1989; 14:188.

Winick M: *Nutrition, Pregnancy, and Early Infancy.* Baltimore: Williams & Wilkins, 1989.

Worthington-Roberts B, Williams SR: *Nutrition in Pregnancy and Lactation,* 4th ed. St. Louis: Mosby, 1989.

Additional Readings

Barness LA: Bases of weaning recommendations. *J Pediatr* 1990; 117(2):S84.

Dusdieker LB et al: Prolonged maternal fluid supplementation in breast-feeding. *Pediatr* 1990; 86:737.

Grossman LK et al: The effect of postpartum lactation counseling on the duration of breast-feeding in low-income women. *AJDC* April 1990; 144:471.

Lauwers J, Woessner C: *Counseling the Nursing Mother,* 2nd ed. Wayne, NJ: Avery Publishing, 1990.

Mathew OP: Determinants of milk flow through nipple units. *AJDC* February 1990; 144:222.

Satter E: The feeding relationship: Problems and interventions. *J Pediatr* August 1990; 117(2):S181.

Walker M: Management of selected early breastfeeding problems seen in clinical pediatrics. *Birth* September 1989; 16(3):148.

Weigley E S: Changing patterns in offering solids to infants. *Pediatric Nursing* September-October 1990; 16(5):439.

CHAPTER 31

The Newborn at Risk:

Conditions Present at Birth

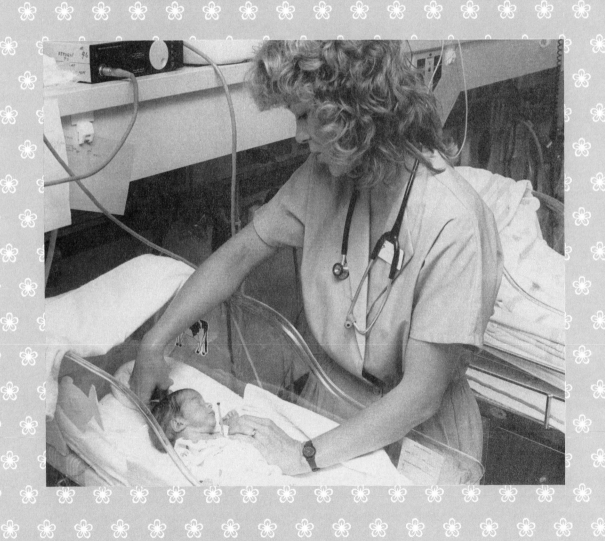

OBJECTIVES

Identify factors which may result in a neonate at risk.

Compare the underlying etiologies of the similar physiologic complications of small-for-gestational-age (SGA) newborns and preterm appropriate-for-gestational-age (AGA) newborns.

Compare the characteristics and potential complications of the postterm newborn and the infant with postmaturity syndrome.

Discuss the physiologic characteristics of the preterm newborn that predispose each body system to various complications of prematurity.

Use supporting data to identify nursing diagnoses required to plan interventions for the care of the AGA preterm newborn.

Identify nursing actions necessary to support family members dealing with the crisis of preterm birth.

Explain the care needed by newborns with acquired immunodeficiency syndrome (AIDS), alcohol- or drug-dependent newborns, and newborns with inborn errors of metabolism.

Delineate interventions to facilitate parent-infant attachment with the at-risk newborn.

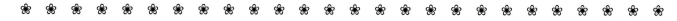

The rhythmic tides of her sleeping and feeding spaciously measured her days and nights. Her frail absorption was a commanding presence, her helplessness strong as a rock. (Laurie Lee, Two Women)

Within the past three decades, the field of neonatology has expanded greatly. Many levels of nursery care have evolved in response to increasing knowledge about the neonate: special care; transitional care; and low-, medium-, and high-risk care. The nurse is an important care giver in all these nurseries. As a member of the multidisciplinary health care team, the nurse has contributed to the high level of perinatal care available today.

In addition to the availability of high-level neonatal care other factors influence the outcome of these at-risk infants. These factors include the following:

- Birth weight
- Gestational age
- Type and length of neonatal illness
- Environmental and maternal factors

Identification of At-Risk Newborns

An at-risk infant is one who is susceptible to illness (morbidity) or even death (mortality) because of dysmaturity, immaturity, physical disorders, or complications of birth. In most cases, the infant is the product of pregnancy involving one or more predictable risk factors, including the following:

- Low socioeconomic level of the mother
- Exposure to environmental dangers such as toxic chemicals
- Preexisting maternal conditions such as heart disease and diabetes
- Obstetric factors such as age or parity
- Medical conditions related to pregnancy such as prenatal maternal infection
- Obstetric complications such as abruptio placentae

Various risk factors and their specific effects on the pregnancy outcome are listed in Table 13–2 on page 322.

Because these factors and the perinatal risks associated with them are known, the birth of at-risk newborns can often be anticipated and prepared for through adequate prenatal care. The pregnancy can be closely monitored, treatment can be instituted as necessary, and arrangements can be made for birth to occur at a facility with appropriate equipment and personnel to care for both mother and child.

Identification of at-risk infants cannot always be made before labor, since the course of labor and birth or how the infant will withstand the stress of labor is not known prior to the actual process. Thus during labor, fetal heart monitoring has played a significant role in detecting fetuses in distress.

Immediately after birth the Apgar score is a useful tool in identifying the at-risk newborn, but it is difficult to predict long-term outcome based solely on Apgar scores. In general, the lower the Apgar score at 5 minutes after birth, the higher the incidence of neurologic abnormalities seen at 1 year of age. Also data has shown that there is a higher mortality rate for infants with an Apgar score of three or less at 15 minutes of age. If these infants survive,

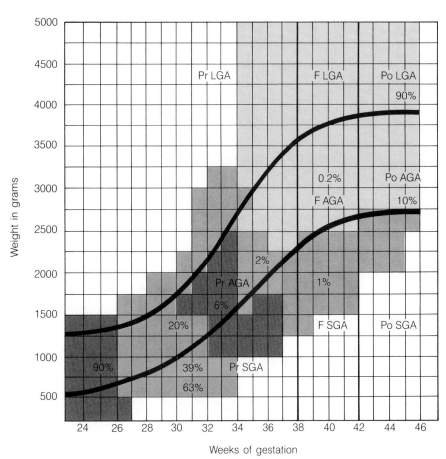

Figure 31–1   Newborn classification and neonatal mortality risk chart (From Koops BL, Morgan LP, Battaglia FC: Neonatal mortality risk in relationship to birth weight and gestational age. J Pediatr 1982; 101(6):969)

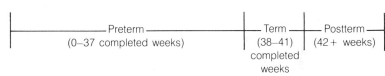

they are at a higher risk for cerebral palsy, but the majority of survivors escape other major neurologic injury (Volpe 1987). Neurologic abnormalities increase significantly as birth weight decreases.

The newborn classification and neonatal mortality risk chart is another useful tool in identifying newborns at risk (Figure 31–1). Before this classification tool was developed, birth weight of less than 2500 g was the sole criterion for determination of immaturity. It was eventually recognized that an infant could weigh more than 2500 g but still be immature. Conversely, an infant less than 2500 g might be functionally at term or beyond. Thus birth weight and gestational age together became the criteria used to assess neonatal maturity and mortality risk.

According to the newborn classification and neonatal mortality risk chart, *gestation* is divided as follows:

- Preterm = 0–37 (completed) weeks
- Term = 38–42 (completed) weeks
- Postterm = greater than 42 weeks

As shown in Figure 31–1, large-for-gestational-age (LGA) infants are those above the curved line labeled 90 percent. Appropriate-for-gestational-age (AGA) infants are those between the lines labeled 10th percentile and 90th percentile. Small-for-gestational-age (SGA) infants are those below the curved line labeled 10th percentile. A newborn is assigned to a category depending on birth weight and gestational age. For example, a newborn classified as Pr SGA is preterm and small for gestational age. The full-term newborn whose weight is appropriate for gestational age is classified F AGA.

Neonatal mortality risk is the chance of death within

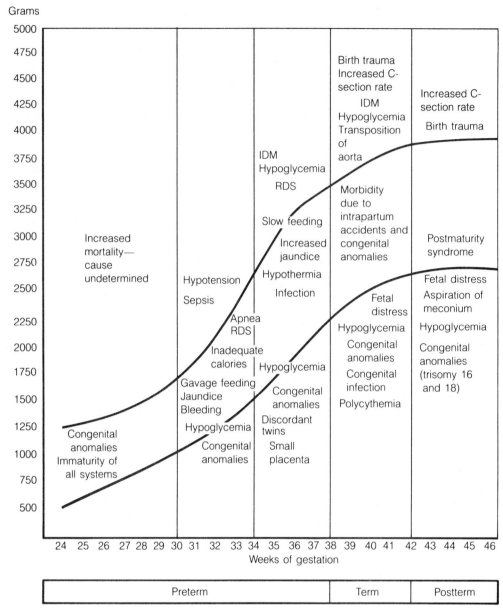

Grams

5000
4750
4500
4250
4000
3750
3500
3250
3000
2750
2500
2250
2000
1750
1500
1250
1000
750
500

Increased mortality— cause undetermined

Congenital anomalies Immaturity of all systems

Hypotension

Sepsis

Apnea RDS

Inadequate calories

Gavage feeding Jaundice Bleeding

Hypoglycemia

Congenital anomalies

IDM Hypoglycemia RDS

Slow feeding

Increased jaundice

Hypothermia

Infection

Hypoglycemia

Congenital anomalies

Discordant twins

Small placenta

Birth trauma Increased C-section rate IDM Hypoglycemia Transposition of aorta

Morbidity due to intrapartum accidents and congenital anomalies

Fetal distress Hypoglycemia Congenital anomalies Congenital infection Polycythemia

Increased C-section rate Birth trauma

Postmaturity syndrome

Fetal distress Aspiration of meconium Hypoglycemia Congenital anomalies (trisomy 16 and 18)

24 25 26 27 28 29 30 31 32 33 34 35 36 37 38 39 40 41 42 43 44 45 46

Weeks of gestation

Preterm	Term	Postterm

Figure 31–2   Neonatal morbidity by birth weight and gestational age (From Lubchenco LO: The High Risk Infant. *Philadelphia: Saunders, 1976, p 122)*

the neonatal period, that is, within the first 28 days of life. As indicated in Figure 31–1, the neonatal mortality risk decreases as both gestational age and birth weight increase. Infants who are preterm and small for gestational age have the highest neonatal mortality risk. The mortality for LGA infants has decreased at most perinatal centers because of improved management of diabetes in pregnancy and increased recognition of potential problems with LGA infants.

Neonatal morbidity can be anticipated based on birth weight and gestational age. In Figure 31–2 the infant's birth weight is located in the vertical column, and the gestational age in weeks is found horizontally. The area where the two meet on the graph identifies commonly occurring problems. This tool assists in determining the needs of particular infants for special observation and care. For example, an infant of 2000 g at 40 weeks' gestation should be carefully assessed for evidence of fetal distress, hypoglycemia, congenital anomalies, congenital infection, and polycythemia.

❀ *USING THE NURSING PROCESS WITH* ❀

At-Risk Newborns

Nursing Assessment

Assessment of the at-risk newborn is an ongoing component of the nursing process. It begins with the history of the newborn, which includes family and maternal history and other factors that may influence development in utero.

In the birthing area, the nurse correlates the Apgar scores and careful observation with information about the duration of labor, maternal analgesia and anesthesia, and complications of the labor and birth process. Assessment continues when the newborn is admitted to the nursery. All previous assessments, Apgar scores, and treatments immediately after birth are evaluated in conjunction with the physical assessment of the newborn. As discussed in Chapter 28, the physical examination includes all of the following:

- Complete head-to-toe assessment, observing for cardiorespiratory function, temperature, and congenital anomalies.
- Clinical determination of gestational age
- Classification of the baby as AGA, SGA, or LGA and correlation with the morbidity risk for the specific classification (Figure 31–2).

Nursing Diagnosis

All of the nursing diagnoses for the at-risk newborn are based on careful analysis of the assessment data and are centered around alteration in physiologic process and the newborn's response to procedures or stimuli. Nursing diagnoses may include the following:

- Impaired gas exchange related to respiratory distress secondary to fluid aspiration or surfactant deficiency
- Alteration in nutrition: less than body requirements related to diminished sucking reflex
- Hypothermia related to inadequate subcutaneous tissue

The psychosocial needs of these newborns and their parents may be addressed in such nursing diagnoses as:

- Ineffective family coping related to birth of potentially ill newborn
- Knowledge deficit related to potential long-term developmental outcomes secondary to at-risk newborn complications
- Anticipatory grieving related to loss of idealized perfect child

Nursing Plan and Implementation

When all the data are gathered and analyzed, the care plan is developed. Nursing care of the at-risk newborn depends on minute-to-minute observations of the changes in the neonate's physiologic status. It is essential to a baby's survival that the neonatal nurse understand the basic physiologic principles that guide nursing management of the at-risk neonate. The organization of nursing care must be directed toward the following:

- Decreasing physiologically stressful situations
- Constantly observing for subtle signs of change in clinical condition
- Interpreting laboratory data and coordinating interventions
- Conserving the infant's energy, especially in frail, debilitated newborns
- Providing for developmental stimulation and sleep cycle
- Assisting the family in attachment behaviors

The at-risk newborn is the newest member of a family, so it is imperative to incorporate the parents into the plan of care. They must be kept informed of their newborn's condition and progress, involved in care, and given frequent opportunities to interact with their newborn and voice their fears and concerns. They should also be assisted in learning about their baby and how to care for their baby.

Evaluation

The success of the care plan is confirmed by continuous assessments of the neonate's behavior, communication with family and health team members, and use of diagnostic measures. The nurse should make every effort to evaluate on an ongoing basis how the family is being incorporated into the care of their newborn and how they are adjusting to this new member of the family.

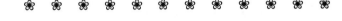

Care of the Small-for-Gestational-Age (SGA) Newborn

A **small-for-gestational-age (SGA)** newborn is any newborn who at birth is at or below the tenth percentile (intrauterine growth curves) on the newborn classification chart (Figure 31–1). It should be noted that intrauterine growth charts are influenced by altitude and ethnicity. There is a high correlation between increase in altitude and decrease in birth weight (Yip 1987). When assigning SGA classification to a newborn, birth weight charts should be based on the local population into which the newborn is born (Lugo & Tominey 1989). An SGA newborn may be preterm, term, or postterm. Other terms used to designate a growth-retarded newborn include *intrauterine growth retarded (IUGR)*, and *dysmature*. For this discussion, **SGA** and **IUGR** will be used interchangeably.

Between 6% and 15% of all pregnancies are complicated by IUGR. Small-for-gestational-age infants have a fivefold greater incidence of perinatal asphyxia and an eightfold higher perinatal mortality than normal infants (Lawrence et al 1990). The incidence of polycythemia and hypoglycemia are also increased in this group of infants (Lugo & Tominey 1989).

Factors Contributing to Intrauterine Growth Retardation (IUGR)

IUGR may be caused by maternal, placental, or fetal factors and may not be apparent antenatally. Intrauterine growth is linear in the normal pregnancy from approximately 28 to 38 weeks' gestation. After 38 weeks, growth is variable, depending on the growth potential of the fetus and placental function. The most common causes of growth retardation are the following:

- *Malnutrition.* Maternal nutrition has not been found to influence the birth weight of the newborn significantly unless starvation occurs during the last trimester of pregnancy. Before the third trimester, the nutritional supply far exceeds the needs of the fetus. Only in the third trimester is maternal nutrition supply a limiting factor to fetal growth.

- *Vascular complications.* Complications associated with pregnancy-induced hypertension (preeclampsia and eclampsia), chronic hypertensive vascular disease, and advanced diabetes mellitus cause diminished blood flow to the uterus.

- *Maternal disease.* Maternal heart disease, substance abuse (drugs and alcohol), sickle cell anemia, phenylketonuria (PKU), and asymptomatic pyelonephritis are associated with SGA.

- *Maternal factors.* SGA is associated with maternal factors such as small stature, primiparity, grand multiparity, smoking, lack of prenatal care, age (<16 or >40), and low socioeconomic class (which can result in poor health care, poor education, and poor living conditions).

- *Environmental factors.* Such factors include high altitude, x rays, and maternal use of drugs, such as antimetabolics, anticonvulsants, and trimethadione, which have teratogenic effects.

- *Placental factors.* Placental conditions such as infarcted areas, abnormal cord insertions, single um-

bilical artery, placenta previa, or thrombosis may affect circulation to the fetus, which becomes more deficient with increasing gestational age.

- *Fetal factors.* Congenital infections (rubella, toxoplasmosis, syphilis, cytomegalic inclusion disease) or malformations, multiple pregnancy (twins or triplets), discordant twins, sex of the fetus (female), chromosomal syndromes, and inborn errors of metabolism can predispose a fetus to IUGR.

Antenatal identification of fetuses with IUGR is the first step in the detection of common disorders of the SGA newborn. The perinatal history of maternal conditions, early serial ultrasound measurements, Doppler velocimetry, and examination of the placenta and newborn are also important in identifying this at-risk newborn.

Patterns of Intrauterine Growth Retardation (IUGR)

Growth occurs in two ways: increase in cell number and increase in cell size. If insult occurs early during the critical period of organ development in the fetus, fewer new cells are formed, organs are small, and organ weight is subnormal. In contrast, growth failure that begins later in pregnancy does not affect the total number of cells but only their size. The organs are normal, but their size is diminished.

Two clinical pictures of SGA newborns have been described. These clinical presentations are classified as either *symmetric* (proportional) IUGR or *asymmetric* (disproportional) IUGR.

Symmetric IUGR is caused by long-term maternal conditions (such as chronic hypertension, severe malnutrition, chronic intrauterine infection, substance abuse, and anemia) or fetal genetic abnormalities (Brar & Rutherford 1988). Symmetric IUGR can be noted by ultrasound in the first half of the second trimester with its onset prior to 32 weeks' gestation. In symmetric IUGR there is chronic prolonged retardation of growth in size of organs, weight, length, and, in severe cases, head circumference.

Asymmetric IUGR is associated with an acute compromise of uteroplacental blood flow. Some associated causes are placental infarcts, pregnancy-induced hypertension (PIH), and poor weight gain in pregnancy. The growth retardation is usually not evident before the third trimester because length and head circumference remain appropriate for that gestational age, although weight is decreased. Asymmetric IUGR can be detected on ultrasound after 36 weeks, when the size of the head of a normal fetus becomes smaller than the abdominal circumference. In asymmetric IUGR, the head circumference remains larger than the abdominal circumference. Thus measuring only the biparietal diameter on ultrasound will cause a failure to detect asymmetric IUGR (Lawrence et al 1990).

Birth weight is reduced below the tenth percentile, whereas head size may be between the 15th and 90th percentiles. Asymmetric SGA neonates are particularly at risk for perinatal asphyxia, pulmonary hemorrhage, hypocalcemia, and hypoglycemia in the neonatal period (Teberg et al 1988).

Despite growth retardation, physiologic maturity develops according to gestational age. Therefore, the SGA newborn may be more physiologically mature than the preterm AGA newborn and less predisposed to complications of prematurity such as respiratory distress syndrome and hyperbilirubinemia. The SGA newborn's chances for survival are better because of organ maturity, although this newborn still faces many other potential difficulties in the newborn period and long-term problems.

Common Complications of the SGA Newborn

The problems occurring most frequently in the SGA newborn include the following:

- *Perinatal asphyxia.* The SGA infant suffers chronic hypoxia in utero, which leaves little reserve to withstand the demands of normal labor and birth. Thus intrauterine asphyxia occurs with its potential systemic problems.

- *Aspiration syndrome.* In utero hypoxia can cause the fetus to gasp during birth, resulting in aspiration of amniotic fluid into the lower airways. It can also lead to relaxation of the anal sphincter and passage of meconium. This results in aspiration of the meconium with the first breaths after birth.

- *Heat loss.* Diminished subcutaneous fat (used for survival in utero), depletion of brown fat in utero, and a large surface area decrease the IUGR newborn's ability to conserve heat. The effect of surface area is diminished somewhat because of the flexed position assumed by the term SGA newborn.

- *Hypoglycemia.* An increase in metabolic rate in response to heat loss and poor hepatic glycogen stores cause hypoglycemia. In addition, the infant is compromised by inadequate supplies of enzymes to activate gluconeogenesis (conversion of nonglucogen sources such as fatty acids and proteins to glucose).

- *Hypocalcemia.* Decreased calcium levels occur secondary to birth asphyxia and preterm birth.

- *Polycythemia.* The number of red blood cells is increased in the SGA newborn. This finding is considered a physiologic response to in utero chronic hypoxic stress.

Infants who have significant IUGR tend to have a poor prognosis, especially when born before 37 weeks' gestation. Factors contributing to poor outcome for these infants are as follows:

- *Congenital malformations.* Congenital malformations occur 10 to 20 times more frequently in SGA infants than in AGA infants. The more severe the IUGR, the greater the chance for malformation as a result of impaired mitotic activity and cellular hypoplasia.

- *Intrauterine infection.* When fetuses are exposed to intrauterine infections such as rubella and cytomegalovirus, they are profoundly affected by direct invasion of the brain and other vital organs by the offending virus resulting in IUGR.

- *Continued growth difficulties.* It is generally agreed that SGA newborns tend to be shorter than newborns of the same gestational age but will have appropriate size growth. A symmetric IUGR infant can be expected to catch up in weight to normal growth infants by 3 to 6 months of age. Symmetric SGA infants reportedly have varied growth potential but tend not to catch up to their peers (Peterson & Frank 1987).

- *Learning difficulties.* Often SGA newborns exhibit poor brain development and subsequent failure to catch up, and learning disabilities are not uncommon. The disabilities are characterized by hyperactivity, short attention span, and poor fine motor coordination (reading, writing, and drawing). Poor scholastic performance is also a common problem (Creasy & Resnik 1989). Some hearing loss and speech defects also occur.

Studies have determined that the quality of the home environment of an SGA infant predicts developmental outcome better than any single biologic risk factor (Watt 1989).

Medical Therapy

The goal of medical therapy is early recognition and implementation of medical management of the potential problems associated with SGA babies.

❀ *APPLYING THE NURSING PROCESS* ❀

Nursing Assessment

The nurse is responsible for assessing gestational age and identifying signs of potential complications associated with SGA infants.

All body parts of the symmetric IUGR infant are in proportion, but they are below normal size for the baby's gestational age. Therefore the head does not appear overly large or the length excessive in relation to the other body parts. These newborns are generally vigorous.

The asymmetric IUGR infant appears long, thin, and emaciated, with loss of subcutaneous fat tissue and muscle mass (Figure 31–3). The baby has loose skin folds; dry, desquamating skin; and a thin and often meconium-stained cord. The head appears relatively large (although it ap-

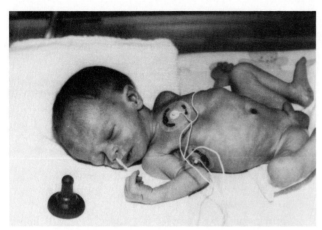

Figure 31–3   The infant with asymmetric IUGR appears long, thin, and emaciated. The gestational age of the infant shown here is 41 weeks. He weighed approximately 1560 g at birth.

proaches normal size) because the chest size and abdominal girth are decreased. The baby may have a vigorous cry and appear deceptively alert.

Nursing Diagnosis

Nursing diagnoses that may apply are included in the Nursing Care Plan for the Small-for-Gestational-Age Newborn.

Nursing Plan and Implementation

Promotion of Physical Well-Being
Hypoglycemia, the most common metabolic complication of IUGR, can produce CNS abnormalities and mental retardation. In addition to hypoglycemia, conditions such as asphyxia, hyperviscosity, and cold stress may also affect the baby's outcome. Meticulous attention to physiologic parameters is essential for immediate nursing management and reduction of long-term disorders (see the Nursing Care Plan for the Small-for-Gestational-Age Newborn).

Provision of Follow-Up Care
The long-term needs of the SGA newborn include careful follow-up evaluation of patterns of growth and possible disabilities that may later interfere with learning or motor functioning. Long-term follow-up care is especially necessary for those infants with congenital malformations, congenital infections, and obvious sequelae from physiologic problems. In addition, the parents of the IUGR baby need support, because a positive atmosphere can enhance the baby's growth potential and the child's ultimate outcome.

Evaluation

Anticipated outcomes of nursing care include the following:

- The small for gestational age newborn is free from apnea.
- The small for gestational age newborn maintains a stable temperature and glucose hemostasis.
- The small for gestational age newborn gains weight and takes nipple feedings without developing fatigue.
- The parents verbalize their concerns surrounding their baby's health problems and understand the rationale behind management of their newborn.

❀ ❀ ❀ ❀ ❀ ❀ ❀ ❀ ❀ ❀ ❀ ❀

Care of the Large-for Gestational-Age (LGA) Newborn

A **large-for-gestational-age (LGA)** neonate is one whose birth weight is at or above the 90th percentile on the intrauterine growth curve (at any week of gestation). The classification of LGA may vary depending on the intrauterine growth curve chart used; therefore, the chart used should correlate with the characteristics of the client population (Katz & Satish 1989). The majority of LGA newborns have been incorrectly categorized as LGA because of miscalculation of the date of conception due to postconceptual bleeding. Careful gestational age assessment is therefore essential to identify the potential needs and problems of such infants.

The best-known condition associated with excessive fetal growth is maternal diabetes (White's classes A–C; see Table 18–2, page 454). However, only a small fraction of LGA newborns are born to diabetic mothers. The cause of the majority of cases of LGA infants is unclear, but certain factors or situations have been found to correlate with their births:

- Genetic predisposition is correlated proportionally to the mother's prepregnancy weight and to weight gain during pregnancy. Large parents tend to have large infants.
- Multiparous women have three times the number of LGA infants as primigravidas.
- Male infants are traditionally larger than female infants.
- Infants with erythroblastosis fetalis, Beckwith-Wiedemann syndrome (genetic condition asso-

(Text continues on p 953.)

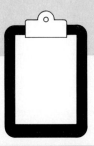

Nursing Care Plan
Small-for-Gestational-Age Newborn

Client Assessment

Nursing History

Maternal factors:
Vascular—PIH, chronic hypertension, advanced diabetes

Preexisting diseases—heart disease, alcoholism, narcotic addiction, sickle cell anemia, PKU

Primiparity, smoking, lack of prenatal care, low socioeconomic level, very young or old

Environmental factors—high altitude, x-rays, maternal drug use (antimetabolics, anticonvulsants)

Placental factors—infarcts, placenta previa

Fetal factors:
Congenital infections

Multiple pregnancy

Inborn errors of metabolism

Chromosomal syndrome

Physical Examination

Large-appearing head in proportion to chest and abdomen

Loose dry skin

Scarcity of subcutaneous fat, with emaciated appearance

Long, thin appearance

Sunken abdomen

Sparse scalp hair

Anterior fontanelle may be depressed

May have vigorous cry and appears alert

Birth weight below tenth percentile

Diagnostic Studies

Blood glucose and Dextrostix/Chemstrip

Hematocrit

Total bilirubin level

Calcium levels

Chest x-rays

Nursing Diagnosis	Nursing Interventions	Rationale	Evaluation
Impaired gas exchange related to aspiration of meconium *Client Goal:* Baby's respirations will be 30–50/min with no periods of apnea, intermittent cyanosis, sternal retractions, grunting, or nasal flaring.	Auscultate breath sounds every four hr. Suction endotracheal tube every three to four hr. Give oxygen prior to suction as needed. Ensure chest physiotherapy is done as indicated. Observe for worsening signs of respiratory distress such as generalized cyanosis; worsening retractions, grunting, and nasal flaring, as evidenced by Silverman respiratory index; sustained tachypnea; apnea episodes; inequality of breath sounds; presence of rales and rhonchi.	In utero, hypoxia causes relaxation of anal sphincter and reflex gasping of meconium. Maintain airway patency.	Baby's respirations are 30 to 50 per minute without apnea, retractions, grunting or nasal flaring.

(continued)

Nursing Care Plan (continued)

Nursing Diagnosis	Nursing Interventions	Rationale	Evaluation
	Administer oxygen per order for relief of respiratory distress signs (see p 1025 for nursing care and treatment of meconium aspiration, infant resuscitation). Implement treatment plan by respiratory distress.		
	Monitor blood glucose levels every eight hours until stable or by Dextrostix/Chemstrip within one to two hr after birth and frequently for two to three days.	Respiratory distress increases consumption of glucose.	
Hypothermia related to decreased subcutaneous fat *Client Goal:* Baby will maintain skin temperature between 36.1 and 36.7C (97–98F).	Provide neutral thermal zone (NTZ) range for infant based on postnatal weight.	Neutral thermal environment charts used for preterm baby must be altered for SGA newborns.	Baby's temperature is maintained between 36.1 and 36.7C.
	Use skin probe to maintain skin temperature at 36.1–36.7C.	Diminished subcutaneous fat and a large body surface compared to body weight predispose SGA baby to thermoregulation problems.	
	Obtain axillary temps and compare to registered skin probe temp every two to three hrs. and PRN. If discrepancy exists, evaluate potential cause.	Discrepancies between axillary and skin probe monitor temp may be due to mechanical causes or the burning of brown fat.	
	Adjust and monitor incubator or radiant warmer to maintain skin temperature.		
	Minimize heat losses and prevent cold stress by: 1. Warming and humidifying oxygen without blowing over face in order to avoid increasing oxygen consumption 2. Keeping skin dry	SGA infant has increased heat loss due to decreased available brown fat stores for heat production and less fat insulation.	

(continued)

Nursing Care Plan (continued)

Nursing Diagnosis	Nursing Interventions	Rationale	Evaluation
	3. Keeping Isolettes, radiant warmers, and cribs away from windows and cold external walls and out of drafts		
	4. Avoiding placing infant on cold surfaces such as metal treatment tables, cold x-ray plates		
	5. Padding cold surfaces with diapers and using radiant warmers during procedures		
	6. Warming blood for exchange transfusions.		
	Monitor for signs and symptoms of cold stress: decreased temperature, lethargy, pallor (for further discussion see p 1035).	Cold stress increases oxygen requirements.	
Injury: High risk to tissues related to decreased glycogen stores and impaired gluconeogenesis	Monitor blood glucose per SGA protocol and report values < 40 mg/dL.	Combined with depletion of glycogen stores, impaired gluconeogenesis predisposes SGA infants to profound hypoglycemia within first two days of life.	Baby's blood glucose is greater than 40 mg/dL, baby is alert and active.
Client Goal: Baby will have blood glucose of greater than 40 mg/dL, no signs of respiratory distress, and will be alert and active.	Observe, record, and report signs of hypoglycemia: cyanosis, lethargy, jitteriness, seizure activity, and apnea.	Hypoglycemia causes CNS irritability.	
	Notify physician if values are low. Monitor vital signs every two hr PRN.		
	Initiate feeding schedule for SGA newborns per agency protocol. Monitor blood glucose.	Frequent monitoring of blood glucose assists in identifying decreasing glucose levels.	
	Provide glucose intake either through early enteral feeding (before four hr) or by IV per physician's order. See further discussion of hypoglycemia on p 1035.	Provision of glucose through early feedings (begin before four hr of age), or IV, maintains needed glucose levels.	
	Record input and output, monitor IV rate and site hourly.	Decreasing glucose is reflected in lethargy, decreased appetite.	

(continued)

Nursing Care Plan (continued)

Nursing Diagnosis	Nursing Interventions	Rationale	Evaluation
Altered nutrition: less than body requirements related to SGA's increased metabolic rate *Client Goal:* Baby will not lose more than 2% weight, will take formula without tiring, and will gain weight.	Initiate test water feeding at one hr of age, then proceed to 5% glucose/water. Move early to formula feeding every two to three hr. Supplement oral feedings with intravenous intake per orders. Monitor intake and output every four hours or more frequently. Use concentrated formulas that supply more calories in less volume, such as Similac 24. Promote growth by providing caloric intake of 120–150 cal/kg/day in small amounts. Monitor and record signs of respiratory distress or fatigue occurring during feedings. Supplement gavage, bottle or breast feedings with intravenous therapy per physician order until oral intake is sufficient to support growth. Begin bottle- or breast-feeding slowly, such as bottle- or breast-feed once per day, bottle- or breast-feed once per shift, and then bottle- or breast-feed every other feeding. Monitor daily weight with anticipation of small amount of weight loss when bottle- or breast-feedings start.	Sterile water is desirable for first feedings because it causes fewer pulmonary complications in the presence of aspiration of feeding. SGA newborns require more calories/kg for growth because of increased metabolic activity and oxygen consumption secondary to increased percentage of body weight made up by visceral organs. Small, frequent feedings of high caloric formula are used because of limited gastric capacity and decreased gastric emptying. Small, frequent feedings decrease fatigue associated with feeding. Adequate nutritional intake promotes growth and prevents such complications as metabolic catabolism and hypoglycemia. Gavage feedings require less energy expenditure on the part of the newborn. Bottle- or breast-feeding, an active rather than passive intake of nutrition, requires energy expenditure, burning of calories, and potential weight loss.	Baby receives 120–150 cal/kg/day, maintains weight with expected gain pattern, takes formula without tiring.

(continued)

Nursing Care Plan (continued)

Nursing Diagnosis	Nursing Interventions	Rationale	Evaluation
Altered tissue perfusion related to increased blood viscosity *Client Goals:* Baby's hemoglobin will be less than 22 g/dL, hematocrit less than 65%; baby will show no signs of respiratory distress, cyanosis, or tachycardia.	Obtain central hematocrit on admission	Exact etiology of polycythemia in SGA is not known but is thought to be a physiologic response to chronic hypoxia with increased erythropoietin production.	Baby's hemoglobin is less than 22 g/dL, hematocrit is less than 65%, and there are no signs of respiratory distress.
	Monitor, record, and report symptoms, including: 1. Decrease in peripheral pulses, discoloration of extremity, alteration in activity or neurologic depression, renal vein thrombosis with decreased urine output, hematuria, or proteinuria in thromboembolic conditions 2. Tachycardia or congestive heart failure 3. Respiratory distress syndrome, cyanosis, tachypnea, increased oxygen need, labored respirations, or hemorrhage in respiratory system	Polycythemia is defined as a central venous hematocrit above 65%–70% in the first week of life. Hyperviscosity is resultant "thickness" of red-cell rich blood so that its ability to perfuse the tissues is disturbed due to thickness and decrease in deformability of cells. Symptoms are caused by poor perfusion of tissues.	
	Watch for other signs of increased hematocrit such as hyperbilirubinemia Monitor bilirubin levels every eight hr.	As the increased red blood cells begin to break down, hyperbilirubinemia may present.	
	Assist with partial plasma exchange.	Partial plasma exchange decreases blood volume and blood viscosity to less than 60%.	

(continued)

Nursing Care Plan (continued)

Nursing Diagnosis	Nursing Interventions	Rationale	Evaluation
Altered parenting: High risk related to prolonged separation of baby and parents secondary to illness *Client Goals:* Baby's parents will touch, hold, and participate in the baby's care and talk about the future of their baby.	Include parents in determining infant's plan of care and encourage their participation. Encourage parents to visit frequently. Provide opportunities for parents to touch, hold, talk to, and care for infant. Determine the type and amount of appropriate sensory stimulation and implement sensory stimulation program.	Parent-infant bonding begins in first few hours or days following birth of an infant. SGA infants experience prolonged periods of separation from their parents, which necessitates intervention to ensure parent-infant bonding. Emotional support of the psychologic well-being of family, including positive parent-infant bonding and sensory stimulation of infant, is important.	Baby's parents have bonded with their infant, are involved in their infant's care, and have realistic expectations about their baby.
Knowledge deficit (parental) concerning care of newborn at home *Client Goals:* Baby's parents will ask about taking her or him home and will participate in discharge planning, attend necessary classes on infant care, and ask about when to call the doctor and follow-up needs.	Prepare for discharge by instructing parents in such areas as feeding techniques, formula preparation (including bottle sterilization), and breast-feeding; bathing, diapering, and hygiene; rectal temperature monitoring; administration of vitamins; sibling rivalry; care of complications and preventing exposure to infections; normal elimination patterns, expected weight gain patterns, normal reflexes and activity, and how to promote normal growth and development without being overprotective; returning for continued medical care; and availability of community resources if indicated.	Parents should receive the same postpartum teaching as any parent taking a new infant home. Parents need to understand the changes to expect in color of the infant's stool and number of bowel movements plus odor from bottle- or breast-feeding in order to avoid unnecessary concern. Preterm infants usually do not require referral to community agencies such as visiting nurse associations unless there is a specific problem requiring assistance. Infants with congenital abnormalities, feeding problems, or resolving complications with infections, or mothers unable to cope with defective infants are examples of conditions requiring referral to community resources.	Baby's parents verbalize how to take care of their baby at home and know when to return for follow-up and when to call their health care provider.

ated with neonatal hypoglycemia and hyperinsulinism), or transposition of the great vessels are usually large.

The increase in the LGA infant's body size is characteristically proportional, although head circumference and body length are in the upper limits of intrauterine growth. The exception to this rule is the infant of the diabetic mother; in these infants, body weight increases only in proportion to length.

Common Complications of the LGA Newborn

Common disorders of the LGA infant include the following:

- *Birth trauma because of cephalopelvic disproportion.* Often these infants have a biparietal diameter greater than 10 cm or are associated with a maternal fundal height measurement greater than 42 cm without the presence of hydramnios. Because of their excessive size, there are more breech presentations and shoulder dystocias. These complications may result in asphyxia, fractured clavicles, brachial plexus palsy, facial paralysis, phrenic nerve palsy, depressed skull fractures, hematomas, and bleeding due to birth trauma.

- *Increased incidence of cesarean births and oxytocin-induced births due to fetal size.* These births are accompanied by all the risk factors associated with these procedures.

- *Hypoglycemia, polycythemia, and hyperviscosity.* These disorders are most often seen with erythroblastosis fetalis and Beckwith-Wiedemann syndrome and in infants of diabetic mothers.

Nursing Care

The perinatal history, in conjunction with ultrasonic measurement of fetal skull and gestational age testing, is important in identifying an at-risk LGA newborn. Nursing care is directed toward early identification and immediate treatment of the common disorders. Essential components of the nursing assessment are monitoring vital signs, screening for hypoglycemia and polycythemia, and observing for signs and symptoms related to birth trauma. The nursing care for the complications associated with LGA newborns is the same as for the infant of a diabetic mother and will be discussed in the next section. Parental concerns about the potential for a continuing overweight pattern and about visual signs of birth trauma must be addressed.

Care of the Infant of a Diabetic Mother (IDM)

Infants of diabetic mothers (IDMs) are considered at risk and require close observation the first few hours to the first few days of life. Mothers with severe diabetes or diabetes of long duration (type 1, or White's classes D–F, associated with vascular complications; see Table 18–2) may give birth to SGA infants. The typical IDM (type 1, or White's classes B and C), however, is LGA. These infants are fat, macrosomic, and plethoric (Figure 31–4). The cord and placenta are also large.

IDMs have decreased total body water, particularly in the extracellular spaces and are therefore not edematous. Their excessive weight is due to increased weight of the visceral organs, cardiomegaly (hypertrophy), and increased body fat. The only organ not affected is the brain (Meyer & Palmer 1990).

The excessive fetal growth of the IDM is caused by exposure to high levels of maternal glucose, which readily crosses the placenta. The fetus responds to these high glucose levels with increased insulin production and hyperplasia of the pancreatic beta cells. The main action of the insulin is to facilitate the entry of glucose into muscle and fat cells in a function similar to a cellular growth hormone. Once in the cells, glucose is converted to glycogen and stored. Insulin also inhibits the breakdown of fat to free fatty acids, thereby maintaining lipid synthesis, increasing the uptake of amino acids and promoting protein synthesis. Insulin is an important regulator of fetal growth and metabolism.

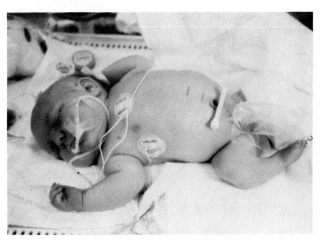

Figure 31–4 Macrosomic infant of diabetic mother. X-ray examination of this infant revealed caudal regression of the spine.

Common Complications of the IDM

Although IDMs are usually large, they are immature in physiologic functions and exhibit many of the problems of the preterm (premature) infant. The complications most often seen in an IDM are the following:

- *Hypoglycemia.* After birth the most common problem of an IDM is hypoglycemia. Even though the high maternal blood sugar supply is lost, this newborn continues to produce high levels of insulin, which deplete the infant's blood glucose within hours after birth. IDMs also have less ability to release glucagon and catecholamines, which normally stimulate glucagon breakdown and glucose release. The incidence of hypoglycemia in IDMs varies from 2% to 75%. The wide range in incidence of hypoglycemia is due to the degree of success in controlling the maternal diabetes, differences in maternal blood sugars at the time of birth, length of labor, the class of maternal diabetes, and late feedings (could increase the incidence of hypoglycemia) of the newborn.

- *Hypocalcemia.* Tremors are the obvious clinical sign of hypocalcemia. This complication may be due to the increased incidence of prematurity and to the stresses of difficult pregnancy, labor, and birth, which predispose any infant to hypocalcemia. Diabetic women tend to have higher calcium levels at term, which causes secondary hypoparathyroidism in their infants (Meyer & Palmer 1990). Other factors may include vitamin D antagonism, which results from elevated corticol levels, hypophosphatemia from tissue catabolism, and decreased serum magnesium levels.

- *Hyperbilirubinemia.* This condition may be seen at 48 to 72 hours after birth. It may be caused by slightly decreased extracellular fluid volume, which increases the hematocrit level. Enclosed hemorrhages resulting from complicated vaginal birth may also cause hyperbilirubinemia. There may also be an increase in the rate of bilirubin production in the presence of polycythemia.

- *Birth trauma.* Since most IDMs are LGA, trauma may occur during labor and birth (see page 946).

- *Polycythemia.* This condition may be caused by the decreased extracellular fluid volume in IDMs. Research has focused on the ability of hemoglobin A$_{1c}$ to bind to oxygen, which decreases the oxygen available to the fetal tissues. This tissue hypoxia stimulates increased erythropoietin production, which increases the hematocrit level.

- *Respiratory distress syndrome (RDS).* This complication occurs especially in newborns of White's classes A–C diabetic mothers. It has been demonstrated that insulin antagonizes the cortisol-induced stimulation of lecithin synthesis that is necessary for lung maturation. Therefore, IDMs may have lungs that are less mature than expected for their gestational age. There is also a decrease in the phospholipid PG that stabilizes surfactant and thereby decreases the incidence of RDS (Meyer & Palmer 1990).

 RDS does not appear to be a problem for infants born of diabetic mothers in White's classes D–F; instead the stresses of poor uterine blood supply may lead to increased production of steroids, which accelerates lung maturation.

- *Congenital birth defects.* Congenital anomalies that may occur in IDMs are transposition of the great vessels, ventricular septal defect, patent ductus arteriosus, small left colon syndrome, limb deformity (femoral hypoplasia) and caudal regression syndrome.

Medical Therapy

The goal of medical therapy is the early detection of and intervention in the problems associated with infants born to diabetic mothers. Prenatal management is directed toward control of maternal hyperglycemia, which minimizes the common complications of IDMs: pulmonary problems, macrosomia, polycythemia, and hypoglycemia.

Because the onset of hypoglycemia occurs between one and three hours after birth in IDMs (with a spontaneous rise to normal levels by four to six hours), blood glucose determinations should be done on cord blood and at 1, 2, and 4 hours of age and then every six hours until resolved (Hoskins 1990).

IDMs who are symptomatic should be given 10% to 15% glucose intravenously immediately after birth at the volume of fluids necessary for the hydration of the infant. The rate of 4 to 6 mg/kg/min usually maintains normoglycemia in the IDM (Avery 1987). Once the blood glucose has been stable for 24 hours, the solution is then decreased in concentration with careful attention to the neonate's blood glucose level. Dextrose (25% to 50%) as a rapid infusion is contraindicated because it may lead to severe rebound hypoglycemia following an initial brief increase in glucose level.

❧ *APPLYING THE NURSING PROCESS* ❧

Nursing Assessment

In caring for the IDM baby, the nurse assesses for signs of respiratory distress, hyperbilirubinemia, birth trauma, and congenital anomalies. Close and ongoing nursing assessments and care are essential in decreasing the potential harmful effects of the problems associated with being an IDM.

CRITICAL THINKING

What information would you provide a diabetic woman prior to conception which could decrease the possible complications for her baby?

Nursing Diagnosis

Nursing diagnoses that may apply to IDMs include the following:

- Alteration in nutrition: less than body requirements related to increased glucose metabolism secondary to hyperinsulinemia
- Impaired gas exchange related to respiratory distress secondary to impaired production of surfactant
- Ineffective family coping related to the illness of the baby

Nursing Plan and Implementation

Promotion of Physical Well-Being

Nursing care of the IDM is directed toward early detection and ongoing monitoring of hypoglycemia (by doing glucose tests) and polycythemia (by obtaining central hematocrits), respiratory distress, and hyperbilirubinemia. For specific nursing interventions for respiratory distress syndrome, hypoglycemia, hyperbilirubinemia, and polycythemia, see Chapter 32.

Promotion of Family Adaptation

The nurse educates parents about prevention of macrosomia and resultant fetal/neonatal problems through early and ongoing diabetic control (Todros 1989). Parents are advised that with early identification and care, most IDMs' neonatal problems have no significant sequelae.

Evaluation

Anticipated outcomes of nursing care include the following:

- The IDM's respiratory and metabolic alteration problems are minimized.
- The parents understand the cause of the baby's health problems and preventative steps they can initiate to decrease the impact of maternal diabetes on subsequent fetuses.
- The parents verbalize their concerns surrounding their baby's health problems and understand the rationale behind management of their newborn.

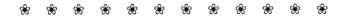

Care of the Postterm Newborn

The **postterm newborn** is any newborn born after 42 weeks' gestation. In the past, the term *postterm* and *postmature* were used interchangeably. The term **postmaturity** is now used only when the infant is born after 42 weeks of gestation and also demonstrates characteristics of the *postmaturity syndrome* (Hendriksen 1985).

Postterm, or prolonged, pregnancy occurs in approximately 3% to 14% of all pregnancies (Phelan 1989). The cause of postterm pregnancy is not completely understood, but several factors are known to be associated with it, including primiparity, high multiparity (five or more pregnancies) and a history of prolonged pregnancies. Many pregnancies classified as prolonged are thought to be a result of inaccurate estimation of the estimated date of birth (EDB) (Scott et al 1990).

Most babies born as a result of prolonged pregnancy are of normal size and health; some keep on growing and are over 4000 g at birth, which supports the premise that the postterm fetus can remain well nourished. Intrapartal problems for these healthy but large fetuses are cephalopelvic disproportion (CPD) and shoulder dystocia. At birth about 5% of postterm newborns show signs of postmaturity syndrome (Oxorn 1986). The major portion of the following discussion will address the fetus who is not tolerating the prolonged pregnancy, is suffering from uteroplacental compromise to blood flow and resultant hypoxia, and is considered to have postmaturity syndrome.

Common Complications of the Newborn with Postmaturity Syndrome

The truly postmature newborn is at high risk for morbidity and has a mortality rate two to three times higher than that of term infants. Although today the percentages are extremely low, the majority of deaths occur during labor, since by that time the fetus has used up necessary reserves. Because of deceased placental function, oxygenation and nutrition transport are impaired, leaving the fetus prone to hypoglycemia and asphyxia when the stresses of labor begin. Problems faced by surviving postmature babies are caused by inadequate placental function, decreased oxygen and glucose reserves, and the stress of labor. The following are the most common disorders of the postmature newborn:

- Hypoglycemia, from nutritional deprivation and resultant depleted glycogen stores.
- Meconium aspiration in response to in utero hypoxia. In the presence of oligohydramnios the danger of aspirating thick meconium is increased. Severe meconium aspiration syndrome increases the baby's chance of developing persistent fetal circulation, pneumothorax and pneumonia (see Chapter 32).
- Polycythemia due to increased production of red blood cells (RBCs) in response to hypoxia.
- Congenital anomalies of unknown cause.
- Seizure activity because of hypoxic insult.

- Cold stress because of loss or poor development of subcutaneous fat.

    The long-term effects of postmaturity syndrome are unclear. At present studies do not agree on the effect of postmaturity syndrome on weight gain and IQ scores.

    Prolonged pregnancy itself is not responsible for the postmaturity syndrome. The characteristics of the postmature newborn are primarily caused by a combination of advanced gestational age, placental insufficiency, and continued exposure to amniotic fluid (Thorp & Creasy 1990).

Medical Therapy

The goal of medical therapy is identification and management of the postmature newborn's potential problems.

    Antenatal management is directed at differentiating the fetus who has postmaturity syndrome from the fetus who at birth is large, well-nourished, and equally alert and who is tolerating the prolonged (postterm) pregnancy.

    Antenatal tests that can be done to evaluate fetal status and determine obstetric management include fetal ultrasound, measurement of serum placental hormones such as human chorionic gonadotropin (hCG) and human placental lactogen (hPL), and the nonstress test (NST) and contraction stress test (CST). These tests and their use in postterm pregnancy are discussed in more depth in Chapters 20 and 25.

    At birth, if the amniotic fluid is meconium stained the baby's airway should be suctioned by the clinician prior to emergence of the chest and trunk and before the baby takes its first breath to minimize the chance of meconium aspiration syndrome. For detailed discussion of medical management and nursing assessments and care, see Chapter 32. Postnatally hypoglycemia is monitored by serial glucose determinations. The baby may be placed on glucose infusions or given early feedings if respiratory distress is not present. Postmature newborns are often voracious eaters.

    As with SGA infants, a hematocrit is used to screen for polycythemia. Oxygen is provided for respiratory distress. A partial exchange transfusion may be necessary to prevent complications such as hyperviscosity.

❀   *APPLYING THE NURSING PROCESS*   ❀

Nursing Assessment

The newborn with postmaturity syndrome appears alert. This wide-eyed, alert appearance is not necessarily a positive sign as it may indicate chronic intrauterine hypoxia.

    The infant has dry, cracking, parchmentlike skin without vernix or lanugo (Figure 31–5). Fingernails are long, and scalp hair is profuse. The infant's body appears long and thin. The wasting involves depletion of previously stored subcutaneous tissue causing the skin to be loose. Fat layers are almost nonexistent.

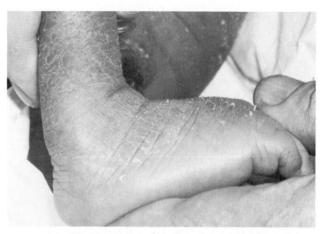

Figure 31–5   Postterm infant has deep cracking and peeling of skin. (From Dubowitz L, Dubowitz V: Gestational Age of the Newborn. *Menlo Park, CA: Addison-Wesley, 1977. Reprinted by permission of Dr V Dubowitz.)*

    Postmature newborns frequently have meconium staining, which colors the nails, skin, and umbilical cord. The varying shades (yellow to green) of meconium staining can give some clue about whether the expulsion of meconium was a recent or chronic, long-standing event.

Nursing Diagnosis

Nursing diagnoses that may apply to the postmature newborn include the following:

- Hypothermia related to decreased liver glycogen and brown fat stores
- Alteration in nutrition: less than body requirements related to increased use of glucose secondary to in utero stress
- Impaired gas exchange in the lungs and at the cellular level related to airway obstruction from potential meconium aspiration in utero.

Nursing Plan and Implementation

Promotion of Physical Well-Being

Nursing interventions are primarily supportive measures. They include the following:

- Observation of cardiopulmonary status, since the stresses of labor are poorly tolerated and severe asphyxia can occur at birth
- Provision of warmth to counterbalance the infant's poor response to cold stress and decreased liver glycogen and brown fat stores
- Frequent monitoring of blood glucose and initiation of early feeding (at 1 or 2 hours of age) or intravenous glucose per physician order

- Observation for the common disorders identified earlier and institution of nursing care and medical management as ordered

Provision of Emotional Support to the Parents

The nurse encourages parents to express their feelings and fears regarding the newborn's condition and potential long-term problems and keeps them informed.

Evaluation

Anticipated outcomes of nursing care include the following:

- The postterm newborn establishes effective respiratory function.
- The postmature baby is free of metabolic alterations (hypoglycemia) and maintains a stable temperature.

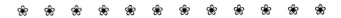

Care of the Preterm (Premature) Newborn

A preterm newborn is any infant born before 38 weeks' gestation. The length of gestation and thus the level of maturity vary even in the "premature" population. Figure 31–6 shows a preterm newborn.

The incidence of preterm births in the United States ranges from 7% of white newborns to 14% to 15% of nonwhites. The causes of preterm labor are poorly understood, but more and more of the variables that influence preterm labor and birth are being identified (see Chapter 25 for a discussion of preterm labor and birth).

With the help of modern technology, some babies under 500 g and between 23 and 26 weeks' gestation are surviving. But the mortality rates are the highest among these newborns.

Physiologic Considerations

The major problem of the preterm newborn is variable immaturity of all systems. The degree of immaturity depends on the length of gestation. For example, newborns of 32 weeks' gestation can be expected to exhibit more immaturity than newborns of 36 weeks' gestation. The degree of immaturity also presents problems of management. Maintenance of the preterm newborn falls within narrow physiologic parameters. "Catch-up care" is usually not possible if ground is lost in initial management. Improper physiologic management (or lack of management) adds stress and feeds the vicious cycle of physiologic deterioration.

The preterm newborn must traverse the same complex, interconnected pathways from intrauterine to extrauterine life as the term newborn. Because of immaturity, the preterm neonate is ill-equipped to make this transition smoothly. This section addresses the physiologic and nutritional factors associated with prematurity.

Respiratory and Cardiac Physiology and Considerations

The preterm newborn is at risk for respiratory problems because the lungs are not fully mature and ready to take over the process of oxygen and carbon dioxide exchange until 37 to 38 weeks' gestation. The length of time needed varies; some infants who are born before 37 to 38 weeks do not develop respiratory distress, and some infants born at 37 weeks experience severe respiratory distress. The most critical influencing factor in the development of respiratory distress is the preterm baby's inability to produce adequate amounts of surfactant. Surfactant prevents alveolar collapse when the baby exhales and increases lung compliance (ability of the lung to fill with air easily). When surfactant is decreased, compliance is also lessened, and the inspiratory pressure needed to expand the lungs with air increases (see Chapter 27 for discussion of respiratory adaption and development).

Besides adequate surfactant production, alveolar sacs must be present in sufficient number to provide the surface area needed to accomplish oxygen and carbon dioxide exchange. The term infant has about 24 million alveoli, while the adult has 200 million to 600 million (Korones 1986).

Lung development begins at around 24 days of fetal life, when the primitive lung bud appears (Figure 31–7). The primitive lung bud branches at about 26 to 28 days to form the major right and left bronchi. Throughout gestation, growth and branching continue, forming terminal

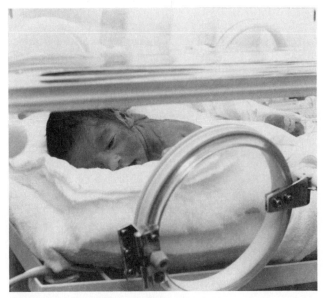

Figure 31–6 Preterm infant

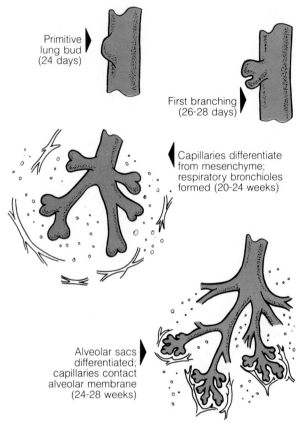

Primitive
lung bud
(24 days)▶

▶First branching
(26-28 days)

◀Capillaries differentiate
from mesenchyme;
respiratory bronchioles
formed (20-24 weeks)

Alveolar sacs
differentiated;
capillaries contact
alveolar membrane
(24-28 weeks)▶

Figure 31–7   Development of primitive lung bud and
subsequent branching into surrounding mesenchyme.
(From Korones SB: High Risk Newborn Infants, *3rd ed. St.*
Louis: Mosby, 1986)

bronchioles to respiratory bronchioles, from which arise alveolar ducts. The alveolar ducts are differentiated by approximately 24 weeks' gestation and give rise to thin-walled terminal air sacs. From 24 weeks until birth, growth and development of these terminal air sacs or premature alveoli are continuous. At about 24 to 26 weeks' gestation, the surface area available for gas exchange is very limited (because of inadequate number and size of alveoli) and inadequate surfactant is produced, making survival at this time unlikely.

By 27 to 28 weeks, more alveolar sacs have developed, and more capillaries are in contact with the alveolar membrane. This allows some exchange of oxygen and carbon dioxide from the alveoli to the capillaries, and from the capillaries to the alveoli. Surfactant production at this time is unstable and inadequate, but with respiratory assistance, survival is possible. The newborn is at risk, however, for many complications, such as RDS, hypoxemia, acidemia, intraventricular hemorrhage, cold stress, and metabolic imbalances, any one of which may compromise ultimate survival.

Between 29 and 30 weeks, additional differentiation of the alveolar sacs occurs and additional surfactant is re-

leased. After 30 weeks' gestation, growth of new primitive alveoli is rapid, and by 34 to 36 weeks, mature alveoli are present (Korones 1986). Also by this time surfactant production increases rapidly as the second pathway of surfactant production begins optimal functioning. If the fetus is unstressed and without iatrogenic complications, adequate amounts of surfactant should be produced for lung expansion and gas exchange at this time. In the presence of asphyxia, hypoxemia, acidemia, or cold stress, surfactant production is impaired, resulting in increased chances of respiratory distress. The more immature the infant, the more devastating the physiologic complications.

In the preterm infant, the muscular coat of the pulmonary arterioles is incompletely developed. This muscular development occurs late in gestation; therefore the more premature the infant, the less muscular the pulmonary arterioles (Avery 1987). Because of decreased pulmonary arteriole musculature, vasoconstriction is not effective in response to decreased oxygen levels. Therefore, the healthy preterm infant has a lower pulmonary vascular resistance than a full-term infant. This lowered resistance leads to increased left-to-right shunting through the ductus arteriosus, which steps up the blood flow back into the lungs. On the other hand, the preterm infant who develops respiratory distress and its complications (acidemia and hypoxemia) is at greater risk for increasing pulmonary vascular resistance because decreased PO_2 triggers vasoconstriction. Increased resistance decreases blood flow through the lungs, causing additional hypoxemia and acidemia. The ductus arteriosus responds to increasing oxygen levels by vasoconstriction; in the preterm infant, who is more susceptible to hypoxia, the ductus may remain open. A patent ductus increases the blood volume to the lungs, causing pulmonary congestion, increased respiratory effort, and higher oxygen consumption.

Thermoregulation

Maintaining a normal body temperature in the preterm baby presents a nursing challenge. One of the greatest threats to the preterm baby is heat loss. However, heat loss is a problem that the nurse can do much to prevent.

Heat production in the preterm infant is primarily a result of normal metabolic functions. Heat is produced by the oxidation of glucose and free fatty acids and also by the metabolism of brown fat. Two limiting factors in heat production, however, are the availability of glycogen in the liver (glycogen stores are primarily laid down during the third trimester) and the amount of brown fat available for metabolism (the preterm newborn does not have a full complement of brown fat). If the baby is chilled after birth, both glycogen and brown fat stores are metabolized rapidly for heat production, leaving the newborn with no reserves in the event of future stress. Since the muscle mass is small and muscular activity is diminished in preterm infants (they are unable to shiver), little heat is produced. Heat loss occurs as a result of several physiologic and anatomic factors:

1. The preterm baby has a much larger ratio of body surface to body weight. This means that the baby's ability to produce heat (body weight) is much less than the potential for losing heat (surface area). The loss of heat in a preterm newborn weighing 1500 g is five times greater per unit of body weight than in an adult (Korones 1986). Without an adequate thermal environment, the preterm baby is at risk for excessive heat loss.

2. The preterm baby has very little subcutaneous fat, which is the human body's insulation. Without adequate insulation, heat is easily conducted from the warmer core of the body to the cooler surface of the body. Heat is lost from the body as the blood vessels (which lie close to the skin surface in a preterm infant) transport blood from the body core to the subcutaneous tissues.

3. The posture of the preterm baby is another important factor influencing heat loss. Flexion of the extremities decreases the amount of surface area exposed to the environment; extension increases the surface area exposed to the environment and thus increases heat loss. The gestational age of the newborn influences the amount of flexion, from completely hypotonic and extended at 28 weeks to strong flexion displayed by 36 weeks (Figure 28–2)

In summary, the more preterm an infant the less capable he or she is of maintaining heat balance because of disproportionate body surface area, decreased subcutaneous fat, and increased heat loss due to body posture. Prevention of heat loss by providing a neutral thermal environment is one of the most important considerations in nursing management of the preterm newborn. Cold stress, with its accompanying severe complications, can be prevented (see Chapter 32).

Digestive Physiology and Considerations

The basic structure of the gastrointestinal (GI) tract is formed early in gestation, so even the very preterm newborn is able to take in some nourishment. Maturation of the digestive and absorptive process is more variable, however, and occurs later in gestation

As a result of GI immaturity, the preterm neonate has the following digestive and absorption problems:

- Limited ability exists to convert certain essential amino acids to nonessential amino acids. Certain amino acids, such as histidine, taurine, and cysteine, are essential to the preterm infant but not to the term infant (American Academy of Pediatrics 1985).

- Kidney immaturity causes an inability to handle the increased osmolarity of formula protein. The preterm infant requires a higher concentration of whey protein than casein.

- Difficulty absorbing saturated fats occurs because of decreased bile salts and pancreatic lipase. Severe illness of the newborn may also prevent intake of adequate nutrients.

- Lactose digestion may not be fully functional during the first few days of a preterm infant's life. The preterm neonate can digest and absorb most simple sugars.

- Deficiency of calcium and phosphorus may exist since two-thirds of these minerals are deposited in the last trimester. As a result the preterm infant is prone to rickets and significant bone demineralization.

Renal Physiology and Considerations

The kidneys of the preterm infant are immature in comparison with those of the full-term infant, which poses clinical problems in the management of fluid and electrolyte balance. Specific characteristics of the preterm infant include the following:

- The glomerular filtration rate (GFR) is lower due to decreased renal blood flow. Since the GFR is directly related to lower gestational age, the more preterm the newborn the lower the GFR. The GFR is also decreased in the presence of diseases or conditions that decrease the renal blood flow and/or oxygen content, such as severe respiratory distress and perinatal asphyxia. Anuria and/or oliguria may be observed in the preterm infant after severe asphyxia with associated hypotension.

- The preterm infant's kidneys are limited in their ability to concentrate urine or to excrete excess amounts of fluid. This means that if excess fluid is administered, the infant is at risk for fluid retention and overhydration. If too little is administered, the infant will become dehydrated, because of the inability to retain adequate fluid.

- The kidneys of the preterm infant begin excreting glucose at a lower serum glucose level than adult kidneys. Therefore, glycosuria with hyperglycemia is common.

- The buffering capacity of the kidney is reduced, predisposing the infant to metabolic acidosis. Bicarbonate is excreted at a lower serum level, and excretion of acid is accomplished more slowly. Therefore, after periods of hypoxia or insult, the preterm infant's kidneys require a longer time to excrete the lactic acid that accumulates. Sodium bicarbonate is frequently required to treat the metabolic acidosis.

- The immaturity of the renal system affects the preterm infant's ability to excrete drugs. Because excretion time is longer, many drugs are given over longer intervals (for example, every 12 hours instead of every 8 hours). Urine output must be carefully monitored when the infant is receiving nephrotoxic drugs such as gentamicin, nafcillin, and others. In the event of poor urine output, drugs can become toxic in the infant much more quickly than in the adult.

Hepatic Physiology and Considerations

Immaturity of the preterm newborn's liver predisposes the infant to several problems. First, glycogen is stored in the liver throughout gestation, reaching approximately 5% of the weight of the liver by term (Klaus & Fanaroff 1986). After birth, the glycogen stores are rapidly used for energy. Glycogen deposits are affected by asphyxia in utero, and after birth by both asphyxia and cold stress. The baby born preterm has decreased glycogen stores at birth because of low gestational age and frequently experiences stress, which uses up the glycogen rapidly. Therefore the preterm newborn is at high risk for hypoglycemia and its complications.

Iron is also stored in the liver, and the amount greatly increases during the last trimester of pregnancy. Therefore, the preterm newborn is born with low iron stores. If subject to hemorrhage, rapid growth, and excess blood sampling, the preterm infant is likely to become iron depleted more quickly than the term infant. Many preterm babies require transfusions of packed cells to replace the blood withdrawn by frequent blood sampling.

Conjugation of bilirubin in the liver is also impaired in the preterm infant until approximately 37 weeks' gestation. Thus, bilirubin levels increase more rapidly and to a higher level than in the full-term infant (Avery 1987). Early clinical assessment of jaundice at nontoxic bilirubin levels is more difficult in preterm newborns, because they lack subcutaneous fat.

Immunologic Physiology and Considerations

The preterm infant is at a much greater risk for infection than the term infant. This increased susceptibility is partially attributable to low gestational age but may also be the result of an infection acquired in utero, which precipitates preterm labor and birth.

In utero, the fetus receives passive immunity against a variety of infections from maternal IgG immunoglobulins, which cross the placenta (see Chapter 27). Because most of this immunity is acquired in the last trimester of pregnancy, the preterm infant has few antibodies at birth, which provide less protection and become depleted earlier than in a full-term infant. This may be a contributing factor in the higher incidence of recurrent infection during the first year of life as well as in the immediate neonatal period (Korones 1986).

The other immunoglobulin significant for the preterm infant is secretory IgA, which does not cross the placenta but is found in breast milk in significant concentrations. Breast-milk's secretory IgA provides immunity to the mucosal surfaces of the GI tract, providing protection from enteric infections such as those caused by *Escherichia coli* and *Shigella.* Ill preterm infants may be unable to have breast milk and thus are at risk for enteric infections.

Another altered defense against infection in the preterm infant is the skin surface. In very small infants the skin is easily excoriated, and this factor, coupled with many invasive procedures, places the infant at great risk for nosocomial infections. It is vital to use good hand-washing techniques in the care of these infants to prevent unnecessary infection.

Hematologic Physiology and Considerations

The normal cord hemoglobin in an infant of 34 weeks' gestation is approximately 16.8 g/dL, and total blood volume ranges from 89 mL/kg to 105 mL/kg (Avery 1987). Because of the small total blood volume, any blood loss is highly significant to the preterm infant. For this reason, all blood taken for sampling must be recorded. Blood is generally replaced when the infant has lost 10% of total blood volume.

Central Nervous System Physiology and Considerations

After the general shape of the brain is formed during the first six weeks of gestation, the complexity of the human nervous system begins an evolution that continues into adult life. Between the second and fourth months of gestation there is proliferation of the brain's total complement of neurons and migration of these neurons to specific sites throughout the central nervous system. Organization of the neurons that establish the nerve impulse pathways occur from the sixth month of gestation to several years after birth. The final step in neurologic development is the covering of these nerves with myelin. Myelination begins in the second trimester of gestation and continues into adult life (Volpe 1987).

Because the period of most rapid brain growth and development occurs during the third trimester of pregnancy, the closer to term an infant is born, the better the neurologic prognosis.

A common interruption of neurologic development in the preterm infant is caused by intraventricular hemorrhage (IVH). For more in-depth discussion, see page 969.

Reactivity Periods and Behavioral States

The newborn infant's response to extrauterine life is characterized by two periods of reactivity, as discussed in Chapter 29. Because of the immaturity of all systems in comparison to those of the full-term neonate, the preterm infant's periods of reactivity are delayed. If the infant is very ill, these periods of reactivity may not be observed at all, as the infant may be hypotonic and unreactive for several days after birth.

As the preterm newborn grows and the condition stabilizes, it becomes increasingly possible to identify behavioral states and traits unique to each infant. This is a very important part of nursing management of the high-risk infant, because it facilitates parental knowledge of their infant's cues for interaction.

In general, stable preterm infants do not demonstrate

Research Note

Clinical Application of Research

Pamela Deiriggi (1990) analyzed the relationship between the use of waterbed flotation and energy expenditure for preterm infants. The variables for energy expenditure included motor activity, heart rate, and behavioral state. Behavioral states consisted of quiet sleep, active sleep, drowse, alert inactivity, waking activity, fussing/crying, and indeterminate state. Each infant served as his/her own control and was randomly assigned to the sequence of on–off or off–on the waterbed.

Analysis of the results of the study by repeated measures ANOVA showed that activity was significantly diminished while the infant was on the waterbed. Use of the waterbed reduced heart rate; however, a significant interaction between sequence of treatment (on the waterbed) and heart rate also resulted. While on the waterbed, the infants demonstrated greater percentages of time spent in sleep states, specifically the state of quiet sleep. In contrast, when infants were off the waterbed, they had more active awake and fussy states. Additionally, during the period on the waterbed, the infants had fewer state changes or they maintained each state for longer periods.

The researcher also found that use of theophylline had a significant main effect on heart rate, activity level, and sleep states. After grouping the infants by theophylline administration (never had it, discontinued at least 5 days prior to study, received it during study), the researcher ran a two-way ANOVA with the two treatments being waterbed use and theophylline administration.

Critical Thinking Applied to Research

Strengths: Excellent conceptual framework, thorough description of tools used with some psychometric properties identified.

Concerns: With only 22 subjects, the group numbers for the two-way ANOVA must have been small, but the researcher did not give n's or a table of results.

Deiriggi P: Effects of waterbed flotation on indicators of energy expenditure in preterm infants. *Nurs Res* 1990; 39(3):140.

the same behavioral states as term infants. Preterm infants are more disorganized in their sleep-wake cycles and are unable to attend as well to the human face and objects in the environment. Neurologically, their responses are weaker (sucking, muscle tone, states of arousal) than full-term infants' responses (Davis & Thomas 1987).

By observing each infant's patterns of behavior and responses, especially the sleep-wake states, the nurse can teach parents optimal times for interacting with their infant. The parents and nurse can plan nursing care around the times when the infant is alert and best able to attend. In addition, the more knowledge parents have about the meaning of their infant's responses and behaviors, the better prepared they will be to meet their newborn's needs and to form a positive attachment with their child.

Management of Nutrition and Fluid Requirements

Providing adequate nutrition and fluids for the preterm infant is a major concern of the health care team. It is now recognized that early feedings are extremely valuable in maintaining normal metabolism and lowering the possibility of such complications as hypoglycemia, hyperbilirubinemia, hyperkalemia, and azotemia. However, the preterm newborn is at risk for complications that may develop because of immaturity of the digestive system.

Nutritional Requirements

Enteral caloric intake necessary for growth in an uncompromised healthy preterm infant is 120 to 150 kcal/kg/day. In addition to these relatively high caloric needs, the preterm infant requires more protein (3 to 4 g/kg/day, as opposed to 2.0 to 2.5 g/kg/day for the full-term infant). To meet these needs, a number of higher-calorie, higher protein formulas are available that meet the preterm infant's nutritional demands yet do not overtax the concentration abilities of the immature kidneys. Feeding regimens are then established based on the weight and estimated stomach capacity of the infant (Table 31–1). In many instances it is necessary to supplement the oral feedings with parenteral fluids to maintain adequate hydration and caloric intake.

In addition to a higher calorie and protein formula, it is recommended that preterm infants receive supplemental multivitamins and vitamin E. The requirement for vitamin E is increased by a diet high in polyunsaturated fats (which are tolerated best by preterm infants). Preterm infants fed iron-fortified formulas have higher red cell hemolysis and lower vitamin E concentrations and thus require additional vitamin E. Vitamin E supplements decrease susceptibility to hemolytic anemia (American Academy of Pediatrics 1985). Serum levels of vitamin E should be monitored if large amounts of oral supplements are used (Phelps 1987).

Since two-thirds of the calcium and phosphorus in the newborn's body is deposited in the last trimester of gestation, the preterm infant is deficient in these minerals. Rickets and significant bone demineralization have been documented in very low-birth-weight infants and otherwise healthy preterm infants. The recommended amount of elemental calcium for a 1000-g premature infant is 210

Table 31–1 Oral Feeding Schedule for the Low-Birth-Weight Infant

Time and substance*	Less than 1000 g Amount	Fre-quency	1001–1500 g Amount	Fre-quency	1501–2000 g Amount	Fre-quency	More than 2000 g Amount	Fre-quency
First "drink"; sterile H$_2$O, 5% glucose	1–2 mL	1 hr	3–4 mL	2 hr	4–5 mL	2–3 hr	10 mL	3 hr
Formula: Subsequent feedings, 12–72 hr	Increase 1 mL every other feeding to maximum 5 mL	1 hr	Increase 1 mL every other feeding to maximum 10 mL	2 hr	Increase 2 mL every other feeding to maximum 15 mL	2–3 hr	Increase 5 mL every other feeding to maximum 20 mL	3 hr
Formula: Final feeding schedule, 150 mL/kg	10–15 mL	2 hr	20–28 mL	2–3 hr	28–37 mL	3 hr	37–50 mL	3–4 hr

Supplemental IV fluids should be given to fulfill fluid requirements of 140–160 mL/kg or to give urine specific gravities of 1.008–1.010 and caloric requirements of 90–130 cal/kg.

Modified from Avery GB (editor): Neonatology, 3rd ed. Philadelphia: Lippincott, 1987, p 1196.

mg/kg/day. For larger preterm infants, 150 to 180 mg/kg/day may be sufficient.

Special formulas available for preterm infants have increased calcium and phosphorus supplementation. These may lead to mineral acquisition similar to that acquired in utero if the infant can tolerate a minimum of 150 mL/kg/day. If other formulas are used, enteral supplements are recommended. In addition to calcium and phosphorus supplementation, vitamin D intake should be at least 500 IU/day to facilitate retention of calcium and increase bone densities (American Academy of Pediatrics 1985).

Formulas for Preterm Newborns

The formula of choice for feeding the preterm infant varies somewhat among institutions and areas of the country. However, most of the formulas contain protein with a whey/casein ratio of 60:40, a similar proportion to that found in breast milk, and a caloric value of 24 calories per ounce (Table 31–2). Initial feedings may be diluted to 12 calories per ounce and gradually increased, as the infant tolerates them, to 24-calorie formulas. Breast milk is widely used to feed preterm infants. Besides its many benefits for the infants, it allows the mother to contribute to the in-

Table 31–2 Commonly Used Preterm Formulas

Formula	Caloric content	Carbohydrate g/dL	Type	Protein g/dL	Whey/casein ratio	Fat g/dL	Type	Osmolality mOsm/kg H$_2$O
Enfamil 24 Premature Formula	81	8.9	60% polycose 40% lactose	2.4	60/40	4.1	40% MCT 40% corn	300
SMA "Preemie"	81	8.6	50% lactose 50% maltodextrins	2.0	60/40	4.4	27% coconut 25% oleic	268
Similac Special Care Infant Formula	81	8.6	50% lactose 50% polycose	2.2	60/40	4.4	50% MCT 30% corn	300
Similac 24 w/Iron	81	8.5	lactose	2.2	18/82	4.3	60% coconut	360
Similac PM 60/40	68	7.6	lactose	1.6	60/40	3.5	60% coconut	260
SMA 24	81	4.2	lactose	1.8	60/40	4.2	oleo, soy, coconut	364

Modified from Avery ME, Taeusch HW (editors): Schaffer's Diseases of the Newborn, 5th ed. Philadelphia: Saunders, 1984, p 974.

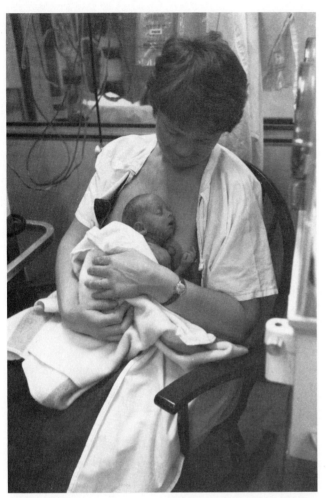

Figure 31–8 Mother visits intensive care unit to breast-feed her preterm infant.

fant's well-being (Figure 31–8) The nurse should inform mothers of their option to breast-feed if they choose to do so. It is important for the nurse to be aware of the advantages and possible disadvantages of breast-feeding, such as decreased growth rate, hyponatremia, lactose intolerance, and rickets if breast milk is the sole source of food.

Methods of Feeding

Various feeding methods are used for the preterm infant, depending on the infant's gestational age, health and physical condition, and neurologic status. The methods, criteria for selection, description, and nursing responsibilities associated with each method are summarized in the following sections.

Nipple Feeding Nipple feeding is used in infants who are 34 weeks' gestation and have a coordinated suck and swallow reflex. Infants who are showing consistent weight gain (20 to 30 g per day) are also nipple fed, since they have the extra strength that sucking requires.

Method The feeding should take no longer than 15 to 20 minutes. A premature infant nipple or regular-sized nipple may be used, depending on the infant's strength and ability (nippling requires more energy than other methods). The infant is fed in a semisitting position and burped gently after each half ounce or ounce. Babies who are progressing from gavage feedings to bottle-feeding should start with one session of bottle-feeding a day and slowly increase the number of times a day a bottle is given until the baby tolerates all feedings from a bottle.

Nursing Care The infant's ability to suck is assessed. Sucking may be affected by age, asphyxia, sepsis, intraventricular hemorrhage or other neurologic insult. Before initiating nipple feeding, the infant is observed for any signs of stress, such as tachypnea (more than 60 respirations/min), respiratory distress, or hypothermia, which may increase the risk of aspiration. During the feeding, the infant should be observed for signs of difficulty with feeding (tachypnea, cyanosis, bradycardia, lethargy, and uncoordinated suck and swallow). After the feeding, the infant is gently burped and positioned on the right side or abdomen.

Breast-Feeding Mothers who wish to breast-feed their preterm infants should be given the opportunity to put the infant to breast as soon as the infant has demonstrated a coordinated suck and swallow reflex, is showing consistent weight gain, and can control body temperature outside of the isolette, regardless of weight. Delaying transition from bottle to breast results in the infant developing a sucking mechanism specific to the artificial nipple that impedes subsequent transfer to the breast (Meier & Pugh 1985). Studies have shown that preterm infants tolerate breast-feeding with higher transcutaneous oxygen pressure and maintenance of body temperature better than during bottle-feeding (Meier 1988).

Method The infant is placed at the mother's breast. It has been suggested that the football hold is a convenient position for preterm babies. Feeding time may take up to 45 minutes, and babies should be burped as they alternate breasts (Meier & Pugh 1985).

Nursing Care Nursing responsibilities are the same as with an infant who is bottle-feeding. In addition, the nurse coordinates a flexible feeding schedule so babies can nurse during alert times and be allowed to set their own pace. A similar regimen should be used for the baby who is progressing from gavage feeding to breast-feeding. The baby should begin with one breast-feeding and gradually increase the number of times during the day that the baby breast-feeds.

Gavage Feeding The gavage feeding method is used with preterm infants (less than 34 weeks' gestation) who lack or have a poorly coordinated suck and swallow reflex or are ill. Gavage feeding may be used as an adjunct to nipple feeding if the infant tires easily or as an alternative if an infant is losing weight because of the energy expenditure required for nippling.

Method and Nursing Care Procedure 31–1 for description.

Transpyloric Nasojejunal or Nasoduodenal Tube Feeding
Transpyloric, nasojejunal, or nasoduodenal feeding by tube is used with very small preterm infants who are ventilator dependent or tachypneic, have chronic lung disease, recurrent aspiration, or repeated residuals with other methods of feeding.

Method Transpyloric, nasojejunal, or nasoduodenal feeding involves a continuous infusion of formula into the duodenum or jejunum of the baby to prevent vomiting. An indwelling feeding tube is passed through the nostril, into the stomach, past the pylorus, and into the small intestine. Tube placement is confirmed by x-ray examination. A constant infusion pump is used to administer small amounts of formula continuously. The tube is left in place and changed every three days.

Potential Risks Although this feeding method has advantages (for example, decreased risk of aspiration), it poses risks of stomach and intestinal perforation and accidental bolus infusion by the pump. In addition, formula bypasses the digestive activity of the stomach. The transpyloric method is never used in some centers, where the risks are believed to outweigh the benefits.

Nursing Care The nurse assists with the passing of the tube, observing the infant's vital signs and watching for any intolerance of the procedure. After the transpyloric feedings have begun, the nurse does the following:

- Observes and records rate of infusion hourly to make sure the correct amount is infusing
- Changes infusion setup every eight hours to decrease chances of bacterial growth in the formula
- Ensures that no more than three hours' worth of formula is hung at one time to prevent "dumping" of excess formula
- Checks all stools for blood and glucose (signs of necrotizing enterocolitis)

Total Parenteral Nutrition
Total parenteral nutrition (TPN) is used in situations that contraindicate feeding the infant through the GI tract. Contraindications include GI anomalies requiring surgical intervention, necrotizing enterocolitis, intolerance of feedings, and extreme prematurity.

Method The TPN method provides complete nutrition to the infant intravenously. Hyperalimentation gives calories, vitamins, minerals, protein, and glucose. Intralipids must also be administered to provide essential fatty acids. Hyperalimentation may be infused through either a central or a peripheral line. Intralipids may only be infused peripherally, and if added as a piggyback to the hyperalimentation, they must be piggybacked as close to the infusion site as possible and not through the filter.

Nursing Care The nurse needs to monitor serum glucose levels carefully during TPN. Urine is checked for protein, sugar, and specific gravity at least every eight hours. The intravenous rate is monitored hourly to maintain accurate intake. The rate should not be increased to "catch up" if behind. The intravenous site should be observed hourly for signs of infiltration—hyperalimentation is extremely caustic and causes severe tissue destruction if it infiltrates. Fluid intake and output are carefully monitored (hyperglycemia causing an osmotic diuresis can lead to dehydration). The nurse observes for signs of reaction to intralipids, such as dyspnea, vomiting, elevated temperature, or cyanosis.

Whichever method of feeding is selected for an infant, the nurse should carefully watch for any signs and symptoms of feeding intolerance, including the following:

- Increasing gastric residuals (more than 2 mL)
- Abdominal distention (measured routinely before feedings)
- Guaiac-positive stools (occult blood in stools)
- Presence of glucose in the stools
- Vomiting
- Diarrhea

Fluid Requirements
Calculation of fluid requirements takes into account the infant's weight and postnatal age. Recommendations for fluid therapy in the preterm newborn are approximately 80 to 100 mL/kg/day for the first day of life; 100 to 120 mL/kg/day for day 2; and 120 to 150 mL/kg/day by day 3 of life. These amounts may be increased up to 200 mL/kg/day if the baby is very small, receiving phototherapy, or under a radiant warmer which may increase fluid loss an additional 50%. The baby may need less fluid if a heat shield is used, the environment is more humid, or humidified oxygen is being provided.

Common Complications of Preterm Newborns and Their Medical Management

The goals of medical therapy are to meet the growth and development needs of the preterm newborn and to anticipate and manage the complications associated with prematurity. Complications associated with prematurity that

PROCEDURE 31–1
Gavage Feeding

Nursing Action

Objective: Ensure smooth accomplishment of the procedure.

Gather necessary equipment including:

1. No. 5 or No. 8 Fr. feeding tube
2. 10–30 mL syringe
3. ¼-in. paper tape
4. Stethoscope
5. Appropriate formula
6. Small cup of sterile water

Explain procedure to parents.

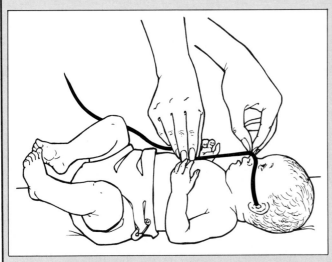

Figure 31–9   Measuring gavage tube length

Objective: Insert tube accurately into stomach.

Position infant on back or side with head of bed elevated.

Take tube from package and measure the distance from the tip of the ear to the nose to the xiphoid process, and mark the point with a small piece of paper tape (Figure 31–9).

If inserting tube nasally, lubricate tip in cup of sterile water. Shake excess drops to prevent aspiration.

Stabilize infant's head with one hand, and pass the tube via the mouth (or nose) into the stomach, to the point previously marked. If the infant begins coughing or choking or becomes cyanotic or aphonic, remove the tube immediately.

Rationale

Considerations in choosing size of catheter include size of the infant, area of insertion (oral or nasal), and rate of flow desired. The very small infant (less than 1600 g) requires a 5 Fr. feeding tube; an infant greater than 1600 g may tolerate a larger tube. Orogastric insertion is preferred over nasogastric insertion as most infants are obligatory nose breathers. If nasogastric insertion is used, a No. 5 catheter should be used to minimize airway obstruction. The size of the catheter will influence the rate of flow. The syringe is used to aspirate stomach contents prior to feeding, to inject air into the stomach for testing tube placement, and for holding measured amount of formula during feeding. Tape is used to mark tube for insertion depth as well as for securing tube during feeding. Stethoscope is needed to auscultate rush of air into stomach when testing tube placement.

Sterile water may be used to lubricate feeding tube when inserted nasally. With oral insertion, there are enough secretions in the mouth to lubricate the tube adequately. The cup of sterile water may also be used to test for placement by placing the end of the tube into the water to check for air bubbles from the lungs. However, this test may not be accurate as air may also be present in the stomach (Avery 1987).

This position allows easy passage of the tube.

This measuring technique ensures enough tubing to enter stomach.

Water should be used, as opposed to an oil-based lubricant, in case the tube is inadvertently passed into a lung.

Any signs of respiratory distress signal likelihood that tube has entered trachea. Orogastric insertion is less likely to result in passage into the trachea than nasogastric insertion.

(continued)

Nursing Action

If no respiratory distress is apparent, lightly tape tube in position, draw up 0.5–1.0 mL of air in syringe, and connect it to tubing. Place stethoscope over the epigastrium and briskly inject the air (Figure 31–10).

Rationale

Nurse should hear a sudden rush of air as it enters stomach.

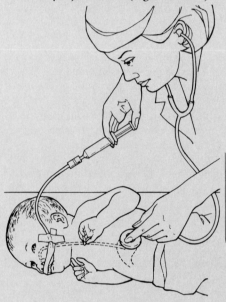

Figure 31–10 Auscultation for placement of gavage tube

Aspirate stomach contents with syringe, and note amount, color, and consistency. Return residual to stomach unless otherwise ordered to discard it.

Residual formula should be evaluated as part of the assessment of infant's tolerance of gavage feedings. It is not discarded, unless particularly large in volume or mucoid in nature, because of the potential for causing an electrolyte imbalance.

If only a clear fluid or mucus is found upon aspiration and if any question exists as to whether the tube is in the stomach, the aspirate can be tested for pH.

Stomach aspirate tests in the 1–3 range for pH.

Objective: Introduce formula into stomach without complication.

Hold infant for feeding or position on right side if infant cannot be held.

Positioning on side decreases the risk of aspiration in case of emesis during feeding.

Separate syringe from tube, remove plunger from barrel, reconnect barrel to tube, and pour formula into syringe.

Feeding should be allowed to flow in by gravity. It should not be pushed in under pressure with a syringe.

Elevate syringe 6–8 in. over infant's head. Allow formula to flow at slow, even rate.

Raising column of fluid increases force of gravity. Nurse may need to initiate flow of formula by inserting plunger of syringe into barrel just until formula is seen to enter feeding tube. Rate should be regulated to prevent sudden stomach distention, with possibility of vomiting and aspiration.

Continue adding formula to syringe until desired volume has been absorbed. Then rinse tubing with 2–3 mL sterile water.

Rinsing tube ensures that infant receives all of formula. It is especially important to rinse tube if it is going to be left in place, because this decreases risk of clogging and bacterial growth in tube.

Remove tube by loosening tape, folding the tube over on itself, and quickly withdrawing it in one smooth motion. If tube is to be left in, position it so that infant is unable to remove it.

Folding tube over on itself minimizes potential for aspiration of fluid, which would otherwise flow from tubing as it passes epiglottis. A tube left in place should be replaced at least every 24 hours.

(continued)

PROCEDURE 31–1 (continued)

Nursing Action	Rationale
Objective: Maximize feeding pleasure of infant.	
Whenever possible hold infant during gavage feeding. If it is too awkward to hold infant during feeding, be sure to take time for holding afterward.	Feeding time is important to infant's tactile sensory input.
Offer a pacifier to infant during feeding.	Infants fed for long periods by gavage can lose their sucking reflex. Sucking during feeding comforts and relaxes infant, making formula flow more easily. One study showed that infants allowed to suck during feedings were able to nipple sooner and were discharged earlier than a control group of infants who did not suck during tube feedings.

---

require medical intervention are respiratory distress syndrome (RDS), patent ductus arteriosus (PDA), apnea, and intraventricular hemorrhage (IVH). Long-term problems include retinopathy of prematurity (ROP) and bronchopulmonary dysplasia (BPD).

An in-depth discussion of RDS and BPD, including pathophysiology, medical management, and nursing care, is contained in Chapter 32. Patent ductus arteriosus, apnea, intraventricular hemorrhage, retinopathy of prematurity, and other complications are discussed in this section.

Patent Ductus Arteriosus

Spontaneous closure of the connection between the aorta and pulmonary artery is often delayed in preterm infants. The incidence of symptomatic patent ductus arteriosus is related to birth weight in preterm infants and has been shown to decrease with increase in birth weight (Bhatt & Nahata 1989).

Symptomatic PDA is often seen around the third day of life when the premature infant is recovering from RDS. Initially, when the preterm neonate is hypoxic secondary to RDS, the pulmonary vascular resistance (PVR) can be higher than the systemic vascular resistance, and right-to-left shunting through the ductus will occur. However, as the RDS improves and adequate oxygenation is maintained, the lungs open up and more blood flows into them, leading to left ventricular volume overload, pulmonary edema, and congestive failure. Oxygenation is again compromised and ventilator requirements will increase, leading to the possibility of long-term pulmonary sequelae.

Ductal patency with left-to-right shunting is manifested with a continuous or systolic murmur, active precordium (visible heart pulsation), bounding pulses (increased pulse pressure), tachycardia, tachypnea, hepatomegaly, and pulmonary edema. These problems lead to signs of respiratory distress and continued oxygen and ventilator requirements. Chest radiographs reveal cardiomegaly with increased pulmonary vascularity.

Patency of the ductus arteriosus can be determined by aortic contrast echocardiography. This technique visualizes microbubbles that result when saline is injected into an umbilical artery catheter. In the presence of a PDA, the bubbles pass left-to-right through the patent ductus. Since the left atrium and aorta are usually the same size, regular echocardiography can also demonstrate a patent ductus by determining an increase in left atrial size compared to the aortic root dimension.

The goal of medical therapy is to achieve ductal closure. Early identification of symptomatic infants and prompt intervention will minimize long-term complications. The following three methods are currently used, separately or in combination, to effect closure:

1. *Medical therapy.* Initial medical management consists of providing adequate respiratory support, maintaining a relatively high hematocrit (greater than 40%), restricting fluids, and using diuretics (to decrease pulmonary edema) and perhaps digoxin while waiting for spontaneous closure of the ductus to occur (Bhatt & Nahata 1989).

2. *Pharmacologic therapy.* Administration of prostaglandin synthetase inhibitors such as indomethacin impairs synthesis of the E series prostaglandins responsible for dilatation of the ductus and can cause ductal closure. Indomethacin is effective, but it is not without side effects and must be used cautiously. Side effects include decreased platelet aggregation, association with intracranial bleeding, gastrointestinal hemorrhage, and transient renal dysfunction. Aminoglycoside levels should be monitored during indomethacin use, because high serum aminoglycoside concentrations may result from the decline in renal function associated with indomethacin (Bhatt & Nahata 1989).

3. *Surgical therapy.* The ductus may be surgically ligated.

A national collaborative study showed the preferable mode of therapy in infants with symptomatic PDA to be a trial of medical therapy alone at the time of diagnosis followed by intravenous administration of indomethacin as back-up therapy if indicated. No significant differences in outcome (at one year of age) were identified with any of the three therapies.

Patent ductus arteriosus will often prolong the course of illness in a preterm newborn and lead to chronic pulmonary dysfunction. Early identification is essential for prompt treatment to minimize the complications that may have long-term effects.

Apnea

Apnea of prematurity refers to cessation of breathing for 20 seconds or longer or for less than 20 seconds when associated with cyanosis, bradycardia, and/or limpness (Grisemer 1990). Apnea is a common problem in the preterm infant (of less than 36 weeks' gestation) and is thought to be primarily a result of neuronal immaturity, a factor that contributes to the preterm infant's irregular breathing patterns. The immaturity of the preterm's CNS increases the baby's vulnerability to any adverse factors affecting nerve cell metabolism. Impaired nerve cell metabolism in turn can impair respiratory neurons in the brain stem. Factors that adversely affect brain nerve cells include hypoxia, acidosis, edema, intracranial bleeding, hyperbilirubinemia, hypoglycemia, hypocalcemia, and sepsis.

Nursing Care

Apneic onset is often insidious; cardiorespiratory monitoring allows for early recognition and intervention, thus decreasing the need for resuscitative efforts. The nurse checks during each shift to make sure alarms are set and working properly. Apnea may occur during feeding, suctioning, or while stooling. On the other hand, there may be no observable activity related to apnea. All episodes of apnea are documented. The documentation includes activity at the time of apnea, length of episode, along with any bradycardia, color change, or desaturation on pulse-oximeter associated with apneic episodes, and treatment required to bring the baby out of the apneic spell. This data is useful in determining etiology and possible treatment.

The nurse needs to make careful observations and quickly assess the need for intervention. The intervention required depends on the severity of the apneic episode and the baby's response. If an apneic episode occurs the nurse may do the following:

1. Observe the infant briefly to see if treatment is necessary or if the infant is having periodic breathing and begins to breathe spontaneously.

2. Begin stimulation by gently rubbing the soles of the feet, the ankles, and the infant's back. Rubbing bony prominences is uncomfortable to the infant and therefore more stimulating than rubbing other areas of the body.

3. Suction nasopharynx and oropharynx, provide additional oxygen, and prepare for bag and mask ventilation if the infant is dusky, cyanotic, or bradycardic. Obstruction of the airway by mucus or formula may result in apnea and bradycardia. Clearing the airway while providing increased oxygen concentration and stimulation may resolve apneic episodes. If the infant does not respond, bag and mask ventilation may be required to relieve cyanosis and return heart rate to normal.

4. Administer oxygen and warm humidified air per physician order to control dyspnea and cyanosis. Increased oxygen may alleviate episodes of apnea and bradycardia. Monitor and record the oxygen concentration every two hours.

5. Prepare for septic workup if the infant is not already on antibiotics.

6. Prepare for intubation and use of the respirator for ventilation if the infant has frequent apneic episodes that require bag and mask ventilation. Ventilatory assistance may be necessary to prevent possible sequelae of frequent apneic spells with resulting hypoxemia.

7. Report and assess variations in blood gases and laboratory reports. Apnea is associated with elevated PCO_2, decreased PO_2, and other electrolyte imbalances.

8. Maintain thermal neutrality. Temperature instability may precipitate apnea.

9. Use methylxanthine drugs (aminophylline, theophylline, or caffeine) to treat apnea of prematurity. Advantages of caffeine over theophylline include a larger therapeutic index, once-daily administration, a small fluctuation in plasma concentrations, a potent central respirogenic effect, and fewer peripheral adverse effects (Kriter & Blanchard 1989).

The general care given an apneic baby should include gentle handling to prevent unnecessary stress on the baby. Keeping the airway clear is very important, but nasopharyngeal suctioning should be done gently and only as necessary, since it can cause apnea. Use of indwelling orogastric or nasogastric tubes is preferred to intermittent passage of feeding tubes. The nurse provides IV fluids as ordered to maintain adequate fluid and electrolyte balance. Severe apnea may preclude oral feeding for a time, and the infant may require nutritional maintenance with intravenous therapy. Adequate nutrition prevents catabolism of body tissues, as well as biochemical aberrations such as hypoglycemia, hyperglycemia, acidosis, or electrolyte imbalance. Following feedings, the baby should be positioned prone or supported on the right side with the head of the bed elevated.

Intraventricular Hemorrhage

Intraventricular hemorrhage (IVH) is the most common type of intracranial hemorrhage in the small preterm infant. Those most susceptible to IVH are infants weighing less than 1500 g or of less than 34 weeks' gestation. The incidence of intracranial hemorrhage in these newborns is between 34% and 49% (Volpe 1989).

An IVH frequently occurs after an insult to the infant that results in hypoxia such as respiratory distress, birth trauma, and birth asphyxia, with the more immature infants being at higher risk for these complications.

The most common site of hemorrhage is in the periventricular subependymal germinal matrix, where there is a rich blood supply and the capillary walls are thin and fragile. The matrix provides little supportive tissue for the fragile blood vessels. Before 32 weeks' gestation, an infant is much more susceptible to hemorrhage of these tiny vessels, because they are vulnerable to hypoxic events that damage vessel walls and cause them to rupture. Computerized axial tomography (CT) or ultrasound scanning can be used to identify both the site and the extent of hemorrhage.

The clinical signs observed in an infant with IVH are variable. The infant may suddenly "crash" (characterized by pallor and shocklike appearance) and die or may show very subtle or no signs at all. The most common manifestations are neurologic signs (hypotonia, lethargy, temperature instability, nystagmus, bulging fontanelle, falling hematocrit, apnea, bradycardia, hypotension, and a worsening in the respiratory condition (increasing hypoxia) with metabolic acidosis. Seizures may occur, and decerebrate posturing may be observed.

Prevention of IVH remains an important goal. Prenatal interventions include prevention of premature birth and maternal transport to a tertiary care center. Administration of phenobarbital and vitamin K to the mother is being studied for their preventive effect. Postnatal preventive interventions include careful resuscitation, correction or prevention of major hemodynamic disturbances, and correction of coagulation abnormalities. Postnatal preventive pharmacologic interventions include phenobarbital to control seizures, indomethacin to decrease the hemodynamics resulting from PDA, and vitamin E for its antioxidant abilities (Volpe 1989).

Therapeutic efforts include supportive care of the infant with an IVH and prevention of early recognition of posthemorrhagic hydrocephalus. Placement of a ventriculoperitoneal shunt may be required if progressive ventricular dilatation is documented.

The outcome for the infant depends on the size of the intracerebral bleed and the gestational age of the infant. The most severe hemorrhages may cause motor deficits, hydrocephalus, hearing loss, and blindness. Less severe bleeds may have no observable effects (Volpe 1987).

Nursing Care Nursing care of a newborn with IVH is mainly observational and supportive. Vital signs, fontanelle tenseness, seizure activity, hematocrit, blood pressure, and changes in muscle tone or activity should be monitored closely. The nurse prepares the infant and assists with lumbar puncture for spinal fluid analysis. While administering replacement whole blood or albumin, the nurse monitors blood pressure. Thermal neutrality must be maintained. After a suspected bleed, the occipital frontal circumference is checked closely, as hydrocephalus may occur. The nurse also monitors for signs of increased intracranial pressure (apnea, bradycardia, hypotension). Serial head ultrasound may be done. The treatment of infants with severe hemorrhagic intracerebral involvement brings up complex ethical issues for parents and health care providers.

In caring for the infant with an IVH, the nurse provides support for the parents identifying their level of understanding and facilitating interdisciplinary communication with them. As a member of the interdisciplinary team, the nurse can identify the parents' needs and provide continuing supportive care.

Retinopathy of Prematurity

Premature neonates are particularly susceptible to characteristic retinal changes known as retinopathy of prematurity (ROP). This disease has previously been referred to as retrolental fibroplasia (RLF).

Until recently ROP was thought to be exclusively the result of excessive use of oxygen in the treatment of premature infants. However, ROP has also occurred in premature infants who never received oxygen, in full-term infants with cyanotic congenital heart disease, and in certain other congenital anomalies. The disease is now viewed as multifactorial in origin.

Increased survival of very-low-birth-weight (VLBW) infants may be the most important factor in the increased incidence of ROP. In those with birth weights below 1000 g, the incidence can be as high as 88%. The susceptibility of these infants is thought to be due to many factors, including immaturity, a wide range of medical problems, and associated therapies (Fanaroff & Martin 1987).

An international classification of ROP has been developed to describe the disease and the extent of retinal changes (Committee for the Classification of Retinopathy of Prematurity 1984).

The fetal retina is unique in that its vascularization does not begin until the fourth month of gestation, with the temporal peripheral area of retinal vasculature lagging in development. Vascularization is not completed until term. Consequently, the immature vascular system is susceptible to damage in the preterm neonate and occasionally in the term neonate. In the early, acute stages of ROP, immature retinal vessels constrict. If the vasoconstriction is sustained, vascular closure follows and irreversible capillary endothelial damage occurs. This disintegration of vessels is called vaso-obliteration. New vessels will eventually emerge from the point of vaso-obliteration, but they will lack normal structural integrity. In the later stages of ROP, vasoproliferation occurs as the new vessels erupt through the retina to proliferate into the vitreous body. The fragile vessels often rupture to produce retinal and vitreous hemorrhage. Scar tissue forms and traction may occur, leading to retinal detachment and subsequent blindness.

The goal of therapy is early identification and selective intervention. In the absence of therapeutic intervention, detection will at least enable early counseling and support of the parents when visual defects are suspected. An initial fundal examination with an indirect ophthalmoscope should be performed between 4 and 8 weeks of age (Cryotherapy Retinopathy of Prematurity [Cryo-ROP] Cooperative Group 1988). The American Academy of Pediatrics recommends eye examinations for all infants of less than 36 weeks' gestation or all infants who weighed less than 2000 g and received oxygen therapy. Frequency of repeat examinations depends on the rapidity of progression or the severity of the disease.

Preventive care is aimed at maintaining the small premature infant in as stable a physiologic condition as possible. Treatment of the acute stages of ROP with laser or cryotherapy is an option. The results of a multi-center randomized trial of cryotherapy support the efficacy of cryotherapy in reducing by approximately one-half the risk of unfavorable outcome. Unfavorable outcome was defined as a retinal fold involving the posterior pole or total retrolental mass (CRYO-ROP Cooperative Group 1988). Cryotherapy obliterates the neovascularization (new vessel formation) and reduces the traction that causes retinal detachment. Since most acute cases of ROP regress spontaneously with no long-term visual impairment, the possibility of regression must be weighed against the risk of an unfavorable outcome.

For infants with bilateral traction and retinal detachment, surgical vitrectomy and scleral buckling have been used experimentally. These surgeries are technically difficult due to the small size of the infant's eye. Since they are experimental, further follow-up is required for evaluation.

Nursing Care

Nursing care for the visually impaired infant must concentrate on parental support and education. When the crisis of premature birth is quickly followed by the devastating news of suspected visual impairment or blindness, the parents will need extensive support by all members of the management team. The parents again experience overwhelming anxiety and uncertainty about their infant's future abilities.

Premature infants with blindness due to ROP may be at increased risk of cognitive and emotional problems. The evidence suggests that this increased risk may be due to environmental factors rather than to inherent intellectual or neurologic factors. Isolation, overprotectiveness, understimulation, and parental despair or emotional withdrawal may accentuate the problems of blindness (Teplin 1983). Figure 31–11 demonstrates the "vicious cycle" leading to emotional and developmental problems that may arise when the problems of parental attachment to a premature infant are compounded by the news of visual impairment.

Nurses can prevent the development of this cycle by helping parents develop appropriate attachment behaviors. Parents can be assured that their infant will be able to recognize them by voice and touch. They must also be told that visually impaired infants may not show recognition or feeling by changes in facial expressions. They will need to look for other cues or body language that their infant uses for self-expression.

In caring for the infant, the nurse can model specific developmental intervention activities and give the parents information on normal developmental milestones. Since the visually impaired child uses the other senses for exploration, parents can be taught specific activities to enhance their child's learning.

Prior to discharge, the management team should provide detailed information about and contacts with available community services and resource groups. Community agencies can provide support and direction for the parents as their child grows and new problems are encountered.

Sensorineural Hearing Loss

High-risk infants have a 2.5% to 5% incidence of moderate to profound hearing loss and should be screened for hearing problems between the ages of 3 and 6 months. Those at increased risk include infants with congenital viral infections, hyperbilirubinemia, perinatal asphyxia, and birth trauma. Damage from ototoxic drugs such as gentamicin and furosemide (Lasix) is variable and related to multiple factors, including renal function, age, duration of treatment, and concomitant administration of other ototoxic agents. If evidence of hearing loss is found during screening, the infant should be referred for diagnostic testing with the goal of getting the infant involved in rehabilitation by 6 months of age (Casey & Bradley 1987).

Speech Defects

The most frequently observed speech defects involve delayed development of receptive and expressive ability that may persist into the school-age years.

Neurologic Defects

The most common neurologic defects include cerebral palsy, hydrocephalus, seizure disorders, lower IQ scores, and learning disabilities. However, the socioeconomic climate and family support systems have been shown to be important factors influencing the child's ultimate school performance in the absence of major neurologic defects. Families can be reminded that risk does not equal injury, injury does not equal damage, and description of damage does not allow a precise prediction about recovery or outcome (Casey & Bradley 1987).

When evaluating the infant's abilities and disabilities, it is important for parents to understand that the developmental level cannot be evaluated based on chronologic

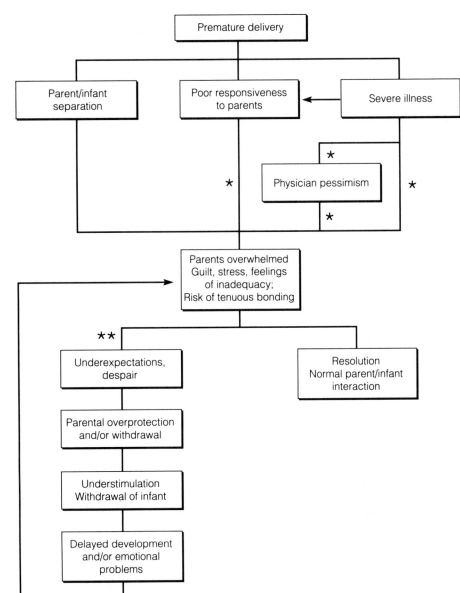

Figure 31–11   Suggested causes and outcomes of altered parental attachment to premature infants with blindness due to ROP. A single asterisk indicates factors affecting attachment in all premature babies that are exacerbated by discovery of blindness. A double asterisk indicates onset of "vicious cycle" leading to emotional/developmental problems (pseudoretardation). (From Teplin SW: Development of blind infants and children with retrolental fibroplasia: Implications for physicians. Pediatrics *1983; 71:6)*

age. Developmental progress must be evaluated from the expected date of birth, not from the actual date of birth. In addition, the parents need the consistent support of health care professionals in the long-term management of their infant. Many new and ongoing concerns arise as the high-risk infant grows and develops; the goal is to promote the highest quality of life possible.

Long-Term Needs and Outcome
The care of the preterm infant and the family is not complete upon discharge from the nursery. Follow-up care is extremely important because many developmental problems are not noted until the infant is older and begins to demonstrate motor delays or sensory disability.

Within the first year of life, low-birth-weight preterm infants face higher mortality than term infants. Causes of death include sudden infant death syndrome (SIDS), which occurs about five times more frequently in the low-birth-weight infant, and respiratory infections and neurologic defects. Morbidity is also much higher among preterm infants, with those weighing less than 1500 g at highest risk for long-term complications.

❋   *APPLYING THE NURSING PROCESS*   ❋
Nursing Assessment

Accurate assessment of the physical characteristics and gestational age of the preterm newborn is imperative to anticipate the special needs and problems of this baby. Physical characteristics vary greatly depending on the gestational age, but the following characteristics are frequently present:

- Color—usually pink or ruddy but may be acrocyanotic; cyanosis, jaundice, pallor, or plethora should be noted.
- Skin—reddened, translucent, blood vessels readily apparent, lack of subcutaneous fat
- Lanugo—plentiful, widely distributed
- Head size—appears large in relation to body
- Skull—bones pliable, fontanelle smooth and flat
- Ears—minimal cartilage, pliable, folded over
- Nails—soft, short
- Genitals—small; testes may not be descended
- Resting position—flaccid, froglike
- Cry—weak, feeble
- Reflexes—poor sucking, swallowing, and gag
- Activity—jerky, generalized movements (seizure activity is abnormal)

Determination of gestational age in preterm newborns requires knowledge and experience in administering gestational assessment tools. The tool used should be specific, reliable, and valid. For a discussion of gestational age assessment tools, see Chapter 28.

Nursing Diagnosis

Nursing diagnoses that may apply to the preterm newborn include the following:

- Impairment of gas exchange related to newborn respiratory distress secondary to immature pulmonary vasculature
- Ineffective breathing patterns: apnea related to immature central nervous system
- Alteration in metabolic processes related to cold stress
- Alteration in nutrition: less than body requirements related to weak suck and swallow reflexes
- Fluid volume deficit related to dehydration secondary to high insensible water losses
- Ineffective parental coping related to anger/guilt at giving birth to a premature baby

Nursing Plan and Implementation

Maintenance of Respiratory Function
There is increased danger of respiratory obstruction in preterm newborns because their bronchi and trachea are so narrow that mucus can obstruct the airway. The nurse

needs to use suctioning judiciously to maintain airway patency.

Positioning of the newborn can also affect respiratory function. The nurse should slightly elevate the infant's head to maintain the airway. Because the newborn has weak neck muscles and cannot control head movement, the nurse should ensure that this head position is maintained. The nurse should avoid placing the infant in the supine position because the newborn has difficulty raising the chest due to weak chest and abdominal muscles. The prone position is best for facilitating chest expansion. Weak or absent cough or gag reflexes increase the chance of aspiration in the premature newborn. The nurse should ensure that the infant's position facilitates drainage of mucus or regurgitated formula.

The nurse monitors heart and respiratory rates with cardiorespiratory monitors and observes the newborn to identify alterations in cardiopulmonary status. Nursery nurses must be alert to signs of respiratory distress, including the following:

- Cyanosis—serious sign when generalized
- Tachypnea—sustained respiratory rate greater than 60/min after first four hours of life
- Retractions
- Expiratory grunting
- Flaring nostrils
- Apneic episodes
- Presence of rales or rhonchi on auscultation
- Inadequate breath sounds.

The nurse who observes any of these alterations records and reports them for further evaluation. If respiratory distress occurs, the nurse administers oxygen per physician order to relieve hypoxemia. If hypoxemia is not treated immediately, it may result in patent ductus arteriosus or metabolic acidosis. If oxygen is administered to the newborn, the nurse monitors the oxygen concentration with devices such as the transcutaneous oxygen monitor ($tcPO_2$) or the pulse-oximeter. Monitoring of oxygen concentration in the baby's blood is essential since hyperoxemia can lead to blindness (see discussion of ROP, page 969).

The nurse also needs to consider respiratory function during feeding. To prevent aspiration and increased energy expenditure and oxygen consumption, the nurse needs to ensure that the infant's gag and suck reflexes are intact before initiating oral feedings. To minimize oxygen consumption, the body temperature is maintained around 36.5C± 0.2C (97.7F±0.5F).

Maintenance of Neutral Thermal Environment
A neutral thermal environment minimizes the oxygen consumption expended to maintain a normal core temperature; it also prevents cold stress and facilitates growth by

decreasing the calories needed to maintain body temperature. The preterm infant's immature central nervous system provides poor temperature control, and stores of brown fat are decreased. A small infant (<1200 g) can lose 80 cal/kg/day through radiation of body heat.

To minimize heat loss and temperature instability effects, the nurse should do the following:

1. Warm and humidify oxygen without blowing it over the infant's face to avoid increasing oxygen consumption.

2. Place the baby in a double-walled Isolette, and use a heat shield over small preterm infants.

3. Avoid placing the baby on cold surfaces such as metal treatment tables and cold x-ray plates; pad cold surfaces with diapers and use radiant warmers during procedures; and warm hands before handling the baby to prevent heat transfer via convection/conduction.

4. Warm the blood before exchange transfusions.

5. Keep the skin dry and place a cap on the baby's head to prevent heat loss via evaporation. (The head makes up 25% of the total body size.)

6. Keep Isolettes, radiant warmers, and cribs away from windows and cold external walls and out of drafts to prevent heat loss by radiation.

7. Use a skin probe to monitor the baby's skin temperature. The temperature should be 36C to 37C (96.8F to 97.7F). Temperature fluctuations indicate hypothermia or hyperthermia.

Maintenance of Fluid and Electrolyte Status

Maintenance of hydration is accomplished by providing adequate intake based on the neonate's weight, gestational age, chronologic age, and volume of sensible and insensible water losses. Adequate fluid intake should provide sufficient water to compensate for increased insensible losses and to provide the amount needed for renal excretion of metabolic products. Insensible water losses can be minimized by providing a high ambient humidity, humidifying oxygen, using heat shields, covering the skin with plastic wrap, and placing the infant in a double-walled Isolette.

The nurse evaluates the hydration status of the baby by assessing and recording signs of dehydration. Signs of dehydration include sunken fontanelle, loss of weight, poor skin turgor (skin returns to position slowly), dry oral mucous membranes, decreased urine output, and increased specific gravity (>1.013). The nurse must also identify signs of overhydration by observing the newborn for edema or excessive weight gain and by comparing urine output with fluid intake.

The preterm infant should be weighed at least once daily at the same time each day. Weight change is one of the most sensitive indicators of fluid balance.

Intake and output is measured accurately. A comparison of intake and output measurements over an 8-hour or 24-hour period provides important information about renal function and fluid balance. Assessment of patterns and whether they show a net gain or loss over several days is also essential to fluid management. Blood serum levels and pH should be monitored to evaluate for electrolyte imbalances.

Accurate hourly intake calculations should be maintained when administering intravenous fluids. Since the preterm infant is unable to excrete excess fluid, it is important to maintain the correct amount of intravenous fluid to prevent fluid overload. This can be accomplished by using neonatal or pediatric infusion pumps. To prevent electrolyte imbalance and dehydration, care must be taken to give the correct IV solutions and volumes and concentrations of formulas. Urine specific gravity and pH are obtained periodically. Urine osmolality provides an indication of hydration, although this factor must be correlated with other assessments (for example, serum sodium). Hydration is considered adequate when the urine output is 1 to 3 mL/kg/hr.

Prevention of Infection

The nurse is responsible for minimizing the preterm newborn's exposure to pathogenic organisms. The preterm newborn is susceptible to infection because of an immature immune system and thin, permeable skin. Invasive procedures, techniques such as umbilical catheterization and mechanical ventilation, and prolonged hospitalization place the infant at greater risk for infection.

Strict hand washing, reverse isolation, and using separate equipment for each infant help minimize exposure of the preterm newborn to infectious agents. Many intensive care nurseries require a two- to three-minute scrub using iodined antibacterial solutions, which inhibit the growth of gram-positive cocci and gram-negative rod organisms. Other specific nursing interventions include limiting visitors; requiring visitors to wash their hands; and maintaining strict aseptic practices when changing intravenous tubing and solutions (IV solutions and tubing should be changed every 24 hours), administering parenteral fluids, and assisting with sterile procedures. Isolettes and radiant warmers should be changed weekly. There should be minimal use or avoidance of chemical skin preps and tape, which may cause skin trauma.

If infection (sepsis) occurs in the preterm newborn, the nurse may be the first to identify the subtle clinical signs associated with infection. The nurse informs the clinician of the findings immediately and implements the treatment plan per clinician orders in the presence of infection. For specific nursing care required for the newborn with an infection, see Chapter 32.

Provision of Adequate Nutrition and Prevention of Fatigue During Feeding

The first feeding may be sterile water in small amounts given every two to three hours. These small amounts are increased slowly by 1 to 2 mL. Formula or breast milk (with or without fortifiers to increase caloric content) is incorporated into the feedings slowly. Initial feedings may be at a quarter strength and slowly increased to full strength. This is done to avoid overtaxing the digestive capacity of the preterm newborn.

Special formulas (eg, Similac Special Care, Preemie Enfamil) are used to meet the caloric needs of the preterm newborn. These special formulas are concentrated to supply more calories in less volume. Small, frequent feedings of high-calorie formula are used because the newborn has limited gastric capacity and decreased gastric emptying.

The feeding method depends on the feeding abilities and health status of the preterm newborn; see the discussion of various feeding methods on page 963. Nipple and gavage methods are initially supplemented with intravenous therapy until oral intake is sufficient to support growth. Growth usually occurs when 120 to 150 cal/kg/day are provided, and this prevents metabolic catabolism and hypoglycemia. Growth is evaluated by an increase in weight, length, and body measurements such as continued weight gain of 20 to 30 g per day (initially, no gain may be noted for several days, but total weight loss should not exceed 15% of the total body weight or more than 1% to 2% per day). Some institutions add the criteria of head circumference growth and increase in body length of 1 cm/week, once the infant is stable.

The nurse watches for signs of respiratory distress or fatigue during feedings. Prior to each feeding, the nurse measures abdominal girth and auscultates the abdomen to determine the presence and quality of bowel sounds. Such assessments promote early detection of abdominal distention and decreased peristaltic activity, which may indicate necrotizing enterocolitis (NEC) or paralytic ileus. The nurse also checks for residual formula in the stomach via orogastric tube prior to feeding. This is done when the newborn is fed by gavage or transpyloric method or in the presence of abdominal distention in a nipple-fed newborn. The presence of residual formula is an indication of intolerance to the type or amount of feeding or the increase in amount of feeding. Residual formula is usually readministered because digestive processes have already been initiated.

Preterm newborns who are ill or fatigue easily with nipple feedings are usually fed by gavage or transpyloric feeding. The infant is essentially passive with these methods, thus conserving energy and calories. As the baby matures, gavage feedings are replaced with nipple feedings to assist in strengthening the sucking reflex and meeting oral and emotional needs. Daily weights are monitored because often there is a small weight loss when nipple feedings are started. After feedings, the baby is placed on the right side (with support to maintain this position) or on the abdomen. These positions enhance gastric emptying and decrease the chance of aspiration if regurgitation occurs. Gastroesophageal reflux is *not* uncommon in preterm newborns.

The nurse involves the parents in feeding their preterm baby. This is essential to the development of attachment between parents and infant. In addition, such involvement increases parental knowledge about the care of their infant and helps them cope with the situation.

Promotion of Parent-Infant Attachment

Preterm newborns are generally separated from their parents for prolonged periods. Illness or complications may be detected in the first few hours or days following birth. The resultant interruption in parent-newborn bonding requires intervention to ensure successful attachment of parent and infant.

Nurses should take measures to promote positive parental feelings toward the newborn. Photographs of the baby are given to parents to have at home or to the mother if she is in a different hospital. The infant's name is placed on the Isolette as soon as it is known to help the parents feel that their infant is a unique and special person. The telephone number of the nursery and/or intensive care unit and names of staff members are given to parents so that they have access to information about their baby at any time of day or night. Equipment and therapies are explained to parents, and the explanations are repeated as often as necessary to familiarize them with the treatment and decrease their anxiety.

Parents are included in determining the baby's plan of care. Early involvement in the care and decisions regarding their baby provide parents with realistic expectations. Their daily participation (if possible) is encouraged, as are early and frequent visits. The nurse provides opportunities for parents to touch, hold, talk to, and care for the baby. Parents start with simple tasks, based on the nurse's assessment of the parent's skill and coping abilities. Early success in performing simple tasks builds parents' confidence in their care-taking abilities.

Promotion of Sensory Stimulation

Within the past 25 years, increased attention has been given to the infant's need for sensory stimulation. Evidence suggests that the infant who receives tactile, kinesthetic, and auditory stimulation has fewer apneic spells, decreased stooling, improved weight gain, and advanced CNS functioning (Klaus & Kennell 1982).

With prolonged separation and the neonatal intensive care unit (NICU) environment, individualized baby sensory (visual, tactile, and auditory) stimulation programs are necessary. The nurse plays a key role in determining the appropriate type and amount of sensory stimulation.

Research into the unique behavioral characteristics of the preterm infant highlight many responses that reflect disorganization of the autonomic nervous system. This work suggests that some preterm infants are not developmentally able to deal with more than one sensory input at a time. The Assessment of Preterm Infant Behavior (APIB) scale (Als et al 1982) identifies the individual preterm newborn behaviors according to five areas of development. The preterm baby's behavioral reactions to stimulation are observed, and developmental interventions are aimed at reducing detrimental environmental stimuli to the lowest possible level and providing appropriate opportunities for development.

In the NICU environment, there are many detrimental stimuli that the nurse can help reduce. Noise levels can be reduced by responding to and silencing alarms quickly and keeping conversations away from the baby's bedside. Bright lights can be modified by shielding the baby's eyes with blankets over the top portion of the Isolette. Nursing care should be planned to decrease the number of times the baby is disturbed and to allow the baby some periods of uninterrupted sleep (Lott 1989).

Parents are ideally equipped to meet the baby's need for stimulation. Stroking, playing music, rocking, cuddling, singing, and talking can all be an integral part of the baby's care. Visual stimulation in the form of mobiles and en face interaction with the care giver are also important. Teaching the parents to read behavioral cues will help them move at their infant's own pace when providing stimulation.

Preparation for Discharge

Parents of preterm babies should receive the same postpartal teaching as any parent taking a new infant home. In preparing for discharge, parents are encouraged to spend time just before discharge caring directly for their baby. This familiarizes the parents with their baby's behavior patterns and helps them establish realistic expectations about the infant.

Discharge instruction includes breast- and bottle-feeding techniques, formula preparation, and vitamin administration. For mothers planning to breast-feed, pumping allows breast-feeding after discharge from the hospital. Information on bathing, diapering, hygiene, and normal elimination patterns is given. Parents should be told to expect changes in the color of the baby's stool, number of bowel movements, and timing of elimination if the infant is switched from formula to breast-milk. This information can prevent unnecessary concern by the parents. The nurse should also discuss normal growth and development patterns, reflexes, and activity for preterm infants. Care of the preterm infant with complications, prevention of infections, and the need for continued medical follow-up are emphasized.

Referral of families to community agencies at the time of discharge may be necessary if the infant has severe congenital abnormalities, feeding problems, or complications with infections or respiratory problems, or if the parents seem unable to cope with an at-risk baby. Parents of preterm infants can benefit from meeting with others in a similar situation to share common experiences and concerns. Nurses can refer parents to support groups sponsored by the hospital or by others in the community.

Evaluation

Anticipated outcomes of nursing care include the following:

- The preterm newborn is free of respiratory distress and establishes effective respiratory function.

- The preterm newborn gains weight and shows no signs of fatigue and/or aspiration during feedings.

- The parents are able to verbalize their anger and guilt feelings about the birth of a preterm baby and show attachment behavior such as frequent visits and growing confidence in their participatory care activities.

❀ ❀ ❀ ❀ ❀ ❀ ❀ ❀ ❀ ❀ ❀ ❀

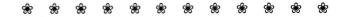

CRITICAL THINKING

What ethical issues arise from the birth and survival of increasing numbers of very-low-birth-weight infants?

Care of the Newborn of a Substance-Abusing Mother

The newborn of an alcoholic or drug-addicted woman will also be alcohol- or drug-dependent. After birth, when an infant's connection with the maternal blood supply is severed, the baby suffers withdrawal. In addition, the drugs ingested by the mother may be teratogenic, resulting in congenital anomalies.

Alcohol Dependency

Infants born to alcohol-dependent mothers can suffer long-term complications in addition to suffering withdrawal symptoms.

The fetal alcohol syndrome (FAS) includes a series of malformations frequently found in infants born to women who have been severe alcoholics (Little et al 1990). It has been estimated that complete FAS syndrome occurs in 1 to 3 live births per 1000. Fetal alcohol effects (FAE) are less severe effects of maternal alcohol use during pregnancy and include mild to moderate mental and physical growth retardation.

Controversy surrounds the exact cause of FAS. Although it is known that ethanol freely crosses the placenta to the fetus, it is still not known whether the alcohol alone or the break-down products of alcohol cause the damage. For in-depth discussion of alcohol abuse in pregnancy, see Chapter 18. The effects of other substances often combined with alcohol, such as nicotine, diazepam (Valium), marijuana, and caffeine, as well as poor diet enhance the likelihood of FAS (Chasnoff 1988).

Long-Term Complications

The long-term prognosis for the FAS neonate is less than favorable. Most infants with FAS are growth-deficient at birth, and few infants have demonstrated postnatal catch-up growth. In fact most FAS infants are evaluated for failure to thrive. It has been found that decreased adipose tissue is a constant problem in individuals with FAS.

Feeding problems are frequently present during infancy and preschool years. These infants have a delay in the normal progression of oral feeding development but have a normal progression of oral motor function. Many FAS infants nurse poorly and have persistent vomiting until 6 to 7 months of age. They have difficulty adjusting to solid foods and show little spontaneous interest in food. They continue to have feeding problems into adolescence, including eustachian tube dysfunction and malocclusion, which may result from midface malformation in utero (Streissguth & LaDue 1985).

Central nervous system dysfunctions are the most common and serious problem associated with FAS. Most children exhibiting FAS are mildly to severely mentally retarded. The more dysmorphic the facial features, the lower the IQ scores. However, cases of infants of chronic alcoholics in whom neurologic disturbance appeared to be the only apparent abnormality are well documented (Volpe 1987).

Providing a better environment for infants with FAS has been found to have no remarkable influence on IQ, which indicates that the brain damage occurred prenatally. These children are often hyperactive and show a high incidence of speech and language abnormalities indicative of CNS disorders. The brain is the organ most sensitive to damage from alcohol in the fetus. (Volpe 1987).

Medical Therapy

Prevention of alcohol-induced complications is the foremost goal of medical therapy. This can be accomplished by educating the pregnant woman about the risks of alcohol ingestion and having the woman eliminate, or at least significantly reduce, her alcohol intake. Reducing alcohol intake during midpregnancy can prevent growth retardation, although malformations may still occur (Waldman 1989).

The medical goal during the neonatal period is the management of CNS dysfunction and withdrawal. Seizures are treated with phenobarbital or diazepam.

❀ *APPLYING THE NURSING PROCESS* ❀

Nursing Assessment

Newborns with FAS show the following characteristics:

- *Abnormal structural development and CNS dysfunction.* This may include mental retardation, microcephaly, and hyperactivity.

- *Growth deficiencies.* Infants with FAS are often IUGR with weight, length, and head circumference being affected. These infants continue to show a persistent postnatal growth deficiency with weight being more affected than linear growth.

- *Distinctive facial abnormalities.* These include short palpebral fissures, midfacial and maxillary hy-

poplasia, micrognathia, hypoplastic upper lip, and diminished or absent philtrum.

- *Associated anomalies.* Abnormalities affecting cardiac (primarily septal defects), ocular, renal, and skeletal (especially involving joints such as congenital dislocated hips) systems are often noted.

Withdrawal symptoms of the alcohol-dependent neonate have been documented in children with normal facial features as well as in those with the typical features of FAS (Coles et al 1984). These symptoms include tremors, seizures, sleeplessness, unconsolable crying, abnormal reflexes, activeness with little ability to maintain alertness and attentiveness to environment, abdominal distention, and exaggerated mouthing behaviors such as hyperactive rooting and increased nonnutritive sucking (Chasnoff 1988).

Signs and symptoms of withdrawal often appear within 6 to 12 hours and at least within the first three days of life. Seizures after the neonatal period are rare. Alcohol dependence in the infant is physiologic, not psychologic.

Nursing Diagnosis

Nursing diagnoses that may apply to the FAS newborn include the following:

- Alteration in nutrition: less than body requirements related to decreased food intake and hyperirritability

- Injury: High risk related to seizure activity secondary to CNS dysfunction or chemical dependence

- Ineffective family coping related to potential developmental delay and/or guilt over the diagnosis

Nursing Plan and Implementation

Promotion of Physical Well-Being

The nurse's awareness of the signs and symptoms of fetal alcohol effects is important in structuring and guiding nursing care. Nursing care of the FAS newborn is aimed at avoiding heat loss, protecting the infant from injury during seizures, administering medications such as phenobarbital or diazepam to limit convulsions, monitoring intravenous fluid therapy, and reducing environmental stimuli. The FAS baby is most comfortable in a quiet, dimly lit environment. Because of their feeding problems, these infants require extra time and patience during feedings.

Mothers should be informed that breast-feeding is not contraindicated but that excessive alcohol consumption may intoxicate the newborn and inhibit the letdown reflex. The nurse should monitor the newborn's vital signs closely and observe for evidence of seizure activity and respiratory distress.

Promotion of Family Adaptation

Infants affected by maternal alcohol abuse are also at risk psychologically. Restlessness, sleeplessness, agitation, resistance to cuddling or holding, and frequent crying can be frustrating to parents as their efforts to relieve the distress are unrewarded. Feeding dysfunction can also result in frustrations for the care giver and digestive upsets for the infant. Frustration may cause the parents to punish the baby or result in the unconscious desire to "stay away from the infant." Either outcome may create an unstable family environment and result in the infant's failure to thrive.

The nurse should focus on providing support for the parents and reinforcing positive parenting activity. Prior to discharge, parents should be given opportunities to provide baby care so that they can feel confident in their interpretations of their baby's cues and their ability to meet the baby's needs. Referring the family to social services and visiting nurse or public health nurse associations is essential for the well-being of the infant. Follow-up care and teaching can strengthen the parents' skills and coping abilities and help them create a stable, healthy environment for their family.

Evaluation

Anticipated outcomes of nursing care include the following:

- The FAS newborn is able to tolerate feedings and gain weight.
- The FAS infant's hyperirritability and/or seizures are controlled and the baby has suffered no physical injuries.
- The parents are able to identify the special needs of their newborn and accept outside assistance as needed.

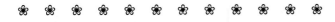

Drug Dependency

Almost all drugs ingested by a pregnant woman cross the placenta and enter the fetal circulation. Thus the fetus can develop drug-associated problems in utero or soon after birth.

During the antenatal period, the greatest risk to the fetus is intrauterine asphyxia. This is often a direct result of fetal withdrawal, secondary to maternal withdrawal. Fetal withdrawal is accompanied by hyperactivity with increased oxygen consumption, which, if not adequately compensated, can lead to fetal asphyxia. Moreover, narcotic-addicted women tend to have a higher incidence of PIH, abruptio placentae, and placenta previa, which lead to placental insufficiency and fetal asphyxia.

The birth weights of newborns of narcotic-addicted women are significantly lower than those of drug-free newborns.

Addicted newborns often have low Apgar scores at birth. Low scores may be related to the intrauterine as-

phyxia or the medication the woman received during labor. The use of a narcotic antagonist (naloxone and levallorphan) to reverse respiratory depression in the newborn is contraindicated. These drugs may precipitate acute withdrawal in the baby. After birth, the infant born to a drug-dependent mother may also be subject to neglect and/or abuse.

While patterns of abuse of alcohol, marijuana, and heroin in childbearing women have changed very little, the incidence of cocaine (especially "crack") use has risen dramatically (see Chapter 18 for more in-depth discussion of maternal substance abuse). Marijuana, alcohol, and nicotine are sometimes used in conjunction with cocaine. Therefore, the effects of secondary drugs on the newborn must also be taken into consideration. A high rate of perinatal complications has been noted for cocaine-exposed infants, including cerebral infarctions; genitourinary, cardiac, and central nervous system malformations; and increased incidence of apnea. These infants also exhibit a high degree of irritability and tremulousness with poor state organization (rapid shifts between irritability and lethargy) (Howard 1989).

Common Complications of the Drug-Addicted Newborn

The newborn of a woman who abused drugs during her pregnancy is predisposed to the following problems:

- *Respiratory distress.* The heroin addicted newborn frequently suffers respiratory stress, mainly meconium-aspiration pneumonia and transient tachypnea. Meconium aspiration is usually secondary to increased oxygen consumption and activity experienced by the fetus during intrauterine withdrawal. Transient tachypnea may develop secondary to the inhibitory effects of narcotics on the reflex responsible for clearing the lungs. Respiratory distress syndrome occurs less in heroin-addicted newborns even in the presence of prematurity because they have tissue-oxygen unloading capabilities comparable to those of a 6-week-old term infant. In addition, heroin stimulates production of glucocorticoids via the anterior pituitary gland.

- *Jaundice.* Newborns of methadone-addicted women may develop jaundice due to prematurity. Heroin contributes to early maturity of the liver, leading to a lower incidence of hyperbilirubinemia in these babies.

- *Congenital anomalies and growth retardation.* The incidence of anomalies of the genitourinary and cardiovascular systems is slightly increased in infants of heroin-addicted mothers. Infants of cocaine-addicted mothers exhibit congenital malformations involving bony skull defects such as microencephaly (Hadeed & Siegel 1989) and symmetric intrauterine growth retardation (Dattel 1990).

- *Behavioral abnormalities.* Babies exposed to cocaine have poor state organization and decreased interactive behaviors when tested with the Brazelton Neonatal Behavioral Assessment Scale (Chasnoff 1988).

- *Withdrawal.* The most significant postnatal problem of the drug-addicted newborn is that of narcotic withdrawal. The onset of the withdrawal manifestations usually occurs within the first 72 hours after birth. For heroin-addicted newborns a majority of withdrawal symptoms are seen within the first 24 to 48 hours. For newborns exposed to barbiturates, symptoms may be delayed for several days. Withdrawal for cocaine-addicted infants may occur four to five days after birth (Dattel 1990). For methadone-addicted infants, withdrawal symptoms may appear immediately after birth (Verklan 1989). In most cases, the withdrawal manifestations peak in the newborn about the third day and subside by the fifth to seventh day.

Long-Term Complications

During the first two years of life, many cocaine-exposed infants demonstrate deviant psychologic behavior. This is attributed to the irreversible damage to dopamine neurons caused by long-term administration of cocaine. This damage is manifested by susceptibility to behavior lability and the inability to express strong feelings such as pleasure, anger, or distress or even a strong reaction to being separated from their parents (Howard 1989).

Infants of drug-addicted mothers often demonstrate a higher incidence of gastrointestinal and respiratory illnesses; it is believed these are related not to narcotic addiction but to lack of education regarding proper infant care, feeding, and hygiene.

Another important long-term complication is the five- to tenfold incidence of sudden infant death syndrome (SIDS) in infants born to opiate-abusing mothers when compared to those in the general population (Ward et al 1990). Some studies have shown that infants of cocaine-addicted mothers have even higher rates of SIDS; this may be related to Chasnoff's (1989) findings of abnormal sleeping ventilatory patterns in cocaine-exposed infants. The occurrence of SIDS may be even higher in those infants who have had moderate-to-severe postnatal withdrawal.

Medical Therapy

The goal of medical therapy is early prenatal management of drug-addicted women (see Chapter 18) and pharmacologic management of neonatal narcotic withdrawal. For optimal fetal and neonatal outcome, the narcotic-addicted woman should receive complete prenatal care as soon as possible. She should be started on a methadone program with a reduction in dosage to 20 mg or less, if possible. The aim of methadone maintenance during pregnancy is the prevention of heroin use. Thus the dose of methadone used for maintenance should be sufficient to ensure this goal

even if the dose is greater than 20 mg. It is not recommended that the woman be withdrawn completely from narcotics while pregnant since this induces fetal withdrawal with poor newborn outcomes.

About 50% of newborns of addicted mothers experience withdrawal symptoms severe enough to require treatment. Drugs used to control withdrawal symptoms are phenobarbital or paregoric. Attention to nutritional support is important in light of the increase in energy expenditure that withdrawal may entail. The American Academy of Pediatrics (1983) recommends use of a formula that supplies 24 calories per ounce to provide 150 to 250 cal/kg/day.

❀ *APPLYING THE NURSING PROCESS* ❀

Nursing Assessment

Early identification of the newborn needing medical or pharmacologic interventions decreases the incidence of mortality and morbidity. During the newborn period, nursing assessment focuses on the following:

- Discovering the mother's last drug intake and dosage level. This is accomplished through the perinatal history and laboratory tests. It must be remembered that women may be reluctant to disclose this information; therefore, a nonjudgmental interview technique is essential.

- Assessing the complications related to intrauterine withdrawal such as SGA, intrauterine asphyxia, and prematurity. (For nursing care of SGA newborns, see page 946; for nursing care of premature newborns, see page 972; for nursing care of the infant who suffered intrauterine asphyxia, see Chapter 32.)

- Identifying the signs and symptoms of newborn withdrawal or neonatal abstinence syndrome. The signs and symptoms of newborn withdrawal can be classified in five groups:

  1. Central nervous system signs
     a. Hyperactivity
     b. Hyperirritability (persistent high-pitched cry)
     c. Increased muscle tone
     d. Exaggerated reflexes
     e. Tremors, seizures
     f. Sneezing, hiccups, yawning
     g. Short, unquiet sleep
     h. Fever
  2. Respiratory signs
     a. Tachypnea
     b. Excessive secretions
  3. Gastrointestinal signs
     a. Disorganized, vigorous suck
     b. Vomiting
     c. Drooling
     d. Sensitive gag reflex
     e. Hyperphagia

f. Diarrhea
g. Abdominal cramping
4. Vasomotor signs
    a. Stuffy nose, yawning, sneezing
    b. Flushing
    c. Sweating
    d. Sudden, circumoral pallor
5. Cutaneous signs
    a. Excoriated buttocks
    b. Facial scratches
    c. Pressure point abrasions

Although many of the signs and symptoms of narcotic withdrawal are similar to those seen with hypoglycemia and hypocalcemia, glucose and calcium values are reported to be within normal limits for this group of infants.

Nursing Diagnosis

Nursing diagnoses that may apply to drug-dependent newborns include the following:

- Alteration in nutritional and fluid requirements: less than body requirements related to vomiting and diarrhea, uncoordinated suck and swallow reflex, hypertonia secondary to withdrawal
- Alteration in comfort related to skin excoriation over bony prominences secondary to constant activity
- Alteration in parenting related to hyperirritable behavior of the infant
- Ineffective family coping related to drug abuse, poverty, and lack of education

Nursing Plan and Implementation

Promotion of Physical and Psychological Well-Being   Care of the drug-dependent newborn is based on reducing withdrawal symptoms and promoting adequate respiration, temperature, and nutrition. See the Nursing Care Plan for the Infant of Substance-Abusing Mother for specific nursing care measures. Some general nursery care measures include the following:

- Temperature regulation.
- Careful monitoring of pulse and respirations every 15 minutes until stable; stimulation if apnea occurs.
- Small frequent feedings, especially in the presence of vomiting, regurgitation, and diarrhea.
- Intravenous therapy as needed.
- Medications as ordered, such as phenobarbital, paregoric, diazepam (Valium), or chlorpromazine hydrochloride (Thorazine). Methadone should not be given because of possible neonatal addiction to it.
- Proper positioning on the right side to avoid possible aspiration of vomitus or secretions.

- Observation for problems of SGA or LGA newborns.
- Swaddling to minimize injury.

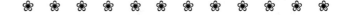

CRITICAL THINKING

What issues need to be addressed to meet the needs of babies of substance-abusing mothers?

Promotion of Family Adaptation

Parents should be prepared for what they can expect for the first few months at home. At the time of discharge the mother should be instructed to anticipate mild jitteriness and irritability in the newborn, which may persist from 8 to 16 weeks, depending on the initial severity of the withdrawal. The nurse should help the mother learn feeding techniques and comforting measures. Parents are to be counseled regarding available resources, such as support groups, and signs and symptoms that require further care. Ongoing evaluation is necessary because of the potential for long-term problems.

Evaluation

Anticipated outcomes of nursing care include the following:

- The newborn tolerates feedings, gains weight, and has a decreased number of stools.
- The parents learn ways to comfort their newborn.
- The parents are able to cope with their frustrations and begin to use outside resources as needed.

❀   ❀   ❀   ❀   ❀   ❀   ❀   ❀   ❀   ❀   ❀   ❀

Care of the Newborn with AIDS

There is an increase in the number of newborns being born with AIDS or acquiring AIDS in the neonatal period of early infancy. Perinatal and neonatal modes of transmission have been identified as transplacental (vertical transmission), breast-feeding, and/or infusion of contaminated blood. Ongoing prospective studies indicate the vertical transmission rate ranges from 24% to 35% (Husson et al 1990).

Early identification of babies with AIDS and those at risk for AIDS is essential in the newborn period. Diagnosis may be made by doing an ELISA (enzyme-linked immunosorbent assay) test followed by the Western Blot test (immunoblot). These tests show antibodies to the AIDS virus; some false positives can occur in infants who still have maternal antibodies in their blood. Therefore, babies should have serial tests through 15 months of age. New diagnostic tests, such as those detecting the infant's specific antibody (IgG or IgM) responses to the human immunodeficiency virus (HIV), are being investigated (Husson et al

(Text continues on p 983.)

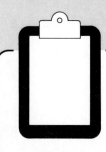

Nursing Care Plan:
Newborn of a
Substance–Abusing Mother

Nursing History

Type and amount of drug(s) consumed by mother during each month of pregnancy

Type and amount of prenatal care

Prior history of addiction and treatment

Maternal disease/infection such as placenta previa, hypertension, bacterial and TORCH infections, HIV seropositive and sexually transmitted diseases

Preterm labor and birth

Physical Examination

Withdrawal symptoms: hyperactivity, jitteriness, irritability, shrill high-pitched cry, vomiting, diarrhea, weak suck, stuffy nose, frequent sneezing, yawning, tachycardia, hypertension, apnea. With cocaine, withdrawal pattern may be unpredictable or may be asymptomatic with only subtle behavioral state organization problems. Disturbed sleep-wake cycle and rhythm at 24 to 28 hr.

Diagnostic Studies

Toxicology screen—Identify drug(s) and drug levels in mother and infant blood and urine

Serum electrolyte (Na, K, Ca)—Detect losses from vomiting, diarrhea, detect causes of neurologic symptoms or seizures

Glucose

Serial capillary gases

CBC and blood culture—Detect sepsis

Urine specific gravity—high due to dehydration.

Nursing Diagnosis	Nursing Interventions	Rationale	Evaluation
Altered sleep pattern disturbance related central nervous system excitation secondary to drug withdrawal *Client Goal:* Babies at risk for withdrawal will be identified early and normal rest/sleep patterns will be established throughout withdrawal period.	Assess for withdrawal symptoms including: frequent sneezing and yawning, restlessness, high-pitched shrill cry, hypertonicity, vomiting or diarrhea, wakefulness Provide calming techniques including: Swaddle infant tightly in side-lying or prone position with small pillow supporting back. Provide quiet, dim environment for rest Schedule tests or treatments to avoid stress.	Most addicted newborns will show symptoms of withdrawal as early as 12 hr after birth. Begins with jitteriness, hyperactivity and wakefulness; progressing to GI symptoms and seizures. Early identification allows for early intervention and prevention of complications. Positioning provides for rest and discourages hyperactivity and increases comfort while reducing stimuli. Quiet environment decreases external stimuli and therefore infant's irritability Planned care allows for maximum rest and reduce external stimuli.	Baby is free from jitteriness and has normal sleep-wake behaviors.

(continued)

Nursing Care Plan (continued)

Nursing Diagnosis	Nursing Interventions	Rationale	Evaluation
	Hold, rock, and cuddle infant. Use touching, patting, smiling, and talking to infant. Use infant snugglies for closeness.	Holding infant as often as possible promotes comfort and cuddling quiets and comforts infant. These activities promote close contact.	
	Provide pacifier or position baby so that baby can get hand to mouth.	Hand to mouth activity or pacifier satisfies increased need to suck during withdrawal.	
	Administer medications for withdrawal as ordered such as paregoric, chlorpromazine, valium, phenobarbital; observe for effectiveness and side effects.	Pharmacologic agents alleviate withdrawal symptoms	
Altered nutrition: less than body requirements related to withdrawal symptoms *Client Goal:* Baby will not lose more than 2% weight, will take feeding without vomiting, aspiration or fatigue, and will gain weight.	Assess for increased nutritional needs because of gestational age, weight, uncoordinated suck and swallow, vomiting, diarrhea, and regurgitation. Provide appropriate nutrition: Initiate IV feedings until stable.	Infants of drug-addicted mothers tend to be SGA and premature. CNS stimulation causes hyperactivity leading to poor feeding, GI hypermotility and irritation leading to inability to retain or absorb nutrients. Oral feeding an irritable infant with possible seizures may foster aspiration.	Infant gains approximately 1 oz per day and has vigorous suck reflex.
	Supplement oral or gavage feedings with intravenous intake per orders. Give small, frequent feedings of high caloric formula, may start feedings at one-half strength every 3 hours.	SGA infants need 110–120 cal/kg/day for optimal nutrition. Smaller feedings facilitate nutritional intake.	
	Check for residuals after oral or gavage feedings; reduce feeding volume if residuals are high. As hyperactivity decreases, increase feedings as tolerated. Place on right side with back support or on abdomen after feedings.	Prevents vomiting from overfeeding while still providing IV fluids according to infant's tolerance. Position decreases vomiting, regurgitation and distention.	

(continued)

Nursing Care Plan (continued)

Nursing Diagnosis	Nursing Interventions	Rationale	Evaluation
Knowledge deficit related to feelings of inadequacy or inability to care for infant. *Client Goal:* Mother will touch, hold infant and develop confidence in her ability to provide safe newborn care.	Identify mother's knowledge needs and readiness for learning. Provide information including: 1. Signs and symptoms of baby's withdrawal, current condition, and rationale for treatment 2. Newborn capabilities and developmental behaviors 3. Newborn's need for appropriate stimulation as well as rest depending on infant's cues 4. Physical care needs such as feeding, bathing, clothing, and holding Encourage and support positive mothering behaviors with infant.	Assessment provides information regarding mother's ability to care for infant. Provides information about parent's understanding of baby's behavior and how to care for the baby with symptoms. Assists parents to be realistic about infant's progress. Mother needs to adjust infant interaction based on infant's cues to foster development. This information helps mother provide for safe infant care. Increases mother's feelings of competence in her parenting abilities.	Mother has bonded with infant; parents are involved in care and have realistic expectations for their baby.

1990). Opportunistic diseases such as gram-negative sepsis and problems associated with prematurity are the primary causes of mortality.

❀ *APPLYING THE NURSING PROCESS* ❀
Nursing Assessment

Many newborns with AIDS are premature and/or SGA and show failure to thrive during neonatal and infant life. They can show signs and symptoms of disease within days of birth. Signs that may be seen in the newborn period include: failure to thrive, enlarged spleen and liver, swollen glands, interstitial pneumonia (rarely seen in adults), recurrent GI (diarrhea and weight loss) and urinary system infections, chronic cough, seborrheic rash, developmental delays, neurologic deficits, and/or microcephaly (Johnson et al 1989). Some cranial and facial stigmas have been associated with AIDS contracted in utero (Klug 1986). These features are: prominent boxlike forehead, increased distance between inner canthuses of the eyes, mild obliquity of the eyes, flattened nasal bridge, prominent triangular philtrum, and patulous (distended) lips.

Nursing Diagnosis

Nursing diagnoses that may apply to the infant with AIDS include the following:

- Altered nutrition: less than body requirements related to formula intolerance and inadequate intake
- Impaired skin integrity related to chronic diarrhea
- Infection: High risk related to AIDS immuno-suppression
- Impaired physical mobility related to decreased neuromuscular development
- Altered growth and development related to lack of attachment and stimulation
- Altered parenting related to diagnosis of AIDS
- Ineffective family coping related to diagnosis of AIDS

Nursing Plan and Implementation

 AIDS newborn nursing care involves normal newborn care or the care required for a newborn in a NICU. In addition, the nurse must include care for a newborn suspected of having a blood-borne infection, as with hepatitis B. Universal precautions should be used when caring for the newborn immediately after birth and when obtaining blood samples via vein puncture or heel stick. The blood of all newborns must be considered potentially infectious because knowledge of the status of the infant's blood is often not known until after the infant is discharged. The major goals of nursing care involve providing for comfort, keeping the newborn well nourished and protected from oppor-

tunistic infections, and facilitating growth, development, and attachment. See the Nursing Care Plan for Infant with Acquired Immunodeficiency Syndrome for specific nursing care measures.

Parents and family members need to be reassured that there are no documented cases of people contracting AIDS from routine care of infected babies. Emotional support for the family is essential because of the stress and social isolation they may face. Because of these stresses, attachment may not occur and/or the infant may suffer from lack of sensory and tactile stimulation. Babies should be held for feedings and benefit from frequent, gentle touch. Auditory stimulation may also be provided using music or tapes of parents' voices. Families should be informed about support groups, available counseling, and information resources (Klindworth et al 1989).

Evaluation

Anticipated outcomes of nursing care include the following:

- The parents are able to bond with their infant and have realistic expectations about the baby.
- Early identification and treatment of potential opportunistic infections is provided.
- The parents verbalize their concerns surrounding their baby's existing and potential health problems and accept outside assistance as needed.

❀ ❀ ❀ ❀ ❀ ❀ ❀ ❀ ❀ ❀ ❀ ❀

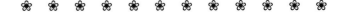

Care of the Newborn with Congenital Anomalies

The birth of a baby with a congenital defect places both newborn and family at risk. Many congenital anomalies can be life-threatening if not corrected within hours after birth; others are very visible and cause the families emotional distress. Table 31–3 identifies some of the more common anomalies and their early management and nursing care in the neonatal period.

Care of the Newborn with Congenital Heart Defect

The incidence of congenital heart defects is 4 to 5 per 1000 live births (Lin & Garver 1988). They account for one-third of the deaths caused by congenital defects in the first year of life. Because accurate diagnosis and surgical treatment are now available, many such deaths can be prevented. It is now possible to do corrective surgery at an earlier age; for example, more than one-half of the children

(Text continues on p 988)

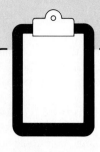

Nursing Care Plan
Infant with Acquired
Immunodeficiency Syndrome

Client Assessment

Nursing History

Maternal
History of drug abuse or needle sharing

Sexual partner or partners with a positive HIV antibody test or ELISA test

Physical Examination

Complete physical examination—Variable findings and symptoms depending on the type of infection

Diagnostic Studies

ELISA—Detects HIV antibody. May take six months to convert to seropositive.

Newborns may have HIV antibodies from maternal infection

Western Blot test—To confirm ELISA test

Immunoglobin studies—to detect increased levels of IgG and IgM, depressed levels of T4 and T4:T8 ratio

Hemoglobin and hematocrit—Detect anemia

Nursing Diagnosis	Nursing Interventions	Rationale	Evaluation
Infections: High risk related to perinatal exposure and immunoregulation suppression *Client Goal:* Infant will not develop infection while in birthing area	Assess infant for signs of ongoing infection such as: ● Failure to thrive ● Weight loss over 10% at time of diagnosis ● Temperature instability ● More than three diarrheal episodes a day ● Hepatosplenomegaly-palpate once a day for continued enlargement ● Lethargy Assess for opportunistic diseases such as: Herpes simplex lasting more than one month Cytomegalovirus disease Lymphoid interstitial pneumonia Viral, fungal, or protozoal infections	Signs and symptoms of infection and inflammation may persist prior to definitive AIDS diagnosis. Decrease activity and lethargy can indicate sepsis. Opportunistic infections occur because of immune system suppression.	At-risk infant is identified and remains free of opportunistic infections.

(continued)

Nursing Care Plan (continued)

Nursing Diagnosis	Nursing Interventions	Rationale	Evaluation
	Maintain universal precautions—especially until baby has had first bath—when changing diapers, drawing blood or doing heel sticks, and suctioning newborn.	Universal precautions protect care givers from infant's body secretions. Also newborn is protected from other infectious agents.	
Altered nutrition: less than body requirements related to formula intolerance and inadequate intake. *Client Goal:* Baby will gain weight and progress on normal growth curve.	Assess for residuals, abdominal distention (abdominal girth measurements) prior to each feeding. Obtain accurate intake and output (weigh diapers). Monitor stools for amount, type, consistency, and any change in pattern. Check stools for occult blood and reducing substances. Provide small frequent feedings.	Feeding intolerance causes gastric residuals, increasing abdominal girth and dehydration. Loose stools and presence of reducing substances may indicate feeding intolerance. Occult blood indicates irritation or ulceration of bowel mucosa.	Baby has steady weight gain and follows normal growth curve.
Altered parenting related to diagnosis of AIDS and fear of future outcome *Client Goal:* Parents will express fears and begin to bond with their infant.	Assess cause of parents' fear by • Providing time for expression of concerns • Determine parents' understanding about AIDS Provide information about AIDS as to cause, signs of HIV in infants, current and experimental treatment modalities, support groups, and community resources.	Lack of information and distorted perception about AIDS may increase parents' fears. Accurate information about AIDS reduces fear. Access to community services and participation in support groups provides assistance with coping with a potentially critically ill child.	Parents verbalize their fears, hold and talk with newborn, and carry out infant caretaking activities.

Table 31–3 Congenital Anomalies: Identification and Care in Newborn Period

Congenital anomaly	Nursing assessments	Nursing goals and interventions
Congenital hydrocephalus	Enlarged head Enlarged or full fontanelles Split or widened sutures "Setting sun" eyes Head circumference > 90% on growth chart	Assess presence of hydrocephalus: Measure and plot occipital-frontal baseline measurements, then measure head circumference once a day. Check fontanelle for bulging and sutures for widening. Assist with head ultrasound and transillumination. Maintain skin integrity: Change position frequently. Clean skin creases after feeding or vomiting. Use sheepskin pillow under head. Postoperatively, position head off operative site. Watch for signs of infection.
Choanal atresia	Occlusion of posterior nares Cyanosis and retractions at rest Snorting respirations Difficulty breathing during feeding Obstruction by thick mucus	Assess patency of nares: Listen for breath sounds while holding baby's mouth closed and alternately compressing each nostril. Assist with passing feeding tube to confirm diagnosis. Maintain respiratory function: Assist with taping airway in mouth to prevent respiratory distress. Position with head elevated to improve air exchange.
Cleft lip	Unilateral or bilateral visible defect May involve external nares, nasal cartilage, nasal septum, and alveolar process Flattening or depression of midfacial contour (Figure 31–12)	Provide nutrition: Feed with special nipple. Burp frequently (increased tendency to swallow air and reflex vomiting). Clean cleft with sterile water (to prevent crusting on cleft prior to repair). Support parental coping: Assist parents with grief over loss of idealized baby. Encourage verbalization of their feelings about visible defect. Provide role model in interacting with infant. (Parents internalize others' responses to their newborn.)

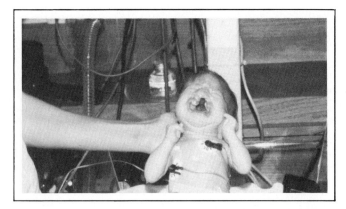

Figure 31–12   Cleft abnormality involving both hard and soft palate and unilateral cleft lip

Cleft palate	Fissure connecting oral and nasal cavity May involve uvula and soft palate May extend forward to nostril involving hard palate and maxillary alveolar ridge Difficulty in sucking Expulsion of formula through nose (Figure 31–12)	Prevent aspiration/infection: Place prone or in side-lying position to facilitate drainage. Suction nasopharyngeal cavity (to prevent aspiration or airway obstruction). During neonatal period, feed in upright position with head and chest tilted slightly backward (to aid swallowing and discourage aspiration). Provide nutrition: Feed with special nipple that fills cleft and allows sucking. Also decreases change of aspiration through nasal cavity. Clean mouth with water after feedings. Burp after each ounce (tend to swallow large amounts of air). Thicken formula to provide extra calories. Plot weight gain patterns to assess adequacy of diet. Provide parental support: Refer parents to community agencies and support groups. Encourage verbalization of frustrations as feeding process is long and frustrating. Praise all parental efforts. Encourage parents to seek prompt treatment for upper respiratory infection (URI) and teach them ways to decrease URI.
Tracheoesophageal fistula (type 3)	History of maternal hydramnios Excessive mucous secretions Constant drooling Abdominal distention beginning soon after birth	Maintain respiratory status and prevent aspiration: Withhold feeding until esophageal patency is determined. Quickly assess patency before putting to breast in birth area. Place on low intermittent suction to control saliva and mucus (to prevent aspiration pneumonia).

(continued)

Table 31-3 (continued)

Congenital anomaly	Nursing assessments	Nursing goals and interventions
	Periodic choking and cyanotic episodes Immediate regurgitation of feeding Clinical symptoms of aspiration pneumonia (tachypnea, retractions, rhonchi, decreased breath sounds, cyanotic spells) Failure to pass nasogastric tube (Figure 31–13)	Place in warmed, humidified Isolette (liquefies secretions facilitating removal). Elevate head of bed 20°–40° (to prevent reflux of gastric juices). Keep quiet (crying causes air to pass through fistula and to distend intestines causing respiratory embarrassment). Maintain fluid and electrolyte balance: Give fluids to replace esophageal drainage and maintain hydration. Provide parent education: Explain staged repair—provision of gastrostomy and ligation of fistula, then repair of atresia. Keep parents informed; clarify and reinforce physician's explanations regarding malformation, surgical repair, pre- and postoperative care, and prognosis (knowledge is ego strengthening). Involve parents in care of infant and in planning for future; facilitate touch and eye contact (to dispel feelings of inadequacy, increase self-esteem and self-worth, and promote incorporation of infant into family).

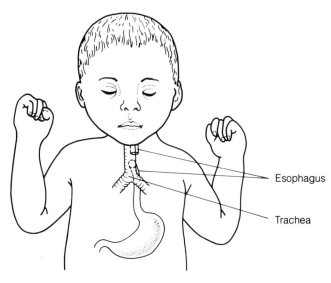

Esophagus

Trachea

Figure 31–13   The most frequently seen type of congenital tracheoesophageal fistula and esophageal atresia

Congenital anomaly	Nursing assessments	Nursing goals and interventions
Diaphragmatic hernia	Difficulty initiating respirations Gasping respirations with nasal flaring and chest retraction Barrel chest and scaphoid abdomen Asymmetric chest expansion Breath sounds may be absent, usually on left side Heart sounds displaced to right Spasmodic attacks of cyanosis and difficulty in feeding Bowel sounds may be heard in thoracic cavity (Figure 31–14)	Maintain respiratory status: Immediately administer oxygen. Initiate gastric decompression. Place in high semi-Fowler's position (to use gravity to keep abdominal organs' pressure off diaphragm). Turn to affected side to allow unaffected lung expansion. Carry out interventions to alleviate respiratory and metabolic acidosis. Assess for increased secretions around suction tube (denotes possible obstruction). Aspirate and irrigate tube with air or sterile water.

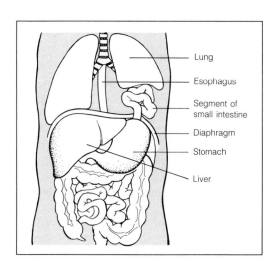

Lung

Esophagus

Segment of small intestine

Diaphragm

Stomach

Liver

Figure 31–14   Diaphragmatic hernia. Note compression of the lung by the intestine on the affected side

(continued)

Table 31–3 (continued)

Congenital anomaly	Nursing assessments	Nursing goals and interventions
Omphalocele	Herniation of abdominal contents into base of umbilical cord May have an enclosed transparent sac covering	Maintain hydration and temperature: Provide D_5LR and albumin for hypovolemia. Place infant in sterile bag up to above defect. Cover sac with moistened sterile gauze and place plastic wrap over dressing (to prevent rupture of sac and infection). Initiate gastric decompression by insertion of nasogastric tube attached to low suction (to prevent distention of lower bowel and impairment of blood flow). Prevent infection and trauma to defect. Position to prevent trauma to defect. Administer broad-spectrum antibiotics.
Myelomeningocele	Saclike cyst containing meninges, spinal cord, and nerve roots in thoracic and/or lumbar area (Figure 31–15). Myelomeningocele directly connects to subarachnoid space so hydrocephalus often associated No response or varying response to sensation below level of sac May have constant dribbling of urine Incontinence or retention of stool Anal opening may be flaccid	Prevent trauma and infection. Position on abdomen or on side and restrain (to prevent pressure and trauma to sac). Meticulously clean buttocks and genitals after each voiding and defecation (to prevent contamination of sac and decrease possibility of infection). May put protective covering over sac (to prevent rupture and drying). Observe sac for oozing of fluid or pus. Credé bladder as ordered (to prevent urinary stasis). Assess amount of sensation and movement below defect. Observe for complications: Obtain occipital-frontal circumference baseline measurements, then measure head circumference once a day (to detect hydrocephalus). Check fontanelle for bulging.
Imperforate anus, congenital dislocated hip, and clubfoot	See discussion in Chapter 28, pp 856–857	Identify defect and initiate appropriate referral early.

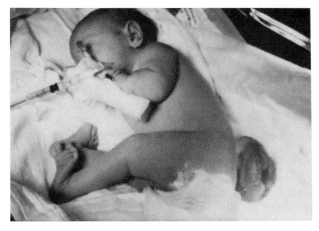

Figure 31–15   Newborn with lumbar meningocele (Courtesy of Dr Paul Winchester)

undergoing surgery are less than 1 year of age, and one-fourth are less than 1 month old (Benson 1989). It is crucial for the nurse to have comprehensive knowledge of congenital heart disease to detect deviations from normal and to initiate interventions.

Overview of Congenital Heart Defects

Factors that might influence development of congenital heart malformation can be classified as environmental or genetic. Infections of the pregnant woman, such as rubella, coxsackie B, and influenza, have been implicated. Thalidomide, steroids, alcohol, lithium, and some anticonvulsants have been shown to cause malformations of the heart. Seasonal spraying of pesticides has also been linked to an increase in congenital heart defects. Clinicians are also beginning to see cardiac defects in infants of mothers with phenylketonuria (PKU) who do not follow their diets.

Twelve percent of all infants with congenital heart disease were found to have chromosomal abnormalities (Lin & Garver 1988). Infants with Down syndrome and trisomy 13/15 and 16/18 frequently have heart lesions. Increased incidence and risk of recurrence of specific defects occur in families.

It is customary to describe congenital malformations of the heart as either *acyanotic*—those that do not present with cyanosis—or *cyanotic*—those that do present with cyanosis. If an opening exists between the right and left sides of the heart, blood will normally flow from the area of greater pressure (left side) to the area of lesser pressure (right side). This process is referred to as left-to-right shunt and does not produce cyanosis because oxygenated blood is being pumped out to the systemic circulation. If pressure in the right side of the heart, due to obstruction of normal flow, exceeds that in the left side, unoxygenated blood will flow from the right side to the left side of the heart and out into the system. This right-to-left shunt causes cyanosis. If the opening is large, there may be a bidirectional shunt with mixing of blood in both sides of the heart, which also produces cyanosis.

The common cardiac defects seen in the first six days of life are left ventricular outflow obstructions (mitral stenosis, aortic stenosis, or atresia), hypoplastic left heart, coarctation of the aorta, patent ductus arteriosus (PDA, the most common defect), transposition of the great vessels, tetralogy of Fallot, and large ventricular septal defect or atrial septal defects (see Figure 31–16). Table 31–4 presents the clinical manifestations and medical/surgical management of these cardiac defects.

❁ *APPLYING THE NURSING PROCESS* ❁
Nursing Assessment

The primary goal of the neonatal nurse is early identification of cardiac defects and initiation of referral to the physician. The three most common manifestations of cardiac defect are cyanosis, detectable heart murmur, and congestive heart failure signs (tachycardia, tachypnea, diaphoresis, hepatomegaly, and cardiomegaly).

Nursing assessment of the following signs and symptoms assists in identifying the newborn with a cardiac problem:

1. Tachypnea—reflects increased pulmonary blood flow
2. Dyspnea—caused by increased pulmonary venous pressure and blood flow; can also cause chest retractions, wheezing
3. Color—ashen, gray, or cyanotic because of decreased peripheral circulation or low oxygen saturation of the blood
4. Difficulty in feeding—requires many rest periods before finishing even 1 or 2 ounces
5. Diaphoresis—beads of perspiration over the upper lip and forehead; may accompany feeding fatigue
6. Stridor or choking spells
7. Failure to gain weight
8. Heart murmur—may not be heard in left-to-right shunting defects since the pulmonary pressure in the newborn is greater than pressure in the left side of the heart in the early newborn period
9. Hepatomegaly—in right-sided heart failure caused by venous congestion in the liver
10. Tachycardia—pulse over 160, may be as high as 200 as heart attempts to increase cardiac output
11. Cardiac enlargement

Nursing Diagnosis

Nursing diagnoses that may apply to the newborn with cardiac defect include the following:

- Altered tissue perfusion related to decrease in circulating oxygen
- Ineffective breathing pattern related to fatigue
- Altered nutrition: less than body requirements related to increased energy expenditure
- Knowledge deficit of parents related to cardiac anomaly and future implications for care

Nursing Plan and Implementation
Maintenance of Cardiopulmonary Status
When the baby has dyspnea or cyanosis, oxygen is to be given by an oxygen hood, tent, mask, cannula, or oxygen prongs. Mist is often ordered, which requires the use of an oxygen hood or tent. Oxygen administration should always be accompanied by humidity, and the air should be warmed to decrease the drying effects of cold, dry oxygen. Vital signs are carefully monitored for evidence of tachycardia, tachypnea, expiratory grunting, and retractions.

Morphine sulfate, a dose of 0.05 mg/kg of body weight, can be used if the infant is markedly irritable. Morphine is thought to decrease peripheral and pulmonary vascular resistance, which results in decreased tachypnea. Infants in congestive heart failure are more comfortable in a semi-Fowler's position.

The nurse provides for rest by administering a sedative as required. Organizing nursing care is a key to decreasing energy requirements and providing periods of rest.

Family Education
After the baby is stabilized and gaining weight, decisions are made about ongoing care and surgical interventions. The parents need careful and complete explanations and the opportunity to take part in decision making. They also require ongoing emotional support.

Evaluation

Anticipated outcomes of nursing care of newborns with congenital heart defects include the following:

- The newborn's oxygen consumption and energy expenditure are minimal while at rest and during feedings.
- The newborn is protected from additional stresses such as infection, cold stress, and dehydration.
- The parents verbalize their concerns surrounding

Table 31–4 Cardiac Defects of the Early Newborn Period

Congenital heart defect	Clinical findings	Medical/surgical management
Acyanotic		
Patent ductus arteriosus (PDA) ↑ in females, maternal rubella, RDS, <1500 g preterm newborns, high-altitude births	Harsh grade 2–3 machinery murmur upper left sternal border (LSB) just beneath clavicle ↑ difference between systolic and diastolic pulse pressure Can lead to right heart failure and pulmonary congestion ↑ left atrial (LA) and left ventricular (LV) enlargement, dilated ascending aorta ↑ pulmonary vascularity	Indomethacin—0.2 mg/kg orally (prostaglandin inhibitor) Surgical ligation Use of O₂ therapy and blood transfusion to improve tissue oxygenation and perfusion Fluid restriction and diuretics

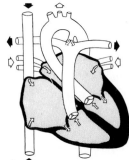

Figure 31–16 (A)   The patent ductus arteriosus is a vascular connection that, during fetal life, short-circuits the pulmonary vascular bed and directs blood from the pulmonary artery to the aorta.

Congenital heart defect	Clinical findings	Medical/surgical management
Atrial septal defect (ASD) ↑ in females and Down syndrome	Initially frequently asymptomatic Systolic murmur 2nd left intercostal space (LICS) With large ASD, diastolic rumbling murmur lower left sternal (LLS) border Failure to thrive, upper respiratory infection (URI), poor exercise tolerance	Surgical closure with patch or suture
Ventricular septal defect (VSD) ↑ in males	Initially asymptomatic until end of first month or large enough to cause pulmonary edema Loud, blowing systolic murmur 3rd–4th intercostal space (ICS) pulmonary blood flow Right ventricular hypertrophy Rapid respirations, growth failure, feeding difficulties Congestive right heart failure at 6 weeks–2 months of age	Follow medically—some spontaneously close Use of lanoxin and diuretics in congestive heart failure (CHF) Surgical closure with Dacron patch
Coarctation of aorta Can be preductal or postductal	Absent or diminished femoral pulses Increased brachial pulses Late systolic murmur left intrascapular area Systolic BP in lower extremities Enlarged left ventricle Can present in CHF at 7–21 days of life	Surgical resection of narrowed portion of aorta

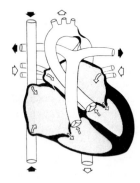

Figure 31–16 (B)   Coarctation of the aorta is characterized by a narrowed aortic lumen. The lesion produces an obstruction to the flow of blood through the aorta, causing an increased left ventricular pressure and work load.

Congenital heart defect	Clinical findings	Medical/surgical management
Cyanotic		
Tetralogy of Fallot (Most common cyanotic heart defect) Pulmonary stenosis Ventricular septal defect (VSD) Overriding aorta Right ventricular hypertrophy	May be cyanotic at birth or within first few months of life Harsh systolic murmur LSB Crying or feeding increases cyanosis and respiratory distress X-ray: Boot-shaped appearance secondary to small pulmonary artery Right ventricular enlargement	Prevention of dehydration intercurrent infections Alleviation of paroxysmal dyspneic attacks Palliative surgery to increase blood flow to the lungs Corrective surgery—resection of pulmonic stenosis, closure of VSD with Dacron patch

(continued)

Table 31–4 (continued)

Congenital heart defect	Clinical findings	Medical/surgical management

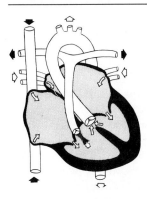

Figure 31–16 (C)   Tetralogy of Fallot. The severity of symptoms depends on the degree of pulmonary stenosis, the size of the ventricular septal defect, and the degree to which the aorta overrides the septal defect.

Transposition of great vessels (TGA) (↑ females, IDMs, LGAs)	Cyanosis at birth or within three days Possible pulmonic stenosis murmur Right ventricular hypertrophy Polycythemia "Egg on its side" x-ray	Prostaglandin E to vasodilate ductus to keep it open Initial surgery to create opening between right and left side of heart if none exists Total surgical repair—usually the arterial switch procedure

Figure 31–16 (D)   Complete transposition of great vessels. This anomaly is an embryologic defect caused by a straight division of the bulbar trunk without normal spiraling. As a result, the aorta originates from the right ventricle, and the pulmonary artery from the left ventricle. An abnormal communication between the two circulations must be present to sustain life. (All illustrations from Congenital Heart Abnormalities. *Clinical Education Aid No. 7. Ross Laboratories, Columbus, Ohio.)*

Hypoplastic left heart syndrome	Normal at birth—cyanosis and shocklike congestive heart failure develop within a few hours to days Soft systolic murmur just left of the sternum Diminished pulses Aortic and/or mitral atresia Tiny, thick-walled left ventricle Large, dilated, hypertrophied right ventricle X-ray: Cardiac enlargement and pulmonary venous congestion	Currently no effective corrective treatment

their baby's health maintenance and surgical intervention, and they understand the rationale for follow-up care.

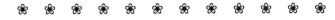

Care of the Newborn with Inborn Errors of Metabolism

Inborn errors of metabolism are a group of hereditary disorders that are transmitted by mutant genes and result in an enzyme defect that blocks a metabolic pathway and leads to an accumulation of metabolites that are toxic to the infant. Most of the disorders are transmitted by an autosomal recessive gene, requiring two heterozygous parents to produce a homozygous infant with the disorder. Heterozygous parents carrying some inborn errors of metabolism disorders can be identified by special tests, and some inborn errors of metabolism can be detected in utero.

The detection of many inborn errors of metabolism is now accomplished neonatally through newborn screening programs. These programs principally test for disorders associated with mental retardation.

Phenylketonuria (PKU) is the most common of the amino acid disorders. Newborn screenings have set its incidence at about one in 12,000 live births worldwide (Levy 1990). The highest incidence is noted in white populations from northern Europe and the United States. It is rarely observed in African, Jewish, or Japanese people.

Phenylalanine is an essential amino acid used by the body for growth, and in the normal individual any excess is converted to tyrosine. The newborn with PKU lacks this converting ability, which results in an accumulation of phenylalanine in the blood. Phenylalanine produces two abnormal metabolites, phenylpyruvic acid and phenylacetic acid, which are eliminated in the urine, producing a musty odor. Excessive accumulation of phenylalanine and its abnormal metabolites in the brain tissue leads to progressive mental retardation.

Maple syrup urine disease (MSUD) is an inborn error of metabolism and, when untreated, is a rapidly progressing and often fatal disease caused by an enzymatic defect in the metabolism of the branched chain amino acids leucine, isoleucine, and valine.

Homocystinuria is a disorder caused by a deficiency of the enzyme cystathionine B synthase, which produces a block in the normal conversion of methionine to cystine.

Galactosemia is an inborn error of carbohydrate metabolism in which the body is unable to use the sugars galactose and lactose. Enzyme pathways in liver cells normally convert galactose and lactose to glucose. In galactosemia, one step in that conversion pathway is absent, either because of the lack of the enzyme galactose 1-phosphate uridyl transferase, or because of the lack of the enzyme galactokinase. High levels of unusable galactose circulate in the blood, which causes cataracts, brain damage, and liver damage (Levy 1990).

Another disorder frequently included in mandatory newborn screening blood tests is *congenital hypothyroidism.* An inborn enzymatic defect, lack of maternal dietary iodine, or maternal ingestion of drugs that depress or destroy thyroid tissue can cause congenital hypothyroidism.

The incidence of metabolic errors is relatively low, but for affected infants and their families these disorders pose a threat to survival and frequently require lifelong treatment.

Medical Therapy

Identification via newborn screening and early medical intervention for inborn errors of metabolism has become more difficult with the advent of early discharge of newborns. In most states, the Guthrie blood test for PKU is required for all newborns. The test, done before discharge, is a simple screening tool that uses a drop of blood collected from a heel stick and placed on filter paper. The Guthrie test should be done at least 24 hours, but preferably 72 hours, after the initiation of feedings containing the usual amounts of breast milk or formula. Phenylalanine is found in milk, so its metabolites begin to build up in the PKU baby once milk feedings are initiated.

High-risk newborns should be receiving a 60% milk intake with no more than 40% of their total intake coming from nonprotein intravenous fluids. The PKU testing of high-risk newborns should be deferred for at least 48 hours after hyperalimentation is initiated. Hospitals and birthing centers frequently discharge mother and infant 24 to 48 hours after birth. It is vital that the parents understand the need for the screening procedure, and a follow-up check is necessary to confirm that the test was done.

Because it is possible to do the testing on an infant with PKU before the phenylalanine concentration rises and thus miss the diagnosis, some states routinely request a repeat test at 10 to 14 days. When the Guthrie blood test is performed early, during the first three to four days of life, a phenylalanine blood level of about 4 to 6 mg/dL is considered a presumptive positive; but only one in 20 to 30 infants with this level are true positives (Seashore 1990). Treatment involves stringent restriction of phenylalanine intake. See later discussion of family education.

Some states simultaneously test all hospitalized newborns for MSUD, homocystinuria, and PKU during the first three to four days of life. Diagnosis of MSUD is made by analyzing blood levels of leucine, isoleucine, and valine. Confirmation of the diagnosis depends on blood assay for the enzyme oxidative decarboxylase. Dietary treatment prior to 12 days of life has been reported to result in normal intelligence (AAP 1989).

In several states newborn screening includes an enzyme assay for galactose 1-phosphate uridyl transferase; this test, however, does not detect galactosemia if it is caused by a deficiency of the enzyme galactokinase. Treatment involves a galactose-free diet. Even with early treatment, children may have learning disabilities, speech problems, and ovarian failure (Seashore 1990).

For hypothyrodism, immediate and appropriate thyroid replacement therapy is established based on newborn screening and laboratory data. Frequently, premature infants of less than 30 weeks' gestation have low T4 or thyroid-stimulating hormone (TSH) values when compared with normal values of term infants. This may reflect the premature infant's inability to bind thyroid. Management includes frequent laboratory monitoring and adjustment of thyroid medication to accommodate growth and development of the infant. With adequate treatment, children remain free of symptoms, but if the condition is untreated, stunted growth and mental retardation occur.

❀ *APPLYING THE NURSING PROCESS* ❀

Nursing Assessment

The clinical picture of a PKU baby involves a normal-appearing newborn, most often with blond hair, blue eyes, and fair complexion. Decreased pigmentation may be related to the competition between phenylalanine and tyrosine for the available enzyme, tyrosinase. Tyrosine is needed for the formation of melanin pigment and the hormones epinephrine and thyroxin. Without treatment, the infant fails to thrive and develops vomiting and eczematous rashes. By about six months of age, the infant exhibits behaviors indicative of mental retardation and other CNS involvement, including seizures and abnormal electroencephalogram (EEG) patterns.

Newborns with MSUD have feeding problems and neurologic signs (seizures, spasticity, opisthotonus) during the first week of life. A maple syrup odor of the urine is noted and, when ferric chloride is added to the urine, its color changes to gray-green.

Homocystinuria varies in its presentation, but the more common characteristics are skeletal abnormalities, dislocation of ocular lenses, intravascular thromboses, and mental retardation. Abnormalities occur because of the toxic effects of the accumulation of methionine and the metabolite homocystine in the blood.

Clinical manifestations of galactosemia include vomiting, diarrhea, failure to thrive (Greenberg et al 1989), hepatosplenomegaly, jaundice, and mental retardation. The condition is frequently associated with anemia, sepsis, and cataracts in the neonatal period. Except for cataracts and mental retardation, those findings are reversible when galactose is excluded from the diet. Developmental disabilities are seen in many children despite treatment with a galactose-free diet (Seashore 1990).

A large tongue, umbilical hernia, cool and mottled skin, low hairline, hypotonia, and large fontanelles are frequently associated with congenital hypothyroidism. Early symptoms include prolonged neonatal jaundice, poor feeding, constipation, low-pitched cry, poor weight gain, inactivity, and delayed motor development.

Nursing Diagnosis

Nursing diagnoses that may apply to the newborn with an inborn error of metabolism include the following:

- Knowledge deficit related to special dietary management required secondary to inborn error of metabolism
- Compromised family coping related to parental guilt secondary to hereditary nature of disease

Nursing Plan and Implementation

Newborn Screening

Newborn screening for several inborn errors of metabolism is mandatory in many states. It is the nurse's responsibility to obtain the heel stick blood on the filter paper prior to discharge of the baby. The first filter paper test screens for PKU, homocystinuria, MSUD, galactosemia, and sickle cell anemia. A second blood specimen is usually required at 7 to 14 days after birth, but the nurse needs to remember that this second blood specimen tests only for PKU.

Some clinicians have the parents perform a diaper test for PKU. At about six weeks of age, the parent should take a freshly wet diaper and press the prepared test stick against the wet area. They note the color of the test stick, record the color on the prepared sheet, and mail the form back to the physician. A green color reaction is positive and indicates probable PKU.

Family Education—Dietary Management

Nursing responsibilities include prompt and appropriate dietary management of the newborn with an inborn error of metabolism. Once identified, an afflicted PKU infant can be treated by a special diet that limits ingestion of phenylalanine. Special formulas low in phenylalanine, such as Lofenalac, are available. Special food lists are helpful for parents of a PKU child. If treatment is begun before three months of age, CNS damage can be minimized.

Controversy exists about when, if ever, the special diet should be terminated. Because of the rigidity and severe limitations of the low phenylalanine diet, many clinicians terminate the special diet at six years of age. Brain size does not dramatically increase after age 6, but myelination continues actively through adolescence and to some extent possibly through 40 years of age. Recent studies have shown loss of intellectual function some years after relaxation of dietary restriction (Seashore 1990). Most centers now recommend keeping blood phenylalanine levels below 20 mg/dL, or even below 15 mg/dL, for life.

Female children with PKU are now living longer and may bear children. There is a 95% risk of producing a child with mental retardation if the mother with PKU is not on a low-phenylalanine diet during pregnancy. It is recommended that the woman reinstate her low phenylalanine diet a few months before becoming pregnant (Seashore 1990).

Dietary management of MSUD must be initiated immediately with a formula that is low in the branched-chain amino acids, leucine, isoleucine, and valine, which must be continued indefinitely (AAP 1989).

Infants with homocystinuria are managed on a diet that is low in methionine but supplemented with cystine and pyridoxine (vitamin B_6). With early diagnosis and careful management, mental retardation may be prevented.

Galactosemia is treated by the use of a galactose-free formula, such as Nutramigen (a protein hydrolysate process formula), a meat-base formula, or a soybean formula. As the infant grows, parents must be educated not only to avoid giving their child milk and milk products but also to read all labels carefully and avoid any foods containing dry milk products.

Parent of affected newborns should be referred to support groups. The nurse should also ensure that parents are informed about centers that can provide them with information about biochemical genetics and dietary management.

Evaluation

Anticipated outcomes of nursing care include the following:

- The risk of inborn errors of metabolism is promptly identified, and early intervention is initiated.

- The parents verbalize their concerns about their baby's health problems, long-term care needs, and potential outcomes.
- The parents are aware of available community health resources and use them as indicated.

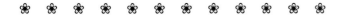

Care of the Family of the At-Risk Newborn

The Effects of Maternal-Infant Separation on Attachment

Studies of maternal-infant interactions in most human cultures have found that mother and infant remain together, usually for three to seven days after birth, without prolonged periods of separation. Only in the high-risk and preterm nurseries of the Western world are mothers and infants separated after birth.

This separation has a historical basis. In the early 1900s, it was discovered that newborn survival rates were improved if strict isolation procedures and visitor restrictions were enforced for all newborns. Of course, infection-preventing practices have rendered such isolation practices relatively obsolete for the normal newborn. The health of infants at risk, however, is extremely fragile, and separation from parents is necessary to allow treatment of complications.

The question that arises is whether interruptions in maternal contact and care giving can disrupt the process of maternal-infant attachment. The evidence seems to indicate that such interruptions may have a negative effect on bonding. It has been found, for example, that a disproportionately high number of battered or neglected children were born prematurely and stayed in an intensive care nursery for prolonged periods following birth.

What exactly in the attachment process is being interrupted by early maternal-infant separation? The period immediately after birth has been described as the *maternal sensitive period.* During this period certain behaviors have been identified as specific for development of attachment, bonding, and effective mothering. These behaviors include seeing and touching the newborn. Immediate performance of these behaviors is often impossible if the infant is preterm or has a congenital anomaly.

Parental Adjustments to the At-Risk Newborn

The events of premature labor and birth abruptly terminate the normal adaptive processes to pregnancy. Taylor and Hall (1979) have devised a schematic representation inter-

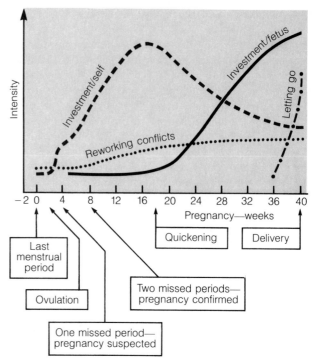

Figure 31–17   Relationship between basic psychologic processes and milestones of pregnancy. General agreement exists about the sequence and time courses of the process of investment in self, investment in fetus, and letting go, as represented here. The process of reworking unresolved conflicts with the woman's own mother is represented only tentatively. (From Taylor PM, Hall BL: Parent-infant bonding problems and opportunities in a perinatal center. Semin Perinatol 1979; 3:375)

relating the initiation-to-end course of the main psychologic processes that occur during pregnancy (Figure 31–17). Because pregnancy can be viewed as a developmental crisis, the pregnant woman spends much energy reworking unresolved conflicts she may have with her mother. In addition, as the pregnancy progresses to term, the mother-to-be begins voicing a desire to have the pregnancy end; these feelings usually coincide with a fetal gestation age that is maximal for extrauterine survival. It is believed that the mother's desire either to retain the pregnancy or to "let it go" might affect her attitude toward birth and her infant. When an infant is born prior to term, the mother may not have had sufficient time to rework conflicts or be prepared to let the pregnancy go. As a result, the mother harbors feelings not only of anxious concern over the labor and birth and survival of the infant, but also of separation, helplessness, failure, and loss of control over the ability to produce the desired outcome.

Feelings of guilt and failure also often plague the mothers of preterm newborns. They may ask themselves "Why did labor start? What did I do (or not do)?" A woman may have guilt fantasies, and wonder "Was it because I had sexual intercourse with my husband (a week, three days, a day) ago?" "Was it because I carried three loads of wash up from the basement?" "Am I being punished for something done in the past—even in childhood?"

The birth of the newborn with congenital abnormalities also engenders feelings of guilt and failure. As in the birth of a preterm infant, the woman may entertain ideas of personal guilt: "What did I do (or not do) to cause this?" "Am I being punished for something?"

Parental reactions and steps of attachment are altered by the birth of a preterm infant or one with a congenital anomaly. A variety of new feelings, reactions, and stresses must be recognized and dealt with before the family can work toward the establishment of a healthy parent-infant relationship.

Kaplan and Mason (1974) view maternal reactions to preterm births as an acute emotional disorder. They have identified four psychologic tasks as essential for coping with the stress and for providing a basis for the maternal-infant relationship:

1. Anticipatory grief as a psychologic preparation for possible loss of the child, while still hoping for his or her survival.

2. Acknowledgment of maternal failure to produce a term infant, expressed as anticipatory grief and depression and lasting until the chances for survival seem secure.

3. Resumption of the process of relating to the infant, which was interrupted by the threat of nonsurvival. This task may be impaired by continuous threat of death or abnormality, and the mother may be slow in her response of hope for the infant's survival.

4. Understanding of the special needs and growth patterns of the preterm infant, which are temporary and yield to normal patterns.

Most authorities agree that the birth of a preterm infant or a less-than-perfect infant does require major adjustments as the parents are forced to surrender the image they had nurtured for so long of their ideal child.

Solnit and Stark (1961) postulate that grief and mourning of the loss of the loved object—the idealized child—mark parental reactions to an infant with abnormalities. The parents must grieve the loss of the valued object—their wished-for perfect child. Simultaneously, they must adopt the imperfect child as the new love object. Parental responses to an infant with health problems may also be viewed as a five-staged process (Klaus & Kennell 1982):

1. *Shock* is felt at the reality of the birth of this baby. This stage may be characterized by forgetfulness, amnesia of the situation, and a feeling of desperation.

2. There is disbelief (*denial*) of the reality of the situation, characterized by a refusal to believe the child is defective. This stage is exemplified by assertions that "It didn't really happen!" "There has been a mistake; it's someone else's baby."

3. *Depression* over the reality of the situation and a corresponding grief reaction follows acceptance of the situation. This stage is characterized by much crying and sadness. Anger about the reality of the situation may also occur at this stage. A projection of blame on others or on self and feelings of "not me" are characteristic of this stage.

4. Equilibrium and *acceptance* are characteristic of a decrease in the emotional reactions of the parents. This stage is variable and may be prolonged because of a prolongation of the threat to the infant's survival. Some parents experience chronic sorrow in relation to their child.

5. *Reorganization* of the family is necessary to deal with the child's problems. Mutual support of the parents facilitates this process, but the crisis of the situation may precipitate alienation between the parental partners.

These stages of parental adjustment are similar to the stages of dying and grieving. Indeed, reorganization is necessary to deal with a crisis concerning an infant at risk.

In the birth of either a child with an anomaly or a preterm infant, the process of mourning is necessary for attachment to the less-than-perfect baby. *Grief work*, the emotional reaction to significant loss, must occur before adequate attachment to the actual baby is possible. Parental detachment precedes parental attachment.

It is essential that the mother be reunited with her infant as soon as possible after birth so that:

1. She knows that her infant is alive.

2. She knows what the infant's real problems are. Fantasies of the infant's problems may be more devastating than the reality of the problem. Early acquaintance between mother and infant allows a realistic perspective of the baby's condition.

3. She can begin the grief work over the loss of the idealized infant and begin the process of attachment to the actual infant.

4. She can share the experience of the infant's problems with the father, and other family members who may have already seen and touched the infant.

The intensive care environment can be frightening and overwhelming and interfere with the adjustment of the parents to their at-risk infant. Strange sounds, sights, activity, and lack of privacy can impede parental feelings and behavior. Admission to a neonatal intensive care unit (NICU) creates at least two kinds of separation that interfere with parental attachment. The first type of separation is distance. Either the NICU is away from the obstetric unit or the baby needs to be transported to a different hospital where NICU care is available. The second type of separation is mechanical. The baby is often surrounded by equipment that is unfamiliar to the parents and touching the baby is difficult. Noise from monitors and equipment needed to care for the baby also contribute to mechanical separation (Johnson 1986).

It is not unusual for parents to be so overwhelmed by the environment that it is difficult for them to concentrate on their baby. Steps should be taken by the nurse to orient the parents to the NICU. Their attention should first be focused toward the baby, and then simple explanations of the equipment attached to and surrounding the baby should be given.

The nurse should guard against indiscriminate admission of normal newborns to the intensive care unit because of prior high-risk conditions, such as cesarean birth, fetal bradycardia, or short periods of rapid breathing after birth. While these unjustified short-term admissions to special care nurseries cause no long-term maternal-infant attachment problems, they do cause unnecessary anxiety and unhappiness for the parents and stress in the newborn.

❀ *APPLYING THE NURSING PROCESS* ❀
Nursing Assessment

Development of a nurse-family relationship facilitates information gathering in areas of concern. A concurrent illness of the mother or other family members or other concurrent stress (lack of hospitalization insurance, loss of job, age of parents) may alter the family response to the baby. Feelings of apprehension, guilt, failure, and grief that are verbally or nonverbally expressed are important aspects of the nursing history. These observations enable all professionals to be aware of the parental state, coping behaviors, and readiness for attachment, bonding, and caretaking. Appropriate nursing observations during interviewing and relating to the family include the following:

1. *Level of understanding.* Observations concerning the ability to assimilate information given and to ask appropriate questions; the need for constant repetition of "the same" information.
2. *Behavioral responses.* Appropriateness of behavior in relation to information given; lack of response; "flat" affect.
3. *Difficulties with communication.* Deafness (reads lips only); blindness; dysphagia; understanding only a foreign language.
4. *Paternal and maternal education level.* Parents unable to read or write; only eighth grade completed; mother an MD, RN, or PhD; and so on.

Documentation of such information, obtained by the nurse through continuing contact and development of a therapeutic family relationship, enables all professionals to understand and use the nursing history in providing continuous individual care.

Visiting and care-giving patterns give an indication of the level or lack of parental attachment. A record of visits, caretaking procedures, affect (in relating to the newborn), and telephone calls is essential. Serial observations must be obtained, rather than just isolated instances of concern. Grant (1978) has developed a conceptual framework depicting adaptive and maladaptive responses to parenting of a preterm or less-than-perfect infant (Figure 31–18).

If a pattern of distancing behaviors evolves, appropriate intervention should be instituted. Follow-up studies have found that a statistically significant number of preterm, sick, and congenitally defective infants suffer from failure to thrive, battering, or other disorders of mothering. Early detection and intervention will prevent these aberrations in mothering behaviors from leading to irreparable damage or death.

Nursing Diagnosis

Nursing diagnoses that may apply to the family of a newborn at risk include the following:

- Grief related to loss of idealized newborn
- Fear related to emotional involvement with an at-risk newborn
- Altered parenting related to impaired bonding secondary to feelings of inadequacy about caretaking activities

Nursing Plan and Implementation

Preparation of Parents for Initial Viewing of Newborn

Before parents see their child, the nurse must prepare them for the viewing. It is important that a positive, realistic attitude regarding the infant be presented to the parents.

In preparing parents for the first view of their infant, it is important for a professional to have looked at the baby. The parents should be prepared to see both the deviations and the normal aspects of their infant. All infants exhibit strengths as well as deficiencies. The nurse may say, "Your baby is small, about the length of my two hands. She weighs 2 lb, 3 oz but is very active and cries when we disturb her. She is having some difficulty breathing but is breathing without assistance and in only 35% oxygen."

The equipment being used for the at-risk newborn and its purpose should be described before the parents enter the intensive care unit. Many intensive care units have booklets for parents to read before entering the unit. Through explanations and pictures, the parents can be better prepared to deal with the feelings they may experience when they see their infant for the first time.

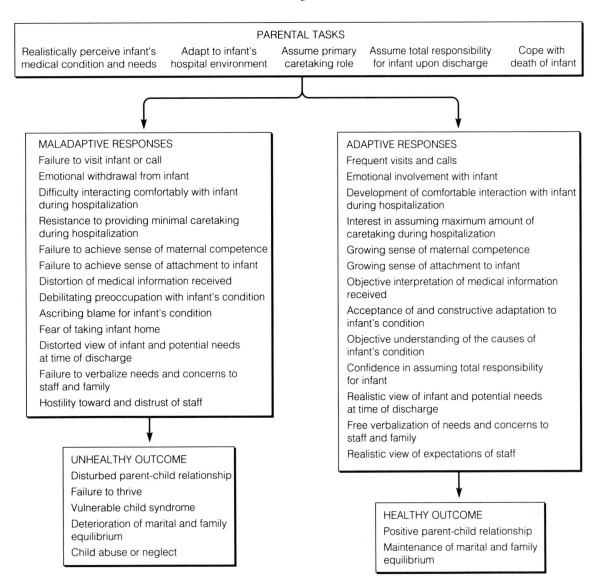

Figure 31–18   Maladaptive and adaptive parental responses during crisis period showing unhealthy and healthy outcomes (Reprinted from Family & Community Health *1978; 1(3): 93, by permission of Aspen Publishers, Inc.)*

Support of Parents During Their Initial Viewing of the Newborn

Upon entering the unit, parents may be overwhelmed by the sounds of monitors, alarms, and respirators, as well as by the unfamiliar language and "foreign atmosphere. It is more reassuring when parents are prepared and accompanied to the unit by the same person(s). The primary physician and primary nurse caring for the newborn should be with the parents when they first visit their baby. Parental reactions are varied, but there is usually an element of initial shock. Provision of chairs and time to regain composure will assist the parents. Slow, complete, and simple explanations—first about the infant and then about the equipment—allay fear and anxiety.

As parents attempt to deal with the initial stages of shock and grief at the birth of a premature or less-than-perfect baby, they may fail to assimilate new information. They may require constant repetition by the nurse to accept the reality of the situation, procedures, equipment, and the infant's condition on subsequent visits.

Misconceptions about equipment and its placement on the infant and about its potential harm are common. Such questions as "Does the fluid go into the brain?" "Does the white wire on the abdomen go into the stomach?" and

"Does the monitor make the baby's heart beat?" imply much fear for the infant's safety and misconception about the machines. These worries are easily overcome by simple explanations of all equipment being used.

Concern about the infant's physical appearance is common yet may remain unvoiced. Parents may express such concerns as "He looks so small and red—like a drowned rat." "Why do her genitals look so abnormal?" "Will that awful looking mouth [cleft lip and palate] ever be normal?" Such questions need to be anticipated by the nurse and addressed. Use of pictures, such as of an infant after cleft lip repair, may be reassuring to doubting parents. Knowledge of the development of a "normal" preterm infant will allow the nurse to make reassuring statements such as "The baby's labia may look very abnormal to you, but they are normal for her maturity. As she grows, the outer lips of the labia will become larger and the clitoris will be covered and the genitals will then look as you expect them to. She is normal for her level of maturity."

The tone of the neonatal intensive care unit is set by the nursing staff. Development of a safe, trusting environment depends on viewing the parents as essential care givers and not as "visitors" or "nuisances" in the unit. Pleasant, relaxed physical surroundings convey the sense of hospitality and encourage parents to "be at home." Provision of chairs, privacy when needed, and easy access to staff and facilities are all important in developing an open, comfortable environment. An uncrowded and welcoming atmosphere lets parents know "You are welcome here." However, even in crowded physical surroundings, an attitude of openness and trust can be conveyed by the nursing staff.

A trusting relationship is essential for collaborative efforts in caring for the infant. Nurses must therapeutically use their own responses to relate on a one-to-one basis with the parents. Each individual has different needs, different ways of adapting to crisis, and different means of support. Professionals must use techniques that are real and spontaneous to them and avoid adopting words or actions that are foreign to them. Nurses must also gauge their interventions to match the parents' pace and needs.

Facilitation of Attachment If Neonatal Transport Occurs

Smaller hospitals may be unable to care for sick infants. Transport to a regional referral center may be necessary. These centers may be as far as 500 miles from the parents' community; it is therefore essential that the mother see and touch her infant before the infant is transported. Facilitation of this important contact may be the responsibility of the referring hospital staff as well as the transport team. Bringing the mother to the nursery or taking the infant in a warmed transport incubator to the mother's bedside will allow her to see the infant before transportation to the center.

Once the infant has reached the referral center, parents also appreciate a telephone call relaying the infant's condition during the transport, safe arrival at the center, and present condition. A member of the transport team is often the best person to make the call, as the team has already begun a trusting relationship with the parents and are most knowledgeable about the infant.

Support of parents, with explanations from the professional staff, is crucial. Occasionally the mother may be unable to see the infant before transport, for example, if she is still under general anesthesia or experiencing complications such as shock, hemorrhage, or seizures. In these cases, before the infant is transported a photograph of the infant should be taken to be given to the mother, along with an explanation of the infant's condition, problems, and a detailed description of the infant's characteristics, to facilitate the attachment process until the mother can visit. An additional photograph is also helpful for the father to share with siblings and/or the extended family. With the increased attention to improved fetal outcome, maternal transports, rather than neonatal transports, are occurring more frequently. This practice gives the mother of a high-risk infant the opportunity to visit and care for her infant during the early postpartal period.

Promotion of Touching

Mothers visiting a small or sick infant may need several visits to become comfortable and confident in their abilities to touch the infant without injuring him or her. Barriers such as incubators, incisions, monitor electrodes, and tubes may delay the mother's confidence. Knowledge of this "normal" delay in touching behavior will enable the nurse to understand parental behavior.

Klaus and Kennell (1982) have demonstrated a significant difference in the amount of eye contact and touching behavior of mothers of preterm infants. Whereas mothers of normal newborns progress within minutes to palm contact of the infant's trunk, the mother of a preterm infant is slower in her progression from fingertip to palm contact and from the extremities to the trunk. The progression to palm contact with the infant's trunk may take several visits.

Through support, reassurance, and encouragement, the nurse can facilitate the mother's positive feelings about her ability and her importance to her infant. Touching facilitates "getting to know" the infant and thus establishes a bond with the infant. Touching as well as seeing the infant helps the mother to realize the "normals" and potentials of her baby.

Facilitation of Parental Caretaking

Bonding can be facilitated by encouraging parents to visit and become involved in their baby's care (Figure 31–19). When visiting is impossible, the parents should feel free to phone whenever they wish to receive information about their baby. A warm, receptive attitude is very supportive. Nurses can also facilitate parenting by personalizing a baby to the parents, by referring to the infant by name, or by relating personal behavioral characteristics to the parents. Remarks such as "Jenny loves her pacifier" help make the infant more individual and unique.

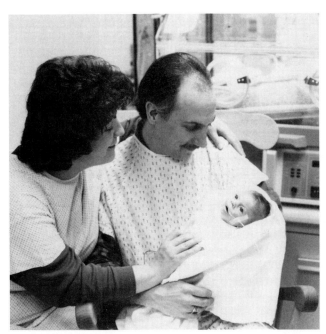

Figure 31–19 It is important that the parents of high-risk infants be given the opportunity to get acquainted with their children. Physical contact is extremely important in the bonding process and should be encouraged whenever possible.

Caretaking may be delayed for the mother of a preterm, defective, or sick infant. The variety of equipment needed for life support is hardly conducive to anxiety-free caretaking by the parents. However, even the sickest infant may be cared for, if even in a small way, by the parents. As a facilitator of parental caretaking, it is the responsibility of the nurse to promote the parents' success. Demonstration and explanation, followed by support of the parents in initial caretaking behaviors, positively reinforce this behavior. Changing the infant's diaper, giving their infant skin care or oral care, or helping the nurse turn the infant may at first be anxiety-provoking for the parents, but they will become more comfortable and confident in caretaking and receive satisfaction from the baby's reactions and their ability "to do something." Complimenting the parents' competence in caretaking also increases their self-esteem, which has received recent "blows" of guilt and failure. It is vitally important that the parents never be given a task if there is any possibility that they will not be able to accomplish it.

Often mothers have ambivalent feelings toward the nurse, in the face of their own inability to provide the sophisticated care needed by the infant. As the mother watches the nurse competently perform the caretaking tasks, she feels both grateful to the nurse for the skill and expertise and jealous of the nurse's ability to care for her infant. These feelings may be acted out in criticism of the care being received by her infant, in manipulation of staff, or in personal guilt about such feelings. Instead of fostering (by silence) these inferiority feelings within mothers, nurses are in a special position to recognize these feelings and to intervene appropriately to facilitate mother-infant attachment.

Nurses who are understanding and secure will be able to support the parents' egos instead of collecting rewards for themselves. To reinforce positive parenting behaviors, professionals must first believe in the importance of the parents. The nurse could hardly convince a doubting parent of her or his importance to the infant unless the nurse really believes it. The attitude of the professionals communicates acceptance or rejection to the parents, regardless of what is said. During this crisis period, it is essential that attitudes *and* words say: "You are a good mother/father. You are a good person. You have an important contribution to make to the care of your infant." Unless as much care is taken in facilitating parental attachment as in providing physiologic care, the outcome will not be a healthy family.

Verbalizations by the nurse that improve parental self-esteem are essential and easily shared. Breast-feeding is possible and in many centers this is recommended for preterm or sick infants for nutrition as well as for defense against the development of necrotizing enterocolitis. In addition to physiologic use, breast milk is important because of the emotional investment of the mother. Pumping, storing, labeling, and delivering quantities of breast milk is time-consuming and a "labor of love" for mothers. Positive remarks regarding breast milk reinforce the maternal behavior of caretaking and providing for her infant: "Breast milk is something that only you can give your baby" or "You really have brought a lot of milk today" or "Look how rich this breast milk is" or "Even small amounts of milk are important, and look how rich it is."

If the infant begins to gain weight while being fed breast milk, it is important to point this out to the mother. Parents should also be advised that initial weight loss with beginning breast- or bottle-feedings is common because of the increased energy expended when the infant begins active rather than passive nutritional intake.

Provision of care by the parents is appropriate even for very sick or defective infants who are likely to die. It has been found that detachment is easier after attachment, because the parents are comforted by the knowledge that they did all they could for their child while he or she was alive.

Provision of Continuity in Information Giving

During crisis, maintenance of interpersonal relationships is difficult. Yet in a newborn intensive care area, the parents are expected to relate to many different care providers. It is important that parents have as few professionals as possible relaying information to them. A primary nurse should coordinate and provide continuity in giving information to parents. Care providers are individuals and thus will use different terms, inflections, and attitudes. These subtle differences are monumental to parents and only confuse, confound, and produce anxiety. Several relationships with trusted professionals minimize unnecessary anxiety and concern and facilitate open communication. The nurse not only functions as a liaison between the parents and the wide variety of professionals interacting with the infant and parents but also offers clarification, explanation, interpretation of information, and support to the parents.

Use of Family's Support System

The parents should be encouraged to deal with the crisis with help from their support system. The support system attempts to meet the emotional needs and provide support for the family members in crisis and stress situations. Biologic kinship is not the only valid criterion for a support system; an emotional kinship is the most important factor. In our mobile society of isolated nuclear families, the support system may be a next-door neighbor, a best friend, or perhaps a school chum.

The nurse can search out the significant others in the lives of the parents and help them understand the problems so that they can be a constant parental support.

Facilitation of Family Adjustment

The impact of the crisis on the family is individual and varied. Information about the ability of the family to adapt to the situation is obtained through the nurse-family relationship. The event itself (normal newborn, preterm infant, infant with congenital anomaly) can then be viewed as it is defined by the family, and appropriate intervention can be instituted.

Because the family is a unit composed of individuals who must deal with the situation, it is important to encourage open intrafamily communication. Secret-keeping should not be encouraged, especially between spouses, because secrets undermine the trust of their relationship. Well-meaning rationales such as "I want to protect her," "I don't want him to worry about it," and so on can be destructive to open communication and to the basic element of a relationship—trust.

The nurse should be particularly sensitive to open communication when the mother is in an institution separate from the infant. The father is the first to visit the infant and relays information regarding the infant's care and condition to the mother. In this situation, the mother has had minimal contact, if any, with her infant. Because of her anxiety and isolation, she may mistrust all those who provide information (the father, nurse, physician, or extended family) until she can see for herself. This alone can put tremendous stress on the relationship between the spouses. The parents (and family) should be given information together. This practice helps overcome misunderstandings and misinterpretations and helps to promote "working through" together.

The entire family—siblings as well as relatives—should be encouraged to visit and receive information about the baby. Methods of intervention in assisting the family to cope with the situation include providing support, confronting the crisis, and understanding the reality.

Support, explanations, and the helping role must extend to the kin network, as well as to the nuclear family, in an attempt to aid them in communication and support ties with the nuclear family.

It is also essential to meet the needs of the individuals involved. Desires and needs of the individuals must be respected and facilitated; differences are tolerable and able to exist side by side. Eliciting the parents' feelings is easily accomplished with the question: "How are you doing?" The emphasis is on *you,* and the interest must be sincere.

Families with children in the newborn intensive care unit become friends and support one another. To encourage the development of these friendships and to provide support, many units have established parent groups. The core of the groups consists of parents who previously have had an infant in the intensive care unit. Most groups make contact with families within a day or two of the infant's admission to the unit, either through phone calls or visits to the hospital. Early one-on-one parent contacts help families work through their feelings better than discussion groups. This personalized method gives the grieving parents an opportunity to express personal feelings about the pregnancy, labor, and birth and their "different than expected" infant with others who have experienced the same feelings and with whom they can identify.

Provision of Predischarge Teaching

Predischarge planning begins once the infant's condition becomes stable and indications suggest the newborn will survive. Through adequate predischarge teaching, the parents are able to transform their feelings of inadequacy and competition with the nurse into feelings of self-assurance and attachment. From the beginning the parents should be included in the infant's care and taught about the infant's special needs and growth patterns. This teaching and involvement is best facilitated by a nurse who is familiar with the infant and his or her family over a period of time and who has developed a comfortable and supportive relationship with them.

The nurse's responsibility is to provide instructions in an optimal environment for parental learning. Learning should take place over time, to avoid the necessity of bombarding the parents with instructions in the day and or hour before discharge.

Routine well-baby care, such as bathing, temperature taking, formula preparation, and breast-feeding are learned by the parents. Parents are also trained in the special procedures specific for their newborn. These procedures may include gavage or gastrostomy feedings, tracheostomy or enterostomy care, administration of medications, and cardiopulmonary resuscitation. Before discharge, the parents should be as comfortable as possible with these tasks and should demonstrate independence. Written tools and instructions are useful for parents to refer to once they are home with the infant, but these should not replace actual participation in the infant's care.

Teaching and learning methods are used in assessment of parental readiness to learn. Parents often enjoy doing minimal caretaking tasks with gradual expansion of their role. Many intensive care units provide facilities for parents to room-in with their infants for a few days before discharge. This allows parents a degree of independence in the care of their infant with the security of nursing help nearby. This practice is particularly helpful for anxious parents, parents who have not had the opportunity to spend extended time with their infant, or parents who will be giving a high level of physical care at home, such as tracheostomy care.

Referrals to community health services are done before discharge. The visiting nurses' association, public health nurses, or social services can assist the parents in the stressful transition from hospital to home by providing the necessary home teaching and support. Some intensive care nurseries have their own parent support groups to help bridge the gap between hospital and home care. Parents can also find support from a variety of community support organizations, such as mother of twins groups, or trisomy 13 clubs, March of Dimes Birth Defects Foundation, handicapped children services, and teen mother and child programs. Each community has numerous agencies capable of assisting the family in adapting emotionally, physically, and financially to the chronically ill infant. The nurse should be familiar with community resources and help the parents identify which agencies may benefit them.

The nurse helps parents recognize the growth and development needs of their infant. A development program begun in the hospital can be continued at home, or parents may be referred to an infant development program in the community.

Arrangements are made for medical follow-up care before discharge. The infant may need to be followed up by a family pediatrician, a well-baby clinic, or a specialty clinic. The first appointment should be made before the infant is discharged from the hospital

The nurse evaluates the need for special equipment for infant care (such as a respirator, oxygen, apnea monitor) in the home. Any extra equipment or supplies should be placed in the home before the infant's discharge. The nurse can be instrumental in helping the parents assess the newborn's needs and coordinate services.

Evaluation

Anticipated outcomes of nursing care include the following:

- The parents are able to verbalize their feelings of grief and loss.
- The parents verbalize their concerns about their baby's health problems, care needs, and potential outcome.
- The parents are able to participate in their infant's care and show attachment behaviors.

❀ ❀ ❀ ❀ ❀ ❀ ❀ ❀ ❀ ❀ ❀ ❀

Considerations for the Nurse Who Works with At-Risk Newborns

Support cannot be given unless it can be received. Working in an emotional environment of "lots of living and lots of dying" takes its toll on staff. Neonatal intensive care units are among the most stressful areas in health care for patients, families, and nurses. Nurses bear most of the stress and largely determine the atmosphere of the NICU. The nurse's ability to cope with stress is the key to creating an emotionally healthy environment and a positive working atmosphere. The emotional needs and feelings of the staff must be recognized and dealt with in order to enable them to support the parents. An environment of openness to feelings and support in dealing with their own human needs and emotions is essential for staff. Such techniques as group meetings, individual support, and primary care nursing may assist in maintaining staff mental health.

The staff NICU nurses may never see the long-term results of the specialized, sensitive care they give to parents and their newborns. Their immediate evidence of effective care may be only the beginning of resolution of parental grief, discharge of a recovered thriving infant to the care of happy parents, and reintegration of family life.

❀ ❀

KEY CONCEPTS

Early identification of potential high-risk fetuses through assessment of prepregnant, prenatal, and intrapartal factors facilitates strategically timed nursing observations and interventions.

High-risk neonates, whether they are premature, SGA, LGA, postterm, or infant of a diabetic or substance-

addicted mother, have many similar problems, although their problems are based on different physiologic processes.

Small-for-gestational-age newborns are associated with perinatal asphyxia and resulting aspiration syndrome, hypothermia, hypoglycemia, hypocalcemia, polycythemia, congenital anomalies, and intrauterine infections. Long-term problems include continued growth and learning difficulties.

Large-for-gestational-age newborns are at risk for birth trauma as a result of cephalopelvic disproportion, hypoglycemia, polycythemia, and hyperviscosity.

Infants of diabetic mothers are at risk for hypoglycemia, hypocalcemia, hyperbilirubinemia, polycythemia, and respiratory distress due to delayed maturation of their lungs.

Postterm newborns frequently encounter the following intrapartal problems: CPD (shoulder dystocia) and birth traumas, hypoglycemia, polycythemia, meconium aspiration, cold stress, and possible seizure activity. Long-term complications may involve poor weight gain and low IQ scores.

The common problems of the preterm newborn are a result of the baby's immature body systems. Potential problem areas include respiratory distress (respiratory distress syndrome), patent ductus arteriosus, hypothermia and cold stress, feeding difficulties and necrotizing enterocolitis, marked insensible water loss and loss of buffering agents through the kidneys, infection, anemia of prematurity, apnea and intraventricular hemorrhage, retinopathy of prematurity, and behavioral state disorganization. Long-term needs and problems include bronchopulmonary dysplasia, speech defects, sensorineural hearing loss, and neurologic defects.

Newborns of alcohol-dependent mothers are at risk for physical characteristic alterations and the long-term complications of feeding problems; CNS dysfunction, including lower IQ, hyperactivity, and language abnormalities; and congenital anomalies.

Newborns born to drug-dependent mothers experience drug withdrawal as well as respiratory distress, jaundice, congenital anomalies, and behavioral abnormalities. With early recognition and intervention, the potential long-term physiologic and emotional consequences of these difficulties can be avoided or at least lessened in severity.

Newborns born to mothers with AIDS require early recognition and treatment so that the physiologic and emotional consequences may be lessened in severity and CDC guidelines implemented.

Cardiac defects are a significant cause of morbidity and mortality in the newborn period. Early identification and nursing and medical care of newborns with cardiac defects is essential to the improved outcome of these infants. Care is directed toward lessening the work load of the heart and decreasing oxygen and energy consumption.

Inborn errors of metabolism such as galactosemia, PKU, homocystinuria, and maple syrup urine disease are usually included in a newborn screening program designed to prevent mental retardation through dietary management and medication.

The nursing care of the neonate with special problems involves the understanding of normal physiology, the pathophysiology of the disease process, clinical manifestations, and supportive or corrective therapies. Only with this theoretical background can the nurse make appropriate observations concerning responses to therapy and development of complications.

Neonates communicate needs only by their behavior; the neonatal nurse, through objective observations and evaluations, interprets this behavior into meaningful information about the infant's condition.

The nurse is the facilitator for interdisciplinary communication with the parents, identifying their understanding of their infant's care and their needs for emotional support.

Parents of at-risk newborns need support from nurses and health care providers to understand the special needs of their baby and to feel comfortable in an overwhelmingly strange environment.

❀ ❀

References

Als H et al: Assessment of preterm infant behavior (APIB). In: *Theory and Research in Behavioral Pediatrics,* Vol. 1. Fitzgerald HE, Lester BM, Yogman MW (editors). New York: Plenum, 1982.

American Academy of Pediatrics Committee on Nutrition: Nutritional needs of low-birthweight infants. *Pediatrics* 1985; 75(5):976.

American Academy of Pediatrics: Report: Neonatal drug withdrawal. *Pediatrics* 1983; 72:895.

American Academy of Pediatrics Committee on Pediatrics and Committee on Genetics: Newborn screening fact sheets. *Pediatrics* 1989; 83(3):449.

Avery GB (editor): *Neonatalogy,* 3rd ed. Philadelphia: Lippincott, 1987.

Benson DW: Changing profile of congenital heart disease. *Pediatrics* 1989; 83(5):790.

Bhatt V, Nahata MC: Pharmacologic management of patent ductus arteriosus. *Clin Pharm* 1989; 1:17.

Brar HS, Rutherford SE: Classification of intrauterine growth retardation. *Semin Perinatol* January 1988; 12:2.

Casey PH, Bradley RH: The home environment. In: *Follow-up Management of the High-Risk Infant.* Taeusch HW, Yogman MW (editors). Boston: Little Brown, 1987.

Chasnoff IJ et al: Prenatal cocaine exposure is associated with respiratory pattern abnormalities. *Am J Dis Child* 1989; 143:583.

Chasnoff IR: Drug use in pregnancy: Parameters of risk. *Pediatr Clin North Am* 1988; 35(6):1403.

Coles CD et al: Neonatal ethanol withdrawal: Characteristics in clinically normal, nondysmorphic neonates. *J Pediatr* 1984; 105(3):445.

The Committee for the Classification of Retinopathy of Prematurity: An international classification of retinopathy of prematurity. *Arch Ophthalmol* 1984; 102:1130.

Creasy RK, Resnik R: *Maternal Fetal Medicine: Principles and Practice,* 2nd ed. Philadelphia: Saunders, 1989.

Casey PH, Bradley RH: The home environment. In: *Follow-up Management of the High-Risk Infant.* Taeusch HW, Yogman MW (editors). Boston: Little Brown, 1987.

Dattel BJ: Substance abuse in pregnancy. *Seminars Perinatol* 1990; 14(2):179.

Davis DH, Thomas EB: Behavioral states of premature infants: Implications for neural and behavioral development. *Dev Psychobiol* 1987; 20(1):25.

Fanaroff AA, Martin RJ: *Neonatal-Perinatal Medicine: Diseases of the Fetus and Infant,* 4th ed. St. Louis: Mosby, 1987.

Grant P: Psychosocial needs of families of high-risk infants. *Fam Com Health* November 1978; 1:91.

Greenberg CR: Newborn screening for galactosemia: A new method used in Manitoba. *Pediatrics* 1989; 84(2):331.

Grisemer AN: Apnea of prematurity: Current management and nursing implications. *Pediatr Nurs* 1990; 16(6):606.

Hadeed AJ, Siegel SR: Maternal cocaine use during pregnancy: Effect on the newborn infant. *Pediatrics* 1989; 84(2):205.

Hall Johnson S: *Nursing Assessment and Strategies for the Family at Risk, High Risk Parenting,* 2nd ed. Philadelphia: Lippincott, 1986.

Hendriksen A: Prolonged pregnancy: A literature review. *J Nurse-Midwifery* 1985; 39(1):33.

Hoskins SK: Nursing care of the infant of a diabetic mother: An antenatal, intrapartal, and neonatal challenge. *Neonatal Netw* 1990; 9(4):39.

Howard J: Cocaine and its effects on the newborn. *Dev Med Child Neuro* 1989; 31:255.

Husson RN, Comeau AM, Hoff R: Diagnosis of human immunodeficiency virus infection in infants and children. *Pediatrics* 1990; 86(1):2.

Johnson JP et al: Natural history and serologic diagnosis of infants born to human immunodeficiency virus-infected women. *Am J Dis Child* 1989; 143:1147.

Kaplan DM, Mason EA: Maternal reactions to premature birth viewed as an acute emotional disorder. In: *Crisis Interventions,* Parad HJ (editor). New York: Family Services Association of America, 1974.

Katz GH, Satish M: Screening term LGA neonates for hypoglycemia: The Colorado vs. the Portland intrauterine growth chart. *J Perinatol* 1989; 7:44.

Klaus MH, Fanaroff AA: Care of the High-Risk Neonate. Philadelphia: Saunders, 1986.

Klaus MH, Kennell JH: *Maternal-Infant Bonding,* 2nd ed. St. Louis: Mosby, 1982.

Klindworth LM et al: Pediatric AIDS, developmental disabilities, and education: A review. *AIDS Educ Preven* 1989; 1(4):291.

Klug RM: AIDS beyond the hospital. *Am J Nurs* October 1986; (Part 2):1126.

Korones SB: *High-Risk Newborn Infants: The Basis for Intensive Care Nursing,* 4th ed. St. Louis: Mosby, 1986.

Kriter KE, Blanchard J: Management of apnea in infants. *Clin Pharm* 1989; 8:577.

Lawrence RA: Breast feeding: A guide for the medical profession. 3rd ed., St. Louis: Mosby, 1989.

Levy HL: Problems of newborn screening for inborn errors of metabolism. *Metabol Curr-Ross Laboratories* 1990; 3(2):5.

Lin AE, Garver KL: Genetic counseling for congenital heart defects. *J Pediatr* 1988; 113(6):1105.

Lindo, M: Drug addiction: Its effects on mother and baby. *Midwifery* 1987; 3(2):82.

Little BR et al: Failure to recognize fetal alcohol syndrome in newborn infants. *Am J Dis Child* October 1990; 144:1142.

Lott JW: Developmental care of the preterm infant. *Neonatal–Netw* 1989; 7(4): 21.

Lugo ES, Tominey TM: The adverse effects of utilizing altitude-inappropriate fetal growth curves. *J Perinatol* 1989; 9(2):147.

Meier P: Bottle and breast feeding: Effects on transcutaneous oxygen pressure and temperature in preterm infants. *Nurs Res* 1988; 37(1):36.

Meier P, Pugh EJ: Breast feeding behavior of small preterm infants. *MCN* 1985; 10:396.

Meyer BA, Palmer SM: Pregestational Diabetes. *Semin Perinatol* 1990; 14(1):12.

Oxorn, H: Human labor and birth. 5th ed., Norwalk, CT: Appleton-Century-Crofts, 1986.

Peterson KE, Frank DE: Feeding and growth of premature and small for gestational age infants. In: *Follow-up Management of the High Risk Infant.* Taeusch HW, Yogman MW (editors). Boston: Little Brown, 1987.

Phelan JP: The postdate pregnancy: An overview. *Clin Obstet Gynecol* 1989; 32(2):221.

Phelps DL: Current perspectives on vitamin E in infant nutrition. *Am J Clin Nutr* 1987; 46:187.

Scott JR et al: *Obstetrics and Gynecology,* 6th ed. Philadelphia: Lippincott, 1990.

Seashore MR: Neonatal screening for inborn errors of metabolism: Update. *Semin Perinatol* 1990; 14(6):431.

Streissguth & LaDue 1985, ms p 31-063

Taylor PM, Hall BL: Parent-infant bonding: Problems and opportunities in perinatal center. *Semin Perinatol* 1979; 3(1):75.

Teberg AJ, Walther FJ, Pena IC: Mortality, morbidity, and outcome of the small-for-gestational age infant. *Semin Perinatol* January 1988; 12(1):84.

Teplin SW: Development of blind infants and children with retrolental fibrolasia: Implications for physicians. *Pediatrics* 1983; 71:6.

Thorp JA, Creasy RK: Postdate pregnancy. In: *Current Therapy in Neonatal-Perinatal Medicine,* 2nd ed. Nelson NM (editor). Philadelphia: Dekker 1990.

Todros et al: Growth of fetuses of diabetic mothers. *J Clin Ultrasound* 1989; 17:333.

Verklan MT: Safe in the womb? Drug and chemical effects on the fetus and neonate. *Neonatal Netw* 1989; 8(1):59.

Volpe JJ: Hemorrhage and brain injury. *Clin Perinatol* 1989; 16(2):361.

Volpe JJ: *Neurology of the Newborn,* 2nd ed. Philadelphia: Saunders, 1987.

Waldman HB: Fetal alcohol syndrome and the realities of our time. *J Dent Child* 1989; 56(6):435.

Ward SL et al: Sudden infant death syndrome in infants of substance-abusing mothers. *J Pediatr* 1990; 117(6):876.

Watt J: The consequences of intrauterine growth retardation: What do we know? *Aust NZ Obstet Gynaecol* 1989; 29(3):279.

Yip R: Altitude and birth weight. *J Pediatr* 1987; 111(6):869.

Additional Readings

Balcazar H, Haas J: Classification schemes of small-for-gestational age and type of intrauterine growth retardation and its implications to early neonatal mortality. *Early Human Development* 1990; 24:219.

Bushy A, Rohr KM: The Plains Indians: Cultural considerations in the Use of Apnea Monitors. *Neonatal Network* 1990; 8(4):59.

Gottwald SR, Thurman SK: Parent-infant interaction in neonatal intensive care units: Implications for research and service delivery. *Inf Young Children* 1990; 2(3):1.

McLean FH, Boyd ME, Usher RH, Kramer MS: Postterm infants: Too big or too small. *Am J Obstet Gynecol* 1991; 164:619.

Mendez H, Jule JE: Care of the infant born exposed to human immunodeficiency virus. *Obstet and Gynecology Clinics of North America.* 1990; 17(3):637.

Mendoza JC, Wilkerson SA, Reese AH: Follow-up of patients who underwent arterial switch repair for transposition of the great arteries. *AJDC* 1991; 145:40.

Neuspiel DR, Hamel SC: Cocaine and infant behavior. *J Dev Behav Pediatr* 1991; 12:55.

Rostrand A, Kaminski M, LeLong N, Dehaene P, Delestret I, Klein-Bertrand C, Querleu D, Crepin, G: Alcohol use in pregnancy, craniofacial features, and fetal growth. *J Epidemiol Community Health* 1990; 44:302.

Roth KS: Inborn errors of metabolism: The essentials of clinical diagnosis. *Clinical Pediatrics* 1991; 30(3):183.

CHAPTER 32

The Newborn at Risk:

Birth-Related Stressors

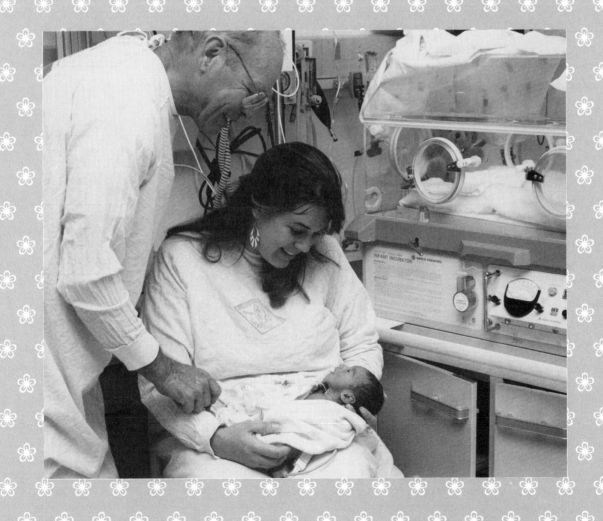

OBJECTIVES

Based on the labor record, Apgar score, and observable physiologic indicators describe the appropriate method of resuscitation for the infant in need of resuscitation.

Differentiate the various types of respiratory distress patterns seen in newborns.

Apply the nursing process to caring for the infant with respiratory distress syndrome.

Explain the relationship between the disease process and the clinical manifestations of an infant with persistent pulmonary hypertension of the newborn.

Correlate the clinical manifestations of bronchopulmonary dysplasia with the underlying disease process.

Differentiate between physiologic and pathologic jaundice based on onset, etiology, severity, and duration of disease.

Use nursing assessment and diagnosis to identify nursing responsibilities in caring for the neonate receiving phototherapy or an exchange transfusion.

Discuss selected metabolic abnormalities (including cold stress and hypoglycemia), their effects on the neonate, and the nursing implications.

Discuss selected hematologic problems such as anemia and the nursing implications for each problem.

Summarize the nurse's role in the care of an infant with hemolytic disease.

Describe the nursing assessment of clinical manifestations that would lead the nurse to suspect neonatal sepsis.

Relate the consequences of maternal syphilis, gonorrhea, or herpesvirus to the management of the infant in the neonatal period.

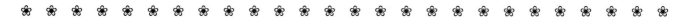

I watched her breathe every precious breath on the respirator. I saw her covered with wires and tubes. I kept watch. She was special to me and I would tell her over and over, "Daddy is here. Daddy loves you." The three days she lived were hell— not knowing if she would make it, uncertain about what plans we should make. Somehow I thought she would live; I was hopeful. When she died, at least I was there with her. The grief was unbearable. But there was also a sense of relief. The uncertainty, the waiting were finally over. (When Pregnancy Fails).

Marked homeostatic changes occur during the transition from fetal to neonatal life. The most rapid anatomic and physiologic changes of this period occur in the cardiopulmonary system. Thus the major problems of the newborn are usually related to this system. These problems include cold stress, asphyxia, respiratory distress, jaundice, hemolytic disease, and anemia. Ideally, problems are anticipated and identified prenatally, and appropriate intervention measures are begun at that time.

Care of the Newborn at Risk Due to Asphyxia

Neonatal asphyxia results from circulatory, respiratory, and biochemical factors. Circulatory patterns that accompany asphyxia are in effect a return to fetal-like circulatory patterns. They represent an inability to make the transition to extrauterine circulation. Failure of lung expansion and establishment of respiration rapidly produces hypoxia (decreased PaO_2), acidosis (decreased pH), and hypercarbia (increased PCO_2). These biochemical changes result in pulmonary vasoconstriction and high pulmonary vascular resistance, hypoperfusion of the lungs, and a large right-to-left shunt through the ductus arteriosus. As right atrial pressure exceeds left atrial pressure, the foramen ovale opens and blood flows from right to left.

Biochemical changes that occur in asphyxia contribute to these circulatory changes. The most serious biochemical abnormality is a change from aerobic to anaerobic metabolism when hypoxia is present. This change results in the accumulation of lactate and the development of metabolic acidosis. Respiratory acidosis may also occur due to a rapid increase in PCO_2 during asphyxia. In response to hypoxia and anaerobic metabolism, the amounts of free fatty acids (FFA) and glycerol in the blood increase. Glycogen stores are mobilized to provide a continuous glucose source for the brain. Rapid use of hepatic and cardiac stores of glycogen may occur during an asphyxial attack.

The neonate is supplied with protective mechanisms against hypoxial insults. These mechanisms include a relatively immature brain and a resting metabolic rate lower than that observed in the adult; an ability to mobilize substances within the body for anaerobic metabolism and use the energy more efficiently; and an intact circulatory system able to redistribute lactate and hydrogen ion in tissues still being perfused. Unfortunately, severe prolonged hypoxia will overcome these protective mechanisms, resulting in brain damage or death of the neonate.

The newborn who is apneic at birth requires immediate resuscitative efforts. The need for resuscitation can be anticipated if specific risk factors are present during the pregnancy or labor and birth period.

Risk Factors Predisposing to Asphyxia

Need for resuscitation may be anticipated in antepartal, intrapartal or neonatal situations.

Antepartal risk factors for resuscitation include the following:

1. Previous obstetric history of fetal or neonatal death; premature or growth-retarded infant; history of large-for-gestational-age infant (infant weighing 10 lb or more).
2. Maternal conditions that affect the placenta or fetus—pregnancy-induced hypertension (PIH), postterm (more than 42 weeks), preexisting hypertension, diabetes, infection, chronic renal disease, maternal obesity, and cardiac disease
3. Maternal age—younger than 15 or over 35 years
4. Isoimmunization
5. Abruptio placentae or placenta previa
6. Multiple gestation
7. Abnormal presentation
8. Preterm infant
9. Prolonged rupture of the membranes
10. Hydramnios or oligohydramnios
11. Abnormal estriol levels
12. Less-than-mature L/S ratio
13. Maternal drug usage (narcotic, barbiturate, tranquilizer, or alcohol)
14. Anemia (hemoglobin less than 10 mg/dL)

Intrapartal risk factors for resuscitation are as follows:

1. Abnormal labor pattern—dystocia, precipitous birth
2. Meconium-stained amniotic fluid
3. Fetal heart rate (FHR) patterns—tachycardia (greater than 160/min without maternal temperature elevation); bradycardia (less than 120/min, particularly associated with smooth baseline, an ominous sign); irregular rate; lack of baseline variability of FHR (smooth or fixed); lack of significant variability with fetal movement; ominous patterns (moderate to severe variable deceleration and late deceleration of any magnitude)
4. Abnormal fetal presentation—breech, transverse lie, shoulder
5. Prolapsed cord
6. Abruptio placentae or placenta previa
7. Indications for cesarean birth (see Chapter 26)

Neonatal risk factors for resuscitation include the following:

1. Difficult birth
2. Fetal blood loss
3. Apneic episode unresponsive to tactile stimulation
4. Cardiac arrest
5. Inadequate ventilation

Medical Therapy

The initial goal of medical management is to identify the fetus at risk for asphyxia, so that resuscitative efforts can begin at birth.

Fetal biophysical assessment and monitoring (fetal and maternal pH and blood gases) during the intrapartal period may help identify fetal distress. If fetal distress is present, appropriate measures can be taken to proceed with the birth of the fetus immediately, before major damage occurs, and to treat the asphyxiated newborn.

The fetal biophysical profile includes tests for heart rate accelerations associated with fetal movement, sustained fetal breathing movements, fetal limb or trunk movements, extension and flexion movements, and measurement of amniotic fluid volume. Use of this testing procedure improves the ability to predict an abnormal perinatal outcome (see Chapter 20). Fetal scalp blood sampling may indicate asphyxic insult and related degree of fetal acidosis if considered in relation to stage of labor, uterine contractions, and ominous FHR patterns. Normal fetal pH ranges from 7.30 to 7.35. The pH falls gradually during the first stage of labor. During the second stage and birth, it decreases more drastically. The stress of labor causes an intermittent decrease in exchange of gases in the placental intervillous space, which causes a fall in pH and fetal acidosis. The acidosis is primarily metabolic rather than respiratory, because exchange of CO_2 is more rapid than exchange of hydrogen ions in the placenta.

During labor, a fetal pH of 7.25 or higher is considered normal. A pH value of 7.21–7.24 is considered "preacidosis." A pH value of 7.20 or less is considered an ominous sign of fetal asphyxia. However, low fetal pH without associated hypoxia can be caused by maternal acidosis resulting from prolonged labor, dehydration, and maternal lactate production. Simultaneous testing of maternal venous pH and fetal pH may help rule out maternal acidosis as a contributing factor or to identify maternal alkalosis, which might result in a false normal fetal pH finding when the fetus has actually been compromised.

The treatment of fetal/neonatal asphyxia is resuscitation. The goal of resuscitation is to provide an adequate airway with expansion of the lungs, to decrease the PCO_2 and increase the PO_2, to support adequate cardiac output, and to minimize oxygen consumption by reducing heat loss.

Initial resuscitative management of the neonate is extremely important. The baby should be kept in a head-down position prior to the first gasp to avoid aspiration of the oropharyngeal secretions. The oropharynx and nasopharynx must be suctioned immediately. Clearing the nasal and oral passages of fluid that may obstruct the airway establishes a patent airway. Suction is always performed before resuscitation so that mucus, blood, meconium, or formula is not aspirated into the lungs.

After the first few breaths, the infant is kept in a flat position under a radiant heat source and is dried quickly with towels to maintain skin temperature at about 36.5C (97.7F). Drying is also a good stimulation to breathing. Heat loss through evaporation is tremendous during the first few minutes of life. The temperature of a wet 1500 g baby in a 16C (62F) room drops 1C every 3 minutes. Hypothermia increases oxygen consumption and in an asphyxiated infant increases the hypoxic insult and may lead to severe acidosis and development of respiratory distress.

Assessment of the infant's need for resuscitation begins at the time of birth. The time of the first gasp, first cry, and onset of sustained respirations should be noted in order of occurrence. The Apgar score (page 677) can be helpful in determining the severity of neonatal depression and the immediate course of action.

Breathing is established by employing the simplest form of resuscitative measures initially, with progression to more complicated methods as required.

1. Simple stimulation is provided by rubbing the back.

2. If respirations have not been initiated or are inadequate (gasping or occasional respirations), the lungs must be inflated with positive pressure. The mask is positioned securely on the face (over nose and mouth; avoiding the eyes) with the head in "sniffing" or neutral position (Figure 32–1). Hyperextension of the infant's neck will obstruct the trachea. An airtight connection is made between the baby's face and the mask (thus allowing the bag to inflate). The lungs are inflated rhythmically by squeezing the bag. Oxygen can be delivered at 100% with an anesthesia or Laerdal bag and adequate liter flow, whereas an Ambu or Hope bag delivers only 40% oxygen, unless it has been

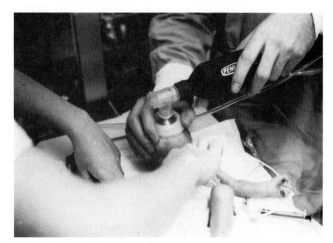

Figure 32–1 Resuscitation of infant with bag and mask. The mask covers the nose and mouth and the head is in a neutral position. Note: The resuscitation bag is placed to the side of the baby so that chest movement may be seen. In birthing room, gloves would be worn.

adapted. In addition, it may not be possible to maintain adequate inspiratory pressure with Ambu or Hope bags. In a crisis situation it is crucial that 100% O_2 be delivered with adequate pressure.

3. The rise and fall of the chest is observed for proper ventilation. Air entry and heart rate are checked by auscultation. Manual resuscitation is coordinated with any voluntary efforts. The rate of ventilation should be between 40 and 60 breaths per minute. Pressure should be less than 30 cm of H_2O. If ventilation is adequate, the chest moves with each inspiration, bilateral breath sounds are audible, and the lips and mucous membranes become pink. If color and heart rate fail to respond to ventilatory efforts, poor or improper placement of an endotracheal tube may be the cause; if the baby is intubated properly, pneumothorax, diaphragmatic hernia, or hypoplastic lungs (Potter's syndrome) may exist. Distention of the stomach is controlled by inserting a nasogastric tube for decompression.

4. Intubation (Figure 32–2) is rarely needed. Most newborns, except for very-low-birth-weight (VLBW) infants, can be resuscitated by bag and mask ventilation.

Once breathing has been established, the heart rate should increase to over 100 beats per minute. If the heart rate is less than 60 beats per minute or between 60 and 80 beats per minute and is not increasing despite 15 to 30 seconds of ventilation with 100% oxygen, external cardiac massage (chest compression) is begun. Chest compressions are started immediately if there is no detectable heart beat.

1. The infant is positioned *properly* on a firm surface.

2. The resuscitator uses the two-fingers method (Fig-

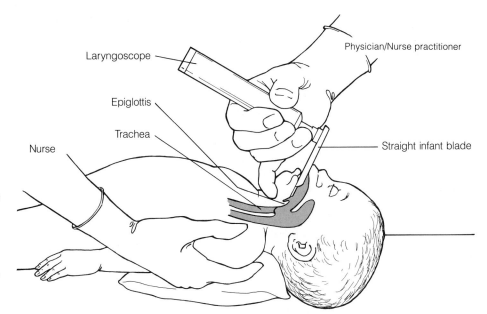

Figure 32–2 Endotracheal intubation is accomplished with the infant's head in the "sniffing" position. The clinician places the fifth finger under the chin, to hold the tongue forward, and inserts the laryngoscope blade. Once the blade is in position as shown, an endotracheal tube is inserted through the groove in the laryngoscope blade. The endotracheal tube is not seen in this figure.

ure 32–3) or may stand at the foot of the infant and place both thumbs over the lower third of the sternum (just below an imaginary line drawn between the nipples) with the fingers wrapped around and supporting the back.

3. The sternum is depressed approximately two-thirds of the distance to the vertebral column (1/2 to 3/4 inch or 1 to 2 cm) at a rate of 120 beats per minute or 10 in 5 seconds (Bloom & Cropley 1987).

4. A 3:1 ratio of heartbeat to assisted ventilation is used.

Drugs that should be available in the birthing area include those needed in the treatment of shock, cardiac arrest, and narcosis. Oxygen, because of its effective use in ventilation, is the drug most often used.

If by 5 minutes after birth the neonate has not responded to the resuscitation with spontaneous respirations and a heart rate above 100 beats per minute, it may be necessary to correct the acidosis and provide the myocardium with glucose. The most accessible route for administering medications is the umbilical vein. In a severely asphyxiated newborn, sodium bicarbonate (2 to 4 mEq/kg of 4.2% solution) is given slowly, at a rate of 1 mEq/kg/min to correct

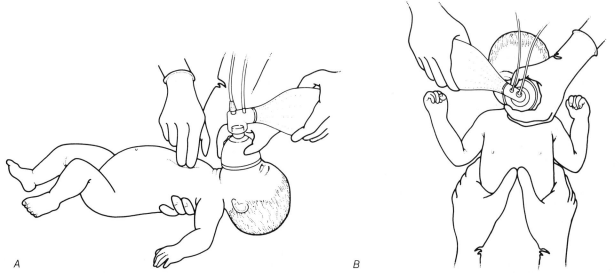

A   *B*

Figure 32–3 External cardiac massage. The lower third of the sternum is compressed with two fingertips or thumbs at a rate of 120 beats/min. A The two-fingers method uses the tips of two fingers of one hand to compress the sternum and the other hand or a firm surface to support the infant's back. B The thumb method uses the fingers to support the infant's back and uses both thumbs to compress the sternum.

metabolic acidosis, but only after adequate ventilation is established. If bradycardia is profound, epinephrine (0.1 to 0.3 mL/kg of a 1:10,000 solution) is given through the umbilical vein catheter, the peripheral IV, or the endotracheal tube (if an IV has not yet been started). Dextrose is given to correct hypoglycemia. Usually a 10% dextrose in water intravenous solution is sufficient to prevent or treat hypoglycemia in the birthing area. Naloxone hydrochloride (0.02 mg/mL neonatal solution intravenously, intramuscularly, or via endotracheal tube), a narcotic antagonist, is used to reverse narcotic depression. See the Drug Guides for Sodium Bicarbonate and Naloxone.

Calcium gluconate (1 or 2 mL/kg of a 10% solution) intravenously is used for arrhythmias, poor cardiac output despite adequate ventilation, and severe hypocalcemia or hyperkalemia but is *not* usually used in birthing area resuscitation.

In the advent of shock (low blood pressure or poor peripheral perfusion) the baby may be given a volume expander such as 5% albumin or lactated Ringer's. Whole blood, fresh frozen plasma, plasminate, and packed red blood cells can also be used for volume expansion and treatment of shock.

✿   *APPLYING THE NURSING PROCESS*   ✿

Nursing Assessment

Communication between the obstetric office or clinic and the birthing area nurse facilitates the identification of newborns who may be in need of resuscitation. Upon arrival of the woman in the birthing area, the nurse should have the antepartal record and should note any contributory perinatal history factors and assess present fetal status. As labor progresses, nursing assessments include ongoing monitor-

DRUG GUIDE
Sodium Bicarbonate

Overview of Neonatal Action

Sodium bicarbonate is an alkalizing agent. It buffers hydrogen ions caused by accumulation of lactic acid from anaerobic metabolism occurring during hypoxemia. Sodium bicarbonate thereby raises the blood pH, reversing the metabolic acidosis. Sodium bicarbonate should *only* be used to correct severe metabolic acidosis in asphyxiated newborns once adequate ventilation has been established.

Note: Sodium bicarbonate dissociates in solution into sodium ion and carbonic acid, which can split into water and carbon dioxide. The carbon dioxide must be eliminated via the respiratory tract.

Route, Dosage, Frequency

For resuscitation and severe asphyxiation: intravenous push via umbilical vein catheter for quick infusion. Dosage is 2 mEq/Kg: 4 mL of 0.5 mEq/mL (4.2%) or 2 mL of mEq/mL (8.4%). 8.4% solution diluted at least 1:1 with sterile water to decrease the osmolarity; infuse at rate no faster than 1 mEq/kg/min. Can repeat every 15 minutes if needed for total of 4 doses. For marked metabolic acidosis: a pH of less than 7.05 and a base deficit of 15 mEq/L or more should be corrected using a 0.5 mEq/mL solution of sodium bicarbonate at a rate of 1 mEq/kg/min or slower. Calculate total dosage by the following formula:

$$mEq = 0.3 \times weight\ (kg) \times base\ deficit\ in\ mEq/L$$

Neonatal Contraindications

Inadequate respiratory ventilation that causes a rise in PCO_2 and a decrease in pH

Presence of edema; metabolic or respiratory alkalosis; and hypocalcemia, anuria, or oliguria

Neonatal Side Effects

Hypernatremia, hyperosmolarity, fluid overload

Intracranial hemorrhage (rapid infusion of bicarbonate increases serum osmolarity, causing a shift of interstitial fluid into the blood and capillary rupture)

Nursing Considerations

Assess for any contraindications.

Monitor intake and output rates.

Assess adequacy of ventilation by monitoring respiratory status, rate, and depth; ventilate as necessary.

Dilute bicarbonate prior to administration into umbilical vein catheter (for resuscitation) or peripheral IV to prevent sloughing of tissue.

Evaluate effectiveness of drug by monitoring arterial blood gases for PCO_2, bicarbonate concentration, and pH determination.

Incompatible with acidic solutions.

Administration with calcium creates precipitates.

DRUG GUIDE
Naloxone Hydrochloride (Narcan)

Overview of Neonatal Action

Naloxone hydrochloride (Narcan) is used to reverse respiratory depression due to acute narcotic toxicity. It displaces morphinelike drugs from receptor sites on the neurons; therefore, the narcotics can no longer exert their depressive effects. Naloxone reverses narcotic-induced respiratory depression, analgesia, sedation; hypotension, and pupillary constriction.

Route, Dosage, Frequency

Intravenous dose is 0.01 mg/kg, usually through umbilical vein, although naloxone can be given intramuscularly. Neonatal dose is supplied as 0.02 mg/mL solution (0.5–1.0 mL for preterms and 2 mL for full-terms). Reversal of drug depression occurs within 1 to 2 minutes. The duration of action is variable (minutes to hours) and depends on amount of drug present and rate of excretion. Dose may be repeated in 5 minutes. If no improvement after two or three doses, naloxone administration should be discontinued. If initial reversal occurs, repeat dose as needed. Some institutions use 0.1 mg/kg of 0.4 mg/mL Narcan preparation.

Neonatal Contraindications

Must be used with caution in infants of narcotic-addicted mothers as it may precipitate acute withdrawal syndrome. Respiratory depression resulting from nonmorphine drugs such as sedatives, hypnotics, anesthetics, or other nonnarcotic CNS depressants.

Neonatal Side Effects

Excessive doses may result in irritability and increased crying, and possibly prolongation of PTT

Tachycardia

Nursing Considerations

Monitor respirations closely—rate and depth.

Assess for return of respiratory depression when naloxone effects wear off and effects of longer-acting narcotic reappear.

Have resuscitative equipment, O_2, and ventilatory equipment available.

Monitor bleeding studies.

Note that naloxone is incompatible with alkaline solutions.

---

ing of fetal heartbeat and its response to contractions, assisting with fetal scalp blood sampling, and observing the presence of meconium in the amniotic fluid to thereby identify fetal asphyxia. In addition, the nurse should alert the resuscitation team and the practitioner responsible for the care of the newborn of any potential high-risk laboring women.

Nursing Diagnosis

Nursing diagnoses that may apply to the newborn with asphyxia include the following:

- Ineffective breathing pattern related to lack of spontaneous respirations at birth secondary to in utero asphyxia
- Decreased cardiac output related to impaired oxygenation
- Ineffective parental coping related to baby's lack of spontaneous respirations at birth and fear of losing the baby

Nursing Plan and Implementation

Preparation of Resuscitation Equipment

In preparation for possible high-risk situations, the nurse assembles the necessary equipment and ensures proper functioning (see Table 32–1). It is desirable to provide for pH and blood gas determinations as well. Necessary equipment includes a radiant warmer that provides an overhead radiant heat source (a thermostatic mechanism that is taped to the infant's abdomen triggers the radiant warmer to turn on or off in order to maintain a level of thermoneutrality) and an open bed for easy access to the newborn. It is essential that the nurse keep the infant warm. The infant is dried quickly with warmed towels or blankets to prevent evaporative heat loss and is placed under the radiant warmer.

Resuscitative equipment in the birthing room must be sterilized after each use. In the high-risk nursery the need for resuscitation may occur at any time.

Equipment reliability must be maintained before an emergency arises. Inspect all equipment—bag and mask, oxygen and flow meter, laryngoscope, suction equipment—

Table 32-1 Newborn Resuscitation Equipment

1. Radiant warmer
2. Stethoscope
3. Bag (that can deliver 100% oxygen)
4. Mask (two mask sizes: one preterm and one newborn)
5. Tubing and pressure gauges for bag
6. Oxygen, flow meter, and provision for warmth and humidification
7. Suction equipment
    a. DeLee suction trap
    b. Mechanical suction apparatus
    c. Suction catheters (No. 5, 6, and 8 Fr.)
8. Intubation equipment
    a. Magill forceps
    b. Endotracheal tubes—sizes 2.5, 3.0, 3.5, 4.0 mm (fitted with adapter)
    c. Wire stylets for tubes
    d. Laryngoscope handle with two blades—size 0 (premature), size 1 (newborn)
    e. Four extra batteries
    f. Two extra bulbs
9. Nasogastric tube (for decompression of stomach)
10. Infant plastic airway
11. K-Y lubricating jelly
12. Benzoin
13. Cotton applicators
14. Adhesive tape
15. Scissors
16. Safety pins (for attachments)
17. Syringes (tuberculin, 3, 5, and 10 mL)
18. Umbilical artery catheter tray (No. 3.5 and 5 Fr. catheters)
19. IV solution and tubing
20. Drugs (solutions)
    a. Sodium bicarbonate (0.5 mEq/mL)
    b. Epinephrine (0.01 mL/kg of 1:10,000 solution)
    c. Dextrose and water (D/W) (10% D/W for IV for hypoglycemia)
    d. Calcium gluconate (10% solution)
    e. Narcan (0.02 mg/mL neonatal solution or 0.4 mg/mL.)
    f. Volume expanders (plasma or human plasma protein fraction [plasminate])
    g. Normal saline (for suctioning)
    h. Atropine (0.4 mg/0.5 mL)
21. Blood pressure cuff and gauge or pressure transducer
22. Doppler (to measure blood pressure)
23. ECG electrodes and heart rate monitor

for damaged or nonfunctioning parts before a birth or before assembly at the infant's bedside. A systematic check of the emergency cart and equipment should be a routine responsibility of each shift.

Provision and Documentation of Resuscitation

Training and knowledge about resuscitation are vital to personnel in the birth setting for both normal and high-risk births. Since resuscitation is at least a two-person effort, the nurse should call for assistance so that there is adequate staff available. The resuscitative efforts are recorded on the newborn's chart so that all members of the health care team will have access to this information.

Parent Education

Resuscitation in the birthing area is particularly distressing for the parents. If the need for resuscitation is anticipated, the parents should be assured that a team will be present at the birth to care specifically for their infant. As soon as stabilization is accomplished, a member of the interdisciplinary team needs to discuss the baby's condition with the parents. The parents may have many fears about the reasons for resuscitation and the condition of their baby following the resuscitation.

Evaluation

Anticipated outcomes of nursing care include the following:

- The risk of asphyxia is promptly identified, and intervention is started early.
- The newborn's metabolic and physiologic processes are stabilized, and recovery is proceeding without complications.
- The parents can describe the reason for resuscitation and what was done to resuscitate their newborn.
- The parents discuss their fears about the resuscitation process and potential implications for their baby's future.

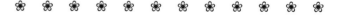

Care of the Newborn with Respiratory Distress

One of the severest conditions to which the newborn may fall victim is respiratory distress—an inappropriate respiratory adaptation to extrauterine life. The nursing care of a baby with respiratory distress requires understanding of the normal pulmonary and circulatory physiology (Chapter 27), the pathophysiology of the disease process, clinical manifestations, and supportive and corrective therapies. Only with this knowledge can the nurse make appropriate observations concerning responses to therapy and development of complications. Unlike the verbalizing adult client, the newborn communicates needs only by behavior. The neonatal nurse interprets this behavior as clues about the individual baby's condition.

Idiopathic Respiratory Distress Syndrome (Hyaline Membrane Disease)

Respiratory distress syndrome (RDS), also referred to as *hyaline membrane disease (HMD),* is a complex disease affecting primarily preterm infants and accounts for approximately 7000 deaths per year in the United States alone. The syndrome occurs more frequently in premature white infants than in black infants and almost twice as often in males as in females.

The factors precipitating the pathologic changes of RDS have not been determined, but two main factors are associated with its development:

1. *Prematurity.* All preterm newborns—whether average-for-gestational-age (AGA), small-for-gestational-age (SGA), or large-for-gestational-age (LGA)—and especially infants of diabetic mothers (IDMs) are at risk for RDS. The incidence of RDS increases with the degree of prematurity, with most deaths occurring in newborns weighing less than 1500 g. The maternal and fetal factors resulting in preterm labor and birth, complications of pregnancy, indications for cesarean birth, and familial tendency are all associated with RDS.

2. *Asphyxia.* Asphyxia, with a corresponding decrease in pulmonary blood flow, may interfere with surfactant production.

Development of RDS indicates a failure to synthesize lecithin, which is required to maintain alveolar stability. Upon expiration this instability increases atelectasis, which causes hypoxia and acidosis. These conditions further inhibit surfactant production and cause pulmonary vasoconstriction. Thus the central pathophysiologic defect, lung instability due to this abnormality in the surfactant system, leads to the biochemical problems of hypoxemia (decreased PO_2), hypercarbia (increased PCO_2), and acidemia (decreased pH), which further increases pulmonary vasoconstriction and hypoperfusion. The cycle of events of RDS leading to eventual respiratory failure is diagrammed in Figure 32–4.

Because of these pathophysiologic conditions, the neonate must expend increasing amounts of energy to reopen the collapsed alveoli with every breath, so that each breath becomes as difficult as the first. The progressive atelectasis with each expiration upsets the physiologic homeostasis of the pulmonary and cardiovascular systems and prevents adequate gaseous exchange. Lung compliance decreases, and stiff lungs, which account for the difficulty of inflation, labored respirations, and the increased work of breathing, are the result.

The physiologic alterations of RDS produce the following complications:

1. *Hypoxia.* As a result of hypoxia, the pulmonary vasculature constricts, pulmonary vascular resistance increases, and pulmonary blood flow is reduced. Increased pulmonary vascular resistance may cause a return to fetal circulation as the ductus opens and blood flow is shunted around the lungs. This increases the hypoxia and decreases pulmonary perfusion. Hypoxia also causes impairment or absence of metabolic response to cold, reversion to anaerobic metabolism resulting in lactate accumulation (acidosis), and impaired cardiac output, which decreases perfusion to vital organs.

2. *Respiratory acidosis.* Increased PCO_2 and decreased pH are results of alveolar hypoventilation. Carbon dioxide retention and the respiratory acidosis that results are the measure of ventilatory inadequacy, so that persistently rising PCO_2 and decrease in pH are poor prognostic signs of pulmonary function and adequacy.

3. *Metabolic acidosis.* Decreased pH and decreased bicarbonate levels may be results of impaired delivery of oxygen at the cellular level. Because of the lack of oxygen, the neonate begins an anaerobic pathway of metabolism, with an increase in lactate levels and a resultant base deficit (loss of bicarbonate). As the lactate levels increase, the pH decreases and the buffer base decreases in an attempt to maintain acid-base homeostasis.

The classic radiologic picture of RDS is diffuse reticulogranular density that occurs bilaterally, with portions of the air-filled tracheobronchial tree (air bronchogram) outlined by the opaque lungs. Opacification of the lungs on x-ray ("white-out") may be due to massive atelectasis, diffuse alveolar infiltrate, or pulmonary edema. The progression of x-ray findings parallels the pattern of resolution, which occurs in four to seven days, and the time of surfactant reappearance.

If death occurs an autopsy would reveal that the lungs of the RDS infant are dark red-purple, airless, and liverlike in consistency. Atelectasis is widespread, and the lungs are difficult to inflate. The presence of hyaline membranes in overdistended terminal bronchioles and alveoli reveals destruction and damage to the basement membrane of the alveolar cells.

Medical Therapy

The primary goal of prenatal medical management is the prevention of preterm birth through aggressive treatment of premature labor and possible administration of glucocorticoids to enhance fetal lung development (see page 497). The goals of postnatal therapy are maintenance of adequate oxygenation and ventilation, correction of acid-base abnor-

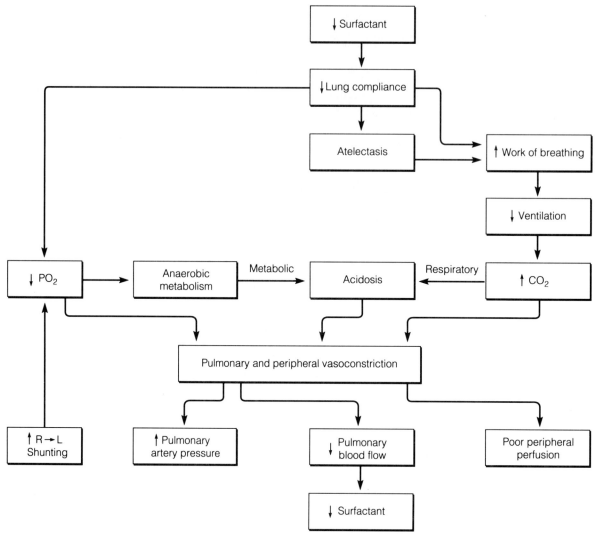

Figure 32–4   Cycle of events of RDS leading to eventual respiratory failure. (Modified from Gluck L, Kulovich MV: Fetal lung development. Pediatr Clin North Am *1973; 20:375)*

malities, and provision of the supportive care required to maintain homeostasis.

Supportive medical management consists of ventilatory therapy, transcutaneous oxygen and carbon dioxide monitoring, correction of acid-base imbalance, environmental temperature regulation, adequate nutrition, and protection from infection. Ventilatory therapy is directed toward prevention of hypoventilation and hypoxia. Infants with mild cases of RDS may require only increased humidified oxygen concentrations. Use of continuous positive airway pressure (CPAP) may be required in moderately afflicted infants. Babies with severe cases of RDS require mechanical ventilatory assistance, with positive end-expiratory pressure (PEEP) (Figure 32–5). Surfactant

replacement therapy is now available for infants to decrease the severity of RDS, especially in low-birth-weight infants.

❀   *APPLYING THE NURSING PROCESS*   ❀

Nursing Assessment

Characteristics of RDS the nurse should look for are increasing cyanosis, tachypnea, grunting respirations, nasal flaring, and significant retractions. Table 32–2 reviews clinical findings associated with respiratory distress. The Silverman-Andersen index (Figure 32–6) may be helpful in evaluating the signs of respiratory distress and can be done in the birth area.

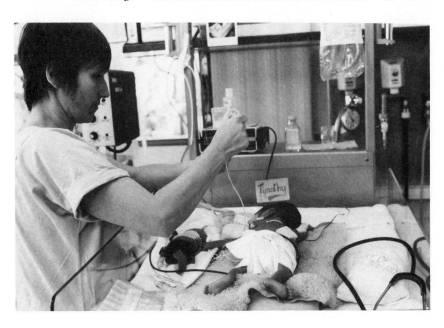

Figure 32–5   Infant on a respirator

Nursing Diagnosis

Nursing diagnoses that may apply are included in the Nursing Care Plan for Respiratory Distress Syndrome, page 1017.

Nursing Plan and Implementation

Based on clinical parameters nursing care is focused on maintaining physiologic homeostasis and providing supportive care to the newborn with RDS (see the Nursing Care Plan for Respiratory Distress Syndrome).

Provision of Mechanical Ventilatory Assistance

Nursing interventions and criteria for instituting mechanical ventilatory assistance are done per institutional protocol. Methods of transcutaneous monitoring and nursing interventions are included in Table 32–3. Ventilatory

(Text continues on p 1025.)

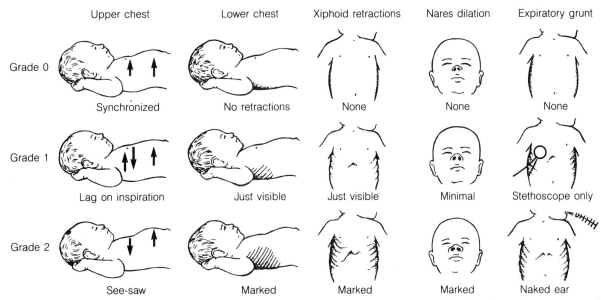

Figure 32–6   Evaluation of respiratory status using the Silverman-Andersen index. The baby's respiratory status is assessed, and a grade of 0, 1, or 2 is determined for each area and a total score is charted in the baby's record—or on a copy of this tool—and placed in the chart. (From Ross Laboratories, Nursing Inservice Aid No. 2, Columbus, OH, and Silverman WA, Andersen DH: Pediatrics 1956; 17:1, Copyright 1956, American Academy of Pediatrics)

Table 32–2   Clinical Assessments Associated with Respiratory Distress

Clinical picture	Significance
Skin	
Color	
Pallor or mottling	Represents poor peripheral circulation due to systemic hypotension and vasoconstriction and pooling of independent areas (usually in conjunction with severe hypoxia).
Cyanosis (bluish tint)	Depends on hemoglobin concentration, peripheral circulation, intensity and quality of viewing light, and acuity of observer's color vision; frankly visible in advanced hypoxia; central cyanosis is most easily detected by examination of mucous membranes and tongue.
Jaundice (yellow discoloration of skin and mucous membranes due to presence of unconjugated [indirect] bilirubin)	Metabolic aberrations (acidosis, hypercarbia, asphyxia) of respiratory distress predispose to dissociation of bilirubin from albumin-binding sites and deposition in the skin and central nervous system.
Edema (presents as slick, shiny skin)	Characteristic of preterm infant because of low total protein concentration with decrease in colloidal osmotic pressure and transudation of fluid; edema of hands and feet frequently seen within first 24 hours and resolved by fifth day in infant with severe RDS.
Respiratory System	
Tachypnea (normal respiratory rate 30–50/min; elevated respiratory rate 60+/min)	Increased respiratory rate is the most frequent and easily detectable sign of respiratory distress after birth; a compensatory mechanism that attempts to increase respiratory dead space to maintain alveolar ventilation and gaseous exchange in the face of an increase in mechanical resistance. As a decompensatory mechanism it increases work load and energy output (by increasing respiratory rate), which causes increased metabolic demand for oxygen and thus increase in alveolar ventilation (of already over-stressed system). During shallow, rapid respirations, there is increase in dead space ventilation, thus decreasing alveolar ventilation.
Apnea (episode of nonbreathing of more than 20 sec in duration; periodic breathing, a common "normal" occurrence in preterm infants, is defined as apnea of 5–10 sec alternating with 10–15 sec periods of ventilation)	Poor prognostic sign; indicative of cardiorespiratory disease, CNS disease, metabolic alterations, intracranial hemorrhage, sepsis, or immaturity; physiologic alterations include decreased oxygen saturation, respiratory acidosis, and bradycardia.
Chest	Inspection of thoracic cage includes shape, size, and symmetry of movement. Respiratory movements should be symmetric and diaphragmatic; asymmetry reflects pathology (pneumothorax, diaphragmatic hernia). Increased anteroposterior diameter indicative of air-trapping (meconium aspiration syndrome).
Labored respirations (Silverman-Andersen chart in Figure 32–6 indicates severity of retractions, grunting, and flaring, which are signs of labored respirations)	Indicative of marked increase in work of breathing.
Retractions (inward pulling of soft parts of chest cage—suprasternal, substernal, intercostal, subcostal—at inspiration)	Reflect significant increase in negative intrathoracic pressure necessary to inflate stiff, noncompliant lung; infants attempt to increase lung compliance by using accessory muscles; markedly decreases lung expansion; seesaw respirations are seen when chest flattens with inspiration and abdomen bulges; retractions increase work and O_2 need of breathing, so that assisted ventilation may be necessary due to exhaustion.
Flaring nares (inspiratory dilation of nostrils)	Compensatory mechanism that attempts to lessen resistance of narrow nasal passage.
Cardiovascular System	
Continuous systolic murmur may be audible	Patent ductus arteriosus is common occurrence with hypoxia, pulmonary vasoconstriction, right-to-left shunting, and congestive heart failure.
Heart rate usually within normal limits (fixed heart rate may occur with a rate of 110–120/min)	Fixed heart rate indicates decrease in vagal control.
Point of maximal impulse usually located at fourth to fifth intercostal space, left sternal border.	Displacement may reflect dextrocardia, pneumothorax, or diaphragmatic hernia.
Hypothermia	Inadequate functioning of metabolic processes that require oxygen to produce necessary body heat.
Muscle Tone	
Flaccid, hypotonic, unresponsive to stimuli	May indicate deterioration in neonate's condition and possible CNS damage due to hypoxia, acidemia, or hemorrhage.
Hypertonia and/or seizure activity	

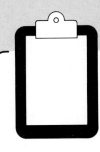

Nursing Care Plan
Newborn with
Respiratory Distress Syndrome

Client Assessment

Nursing History

Preterm delivery

Gestational history: Recent episodes of fetal or intrapartal stress (maternal hypotension, bleeding, maternal and resultant fetal oversedation), severe fetal lung circulation compromise

Neonatal history: Birth asphyxia resulting in acute hypoxia, exposure to hypothermia

Familial tendency

Low Apgar score, requiring bag and mask resuscitation in birthing area

Physical Examination

At birth or within two hours, rapid development initially of tachypnea (over 60 respirations/min), expiratory grunting (audible), or subcostal/intercostal retractions

Followed by flaring of nares on inspiration, cyanosis and pallor, signs of increased air hunger (apneic spells, hypotonus), rhythmic movement of body and labored respirations, chin tug

Auscultation: Initially breath sounds may be normal; then decreased air exchange with harsh breath sounds and, upon deep inspiration, rales; later a low-pitched systolic murmur indicates patent ductus

Increasing oxygen concentration requirements to maintain adequate PO$_2$ levels

Diagnostic Studies

Lung profile to determine lung maturity is done on amniotic fluid (for fetuses predisposed to RDS) as follows:

- Lecithin/Sphingomyelin: Ratio of 2:1 or more indicates pulmonary maturity.
- Phosphatidylglycerol (PG): Elevated at 35 weeks' gestation

Arterial blood gases (indicating respiratory failure): PaO$_2$ less than 50 mm Hg while breathing 100% O$_2$, and PCO$_2$ above 60 mm Hg

Potassium levels increase as potassium is released from injured alveolar cells.

X-ray: Diffuse reticulogranular density bilaterally, with air-filled tracheobronchial tube outlined by opaque lungs (air bronchogram); atelectasis/hypoexpansion in severe cases.

Clinical course worsens first 24–48 hours after birth and persists for more than 24 hours

Dextrostix

Nursing Diagnosis	Nursing Interventions	Rationale	Evaluation
Nursing Diagnosis: Impaired gas exchange related to inadequate lung surfactant *Client Goals:* Baby's respirations will be 30–50/min, regular, and without apneic periods. Baby's oxygen requirement and work of breathing will diminish.	Determine baseline of respiratory effort, ventilatory adequacy—observation of chest wall movement, skin, mucous membranes, color; estimation of degree and equality of air entry by auscultation, arterial blood gases, and pH determination.	Alveoli of normal infant remain stable during expiration due to presence of surfactant. Alveoli of infant with RDS lack surfactant and collapse with expiration. Values used to determine adequate oxygenation—normal PaO$_2$ 50–70 mm Hg. Adequate ventilation—normal PaCO$_2$ 35–45 mm Hg. Acid-base balance—normal pH 7.35–7.45.	Baby's respirations are 30–50 per minute without apnea, PaO$_2$ is between 50–70 mm Hg.

(continued)

Nursing Care Plan (continued)

Nursing Diagnosis	Nursing Interventions	Rationale	Evaluation
Baby's need for assisted ventilation will be noted early.	Maintain on respiratory and cardiac monitors—note rates every 30–60 min or more often as indicated by the severity of infant's distress. Check and calibrate all monitoring and measuring devices every eight hr. Calibrate oxygen devices to 21% and 100% O_2 concentrations.	Alveolar atelectasis and intrapulmonary shunting results in poor gas exchange, hypoxemia, hypercarbia, and acid-base derangements. Grunting, a compensatory mechanism, increases transpulmonary pressure, overcomes high surface tension, forces and prevents atelectasis, and thus enables improved oxygenation and a rise in PaO_2. It is the sound of the glottis closing to stop exhalation of air by forcing it against the vocal cords.	
	Provide warmed air (89 to 93F) 31.7 to 33.9C and humidified (40% to 60%) oxygen.	Humidified oxygen prevents mucosal dryness.	
	Monitor oxygen concentrations at least every hour.	Maintains constant level.	
	Administer oxygen by oxygen hood (a small transparent head hood that contains an inlet and carbon dioxide outlet) (Figure 32–7).	Provides a constant oxygen environment. Incubators are not recommended for long-term oxygen delivery since the concentration is difficult to regulate and fluctuates when portholes are opened for care giving.	

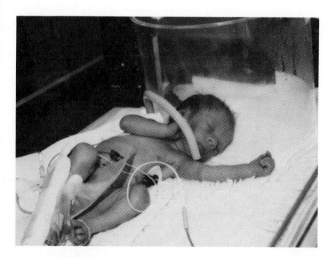

Figure 32–7 Infant in oxygen hood

(continued)

Nursing Care Plan (continued)

Nursing Diagnosis	Nursing Interventions	Rationale	Evaluation
	Avoid hood touching infant's face.	Contact with infant's face may cause apnea by stimulating facial nerve.	
	Maintain stable oxygen concentration by increasing or decreasing oxygen by 5%–10% increments and then obtain arterial blood gases.	Stable concentration of oxygen is necessary to maintain PaO_2 within normal limits (50–70 mm Hg). Sudden increase or decrease in O_2 concentration may result in disproportionate increase or decrease in PaO_2 due to vasoconstriction in response to hypoxemia.	
	Monitor: 1. Color (pink), cyanosis (central or acrocyanosis), duskiness, pallor 2. Respiratory effort (evaluation at rest), rate of respirations, patterns (apnea, periodic breathing), quality (easy, unlabored; abdominal, labored), auscultation (site of breath sounds—overall or part of lung fields—describe quality of breath sounds every one to two hr), accompanying sounds with respiratory effort (change from previous observations) 3. Activity—less active, flaccid, lethargic, unresponsive, increased activity, restless, irritable; inability to tolerate exertion, crying, sucking, or nursing care activity 4. Circulatory response (evaluate at rest); rate, regularity, and rhythm of heart rate; periods of bradycardia; alterations of blood pressure	Observations of clinical condition are taken serially for comparison and changes. Observations should be taken while infant is receiving oxygen and with any oxygen adjustment.	

(continued)

Nursing Care Plan (continued)

Nursing Diagnosis	Nursing Interventions	Rationale	Evaluation
	Return O_2 concentration to previous levels if there is deterioration in neonate's condition or drop below desired transcutaneous oxygen monitor (TCM) levels.	Any deterioration of clinical condition with oxygen adjustments (usually a decrease in ambient oxygen concentration) indicates inability of neonate to compensate for hypoxia.	
	Repeat arterial blood gases (keep PaO_2 50–70 mm Hg). Gases should be done within 15–20 min after any change in ambient O_2 concentration or after inspiratory or expiratory pressure changes.		
	Record and report clinical observations and action taken.		
	Maintain stable environment prior to collection of arterial blood gas sample:		
	1. Maintain constant O_2 concentration at least 15–20 min before sample.	Accurate arterial blood determinations are essential in management of any infant receiving oxygen, because presence or absence of cyanosis is unreliable.	
	2. Avoid any disturbances of infant 15 min before gases are drawn.	Crying or struggling may cause hyperventilation or breath holding and may increase shunting of blood.	
	Do not suction; if suction is absolutely necessary, delay blood sample.		
	Maintain temperature of sample (pH should be measured at body temperature).	Use of temporal, radial, or brachial arteries takes skill, is time-consuming, and may have serious consequences; therefore, most common technique for sampling is through umbilical artery catheter.	
	Provide arterial blood gas setup (a 3-mL syringe with heparinized solution and a heparinized tuberculin syringe) to obtain blood sample.		

(continued)

Nursing Care Plan (continued)

Nursing Diagnosis	Nursing Interventions	Rationale	Evaluation
	After blood sample is taken, recheck flow through line to assure patency and prevent establishment of clot.		
	Replace blood used to clear line.	Total blood volume of infant is small; blood removed to clear catheter must be returned to prevent hypovolemia, anemia.	
	Use heparinized flush solution before restarting IV solution to prevent clots in the line.		
	With transcutaneous PO_2 or pulse oximeter, monitor continuously or every hour and record. Calibrate sensor each shift and rotate sensor position every 3–4 hr.	Transcutaneous monitors and pulse oximeter measure percentage of oxygen in inspired air, ensures FIO_2 concentrations and accuracy of readings. Rotating sensor prevents skin burns. Electrode sites include chest, abdomen, and inner thigh. Oxygen diffuses through the skin from capillaries directly beneath the skin and can then be measured. Oximeter is preferred because it doesn't produce heat.	
	Assess need for assisted ventilatory measures. Criteria for assisted ventilation: 1. Apnea 2. Hypoxia (PaO_2 <50 mm Hg) 3. Hypercarbia ($PaCO_2$ >60 mm Hg) 4. Respiratory acidosis (pH <7.20)	Application of CPAP or PEEP produces same stabilization force on alveoli as grunting does and produces same effect—improved oxygenation and rise in PaO_2.	
	Have ventilatory support equipment available.		
	Administer ventilator care per agency protocol.	Delivery of CPAP or PEEP can only be done by use of nasal prongs, nasopharyngeal tube, or oral intubation.	
Altered nutrition: less than body requirements related to increased metabolic needs of stressed infant	Maintain IV rate at prescribed levels, usually 65 to 80 mL/kg/day	This is the needed rate for initial caloric intake.	Baby maintains normal glucose levels, follows normal weight curves, and is tolerating oral feedings.

(continued)

Nursing Care Plan (continued)

Nursing Diagnosis	Nursing Interventions	Rationale	Evaluation
Client Goals: Baby will not have greater than 2% weight loss, will have greater than 40 mg % glucose, and will progress to oral feedings.	Maintain IV rate at prescribed level; record type and amount of fluid infused hourly. Use infusion pump. Observe vital signs for signs of too-rapid infusion. Maintain normal urine output (1–3 mL/kg/hr). Maintain specific gravity of urine between 1.006 and 1.012. Take daily weights.	Fluids are provided to sick neonate by intravenous route and are calculated to replace sensible and insensible water losses as well as evaporative losses due to tachypnea. Overload of circulatory system by too much or too rapid administration of fluid causes pulmonary edema and cardiac embarrassment that may be fatal.	
	Manage route of IV administration. With umbilical catheter: Protect catheter from strain or tension. Restrain as necessary. Prevent dislodgement of catheter. Always keep catheter and stopcock on top of bed linens so they are easily visible.	Greater nutritional fluid is required because of energy needed to cope with stress. Stressed infants are predisposed to hypoglycemia because of increased metabolic demands as well as reduced glycogen stores and decreased ability to convert fat and protein to glucose.	
	Observe for occlusion of vessels by clot and for vasospasm—discoloration of skin, discoloration of toes or feet (blanching or cyanosis). If discoloration occurs, contralateral foot may be wrapped with warm cloth, but this is controversial. Removal of catheter is preferred.	Vasospasm in unwrapped foot will be relieved by treatment, and the discoloration will disappear and toes will be pink. If discoloration persists, clot may be occluding vessel—catheter must be removed, or loss of extremity is possible.	
	Observe for signs of infection or sepsis: temperature instability, drainage, redness or foul odor from cord, lethargy, irritability, vomiting, poor feeding, hypotonia.		
	Peripheral IV in scalp or extremity vein: Prepare equipment, insert IV in vein, and restrain infant.		
	If vessel chosen is an artery, it pulsates. Place peripheral IV in vein (which doesn't pulsate).	Very small arteries may not pulsate and arterial area will blanch if saline is infused.	

(continued)

Nursing Care Plan (continued)

Nursing Diagnosis	Nursing Interventions	Rationale	Evaluation
	Maintain proper placement of IV.	Ability to aspirate blood and/or easily inject small amount of saline indicates patent IV. Infiltration is evaluated by area of edema and redness about site, inability to obtain blood on aspiration, or difficulty in injecting solution.	
	Provide total parenteral nutrition (TPN) when indicated.	TPN is used as nutritional alternative if bowel sounds are not present and infant remains in acute distress.	
	Advance as soon as possible from intravenous to oral feedings. Gavage or nipple feedings are used, and IV is used as supplement (discontinued when oral intake is sufficient) (see Procedure 31–1).		
	Provide adequate caloric intake: amount of intake, type of formula, route of administration, and need for supplementation of intake by other routes.	Calories are essential to prevent catabolism of body proteins, and metabolic acidosis due to starvation or inadequate caloric intake.	
	Monitor for hypocalcemia. Monitor for hypoglycemia: Dextrostix below 45 mg/dL, urine screening for glucose.	Hypocalcemia and hypoglycemia result from delayed or inadequate caloric intake and stress.	
Infection: High risk related to invasive procedures *Client Goals:* Baby will maintain a stable temperature and blood pressure and will be free from infection.	See section on sepsis nursing care.	Decreased lung expansion predisposes to atelectasis and secondary superimposed infections.	Baby's temperature and blood pressure are within normal limits and are stable; no signs of infection are present.
	Pay careful attention to infection control by cleaning and replacing nebulizers/humidifiers at least every 24 hr; use sterile tubing and replace ever 24 hr; use sterile distilled water.	The warm, moist environment found in Isolettes and with O_2 equipment promotes growth of microorganisms.	

(continued)

Nursing Care Plan (continued)

Nursing Diagnosis	Nursing Interventions	Rationale	Evaluation
Ineffective thermoregulation related to increased respiratory effort secondary to RDS *Client Goals:* Baby will maintain a stable temperature. Baby will not become hypoglycemic, cyanotic, or have periods of bradycardia or apnea.	Observe infant for temperature instability and signs of increased oxygen consumption (need for increased O_2 concentration) and metabolic acidosis. Maintain neutral thermal environment.	Cold stress increases oxygen consumption and promotes pulmonary vasoconstriction. This leads to hypoxia and acidosis, which further depress surfactant production. Cold stress leads to chemical thermogenesis (burning brown fat to maintain body temperature), which increases O_2 needs in an already compromised infant.	Baby's temperature was within normal limits. Signs of cold stress are absent or minimized.
	Use servocontrol to maintain constant temperature regulation.		
	Warm all inspired gases. Place a thermometer in the oxygen hood and document the temperature of the delivered gas with vital signs. Oxyhood and Isolette temperature should be maintained in the infant's neutral thermal range. Place thermometer in-line of ventilatory circuit and maintain inspired gas at 34 to 35C.	Cold air/oxygenation blown in face of newborn is source of cold stress and is stimulus for increased consumption of oxygen and increased metabolic rate.	
	Use heat shields for small infants.	Heat shields will prevent heat loss by convection and reduce insensible water losses.	

Table 32-3   Transcutaneous Monitors

Type	Function and rationale	Nursing interventions
TCPO$_2$ Measures oxygen diffusion across the skin Clark electrode is heated to 44C (preterm) or 45C (term) to warm the skin beneath the electrode and promote diffusion of oxygen across the skin surface. PO$_2$ is measured when oxygen diffuses across the capillary membrane, skin, and electrode membrane (Gunderson & Kenner 1988).	When transcutaneous monitors are properly calibrated and electrodes are appropriately positioned they will provide reliable, continuous, noninvasive measurements of PO$_2$, PcO$_2$, and oxygen saturation. Readings vary when skin perfusion is decreased. Reliable as trend monitor. Frequent calibration necessary to overcome mechanical drift. Following membrane change, machine must "warm-up" one hour prior to initial calibration; otherwise, after turning it on, it must equilibrate for 30 min prior to calibration. When placed on infant values will be low until skin is heated; approximately 15 min required to stabilize. Second-degree burns are rare but can occur if electrodes remain in place too long. Decreased correlations noted with older infants (related to skin thickness); with infants with low cardiac output (decreased skin perfusion); and with hyperoxic infants. The adhesive that attaches the electrode may abrade the fragile skin of the preterm infant. May be used for both pre- and postductal monitoring of oxygenation for observations of shunting.	Use TCPO$_2$ to monitor trends of oxygenation with routine nursing care procedures. Clean electrode surface to remove electrolyte deposits; change solution and membrane once a week. Allow machine to stabilize before drawing arterial gases; note reading when gases are drawn and use values to correlate. Ensure airtight seal between skin surface and electrode; place electrodes on clean, dry skin on upper chest, abdomen, or inner aspect of thigh; avoid bony-prominences or excessive fatty areas. Change skin site and recalibrate at least every four hours; inspect skin for burns; if burns occur, use lowest temperature setting and change position of electrode more frequently. Adhesive discs may be cut to a smaller size or skin prep may be used under the adhesive circle only; allow membrane to touch skin surface at center.
Pulse Oximeter Monitors beat-to-beat arterial oxygen saturation. Microprocessor measures saturation by the absorption of red and infrared light as it passes through tissue. Changes in absorption related to blood pulsation through vessel determine saturation and pulse rate (Harbold 1989).	Calibration is automatic. Less dependent on perfusion than TCPO$_2$ and TCPCO$_2$; however, functions poorly if peripheral perfusion is decreased due to low cardiac output. Much more rapid response time than TCPO$_2$—offers "real-time" readings. Can be located on extremity, digit, or palm of hand leaving chest free, not affected by skin characteristics. Requires understanding of oxyhemoglobin dissociation curve. Pulse oximeter reading of 85%–90% reflects clinically safe range of saturation. Extreme sensitivity to movement; decreases if average of seventh or fourteenth beat is selected rather than beat-to-beat. Poor correlation with extreme hyperoxia.	Understand and use oxyhemoglobin dissociation curve. Monitor readings and correlate with arterial blood gases. Use disposable cuffs (reusable cuffs allow too much ambient light to enter and readings may be inaccurate).

assistance with high-frequency jet ventilations is a new therapeutic intervention that shows positive results.

Evaluation

Anticipated outcomes of nursing care include the following:

- The risk of RDS is promptly identified and early intervention is initiated.

- The newborn is free of respiratory distress and metabolic alterations.

- The parents verbalize their concerns about their baby's health problem/survival and understand the rationale behind management of their newborn.

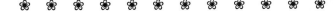

Transient Tachypnea of the Newborn (Type II Respiratory Distress Syndrome)

Some newborns, primarily AGA and near-term infants, develop progressive respiratory distress that resembles classic RDS. These infants have usually had some intrauterine or intrapartal asphyxia due to maternal oversedation, cesarean birth, maternal bleeding, prolapsed cord, breech birth, or maternal diabetes. The result is failure by the newborn to clear the airway of lung fluid, mucus, and other debris or an excess of fluid in the lungs due to aspiration of amniotic or tracheal fluid.

Usually little or no difficulty is experienced at the onset of breathing. However, shortly after admission to a nursery, expiratory grunting, flaring of the nares, and mild cynosis may be noted in room air. Tachypnea is usually present by 6 hours of age, with respiratory rates as high as 100 to 140 breaths per minute.

Medical Therapy

The goal of medical management is to identify the type of respiratory distress and to institute treatment.

Initial x-ray findings may be identical to those showing RDS within the first three hours. However, radiographs of infants with transient tachypnea usually reveal a generalized overexpansion of the lungs (hyperaeration of alveoli), which is identifiable principally by flattened contours of the diaphragm. Dense streaks (increased vascularity) radiate from the hilar region and represent engorgement of the lymphatics which are needed to clear alveolar fluid upon initiation of air breathing.

Ambient oxygen concentrations as high as 70% may be required to correct the cyanosis initially. Thereafter, oxygen requirements usually decrease over the first 48 hours, unlike in infants with RDS, whose oxygen needs increase during this time.

The infant should be improving by 24 to 48 hours, except for modest O_2 dependence (less than 30%). The duration of the clinical course of transient tachypnea is approximately four days (96 hours). Early respiratory and metabolic acidosis (with moderate elevations of PCO_2) is easily corrected. Ventilatory assistance is rarely needed, and most of these infants survive.

Radiographs are usually normal within a week and the infant is well within two to five days. If progressive deterioration occurs to the extent that assisted ventilation is required, a diagnosis of superimposed sepsis must be considered and treatment measures initiated. For nursing actions, see the Nursing Care Plan for Respiratory Distress Syndrome, page 1017.

Care of Newborn with Meconium Aspiration Syndrome

The presence of meconium in amniotic fluid indicates an asphyxial insult to the fetus before or during labor. The physiologic response to asphyxia is increased intestinal peristalsis, relaxation of the anal sphincter, and passage of meconium into the amniotic fluid.

Approximately 10% of all pregnancies will have meconium-stained fluid (Hudak & Jones 1990). This fluid may be aspirated into the tracheobronchial tree by the fetus in utero or during the first few breaths taken by the newborn. This aspiration is called **meconium aspiration syndrome** (MAS). This syndrome primarily affects term, SGA, and postterm newborns and those that have experienced a long labor.

Presence of meconium in the lungs produces a ball-valve action (air is allowed in but not exhaled), so that alveoli overdistend; rupture with pneumomediastinum or pneumothorax is a common occurrence. The meconium also initiates a chemical pneumonitis in the lung with oxygen and carbon dioxide trapping and hyperinflation. Secondary bacterial pneumonias are common. Clinical manifestations of MAS include: (a) fetal hypoxia in utero a few days or a few minutes prior to birth indicated by a sudden increase in fetal activity followed by diminished activity, slowing of fetal heart rate or weak and irregular heartbeat, loss of beat-to-beat variability and meconium staining of amniotic fluid; and (b) presence of signs of distress at birth, such as pallor, cyanosis, apnea, slow heartbeat, and low Apgar scores (below 6) at one and five minutes. Because of intrauterine asphyxia, meconium-stained neonates who have aspirated meconium are often depressed at birth and require resuscitative efforts to establish adequate respiratory effort.

After the initial resuscitation, the severity of clinical symptoms correlates with the extent of aspiration. These infants frequently require mechanical ventilation from birth due to immediate signs of distress (generalized cyanosis, tachypnea, and severe retractions). Later an overdistended, barrel-shaped chest with increased anteroposterior diameter is common. Auscultation reveals diminished air movement with prominent rales and rhonchi. Palpation of the infant's abdomen may reveal a displaced liver caused by diaphragmatic depression resulting from the overexpansion of the lungs. Staining of the skin, nails, and umbilical cord is usually present.

The chest x-ray film for neonates with MAS reveals nonuniform, coarse, patchy densities and hyperinflation (9- to 11-rib expansion). The densities are associated with focal areas of irregular aeration, some of which appear atelectatic or consolidated, while others appear emphysemic. Evidence of pulmonary air leak is frequently present. These infants have serious biochemical alterations, which include: (a) extreme metabolic acidosis resulting from the cardiopulmonary shunting and hypoperfusion; (b) extreme respiratory acidosis due to shunting and alveolar hypoventilation; and (c) extreme hypoxia, even in 100% O_2 concentrations and with ventilatory assistance. The extreme hypoxia is also caused by the cardiopulmonary shunting and resultant failure to oxygenate and can lead to persistent pulmonary hypertension (see page 1028).

Medical Therapy

The combined efforts of the obstetrician and pediatrician are needed to prevent MAS. The most effective form of preventive management is outlined as follows:

1. After the head of the newborn is born and the shoulders and chest are still in the birth canal the baby's oropharynx first then the nasopharynx are suctioned. (The same procedure is followed with a cesarean birth.) To decrease the possibility of acquired immunodeficiency syndrome (AIDS) transmission, wall suction is used rather than just a DeLee device, which the physician places in his or her mouth to create suction.

2. If the infant is vigorous and there is only thin meconium in the amniotic fluid, no special resuscitation is indicated.

3. If the infant is vigorous and there is thick meconium in the amniotic fluid, the glottis is visualized and suctioning of meconium from the trachea is done.

4. Any depressed infant (heart rate less than 100 beats per minute or poor respiratory effort with meconium staining), the glottis is visualized and the trachea suctioned (Hudak & Jones 1990).

If the newborn's head is not adequately suctioned on the perineum, respiratory or resuscitative efforts will push meconium into the airway and into the lungs. Stimulation of the newborn should be avoided to minimize respiratory movements. Further resuscitative efforts are undertaken as indicated, following the same principles mentioned earlier in this chapter, page 1008. Resuscitated neonates should be immediately transferred to the nursery for closer observation. An umbilical arterial line may be used for direct monitoring of arterial blood pressures; blood sampling for pH, and blood gases; and infusion of intravenous fluids, blood, or medications.

Treatment of the infant with MAS usually involves delivery of high ambient concentration and controlled ventilation. Low positive end-expiratory pressures (PEEP) are desired to avoid air leaks. Unfortunately, high pressures may be needed to cause sufficient expiratory expansion of obstructed terminal airways or to stabilize airways that are weakened by inflammation so that the most distal atelec-

tatic alveoli are ventilated. Systemic blood pressure and pulmonary blood flow must be maintained. Intravenous tolazoline (Priscoline) or isoproterenol (Isuprel) may be used to increase the pulmonary blood flow by overcoming the arterioles' vasoconstriction and pulmonary vasospasm, which has created a right-to-left cardiopulmonary shunt. Tolazoline must be used with extreme *caution,* as dramatic falls in blood pressure can occur. Tolazoline is usually used in conjunction with dopamine or dobutamine and/or volume expanders to maintain systemic blood pressure.

Treatment also includes chest physiotherapy (chest percussion, vibration, and drainage) to remove the debris. Prophylactic antibiotics are frequently given. Bicarbonate may be necessary for several days for severely ill newborns. Mortality in term or postterm infants is very high, because they are so difficult to oxygenate.

❀   *APPLYING THE NURSING PROCESS*   ❀

Nursing Assessment

During the intrapartal period, the nurse should observe for signs of fetal hypoxia and meconium staining of amniotic fluid. At birth, the nurse assesses the newborn for signs of distress. During the ongoing assessment of the newborn, the nurse carefully observes for complications such as pulmonary air leaks; anoxic cerebral injury manifested by cerebral edema and/or convulsions; anoxic myocardial injury evidenced by congestive heart failure or cardiomegaly; disseminated intravascular coagulation (DIC) resulting from hypoxic hepatic damage with depression of liver-dependent clotting factors; anoxic renal damage demonstrated by hematuria, oliguria, or anuria; fluid overload; sepsis secondary to bacterial pneumonia; and any signs of intestinal necrosis from ischemia, including gastrointestinal obstruction or hemorrhage.

Nursing Diagnosis

Nursing diagnoses that may apply to the newborn with meconium aspiration syndrome include the following:

- Ineffective gas exchange related to presence of respiratory distress secondary to aspiration of meconium and amniotic fluid during birth

- Alteration in nutrition: less than body requirements related to respiratory distress and increased energy requirements

- Ineffective family coping related to life-threatening illness in a full-term infant

Nursing Plan and Implementation

Initial interventions are primarily aimed at prevention of the aspiration by assisting with the removal of the meconium from the infant's oro- and nasopharynx prior to the first extrauterine breath to prevent aspiration.

When significant aspiration occurs, therapy is supportive with the primary goals of maintaining appropriate gas exchange and minimizing complications. Nursing interventions for the newborn after resuscitation should include: maintenance of adequate oxygenation and ventilation, temperature regulation, glucose strip test at 2 hours of age to check for hypoglycemia, observation of intravenous fluids, calculation of necessary fluids (which may be restricted in first 48 to 72 hours due to cerebral edema), and provision of caloric requirements.

Evaluation

Anticipated outcomes of nursing care include the following:

- The risk of MAS is promptly identified and early intervention is initiated.

- The newborn is free of respiratory distress and metabolic alterations.

- The parents verbalize their concerns about their baby's health problem/survival and understand the rationale behind management of their newborn.

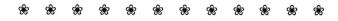

Care of the Newborn with Persistent Pulmonary Hypertension

Persistent pulmonary hypertension of the newborn (PPHN) is a serious disorder that may affect near-term, term, or postterm neonates. It has been called persistent fetal circulation (PFC) because the problems that occur are a result of right-to-left (R–L) shunting of blood away from the lungs and through the fetal ductus arteriosus and patent foramen ovale.

The disease was originally described only in newborns who had suffered severe perinatal asphyxia. It has since been associated with several events causing hypoxemia and acidosis: postmaturity syndrome, RDS, MAS, intrapartal asphyxia, pneumonia, Group B streptococcal sepsis, and diaphragmatic hernia. Many fetuses have problems that compromise fetal oxygenation prior to the onset of labor (Ward 1990).

During pregnancy, the fetal pulmonary vascular resistance (PVR) is high due to the lack of air and collapsed position of the lungs. After initiation of respiration at birth, the cord is clamped and systemic vascular resistance increases with the removal of the placental vascular bed. Expansion of the lungs opens the pulmonary circulation. The resulting decrease in the resistance of the pulmonary vasculature encourages flow of blood into the pulmonary vas-

cular bed and initiates the disappearance of the fetal R–L shunt. With oxygenation of the blood, the pulmonary circulation dilates further, the ductus narrows, and within a very short time, the adult circulatory pattern is established.

Depending on the cause, PPHN is classified as primary or secondary. Primary disease results from vascular changes prior to birth, which causes abnormally high PVR. The small arteries develop in the lung periphery as alveolar development occurs. These arteries, which develop along with the alveoli, are normally free of muscular coats. Muscular development progresses between birth and adolescence until full muscularization is present during adult life. Alveolar hypoxia in utero, regardless of the cause, can stimulate precocious muscularization. This early abnormal reconstruction of the arteries results in increased PVR, which interrupts the normal sequence of events that take place with the onset of respiration.

Secondary PPHN occurs when the initial sequences of respiration and change in circulation after birth are interrupted by events that increase the PVR. The increased vascular resistance causes a reversal of the blood flow, which opens the fetal shunts. Once this process has begun, it is self-perpetuating: Increased PVR leads to R–L shunting across the ductus, which leads to increased hypoxemia, further increasing the PVR. The cycle is difficult to interrupt, and clinical deterioration is rapid.

Medical Therapy

The first goal of medical management is early diagnosis of this disorder to halt the progressive worsening of the R–L shunt. Certain diagnostic tests are often used to evaluate the increased PVR and shunting:

1. *Simultaneous preductal and postductal blood gases.* The ductus enters the aorta below the area of the right subclavian and carotid arteries; thus preductal blood samples will have a higher oxygen content than postductal samples in infants with significant R–L shunting. Simultaneous pre- and postductal arterial blood gases demonstrate a 10% difference between the two PaO_2 values (>15 torr difference). Pre- and postductal transcutaneous monitors can also demonstrate ductal shunting.

2. *Hyperoxia-hyperventilation test.* Most PPHN infants have a "critical" PCO_2 level at which vasodilatation occurs. This PCO_2 level may be less than 20 torr in some infants. Once the critical PCO_2 is reached by manual hyperventilation, the resulting metabolic alkalosis causes pulmonary vasodilatation, which reverses the R–L shunt and improves oxygenation. A positive response to the hyperoxia-hyperventilation test is a rise in PaO_2 to greater than 100 torr with hyperventilation. The improved oxygenation can be noted clinically if the infant's mucus membranes turn pink. Arterial gases or

transcutaneous monitoring can be used to document the increased PaO_2.

3. *Echocardiography.* This procedure will demonstrate R–L shunting and a prolonged ratio of right ventricular ejection period to right ventricular ejection time in infants with PPHN.

The goal of therapeutic intervention is to lower the PVR and reverse the process of shunting. Maintenance of tissue oxygenation in the presence of R–L shunting presents the greatest therapeutic challenge but is essential to minimize complications.

Initial therapeutic efforts are directed at relieving the precipitating factors, if identified, to reverse the hypertension. In addition, aggressive ventilatory management is undertaken to decrease the PVR and increase oxygenation. Hyperventilation to achieve respiratory alkalosis (pH >7.55) will cause pulmonary vasodilatation, which increases oxygenation. To prevent respiratory interference and achieve hypocarbia, most infants require paralysis with a neuromuscular blocking agent such as pancuronium (Pavulon).

If hyperventilation alone does not lead to a decrease in the PVR, pharmacologic vasodilatation may be attempted by administration of intravenous tolazoline. Since tolazoline also induces systemic vasodilatation, dopamine and/or dobutamine may be required to maintain an adequate cardiac output to maintain the blood pressure.

Oxygenation and ventilation efforts continue until the PaO_2 can be consistently maintained greater than 100 torr. Even when this level is achieved, the improvement may be unstable, and reduction of ventilatory support must be made in extremely small increments with intensive surveillance to detect rapid negative responses. Alkalosis and hyperoxia may have to be maintained for several days to avoid sudden return to hypoxemia and increased PVR. Extracorporal membrane oxygenation (ECMO) has developed over the past five years and is now a therapeutic option for the newborn with PPHN who fails to respond to more conventional therapy.

❀ *APPLYING THE NURSING PROCESS* ❀

Nursing Assessment

The nurse assesses for the onset of symptoms, which usually occur in the first 12 to 24 hours of life. Affected newborns exhibit signs of respiratory distress (grunting, nasal flaring, tacypnea), with increased anteroposterior diameter and cyanosis. They typically fail to respond to conventional methods of oxygenation and ventilation. There is significant unexplained hypoxemia in the absence of congenital heart disease. The chest radiograph might show no evidence of pulmonary parenchymal disease (depending on the underlying disease). The hypoxemia and cyanosis associated with PPHN are characteristic of extreme changeability. Marked, rapid changes in PaO_2 and color are seen with agitation, stimulation, or therapeutic intervention (suctioning).

Nursing Diagnosis

The following diagnoses may apply to a newborn with PPHN:

- Alteration in oxygen and carbon dioxide exchange related to airway obstruction
- Alteration in cardiac output related to hypotension
- Ineffective family coping related to life-threatening illness in their full-term infant

Nursing Plan and Implementation

Prevention of Complications

Infants with PPHN are critically ill and require experienced, skilled nurses to provide optimal care with minimal manipulation. Any disturbance may cause agitation, which leads to hypoxemia. Therefore goals and priorities of care must be established. If a paralyzing agent is used, nursing care includes monitoring the newborn's response to artificial oxygenation and mechanical ventilation. The nurse ensures that the oxygen is delivered in correct amounts and route and records the percentage of oxygen flow. The ventilator settings are checked frequently and recorded every two hours. The nurse carefully suctions the endotracheal tube every two hours or as necessary while assessing the effect of the procedure on the baby's oxygenation and perfusion (see Procedure 32–1). The amount and type of secretions are noted. The nurse carefully assesses arterial blood gases and notifies the clinician if the results are out of the acceptable range. Trancutaneous monitoring is essential for identification of activities that may compromise the infant's status. (See Table 32–3 for nursing interventions required for transcutaneous monitoring.) Continuous monitoring of vital signs and blood pressure is required, and careful inspection of the skin during positioning is necessary to avoid pressure necrosis.

Pharmacologic vasodilation may lead to precipitous central hypotension, which must be quickly identified and corrected. The infant is monitored for other side effects of tolazoline therapy (increased gastric secretion, gastrointestinal bleeding, and oliguria).

With aggressive ventilation, potential for pneumothorax exists. The nurse can best prevent complications by advanced preparation and close monitoring for signs of compromise. (See discussion of pneumothorax, page 1033, for appropriate nursing interventions.)

Parent Education

Many infants suffering PPHN are born at or near term at a time when parents least expect problems—especially life-threatening problems—to occur. The magnitude of the infant's illness and the rapid deterioration may be overwhelming to parents. The nurse should assess their level of understanding and assist them by providing information

Endotracheal Suctioning

Nursing Action

Objective: Minimize potential for pulmonary infection through cross-contamination.

Assess respiratory status to determine necessity for suctioning.

Gather all necessary equipment: catheters, suction machine, disposable sterile suction tubing, saline (no preservatives), sterile syringe/needle, and gloves (not powdered). Ensure that gloves, catheters, and liquefying solutions are sterile.

Maintain sterile technique throughout entire suctioning procedure.

Discard catheter, glove, and saline after each procedure.

Set wall suction for not more than 80 mm Hg.

Objective: Alleviate partial or total airway obstruction in support of cell oxygenation.

Monitor transcutaneous readings during suctioning procedure and supplement with increased oxygen as needed.

Position and immobilize infant.

Using sterile technique, don sterile glove; hook up appropriate suction catheter; lubricate tip.

Place sterile normal saline in a sterile specimen cup or unit dose plastic container.

If infant is intubated:

1. Disconnect source of oxygenation from newborn just prior to entry of suction catheter.
2. Assistant should stabilize endotracheal tube while suctioning.

3. Insert catheter without applied suction into tube the distance from the proximal airway to no more than 1 cm below the end of the endotracheal tube. (This can be determined by noting cm markings on tube or by using calculations for oral-carinal distance.)

Rationale

Infant should be suctioned only as often as necessary to maintain patent airway and adequate oxygenation.

In healthy individual, lower respiratory tract is free of pathogenic organisms.

Once equipment is moistened and contaminated with body flora and mucus, it becomes a culture bed for noxious organism growth.

Mucosal hemorrhages and tissue invagination occur more frequently when higher pressure is used.

Suctioning physically removes oxygen from airways. In addition, it mechanically occludes airways and therefore diminishes potential for oxygenation. It usually stimulates coughing and increases work of breathing, thereby increasing tissue demand for oxygen.

It is quite difficult to suction alert infant successfully without restraint. An assistant should be employed to ensure effective, atraumatic suctioning in infants.

"Whistle-tip" catheter should be used for respiratory tract suctioning, because it tends to be less traumatizing to tissues.

Catheter size should be no more than ½ the size of lumen to be suctioned in order to minimize hypoxemia due to airway obstruction.

Prelubrication of catheter is essential to minimize tissue trauma with subsequent obstructive edema.

Suction applied while entering airway increases removal of oxygen from airways.

During suctioning, tube can be easily dislodged and increases potential for tissue invagination once catheter tip passes end of tube. Passing the suction catheter more than 1 cm beyond the endotracheal tube risks damaging the carina and creating pneumothoraces (Figure 32–8).

(continued)

PROCEDURE (continued)

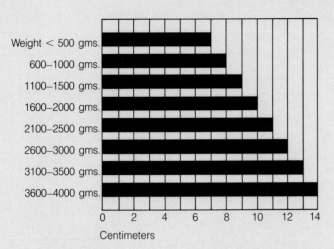

Weight < 500 gms.		
600–1000 gms.		
1100–1500 gms.		
1600–2000 gms.		
2100–2500 gms.		
2600–3000 gms.		
3100–3500 gms.		
3600–4000 gms.		

Centimeters: 0 2 4 6 8 10 12 14

Note: Measure catheter along appropriate line for weight. Add length E-T tube that is sticking out of mouth. This is the maximum safe distance for insertion of suction catheter through E-T tube.

Figure 32–8 Safe length for endotracheal suctioning (From Anderson D, Chandra R: Pneumothorax secondary to perforation of sequential bronchi by suction catheter. J Pediatr Surg 1976; 11:687)

Nursing Action

4. Apply suction by placing thumb of assistive hand over vent port or Y-connector (Figure 32-9).

Rationale

Placing thumb over venting device closes negative pressure system, which allows atmospheric pressure to push secretions and debris into catheter, facilitating their removal.

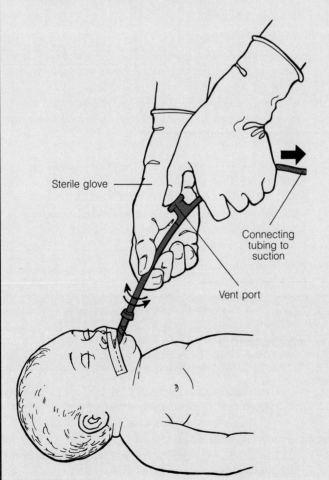

Sterile glove

Connecting tubing to suction

Vent port

Figure 32–9 Suctioning with endotracheal tube

(continued)

PROCEDURE (*continued*)

Nursing Action	Rationale
5. Slowly withdraw catheter in a pill-rolling rotation.	Rotating catheter in a slow, steady fashion maximizes catheter access to secretions while minimizing potential for tissue invagination.
6. Clear catheter with sterile saline.	
7. After each suction attempt, ventilate for a few breaths to reinflate atelectatic areas.	Hypoxia insult with a drop in PaO_2 occurs during suction efforts. Suction, the application of negative pressure to the airway, decreases by 50% the pulmonary compliance and tidal volume. Suction creates pulmonary atelectasis.
8. If tenacious secretions are encountered, instill normal saline with syringe (needleless) into tube prior to suctioning.	Instillation of normal saline liquefies and loosens secretions.
If infant is not intubated: After having failed to get infant to cough voluntarily in effective manner, follow procedure for suctioning intubated infant with these exceptions:	Suctioning to clear airways should be employed only when infant is unable to clear own airways effectively by use of cough reflex. It should be considered a last resort.
1. Enter airway via nasopharynx, advancing catheter into trachea on inspiration.	Inspiration opens glottis and tends to entrain catheter along with inspired air. Achieving coordination with inspiration is often quite easy with pediatric clients, because they are frequently crying involuntarily during procedure. Instillation of liquefying agents directly into trachea in unintubated infant is not possible. Indirect means must be used.
2. Attempt to liquefy tenacious secretions by humidification via mist tent, face mask, or hand-held nebulizer.	
Objective: Minimize iatrogenic hypoxemia secondary to suctioning.	
Suction only when absolutely necessary.	Always assess need for suctioning. There should never be standing orders such as "Suction every hour."
Limit each catheter insertion to no more than 10 sec. Reoxygenate newborn (monitoring transcutaneous readings) between each insertion and at conclusion of procedure.	Limiting suction time and frequent reoxygenation counterbalance the mechanical obstruction of airway and removal of available oxygen.
Remove catheter with suction applied as soon as infant begins to cough.	Holding catheter in airway while infant coughs can deprive infant of needed inspiratory volume at end of cough because of airway obstruction by catheter.
During procedure, assess infant for signs of bradycardia.	Suctioning can cause vagal response in form of bradycardia, which, if unchecked, can lead to asystole.
Objective: Record information on infant's record.	
Record infant's response during and after the procedure. Also record amount and type of secretions obtained.	Provides record of infant's response to procedure.

about their baby's condition and therapies in easily understandable terms.

Attachment becomes difficult when the infant responds poorly to touching (as seen by decreased PaO_2). Parents can be encouraged to talk very softly to their infant since this will usually not compromise the baby's condition. Continuity of nursing care is helpful since it will be less threatening for the parents to relate to a smaller group of nurses.

Evaluation

Anticipated outcomes of nursing care include the following:

- The risks for development of persistent pulmonary hypertension (PPHN) are identified early, and immediate action is taken to minimize the development of sudden, severe illness.

- The newborn is free of respiratory distress and establishes effective respiratory function.

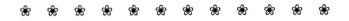

- The parents verbalize their concerns about their baby's illness and understand the rationale behind the management of their newborn.

Care of the Newborn with Complications Due to Respiratory Therapy

Oxygen and mechanical ventilation, while required as therapeutic interventions to reduce hypoxia, hypercarbia, ischemia, and infarction to vital organs, may also have harmful effects. The concentrations of ambient oxygen administered to the neonate must be titrated according to oxygen tension within arterial blood. Pulmonary air leaks occur in approximately 15% of mechanically ventilated newborns. In many cases the air leaks are a consequence of injury due to the disease rather than the mechanical ventilation.

Pulmonary Interstitial Emphysema

Pulmonary interstitial emphysema (PIE) is the accumulation of air in the tissues of the lungs. Extraalveolar air collections are most common with use of positive pressure ventilation. Air collections outside the lung are a function of compliance of the lung and use of increased pressures to ventilate. Overdistention of alveolar air spaces may progress to PIE when rupture occurs and air escapes into the interstitial spaces. Air dissects along perivascular spaces but not into the pleural space or mediastinum. This condition is a precursor of pneumothorax or pneumomediastinum.

Pneumothorax

Pneumothorax, a common complication of respiratory therapy, is an accumulation of air in the thoracic cavity between the parietal and visceral pleura. Pneumothorax occurs when alveoli are overdistended, usually by excessive intraalveolar pressure and rupture; air then leaks into the thoracic cavity. Excessive intraalveolar pressure is a result of stiff, noncompliant lungs and the use of assisted positive pressure ventilation with high inspiratory pressure. Meconium aspiration with subsequent obstruction of the airway and a ball-valve phenomenon produces poor lung compliance and trapping of air in the alveoli. Pneumothorax frequently develops as a complication.

Pneumothorax in the newborn causes several physiologic changes: collapse of the lung; compression of the heart and lungs and compromise of venous return to the right heart with mediastinal air; and development of tension in the pleural space. Symptoms of pneumothorax include a sudden unexplained deterioration in the newborn's condition; decreased breath sounds; apnea; bradycardia; cyanosis; increased oxygen requirements; higher PCO_2; decrease in pH; mottled, asymmetric chest expansion; decreased arterial blood pressure; shocklike appearance; and a shift in the apical cardiac impulses to the side opposite the pneumothorax.

X-ray examination is the main method of diagnosing a pneumothorax. Transillumination of the chest can be used when it is not possible to obtain an x-ray series rapidly. Transillumination is the visualization of light transmitted through the air in the affected side of the chest. Follow-up radiographs should always be done to confirm the diagnosis and extent of the pneumothorax.

Pneumothorax is a life-threatening situation for the neonate and demands immediate removal of the accumulated air. The air is aspirated with a syringe attached to an 18-gauge intercath or 23-gauge butterfly needle and inserted into the second or third intercostal space midclavicular line when the newborn is supine. This procedure is done only as an emergency and carries a risk of damaging the myocardium with needle tracks as the air is evacuated. The procedure must be done only by skilled and specifically trained personnel.

For complete resolution of the pneumothorax a No. 10 Fr. chest tube will be placed and connected to continuous negative pressure (10 to 15 cm H_2O) suction with an underwater seal.

Bronchopulmonary Dysplasia

Bronchopulmonary dysplasia (BPD) typically occurs in very compromised low-birth-weight (LBW) infants who require oxygen therapy and assisted mechanical ventilation for the treatment of respiratory distress syndrome. It has only rarely been associated with neonatal pneumonia, MAS, PPHN, congenital cardiac disease, and other congenital anomalies. The incidence of BPD is approximately 15% to 38%, with individual reports ranging widely due to varying methods of grading the severity of the disease (Houska Lund 1990). The cause is multifactorial, with oxygen, endotracheal ventilation, barotrauma (leads to inflammatory changes and leakage of fluid into the interstitial spaces), mechanical ventilation, patent ductus arteriosus (PDA), overhydration, PIE, LGA, and LBW all being implicated.

The pulmonary pathology of BPD has been historically described by Northway et al (1967) as having four progressive stages according to radiographic findings and clinical findings (Houska Lund 1990). Stage 1 is clinically and radiographically indistinguishable from RDS. Lacking surfactant, the alveoli collapse; the resultant ischemia leads to necrosis of the surrounding tissue and capillaries. The sloughed necrotic material fills the terminal bronchioles, causing mucosal and ciliated cell damage. In stage 2, severe lung disease, the radiographs progress to a characteristic "white-out" with opacification of lung fields and indistinguishable cardiac borders. This clinical picture is similar to severe RDS with the complications of PDA and pulmonary edema. During stage 3, or transition to chronic lung disease, regeneration begins in the lining cells of the bronchioles. Fibrous tissue forms as connective tissue cells proliferate. This leads to distortion and eventual rupture of the alveoli with small amounts of air being trapped in the interstitium. These emphysematous areas surrounded by collapsed alveoli are seen as small cystic light areas on x-ray films. Increasing PCO_2 despite adequate mechanical ventilation. Stage 4 is characterized by hypertrophy of the smooth muscles surrounding the bronchi and bronchioles, which leads to narrowing of the airways. During this period, the mucus-producing cells also hypertrophy, and the increase in mucus production leads to further airway obstruction. Thickening of the pulmonary arteries and capillary membranes leads to narrowing of these vessels, which causes pulmonary hypertension. Cor pulmonale with right ventricular hypertrophy and cardiomegaly may occur secondary to the pulmonary hypertension. Radiographs show enlargements of the emphysematous areas.

Medical Therapy

Prevention of all the factors associated with BPD is not possible. However, optimal physiologic maintenance will minimize the complications. The goals of therapeutic intervention for the newborn with BPD are to provide adequate oxygenation and ventilation, optimal nutrition, and supportive care to ensure adequate rates of growth and development.

Because of the chronic nature of this disease, therapeutic intervention must be individualized to meet the specific needs of the infant. Of prime importance is maintenance of adequate gas exchange. At each stage of BPD, pulmonary pathologic changes interfere with adequate oxygenation and normal ventilation. Ventilatory assistance and increased ambient (environmental) oxygen must be regulated precisely by close monitoring of blood gases to prevent episodic hypoxemia or hyperoxemia and hypercarbia. Antibiotics are indicated for secondary infections. Diuretics and fluid restriction are frequently used to control pulmonary fluid retention and to improve lung function (Houska Lund 1990); electrolyte supplements are necessary to offset the results of chronic diuretic therapy. In addition, bronchodilators are indicated to decrease airway resistance and to control bronchospasm. Serial echocardiography is used to monitor cardiac response to the chronic pulmonary disease. Periodic digitalization may be required if cor pulmonale develops.

❀   *APPLYING THE NURSING PROCESS*   ❀

Nursing Assessment

At each stage of BPD, the infant exhibits recognizable clinical signs that reflect the pulmonary pathologic changes. Nursing assessment is based on a knowledge of these stages.

In stage 1, the infant exhibits typical signs of RDS with audible grunting, nasal flaring, and retractions. Due to the extensive alveolar damage, the infant is hypoxic and requires supplemental oxygen and assisted ventilation.

During stage 2, when the cellular debris fills the lumens of the bronchi and bronchioles, the infant has increased pulmonary secretions that may interfere with extubation. With progression to stage 3, the alveoli rupture and the capillary membranes thicken. This leads to separation of the capillaries from the alveoli and impairment of oxygen and carbon dioxide exchange. The infant's oxygen dependency becomes apparent and he or she begins to retain carbon dioxide, which prevents extubation. Lymphatic distortion leads to pulmonary interstitial fluid retention and evidence of diffuse rales with auscultation.

The hypertrophy of the bronchiolar smooth muscles characteristic of stage 4 increases the airway resistance and the risk of bronchospasm. During this stage infants will manifest bronchospasm by intermittent wheezing respirations, cyanosis, and continued supplemental oxygen requirements. Marked carbon dioxide retention continues to be a problem and ventilator dependency may result. Pulmonary fluid retention and mucus production will be manifested by audible rales and rhonchi, secretions, and chronic cough.

Nursing Diagnosis

Nursing diagnoses that may apply to a baby with BPD include the following:

- Impaired gas exchange related to chronic retention of carbon dioxide and borderline oxygenation secondary to fibrosis of lungs
- Ineffective airway clearance related to chronic intubation and increased secretion secondary to BPD
- Ineffective parental coping related to prolonged hospitalization and decreased opportunities to hold the baby

Nursing Plan and Implementation

Maintenance of Oxygenation   The nurse observes carefully any changes in the newborn's oxygenation. Special attention must be given to maintaining the prescribed oxygen concentration during all activities. Since the infant is oxygen dependent, the oxygen level must be maintained, especially during periods of stress, such as when the infant is crying; when blood is drawn; while starting an IV; and during an LP, suctioning, chest physiotherapy (CPT), and feeding.

A decrease in the arterial oxygen levels will increase the risk of pulmonary hypertension or cor pulmonale. The nurse obtains blood gases based on the institution's chronic blood gas protocol—for example, every three days, 20 minutes after a permanent change in ambient oxygen concentration (FiO_2), or more frequently if the infant experiences increasing respiratory distress or increasing lethargy.

Postural drainage, CPT, and vibration followed by suctioning are carried out with close attention to the baby's tolerance. It is essential to time the care activities with rest periods to avoid fatiguing the infant. The nurse maintains the infant's body temperature, as hypothermia or hyperthermia will increase oxygen consumption and may increase oxygen requirements. Positioning on the abdomen helps the baby maintain higher transcutaneous oxygen saturation ($TcPO_2$) and improved ventilation. Providing for adequate nutrition enhances formation of new alveoli and enlargement of the airway diameter.

Prevention of Infection Infants with BPD are very susceptible to infection; therefore, it is important to discourage anyone with early signs of infectious disease from having contact with the baby. The infant's behavior and vital signs should be monitored for changes that might indicate early developing infection. Changes in color, quantity, or quality of pulmonary secretions are noted and reported. The frequency of CPT and suctioning may need to be increased.

Provision of Adequate Nutrition The nurse assists in providing adequate nutrition and monitors the amount of calories the newborn ingests and the energy expended during the feeding process. If possible, at least 90 cal/kg/day should be given to the infant, with increases daily until at least 130 cal/kg/day are taken. As soon as tolerated, a 24-calorie formula for preterm infants is started, especially if the baby is on fluid restriction. More oxygen may be required during feeding, and the least energy-consuming feeding method should be used. If the feeding schedule is too stressful, smaller, more frequent feedings may be initiated (see Chapter 31).

Providing adequate nutritional intake becomes a major nursing task. Infants with BPD frequently experience negative oral sensations due to suctioning and intubation, which can adversely affect their transition to nipple or spoon feeding. In addition, most infants receive numerous, possibly unpalatable, medications with meals. Attempts must be made to include pleasurable activities such as cuddling at mealtime to develop positive associations with appropriate feeding behaviors (Figure 32–10).

Monitoring of Medications Bronchodilators, diuretics, electrolyte supplements, and high-calorie supplements may be used in the medical management of the BPD infant. Appropriate timing of administration is essential to maintain adequate blood levels. The nurse must monitor the infant for toxic effects of the medication and adverse effects of the therapy (for example, electrolyte imbalance, such as hypokalemia, and fractures as a result of diuretic therapy).

Provision of Sensory Stimulation Since BPD infants require prolonged hospitalization, the nurse should give special attention to formulating a program of early stimulation activities. Psychomotor delays are seen frequently in these infants and are most likely due in part to prolonged exposure to the hospital environment. Since their tolerance level for activity is limited due to their illness, activities must be individualized for each baby.

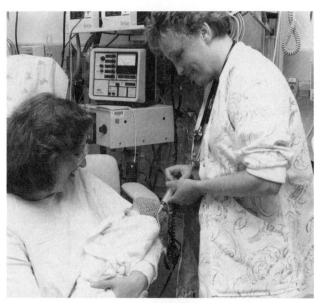

Figure 32–10 The baby with BPD has ongoing oxygen and nutritional needs as well as the need for gentle individualized care

Parent Education The birth of a premature infant causes significant stress to the family. When the infant develops BPD and the family becomes aware of the implications of chronic illness and prolonged hospitalization, they may experience despair and find it difficult to cope with this added burden. The nurse can help the family cope by encouraging them to take an active role in their infant's daily activities. Their involvement will help dispel feelings of inadequacy and prepare them to perform the unique tasks necessary to meet their infant's needs (Houska Lund 1990). Prior to discharge, parents must be taught to evaluate their infant's tolerance of activities and to recognize signs of distress due to poor oxygenation, inadequate ventilation, infection, fluid retention, and bronchospasm. The process of learning about the treatment of their infant's BPD can best be accomplished by a program of parent-infant caretaking activities supervised by the nurse while the infant is hospitalized. The chronicity of the disease requires that the parents be taught the essentials of problem recognition so that they can cope with the infant's special problems after discharge.

Evaluation

Anticipated outcomes of nursing care include the following:

● The parents understand the causes, risks, therapy options, and nursing care involved in the care of their newborn with BPD.

● The parents participate in their newborn's care and show attachment behaviors.

● The parents are able to cope with their frustrations and begin to use outside resources as needed.

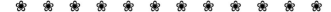

Care of the Newborn with Cold Stress

Cold stress is excessive heat loss resulting in the use of compensatory mechanisms (such as increased respirations and nonshivering thermogenesis) to maintain core body temperature. Heat loss that results in cold stress occurs in the newborn through the mechanisms of evaporation, convection, conduction, and radiation. (See Chapter 27 for a detailed discussion of thermoregulation.) Heat loss at birth that leads to cold stress can play a significant role in the severity of RDS and the ultimate outcome for the infant.

The amount of heat lost by an infant depends to a large extent on the actions of the nurse or care giver. Both preterm and SGA newborns are at risk for cold stress because they have decreased adipose tissue, brown fat stores, and glycogen available for metabolism.

As discussed in Chapter 27, the newborn infant's major source of heat production in nonshivering thermogenesis (NST) is brown fat metabolism. The ability of an infant to respond to cold stress by NST is impaired in the presence of several conditions:

- Hypoxemia (PO_2 less than 50)
- Intracranial hemorrhage or any CNS abnormality
- Hypoglycemia (blood glucose < 40 mg/dL)

When these conditions occur, the infant's temperature should be monitored more closely and the neutral thermal environment conscientiously maintained. It is important for the nurse to recognize these conditions and treat them as soon as possible.

The metabolic consequences of cold stress can be devastating and potentially fatal to an infant. Oxygen requirements are raised, glucose use increases, acids are released into the bloodstream, and surfactant production decreases. The effects are graphically depicted in Figure 32–11.

Nursing Care

The nurse observes for signs of cold stress. These include increased respirations, decrease in skin temperature, de-

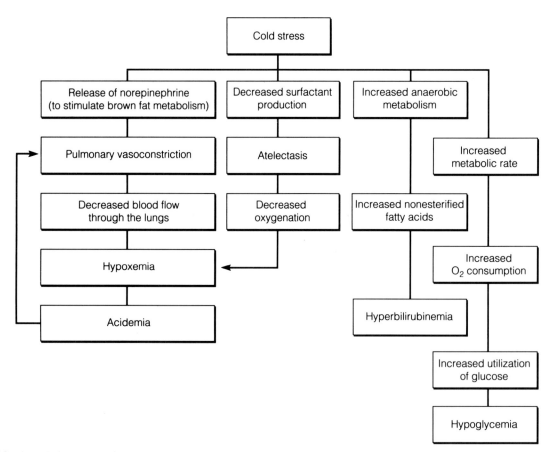

Figure 32–11 Cold stress schematic

crease in peripheral perfusion, appearance of hypoglycemia, and the possible development of metabolic acidosis.

Skin temperature assessments are used because initial response to cold stress is vasoconstriction, resulting in a decrease in skin temperature; therefore, monitoring rectal temperature is not satisfactory. A decrease in rectal temperature means that the infant has long-standing cold stress with a decreased ability to maintain core body temperature.

If a decrease in skin temperature is noted, the nurse determines whether hypoglycemia is present. Hypoglycemia is a result of the metabolic effects of cold stress and is suggested by glucose strip values below 45 mg/mL, tremors, irritability or lethargy, apnea, or seizure activity.

If cold stress occurs, the following nursing interventions should be initiated:

- The newborn is warmed slowly since rapid temperature elevation may cause apnea.
- Skin temperature is monitored every 15 minutes to determine if the infant's temperature is increasing.
- The infant is placed and maintained in a neutral thermal environment.

The presence of anaerobic metabolism is assessed and interventions initiated for the resulting metabolic acidosis. Attempts to burn brown fat increase oxygen consumption, lactic acid levels, and metabolic acidosis. Hypoglycemia may be reversed by adequate glucose intake. See the section on Care of the Newborn with Hypoglycemia for interventions.

Care of the Newborn with Hypoglycemia

Hypoglycemia is the most common metabolic disorder occurring in IDM, SGA, and preterm AGA newborns. The pathophysiology of hypoglycemia differs for each classification.

AGA preterm infants have not been in utero a sufficient time to store glycogen and fat. Therefore, they have very low glycogen and fat stores and a decreased ability to carry out gluconeogenesis. This situation is further aggravated by increased use of glucose by the tissues (especially the brain and heart) during stress and illness (chilling, asphyxia, sepsis, and RDS).

Infants of White's class A–C or type I diabetic mothers (women with diagnosed, suspected, or gestational diabetes) have increased stores of glycogen and fat. Circulating insulin and insulin responsiveness are higher when compared with other newborns. Because the high glucose loads present in utero stop at birth, the neonate experiences rapid and profound hypoglycemia. The SGA infant has used up glycogen and fat stores because of intrauterine malnutrition and has a blunted hepatic enzymatic response with which to produce and use glucose. Any newborn who is stressed at birth (from asphyxia or cold) also quickly uses up available glucose stores and becomes hypoglycemic.

Hypoglycemia is defined as a blood glucose below 30 mg/dL in the first 72 hours and below 40 mg/dL after the first three days. It may also be defined as a glucose strip result below 45 mg/dL when corroborated with laboratory blood glucose value (Yeh 1991). (See Procedure 32–2.)

Medical Therapy

The goal of medical management includes early identification of hypoglycemia through observation and screening of newborns at risk. The baby may be asymptomatic, or any of the following may occur:

- Lethargy, jitteriness
- Poor feeding
- Vomiting
- Pallor
- Apnea, irregular respirations, respiratory distress, cyanosis
- Hypotonia, possible loss of swallowing reflex
- Tremors, jerkiness, seizure activity
- High-pitched cry

Differential diagnosis of an infant with nonspecific hypoglycemic symptoms includes determining if the infant has any of the following:

- CNS disease
- Sepsis
- Metabolic aberrations
- Polycythemia
- Congenital heart disease
- Drug withdrawal
- Temperature instability
- Hypocalcemia

Aggressive treatment is recommended after a single low blood glucose value if the infant shows any of these symptoms.

Provision of adequate caloric intake is important. Early breast or formula feeding is one of the major preventive approaches. If early feeding or intravenous glucose is started to meet the recommended fluid and caloric needs, the blood glucose is likely to remain above the hypoglycemic level. Intravenous infusions of a dextrose solution (5% to 10%) begun immediately after birth should prevent hypoglycemia. However, in the very small AGA infant infusions of 10% dextrose solution may cause *hyper*glycemia to develop, requiring an alteration in the glucose concentration. Infants require 6 to 10 mg/kg/min of glucose to maintain normal glucose concentrations (Yeh 1991). There-

Glucose Chemstrip Test Using Accu-Check II Machine

Nursing Action

Objective: Assemble equipment

Gather the following equipment:

1. Lancet (do not use needles)
2. Alcohol swabs
3. 2 × 2 sterile gauze squares
4. Small Band-Aid ™
5. Glucose strips and bottle
6. Gloves

Wash hands before and after touching infant and equipment; then apply gloves.

Objective: Prepare infant's heel for procedure

Select clear, previously unpunctured site. Clean site by rubbing vigorously with 70% isopropyl alcohol swab, followed by dry gauze square. Grasp lower leg and heel so as to impede venous return slightly.

Objective: Minimize trauma at puncture site.

Blot dry site completely before lancing.

With quick piercing motion, puncture lateral heel with microlancet, being careful not to puncture too deeply (Figure 32–12). Toes are acceptable sites if necessary.

Rationale

All necessary equipment must be ready to ensure that blood sample is collected at time and in manner necessary. Do not use needles because of danger of nicking periosteum. Warm heel for five to ten sec prior to heel stick with a warm wet wrap or specially designed chemical heat pad to facilitate flow of blood.

To implement universal precautions and prevent nosocomial infections.

Selection of previously unpunctured site minimizes risk of infection and excessive scar formation. Friction produces local heat, which aids vasodilation.
Impeding venous return facilitates extraction of blood sample from puncture site.

Alcohol is irritating to injured tissue and may also produce hemolysis.

The lateral heel is the site of choice because it precludes damaging the posterior tibial nerve and artery, plantar artery, and important longitudinally oriented fat pad of the heel, which in later years could impede walking.
This is especially important for infant undergoing multiple heel stick procedures. Optimal penetration is 4 mm.

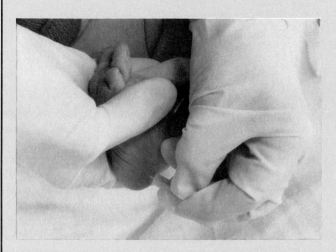

Figure 32–12   Glucose chem. strip test (heel stick)

(continued)

Nursing Action

Objective: Ensure accurate blood sampling.

After puncture is made, allow first drop of blood to touch both test pads on Chemstrip, making sure to cover both yellow and white squares completely (Figure 32–13).

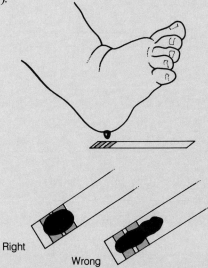

Right

Wrong

If Dextrostix reagent strip was used, first drop of blood would be discarded.

Objective: Read reagent strip via Accu-Check II machine.

If using Accu-Check II machine,

Immediately press the TIME button. The meter will count to 60 but emit 3 high beeps on 57, 58, 59 then one low beep on 60. This is a warning to prepare for wiping the blood from the test strip. Wipe blood from test strips with clean dry cotton ball using moderate pressure when display reads 60. Do not leave any blood on test pad.

Machine will continue to count to 120 seconds. While meter is counting, turn test strip on side, with the test pads facing the On/Off button, and insert the reacted test strip into the test strip adaptor. *The strip must be inserted before the display reads* 120.

When the display reads 120, a high beep will be emitted, followed by the blood sugar value on the display screen in mg/dL. Read the blood sugar value on the display screen.

HHH = blood sugar > 500 mg/dL. Wait an additional minute and take the reacted test strip out of the meter and compare it to the color chart on the side of the Chemstrip bG vial to estimate results up to 800 mg/dL.

LLL = blood sugar is lower than the reading range of the instrument (less than 10 mg/dL). Values below 20 mg/dL have not been confirmed clinically.

Rationale

The first drop of blood is used for accuracy.

Figure 32–13   Glucose strip drop of blood

The first drop is usually discarded because it tends to be minutely diluted with tissue fluid from puncture.

For accurate results, directions must be followed closely, and reagent strips must be fresh. False low readings may be caused by the following:

1. Timing
2. Blood left on test strip

(continued)

PROCEDURE 32–2(continued)

Nursing Action	Rationale
Objective: Prevent excessive bleeding.	
Apply folded gauze square to puncture site and secure firmly with bandage.	A pressure dressing should be applied to puncture site to stop bleeding.
Check puncture site frequently for first hour after sample.	Active infants sometimes kick or rub their dressings off and can bleed profusely from puncture site, especially if bandage becomes moist or is rubbed excessively against crib sheet.
Objective: Record findings on infant's record.	
Record test results. Report immediately any results under 45 mg/dL or over 175 mg/dL.	Recording of infant's results assists in identifying possible complications.

---

fore, an intravenous glucose solution should be calculated based on body weight of the infant, with blood glucose tests to determine adequacy of the infusion treatment.

A rapid infusion of 25% to 50% dextrose *is contraindicated* because it may lead to profound rebound hypoglycemia following an initial brief increase. Hypoglycemia resulting from hyperinsulinemia may be helped by administration of long-acting epinephrine. Epinephrine promotes glycogen conversion to glucose; it is also an antiinsulin agent. In more severe cases of hypoglycemia, corticosteroids may be administered. It is thought that steroids enhance gluconeogenesis from noncarbohydrate protein sources (Yeh 1991).

The prognosis for untreated hypoglycemia is poor. It may result in permanent, untreatable CNS damage or death (see Research Note).

❀ *APPLYING THE NURSING PROCESS* ❀

Nursing Assessment

The objective of assessment is to identify newborns at risk and to screen symptomatic infants. For newborns who are diagnosed as having hypoglycemia, assessment is ongoing with careful monitoring of glucose values. Glucose strips, urine dipsticks, and urine volume (above 1 to 3 mL/kg/hr) are evaluated frequently for osmotic diuresis and glycosuria.

Nursing Diagnosis

The following diagnoses may apply to the newborn with hypoglycemia:

- Alteration in nutrition: less than body requirements related to increased glucose use secondary to physiologic stress
- Ineffective breathing pattern related to tachypnea and apnea

- Pain related to frequent heel sticks for glucose monitoring

Nursing Plan and Implementation

Monitoring of Glucose Levels

When caring for a preterm AGA infant, blood glucose levels should be monitored using glucose strips or laboratory determinations every four to eight hours for the first day of life, and daily or as necessary thereafter. The IDM should be monitored hourly for the first several hours after birth, as this is the time when precipitous falls in glucose are most likely. In the SGA newborn, symptoms usually appear between 24 and 72 hours of age; occasionally they may begin as early as 3 hours of age. Infants who are below the tenth percentile on the intrauterine growth curve should have blood sugar assessments at least every eight hours until four days of age or more frequently if any symptoms develop.

Calculation of glucose requirements and maintenance of intravenous glucose will be necessary for any symptomatic infant with low serum glucose levels. Careful attention to glucose monitoring is again required when the transition from intravenous to oral feedings is attempted. Titration of intravenous glucose may be required until the infant is able to take adequate amounts of formula or breast milk to maintain a normal blood sugar level.

Decreasing Physiologic Stress

The method of feeding greatly influences glucose and energy requirements. In addition, the therapeutic nursing measure of nonnutritive sucking during gavage feedings has been reported to increase the baby's daily weight gain and lead to earlier bottle/breast feeding and discharge (Gill et al 1988). *Nonnutritive sucking* may also lower activity levels, which allows newborns to conserve their energy stores. Activity can increase energy requirements; crying

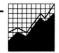

Research Note

Clinical Application of Research

Claudia Beckman (1990) designed a study to compare term and postterm infants on their ability to regulate their temperature and glucose for the first 24 hours. The study theorized that the placenta may become dysfunctional with postmaturity. The fetus's glycogen and fat stores may become depleted, compromising the newborn's ability to regulate glucose. Difficulty with glucose control may lead to problems with temperature regulation. Hypothermia was defined as below 36.1C, and hypoglycemia was a blood glucose level of 40 mg/dL or below.

Results of the study demonstrated that while the two groups of mothers did not differ by age, number of previous pregnancies, total weight gain, and other variables, the postterm mothers had a longer average length of labor—17 hours as compared to 13 hours for the term mothers. Also, labor for the postterm mothers was more likely to fail to progress than the term comparison mothers. Postterm infants exhibited more meconium-stained amniotic fluid, wasting, and neonatal peeling of the skin, they weighed more and were longer, but no difference was found in placental weight and head circumference.

No relationship was found between gestational age and temperature regulation. Although there was a statistically significant difference between the term and postterm infants at 1 and 8 hours post birth, there were no clinically significant differences between the two groups for glucose control at any data collection point. The author attributed these findings to acceptable antepartal care and appropriate intrapartum and postpartum intervention.

Critical Thinking Applied to Research

Strengths: Thorough description of sample for both infants and mothers and their demographic characteristics. Comprehensive description of instruments used to obtain data as well as the procedures followed for data collection.

Beckman C: Postterm pregnancy: Effects on temperature and glucose regulation. *Nurs Res* 1990; 39(1):21.

---

and received calories and weighs the newborn daily at consistent times, preferably before a feeding. Only then can findings of unusual losses or gains, as well as the pattern of weight gain, be considered reliable.

Evaluation

Anticipated outcomes of nursing care include the following:

- The risk of hypoglycemia is promptly identified, and intervention is started early.
- The newborn's metabolic and physiologic processes are stabilized, and recovery is proceeding without sequelae.
- The parents express their concerns about their baby's health problem and understand the rationale behind management of their newborn.

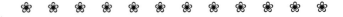

Care of the Newborn with Jaundice

The most common abnormal physical finding in neonates is **jaundice** (icterus). Jaundice develops from deposit of the yellow pigment *bilirubin* in lipid tissues. Unconjugated bilirubin is a break-down product derived primarily from hemoglobin that is released from lysed red blood cells and heme pigments found in cell elements (nonerythrocyte bilirubin).

Fetal unconjugated bilirubin is normally cleared by the placenta in utero, so total bilirubin at birth is usually less than 3 mg/dL unless an abnormal hemolytic process has been present. Postnatally, the infant must conjugate bilirubin (convert a lipid-soluble pigment into a water-soluble pigment) in the liver, producing a rise in serum bilirubin in the first days of life.

The rate and amount of conjugation depend on the rate of hemolysis, on the maturity of the liver, and on albumin-binding sites. See Chapter 27, page 829, for discussion of conjugation of bilirubin. A normal, healthy, full-term infant's liver is usually mature enough and producing enough glucuronyl transferase that total serum bilirubin levels do not reach pathologic levels (above 12 mg/dL in the blood).

Pathophysiology

Serum albumin-binding sites are usually sufficient to meet normal demands. However, certain conditions tend to decrease the sites available. Fetal or neonatal asphyxia decreases the binding affinity of bilirubin to albumin as acidosis impairs the capacity of albumin to hold bilirubin. Hypothermia and hypoglycemia release free fatty acids that

---

alone can double the baby's metabolic rate. Establishment and maintenance of a neutral thermal environment has a potent influence on the newborn's metabolism. The nurse pays careful attention to environmental conditions, physical activity, and organization of care and integrates these factors into delivery of nursing care. The nurse identifies any discrepancies between the baby's caloric requirements

dislocate bilirubin from albumin. Maternal use of sulfa drugs or salicylates interferes with conjugation or interferes with serum albumin-binding sites by competing with bilirubin for these sites.

A number of bacterial and viral infections (cytomegalic inclusion disease, toxoplasmosis, herpes, syphilis) can affect the liver and produce jaundice. **Hyperbilirubinemia** (elevation of bilirubin level) may also result from blood disorders such as polycythemia (due to twin-to-twin transfusion, large placental transfer of blood), or enclosed hemorrhage (cephalhematoma, bleeding into internal organs, ecchymoses). Increased hemolysis due to conditions such as sepsis, hemolytic disease of the newborn, or an excessive dose of vitamin K may also cause elevated bilirubin levels.

The bilirubin level at which an infant is harmed varies, but at that level the infant may suffer neurologic defects and eventually death. While the mechanism of bilirubin-produced neuronal injury is uncertain, evidence indicates that high concentrations of unconjugated bilirubin can be neurotoxic (Connolly & Volpe 1990). Unconjugated bilirubin has a high affinity for extravascular tissue such as fatty tissue (subcutaneous tissue) and the brain. Thus bilirubin not bound to albumin can cross the blood-brain barrier and damage the cells of the CNS and produce kernicterus. **Kernicterus** (meaning "yellow nucleus") refers to the deposition of unconjugated bilirubin in the basal ganglia of the brain and to the symptoms of neurologic damage that follow untreated hyperbilirubinemia. The classic bilirubin encephalopathy of kernicterus most commonly found with Rh and ABO blood group incompatibility is virtually unknown today due to aggressive treatment with phototherapy and exchange transfusions.

Kernicterus, usually associated with unconjugated bilirubin levels of over 20 mg/dL in normal term infants and over 12 mg/dL in *sick* preterm newborns, has been noted at autopsy in both types of babies at lower levels. The risk of kernicterus at lowered bilirubin levels has been associated with asphyxia, acidosis, and low serum albumin levels. Current therapy can reduce the incidence of kernicterus encephalopathy but cannot distinguish all infants who are at risk.

Complications associated with kernicterus include athetosis, hearing loss, limited upward gaze, and—in some—intellectual deficits (Connolly & Volpe 1990).

Causes of Hyperbilirubinemia

A primary cause of hyperbilirubinemia is **hemolytic disease of the newborn** secondary to Rh incompatibility. Thus the pregnant woman who is Rh negative or who has blood type O should be asked about outcomes of any previous pregnancies and her history of blood transfusion. Prenatal amniocentesis with spectrophotographic examination may be indicated in some cases. Cord blood from neonates is evaluated for bilirubin level, which should not exceed 5 mg/dL. Neonates of Rh negative and O-blood type mothers are carefully assessed for appearance of jaundice and levels of serum bilirubin.

Isoimmune hemolytic disease, also known as **erythroblastosis fetalis**, occurs after transplacental passage of a maternal antibody that predisposes fetal and neonatal red blood cells to early destruction. Jaundice, anemia, and compensatory erythropoiesis result. Immature red blood cells—erythroblasts—are found in large numbers in the blood, hence the designation erythroblastosis fetalis. **Hydrops fetalis**, the most severe form of erythroblastosis fetalis, occurs when maternal antibodies attach to the Rh antigen of the fetal red blood cells, making them susceptible to destruction by phagocytes. The fetal system responds by increased erythropoiesis within foci in the placenta and extramedullary sites, and hyperplasia of the bone marrow. Rapid and early destruction of erythrocytes results in a marked increase of immature red blood cells (erythroblasts) that do not have the functional capabilities of mature cells.

If anemia is severe, as seen in infants with hydrops fetalis, cardiomegaly with severe cardiac decompensation and hepatosplenomegaly occur. Severe generalized massive edema (*anasarca*) and generalized fluid effusion into the pleural cavity (hydrothorax), pericardial sac, and peritoneal cavity (ascites) develop. Jaundice is not present until later because the bili pigments are being excreted through the placenta into the maternal circulation. Severe anemia is also responsible for hemorrhage in pulmonary and other tissues. The hydropic hemolytic disease process is also characterized by hyperplasia of the fetal zone of the adrenal cortex and pancreatic islets. Hyperplasia of the pancreatic islets predisposes the infant to neonatal hypoglycemia similar to that of IDMs. These infants also have increased bleeding tendencies due to associated thrombocytopenia and hypoxic damage to the capillaries. Hydrops is a frequent cause of intrauterine death among infants with Rh disease. In rare cases, the grossly enlarged edemic fetus and placenta may cause uterine rupture.

ABO incompatibility may result in jaundice, although it rarely results in hemolytic disease severe enough to be clinically diagnosed and treated. Hepatosplenomegaly may be found occasionally in newborns with ABO incompatibility, but hydrops fetalis and stillbirth are rare.

The best treatment for hemolytic disease is prevention. Prenatal identification of the fetus at risk for Rh or ABO incompatibility will allow prompt treatment. See Chapter 19 for discussion of in utero management of this condition.

Certain prenatal and perinatal factors in the mother predispose the newborn to hyperbilirubinemia. During pregnancy, maternal conditions that are associated with neonatal hyperbilirubinemia include hereditary spherocytosis, diabetes, intrauterine infections (TORCH and gram-negative bacilli) that stimulate production of maternal isoimmune antibodies, and drug ingestion (sulfas, salicylates, novobiocin, diazepam, oxytocin).

Certain neonatal conditions predispose to hyperbilirubinemia; polycythemia (central hematocrit 65% or more), pyloric stenosis, obstruction or atresia of the biliary duct or of the lower bowel, low-grade urinary tract infection, sepsis, hypothyroidism, enclosed hemorrhage (cephalhematoma, large bruises), asphyxia neonatorum, hypothermia, acidemia, and hypoglycemia. Hepatitis from intrauterine infections or metabolic liver disease elevates the level of conjugated bilirubin.

Neonates born with congenital biliary duct atresia have a poor prognosis; about two-thirds have an inoperable lesion and die during the first three years of life. The prognosis for a newborn with hyperbilirubinemia depends on the extent of the hemolytic process and the underlying cause. Severe hemolytic disease results in fetal and early neonatal death from the effects of anemia—cardiac decompensation, edema, ascites, and hydrothorax. Hyperbilirubinemia that is not aggressively treated may lead to kernicterus. The resultant neurologic damage is responsible for death, cerebral palsy, mental retardation, sensory difficulties, or to a lesser degree, perceptual impairment, delayed speech development, hyperactivity, muscle incoordination, or learning difficulties.

Medical Therapy

The goals of medical management are prompt identification of infants at risk for jaundice based on perinatal and neonatal history, laboratory tests to identify the cause of the jaundice, and prompt treatment to prevent the neurologic damage that can result from hyperbilirubinemia.

When one or more of the predisposing factors is present, laboratory determination should be made of the maternal and neonatal blood types for Rh or ABO incompatibility. Other necessary laboratory evaluations are Coombs' test, serum bilirubin levels (direct, indirect, and total), hemoglobin, reticulocyte percentage, and white cell count.

Neonatal hyperbilirubinemia of any origin must be considered pathologic (Avery & Taeusch 1984) if any of the following criteria are met:

1. Clinically evident jaundice in the first 24 hours of life

2. Serum bilirubin concentration rising by more than 5 mg/dL per day

3. Total serum bilirubin concentrations exceeding 12.9 mg/dL in term infants or 15 mg/dL in preterm babies (since preterm newborns have less subcutaneous fat, bilirubin may reach higher levels before it is visible)

4. Conjugated bilirubin concentrations greater than 2 mg/dL

5. Persistence of clinical jaundice beyond seven days in term infants or beyond 14 days in preterm infants

Initial diagnostic procedures are aimed at differentiating jaundice resulting from increased bilirubin production, impaired conjugation or excretion, increased intestinal reabsorption, or a combination of these factors. The Coombs' test is performed to determine whether jaundice is due to hemolytic disease.

If the hemolytic process is due to Rh sensitization, laboratory findings reveal the following: (a) an Rh positive neonate with a positive Coombs' test, (b) increased erythropoiesis with many immature circulating red blood cells (nucleated blastocysts), (c) anemia, in most cases, (d) elevated levels (5 mg/dL or more) of bilirubin in cord blood, and (e) a reduction in albumin-binding capacity. Maternal data may include an elevated anti-Rh titer and spectrophotometric evidence of fetal hemolytic process.

The Coombs' test can be either indirect or direct. The indirect Coombs' test measures the amount of Rh positive antibodies in the mother's blood. Rh positive red blood cells are added to the maternal blood sample. If the mother's serum contains antibodies, the Rh positive red blood cells will agglutinate (clump) when rabbit immune antiglobulin is added, and the test results are labeled positive.

The direct Coombs' test reveals the presence of antibody-coated (sensitized) Rh positive red blood cells in the neonate. Rabbit immune antiglobulin is added to the neonatal blood cells specimen. If the neonatal red blood cells agglutinate, they have been coated with maternal antibodies, and the test result is positive.

If the hemolytic process is due to ABO incompatibility, laboratory findings reveal an increase in recticulocytes. The resulting anemia is usually not significant during the neonatal period and is rare later on. The direct Coombs' test may be negative or mildly positive, while the indirect Coombs' test may be strongly positive. Infants with a positive direct Coombs' test have increased incidence of jaundice with bilirubin levels in excess of 10 mg/dL. Increased numbers of spherocytes (spherical, plump, mature erythrocytes) are seen on a peripheral blood smear. Increased numbers of spherocytes are not seen on smears from Rh disease infants.

Regardless of the cause of hyperbilirubinemia, management of these infants is directed toward preventing anemia and minimizing the consequences of hyperbilirubinemia.

Treatment has four goals:

- Alleviating the anemia
- Removing maternal antibodies and sensitized erythrocytes
- Increasing serum albumin levels
- Reducing the levels of serum bilirubin

Therapeutic methods of management of hyperbilirubinemia include phototherapy, exchange transfusion, infusion of albumin, and drug therapy. If hemolytic disease is present, it may be treated by phototherapy, exchange transfusion, and drug therapy. When determining the appropriate management of hyperbilirubinemia due to hemolytic disease, the three variables that must be taken into account are the newborn's (1) serum bilirubin level, (2) birth weight, and (3) age in hours. If a neonate has hemolysis with an unconjugated bilirubin level of 14 mg/dL, weighs less than 2500 g (birth weight), and is 24 hours old or less, an exchange transfusion may be the best management. However, if that same neonate is over 24 hours of age, phototherapy may be the treatment of choice to prevent the possible complication of kernicterus.

Phototherapy

Phot\therapy may be used alone or in conjunction with exchange transfusion to reduce serum bilirubin levels. Exposure of the baby to high-intensity light (a bank of fluorescent light bulbs or bulbs in the blue-light spectrum) decreases serum bilirubin levels in the skin. Phototherapy reduces serum bilirubin by facilitating biliary excretion of unconjugated bilirubin. This occurs when light absorbed by the tissue converts unconjugated bilirubin to two isomers called photobilirubin. The photobilirubin moves from the tissues to the blood by a diffusion mechanism. In the blood it is bound to albumin and transported to the liver. It moves into the bile and is excreted with the feces without requiring conjugation by the liver (Ennever 1990). The photodegradation products formed when light oxidizes bilirubin can be excreted in the urine. Phototherapy plays an important role in preventing a rise in bilirubin levels but does not alter the underlying cause of jaundice, and hemolysis may continue to produce anemia.

It is generally accepted that phototherapy should be started at 4 to 5 mg/dL below the calculated exchange level for each infant. Sick neonates of less than 1000 g should have phototherapy instituted at a bilirubin concentration of 5 mg/dL. Many authors have recommended initiating phototherapy "prophylactically" in the first 24 hours of life in high-risk, very-low-birth-weight infants (Yeh 1991). Sick preterm infants who are at least 1500 g should have phototherapy instituted when the bilirubin level is 10 mg/dL.

Any neonate with a bilirubin level of 20 mg/dL or above may need an exchange transfusion if illness or associated conditions are present (Yeh 1991) (see Table 32–4). It is generally accepted that phototherapy is started at 4 to 5 mg/dL below the calculated exchange level for each infant (the level at which an exchange transfusion would be done).

Exchange Transfusion

Exchange transfusion is the withdrawal and replacement of the neonate's blood with donor blood.

Exchange transfusion is used to treat anemia with red blood cells that are not susceptible to maternal antibodies, remove sensitized red blood cells that would be lysed soon, remove serum bilirubin, and provide bilirubin-free albumin and increase the binding sites for bilirubin. In Rh incompatibility, fresh (under two days old) group O, Rh negative "low-titer" whole blood, or washed packed red blood cells reconstituted with fresh frozen plasma is chosen. This type of blood contains no A or B antigens or Rh antigens; therefore the maternal antibodies still present in the neonate's blood will not cause hemolysis of the transfused blood. Packed cells are used if the infant is anemic. Citrate-phosphate-dextrose (CPD) blood is preferred because it presents less of an acid load to the infant.

In case of ABO incompatibility, group O with Rh specific cells and low titers of anti-A and anti-B donor blood is used, not the infant's blood type, since donor blood contains no antigens to further stimulate maternal antibodies.

Every four to eight hours after the transfusion, serum bilirubin determinations are made. Repeat exchange may be necessary if the bilirubin level exceeds 20 mg/dL or the exchange level for that infant. Daily hemoglobin estimates should be obtained until stable, and hemoglobin determinations done every two weeks for two months are valuable.

Table 32–4　Management of Jaundice in Low-Birth-Weight Infants

	Indirect Bilirubin Concentrations					
Birth Weight	**5–6 mg/dL**	**7–9 mg/dL**	**10–12 mg/dL**	**12–15 mg/dL**	**15–20 mg/dL**	**>20 mg/dL**
≤1000 g	Phototherapy	⟶	Exchange transfusion*	⟶		
1001–1500 g	Observe and repeat BR	Phototherapy	⟶	Exchange transfusion	⟶	
1501–2000 g	Observe and repeat BR	⟶	Phototherapy	⟶	Exchange transfusion	⟶
>2000 g	Observe	Observe and repeat BR	Phototherapy (<2500 g)	Phototherapy (>2500 g)	⟶	Exchange transfusion

Exchange if albumin binding is saturated, or if serum indirect BR continues to rise. BR = bilirubin
From Cashore W, Stern L: The management of hyperbilirubinemia. Clin Perinatol June 1984; 11(2): 353.

❀ *APPLYING THE NURSING PROCESS* ❀

Nursing Assessment

Assessment is aimed at identifying prenatal and perinatal factors that predispose to development of jaundice and identifying jaundice as soon as it is apparent. Clinically, ABO incompatibility presents as jaundice and occasionally as hepatosplenomegaly. Hydrops is rare. Hemolytic disease of the newborn is suspected if the placenta is enlarged, if the newborn is edematous with pleural and pericardial effusion plus ascites, if pallor or jaundice is noted during the first 24 to 36 hours, if hemolytic anemia is diagnosed, or if the spleen and liver are enlarged. The nurse carefully notes changes in behavior and observes for evidence of bleeding. If laboratory tests indicate elevated bilirubin levels, the nurse checks the newborn for jaundice about every two hours and records observations.

To check for jaundice, the nurse should blanch the skin over a bony prominence (forehead, nose, or sternum) by pressing firmly with the thumb. After pressure is released, if jaundice is present, the area appears yellow before normal color returns. The nurse should check oral mucosa and posterior portion of the hard palate and conjunctival sacs for yellow pigmentation in darker-skinned babies. Assessment in daylight gives best results as pink walls and surroundings may mask yellowish tints and yellow light makes differentiation of jaundice difficult. The time of onset of jaundice is recorded and reported. If jaundice appears, careful observation of the increase in depth of color and the infant's behavior is mandatory.

The newborn's behavior is assessed for neurologic signs of kernicterus, which are rare but may include hypotonia, diminished reflexes, lethargy, seizures, or opisthotonic posturing.

Nursing Diagnosis

Nursing diagnoses that may apply are included in the Nursing Care Plan for the Newborn with Jaundice.

Nursing Plan and Implementation

Promotion of Effective Phototherapy

Ideally the entire skin surface of the newborn is exposed to the light. Minimal covering is applied over the genitals and buttocks to expose maximum skin surface while protecting the bedding. Genitals are covered with a diaper since phototherapy may produce DNA strand breaks and possible mutations (Page 1989). Phototherapy success is measured every 12 hours or with daily serum bilirubin levels. The lights must be turned off while drawing blood for serum bilirubin levels. Because it is not known if phototherapy injures the delicate eye structures, particularly the retina, the nurse applies eye patches over the newborn's closed eyes during exposure (Figure 32–14). Phototherapy is discon-

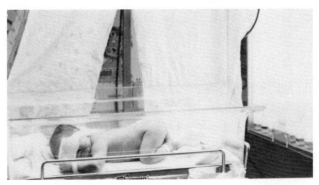

Figure 32–14 Infant receiving phototherapy. The phototherapy light is positioned over the Isolette. The infant is undressed to expose as much skin as possible. Bilateral eye patches are always used during phototherapy to protect the baby's eyes.

tinued and the eye patches are removed at least once per shift to assess the eyes for the presence of conjunctivitis. Patches are also removed to allow eye contact during feeding (for social stimulation) or when parents are visiting (to promote parental attachment).

The irradiance level at the skin determines the effectiveness of the phototherapy. The desired level of irradiance is 5 to 6 microwatts per square centimeter per nanometer. Most phototherapy units will provide this level of irradiance 42 to 45 cm below the lamps. Irradiance levels can be increased slightly as indicated. The nurse can use a photometer to measure and maintain desired levels (King & Jung 1990).

The neonate's temperature is monitored to prevent hyperthermia or hypothermia. The newborn will require additional fluids to compensate for the increased water loss through the skin and loose stools. Loose stools and increased urine output are the results of increased bilirubin excretion. The infant is observed for signs of dehydration and perianal excoriation (Page 1989).

A transient bronze discoloration of the skin may occur with phototherapy when the infant has elevated direct serum bilirubin levels or liver disease. As a side effect of phototherapy, some newborns develop a maculopapular rash. In addition to assessing the neonate's skin color for jaundice and bronzing, the nurse examines the skin for developing pressure areas. The neonate should be repositioned at least every two hours to permit the light to reach all skin surfaces, to prevent pressure areas, and to vary the stimulation to the infant. The nurse keeps track of the number of hours each lamp is used so that each can be replaced before its effectiveness is lost.

Phototherapy can also be carried out in the parents' room if the only problem is hyperbilirubinemia. The parent must be willing to keep the baby in the room for 24 hours a day, able to take emergency action as for choking if necessary, and complete instruction checklists. Some institutions

(Text continues on p 1052.)

Nursing Care Plan
Newborn with Jaundice

Nursing History

Maternal

ABO incompatibility

Rh negative

Diabetes

Presence of infection, such as syphilis, cytomegalovirus, rubella, toxoplasmosis

Presence of familiar blood dyscrasias such as spherocytosis, G-6-PD deficiency

Medications: Novobiocin, sulfonamides, and salicylates interfere with conjugation or compete for serum albumin-binding sites

Number and outcome of previous pregnancies

Condition at birth and current health status of other children

Paternal

Rh factor—negative or positive

Birth

Enlarged placenta (larger than one-seventh of neonate's weight)

Delayed clamping of umbilical cord

Traumatic birth

Neonate

Enclosed hemorrhage, hematoma, large bruises, intracranial bleeding

Bacterial and/or viral infections can affect liver and thus decrease glucuronyl transferase activity

Polycythemia (central hematocrit of 65% or more)

Biliary atresia, cystic fibrosis (inspissated bile)

Congenital hypothyroidism

Conditions that decrease available albumin-binding sites:

1. Fetal or neonatal asphyxia decreases binding affinity of bilirubin to albumin.

2. Chilling and hypoglycemia create fatty acids to compete for binding sites.

3. Preterm neonates tend to have lower serum albumin levels and therefore less albumin to bind to.

Physical Examination

Generalized edema with pleural and pericardial effusion

Pallor or jaundice noted in first 24–36 hours

May have enlargement of spleen or liver

Changes in behavior (lethargy, irritability), tremors

Dark, concentrated urine

Hypoactive bowel sounds

Hypotonia

Presence of hematomas or large bruises (assess for other signs of enclosed bleeding)

Excessive ecchymosis or petechiae

Meconium passage may be delayed

Diagnostic Studies

Coombs' test—direct on baby, indirect on mother's blood

Total bilirubin level

Indications for exchange transfusion:
In ABO incompatibility, serum bilirubin levels greater than 20 mg/dL (full-term) and 15 mg/dL (preterm)
In Rh incompatibility, serum bilirubin greater than 20 mg/dL (term) greater than 15 mg/dL (large preterms), and greater than 13 mg/dL (less than 1250 g preterms)

Total serum protein (provides measure of binding capacity)

Complete blood cell count (CBC)—assess anemia and polycythemia

Peripheral smear—evaluate red blood cells for immaturity or abnormality

Blood glucose

CO_2 combining power

Reticulocyte count

Kleihauer-Betke test

Transcutaneous jaundice meter

(continued)

Nursing Care Plan (continued)

Nursing Diagnosis	Nursing Interventions	Rationale	Evaluation
Impaired tissue integrity related to predisposing factors associated with hyperbilirubinemia *Client Goal:* Babies at risk for jaundice and early signs of jaundice will be identified.	Evaluate baby's history for predisposing factors for hyperbilirubinemia.	Early identification of risk factors enables the nurse to monitor babies for early signs of hyperbilirubinemia. Acidosis, hypoxia, hypothermia, etc increase the risk of hyperbilirubinemia at lower bilirubin levels.	Baby's jaundice is identified early.
	Observe color of amniotic fluid at time of rupture of membranes.	Amber-colored amniotic fluid is indicative of hyperbilirubinemia.	
	Assess baby for developing jaundice in daylight if possible.	Early detection is affected by nursery environment. Artificial lights (with pink tint) may mask beginning of jaundice.	
	1. Observe sclera.	Most visible sign of hyperbilirubinemia is jaundice noted in skin, sclera, or oral mucosa. Onset is first seen on face.	
	2. Observe skin color and assess by blanching.	Blanching the skin leaves a yellow color to the skin immediately after pressure is released.	
	3. Check oral mucosa, posterior portion of hard palate, and conjunctival sacs for yellow pigmentation in dark-skinned newborns.	Underlying pigment of dark-skinned people may normally appear yellow.	
	Report jaundice occurring within 24 hours of birth.		
Injury: High risk related to reabsorption of bilirubin secondary to decreased stooling *Client Goal:* Baby will start feedings within four to six hr after birth, have active bowel sounds, and begin to pass meconium stools.	Initiate feedings as soon as possible, at least within four to six hr after birth or per protocol.	Early feeding stimulates digestive enzymes involved in establishing gut bacterial flora and decreased enterohepatic circulation.	Baby tolerates feedings with minimal regurgitation; active bowel sounds are present in all four quadrants; meconium stool is passed within 24 hours.

(continued)

Nursing Care Plan (continued)

Nursing Diagnosis	Nursing Interventions	Rationale	Evaluation
Fluid volume deficit secondary to phototherapy *Client Goal:* Baby will have good skin turgor, clear amber urine output of 1–3 mL/kg/hr, six to eight wet diapers/day, and will maintain weight.	Offer feedings every two to four hr. Do not skip feedings Provide 25% extra fluid intake. Offer water between breast- or bottle-feedings. Assess for dehydration: **1.** Poor skin turgor **2.** Depressed fontanelles **3.** Sunken eyes **4.** Decreased urine output **5.** Weight loss **6.** Changes in electrolytes Monitor intake and output. Weigh diapers before discarding. Check specific gravity every eight hr. Record urine color and frequency. Record number and characteristics of stools. Weigh daily. Report signs of dehydration. Administer IV fluids **1.** Monitor flow rates. **2.** Assess insertion site for signs of infection.	Adequate hydration increases peristalsis and excretion of bilirubin. Replace fluid losses due to watery stools, if under phototherapy. Phototherapy treatment may cause liquid stools and increased insensible water loss, which increases risk of dehydration. Prevents fluid overload. IV fluids may be used if baby is dehydrated or in presence of other complications. IV may be started if exchange transfusion is to be done.	Baby tolerates oral feedings and is adequately hydrated as indicated by good skin turgor, six to eight wet diapers per day, and maintenance of weight.
Injury: High risk related to use of phototherapy *Client Goal:* Baby will not have any corneal irritation/drainage, skin breakdown, or major fluctuations in temperature.	Cover baby's eyes with eye patches while under phototherapy lights. Cover testes/penis in male infants. Make certain that eyelids are closed prior to applying eyepatches. Ensure patches do not slip down over nose. Remove baby from under phototherapy and remove eye patches during feedings.	Protects retina from damage due to high intensity light and testes from damage from heat. Prevents corneal abrasions. Blocked nose causes upper airway obstruction and apnea. Provides visual stimulation and facilitates attachment behaviors.	Baby's eyes are protected at all times while under the phototherapy lights, no corneal irritation occurs; baby maintains a stable temperature.

(continued)

Nursing Care Plan (continued)

Nursing Diagnosis	Nursing Interventions	Rationale	Evaluation
	Inspect eyes every eight hours for conjunctivitis, drainage, and corneal abrasions due to irritation from eye patches.	Prevents or facilitates prompt treatment of purulent conjunctivitis.	
	Administer thorough perianal cleansing with each stool or change of perianal protective covering.	Frequent stooling increases risk of skin breakdown. Prevents infection.	
	Provide minimal coverage—only of diaper area.	Provides maximal exposure. Shielded areas become more jaundiced, so maximum exposure is essential.	
	Use paper face mask after removing nose strip.	Metal strip can burn baby's skin when heated by the lights.	
	Avoid the use of oily applications on the skin.		
	Reposition baby every two hours.	Provides equal exposure of all skin areas and prevents pressure areas.	
	Observe for bronzing of skin.	Bronzing is related to use of phototherapy with increased direct bilirubin levels or liver damage; may last for two to four months.	
	Place baby approximately 18 inches from light source.	Ensures correct exposure to the phototherapy lights.	
	Place Plexiglas™ shield between baby and light.		
	Monitor baby's skin and core temperature frequently until temperature is stable.	Hypothermia and hyperthermia are common complications of phototherapy. Hypothermia results from exposure to lights, subsequent radiation, and convection losses.	
	Check axillary temperature with readings on servo-controlled unit on Isolette.	Hyperthermia may result from the increased environmental heat.	
	Regulate Isolette temperature as needed.	Additional heat from phototherapy lights frequently causes a rise in the baby's and the Isolette's temperatures. Fluctuations in temperature may occur in response to radiation and convection.	

(continued)

Nursing Care Plan (continued)

Nursing Diagnosis	Nursing Interventions	Rationale	Evaluation
Sensory/perceptual alterations related to neurologic damage secondary to kernicterus *Client Goal:* Baby will not show signs of altered biorhythms, hypotonia, temperature instability, spasticity, lethargy, poor sucking reflex.	Monitor any neurologic/behavioral changes in baby by taking vital signs every two hr. Report any changes promptly. Closely assess infant's daily patterns to detect notable changes in food ingestion, bowel and urine and sleeping and waking rhythms, irritability. Report signs of worsening condition (kernicterus): 1. Hypotonia, lethargy, poor sucking reflex, hypertonicity 2. Spasticity and opisthotonus 3. Temperature instability 4. Gradual appearance of extrapyramidal signs 5. Impaired or absent hearing Monitor laboratory studies as indicated: 1. Direct and indirect bilirubin 2. CO_2 3. Reticulocyte count 4. Hematocrit and hemoglobin (H&H), total serum protein	Baby may develop green, watery stools and green urine due to excretion of bilirubin byproducts. Changes in biologic rhythms caused by phototherapy are unclear and may indicate signs of worsening condition. Deposition of bilirubin in brain leads to development of symptoms of kernicterus. Note: Treatment may be more aggressive in presence of neonatal complications such as asphyxia, respiratory distress, metabolic acidosis, hypothermia, low serum protein, sepsis, signs of CNS deterioration (Avery 1987).	Baby's neurologic status is within normal limits.
Knowledge deficit related to causes of and care of baby with hyperbilirubinemia *Client Goals:* Parents will be informed of baby's disease process, rationale for treatments, and expected outcome. Mother will understand the reason for temporary discontinuation of breast-feeding, how to pump her breasts, and how to reinstate breast-feeding.	Provide explanation of: 1. Infant's condition 2. Treatment modalities, causative and contributing factors of jaundice and hyperbilirubinemia 3. Reasons that mother may be asked to cease breast-feeding temporarily	Parents may not understand what is happening or why. Physician preference of treatment modalities may vary. Parents may not understand why their newborn is not receiving a treatment that another with the same condition is receiving. The etiology of breast milk jaundice remains uncertain. The serum bilirubin levels begin to fall within 48 hr after discontinuation of breast-feeding.	Parents understand the process and treatment of jaundice and reasons for interruption of breast-feeding.

(continued)

Nursing Care Plan (continued)

Nursing Diagnosis	Nursing Interventions	Rationale	Evaluation
		Opinion of physicians varies regarding the need for discontinuing breast-feeding.	
	Assist mother to pump her breasts to maintain her milk supply.	Mother may need support and information to restart breast-feeding.	
	Give explanation of equipment being used and changes in bilirubin levels. Allow parents an opportunity to ask questions; reinforce or clarify information as needed.	If breast-feeding is temporarily discontinued, assess mother's knowledge of pumping her breasts and provide information and support as needed.	
	Teach parents signs of jaundice (example: yellow tinge to skin or sclera) and to report them to the health care team.	Parents know when to report recurrence of jaundice and importance of follow-up.	
Altered parenting: High risk related to parenting a baby with jaundice	Encourage parents to provide tactile stimulation during feeding and diaper changes.	Neonate has normal needs for tactile stimulation.	Parents are involved in the care of their baby and the bonding process occurs.
Client Goals: Parents will provide care and stimulation for their baby.	Provide cuddling and eye contact during feedings and talk to baby frequently.	Provides comforting and decreases sensory deprivation.	
	Encourage parents to come into nursery or bring baby to mother's room for feedings and to touch their baby. Provide opportunities for parents to express feelings.	Presence of equipment may discourage parents from interacting with neonate.	

Table 32–5 Instructional Checklist for In-Room Phototherapy
The nurse
1. Explains and demonstrates the placement of eye patches and states that they must be in place when the infant is under the lights.
2. Explains the clothing to be worn (diaper under lights, dress and wrap when away from the lights).
3. Explains the importance of taking the infant's temperature regularly.
4. Explains the importance of adequate fluid intake.
5. Explains the charting flowsheet (intake, output, eyes covered).
6. Explains how to position the lights at a proper distance.
7. Explains the need to keep the infant under phototherapy, except during feeding and diaper changes.

require that parents sign a consent form (King & Jung 1990). The nurse gives the instructions to the parents but also continues to monitor the infant's temperature, activity, intake and output, and positioning of eye patches at regular intervals (see Table 32–5).

Promotion of Effective Exchange Transfusion

The nurse's responsibilities during exchange transfusion are to assemble equipment, prepare the baby, assist the physician during the procedure, and maintain a careful record of all events. After the procedure the nurse observes the newborn for complications from the transfusion and clinical signs of hyperbilirubinemia and neurologic damage (Procedure 32–3).

Provision of Teaching and Emotional Support to Families

Many parents must face the mother's discharge while the neonate remains in the hospital for treatment of hyperbilirubinemia. The terms *jaundice, hyperbilirubinemia, exchange transfusion,* and *phototherapy* may sound frightening and threatening. Some parents may feel guilty and think they have caused the problem. On occasion, a multidisciplinary team (nurse, obstetrician, pediatrician, clergyman, genetic counselor, psychologist) may collaborate to help the parents cope with the situation. Under stress, parents may not be able to understand the physician's first explanations. The nurse must expect that the parents will

---

PROCEDURE 32–3
Nursing Responsibilities During Exchange Transfusion *

Nursing Action	Rationale
Objective: Prepare infant.	
1. Identify baby.	To prepare correct infant.
2. Keep newborn NPO for four hr preceding exchange transfusion or aspirate stomach.	To decrease chance of regurgitation and aspiration by neonate.
3. May administer salt-poor albumin (1 g/kg body weight) one hr before exchange transfusion.	To increase binding of bilirubin. Do not give to severely anemic or edemic neonate or to neonate with congestive heart failure, because of hazard of hypervolemia.
4. Assess vital signs.	To provide a baseline.
5. Position neonate in supine position, soft restraints; provide warmth under radiant warmer and have warm blankets available.	To provide maximum visualization, thermoregulation and prevent chilling.
6. Clean abdomen by scrubbing.	To reduce number of bacteria present.
7. Attach monitor leads to infant.	To assess pulse and respiration.
Objective: Prepare equipment.	
1. Have resuscitation equipment available (oxygen, bag and mask, intubation equipment, 10% glucose IV solution and sodium bicarbonate).	To provide life support measures if necessary.

(continued)

PROCEDURE 32–3 (continued)

Nursing Action	Rationale
2. Obtain blood and check it with physician for type, Rh, and age.	To ensure using correct blood.
3. Attach blood tubing.	To allow infusion.
4. Apply blood warmer.	To reduce chill.
5. Open exchange transfusion and umbilical vein trays. Pour prep solution into basins.	To maintain sterility
6. Prepare gown and gloves for physician.	

Objective: Monitor infant status before and during procedure.

Assess pulse, respirations, color, and activity state.	To recognize possible problems such as apnea, bradycardia, cardiac arrhythmia, or arrest and provide data on neonate's response to treatment.

Objective: Record blood exchange and medications used.

1. Using blood exchange sheet, record time, amount of blood in, amount of blood out, medications and baby's response, and any other pertinent information.	Donor blood is given at rate of 170 mL/kg of body weight. It replaces 85% of infant's own blood.
2. Inform physician when 100 mL of blood has been used.	Calcium gluconate is given IV after each 100 mL of blood if indicated to decrease cardiac irritability.

Objective: Assess neonate response after transfusion.

After the exchange, carefully monitor the following for 24–48 hr:	To provide information on status of neonate and identification of complications such as hypocalcemia, hyperkalemia, hypernatremia, hypoglycemia and acidosis, sepsis, shock, thrombus formation, and transfusion mismatch reaction.

1. Vital signs
2. Neurologic signs (lethargy, increased irritability, jitteriness, convulsion)
3. Amount and color of urine (hematuria)
4. Presence of edema
5. Signs of necrotizing enterocolitis
6. Infection or hemorrhage at infusion site
7. Signs of increasing jaundice
8. Neurologic signs of kernicterus
9. Calcium, glucose, and bilirubin levels
10. Other complications such as hypokalemia, septicemia, shock, and thrombosis

Objective: Prepare blood samples.

Label tubes and send to laboratory with appropriate laboratory slips.	To follow routines of your institution.
Retype and cross-match 2 units of blood two hours postexchange.	To provide for possible future exchange.

Objective: Record information on infant's record.

Record infant's response during and after the exchange procedure.	Recording of infant's responses assists in identifying possible complications.

*Exchange transfusion is a therapeutic procedure for hyperbilirubinemia of any etiology.

need explanations repeated and clarified and that they may need help voicing their questions and fears. Eye and tactile contact with the infant is encouraged. The nurse can coach parents when they visit with the baby. Parents are kept informed of their infant's condition and are encouraged to return to the hospital or telephone at any time so that they can be fully involved in the care of their infant. (See the Nursing Care Plan for Newborn with Jaundice.)

Evaluation

Anticipated outcomes of nursing care include the following:

* The risks for development of hyperbilirubinemia are identified and action is taken to minimize the potential impact of hyperbilirubinemia.

* The baby will not have any corneal irritation or drainage, skin breakdown, or major fluctuations in temperature.

* Parents will understand rationale for, goal of, and expected outcome of therapy. Parents verbalize their concerns about their baby's condition and identify how they can facilitate their baby's improvement.

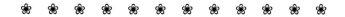

Care of the Newborn with Potential Hemorrhagic Disease

Several transient coagulation-mechanism deficiencies normally occur in the first several days of a newborn's life. Foremost among these is a slight decrease in the level of prothrombin, resulting in a prolonged clotting time during the initial week of life. Vitamin K is required for the liver to form prothrombin (factor II) and proconvertin (factor VII) for blood coagulation. Vitamin K, a fat-soluble vitamin, may be obtained from food, but it is usually synthesized by bacteria in the colon, and consequently a dietary source is unnecessary. However, intestinal flora are practically nonexistent in newborns, so they are unable to synthesize vitamin K.

Bleeding due to vitamin K deficiency generally occurs on the second or third day of life, but it may occur earlier in babies of mothers treated with phenytoin sodium (Dilantin) or phenobarbital. These drugs impair vitamin K activity, and bleeding may be seen at birth. Coumarin compounds are vitamin K antagonists that can cross the placenta. Thus the baby exposed to maternal coumarin can also manifest bleeding in the first 24 hours of life. Bleeding may also occur in babies receiving parenteral nutrition without adequate vitamin K additives (1 mg/week).

Bleeding from the nose, umbilical cord, circumcision site, gastrointestinal tract, and scalp, as well as generalized ecchymoses may be seen. Internal hemorrhage may occur.

This disorder can be completely prevented by the prophylactic use of an injection of vitamin K. A dose of 1 mg of

AquaMEPHYTON is given as part of newborn care immediately following birth, and consequently the disease is rarely seen today (see Drug Guide, Chapter 29). Larger doses are contraindicated because they may result in the development of hyperbilirubinemia.

Care of the Newborn with Anemia

Neonatal anemia is often difficult to recognize by clinical evaluation alone. Mean hemoglobin in a full-term newborn is 17 g/dL, slightly higher than in premature infants, in whom the mean hemoglobin is 16 g/dL. Infants with hemoglobin values of less than 14 mg/dL (term) and 13 g/dL (preterm) are usually considered anemic. The most common causes of neonatal anemia are blood loss, hemolysis, and impaired red blood cell production.

Blood loss (hypovolemia) occurs in utero from placental bleeding (placenta previa or abruptio placentae). Intrapartal blood loss may be fetomaternal, fetofetal, or the result of umbilical cord bleeding. Birth trauma to abdominal organs or the cranium may produce significant blood loss, and cerebral bleeding may occur due to hypoxia.

Excessive hemolysis of red cells is usually a result of blood group incompatibilities but may be due to infections. The most common cause of impaired red cell production is a deficiency in G-6-PD, which is genetically transmitted. Anemia and jaundice are the presenting signs.

A condition known as **physiologic anemia** exists as a result of the normal gradual drop in hemoglobin for the first 6 to 12 weeks of life. Theoretically, the bone marrow stops production of red blood cells as a response to the elevated oxygenation of extrauterine respirations. When the amount of hemoglobin becomes lower, reaching levels of 10 to 11 g/dL at about 6 to 12 weeks of age, the bone marrow begins production of RBCs again, and the anemia disappears.

Anemia in preterm newborns occurs earlier and reversal by bone marrow is initiated at lower levels of hemoglobin (7 to 9 g/dL). The preterm baby's hemoglobin reaches a low sooner (four to eight weeks after birth) than does a term newborn's (6 to 12 weeks) because red blood cell survival time is shorter in the preterm infant than in the term newborn, because the rate of growth in preterm infants is relatively rapid, and because a vitamin E deficiency is common in small preterm newborns.

Medical Therapy

The goal of management is early identification and correction of anemia. Hematologic problems can be anticipated based on the obstetric history and clinical manifestations. The age at which anemia is first noted is also of diagnostic value.

Clinically, anemic infants are very pale in the absence of other symptoms of shock and usually have abnormally low red blood cell counts. In *acute* blood loss, symptoms of shock may be present, such as pallor, low arterial blood pressure, and a decreasing hematocrit value. The initial laboratory workup should include hemoglobin and hematocrit measurements, reticulocyte count, examination of peripheral blood smear, bilirubin determinations, direct Coombs' test of infant's blood, and examination of maternal blood smear for fetal erythrocytes (Kleihauer-Betke test). Medical management depends on the severity of the anemia and whether blood loss is acute or chronic. The baby should be placed on constant cardiac and respiratory monitoring. Mild or slow chronic anemia may be treated adequately with iron supplements alone or with iron-fortified formulas. Frequent determinations of hemoglobin, hematocrit, and bilirubin levels (in hemolytic disease) are essential. In severe cases of anemia, transfusions are the preferred method of treatment.

Nursing Care

The nurse assesses the newborn for symptoms of anemia (pallor). If the blood loss is acute, the baby may exhibit signs of shock. Continued observations will be necessary to identify physiologic anemia as the preterm newborn grows. Signs of dysfunction include poor weight gain, tachycardia, tachypnea, and apneic episodes. The nurse promptly reports any symptoms indicating anemia or shock. The amount of blood drawn for all laboratory tests is recorded so that total blood removed can be assessed and replaced by transfusion when necessary. If the newborn exhibits signs of shock, the nurse may need to begin necessary interventions.

Care of the Newborn with Polycythemia

Polycythemia is a condition in which blood volume and hematocrit values are increased. A common problem in low-risk nurseries, polycythemia affects 2% to 17% of newborns (Nantze 1985). It is observed more commonly in SGA and full-term infants than in preterm neonates. An infant is considered polycythemic when the central venous hematocrit value is greater than 65% to 70% or the venous hemoglobin level is greater than 22 g/dL during the first week of life (Avery 1987).

Several conditions predispose the neonate to polycythemia:

1. At the time of birth an excessive volume of placental blood may transfuse into the infant before the cord is clamped ("cord stripping"), resulting in a blood volume increase.

2. During gestation an increased amount of blood may cross the placenta to the infant (maternofetal transfusion), resulting in increased blood volume after birth.

3. A twin-to-twin transfusion may occur, in which one twin receives less blood and becomes anemic, and the other twin receives an excess amount of blood and becomes polycythemic.

4. Increased red blood cell production may occur in utero in response to chronic fetal distress in SGA, IDM, or postmature infants and secondary to conditions of PIH and placenta previa.

Other conditions that present with polycythemia are chromosomal anomalies such as trisomy 21, 18, and 13; endocrine disorders such as hypoglycemia and hypocalcemia; and births at altitudes over 5000 feet.

Medical Therapy

The goal of therapy is to reduce the central venous hematocrit to less than 60% in symptomatic infants. Treatment of asymptomatic infants is more controversial, but many authorities agree that these newborns benefit from prophylactic exchanges (Merestein & Gardner 1989). To decrease the red cell mass, the symptomatic infant receives a partial exchange transfusion in which blood is removed from the infant and replaced millimeter for millimeter with fresh plasma, plasmanate, or 5% albumin (Merenstein & Gardner 1989). Supportive treatment of presenting symptoms is required until resolution which usually occurs spontaneously following the partial exchange transfusion.

Nursing Care

The nurse assesses, records, and reports symptoms of polycythemia. The nurse also does an initial screening of the newborn's hematocrit on admission to the nursery. It is important to remember that if a capillary hematocrit is done, warming the heel prior to obtaining the blood helps to decrease falsely high values. Peripheral venous hematocrit samples are usually obtained from the antecubital fossa.

Many infants are asymptomatic, but as symptoms develop they are related to the increased blood volume, hyperviscocity (thickness) of the blood, and decreased deformability of red blood cells, all of which result in poor perfusion of tissues. The infants have a characteristic plethoric (ruddy) appearance. The most common symptoms observed include the following:

- Tachycardia and congestive heart failure due to the increased blood volume

- Respiratory distress with grunting, tachypnea, and cyanosis; increased oxygen need; or hemorrhage in respiratory system due to pulmonary venous congestion, edema, and hypoxemia
- Hyperbilirubinemia due to increased numbers of red blood cells hemolysed
- Decrease in peripheral pulses, discoloration of extremities, alteration in activity or neurologic depression, renal vein thrombosis with decreased urine output, hematuria, or proteinuria due to thromboembolism
- Seizures due to decreased perfusion of the brain and increased vascular resistance secondary to sluggish blood flow, which can result in neurologic or developmental problems

The nurse observes closely for signs of distress or change in vital signs during the partial exchange. The nurse assesses carefully for potential complications resulting from the exchange such as transfusion overload (which can result in congestive heart failure), irregular cardiac rhythm, bacterial infection, hypovolemia (because of decreased plasma volume) and anemia.

Parents need specific explanations about polycythemia and its treatment. The newborn needs to be reunited with the parents as soon after the exchange as the baby's status permits.

Care of the Newborn with Infection

Newborns up to one month of age are particularly susceptible to infection, referred to as **sepsis neonatorum**, caused by organisms that do not cause significant disease in older children. Incidence of severe infection is 0.5 to 2 per 1000 live newborns.

One predisposing factor is prematurity. The general debilitation and underlying illness often associated with prematurity necessitates invasive procedures such as umbilical catheterization, intubation, resuscitation, ventilatory support, and monitoring. Even full-term infants are susceptible because their immunologic systems are immature. They lack the complex factors involved in effective phagocytosis and the ability to localize infection or to respond with a well-defined recognizable inflammatory response.

Maternal antepartal infections such as rubella, toxoplasmosis, cytomegalic inclusion disease, and herpes may cause congenital infections and resulting disorders in the newborn. Intrapartal maternal infections, such as amnionitis and those resulting from premature rupture of membranes and precipitous birth, are sources of neonatal infection. Passage through the birth canal and contact with the vaginal flora (β-hemolytic streptococci, herpes, listeria, and gonococci) expose the infant to infection (see Table 32–6). With infection anywhere in the fetus or newborn, the adjacent tissues or organs are very easily penetrated, and the blood-brain barrier is ineffective. Septicemia is more common in males, except for those infections caused by group B β-hemolytic streptococcus.

At present, gram-negative organisms (especially *Escherichia coli,* Aerobacter, *Proteus,* and *Klebsiella*) and the gram-positive organism β-hemolytic streptococcus are the most common causative agents. Pseudomonas is a common fomite contaminant of ventilatory support and oxygen therapy equipment. *Staphylococcus* (*S aureus* and *S epidermidis*) is becoming an increasingly prevalent infecting organism for babies with prolonged hospitalization.

Protection of the newborn from infections starts prenatally and continues throughout pregnancy and birth. Prenatal prevention should include maternal screening for sexually transmitted disease and monitoring of rubella titers in women who test negative. Intrapartally, sterile technique is essential, smears from genital lesions are taken,

Table 32–6 Maternally Transmitted Newborn Infections		
Infection	**Nursing assessment**	**Nursing plan and implementation**
Group B Streptococcus		
1–2% colonized with one in ten developing disease Early onset—usually within hours of birth or within first week Late onset—one week to three months	Severe respiratory distress (grunting and cyanosis). May become apneic or demonstrate symptoms of shock. Meconium-stained amniotic fluid seen at birth.	Early assessment of clinical signs necessary. Assist with x-ray—shows aspiration pneumonia or hyaline membrane disease. Immediately obtain blood, gastric aspirate, external ear canal and nasopharynx cultures. Administer antibiotics, usually aqueous penicillin or ampicillin combined with gentamicin as soon as cultures are obtained. Early assessment and intervention are essential to survival. Initiate referral to evaluate for blindness, deafness, learning or behavioral problems.

(continued)

Table 32−6 (continued)

Infection	Nursing assessment	Nursing plan and implementation

Syphilis
 	
Spirochetes cross placenta after 16−18th week of gestation
	Check perinatal history for positive maternal serology.
	Assess infant for:
	  Elevated cord serum IgM and FTA-ABS IgM
	  Rhinitis (snuffles)
	  Fissures on mouth corners and excoriated upper lip
	  Red rash around mouth and anus
	  Copper-colored rash over face, palms, and soles
	  Irritability
	  Generalized edema, particularly over joints; bone lesions; painful extremities
	  Hepatosplenomegaly, jaundice
	  Congenital cataracts
	  SGA and failure to thrive
		Initiate isolation techniques until infants have been on antibiotics for 48 hours.
		Administer penicillin.
		Provide emotional support for parents because of their feelings about mode of transmission and potential long-term sequelae.

Gonorrhea	Assess for:
	  Ophthalmia neonatorum (conjunctivitis)
	  Purulent discharge and corneal ulcerations
	  Neonatal sepsis with temperature instability, poor feeding response, and/or hypotonia, jaundice
		Administer 1% silver nitrate solution or ophthalmic antibiotic ointment (see Drug Guide—Erythromycin [Ilotycin]) or, in lieu of silver nitrate, penicillin.
		Initiate follow-up referral to evaluate any loss of vision.

Herpes Type 2	Small cluster vesicular skin lesions over all the body. Check perinatal history for active herpes genital lesions. Disseminated form—DIC, pneumonia, hepatitis with jaundice, hepatosplenomegaly, and neurologic abnormalities. Without skin lesions, see fever or subnormal temperature, respiratory congestion, tachypnea and tachycardia.	Carry out careful hand washing and gown and glove isolation with linen precautions. Administer intravenous vidarabine (Vira A) or acyclovir (Zovirax). Initiate follow-up referral to evaluate potential sequelae of microcephaly, spasticity, seizures, deafness, or blindness. Encourage parental rooming-in and touching of their newborn. Show parents appropriate hand-washing procedures and precautions to be used at home if mother's lesions are active. Obtain throat, conjunctiva, cerebral spinal fluid (CSF), blood, urine, and lesion cultures to identify herpesvirus type 2 antibiotics in serum IgM fraction. Cultures positive in 24−48 hours.
Monilial Infection (Thrush)	Assess buccal mucosa, tongue, gums, and inside the cheeks for white plaques (seen five to seven days of age). Check diaper area for bright red, well-demarcated eruptions. Assess for thrush periodically when newborn is on long-term antibiotic therapy.	Differentiate white plaque areas from milk curds by using cotton tip applicator (if it is thrush, removal of white areas causes raw bleeding areas). Maintain cleanliness of hands, linen, clothing, diapers and feeding apparatus. Instruct breast-feeding mothers on treating their nipples with nystatin. Administer gentian violet (1%−2%) swabbed on oral lesions one hour after feeding, or nystatin instilled in baby's oral cavity and on mucosa. Swab skin lesions with topical nystatin. Discuss with parents that gentian violet stains mouth and clothing. Avoid placing gentian violet on normal mucosa; causes irritation.
Chlamydia Trachomatis	Assess for perinatal history of preterm birth. Symptomatic newborns present with pneumonia—conjunctivitis after three to four days. Chronic follicular conjunctivitis (corneal neovascularization and conjunctival scarring).	Instill ophthalmic erythromycin (See Drug Guide—Erythromycin [Ilotycin]). Initiate follow-up referral for eye complications.

and placenta and amniotic fluid cultures are obtained if amnionitis is suspected. If genital herpes is present toward term, cesarean birth may be indicated. Local eye treatment with silver nitrate or an antibiotic ophthalmic ointment is given to all newborns to prevent damage from gonococcal infections.

Medical Therapy

Infants with a history of possible exposure to infection in utero (for example, premature rupture of membranes more than 24 hours before birth or questionable maternal history of infection) should have cultures (gastric aspirate and ear canal) taken as soon after birth as possible. Cultures are obtained before antibiotic therapy is begun.

1. Two blood cultures are obtained from different peripheral sites. They are taken from a peripheral rather than an umbilical vessel, because catheters have yielded false positives resulting from contamination. The skin is prepared by cleaning with an antiseptic solution, such as one containing iodine, and allowed to dry; the specimen is obtained with a sterile needle/syringe.

2. Spinal fluid culture is done following a spinal tap.

3. Urine culture is best obtained from a specimen obtained by a suprapubic bladder aspiration.

4. Skin cultures are taken of any lesions or drainage from lesions or reddened areas.

5. Nasopharyngeal, rectal, ear canal, and gastric aspirate cultures may be obtained.

Other laboratory investigations include a complete blood count, chest x-ray examination, serology, and Gram stains of cerebrospinal fluid, urine, skin exudate, and umbilicus. White blood count (WBC) with differential may indicate the presence or absence of sepsis. A level of 30,000 WBC may be normal in the first 24 hours of life, while low WBC may be indicative of sepsis. A low neutrophil count and high band (immature white cells) count indicate that an infection is present. Stomach aspirate should be sent for culture and smear if a gonococcal infection or amnionitis are suspected. Serum IgM levels are elevated (normal level less than 20 mg/dL) in response to transplacental infections. If available, counterimmuno-electrophoresis tests for specific bacterial antigens are done. Evidence of congenital infections may be seen on skull x-ray films for cerebral calcifications (cytomegalovirus, toxoplasmosis), on bone x-ray films (syphilis, cytomegalovirus), and in serum-specific IgM levels (rubella). Cytomegalovirus infection is best diagnosed by urine culture.

Because neonatal infection causes high mortality, therapy is instituted before results of the septic workup are obtained. A combination of two broad-spectrum antibiotics, such as ampicillin and gentamicin, is given in large doses until a culture with sensitivities is obtained.

After the pathogen and its sensitivities are determined, appropriate specific antibiotic therapy is begun. Combinations of penicillin or ampicillin and kanamycin have been used in the past, but new kanamycin-resistant enterobacteria and penicillin-resistant staphylococcus necessitate increasing use of gentamicin.

The possibility of rotating aminoglycosides has been suggested to prevent development of resistance. Use of cephalosporins and, in particular, cefotaxime, has emerged as an alternative to aminoglycoside therapy in the treatment of neonatal infections. Duration of therapy varies from 7 to 14 days (Table 32–7). If cultures are negative and symptoms subside, antibiotics may be discontinued after three days. Supportive physiologic care may be required to maintain respiratory, hemodynamic, nutritional, and metabolic homeostasis.

❈ *APPLYING THE NURSING PROCESS* ❈

Nursing Assessment

Symptoms are most often noticed by the nurse during daily care of the neonate rather than during the infant's sporadic contact with the physician. The infant may deteriorate rapidly in the first 12 to 24 hours after birth if β-hemolytic streptococcal infection is present, with signs and symptoms mimicking RDS. On the other hand, the onset of sepsis may be more gradual with more subtle signs and symptoms. The most common symptoms observed include the following:

1. Subtle behavioral changes—the infant "isn't doing well" and is often lethargic or irritable (especially after first 24 hours) and hypotonic. Color changes may include pallor, duskiness, cyanosis, or a "shocky" appearance. Skin is cool and clammy.

2. Temperature instability, manifested by either hypothermia (recognized by a decrease in skin temperature) or hyperthermia (elevation of skin temperature) necessitating a corresponding increase or decrease in Isolette temperature to maintain neutral thermal environment

3. Poor feeding, evidenced by a decrease in total intake, abdominal distention, vomiting, poor sucking, lack of interest in feeding, and diarrhea

4. Hyperbilirubinemia

5. Onset of apnea

Signs and symptoms may suggest CNS disease (jitteriness, tremors, seizure activity), respiratory system disease (tachypnea, labored respirations, apnea, cyanosis), hematologic disease (jaundice, petechial hemorrhages, hepatosplenomegaly), or gastrointestinal disease (diarrhea, vomiting, bile-stained aspirate, hepatomegaly). A differential diagnosis is necessary because of the similarity of symptoms to other more specific conditions.

Table 32–7 Neonatal Sepsis Antibiotic Therapy

Drug	Dose	Route	Schedule	Comments
Ampicillin	50–100 mg/kg/day	IM or IV	Every 12 hours* Every 8 hours†	Effective against gram-positive microorganisms and majority of *E coli* strains.
Cefotaxime	100–150 mg/kg/day	IM or IV	Every 12 hours* Every 8 hours†	Active against most major pathogens in infants; effective against aminoglycoside-resistant organisms; achieves CSF bactericidal activity; lack of ototoxicity and nephrotoxicity; wide therapeutic index (levels not required); resistant organisms can develop rapidly if used extensively; ineffective against pseudomonas, listeria.
Gentamicin	5.0–7.5 mg/kg/day	IM or IV	Every 12 hours* Every 8 hours†	Effective against gram-negative rods and staphylococci; may be used instead of kanamycin against penicillin-resistant staphylococci and *E coli* strains and *Pseudomonas aeruginosa.* May cause ototoxicity and nephrotoxicity. Need to follow serum levels. Must never be given as IV push. Must be given over at least 30–60 min. In presence of oliguria or anuria, dose must be decreased or discontinued. In infant less than 1000 g, dosage interval may be as long as 24 hours. Monitor serum levels before administration of second dose.
Methicillin	50–100 mg/kg/day	IM or IV	Every 12 hours* Every 6–8 hours†	Effective against penicillinase-resistant staphylococci
Nafcillin	50–100 mg/kg/day	IM or IV	Every 12 hours* Every 6 hours†	Effective against penicillinase-resistant staphylococci.
Penicillin G (aqueous crystalline)	50,000–125,000 U/kg/day	IM or IV	Every 12 hours* Every 8 hours†	Initial sepsis therapy effective against most gram-positive microorganisms except resistant staphylococci; can cause heart block in infants.
Vancomycin	30 mg/kg/day	IV	Every 12 hours* Every 8 hours†	Effective for methicillin-resistant strains (*S epidermidis*); must be administered by slow intravenous infusion to avoid prolonged cutaneous eruption. For smaller infants <1200 g; smaller dosages and longer intervals between doses. Nephrotoxic, especially when given in combination with aminoglycosides.

† *Greater than seven days of age.*
* *Up to seven days of age.*

Nursing Diagnosis

Nursing diagnoses that may apply to the infant with sepsis neonatorum include the following:

- Infection: High risk related to immature immunologic system
- Fluid volume deficit related to feeding intolerance
- Ineffective family coping related to present illness resulting in prolonged hospital stay for the newborn

Nursing Plan and Implementation

Prevention of Infection

In the nursery, environmental control and prevention of acquired infection is the responsibility of the neonatal nurse. The nurse must promote strict hand-washing technique for all who enter the nursery, including nursing colleagues; physicians; laboratory, x-ray, and inhalation technicians; and parents. The nurse must be prepared to assist in the aseptic collection of specimens for laboratory investigations. Scrupulous care of equipment—changing and clean-

ing of incubators at least every seven days, removal and sterilization of wet equipment every 24 hours, prevention of cross-use of linen and other equipment, periodic cleaning of sinkside equipment such as soap containers, and special care with the open radiant warmers (access without prior hand washing is much easier than with the closed incubator)—will prevent fomite contamination or contamination through improper hand washing of debilitated, infection-prone newborns. An infected neonate can be effectively isolated in an incubator and receive close observation. Visiting of the nursery area by unnecessary personnel should be discouraged.

Provision of Antibiotic Therapy

The nurse administers antibiotics as ordered by the clinician. It is the nurse's responsibility to be knowledgeable about the following:

- The proper dose to be administered, based on the weight of the newborn and desired peak and trough levels
- The appropriate route of administration, as some antibiotics cannot be given intravenously

- Admixture incompatibilities, since some antibiotics are precipitated by intravenous solutions or by other antibiotics
- Side effects and toxicity

Promotion of Physical Well-Being

In addition to antibiotic therapy, physiologic supportive care is essential in caring for a septic infant. The nurse should do the following:

- Observe for resolution of symptoms or development of other symptoms of sepsis.
- Maintain neutral thermal environment with accurate regulation of humidity and oxygen administration.
- Provide respiratory support: Administer oxygen and observe and monitor respiratory effort.
- Provide cardiovascular support: Observe and monitor pulse and blood pressure; observe for hyperbilirubinemia, anemia, and hemorrhagic symptoms.
- Provide adequate calories, because oral feedings may be discontinued due to increased mucus, abdominal distention, vomiting, and aspiration.
- Provide fluids and electrolytes to maintain homeostasis. Monitor weight changes and urine output and specific gravity.
- Detect and treat metabolic disturbances, a common occurrence.
- Observe for the development of hypoglycemia, hyperglycemia, acidosis, hyponatremia, and hypocalcemia.

Provision of Support and Education to Parents

Restriction of parent visits has not been shown to have any effect on the rate of infection and may indeed be harmful to the newborn's psychologic development. With instruction and guidance from the nurse, both parents should be allowed to handle the baby and participate in daily care. Support to the parents is crucial. They need to be informed of the newborn's prognosis as treatment continues and to be involved in care as much as possible. They also need to understand how infection is transmitted.

Evaluation

Anticipated outcomes of nursing care include the following:

- The risks for development of sepsis are identified early, and immediate action is taken to minimize the development of the illness.
- Appropriate use of aseptic technique protects the newborn from further exposure to illness.
- The baby's symptoms are relieved, and the infection is treated.

- The parents verbalize their concerns about their baby's illness and understand the rationale behind the management of their newborn.

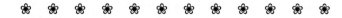

Care of the Family of a Newborn with a Complication

Adaptation of the Family

The birth of a baby with a problem or disorder is a traumatic event with the potential for either total disruption or growth of the involved family. Throughout the pregnancy both parents, together and separately, have felt excitement, experienced thoughts of acceptance, and pictured what their baby would look like. Both parents have wished for a perfect baby and feared a damaged, unhealthy one. Each parent and family member must accept and adjust when the fantasized fears become a reality.

Grieving for the loss of the hoped-for perfect child is necessary before the development of a positive relationship to the existing child can begin. Grief is expressed as shock and disbelief, denial of reality, anger toward self and others, guilt, blame, and concern for the future. Self-esteem and feelings of self-worth are jeopardized.

Fear, separation, and grief begin during the birth, when the newborn requires immediate resuscitation or special treatment. Instead of being handed to its mother, the baby is given to a nurse or a pediatrician who rushes it to a special care area. The joyful cries of "It's a boy!" or "It's a girl!" are absent; there is only the mother's pleading question, "What's wrong with my baby?" If no answer is given to the mother, she frequently fantasizes the worst and assumes that the baby is dead. It is extremely important for the mother's health and the mother-infant relationship that some immediate answer be given to the parents. Honest, simple, and positive facts can be shared: "Your baby is alive"; "Your baby is a girl"; "Your baby has a strong heartbeat but needs some help with breathing"; "Your baby is alive but needs some special care right now"; "The pediatrician is helping your baby now and will talk with you soon." The information that nurses share with parents must always be honest data that nurses can observe and document. Nurses should not make promises that they cannot fulfill and should refrain from offering empty reassurances that everything will be all right.

The period of waiting between suspicion and confirmation of abnormality or dysfunction is a very anxious one for parents because it is difficult, if not impossible, to begin attachment to the infant if the newborn's future is questionable. During the "not knowing period," parents need support and acknowledgment that this is an anxious time and must be kept informed about efforts to gather additional data and maintain the infant's livelihood. It is helpful to tell both parents about the problem at the same time, with the baby present. An honest discussion of the problem and anticipatory management at the earliest possible time by health professionals help the parents (a) maintain trust in the physician and nurse, (b) appreciate the reality of the situation by dispelling fantasy and misconception, (c) begin the grieving process, and (d) mobilize internal and external support.

Nurses need to be aware that anger is a universal response and that it is best directed outward, because holding it in check requires great energy, which is diverted away from grieving and physical recovery from pregnancy and giving birth. Anger may be directed unjustifiably at the physician and/or nurse, at the food, at nursing care, or at hospital regulations and routines. Anger with the baby is rarely demonstrated by parents and can precipitate guilt feelings.

A heightened concern for self may be misinterpreted by health professionals as rejection of the newborn. Both parents need time and understanding to deal with their own feelings before they can direct concern toward the baby. In a short span of time, the parent is confronted with the loss of the idealized child, the need to accept a child who deviates from normal, and a sense of personal failure. In addition, the new mother may be suffering from fatigue and sleep deprivation from her pregnancy and labor and from discomforts arising from cesarean birth, episiotomy, inability to void, hemorrhoids, and afterpains. In the postpartal period concern for self and dependency are normal events.

In their sensitive and vulnerable state, parents are acutely perceptive of others' responses and reactions (particularly nonverbal) to the child. Parents can be expected to identify with the responses of others. Therefore, it is imperative that medical and nursing staff be fully aware of their feelings and come to terms with those feelings so that they are comfortable and at ease with the baby and the grieving family.

Nurses may feel uncomfortable not knowing what to say to parents or may fear confronting their own feelings as well as those of the parents. Each nurse must work out personal reactions with instructors, peers, clergy, parents, or significant others. It is helpful to have a stockpile of therapeutic questions and statements to initiate meaningful dialogue with parents. Opening statements can be as follows: "You must be wondering what could have caused this"; "Are you thinking you (or someone else) may have done something?"; "How can I help?"; "Go ahead and cry. It's worth crying about"; or "Are you wondering how you are going to manage?" Avoid statements such as "It could have been worse"; "It's God's will"; "You have other children"; "You are still young and can have more"; and "I understand how you feel." *This* child is important *now.*

Some nurses find relief for themselves or a means of escape from painful circumstances by overzealous and unrealistic reassurance that "everything will be all right" and by avoidance of the newborn and family. Other medical and nursing staff take refuge in technical jargon and in-

volvement in the technical aspects of the mother's care rather than taking time to talk about the situation. These approaches confuse the parents at a time when they need most to be understood and to understand.

Nurses show concern and support by planning time to spend with the parents, by being psychologically as well as physically present, by encouraging open discussion and grieving, by repetitious explanations (as necessary), by providing privacy as needed, and by encouraging contact with the newborn. Identification and clarification of feelings and fears decrease distortions in perception, thinking, and feeling. Nurses invest the baby with value in the eyes of the parents when they provide meticulous care to the newborn, talk and coo (especially in the face-to-face position) while holding or providing care to the newborn, refer to the child by gender or name, and relate the newborn's activities ("He took a whole ounce of formula"; "She burped so loud that . . ."; "He took hold of the blanket and just wouldn't let go"; "He voided all over the doctor"). Nurses should note the "normal" characteristics and capabilities of each newborn as well as the newborn's needs. The nurse should also learn the baby's name and refer to him or her by name.

Many physicians show parents "before" and "after" photographs of conditions requiring surgical intervention. Parents also may benefit from meeting other parents who have faced the same problem through a parental support group or organization that is specific to that problem. Specialists (plastic surgeons, perinatal clinic nurse specialists, neurosurgeons, orthopedists, oral surgeons, dentists, and rehabilitation therapists) can be reassuring and supportive of parents in their short- and long-term goals. However, these types of interventions must be carefully timed to the readiness of the parents.

Cues that the parents are ready to become involved with the child's care or planning for the future include their reference to the baby as "she" or "he" or by name and their questioning as to amount of feeding taken, appearance today, and the like.

Mothers may feel inadequate or guilty when they do not feel motherly toward their baby. One mother, looking at her child born with a severe cleft lip and palate, said, "God help me. I can't stand looking at her. I wish she wasn't mine. What a horrid thing to say, but I can't . . . I just can't." She could not bring herself to hold or touch the infant prior to cleft lip repair. She needed considerable assistance to talk of these feelings in a nonjudgmental and accepting atmosphere before she was able to hold the infant after surgery. She proceeded to learn to feed her daughter (whose cleft palate was not yet repaired) and become very "motherly" before the infant was discharged. Her husband, fortunately, facilitated the whole process by his continued love for and acceptance of his wife throughout the experience.

Occasionally a mother may become overprotective and overoptimistic shortly after the baby's birth. The nurse should accept her behavior but continue to remind her that it is okay and natural to feel disappointment, a sense of

Contemporary Issue
When the Newborn Isn't Perfect

The issue of who is responsible and what should be done for a child with a congenital anomaly or severe handicap has recently been raised. What is the impact on the child and/or the family at the time of the birth and in the future? Severe disability in a newborn also raises questions of evaluating the distress the newborn is going through or will suffer during a lifetime.

A legal term being introduced is "wrongful life" or "wrongful birth" cases. A wrongful life case is a lawsuit brought by a child with a birth defect, which alleges that the physician failed to advise the parents of the risk of birth defects or failed to perform tests that would have indicated the presence or likelihood of birth defects. In addition the suit claims that because the child's parents were deprived of medical information to make an informed choice, the mother conceived and carried to term a child suffering from birth defects. A wrongful birth case is identical to a wrongful life case, with the exception that it is usually brought by the parents rather than the child. Courts have recognized wrongful birth cases over the past decade but have been perplexed by the wrongful life claims because of the traditional view that the involved handicapped child is arguing that he or she would have

been better off not being born rather than being born with a birth defect. The courts were unwilling to "weigh the value of life with impairments against the nonexistence of life itself." The courts are now addressing these cases with the focus on the child's right to be compensated for injuries caused by the physician's negligence. This dilemma has prompted philosophical, ethical, moral, legal, and economic questions. The questions and concerns that are being raised include the following:

● How does one measure the emotional impact of the birth of a severely disabled infant?

● Is not being born preferable to being born with a serious handicap or birth defect?

● Who or what determines quality of life?

● Is a certain quality of life guaranteed?

● What is the social and economic impact on the child and family over the lifetime of the child born with a birth defect/severe handicap?

● What constitutes a "defect"? Should we as a society reevaluate our insistence on "perfection" and widen our acceptance of "disability"?

---

failure, helplessness, or anger. The overprotectiveness and overoptimism are defense mechanisms. To deny the negative feelings only entrenches them further, delays their resolution, and delays realistic planning.

Developmental Consequences

The baby who is born prematurely, is ill, or has a malformation or disorder is at risk in emotional and intellectual, as well as physical, development. The risk is directly proportional to the seriousness of the problem and the length of treatment. For example, resolution of a meconium plug syndrome during the expected hospital stay, allowing the infant to be discharged with the mother, is not expected to alter the child's developmental course. However, the physical appearance, immediate and repeated surgeries, and complex rehabilitation problems of exstrophy of the bladder or meningomyelocele preclude a normal developmental course for the child.

Medical, surgical, and technical advances in recent years have been responsible for salvaging increasing numbers of preterm and ill neonates. The necessary physical separation of family and infant and the tremendous emo-

tional and financial burden have adversely affected the parent-child relationship. A considerable percentage of these children have been rescued only to be emotionally or physically battered by the parents. The most recent trend in many hospitals is to involve the parents with the neonate early, repeatedly, and over protracted periods of time. Early and continued involvement may only mean opportunities to look at or stroke the baby. Later, when the mother's and baby's conditions warrant it, the mother participates in her baby's care (to the extent she is willing) and in planning for the future. This type of involvement facilitates early bonding, attachment, and emotional investment. The parents need a sense of personal success, self-worth, self-esteem, and confidence from knowledge that they can cope with the situation. This atmosphere aids the baby as well—the child may escape battering and may instead be assisted toward self-actualization (Figure 32–15).

Mothers of newborns who are gravely ill are often unable to chance an emotional investment in their child. These mothers need assistance in perceiving the cues and hearing the words that indicate the baby is going to survive. They need time and support to establish a positive relationship with the newborn. A mother who is unable to

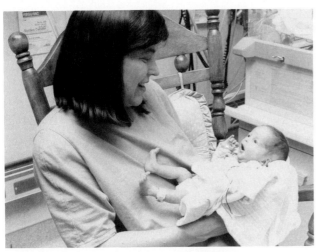

Figure 32–15 Parents and children thrive when parents have realistic expectations of the child's long-term developmental need.

develop maternal feelings may reject the baby or overcompensate because of underlying guilt feelings; in either case an unproductive relationship may develop. The child may then be further handicapped by inability to relate well to others and by seeing the world as unsatisfying and painful.

The parents must have a clear picture of the reality of the handicap and the types of developmental hurdles ahead. Unexpected behaviors and responses from the baby due to his or her defect or disorder can be upsetting and frightening. For example, parents find it difficult to cope with a baby's lack of motor or social responsiveness and tend to interpret the lack as a form of rejection. The parents may in return respond with rejection, and an unfortunate cycle is begun.

The demands of care of the child and disputes regarding management or behavior stress family relationships. One or more members of the family may make a scapegoat of the child. Another may become the youngster's champion to the exclusion of others. One or the other spouse may feel pushed aside or denied attention and thus may withdraw or leave the family unit. Parents or siblings may feel that their own needs (schooling, material goods, freedom of movement) are being set aside while all assets (financial and other) go to support the one child's needs.

The entire multidisciplinary team may need to pool their resources and expertise to help parents of children born with problems or disorders so that both parents and children can thrive.

❀ ❀

KEY CONCEPTS

The sick neonate—whether preterm, term, or postterm—must be managed within narrow physiologic parameters.

These parameters (respiratory and thermal regulation) will maintain physiologic homeostasis and prevent introduction of iatrogenic stress to the already stressed infant.

Maintenance of this physiologic environment must begin immediately, because lost ground is difficult or impossible to recover.

The nursing care of the neonate with special problems involves the understanding of normal physiology, the pathophysiology of the disease process, clinical manifestations, and supportive or corrective therapies. Only with this theoretical background can the nurse make appropriate observations concerning responses to therapy and development of complications.

Neonates communicate needs only by their behavior; the neonatal nurse, through objective observations and evaluations, interprets this behavior into meaningful information about the infant's condition.

The nurse is the facilitator for interdisciplinary communication with the parents, identifying their understanding of their infant's care and their needs for emotional support.

Newborn conditions that commonly present with respiratory distress and require oxygen and ventilatory assistance are respiratory distress syndrome, meconium aspiration syndrome, transient tachypnea of the newborn, and persistent pulmonary hypertension of the newborn.

Cold stress sets up the chain of physiologic events of hypoglycemia, pulmonary vasoconstriction, hyperbilirubinemia, respiratory distress, and metabolic acidosis. Nurses are responsible for early detection and initiation of treatment for hypoglycemia.

Differentiation between pathologic and physiologic jaundice is the key to early and successful intervention.

Nursing assessment of the septic newborn involves identification of very subtle clinical signs that are also seen in other clinical disease states.

❀ ❀

References

Avery GB (editor): *Neonatology,* 3rd ed. Philadelphia: Lippincott, 1987.

Avery ME, Taeusch HW (editors): *Schaffer's Diseases of the Newborn,* 5th ed. Philadelphia: Saunders, 1984.

Bloom RS, Cropley C: *Textbook of Neonatal Resuscitation.* Los Angeles: American Heart Association and American Academy of Pediatrics, 1987.

Connolly AM, Volpe JJ: Clinical features of bilirubin encephalopathy. *Clin Perinatol* 1990; 17(2):371.

Ennever JF: Blue light, green light, white light, more light: Treatment of neonatal jaundice. *Clin Perinatol* 1990; 17(2):467.

Gill NE, Behnke M, Conlon M et al: Effect of nonnutritive sucking on behavioral state in preterm infants before feeding. *Nurs Res* 1988; 37(8):344.

Gunderson LP, Kenner C: Transcutaneous oxygen monitoring. *Neonatal Netw* 1988; 6(6):7.

Harbold LA: A protocol for neonatal use of pulse oximetry. *Neonatal Netw* 1989; 8(1):41.

Houska Lund C: *Bronchopulmonary Dysplasia: Strategies for Total Patient Care.* Petaluma, CA: Neonatal Network, 1990.

Hudak BB, Jones MD: Meconium aspiration. In *Current Therapy in Neonatal-Perinatal Medicine-2.* Nelson NM (editor). Philadelphia: Decker, 1990.

King JD, Jung AL: Phototherapy. In: *Current Therapy in Neonatal-Perinatal Medicine-2.* Nelson NM (editor). Philadelphia: Decker, 1990.

Merenstein GB, Gardner SL: *Handbook of Neonatal Intensive Care,* 2nd ed. St. Louis: Mosby, 1989.

Northway WH et al: Pulmonary disease following respiratory therapy of hyaline membrane disease: Bronchopulmonary dysplasia. *N Engl J Med* 1967; 276:357.

Page S: Rh hemolytic disease of the newborn. *Neonatal Netw* 1989; 7(6):31.

Ward RM: Persistent pulmonary hypertension. In: *Current Therapy in Neonatal-Perinatal Medicine-2.* Nelson NM (editor). Philadelphia: Decker, 1990.

Yeh TF: *Neonatal Therapeutics,* 2nd ed. St. Louis: Mosby/Year Book, 1991.

Additional Readings

Auten RL et al: Surfactant treatment of full-term newborns with respiratory failure. *Pediatrics* 1991; 87(1):101.

Ballard RA: *Pediatric Care of the ICN Graduate.* Philadelphia: Saunders, 1988.

Blayney M et al: A new system for location of endotracheal tube in preterm and term neonates. *Pediatrics* 1991; 87(1):44.

Fox MD, MG Molesky: The effects of prone and supine positioning on arterial oxygen pressure. *Neonatal Netw* 1990; 8(4):25.

Hodge D: Endotracheal suctioning and the infant: A nursing care protocol to decrease complications. *Neonatal Netw* 1991; 9(5):7.

Langer VS: Minimal handling protocol for the intensive care nursery. *Neonatal Netw* 1990; 9(3):231.

Morrow CJ et al: Transcutaneous oxygen tension in preterm neonates during neonatal behavior assessments and heelsticks. *Journal of Developmental and Behavioral Pediatrics* 1990; 11(6):312.

Rose BS: Phototherapy: All wrapped up? *Pediatr Nurs* 1990; 16(1):57.

Rosenberg AL: The return of congenital syphilis. *Neonatal Netw* 1991; 9(5):17.

Sterling YM: Resource needs of mothers managing chronically ill infants at home. *Neonatal Netw* 1990; 9(1):55.

PART SEVEN

Postpartum

CHAPTER 33

Postpartal Adaptation and Nursing Assessment

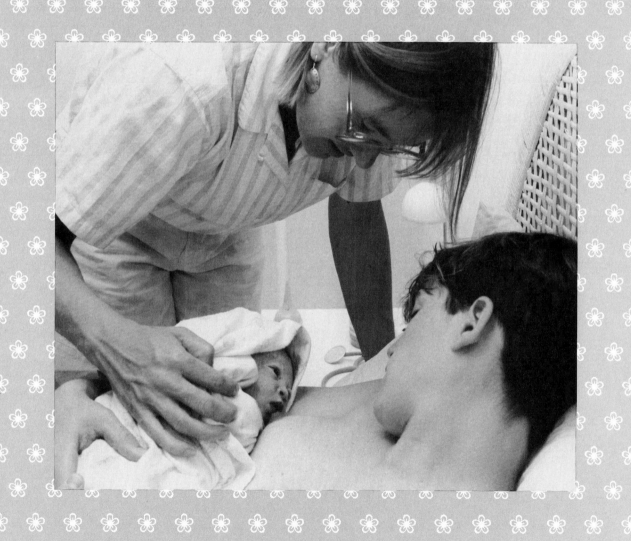

Summarize the physical and psychologic adaptations that occur postpartally as a woman's body returns to its prepregnant state.

Relate the physiologic changes that occur postpartally to an appropriate nursing assessment.

Discuss nursing assessment of the psychologic changes that occur in the childbearing woman during the postpartal period.

❊ ❊

I had heard about the negatives—the fatigue, the loneliness, loss of self. But nobody told me about the wonderful parts: holding my baby close to me, seeing her first smile, watching her grow and become more responsive day by day. How can I describe the way I felt when she stroked my breast while nursing, or looked into my eyes or arched her eyebrows like an opera singer? This was the deepest connection I'd felt to anybody. Sometimes the intensity almost frightened me. For the first time I cared about somebody else more than myself, and I would do anything to nurture and protect her. (The New Our Bodies, Ourselves)

The **puerperium (postpartum)** is the period of time during which the body adjusts, both physically and psychologically, to the process of childbearing. It begins immediately after childbirth and proceeds for approximately six weeks or until the body has completed its adjustment and has returned to a near prepregnant state. Some have referred to the puerperium as "the fourth trimester," and whereas the time span does not necessarily cover three months, this terminology demonstrates the idea of continuity.

This chapter first describes the physical and psychologic changes that occur postpartally. Using this information as a base, the second portion of the chapter focuses on a thorough postpartal assessment.

Postpartal Physical Adaptations

Comprehensive nursing assessment is based on a sound understanding of the normal anatomic and physiologic processes of the puerperium. These processes involve the reproductive organs and other major body systems.

Reproductive Organs

Involution of the Uterus

The term **involution** is used to describe the rapid reduction in size of the uterus and its return to a condition similar to its prepregnant state.

Immediately following the expulsion of the placenta, the uterus contracts firmly to the size of a large grapefruit. The fundus is situated in the midline, one-half to two-thirds of the way between the symphysis pubis and the umbilicus (Figure 33–1). The walls of the contracted uterus, each about 4 to 5 cm thick, are close together, and the uterine blood vessels are firmly compressed by the myometrium. Within a few hours after birth the fundus of the uterus rises to the level of the umbilicus. A fundus that is above the umbilicus and **boggy** (feels soft and spongy rather than firm and well-contracted), is associated with excessive uterine bleeding. As blood collects and forms clots within the uterus, the fundus rises; firm contractions of the uterine muscle are interrupted, causing a boggy uterus. When the fundus is higher than expected and deviated from the midline (usually to the right), bladder distention should be suspected. Because the uterine ligaments are still stretched, a full bladder can move the uterus.

The uterus remains at the level of the umbilicus for about a day and then on each succeeding postpartal day descends into the pelvis approximately one fingerbreadth. This descent occurs so rapidly that within ten days to two weeks the uterus is again a pelvic organ and cannot be palpated abdominally. If the woman is breast-feeding, the release of oxytocin from the posterior pituitary, which is a response to suckling, may cause the uterus to descend more rapidly into the pelvis.

Barring complications such as infection or retained placental fragments, the uterus approaches the nonpregnant size by four to six weeks. Changes in the weight of the uterus are equally dramatic. Although it weighs about 1000 g at term, the uterus decreases to 500 g at one week, 300 g at two weeks, and 100 g after the third week (Cunningham et al 1989).

With the dramatic decrease in the levels of circulatory estrogen and progesterone following placental separation, the uterine cells atrophy, and the hyperplasia of preg-

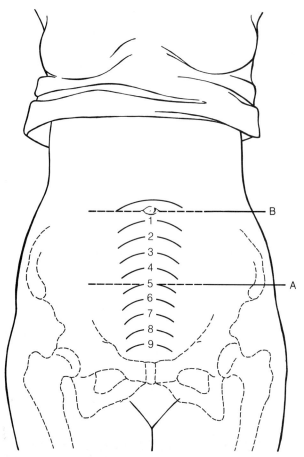

Figure 33–1 Involution of the uterus. A Immediately after expulsion of the placenta the uterine fundus is positioned in the midline about one-half to two-thirds of the way between the symphysis pubis and the umbilicus. B Within two to four hours after birth, the fundus is at the level of the umbilicus. The height of the fundus then decreases approximately one fingerbreadth (about 1 cm) each day.

nancy begins to reverse. The process is basically one of cell size reduction rather than a radical decrease in cell number. Proteolytic enzymes are released, and macrophages migrate to the uterus to promote autolysis (self-digestion). Protein material in the uterine wall is broken down and absorbed.

Following separation of the placenta, the decidua of the uterus is irregular, jagged, and varied in thickness. The spongy layer of the decidua is cast off as lochia, and the basal layer of the decidua remains in the uterus to become differentiated into two layers within the first 48 to 72 hours after birth. The outermost layer becomes necrotic and is sloughed off in the lochia. The layer closest to the myometrium contains the fundi of the uterine endometrial glands, and these glands lay the foundation for the new endometrium. Except at the placental site, this process is completed in approximately three weeks.

Involution of the placental site is a similar process but takes up to six weeks for completion. Following separation, the placental site contracts to an area 8 to 9 cm in diameter that appears raised and irregular. Bleeding from the larger uterine vessels is controlled by compression of the retracted uterine muscle fibers. The placental site consists of multiple thrombosed vascular sinusoids that are treated by the body as any other vascular clot. Some of these vessels are eventually destroyed and replaced by new vessels with smaller lumens.

Rather than forming a fibrous scar in the decidua, the placental site heals by a process of exfoliation. The placental site is undermined by the growth of the endometrial tissue both from the margins of the site and from the fundi of the endometrial glands left in the basal layer of the site. The infarcted superficial tissue then becomes necrotic and is sloughed off. *Exfoliation* is one of the most important aspects of involution. If the healing of the placental site left a fibrous scar, the area available for future implantation would be limited, as would the number of possible pregnancies.

Factors that retard uterine involution and the rationale are listed in Table 33–1. Some factors that enhance involution include an uncomplicated labor and birth, complete expulsion of the products of conception, breast-feeding, and early ambulation.

Lochia

One of the unique capabilities of the uterus is its ability to rid itself of the debris remaining after birth. This discharge, termed **lochia**, is classified according to its appearance and contents. **Lochia rubra** is dark red in color. This discharge occurs for the first two to three days and contains epithelial cells, erythrocytes, leukocytes, shreds of the decidua, and occasionally fetal meconium, lanugo, and vernix caseosa. Lochia should not contain large clots; if it does, the cause should be discovered without delay. A few small clots (no larger than a nickel) are considered normal. **Lochia serosa** follows from about the third until the tenth day. It is a pinkish to brownish color and is composed of serous exudate (hence the name), shreds of degenerating decidua, erythrocytes, leukocytes, cervical mucus, and numerous microorganisms.

The blood cell component decreases gradually, and a creamy or yellowish discharge persists for an additional week or two. This final discharge is termed **lochia alba** and is composed primarily of leukocytes, decidual cells, epithelial cells, fat, cervical mucus, cholesterol crystals, and bacteria. When the lochia stops, the cervix is considered closed, and chances of infection ascending from the vagina to the uterus decrease.

Like menstrual discharge, lochia has a musty, stale odor that is not offensive. Microorganisms are always present in the vaginal lochia, and by the second day following birth the uterus is contaminated with the vaginal bacteria. Researchers speculate that infection does not develop because the organisms involved are relatively nonvirulent. In addition, by the time the bacteria reach the raw, exposed

Table 33-1 Factors That Retard Uterine Involution

Factor	Rationale
Prolonged labor	Relaxation of muscles due to prolonged time of contraction during labor
Anesthesia	Results in muscle relaxation
Difficult birth	Excessive manipulation of uterus
Grandmultiparity	Repeated distention of uterus during pregnancy and labor leads to muscle stretching, diminished tone, and muscle relaxation.
Full bladder	Pushes uterus up and to right; pressure on uterus interferes with effective uterine contraction.
Incomplete expulsion of placenta and/or membranes	Presence of even small amounts of tissue interferes with ability of uterus to remain firmly contracted.
Infection	Inflammation interferes with ability of uterine muscle to contract effectively.

surface of the uterus the process of granulation has begun, forming a protective barrier. Any foul smell to the lochia or used peri-pad suggests infection and the need for prompt assessment.

The total volume of lochia is approximately 240 to 270 mL (8 to 9 oz) and the volume decreases gradually. Discharge is heavier in the morning than at night because lochia tends to pool in the vagina and uterus when the woman is recumbent and is discharged when she arises. The amount of lochia may also be increased by exertion or breast-feeding.

Evaluation of lochia is necessary not only to determine the presence of hemorrhage but also to assess uterine involution. The type, amount, and consistency of lochia determine the state of healing of the placental site, and a progressive change from bright red at birth to dark red to pink to white/clear discharge should be observed. Persistent discharge of lochia rubra or a return to lochia rubra indicates subinvolution or late postpartal hemorrhage (see Chapter 36).

Caution should be exercised in the evaluation of bleeding immediately after birth. The continuous seepage of blood is more consistent with cervical or vaginal lacerations and may be effectively diagnosed when the bleeding is evaluated in conjunction with the consistency of the uterus. Lacerations should be suspected if the uterus is firm, of expected size, and if no clots can be expressed.

Cervical Changes

Following birth the cervix is spongy, flabby, and formless and may appear bruised. The external os is markedly irregular and closes slowly. It admits two fingers for a few days following birth, but by the end of the first week only a fingertip opening remains.

The shape of the external os is permanently changed following the first childbearing. The characteristic dimple-like os of the nullipara changes to the lateral slit (fish mouth) os of the multipara. After significant cervical laceration or several lacerations, the cervix may appear lopsided.

Vaginal Changes

Following birth the vagina appears edematous and may be bruised. Small superficial lacerations may be evident, and the rugae have been obliterated. The apparent bruising of the vagina is due to pelvic congestion and will quickly disappear. The hymen, torn and jagged, heals irregularly, leaving small tags called the *carunculae myrtiformes.*

The size of the vagina decreases and vaginal rugae begin to return by three weeks. This facilitates the gradual return to smaller, although not nulliparous, dimensions. Tone and contractibility of the vaginal opening may be improved by perineal tightening exercises (Kegel's exercises), which may begin soon after birth. The labia majora and labia minora are flabbier in the woman who has borne a child than in the nullipara.

Perineal Changes

During the early postpartal period the soft tissue in and around the perineum may appear edematous with some bruising. If an episiotomy or laceration is present, the edges should be approximated. Occasionally ecchymosis occurs, and this may delay healing.

Recurrence of Ovulation and Menstruation

Approximately 40% of nonnursing mothers resume menstruation in six weeks, while 90% resume within 24 weeks after birth. Of these, approximately 50% ovulate during the first cycle. At 12 weeks after birth about 45% of lactating primiparas are menstruating. Among nursing mothers 80% have one or more anovulatory cycles before the first ovulatory one (Easterling & Herbert 1986).

Abdomen

The uterine ligaments (notably the round and broad ligaments) are stretched and require time to recover. The abdominal wall itself has also been stretched and will appear loose and somewhat flabby for a time. With exercise, abdominal muscle tone will improve greatly within two to three months. In the grandmultipara, in the woman in whom overdistention of the abdomen has occurred, or in the woman with poor muscle tone before pregnancy, the abdomen may fail to regain good tone and may remain flabby. **Diastasis recti abdominis**, a separation of the rectus abdominis muscles, may occur with pregnancy, especially in women with poor abdominal muscle tone. If diastasis occurs, part of the abdominal wall has no muscular support but is formed only by skin, subcutaneous fat, fascia, and peritoneum. Diastasis recti abdominis and poor muscle tone respond well to abdominal exercises. Improvement also depends on the physical condition of the mother, the total number of pregnancies, and the type and amount of physical exercise. See page 1103 for a discussion of postpartal exercises. If rectus muscle tone is not regained, support may be inadequate during future pregnancies. This may result in a pendulous abdomen and increased maternal backache.

The striae (stretch marks), which occurred as a result of stretching and rupture of the elastic fibers of the skin, are red to purple at the time of birth. They gradually fade and after a time appear as silver or white streaks.

Lactation

During pregnancy, the breasts develop in preparation for lactation as a result of the influence of both estrogen and progesterone. After birth, the interplay of maternal hormones leads to the establishment of milk production. This process is described in detail in the section on breast-feeding in Chapter 30.

Gastrointestinal System

Hunger following birth is common, and the mother may enjoy a light meal. Frequently she is quite thirsty and will drink large amounts of fluid. Drinking fluids helps replace fluid lost during labor, in the urine, and through perspiration.

The bowel tends to be sluggish after birth due to the lingering effects of progesterone and decreased abdominal muscle tone. The practice of omitting solid food during labor may cause a delay in the first bowel movement.

The pain from an episiotomy, any lacerations, and hemorrhoids may lead the woman to delay elimination for fear of increasing the pain or tearing her stitches. In most instances the initial bowel movement is not uncomfortable. However, refusing or delaying the bowel movement may cause constipation and more discomfort when elimination finally occurs.

Fluids and solid foods are delayed for the woman who has had a cesarean birth until bowel sounds return. Clear liquids are generally begun by the day after surgery (first postoperative day), and the diet is quickly advanced to solid food. The woman may experience some discomfort from flatulence initially. This is relieved by early ambulation and use of antiflatulent medications. It may take a

few days for the bowel to regain its tone. The woman who had a cesarean or a difficult birth may benefit from stool softeners. In some cases it may be necessary to administer an enema or suppository to promote elimination.

Urinary Tract

Increased bladder capacity, swelling and bruising of the tissues around the urethra, decreased sensation of bladder filling, and inability to void in the recumbent position put the puerperal woman at risk for overdistention, incomplete emptying, and buildup of residual urine. In addition, women who have had conductive anesthesia have inhibited neural functioning of the bladder and are more susceptible to bladder complications.

Urinary output increases during the early postpartal period (first 12 to 24 hours) due to *puerperal diuresis.* The kidneys must eliminate an estimated 2000 to 3000 mL of extracellular fluid associated with a normal pregnancy. With pregnancy-induced hypertension (PIH), chronic hypertension, and diabetes, even greater fluid retention is experienced, and postpartal diuresis is increased accordingly.

Bladder elimination presents an immediate problem. If stasis exists, chances increase for urinary tract infection because of bacteriuria and the presence of dilated ureters and renal pelves, which persist for about six weeks after birth. A full bladder may also increase the tendency of relaxation of the uterus by displacing the uterus and interfering with its contractility, leading to hemorrhage.

Hematuria, resulting from bladder trauma, may occasionally occur after birth, but the presence of lochia may mask this sign. If hematuria occurs in the second or third postpartal week, there may be a bladder infection. Acetone may be present in the urine of women with diabetes or of women with prolonged labor and dehydration. Slight (1+) proteinuria may occur during the first week following birth. However, since proteinuria may be associated with an infectious process (cystitis, pyelitis), it should be further evaluated. A urine specimen contaminated with lochia may be the cause of proteinuria, so any specimen should be obtained as a midstream or a catheterized specimen.

Vital Signs

During the postpartal period, with the exception of the first 24 hours, the woman should be afebrile. A temperature of up to 100.4F (38C) may occur after birth as a result of the exertion and dehydration of labor. Infection must be considered in the woman with a temperature of 100.4F or above after the first 24 hours.

Blood pressure readings should remain stable and normal following the birth. A decrease may indicate physiologic readjustment to decreased intrapelvic pressure, or it may be related to uterine hemorrhage. Blood pressure elevations, especially when accompanied by headache, suggest PIH, and the woman should be evaluated further.

Puerperal bradycardia with rates of 50 to 70 beats per minute commonly occurs during the first six to ten days of the postpartal period. It may be related to decreased cardiac strain, the decreased blood volume following placental separation, contraction of the uterus, and increased stroke volume. Tachycardia occurs less frequently and is related to increased blood loss or difficult, prolonged labor and birth.

Blood Values

The blood values should return to the prepregnant state by the end of the postpartal period. Pregnancy-associated activation of coagulation factors may continue for variable amounts of time. This condition, in conjunction with trauma, immobility, or sepsis, predisposes the woman to development of thromboembolism. Plasma fibrinogen is maintained at pregnancy levels for a week, accounting for the higher sedimentation rate observed in the early postpartum period.

Leukocytosis often occurs with white blood cell counts of 15,000 and 20,000 μL.

Blood loss averages 200 to 500 mL with a vaginal birth and 700 to 1000 mL with cesarean birth. Hemoglobin and erythrocyte values vary during the early puerperium, but they should approximate or exceed prelabor values within two to six weeks as normal concentrations are reached. As extracellular fluid is excreted, hemoconcentration occurs, with a concomitant rise in hematocrit. A drop in values indicates an abnormal blood loss. The following is a convenient rule of thumb: a 2-point drop in hematocrit equals 1 pint of blood loss (Varney 1987).

Weight Loss

An initial weight loss of 10 to 12 lb occurs as a result of the birth of infant, placenta, and amniotic fluid. Puerperal diuresis accounts for the loss of an additional 5 lb during the early puerperium. By the sixth to eighth week after birth, the woman has returned to approximately her prepregnant weight if she has gained the average 25 to 30 lb.

Postpartal Chill

Frequently the mother experiences a shaking chill immediately after birth, which may be related to a neurologic response or to vasomotor changes. If not followed by fever, it is not of clinical concern, but it is uncomfortable for the woman. Covering the woman with warmed bath blankets will help alleviate the chill. The mother may also find a warm beverage helpful. Later in the puerperium, chills and fever indicate infection and require further evaluation.

Postpartal Diaphoresis

The elimination of excess fluid and waste products via the skin during the puerperium greatly increases perspiration. Diaphoretic episodes frequently occur at night, and the woman may awaken drenched with perspiration. This perspiration is not significant clinically, but the mother should be protected from chilling.

Afterpains

Afterpains occur more commonly in multiparas than in primiparas and are caused by intermittent uterine contractions. Although the uterus of the primipara usually remains consistently contracted, the lost tone of the uterus of the multipara results in alternate contraction and relaxation. This phenomenon also occurs if the uterus has been markedly distended, as with multiple pregnancies or hydramnios, or if clots or placental fragments were retained. These afterpains may cause the mother severe discomfort for two to three days following birth. The administration of oxytocic agents stimulates uterine contraction and increases the discomfort of the afterpains. Because oxytocin is released when the infant suckles, breast-feeding also increases the severity of the afterpains. Some women obtain relief by lying on the abdomen with a pillow placed under it to apply abdominal pressure; others prefer rocking in a rocking chair. The nursing mother may find it helpful to take a mild analgesic approximately one hour before feeding her infant. An analgesic is also helpful at bedtime if the afterpains interfere with the mother's rest.

Postpartal Psychologic Adaptations

The postpartal period is a time of readjustment and adaptation for the entire childbearing family but especially for the mother. The woman experiences a variety of responses as she adjusts to a new family member, postpartum discomforts, changes in her body image, and the reality that she is no longer pregnant. One young mother described her responses well:

I feel like it's the day after Christmas. I'm relieved that everything went well and I have a fine baby, but I feel so let down. I had an image of what my delivery would be like, and everything was a little different. I figured that as soon as I delivered I would feel fine. Why didn't someone tell me I would still be sore; the pain didn't magically disappear! When I was pregnant everyone treated me as though I was a little fragile. Now when people call or visit all they talk about is the baby. I don't think I'm really jealous, but I do miss the attention. During this past day I've started to realize that my life will never, ever be the same again. I've always wanted to be a mother, but I'm not really sure how to do it. Isn't that strange?

During the first day or two following birth the woman tends to be passive and somewhat dependent. The new mother follows suggestions, is hesitant about making decisions, and is still rather preoccupied with her needs. She may have a great need to talk about her perceptions of her labor and birth. This helps her work through the process, sort out the reality from her fantasized experience, and clarify anything that she did not understand.

During this time food and sleep are major focuses for her. The woman is talkative but passive. In Rubin's early work (1961) she labeled this the *taking-in* period.

By the second or third day after birth, the new mother has had time to relive her experiences, adjust to her new life, rest, and recover from childbirth. She is then ready to resume control of her life. The new mother may be concerned about controlling bodily functions such as elimination. If she is breast-feeding, she may worry about the quality of her milk and her ability to nurse her baby. She requires assurance that she is doing well as a mother. If her baby spits up following feeding she may view it as a personal failure. She may also feel demoralized by the fact that the nurse handles her baby proficiently while she feels unsure and tentative. Rubin (1961) labeled this phase as *taking-hold*.

Today's mothers seem to be more independent and better able to adjust to motherhood early in the postpartum period. Gay et al (1988) and Martell and Mitchell (1984) suggest that nurses should examine Rubin's concepts carefully and more skeptically in light of changing trends in maternity care. Ament (1990) found that women did exhibit behavior characteristic of "taking-in" and "taking-hold" but found that the time frames were shorter than those cited by Rubin. Ament found that taking-in occurred only during the first 24 hours after childbirth. It will be interesting to see what further study brings to this subject.

Postpartally the woman must adjust to a changed body image. Often women, especially primiparas, are surprised and rather dismayed to discover that they do not return to their prepregnant weight and shape as soon as the baby is born. Women often express dissatisfaction about their appearance and concern with the return of their weight and figure to normal. Multiparas tend to be more positive about their appearance postpartally than primiparas. This may be because the multipara's previous experience has prepared her for the fact that the body does not immediately return to a prepregnant state.

The psychologic outcomes of the postpartal period are far more positive when the parents have access to a support network. Women and their partners may find that family relationships become increasingly important, and the attention that their infant receives from family members is a source of satisfaction to the new parents (Belsky & Rovine 1984). In many cases the ties to the woman's family become especially good. Many fathers report that their re-

lationships with their in-laws become far more positive and supportive (Cronenwett 1985). On the other hand, the increased family interaction can be a source of stress, especially for the new mother, who tends to have more contact with the families.

Research Note

Clinical Application of Research

Lorraine Tulman and her associates (1990) developed a longitudinal study to determine the functional status of women after childbirth. Functional status activities included infant care, household and community activities, self-care, and job-related activities.

Data regarding functional status were collected at three weeks, six weeks, three months, and six months postpartum from 97 women. Additional data were collected related to psychosocial variables such as life satisfaction, maternal perception of father's participation in child care, quality of relationship with husband. Infant temperament data were compiled with the temperament rated as fussy-difficult, inadequate, unpredictable, and dull.

At the 6-week postpartum collection point, the traditional time period identified as complete recovery from birth, only 29% of the women had fully resumed previous levels of function regarding household activities or social and community activities. Seventy-five percent had assumed full infant care, 3% self-care, and of the 15 who had returned to work, only three reported resumption of full occupational status.

Canonical analysis of each time period showed that different functional components formed one or two variates at each period. Each variate had different associated variables. For example, at six weeks, household, social, and self-care activities formed a variate that explained 43% of the variance. Associated variables included degree of physical energy, occupational status other than housewife, and vaginal delivery.

Critical Thinking Applied to Research

Strengths: Use of a nursing theory, Roy's adaptation model, as a partial basis for conceptual framework of role theory. Reported psychometric properties of internal consistency, subscale and total scale correlations, test-retest reliability, and content validity. Identified limitations of the study regarding generalizability.

Tulman L, Fawcett J, Groblewski L et al: Changes in functional status after childbirth. *Nurs Res* 1990; 39(2):70.

Childbearing couples often change their social network somewhat following the birth of their child. Once the new parents have made the transition to parenthood, they both tend to have more contact with other parents of small children. For the woman, interaction with coworkers often declines postpartally, but contact with friends increases. Thus, the woman maintains the size of her support group but alters it to meet the changes that have occurred in her life-style.

Perhaps the greatest concern involves women and their partners who have no family available and no friends to form a social network. Isolation at a time when the woman feels an increased need for support can result in tremendous stress and is often a contributing factor in situations of child neglect or abuse.

A prime focus of research in recent years has been maternal role attainment. **Maternal role attainment** is the process by which a woman learns mothering behaviors and becomes comfortable with her identity as a mother. The formation of a maternal identity indicates that the woman has attained the maternal role. Formation of a maternal identity occurs with each child a woman bears. As the mother grows to know this child and forms a relationship with her or him, the mother's maternal identity gradually, systematically evolves and she "binds in" to the infant (Rubin 1984).

Maternal role attainment occurs in four stages (Mercer 1985). (The formal and informal stages of maternal role attainment correspond with the taking-in and taking-hold stages previously identified by Rubin [1961]):

1. The *anticipatory stage* occurs during pregnancy. The woman looks to role models, especially her own mother, for examples of how to mother.

2. The *formal stage* begins when the child is born. The woman is still influenced by the guidance of others and tries to act as she believes others expect her to act.

3. The *informal stage* begins when the mother begins to make her own choices about mothering. The woman begins to develop her own style of mothering and finds ways of functioning that work well for her.

4. The *personal stage* is the final stage of maternal role attainment. When the woman reaches this stage, she is comfortable with the notion of herself as "mother."

In most cases maternal role attainment occurs within three to ten months following birth. Social support, the woman's age and personality traits, the temperament of her infant, and the family's socioeconomic status all influence the woman's success in attaining the maternal role.

The postpartum woman faces a number of challenges as she adjusts to her new role. For many women, finding time for themselves is one of the greatest challenges. It is often difficult for the new mother to find time to read a book, talk to her partner, or even eat a meal without interruption! Women also report feelings of incompetence because they have not mastered all aspects of the mothering role. The next greatest challenge involves fatigue due to sleep deprivation. The demands of nighttime care are tremendously draining, especially if she has other children at home. One challenge faced by the new mother involves the feeling of responsibility that having a child brings. Women experience a sense of lost freedom, an awareness that they will never again be quite as carefree as they were before becoming mothers. Finally mothers cite the infant's behavior as a problem, especially when the child is about 8 months old. Stranger anxiety may be developing, the infant may begin crawling and getting into things, teething may cause fussiness, and the baby's tendency to put everything in his or her mouth requires constant vigilance by the parent (Mercer 1985).

All too often postpartum nurses are unaware of the long-term adjustments and stresses that the childbearing family faces as its members adjust to new and different roles. Nurses can help by providing anticipatory guidance about the realities of being a mother. Agencies should have literature available for reference at home. Ongoing parenting groups also give parents an opportunity to discuss problems and become comfortable in new roles.

Postpartum Blues

The **postpartum blues** consist of a transient period of depression that occurs during the first week or two after birth in up to 70% of women (Theesen et al 1989). It may be manifested by mood swings, anger, weepiness, anorexia, difficulty sleeping, and a feeling of letdown. Because of the practice of early postpartum discharge, the depression often occurs at home. Psychologic adjustments and hormonal changes are thought to be the main cause, although fatigue, discomfort, and overstimulation may play a part. The postpartum blues usually resolve naturally, especially if the woman receives understanding and support. If symptoms persist or intensify, the woman may require evaluation for postpartum depression. (see Chapter 36).

Cultural Influences

Many cultures emphasize certain postpartal routines or rituals for mother and baby. These are frequently designed to restore harmony or the hot-cold balance of the body. For many Mexican Americans, black Americans, and Asians, cold is avoided after birth. This prohibition includes cold air, wind, and all water (even if heated). Dietary changes also reflect the need to avoid cold foods and restore the balance between hot and cold (Horn 1981).

The diet of the traditional Mexican American reflects this concern about hot-cold balances. Chamomile tea, chicken soup, and corn gruel are offered in the first days. Fruits, vegetables, pork, chili, garlic, beans, and chocolate are avoided (Clark 1978).

Many Japanese women do not have rooming-in because it interferes with the mother's rest. They are advised not to wash their hair for a week following birth and not to bathe until their lochia serosa stops (Engel 1989). The Hmong woman from Laos wants the head of the bed elevated following birth. The woman must be kept warm and given only warm beverages to drink. In keeping with cultural tradition, most Hmong women prefer a diet of poached or stewed chicken served with its broth, rice, and coarsely ground black pepper (LaDu 1985). Korean mothers may prefer a traditional diet of seaweed (tangle) soup and rice, although some may choose to eat both the traditional diet and a more nutritionally balanced diet (Choi 1986).

The black American new mother is traditionally offered chicken soup and sassafras tea in the early weeks to aid healing. Liver and hog chitterlings are restricted (liver has a high blood-producing function and is believed to increase lochial flow). Onions and alcohol are avoided because they affect breast milk. The mother may have a two- to six-week period of confinement. Showers, tub baths, and shampoos are restricted during the "sick time" while the lochia flows.

The Mexican-American family is concerned with a balance of humors during the postpartal period. The new mother remains in bed for three days, begins to walk about her home after eight days, and may go outside after 15 days. She is helped at home by family members. She avoids bathing for 15 days and carefully covers her head, body, and feet to avoid cold air because she believes that it may cause mastitis, a sudden infection (*pasmo*), a distended belly, frigidity, or sterility. A binder is worn about the abdomen and perineum to protect the body from cold (Clark 1978).

A variety of traditions and rituals also exist in Native American and other cultural groups. The nurse caring for a mother during the postpartal period carefully assesses the family's beliefs and practices and adapts to them whenever possible. Family members can be encouraged to bring in preferred food and drink and some modifications in client care may be made to follow traditional beliefs.

The extended family frequently plays an essential role during the puerperium. The grandmother is often the primary helper to the mother and newborn. She brings wisdom and experience, allowing the new mother time to rest as well as giving her ready access to someone who can help with problems and concerns as they arise. It is imperative to include members who have authority in the family. Visiting rules may be waived to allow family members or authority figures access to the mother and newborn. These practices show respect, and the nurse may gain an ally in the care of the mother and baby, especially if the mother follows the advice of her cultural mentor. Often younger members of a specific cultural group have been acculturated by the dominant culture (American, Canadian, etc) and no longer follow traditional practices. In other instances they follow some practices but not others. Nurses can work for a blending of behaviors—the old and the new—to meet the goals of all concerned.

Development of Attachment

During the postpartal period the parents begin to develop close bonds with their new infant. This process of attachment has been the focus of significant research in recent years. It is described in depth in Chapter 35.

Postpartal Nursing Assessment

Comprehensive care is based on a thorough assessment, with identification of individual needs or potential problems.

Risk Factors

The emphasis on ongoing assessment and client education during the puerperium is designed to meet the needs of the childbearing family and to detect and treat possible complications. Table 33–2 identifies factors that may place the new mother at risk during the postpartal period. The nurse uses this knowledge during the assessment and is particularly alert for possible complications that may occur in an individual because of identified risk factors.

CRITICAL THINKING

Using your knowledge of general physical assessment, plan a logical approach to postpartum physical assessment.

Physical Assessment

Several principles should be remembered in preparing for and completing the assessment of the postpartal woman:

1. The nurse selects the time that will provide the most accurate data. Palpating the fundus when the woman has a full bladder, for example, will not result in a true indication of involution.

2. The nurse should explain the purpose of regular assessment to the woman.

Table 33–2 Postpartal High-Risk Factors

Factors	Maternal implications
PIH	↑ Blood pressure ↑ CNS irritability ↑ Need for bed rest → ↑ risk thrombophlebitis
Diabetes	Need for insulin regulation Episodes of hypoglycemia or hyperglycemia ↓ Healing
Cardiac disease	↑ Maternal exhaustion
Cesarean birth	↑ Healing needs ↑ Pain from incision ↑ Risk of infection ↑ Length of hospitalization
Overdistention of uterus (multiple gestation, hydramnios)	↑ Risk of hemorrhage ↑ Risk of anemia ↑ Stretching of abdominal mucles ↑ Incidence and severity of afterpains
Abruptio placentae—placenta previa	Hemorrhage → anemia ↓ Uterine contractility after birth → ↑ infection risk
Precipitous labor (<3 hours)	↑ Risk of lacerations to birth canal → hemorrhage
Prolonged labor (>24 hours)	Exhaustion ↑ Risk of hemorrhage Nutritional and fluid depletion ↑ Bladder atony and/or trauma
Difficult birth	Exhaustion ↑ Risk of perineal lacerations ↑ Risk of hematomas ↑ Risk of hemorrhage → anemia
Extended period of time in stirrups at birth	↑ Risk of thrombophlebitis
Retained placenta	↑ Risk of hemorrhage ↑ Risk of infection

3. The woman should be relaxed, and the procedures should be accomplished as gently as possible to avoid unnecessary discomfort.

4. The data obtained during the assessment should be recorded and reported clearly.

A sample assessment form is shown in Figure 33–2. This form assists the nurse in organizing and charting the postpartal physical assessment.

While the nurse is performing the physical assessment, she should also be teaching the woman. For example, assessing the breast provides an optimal time to discuss milk formation, the letdown reflex, and breast self-examination. Mothers are very receptive to instruction on postpartal abdominal tightening exercises when the nurse assesses the woman's fundal height and diastasis. The assessment also provides an excellent time to teach her about the body's physical and anatomic changes postpartally as well as danger signs to report. A Postpartal Assessment Guide can be found on page 1077. Since the time the woman spends on the postpartum unit often is limited, nurses should use every opportunity for client teaching. To assist nurses in recognizing these opportunities, examples of client teaching during the assessment have been included in the narrative.

Breasts

Beginning with the breasts, the nurse should first assess the fit and support provided by the bra. The nurse provides information about how to select a supportive bra. A properly fitting bra provides support to the breasts and helps maintain the shape of the breasts by limiting stretching of connective tissue and ligaments. If the mother is breast-feeding, the straps of the bra should be cloth, not elastic, and easily adjustable. The back should be wide and have at least three rows of hooks to adjust for fit. Underwires are not necessary unless the breast is large (C cup or larger). Traditional nursing bras have a fixed inner cup and a separate half cup or flap that can be unhooked for breast-feeding while continuing to support the breast. Some companies have designed the nursing flap to open and close with a plastic snap or with Velcro rather than the traditional loop and hook. Some women find these easier to use.

NAME _____

ROOM _____

FEEDING METHOD _____

DATE _____

POSTPARTUM DAY_____

VITAL SIGNS _____

1. LUNGS _____

2. BREASTS
    a. General appearance _____
    b. Nipples _____

3. DIASTASIS   Rectus abdominis
    a. Length (cm) _____
    b. Width (cm) _____

4. FUNDUS
    a. Height in finger breadths in relationship to

       umbilicus _____
    b. Position _____
    c. Tenderness _____
        (1) with touch _____
        (2) constant _____

5. LOCHIA
    a. Amount _____
    b. Color _____
    c. Consistency _____
    d. Odor _____

6. PERINEUM
    a. Intact _____
    b. Episiotomy _____
        (1) type _____
        (2) healing _____
            (a) REEDA scale _____
    c. Hygiene _____
    d. Lacerations _____
    e. Hemorrhoids _____

7. CESAREAN INCISION _____
    a. Healing (REEDA) _____

8. CVA TENDERNESS _____

9. HOMAN'S SIGN _____
    a. Superficial varicosities _____

10. BOWEL AND BLADDER HABITS _____

    _____

11. SLEEP PATTERNS _____

    _____

12. PSYCHOLOGIC ADAPTATION _____

    _____

13. NUTRITIONAL INTAKE _____

    _____

14. ADJUSTMENT TO INFANT _____

    _____

15. DISCOMFORT _____
    a. Site _____
    b. Relief measures _____

Figure 33–2 Postpartal assessment form

Some women prefer a standard bra that hooks in front, and if the breast is not heavy this is acceptable. Purchasing a nursing bra with a cup one size too large during pregnancy will usually result in a good fit because the breasts increase in size with milk production.

The bra is removed to examine the breasts. The nurse notes the size and shape of the breasts and any abnormalities, reddened areas, or engorgement. The nurse palpates the breasts lightly, checking for softness, slight firmness associated with filling, firmness associated with engorgement, heat, edema, and caking (swelling of the lobules due to a blockage of the duct). Any areas of tenderness should be examined carefully. The nipples are checked for fissures, cracks, soreness, or inversion.

The nursing mother needs to be reminded to keep the nipples cleaned with water to avoid a buildup of secre-

tions that could irritate the nipples (see discussion of nipple care, page 928). The nonnursing mother is assessed for evidence of breast discomfort and relief measures taken if necessary (see discussion of lactation suppression in the nonnursing mother, page 1102). Breast assessment findings for a nursing woman may be recorded as follows: Breasts soft, filling, no evidence of nipple tenderness or cracking.

Abdomen and Fundus

Having the woman void before doing the assessment ensures that a full bladder is not causing any uterine atony; if atony is present, other causes must be investigated.

The nurse assesses fundal height by determining the relationship of the fundus to the umbilicus. The nurse notes whether the fundus is in the midline or displaced to either side of the abdomen. The most common cause of dis-

POSTPARTAL ASSESSMENT GUIDE

Assess/Normal Findings	Alterations and Possible Causes*	Nursing Responses to Data†
Vital Signs		
Blood pressure: Should remain consistent with baseline BP during pregnancy	High BP (PIH, essential hypertension, renal disease, anxiety) Drop in BP (may be normal; uterine hemorrhage)	Evaluate history of preexisting disorders and check for other signs of PIH Assess for other signs of hemorrhage. (↑ pulse, cool clammy skin)
Pulse: 50–90 beats/min May be bradycardia of 50–70 beats/min during first 6–10 days	Tachycardia (difficult labor and birth, hemorrhage)	Evaluate for other signs of hemorrhage. (↓ BP, cool clammy skin)
Respirations: 16–24/min	Marked tachypnea (respiratory disease)	Assess for other signs of respiratory disease.
Temperature: 36.2–38C (98–100.4F)	After first 24 hr, temperature of 38C (100.4F) or above suggests infection	Assess for other signs of infection; notify physician/nurse-midwife.
Lungs		
All lobes clear to percussion and auscultation	High diaphragm (atelectasis or paralysis) Adventitious sounds (infection, reactive airway disease [RAD])	Refer to physician.
Breasts		
General appearance: Smooth, even pigmentation, changes of pregnancy still apparent; one may appear larger	Reddened area (mastitis)	Assess further for signs of infection.
Palpation: Depending on postpartal day—may be soft, filling, full or engorged	Palpable mass (caked breast, mastitis) Engorgement (venous stasis) Tenderness, heat, edema (engorgement, caked breast, mastitis)	Assess for other signs of infection: if blocked duct consider heat, massage, position change for breast-feeding. See interventions for engorgement on p 929. Assess for further signs. Report mastitis to physician/nurse-midwife.
Nipples: Supple, pigmented, intact; become erect when stimulated	Fissures, cracks, soreness (problems with breast-feeding), not erectile with stimulation (inverted nipples)	Reassess technique; recommend appropriate interventions. See p 927 for appropriate interventions for nursing mothers.
Abdomen		
Musculature: Abdomen may be soft, have a "doughy" texture; rectus muscle intact	Separation in musculature (diastasis rectus abdominis)	Evaluate size of diastasis; teach appropriate exercises for decreasing the separation.
Fundus: Firm, midline; following appropriate schedule of involution Cesarean birth woman—assess fundus for firmness gently	Boggy (full bladder, uterine bleeding)	Massage until firm; assess bladder and have woman void; attempt to express clots when firm. If bogginess remains or recurs, report to physician/nurse-midwife.

(continued)

POSTPARTAL ASSESSMENT GUIDE (continued)

Assess/Normal Findings	Alterations and Possible Causes*	Nursing Responses to Data†
May be tender when palpated	Constant tenderness (infection)	Assess for evidence of endometritis.
Distention: Cesarean birth women should have no distention or only slight distention. Bowel sounds present by 1st or 2nd postoperative day	Absent bowel sounds, marked distention (decreased or absent peristalsis, paralytic ileus)	Encourage ambulation, obtain order for anti-flatulent; report to physician.
Lochia		
Scant to moderate amount, earthy odor; no clots	Large amounts, clots (hemorrhage) Foul-smelling lochia (infection)	Assess for firmness, express additional clots; begin peri-pad count. Assess for other signs of infection; report to physician/nurse-midwife.
Normal progression: First 1–3 days—rubra Days 3–10—serosa (Alba seldom seen in hospital)	Failure to progress normally or return to rubra from serosa (subinvolution)	Report to physician/nurse-midwife.
Perineum		
Slight edema and bruising in intact perineum	Marked fullness, bruising, pain (vulvar hematoma)	Assess size; apply ice glove or ice pack; report to physician/nurse-midwife.
Episiotomy: No redness, edema, ecchymosis, discharge, edges well-approximated (REEDA)	Redness, edema, ecchymosis, discharge, or gaping stitches (infection)	Encourage sitz baths, review perineal care, appropriate wiping techniques.
Hemorrhoids: None present; if present, should be small and nontender	Full, tender, inflamed hemorrhoids	Encourage sitz baths, side-lying position; tucks pads, anesthetic ointments, manual replacement of hemorrhoids; stool softeners, increased fluid intake.
Costovertebral Angle (CVA) Tenderness		
None	Present (kidney infection)	Assess for other symptoms of UTI; obtain clean-catch urine; report to physician/nurse-midwife.
Lower Extremities		
No varices or only superficial ones on inspection. No pain with palpation; negative Homan's sign	Positive findings (thrombophlebitis)	Report to physician/nurse-midwife.
Patellar reflexes 1+ to 2+.	Reflexes 3+ or 4+ (PIH)	Report to physician/nurse-midwife.

(continued)

POSTPARTAL ASSESSMENT GUIDE *(continued)*

Assess/Normal Findings	Alterations and Possible Causes*	Nursing Responses to Data†
Elimination		
Urinary output: Voiding in sufficient quantities at least every 4–6 hr; bladder not palpable	Inability to void (urinary retention) Symptoms of urgency, frequency, dysuria (UTI)	Employ nursing interventions to promote voiding; if not successful obtain order for catheterization. Report symptoms of UTI to physician/nurse-midwife.
Bowel elimination: Should have normal bowel movement by second or third day after birth	Inability to pass feces (constipation due to fear of pain from episiotomy, hemorrhoids, perineal trauma)	Encourage fluids, ambulation, roughage in diet; sitz baths to promote healing of perineum; obtain order for stool softener.
Psychologic Adaptation		
During first 24 hours: Somewhat passive, preoccupied with own needs; may talk about her labor and birth experience. *By 24–48 hours:* Beginning to assume responsibility; eager to learn, easily feels overwhelmed.	Very quiet and passive; sleeps frequently (fatigue from long labor; feelings of disappointment about some aspect of the experience) Excessive weepiness, mood swings, pronounced irritability (postpartum blues, feelings of inadequacy)	Provide opportunities for adequate rest; provide nutritious meals and snacks; provide opportunities to discuss birth experience in nonjudgmental atmosphere. Explain postpartum blues; provide supportive atmosphere; consider referral for excessive depression.
Attachment		
Enface position; holds baby close; cuddles and soothes; calls by name; identifies characteristics of family members in infant; may be awkward in providing care. Initially may express disappointment over sex or appearance of infant but within 1–2 days demonstrates appropriate attachment behaviors.	Continued expressions of disappointment in sex, appearance of infant; refusal to care for infant; derogatory comments; lack of bonding behaviors (failure of attachment)	Provide reinforcement for positive behaviors; teach necessary infant care skills; give woman opportunity to express her feelings; consider social service home referral for continued high-risk behaviors.
Client education		
Has basic understanding of self-care activities and infant care needs; can identify signs of complications that should be reported.	Cannot demonstrate basic self-care and infant care activities (knowledge deficit; postpartum blues)	Continue appropriate teaching and guidance; provide written information and telephone number for questions; consider home follow-up.

*Possible causes of alterations are placed in parentheses.

†This column provides guidelines for further assessment and initial nursing actions.

placement is a full bladder. Usually the nurse ascertains tone when first palpating the fundus (see Procedure 33–1). The results of the assessment should then be recorded.

Modifications in technique are required for cesarean birth mothers. If a vertical skin incision is made, firmness and position are determined by gently palpating on each side of the incision. With the cesarean birth woman, it is essential to observe the amount of lochia to assess for relaxation of the uterus.

A well-contracted uterus feels as firm as the uterus does during a strong labor contraction. If handled gently, the uterus should not be overly tender. Excessive pain in the uterus during postpartal examination should alert the nurse to possible uterine infection. If the uterus is not firm,

Assessing the Fundus

Nursing Action

Objective: Prepare woman.

Explain procedure; have the woman void; position woman flat in bed with head comfortably positioned on a pillow; if the procedure is uncomfortable, woman may flex legs.

Objective: Determine uterine firmness.

Gently place one hand on the lower segment of the uterus; using the side of the other hand, palpate the abdomen until the top of the fundus is located. Determine whether the fundus is firm. If it is not firm, massage until firm.

Objective: Determine the height of the fundus.

Measure the height of the top of the fundus in finger-breadths. (See Figure 33–3.)

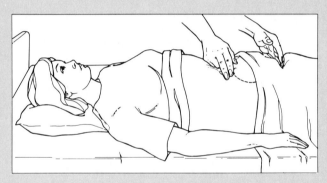

Rationale

Having the woman void assures that a full bladder is not causing any uterine atony. Having woman flat prevents falsely high assessment of fundal height.
Flexing the legs relaxes the abdominal muscles. The uterus may be tender if frequent massage has been necessary.

Provides support for uterus.
Provides a larger surface for palpation and is less uncomfortable for the woman. A firm fundus indicates that the muscles are contracted and bleeding will not occur.

Fundal height gives information about the progress of involution.

Figure 33–3 Measurement of descent of fundus: The fundus is located two fingerbreadths below the umbilicus.

Objective: Ascertain position.

Determine whether fundus is deviated from the midline. If not in midline, locate position. Evaluate bladder for distention. Ascertain voiding pattern; use measuring device to measure urine output for next few hours (until normal elimination status is established).

Objective: Correlate uterine status with lochia.

Observe lochia for amount, presence of clots, color, and odor.

Fundus may be deviated when bladder is full.

As normal involution occurs, the lochia decreases in amount and changes from rubra to serosa. Increased amounts of lochia may be associated with uterine relaxation; failure to progress to next type of lochia may indicate uterine relaxation or infection.

Objective: Record findings.

Fundal height is recorded in fingerbreadths; example: 2 FB ↓ U; 1 FB ↑ U.

If massage had been necessary it could be recorded as: Uterus: Boggy → firm c̄ light massage.

A complete note illustrating normal findings might be: Fundus firm, 1 FB ↓ U, lochia rubra, scant amount.

Allows for consistency of reporting among care givers.

DRUG GUIDE
Methylergonovine Maleate (Methergine)

Overview of Obstetric Action

Methylergonovine maleate is an ergot alkaloid that stimulates smooth muscle tissue. Because the smooth muscle of the uterus is especially sensitive to this drug, it is used postpartally to stimulate the uterus to contract. This contraction clamps off uterine blood vessels and prevents hemorrhage. In addition, the drug has a vasoconstrictive effect on all blood vessels, especially the larger arteries. This may result in hypertension, particularly in a woman whose blood pressure is already elevated.

Route, Dosage, and Frequency

Methergine has a rapid onset of action and may be given intramuscularly, orally, or intravenously.

Usual IM dose: 0.2 mg following expulsion of the placenta. The dose may be repeated every 2–4 hours if necessary.

Usual oral dose: 0.2 mg every 4 hours (six doses).

Usual IV dose: Because the adverse effects of Methergine are far more severe with IV administration, this route is seldom used. If Methergine is given intravenously, the rate should *not* exceed 0.2 mg/min, and the client's blood pressure should be monitored prior to administration and frequently afterward until it is stable.

Maternal Contraindications

Pregnancy, hepatic or renal disease, cardiac disease and hypertension, contraindicate this drug's use (Karch & Boyd 1989).

Maternal Side Effects

Hypertension (particularly when administered IV), nausea, vomiting, headache, bradycardia, dizziness, tinnitus, abdominal cramps, palpitations, dyspnea, chest pain, and allergic reactions may be noted.

Effects on Fetus/Neonate

Because Methergine has a long duration of action and can thus produce tetanic contractions, it should never be used during pregnancy as it may result in fetal trauma or death.

Nursing Considerations

1. Monitor fundal height and consistency and the amount and character of the lochia.
2. Assess the blood pressure before administration.
3. Observe for adverse effects or symptoms of ergot toxicity.

---

the nurse should gently massage the fundus with the fingertips of the examining hand, then assess the results. If the uterus becomes firm, the chart should read "Uterus: boggy → firm c̄ light massage." A good habit for the nurse to develop during the postpartal examination is to have the woman lie flat on her back with her head on a pillow and legs flexed. Then the nurse can release the perineal pad to observe the results of uterine massage based on the amount of expelled blood. Occasionally, oxytocic agents such as IV Pitocin, ergonovine maleate (Ergotrate), and methylergonovine maleate (Methergine) are administered postpartally to maintain uterine contraction and prevent hemorrhage (see Drug Guide—Methylergonovine Maleate (Methergine), above).

The boggy uterus that does not contract with light, gentle massage may need more vigorous massage. The amount and character of any expelled blood obtained while massaging the fundus is assessed. When a woman has postpartal uterine atony, the nurse should do the following:

1. Reevaluate for full bladder; if the bladder is full, have the woman void.
2. Question the woman on her bleeding history since the birth or last examination. How heavy does her flow seem? Has she passed any clots? How frequently has she changed pads?
3. For the nursing mother, put the newborn to the mother's breast to stimulate oxytocin production.
4. Reassess the fundus; if the fundus is still boggy, alert the certified nurse-midwife or physician, as further intervention is now needed.

The nurse assesses for diastasis recti abdominis following the uterine assessment and before assessing the lochia. The separation in the rectus abdominous muscles is evaluated according to its length and width. The separation is palpated first just below the umbilicus, and the width is ascertained. Then the separation is palpated for length toward the symphysis pubis and toward the xiphoid process. If palpation is difficult due to abdominal relaxation, the woman is asked to lift her head unassisted by the nurse. This action contracts the rectus muscles and more clearly defines their edges.

Methods of charting these results vary from institution to institution. Some prefer recording the diastasis measured from the umbilicus down and then from the umbilicus up:

Diastasis U ↓ 4 cm by 1 cm
U ↑ 2 cm by 1 cm

Others prefer recording the entire length:

Diastasis: 6 cm by 1 cm

Either method is acceptable.

In the woman who has had a cesarean birth, the abdominal incision should be inspected for evidence of separation and for any signs of infection, including drainage, foul odor, or redness. During the assessment, the nurse teaches the woman about her incision, signs of normal healing, and characteristics of infection.

Lochia

The next aspect to be evaluated is the lochia, which is assessed for character, amount, odor, and the presence of clots. During the first one to three days the lochia should be dark red, similar in appearance to menstrual flow (lochia rubra). A few small clots are normal and occur as a result of blood pooling in the vagina. However, the passage of numerous or large clots is abnormal, and the cause should immediately be investigated. After two to three days the lochia changes to lochia serosa.

Lochia should never exceed a moderate amount, such as four to eight perineal pads daily, with an average of six. However, because this is influenced by an individual woman's pad-changing practices, she should be questioned about the length of time the current pad has been in use, and whether any clots were passed prior to this examination, such as during voiding. If heavy bleeding is reported but not seen, the woman is asked to put on a clean perineal pad and is reassessed in one hour. Figure 33–4 provides suggested guidelines for assessing lochia volume. If clots are reported but not seen, the woman is asked to save all pads with clots or not flush the toilet if clots were expelled during urination. Clots and heavy bleeding may be caused by uterine atony or retained placental fragments and require further assessment. Because of the evacuation of the uterine cavity during cesarean birth, women with such surgery have less lochia after the first 24 hours than mothers who gave birth vaginally. Therefore, amounts of lochia that would be normal in women who had vaginal births are suspect in women who have undergone cesarean birth. Research suggests that estimations of blood loss are influenced by the brand of peri-pad used (Luegenbiehl et al 1990). Consequently if standards for estimating blood loss are established in a clinical facility, they should be brand-specific.

In situations where a more accurate assessment of blood loss is needed, the perineal pads can be weighed. When pads are weighed, 1 g is considered equivalent to 1 mL blood.

The odor of the lochia is nonoffensive and never foul. If foul odor is present, so is an infection.

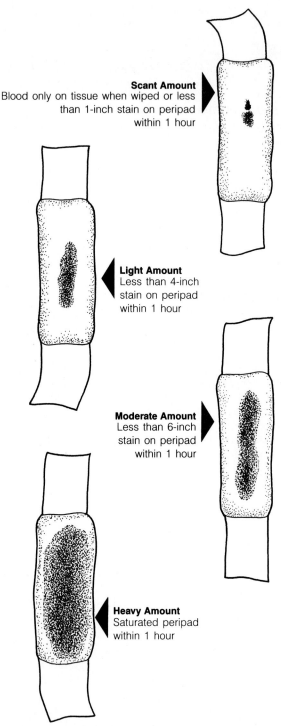

Scant Amount
Blood only on tissue when wiped or less than 1-inch stain on peripad within 1 hour

Light Amount
Less than 4-inch stain on peripad within 1 hour

Moderate Amount
Less than 6-inch stain on peripad within 1 hour

Heavy Amount
Saturated peripad within 1 hour

Figure 33–4 Suggested guidelines for assessing lochia volume. (From Jacobson H: A standard for assessing lochia volume. Am J Mat Child Nurs May/June 1985; 10:175. American Journal of Nursing Company. Used with permisison. All rights reserved.

The amount of lochia is charted first, followed by character. For example:

● Lochia: moderate amount rubra
● Lochia: small amount rubra/serosa

Client teaching that may be addressed during assessment of the lochia may center on normal changes that can be expected in the amount and color of the flow. Hygienic measures may be reviewed if appropriate. When the nurse approaches the teaching with the goals of promoting comfort, enhancing tissue healing, and preventing infection, value-laden statements regarding personal beliefs about the need for cleanliness or control of body odor can be avoided.

Perineum

The perineum is inspected with the woman lying in a Sims' position. The buttock is lifted to expose the perineum and anus (Figure 33–5). If an **episiotomy** was done or a laceration required suturing, the wound is assessed. The state of healing is evaluated by observing for redness, edema, ecchymosis, discharge, and approximation—the REEDA scale (Davidson 1974) (see Table 36–3).

After 24 hours some edema may still be present, but the skin edges should be "glued' together (well approximated) so that gentle pressure does not separate them. Gentle palpation should elicit minimal tenderness and there should be no hardened areas suggesting infection. The perineum may be somewhat edematous even if no epi-

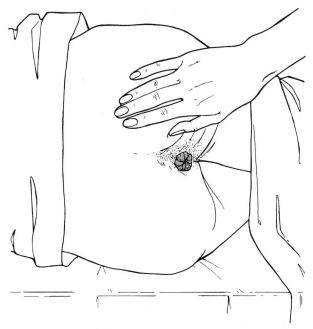

Figure 33–5 Intact perineum with hemorrhoids. Note how the examiner's hand raises the upper buttocks to fully expose the anal area.

siotomy was performed, but marked swelling may indicate hematoma formation and requires further assessment. Ecchymosis interferes with normal healing, as does infection.

The nurse next assesses the state of any hemorrhoids present around the anus for size, number, and pain or tenderness.

During the assessment, the nurse talks with the woman to determine the effectiveness of comfort measures that have been used. The nurse provides teaching about the episiotomy. As the nurse explains the findings of her assessment, information about the episiotomy, its location, and signs that are being assessed can be addressed. In addition, the nurse can casually add that the sutures are special and that they will dissolve slowly over the next few weeks as the tissues heal. By the time the sutures are dissolved the tissues are strong and the incision edges will not separate. This is also an opportunity to teach comfort measures that may be used (see Chapter 34).

Lower Extremities

If thrombophlebitis occurs, the most likely site will be in the woman's legs. To assess for this condition, her legs should be stretched out, with the knees slightly flexed, and should be relaxed. The foot is then grasped and sharply dorsiflexed. No discomfort or pain should be present. If pain is elicited, the nurse-midwife or physician is notified that the woman has a positive Homan's sign (Figure 36–2). The pain is caused by inflammation of the vessel. The legs are also evaluated for edema. This may be done by comparing both legs, since usually only one leg is involved. Any areas of redness, tenderness, and increased skin temperature should be noted.

Early ambulation is an important aspect in the prevention of thrombophlebitis. Most women are able to get up shortly after birth. The cesarean birth client requires passive range of motion exercises until she is ambulating more freely.

Client teaching associated with assessment of the lower extremities focuses on the signs and symptoms of thrombophlebitis. In addition, the nurse may review self-care measures to promote circulation and measures to prevent thrombophlebitis, such as ambulation, avoiding pressure behind the knees, and avoiding using the knee gatch on the bed and crossing the legs.

Results of the assessment are usually contained in a summary nursing note. If tenderness and warmth have been noted, they might be recorded as follows: Tenderness, warmth, and slight redness noted on posterior aspect of left calf—positive Homan's. Woman advised to avoid pressure to this area; lower leg elevated and moist heat applied per agency protocol. Call placed to Dr Smith to report findings.

Vital Signs Assessment

Alteration in vital signs may indicate complications, so they are assessed at regular intervals. The blood pressure should remain stable, while the pulse often shows a characteristic slowness that is no cause for alarm. Pulse rates return to prepregnant norms very quickly unless complications arise.

Temperature elevations (less than 38C [100.4F]) due to normal processes should last for only a few days and should not be associated with other clinical signs of infection. Any elevation should be evaluated in light of other signs and symptoms. The woman's history should also be carefully reviewed to identify other factors, such as premature rupture of membranes (PROM) or long labor, which might increase the incidence of infection in the genital tract.

The nurse informs the woman of the results of the vital signs assessment. Information regarding the normal changes in blood pressure and pulse can be provided. This may be an opportunity to assess whether the mother knows how to assess her own and her infant's temperature and how to read a thermometer.

Nutritional Status

Determination of postpartal nutritional status is based primarily on information provided by the mother and on direct assessment. This is discussed in more detail in Chapter 16.

Elimination

During the hours after birth the nurse carefully monitors a new mother's bladder status. A boggy uterus, a displaced uterus, or a palpable bladder are signs of urinary distention and require nursing intervention.

The postpartal woman should be encouraged to void every two to four hours. A careful monitoring of intake and output should be maintained, and the bladder should be assessed for distention until the woman demonstrates complete emptying of the bladder with each voiding. The nurse may employ techniques to facilitate voiding, such as helping the woman out of bed to void or pouring warm water on the perineum to promote relaxation.

Catheterization is required if the bladder is distended and the woman cannot void or if no voiding has occurred in eight hours. Nurses must be alert for the problem of urinary retention with overflow. In this case the woman voids small amounts (usually less than 100 mL) frequently but never actually empties the distended bladder. When the catheter is removed, accurate measuring of the amount of urine is essential until voiding is no longer a problem. The cesarean birth woman may have an indwelling catheter inserted prophylactically. The same considerations should be made in evaluating bladder emptying once the catheter is removed.

During the assessment, the nurse elicits information from the woman regarding the adequacy of her fluid intake, whether she feels she is emptying her bladder completely when she voids, and any signs of urinary tract infection she may be experiencing. The nurse asks specifically about signs such as urgency, frequency, and dysuria. The nurse also provides information about postpartum diuresis.

The nurse obtains information about the new moth-er's intestinal elimination and any concerns she may have about it. Many mothers fear that the first bowel movement will be painful and possibly even damaging if an episiotomy has been done. Information must be provided about ways of keeping the stool soft to avoid discomfort and constipation. Often a frank discussion with the nurse does much to alleviate a new mother's anxieties about this subject.

Rest and Sleep Status

As part of the postpartal assessment, the nurse evaluates the amount of rest a new mother is getting. If the woman reports difficulty sleeping at night, the cause should be determined. If it is simply the strange hospital environment, a warm drink, back rub, or mild sedative may prove helpful. Appropriate nursing measures are indicated if the woman is bothered by normal postpartal discomforts such as afterpains, diaphoresis, episiotomy, or hemorrhoidal pain. A daily rest period should be encouraged, and hospital activities should be scheduled to allow time for napping.

CRITICAL THINKING

What techniques might you use to accurately assess the woman's psychologic status?

Psychologic Assessment

Adequate assessment of the mother's psychologic adjustment is an integral part of postpartal evaluation. This assessment focuses on the mother's general attitude, feelings of competence, available support systems, and care-giving skills. It also evaluates her fatigue level, sense of satisfaction, and ability to accomplish her developmental tasks.

Often fatigue is a significant factor in a new mother's apparent disinterest in her newborn. Frequently the woman is so tired from a long labor and birth that everything seems to be an effort. To avoid inadvertently classifying a very tired mother as one with a potential bonding problem, the nurse should do the psychologic assessment on more than one occasion. After a nap the new mother is often far more receptive to her infant and her surroundings.

Some new mothers have little or no experience with infants and may feel totally overwhelmed. Women may show these feelings by asking questions and reading all available material or by becoming passive and quiet because they simply cannot deal with their feelings of inadequacy. Unless a nurse questions the woman about her plans and previous experience in a supportive, nonjudgmental way, one might conclude that the woman was disinterested, withdrawn, or depressed. Problem clues might include excessive continued fatigue, marked depression, excessive preoccupation with physical status and/or discomfort, evidence of low self-esteem, lack of support systems, marital problems, inability to care for or nurture the newborn, and current family crises (such as illness, unemployment, and so on). These characteristics frequently indicate a potential for maladaptive parenting, which may lead to child abuse or neglect (physical, emotional, intellectual) and cannot be ignored. Public health nurses or other available community resources may provide greatly needed assistance and may alleviate potentially dangerous situations.

Assessment of Early Attachment

Attachment is a desired outcome of maternal-infant interactions during the postpartum period. The nurse in the postpartum setting can periodically observe and note progress toward attachment. This content is discussed in detail in Chapter 35.

Data Base: the Fourth Trimester

The first several postpartal weeks have been termed the **fourth trimester** to stress the idea of continuity as the family adjusts to having a new member and as the woman's body returns to a prepregnant state. During this period the woman must accomplish certain physical and developmental tasks:

- Restoring physical condition
- Developing competence in caring for and meeting the needs of her infant
- Establishing a relationship with her new child
- Adapting to altered life-styles and family structure resulting from the addition of a new member

The new mother and her family may have an inadequate or incorrect understanding of what to expect during the early postpartal weeks. She may be concerned with restoring her figure and surprised because of continuing physical discomfort from sore breasts, episiotomy, or hemorrhoids. Fatigue is perhaps her greatest yet most underestimated problem during the early weeks. This may be aggravated if she has no extended family support or if there are other young children at home.

Developing skill and confidence in caring for an infant may be especially anxiety provoking for a new mother. As she struggles to establish a mutually acceptable pattern with her baby, small unanticipated concerns may seem monumental. The woman may begin to feel inadequate and, if she lacks support systems, isolated.

Many obstetricians and nurse practitioners now routinely see all postpartal women one to two weeks after birth in addition to the routine six-week checkup. This extra visit provides an opportunity for physical assessment as well as assessment of the mother's psychologic and informational needs.

Assessment of Family Wellness

A trend toward early discharge following birth has evolved over the past few years, and many women and their new-borns leave the hospital or birthing center within 6 to 48 hours following birth. Proponents cite decreased cost, less exposure of mother and baby to iatrogenic infection, enhanced parent-infant attachment, and decreased disruption of family life as advantages of this practice. However, this practice does raise questions about possible health risks if follow-up care is not provided.

Follow-up care for the postpartal family may be accomplished by home visits, postpartal classes, or follow-up phone calls. In some areas self-help support groups for new mothers are also available (Gosha & Bruckner 1986).

Home visits are becoming increasingly popular. Many health maintenance organizations (HMOs), group practices, and nurse-midwives have included home visits as part of their maternity care package. Home visits have long been part of the care provided to high-risk clients by community health nurses. A home visit should include a health assessment of the mother and baby in addition to the completion of necessary teaching or other nursing interventions. A subsequent visit can be scheduled if necessary. Figure 33–6 is a sample form the nurse can complete about the childbearing family when making a home visit.

Postpartal classes are becoming more common as care givers recognize the continuing needs of the childbearing family. A series of structured classes may focus on topics such as parenting, postpartal exercise, or nutrition, or there may be loosely structured group sessions that address concerns of mothers as they arise. Such classes offer chances for the new mother to socialize, share her concerns, and receive encouragement.

Two- and Six-Week Examinations

The routine physical assessment, which can be made rapidly, focuses on the woman's general appearance, breasts, reproductive tract, bladder and bowel elimination, and any specific problems or complaints. In addition, conversation is used to determine nutrition patterns, fatigue level, family adjustment, and psychologic status of the mother (see the Postpartal Assessment Guide—Two Weeks and Six Weeks After Birth). Any problems with child care are explored, and referral to a pediatric nurse-practitioner or pediatrician is made if needed. Available community resources, including Public Health Department follow-up visits, are mentioned when appropriate. If not already discussed, teaching about family planning is appropriate at this time, and information regarding birth control methods is provided.

In ideal situations a family approach involving the father, infant, and possibly other siblings would permit a total evaluation and provide an opportunity for all family members to ask questions and express concerns. In addition, disturbed family patterns might be more readily diagnosed so that therapy could be instituted to prevent future problems of neglect or abuse.

POSTPARTUM FOLLOW-UP GUIDE
General Information and Significant History

Date _____

Mother's Name _____

Address _____

Phone _____

Marital Status _____ Para _____ Gravida _____ Age _____

Education _____ Employment _____

Prenatal Care _____ Childbirth Education _____

Name(s) of Significant Other(s) _____

Primary Nurse _____

Obstetric Physician _____

Pediatric Physician _____

Other _____

Describe initial postpartum follow-up contact:
(telephone, home visit, clinic)

Significant Personal History:

Significant Antepartal History:

Significant Family History:

Assessment		Intervention	Evaluation	Follow-up
Maternal	**Self-care**	**Maternal**		
Physiologic	Nutrition	Discomfort		
Breasts	Basic four tid plus	Rest		
Engorgement	Fluids	Medication		
Nipples	Vitamins	Nutrition		
Other	Rest/nocturnal	Fluids		
Perineum	Naps	Exercise		
Episiotomy	Breasts	Breasts		
Lacerations	Nipple care	Nipple care		
Hemorrhoids	Massage	Clothing		
Eliminations	Self breast exam	Hygiene		
Bladder	Perineum	Technique		
Bowel	Episiotomy care	Perineum		
Cesarean incision	Hygiene regimen	Hygiene		
Appearance	Rx of pain	Treatment regimen		
Drainage	Sexuality	Sexuality		
Care and cleansing	Vaginal rest	Family planning		
Discomforts and	Family planning	Resumption of intercourse		
concerns	Exercise			
	Appropriate to			
	puerperium			
	Postpartum exercise			
	regimen			
	Mobilization of supports	Using support system		
	Family	Exploring supports		
	Friends	Strategies to use support		
	Other assistance	Handling unwelcome interference		
Maternal role-taking				
Expectations		Coping strategies		
Labor and birth (length, pain, support, etc.)		Adaptability		
Related to newborn (gender, appearance, size)		Information seeking		
Related to mothering (fantasy/reality, ability, etc.)		Increased flexibility		
Experience		Reorganizing		
Previous mothering		Expanding and use supports		
Preparation for parenthood		Bibliotherapy recommended		
Confidence/competence		reading		
Infant feeding				
Infant comforting				
Care and hygiene				
Infant bath				
Umbilical care				
Circumcision care				
Diapering and perineal care				
Verbal identifying		Parent-Infant Interaction		
Name _____ (s/he, it)		Infant states		
Describes infant behaviors, cues, and rhythms		Infant behavioral characteristics		
		Specific cues (hunger,		
Verbal expression of affection "_____"		fatigue, distress, etc.)		
Physical expressions of affection (en face,		Sensory stimulation		
positioning, caress, kiss, etc.)		Contingent caregiving		
Infant				
Physiologic		Essentials of infant care		
Physical assessment:		Feeding		
		Method		
Via report _____		Frequency		
(source and circumstance)		Duration		
Via exam _____				

Figure 33–6   Sample health assessment form to be completed by the nurse on all members of the childbearing family (Used with permission of NAACOG)

Assessment	Intervention	Evaluation	Follow-up

Vital Signs
  Temp
  Pulse
  Respirations
Color
  Jaundice
  Cyanosis
Skin
  Rashes
  Ecchymosis
  Inflammation
Eyes
Fontanelles
Central nervous system
  Reflexes observed/reported
Genitals
Elimination
  Bladder (frequency, color)
  Bowel (frequency, color, consistency)
Nutrition
  Feeding (method, frequency, quantity, satiation)
Hygiene
  Bathing (method, frequency, safety)
  Umbilicus
  Circumcision
  Perineal cleansing
  Diapering regimen
Sleep/activity patterns
  Sleep/wake pattern (typical 24-hour)
  Irritability
  Consolability (methods and effectiveness)
  Self-comforting (methods and effectiveness)
  Cuddliness
  Responsiveness to caregiver
    Visual
    Auditory
    Smile
  Clarity of cues
	Pre-feeding infant care
	  Satiation cues
	  Bubbling
	Hygiene
	  Bathing
	    Method
	    Safety
	    Organization
	  Eyes
	  Ears
	  Umbilicus
	  Perineum
	    Genitals
	    Diapering
	
	Knowledge of development needs
	Knowledge regarding safety and
	  signs of illness		

Father
Involvement
  Past Experience
  Preparation for this birth
  Style of involvement during pregnancy/birth
  Involvement postpartum
  Support to mother (psychologic/practical)
  Participation in care of siblings
Self-Care
  Rest
  Nutrition
	Expectations and reality
	  Exploring expectations and
	    myths
	  Identifying primary stressors
	
	Parent growth and development
	
	Importance of father in care of
	  mother and infant		

Father role-taking
  Expectations vs. reality
  Participation in infant care
    Feeding
    Diapering
    Bathing
    Comforting
    Entertaining
	Common stressors of fourth
	  trimester
	
	Crisis balancing factors
	
	Discuss smoking, alcohol, and
	  medications related to
	  breastfeeding		

Siblings
  Age(s)
  Gender(s)
  Preparation
  Expectations
  Initial responses to mother/parents
  Initial responses to infant
  Participation in infant care
  Parent actions to support siblings
  Role of extended family/friends
	Siblings
	  Needs and fears related to
	    new baby
	  Age appropriate regression
	  Strategies for meeting
	    sibling special needs
	  Books for sibling		

POSTPARTAL ASSESSMENT GUIDE
Two Weeks and Six Weeks After Birth

Assess/Normal Findings	Alterations and Possible Causes*	Nursing Responses to Data*
Vital Signs		
Blood pressure: Return to normal prepregnant level	Elevated blood pressure (anxiety, essential hypertension, and renal disease)	Review history, evaluate normal baseline; refer to physician/nurse-midwife if necessary.
Pulse: 60–90 beats/min (or prepregnant normal rate)	Increased pulse rate (excitement, anxiety, cardiac disorders)	Count pulse for full minute, note irregularities; marked tachycardia or beat irregularities require additional assessment and possible physician/nurse-midwife referral.
Respirations: 16–24/min	Marked tachypnea or abnormal patterns (respiratory disorders)	Evaluate for respiratory disease; refer to physician/nurse-midwife if necessary.
Temperature: 36.2C–37.6C (98F–99.6F)	Increased temperature (infection)	Assess for signs and symptoms of infection or disease state.
Weight		
Two weeks: Probable weight loss of 14–20+ lb	Little or no weight loss (fluid retention, subinvolution, excessive caloric intake)	Evaluate dietary habits and nutritional state; review blood pressure to evaluate fluid retention or blood losses.
Six weeks: Returning to normal prepregnant weight	Retained weight (excessive caloric intake)	Determine amount of daily exercise. Provide dietary teaching. Refer to dietitian if necessary for additional dietary counseling.
	Extreme weight loss (inadequate caloric intake)	Discuss appropriate diets; refer to dietitian for additional counseling if necessary.
Breasts		
Nonnursing:		
Two weeks: May have mild tenderness; small amount of milk may be expressed; breasts returning to prepregnant size	Some engorgement (incomplete suppression of lactation)	Engorgement usually seen when no medication has been given to suppress lactation or may occur after lactation suppression medication is stopped. Advise client to wear a supportive well-fitted bra, avoid hot showers, etc; evaluate for signs and symptoms of mastitis (rare in nonnursing mothers).
Six weeks: Soft, with no tenderness; return to prepregnant size	Redness; marked tenderness (mastitis)	
	Palpable mass (tumor)	
Nursing:		
Full, with prominent nipples; lactation established	Cracked, fissured nipples (feeding problems)	Counsel about nipple care. Evaluate client condition, evidence of fever; refer to physician/nurse-midwife for initiation for antibiotic therapy, if indicated.
	Redness, marked tenderness, or even abscess formation (mastitis)	
	Palpable mass (full milk duct, tumor)	

(continued)

POSTPARTAL ASSESSMENT GUIDE (*continued*)

Assess/Normal Findings	Alterations and Possible Causes*	Nursing Responses to Data*
Breasts		Opinion varies as to value of breast examination for nursing mothers; some feel a nursing mother should examine her breasts monthly, after feeding, when breasts are empty; if palpable mass is felt, refer to physician for further evaluation.
		For breast inflammation instruct the mother to:
		1. Keep breast empty by frequent feeding.
		2. Rest when possible.
		3. Take aspirin for pain.
		4. Increase fluids to at least 2000 mL/day.
		If symptoms persist for more than 24 hours, instruct her to call her physician/nurse-midwife.
Abdominal Musculature		
Two weeks: Improved firmness, although "bread dough" consistency is not unusual, especially in multipara	Marked diastasis recti abdominis (relaxation of muscles)	Evaluate exercise level; provide information on appropriate exercise program.
Striae pink and obvious		
Cesarean incision healing	Drainage, redness, tenderness, pain, edema (infection)	Evaluate for infection; refer to physician/nurse-midwife if necessary.
Six weeks: Muscle tone continues to improve; striae may be beginning to fade, may not achieve a silvery appearance for several more weeks; linea nigra fading		
Elimination Pattern		
Urinary tract:		
Return to prepregnant urinary elimination routine	Urinary incontinence, especially when lifting, coughing, laughing, and so on (urethral trauma, cystocele)	Assess for cystocele; instruct in appropriate muscle tightening exercises; refer to physician/nurse-midwife.
	Pain or burning when voiding, urgency and/or frequency, pus or white blood cells (WBC) in urine, pathogenic organisms in culture (urinary tract infection)	Evaluate for urinary tract infection; obtain clean catch urine; refer to physician/nurse-midwife for treatment if indicated.
Routine urinalysis within normal limits (proteinuria disappeared)	Sugar or ketone in urine—may be some lactose present in urine of breast-feeding mothers (diabetes)	Evaluate diet; assess for signs and symptoms of diabetes; refer to physician/nurse-midwife.

(*continued*)

POSTPARTAL ASSESSMENT GUIDE (continued)

Assess/Normal Findings	Alterations and Possible Causes*	Nursing Responses to Data†
Elimination Pattern *Bowel habits:* *Two weeks:* May still be some discomfort with defecation, especially if client had severe hemorrhoids or 3° or 4° extension	Severe constipation or pain when defecating (trauma or hemorrhoids)	Discuss dietary patterns; encourage fluid, adequate roughage. Continue use of stool softener if necessary to prevent pain associated with straining; continue sitz baths, periods of rest for severe hemorrhoids; assess healing of episiotomy and/or lacerations; severe constipation may require administration of laxatives, stool softeners, and an enema.
Six weeks: Return to normal prepregnant bowel elimination	Marked constipation	See above.
	Fecal incontinence or constipation (rectocele)	Assess for evidence of rectocele; instruct in muscle tightening exercises; refer to physician/nurse-midwife.
Reproductive Tract *Lochia:* *Two weeks:* Lochia alba, scant amounts, fleshy odor	Foul odor, excessive in amounts (infection) Return to lochia rubra or persistence of lochia rubra or serosa	Assess for evidence of infection and/or subinvolution; culture lochia; refer to physician/nurse-midwife.
Six weeks: No lochia, or return to normal menstruation pattern *Pelvic examination:*	See above.	See above.
Two weeks: Uterus no longer palpable abdominally; external os closed; uterine muscles still somewhat lax and uterus may be displaced; introitus of vagina still lacking tone—gapes when intra-abdominal pressure is increased by coughing or straining Episiotomy and/or lacerations healing; no signs of infection	External cervical os open, uterus not decreasing appropriately (subinvolution, infection) Evidence of redness, tenderness, poor tissue approximation in episiotomy and/or laceration (wound infection)	Assess for evidence of subinvolution and/or infection; refer to physician/nurse-midwife if indicated.
Six weeks: Almost returned to prepregnant size with almost completely restored muscle tone	Continued flow of lochia, some opening of cervical os, failure to decrease appropriately in size (subinvolution)	Assess for evidence of subinvolution and/or infection; refer to physician for further evaluation and for dilatation and curettage if necessary. Cervix completely closed with only transverse slit apparent
Good return of muscle tone to pelvic floor	Marked relaxation of pelvic floor muscles (uterine prolapse)	Assess for evidence of uterine prolapse; discuss appropriate perineal exercises; refer to physician/nurse-midwife if indicated.
Papanicolaou test: Negative	Test results show atypical cells	Refer to physician/nurse-midwife for further evaluation and treatment.

(continued)

POSTPARTAL ASSESSMENT GUIDE (*continued*)

Assess/Normal Findings	Alterations and Possible Causes*	Nursing Responses to Data†
Hemoglobin and Hematocrit Levels *Six weeks:* Hb 12 g/dL Hct 37% ± 5%	Hb < 12 g/dL Hct 32% (anemia)	Assess nutritional status, begin (or continue supplemental iron; for marked anemia (Hb 9g/dL) additional assessment and/or physician/nurse-midwife referral may be necessary.

POSTPARTAL PSYCHOLOGIC ASSESSMENT GUIDE

Assess/Normal Findings	Alterations and Possible Causes*	Nursing Responses to Data ⁴
Attachment Bonding process demonstrated by soothing, cuddling, and talking to infant; appropriate feeding techniques; eye-to-eye contact; calling infant by name.	Failure to bond demonstrated by lack of behaviors associated with bonding process, calling infant by nickname that promotes ridicule, inadequate infant weight gain, infant is dirty, hygienic measures are not being maintained, severe diaper rash, failure to obtain adequate supplies to provide infant care (malattachment).	Provide counseling; talk with the woman about her feelings regarding the infant; provide support for the caretaking activities that are being performed; refer to public health nurse for continued home visits.
Parent interacts with infant and provides soothing, caretaking activities.	Parent is unable to respond to infant needs (inability to recognize needs, inadequate education and support, fear, family stress).	Provide support for caretaking activities observed; provide information regarding caretaking activities, such as responding to infant cry; methods of wrapping infant; methods of soothing the infant such as swaddling, rocking, increasing stimuli by singing to the infant or decreasing stimuli by putting infant to rest in quiet room; methods of holding the infant; differences in the cry. Identify support system such as friends, neighbors; provide information regarding community resources and support groups.

(continued)

POSTPARTAL PSYCHOLOGIC ASSESSMENT GUIDE (cont.)

Assess/Normal Findings	Alterations and Possible Causes*	Nursing Responses to Data†
Attachment		
Parents are feeling more comfortable and successful with the parent role.	Evidence of stress and anxiety (difficulty moving into or dealing with the parent role).	Provide support and encouragement; provide information regarding progression into parent role and assist parents in talking through their feelings; refer to community resources and support groups.
Woman is in the informal or personal stage of maternal role attainment.	Woman is still greatly influenced by others, has not developed an image or style of her own (woman remains in the anticipatory stage).	Provide role modeling for the woman in working through problem solving with the infant; provide encouragement as she thinks through decisions and develops her sense of problem solving; encourage her to make decisions regarding infant care.
Adjustment to Parental Role		
Parents are coping with new roles in terms of division of labor, financial status, communication, readjustment of sexual relations, and adjusting to new daily tasks.	Inability to adjust to new roles (immaturity, inadequate education and preparation, ineffective communication patterns, inadequate support, current family crisis).	Provide counseling; refer to parent groups.
Education		
Mother understands self-care measures.	Inadequate knowledge of self-care (inadequate education).	Provide education and counseling.
Parents are knowledgeable regarding infant care.	Inadequate knowledge of infant care (inadequate education).	
Siblings are adjusting to new baby.	Excessive sibling rivalry.	
Parents have chosen a method of contraception.	Birth control method not chosen.	

*Possible causes of alterations are placed in parentheses.

†This column provides guidelines for further assessment and initial nursing interventions.

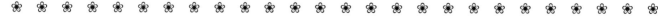

KEY CONCEPTS

The uterus involutes rapidly, primarily through a reduction in cell size.

Involution is assessed by measuring fundal height. The fundus is at the level of the umbilicus within a few hours after birth and should decrease by approximately one fingerbreadth per day.

The placental site heals by a process of exfoliation, so no scar formation occurs.

Lochia progresses from rubra to serosa to alba and is assessed in terms of type, quantity, and characteristics.

The abdomen may be flabby initially. Diastasis recti abdominis should be measured.

Constipation may develop postpartally due to decreased tone, limited diet, and denial of the urge to defecate due to fear of pain.

Decreased bladder sensitivity, increased capacity, and postpartal diuresis may lead to problems with bladder elimination. Frequent assessment and prompt intervention are indicated. A fundus that is boggy but does not respond to massage, is higher than expected, or deviates to the side usually indicates a full bladder.

Postpartally a healthy woman should be normotensive and afebrile. Bradycardia is common.

Postpartally the WBC is often elevated. Activation of clotting factors predisposes the woman to thrombus formation.

The REEDA scale provides criteria for evaluating the episiotomy or a cesarean incision.

Psychologic adaptions are traditionally described as taking-in and taking-hold.

Postpartal cultural practices are often based on a belief in a balance between hot and cold.

Postpartal assessment should be completed in a systematic way, usually cephalocaudally. It provides a tremendous opportunity for informal client teaching.

Because of the trend toward early discharge, follow-up care is more important than ever. Many approaches are used, especially home visits and telephone follow-up.

❀ ❀

References

Ament LA: Maternal tasks of the puerperium reidentified. *JOGGN* July/August 1990; 19:330.

Belsky J, Rovine M: Social-network contact, family support, and the transition to parenthood. *J Marriage Fam* 1984; 46:455.

Choi EC: Unique aspects of Korean-American mothers. *JOGNN* September/October 1986; 15:394.

Clark AL: *Culture, Childbearing, Health Professionals.* Philadelphia: Davis, 1978.

Cronenwett LR: Parental network structure and perceived support after birth of first child. *Nurs Res* November/December 1985; 34:347.

Cunningham FG et al: *Williams Obstetrics,* 18th ed. Norwalk CT: Appleton & Lange, 1989.

Davidson N: REEDA: Evaluating postpartum healing. *J Nurse-Midwifery* 1974; 9(2):6.

Engel NS: An American experience of pregnancy and childbirth in Japan. *Birth* June 1989; 16:2.

Gay JT et al: Reva Rubin revisited. *JOGNN* November/December 1988; 17:394.

Gosha J, Bruckner MC: A self-help group for new mothers: An evaluation. *MCN* January/February 1986; 11:20.

Horn BM: Cultural concepts and postpartal care. *Nurs Health Care* 1981; 2:516.

Jacobson H: A standard for assessing lochia volume. *MCN* May/June 1985; 10:174.

Karch A, Boyd E: *Handbook of Drugs.* Philadelphia: Lippincott, 1989.

LaDu EB: Childbirth care for Hmong families. *MCN* November/December 1985; 10:382.

Luegenbiehl DL et al: Standardized assessment of blood loss. *MCN* July/August 1990; 15:241.

Martell LK, Mitchell SK: Rubin's puerperal change reconsidered. *JOGNN* May/June 1984; 13:145.

Mercer RT: The process of maternal role attainment over the first year. *Nurs Res* July/August 1985; 34:198.

Rubin R: *Maternal Identity and the Maternal Experience.* New York: Springer, 1984.

Rubin R: Puerperal change. *Nurs Outlook* 1961; 9:753.

Strang VR, Sullivan PL: Body image attitudes during pregnancy and the postpartum period. *JOGNN* July/August 1985; 14:332.

Theesen K et al: Caring for the depressed obstetric patient. *Contemp OB/GYN* February 1989; 33:122.

Tulman L, Fawcett J: Return of functional ability after childbirth. *Nurs Res* March/April 1988; 37:77.

Varney H: *Nurse Midwifery,* 2nd ed. Boston: Blackwell Scientific Publications, 1987.

Additional Readings

Boissonnault JS, Blaschak MJ: Incidence of diastasis recti abdominis during the childbearing year. *Phys Ther* 1988; 68(7):1082.

Flagler S: Maternal role competence. *West J Nurs Res* 1988; 10(3):274.

Johnston PK: Counseling the pregnant vegetarian. *Am J Clin Nutr* 1988; 48(3 Suppl):901.

Lindell SG: Education for childbirth: A time for change. *JOGNN* 1988; 17(2):108.

Lutwak RA, Ney AM, White JE: Maternity nursing and Jewish law. *MCN* January/February 1988; 13:44.

McInerney PA: European cultural childbirth practices. *Nurs RSA* 1988; 3(3):35.

Mercer RT et al: Effect of stress on family functioning during pregnancy. *Nurs Res* 1988; 37(5):268.

Specker BL, et al: Changes in calcium homeostasis over the first years postpartum: Effect of lactation and weaning. *Obstet Gynecol* July 1991; 78(1):56.

Tulman L, Fawcett J: Functional status during pregnancy and the postpartum: A framework for research. *Image* Fall 1990; 22(3):191.

CHAPTER 34

The Postpartal Family:
Needs and Care

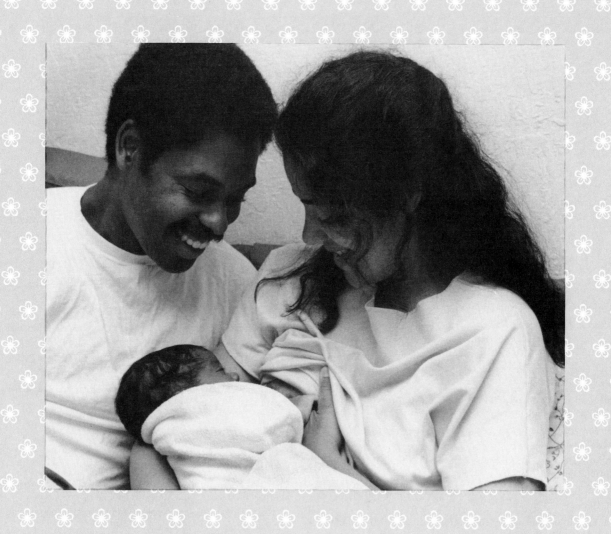

OBJECTIVES

Relate the use of nursing diagnoses to the findings of the "normal" postpartum assessment and analysis.

Delineate nursing responsibilities for client education during the early postpartum period.

Discuss appropriate nursing interventions to meet identified nursing goals for the childbearing family.

Compare the nursing needs of a woman who experienced a cesarean birth with the needs of a woman who gave birth vaginally.

Summarize the nursing needs of the childbearing adolescent during the postpartum period.

Describe possible approaches to follow-up nursing care for the childbearing family.

❀ ❀

Not long ago my husband, my sons, and I sat out on the deck enjoying a summer evening and reminiscing. We talked about earlier camping trips, family vacations, and Christmas festivities. Suddenly my nine year old said, "It's fun talking about the olden days, isn't it!" My husband and I laughed but we realized our son was saying something important about the experiences that a family shares, about the memories we build together. I remember so clearly the day I brought my firstborn home from the hospital. My husband dropped me off and then had to return to work. I sat in the living room with my new son and tried to envision the future. How would this small person change our lives? I know now that, though it is sometimes frustrating to be a parent, it is infinitely enriching, too. Our boys have brought great meaning to our lives. When we talk about the "olden days" I realize how many memories we have as a family and how many more we will build in the years to come.

Certain premises form the basis of effective nursing care during the postpartal period.

- The best postpartal care is family centered and disrupts the family unit as little as possible. This approach uses the family's resources to support an early and smooth adjustment to the newborn by all family members.
- Knowledge of the range of normal physiologic and psychologic adaptations occurring during the postpartal period allows the nurse to recognize alterations and initiate interventions early. Communicating information about postpartal adaptations to the family facilitates their adjustment to the new situation.
- Nursing care is aimed at accomplishing specific goals that ultimately meet individual needs. These goals are formulated after careful assessment and consideration of factors that could influence the outcome of care.

This chapter describes how the nurse can use the nursing process effectively to plan and provide care. Specific nursing responses to the mother's physical needs and the family's psychosocial needs are described at length.

❀ *USING THE NURSING PROCESS WITH* ❀

The Postpartal Family

Often standardized nursing care plans provide the written guidelines for a nurse's action during the postpartal period. Each family is different, however, and the nurse needs to modify interventions to meet a family's needs. Whether a predetermined care plan exists or not, using the nursing process can help the nurse individualize the approach to families and determine priorities.

Nursing Assessment

The postpartal assessment focuses on three interrelated areas of concern—the mother's physical changes and psychologic adjustments, the educational needs of the parents, and the family's adjustment to the new baby. During the postpartal assessment, the nurse identifies the strengths of the woman or family as well as actual and potential problems that may influence maternal or family well-being. Ultimately, the assessment findings influence the plan of care.

The assessment period can also be used as a forum for client education. For example, as the postpartal nurse identifies physical changes in the mother, he or she explains them to the woman and her partner. As the nurse assesses the parents' skill in handling the new baby, he or she offers information or provides demonstrations that will enhance the parents' competence in caring for their new infant.

Nursing Diagnosis

For most postpartal women, physical recovery goes smoothly and is considered a healthy process. Because of this perception, it is all too common for care givers to think that the woman and her family have no "real" needs and thus that no care plan is needed. Nothing could be further from the truth.

The postpartal family's needs, which should be identified during assessment, are the basis for developing nursing diagnoses. Once a nursing diagnosis is made and recorded, systematic action, as delineated in a nursing care plan, can be taken to meet the identified need.

Many nurses have suggested that nursing diagnoses are difficult to make in a wellness setting because of their emphasis on "problems." Nurses involved in the effort to formulate standardized diagnoses recognize this difficulty and are working to develop diagnoses that are more useful in wellness settings.

Many agencies that use nursing diagnoses prefer to use the North American Nursing Diagnosis Association (NANDA) list exclusively. Consequently, physiologic alterations form the basis of many postpartal diagnoses. Examples of such diagnoses are as follows:

- Constipation related to fear of tearing stitches and/or pain.
- Altered patterns of urinary elimination related to dysuria.

Nursing Plan and Implementation

Many women remain on a postpartum unit for only a short time, so it is often possible to assign a woman's care to the same nurse. However, time off and shift changes still make it essential to develop and record a specific care plan. Implementation of the plan by all personnel caring for the postpartal woman promotes consistency, progress in client education, and more effective ongoing assessment and evaluation. An important component of nursing care is client teaching, which is given high priority by many agencies. Sophisticated, detailed forms and guidelines are often available to assist in health teaching. Such tools are a useful adjunct but cannot take the place of the nurse's client-specific plan.

Evaluation

Nursing evaluation on the postpartum unit enables the nurse to refine or modify the care plan based on its effectiveness and/or changes in the woman's status. Evaluation tends to be the most overlooked step of the nursing process, yet the nurse cannot provide quality care without determining whether interventions have been effective.

❀ ❀ ❀ ❀ ❀ ❀ ❀ ❀ ❀ ❀ ❀ ❀ ❀ ❀

Care of the Postpartal Family

❀   *APPLYING THE NURSING PROCESS*   ❀

Nursing Assessment

The nurse completes assessments of the new family and analyzes the data obtained. Cues are identified and additional assessments may be made as needed. See Chapter 33 for thorough discussion of the postpartal assessment.

Nursing Diagnosis

The nurse can anticipate that for many women with a low-risk postpartal period, certain nursing diagnoses such as those discussed previously and possibly those presented in the Key Nursing Diagnoses to Consider—The Postpartal Period will be used. After completing the assessment and diagnosis steps of the nursing process, the nurse creates a plan of care arranged around nursing goals.

Nursing Plan and Implementation During the Postpartal Period

Promotion of Maternal Physical Well-Being
Maternal physical well-being is promoted by monitoring the status of the uterus, monitoring vital signs on a regular schedule, and providing medications as needed for women with problems involving the Rh factor, women who are not rubella immune, and women with some degree of anemia following childbirth.

Monitoring Uterine Status   The nurse completes an assessment of the uterus as discussed in Chapter 33. The

Dx

Key Nursing Diagnoses to Consider
The Postpartal Period

Altered family processes	Family coping: Potential for growth
Altered patterns of urinary elimination: Urinary retention	Impaired physical mobility
Altered tissue perfusion	Ineffective individual coping
Anxiety	Knowledge deficit
Bathing/hygiene self-care deficit	Pain
Constipation	Infection: High risk
	Fluid volume deficit: High risk

Table 34–1 Changes in Lochia That Cause Concern

Change	Possible problem	Nursing actions
Presence of clots	Inadequate uterine contractions that allow bleeding from vessels at the placental site	Assess location and firmness of fundus. Assess voiding pattern. Record and report findings.
Persistent lochia rubra	Inadequate uterine contractions; retained placental fragments; infection	Assess location and firmness of fundus. Assess activity pattern. Assess for sign of infection. Record and report findings.

assessment interval is every 15 minutes for the first hour after childbirth, every 30 minutes for the next hour, and then hourly for approximately two hours. After that, the nurse monitors uterine status at the beginning of each shift (every eight hours) or more frequently if problems arise such as bogginess, positioning out of midline, heavy lochia flow, or the presence of clots.

Medications may be ordered to promote uterine contractions. See Drug Guide—Methylergonovine Maleate (Methergine) in Chapter 33.

The amount, consistency, color, and odor of the lochia is monitored on an ongoing basis. Changes in lochia that need to be assessed further, documented, and reported to the physician/nurse-midwife are presented in Table 34–1.

Rubella Vaccine Women who have a rubella titer of less than 1:10 are usually given rubella vaccine in the postpartal period. If the woman is not rubella immune and is also Rh negative and receives RhoGAM, there is some question as to whether the RhoGAM will interfere with the production of antibodies to rubella (Varney 1987). At this time, most physicians/nurse-midwives would continue to order rubella vaccine and would repeat the rubella titer in a few weeks to determine immunity. (See Table 34–2.)

Education for Self-Care The nurse needs to ensure that the woman understands the purpose of the vaccine and that she must avoid becoming pregnant in the next three months. Because the avoidance of pregnancy is so important, counseling regarding contraception is suggested.

RhIgG (Rhogam) All Rh negative women who meet specific criteria should receive RhIgG (RhoGAM) within 72 hours after childbirth. See discussion of criteria on page 526.

Education for Self-Care The Rh negative woman needs to understand the implications of her Rh negative status in future pregnancies. The nurse provides opportunities for questions.

Promotion of Comfort and Relief of Pain

Relief of Perineal Discomfort Many nursing interventions are available for the relief of perineal discomfort. Before selecting a method, the nurse should assess the perineum to determine the degree of edema and so forth. The nurse can ask the woman which comfort measures she believes will be most effective or offer her choices when possible. Handwashing is important both before and after all relief measures.

If an episiotomy is done at the time of birth, an ice pack is often applied to reduce edema and relieve discomfort by numbing the tissue. In some agencies, chemical ice bags are used. These are usually activated by folding both ends toward the middle. Inexpensive ice bags may be made by filling a disposable glove with ice chips or crushed ice and then taping the top of the glove. The disposable glove needs to first be rinsed under running water to remove any powder that may be present, and then wrapped in an absorbent towel or washcloth before placing it against the perineum. To attain the maximum effect of this cold treatment, the ice pack should remain in place approximately 20 minutes and then be removed for about ten minutes before replacing it. Care needs to be taken to protect the perineum from burns caused by contact with the ice pack.

After the first few hours have passed, perineal discomfort may be relieved by a variety of approaches, including routine perineal care, sitz baths, heat lamps, topical application of anesthetic ointments or sprays, and administration of analgesics. The woman may also find it helpful to tighten her buttocks before sitting to avoid direct trauma to the perineum. For similar reasons lateral positions may be more comfortable.

Education for Self-Care Perineal care should be encouraged after each elimination to clean the perineum and promote comfort. Some agencies provide "peri-bottles," which the woman fills with warm water that is squirted over the perineum following elimination. She should be instructed to cleanse from front to back to prevent con-

Table 34-2 Key Information for Common Postpartum Drugs

Drug	Indication	Adverse effects	Nursing implications
Deladumone OB (contains 360 mg testosterone enanthate and 16 mg estradiol valerate) Drug class: Androgen, hormone Dose/Route: 2 mL deep IM at the beginning of the second stage of labor or just prior to the birth of the baby.	Suppress lactation	Hirsutism, hoarseness, deepening of voice, facial hair growth, discomfort at injection site	Determine if woman has known sensitivity to androgens; presence of liver, cardiac, or kidney disease. Administer deep IM. *Possible Nursing Diagnoses Related to Drug Therapy* Knowledge deficit regarding the drug therapy Body image disturbance related to androgenic effects of drug
TACE (chlorotrianisene) Drug class: Nonsteroidal synthetic estrogen, hormone Dose/Route: One of the following regimens: 12 mg PO TID for seven days or 50 mg PO every six hours for six doses or 72 mg PO BID for two days Administer first dose within eight hours of birth	Suppress lactation	Nausea and vomiting, abdominal cramps, headache, thrombophlebitis, photosensitivity, migraine headache, depression, pulmonary emboli	Determine if woman has sensitivity or prior problems with estrogens or contraindications to the use of estrogens (hypertension, history of migraine headaches). Observe diabetic women closely (may increase insulin requirements); observe women at risk for thrombophlebitis. *Client Teaching* Inform client about name of drug, expected action, possible side effects, that drug is excreted in breast milk, need to take all pills that are ordered, possibility that engorgement may occur a few days after she finishes taking the pills (Varney 1987). *Possible Nursing Diagnoses Related to Drug Therapy* Knowledge deficit regarding drug therapy Personal identity disturbance related to androgenic effects of drug
Empirin #3 (325 mg aspirin and 30 mg codeine) Drug class: Narcotic analgesic Dose/Route: Usual adult dose: One to two tablets PO every four hours PRN	For relief of mild to moderate pain	Aspirin: Nausea, dyspepsia, epigastric discomfort, dizziness Codeine: respiratory depression, apnea, lightheadedness, dizziness, nausea, sweating, dry mouth, constipation, facial flushing, suppression of cough reflex, ureteral spasm, urinary retention, pruritis	Determine if woman is sensitive to aspirin or codeine; has history of impaired hepatic or renal function. Monitor bowel sounds, respirations, urine output. Administer with food or after meals if GI upset occurs; encourage woman to drink one full glass (240 mL) with the tablet to reduce the risk of the tablet lodging in the esophagus. *Client Teaching* Inform client about name of drug, expected action, possible side effects, that it is secreted in breast milk (Note: Some physician/nurse-midwives may avoid ordering this medication for nursing mothers), and review safety measures (assess for dizziness, use side rails, call for assistance when getting out of bed and ambulating, report to nurse any signs of adverse effects); ask if she has any questions. *Possible Nursing Diagnoses Related to Drug Therapy* Knowledge deficit regarding the drug therapy Injury: High risk related to dizziness secondary to effect of drug
Percoset (contains 325 mg acetaminophen and 5 mg oxycodone) Drug class: Narcotic analgesic Dose/Route: One to two tablets PO every four hours PRN	For moderate to moderately severe pain Can be used in aspirin-sensitive women	Acetaminophen: Hepatotoxicity, headache, rash, hypoglycemia Oxycodone: Respiratory depression, apnea, circulatory depression, euphoria, facial flushing, constipation, suppression of cough reflex, ureteral spasm, urinary retention	Determine if woman is sensitive to acetaminophen or codeine; has bronchial asthma, respiratory depression, convulsive disorder. Observe woman carefully for respiratory depression if given with barbiturates or sedative/hypnotics. Consider that postcesarean-birth woman may have depressed cough reflex, so teaching and encouragement to deep breathe and cough is needed. Monitor bowel sounds, urine and bowel elimination. *Client Teaching* Teaching should include name of drug, expected effect, possible adverse effects, that drug is secreted in the breast milk, encouragement to report any signs of adverse effects immediately.

(continued)

Table 34–2 (continued)

Drug	Indication	Adverse effects	Nursing implications
			Possible Nursing Diagnoses Related to Drug Therapy Altered breathing patterns Depression Constipation Urinary retention
Rubella virus vaccine, live (Meruvax 2) Dose/Route: Single-dose vial, inject subcutaneously in outer aspect of the upper arm	Stimulate active immunity against rubella virus	Burning or stinging at the injection site; about two to four weeks later may have rash, malaise, sore throat, or headache	Determine if woman has sensitivity to neomycin (vaccine contains neomycin); is immunosuppressed, or has received blood transfusions (not to be administered within three months of blood transfusion, plasma transfusion, or serum immune globulin). Note: If a woman is to receive both RhIgG and rubella, there is a possibility that the formation of antibodies to rubella may be suppressed by the RhIgG injection. Most physicians will go ahead and order both injections and retest for maternal rubella immune status in about three months (Varney 1987). *Client Teaching* Name of drug, expected effect, possible adverse effects, possible comfort measures to use if adverse effects occur; rubella titer will be assessed in about three months. Instruct woman to AVOID PREGNANCY FOR THREE MONTHS following vaccination. Provide information regarding contraceptives and their use. *Possible Nursing Diagnoses Related to Drug Therapy* Knowledge deficit regarding drug therapy Knowledge deficit regarding types and use of contraceptives Pain related to rash and malaise
RhIgG (RhoGAM) (Rh immune globulin specific for D antigen) Dose/Route: Postpartum: One vial IM within 72 hours of birth Antepartal: One vial microdose RhoGAM IM at 28 weeks in Rh negative women; after amniocentesis, spontaneous or therapeutic abortion, or ectopic pregnancy	Prevention of sensitization to the Rh factor in Rh negative women and to prevent hemolytic disease in the newborn in subsequent pregnancies Mother must be: Rh negative Not previously sensitized to Rh factor Infant must be: Rh positive Direct antiglobulin negative	Soreness at injection site	Confirm criteria for administration are present. Ensure correct vial is used for the client (each vial is cross-matched to the specific woman and must be carefully checked). Inject entire contents of vial. *Client Teaching* Name of drug, expected action, possible side effects, report soreness at injection site to nurse; woman should carry information regarding Rh status and dates of RhoGAM injections with her at all times; explain use of RhoGAM with subsequent pregnancies. *Possible Nursing Diagnoses Related to Drug Therapy* Knowledge deficit related to the need for RhoGAM and future implications Pain related to soreness at injection site
Seconal Sodium (secobarbital sodium) Drug Class: Sedative, short-acting barbiturate Dose/Route: 100 mg PO at bedtime	Promote sleep	Somnolence, confusion, ataxia, vertigo, nightmares, hypoventilation, bradycardia, hypotension, nausea, vomiting, rashes	Determine if woman has sensitivity to barbiturates, or respiratory distress. Monitor respirations, blood pressure, pulse. Modify environment to increase relaxation and promote sleep. Monitor for drug interaction if woman also is taking tranquilizers, or TACE. *Client Teaching* Name of drug, expected effect, possible adverse effects, safety measures (side rails, use call bell, ask for assistance when out of bed); medication is secreted in breast milk. *Possible Nursing Diagnoses Related to Drug Therapy* Injury: High risk related to possible ataxia or vertigo Altered thought processes related to drug-induced confusion Knowledge deficit regarding drug therapy

TEACHING GUIDE
Care of an Episiotomy

Assessment During the time following labor and birth, the nurse assesses the woman's understanding of the purpose of the episiotomy, factors that contribute to wound healing, and comfort measures available if the woman experiences discomfort. The woman's level of knowledge may be influenced by several factors including, for example, childbirth preparation activities and previous childbirth experience.

Nursing Diagnosis The key nursing diagnosis will probably be: Knowledge deficit related to self-care measures to promote episiotomy healing and personal comfort.

Nursing Plan and Implementation The teaching will focus on the process of healing, factors that increase the risk of infection, and steps the woman can take to promote healing and increase her personal comfort.

Client Goals At the completion of the teaching the woman will be able to do the following:

1. Identify factors that promote wound healing and those that interfere with healing.
2. Summarize self-care activities to promote healing and increase personal comfort.
3. Demonstrate the correct procedure for taking a sitz bath.
4. Discuss the judicious use of prescribed analgesics as needed.

Teaching Plan

Content Describe the process of wound healing including the value of healing by first intention as opposed to a jagged tear. Discuss the risk of contamination of the episiotomy by bacteria from the anal area.

Explain techniques that are used to keep the episiotomy clean and promote healing such as:

- Sitz bath
- Use of peri-bottle or surgigator following each voiding or defecation
- Pad change following each elimination and at regular intervals
- Use of sanitary belt with snugly applied pad
- Heat lamp

Describe comfort measures:

- Ice pack or glove immediately following birth
- Sitz bath
- Judicious use of analgesics or topical anesthetics
- Tightening buttocks before sitting

Identify signs of episiotomy infection. Advise the woman to contact care giver if infection develops.

Evaluation At the end of the teaching session the woman will be able to verbalize principles of wound healing and episiotomy care. She also will be able to demonstrate self-care measures such as peri-care, taking a sitz bath, and so forth.

Teaching Method Many women fail to consider the episiotomy a surgical incision. Discussion helps them understand the importance of good wound care.

Discussion and demonstration as indicated. Many young women today are not familiar with a sanitary belt and may require explanation.
Demonstration may also be necessary for sitz bath or surgigator.

Discussion and opportunity for questions.

Discussion and printed handouts. Some of this content may also be covered during a small postpartum class.

tamination of the vulva from the anal area. Other agencies have wall-mounted surgigators with soap cartridges to cleanse the perineum. The steady stream of warm, soapy water they provide is especially effective for cleaning. When toilet tissue is used, the woman will be more comfortable if she uses a blotting motion. She is also instructed to apply the perineal pad from front to back to prevent contamination from the anal area. The perineal pad should fit snugly against the perineum. If it is too loose, it may rub back and forth, irritating the tissues and causing contamination between the anal and vaginal areas.

Sitz baths are particularly useful if the perineum has been severely traumatized, as moist heat not only increases circulation to promote healing but also relaxes the tissue to promote comfort and decrease edema.

When assisting a woman into a sitz bath, the nurse should be certain the water temperature is comfortable. Most women find a temperature of 105F comfortable, although recent research suggests that a cool sitz bath may be more effective in decreasing perineal edema. Until definite research supports one temperature (warm or cold) as more effective, it may be best to offer women a choice according to personal preference (La Foy & Geden 1989; Ramler & Roberts 1986).

The sitz tub should be cleansed before each use. While in a sitz tub, the woman may wear a hospital gown and drape it over the edge of the tub to prevent chilling and provide privacy. A call light should be within reach. The position and warmth of a sitz bath can make a woman become faint; the nurse should check on her frequently. Once the woman is familiar with the use of the sitz bath, she should be encouraged to use it as frequently as she wishes, generally for about 20 minutes three or four times a day. Many agencies are now using disposable sitz baths that fit inside the toilet. These are convenient for the woman to use as often as she wishes both in the hospital and when she goes home.

Dry heat in the form of heat lamps is sometimes used. The perineum should be cleaned to prevent drying of secretions on the perineum. Heat lamps generally are used for 20 minutes two or three times daily. The heat source should contain a 60-watt bulb and should be placed approximately 12 inches from the perineum to avoid burns.

Topical anesthetics such as Dermoplast Aerosol Spray or Nupercainal ointment may be used to relieve perineal discomfort. The woman is advised to apply the anesthetic following a sitz bath or perineal care. Because of the danger of tissue burns she must be cautioned not to apply anesthetic before using a heat lamp.

Relief of Hemorrhoidal Discomfort

Some mothers experience hemorrhoidal pain after giving birth. Relief measures include the use of sitz baths two or three times per day and anesthetic ointments, rectal suppositories, or witch hazel pads applied directly to the anal area. The woman may be taught to digitally replace external hemorrhoids in her rectum (see Chapter 14). She may also find it helpful to maintain a side-lying or prone position when possible and to avoid prolonged sitting. The mother is encouraged to maintain an adequate fluid intake and to take stool softeners or laxatives to ensure greater comfort with bowel movements. The hemorrhoids usually disappear a few weeks after the birth if the woman did not have them prior to this pregnancy.

Relief of Discomfort from Afterpains

Afterpains are the result of intermittent uterine contractions. A primipara may not experience afterpains because her uterus is able to maintain a contracted state. Multiparous women and those who have had a multiple pregnancy or hydramnios frequently experience discomfort from afterpains as the uterus intermittently contracts. The nurse can suggest the woman lie prone with a small pillow under the lower abdomen. The woman needs to be told that the discomfort may feel intensified for about five minutes but then will diminish greatly if not completely. The prone position applies pressure to the uterus and therefore stimulates contractions. When the uterus maintains a constant contraction, the afterpains cease. Additional nursing interventions may be to encourage a sitz bath (for warmth), positioning, ambulation, or administration of an analgesic agent. For breast-feeding mothers, a mild analgesic administered an hour before feeding will promote comfort and enhance maternal-infant interactions.

Education for Self-Care   The nurse provides information about the cause of afterpains and methods to decrease discomfort. Any medications that are ordered are explained, along with expected effect, benefits and possible side effects, and any special considerations such as the possibility of dizziness or sleepiness with particular medications.

Relief of Discomfort from Immobility

Discomfort may also be caused by immobility. The woman who has been in stirrups for any length of time may experience muscular aches from such extreme positioning. It is not unusual for women to experience joint pains and muscular pain in both arms and legs, depending on the effort they exerted during the second stage of labor.

Early ambulation is encouraged to help reduce the incidence of complications such as constipation and thrombophlebitis. It also helps promote a feeling of general well-being.

The nurse assists the woman the first few times she gets up during the postpartal period. Fatigue, effects of medications, loss of blood, and possibly even lack of food intake may result in feelings of dizziness or faintness when the woman stands up. Because this may be a problem during the woman's first shower, the nurse should remain in the room, check the woman frequently, and have a chair close by in case she becomes faint. Dizziness may be aggravated by standing still and by the warmth of the water, so it is best to keep the first shower somewhat brief. Many postpartal units tape ammonia inhalants to the bathroom door for use in case of fainting. During this first shower the nurse instructs the woman in the use of the emergency call button in the bathroom; if she becomes faint during a future shower, she can call for assistance.

Relief of Discomfort from Excessive Perspiration Postpartal diaphoresis may cause discomfort for new mothers. The nurse can offer a fresh dry gown and bed linens to enhance comfort. Some women may feel refreshed by a shower. It is important to consider cultural practices and realize that some Mexican American and Asian women may prefer not to shower in the first few days following birth. Because diaphoresis also may lead to increased thirst, the nurse can offer fluids as the woman desires. Again, cultural practices are important to consider. Caucasian women may prefer iced water and Asian women may prefer water at room temperature. Thus the nurse may ascertain the woman's wishes rather than operate solely from the nurse's own value/cultural belief system.

Suppression of Lactation in the Nonnursing Mother Lactation may be suppressed through drug therapy and mechanical inhibition. The drugs used are hormones that inhibit the secretion of prolactin. However, because many of these drugs, such as chlorotrianisene (TACE), are estrogen-based medications and are associated with an increased incidence of thromboembolic disease, most practitioners prescribe them much less frequently than formerly. A newer, nonhormonal lactation suppressant, bromocriptine mesylate (Parlodel) is sometimes used. See the accompanying Drug Guide—Bromocriptine (Parlodel).

Because bromocriptine is expensive and not always completely successful in suppressing lactation, mechanical methods of lactation suppression are becoming increasingly popular. Although signs of engorgement do not usually occur until the second or third postpartum day, prevention of engorgement is best accomplished by beginning nonpharmaceutical methods of lactation suppression as soon as possible after birth. Ideally this involves having the woman begin wearing a supportive, well-fitting bra within six hours after birth. The bra is worn continuously until lactation is suppressed (usually about five days) and is removed only for showers (Wong & Stepp-Gilbert 1985). The bra provides support and eases the discomfort that can occur with tension on the breasts because of fullness. A snug breast binder may be used if the woman does not

---

DRUG GUIDE
Bromocriptine (Parlodel)

Overview of Obstetric Action

Bromocriptine is a dopamine agonist that acts to suppress lactation by stimulating the production of prolactin-inhibiting factor at the hypothalmic level. This results in decreased secretion of prolactin by the pituitary gland. The drug may also directly inhibit the pituitary by preventing the release of prolactin from the hormone-producing cells (Foster 1982). When administered postpartally it helps suppress milk production and decrease breast leakage and pain. It may also be used for suppression after lactation has already begun.

Route, Dosage, and Frequency

The usual dose is 2.5 mg orally two times per day. The total daily dose generally does not exceed 7.5 mg. The medication is usually taken for 2–3 weeks. Research regarding the efficacy of parenteral administration suggests that a single intramuscular dose of a microencapsulated form of bromocriptine may be effective in suppressing lactation when administered following birth. This would be useful following obstetric surgery or for women experiencing severe vomiting (Peters et al 1986).

Maternal Contraindications

Maternal hypotension, desire to breast-feed, pregnancy.

Maternal Side Effects

Hypotension is the primary side effect. To prevent problems associated with hypotension, administration should be delayed until the new mother's vital signs are stable. Other side effects include nausea, headache, dizziness, and occasionally faintness and vomiting.

Nursing Considerations

Administration should be delayed until maternal blood pressure is stable. Blood pressure should be carefully monitored if bromocriptine is administered concurrently with any antihypertensives. Taking bromocriptine with meals may help decrease the possibility of nausea. Early resumption of ovulation has occurred in women taking bromocriptine; the woman should be informed of this and receive information about contraceptives (Foster 1982). The woman should be advised that engorgement may occur when medication is stopped.

have a bra available or if she finds the binder more comfortable. Ice packs should be applied over the axillary area of each breast for 20 minutes four times daily. This, too, should be begun soon after birth. Ice is also useful in relieving discomfort if engorgement occurs.

 Education for Self-Care   The mother is advised to avoid any stimulation of her breasts by her baby, herself, breast pumps, or her sexual partner until the sensation of fullness has passed (usually about one week). Such stimulation will increase milk production and delay the suppression process. Heat is avoided for the same reason, and the mother is encouraged to let shower water flow over her back rather than her breasts. Suppression takes only a few days in most cases, but small amounts of milk may be produced up to a month after birth. In some instances, lactation is suppressed until the woman stops taking bromocriptine, and then engorgement occurs.

Relief of Breast Discomfort

Breast engorgement may be a source of pain for the postpartal woman. Specific nursing interventions for the bottle-feeding mother are discussed in Chapter 30.

Promotion of Rest and Graded Activity

Following birth some women feel exhausted and in need of rest. Other women are euphoric and full of psychic energy, ready to retell their experience of birth repeatedly. The nurse evaluates individual needs, always with the goal of providing opportunities for rest. The nurse can provide time for the excited, euphoric woman to air her feelings and then can encourage a period of rest.

Physical fatigue often influences many other adjustments and functions with the new mother. It may also reduce milk flow, thereby increasing problems with breastfeeding. The mother requires energy to make the psychologic adjustments to a new infant and to assume new roles. She makes these adjustments more smoothly when she gets adequate rest.

The nurse may encourage rest by organizing activities to avoid frequent interruptions for the woman. If the new mother chooses, rest times may be provided before encounters with the newborn if rooming-in is not used.

Postpartal Exercises

The woman is encouraged to begin simple exercises and continue them at home. She is advised that increased lochia or pain means she should re-evaluate her activity and make necessary alterations. Most agencies provide a booklet describing suggested postpartal activities. (Exercise routines vary for women undergoing tubal ligation following birth or for cesarean birth clients.) See Figure 34–1 for a description of some common exercises.

Resumption of Activities

Activity may increase gradually after discharge. The new mother should avoid heavy lifting, excessive stair climbing, and strenuous activity. One or two daily naps are essential and are most easily achieved if the mother sleeps when her baby does.

By the second week at home, light housekeeping may be resumed. Although it is customary to delay returning to work for six weeks, most women are physically able to resume practically all activities by four to five weeks. Delaying returning to work until after the final postpartal examination will minimize the possibility of problems.

Promotion of Maternal Psychologic Well-Being

The birth of a child, with the role changes and increased responsibilities it produces, is a time of emotional stress for the new mother. This stress is increased by the tremendous physiologic changes as her body adjusts to a nonpregnant state. During the early postpartal days mood swings and tearfulness are common.

At first the mother may repeatedly discuss her experiences in labor and birth. This allows her to integrate her experiences. If she feels that she did not cope well with labor, she may have feelings of inadequacy and may benefit from reassurance that she did well.

Open discussion of feelings is possible only if the postpartum nurse has established a warm, supportive relationship with the woman. Follow-up visits from the nurse who assisted her in labor and birth provide additional opportunities for the mother to relive her experiences and come to terms with them.

During the postpartal period, the mother must adjust to the loss of her fantasized child and accept the child she has borne. This may be more difficult if the child is not of the desired sex or if she or he has birth defects.

Immediately following the birth (the *taking-in* period) the mother is focused on bodily concerns, and teaching may not be totally effective. Because early discharge is common, however, classes and information should be offered, and printed handouts provided for reference as questions arise at home.

Following the initial dependent period, the mother becomes very concerned about her ability to be a successful parent (the *taking-hold* period). Skillful intervention by the nurse, with constant reassurance that the woman is a successful mother, is vital. During this time the mother is most receptive to teaching, and tactful instruction and demonstration assist her in mothering effectively. The nurse must carefully avoid "taking over" the infant. By functioning as an advisor and allowing the mother to perform the actual care, the nurse demonstrates confidence in the mother's skill and ability, which in turn increases the mother's self-confidence about her effectiveness as a parent.

The depression, weepiness, and "let down feeling" that characterize the postpartum blues are often a surprise for the new mother. She and her family may require reassurance that these feelings are normal and an explanation about why they occur. It is vital to provide a supportive environment that permits the mother to cry without feeling guilty.

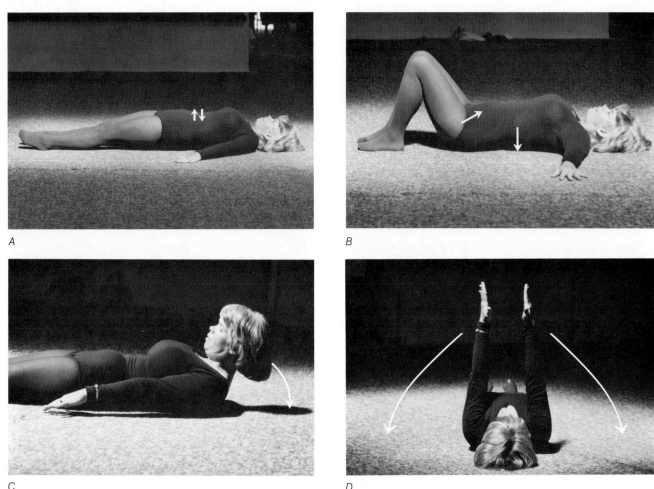

A

B

C

D

Figure 34–1 Postpartal exercises. Begin with five repetitions two or three times daily and gradually increase to ten repetitions. First day: A Abdominal breathing. Lying supine, inhale deeply using the abdominal muscles. The abdomen should expand. Then exhale slowly through pursed lips, tightening the abdominal muscles. B Pelvic rocking. Lying supine with arms at sides, knees bent, and feet flat, tighten abdomen and buttocks and attempt to flatten back on floor. Hold for a count of ten, then arch back, causing the pelvis to "rock." On second day add: C Chin to chest. Lying supine with no pillow and legs straight, raise head and attempt to touch chin to chest. Slowly lower head. D Arm raises. Lying supine with arms extended at 90° angle from body, raise arms so they are perpendicular to the floor. Lower slowly. On fourth day add: E Knee rolls. Lying supine with knees bent, feet flat, and arms extended to the side, roll knees slowly to one side, keeping shoulders flat. Return to original position and roll to opposite side. F Buttocks lift. Lying supine, with arms at sides, knees bent, and feet flat, slowly raise buttocks and arch the back. Return slowly to starting position. On sixth day add: G Abdominal tighteners. Lying supine with knees bent and feet flat, slowly raise head toward knees. Extend arms along either side of knees. Return slowly to original position. H Knee to abdomen. Lying supine with arms at sides, bend one knee and thigh until foot touches buttocks. Straighten leg and lower it slowly. Repeat with other leg. After two to three weeks, more strenuous exercises such as sit ups with knees flexed and side leg raises may be added as tolerated. Kegel exercises, begun antepartally, should be done many times daily during postpartum to restore vaginal and perineal tone.

I had my first son several years ago before rooming-in was popular. Postpartally I was in a four-bed room. As a maternity nurse myself, I found it interesting to watch how other nurses interacted with patients. One nursery nurse was especially tactless and at one time or another reduced all three of my roommates to

tears. To one she said, "Your baby has cried almost continuously since the last feeding. Try to get him to eat better this time." My roommate was breast-feeding, and cried because she felt like a failure. To another the nurse said, "Boy, your baby really is a little baldy." This roommate cried because her baby was "ugly." To the third the nurse said, "Your baby sure needs lessons in

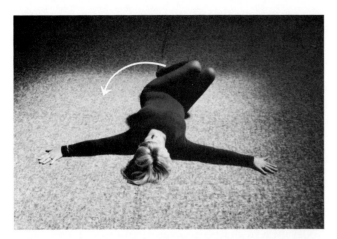

E

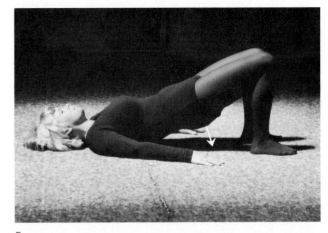

F

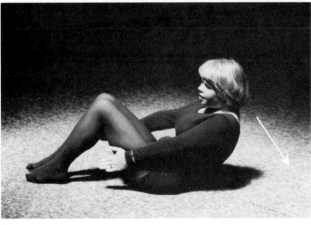

G

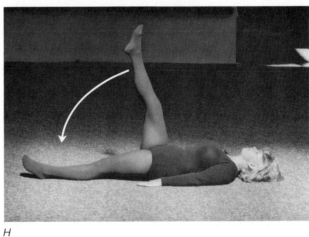

H

manners. He sprayed all over when I changed him!" I think the nurse was trying to joke but my roommate was in a tizzy thinking her baby would be neglected because of his "rudeness." It's amazing how such little, tactless comments can hurt when a woman's emotions are so topsy-turvy.

Provision of Effective Parent Education

Meeting the educational needs of the new mother and her family is one of the primary challenges facing the postpartum nurse. Effective education provides the childbearing family with sufficient knowledge to meet many of their own health needs and seek assistance if necessary.

Educational assessment may be accomplished through observation, sensitivity to nonverbal clues, and tactfully phrased questions. For example, asking "What plans have you made for handling things when you get home?" will elicit a more detailed response than, "Will someone be available to help you at home?"

To assess learning needs some agencies provide a client handout listing the most frequently identified areas of concern for new mothers. The mother checks those that apply to her or writes in concerns not included.

In many educational settings, planning primarily involves the development of objectives that clarify what is to be taught and describe how the learner will demonstrate achievement of each objective. In planned postpartal classes, objectives are predetermined and generalized to meet the needs of most of the participants. Even in nonstructured, individualized situations, however, objectives can be identified by the nurse—"Mrs Warren, when we are finished, you will be able to demonstrate the procedure for manually expressing your breast milk and describe appropriate methods of storing it."

The educational method chosen to implement the objectives varies. Agencies with many clients and limited staff may rely heavily on structured classes while smaller units may provide more individualized instruction. Because more effective learning occurs when there is sensory involvement and active participation, television and movies (sight and hearing) are more helpful than lecture (hearing only), and demonstration-return demonstration (sight, touch, hearing, and possibly smell and taste) is even more effective.

Postpartal units use a variety of approaches—scheduled classes or demonstrations, handouts, group discussions, movies, videotapes, and individual interaction. Some agencies have access to a television channel and can show instructional films at scheduled times during the day. Women should have pencils and paper provided to jot down questions that arise as they view the material. Afterward nurses are available to clarify material or answer any questions about the content.

Timing is important in implementing educational activities. The new mother is more receptive to teaching after the first 24 to 48 hours when she is ready to assume responsibility for her own care and that of her newborn. However, many women are discharged in the early, dependent phase. Because of this, teaching should be done, and handouts should be provided for future reference. Some clinicians suggest that client education in early postpartum discharge programs is most effective if based on comprehensive assessment, home follow-ups, and individualized teaching (Harrison 1990).

Timing is also important for new fathers, who are more likely to attend sessions planned for them if they are scheduled in the evening after visiting hours. If material is planned for siblings, late afternoon teaching, after school or naps, might be most effective.

Demonstration-return demonstration techniques offer opportunities for an individual to practice in a supervised situation. Emphasizing understanding of principles rather than simply mimicking of techniques facilitates transfer of the learning to the home situation.

Teaching should not be limited to "how to" activities, however. Anticipatory guidance is essential in assisting the family to cope with role changes and the realities of a new baby. Small group discussions provide a chance for the new parents to talk about fears and expectations. Questions may arise regarding sexuality, contraception, child care, and even the grief associated with giving up the fantasized infant in order to accept the actual one.

Information is also essential for individuals with specialized educational needs—the mother who had a cesarean birth, the adolescent mother, the parents of an infant with congenital anomalies, and so on. They may feel overwhelmed, have difficult feelings to work through, and not even realize what it is they need to know. Nurses who are attuned to these individual problems can begin providing guidance as soon as possible.

Methods for evaluating learning vary according to the objectives and teaching methods. Return demonstrations, question-and-answer sessions, and even programmed instruction are opportunities for evaluating learning, as are formal evaluation tools.

Evaluation of attitudinal or less concrete learning is more difficult. For example, a mother's ability to express her frustrations over an unanticipated cesarean birth or a new mother's decision to delay for several weeks a family dinner originally scheduled for the first weekend after she arrives home, may be the nurse's only clues that learning

has occurred. Follow-up phone calls after discharge may provide additional evaluative information and continue the helping process as the nurse assesses the family's current educational status and begins planning accordingly.

Promotion of Family Wellness

A satisfactory maternity experience may have a positive impact on the entire family. The new or expanding family that receives appropriate information and has adequate time to interact with its newest member in a supportive environment will feel more comfortable and secure at home.

Mother-Baby Units   In the past, newborns were typically separated from their parents immediately after birth. Today most facilities encourage parents to spend time with their infants. Some facilities offer the option of **mother-baby units** (also called mother-baby primary nursing, mother-infant nursing, combined care, and family-centered maternity care). This concept works very well when combined with the practice of single room maternity care (LDRP, ie, labor, delivery, recovery, postpartum). A mother-baby unit is based on the concept that mother and infant will both benefit from time spent together, so the infant remains at the mother's bedside and both are cared for by the same nurse. Some agencies call this option *rooming-in*. In other facilities the rooming-in policy varies slightly in that nursery personnel remain responsible for the child at the mother's bedside, while postpartum staff care for the mother.

In a mother-baby unit, the newborn's crib is placed near the mother's bed where she can see her baby easily. The crib should be a self-contained unit stocked with items the mother might require in providing care. A bulb syringe for suctioning the mouth or nares should always be accessible and the mother should be familiar with its use.

Mothers are frequently very tired after birth, so the responsibility for providing total infant care could be overwhelming. The mother-baby policy must be flexible enough to permit the mother to return the baby to the nursery if she finds it necessary because of fatigue or physical discomfort. Many agencies return the infant to the central nursery at night, allowing the mother more time for uninterrupted rest.

The mother-baby unit is conducive to a self-demand feeding schedule for both breast-feeding and bottle-feeding infants. The lactating mother may find it especially beneficial to be able to nurse her child every $1\frac{1}{2}$ to 3 hours if necessary.

Many agencies have unlimited visiting hours for the father. Fathers, after washing their hands, are able to care for their infant in a mother-baby unit. These opportunities to hold and care for the child promote paternal self-confidence and foster paternal attachment.

Sibling Visitation   **Sibling visitation** helps meet the needs of both the siblings and their mother. A visit to the hospital reassures children that their mother is well and

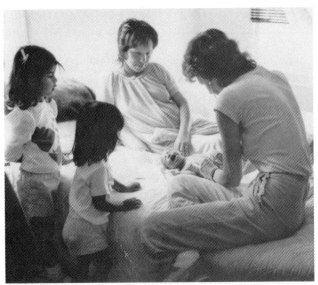

Figure 34–2 The sisters of this newborn become acquainted with the new family member during a nursing assessment.

still loves them. It also provides an opportunity for the children to become familiar with the new baby. For the mother the pangs of separation are lessened as she interacts with her children and introduces them to the newest family member.

Most agencies now recognize the importance of providing siblings with opportunities to see their mother and meet the infant during the early postpartal period (Figure 34–2). Approaches to this issue vary from specified visiting hours for siblings to unlimited visiting privileges.

Education for Self-Care Although the parents have prepared the child for the presence of a new brother or sister, the actual arrival of the infant requires some adjustments. If the woman gives birth in a birthing center, her children may be present for the birth. They then have an opportunity to spend time with their new sibling and their parents. They may even remain throughout the woman's hospitalization, especially if it is brief, and all go home as a family.

For the mother who is returning home to small children, it is often helpful to have the father carry the new baby inside. This practice keeps the mother's arms free to hug and hold her older children. She thereby reaffirms her love for them before introducing them to their new sibling. Many mothers have found that bringing a doll home with them for the older child is helpful. The child cares for the doll alongside his or her parents, thereby identifying with the parent. This identification helps decrease anger and the need to regress to get attention.

Often older children enjoy working with the parents to care for the newborn. Involvement in care helps the older child develop a sense of closeness to the baby. It also helps the child learn acceptable behavior toward the newborn, feel a sense of accomplishment, and develop tenderness and caring—qualities that are appropriate for both males and females. With constant supervision and assistance as necessary, even very young children can hold the baby or a bottle during feeding. Breast-feeding mothers may allow siblings to help give the new infant an occasional bottle of water.

Regression is a common occurrence even when siblings have been well prepared. The nurse can provide anticipatory guidance so that parents do not become overly upset if their previously toilet-trained child begins to have accidents or requests a bottle to feed from.

Regardless of age, an older sibling needs reassurance that he or she is still special to the parents, a truly loved and valued family member. Words of love and praise coupled with hugs and kisses are very important. So, too, is special parent-child time. Both parents should spend quality time in a one-to-one experience with each of their older children. This may require some careful planning, but its worth cannot be overestimated. It confirms the parents' love for the child and often helps the child accept the new baby.

The child, especially one of the opposite sex from the newborn, may raise queries about the appearance of the genitals as compared to his or her own. A simple explanation, such as, "That's what little girls (boys) look like," is often sufficient.

Resumption of Sexual Activity Nursing interventions in the postpartal period acknowledge that the parent is also a sexual being. Couples were formerly discouraged from engaging in sexual intercourse until six weeks postpartum. Currently the couple is advised to abstain from intercourse until the episiotomy is healed and the lochial flow has stopped (usually by the end of the third week). Because the vaginal vault is still "dry" (hormone-poor), some form of lubrication, such as K-Y jelly, may be necessary during intercourse. The female-superior or side-by-side positions for coitus may be preferable because they enable the woman to control the depth of penile penetration.

Breast-feeding couples should be forewarned that during orgasm milk may spout from the nipples due to the release of oxytocin. Some couples find this pleasurable or amusing; other couples choose to have the woman wear a bra during sex. Nursing the baby prior to lovemaking may reduce the chance of milk release.

Other factors may inhibit satisfactory sexual experience: The baby's crying may "spoil the mood"; the woman's changed body may be unattractive to her or to her partner; and maternal sleep deprivation may interfere with a mutually satisfying experience. Couples may also be frustrated if there are changes in the woman's physiologic response to sexual stimulation. These changes are due to hormonal changes and may persist for several months. Many couples report that even four months following childbirth, they continue to experience a decline in sexual activity due to the woman's lingering discomfort (often related to episi-

Resumption of Sexual Activity After Childbirth

Assessment The nurse recognizes that couples, especially if they have become parents for the first time, may have questions about resuming sexual activity. Although the woman may initiate this discussion, often the nurse can best assess the woman's (and her partner's) understanding by providing some general information followed by some tactful questions.

Nursing Diagnosis The key nursing diagnosis will probably be: Knowledge deficit related to changes in sexual activity that commonly occur postpartally.

Nursing Plan and Implementation For the teaching plan to be effective, the nurse must first establish rapport with the couple and should promote an environment that is conducive to teaching and discussion. It is helpful to provide privacy during the session so that the couple feel free to ask questions without fear of interruption. The format is generally a question and answer or discussion approach.

Client Goals At the completion of the teaching the couple will be able to do the following:

1. Discuss the changes in the woman's body that affect sexual activity.
2. Formulate alternative approaches to sexual activity based on an understanding of these changes.
3. Identify the length of time that is advisable to wait before resuming sexual activity.
4. Discuss information needed to make contraceptive choices.

Teaching Plan

Content Present information about changes that may affect sexual activity including the following:

- Tenderness of the vagina and perineum
- Presence of lochia and the healing process
- Dryness of the vagina
- Breast engorgement and tenderness
- Escape of milk during sexual activity

The nurse discusses healing at the placental site and stresses that the presence of lochia indicates that healing is not yet complete. The nurse points out that because the vagina is "hormone-poor" postpartally, vaginal dryness may be problematic. This can be avoided by using a water-soluble lubricant. Escape of milk during sexual activity can be minimized by having the breast-feeding mother nurse immediately beforehand.

Discuss the importance of contraception even during the early postpartal period. Provide information on the advantages and disadvantages of different methods. The woman's body needs adequate time to heal and recover from the stress of pregnancy and childbirth. Couples who are opposed to contraception may choose abstinence at this time.

Discuss impact of fatigue and the new baby's schedule on the woman's feelings of desire. Refer to physician/nurse-midwife for additional information if needed.

Evaluation The nurse determines the couple's learning by providing time for discussion and questions. If the couple indicates that they plan to use a particular contraceptive method, the nurse may ask them about aspects of the method to ascertain that they have correct and complete information.

Teaching Method Discussion is a logical approach. It may be useful to make a universal statement and link it with a question to determine a couple's initial level of knowledge. For example, "Many women experience vaginal dryness when they resume intercourse for the first several weeks after childbirth. Are you familiar with this change and the cause for it?"
Use the information gained during this discussion to determine the depth with which to cover the material.

Provide printed information to clarify content and serve as a resource for the couple following discharge.

Have samples of different types of contraceptives available.
Provide literature on specific contraceptive methods.

Many couples are unprepared for the impact of fatigue and the baby on lovemaking. Information enables the couple to anticipate this impact.

otomy pain), fatigue, decreased physical strength, and dissatisfaction with personal appearance (Fishman et al 1986).

🍎 **Education for Self-Care**   Anticipatory guidance during the prenatal and postnatal period can forewarn the couple of these eventualities and of their temporary nature. See Teaching Guide—Resumption of Sexual Activity After Childbirth.

Couples can be encouraged to express their affection and love through kissing, holding, and talking. Because the man's level of desire does not show the same decrease as the woman's, he requires forewarning that he may experience a decrease in sexual intercourse for up to a year following childbirth (Fishman et al 1986).

Contraception   Because many couples resume sexual activity before the postpartal examination, family-planning information should be made available before discharge. A couple's decision to use a contraceptive is often motivated by a desire to gain control over the number of children they will conceive or to determine the spacing of future children. In choosing a specific method, consistency of use outweighs the absolute reliability of a given method. Risk factors and contraindications of the various methods must be identified by the nurse to help the couple select a contraceptive method that has practical application and is compatible with the couple's health and physical needs.

Often different methods of contraception are appropriate at different times in the couple's life. Thus they should have a clear understanding of the methods available to them so that they can make an appropriate choice. The currently available contraceptive methods are discussed in detail in Chapter 7.

Nursing Plan and Implementation for Cesarean Birth

After a cesarean birth the new mother has postpartal needs similar to those of women who gave birth vaginally. Because she has undergone major abdominal surgery, however, the woman who has had a cesarean also has nursing care needs similar to those of other surgical clients.

Promotion of Maternal Physical Well-Being

The chances of pulmonary infection are increased due to immobility after the use of narcotics and sedatives, and because of the altered immune response in postoperative clients. For this reason, the woman is encouraged to cough and deep breathe and to use incentive spirometry every two to four hours while awake for the first few days following cesarean birth.

Leg exercises are carried out every 15 minutes in conjunction with the postpartal check in the recovery room. The exercises should be continued every two hours until the woman is ambulatory. The leg exercises increase circulation, help prevent thrombophlebitis, and aid in the

improvement of abdominal motility by tightening abdominal muscles.

Monitoring and management of the woman's pain are carried out during the postpartum period. Sources of pain include incisional pain, gas pain, referred shoulder pain, periodic uterine contractions (afterbirth pains), and pain from voiding, defecation, or constipation.

Nursing interventions are oriented toward preventing or alleviating pain or helping the woman cope with pain. The nurse should undertake the following measures:

- Administer analgesics as needed, especially during the first 24 to 72 hours. Their use will improve the woman's outlook and enable her to be more mobile and active.

- Offer comfort through proper positioning, back rubs, oral care, and the reduction of noxious stimuli such as noise and unpleasant odors.

- Encourage the presence of significant others, including the newborn. This practice provides distraction from the painful sensations and helps reduce the woman's fear and anxiety.

- Encourage the use of breathing, relaxation, and distraction techniques (for example, stimulation of cutaneous tissue) taught in childbirth preparation class.

CRITICAL THINKING

Can you identify some of the advantages of patient-controlled analgesia (PCA)? What about the disadvantages?

The use of **patient-controlled analgesia** (PCA) following cesarean birth is becoming increasingly popular. With this approach, the woman is given a bolus of analgesia, usually morphine or meperidine, at the beginning of therapy. Using an IV pump system, the woman presses a button to self-administer small doses of the medication as needed. For safety the pump is preset with a time lock-out so that the woman cannot deliver another dose before a specified time has elapsed. Women using PCA feel less anxious, have a greater sense of control with less dependence on the nursing staff, experience rapid pain relief without grogginess and a drugged feeling, sleep better, and avoid the discomfort of injections (Bucknell & Sikorski 1989). Other agencies report good pain relief using epidural morphine (Inturrisi et al 1988) or transcutaneous electrical nerve stimulation therapy (TENS).

The accumulation of gas in the intestines may produce discomfort for the woman during the first postpartal days. Measures to prevent or minimize gas pains include leg exercises, abdominal tightening, ambulation, avoiding carbonated or very hot or cold beverages, avoiding the use of straws, and providing a high-protein liquid diet for the first 24 to 48 hours.

The woman may find it helpful to lie prone or on her left side. Lying on the left side allows gas to rise from the descending colon to the sigmoid colon so that it can be expelled more readily. Other women report that a rocking chair helps them obtain relief. Medical interventions for gas pain include the use of antiflatulents (such as Mylicon), suppositories, and enemas.

Preventive measures to avoid pain secondary to constipation include encouraging fluids and administering a stool softener or mild cathartic.

The nurse can minimize discomfort and promote satisfaction as the mother assumes the activities of her new role. Instruction and assistance in assuming comfortable positions when holding and/or breast-feeding the infant will do much to increase her sense of competence and comfort. Sitting in a chair or tailor fashion in bed, leaning slightly forward with the infant propped on a pillow in her lap will prevent irritation to the incision. Another preferred position for breast-feeding during the first postoperative days is lying on the side with the newborn positioned along the mother's body.

By the second or third day the cesarean birth mother is usually receptive to learning how to care for herself and her infant. Special emphasis should be given to home management. She should be encouraged to let others assume responsibility for housekeeping and cooking. Fatigue not only prolongs recovery but also interferes with breast-feeding and mother-infant interaction. Demonstration of proper body mechanics in getting out of bed without the use of a side rail and ways of caring for the infant that prevent strain and torsion on the incision are also indicated.

The cesarean birth woman usually does extremely well postoperatively. If birth was accompanied by spinal anesthesia, the side effects of general anesthesia are avoided. Even after general anesthesia, however, most women are ambulating by the day after the surgery. Usually by the second or third postpartal day the incision can be covered with plastic wrap so the woman can shower, which seems to provide a mental as well as physical lift. If staples have been used, the incision is sometimes left open to the air and showering is permitted without covering it. Most women are discharged by the third or fourth postoperative day.

Promotion of Parent-Infant Interaction After Cesarean Birth

Many factors associated with cesarean birth may hinder successful and frequent maternal-infant interaction. These include the physical condition of the mother and newborn and maternal reactions to stress, anesthesia, and medications. The mother and her infant may be separated after birth because of hospital routines, prematurity, or neonatal complications. A healthy infant born by an uncomplicated cesarean birth is no more fragile than an infant born vaginally. Many agencies are beginning to provide time for the family together in the operating room if the mother's and infant's conditions permit, but some agencies still auto-

matically place cesarean birth newborns in a high-risk nursery for a time.

Signs of depression, anger, or withdrawal in the cesarean birth mother may indicate a grief response to the loss of the fantasized vaginal birth experience. Fathers as well as mothers may experience feelings of "missing out," guilt that the surgery was the result of something they did "wrong," and even jealousy toward another couple who had a vaginal birth. The couple may also feel guilty that they are considering their personal needs and not simply the welfare of the infant.

The nurse can support the parents in a variety of ways. Initially nurses must work through their own feelings about cesarean birth. The nurse who considers a vaginal birth "normal" and refers to it as such, indicates that a cesarean birth is, therefore, "abnormal" rather than simply an alternative method. By the same token, referring to a woman as "the section" turns her into an object. Thus language and terminology, though seemingly insignificant, can convey to the couple negative messages about their cesarean birth experience.

The nurse should offer positive support to the couple. The cesarean birth couple needs the opportunity to tell their story repeatedly to work through their feelings. The nurse can provide factual information about their situation and support the couple's effective coping behaviors. The nurse should provide the parents with choices by allowing them to participate in decision making about the options available to them (for example, participating in rooming-in).

The perception of and reactions to a cesarean birth experience depend on how the woman defines that experience. Her reality is what she perceives it to be. If the woman's attitude is more positive than negative, successful resolution of subsequent stressful events is more likely. Because the definition of events is transitory in nature, the possibility of change and growth is present. Often the mothering role is perceived as an extension of the childbearing role, and inability to fulfill expected childbearing behavior (vaginal birth) may lead to parental feelings of role failure and frustration. The nurse can help families alter their negative definitions of cesarean birth and bolster and encourage positive perceptions.

Nursing Plan and Implementation for the Postpartal Adolescent

The adolescent may have special postpartal needs, depending on her level of maturity, support systems, and cultural background. The nurse needs to assess maternal-infant interaction, roles of support people, plans for discharge, knowledge of childrearing, and plans for follow-up care. It is imperative to have a community health service be in touch with the young woman shortly after discharge.

Contraception counseling is an important part of teaching. The incidence of repeat pregnancies during adolescence is high and the younger the adolescent, the more likely she is to become pregnant again. Often the young woman tells the nurse that she does not plan on engaging in sex again. This denial mechanism is unrealistic, and the nurse must help the young woman realize this. The nurse should make sure that the woman has some method of birth control available to her and that she understands ovulation and fertility in relation to her menstrual cycle. This is an excellent opportunity for sex education.

Promotion of Parenting Skills

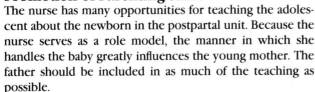

The nurse has many opportunities for teaching the adolescent about the newborn in the postpartal unit. Because the nurse serves as a role model, the manner in which she handles the baby greatly influences the young mother. The father should be included in as much of the teaching as possible.

A newborn physical exam done at the bedside gives the adolescent immediate feedback about the newborn's health and shows her the proper methods of handling an infant. The nurse can teach as the examination progresses, giving the new mother information about the fontanelles, cradle cap, shampooing the newborn's hair, and so on. The nurse might also use this time to teach the young mother about infant stimulation techniques, Because adolescent mothers tend to concentrate their interactions in the physical domain, they need to comprehend the importance of verbal, visual, and auditory stimulation for newborns as well.

Performing an examination at the bedside also gives the adolescent permission to explore her baby, which she may have been hesitant to do. A Brazelton neonatal assessment (see Chapter 28) will help the mother understand her newborn's response to stimuli, a key factor in the adolescent's response to the individuality of her newborn once she goes home. Parents who have some idea of what to expect from their infants will be less frustrated with the newborn's behavior.

The adolescent mother appreciates positive feedback about her fine newborn and her developing maternal responses. This praise and encouragement will increase her confidence and self-esteem.

Group classes for adolescent mothers should include infant care skills, information about growth and development, infant feeding, well-baby care, and danger signals in the ill newborn.

Lunch groups can be organized around discussions of topics that interest adolescents. These are ideal times to explore the young mothers' ideas about cuddling and rocking their newborns, ways to handle crying, misbehavior, and "spoiling." The nurse can correct misconceptions and unrealistic expectations about growth and development.

Ideally, teenage mothers should visit adolescent clinics where mother and baby are assessed for several years after birth. In this way, classes on parenting, vocational guidance, and school attendance can be followed closely.

School systems' classes for young mothers are an excellent way of helping adolescents finish school and learn how to parent at the same time.

Nursing Plan and Implementation for the Woman with an Unwanted Pregnancy

Sometimes a pregnancy is unwanted. The expectant woman may be an adolescent, unmarried, or economically restricted. She may dislike children or the idea of being a mother. She may feel that she is not emotionally ready for the responsibilities of parenthood. Her partner may disapprove of the pregnancy. These and many other reasons may cause the woman to continue to reject the idea of her pregnancy. An emotional crisis arises as she attempts to resolve the problem. She may choose to have an abortion, to carry the fetus to term and keep the baby, or to have the baby and relinquish it for adoption.

Many mothers who choose to give their infants up for adoption are young and/or unmarried. More young women choose to keep the child than to give it up, however. Approximately two-thirds of children born to single women are raised by their mothers alone.

The decision of a mother to relinquish her infant is an extremely difficult one. There are social pressures against giving up one's child. Some women may want to prove to themselves that they can manage on their own by keeping their infants.

The mother who chooses to let her child be adopted usually experiences intense ambivalence. These feelings may heighten just before birth and upon seeing her baby. After childbirth, the mother will need to complete a grieving process to work through her loss.

CRITICAL THINKING

How have attitudes toward single mothers and their children changed over the years? What impact do you think these changes have had on relinquishment as an option?

Provision of Support to the Woman Relinquishing Her Infant

The mother who decides to relinquish her child usually has made considerable adjustments in her life-style to give birth to this child. She may not have told friends and relatives about the pregnancy and so lacks an extended support system. During the prenatal period, the nurse can help her by encouraging her to express her grief, loneliness, guilt, and other feelings.

When the relinquishing mother is admitted to the maternity unit, the staff should be informed about the mother's decision to relinquish the infant. Any special re-

Patient Name:

Medical Record Number:

(addressograph stamp)

STANFORD UNIVERSITY HOSPITAL
Stanford University Medical Center
Stanford, California 94305

TEACHING FLOW SHEET AND DISCHARGE PLANNING
INFANT CARE AND POSTPARTUM

KNOWLEDGE AND SKILLS TO BE TAUGHT	INSTRUCTIONS/ INITIALS		PATIENT / AND OR SIGNIFICANT OTHER VERBALIZES AND / OR DEMONSTRATES UNDERSTANDING		POST TEACHING COMMENTS / FOLLOW—UP
	Verbal	Demon.	Return Demon.	Assessment	
FAMILY PLANNING INFORMATION					
EMOTIONAL CHANGES FOR NEW PARENTS		xxxx	xxxx		
OTHER CHILDREN AT HOME		xxxx	xxxx		
BODY MECHANICS AND EXERCISES					
OTHER					

The content of each item with added detail is listed in the Master Teaching Guide.

Assessment Code: V - Verbalizes concept accurately
D - Demonstrates concept safely
C - Confidence building needed (V and D accomplished)
R - Repeat, Redemonstrate, Remind
O - Offered, but refused teaching
N/A - Not Applicable

DISCHARGE PLANNING

Public Health Referral: (All Clinic patients must have a referral)

Written _____

Sent _____

Follow-Up Appointment Made:

Clinic Appt. - Mother _____

Clinic Appt. - Baby _____

Private M.D. Appt. _____

Social Worker Consult _____

Other follow-up:

Home Assistance _____

Child Protective Services _____

_____ _____

_____ _____

Figure 34–3   A teaching flow sheet and discharge planning guide helps focus health teaching. (Courtesy of Stanford University Hospital, Stanford, California)

Patient Name:

Medical Record Number:

(addressograph stamp)

STANFORD UNIVERSITY HOSPITAL
Stanford University Medical Center
Stanford, California 94305

TEACHING FLOW SHEET AND DISCHARGE PLANNING
INFANT CARE AND POSTPARTUM

Para_____ DD_____ Fdg _____ Other _____

KNOWLEDGE AND SKILLS TO BE TAUGHT	INSTRUCTIONS/ INITIALS		PATIENT/AND OR SIGNIFICANT OTHER VERBALIZES AND/OR DEMONSTRATES UNDERSTANDING		POST-TEACHING COMMENTS/FOLLOW-UP
	Verbal	Demon.	Return Demon.	Assessment	
OBSERVING BABY					
1. General Appearance			xxxx		
2. Senses		xxxx	xxxx		
3. Protective Reflexes		xxxx	xxxx		
4. Vital Signs -including Temp. Taking					
5. Circulation		xxxx	xxxx		
6. Rashes		xxxx	xxxx		
7. Reflexes of Newborn			xxxx		
8. Stool Cycle		xxxx	xxxx		
9. Emotional Needs		xxxx	xxxx		
BATHING BABY					
1. Shampoo					
2. Bath					
DIAPERING					
WRAPPING					
HOLDING BABY					
1. Cradle					
2. Football					
FEEDING					
1. Schedule		xxxx			
2. Reflexes					
3. Bottle					
4. Breast		xxxx			
5. Bubble or Burp					
LAYETTE-LISTS OF SUGGESTIONS		xxxx	xxxx		
PERI-CARE					
1. Hospital (e.g., Sitz Bath)		xxxx			
2. Home		xxxx			
3. Episiotomy		xxxx			
BREAST CARE					
1. If Breast Feeding		xxxx			
2. If Not Breast Feeding		xxxx			
LOCHIAL CHANGES		xxxx	xxxx		
UTERINE INVOLUTION		xxxx	xxxx		
BLADDER FUNCTION		xxxx	xxxx		
AFTERCONTRACTIONS		xxxx	xxxx		
REST		xxxx	xxxx		
DIET		xxxx	xxxx		
EARLY AMBULATION ADVANTAGES		xxxx	xxxx		

Assessment Code:
V - Verbalizes concept accurately
D - Demonstrates concept safely
C - Confidence building needed (V and D accomplished)
R - Repeat, Redemonstrate, Remind
O - Offered, but refused teaching
N/A - Not Applicable

quests regarding the birth should be respected, and the woman should be encouraged to express her emotions.

After the birth the mother should be able to decide whether she wants to see the newborn. Seeing the newborn often facilitates the grieving process. When the mother sees her baby, she may feel strong attachment and love. The nurse needs to assure the woman that these feelings do not mean that her decision to relinquish the child is a wrong one; relinquishment is often a painful act of love (Arms 1990). Postpartal nursing management also includes arranging ongoing care for the relinquishing mother.

Promotion of Acceptance When a Woman Denies Pregnancy

Initial denial of pregnancy by women usually progresses to acceptance of the pregnant state. Occasionally, however, a nurse may encounter a woman who denies she is pregnant even as she is admitted to the maternity unit. It may seem impossible that a woman who is so obviously pregnant could maintain this delusion. Because of this denial, the woman has not sought prenatal care. Preparation for the birth experience may be incomplete, and the mother and infant may be at risk.

The nurse must establish a trusting relationship with this woman. While building rapport with the woman, the nurse should gently guide the woman to accept reality.

Promotion of Family Wellness

In the event that a woman decides to keep an unwanted child, the nurse should be aware of the potential for parenting problems. Families with unwanted children are more prone to crisis than others, although in many cases, parents grow to love their child after attachment occurs. The nurse should be ready to initiate crisis strategies or make appropriate referrals as the need arises.

Nursing Plan and Implementation Regarding Discharge Information

Ideally, preparation for discharge begins from the moment a woman enters the hospital or birthing center to give birth. Nursing efforts should be directed toward assessing the couple's knowledge, expectations, and beliefs and then providing anticipatory guidance and teaching accordingly. Because many women remain hospitalized for such a brief time postpartally, it is vital for postpartum nurses to approach health teaching and education for self-care in a systematic way. Most agencies have developed flow sheets such as the one in Figure 34–3. The use of such a tool helps nurses complete teaching and identify any areas of knowledge deficit so that follow-up teaching can be planned.

Before the actual discharge the nurse should spend time with the couple to determine if they have any last-minute questions. In general, discharge teaching should include at least the following information:

1. The woman should contact her care giver if she develops any of the signs of possible complications:
   - Sudden persistent or spiking fever
   - Change in the character of the lochia—foul smell, return to bright red bleeding, excessive amount
   - Evidence of mastitis, such as breast tenderness, reddened areas, malaise
   - Evidence of thrombophlebitis, such as calf pain, tenderness, redness
   - Evidence of urinary tract infection, such as urgency, frequency, burning on urination
   - Continued severe or incapacitating postpartal depression
   - Evidence of infection in an incision (either episiotomy or cesarean), such as redness, edema, bruising, discharge, or lack of approximation

2. The woman should review the literature she has received that explains recommended postpartum exercises, the need for adequate rest, the need to avoid overexertion initially, and the recommendation to abstain from sexual intercourse until lochia has ceased. The woman may take either a tub bath or shower and may continue sitz baths at home if she desires.

3. The woman should be given the phone numbers of the postpartum unit and nursery and encouraged to call if she has any questions, no matter how simple.

4. The woman should receive information on local agencies and/or support groups, such as La Leche League and Mothers of Twins, that might be of particular assistance to her.

5. Both breast-feeding and bottle-feeding mothers should receive information geared to their specific nutritional needs. They should also be told to continue their vitamin and iron supplements until their postpartal examination.

6. The woman should have a scheduled appointment for her postpartal examination and for her infant's first well-baby examination before they are discharged.

7. The mother should clearly understand the correct procedure for obtaining copies of her infant's birth certificate.

8. The new parents should be able to provide basic care for their infants and should know when to anticipate that the cord will fall off; when the infant can have a tub bath; when the infant will need his or her first immunizations; and so on. They should also be comfortable feeding and handling the baby

Research Note

Clinical Application of Research

Margaret Harrison (1990) evaluated the interactions of mothers and fathers with their infant three months after the infant's discharge from the hospital. To determine if interactions with term infants differed from those with premature infants, the researcher obtained a convenience sample of 31 term infants and 28 premature infants and their parents.

During the home visit, observers recorded behaviors of the infant and each parent while the parent, without the other parent present, interacted with the child to teach an age-appropriate task. Parents also answered questions about the father's participation in the care of the infant.

Results showed that preterm infants were less responsive to their mothers than term infants, but the response for preterm infants to their fathers was comparable to that of term infants to their fathers. Scores for the mother's interaction with her infant were similar for both groups; however, the fathers of preterm infants had a significantly higher interaction score than did fathers with their term infants. No difference was found between the two groups in the terms of frequency of father's participation with child care activities or in education, age, or socioeconomic class.

Critical Thinking Applied to Research

Strengths: Although subjects were not matched, several statistical tests were done to ensure that the groups did not differ on selected demographic variables. Sample loss was described.

Concerns: Only prior psychometric properties about reliability were reported on one tool. No current validity or reliability measurements were included.

Harrison M: A comparison of parental interactions with term and preterm infants. *Res Nurs Health* 1990; 13:173.

and should be aware of basic safety considerations, including the need to use a car seat whenever the infant is in a car.

9. The parents should also be aware of signs and symptoms in the infant that indicate possible problems and who they should contact about them (see page 901).

The nurse can also use this final period to reassure the couple of their ability to be successful parents. She can stress the infant's need to feel loved and secure. She can also urge parents to talk to each other and work together to solve any problems that may arise.

Evaluation

Anticipated outcomes of nursing care include the following:

- The woman experiences minor discomfort at most and has a clear understanding of measures she can employ to enhance her comfort.

- The woman is able to verbalize the need for adeqate rest and has developed a plan (with the support of her family) to begin graded activity.

- The woman has had an opportunity to discuss her perceptions of her childbearing experience with an empathetic nurse and has some anticipatory knowledge of potential mood changes and emotions she may experience.

- The chosen infant feeding method is successful and the parents seem able to care for their child.

- There is evidence of positive parent-infant attachment.

- The couple clearly understand the available family planning methods and have chosen an option they find suitable for them.

- The woman clearly understands the discharge information she was given and is able to state the actions she will take if any complications develop.

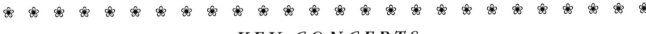

KEY CONCEPTS

Postpartum discomfort may be due to a variety of factors, including engorged breasts, an edematous perineum, an episiotomy or extension, engorged hemorrhoids, or hematoma formation.

Lactation suppression may be accomplished by mechanical techniques or by administering the medication bromocriptine. Because of the increased risk of

thrombus formation, estrogen-based medications are rarely used.

The first day or two following birth are marked by maternal behaviors that are more dependent and comfort oriented. Then the woman becomes more independent and ready to assume responsibility.

Mother-baby units provide the childbearing family with opportunities to interact with their new member during the first hours and days of life. This enables the family to develop some confidence and skill in a "safe" environment.

Sexual intercourse may resume once the episiotomy has healed and lochia has stopped. Couples should be forewarned of possible changes; for example, the vagina may be "dry," the level of desire may be influenced by fatigue, or the woman's breasts may leak milk during orgasm.

The couple's decision regarding contraception should be made voluntarily, with full knowledge of options, advantages, disadvantages, and side effects of all the forms of birth control

Prior to discharge the couple should be given any information necessary for the woman to provide appropriate self-care. They should have a beginning skill in

caring for their newborn and should be familiar with warning signs of possible complications for mother or baby. Printed information is valuable in helping couples deal with questions that may arise at home.

Following cesarean birth a woman has the nursing care needs of a surgical client in addition to her needs as a postpartum client. She may also require assistance in working through her feelings if the cesarean birth was unexpected.

Postpartally the nurse evaluates the adolescent mother in terms of her level of maturity, available support systems, cultural background, and existing knowledge and then plans care accordingly.

The mother who decides to relinquish her baby needs emotional support. She should be able to decide whether to see and hold her baby and should have any special requests regarding the birth honored.

❀ ❀

References

Arms S: *Adoption: A Handful of Hope.* Berkeley CA: Celestial Arts, 1990.

Bucknell S, Sikorski K: Putting patient-controlled analgesia to the test. *MCN* January/February 1989; 14:37.

Fishman SH et al: Changes in sexual relations in postpartum couples. *JOGNN* January/February 1986; 15:58.

Foster S: Bromocriptine: Suppressing lactation. *MCN* March/April 1982; 7:99.

Gosha J, Brucker MC: A self-help group for new mothers: An evaluation. *MCN* January/February 1986; 11:20.

Harrison LL: Patient education in early postpartum discharge programs. *MCN* January/February 1990; 15:39.

Inturrisi M et al: Epidural morphine for relief of postpartum, postsurgical pain. *JOGNN* July/August 1988; 17:238.

Jansson P: Early postpartum discharge. *Am J Nurs* May 1985; 85:547.

LaFoy J, Geden EA: Postepisiotomy pain: Warm versus cold sitz bath. *JOGNN* September/October 1989; 18:399.

Peters F et al: Inhibition of lactation by long-acting bromocriptine. *Obstet Gynecol* 1986; 67:82.

Ramler D, Roberts J: A comparison of cold and warm sitz baths for relief of postpartum perineal pain. *JOGNN* November/December 1986; 15:471.

Varney H: *Nurse Midwifery,* 2nd ed. Boston, Blackwell Scientific Publications, 1987.

Wong S, Stepp-Gilbert E: Lactation suppression: Nonpharmaceutical versus pharmaceutical method. *JOGNN* July/August 1985; 14:302.

Additional Readings

Aderhold KJ, Perry L: Jet hydrotherapy for labor and postpartum pain relief. *MCN* March/April 1991; 16(2):97.

Anderson GC: Risk in mother-infant separation postbirth. *Image* Winter 1989; 21(4):196.

Blackburn S et al: Patients' and nurses' perceptions of patient problems during the immediate postpartum period. *Appl Nurs Res* November 1988; 1:141.

Flagler S: Maternal role competence. *West J Nurs Res* 1988; 10(3):274.

Friedman LH et al: Cost-effectiveness of a self-care program. *Nurs Econ* July/August 1988; 6:173.

Mercer RT et al: Effect of stress on family functioning during pregnancy. *Nurs Res* 1988; 37(5):268.

Morales-Mann ET: Comparative analysis of the perceptions of patients and nurses about the importance of nursing activities in a postpartum unit. *J Adv Nurs* June 1989; 14:478.

Popkess-Vawter S: Wellness nursing diagnosis: To be or not to be. *Nurs Diagnosis* January/March 1991; 2(1):19.

CHAPTER 35

Attachment

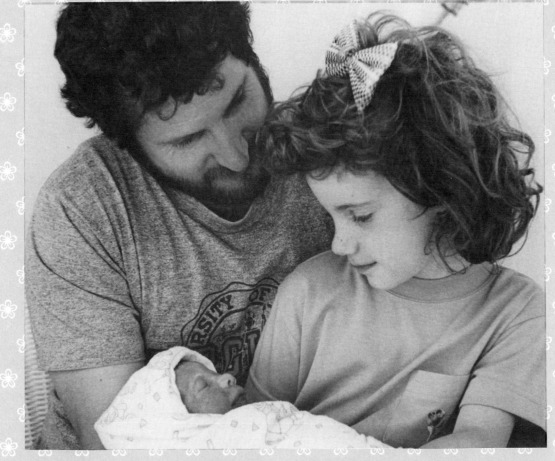

OBJECTIVES

Describe the attachment process, including the phases of maternal-infant interaction.

Compare the factors influencing the first maternal-infant interaction.

Explore the factors affecting family member interactions with the infant.

Explain the types of questions used for evaluating the maternal-infant relationship.

Select methods the nurse can use to facilitate a positive attachment process.

Identify complications that can affect the maternal-infant attachment process.

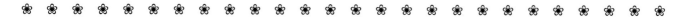

It's one of those "grass-is-greener" things—I envied, sometimes even hated Sam when he went out to work. I don't know what I was imagining—that he hung around talking, went out to lunch, did interesting things. One time he was watching me bathe Annie in the sink. He asked if he could do it—he stood there, soaping her back over and over like he couldn't get enough of it, and he talked about how he hated to leave us in the morning and how he worried he would be closed out, left looking in at what she and I had together. (The New Our Bodies, Ourselves)

There has been a great deal of research on attachment in recent years. The goals of the research have been to describe, operationally define, and relate attachment to cognitive and social outcomes; to support or refute psychologic theories; and to determine public child-care policy.

The early literature on attachment related primarily to the infant's tie to her or his mother, which was understood to occur in the second half of the first year of life when the infant was capable of recognizing the mother. This literature was derived in part from experience with maternally deprived infants. More recently, and motivated in part by disorders and failures in mothering, researchers have investigated the attachment of mothers to infants. The importance of attachment of fathers and siblings continues to be explored. Attachment to the fetus has also received attention.

This chapter begins by exploring the nature and operation of attachment. Having established this knowledge base, the chapter concludes by discussing nursing assessment and interventions related to attachment.

Nature of Attachment

Attachments are enduring bonds or relationships of affection between persons. Affectional ties exist in families between parents, between parents and their children, and between siblings.

Attachment originally referred to a child's tie to his or her mother, although it was recognized that the tie was to a mother figure, a primary care giver, who was usually, although not necessarily, the biologic mother. Attachment may now refer to an infant's tie to a parent or a parent's tie to the child. The essence of infant attachment is organization and patterning of behavior that results in feelings of closeness to the attachment figure. Elements of this behavior are clinging, crying, smiling, sucking, following, and eye-to-eye contact.

Bonding is considered a process of mother-infant attachment that occurs at or soon after birth, but it is only one brief phase in the development of the enduring reciprocal emotional relationship between mother and child called attachment (Taylor 1990).

Perspectives on Attachment

Attachment is viewed from three major perspectives: psychoanalytic, ethologic, and learning theory.

From a psychoanalytic perspective, attachment is explained by instinctual responses and object relations. Attachment is innate, an instinctual drive. The mother is the object of the drive. Fathers are important as support for the mother, but attachment with anyone other than the mother is thought to interfere with and be detrimental to the child's development. Other attachments will follow once attachment to the mother is assured. The quality of later attachments depends on the quality of attachment to the mother.

Within an ethologic framework, attachment consists of species specific behaviors. Examples of such behaviors are ducklings imprinting on the first moving object seen after hatching, primates clinging when alarmed, and cats licking newborn kittens to stimulate respiratory and gastrointestinal functioning. Sucking, clinging, crying, smiling, and following are attachment behaviors promoting closeness in the human species.

According to learning theory framework, attachment is formed through secondary drives. The mother meets her infant's needs and the infant associates need satisfaction, comfort, and love with the mother.

Questions about the origin of attachment, behaviors denoting attachment, and interventions to promote attachment may differ depending on the theoretical perspective taken.

What the Mother Brings to the First Interaction

Prenatal Influences

A mother has a specific genetic makeup of intelligence, personality and temperament, body structure, physical health, and biochemical/hormonal status. Each of these factors influences the environment the mother can provide for the fetus and newborn and affects her ability to relate well to her child. Her cultural and ethnic background will influence her attitudes, behaviors, and practices related to pregnancy and childbirth. Her experiences in infancy and childhood, the mothering she received, and her exposure to appropriate role models will shape her own mothering practices.

The mother's current developmental level and relationships with significant others will provide the foundation for the developing relationship with her fetus and the newborn. Often she will "rework" the relationship with her own mother and develop a closer relationship to her mother as a result.

Family readiness for pregnancy is crucial for providing an environment in which attachment to the fetus and newborn can occur. The optimum environment is created when the baby is planned and wanted, and the family has the necessary resources to provide for the infant.

Present Pregnancy

Each mother brings to her first visual contact with her newborn her reactions to that particular pregnancy, from conception through birth. A variety of factors may influence her response to the pregnancy and the baby: whether the pregnancy was planned and a baby wanted (Brazelton & Cramer 1990), complications she experienced in pregnancy, and the support she received from family and friends. Life events essentially unrelated to her pregnant condition may have enhanced a woman's response to pregnancy or depleted the energy reserves and coping ability necessary to pregnancy adjustments. Stress during pregnancy can interfere with attachment, but support from family and others can offset some of the adverse effects of such stress (Cranley 1981b).

By the time of birth, each mother has developed an emotional orientation of some kind toward the fetus. This attachment is based on a tactile-kinesthetic awareness combined with fantasy images and perceptions. For many women, an emotional bond to the fetus develops soon after conception and deepens during pregnancy.

By the third trimester, significant attachment has occurred as evidenced by nesting behaviors such as preparing the baby's room, expectations about gender, appearance, and temperament, and selection of names (Taylor 1990). Fathers, too, become attached to the fetus.

Events such as hearing the fetal heart or visualizing the fetus on a screen through sonography affect the mother's perception of her fetus and appear to increase her feelings of attachment. However, research indicates that knowledge of whether the fetus is male or female does not affect attachment (Grace 1984).

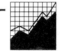

Research Note

Clinical Application of Research

Judith Fuller (1990) studied the relationship between prenatal maternal attachment, or the commitment and affection a woman feels for her unborn child, and maternal-infant interactions postpartum. The maternal-fetal attachment scale measured the mother's interactions with and attribution of characteristics to the fetus as well as role taking. The nursing child assessment feeding scale (NCAFS), one of two scales used to examine maternal infant interactions postpartum, looked at such items as sensitivity to cues, response to distress, and growth fostering. The second scale, the Funke mother-infant interaction assessment (FMII), explored eye contact, physical closeness, and verbal stimulation.

The maternal-infant attachment scale was predictive of total scale results and subscales for both the NCAFS and the FMII. Attachment of mother to her unborn fetus was highly correlated to postpartum interactions between mother and baby.

Critical Thinking Applied to Research

Strengths: Use of triangulation across methods of data collection with both quantitative and qualitative methodologies employed. Cronbach's alpha coefficients were reported for all the quantitative tools.
Concerns: The study is not clear about who obtained the antepartal interview and who collected the observational data postpartum. If either or both were collected by the researcher, this procedure would create an internal validity issue related to experimenter expectations. Test-retest reliability determinations were only one day apart.

Fuller J: Early patterns of maternal attachment. *Health Care Women Internat* 1990; 11:433.

Pascoe and French (1989) found that women who did not plan to become pregnant or who conceived for reasons of status or security were frequently among those who had minimal feelings of closeness to the fetus throughout the pregnancy. Those who felt well adjusted in their marriage and emotionally ready to have a baby were able to develop strong affectionate feelings.

What the Newborn Brings to the First Interaction

Each partner in an interpersonal interaction contributes in some way to the process. In years past, the newborn's influence on the beginning mother-infant relationship was ignored. More recently, research on the capacities of newborns and very young neonates has shown that they are indeed active partners in the exchange and take part shaping their own human environment from the moment of birth. Newborns do this by virtue of who they are and what they do—their appearance and behavior.

Appearance

At the moment of birth certain information about the newborn's external appearance is available. Each characteristic may have a special meaning for the parents as it relates to their hopes, fears, and expectations. The relatively obvious things are usually noted first: sex, size, shape, color, and presence or absence of abnormality or injury. The eyes are a particularly important feature.

Behaviors

The newborn has, and may demonstrate at birth, certain functional behaviors, such as crying, sucking, eliminating, looking, listening, and startling. In the very first days of life, the infant selectively attends to the human face, prefers the human voice over other sounds, and becomes quiet and alert when picked up and held over the shoulder.

In addition to having behaviors in common with other neonates, each newborn, like the parent, is already a unique combination of genetic potential and life experience. The newborn's life experience is shorter and more limited in scope, of course, but it can have a powerful effect on behavior. The past history and present personality of each mother and father combine with the characteristics and behavior of their infant to influence the quality and direction of the parent-infant relationship.

The Setting

The physical environment, human environment, and condition of the mother and newborn at first contact may influence the opportunities for interaction.

Physical Environment

Childbirth may occur in a variety of settings. The most frequent setting by far is a maternity unit in a hospital. The physical surroundings are usually relatively strange to the woman as she moves from the admitting area to the labor room, birthing area, recovery area, and her room in the postpartal unit.

She may encounter a variety of unfamiliar equipment and procedures. Noise levels are often high. Food is usually withheld until after the birth. The stress of accommodating to the physical environment can interfere with the progress of labor and birth and with the comfort of mother-infant interaction. In addition, the parents may be separated from the newborn.

Consumer and professional efforts to increase the comfort of hospital births while decreasing the risks sometimes associated with home birth have produced an intermediate type of setting: hospital-independent birth centers or hospital birthing rooms. These facilities are more home-like in appearance and do not require moves from one area to another during the progression from labor through early recovery. The newborn remains with the parents in this setting and provides the environment for facilitating early parent-infant contact and flexible rooming-in. Many institutions are also offering an early discharge program for families with support at home (Taylor 1990).

Human Environment

Labor and birth usually occur in a social setting. Very few women express the wish to be alone during childbirth; most respond with distress to the idea of abandonment at such a time. Hospitals generally provide for fairly constant nursing supervision of women in active labor, in the course of the birth, and in the early postpartum period. Usually, however, there is a different caretaker present in each phase of the childbearing activities. This requires the woman to relate to a variety of nurses—each with advice, expectations, and attitudes—at a very vulnerable time.

In almost all settings the laboring woman is able to have any support person she desires with her during labor and birth. This practice increases the possibility that a woman will have the support of one trusted person for the whole childbirth experience. The quality of support available from professionals or laypersons varies considerably according to their clinical and psychosocial skills. There are indications that a woman's perceptions of her physical care and emotional support and her reactions to the nonhuman elements of the environment can influence her mothering responses.

Condition of the Interactors

When the postbirth conditions are optimal, mother and newborn are ready to relate effectively to each other and to benefit from the interaction. The mother is emotionally high and alert, primed for maternal responsiveness by her hormonal state. The newborn is in a quiet, alert state, capable of attending to the mother's face and voice. However, several common conditions diminish or divert the mother's physical and psychologic energies. Fatigue, pain, cold, chills and shaking, hunger, and thirst are frequently reported by mothers after childbirth. The mother may also have received medication for relaxation and pain relief and may be encumbered in her movements by intravenous tubing.

Certain conditions may also lower the newborn's potential for human interaction. In addition to the physiologic adaptations necessary for extrauterine existence, physical maturity, nutritional adequacy, neurologic intactness, bodily discomfort, suctioning, extremes of temperature, and levels of analgesic and anesthetic agents have all been related to the infant's behavioral responses in the first hours of life—as well as later. Prophylactic eye treatments interfere with newborns' ability to keep their eyes open and focused on the mother's face. Generally speaking, any situation, condition, or stimulus that detracts from the energy either partner can use to attend to the other diminishes the probability of optimal interaction between the two.

Mother-Infant Interactions

Introductory Phase

Observers of very early mother-newborn interactions in hospital settings have presented evidence that a fairly regular pattern of maternal behaviors is exhibited at first contact with the normal newborn (Rubin 1963; Klaus et al 1970). In a progression of touching activities, the mother proceeds from fingertip exploration of the newborn's extremities toward palmar contact with the larger body areas and finally to enfolding the infant with the whole hand and arms. The time taken to accomplish these steps varies from minutes to days, depending, it appears, on the timing of the first contact, the clothing barriers present, and the physical condition of the baby. There also may be ethnic or cultural differences in patterns of interaction. Maternal excitement and elation tend to increase during the time of the initial meeting (Figure 35–1). The mother also increases the proportion of time spent in the *en face* position (Figure 35–2). She arranges herself or the newborn to facilitate direct face-to-face and eye-to-eye contact. The majority of women cradle their infant in their left arm (de Chateau 1987). There is an intense interest in having the infant's eyes open. When the eyes are open, the mother characteristically greets the baby and talks in high-pitched tones to her or him.

Clinical observations indicate that behaviors differ somewhat in unconventional birth situations. Home and LeBoyer births seem to speed up the behaviors described. Often after a home birth the mother turns almost immediately to pick up and hold the newborn and to rub the infant's cheek with her fingertip. The newborn is often of-

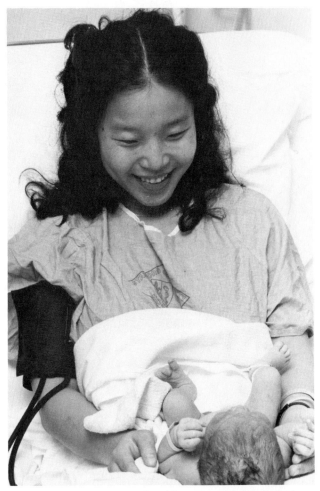

Figure 35–1   A new mother interacts with her infant.

fered the breast before the placenta is expelled. In a birth patterned after the LeBoyer method, the mother, and sometimes the father, is encouraged to gently massage the infant's whole body while waiting for the placenta to be expelled.

In most instances the mother relies heavily on her senses of sight, touch, and hearing in getting to know what her baby is really like. She tends also to respond verbally to any sounds emitted by the newborn, such as cries, coughs, sneezes, and grunts. Mothers are able to distinguish their infant's odor, and the sense of smell may be involved in the acquaintance process.

While interacting with the newborn, the mother is undergoing her own emotional reactions to the labor and birth and to the baby. Sometimes direct comments and nonverbal cues clearly reflect her emotions; sometimes the mother reports only later on her feelings at the time. An expression of "I can't believe it" and a feeling of emotional distance from the newborn are quite common: "I felt he was a stranger." On the other hand, feelings of connectedness between the newborn and the rest of the family can be expressed in positive or negative terms: "He's got your

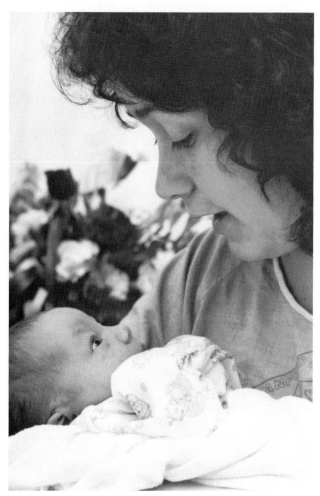

Figure 35–2 En face *position*

cute nose, Daddy" or "Oh, no! She looks just like the first one, and she was an impossible baby." A mother's facial expressions or the frequency and content of her questions may demonstrate concerns about the infant's general condition or normality, especially if her pregnancy was complicated or if a previous baby was not normal.

During the initial mother-newborn interaction the neonate, too, is continuously communicating. Elements of the newborn's appearance and behavior may be perceived by the mother as if they represented intentionality and interpersonal dialogue, and they do influence her responses. The newborn's size says to the mother, "You nourished me well—you did a good job." Individual features say, "I am a part of you, or of my father. I belong with you." Even the time of birth can be read as a message: "I'm cooperative—or uncooperative." The intensity, timing, configuration, and other elements of the newborn's observable activity, however reflexive, are regularly responded to as a very personal communication from the baby to the mother.

When newborns no longer need to concentrate most of their energy in physical and physiologic response to the immediate crisis of birth, they are able to lie quietly with their eyes open, looking about, moving occasionally, making sucking motions, possibly attempting to get hand to mouth. Placed in appropriate proximity to the mother, the baby appears to focus briefly on her face and to attend to her voice repeatedly in the first moments. When their mother is talking and they are attending, babies are likely to move arms, legs, fingers, or eyelids in an exact synchrony with their mother's minute voice changes.

The significant behavioral cues that shape the interaction at the first and subsequent contacts and factors that influence the mother and infant are illustrated in Figure 35–3.

In studies of maternal responsiveness some groups of mothers were given earlier and/or more extended contact with their baby than was the routine for control groups of similar mothers and then were observed in later interactions with their newborns. Mothers who were allowed earlier contact and/or increased in-hospital contact smiled more at their infants, showed more face-to-face behavior, and were quicker to use soothing and comforting behaviors when their infants exhibited distress. They appeared to enjoy subsequent contact with their infants more than the control group of mothers did. Differences between the groups were still observable two years later. However, other studies have found that extra contact makes no difference in maternal behaviors (Curry 1982), or that the differences were apparent only in those mothers who were lacking in support (Anisfeld & Lipper 1983).

During the introductory contact after birth, the mother gathers a certain amount of information about her baby. This learning about the partner is the first step in any interpersonal acquaintance. From the remarks, questions, and activities of a new mother in the earliest postpartal days, it is apparent that she is applying herself to the task of getting acquainted with her newborn. She wants to know what kind of baby she is taking into her family system and what the infant's reaction to her is. She is also consciously involved in clarifying the nature of her own developing feelings toward the newborn. In part she is becoming acquainted with herself as the mother of this particular infant. Gottlieb (1978) described a discovery process in which a mother *identifies* the infant as her own, pointing out what the infant looks like and what the baby can do. Next she *relates* the behavior or appearance to someone or something familiar: "Her nose is just like her daddy's." A third step in the process is *interpreting* or giving meaning to the infant's behavior or appearance: "Look at that face, he's going to be a feisty one!"

There is some indication that the degree to which a mother develops feelings of affectionate closeness or attachment to the fetus before birth is generally predictive of the course of maternal feelings toward the baby immediately after birth and in the acquaintance phase. Minimal closeness before birth seems to lead to less enjoyment of the newborn, less responsiveness to needs, and less empathy when the infant is in distress. Women who feel an intense attachment and interaction before birth appear to

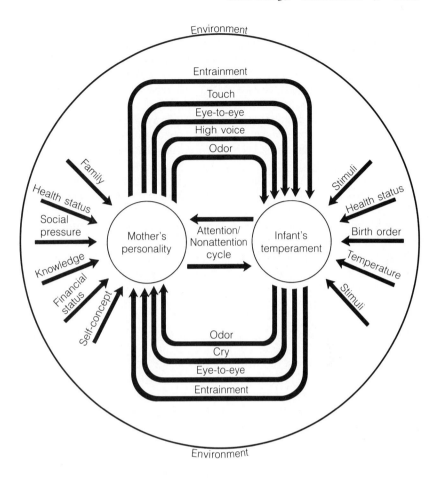

Figure 35–3   Reciprocity system

pick up the relationship at that level after birth and to develop increased feelings of closeness in the acquaintance phase. They eagerly respond to the newborn's needs and are gratified by the baby's apparent well-being. In addition, they are likely to be more successful at initiating and maintaining breast-feeding than are minimally attached mothers. Liking the infant at the start apparently contributes to the woman's understanding of her newborn as an individual with unique needs and adds to her willingness to respond to those needs. The positive orientation at the beginning of contact probably also influences the woman to believe that her baby appreciates her.

The newborn plays an important part in determining the outcome of the mother-infant relationship. If infants respond in an organized way to the usual caretaking stimuli and are regular in biologic rhythms, they tend to be easy to understand. If infants give clear behavioral cues about needs, their responses to mothering will be predictable. Such predictability makes a mother feel effective and competent. If the newborn responds to the mother's care with a predominantly positive mood rather than with irritability, and if the baby has relatively long periods of being quietly awake and attentive, the infant is pleasant to be near and to interact with. Other behaviors that make an infant more attractive to caretakers are smiling, grasping a finger, nursing eagerly, cuddling, and being easy to console.

The newborn is also becoming acquainted with his or her mother. Newborns gather what information they can about their new world. They attend to sights, sounds, tastes, and smells, and experience different tactile and kinesthetic sensations. Within a few days after birth, infants show signs of recognizing recurrent situations and responding to changes in routine.

Phase of Mutual Regulation

In performing of the necessary tasks of newborn care, such as feeding, bathing, and comforting, the new mother develops awareness that there is some discrepancy between her wishes and needs and her baby's needs and desires. This awareness ushers in a phase of mutual regulation of behaviors. The degree of control to be exerted by each partner in the interpersonal adjustment is an issue in the early postpartal weeks. Maternal goals in resolving this issue of control are, of course, variable, both among different mothers and in the same mother at different times. In some mother-infant pairs, the maternal goal is primarily to change the infant to meet the mother's needs. In other pairs it is quite apparent that the mother's intent is primarily to interpret correctly and to gratify completely all of her baby's needs. Either of those approaches is likely to result in relational disturbances, the degree of distress and tension depending to a large extent on the newborn's reactions to the maternal behaviors used to reach the goal. For example, the mother who wishes to adjust her baby rather than adjust to him or her will have a smoother postpartal course if she is blessed with a highly adaptive infant who is positive in mood. The mother who is intent on meeting every need of her child at the same moment it arises will meet with failure very quickly if the newborn is unpredictable, is irregular in daily rhythms, and presents behavioral cues that are difficult to interpret.

The ideal solution to the control issue would be somewhere between the two extremes. A mother who realizes that she is a person with her own needs will be less vulnerable to the buildup of anger, frustration, anxiety, and guilt. In all but the most ideal situations, each partner must undergo disappointments, and each must at some time subordinate his or her own needs to the needs of the other. The most important consideration is that each should obtain a good measure of enjoyment from the ongoing interactions.

Generally speaking, enjoyment is enhanced during the early months if the infant can make clear her or his needs behaviorally and if the mother's personality allows her to let the infant lead the interaction. Mutual maternal-infant regulation is never instantaneous; it is a process that continues throughout infancy and childhood. Fortunately, there appears to be a tendency toward improved organization of behavior in the newborn period and an increasing ability to nurture in the mother during the same time.

It is during the mutual adjustment phase that negative maternal feelings are likely to surface or intensify. Because "everyone knows that mothers love their babies," these negative feelings often go unexpressed and are allowed to build up. If they are expressed, the response of friends, relatives, or health care personnel is often to deny the feeling to the mother: "You don't mean that"; "You can't feel that way"; "Your baby is not ugly, he is beautiful." Some negative feelings are normal in the first few days following birth, and the nurse should be supportive when the mother vocalizes these feelings.

When mother and baby enjoy each other's company, it is usually obvious to an observer that the relationship is good. It may be said that reciprocity has been achieved. A high degree of reciprocity is characteristic of successful mutual regulation.

Reciprocity

Reciprocity within a mother-infant system may be described as an interactional cycle that occurs simultaneously between the mother and the infant (Brazelton & Cramer 1990). It involves mutual cuing behaviors, expectancy, rhythmicity, and synchrony. There are intimations of reciprocity in the early hours of life. The mother and her infant respond to each other's cues. They develop rhythms in interaction that form the basis for communication. During several weeks of interaction, they establish a pattern of

behavior in which they mesh with each other. When this meshing or synchrony is attained, the mother and infant perform a reciprocal process of cyclic attention and non-attention. Brazelton and his colleagues (1974) have studied this reciprocal process in the laboratory and have carefully analyzed the component parts. They have described five phases of the cycle: (1) initiation, (2) orientation, (3) acceleration, (4) deceleration, and (5) turning away. The first two phases establish the partners' expectations regarding the interaction. Both mother and infant use clusters of behaviors as the interaction develops. Feedback between partners enables them to modulate their behaviors. Sensitivity and adjustment by the mother allows the infant to maintain a homeostatic state and to develop an expanding attention cycle. The infant may begin to develop recognizable patterns of behavior by about 2 weeks of age, and patterns are often well established by 6 weeks.

If the observer is aware of what to look for, the segments of an interactional cycle can be described as they are observed. The following is a hypothetical example of an interactional period, as it is likely to appear when things are going well:

Initiation: The infant is held on the mother's knee, facing her. He looks toward her with a relaxed expression and makes slow movements with his arms and hands.

Orientation: As the infant makes eye contact with his mother, his eyes brighten and become alert, and he turns his whole body toward her, extending arms and legs in her direction. He reaches toward the mother.

State of attention: The mother smiles and talks to the infant, and he responds by smiling, moving his arms and legs in pedaling motions, cooing, and making other sounds. The eyes alternately become alert and dull as he responds to the smiles and words of his mother. The limbs move rhythmically, in time with the mother's voice. There is a constant slow smooth reaching and circular movement occurring as the tension within the infant's body rises and falls. The infant assumes the look of expectancy.

Acceleration: The infant continues to move, to wave his hands and feet about, and to increase his smiling activity. His eyes are bright and alert. He strains toward his mother in the intensity of the interaction, all the time watching her and cuing to her smile. For the most part, the body movement is smooth, but there may be occasional jerkiness.

Peak of excitement: As the infant becomes wholly involved in the interaction, his movements may become jerky and intense. He brings his hand to his mouth and tries to insert his thumb while still smiling and cooing. The other hand clutches his thigh and he leans forward to his mother as she continues to smile at him. As he endeavors to reach forward, his back arches and his body tends to twist toward one side.

Deceleration: The excitement begins to pass and the infant's movements slow. There is a gradual decrease in body movement, the bright look dims, the eyes become dull, and the lids appear to droop. The smiles fade, and vocalization decreases. Suddenly the infant yawns and begins to suck his thumb as he leans away from his mother. His hands drop to his lap with the fingers widespread, and he appears to be relaxing.

Withdrawal or turning away: The infant's activity slows down almost completely. He slumps against his mother's hands with his body half turned away from her. His eyes are dull and focused in the direction of an object to the side. There is a faint smile on his face. The mother stops smiling and talking to the infant. She just sits holding him quietly, waiting for his next cue. The mother briefly raises her head and glances beyond the infant. This prompts a reaction in the infant. He looks toward his mother, smiles briefly, and looks away again, then turns back to the mother, ready to resume another period of interaction.

The responsibility for monitoring cues and for sensitively initiating or maintaining the interaction rests primarily with the mother. The infant uses the nonattention time to recover from the tension of interaction, to organize behavior, and to process what has been taken in during the attentive periods.

The development of reciprocity between a mother and her infant is evidence of the bond or attachment that has formed between them. It enables the mother to let go of the infant she knew as a fetus during pregnancy. A new relationship now develops with an individual who has a unique character and who evokes a response entirely different from the fantasy response of pregnancy. When reciprocity is synchronous, the interaction between mother and infant is mutually gratifying and is sought and initiated by both partners. Pleasure and delight develop in each other's company, and there is mutual development of love and growth.

Reciprocity may take weeks to develop, and it usually requires sensitive stimuli from both partners. As infants become more organized in their behavior and as senses develop, they are able to give positive feedback to their mothers. As they transmit the appearance of listening, they follow voice and movements and respond with intentionality to the mother as an individual whom they recognize and with whom they seek to communicate. In cases in which either the mother or the newborn is sick and the initial acquaintance is delayed, a delay in the development of reciprocity is also likely.

Overstimulation or inappropriate stimulation by the mother may interfere with the synchrony of the interaction. In the resultant asynchrony, the mother may be in the attention phase of the reciprocal process when the infant is in the nonattention phase. This asynchrony can lead to frustration on the part of either partner or both and may lead to a disharmonious relationship as both become established in their interactional patterns. In extreme instances mother and infant may cease to communicate with each other.

Infants vary in their strategies for dealing with an overload of stimulation. Four types of reaction have been described in infants responding to unpleasant and inappropriately timed stimuli (Brazelton & Cramer 1990): (1) active physical withdrawal, (2) rejection, (3) decreased sensitivity, and (4) communication of distress. An infant can move away from the source of stimulation, can push the stimulus away, can lapse into drowsiness or sleep, or can fuss and cry. Some of these strategies, if they become characteristic of an infant's behavior, are easier to live with than others; they interact with a mother's expectations and her personality.

The nurse may have the opportunity to observe reciprocity developing between a mother and her newborn in the early weeks of life. If nurses recognize the appearance of asynchrony, they may be able to initiate intervention before the asynchronous behaviors become firmly established.

Attachment

The ultimate goals of maternity nursing care are the continuation of life and the enhancement of the quality of that life in terms of physical and mental health. There is reason to believe that a state of mutual attachment or an enduring emotional bond between a parent (or parent surrogate) and an infant is essential to the infant's optimum health. A new mother's feelings of closeness or attachment to her infant also seem to have a positive effect on her own continued personal growth. The same is true of a new father. Therefore, the facilitation of parent-infant attachment is a significant goal to pursue.

Attachment is a bond of affection and, as such, is invisible. Behavioral cues must be observed for indications of the presence or absence of the bond. Researchers have used a variety of behaviors as indicators of attachment. In the immediate newborn period, smiling at the infant and addressing him or her by name or in affectionate terms; kissing, touching, and enfolding the infant close to the body; cradling the infant in the left arm and assuming the *en face* position; making positive comments about the appearance and behavior of the infant; finding family resemblances; and expressing positive feelings to the spouse are important behaviors. Later, expressions of enjoying caring for the infant, feeling the infant belongs to the parents, thinking about the infant when away from him or her, making warm comments about the infant, and responding appropriately to infant cues indicate that the parent has developed a bond with the infant.

The maternal role includes both emotional and physical tasks. The emotional component includes qualities that enable the mother to feel warmth, affection, attachment, protectiveness, and devotion to the child. The physical tasks include the knowledge and skill to provide care for the infant, that is, to feed, diaper, bathe, and provide a safe environment.

Whether and how soon a parent displays behaviors indicating attachment depend on many factors; the process is believed to be facilitated by a warm, supportive environment.

Attachment Behaviors in the Adolescent Mother

Adolescents demonstrate attachment behaviors toward their infants, although differences in attachment behaviors have been observed in adolescent mothers compared with older mothers. Adolescent mothers had fewer complications during pregnancy and birth but reported being more scared during labor and having a poorer perception of the experience than older mothers. These perceptions were related to later mothering behaviors in teenagers. Young mothers were more anxious, had lower attachment scores, and interacted less favorably than older mothers (von Wendeguth & Urbano 1989). The younger the adolescent, the less likely she is to display typical adult maternal behaviors of touching, synchrony with her newborn, vocalization, and proximity of mother and newborn (Porter & Sobong 1990). It also appears that the most important areas of interaction in the early postpartal period for the adolescent are physical and motor. These mothers appear to be more attuned to these behaviors than to auditory and visual interaction.

Strong ego functioning, as demonstrated by the mother's ability to adapt to pregnancy and to plan for her future, appears to affect the mother's interaction with her newborn. The response of the newborn is also critical. Infants who are healthy are more likely to affect the relationship positively. Adolescents may have problems with parenting because they tend to have less realistic expectations of what an infant can do at a given age. In addition, cognitively immature adolescents may not foresee the consequences of their actions. Neglectful parenting may become a problem. However, many adolescent mothers live with their mothers, who provide support during pregnancy and provide a significant proportion of the care of the infant.

With these considerations in mind the nurse must be attentive to the early maternal-infant interaction, use appropriate modeling and teaching techniques, include the adolescent's mother when appropriate, and refer adolescent mothers for follow-up care and early intervention programs when indicated (Panzarine 1988).

Father-Infant Interactions

The father has traditionally been seen only as a source of support for the pregnant woman. He contributed to the growth and development of his newborn indirectly by nurturing and supporting his partner through the pregnancy and the early postpartal weeks. As fathers have become more involved in the pregnancy and birth experience, researchers have begun to study their experiences and feelings about the fetus and newborn.

The majority of fathers demonstrate attachment behaviors toward the fetus during pregnancy; that is, they talk to the fetus, refer to it by name, enjoy watching their partner's abdomen move as the fetus moves, think about the baby, and show other similar behaviors (Longobucco & Freston 1989). A father's attachment to the fetus is more likely to occur when the marital relationship is strong. Fathers who identify with the pregnancy by having physical symptoms similar to pregnancy symptoms also have higher attachment scores.

A father experiences feelings toward his newborn that are similar to the mother's feelings of attachment. In the past the significance of any psychologic response called fatherliness was minimized. It was implied that, because the man did not have deep physiologic roots of fatherliness, his feelings were somehow of less importance than the mother's and were weaker and longer in developing. Evidence is increasing that a father does have a strong attraction to his newborn and highly positive emotional reactions to first contact. The first hours after birth appear to be significant in the development of the father-mother-infant bond.

The pregnancy and birth experience is important for fathers as well as mothers. When fathers are involved in pregnancy through a close marital relationship, they have a more positive report of the birth and new baby (Nicholson et al 1983). A positive birth experience also leads to greater levels of attachment in fathers.

Greenberg and Morris (1974) noted the reactions of first-time fathers to early contact with their newborns. They used the term **engrossment** to label characteristics of the effect of the newborn on the father—his sense of absorption, preoccupation, and interest in the infant.

The father's emotional reaction to the first sight of the baby and to later contacts is very positive. The intensity of his feelings may come as a surprise to him. The new father's involvement with his newborn can draw time and energy away from the ongoing couple relationship. The man who has been encouraged to support his partner in her new mothering role may feel some guilt about preoccupation with the baby, and the woman may feel ignored or excluded from a significant relationship. It seems likely that couples who shared experiences, relationships, and material things before the birth will also be able to share their infant's attention and the responsibilities of parenting.

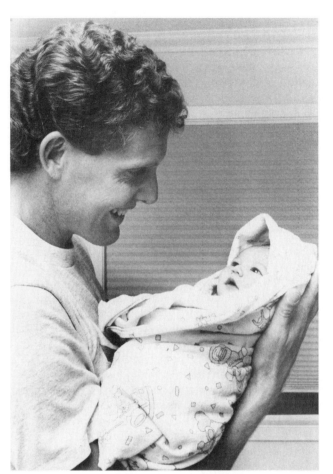

Figure 35–4   A bond develops between father and infant.

When the new father initiates interaction, the newborn responds (Figure 35–4). As with the mother-newborn interaction, the baby contributes his or her part. The infant cries and moves, indicating alertness and well-being. Spontaneous and reflexive movements and grimaces are emitted and the father responds by voice and touch. From the beginning, the father's interactive behaviors are different from the mother's, and these differences are perceptible to the infant. A father's odor, voice pitch, appearance, and touch qualities are all different from a mother's. In a face-to-face "play situation," a mother tends to use her hands to enfold and enclose her baby's body and limbs with gentle molding and smoothing motions, whereas the father punctuates his conversation with finger pokes and more exaggerated changes in facial expression, which act to increase the baby's excitement level. Observers have noted differences in an infant's responses to interaction with mother or father as early as two weeks after birth.

Mothers, too, appear to notice a difference. Often in the early weeks, when asked if they play with the baby, mothers say, "No, but my husband does." It seems as if one function of the father-infant interaction is to further acquaint the mother with her baby's range of possible behaviors in the context of a shared relationship.

It might be helpful if, during the pregnancy, nurses explain the potential for engrossment of the father after birth. If both parents are aware that each has needs at this time, they may be better able to support each other's growing relationship to this new family member. To make nursing goals appropriate and intervention effective, more knowledge is needed about the long-term effects of different levels of direct paternal involvement on the quality of the father-child relationship and other family relationships.

Siblings and Others

Most parents try to prepare their children for the arrival of a new baby. Many hospitals are including sibling classes to help children learn about newborns and become involved in the socialization of the new baby into the family. The type and extent of the preparation may depend on the age of the children and the type of relationships that exist in the home. If the new baby is seen as nonthreatening to the relationships the children have with their parents, there will probably be less disruption, and the new baby will be accepted without serious problems.

Common reactions of a child to the birth of a sibling are negative behaviors toward the mother, withdrawal, sleeping problems, aggressiveness, changes in toileting, and increased attention-seeking (Field & Reite 1984).

The conventional view of the bonding or attachment process has been that the infant was capable of forming only one bond at a time and that this bond should be to the mother. Bowlby (1958) called this tie *monotropy.* More recent work with infants has shown that they are capable of maintaining a number of attachments. These attachments may include siblings, grandparents, aunts, and uncles. Some infants were found to be capable of forming attachments with five or more people simultaneously without loss of quality. The social setting and personalities of the individuals appear to be significant factors in permitting the development of multiple attachments. In addition, the advent of open visiting hours and rooming-in facilitates participation of siblings and grandparents in the attachment process.

Attachment with Adopted Children

Attachment with adopted children occurs even though many factors thought to be important in the attachment process, such as early contact, may not be possible. Smith and Sherwen (1984) identified factors that adoptive mothers described as aiding the attachment process. These factors included physical contact, such as touching, kissing, or feeding, and shared activities. Factors that interfered were the child's negative behaviors and rejection by the (older) child. More problems seemed to occur when the child was over the age of four when the placement occurred. Some mothers mentioned lack of energy and resources and conflicts in roles, factors that also affect biologic mothers. As with biologic mothers, the support system of partner, relatives, and friends was very important.

The quality of attachment in adoptive mother-infant pairs is no different from that in nonadoptive situations, at least in middle-class families (Singer et al 1985). Early contact does not seem to be necessary for attachment to develop. It appears that a warm, supportive environment with competent and confident parents promotes the formation of affectionate bonds.

In some situations, adoptive parents are permitted to be present at the birth and to experience early contact and provide initial care. Some hospitals are allowing adoptive parents to room-in and receive instruction and practice in infant care under supervision of hospital staff. In other situations, the child may be older and may have developed a relationship with another care giver. In these situations, the adoptive parents need assistance and support to allow time for the acquaintance process to occur, to become sensitive to each other's cues, and to develop reciprocity. With appropriate adjustments for time of placement, similar assessments of attachment and interventions to promote attachment can be used in adoptive and biologic families.

Attachment with Severely Handicapped Children

An anomaly in the infant may affect the attachment process. Because reciprocity is an important part of the process of attachment, the process may be at risk when one of the interactors is unable to perform her or his role. When a mother interacts with a nonhandicapped child, the more the child smiles, looks, or vocalizes, the more responsive the mother becomes. When the child is blind, deaf, or mentally retarded, the mother must adapt her interactive behaviors. However, she may not know how to compensate for the child's deficits and may need instruction and role modeling (Landry & Chapieski 1989). This is especially true with severely retarded children.

Severely handicapped children do exhibit attachment behaviors. The nurse can promote attachment in families with handicapped children in a variety of ways such as enhancing the parent's sensitivity to subtle cues. For example, a head turn or ceasing self-stimulatory behavior may be the child's way of recognizing the mother or father. Parents may be either positively or negatively unrealistic about the child's capabilities. Parents can be helped to think realistically about the child's abilities and to re-

spond to the child's signals. Because attachment does occur with severely handicapped children, the implications of separation may be considered when recommending placement of such children. When neither parental attachment nor ability of the child to form an attachment exists, placement of the child outside the home is more likely to be an acceptable appropriate option. When the parents choose to keep the child at home, professionals should help foster attachment.

Assessment and Interventions in Mother-Infant Relationships

Nurses come into professional contact with women and their families at any point in the maternity cycle in public health offices, hospitals, doctor's offices, child protection centers, or in childbirth education classes. Facilitating a mother-infant relationship is usually only one of a number of concurrently operating goals of health care. Much can be done during the performance of other nursing tasks to support the development of maternal attachment.

Usually a maternity or public health nurse is concerned with the care of a specific woman and her baby at a given point in time. The nurse can draw on general knowledge of norms, averages, and risk factors, but must apply what is pertinent from that store of information to a mother with a specific history and personality, in a relationship with a specific infant, and within a specific environment. It is well known that individuals classified as high risk are sometimes able to cope effectively with whatever risks are involved and to relate affectionately to a particular newborn. It also happens that what appears to be a perfect image of a potential mother can be shattered by unpredictable events occurring after the image was created.

Effective evaluation of a mother-infant relationship requires a broad understanding of a mother and newborn pair as it exists within a family and a wider social setting. The manner in which the nurse evaluates a mother-newborn relationship can be concurrently diagnostic, preventive, and therapeutic. While interacting with a maternity client, the nurse can assess the woman's ability to trust people and to enjoy relationships, her skills in communication, and her feeling tone. At the same time the nurse can work to develop a mutually trusting relationship and an increase in maternal self-esteem and self-confidence. Through direct interaction, the nurse can also model appropriate behaviors such as nurturing, communicating, and problem solving that can be unconsciously picked up and imitated or consciously studied and tested by the mother. When feelings are expressed, the nurse can accept them nonjudgmentally. This practice enables the client to accept her feelings and perhaps to examine and understand them. It also encourages the further expression of feelings. As the nurse reaches tentative conclusions in the evaluation of a mother-infant relationship, it is often appropriate to share ideas with the mother, both because the mother is a source of validation of the nurse's observation and because being included in the process of assessment can be ego-enhancing for the mother. Some mothers can be very accurate in predicting their own postpartal adjustment and the quality of their support network.

Assessment of Early Attachment

If attachment is accepted as a desired outcome of nursing care, a nurse in any of the various postpartal settings can periodically observe and note progress toward attachment. The following questions can be addressed in the course of nurse-client interaction:

1. *Is the mother attracted to her newborn?* Does she seek face-to-face contact and eye contact? Is she actively reaching out or only passively holding her newborn? Has she progressed from fingertip touch to palmar contact to enfolding the infant close to her body? Is attraction increasing or decreasing? If the mother does not exhibit increasing attraction, why not? Do the reasons lie primarily within her, the baby, or the environment?

2. *Is the mother inclined to nurture her infant?* Is she progressing in her interactions with her infant? Has she selected a rooming-in arrangement if it is available?

3. *Does the mother act consistently?* Is she developing a consistent and predictable approach to the care of her infant? Does she tend to respond to the same situation in the same way from day to day? If not, is the source of unpredictability within her or her infant?

4. *Does the mother seek information as needed?* Does she seek information and evaluate it objectively? Does she develop solutions based on adequate knowledge of valid data? How did she prepare herself for the parenting role? Does she evaluate the effectiveness of her maternal care and make appropriate adjustment?

5. *Is she sensitive to the newborn's needs as they arise?* How quickly does she interpret her infant's behavior and react to cues? Does she respond when the baby cries or fusses? Does she seem happy and satisfied with the infant's responses to her efforts? Is she pleased with feeding behaviors? How much of this ability and willingness to respond is related to the baby's nature and how much to her own?

6. *Does she seem pleased with her baby's appearance and sex?* Is she experiencing pleasure in interaction with her infant? What times are the most and least enjoyable? What interferes with the enjoyment? Does she speak to the baby frequently and affectionately? Does she call him or her by name? Does she point out family traits or characteristics she sees in the newborn?

7. *Are there any cultural factors that might modify the mother's response?* For instance, is it customary for the grandmother to assume most of the child-care responsibilities while the mother recovers from childbirth?

When these questions are addressed and the facts have been assembled by the nurse, the nurse's intuitive feelings and formal background of knowledge should combine to answer three more questions: Is there a problem in attachment? What is the problem? What is its source? Each nurse can then devise a creative approach to the problem in the context of a unique developing mother-infant relationship.

Assessment of attachment behaviors has become increasingly important in light of current theories that correlate malattachment with an increased incidence of parenting problems, failure to thrive, and child neglect or abuse. When assessing attachment behaviors, the nurse should be careful not to generalize or give too much importance to any one factor. Adaptive behavior may vary from one situation to the next. Cultural factors such as decreased eye contact should also be considered. All cultures may not recognize or value the same behaviors that are valued by Western culture.

Assessment of the mother-infant (or father-infant) interaction should be made on various occasions to avoid attaching too much significance to one behavior on a given occasion. Some behaviors that may indicate a maladaptive attachment process include refusal by the mother to see her newborn, failure to progress from fingertip to palm when holding or exploring the infant, making no attempt to establish eye-to-eye contact, inability to choose a name, or choosing a name that is so unusual that it implies hostility or ridicule (such as "Jim Beam," "Spirits," "Tornado," or the like).

An attachment assessment form is reproduced in Figure 35–5. It provides for recording observations during the prenatal period through six weeks of life. Those involved in care of the family can become aware of potential problems and provide interventions to enhance attachment

Guidelines for Intervention

Actions that minimize mental distress and physical discomfort or maximize feelings of well-being and pleasure have the potential of enhancing the quality of mother-infant interaction. Following are some suggested objectives and ways of achieving them:

1. Determine the childbearing and childrearing goals of the infant's mother and father and use them wherever possible in planning nursing care for the family. This includes giving the parents choices about their labor and birth experience and their initial time with their new infant.

NAME _____ AGE_____ MARITAL STATUS: Single _____ Married _____ Separated _____
GRAVIDA _____ PARA _____ AB _____ DATE OF BIRTH _____
EXPECTED DATE OF CONFINEMENT _____ METHOD OF FEEDING _____
SUMMARY OF LABOR AND BIRTH (anesthesia, complications, presence of a supportive person):
_____

DIRECTIONS: *This form is provided to systematically assess and record the components of the attachment process based on information obtained from available records, observations, and interviews with the parent(s) and other health care providers.*

PRENATAL PERIOD   YES   NO

Planned the pregnancy _____ _____
COMMENTS _____

Confirmed the pregnancy _____ _____
COMMENTS _____

Accepted the pregnancy _____ _____
COMMENTS _____

Received early prenatal care _____ _____
COMMENTS _____

Described fetal movement _____ _____
COMMENTS _____

Personalized the fetus _____ _____
COMMENTS _____

Asked what the fetus was like in utero _____ _____
COMMENTS _____

Attended prenatal classes _____ _____
COMMENTS _____

Planned for infant's needs _____ _____
COMMENTS _____

Thought of possible names _____ _____
COMMENTS _____

Client in good health _____ _____
COMMENTS _____

Father of infant involved _____ _____
COMMENTS _____

AREAS OF CONCERN _____

FIRST POSTPARTUM DAY (*From birth through first day*)
                                        YES   NO
Calls infant by name _____ _____
COMMENTS _____

Describes infant in affectionate terms _____ _____
COMMENTS _____

Offers positive comments about infant's physi- _____ _____
cal appearance
COMMENTS _____

Finds family resemblances _____ _____
COMMENTS _____

Looks and reaches out to infant _____ _____
COMMENTS _____

Hugs and touches infants _____ _____
COMMENTS _____

Kisses infant _____ _____
COMMENTS _____

Smiles at infant _____ _____
COMMENTS _____

Expresses positive emotional feelings to in- _____ _____
fant's father or significant other
COMMENTS _____

Experiences average discomfort _____ _____
COMMENTS _____

Welcomes visitors _____ _____
COMMENTS _____

AREAS OF CONCERN _____

DELIVERY PERIOD (*Birth through 4 hours*)
                                        Yes   No
Accepts sex of infant _____ _____
COMMENTS _____

Calls infant by name _____ _____
COMMENTS _____

Calls infant by affectionate terms _____ _____
COMMENTS _____

Comments on beauty of infant _____ _____
COMMENTS _____

Realistically appraises the physical appearance _____ _____
of the infant
COMMENTS _____

Looks and reaches out to infant _____ _____
COMMENTS _____

Touches infant _____ _____
COMMENTS _____

Smiles at infant _____ _____
COMMENTS _____

AREAS OF CONCERN: _____

POSTPARTUM PERIOD (*From second day to 6 weeks*)
                                        YES   NO
Want to be near infant _____ _____
COMMENTS _____

Enjoys caring for infant _____ _____
COMMENTS _____

Holds infant close _____ _____
COMMENTS _____

Feels infant belongs to her _____ _____
COMMENTS _____

Feels infant notices her _____ _____
COMMENTS _____

When away, thinks about infant _____ _____
COMMENTS _____

Verbalizes warm comments about infant _____ _____
COMMENTS _____

Recuperates with little difficulty _____ _____
COMMENTS _____

Responds sensitively and appropriately to _____ _____
infant
COMMENTS _____

AREAS OF CONCERN: _____

Figure 35–5 Attachment assessment form with provision for continuity from the prenatal period through birth and the first postpartum day to six weeks postpartum (Adapted from Early Parent-Infant Relationships. *National Foundation/ March of Dimes, 1978, p 74. Courtesy of the March of Dimes Birth Defects Foundation.)*

2. Arrange the health care setting so that individual nurse-client professional relationships can be developed and maintained throughout a pregnancy and during the first months of mother-infant adaptation. A consistent care giver during the mother's prenatal experience allows a comfortable trusting relationship to develop in which the mother feels free to express concerns, ask questions, and explore choices. In the hospital a primary nurse can develop rapport and assess the mother's strengths and needs.

3. Enhance the couple's relationship and increase their communication capacity during the pregnancy. A feeling of closeness and personal satisfaction often results when the father plays an active role in the labor and birth process by acting as the woman's coach and support person. Comfort with such a role will develop most easily if the parents attend prenatal classes. As they learn about pregnancy and birth, anxiety decreases.

4. Use anticipatory guidance from conception through the postpartal period to prepare the parents for expected problems of adjustment. Prenatal classes often focus on possible problems a new family might encounter. In addition, literature on a variety of concerns, from feeding to sibling rivalry to infant stimulation, helps the new parents cope. If such information is available in the hospital and at the office or clinic, parents can choose according to their need.

5. Include parents in any nursing intervention planning and evaluation. Give choices whenever possible.

6. Remove barriers to voluntary contact among family members and the infant. This may be accomplished by providing time in the first hour after birth for the new family to become acquainted with as much privacy as possible. Warmth may be maintained by placing the infant against the mother's bare chest and covering both with a warmed blanket. When the father is holding his new daughter or son, the baby may be wrapped in two or three warmed blankets. Postponing eye prophylaxis facilitates eye contact between parents and their newborn. Sibling attendance at the birth or sibling visits also play a role in integrating the newest family member.

7. Initiate and support measures to alleviate parental fatigue.

8. Help parents to identify, understand, and accept both positive and negative feelings related to the overall parenting experience.

9. Support and assist parents in determining the personality and unique needs of their infant. Whenever possible, rooming-in should be available. This practice gives the mother a chance to learn her infant's normal patterns and develop confidence in caring for him or her. It also allows the father more uninterrupted time with his infant in the first days of life. If the mother and baby are doing well and if help is available for the mother at home, early discharge permits the family to begin establishing their life together.

The following are specific strategies to promote the role of the father in pregnancy and childbirth (Kunst-Wilson & Cronenwett 1981):

1. Include the father in all prenatal visits.

2. Encourage his participation in prenatal and parenting classes.

3. Provide educational material depicting active, involved fathers.

4. Address concerns of fathers related to childbirth and infant care.

5. Have a prenatal session for fathers only, with involved fathers as discussion leaders.

6. Encourage discussion of changes in role and parenting issues.

7. Facilitate the father's presence at labor and birth and provide support for the role he wishes.

8. Encourage the father to hold his newborn.

9. Allow the parents to have time alone with their infant after birth.

10. Give the father the opportunity to room-in with the mother.

11. Encourage the father's participation in feeding, holding, and diapering the infant.

12. Include the father in well-baby checks.

13. Provide postpartum classes that include both parents.

14. Facilitate discussion of difficulties in sharing responsibilities for infant care.

15. Encourage formation of parent support groups.

The importance of attachment is widely recognized, as are the adverse effects that may result when attachment does not occur. Formation of the attachment bond depends on numerous factors, and the bond may be enhanced by the sensitive approach of a health care provider in a humanistic environment in which parental preferences are given primary consideration. See Teaching Guide—Enhancing Attachment.

Complications in Maternal-Infant Attachment

The mother who experienced a high-risk labor and birth or who has complications in the immediate postpartal period

TEACHING GUIDE
Enhancing Attachment

Assessment The nurse provides maximum opportunity for parents to interact with their infant immediately after birth and while in the birthing unit. Observation and documentation of these interactions will assist nurse in determining family's needs for teaching, support, or interventions.

Nursing Diagnosis The nursing diagnoses will probably be: Alteration in family process related to addition of a new baby to family or knowledge deficit related to emotional needs of newborn.

Nursing Plan and Implementation The teaching plan includes information about the infant's physical status, normal characteristics, comforting techniques, and emotional needs immediately after birth and during the newborn period. Parents are encouraged to maintain continuous contact through rooming-in.

Parent Goals At the completion of the teaching, the parents will be able to do the following:

1. Demonstrate appropriate nurturing behaviors such as touching, bonding, talking to, kissing, and holding their baby.
2. Discuss normal characteristics and emotional needs of the newborn.
3. List at least three comforting techniques.

Teaching Plan

Content	Teaching Method Discussion
Content Present information on periods of reactivity and expected newborn responses.	
Describe normal physical characteristics of newborn.	Discussion and presentation of slides showing newborn characteristics
Explain the bonding process, its gradual development, and the reciprocal interactive nature of the process.	
Discuss infant's capabilities for interaction, such as non-verbal communication abilities. The nonverbal communications include movement, gaze, touch, facial expressions, and vocalizations—including crying. Emphasis that eye contact is considered one of the cardinal factors in developing infant-parent attachment and will be integrated with touching and vocal behaviors. (Figure 35–6)	Show video on interactive capabilities of newborns.
Discuss that touching, including stroking, patting, massaging, and kissing, will progress to interactive touch between parent and infant; discuss need to assimilate these behaviors into daily routine with baby.	Discussion, demonstration, and handouts
Describe and demonstrate comforting techniques, including use of sound, swaddling, rocking, and stroking.	Demonstration and return demonstration
Discuss progression of the infant's behaviors as infant matures and importance of parents' consistent response to infant's cues and needs.	Discussion, time for questions
Provide information about available pamphlets, videos, and support groups in the community.	
Evaluation The nurse may evaluate the learning by providing time for discussion, questions, and return demonstrations. Continued observation of parent's positive interaction with their baby during remainder of stay in birthing unit also provides a means of evaluating learning.	

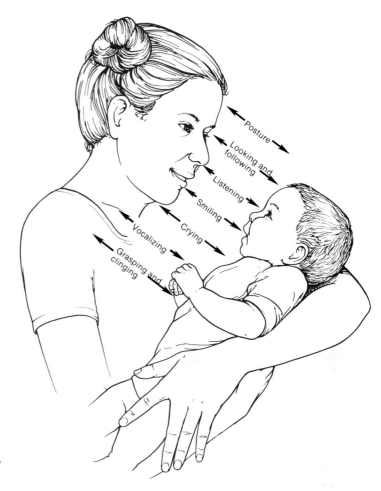

Figure 35–6 Behaviors that enhance parent-infant communication (From Mott SR, James SR, Sperhac AM: Nursing Care of Children and Families, 2nd ed. 1990, p 183)

has an increased risk of encountering difficulties in attachment. She is more likely to have had medications, analgesia, or anesthesia during the intrapartal period, which may influence early interaction with her newborn. In the immediate postpartal period she may be more likely to receive medications or analgesics or to face problems that limit her energy. Complications involving the mother or infant may necessitate separation during the early stages of attachment. Although these are only a few of the factors that may be present, they may be significant if they interfere with the bonding or attachment process.

Malattachment

The most common element in the lives of parents who neglect or abuse their children is a "lack of empathic mothering" in their own lives (Steele & Pollack 1968). This phrase describes inadequate responses of the caretaker to the infant, frequently beginning in the perinatal period and related to poorly developed maternal-infant attachment or insufficient bonding (Kempe & Kempe 1984). Because of this finding, attention has been given to the promotion of adequate parent-infant bonding to prevent malattachment and its related complications. Factors that may retard the

formation of maternal-infant attachment include an abnormal pregnancy, an abnormal labor or birth, neonatal separation, other separation in the first six months, illnesses in the infant during the first year of life, and illnesses in the mother during the first year of life.

In the prenatal period, warning signs that may indicate lack of acceptance of the pregnancy and a potential for malattachment include: negative maternal self-perception, excessive mood swings or emotional withdrawal, failure to respond to quickening, excessive maternal preoccupation with appearance, numerous physical complaints, and failure to prepare for the infant during the last trimester (Kempe & Kempe 1984).

At birth, signs of maladaptive responses may include lack of interest in seeing the newborn; withdrawal, sadness, or disappointment; negative comments such as "She's such an ugly thing"; or expressions of marked disappointment when told of the infant's sex. When shown the infant, the mother may avoid looking at the child or may regard the child without expression. She may decline to hold the infant, or if she does agree to do so, she may not touch or stroke the infant's face or extremities. The mother may also avoid asking questions or talking to the infant and may suddenly decide she does not want to breast-feed.

During the early postpartal period, evidence of maladaptive mothering may include limited handling of or smiling at the infant, lack of preparation or questions about infant needs and care, and failure to snuggle the newborn to her neck and face. The mother may also describe her infant negatively or use animal characteristics in a hostile manner when referring to the infant: "He looks just like a withered old monkey to me!"

The father, too, may exhibit signs of malattachment to his infant. Examples of maladaptive paternal behaviors include inattentiveness and indifference toward the child, rough, unrelaxed handling, and tense, rigid posture. The father may also choose inappropriate types of play and exhibit no protective behavior toward his child.

When maladaptive behaviors are identified, various interventions can be used. A team approach involving all nursing shifts is advised. Any positive behaviors are communicated so that each staff member can continue to offer support and stimulate further development of such strengths.

Hospital practices should be examined for factors that may inhibit or exaggerate the maladaptive behaviors. Hospital practices such as strict adherence to four-hour feedings, discouraging the mother from unwrapping and looking at her newborn, or prolonged separation, although far less common today, may create a problem for some mothers.

The mother needs a supportive, understanding person she can interact with as she works through her feelings about her baby. Personal or telephone contact may be maintained after discharge so that the mother can continue to have contact with a supportive person with whom she is already acquainted. The mother should be encouraged to call the postpartal unit or newborn nursery if she has questions.

When the Newborn Is Hospitalized

Disorders in attachment may occur after separation due to prolonged hospitalization of the infant. Many mothers and fathers appear to be close to their infants and nurture them in a normal, adaptive way, despite separation. When disorders do occur, the mother's affective state and the father's role are critical components (Weingarten et al 1990). It is possible that when a mother is separated from her infant, she needs extra nurturing in order to provide the neces-

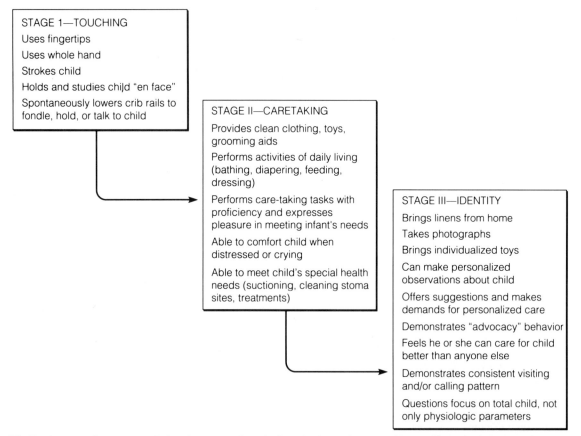

Figure 35–7 Stages of parenting behavior toward an infant in intensive care (From Shraeder BD: Attachment and parenting despite lengthy intensive care Am J Mat Child Nurs January/February 1980; 5:38. (c) 1980 American Journal of Nursing Company. Used with permission. All rights reserved.)

sary nurturing for the infant. Thus it may be that an important role for the father is to nurture his partner so that she can nurture the infant.

When infants require lengthy intensive care, special efforts by the nurse may facilitate attachment. It is important that parents believe that the child "belongs" to them rather than to the medical team. Parents are encouraged to participate in care and to give suggestions about care. A care plan, which includes specific nursing diagnoses such as "alteration in the parent-child relationship" or "impairment of the parent-infant bond" provides for nursing interventions that are established according to the stages of parenting behaviors outlined in Figure 35–7. For example, if the mother entered the nursery, lowered the crib rail, and established an *en face* position while talking to the infant, she would be ready to move into stage II. If there is a specific problem, with the feeding schedule or technique, for example, the parents might be encouraged to work with the nurses to help establish the care plan.

Jenkins and Tock (1986) describe sending an informative letter to the parents "from the baby" on a weekly basis to promote proximity. The letter describes the competencies of the infant and behaviors such as "I like to open my eyes when I eat, but I get so tired that I soon close them" (p 34).

During the postpartal period, continued family interaction should be encouraged through supportive staff, liberal visiting policies, and educational offerings for both father and mother. Staff should be trained in assessment techniques and alert for evidence of malattachment, so that appropriate interventions may be initiated. If necessary, referrals to the community health nurse or social services may provide the ongoing assistance needed. Telephone hotlines may provide a useful resource for a frustrated or worried parent, as may classes or parents' groups during the early weeks after birth.

✱ ✱

KEY CONCEPTS

The three major perspectives on attachment are psychoanalytic, ethologic, and learning theories.

A mother's genetic makeup and background influences the environment she can provide for the fetus and newborn.

Attachment to the fetus develops during pregnancy.

The infant is a significant partner in the attachment interaction.

The childbirth setting is important in creating an environment for early parent-infant interaction.

Mother-infant interaction proceeds through phases: introductory, acquaintance, mutual regulation, reciprocity and rhythmicity, and attachment.

Attachment behaviors may differ in adolescent mothers.

Fathers, siblings, and others also become attached to the fetus and newborn.

Attachment occurs with adopted children and with handicapped children.

Attachment can be systematically assessed.

Interventions can facilitate attachment.

Complications in parent-infant attachment can occur because of maternal illness or hospitalization of the infant.

✱ ✱

References

Anisfeld E, Lipper E: Early contact, social support, and mother-infant bonding. *Pediatrics* 1983; 72:79.

Bowlby J: The nature of the child's tie to his mother. *Int J Psychoanal* 1958; 39:350.

Brazelton TB et al: The origins of reciprocity: The early mother-infant interaction. In: Lewis M, Rosenblum LA (editors). *The Effect of the Infant on Its Caregiver.* New York: Wiley, 1974.

Brazelton TB, Cramer BG: *The Earliest Relationship.* Reading, MA: Addison-Wesley, 1990.

Cranley MS: Roots of attachment: The relationship of parents with their unborn. *Birth Defects* 1981b; 17:59.

Curry MA: Maternal attachment behavior and the mother's self-concept: The effect of early skin-to-skin contact. *Nurs Res* 1982; 31:73.

de Chateau P: Left side preference in holding and carrying newborn infants. A three year follow-up study. *Acta Psychiatr Scand* 1987; 75:283.

Field T, Reite M: Children's responses to separation from mother during the birth of another child. *Child Dev* 1984; 55:1308.

Gottlieb L: Maternal attachment in primiparas. *JOGNN* 1978; 7:39.

Grace JT: Does a mother's knowledge of fetal gender affect attachment? *MCN* 1984; 9:42.

Greenberg M, Morris N: Engrossment: The newborn's impact upon the father. *Am J Orthopsychiatry* 1974; 44:520.

Johnson SH: *High Risk Parenting: Nursing Assessment and Strategies for the Family at Risk.* Philadelphia: Lippincott, 1979.

Kempe RS, Kempe CH: *Child Abuse.* Cambridge, MA: Harvard University Press, 1984.

Klaus MH et al: Human maternal behavior at first contact with her young. *Pediatrics* 1970; 46:187.

Kunst-Wilson W, Cronenwett L: Nursing care for the emerging family: Promoting paternal behavior. *Res Nurs Health* 1981; 4:201.

Landry SH, Chapieski ML: Joint attention and infant toy exploration: Effects of Down syndrome and prematurity. *Child Dev* 1989; 60:103.

Longobucco DC, Freston MS: Relation of somatic symptoms to degree of paternal-role preparation to first-time expectant fathers. *JOGNN* 1989; 18 (6):482.

Nicholson J et al: Outcomes of father involvement in pregnancy and birth. *Birth* 1983; 10:5.

Panzarine S: Teen Mothering. *J Adolesc Health Care* 1988; 9:443.

Pascoe JM, French J: Development of positive feelings in primiparous mothers toward their normal newborns. *Clin Pediatr* 1989; 28 (10):452.

Porter RH, Cernoch JM, McLaughlin FJ: Maternal recognition of neonates through olfactory cues. *Physiol Behav* 1983a; 30:151.

Porter RH, Cernoch JM, Perry S: The importance of odors in maternal-infant interactions. *Mat Child Nurs J* 1983b; 12:147.

Porter LS, Sobong LC: Differences in maternal perception of the newborn among adolescents. *Pediatr Nurs* January/February 1990; 16:101.

Rubin R: Maternal touch. *Nurs Outlook* 1963; 11:828.

Singer LM et al: Mother-infant attachment in adoptive families. *Child Dev* 1985; 56:1543.

Smith DW, Sherwen LN: The bonding process of mothers and adopted children. *Top Clin Nurs* 1984; 6:38.

Steele B, Pollock C: A psychiatric study of parents who abuse infants and small children. In: *The Battered Child.* Helfer R, Kempe CH (editors). Chicago: University of Chicago Press, 1968.

Taylor PM: Bonding and Attachment. In: *Current Therapy in Neonatal-Perinatal Medicine-2.* Nelson NM (editor). Philadelphia: Decker, 1990.

Toney L: The effects of holding the newborn at delivery on paternal bonding. *Nurs Res* 1983; 32:16.

von Windeguth B, Urbano R: Teenagers and the mothering experience. *Pediatr Nurs* 1989; 15 (5):517.

Weingarten CT et al: Married mothers' perceptions of their premature or term infants and the quality of their relationships with their husbands. *JOGNN* 1990; 19 (1):64.

Additional Readings

Anderson A, Anderson B: Toward a substantive theory of mother-twin attachment. *MCN* 1990; 15(6):373.

Dormire SL, Strauss SS, Clarke BA: Social support and adaptation to the parent role in first-time adolescent mothers. *JOGNN* 1989; 18(4):327.

Elsters AB, Lamb ME, Kimmerly N: Perceptions of parenthood among adolescent fathers. *Pediatrics* 1989; 83(5):758.

Fuller JR: Early patterns of maternal attachment. *Health Care Women Int.* 1990; 11(4):433.

Goldberg S: Attachment in infants at risk: Theory, research, and practice. *Infants Young Child* 1990; 2(4):11.

Porter CP: Clinical and research issues related to teen mothers' childrearing practices. *Issues in Comprehensive Pediatric Nursing* 1990; 13:41.

Zahr L: Correlates of mother-infant interaction in premature infants from low socioeconomic backgrounds. *Pediatr Nurs* 1991: 17(3):259.

CHAPTER 36

The Postpartal Family at Risk

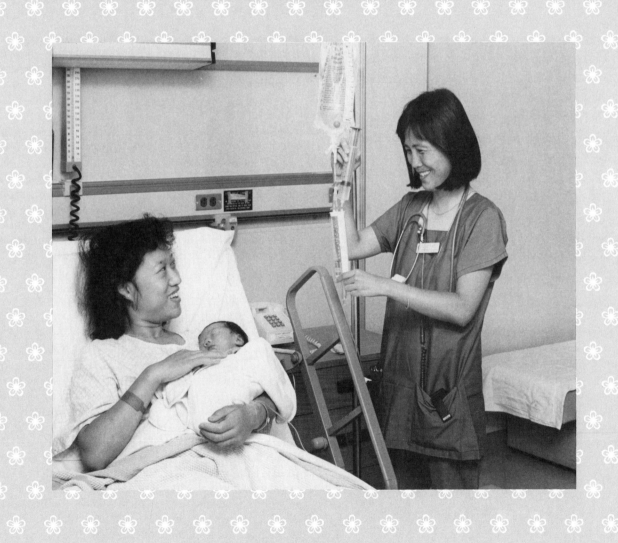

OBJECTIVES

Assess the postpartum woman for predisposing factors, signs, and symptoms of various postpartum complications to facilitate early and effective management of complications.

Incorporate preventive measures for various complications of the postpartum period into nursing care of the postpartum woman.

List the causes of and appropriate nursing interventions for hemorrhage during the postpartal period.

Develop a nursing care plan which reflects a knowledge of etiology, pathophysiology, and current medical management for the woman experiencing postpartum hemorrhage, reproductive tract infection, thrombo-embolic disease, urinary tract infection, mastitis, or a postpartal psychiatric disorder.

Evaluate the mother's knowledge of self-care measures, including measures to prevent recurrence of complications.

❀ ❀

We are surviving. Just. Why don't they give Croix de Guerre to people who can go without more than two hours total daily sleep for five weeks? I thought babies ate at six-ten-two-six-ten-two—mine does. He also eats at five-seven-nine-eleven and four-eight-twelve. I am getting rather used to going around with my breasts hanging out. They are either drying from the last feed or getting ready for the next one. But the love—I never knew, never imagined that I would love him like this. This incredible feeling of boundless, endless love—a wish to protect his innocence from ever being hurt or wounded or scratched. And that awful, horrible, mad feeling in the first week that you'll never be able to keep anything so precious and so vulnerable alive. (The New Our Bodies, Ourselves)

The postpartal period is often seen as a smooth, uneventful time that follows the anticipation of pregnancy and the excitement and work of labor and birth—and often it is. However, it is important for the nurse to be aware of problems that may develop postpartally and their implications for the childbearing family.

❀ *USING THE NURSING PROCESS WITH* ❀

Women at Risk During the Postpartal Period

When providing care to the childbearing woman during the postpartal period, the nurse uses the nursing process to make ongoing assessments, institute preventive measures, and detect, as early as possible, the development of any complications. When a potential problem is noted, the nurse analyzes the data; formulates appropriate nursing diagnoses;

and develops, implements, and evaluates a plan of care. Often the care will be provided in a collaborative way as the nurse works with other members of the health care team.

Nursing Assessment

Complications can develop early in the postpartal period (for example, hemorrhage, PIH, or bladder distention) or later (endometritis, thrombophlebitis). Therefore, ongoing assessment should be a major priority of the postpartum nurse. Such assessment is especially important because the nurse is often the first person to detect a developing complication. If a complication does develop, assessment remains important to determine the effectiveness of therapy and to detect any signs that the problem is worsening.

Analysis and Nursing Diagnosis

The nurse analyzes the information gained from assessment, formulates appropriate nursing diagnoses, and develops with the woman appropriate goals. If, for example, the nurse is caring for a woman who complains of dysuria, the nurse first reviews the woman's history. The nurse learns that the woman was catheterized twice during labor for bladder distention and was also catheterized during the third hour after childbirth. The woman reports that she does not feel that she is fully emptying her bladder. The nurse cannot palpate the bladder suprapubically. The woman has no costovertebral angle (CVA) tenderness but her temperature is 100.8F. She is unable to produce another urine specimen so the nurse offers her additional fluids. The nurse then formulates the nursing diagnosis, "alteration in urinary elimination related to dysuria secondary to possible bladder infection."

Nursing Plan and Implementation

Once the data have been analyzed and the diagnosis established, the nurse develops and implements a care plan. In the case of the woman with dysuria, the nurse notifies the physician of her assessment findings and obtains an order for a clean-catch urine specimen for culture. The nurse explains what is occurring to the woman and may provide increased fluid intake, administer a mild analgesic, or obtain an order for an antispasmodic if the woman is also experiencing bladder spasms.

Evaluation

The nurse evaluates the effectiveness of the plan of care. For example, in the preceding situation the woman was relieved to learn that the nurse took her problem seriously. After receiving the antispasmodic, the woman was able to provide a clean-catch urine specimen, which revealed that the woman did have a bladder infection. Antibiotic therapy was begun. The nurse concluded that the plan had been effective thus far, but discussions with the woman revealed that a new nursing diagnosis was necessary: knowledge deficit related to a lack of understanding of self-care measures to help prevent urinary tract infection (UTI). The nurse then began planning an approach to meet this newly identified need.

Thus the process is cyclic, building on assessment, logical analysis, and well-planned and implemented intervention, followed by evaluation and modification as necessary.

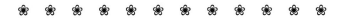

Care of the Woman with Postpartal Hemorrhage

Hemorrhage in the postpartal period is described as either early or late postpartal hemorrhage. **Early postpartal hemorrhage** (or immediate postpartal hemorrhage) occurs in the first 24 hours after birth. **Late postpartal hemorrhage** (delayed postpartal hemorrhage) occurs after the first 24 hours. Postpartal hemorrhage is defined as blood loss greater than 500 mL even though quantitative studies indicate the loss for a normal birth is between 500 and 600 mL. Since the amount of blood lost during birth is often underestimated, blood loss occurring with a postpartal hemorrhage is usually well in excess of 500 mL (Cunningham et al 1989).

Early Postpartal Hemorrhage

The main causes of early postpartal hemorrhage are uterine atony (relaxation of the uterus), laceration of the genital tract, retained placental fragments, and blood coagulation problems. Certain factors predispose to hemorrhage: (a) overdistention of the uterus due to hydramnios, a large infant, or multiple gestation; (b) grand multiparity; (c) use

of anesthetic agents (especially halothane) to relax the uterus; (d) trauma due to obstetric procedures such as midforceps delivery, intrauterine manipulation, or forceps rotation; (e) a prolonged labor or a very rapid labor; (f) use of oxytocin to induce or to augment labor; (g) uterine infection; and (h) maternal malnutrition, anemia, pregnancy-induced hypertension (PIH), history of hemorrhage, or history of blood coagulation problems.

Uterine Atony

Uterine atony can frequently be anticipated in the presence of (a) overdistention of the uterus; (b) dysfunctional labor that has already indicated the uterus is contracting in an abnormal pattern; (c) oxytocin use during labor; and (d) the use of anesthesia that produces uterine relaxation. Hemorrhage from uterine atony may be slow and steady or sudden and massive. The blood may escape the vagina or collect in the uterus. Changes in maternal blood pressure and pulse may not occur until blood loss has been significant because of the increased blood volume associated with pregnancy.

In most cases the clinician can predict when a woman is at risk for hemorrhage. The key to successful management is prevention. Prevention begins with adequate nutrition, good prenatal care, and early diagnosis and management of any complications that may arise. Traumatic procedures should be avoided, and the birth should take place in a facility that has blood immediately available. Any woman at risk should be typed and cross-matched for blood and have intravenous lines in place. Excellent labor management and childbirth technique is imperative.

After expulsion of the placenta, the fundus should be palpated to ensure that it is firm and well contracted. If it is not firm (if it is boggy), fundal massage should be performed until the uterus contracts. If bleeding is excessive, the clinician undertakes bimanual uterine compression (Figure 36-1A) while ordering the administration of intravenous oxytocin (Pitocin) at a rapid rate. (An undiluted bolus of oxytocin *should not* be given because it can cause hypotension.) Oxygen is also administered by mask. The combination of bimanual compression and oxytocin is usually effective in treating uterine atony.

If bleeding persists, the cervix and vagina should be inspected for lacerations. The physician may manually examine the uterine cavity for retained placental fragments or may perform a curettage. If the atony does not respond to these measures, 250 µg of 15-methyl prostaglandin F_2 (Prostin 15M) may be administered intramuscularly. The dose may be repeated at 15- to 90-minute intervals, if necessary. The side effects, such as nausea, vomiting, and diarrhea, are unpleasant and are often treated with medication. Other side effects include fever, flushing, and elevated diastolic blood pressure (Few 1987). If the hemorrhage has not been severe, the need for blood transfusion will be decided after blood values have been obtained and the true extent of the hemorrhage determined. Severe, uncontrolled hemorrhage, in addition to

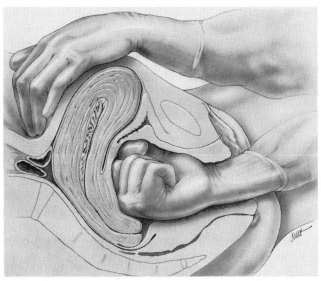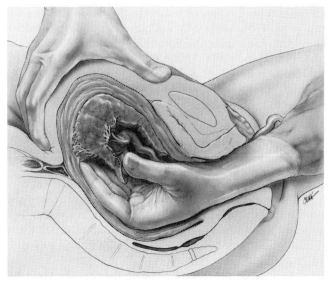

Figure 36–1   A Manual compression of the uterus and massage with the abdominal hand usually will effectively control hemorrhage from uterine atony. B Manual removal of placenta. The fingers are alternately abducted, adducted, and advanced until the placenta is completely detached. Both these procedures are done only by the medical clinician. (Adapted from Cunningham FG, MacDonald PC, Gant NF (editors): Williams Obstetrics, 18th ed. Norwalk, CT: Appleton & Lange, 1989. Fig 24–1, Fig 24–2, pp 417–418.)

the above measures, may require immediate blood transfusion, inspection for uterine rupture, blood coagulation studies, curettage, bilateral internal iliac artery ligation, angiographic embolization, or hysterectomy.

Retained Placenta

Hemorrhage may also occur if the placenta is only partially separated. The most common cause of partial separation is massage of the fundus *prior* to placental separation, so this practice should be avoided. Management of hemorrhage due to a partial separation, once it has occurred, includes uterine massage and manual removal of the placenta (Figure 36-1B). After expulsion of the placenta, the consistency of the fundus is assessed. Rarely, placenta accreta, an abnormal adherence of the placenta to the uterine wall, is the cause of the hemorrhage and may require curettage or emergency hysterectomy.

Late Postpartal Hemorrhage

Late postpartal hemorrhage is most frequently caused by retained placental fragments. Hemorrhage may occur in the hours following the fourth stage of labor or may not develop for a day or two or later. Placental fragments are occasionally retained for a week or longer. In such cases, they may become necrosed, fibrin may be deposited, and the fragments form a so-called placental polyp. Sloughing of the polyp may cause sudden bleeding (Cunningham et al 1989).

Medical Therapy

Careful examination of the placenta after birth for missing pieces or cotyledons is the best preventive measure for late postpartal hemorrhage. The membranes should be inspected for missing sections or for vessels that are transverse from the edge of the placenta outward along the membranes, which may indicate succenturiate placenta and a retained lobe. If retained placental fragments or membranes are suspected, the uterine cavity may also be checked.

Often a boggy uterus is the first indication of the possibility of late postpartal hemorrhage. Bleeding is controlled by intravenous oxytocin, methylergonovine maleate (Methergine) (usual dosage is 0.2 mg every four hours for six doses), ergotrate, or prostaglandins. Antibiotics are also used to prevent infection. Volume expanders and/or blood products are used if large amounts of blood are lost. Sonography is used to determine the presence of retained placental fragments. Curettage, formerly standard treatment, is now thought by some to traumatize the implantation site and thereby increase bleeding (Cunningham et al 1989).

❀   *APPLYING THE NURSING PROCESS*   ❀

Nursing Assessment

Careful and ongoing assessment of the woman during labor and birth and evaluation of her prenatal history will help identify factors that put the woman at risk for postpartal hemorrhage. Following birth, periodic assessment for evidence of bleeding is a major nursing responsibility. Careful observation and documentation of vaginal bleeding is important to determine if further medical intervention is needed. This assessment can be done visually, by pad counts, or by weighing the perineal pads.

Nursing Diagnosis

Nursing diagnoses that may apply when a woman experiences postpartal hemorrhage include the following:

- Knowledge deficit related to signs of delayed postpartal hemorrhage
- Fluid volume deficit related to blood loss secondary to uterine atony, lacerations, or retained placental fragments

For other possible diagnoses, see the Key Nursing Diagnoses—Postpartal Hemorrhage.

Nursing Plan and Implementation

Effective Assessment and Intervention to Ensure Client Well-Being

Regular and frequent assessment of fundal height and firmness will alert the nurse to the possible development or recurrence of hemorrhage. The nurse massages a boggy uterus until it is firm and, if it appears larger than anticipated, attempts to express clots. If the woman seems to

have a slow, steady, free flow of blood the nurse begins weighing the perineal pads (approximately 500 mL fluid weighs 1 lb or 454 grams) and monitors the woman's vital signs at least every 15 minutes—more frequently if indicated. If the fundus is displaced upward or to one side due to a full bladder, the nurse encourages the woman to empty her bladder—or catheterizes her if she is unable to void—to allow for efficient uterine contractions (Barger 1988).

The nurse assesses the woman for signs of anemia, such as fatigue, pallor, headache, thirst, and orthostatic changes in pulse or blood pressure, and reviews the results of all hematocrit determinations. All medical interventions, intravenous infusions, blood transfusions, oxygen therapy, and medications such as methylergonovine maleate are monitored and evaluated for effectiveness. Urinary output should be monitored to determine adequacy of fluid replacement and renal perfusion. The nurse also encourages the woman to obtain adequate rest and helps her plan activities so that rest is possible.

Facilitation of Parent-Infant Attachment

The mother may find it difficult to care for her baby because of the fatigue associated with blood loss. The nurse can often find ways to promote attachment while still recognizing the health needs of the mother. The mother may require additional assistance in caring for her infant. If she has intravenous lines in place, even carrying the newborn may be awkward. For the mother who feels compelled to do as much as possible, the nurse may also need to "give permission" to the mother to return her infant to the nursery so she can have adequate periods of uninterrupted rest. The nurse may also work with the woman's partner and family to find ways to help the mother cope.

Education for Self-Care

Because of current trends toward early discharge, the mother may be sent home any time after four hours post birth. She and her family or support persons should receive clear, preferably written, explanations of the normal postpartal course, including changes in the lochia and fundus and signs of abnormal bleeding. Instruction for the prevention of bleeding should include fundal massage, ways to assess the fundal height and consistency, and inspection of the episiotomy and lacerations, if present. The woman should receive instruction in perineal care. The woman and her family are advised to contact their care giver if any of the following occur: excessive or bright red bleeding (saturation of more than one pad per hour), a boggy fundus that does not respond to massage, abnormal clots, leukorrhea, high temperature, or any unusual pelvic or rectal discomfort or backache. If iron supplementation is ordered, instructions for proper dosage are taught to enhance absorption and avoid constipation and stomach upset. The nurse stresses the importance of reexamination of uterine size in two weeks. See Table 36-1.

Dₓ

Key Nursing Diagnoses to Consider
Postpartal Hemorrhage

Altered tissue perfusion

Decreased cardiac output

Fatigue

Fear

Fluid volume deficit

Impaired gas exchange

Ineffective breast-feeding

Knowledge deficit

Activity intolerance: High risk

Injury: High risk

Table 36–1	Signs of Postpartal Hemorrhage

The nurse must suspect postpartal hemorrhage or hematoma formation if a woman shows any of the following signs:

Excessive or bright red bleeding

A boggy fundus that does not respond to massage

Abnormal clots

Any unusual pelvic discomfort or backache

High temperature

Evaluation

Anticipated outcomes of nursing care include the following:

- Signs of postpartal hemorrhage are detected quickly and managed effectively.
- Maternal infant attachment is maintained successfully.
- The woman is able to identify abnormal changes that might occur following discharge and understands the importance of notifying her care giver if they develop.

❀ ❀ ❀ ❀ ❀ ❀ ❀ ❀ ❀ ❀ ❀ ❀

Hematomas

Hematomas occur as a result of injury to a blood vessel, often without noticeable trauma to the superficial tissue. The soft tissue in the area offers no resistance, and hematomas containing 250 to 500 mL of blood may develop rapidly. Predisposing factors include the increased vascularity and pelvic congestion of pregnancy, PIH, genital varicosities, use of pudendal block anesthesia, primigravidity, precipitous labor, prolonged second stage of labor, infant size greater than 4000 g, blood dyscrasias, and forceps-assisted birth. Hematomas may be vulvar, vaginal (especially in the area of the ischial spines), or subperitoneal. Signs and symptoms vary somewhat with the type of hematoma.

Medical Therapy

Small vulvar hematomas may be treated with the application of ice packs and continued observation. Large hematomas or those increasing in size require surgical intervention to evacuate the clot and achieve hemostasis. Antibiotics, replacement of blood and coagulation factors, and vaginal packing may also be indicated. Infrequently, a pelvic hematoma that is extensive or difficult to control may require angiographic embolization, hypogastric artery ligation, or hysterectomy (Heffner et al 1985).

❀ *APPLYING THE NURSING PROCESS* ❀

Nursing Assessment

Often the first clue that a hematoma is forming is the woman's complaints of severe vulvar pain (pain that seems out of proportion or excessive), usually from her "stitches," or of severe rectal pressure. On examination, the large hematoma appears as a unilateral tense, fluctuant, bulging mass at the introitus or within the labia majora. With smaller hematomas, the nurse checks for unilateral bluish or reddish discoloration of skin of the perineum and buttocks. The area feels firm and is painful to the touch. The nurse should estimate the size of the hematoma carefully with the first assessment to better identify increases in size and the potential blood loss. Frequent visualization of the perineum in women who are still under the effect of regional anesthesia is especially important.

Hematomas that develop in the upper portion of the vagina may cause difficulty voiding because of pressure on the urethra or meatus. Diagnosis is confirmed through careful vaginal examination.

Hematomas that occur upward into the broad ligament may be more difficult to detect. The woman may complain of severe lateral uterine pain, flank pain, or abdominal distention. Occasionally the hematoma can be discovered with high rectal examination or with abdominal palpation although these procedures may be quite uncomfortable for the woman. Signs and symptoms of shock in the presence of a well-contracted uterus and no visible vaginal blood loss should alert the nurse to the possibility of a hematoma.

Continuous assessment of vaginal bleeding after surgery to control a hematoma is required to detect a recurrence.

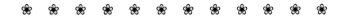

CRITICAL THINKING

If hypovolemic shock is present, what signs might you see?

Nursing Diagnosis

Nursing diagnoses that may apply when a woman develops a hematoma postpartally include the following:

- Injury: High risk related to tissue damage secondary to prolonged pressure from a large vaginal hematoma
- Pain related to tissue trauma secondary to hematoma formation

Nursing Plan and Implementation

If birth required the use of forceps or a vacuum extractor, or if it was traumatic because of the infant's size or position, the postpartal nurse can promote comfort and decrease the possibility of hematoma formation by applying an ice pack to the woman's perineum during the first hour after birth and intermittently thereafter for next 24 hours.

The discomfort experienced by a woman who develops a hematoma cannot be overlooked. If a hematoma develops despite preventive measures, a sitz bath after the first 24 hours will aid fluid absorption once the bleeding has stopped and will promote comfort, as will the judicious use of analgesics.

Evaluation

Anticipated outcomes of nursing care include the following:

- Hematoma formation is detected quickly and managed successfully.
- The woman's discomfort is relieved effectively.
- Tissue damage is avoided or minimized.

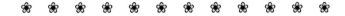

Subinvolution

Subinvolution of the uterus occurs when the uterus fails to follow the normal pattern of involution but instead remains enlarged. Retained placental fragments or infection are the most frequent causes of subinvolution. With subinvolution the fundus is higher in the abdomen than expected. In addition, lochia often fails to progress from rubra to serosa to alba. Lochia may remain rubra or return to rubra several days postpartum. Leukorrhea and backache may occur if infection is the cause. Subinvolution is most commonly diagnosed during the routine postpartal examination at four to six weeks. The woman may relate a history of irregular or excessive bleeding, or describe the symptoms listed previously. An enlarged, softer-than-normal uterus when palpated with bimanual examination indicates subinvolution. Treatment involves oral administration of methylergonovine (Methergine) 0.2 mg orally every three to four hours for 24 to 48 hours. When metritis (inflammation of the uterus) is present, antibiotics are also administered. If this treatment is not effective or if the cause is believed to be retained placental fragments, curettage is indicated (Cunningham et al 1989).

Care of the Woman with a Reproductive Tract Infection

Puerperal infection is an infection of the reproductive tract associated with childbirth that can occur any time from birth to six weeks postpartum. The most common infection is metritis/endometritis and is limited to the uterine cavity. However, infection can spread by way of the lym-

phatics and blood vessels to become a progressive disease resulting in peritonitis or pelvic cellulitis. The woman's prognosis is directly related to the stage of the disease at the time of diagnosis, the invading organism, and the woman's state of health and ability to resist the disease state.

The standard definition of puerperal morbidity established in the 1930s by the Joint Committee on Maternal Welfare is a temperature of 100.4F (38.0C) or higher, with the temperature occurring on any two of the first ten postpartum days, exclusive of the first 24 hours, and when taken by mouth by a standard technique at least four times a day. However, serious infections can occur in the first 24 hours or may cause only persistent low-grade temperatures. Therefore careful assessment of all postpartum women with elevated temperatures is essential.

Antibiotic therapy alone has not caused the decrease in postpartum morbidity and mortality that is seen today. Aseptic technique, fewer traumatic operative births, a better understanding of labor dystocia, improved surgical intervention, and a population that is generally at less risk from malnutrition and chronic debilitative disease have also contributed to this reduction.

Causative Factors

The vagina and cervix of approximately 70% of all healthy pregnant women contain pathogenic bacteria that, alone or in combination, are sufficiently virulent to cause extensive infections. Why the organisms do not cause infection during pregnancy is not altogether clear; however, recent studies indicate that more than the presence of a pathogen in the woman's genital tract is necessary for infection to begin.

Although the uterus is considered a sterile cavity prior to rupture of the fetal membranes, bacterial contamination of amniotic fluid with the membranes still intact at term is more common than previously believed and may contribute to premature labor. Following rupture of the membranes and during labor, contamination of the uterine cavity by vaginal or cervical bacteria can easily occur. Chorioamnionitis and cesarean birth after the onset of labor are the most significant factors in the development of postpartal uterine infection. The relationship between puerperal infection and duration of ruptured membranes, multiple vaginal examinations, and internal fetal monitoring is not well documented and remains controversial. Poor nutritional status; anemia; vaginal infection with group B streptococcus; endocervical infections with *Chlamydia trachomatis* and *Mycoplasma hominis;* underlying disease, such as diabetes; and lacerations of the reproductive tract increase the risk of puerperal infection (Soper 1988). Most infections are polymicrobial (caused by more than one organism) and include both aerobes and anaerobes.

Infectious Agents

The most common aerobic bacteria found in women with postpartal infection are group B β-hemolytic streptococci, other streptococci, and *Gardnerella vaginalis*. Other aerobic bacteria implicated in puerperal infections include *Escherichia coli* and *Staphylococcus aureus* (associated with an increasing number of cases of postpartum toxic shock). *E coli* may be introduced as a result of contamination of the vulva or reproductive tract from feces during labor and birth. Group A β-hemolytic streptococci may be transmitted from the skin or nasopharynx of the woman herself, or more probably from an external source such as personnel and equipment; thus, aseptic technique is essential.

Anaerobic bacteria most frequently isolated from women with postpartal infection include *Bacteroides* species, *Peptostreptococcus* species, and occasionally, *Clostridium perfringens*.

Genital mycoplasmas, *Ureaplasma urealyticum* and *Mycoplasma hominis*, are found in as many as 75% of women with postpartal endometritis (Soper 1988; Watts 1989). Late-onset postpartal endometritis is most commonly associated with the genital mycoplasmas and *Chlamydia trachomatis*. *C. trachomatis* has a longer replication time and latency period than other bacteria and is not consistently eradicated by antibiotics used for early postpartum infections.

Types of Infections

Localized Infections

Localized infections of the episiotomy or of lacerations to the perineum, vagina, or vulva are usually not severe. However, necrotizing fasciitis, an infection of the superficial fascia and subcutaneous tissue arising in an episiotomy site, is an uncommon but rapidly developing, life-threatening infection. Early recognition is essential to successful treatment. Early signs are erythema, edema, and induration at the episiotomy site with later development of skin discoloration and systemic shock. Treatment includes intravenous and/or oral antibiotics, aggressive surgical debridement, and volume resuscitation (Sutton 1985).

Wound infection of the abdominal incision site following cesarean birth is also possible. The skin edges become reddened, edematous, firm, and tender. The skin edges then separate, and purulent material, sometimes mixed with bloody liquid, drains from the wound. The woman may complain of localized pain and dysuria and may have a low-grade fever (less than 101F or 38.3C). If the wound abscesses or is unable to drain, high temperature and chills may result.

Endometritis (Metritis)

Endometritis, an inflammation of the endometrium, may occur postpartally. After expulsion of the placenta, the placental site provides an excellent culture medium for bacterial growth. The site (in the contracted uterus) is a 4-cm round, dark red, elevated area with a nodular surface composed of numerous veins, many of which become occluded due to clot formation. The remaining portion of the decidua is also susceptible to infection because of its thinness (approximately 2mm) and its large blood supply. The cervix may also present a bacterial breeding ground because of the multiple small lacerations attending normal labor and spontaneous birth.

Pathogenic bacteria deposited at the cervix during vaginal examination and those already present infect the decidua and eventually involve the entire mucosa. If the infection is confined to the surface of the mucosa, this area will become necrotic and be sloughed off within three to five days.

In mild cases of endometritis the woman will generally have discharge that is scant (or profuse), bloody, and foul smelling. In more severe cases, symptoms may include uterine tenderness and jagged, irregular temperature elevation, usually between 38.3C (101F) and 40C (104F). Tachycardia, chills, and evidence of subinvolution may be noted. Foul-smelling lochia generally is cited as a classic sign of endometritis, but in the case of infection with β-hemolytic streptococcus, the lochia may be scant and odorless (Cunningham 1989).

Pelvic Cellulitis (Parametritis) and Peritonitis

Pelvic cellulitis (parametritis) refers to infection involving the connective tissue of the broad ligament and, in more severe forms, the connective tissue of all the pelvic structures. It is generally spread by way of the lymphatics in the uterine wall but may also occur if pathogenic organisms invade a cervical laceration that extends upward into the connective tissue of the broad ligament. This laceration then serves as a direct pathway that allows the pathogens already in the cervix to spread into the pelvis. **Peritonitis** refers to infection involving the peritoneum.

A pelvic abscess may form in the case of postpartal peritonitis and most commonly is found in the uterine ligaments, cul-de-sac of Douglas, and the subdiaphragmatic space. Pelvic cellulitis may be a secondary result of pelvic vein thrombophlebitis. This condition occurs when the clot, usually in the right ovarian vein, becomes infected and the wall of the vein breaks down from necrosis, spilling the infection into the connective tissues of the pelvis.

As the course of pelvic cellulitis advances, a mass of exudate develops along the base of the broad ligament that may push the uterus toward the opposite wall (if the infection is unilateral), where it will become fixed. If the exudate spreads into the rectocervical septum, a firm mass develops behind the cervix instead. The abscess that results should be drained or resolved through appropriate antibiotic therapy to avoid rupture of the abscess into the peritoneal cavity and development of a possibly fatal peritonitis.

A woman suffering from parametritis may demonstrate a variety of symptoms, including marked high temperature (102F–104F or 38.9C–40C), chills, malaise, lethargy, abdominal pain, subinvolution of the uterus, tachycardia, and local and referred rebound tenderness. If peritonitis develops, the woman will be acutely ill with severe pain; marked anxiety; high fever; rapid, shallow respirations; pronounced tachycardia; excessive thirst; abdominal distention; nausea; and vomiting.

Medical Therapy

Diagnosis of the infection site and causative organism is accomplished by careful history and complete physical examination, blood tests, cultures of the endometrium (although this may be of limited value since multiple organisms are usually present), and urinalysis to rule out urinary tract infection. When a localized infection develops it is treated with antibiotics, sitz baths, and analgesics as necessary for pain relief. If an abscess has developed or a stitch site is infected, the suture is removed and the area is allowed to drain.

Endometritis is treated by the administration of antibiotics. The route and dosage are determined by the severity of the infection. Careful monitoring is also necessary to prevent the development of a more serious infection.

Parametritis and peritonitis are treated with intravenous antibiotics. Broad-spectrum antibiotics effective against the most commonly occurring causative organisms are chosen initially until the results of culture and sensitivity reports are available. If multiple organisms are present, the approach to antibiotic therapy is continued unless no improvement is observed; then the antibiotic is changed.

The development of an abscess is frequently manifested by the presence of a palpable mass and may be confirmed with ultrasound. An abscess usually requires incision and drainage to avoid rupture into the peritoneal cavity and the possible development of peritonitis. Follow-

ing drainage of the abscess, the cavity may be packed with iodoform gauze to promote drainage and facilitate healing.

The woman with a severe systemic infection is acutely ill and may require care in an intensive care unit. Supportive therapy includes maintenance of adequate hydration with intravenous fluids, analgesics, ongoing assessment of the infection, and possibly continuous nasogastric suctioning if paralytic ileus develops.

❀ *APPLYING THE NURSING PROCESS* ❀

Nursing Assessment

The woman's perineum should be inspected every eight hours or at least twice daily for signs of early developing infection. The REEDA scale helps the nurse to remember to consider redness, edema, ecchymosis, discharge, and approximation (see Table 36-2). Any degree of induration (hardening) should be immediately reported to the clinician.

Fever, malaise, abdominal pain, foul-smelling lochia, larger than expected uterus, tachycardia, and other signs of infection should be noted and reported immediately so that treatment can begin.

Nursing Diagnosis

For nursing diagnoses that might apply see the Nursing Care Plan for Puerperal Infection.

Nursing Plan and Implementation

Prevention of Infection

Careful attention to aseptic technique during labor, birth, and postpartum is essential.

The nurse caring for a woman during the postpartal period is responsible for teaching the woman self-care

(Text continues on p 1150.)

Table 36-2 REEDA Scale Used to Evaluate Healing

Points	Redness	Edema	Ecchymosis	Discharge	Approximation
0	None	None	None	None	Closed
1	Within 0.25 cm of incision bilaterally	Perineal, less than 1 cm from incision	Within 0.25 cm bilaterally or 0.5 cm unilaterally	Serum	Skin separation 3 mm or less
2	Within 0.5 cm of incision bilaterally	Perineal and/or vulvar, between 1 to 2 cm from incision	Between 0.25 to 1 cm bilaterally or between 0.5 to 2 cm unilaterally	Serosanguineous	Skin and subcutaneous fat separation
3	Beyond 0.5 cm of incision bilaterally	Perineal and/or vulvar, greater than 2 cm from incision	Greater than 1 cm bilaterally or 2 cm unilaterally	Bloody purulent	Skin, subcutaneous fat, and fascial layer separation
Score:	_____	_____	_____	_____	_____
					Total _____

From Davidson N: REEDA: Evaluating postpartum healing. J Nurse-Midwifery 1974; 19:7.

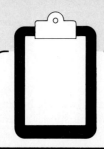

Nursing Care Plan
Puerperal Infection

Nursing History

1. Predisposing health factors include the following:
   a. Malnutrition
   b. Anemia
   c. Debilitated condition
2. Predisposing factors associated with labor and birth including the following:
   a. Prolonged labor
   b. Hemorrhage
   c. Premature and/or prolonged rupture of membranes
   d. Soft tissue trauma
   e. Invasive techniques (eg, internal monitoring, frequent vaginal exams)
   f. Operative procedures
   g. Maternal exhaustion

Physical Examination

1. Localized episiotomy infections may present with the following signs and symptoms:
   a. Complaints of unusual degree of discomfort, localized pain
   b. Reddened edematous lesion
   c. Purulent drainage, sanguineous drainage
   d. Failure of skin edges to approximate
   e. Fever (generally below 38.3C or 101F)
   f. Dysuria with or without dysuria
2. Endometritis
   a. Mild case may be asymptomatic or characterized only by low-grade fever, anorexia, and malaise
   b. More severe cases may demonstrate:
      (1) Fever of 101–103F+ (38.3 to 39.4C)
      (2) Anorexia, extreme lethargy
      (3) Chills

(4) Rapid pulse (tachycardia)
(5) Lower abdominal pain or uterine tenderness
(6) Lochia—appearance varies depending on causative organism: may appear normal, be profuse, bloody, and foul smelling, may be scant and serosanguineous to brownish and foul smelling
(7) Severe afterpains
(8) Vomiting, diarrhea
(9) Uterine subinvolution

3. Pelvic cellulitis (parametritis)
   a. Signs and symptoms of severe infection (see previous discussion of endometritis)
   b. Severe abdominal pain, usually lateral to the uterus on one or both sides and apparent with both abdominal palpation and pelvic examination
   c. Possible abscess formation; dependent on location; may be palpated vaginally, rectally, or abdominally
4. Puerperal peritonitis
   a. Symptoms just described plus severe abdominal pain
   b. Abdominal rigidity, guarding, rebound tenderness
   c. Possible vomiting and diarrhea
   d. Tachycardia, shallow respirations, anxiety, restlessness
   e. Marked bowel distention if paralytic ileus develops, absent bowel sounds

Diagnostic Studies

1. Elevated white blood count (WBC), although it may be within normal puerperal limits ($15,000-30,000/mm^3$) initially
2. Culture of intrauterine material to reveal causative organism
3. Urine culture to rule out an asymptomatic urinary tract infection (should be normal)
4. Elevated sedimentation rate
5. Bimanual examination
6. Ultrasonography

Nursing Diagnosis	Nursing Interventions	Rationale	Evaluation
Injury: High risk related to the spread of infection	Evaluate history for factors that would retard wound healing.	Careful evaluation of client history enables the nurse to identify those women who are at risk for infection and for delayed wound healing.	Therapy and supportive measures are effective and woman does not suffer injury from infection.

(continued)

Nursing Care Plan (continued)

Nursing Diagnosis	Nursing Interventions	Rationale	Evaluation
Client Goal: Woman will not suffer injury from infection as evidenced by: return of temperature to normal range, WBC count in normal range for post-partum client. If localized infection—decreased redness, edema, ecchymosis, drainage; wound edges approximated. If systemic infection—absence of malaise, uterine tenderness, foul-smelling lochia, fever, elevated WBC, abdominal pain, chills, lethargy, tachycardia, abdominal rigidity.	Employ principles of medical asepsis in hand washing and disposal of contaminated material by client and care giver. Promote normal wound healing by using: 1. Sitz baths two to four times daily for 10–15 min or surgigator 2. Peri-care following elimination 3. Frequent changing of peri-pads 4. Early ambulation 5. Diet high in protein and vitamin C, iron 6. Fluid intake to 2000 mL/day Evaluate degree of healing using the REEDA scale (Table 36–2). Report signs and symptoms of wound infection, including: 1. Redness 2. Edema 3. Excessive pain 4. Inadequate approximation of wound edges 5. Purulent drainage 6. Fever, anorexia, malaise Obtain culture from wound site and administer antibiotics, per physician order. Increase wound drainage by: 1. Assisting physician in opening wound for drainage, when indicated 2. Anticipating packing of a cavity greater than 2–3 cm with iodoform gauze Report signs of progressive infection such as uterine subinvolution, foul-smelling lochia, uterine tenderness, severe lower abdominal pain, fever, elevated WBC, malaise, chills, lethargy, tachycardia, nausea and vomiting, abdominal rigidity.	Infection may be spread through direct contact with bacteria on hands, contaminated material, etc. Warm water is cleansing, promotes healing through increased vascular flow to affected area, and is soothing to woman. Peri-care promotes removal of urine and fecal contaminants from perineum. Changing pads frequently decreases the media for bacterial growth. Ambulation promotes drainage of lochia. These nutrients are essential for satisfactory wound healing. REEDA scale provides consistent, objective tool for evaluation of wound healing. Wound infection produces characteristic signs and symptoms that reflect the body's response to the invading organism. Antibiotic therapy based on knowledge of causative organism is treatment of choice for localized infection. Abscesses may develop when infected material accumulates in closed body cavity. Iodoform packing maintains patency of opening so drainage can continue. More severe infections such as endometritis, pelvic cellulitis, or peritonitis can develop and produce characteristic signs as the body responds systematically to the invading pathogens.	

(continued)

Nursing Care Plan (continued)

Nursing Diagnosis	Nursing Interventions	Rationale	Evaluation
	Administer IV fluids and antibiotics as ordered	IV fluids maintain adequate hydration; antibiotics are the treatment of choice to combat the infection.	
	Maintain semi-Fowler's position.	Promotes comfort and helps prevent spread of infection.	
	Monitor vital signs, especially temperature, every four hr and more frequently if they are significantly abnormal. Note temperature trends.	Tachycardia and fever occur because the body's metabolic rate increases in response to its efforts to combat infection. A profound systemic infection can produce septic shock with ↓ blood pressure (BP) and ↑ respirations.	
	Monitor intake and output, urine specific gravity, and level of hydration as ordered.	Vigorous fluid and electrolyte therapy is necessary not only because of vomiting and diarrhea, but also because both fluid and electrolytes become sequestered in lumen and wall of bowel.	
	Maintain continuous nasogastric suction per physician order and assess bowel sounds.	Continuous nasogastric suction is used to decompress the bowel when paralytic ileus complicates the course and results in cessation of gastrointestinal (GI) motility.	
	Transfer woman to intensive care if indicated by her condition.	Woman with peritonitis is in critical condition, and quality of nursing care this patient receives will weigh the balance between recovery and demise.	
Pain related to the presence of infection *Client Goal:* Woman will obtain relief of pain as evidenced by her verbal expressions of comfort, ability to sleep, reduction in tachycardia.	Promote comfort by: 1. Ensuring adequate periods of rest 2. Minimizing disturbing environmental stimuli 3. Judicious use of analgesics and antipyretics 4. Providing emotional support 5. Using supportive nursing measures such as back rubs, instruction in relaxation techniques, maintenance of cleanliness, provision of diversional activities	Comfort is essential to enable the woman to rest and recover. External environmental stimuli may increase pain perceptions. Plan rest periods to increase client's emotional reserve.	Woman states she is free of pain. She is able to rest well and is coping emotionally with her infection.

(continued)

Nursing Care Plan (continued)

Nursing Diagnosis	Nursing Interventions	Rationale	Evaluation
Altered parenting: High risk related to delayed parent-infant attachment secondary to woman's malaise and other symptoms of infection *Client Goal:* Woman will bond with her infant as evidenced by her ability to feed her infant successfully, her involvement in her infant's care, her demonstration of affectionate behaviors, and her expressions of positive thoughts about her baby.	Promote and maintain mother-infant interaction: 1. Provide opportunities for the mother to see and hold her infant. 2. Encourage the mother to feed the infant if she feels able. Assist mother with feeding when IV is in place. 3. If breast-feeding mother is unable to nurse, assist her in pumping her breasts to maintain milk production. 4. Encourage partner/support person to discuss infant with woman and to become involved in infant's care if the woman is not able to do so. 5. Provide pictures of the infant for the mother's bedside. 6. Encourage verbalization of anxieties, fears, and concerns.	Critically ill woman may become very depressed not only from disease process but also because her anticipated post-partal course is now denied to her, and she may interpret this as a failure of her ability to mother her infant. Success at infant feeding generally enhances the woman's outlook and encourages mother-infant interaction. Assists woman to feel involved with her infant and reassures her that her baby is receiving care and love.	The woman bonds well with her newborn and altered parenting is avoided.
	Assess breast-feeding infant's mouth for signs of thrush, a common side effect of antibiotics taken by the mother. Treatment should be initiated, but breast-feeding need not be stopped.	Thrush, a monilial infection caused by *Candida albicans,* often occurs when normal oral flora are destroyed by antibiotic therapy.	
Knowledge deficit related to a lack of understanding of condition and its treatment *Client Goal:* Woman will be able to discuss her condition, its treatment, and her care needs following discharge.	Provide information regarding predisposing factors, signs and symptoms, and treatment. Discuss the value of a nutritious diet in promoting healing Review hygiene practices such as correct wiping after voiding, hand washing, etc, to prevent the spread of infection. Discuss home care routines following postpartal infection.	Women have the right and responsibility to be actively involved in their own health care to the extent that they are able. To be an active participant the woman needs appropriate information.	Woman is able to describe her condition and its implications. She cooperates with therapy and asks appropriate questions.

measures that are helpful in preventing infection. The woman should understand the importance of good perineal care, hygiene practices to prevent contamination of the perineum (such as wiping from front to back and changing the perineal pad after voiding, and thorough handwashing. Once edema and perineal pain are under control, the nurse can also encourage sitz baths, which are cleansing and promote healing. Adequate fluid intake coupled with a diet high in protein and vitamin C, which are necessary to promote wound healing, also helps prevent infection.

Provision of Effective Care

If the woman is seriously ill, ongoing assessment of urine specific gravity and intake and output are necessary. The nurse also carefully administers antibiotics as ordered and regulates the intravenous fluids. Ongoing assessment of the woman's condition is vital to detect subtle changes in her health status. The nurse also recognizes the woman's comfort needs related to hygiene, positioning, oral hygiene, and pain relief.

Promoting maternal-infant attachment can be difficult with the acutely ill woman. The nurse may provide pictures of the infant and keep the mother informed of the infant's well-being. If she feels up to it, the new mother will also benefit from brief visits with her infant.

Preparation for Discharge

The woman with a puerperal infection needs assistance when she is discharged from the hospital. If the family cannot provide this home assistance, a referral to home care services is needed. Home care services should be contacted as soon as puerperal infection is diagnosed so that the nurse can meet with the woman for a family and home assessment and development of a home care plan.

The family needs instruction in the care of a newborn, including feeding, bathing, cord care, immunizations, and significant observations that should be reported. A well-baby appointment should be scheduled. Breast-feeding mothers should be instructed to inspect the infant's mouth for signs of thrush and to report the finding to their physician.

The mother should be instructed regarding activity, rest, medications, diet, and signs and symptoms of complications, and she should be scheduled for a return medical visit.

Evaluation

Anticipated outcomes of nursing care include the following:

- The infection is quickly identified and treated successfully without further complications.

- The woman understands the infection and the purpose of therapy; she carries out any ongoing antibiotic therapy if indicated following discharge.

- Maternal-infant attachment is maintained.

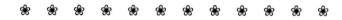

Care of the Woman with Thromboembolic Disease

Thromboembolic disease may occur antepartally, but it is generally considered a postpartal complication. **Venous thrombosis** refers to thrombus formation in a superficial or deep vein with the accompanying risk that a portion of the clot might break off and result in pulmonary embolism. When the thrombus is formed in response to inflammation in the vein wall, it is termed *thrombophlebitis*. In this type of thrombosis the clot tends to be more firmly attached and therefore is less likely to result in embolism. In **noninflammatory venous thrombosis** (also called phlebothrombosis) the clot tends to be more loosely attached and the risk of embolism is greater. The primary factor responsible for noninflammatory deep vein thrombosis is venous stasis (Cunningham 1989).

Factors contributing directly to the development of thromboembolic disease postpartally include (a) increased amounts of certain blood clotting factors; (b) postpartal thrombocytosis (increased quantity of circulating platelets) and their increased adhesiveness; (c) release of thromboplastin substances from the tissue of the decidua, placenta, and fetal membranes; and (d) increased amounts of fibrinolysis inhibitors. Predisposing factors are (a) obesity, increased maternal age and high parity; (b) anesthesia and surgery with possible vessel trauma and venous stasis due to prolonged inactivity; (c) previous history of venous thrombosis; (d) maternal anemia, hypothermia, or heart disease; (e) use of estrogen for suppression of lactation; (f) endometritis; and (g) varicosities.

Superficial Leg Vein Disease

Superficial thrombophlebitis is far more common postpartally than during pregnancy. Often the clot involves the saphenous veins. This disorder is more common in women with preexisting varices (enlarged veins) although it is not limited to these women. Symptoms usually become apparent about the third or fourth postpartal day: tenderness in a portion of the vein, some local heat and redness, absent or low-grade fever, and occasionally slight elevation of the pulse. Treatment involves application of local heat, elevation of the affected limb, bed rest and analgesics, and the use of elastic support hose. Anticoagulants are usually not necessary unless complications develop. In most cases pulmonary embolism is extremely rare. Occasionally the involved veins have incompetent valves, and as a result, the problem may spread to the deeper leg veins, such as the femoral vein.

Deep Vein Thrombosis (DVT)

Deep venous thrombosis/thrombophlebitis is more frequently seen in women with a history of thrombosis. Certain obstetric complications such as hydramnios, PIH, and operative birth are associated with an increased incidence.

Clinical manifestations may include edema of the ankle and leg and an initial low-grade fever often followed by high temperature and chills. Depending on the vein involved, the woman may complain of pain in the popliteal and lateral tibial areas (popliteal vein), entire lower leg and foot (anterior and posterior tibial veins), inguinal tenderness (femoral vein), or pain in the lower abdomen (iliofemoral vein). The Homan's sign (Figure 36–2) may or may not be positive, but pain often results from calf pressure. Because of reflex arterial spasm, sometimes the limb is pale and cool to the touch—the so-called milk leg or *phlegmasia alba dolens*—and peripheral pulses may be decreased.

Septic pelvic thrombophlebitis may develop in conjunction with infections of the reproductive tract and is more common in women who have had a cesarean birth. The classic sign is fever of unknown origin. However, when the ovarian vein is involved, lower abdominal pain also occurs. If untreated, tachycardia, nausea, ileus, and elevated white count usually develop (Fagnant & Monif 1987).

Medical Therapy

Because cases are seldom clear-cut, diagnosis involves a variety of approaches, such as client history and physical examination, occlusive cuff impedence plethysmography (IPG), Doppler ultrasonography, and contrast venography. In questionable cases, contrast venography provides the most accurate diagnosis of deep vein thrombosis. Unfortunately, venography is not practical for multiple examinations or prospective screening and may itself induce phlebitis.

Treatment involves the administration of intravenous heparin, using an infusion pump to permit continuous, accurate infusion of medication. Strict bed rest and elevation of the legs is required, and analgesics are given as necessary to relieve discomfort. If fever is present, deep thrombophlebitis is suspected and the woman is also given antibiotic therapy. In most cases thrombectomy is not necessary.

Once the symptoms have subsided (usually in several days), the woman may begin walking while wearing elastic support stockings. Intravenous heparin is continued and in addition sodium warfarin (Coumadin) is begun. When prothrombin time reaches 1.5 to 1.7, the heparin is discontinued. The woman will continue on Coumadin for two to six months at home. While on warfarin, prothrombin times are assessed periodically to maintain correct dosage levels.

❀   *APPLYING THE NURSING PROCESS*   ❀

Nursing Assessment

The nurse carefully assesses the woman's history for factors predisposing to development of thrombosis and/or thrombophlebitis. In addition, as part of regular postpartal assessment, the nurse is alert to any client complaints of pain in the leg, inguinal area, or lower abdomen because such pain may indicate deep venous thrombosis. The nurse also assesses the woman's legs for evidence of edema, temperature change, or pain with palpation.

Nursing Diagnosis

Nursing diagnoses that may apply to a postpartal woman with thromboembolic disease are found in the Nursing Care Plan for Thromboembolic Disease.

Nursing Plan and Implementation

Prevention of Thrombosis and/or Thrombophlebitis

Women with varicosities should be evaluated for the need for support hose during labor and the postpartum period. Adequate hydration is necessary during labor to avoid dehydration. Because trauma is often a factor in the development of thrombophlebitis, the nurse avoids keeping the woman's legs elevated in stirrups for prolonged periods. If stirrups are used, they should be comfortably padded and

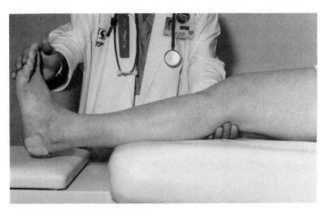

Figure 36–2   Homan's sign. With the client's knee flexed to decrease the risk of embolization, the nurse dorsiflexes the client's foot. Pain in the foot or leg is a positive Homan's sign.

(Text continues on p 1157.)

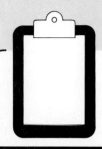

Nursing Care Plan
Thromboembolic Disease

Client Assessment

Nursing History

1. Predisposing factors include the following:
   a. Increased maternal age
   b. Obesity
   c. Increased parity
   d. Prolonged labor with associated pressure of the fetal head on the pelvic veins
   e. PIH
   f. Heart disease
   g. Hypercoagulability of the early puerperium
   h. Anemia
   i. Immobility
   j. Hemorrhage
   k. Previous history of venous thrombosis
2. Initiating factors may include the following:
   a. Trauma to deep leg veins due to faulty positioning for delivery
   b. Operative delivery, including cesarean birth
   c. Abortion
   d. Postpartal pelvic cellulitis

Physical Examination

1. Superficial thrombophlebitis
   a. Tenderness along the involved vein
   b. Areas of palpable thrombosis
   c. Warmth and redness in the involved area
2. Deep venous thrombosis (DVT)
   a. Positive Homan's sign (pain occurs when foot is dorsiflexed while leg is extended)
   b. Tenderness and pain in affected area
   c. Fever (initially low, followed by high fever and chills)
   d. Edema in affected extremity
   e. Pallor and coolness in affected limb
   f. Diminished peripheral pulses
   g. Increased potential for pulmonary embolus

Diagnostic Studies

Thrombophlebitis

   a. Doppler ultrasonography demonstrates increased circumference of affected extremity
   b. Occlusive cuff IPG
   c. Venography confirms diagnosis

Nursing Diagnosis	Nursing Interventions	Rationale	Evaluation
Injury: High risk related to obstructed venous return *Client Goal:* Client will not experience any injury, as evidenced by absence of pain, edema, and pallor; pulses will be palpable; ambulation will be possible; and anticoagulant overdose will be avoided.	Report signs and symptoms of developing thrombophlebitis (see client assessment section of nursing care plan). Maintain bed rest and warm, moist soaks as ordered, with legs elevated. For DVT, administer intravenous heparin as ordered, by continuous intravenous drip, heparin lock, or subcutaneously including the following:	Early detection of developing thrombophlebitis permits prompt treatment. As the thrombus increases in size, signs of obstruction also increase. Bed rest is ordered to decrease possibility that portion of clot will dislodge and cause pulmonary embolism. Warmth promotes blood flow to affected area. Elevation of legs decreases edema and prevents venous stasis.	The woman recovers fully and injury is avoided.

(continued)

Nursing Care Plan (continued)

Nursing Diagnosis	Nursing Interventions	Rationale	Evaluation

	1. Monitor IV or heparin lock site for signs of infiltration.
	2. Obtain Lee-White clotting times or partial thromboplastin time (PTT) per physician order and review prior to administering heparin.
	3. Observe for signs of anticoagulant overdose with resultant bleeding, including the following:
	  a. Hematuria
	  b. Epistaxis
	  c. Ecchymosis
	  d. Bleeding gums
	4. Provide protamine sulfate, per physician order, to combat bleeding problems related to heparin overdosage.
		Heparin does not dissolve clot but is administered to prevent further clotting. It is safe for breast-feeding mothers because heparin is not secreted in mother's milk.
		
		Protamine sulfate is heparin antagonist, given intravenously, which is almost immediately effective in counteracting bleeding complications caused by heparin overdose.	

	Immediately report the development of any signs of pulmonary embolism, including the following: **1.** Sudden onset of severe chest pain, often located substernally **2.** Apprehension and sense of impending catastrophe **3.** Cough (may be accompanied by hemoptysis) **4.** Tachycardia **5.** Fever **6.** Hypotension **7.** Diaphoresis, pallor, weakness **8.** Shortness of breath **9.** Neck vein engorgement **10.** Friction rub and evidence of atelectasis upon auscultation	Pulmonary embolism is major complication of deep venous thrombosis / thrombophlebitis. Signs and symptoms may occur suddenly and require immediate emergency treatment; prognosis is related to size and location of embolism.	

(continued)

Nursing Care Plan (continued)

Nursing Diagnosis	Nursing Interventions	Rationale	Evaluation
	Initiate or support any emergency treatment.		
	Initiate progressive ambulation following the acute phase; provide properly fitting elastic stockings prior to ambulation for management of superficial thrombophlebitis and DVT. For DVT, obtain prothrombin time (PT) and review prior to beginning warfarin. Repeat periodically per physician order.	Elastic stockings or "TEDs" help prevent pooling of venous blood in lower extremities. PT is the test most commonly used to monitor the blood of clients receiving warfarin. Warfarin sodium (Coumadin) inhibits Vitamin K-dependent activation of clotting factors II, VII, IX, and X. Goal of treatment is to maintain prothrombin time (PT) at 1.5 to 2 times normal.	
Pain related to tissue hypoxia and edema secondary to vascular obstruction *Client Goal:* Woman will obtain relief of pain as evidenced by verbal expressions of comfort and ability to rest and sleep.	Administer analgesics as ordered for relief of pain. Provide supportive nursing comfort measures such as back rubs, provision of quiet time for sleep, diversional activities.	Analgesics act to relieve pain and enable the woman to rest. Aspirin or ibuprofen products are contraindicated, as they inhibit platelet adhesiveness. Acetaminophen may be ordered by the physician.	Woman states that pain is relieved and that she is able to rest comfortably.
	Maintain limb in elevated position.	Elevation of affected limb promotes venous return and helps decrease edema.	
Potential altered parenting related to decreased maternal-infant interaction secondary to bed rest and IVs *Client Goal:* Woman will develop bonds of attachment with her infant as evidenced by her ability to feed her infant successfully, her involvement in her infant's care, her demonstration of affectionate behaviors, and verbal expressions of positive thoughts about her baby.	Maintain mother-infant attachment when mother is on bed rest: 1. Provide frequent contacts for mother and infant; modified rooming-in is possible if the crib is placed close to the mother's bed and nurse checks often to help mother lift or move infant. 2. Encourage mother to feed baby. Breast-feeding mothers may nurse; for acutely ill mothers it may be necessary to pump the breasts. 3. Provide photos of infant if contact is limited.	Maternal-infant attachment is enhanced by frequent contact and opportunities to interact.	Woman successfully develops bonds of attachment with her infant.

(continued)

Nursing Care Plan (continued)

Nursing Diagnosis	Nursing Interventions	Rationale	Evaluation
Altered family processes related to illness of family member *Client Goal:* Woman and her family will cope effectively with her illness as evidenced by frequent visits from partner (and other family members, including siblings), verbalized plans for handling family tasks and for coping when woman is discharged, and expressions of assurance by woman that the family will deal effectively with her illness.	1. Encourage woman to express her concerns to her partner. Assist couple in planning ways to manage while woman is hospitalized and after her discharge. 2. Encourage partner or support person to bring other children to hospital to visit mother and meet new sibling. 3. Encourage partner or support person to bring in family pictures. Encourage phone calls. 4. Contact social services if indicated to obtain additional assistance for family if needed.	Illness of any family member impacts the entire family. This is especially true when the family situation is such that the mother is the primary nurturer and she is absent. Family members attempt to continue their own roles while also assuming the tasks of the missing member. This can result in crisis.	Woman expresses assurance that family misses her but is coping effectively. Family is able to discuss plans for coping following the woman's discharge.
Knowledge deficit related to the DVT/thrombophlebitis, its treatment, preventive measures, and the medication, warfarin *Client Goal:* Woman will understand her condition, its treatment, and long-term implications as evidenced by her ability to discuss the condition and answer questions about her care and responsibilities.	1. Discuss ways of avoiding circulatory stasis such as avoiding prolonged standing or sitting; avoiding crossing legs. 2. Review need to wear support stockings and to plan for rest periods with legs elevated. In the presence of DVT, discuss the following: 1. The use of warfarin, its side effects, possible interactions with other medications, and need to have dosage assessed through periodic checks of the prothrombin time.	Such discussion is essential to help the woman understand the condition, her medication, and its implications. She must have a clear understanding to be able to provide effective self-care.	Woman is able to discuss her condition, its treatment, preventive measures, and long-term implications.

(continued)

Nursing Care Plan (continued)

Nursing Diagnosis	Nursing Interventions	Rationale	Evaluation
	2. Discuss signs of bleeding, which may be associated with warfarin sodium and which need to be reported immediately, including the following: a. Hematuria b. Epistaxis c. Ecchymosis d. Bleeding gums e. Rectal bleeding		
	3. Monitor menstrual flow—bleeding may be heavier.		
	4. Review need for woman to eat a consistent amount of leafy green vegetables (lettuce, cabbage, brussels sprouts, broccoli) every day.	Foods are high in vitamin K and will affect balance between dose of warfarin and PT.	
	5. Instruct woman to report *any* bleeding that continues more than 10 minutes.		
	6. Instruct woman to do the following: a. Routinely inspect body for bruising b. Carry Medic Alert card indicating she is on anticoagulant therapy c. Use electric razor to avoid scratching skin, use *soft* bristle tooth brush d. Avoid alcohol intake or keep intake at minimum e. Not to take any other drugs without checking with physician f. Note that stools may change color to pink, red, or black as a result of anticoagulant use		

adjusted to provide correct support. In addition, early ambulation is encouraged following birth, and the use of the knee gatch on the bed should be avoided. Women confined to bed following a cesarean birth are encouraged to do regular leg exercises to promote venous return.

Promotion of Effective Therapy

Once the diagnosis of deep venous thrombosis is made, the nurse maintains the heparin therapy, provides for appropriate comfort measures, and monitors the woman closely for signs of pulmonary embolism. The nurse also assesses for evidence of bleeding related to heparin and keeps the antagonist for heparin, protamine sulfate, readily available.

Education for Self-Care

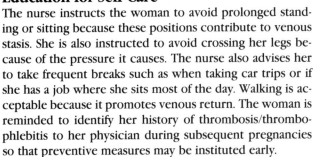

The nurse instructs the woman to avoid prolonged standing or sitting because these positions contribute to venous stasis. She is also instructed to avoid crossing her legs because of the pressure it causes. The nurse also advises her to take frequent breaks such as when taking car trips or if she has a job where she sits most of the day. Walking is acceptable because it promotes venous return. The woman is reminded to identify her history of thrombosis/thrombophlebitis to her physician during subsequent pregnancies so that preventive measures may be instituted early.

Women who are discharged on warfarin must understand the purpose of the medication and be alert to signs of hemorrhage such as bleeding gums, epistaxis, petechiae or ecchymosis, or evidence of blood in the urine or stool. Since careful monitoring is important, the woman should clearly understand the need to keep scheduled appointments for prothrombin time assessment. Certain medications such as aspirin and nonsteroidal antiinflammatory drugs increase anticoagulant activity, so they should be avoided. In fact, the woman should check for possible medication interaction before taking any medication while on warfarin. A woman may choose to carry a Medic Alert card in case of emergency. She should also have vitamin K available in case bleeding occurs. Warfarin is excreted in the breast milk and thus may present problems for breast-feeding mothers. Women who wish to continue nursing may be maintained at home on low doses of subcutaneous heparin, since heparin is not excreted in breast milk.

Evaluation

Anticipated outcomes of nursing care include the following:

- If thrombosis/thrombophlebitis develops, it is detected quickly and managed successfully without further complications.
- At discharge the woman is able to explain the purpose, dosage regimen, and necessary precautions associated with any prescribed medications such as anticoagulants.

- The woman can discuss self-care measures and ongoing therapies (such as the use of elastic stockings) that are indicated.
- The woman has bonded successfully with her newborn and is able to care for the baby effectively.

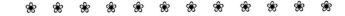

Pulmonary Embolism

A sudden onset of dyspnea accompanied by sweating, pallor, cyanosis, confusion, systemic hypotension, cough (with or without hemoptysis), tachycardia, shortness of breath, fever, and increased jugular pressure may indicate **pulmonary embolism**, a blockage of the pulmonary artery. Chest pain that mimics heart attack, coupled with the woman's verbalized fear of imminent death and complaint of pressure in the bowel and rectum, should alert the nurse to the extensive size of the embolus. A friction rub and evidence of atelectasis may be noted upon auscultation. A gallop (heart) rhythm may be present even if respiratory inspiration is normal, although smaller emboli may present with only transient syncope, tightness of the chest, or unexplained pyrexia.

Even x-ray films and electrocardiographic (ECG) changes and laboratory data are not always reliable. If a case of pulmonary embolism is suspected, prompt treatment should begin even in the absence of corroborative data. If the embolism is small and heparin therapy is begun quickly, the chance of survival is excellent. However, when a large thrombus occludes a major pulmonary vessel, death may occur before therapy can even begin.

Therapy involves the administration of a variety of intravenous medications, such as meperidine hydrochloride to relieve the pain, lidocaine to correct any arrhythmias, and drugs such as papaverine hydrochloride and aminophylline to reduce spasms of the bronchi and coronary and pulmonary vessels. Oxygen is administered and heparin infusion is begun. In severe cases an embolectomy may be necessary, although fibrinolytic therapy with medications (such as streptokinase) that lyse clots may be tried first.

Care of the Woman with a Urinary Tract Infection (UTI)

The postpartal woman is at increased risk of developing urinary tract problems due to the normal postpartal diuresis, increased bladder capacity, decreased bladder sensitivity from stretching and/or trauma, and possible inhibited neural control of the bladder following the use of general or regional anesthesia and contamination from catheterization. The discontinuation of Pitocin may also lead to sudden diuresis, since Pitocin has an antidiuretic effect and therefore overdistends the bladder.

Emptying the bladder is vital. Women who have not sufficiently recovered from the effects of anesthesia cannot void spontaneously, and catheterization is necessary.

Retention of residual urine, bacteria introduced at the time of catheterization, and a bladder traumatized by childbirth combine to provide an excellent environment for the development of cystitis.

Overdistention

Overdistention occurs postpartally when the woman is unable to empty her bladder as a result of the predisposing factors previously identified.

Medical Therapy

Overdistention in the early postpartal period is often managed by draining the bladder with a straight catheter as a one-time measure. If the overdistention recurs or is diagnosed later in the postpartal period, an indwelling catheter is generally ordered for 24 hours.

❀ *APPLYING THE NURSING PROCESS* ❀

Nursing Assessment

The overdistended bladder appears as a large mass, reaching sometimes to the umbilicus and displacing the uterine fundus upward. There is increased vaginal bleeding, the fundus is boggy, and the woman may complain of cramping as the uterus attempts to contract.

Nursing Diagnosis

Nursing diagnoses that may apply when a woman has difficulties due to overdistention include the following:

- Infection: High risk related to urinary stasis secondary to overdistention
- Alteration in patterns of urinary elimination related to overdistention

Nursing Plan and Implementation

Prevention of Overdistention

Diligent monitoring of the bladder during the recovery period and preventive health measures greatly reduce the chance for overdistention of the bladder. Encouraging the mother to void spontaneously and assisting her to use the toilet, if possible, or the bedpan if she has received conductive anesthesia, prevents overdistention in most cases. The woman should be medicated for whatever pain she may be having before attempting to void since pain may cause a reflex spasm of the urethra. Ice packs applied to the perineum immediately postpartum will minimize any edema,

which may interfere with voiding. Pouring warm water over the perineum or having the woman void in a sitz bath may also help.

Promotion of Safe, Effective Catheterization

If catherization becomes necessary, careful, meticulous, aseptic technique should be employed during catheter insertion.

The vagina and vulva are traumatized to some degree by vaginal birth, and edema is common. This edema may obscure the urinary meatus; therefore, the nurse needs to be extremely careful in cleansing the vulva and inserting the catheter. It is imperative to discard a catheter that has inadvertently been introduced into the vagina and thus contaminated. Because catheterization is an uncomfortable procedure due to the postpartal trauma and edema of the tissue, the nurse should be careful and gentle not only in inserting the catheter but also in handling and cleaning the perineal area.

If the amount of urine drained from the bladder reaches 900 to 1000 mL, an indwelling catheter should be clamped, the Foley balloon inflated, and the catheter taped firmly to the woman's leg. The procedure, including taking the woman's vital signs before and after the procedure and noting her responses, should be carefully charted. After an hour, the catheter may be unclamped and placed on gravity drainage. This technique protects the bladder and avoids rapid intraabdominal decompression. When the indwelling catheter is removed, a urine specimen is often sent to the laboratory. The tip of the catheter may also be removed and sent for culture.

Evaluation

Anticipated outcomes of nursing care include the following:

- The woman voids adequately to meet the demands of the increased fluid shifts during the postpartal period.
- The woman doesn't develop infection due to stasis of urine.
- The woman actively incorporates self-care measures to decrease bladder overdistention.

❀ ❀ ❀ ❀ ❀ ❀ ❀ ❀ ❀ ❀ ❀

Cystitis (Lower Urinary Tract Infection)

E coli has been demonstrated to be the causative agent in most cases of postpartal cystitis and pyelonephritis (in both lower and upper UTI). In most cases the infection ascends the urinary tract from the urethra to the bladder and then to the kidneys because vesiculoureteral reflux forces contaminated urine into the renal pelvis.

Medical Therapy

When cystitis is suspected a clean-catch midstream urine sample is obtained for microscopic examination, culture, and sensitivity tests. A catheterized specimen is avoided when possible because of the increased risk of infection. When the bacterial concentration is greater than 100,000 microorganisms per milliliter of fresh urine, infection is generally present; counts between 10,000 and 100,000 are suggestive of infection, particularly if clinical symptoms are noted.

Treatment is theoretically delayed until urine culture and sensitivity reports are available. In the clinical setting, however, antibiotic therapy is often initiated using one of the short-acting sulfonamides, nitrofurantoin (Macrodantin), or, in the case of sulfa allergy, ampicillin. The antibiotic is begun immediately and then can be changed if indicated by the results of the sensitivity report (Cunningham et al 1989). Antispasmodics may be given to relieve discomfort.

Pyelonephritis (Upper Urinary Tract Infection)

Pyelonephritis is an inflammation of the renal pelvis that is usually the result of infection. In most cases the infection has ascended from the lower urinary tract. It occurs more commonly on the right, although both kidneys may be affected. If untreated, the renal cortex may be damaged and kidney function impaired.

Medical Therapy

When pyelonephritis is diagnosed, antibiotic therapy is begun immediately. If sensitivity reports so indicate, the antibiotic can be changed as needed. Bed rest and careful monitoring of intake and output are necessary to detect the development of bacterial shock. Fluids are encouraged; if nausea and vomiting are severe, however, fluids are administered intravenously. Antispasmodics, analgesics, and antipyretics are given to relieve discomfort. The woman usually continues to take antibiotics for two to four weeks after clinical and bacteriologic response. A clean-catch urine culture should be obtained two weeks after completion of therapy and then periodically for the next two years.

Continuation of breast-feeding during therapy is limited only by the degree of the mother's malaise and clinical discomfort. For the breast-feeding mother the antibiotic chosen should be selected carefully to avoid problems for the infant via the milk.

❀   *APPLYING THE NURSING PROCESS*   ❀

Nursing Assessment

Symptoms of cystitis often appear two to three days after birth. The initial symptoms of cystitis may include frequency, urgency, dysuria, and nocturia. Hematuria and su-

prapubic pain may also be present. A slightly elevated temperature may occur, but systemic symptoms are often absent.

When a urinary tract infection progresses to pyelonephritis, systemic symptoms usually occur, and the woman becomes acutely ill. Symptoms include chills, high fever, flank pain (unilateral or bilateral), nausea, and vomiting, in addition to all the signs of lower UTI. Costovertebral pain also may be present. The nurse obtains a urine culture and sensitivity to identify the causative organism.

Nursing Diagnosis

Nursing diagnoses that may apply if a woman develops a UTI postpartally include the following:

- Pain related to dysuria secondary to cystitis
- Knowledge deficit related to long-term effects of pyelonephritis
- Knowledge deficit related to self-care measures to prevent UTI

Nursing Plan and Implementation

Prevention of Urinary Tract Infection

As with other conditions, the nurse plays an important role in preventing the development of UTI. Screening for asymptomatic bacteriuria in pregnancy should be routine. Frequent emptying of the bladder during labor and the postpartum period should be encouraged to prevent overdistention and trauma to the bladder. Nursing actions to prevent overdistention and catheterization technique previously discussed also apply. The woman with pyelonephritis must understand the importance of follow-up care after discharge to prevent recurrence or further complications.

Education for Self-Care

The postpartal woman should be advised to continue good perineal hygiene following discharge. She is also advised to maintain a good fluid intake and to empty her bladder whenever she feels the urge to void, but at least every two to four hours while awake. She can also void following sexual intercourse (to wash any contaminants from the vicinity of the meatus) and to wear cotton-crotch underwear to facilitate air circulation.

A woman diagnosed with pyelonephritis must understand the potential seriousness of the condition and be urged to monitor herself for any symptoms of UTI.

Evaluation

Anticipated outcomes of nursing care include the following:

- Signs of urinary tract infection are detected quickly and the condition is treated successfully.

- The woman incorporates self-care measures to prevent the recurrence of UTI as part of her personal hygiene routine.
- The woman continues with any long-term therapy or follow-up.
- Maternal-infant attachment is maintained and the woman is able to care for her newborn effectively.

Care of the Woman with Mastitis

Mastitis refers to an inflammation of the breast generally caused by *Staphylococcus aureus* and primarily seen in breast-feeding mothers. Symptoms seldom occur before the second to fourth week postpartally, so nurses often are not fully aware of how uncomfortable and acutely ill the woman may be. The most common source of the bacteria is the infant's nose and throat, although other sources include the hands of the mother or of hospital personnel or the woman's circulating blood.

Poor drainage of milk, presence of a pathogenic organism, lowered maternal defenses due to fatigue or stress, poor hygiene practices, or nipple tissue damage make the woman susceptible to mastitis. Tight clothing, missed feedings, poor support of pendulous breasts, a return to work outside the home, or a baby who suddenly begins to sleep through the night can all result in milk stasis, which is a milder inflammatory condition.

Thomsen (1984) has suggested a classification of inflammatory symptoms of the breast based on leukocytes and bacterial counts per milliliter of breast milk: (1) milk stasis; (2) noninfectious inflammation of the breast; and (3) infectious mastitis. Milk stasis is a relatively mild, short-lived condition, usually without fever and not requiring antibiotics. Noninfectious inflammation of the breast presents with more severe inflammatory symptoms that last for several days. Infectious mastitis is a more serious infection with fever, headache, flulike symptoms, and a warm, reddened, painful area of the breast (Figure 36–3).

Medical Therapy

Diagnosis is usually based on symptoms and physical examination, even while waiting for laboratory results. The need for culture and antibody sensitivity of the breast milk remains controversial, although most authors agree on the need for cultures if there is a recurrence of the mastitis. Treatment involves bed rest, increased fluid intake, a supportive bra, feeding the baby frequently, local application of heat, and analgesics for discomfort. Early treatment may prevent the progression of milk stasis and noninfectious inflammation to mastitis. Treatment of mastitis includes all of the measures mentioned previously plus a ten-day course of antibiotics (usually a penicillinase-resistant penicillin). Improved outcome, a decreased duration of symptoms,

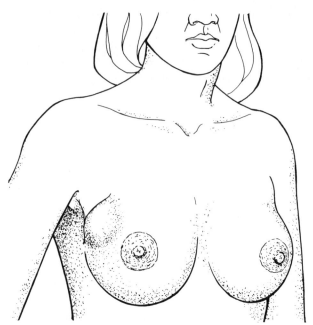

Figure 36–3 Mastitis. Erythema and swelling are present in the upper outer quadrant of the breast. Axillary lymph nodes are enlarged and tender.

and decreased incidence of breast abscess result if the breasts continue to be emptied by either nursing or pumping. Whether to continue nursing or not has been controversial in the past but most experts now recommend continued nursing in most cases. The woman should be contacted within 24 hours of initiation of treatment to ensure that symptoms are subsiding (Lawrence 1989).

Occasionally the process of mastitis may continue and a frank abscess develops. The mother's milk and any drainage from the nipple should be cultured and antibiotic therapy instituted. In addition, it is usually necessary to incise surgically and drain the abscessed area. If multiple abscesses are present, multiple incisions will be necessary, usually under general anesthesia. After incision and drainage, the area is packed with sterile gauze. The packing is gradually decreased to permit proper healing.

Often the breast is covered with a sterile surgical dressing and access to the breast is temporarily inhibited, making breast-feeding impossible. If possible, the dressing should be applied so that the woman can continue to breast-feed or pump her breast, thereby avoiding engorgement.

❀ *APPLYING THE NURSING PROCESS* ❀

Nursing Assessment

Daily assessment of breast consistency, skin color, surface temperature, and nipple condition is essential to detect early signs of problems that may predispose to mastitis. The mother should be observed nursing her baby to ensure use of proper breast-feeding technique.

If an infection has developed, the nurse should assess for contributing factors such as cracked nipples, poor hygiene, engorgement, supplemental feedings, change in routine or infant feeding pattern, abrupt weaning, or lack of proper breast support so that these factors may be corrected as part of the treatment plan.

Nursing Diagnosis

Nursing diagnoses that may apply to the woman with mastitis include the following:

- Knowledge deficit related to appropriate breast-feeding practices
- Altered parenting related to pain secondary to development of mastitis

Nursing Plan and Implementation

Prevention of Mastitis

Prevention of mastitis is far simpler than therapy. Ideally mothers should be instructed in proper breast-feeding technique prenatally. If not, instruction should begin as soon as possible in the postpartal period. The nurse should assist the mother to breast-feed soon after birth and should review correct technique. All women, even those not breast-feeding, are encouraged to wear a good supportive bra at all times to avoid milk stasis, especially in the lower lobes.

Meticulous hand washing by all personnel is the primary measure in preventing epidemic nursery infections and subsequent maternal mastitis. Prompt attention to mothers who have blocked milk ducts eliminates stagnant milk as a growth medium for bacteria. If the mother finds that one area of her breast feels distended, she can rotate the position of her infant for nursing, manually express milk remaining in the breast after nursing (usually only necessary if the infant is not sucking well), or massage the caked area toward the nipple as the infant nurses. Early identification and intervention for sore nipples are also essential.

Education for Self-Care

The nurse stresses to the breast-feeding woman the importance of adequate breast and nipple care to prevent the development of cracks and fissures, a common portal for bacterial entry.

The woman should be aware of the importance of regular, complete emptying of the breasts to prevent engorgement and stasis. She should also understand the role of let-down in successful breast-feeding and the principle of supply and demand. Mothers who will be breast-feeding and returning to work need information on how to do so successfully. Since mastitis tends to develop following discharge, it is important to include information about signs and symptoms in the discharge teaching. All flulike symptoms should be considered a sign of mastitis until proved otherwise. If symptoms develop, the woman should contact her care giver immediately because prompt treatment helps to avoid abscess formation.

Evaluation

Anticipated outcomes of nursing care include the following:

- The woman is aware of the signs and symptoms of mastitis.
- The woman's mastitis is detected early and treated successfully.
- The woman can continue breast-feeding if she chooses.
- The woman understands self-care measures she can employ to prevent the recurrence of the mastitis.

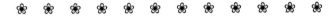

Care of the Woman with a Postpartal Psychiatric Disorder

Many types of psychiatric problems may occur in the postpartum period. The classification of postpartum psychiatric disorders is a subject of some controversy. The *Diagnostic and Statistical Manual of Mental Disorders,* 3rd edition, revised (DSM-IIIR), does not have a separate classification for postpartum psychiatric disorders. In contrast, Inwood (1989) proposes that postpartum psychiatric disorders be considered one diagnosable syndrome with three subclasses: (1) adjustment reaction with depressed mood; (2) postpartum psychosis; and (3) postpartum major mood disorder. The incidence, etiology, symptoms, treatment, and prognosis vary with each subclass.

Adjustment reaction with depressed mood is also known as postpartum, maternal, or "baby" blues. It occurs in at least 50% of all women and is a common, short-lived, early-onset disorder characterized by mild depression, anxiety, crying episodes, headache, fatigue, and irritability. It is more severe in primiparas and seems related to the rapid alteration of estrogen. progesterone, and prolactin levels after birth. Emotional support, information, and reassurance are usually sufficient for recovery.

Postpartum psychosis has an incidence of 1 to 2 per 1000 births. Symptoms include agitation, restlessness, insomnia, mood lability, tearfulness, elation, confusion, irrationality, hallucinations, and delirium. Recovery is usually good, unless schizophrenia is diagnosed. There is a 10% to 50% recurrence rate with subsequent pregnancies. The possibility of suicide or infanticide is highest (up to 10%) in this group (Inwood 1989). Risk factors include: (1) previous puerperal psychosis; (2) manic depressive history;

(3) prenatal stressors such as lack of social support, illegitimacy, and low socioeconomic status; (4) obsessive personality; or (5) a family history of a mood disorder. Treatment consists of hospitalization, antipsychotics, sedatives, electroconvulsive therapy, removal of the infant, social support, psychotherapy, and child care assistance.

Postpartum major mood disorder, major depression, or postpartum neurosis develops in about 10% of all postpartum women. Its onset is later, from four weeks up to one year postpartum. Postpartum blues, socioeconomic status, or obstetric complications such as fetal death, prematurity, or cesarean birth have not been found to be risk factors for postpartum depression. Risk factors include (1) primiparity; (2) ambivalence about maintaining the pregnancy; (3) history of postpartum depression or bipolar illness; (4) lack of social support; (5) lack of a stable relationship with parents or partner; (6) the woman's dissatisfaction with herself; and (7) lack of a supportive relationship with her parents, especially her father, as a child (Inwood 1989). Medication, psychotherapy, support—especially for child care, and hospitalization—if needed—are commonly used in treatment. Prognosis varies from good to continuing recurrences of the problem.

✤ *APPLYING THE NURSING PROCESS* ✤

Nursing Assessment

Assessment for factors predisposing to postpartum depression or psychosis should begin prenatally. Questions designed to detect problems can be included as part of the routine prenatal history interview or questionnaire. Women with a personal or family history of psychiatric disease, particularly postpartum depression or psychosis, need prenatal instruction on the signs and symptoms of depression and additional emotional support. If not done previously, the woman is assessed for predisposing factors during her labor and postpartum stay.

In providing daily care, the nurse observes the woman for signs of depression: anxiety, irritability, poor concentration, forgetfulness, sleeping difficulties, appetite change, fatigue, tearfulness, and statements indicating feelings of failure and self-accusation. Severity and duration of symptoms should be noted. Behavior and verbalizations that are bizarre or seem to indicate a potential for violence against herself or others, including the infant, are reported as soon as possible for further evaluation.

The nurse needs to be aware that many normal physiologic changes of the puerperium are similar to symptoms of depression (lack of sexual interest, appetite change, and fatigue). It is essential that observations be as specific and as objective as possible and that they be carefully documented.

Nursing Diagnosis

Possible nursing diagnoses that may apply to a woman with a postpartum psychiatric disorder include the following:

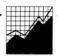

Research Note

Clinical Application of Research

To identify possible predictors of a postpartum emotional reaction (PEREA), Andrea Laizner and Mary Ellen Jeans (1990) used multiple regression analysis. The predictor variables included current health and emotional status, prior psychiatric history, psychosocial assets, locus of control, maternal adaptation to motherhood, and life-change events. State and trait aspects of anxiety, depression, and hostility were measured prenatally, immediately postpartum, and at one month postpartum. The measurements at one month became the dependent variable of PEREA. Fifty-nine percent of the 27 women studied reported an increase in negative affect.

Regression analysis of predictor variables measured prenatally showed that prenatal depression state was significantly related to trait anxiety, trait depression, state anxiety, state depression, and state hostility at one month postpartum. Two of the scales used to evaluate health locus of control, as well as other variables, accounted for significant amounts of variance with one or more of the states and traits.

The in-hospital depression state and in-hospital hostility state both contributed to several of the state and trait aspects used to measure the dependent variable of PEREA. Other important predictors included health locus of control and life-change events.

Critical Thinking Applied to Research

Strengths: Gave specific operational definitions of variables. Gave some psychometric properties of the tools both from prior research studies as well as from current study.

Concerns: Low sample sizes—less than 30 subjects per independent variable—can create high variances, which are actually artifact (Munro et al 1986). A table of measurement findings of the dependent variable (PEREA) would have strengthened the report of the study.

Munro B, Visintainer M, Page E: *Statistical Methods for Health Care Research.* Philadelphia: Lippincott, 1986.

Laizner A, Jeans M: (1990). Identification of predictor variables of postpartum emotional reaction. *Health Care Women Internat* 1990; 11:191.

- Ineffective individual coping related to postpartum depression
- Alteration: in bonding high risk related to child neglect secondary to postpartum psychosis

Nursing Plan and Implementation

Prevention and Provision of Effective Care

The nurse should alert the mother, spouse, and other family members to the possibility of postpartum blues in the early days after birth and reassure them of the short-term nature of the condition. Symptoms of postpartum depression should be described and the mother encouraged to call her health care provider if symptoms become severe, if they fail to subside quickly, or if at any time she feels she is unable to function. Encouraging the mother to plan how she will manage at home and providing concrete suggestions on how to cope will aid in her adjustment to motherhood. Telephone follow-up at three weeks postpartum to ask if the mother is experiencing difficulties is also helpful (Inwood 1989). Home visits, especially for early discharge families, is essential to fostering positive adjustments for the new family constellation.

Women with a history of depression or postpartum psychosis should be referred to a mental health professional for counseling and biweekly visits between the second and sixth week postpartum for evaluation of depression. Medication, social support, and assistance with child care may also be necessary.

The presence of symptoms from four of the following categories that persist daily for two or more weeks is indicative of serious depression. The categories are as follows: (1) appetite or weight change, (2) insomnia or hypersomnia, (3) psychomotor agitation or retardation, (4) loss of interest or pleasure in usual activities, (5) loss of energy, (6) feelings of worthlessness or guilt, (7) difficulty concentrating or making decisions, or (8) thoughts of death or suicide (Garvey 1984). Referral to a mental health professional should be made immediately. Immediate referral should also be made if rejection of the infant or threatened or actual aggression against the infant has occurred.

A diagnosis of postpartum depression or other psychiatric disorder will pose a major problem for the family. Information, emotional support, and assistance in providing or obtaining care for the infant may be needed. The nurse can assist family members by identifying community resources and making referrals to public health nursing services and social services. Postpartum follow-up (home visits, group support, and telephone follow-up), which all postpartum women need, is especially important for the woman at risk for or experiencing postpartum depression (Hampson 1989).

Evaluation

Anticipated outcomes of nursing care include the following:

- Signs of potential postpartal disorders are detected quickly and therapy is implemented.
- The newborn is cared for effectively by the father or another support person until the mother is able to do so.

KEY CONCEPTS

Nursing assessment and intervention play a large role in the prevention of postpartum complications.

The main causes of early postpartal hemorrhage are uterine atony, lacerations of the vagina and cervix, and retained placental fragments.

The most common postpartal infection is endometritis, which is limited to the uterine cavity.

Thromboembolic disease originating in the veins of the leg, thigh, or pelvis may occur in the antepartum or postpartum periods and carries with it the potential for creating a pulmonary embolus.

A postpartal woman is at increased risk for developing urinary tract problems due to normal postpartal diuresis, increased bladder capacity, decreased bladder sensitivity from stretching and/or trauma, and, possibly, inhibited neural control of the bladder following the use of anesthetic agents.

Mastitis is an inflammation of the breast caused by *Staphylococcus aureus* and is primarily seen in breast-feeding women. Symptoms seldom occur before the second to fourth postpartal week.

Although many different types of psychiatric problems may be encountered in the postpartal period, depression is the most common. Episodes occur frequently in the week after birth and are typically transient.

References

Barger MK (editor): *Protocols for Gynecologic and Obstetric Health Care*. Orlando, FL: Grune & Stratton, 1988.

Cunningham FG, MacDonald PC, Gant NF (editors): *Williams Obstetrics*, 18th ed. Norwalk, CT: Appleton & Lange, 1989.

Fagnant RJ, Monif RG: Uncovering and correcting septic pelvic thrombophlebitis. *Contemp OB/GYN* February 1987; 29:129.

Few BJ: Prostaglandin F_2 for treating severe postpartum hemorrhage. *MCN* May/June 1987; 12:169.

Garvey MJ, Tollefson GD: Postpartum depression. *J Reprod Med* 1984; 29(2):113.

Hampson SJ: Nursing interventions for the first three postpartum months. *JOGNN* March/April 1989; 18:116.

Heffner LJ, Mennuti MT, Rudoff JC et al: Primary management of postpartum vulvovaginal hematomas by angiographic embolization. *Am J Perinatol* 1985; 2(3):204.

Inwood DG: Postpartum psychiatric disorders. In: *Comprehensive Textbook of Psychiatry/V*, 5th ed. Vol. 1. Kaplan HI, Sadock BJ (editors). Baltimore: Williams & Wilkins, 1989.

Lawrence RA: *Breastfeeding: A Guide for the Medical Professional*, 3rd ed. St. Louis: Mosby, 1989.

Soper DE: Postpartum endometritis, pathophysiology and prevention. *J Reprod Med* 1988; 33(1) (Suppl):97.

Sutton GP, Smirz LR, Clark DH et al: Group B streptococcal necrotizing fasciitis arising from an episiotomy. *Obstet Gynecol* 1985; 66(5):733.

Thomsen AC, Esperson T, Maigaard S: Course and treatment of milk stasis, noninfectious inflammation of the breast, and infectious mastitis in nursing women. *Am J Obstet Gyencol* 1984; 149(5):492.

Watts DH, Eschenbach DA, Kenny GE: Early postpartum endometritis: the role of bacteria, genital mycoplasmas, and *Chlamydia trachomatis*. *Obstet Gynecol* 1989; 73(1):52.

Additional Readings

Kornblit P, Senderoff J, Davis-Ericksen M, Zenk J: Anticoagulation therapy: Patient management and evaluation of an outpatient clinic. *Nurse Practitioner* 1990; 15(8):22.

McAnarney ER, Stevens-Simon C: Maternal psychological stress/ Depression and low birth weight: Is there a relationship? *Am J Dis Child* July 1990; 144:789.

Puckering C: Annotation: Maternal depression. *J Child Psychol Psychiatr* 1989; 30(6):807.

Robie GF et al: Logothetopulos pack for the management of uncontrollable postpartum hemorrhage. *Am J Perinatol* 1990; 7(4):327.

Rutherford SE, Phelan JP: Deep venous thrombosis and pulmonary embolus. In: *Critical Care Obstetrics*. Clark SL, Phelan J, Cotton DB (editors). Oradell, NJ: Medical Economics Books, 1987.

Weil A, Reyes H, Rottenberg RD et al: Effect of lumbar epidural analgesia on lower urinary tract function in the immediate postpartum period. *Br J Obstet Gynecol* May 1983; 90:428.

Appendices

Common Abbreviations in Maternal-Newborn and Women's Health Nursing

---

ABC	Alternative birthing center *or* airway, breathing, circulation
Accel	Acceleration of fetal heart rate
AC	Abdominal circumference
ACTH	Adrenocorticotrophic hormone
AFAFP	Amniotic fluid alpha fetoprotein
AFP	α-fetoprotein
AFV	Amniotic fluid volume
AGA	Average for gestational age
AID or AIH	Artificial insemination donor (H designates mate is donor)
AIDS	Acquired Immune Deficiency Syndrome
ARBOW	Artificial rupture of bag of waters
AROM	Artificial rupture of membranes
BAT	Brown adipose tissue (brown fat)
BBT	Basal body temperature
BL	Baseline (fetal heart rate baseline)
BMR	Basal metabolic rate
BOW	Bag of waters
BP	Blood pressure
BPD	Biparietal diameter *or* Bronchopulmonary dysplasia
BPM	Beats per minute
BSE	Breast self examination
BSST	Breast self-stimulation test
CC	Chest circumference *or* Cord compression
cc	cubic centimeter
CDC	Centers for Disease Control
C-H	Crown-to-heel length
CHF	Congestive heart failure
CID	Cytomegalic inclusion disease
CMV	Cytomegalovirus
cm	centimeter
CNM	Certified nurse-midwife
CNS	Central nervous system
CPAP	Continuous positive airway pressure
CPD	Cephalopelvic disproportion *or* Citrate-phosphate-dextrose
CPR	Cardiopulmonary resuscitation
CRL	Crown-rump length
C/S	Cesarean section or C-section
CST	Contraction stress test
CT	Computerized tomography
CVA	Costovertebral angle
CVP	Central venous pressure
CVS	Chorionic villus sampling
D&C	Dilatation and curettage
decels	deceleration of fetal heart rate
DFMR	Daily fetal movement response
DIC	Disseminated intravascular coagulation
dil	dilatation
DM	Diabetes mellitus
DRG	Diagnostic related groups
DTR	Deep tendon reflexes
ECHMO	Extracorporal membrane oxygenator
EDC	Estimated date of confinement
EDD	Estimated date of delivery
EFM	Electronic fetal monitoring

EFW	Estimated fetal weight
ELF	Elective low forceps
epis	Episiotomy
FAD	Fetal activity diary
FAS	Fetal alcohol syndrome
FBD	Fibrocystic breast disease
FBM	Fetal breathing movements
FBS	Fetal blood sample *or* fasting blood sugar test
FECG	Fetal electrocardiogram
FFA	Free fatty acids
FHR	Fetal heart rate
FHT	Fetal heart tones
FL	Femur length
FM	Fetal movement
FMAC	Fetal movement acceleration test
FMD	Fetal movement diary
FMR	Fetal movement record
FPG	Fasting plasma glucose test
FRC	Female reproductive cycle
FSH	Follicle-stimulating hormone
FSHRH	Follicle-stimulating hormone-releasing hormone
FSI	Foam stability index
G or grav	Gravida
GDM	Gestational diabetes mellitus
GFR	Glomerular filtration rate
GI	Gastrointestinal
GnRF	Gonadotrophin-releasing factor
GnRH	Gonadotrophin-releasing hormone
GTPAL	Gravida, term, preterm, abortion, living children; a system of recording maternity history
GYN	Gynecology
HA	Head-abdominal rates
HAI	Hemagglutination-inhibition test
HC	Head compression
hCG	Human chorionic gonadotrophin
hCS	Human chorionic somatomammotrophin (same as hPL)
HMD	Hyaline membrane disease
hMG	Human menopausal gonadotrophin
hPL	Human placental lactogen
HVH	Herpes virus hominis
ICS	Intercostal space
IDDM	Insulin-dependent diabetes mellitus (Type I)
IDM	Infant of a diabetic mother
IGT	Impaired glucose tolerance
IGTT	Intravenous glucose tolerance test
IPG	Impedance phlebography
IUD	Intrauterine device
IUFD	Intrauterine fetal death
IUGR	Intrauterine growth retardation
JCAH	Joint Commission on the Accreditation of Hospitals
LADA	Left-acromion-dorsal-anterior
LADP	Left-acromion-dorsal-posterior
LBW	Low birth weight
LDR	Labor, delivery and recovery room
LGA	Large for gestational age
LH	Luteinizing hormone

LHRH	Luteinizing hormone-releasing hormone
LMA	Left-mentum-anterior
LML	Left mediolateral episiotomy
LMP	Last mentrual period *or* Left-mentum-posterior
LMT	Left-mentum-transverse
LOA	Left-occiput-anterior
LOF	Low outlet forceps
LOP	Left-occiput-posterior
LOT	Left-occiput-transverse
L/S	Lecithin/sphingomyelin ratio
LSA	Left-sacrum-anterior
LSP	Left-sacrum-posterior
LST	Left-sacrum-transverse
MAS	Meconium aspiration syndrome *or* Movement alarm signal
MCT	Medium chain triglycerides
mec	Meconium
mec st	Meconium stain
M & I	Maternity and Infant Care Projects
ML	Midline (episiotomy)
MLE	Midline echo
MRI	Magnetic resonance imaging
MSAFP	Maternal serum alpha fetoprotein
MUGB	4-methylumbelliferyl quanidinobenzoate
multip	Multipara
NANDA	North American Nursing Diagnosis Association
NEC	Necrotizing enterocolitis
NGU	Nongonococcal urethritis
NIDDM	Noninsulin-dependent diabetes mellitus (Type II)
NIH	National Institutes of Health
NP	Nurse practitioner
NPO	Nothing by mouth
NSCST	Nipple stimulation contraction stress test
NST	Nonstress test *or* nonshivering thermogenesis
NTD	Neural tube defects
NSVD	Normal sterile vaginal delivery
OA	Occiput anterior
OB	Obstetrics
OCT	Oxytocin challenge test
OF	Occipitofrontal diameter of fetal head
OFC	Occipitofrontal circumference
OGTT	Oral glucose tolerance test
OM	Occipitomental (diameter)
OP	Occiput posterior
p	Para
Pap smear	Papanicolaou smear
PBI	Protein-bound iodine
PDA	Patent ductus arteriosus
PEEP	Positive end-expiratory pressure
PG	Phosphatidyglycerol *or* Prostaglandin
PI	Phosphatidylinositol
PID	Pelvic inflammatory disease
PIH	Pregnancy-induced hypertension
Pit	Pitocin
PKU	Phenylketonuria
PMI	Point of maximal impulse
PPHN	Persistent pulmonary hypertension
Preemie	Premature infant
Primip	Primapara

PROM	Premature rupture of membranes
PTT	Partial thromboplastin test
PUBS	Percutaneous umbilical blood sampling
RADA	Right-acromion-dorsal-anterior
RADP	Right-acromion-dorsal-posterior
REEDA	Redness, edema, ecchymosis, discharge (or drainage), approximation (a system for recording wound healing)
RDA	Recommended dietary allowance
RDS	Respiratory distress syndrome
REM	Rapid eye movements
RIA	Radioimmune assay
RLF	Retrolental fibroplasia
ROA	Right-occiput-anterior
ROP	Right-occiput-posterior
ROP	Retinopathy of prematurity
ROM	Rupture of membranes
ROT	Right-occiput-transverse
RMA	Right-mentum-anterior
RMP	Right-mentum-posterior
RMT	Right-mentum-transverse
RRA	Radioreceptor assay
RSA	Right-sacrum-anterior
RSP	Right-sacrum-posterior
RST	Right-sacrum-transverse
SET	Surrogate embryo transfer
SFD	Small for dates
SGA	Small for gestational age
SIDS	Sudden infant death syndrome
SOAP	Subjective data, objective data, analysis, plan
SOB	Suboccipitobregmatic diameter
SMB	Submentobregmatic diameter
SRBOW	Spontaneous rupture of the bag of waters
SROM	Spontaneous rupture of the membranes
STD	Sexually transmitted disease
STH	Somatotrophic hormone
STS	Serologic test for syphilis
SVE	Sterile vaginal exam
TC	Thoracic circumference
TCM	Transcutaneous monitoring
TNZ	Thermal neutral zone
TORCH	Toxoplasmosis, rubella, cytomegalovirus, herpesvirus hominis type 2
TSS	Toxic shock syndrome
ū	umbilicus
u/a	urinalysis
UA	Uterine activity
UAC	Umbilical artery catheter
UAU	Uterine activity units
UC	Uterine contraction
UPI	Uteroplacental insufficiency
U/S	Ultrasound
UTI	Urinary tract infection
VBAC	Vaginal birth after cesarean
VDRL	Venereal Disease Research Laboratories
WBC	White blood cell
WIC	Supplemental food program for Women, Infants, and Children

NAACOG's Standards for Obstetric, Gynecologic, and Neonatal Nursing

I: NURSING PRACTICE

STANDARD: Comprehensive obstetric, gynecologic, and neonatal (OGN) nursing care is provided to the individual, family, and community within the framework of the nursing process.

INTERPRETATION: The nurse is responsible for decisions and actions within the domain of nursing practice. Comprehensive nursing care includes assisting the person to meet physical, psychosocial, spiritual, and developmental needs. Systematic use of the nursing process which encompasses assessment, nursing diagnosis, planning, implementation, and evaluation will meet the patient's needs. Individualized nursing care is best achieved by collaboration with patient, family, and other members of the health-care team. Complete and accurate documentation of all nursing care and patient response is essential for continuity of care and for meeting legal requirements. The nurse must promote a safe and therapeutic environment for the individual, family, and community.

II: HEALTH EDUCATION

STANDARD: Health education for the individual, family, and community is an integral part of obstetric, gynecologic, and neonatal nursing practice.

INTERPRETATION: The nurse is responsible for providing pertinent information to the individual, family, and community so they may participate in and share responsibility for their own health promotion, maintenance, and restorative care. The nurse plans, implements, and evaluates health education based on principles of teaching and learning. To enhance health care and promote continuity of health education, the nurse uses the educational resources within the community and collaborates with other health-care providers.

Health education should be documented and evaluated. Evaluation is based on individualized goals and set criteria.

III: POLICIES AND PROCEDURES

STANDARD: The delivery of obstetric, gynecologic, and neonatal nursing care is based on written policies and procedures.

INTERPRETATION: Policies and procedures define the boundaries of nursing practice within the health-care setting and indicate the qualifications of personnel authorized to perform OGN nursing procedures. The qualifications may include educational preparation and/or certification. The policies and procedures should be in accordance with the philosophy of the agency, state nurse practice act, governmental regulations, and other applicable standards or regulations.

A multidisciplinary framework should be used in writing policies and procedures. Policies and procedures should be evaluated on an ongoing basis and revised as necessary. The policies and procedures should be readily accessible to the health-care providers within the health-care setting.

IV: PROFESSIONAL RESPONSIBILITY AND ACCOUNTABILITY

STANDARD: The obstetric, gynecologic, and neonatal nurse is responsible and accountable for maintaining knowledge and competency in individual nursing practice and for being aware of professional issues.

INTERPRETATION: Maintaining both the knowledge and skills required to achieve excellence in OGN nursing is incumbent upon the nurse. The nurse should be cognizant of changing concepts, trends, and scientific advances in OGN care. Updating knowledge and skills is achievable through formal education, professional continuing education, and the use of or participation in nursing research. Knowledge of specialty nursing can be recognized through certification.

The nurse should be aware of governmental policies and legislation affecting health care and nursing practice. Participating in legislative and regulatory processes is appropriate for the nurse.

Responsibilities defined in written position descriptions and performance demonstrated by the OGN nurse should be regularly evaluated and documented. In addition, criteria for the evaluation of OGN nursing practice should be drawn from applicable statutes, the ethics of the profession, and current standards of practice.

V: PERSONNEL

STANDARD: Obstetric, gynecologic, and neonatal nursing staff are provided to meet patient care needs.

INTERPRETATION: The obstetric, gynecologic, and neonatal nursing management determines the staff required for the provision of individualized nursing care commensurate with demonstrated patient needs, appropriate nursing interventions, qualifications of available nursing personnel, and other factors which must be considered. These factors may include nursing care needs; number of deliveries; number and types of surgical procedures; average inpatient census; volume of ambulatory patients; percentage of highrisk patients; educational, emotional, and economic needs of the patients; provision for staff continuing education; medical staff coverage; ancillary services available; size and design of facilities; responsibilities of nursing staff; and ongoing research.

Personnel in each OGN unit should be directed by a registered nurse with educational preparation and clinical experience in the specific OGN area of practice. This nurse is responsible for management of nursing care and supervision of nursing personnel.

When nursing, medical, or other specialty students are assigned to the unit for clinical experience, their roles and responsibilities should be clearly defined in writing. Nursing students should not be included in the unit's staffing plan.

Written position descriptions which identify standards of performance of OGN nurses should be developed and used in periodic personnel evaluations. Documentation should reflect each nurse's participation in orientation and verify knowledge and expertise in those skills required for OGN nursing practice. Orientation and evaluation of personnel for whom the registered nurse is held accountable should be documented as well.

Written policies for the reassignment of OGN nursing personnel should exist to accommodate both increases and decreases of inpatient days and ambulatory visits. The policies should include a contingency plan for staffing during peak activity periods.

Cervical Dilatation Assessment Aid

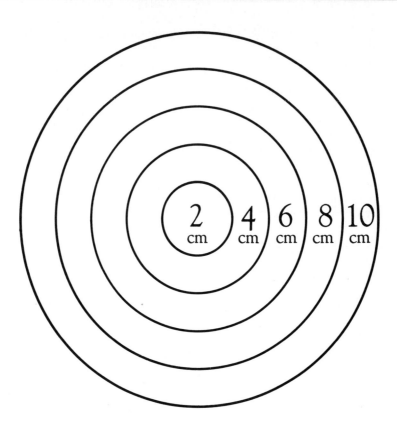

Clinical Estimation of Gestational Age

PATIENT'S NAME _____

▷ **Examination First Hours**

CLINICAL ESTIMATION OF GESTATIONAL AGE
An Approximation Based on Published Data*

PHYSICAL FINDINGS		WEEKS GESTATION																												
		20	21	22	23	24	25	26	27	28	29	30	31	32	33	34	35	36	37	38	39	40	41	42	43	44	45	46	47	48
VERNIX			APPEARS				COVERS BODY, THICK LAYER													ON BACK, SCALP, IN CREASES		SCANT, IN CREASES			NO VERNIX					
BREAST TISSUE AND AREOLA		AREOLA & NIPPLE BARELY VISIBLE NO PALPABLE BREAST TISSUE														AREOLA RAISED		1-2 MM NODULE		3-5 MM	5-6 MM	7-10 MM			?12 MM					
EAR	FORM	FLAT, SHAPELESS														BEGINNING INCURVING SUPERIOR		INCURVING UPPER 2/3 PINNAE		WELL-DEFINED INCURVING TO LOBE									
	CARTILAGE	PINNA SOFT, STAYS FOLDED														CARTILAGE SCANT RETURNS SLOWLY FROM FOLDING		THIN CARTILAGE SPRINGS BACK FROM FOLDING		PINNA FIRM, REMAINS ERECT FROM HEAD									
SOLE CREASES		SMOOTH SOLES s̄ CREASES														1-2 ANTERIOR CREASES	2-3 ANTERIOR CREASES	CREASES ANTERIOR 2/3 SOLE	CREASES INVOLVING HEEL		DEEPER CREASES OVER ENTIRE SOLE									
SKIN	THICKNESS & APPEARANCE	THIN, TRANSLUCENT SKIN, PLETHORIC, VENULES OVER ABDOMEN EDEMA														SMOOTH THICKER NO EDEMA		PINK		FEW VESSELS		SOME DESQUAMATION PALE PINK	THICK, PALE, DESQUAMATION OVER ENTIRE BODY							
	NAIL PLATES	APPEAR													NAILS TO FINGER TIPS							NAILS EXTEND WELL BEYOND FINGER TIPS								
HAIR		APPEARS ON HEAD		EYE BROWS & LASHES			FINE, WOOLLY, BUNCHES OUT FROM HEAD											SILKY, SINGLE STRANDS LAYS FLAT				?RECEDING HAIRLINE OR LOSS OF BABY HAIR SHORT, FINE UNDERNEATH								
LANUGO		APPEARS		COVERS ENTIRE BODY										VANISHES FROM FACE				PRESENT ON SHOULDERS			NO LANUGO								
GENITALIA	TESTES									TESTES PALPABLE IN INGUINAL CANAL								IN UPPER SCROTUM			IN LOWER SCROTUM								
	SCROTUM										FEW RUGAE							RUGAE, ANTERIOR PORTION		RUGAE COVER		PENDULOUS							
	LABIA & CLITORIS										PROMINENT CLITORIS LABIA MAJORA SMALL WIDELY SEPARATED						LABIA MAJORA LARGER NEARLY COVERED CLITORIS		LABIA MINORA & CLITORIS COVERED									
SKULL FIRMNESS		BONES ARE SOFT											SOFT TO 1" FROM ANTERIOR FONTANELLE				SPONGY AT EDGES OF FONTANELLE CENTER FIRM		BONES HARD SUTURES EASILY DISPLACED		BONES HARD, CANNOT BE DISPLACED								
POSTURE	RESTING	HYPOTONIC LATERAL DECUBITUS						HYPOTONIC			BEGINNING FLEXION THIGH		STRONGER HIP FLEXION		FROG-LIKE		FLEXION ALL LIMBS		HYPERTONIC			VERY HYPERTONIC							
	RECOIL - LEG			NO RECOIL							PARTIAL RECOIL										PROMPT RECOIL									
	ARM			NO RECOIL										BEGIN FLEXION NO RECOIL		PROMPT RECOIL MAY BE INHIBITED		PROMPT RECOIL AFTER 30" INHIBITION											
		20	21	22	23	24	25	26	27	28	29	30	31	32	33	34	35	36	37	38	39	40	41	42	43	44	45	46	47	48

Confirmatory Neurologic Examination to be Done After 24 Hours

Confirmatory Neurologic Examination to be Done After 24 Hours

MeadJohnson LABORATORIES

	WEEKS GESTATION																												
PHYSICAL FINDINGS	20	21	22	23	24	25	26	27	28	29	30	31	32	33	34	35	36	37	38	39	40	41	42	43	44	45	46	47	48

TONE

- HEEL TO EAR: NO RESISTANCE — SOME RESISTANCE — IMPOSSIBLE
- SCARF SIGN: NO RESISTANCE — ELBOW PASSES MIDLINE — ELBOW AT MIDLINE — ELBOW DOES NOT REACH MIDLINE
- NECK FLEXORS (HEAD LAG): ABSENT — HEAD IN PLANE OF BODY — HOLDS HEAD
- NECK EXTENSORS: HEAD BEGINS TO RIGHT ITSELF FROM FLEXED POSITION — GOOD RIGHTING CANNOT HOLD IT — HOLDS HEAD FEW SECONDS — KEEPS HEAD IN LINE c̄ TRUNK >40" — TURNS HEAD FROM SIDE TO SIDE
- BODY EXTENSORS: STRAIGHTENING OF LEGS — STRAIGHTENING OF TRUNK — STRAIGHTENING OF HEAD & TRUNK TOGETHER
- VERTICAL POSITIONS: WHEN HELD UNDER ARMS, BODY SLIPS THROUGH HANDS — ARMS HOLD BABY LEGS EXTENDED — LEGS FLEXED GOOD SUPPORT c̄ ARMS
- HORIZONTAL POSITIONS: HYPOTONIC ARMS & LEGS STRAIGHT — ARMS AND LEGS FLEXED — HEAD & BACK EVEN FLEXED EXTREMITIES — HEAD ABOVE BACK

FLEXION ANGLES

- POPLITEAL: NO RESISTANCE — 150° — 110° — 100° — 90° — 80°
- ANKLE: 45° — 20° — 0°
- WRIST (SQUARE WINDOW): 90° — 60° — 45° — 30° — 0°

REFLEXES

- SUCKING: WEAK NOT SYNCHRONIZED c̄ SWALLOWING — STRONGER SYNCHRONIZED — PERFECT
- ROOTING: LONG LATENCY PERIOD SLOW, IMPERFECT — HAND TO MOUTH — BRISK, COMPLETE, DURABLE — PERFECT HAND TO MOUTH
- GRASP: FINGER GRASP IS GOOD STRENGTH IS POOR — STRONGER — CAN LIFT BABY OFF BED INVOLVES ARMS — HANDS OPEN
- MORO: BARELY APPARENT — WEAK NOT ELICITED EVERY TIME — STRONGER — COMPLETE c̄ ARM EXTENSION OPEN FINGERS, CRY — STILL INCOMPLETE — ARM ADDUCTION ADDED — ?BEGINS TO LOSE MORO
- CROSSED EXTENSION: FLEXION & EXTENSION IN A RANDOM, PURPOSELESS PATTERN — EXTENSION BUT NO ADDUCTION — EXTENSION ADDUCTION FANNING OF TOES — COMPLETE
- AUTOMATIC WALK: MINIMAL — BEGINS TIPTOEING GOOD SUPPORT ON SOLE — FAST TIPTOEING — HEEL-TOE PROGRESSION WHOLE SOLE OF FOOT — A PRE-TERM WHO HAS REACHED 40 WEEKS WALKS ON TOES — ?BEGINS TO LOSE AUTO-MATIC WALK

A PRE-TERM WHO HAS REACHED 40 WEEKS STILL HAS A 40° ANGLE

- PUPILLARY REFLEX: ABSENT — APPEARS — PRESENT
- GLABELLAR TAP: ABSENT — APPEARS — PRESENT
- TONIC NECK REFLEX: ABSENT — APPEARS — PRESENT AFTER 37 WEEKS
- NECK-RIGHTING: ABSENT — APPEARS

	20	21	22	23	24	25	26	27	28	29	30	31	32	33	34	35	36	37	38	39	40	41	42	43	44	45	46	47	48

*Brazie, J.V., and Lubchenco, L.O.: The Estimation of Gestational Age Chart, in Kempe, Silver and O'Brien: Current Pediatric Diagnosis and Treatment, ed. 3, Los Altos, California, Lange Medical Publications, 1974, Chapter 3.

Lit. 181, 12/74

Classification of Newborns (Both Sexes) by Intrauterine Growth and Gestational Age[1,2]

NAME _____   DATE OF BIRTH _____   BIRTH WEIGHT _____

HOSPITAL NO. _____   DATE OF EXAM _____   LENGTH _____

RACE _____   SEX _____   HEAD CIRC. _____

GESTATIONAL AGE _____

WEIGHT PERCENTILES

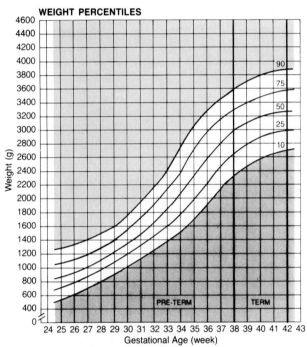

LENGTH PERCENTILES

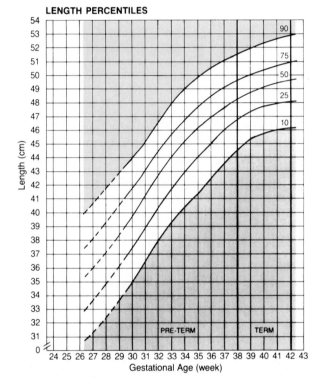

HEAD CIRCUMFERENCE PERCENTILES

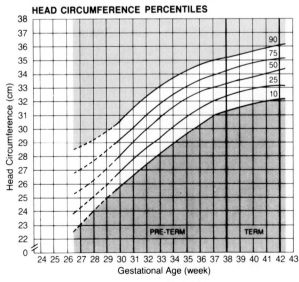

CLASSIFICATION OF INFANT*	Weight	Length	Head Circ.
Large for Gestational Age (LGA) (>90th percentile)			
Appropriate for Gestational Age (AGA) (10th to 90th percentile)			
Small for Gestational Age (SGA) (<10th percentile)			

*Place an "X" in the appropriate box (LGA, AGA or SGA) for weight, for length and for head circumference.

References
1. Battaglia FC, Lubchenco LO: A practical classification of newborn infants by weight and gestational age. *J Pediatr* 71:159-163, 1967.
2. Lubchenco LO, Hansman C, Boyd E: Intrauterine growth in length and head circumference as estimated from live births at gestational ages from 26 to 42 weeks. *Pediatrics* 37:403-408, 1966.

Conversions and Equivalents

Temperature Conversion

(Fahrenheit temperature − 32) × 5/9 = Celsius temperature
(Celsius temperature × 9/5) + 32 = Fahrenheit temperature

Selected Conversions to Metric Measures

Known value	Multiply by	To find
inches	2.54	centimeters
ounces	28	grams
pounds	454	grams
pounds	0.45	kilograms

Selected Conversions from Metric Measures

Known value	Multiply by	To find
centimeters	0.4	inches
grams	0.035	ounces
grams	0.0022	pounds
kilograms	2.2	pounds

Conversion of Pounds and Ounces to Grams

Pounds	Ounces															
S	0	1	2	3	4	5	6	7	8	9	10	11	12	13	14	15
0	—	28	57	85	113	142	170	198	227	255	283	312	340	369	397	425
1	454	482	510	539	567	595	624	652	680	709	737	765	794	822	850	879
2	907	936	964	992	1021	1049	1077	1106	1134	1162	1191	1219	1247	1276	1304	1332
3	1361	1389	1417	1446	1474	1503	1531	1559	1588	1616	1644	1673	1701	1729	1758	1786
4	1814	1843	1871	1899	1928	1956	1984	2013	2041	2070	2098	2126	2155	2183	2211	2240
5	2268	2296	2325	2353	2381	2410	2438	2466	2495	2523	2551	2580	2608	2637	2665	2693
6	2722	2750	2778	2807	2835	2863	2892	2920	2948	2977	3005	3033	3062	3090	3118	3147
7	3175	3203	3232	3260	3289	3317	3345	3374	3402	3430	3459	3487	3515	3544	3572	3600
8	3629	3657	3685	3714	3742	3770	3799	3827	3856	3884	3912	3941	3969	3997	4026	4054
9	4082	4111	4139	4167	4196	4224	4252	4281	4309	4337	4366	4394	4423	4451	4479	4508
10	4536	4564	4593	4621	4649	4678	4706	4734	4763	4791	4819	4848	4876	4904	4933	4961
11	4990	5018	5046	5075	5103	5131	5160	5188	5216	5245	5273	5301	5330	5358	5386	5415
12	5443	5471	5500	5528	5557	5585	5613	5642	5670	5698	5727	5755	5783	5812	5840	5868
13	5897	5925	5953	5982	6010	6038	6067	6095	6123	6152	6180	6209	6237	6265	6294	6322
14	6350	6379	6407	6435	6464	6492	6520	6549	6577	6605	6634	6662	6690	6719	6747	6776
15	6804	6832	6860	6889	6917	6945	6973	7002	7030	7059	7087	7115	7144	7172	7201	7228
16	7257	7286	7313	7342	7371	7399	7427	7456	7484	7512	7541	7569	7597	7626	7654	7682
17	7711	7739	7768	7796	7824	7853	7881	7909	7938	7966	7994	8023	8051	8079	8108	8136
18	8165	8192	8221	8249	8278	8306	8335	8363	8391	8420	8448	8476	8504	8533	8561	8590
19	8618	8646	8675	8703	8731	8760	8788	8816	8845	8873	8902	8930	8958	8987	9015	9043
20	9072	9100	9128	9157	9185	9213	9242	9270	9298	9327	9355	9383	9412	9440	9469	9497
21	9525	9554	9582	9610	9639	9667	9695	9724	9752	9780	9809	9837	9865	9894	9922	9950
22	9979	10007	10036	10064	10092	10120	10149	10177	10206	10234	10262	10291	10319	10347	10376	10404

North American Nursing Diagnosis Association (NANDA) 1990 Approved Nursing Diagnostic Categories

Activity intolerance
Activity intolerance: High risk
Adjustment, Impaired
Airway clearance, Ineffective
Anxiety
Aspiration: High risk
Body image disturbance
Body temperature, Altered: High risk
Bowel incontinence
Breast-feeding, Effective (potential for enhanced)[1]
Breast-feeding, Ineffective
Breathing pattern, Ineffective
Cardiac output, Decreased
Communication, Impaired: Verbal
Constipation
Constipation, Colonic
Constipation, Perceived
Coping, Defensive
Coping, Family: Potential for growth
Coping, Ineffective family: Compromised
Coping, Ineffective family: Disabling
Coping, Ineffective individual
Decisional conflict (specify)
Denial, Ineffective
Diarrhea
Disuse syndrome: High risk
Diversional activity deficit
Dysreflexia
Family processes, Altered
Fatigue
Fear
Fluid volume deficit
Fluid volume deficit: High risk
Fluid volume excess
Gas exchange, Impaired
Grieving, Anticipatory
Grieving, Dysfunctional

Growth and development, Altered
Health maintenance, Altered
Health-seeking behaviors (specify)
Home maintenance management, Impaired
Hopelessness
Hyperthermia
Hypothermia
Infection: High risk
Injury: High risk
Knowledge deficit (specify)
Mobility, Impaired physical
Noncompliance (specify)
Nutrition, Altered: Less than body requirements
Nutrition, Altered; More than body requirements
Nutrition, Altered: High risk for more than body requirements
Oral mucous membrane, Altered
Pain [Acute]
Pain, Chronic
Parental role conflict
Parenting, Altered
Parenting, Altered: High risk
Personal identity disturbance
Poisoning: High risk
Post-trauma response
Powerlessness
Protection, Altered[1]
Rape-trauma syndrome
Rape-trauma syndrome: Compound reaction
Rape-trauma syndrome: Silent reaction
Role performance, Altered
Self-care deficit: Bathing/hygiene
Self-care deficit: Dressing/grooming
Self-care deficit: Feeding

Self-care deficit: Toileting
Self-esteem disturbance
Self-esteem, Low: Chronic
Self-esteem, Low: Situational
Sensory/perceptual alterations: Visual, auditory, kinesthetic, gustatory, tactile, olfactory (specify)
Sexual dysfunction
Sexuality patterns, Altered
Skin integrity, Impaired
Skin integrity, Impaired: High risk
Sleep pattern disturbance
Social interaction, Impaired
Social isolation
Spiritual distress
Suffocation: High risk
Swallowing, Impaired
Thermoregulation, Impaired
Thought processes, Altered
Tissue integrity, Impaired
Tissue perfusion, Altered: Renal, cerebral, cardiopulmonary, gastrointestinal, peripheral (specify type)
Trauma: High risk
Unilateral neglect
Urinary elimination, Altered
Urinary incontinence, Functional
Urinary incontinence, Reflex
Urinary incontinence, Stress
Urinary incontinence, Total
Urinary incontinence, Urge
Urinary retention
Violence, High risk: Self-directed or directed at others

1. Diagnoses accepted in 1990

Universal Precautions

The Centers for Disease Control recommend "*universal blood and body fluid precautions*," now referred to simply as "*universal precautions*," in the care of *all* clients, especially those in emergency care settings, in which the risk of blood exposure is increased and the infection status of the client is unknown. Under universal precautions, blood and certain body fluids of *all* clients are considered potentially infectious for human immunodeficiency virus (HIV), hepatitis B virus (HBV), and other blood-borne pathogens.

The CDC (1989, p. 9) recommends that these precautions apply to blood and to body fluids containing visible blood, as well as semen and vaginal secretions; to tissues, and to the following fluids: cerebrospinal fluid, synovial fluid, pleural fluid, peritoneal fluid, pericardial fluid, and amniotic fluids. **Blood is the single most important source of HIV, HBV, and other blood-borne pathogens in the health care setting**. Universal precautions do not apply to nasal secretions, sputum, saliva (except in the dental setting, where saliva is likely to be contaminated with blood), sweat, tears, urine, feces, and vomitus unless they contain visible blood. However, current infection control practices, already in existence, include the use of gloves for digital examination of mucous membranes and endotracheal suctioning, and hand washing after exposure to saliva. These practices should minimize the risk, if any, for salivary transmission of HIV and HBV (MMWR, 1988, p. 379).

The following specific precautions are recommended to reduce the risk of exposure to potentially infective materials:

- Refrain from all direct client care and from handling client-care equipment if you have exudative lesions or weeping dermatitis. Resume care when the condition is resolved.

Hand Washing Wash your hands thoroughly with warm water and soap (a) immediately, if contaminated with blood or other body fluids to which universal precautions apply, or potentially contaminated articles; (b) between clients; and (c) immediately after gloves are removed, even if the gloves appear to be intact. When hand washing facilities are not available, use a waterless antiseptic hand cleaner in accordance with the manufacturer's directions.

Gloves

- Wear gloves when touching blood and body fluids containing blood, as well as when handling items or surfaces soiled with blood or body fluids as mentioned above.

- Change gloves between client contacts.

- Use sterile gloves for procedures involving contact with normally sterile areas of the body.

- Use examination gloves for procedures involving contact with mucous membranes, unless otherwise indicated, and for other client care of diagnostic procedures that do not require the use of sterile gloves.

- When performing phlebotomy (venipuncture) wear gloves (a) if you have cuts, scratches, or other breaks in the skin; (b) in situations where hand contamination with blood may occur, e.g., with an uncooperative client; and (c) when you are learning phlebotomy techniques.

- Wear gloves when performing finger and/or heel sticks on infants and children.

- Do not wash or disinfect surgical or examination gloves for reuse. Washing with surfactants may cause *wicking*, i.e., the enhanced penetration of liquids through undetected holes in the glove. Disinfecting agents may cause deterioration.

- Use general-purpose gloves (e.g., rubber household gloves) for housekeeping chores involving potential blood contact and for instrument cleaning and decontamination procedures. Utility gloves may be decontaminated and reused, but should be discarded if they are peeling, cracked, or discolored, or if they have punctures, tears, or other evidence of deterioration.

Other Protective Barriers

- Wear masks and protective eyewear (glasses, goggles) or face shields to protect the mucous membranes of your mouth, nose, and eyes during procedures that are likely to generate droplets of blood or other body fluids to which universal precautions apply.
- Wear a disposable plastic apron or gown during procedures that are likely to generate splatters of blood or other body fluid (e.g., peritoneal fluid) and soil your clothing.
- Place mouthpieces, resuscitation bags, or other ventilation devices, in areas where the need for emergency mouth-to-mouth resuscitation is predictable—even though saliva has not been implicated in HIV transmission.
- Wear disposable impervious shoe covering where there is massive blood contamination on floors and wear gloves to remove them.

Needles and Sharps Disposal   To prevent injuries, place used disposable needle-syringe units, scalpel blades, and other sharp items in puncture-resistant containers for disposal. Discard used needle-syringe units **uncapped** and **unbroken**. Place puncture-resistant containers as close as practicable to use areas.

Laundry   Handle soiled linen as little as possible and with minimum agitation to prevent gross microbial contamination of the air and of persons handling the linen. Place linen soiled with blood or body fluids in leakage-resistant bags at the location where it is used.

Specimens   Put all specimens of blood and listed body fluids in well-constructed containers with secure lids to prevent leakage during transport. When collecting specimens, take care to avoid contaminating the outside of the container.

Blood Spills

- Use a chemical germicide that is approved for use as a hospital disinfectant to decontaminate work surfaces after there is a spill of blood or other applicable body fluids. In the absence of a commercial germicide, a solution of sodium hypochlorite (household bleach) in a 1:100 dilution is effective.
- Wear gloves during cleaning and decontaminating procedures. Before decontaminating areas, first remove visible material with disposable towels or other appropriate means that prevent direct contact with the body fluid. Make sure plastic bags are available to remove contaminated items from spill sites.
- Brush-scrub contaminated boots and leather goods with soap and hot water.

Infective Wastes

- Follow agency policies for disposal of infective waste, both when disposing of, and when decontaminating, contaminated materials.
- Carefully pour bulk blood, suctioned fluids, and excretions containing blood and secretions, down drains that are connected to a sanitary sewer.

Sources   U.S. Department of Health and Human Services, Public Health Service, Update: Universal precautions for prevention of transmission of human immunodeficiency virus, hepatitis B virus, and other blood-borne pathogens in health care settings, *Morbidity and Mortality Weekly Report*, June 24, 1988; 37: 377–382, 387–388; *Morbidity and Motality Weekly Report*, June 23, 1989, 38/No. S-6: 9–18.

💧 Blood and Body Fluid Precautions

This logo, used throughout the book, draws attention to the need for blood and body fluid precautions. These precautions are intended to protect the nurse and the client from infection.

Abdominal effleurage Gentle stroking used in massage.

Abortion Loss of pregnancy before the fetus is viable outside the uterus; miscarriage.

Abruptio placentae Partial or total premature separation of a normally implanted placenta.

Abstinence Refraining voluntarily, especially from indulgence in food, alcoholic beverages, or sexual intercourse.

Acceleration Periodic increase in the baseline fetal heart rate.

Acini cells Secretory cells in the human breast that create milk from nutrients in the bloodstream.

Acme Peak or highest point; time of greatest intensity (of a uterine contraction).

Acrocyanosis Cyanosis of the extremities.

Active acquired immunity Formation of antibodies by the pregnant woman in response to illness or immunization.

Acute grief The most severe stage of the grief response; usually resolved within 1–2 months and followed by a gradual return to the pre-loss level of functioning.

Adnexa Adjoining or accessory parts of a structure, such as the uterine adnexa: the ovaries and fallopian tubes.

Adolescence Period of human development initiated by puberty and ending with the attainment of young adulthood.

Afterbirth Placenta and membranes expelled after the delivery of the infant, during the third stage of labor; also called secundines.

Afterpains Cramplike pains due to contractions of the uterus that occur after childbirth. They are more common in multiparas, tend to be most severe during nursing, and last two to three days.

AIDS Autoimmune deficiency syndrome; a sexually transmitted viral disease that so far has proved fatal in 100 percent of cases.

Allele One of a series of alternate genes at the same locus; one form of a gene.

Amenorrhea Suppression or absence of menstruation.

Amniocentesis Removal of amniotic fluid by insertion of a needle into the amniotic sac; amniotic fluid is used to assess fetal health or maturity.

Amnion The inner of the two membranes that form the sac containing the fetus and the amniotic fluid.

Amnionitis Infection of the amniotic fluid.

Amnioscopy Visualization of the amniotic fluid through the membranes with an amnioscope in order to identify meconium staining of the amniotic fluid.

Amniotic fluid The liquid surrounding the fetus in utero. It absorbs shocks, permits fetal movement, and prevents heat loss.

Amniotic fluid embolism Amniotic fluid that has leaked into the chorionic plate and entered the maternal circulation.

Amniotomy The artificial rupturing of the amniotic membrane.

Ampulla The outer two-thirds of the fallopian tube; fertilization of the ovum by a spermatozoon usually occurs here.

Androgen Substance producing male characteristics, such as the male hormone testosterone.

Android pelvis Male-type pelvis.

Antepartum Time between conception and the onset of labor; usually used to describe the period during which a woman is pregnant.

Anterior fontanelle Diamond-shaped area between the two frontal and two parietal bones just above the newborn's forehead.

Anthropoid pelvis Pelvis in which the anteroposterior diameter is equal to or greater than the transverse diameter.

Apgar score A scoring system used to evaluate newborns at 1 minute and 5 minutes after delivery. The total score is achieved by assessing five signs: heart rate, respiratory effort, muscle tone, reflex irritability, and color. Each of the signs is assigned a score of 0, 1, or 2. The highest possible score is 10.

Apnea A condition that occurs when respirations cease for more than 20 seconds, with generalized cyanosis.

Areola Pigmented ring surrounding the nipple of the breast.

AROM Artificial rupture of (amniotic) membranes through use of a device such as an amnihook or allis forceps.

Artificial insemination Introduction of viable semen into the vagina by artificial means for the purpose of impregnation.

Attachment Enduring bonds or relationship of affection between persons.

Atony Lack of normal muscle tone.

Attitude Attitude of the fetus refers to the relationship of the fetal parts to each other.

Autosome A chromosome that is not a sex chromosome.

Bacterial vaginosis A bacterial infection of the vagina, formerly called *Gardnerella vaginalis* or *Hemophilus vaginalis*, characterized by a foul-smelling, grayish vaginal discharge that exhibits a characteristic fishy odor when 10 percent potassium hydroxide (KOH) is added. Microscopic examination of a vaginal wet prep reveals the presence of "clue cells" (vaginal epithelial cells coated with gram-negative organisms).

Bag of waters The membrane containing the amniotic fluid and the fetus (BOW).

Ballottement A technique of palpation to detect or examine a floating object in the body. In obstetrics, the fetus, when pushed, floats away and then returns to touch the examiner's fingers.

Barr body Deeply staining chromatin mass located against the inner surface of the cell nucleus. It is found only in normal females; also called *sex chromatin*.

Basal body temperature (BBT) The lowest waking temperature.

Baseline rate The average fetal heart rate observed during a 10-minute period of monitoring.

Baseline variability Changes in the fetal heart rate that result from the interplay between the sympathetic and the parasympathetic nervous systems.

Battledore placenta Placenta in which the umbilical cord is inserted on the periphery rather than centrally.

Bimanual palpation Examination of the pelvic organs by placing one hand on the abdomen and one or two fingers of the other hand into the vagina.

Biophysical profile Assessment of five variables in the fetus that help to evaluate fetal risk: breathing movement, body movement, tone, amniotic fluid volume, and fetal heart rate reactivity.

Birth rate Number of live births per 1000 population.

Birth center A setting for labor and delivery that emphasizes a family-centered approach rather than for obstetric technology and treatment.

Birthing room A room for labor and delivery with a relaxed atmosphere.

Bishop score A prelabor scoring system to assist in predicting whether an induction of labor may be successful. The total score is achieved by assessing five components: cervical dilatation, cervical effacement, cervical consistency, cervical position, and fetal station. Each of the components is assigned a score of zero to three, and the highest possible score is 13.

Blastocyst The inner solid mass of cells within the morula.

Blending family Families established through remarriage; may include children from previous marriages of each spouse as well as children of the current marriage.

Bloody show Pink-tinged mucous secretions resulting from rupture of small capillaries as the cervix effaces and dilates.

Brachial palsy Partial or complete paralysis of portions of the arm resulting from trauma to the brachial plexus during a difficult delivery.

Bradycardia Slow heart rate.

Bradley method Partner-coached natural childbirth.

Braxton Hicks contractions Intermittent painless contractions of the uterus that may occur every 10 to 20 minutes. They occur more frequently toward the end of pregnancy and are sometimes mistaken for true labor signs.

Brazleton's neonatal behavioral assessment A brief examination used to identify the infant's behavioral states and responses.

Breasts Mammary glands.

Breech presentation A delivery in which the buttocks and/or feet are presented instead of the head.

Broad ligament The ligament extending from the lateral margins of the uterus to the pelvic wall; keeps the uterus centrally placed and provides stability within the pelvic cavity.

Bronchopulmonary dysplasia (BPD) Chronic pulmonary disease of multifactorial etiology characterized initially by alveolar and bronchial necrosis, which results in bronchial metaplasia and interstitial fibrosis. Appears in x-ray films as generalized small, radiolucent cysts within the lungs.

Brown adipose tissue (BAT) Fat deposits in neonates that provide greater heat-generating activity than ordinary fat. Found around the kidneys, adrenals, and neck; between the scapulas; and behind the sternum; also called brown fat.

Calorie Amount of hear required to raise the temperature of 1 g of water 1 degree centigrade.

Caput succedaneum Swelling or edema occurring in or under the fetal scalp during labor.

Cardinal ligaments The chief uterine supports, suspending the uterus from the side walls of the true pelvis.

Cardinal movements of labor The positional changes of the fetus as it moves through the birth canal during labor and delivery. The positional changes are descent, flexion, internal rotation, extension, restitution, and external rotation.

Cardiopulmonary adaptation Adaptation of the neonate's cardiovascular and respiratory systems to life outside the womb.

Caudal block Regional anesthesia used in childbirth in which the anesthetic agent is injected into the caudal area of the spinal canal through the sacral hiatus, affecting the caudal nerve roots and thereby providing anesthesia to the cervix, vagina, and perineum.

Cephalhematoma Subcutaneous swelling containing blood found on the head of an infant several days after delivery, which usually disappears within a few weeks to two months.

Cephalic presentation Delivery in which the fetal head is presenting against the cervix.

Cephalopelvic disproportion (CPD) A condition in which the fetal head is of such a shape or size, or in such a position, that it cannot pass through the maternal pelvis.

Cervical cap A cup-shaped device placed over the cervix to prevent pregnancy.

Cervical dilatation Process in which the cervical os and the cervical canal widen from less than a centimeter to approximately 10 cm, allowing delivery of the fetus.

Cervix The "neck" between the external os and the body of the uterus. The lower end of the cervix extends into the vagina.

Cesarean delivery Delivery of the fetus by means of an incision into the abdominal wall and the uterus; also called *abdominal delivery.*

Chadwick's sign Violet bluish color of the vaginal mucous membrane caused by increased vascularity; visible from about the fourth week of pregnancy.

Chloasma Brownish pigmentation over the bridge of the nose and the cheeks during pregnancy and in some women who are taking oral contraceptives. Also called *mask of pregnancy.*

Chorioamnionitis An inflammation of the amniotic membranes stimulated by organisms in the amniotic fluid, which then becomes infiltrated with polymorphonuclear leukocytes.

Chorion The fetal membrane closest to the intrauterine wall that gives rise to the placenta and continues as the outer membrane surrounding the amnion.

Chromosomes The threadlike structures within the nucleus of a cell that carry the genes.

Chronic grief Grief response involving a denial of the reality of the loss, which prevents any resolution.

Circumcision Surgical removal of the prepuce (foreskin) of the penis.

Circumoral cyanosis Bluish appearance around the mouth.

Circumvallate placenta A placenta with a thick white fibrous ring around the edge.

Cleavage Rapid mitotic division of the zygote; cells produced are called blastomeres.

Client advocacy An approach to client care in which the nurse educates and supports the client and protects the client's rights.

Clitoris Female organ homologous to the male penis; a small oval body of erectile tissue situated at the anterior junction of the vulva.

Coitus interruptus Method of contraception in which the male withdraws his penis from the vagina prior to ejaculation.

Cold stress Excessive heat loss resulting in compensatory mechanisms (increased respirations and nonshivering thermogenesis) to maintain core body temperature.

Colostrum Secretion from the breast before the onset of true lactation; contains mainly serum and white blood corpuscles. It has a high protein content, provides some immune properties, and cleanses the neonate's intestinal tract of mucus and meconium.

Conception Union of male sperm and female ovum; fertilization.

Conceptional age The number of complete weeks since the moment of conception. Because the moment of conception is almost impossible to determine, conceptional age is estimated at 2 weeks less than gestational age.

Condom A rubber sheath that covers the penis to prevent conception or disease.

Condyloma Wartlike growth of skin, usually seen on the external genitals or anus. There are two types, a pointed variety and a broad, flat form usually found with syphilis.

Conduction Loss of heat to a cooler surface by direct skin contact.

Conjugate Important diameter of the pelvis, measured from the center of the promontory of the sacrum to the back of the symphysis pubis. The diagonal conjugate is measured and the true conjugate is estimated.

Conjugate vera The true conjugate, which extends from the middle of the sacral promontory to the middle of the pubic crest.

Conjunctivitis Inflammation of the mucous membrane lining the eyelids.

Contraception The prevention of conception or impregnation.

Contraceptive sponge A small pillow-shaped polyurethane sponge with a concave cupped area on one side, designed to fit over the cervix to prevent pregnancy.

Contraction Tightening and shortening of the uterine muscles during labor, causing effacement and dilatation of the cervix; contributes to the downward and outward descent of the fetus.

Convection Loss of heat from the warm body surface to cooler air currents.

Contraction stress test A method for assessing the reaction of the fetus to the stress of uterine contractions. This test may be utilized when contractions are occurring spontaneously or when contractions are artificially induced by OCT (oxytocin challenge test) or BSST (breast self-stimulation test).

Coombs' test A test for antiglobulins in the red cells. The indirect test determines the presence of Rh-positive antibodies in maternal blood; the direct test determines the presence of maternal Rh-positive antibodies in fetal cord blood.

Cornua The elongated portions of the uterus where the fallopian tubes open.

Corpus The upper two-thirds of the uterus.

Corpus luteum A small yellow body that develops within a ruptured ovarian follicle; it secretes progesterone in the second half of the menstrual cycle and atrophies about three days before the beginning of menstrual flow. If pregnancy occurs, the corpus luteum continues to produce progesterone until the placenta takes over this function.

Cotyledon One of the rounded portions into which the placenta's uterine surface is divided, consisting of a mass of villi, fetal vessels, and an intervillous space.

Couvade In some cultures, the male's observance of certain rituals and taboos to signify the transition to fatherhood.

Crisis Any naturally occurring turning point, such as courtship, marriage, pregnancy, parenthood, or death.

Crisis intervention Actions taken by the nurse to help the client deal with an impending, potentially overwhelming crisis, regain his or her equilibrium, grow from the experience, and improve coping skills.

Crowning Appearance of the presenting fetal part at the vaginal orifice during labor.

Deceleration Periodic decrease in the baseline fetal heart rate.

Decidua Endometrium or mucous membrane lining of the uterus in pregnancy that is shed after delivery.

Decidual basalis The part of the decidua that unites with the chorion to form the placenta. It is shed in lochial discharge after delivery.

Decidua capsularis The part of the decidua surrounding the chorionic sac.

Decidua vera (parietalis) Nonplacental decidua lining the uretus.

Decrement Decrease or stage of decline, as of a contraction.

Desquamation Shedding of the epithelial cells of the epidermis.

Diagonal conjugate Distance from the lower posterior border of the symphysis pubis to the sacral promontory; may be obtained by manual measurement.

Diaphragm A flexible disk that covers the cervix to prevent pregnancy.

Diastasis recti abdominis Separation of the recti abdominis muscles along the median line. In women, it is seen with repeated childbirths or multiple gestations. In the newborn, it is usually caused by incomplete development.

Dilatation of the cervix Expansion of the external os from an opening a few millimeters in size to an opening large enough to allow the passage of the infant.

Dilatation and curettage (D and C) Stretching of the cervical canal to permit passage of a curette, which is used to scrape the endometrium to empty the uterine contents or to obtain tissue for examination.

Diploid number of chromosomes Containing a set of maternal and a set of paternal chromosomes; in humans, the diploid number of chromosomes is 46.

Down syndrome An abnormality resulting from the presence of an extra chromosome number 21 (trisomy 21); characteristics include mental retardation and altered physical appearance. Formerly called Mongolism or Mongoloid idiocy.

Drug-addicted infant The newborn of an alcoholic or drug-addicted woman.

Ductus arteriosus A communication channel between the main pulmonary artery and the aorta of the fetus. It is obliterated after birth by a rising PO_2 and changes in intravascular pressure in the presence of normal pulmonary functioning. It normally becomes a ligament after birth but sometimes remains patent (patent ductus arteriosus), a treatable condition.

Ductus venosus a fetal blood vessel that carries oxygenated blood between the umbilical vein and the inferior vena cava, bypassing the liver; it becomes a ligament after birth.

Duncan's mechanism occurs when the maternal surface of the placenta presents upon delivery rather than the shiny fetal surface.

Duration the time length of each contraction, measured from the beginning of the increment to the completion of the decrement.

Ecchymosis bleeding into tissue caused by direct trauma, serious infection, and bleeding diathesis.

Eclampsia a major complication of pregnancy. Its cause is unknown; it occurs more often in the primigravida and is accompanied by elevated blood pressure, albuminuria, oliguria, tonic and clonic convulsions, and coma. It may occur during pregnancy (usually after the twentieth week of gestation) or within 48 hours after delivery.

Ectoderm outer layer of cells in the developing embryo that give rise to the skin, nails, and hair.

Ectopic in an abnormal position.

Ectopic pregnancy implantation of the fertilized ovum outside the uterine cavity; common sites are the abdomen, fallopian tubes, and ovaries; also called *oocyesis*.

EDD estimated date of delivery.

Effacement thinning and shortening of the cervix that occurs late in pregnancy or during labor.

Ejaculation expulsion of the seminal fluids from the penis.

Ellis-Van Creveld syndrome autosomal recessive syndrome characterized by small stature with disproportionally short extremities, polydactyly of fingers and/or toes, hypoplastic nails, and short upper lip. One half the patients also have a cardiac defect.

Embolus undissolved matter present in a blood vessel brought there by the blood or lymph current; may be solid, liquid, or gaseous.

Embryo the early stage of development of the young of any organism. In humans the embryonic period is from about two to eight weeks of gestation, and is characterized by cellular differentiation and predominantly hyperplastic growth.

Endocervical pertaining to the interior of the canal of the cervix of the uterus.

Endocrine glands glands that secrete special substances (hormones) that regulate body functions.

Endoderm the inner layer of cells in the developing embryo that give rise to internal organs such as the intestines.

Endometriosis ectopic endometrium located outside the uterus in the pelvic cavity. Symptoms may include pelvic pain or pressure, dysmenorrhea, dispareunia, abnormal bleeding from the uterus or rectum, and sterility.

Endometritis infection of the endometrium.

Endometrium the mucous membrane that lines the inner surface of the uterus.

En face an assumed position in which one person looks at another and maintains his or her face in the same vertical plane as that of the other.

Engagement the entrance of the fetal presenting part into the superior pelvic strait and the beginning of the descent through the pelvic canal.

Engorgement vascular congestion or distention. In obstetrics, the swelling of breast tissue brought about by an increase in blood and lymph supply to the breast, preceding true lactation.

Engrossment characteristic sense of absorption, preoccupation, and interest in the infant demonstrated by fathers during early contact with their infants.

Enzygotic developed from one fertilized ovum.

Epicanthus a fold of skin that extends from the top of the nose to the median end of the eyebrow, covering the inner canthus.

Epidural block regional anesthesia effective through the first and second stages of labor.

Episiotomy incision of the perineum to facilitate delivery and to avoid laceration of the perineum.

Epispadias congenital opening of the urethra on the dorsum of the penis, or opening by separation of the labia minora and a fissure of the clitoris (rare).

Epstein's pearls small, white blebs found along the gum margins and at the junction of the hard and soft palates; commonly seen in the newborn as a normal manifestation.

Erb's Duchenne palsy paralysis of the arm and chest wall as a result of a birth injury to the brachial plexus or a subsequent injury to the fifth and sixth cervical nerves.

Erythema toxicum innocuous pink papular rash of unknown cause with superimposed vesicles; it appears within 24 to 48 hours after birth and resolves spontaneously within a few days.

Erythroblastosis fetalis hemolytic disease of the newborn characterized by anemia, jaundice, enlargement of the liver and spleen, and generalized edema. Caused by isoimmunization due to Rh incompatibility or ABO incompatibility.

Estrogen replacement therapy (ERT) Use of estrogen or a progestin to decrease the symptoms of menopause and to prevent osteoporosis.

Estrogens The hormones estradiol and estrone, produced by the ovary.

Ethnocentrism An individual's belief that the values and practices of his or her own culture are the best ones.

Evaporation Loss of heat incurred when water on the skin surface is converted to a vapor.

Exchange transfusion The replacement of 70 percent to 80 percent of circulating blood by withdrawing the recipient's blood and injecting a donor's blood in equal amounts, for the purpose of preventing the accumulation of bilirubin or other byproducts of hemolysis in the blood.

External os The opening between the cervix and the vagina.

Fallopian tubes Tubes that extend from the lateral angle of the uterus and terminate near the ovary; they serve as a passageway for the ovum from the ovary to the uterus and for the spermatozoa from the uterus toward the ovary. Also called oviducts and uterine tubes.

False labor Contractions of the uterus, regular or irregular, that may be strong enough to be interpreted as true labor but that do not dilate the cervix.

False pelvis The portion of the pelvis above the linea terminalis; its primary function is to support the weight of the enlarged pregnant uterus.

Family-centered care An approach to health care based on the concept that a hospital can provide professional services to mothers, fathers, and infants in a homelike environment that would enhance the integrity of the family unit.

Female reproductive cycle (FRC) The monthly rhythmic changes in sexually mature females.

Ferning Formation of a palm-leaf pattern by the crystallization of cervical mucus as it dries at midmenstrual cycle. Helpful in determining time of ovulation. Observed via microscopic examination of a thin layer of cervical mucus on a glass slide. This pattern is also observed when amniotic fluid is allowed to air dry on a slide and is a useful and quick test to determine whether amniotic membranes have ruptured.

Fertility awareness methods Natural family planning.

Fertility rate Number of births per 1000 women aged 15 to 44 in a given population per year.

Fertilization Impregnation of an ovum by a spermatozoon.

Fetal alcohol syndrome (FAS) Syndrome caused by maternal alcohol ingestion and characterized by microcephaly, intrauterine growth retardation, short palpebral fissures, and maxillary hypoplasia.

Fetal death Death of the developing fetus after 20 weeks' gestation. Also called fetal demise.

Fetal blood sampling Blood sample drawn from the fetal scalp (or from the fetus in breech position) to evaluate the acid-base status of the fetus.

Fetal bradycardia A fetal heart rate less than 120 beats/minute during a 10-minute period of continuous monitoring.

Fetal distress Evidence that the fetus is in jeopardy, such as a change in fetal activity or heart rate.

Fetal heart rate (FHR) The number of times the fetal heart beats per minute; normal range is 120 to 160 beats per minute.

Fetal position Relationship of the landmark on the presenting fetal part to the front, sides, or back of the maternal pelvis.

Fetal presentation The fetal body part that enters the maternal pelvis first. The three possible presentations are cephalic, shoulder, or breech.

Fetal tachycardia A fetal heart rate of 160 beats/minute or more during a 10-minute period of continuous monitoring.

Fetoscope An adaptation of a stethoscope that facilitates auscultation of the fetal heart rate.

Fetoscopy A technique for directly observing the fetus and obtaining a sample of fetal blood or skin.

Fetus The child in utero from about the seventh to ninth week of gestation until birth.

Fibrocystic breast disease Benign breast disorder characterized by a thickening of normal breast tissue and the formation of cysts.

Fimbria Any structure resembling a fringe; the fringelike extremity of the fallopian tubes.

Folic acid An important vitamin directly related to the outcome of pregnancy and to maternal and fetal health.

Follicle-stimulating hormone (FSH) Hormone produced by the anterior pituitary during the first half of the menstrual cycle, stimulating development of the graafian follicle.

Fontanelle In the fetus, an unossified space or soft spot consisting of a strong band of connective tissue lying between the cranial bones of the skull.

Foramen ovale Septal opening between the atria of the fetal heart. Normally, the opening closes shortly after birth; if it remains open, it can be repaired surgically.

Forceps Obstetric instruments occasionally used to aid in delivery.

Frequency The time between the beginning of one contraction and the beginning of the next contraction.

Fundus The upper portion of the uterus between the fallopian tubes.

Gametogenesis The process by which germ cells are produced.

Genotype The genetic composition of an individual.

Gestation Period of intrauterine development from conception through birth; pregnancy.

Gestational age The number of complete weeks of fetal development, calculated from the first day of the last normal menstrual cycle.

Gestational age assessment tools Systems used to evaluate the newborn's external physical characteristics and neurologic and/or neuromuscular development to accurately determine gestational age. These replace or supplement the traditional calculation from the mother's last menstrual period.

Gestational trophoblastic disease (GTD) Disorder classified into two types; benign (hydatidiform mole) and malignant.

Goodell's sign Softening of the cervix that occurs during the second month of pregnancy.

Graafian follicle The ovarian cyst containing the ripe ovum; it secretes estrogens.

Gravida A pregnant woman.

Grief An emotional state; a reaction to loss.

Grief work The inner process of working through or managing the bereavement.

Gynecoid pelvis Typical female pelvis in which the inlet is round instead of oval.

Habituation Infant's ability to diminish innate responses to specific repeated stimuli.

Haploid number of chromosomes Half the diploid number of chromosomes. In humans, there are 23 chromosomes, the haploid number, in each germ cell.

Harlequin sign A rare color change that occurs between the longitudinal halves of the newborn's body, such that the dependent half is noticeably pinker than the superior half when the newborn is placed on one side; it is of no pathologic significance.

Hegar's sign A softening of the lower uterine segment found upon palpation in the second or third month of pregnancy.

Hemolytic disease of the newborn *Hyperbilirubinemia* secondary to Rh incompatibility.

Herpesvirus A family of viruses characterized by the development of clusters of small vesicles. The infection is recurring and is frequently found about the lips and nares; a genital form also exists that is primarily sexually transmitted.

Heterozygous A genotypic situation in which two different alleles occur at a given locus on a pair of homologous chromosomes.

Homozygous A genotypic situation in which two similar genes occur at a given locus on homologous chromosomes.

Human chorionic gonadotropin (HCG) A hormone produced by the chorionic villi and found in the urine of pregnant women; also called *prolan*.

Human placental lactogen (HPL) A hormone synthesized by the syncytiotrophoblast that functions as an insulin antagonist and promotes lipolysis to increase the amounts of circulating free fatty acids available for maternal metabolic use.

Hyaline membrane disease Respiratory disease of the newborn characterized by interference with ventilation at the alveolar level, thought to be caused by the presence of fibrinoid deposits lining the alveolar ducts. Also called *respiratory distress syndrome (RDS)*.

Hydatidiform mole Degenerative process in chorionic villi, giving rise to multiple cysts and rapid growth of the uterus with hemorrhage.

Hydramnios An excess of amniotic fluid, leading to overdistention of the uterus. Frequently seen in diabetic pregnant women, even if there is no coexisting fetal anomaly. Also called *polyhydramnios*.

Hydrops fetalis See *erythroblastosis fetalis*.

Hyperbilirubinemia Excessive amount of bilirubin in the blood; indicative of hemolytic processes due to blood incompatibility, intrauterine infection, septicemia, neonatal renal infection, and other disorders.

Hyperemesis gravdarum Excessive vomiting during pregnancy, leading to dehydration and starvation.

Hypnoreflexogenous method A combination of hypnosis and conditioned reflexes used during childbirth.

Hypocalcemia Abnormally low level of serum calcium levels.

Hypoglycemia Abnormally low level of sugar in the blood.

Hysterectomy Surgical removal of the uterus.

Hysterosalpingogram Installation of radiopaque substance into the uterine cavity to visualize uterus and fallopian tubes.

Icterus neonatorum Jaundice in the newborn.

Inborn error of metabolism A hereditary deficiency of a specific enzyme needed for normal metabolism of specific chemicals.

Increment Increase or addition; to build up, as of a contraction.

Induction of labor The process of causing or initiating labor by use of medication or surgical rupture of membranes.

Infant Child under one year of age.

Infant death rate Number of deaths of infants under one year of age per 1000 live births in a given population per year.

Infant of a diabetic mother (IDM) At-risk infant born to a woman previously diagnosed as diabetic, or who develops symptoms of diabetes during pregnancy.

Inferential statistics Statistics that allow an investigator to draw conclusions about what is happening between two or more variables in a population and to suggest or refute causal relationships between them.

Infertility Diminished ability to conceive.

Informed consent A legal concept that protects a person's rights to autonomy and self-determination by specifying that no action may be taken without that person's prior understanding and freely given consent.

Infundibulopelvic ligament Ligament that suspends and supports the ovaries.

Innominate bone The hip bone, ilium, ischium, and pubis.

Intensity The strength of a uterine contraction during acme.

Internal os An inside mouth or opening; the opening between the cervix and the uterus.

Intrapartum The time from the onset of true labor until the delivery of the infant and placenta.

Intrauterine device (IUD) Small metal or plastic form that is placed in the uterus to prevent implantation of a fertilized ovum.

Intrauterine growth retardation (IUGR) Fetal undergrowth due to any etiology, such as intrauterine infection, deficient nutrient supply, or congenital malformation.

Introitus Opening or entrance into a cavity or canal, such as the vagina.

Involution Rolling or turning inward; the reduction in size of the uterus following delivery.

Ischial spines Prominences that arise near the junction of the ilium and ischium and jut into the pelvic cavity; used as a reference point during labor to evaluate the descent of the fetal head into the birth canal.

Isthmus The straight, narrow part of the fallopian tube with a thick muscular wall and an opening into the uterus and an opening (lumen) 2–3 mm in diameter; the site of tubal ligation. Also a constriction in the uterus that is located above the cervix and below the corpus.

Jaundice Yellow pigmentation of body tissues caused by the presence of bile pigments. See also *physiologic jaundice*.

Karyotype The set of chromosomes arranged in a standard order.

Kegel's exercises Perineal muscle tightening that strengthens the pubococcygeus muscle and increases its tone.

Kernicterus An encephalopathy caused by deposition of unconjugated bilirubin in brain cells; may result in impaired brain function or death.

Klinefelter syndrome A chromosomal abnormality caused by the presence of an extra X chromosome in the male; characteristics include tall stature, sparse pubic and facial hair, gynecomastia, small firm testes, and absence of spermatogenesis.

Labor The process by which the fetus is expelled from the maternal uterus; also called childbirth, confinement, or parturition.

Lactation Process of producing and supplying breast milk.

Lacto-ovovegetarians Vegetarians who include milk, dairy products, and eggs in their diets, and occasionally fish, poultry, and liver.

Lactose intolerance A condition in which an individual has difficulty digesting milk and milk products.

Lactovegetarians Vegetarians who include dairy products but no eggs in their diets.

La Leche League Organization that provides information on and assistance with breast-feeding.

Lamaze method A method of childbirth preparation, also known as *psychoprophylaxis*.

Lanugo Fine, downy hair found on all body parts of the fetus, with the exception of the palms of the hands and the soles of the feet, after 20 weeks' gestation.

Large for gestational age (LGA) Excessive growth of a fetus in relation to the gestational time period.

Last menstrual period (LMP) The last normal menstrual period experienced by the mother prior to pregnancy; sometimes used to calculate the infant's gestational age.

Later decelerations Periodic change in fetal heart rate pattern caused by uteroplacental insufficiency; deceleration has a uniform shape and late onset in relation to maternal contraction.

Leboyer method Birthing technique that eases the newborn's transition to extrauterine life wherein lights in the delivery room are dimmed and noise is kept to a minimum.

Leiomyoma A benign tumor of the uterus, composed primarily of smooth muscle and connective tissue. Also referred to as a myoma or a fibroid.

Leopold's maneuvers Series of four maneuvers designed to provide a systematic approach whereby the examiner may determine fetal presentation and position.

Letdown reflex Pattern of stimulation, hormone release, and resulting muscle contraction that forces milk into the lactiferous ducts, making it available to the infant; milk ejection reflex.

Leukorrhea Mucous discharge from the vagina or cervical canal that may be normal or pathologic, as in the presence of infection.

Lie Relationship of the long axis of the fetus and the long axis of the pregnant woman. The fetal lie may be longitudinal, transverse, or oblique.

Lightening Moving of the fetus and uterus downward into the pelvic cavity; engagement.

Linea nigra The line of darker pigmentation extending from the umbilicus to the pubis noted in some women during the later months of pregnancy.

Local infiltration Injection of an anesthetic agent into the subcutaneous tissue in a fanlike pattern.

Lochia Maternal discharge of blood, mucus, and tissue from the uterus; may last for several weeks after birth.

Lochia alba White vaginal discharge that follows lochia serosa and that lasts from about the tenth to the twenty-first day after delivery.

Lochia rubra Red, blood-tinged vaginal discharge that occurs following delivery and lasts two to four days.

Lochia serosa Pink, serous, and blood-tinged vaginal discharge that follows lochia rubra and lasts until the seventh to tenth day after delivery.

Loss A state of being deprived of, or without, something one has had.

L/S ratio The ratio of the phospholipids lecithin and sphingomyelin produced by the fetal lungs; useful in assessing fetal lung maturity.

Luteinizing hormone (LH) Anterior pituitary hormone responsible for stimulating ovulation and for development of the corpus luteum.

Macrosomia Condition seen in neonates of large body size and high birth weight, as those born of prediabetic and diabetic mothers.

Malposition An abnormal position of the fetus in the birth canal.

Malpresentation A presentation of the fetus into the birth canal that is not "normal," that is, brow, face, shoulder, or breech presentation.

Mammogram Soft tissue radiograph of the breast without the injection of a contrast medium.

Mastitis Inflammation of the breast.

Maternal mortality Number of maternal deaths from any cause during the pregnancy cycle per 100,000 live births.

McDonald's sign A probable sign of pregnancy characterized by an ease in flexing the body of the uterus against the cervix.

Meconium Dark green or black material present in the large intestine of a full-term infant; the first stools passed by the newborn.

Meconium aspiration syndrome (MAS) Respiratory disease of term, postterm, and SGA newborns caused by inhalation of meconium or meconium-stained amniotic fluid into the lungs; characterized by mild to severe respiratory distress, hyperexpansion of the chest, hyperinflated alveoli, and secondary atelectasis.

Meiosis The process of cell division that occurs in the maturation of sperm and ova that decreases their number of chromosomes by one half.

Menarche Beginning of menstrual and reproductive function in the female.

Mendelian inheritance A major category of inheritance whereby a trait is determined by a pair of genes on homologous chromosomes; also called *single gene inheritance.*

Menorrhagia Excessive or profuse menstrual flow.

Menstrual cycle Cyclic buildup of the uterine lining, ovulation, and sloughing of the lining occurring approximately every 28 days in nonpregnant females.

Mentum The chin.

Mesoderm The intermediate layer of germ cells in the embryo that give rise to connective tissue, bone marrow, muscles, blood, lymphoid tissue, and epithelial tissue.

Metrorrhagia Abnormal uterine bleeding occurring at irregular intervals.

Middle adolescent The adolescent between 15 and 17 years of age.

Milia Tiny white papules appearing on the face of a neonate as a result of unopened sebaceous glands; they disappear spontaneously within a few weeks.

Miscarriage See *spontaneous abortion.*

Mitleiden A phenomenon in which expectant fathers develop symptoms similar to those of the pregnant woman: weight gain, nausea, and various aches and pains.

Mitosis Process of cell division whereby both daughter cells have the same number and pattern of chromosomes as the original cell.

Modeling The process of teaching behaviors through role playing or having the client talk with a person who has mastered a similar crisis.

Molding Shaping of the fetal head by overlapping of the cranial bones to facilitate movement through the birth canal during labor.

Mongolian spot Dark, flat pigmentation of the lower back and buttocks noted at birth in some infants; usually disappears by the time the child reaches school age.

Moniliasis Yeastlike fungus infection caused by *Candida albicans.*

Mons pubis Mound of subcutaneous fatty tissue covering the anterior portion of the symphysis pubis.

Moro reflex Flexion of the newborn's thighs and knees accompanied by fingers that fan, then clench, as the arms are simultaneously thrown out and then brought together, as though embracing something. This reflex can be elicited by startling the newborn with a sudden noise or movement; also called the *startle reflex.*

Morula Developmental stage of the fertilized ovum in which there is a solid mass of cells.

Mottling Discoloration of the skin in irregular areas; may be seen with chilling, poor perfusion, or hypoxia.

Mucous plug A collection of thick mucus that blocks the cervical canal during pregnancy; also called *operculum.*

Multigravida Female who has been pregnant more than once.

Multipara Female who has had more than one pregnancy in which the fetus was viable.

Multiple pregnancy More than one fetus in the uterus at the same time.

Myometrium Uterine muscular structure.

Nägele's rule A method of determining the estimated date of delivery (EDD): after obtaining the first day of the last menstrual period, one subtracts 3 months and adds 7 days.

Natural childbirth Prepared childbirth, in which the couple attends a prenatal education program and learns exercises and breathing patterns that are used during labor and childbirth.

Neonatal mortality rate Number of deaths of infants in the first 28 days of life per 1000 live births.

Neonate Infant from birth through the first 28 days of life.

Neonatology The specialty that focuses on the management of high-risk conditions of the newborn.

Nevus flammeus Large port-wine stain.

Nevus vasculosus "Strawberry mark"; raised, clearly delineated, dark red, rough-surfaced birth mark commonly found in the head region.

Newborn screening tests Tests that detect inborn errors of metabolism that, if left untreated, cause mental retardation and physical handicaps.

Nipple A protrusion about 0.5 to 1.3 cm in diameter in the center of each mature breast.

Nipple preparation Prenatal activities designed to toughen the nipple in preparation for breast-feeding.

Nonstress test (NST) An assessment method by which the reaction (or response) of the fetal heart rate to fetal movement is evaluated.

Nuchal cord Term used to describe the umbilical cord when it is wrapped around the neck of the fetus.

Nulligravida A female who has never been pregnant.

Nullipara A female who has not delivered a viable fetus.

Nurse-midwife A certified nurse-midwife (CNM) is an RN who has received special training and education in the care of the family during childbearing and the prenatal, labor and delivery, and postpartal periods. After a period of formal education, the nurse-midwife takes a certification test to become a CNM.

Obstetric conjugate Distance from the middle of the sacral promontory to an area approximately 1 cm below the pubic crest.

Older adolescent The adolescent between 17 and 19 years of age.

Oligohydramnios Decreased amount of amniotic fluid, which may indicate a fetal urinary tract defect.

Oogenesis Process during fetal life whereby the ovary produces oogenia, cells that become primitive ovarian eggs.

Oophoritis Infection of the ovaries.

Ophthalmia neonatorum Purulent infection of the eyes or conjunctiva of the newborn, usually caused by gonococci.

Oral contraceptives "Birth control pills" that work by inhibiting the release of an ovum and by maintaining a type of mucus that is hostile to sperm.

orifice Normal outlet of a body cavity.

Orgasm Climax of the sexual experience.

Orientation Infant's ability to respond to auditory and visual stimuli in the environment.

Ortolani's maneuver A manual procedure performed to rule out the possibility of congenital hip dysplasia.

Ovarian ligaments Ligaments that anchor the lower pole of the ovary to the cornua of the uterus.

Ovary Female sex gland in which the ova are formed and in which estrogen and progesterone are produced. Normally there are two ovaries, located in the lower abdomen on each side of uterus.

Ovulation Normal process of discharging a mature ovum from an ovary approximately 14 days prior to the onset of menses.

Ovum Female reproductive cell; egg.

Oxygen toxicity Excessive levels of oxygen therapy that result in pathologic changes in tissue.

Oxytocin Hormone normally produced by the posterior pituitary, responsible for stimulation of uterine contractions and the release of milk into the lactiferous ducts.

Oxytocin challenge test (OCT) See *contraction stress test (CST)*.

Papanicolaou (Pap) smear Procedure to detect the presence of cancer of the uterus by microscopic examination of cells gently scraped from the cervix.

Para A woman who has borne offspring who reached the age of viability.

Paracervical block A local anesthetic agent injected transvaginally adjacent to the outer rim of the cervix.

Parametritis Inflammation of the parametrial layer of the uterus.

Parent-infant attachment Close affectional ties that develop between parent and child. See also *attachment*.

Passive acquired immunity Transferral of antibodies (IgG) from the mother to the fetus in utero.

Pelvic cavity Bony portion of the birth passages; a curved canal with a longer posterior than anterior wall.

Pelvic cellulitis Infection involving the connective tissue of the broad ligament or, in severe cases, the connective tissue of all the pelvic structures.

Pelvic diaphragm Part of the pelvic floor composed of deep fascia and the levator ani and the coccygeal muscles.

pelvic floor Muscles and tissue that act as a buttress to the pelvic outlet.

Pelvic inflammatory disease An infection of the fallopain tubes that may or may not be accompanied by a pelvic abscess; may cause infertility secondary to tubal damage.

Pelvic inlet Upper border of the true pelvis.

Pelvic outlet Lower border of the true pelvis.

Pelvic tilt Also called pelvic rocking; exercise designed to reduce back strain and strengthen abdominal muscle tone.

Penis The male organ of copulation and reproduction.

Perimetrium The outermost layer of the corpus of the uterus; also known as the *serosal layer*.

Perinatal mortality rate The number of neonatal and fetal deaths per 1000 live births.

Perinatology The medical specialty concerned with the diagnosis and treatment of high-risk conditions of the pregnant woman and her fetus.

Perineal body Wedge-shaped mass of fibromuscular tissue found between the lower part of the vagina and the anal canal.

Perineum The area of tissue between the anus and scrotum in the male or between the anus and vagina in the female.

Periodic breathing Sporadic episodes of apnea, not associated with cyanosis, that last for about 10 seconds and commonly occur in preterm infants.

Periods of reactivity Predictable patterns of neonate behavior during the first several hours after birth.

Persistant occiput posterior position Malposition of the fetus in which the fetal occiput is posterior in the maternal pelvis.

Phenotype The whole physical, biochemical, and physiologic makeup of an individual as determined both genetically and environmentally.

Phosphatidylglycerol (PG) A phospholipid present in fetal surfactant after about 35 weeks' gestation.

Phototherapy The treatment of jaundice by exposure to light.

Physiologic anemia of infancy A harmless condition in which the hemoglobin level drops in the first 6 to 12 weeks after birth, then reverts to normal levels.

Physiologic jaundice A harmless condition caused by the normal reduction of red blood cells, occurring 48 or more hours after birth, peaking at the fifth to seventh day, and disappearing between the seventh to tenth day.

Pica The eating of substances not ordinarily considered edible or to have nutritive value.

Placenta Specialized disk-shaped organ that connects the fetus to the uterine wall for gas and nutrient exchange; also called *afterbirth*.

Placenta accreta Partial or complete absence of the decidua basalis and abnormal adherence of the placenta to the uterine wall.

Placenta previa Abnormal implantation of the placenta in the lower uterine segment. Classification of type is based on proximity to the cervical os: *total*—completely covers the os; *partial*—covers a portion of the os; *marginal*—in close proximity to the os.

Platypelloid pelvis An unusually wide pelvis, having a flattened oval transverse shape and a shortened anteroposterior diameter.

Polar body A small cell resulting from the meiotic division of the mature oocyte.

Polycythemia An abnormal increase in the number of total red blood cells in the body's circulation.

Polydactyly A developmental anomaly characterized by more than five digits on the hands or feet.

Positive signs of pregnancy Indications that confirm the presence of pregnancy.

Postdate pregnancy Pregnancy that lasts beyond 42 weeks' gestation.

Postpartal hemorrhage A loss of blood of greater than 500 mL following delivery. The hemorrhage is classified as *early* or *immediate* if it occurs within the first 24 hours and *late* or *delayed* after the first 24 hours.

Postpartum After childbirth or delivery.

Postterm infant Any infant delivered after 42 weeks' gestation.

Postterm labor Labor that occurs after 42 weeks of gestation.

Precipitous delivery (1) Unduly rapid progression of labor; (2) a delivery in which no physician is in attendance.

Precipitous labor Labor lasting less than three hours.

Preeclampsia Toxemia of pregnancy, characterized by hypertension, albuminuria, and edema. See also *eclampsia*.

Pregnancy-induced hypertension (PIH) A hypertensive disorder including preeclampsia and eclampsia as conditions, characterized by the three cardinal signs of hypertension, edema, and proteniuria.

premature infant See *preterm infant*.

Premenstrual syndrome (PMS) Cluster of symptoms experienced by some women, typically occurring from a few days up to two weeks prior to the onset of menses.

Prep Shaving of the pubic area.

presentation The fetal body part that enters the maternal pelvis first. The three possible presentations are cephalic, shoulder, or breech.

presenting part The fetal part present in or on the cervical os.

Presumptive signs of pregnancy Symptoms that suggest but do not confirm pregnancy, such as cessation of menses, quickening, Chadwick's sign, and morning sickness.

Preterm infant Any infant born before 38 weeks' gestation.

Preterm labor Labor occurring between 20 and 38 weeks of pregnancy.

Primigravida A woman who is pregnant for the first time.

Primipara A woman who has given birth to her first child (past the point of viability), whether or not that child is living or was alive at birth.

Probable signs of pregnancy Manifestations that strongly suggest the likelihood of pregnancy, such as a positive pregnancy test, enlarging abdomen, and positive Goodell's, Hegar's, and Braxton Hicks signs.

Progesterone A hormone produced by the corpus luteum, adrenal cortex, and placenta whose function it is to stimulate proliferation of the endometrium to facilitate growth of the embryo.

Prolactin A hormone secreted by the anterior pituitary that stimulates and sustains lactation in mammals.

Prolapsed cord Umbilical cord that becomes trapped in the vagina before the fetus is delivered.

Prolonged labor Labor lasting more than 24 hours.

Prostaglandins Complex lipid compounds synthesized by many cells in the body.

Pseudomenstruation Blood-tinged mucus from the vagina in the newborn female infant; caused by withdrawal of maternal hormones that were present during pregnancy.

Psychoprophylaxis Psychophysical training aimed at preparing the expectant parents to cope with the processes of labor and to avoid concentration on the discomforts associated with childbirth.

Pytalism Excessive salivation.

Pubic Pertaining to the pubes or pubis.

Pudendal block Injection of an anesthetizing agent at the pudendal nerve to produce numbness of the external genitals and the lower one-third of the vagina, to facilitate childbirth and permit episiotomy if necessary.

Puerperal morbidity A maternal temperature of 100.4F (38.0C) or higher on any two of the first 10 postpartal days, excluding the first 24 hours. The temperature is to be taken by mouth at least four times per day.

Puerperium The period after completion of the third stage of labor until involution of the uterus is complete, usually six weeks.

Quickening The first fetal movements felt by the pregnant woman, usually between 16 and 18 weeks' gestation.

Radiation Heat loss incurred when heat transfers to cooler surfaces and objects not in direct contact with the body.

Read method Natural childbirth preparation centered on eliminating the fear-tension-pain syndrome.

Reciprocal inhibition The principle that it is impossible to feel relaxed and tense at the same time; the basis for relaxation techniques.

Recommended dietary allowances (RDA) Government-recommended allowances of various vitamins, minerals, and other nutrients.

Regional anesthesia Injection of local anesthetic agents so that they come into direct contact with nervous tissue.

Relaxin A water-soluble protein secreted by the corpus luteum that causes relaxation of the symphysis and cervical dilatation.

Respiratory distress syndrome See *hyaline membrane disease.*

Retrolental fibroplasia Formation of fibrotic tissue behind the lens; associated with retinal detachment and arrested eye growth, seen with hypoxemia in preterm infants.

Rh factor Antigens present on the surface of blood cells that make the blood cell incompatible with blood cells that do not have the antigen.

RhoGAM An anti-Rh (D) gammaglobulin given after delivery to an Rh-negative mother of an Rh-positive fetus or child. Prevents the development of permanent active immunity to the Rh antigen.

Rhythm method The timing of sexual intercourse to avoid the fertile time associated with ovulation.

Risk factors Any findings that suggest the pregnancy may have a negative outcome, either for the woman or her unborn child.

Rooming-in unit A hospital unit where the infant can reside in the same room with the mother after delivery and during their postpartal stay.

Rooting reflex An infant's tendency to turn the head and open the lips to suck when one side of the mouth or cheek is touched.

Round ligaments Ligaments that arise from the side of the uterus near the fallopian tube insertion to help the broad ligament keep the uterus in place.

Rugae Transverse ridges of mucous membranes lining the vagina, which allow the vagina to stretch during the descent of the fetal head.

Rupture of membranes (ROM) Rupture may be PROM (Premature), SROM (spontaneous), or AROM (artificial). Some clinicians may use the abbreviation RBOW (rupture of bag of water).

Sacral promontory A projection into the pelvic cavity on the anterior upper portion of the sacrum; serves as an obstetric guide in determining pelvic measurements.

salpingitis Infection of the fallopian tubes.

Scarf sign The position of the elbow when the hand of a supine infant is drawn across to the other shoulder until it meets resistance.

Schultze's mechanism Delivery of the placenta with the shiny or fetal surface presenting first.

Self quieting activity Infant's ability to use personal resources to quiet and console him or herself.

Semen Thick whitish fluid ejaculated by the male during orgasm and containing the spermatozoa and their nutrients.

Sepsis neonatorum Infections experienced by a neonate during the first month of life.

Sex chromosomes The X and Y chromosomes, which are responsible for sex determination.

Sexually transmitted disease (STD) Refers to diseases ordinarily transmitted by direct sexual contact with an infected individual.

Show A pinkish mucous discharge from the vagina that may occur a few hours to a few days prior to the onset of labor.

Simian line A single palmar crease frequently found in children with Down syndrome.

Sims Huhner test Postcoital examination to evaluate sperm and cervical mucus.

Sinusoidal pattern A wave form of fetal heart rate where long-term variability is present but there is no short-term variability.

Situational contraceptives Contraceptive methods that involve no prior preparation, for instance, abstinence or coitus interruptus.

Skin turgor Elasticity of skin; provides information on hydration status.

Small for gestational age (SGA) Inadequate weight or growth for gestational age; birth weight below the tenth percentile.

Spermatogenesis The process by which mature spermatozoa are formed, during which the number of chromosomes is halved.

Spermatozoa Mature sperm cells of the male animal, produced by the testes.

Spermicides A variety of creams, foam, jellies, and suppositories, inserted into the vagina prior to intercourse, which destroy sperm or neutralize any vaginal secretions and thereby immobilize sperm.

Spinal block Injection of a local anesthetic agent directly into the spinal fluid in the spinal canal to provide anesthesia for vaginal delivery and cesarean birth.

Spinnbarkeit Describes the elasticity of the cervical mucus that is present at ovulation.

Spontaneous abortion Abortion that occurs naturally; also called *miscarriage.*

Station Relationship of the presenting fetal part to an imaginary line drawn between the pelvic ischial spines.

Sterility Inability to conceive or to produce offspring.

Stillbirth The delivery of a dead infant.

Striae gravidarum Stretch marks; shiny reddish lines that appear on the abdomen, breasts, thighs, and buttocks of pregnant women as a result of stretching the skin.

Subconjunctival hemorrhage Hemorrhage on the sclera of a newborn's eye usually caused by changes in vascular tension during birth.

Subinvolution Failure of a part to return to its normal size after functional enlargement, such as failure of the uterus to return to normal size after pregnancy.

Surfactant A surface-active mixture of lipoproteins secreted in the alveoli and air passages that reduces surface tension of pulmonary fluids and contributes to the elasticity of pulmonary tissue.

Suture (1) fibrous connection of opposed joint surfaces, as in the skull. (2) The uniting of edges of a wound.

Symphysis pubis Fibrocartilaginous joint between the pelvic bones in the midline.

Syndactyly Malformation of the fingers or toes in which there may be webbing or complete fusion of two or more digits.

Telangiectatic nevi (stork bites) Small clusters of pink-red spots appearing on the nape of the neck and around the eyes of infants; localized areas of capillary dilatation.

Teratogens Nongenetic factors that can produce malformations of the fetus.

Testes The male gonads, in which sperm and testosterone are produced.

Testosterone The male hormone; responsible for the development of secondary male characteristics.

Therapeutic abortion Medically induced termination of pregnancy when a mal-

formed fetus is suspected or when the woman's health is in jeopardy.

Thermal neutral zone (TNZ) An environment that provides for minimal heat loss or expenditure.

Thrush A fungus infection of the oral mucous membranes caused by *Candida albicans.* Most often seen in infants; characterized by white plaques in the mouth.

Tonic neck reflex Postural reflex seen in the newborn. When the supine infant's head is turned to one side, the arm and leg on that side extend while the extremities on the opposite side flex; also called the *fencing position.*

TORCH An acronym used to describe a group of infections that represent potentially severe problems during pregnancy. TO = toxoplasmosis, R = rubella, C = cytomegalovirus, H = herpesvirus.

Toxic shock syndrome Infectino caused by *staphylococcus aureus,* found primarily in women of reproductive age.

Transverse diameter The largest diameter of the pelvic inlet; helps determine the shape of the inlet.

Transverse lie A lie in which the fetus is positioned crosswise in the uterus.

Trichomonas vaginalis A parasitic protozoan that may cause inflammation of the vagina, characterized by itching and burning of vulvar tissue and by white, frothy discharge.

Trimester Three months, or one-third of the gestational time for pregnancy.

Trisomy The presence of three homologous chromosomes rather than the normal two.

Trophoblast The outer layer of the blastoderm that will eventually establish the nutrient relationship with the uterine endometrium.

True pelvis The portion that lies below the linea terminalis, made up of the inlet, cavity, and outlet.

Turner syndrome A number of anomalies that occur when a female has only one X chromosome; characteristics include short stature, little sexual differentiation, webbing of the neck with a low posterior hairline, and congenital cardiac anomalies.

Ultrasound High-frequency sound waves that may be directed, through the use of a transducer, into the maternal abdomen.

The ultrasonic sound waves reflected by the underlying structures of varying densities allow various maternal and fetal tissues, bones, and fluids to be identified.

Umbilical cord The structure connecting the placenta to the umbilicus of the fetus and through which nutrients from the woman are exchanged for wastes from the fetus.

Uterosacral ligaments Ligaments that provide support for the uterus and cervix at the level of the ischial spines.

Uterus The hollow muscular organ in which the fertilized ovum is implanted and in which the developing fetus is nourished until birth.

Vagina The musculomembranous tube or passageway located between the external genitals and the uterus of the female.

Variable expressivity The differences in severity of a trait produced by the same gene in different individuals.

Vasectomy Surgical removal of a portion of the vas deferens (ductus deferens) to produce infertility.

Vegan A "pure" vegetarian; one who consumes no food from animal sources.

Vena caval syndrome Symptoms of dizziness, pallor, and clamminess resulting from lowering blood pressure when the pregnant woman lies supine and the enlarging uterus presses on the vena cava; also known as *supine hypotensive syndrome.*

Vernix caseosa A protective cheeselike whitish substance made up of sebum and desquamated epithelial cells that is present on the fetal skin.

Vertex The top or crown of the head.

Vulva The external structure of the female genitals, lying below the mons veneris.

Wharton's jelly Yellow-white gelatinous material surrounding the vessels of the umbilical cord.

Young adolescent The adolescent less than 15 years of age.

Zona pellucida Transparent inner layer surrounding an ovum.

Zygote A fertilized egg.

Epigrams and Featured Quotations

Armstrong, Penny, and Feldman, Sheryl. *A Midwife's Story*. New York: Arbor House, 1986.

Bacall, Lauren. *By Myself*. New York: Alfred A. Knopf, 1978.

Baldwin, Rahima and Palmarini, Terra. *Pregnant Feelings*. Berkeley, CA: Celestial Arts, 1986.

Borg, Susan and Lasker, Judith. *When Pregnancy Fails*. Boston: Beacon Press, 1981.

Boston Women's Health Book Collective, Inc. *The New Our Bodies, Ourselves*. New York: Random House, 1985.

Boston Women's Health Book Collective, Inc. *Ourselves and Our Children*. New York: Random House, 1978.

Danziger, Dennis. *Daddy: The Diary of an Expectant Father*. Tucson, AZ: The Body Press, 1987.

Drabble, Margaret. *The Millstone*. New York: William Morrow, 1966.

Drabble, Margaret. "With All My Love, (Signed) Mama." *The New York Times*. Quoted in Emerson, Sally, ed. *A Celebration of Babies*. New York: Dutton, 1987.

Emerson, Sally, ed. *A Celebration of Babies*. New York: Dutton, 1987.

Hartigan, Harriette. *Women in Birth*. Rochester, NY: Artemis, 1984.

Hoff, Lee Ann. *People in Crisis: Understanding and Helping*, ed. 2. Menlo Park, CA: Addison-Wesley, 1984.

Kenton, Leslie. "All I Ever Wanted Was a Baby." Quoted in Emerson, Sally, ed. *A Celebration of Babies*. New York: Dutton, 1987.

Klaus, Marshall, and Klaus, Phyllis H. *The Amazing Newborn*. Reading, Massachusetts: Addison-Wesley, 1985.

Lazarre, Jane. *The Mother Knot*. Boston: Beacon Press, 1976.

Lederman, Regina. *Psychosocial Adaptation in Pregnancy*. Englewood Cliffs, NJ: Prentice-Hall, 1984.

Ledray, Linda E. *Recovering from Rape*. New York: Henry Holt and Company, 1986.

Lee, Laurie. *Two Women*. Andre Deutsch Ltd. Quoted in Emerson, Sally, ed. *A Celebration of Babies*. New York: Dutton, 1987.

Lessard, Suzannah. "Talk of the Town." *The New Yorker* (August 11, 1980) 22.

Peterson, Gayle, with contributions by Lewis Mehl, M.D. *Birthing Normally: A Personal Growth Approach to Childbirth*. Berkeley, CA: Mind/Body Press, 1981.

Rich, Adrienne. *Of Woman Born*. New York: W. W. Norton, 1976.

Sorel, Nancy Caldwell, ed. *Ever Since Eve: Personal Reflections on Childbirth*. New York: Oxford University Press, 1984.

Photographic Credits

The authors and publisher gratefully acknowledge the following institutions for their kind permission to photograph many of the clients who appear in this book: Alexian Brothers Hospital, San Jose, CA. The Birth Place, Menlo Park, CA. Mayfield Community Clinic, Palo Alto, CA. Merritt Hospital, Oakland, CA. Lucille Salter Packard Children's Hospital, Stanford, CA. Stanford University Hospital, Stanford, CA.

Chapter 1 Opener: Elizabeth D. Elkin. Figures 1–1, 1–2: Amy H. Snyder. Figures 1–3, 1–4: © Suzanne Arms Wimberley.

Chapter 2 Opener: Elizabeth D. Elkin.

Chapter 3 Opener: © Suzanne Arms Wimberley. Figure 3–1 clockwise from upper left: Amy H. Snyder, Amy H. Snyder, Amy H. Snyder, Amy H. Snyder, © Suzanne Arms Wimberley, Amy H. Snyder. Figure 3–2: Amy H. Snyder. Figure 3–3: Judy Braginsky. Figure 3–4: Courtesy of Ed Zierserl, M.D. Figure 3–5: Judy Braginsky.

Chapter 4 Opener: Elizabeth D. Elkin. Figures 4–21, 4–22: Courtesy of Dr. E. S. E. Hafez, Wayne State University, Detroit, Michigan.

Chapter 5 Opener: © Suzanne Arms Wimberley. Figure 5–4: from Speroff, L. et al., *Clinical Gynecologic Endocrinology and Infertility* 4th ed. 1989, p.520 © 1989 Williams & Wilkins Co., Baltimore, MD. Figures 5–6, 5–7, 5–8, 5–9, 5–16: courtesy of Dr. Arthur Robinson, National Jewish Hospital and Research Center, Denver, CO. Figures 5–10, 5–11, 5–12: From Smith D.W.: *Recognizable Patterns of Human Malformations*, 1982. Philadelphia: W. B. Saunders. Figure 5–13: from Lemli

L. Smith D.W., *The XO Syndrome: A Study of the Differentiated Phenotype in 25 Patients*. J PEDIATR 1963;63:577.

Chapter 6 Opener, Figure 6–1: © Suzanne Arms Wimberley.

Chapter 7 Opener: Elizabeth D. Elkin. Figure 7–3: © William Thompson. Condoms courtesy of Planned Parenthood Association, San Mateo County, CA. Figure 7–5: © William Thompson. Cervical caps courtesy of Planned Parenthood Association, San Mateo County, CA. Figure 7–7: © William Thompson. IUD courtesy of Planned Parenthood Association, San Mateo County, CA. Figure 7–8: Photo and illustration courtesy of Wyeth-Ayerst Laboratories, Philadelphia, PA.

Chapter 8 Opener: Amy H. Snyder. Figures 8–4, 8–6: Centers for Disease Control. Figure 8–7: From *Danforth's Obstetrics and Gynecology*, Scott, J.R., DiSaia, P.J., Hammond, C.B., Spellacym W.N. (eds.) 6th ed., 1990, Fig. 47–1, p. 935.

Chapter 9 Opener: Amy H. Snyder.

Chapter 10 Opener: Amy H. Snyder.

Chapter 11 Opener: Elizabeth D. Elkin. Figure 11–5: From Marieb E.N.: *Human Anatomy and Physiology*, 1st ed., Redwood City, CA: Benjamin/Cummings 1989, p.958. Figures 11–14, 11–15, 11–16, 11–17, 11–18, 11–19, 11–20 Landrum B. Shettles, M.D. and Roberts Rugh, M.D..

Chapter 12 Opener: Elizabeth D. Elkin: Figure 12–6: © Suzanne Arms Wimberley.

Chapter 13 Opener, Figures 13–4, 13–6: Amy H. Snyder.

Chapter 14 Opener: Elizabeth D. Elkin. Figures 14–1, 14–3, 14–8, 14–9: © Suzanne Arms Wimberley. Figure 14–6: © William Thompson. Figure 14–7: Amy H. Snyder.

Chapter 15 Opener, Figures 15–1, 15–2: Amy H. Snyder. Figure 15–3: © Suzanne Arms Wimberley.

Chapter 16 Opener: Elizabeth D. Elkin. Figure 16–1: © Suzanne Arms Wimberley.

Chapter 17 Opener, Figures 17–3A, 17–3B, 17–3C: Amy H. Snyder. Figures 17–3D, 17–4, 17–5: © Suzanne Arms Wimberley.

Chapter 18 Opener, Figure 18–1: Amy H. Snyder.

Chapter 19 Opener: Elizabeth D. Elkin. Figures 19–7, 19–8: Amy H. Snyder.

Chapter 20 Opener: Elizabeth D. Elkin. Figures 20–1, 20–2, 20–10: Amy H. Snyder. Figures 20–3, 20–5: Courtesy of Department of Diagnostic Radiology, Section of Diagnostic Ultrasound, Kansas University Medical Center. Figure 20–4: From Jeanty P., Romero R.: *Obstetrical Ultrasound*, New York: McGraw-Hill, 1984, p.53. Figure 20–6: From Hobbins J.C., Winsberg F., Berkowitz R.L.: *Ultrasonography in Obstetrics and Gynecology*, ed. 2. Baltimore: Williams & Wilkins, 1983, p.123. Figure 20–15: © Suzanne Arms Wimberley.

Chapter 21 Opener: Elizabeth D. Elkin. Figures 21–17A, 21–17C, 21–17E, 21–17G, 21–17K, 21–17O: *Birth Atlas*, Maternity Center Association, New York. Figures 21–17I, 21–17J, 21–17M, 21–17N, 21–17Q, last view: © Suzanne Arms Wimberley.

Chapter 22 Opener: Elizabeth D. Elkin. Figures 22–5, 22–11B, 22–11C: © Suzanne Arms Wimberley. Figure 22–6: Courtesy of Corometrics Medical Systems, Inc., Wallingford, CT. Figure 22–8: Courtesy of Utah Medical Products, Inc., Midvale, Utah 84047-1084. Figure 22–11A: © William Thompson.

Chapter 23 Opener: Elizabeth D. Elkin. Figures 23–1, 23–2, 23–3, 23–4, 23–5, 23–6, 23–7, 23–8, 23–10: ©

Suzanne Arms Wimberley. Figure 23–9: George B. Fry III.

Chapter 24 Opener: Elizabeth D. Elkin. Figure 24–4: Courtesy of Baxter Healthcare Corporation, Auto Syringe Division.

Chapter 25 Opener: Elizabeth D. Elkin.

Chapter 26 Opener: Elizabeth D. Elkin.

Chapter 27 Opener, Figures 27–9, 27–10: Elizabeth D. Elkin.

Chapter 28 Opener, Figure 28–12: Elizabeth D. Elkin. Figures 28–2, 28–3, 28–4A, 28–4B, 28–5A, 28–5B, 28–6A, 28–7, 28–8, 28–9, 28–10: Reprinted by permission of V. Dubowitz, M.D., Hammersmith Hospital, London, England. Figures 28–4C, 28–5C, 28–6B, 28–20, 28–23, 28–28, 28–29: © Suzanne Arms Wimberley. Figures 28–15, 28–22: From Korones S.B.: *High Risk Newborn Infants*, ed. 4. St. Louis, C.V. Mosby, 1986. Figures 28–16B, 28–24: Reproduced with permission from Potter E.L., Craig J.M.: *Pathology of the Fetus and Infant*, ed. 3. © 1975 by Year Book Medical Publishers, Chicago. Figures 28–17B, 28–19, 28–21: Courtesy of Mead Johnson Laboratories, Evansville, IN. Figure 28–18: Courtesy of Dr. Ralph Platow, from Potter E.L., Craig J.M.: *Pathology of the Fetus and Infant*, ed 3. © 1975 by Year Book Medical Publishers, Chicago. Figure 28–25: From Smith D.W.: *Recognizable Patterns of Human Deformation*. Philadelphia: W.B. Saunders, 1981.

Chapter 29 Opener, Figures 29–1, 29–2, 29–3, 29–4, 29–6, 29–7, 29–9, 29–10, 29–11: Elizabeth D. Elkin.

Chapter 30 Opener: Elizabeth D. Elkin. Figures 30–1, 30–3, 30–4: © Suzanne Arms Wimberley. Figure 30–6: © Suzanne Arms Wimberley from Renfrow, Arms, Fisher: *Bestfeeding: Getting Breast Feeding Right for You*, Celestial Arts, 1990.

Chapter 31 Opener, Figures 31–6: Elizabeth D. Elkin. Figure 31–5: Reprinted by permission of V. Dubowitz, M.D. from Dubowitz L., Dubowitz V.: *Gestational Age of the Newborn*. Menlo Park, CA: Addison-Wesley, 1977. Figure 31–8: © Suzanne Arms Wimberley. Figure 31–15: Courtesy of Dr. Paul Winchester. Figure 31–19: Judy Braginsky.

Chapter 32 Opener, Figures 32–10, 32–12, 32–15: Elizabeth D. Elkin. Figures 32–1, 32–5, 32–7: © Suzanne Arms Wimberley. Figure 32–14: © William Thompson.

Chapter 33 Opener: Elizabeth D. Elkin.

Chapter 34 Opener: Elizabeth D. Elkin. Figure 34–1: © William Thompson. Figure 34–2: © Suzanne Arms Wimberley.

Chapter 35 Opener, Figure 35–4: Elizabeth D. Elkin. Figures 35–1, 35–2: © William Thompson.

Chapter 36 Opener: Elizabeth D. Elkin. Figure 36–2: Amy H. Snyder.

INDEX

Note: Italicized page numbers refer to figures or tables. A *g* following a page number refers to a glossary term.

Judy . K.

Judy . K.

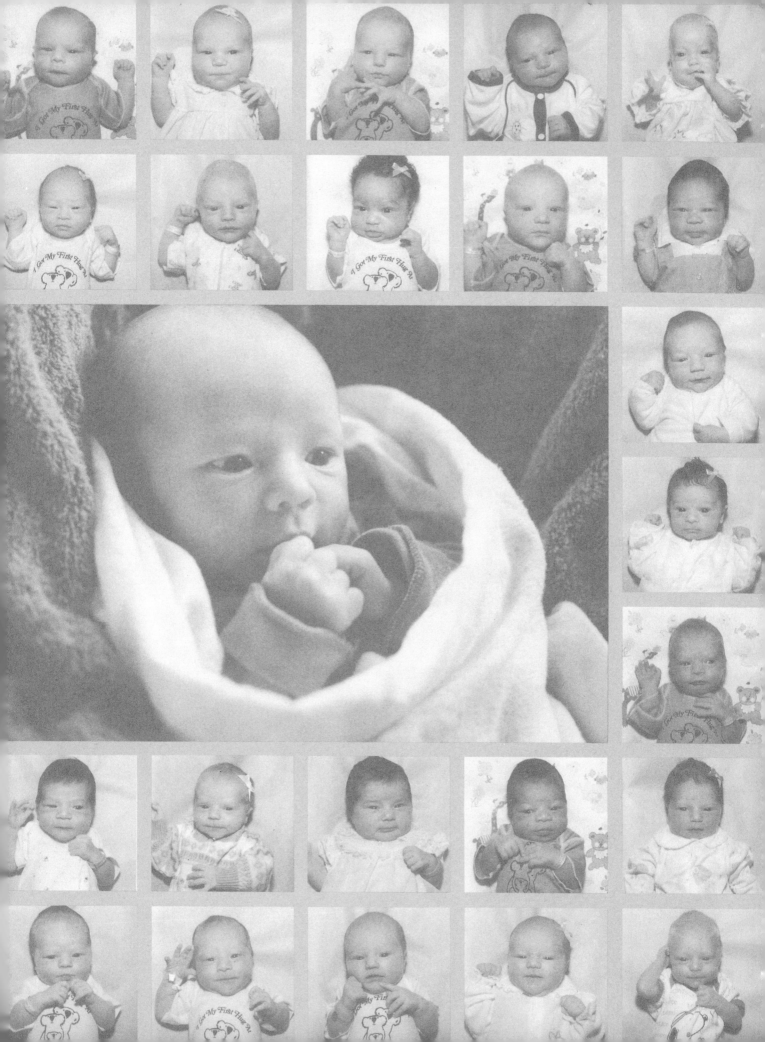